Inflammatory Bowel Diseases

For Churchill Livingstone

Commissioning Editor Sheila Khullar
Project Editor Antonia Seymour
Copy Editor Jennifer Bew
Indexer John Sampson

Inflammatory Bowel Diseases

THIRD EDITION

Medical Editors

Robert N. Allan MD PhD FRCP
Consultant Physician, Queen Elizabeth Hospital, Birmingham, UK

Jonathan M. Rhodes MA MD FRCP
Professor of Medicine (Gastroenterology), Department of Medicine, University of Liverpool, Liverpool, UK

Stephen B. Hanauer MD
Professor of Medicine and Clinical Pharmacology; Director of Clinical IBD Research Center, University of Chicago Hospitals and Clinics, Chicago, USA

Surgical Editors

Michael R. B. Keighley MS FRCS
Professor of Surgery, Barling Professor of Surgery, Queen Elizabeth Hospital, University of Birmingham, Birmingham, UK

John Alexander-Williams MD FRCS
Formerly Professor of Gastrointestinal Surgery, University of Birmingham, Birmingham; Consultant Surgeon, Birmingham Nuffield and Priory Hospitals, Birmingham, UK

Victor W. Fazio MBBS FRACS FACS
Rupert B. Turnbull Jr Chairman, Department of Colorectal Surgery, The Cleveland Clinic Foundation; Professor of Surgery, The Cleveland Clinic Foundation Health Sciences Center of The Ohio State University, Cleveland, Ohio, USA

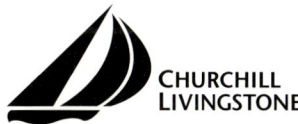

NEW YORK   EDINBURGH   LONDON   MADRID   MELBOURNE   SAN FRANCISCO   AND   TOKYO   1997

CHURCHILL LIVINGSTONE
Medical Division of Pearson Professional Limited

Distributed in the United States of America by Churchill Livingstone Inc., 650 Avenue of the Americas, New York, N.Y. 10011, and by associated companies, branches and representatives throughout the world.

© Pearson Professional Limited 1997

All rights reserved. No part of this publication may be reproduced, stored in a retrieval system, or transmitted in any form or by any means, electronic, mechanical, photocopying, recording or otherwise, without either the prior written permission of the publishers (Churchill Livingstone, Robert Stevenson House, 1–3 Baxter's Place, Leith Walk, Edinburgh EH1 3AF), or a licence permitting restricted copying in the United Kingdom issued by the Copyright Licensing Agency Ltd, 90 Tottenham Court Road, London W1P 9HE.

First edition 1983
Second edition 1990
Third edition 1997

ISBN 0 443 05067 8

British Library Cataloguing in Publication Data
A catalogue record for this book is available from the British Library.

Library of Congress Cataloging in Publication Data
A catalog record for this book is available from the Library of Congress.

Medical knowledge is constantly changing. As new information becomes available, changes in treatment, procedures, equipment and the use of drugs become necessary. The editors and contributors and the publishers have, as far as it is possible, taken care to ensure that the information given in this text is accurate and up to date. However, readers are strongly advised to confirm that the information, especially with regard to drug usage, complies with current legislation and standards of practice.

The publisher's policy is to use **paper manufactured from sustainable forests**

Printed in Hong Kong

Contents

Contributors xi
Preface xvii

SECTION 1
Historical review

1. Historical review 3
   J. Alexander-Williams

SECTION 2
Pathogenesis

2. Genetics of inflammatory bowel disease 13
   I. Koutroubakis and A. S. Peña

3. Molecular implications of genetic studies 27
   W. M. C. Rosenberg

4. Epidemiological overview of inflammatory bowel disease 35
   M. J. S. Langman

5. Epidemiology of inflammatory bowel disease 41
   B. Breuer-Katschinski

6. Epidemiology: smoking and oral contraception 47
   R. Logan

7. Lymphocytes in inflammatory bowel disease 53
   M. J. Zimmerman and D. P. Jewell

8. Humoral immunity in inflammatory bowel disease 63
   M. T. Abreu-Martin and S. R. Targan

9. Role of neutrophils in the pathogenesis of inflammatory bowel disease 73
   M. B. Grisham and P. R. Kvietys

10. Monocytes and macrophages in inflammatory bowel disease 81
    Y. R. Mahida

11. Mast cells and eosinophils in inflammatory bowel disease 87
    S. Bloom

12. Cytokines in inflammatory bowel disease 95
    G. Radford-Smith and D. P. Jewell

13. Platelets and coagulation 101
    M. Hudson and P. Kesteven

14. Inflammatory mediators 107
    D. S. Rampton

15. Infective agents – bacterial and viral 117
    S. Mohammed and W. R. Thayer

16. Infective agents – mycobacteria 125
    H. M. Fidler and J. J. McFadden

17. Infective agents – vascular factors 133
    N. P. Thompson and A. J. Wakefield

18. Mucosal defenses 143
    J. M. Rhodes, B. J. Campbell and R. C. Evans

19. Animal models – naturally occurring 157
    B. F. Warren and P. Watkins

20. Animal models of inflammatory bowel disease – experimental 167
    J. L. Wallace and C. M. Hogaboam

21. Pathophysiology of small-intestinal dysfunction in Crohn's disease 173
    R. C. Spiller

22. Absorption of fluids and electrolytes by the colon – relevance to inflammatory bowel disease 181
    A. M. Levy and S. F. Phillips

23. Pathophysiology of gastrointestinal motor disturbances in inflammatory bowel disease   191
    S. S. C. Rao

24. Mucosal metabolism and proliferation   201
    P. R. Gibson and *D. H. Barkla*

SECTION 3
Clinical diagnosis

25. Radiology – contrast studies   215
    J. R. Lee

26. Radiology – CT, ultrasound and MRI   249
    J. F. C. Olliff

27. Radiology – isotope scanning   261
    A. M. Peters and *J. P. Lavender*

28. Endoscopy – upper gastrointestinal tract   269
    A. I. Morris

29. Endoscopy – lower intestinal tract   273
    E. J. Irvine and *R. H. Hunt*

30. Endoluminal ultrasound   285
    M. S. Bhutani and *R. H. Hawes*

31. Histopathology of ulcerative colitis   291
    R. H. Riddell

32. Histopathology of Crohn's disease   311
    J. R. Goldblum and *R. E. Petras*

33. Histopathology – dysplasia and cancer   317
    J. R. Jass

34. Laboratory markers of inflammatory bowel disease   329
    H. J. F. Hodgson

35. Clinical indices in inflammatory bowel disease   335
    D. T. Spence and *J. F. Mayberry*

36. Ulcerative colitis versus Crohn's disease – one disease or two?   343
    H. J. F. Hodgson

37. Infective colitis   349
    C. A. Hart

38. Acute infectious colitis – diagnostic dilemmas   359
    C. L. Wright and *R. H. Riddell*

39. Collagenous, microscopic and lymphocytic colitis   369
    N. P. Mapstone and *M. F. Dixon*

40. Other granulomatous diseases of the bowel   379
    H. H. Tsai

41. Gastrointestinal Behçet's disease   387
    H. H. Tsai

42. Tuberculosis of the gastrointestinal tract   391
    P. Ghosh

43. Sexually transmitted diseases/HIV   399
    M. S. Kapembwa, P. A. Batman and *G. E. Griffin*

44. Amebic colitis   409
    E. P. Variyam

45. Yersinia-related enteric disease   413
    H. J. Freeman

46. Ischemic colitis   421
    M. G. Thomas

47. Irradiation enterocolitis   425
    G. S. W. Whiteley and *P. F. Schofield*

48. Ulcerative jejunoileitis   431
    G. K. T. Holmes

49. Non-steroidal anti-inflammatory drug-induced enteritis   437
    I. Bjarnason, A. Macpherson and *A. B. Price*

50. Diverticular disease   443
    B. T. Jackson

51. Diversion colitis   449
    R. C. Evans

52. Ileitis in the spondylarthropathies   451
    M. De Vos, H. Mielants and *C. Cuvelier*

SECTION 4
Natural history and prognosis

53. Natural history of ulcerative colitis   463
    H. Debinski and *M. A. Kamm*

54. Natural history of Crohn's disease   475
    A. Brzezinski and *B. A. Lashner*

SECTION 5
Therapeutic options

55. Sulfasalazine and the new salicylates   487
    L. R. Sutherland

56. Corticosteroids   503
    V. Binder and *J. Brynskov*

57. Immunosuppressive drugs in inflammatory bowel disease   513
    A. B. Hawthorne

58. Inflammatory mediators   521
    C. J. Hawkey

59. Dietary manipulations – elemental and enteral   535
    C. O'Morain and M. O'Sullivan

60. Dietary manipulation – parenteral   541
    I. D. A. D'Agata and E. G. Seidman

SECTION 6
Ulcerative colitis

61. Medical management of mild and moderately active ulcerative colitis   549
    J. E. Smithson and D. P. Jewell

62. Management of acute severe colitis   565
    D. Present

63. Treatment of ulcerative colitis in remission   571
    G. Järnerot, H. Sandberg-Gertzén and C. Tysk

SECTION 7
Crohn's disease

64. Crohn's disease of the upper gastrointestinal tract   583
    C. Lamers

65. Crohn's disease of the small intestine – ileum and right colon   589
    R. N. Allan

66. Crohn's disease of the small intestine diffuse jejunal ileitis   597
    R. N. Allan

67. Crohn's disease of the large intestine   601
    J. R. Lowes

68. Perianal Crohn's disease   615
    R. S. McLeod and Z. Cohen

SECTION 8
Inflammatory bowel disease – special problems

69. Extraintestinal manifestations of inflammatory bowel disease   623
    A. Weiss and L. Mayer

70. Oral manifestations of Crohn's disease   633
    J. Hamburger

71. Hepatobiliary disease   637
    R. Chapman

72. Inflammatory bowel disease in childhood   647
    C. M. Evans, R. M. Beattie and J. A. Walker-Smith

73. Inflammatory bowel disease, the oral contraceptive pill and pregnancy   671
    R. N. Allan

74. Cancer risk in ulcerative colitis and Crohn's disease – strategies to avoid cancer deaths   675
    J. E. Lennard-Jones

75. Surgical management of cancer occurring in inflammatory bowel disease   683
    A. J. Greenstein and S. Balasubramanian

SECTION 9
Surgical principles

76. Incisions and surgical approaches in surgery for inflammatory bowel disease   691
    M. R. B. Keighley

77. Antimicrobials and their use in surgery for inflammatory bowel disease   693
    M. R. B. Keighley

78. Thromboembolism in inflammatory bowel disease – etiology, prophylaxis and treatment   697
    W. R. Fleming and W. A. Kmiot

79. A team approach   703
    M. H. Irving and N. Scott

80. Surgical maneuvers in Crohn's disease – a personal guide   707
    J. Alexander-Williams

81. Preserving anorectal function in surgery for inflammatory bowel disease   713
    M. R. B. Keighley

82. The role of laparoscopy   717
    M. J. Hershman and R. S. Kiff

SECTION 10
Surgical treatment of ulcerative colitis

83. Emergency colectomy for fulminant colitis   727
    J. J. Tjandra

84. Ulcerative colitis – indications for elective colectomy   733
    J. J. Murray

85. Surgical treatment of ulcerative coltis – subtotal colectomy and ileorectal anastomosis 741
P. R. Hawley

86. Surgical treatment of ulcerative colitis – proctocolectomy and permanent ileostomy 747
A. P. Meagher and B. G. Wolff

87. Surgical treatment of ulcerative colitis – continent ileostomy 753
J. G. Peiser, Z. Cohen and R. S. McLeod

88. Surgical options – ileoanal pouch 761
P. A. Dean and R. R. Dozois

89. The role of ileoanal anastomosis – patient assessment and counseling 773
L. Hultén, L. W. Köhler and T. Öresland

90. Role of the ileal pouch procedure – pouch construction, and the ileoanal anastomosis 781
P. M. Sagar and J. H. Pemberton

91. Complications after ileal pouch-anal anastomosis 793
D. A. Rothenberger, B. T. Gemlo and K. I. Deen

92. Pouchitis 803
D. P. Jewell and N. J. McC. Mortensen

93. Quality of life after restorative proctocolectomy 811
S. D. Wexner and S. L. Glorsky

SECTION 11
Surgical treatment of Crohn's disease

94. Gastroduodenal Crohn's disease 819
P. L. Roberts

95. Small-bowel Crohn's disease – localized/diffuse disease 823
V. W. Fazio

96. Crohn's disease of the colon – segmental resection 849
S. A. Strong

97. Perianal Crohn's disease 863
I. J. Kodner

98. Perianal Crohn's disease: rectovaginal fistulae 873
T. L. Hull

SECTION 12
Management of surgical complications in inflammatory bowel disease

99. Percutaneous drainage of Crohn's abscesses 877
E. Lee and R. Bleday

100. Enterocutaneous fistula: conservative and surgical management 883
S. T. O'Dwyer

101. Management of the persistent perineal sinus 895
N. A. Scott

102. Management of fecal incontinence complicating inflammatory bowel disease 899
R. D. Madoff

103. Sexual dysfunction in inflammatory bowel disease 905
A. C. Lowry and K. I. Deen

SECTION 13
Stoma management

104. Running a stomaltherapy service 913
P. J. d'E. Stevens

105. Counseling of patients with inflammatory bowel disease 917
J. Alexander-Williams

106. Stoma construction 927
Kong-Weng Eu and J. R. Oakley

107. Complications of stomas and their management 935
J. G. Williams and S. M. Goldberg

SECTION 14
Social and psychological aspects of disease

108. Psychological factors including sexual function 943
F. A. Frizelle and H. Nelson

109. Social consequences of inflammatory bowel disease 947
G. Moody and J. F. Mayberry

110. Inflammatory bowel disease and insurance 951
R. Driscoll

SECTION 15
Follow-up

111. Follow-up in inflammatory bowel disease   957
   R. N. Allan

112. Assuring the quality of care   961
   B. T. Collopy

Index   965

Contributors

M. T. Abreu-Martin MD
Assistant Professor of Medicine, UCLA School of Medicine; Assistant Clinical Director, Inflammatory Bowel Disease Center, Cedars-Sinai Medical Center, Los Angeles, California, USA

J. Alexander-Williams MD FRCS
Formerly Professor of Gastrointestinal Surgery, University of Birmingham, UK; Consultant Surgeon, Birmingham Nuffield and Priory Hospitals, Birmingham, UK

R. N. Allan MD PhD FRCP
Consultant Physician, Queen Elizabeth Hospital, Birmingham, UK

S. Balasubramanian MBBS
Research Assistant, Department of Surgery, Mt Sinai School of Medicine, New York, USA

David H. Barkla BDS MDS PhD
Professor and Head of Department of Anatomy, Monash University, Clayton, Victoria, Australia

P. A. Batman MA MB BChir (Cantab) FRCPath
Consultant Histopathologist, Bradford Royal Infirmary, Bradford, UK

R. M. Beattie MBBS BSc (Hons) MRCP
Consultant Paediatrician, Peterborough District Hospital, Peterborough, UK

Manoop S. Bhutani MD
Chief of Endoscopy, Department of Veterans' Affairs Medical Center; Assistant Professor of Medicine, Wright State University, Dayton, Ohio, USA

V. Binder MD DMedSci
Chief Physician, Department of Medical Gastroenterology, Herlev Hospital, University of Copenhagen, Herlev, Denmark

I. Bjarnason MSc MD MRCPath
Senior Lecturer and Honorary Consultant, Department of Clinical Biochemistry, King's College School of Medicine and Dentistry, London, UK

R. Bleday MD
Assistant Professor of Surgery, Harvard Medical School, Boston, Massachusetts, USA; Chief, Section of Colon and Rectal Surgery, New England Deaconess Hospital, Boston, Massachusetts, USA

S. Bloom DM MRCP (UK)
Lecturer and Senior Registrar in Gastroenterology, Royal Liverpool University Hospital, Liverpool, UK

B. Breuer-Katschinski MD
Privatdozentin, Abt. für Gastroenterologie, Universitätsklinikum Essen, Germany

Jorn Brynskov MD DMSc
Senior Registrar, Department of Gastroenterology, Herlev University Hospital, Herlev, Denmark

Aaron Brzezinski MD FRCP(C)
Department of Gastroenterology, The Cleveland Clinic Foundation, Cleveland, Ohio, USA

B. J. Campbell PhD
Lecturer, Department of Medicine, University of Liverpool, Liverpool, UK

R. W. Chapman BSc (Hons) MD (London) MBBS FRCP
Consultant Gastroenterologist, John Radcliffe Hospital, Oxford, UK; Senior Lecturer (Hon.), University of Oxford Clinical Medical School, UK

Z. Cohen BA MD FRCS(C) FACS
Professor of Surgery, University of Toronto, Ontario, Canada; Surgeon-in-chief, Mount Sinai Hospital, Toronto, Ontario, Canada

B. T. Collopy FRCS FRACS FRACMA
Director, Department of Colon and Rectal Surgery, St Vincent's Hospital, Melbourne, Australia; Clinical Director, ACHS, Care Evaluation Program, Fitzroy, Australia

C. Cuvelier MD PhD
Professor of Pathology, University Hospital, Ghent, Belgium

I. D. A. D'Agata MD
Research Fellow, Department of Paediatric Gastroenterology and Nutrition, Hôpital Ste Justine, Université de Montréal, Canada

Philip A. Dean MD
Assistant Professor of Surgery, Colon and Rectal Surgery, University of Alabama at Birmingham, Birmingham, Alabama, USA

H. Debinski MB BS FRACP
Research Fellow, St Mark's Hospital, London, UK

Kemal I. Deen MD MS FRCS
Colon, Rectal and General Surgeon, University of Kelaniya Medical School, Ragama, Sri Lanka

M. De Vos MD PhD
Professor of Gastroenterology, University Hospital, Ghent, Belgium

M. F. Dixon MD FRCPath
Reader in Gastrointestinal Pathology, University of Leeds, UK; Consultant Histopathologist, Centre for Digestive Diseases, General Infirmary, Leeds, UK

R. R. Dozois MD MS FACS FRCS (Hon) (Glasgow)
Professor of Surgery, Mayo Medical School; Chairman, Division of Colon and Rectal Surgery, Mayo Clinic, Rochester, Minnesota, USA

R. Driscoll BA MLitt MSc
Director, National Association for Colitis and Crohn's Disease, St Albans, UK

Kong Weng Eu MBBS FRCS MMed FICS FAMS
Colon and Rectal Surgeon, Department of Colorectal Surgery, Singapore General Hospital, Singapore

C. M. Evans MB BCh DCH FRCP
Consultant Paediatrician, Royal Surrey County Hospital, Guildford, UK

R. C. Evans MBBS MRCP
Clinical Research Fellow, Department of Medicine, University of Liverpool, UK

Victor W. Fazio MB BS FRACS FACS
Rupert B. Turnbull Jr Chairman, Department of Colorectal Surgery, The Cleveland Clinic Foundation; Professor of Surgery, The Cleveland Clinic Foundation Health Sciences Center of The Ohio State University, Cleveland, Ohio, USA

Helen M. Fidler MD
Senior Registrar, University Department of Medicine, Royal Free Hospital Medical School, London, UK

W. R. Fleming FRACS
Senior Registrar in Surgery, Hammersmith Hospital, London, UK

H. J. Freeman MD CM FRCP(C) FACP FACG
Professor of Gastrointestinal Medicine, University of British Columbia, Vancouver Hospital, Vancouver, Canada

Frank A. Frizelle MBChB MMedSci FRACS
Consultant General and Colorectal Surgeon, Senior Lecturer in Surgery, University Department of Surgery, Christchurch School of Medicine, University of Otago, Christchurch, New Zealand

Brett T. Gemlo MD FACS
Assistant Professor, Division of Colon and Rectal Surgery, Department of Surgery, University of Minnesota, Minneapolis, Minnesota, USA

P. Ghosh MD MRCP
Clinical Assistant Professor, Indiana University Medical School; Consultant Gastroenterologist, Bloomington Hospital, Bloomington, USA

P. R. Gibson MB BS (Hons) MD FRACP
Associate Professor of Medicine, University of Melbourne, Australia; Gastroenterologist, The Royal Melbourne Hospital, Victoria, Australia

Steven L. Glorsky MD
Research Fellow, Department of Colorectal Surgery, Cleveland Clinic Florida, Fort Lauderdale, USA

S. M. Goldberg MD FACS HonFRACS HonFRCS (Eng)
Clinical Professor of Surgery, Colon and Rectal Surgery Associates, Minneapolis, Minnesota, USA

John R. Goldblum MD
Staff Pathologist, Department of Anatomic Pathology, The Cleveland Clinic Foundation, Cleveland, Ohio, USA

A. J. Greenstein MB BCh FACS FRCS
Professor of Surgery, Mount Sinai Medical Center, New York City, USA

G. E. Griffin BSc PhD FRCP FRCP (E)
Professor of Infectious Diseases and Medicine, St George's Hospital Medical School, London, UK

M. B. Grisham PhD
Professor of Physiology, LSU Medical Center, Shreveport, Louisiana, USA

J. Hamburger BDS MSc FFD RCSI
Senior Lecturer and Honorary Consultant in Oral Medicine, The School of Dentistry, University of Birmingham, UK

C. A. Hart MBBS BSc PhD FRCPath
Professor and Head of Department, Department of

Medical Microbiology and Genito-urinary Medicine, University of Liverpool, UK

R. H. Hawes MD
Professor of Medicine and Chief of Endoscopy, Medical University of South Carolina, Charleston, South Carolina, USA

C. J. Hawkey DM FRCP
Professor of Gastroenterology, University Hospital, Nottingham, UK

Peter R. Hawley MS FRCS
Consultant Surgeon, St Mark's Hospital and King Edward VIII's Hospital for Officers, London, UK

A. B. Hawthorne DM MRCP (UK)
Consultant Gastroenterologist, University Hospital of Wales, Cardiff, UK

M. J. Hershman DHMSA MSc MS FRCS (Eng, Edin, Glas & Irel)
Consultant Surgeon, Royal Liverpool University Hospital, Liverpool, UK

H. J. F. Hodgson DM FRCP
Professor of Medicine and Consultant Physician, Royal Postgraduate Medical School, Hammersmith Hospital, London, UK

Cory M. Hogaboam PhD
Research Scientist, McMaster University Intestinal Disease Research Unit, Hamilton, Ontario, Canada

G. K. T. Holmes MD PhD FRCP
Consultant Physician and Gastroenterologist, Derbyshire Royal Infirmary, Derby, UK

Mark Hudson MRCP
Consultant Gastroenterologist, Gastroenterology/Liver Unit, Freeman Hospital, Newcastle upon Tyne, UK

T. L. Hull MD
Staff, Colorectal Surgery, The Cleveland Clinic Foundation, Cleveland, Ohio, USA

L. Hultén MD FRCS (Eng) FACS
Professor of Surgery, Sahlgrenska Hospital, University of Göteborg, Sweden

R. H. Hunt FRCP FRCPEd FRCPC FACG
Professor, Department of Medicine, Division of Gastroenterology, McMaster University Medical Centre, Hamilton, Ontario, Canada

E. Jan Irvine MD FRCPC MSc
Associate Professor of Medicine, Division of Gastroenterology, Department of Medicine, McMaster University, Hamilton, Ontario, Canada

M. Irving MD FRCS
Professor of Surgery and Honorary Consultant Surgeon, Hope Hospital (University of Manchester School of Medicine), Salford, UK

B. T. Jackson MS FRCS
Consultant Surgeon, St Thomas' Hospital, London, UK

G. Järnerot MD PhD
Consultant Gastroenterologist, Division of Gastroenterology, Department of Medicine, Örebro Medical Center Hospital, Örebro, Sweden; Professor of Gastroenterology, Health University, Linköping, Sweden

J. R. Jass BSc MD FRCPath FRCPA
Professor and Head of Department of Pathology, University of Queensland, Brisbane, Australia

D. P. Jewell DPhil FRCP
Consultant Physician, John Radcliffe Hospital, Oxford, UK; Senior Clinical Lecturer, University of Oxford, UK

M. A. Kamm MB BS MD FRCP FRACP
Consultant Gastroenterologist and Director, Physiology Unit, St Mark's Hospital, London, UK

M. S. Kapembwa BSc MB ChB PhD MRCP
Senior Lecturer, Department of Genitourinary Medicine and Infection, Imperial College of Science, Medicine and Technology, St Mary's Hospital Medical School, Northwick Park Hospital, Harrow, UK

M. R. B. Keighley MS FRCS
Professor of Surgery, Barling Professor of Surgery, Queen Elizabeth Hospital, University of Birmingham, UK

Patrick Kesteven FRCP FRCPA PhD
Consultant Haematologist, Freeman Hospital, Newcastle upon Tyne, UK

Robert S. Kiff MS FRCS
Senior Registrar, Department of Surgery, Royal Liverpool University Hospital, Liverpool, UK

W. A. Kmiot MBBS MS FRCS (Gen)
Senior Lecturer in Colorectal Surgery, Hammersmith Hospital, London, UK

I. J. Kodner MD
Professor of Surgery, Washington University School of Medicine, St Louis, Missouri, USA

Lothar W. Köhler MD
Privatdozent, Department of Surgery, University of Cologne, Cologne, Germany

I. Koutroubakis MD
Gastroenterologist, Department of Gastroenterology, University Hospital of Heraklion, Crete, Greece

P. R. Kvietys PhD
Professor of Physiology, Victoria Hospital Research Institute, University of Western Ontario, London, Ontario, Canada

C. B. H. W. Lamers MD PhD
Head, Department of Gastroenterology-Hepatology, University Hospital Leiden, Leiden, The Netherlands

M. J. S. Langman MD FRCP
Professor of Medicine, University of Birmingham, UK

B. A. Lashner MD MPH
Director, Center for Inflammatory Bowel Disease, The Cleveland Clinic Foundation, Cleveland, Ohio, USA

J. P. Lavender MB ChB FRCP FRCR
Emeritus Professor of Diagnostic Radiology, Hammersmith Hospital and Royal Postgraduate Medical School, London, UK; Consultant Radiologist, Ealing Hospital, London, UK

Edward Lee MD
Assistant Professor of Surgery, Albany Medical College, Department of Surgery, Albany, New York, USA

J. R. Lee MB ChB FRCS FRCR
Formerly Consultant Radiologist, The General Hospital, Birmingham, UK; Honorary Senior Lecturer, University of Birmingham, UK

J. E. Lennard-Jones MD FRCP FRCS
Emeritus Professor of Gastroenterology, University of London; Emeritus Consultant Gastroenterologist, St Mark's Hospital, London, UK

A. M. Levy MD
Fellow in Gastroenterology, Mayo Graduate School of Medicine, Mayo Clinic and Foundation, Rochester, Minnesota, USA

R. F. A. Logan BSc MB ChB MSc (Epidemiol) MFPHM FRCP
Reader in Clinical Epidemiology, Department of Public Health and Epidemiology, University of Nottingham, UK

J. R. Lowes MA MD MRCP (UK)
Consultant Gastroenterologist, Torbay Hospital, Torquay, UK

A. C. Lowry MD FACS
Associate Clinical Professor, Division of Colon and Rectal Surgery, Department of Surgery, University of Minnesota, Minneapolis, USA

J. J. McFadden PhD
Reader in Molecular Microbiology, University of Surrey, Guildford, UK

R. S. McLeod MD FRCSC FACS
Professor of Surgery and Head, Colorectal Surgery Program, University of Toronto, Ontario, Canada; Head, Division of General Surgery, Mount Sinai Hospital, Toronto, Ontario, Canada

A. Macpherson PhD MRCP
Senior Lecturer, Honorary Consultant Gastroenterologist, King's College School of Medicine and Dentistry, London, UK

R. D. Madoff MD FACS
Clinical Associate Professor of Surgery and Director of Research, Division of Colon and Rectal Surgery, University of Minnesota Medical School, St Paul, Minnesota, USA

Y. R. Mahida MD MRCP
Senior Lecturer and Consultant Physician & Gastroenterologist, University Hospital, Queen's Medical Centre, Nottingham, UK

Nicholas P. Mapstone MBChB MRCPath
Senior Lecturer in Pathology, University of Leeds, Leeds, UK

J. F. Mayberry DSc MD LIM FRCP FRCP (Irel)
Consultant Physician, Leicester General Hospital, Leicester, UK; Visiting Professor, Loughborough Business School, University of Loughborough, UK

L. Mayer MD
Dorothy and David Merksayer Professor of Medicine and Professor of Microbiology; Chief, Division of Clinical Immunology, Mount Sinai Medical Center, New York City, USA

Alan P. Meagher FRACS
Colorectal Surgeon, St Vincent's Hospital and St Luke's Hospital, Sydney, Australia

H. Mielants MD PhD
Professor of Rheumatology, University Hospital, Ghent, Belgium

Suneel Mohammed MD
Fellow, Division of Gastroenterology, Brown University School of Medicine, Providence, Rhode Island, USA

Gillian Moody MRCP
Senior Registrar in Medicine and Gastroenterology, Leicester General Hospital, Leicester, UK

A. I. Morris MSc MD FRCP
Consultant Physician and Clinical Director of Gastroenterology, Royal Liverpool University Hospital, Liverpool, UK

N. J. McC. Mortensen MA MD FRCS
Consultant Surgeon and Clinical Reader in Colorectal Surgery, John Radcliffe Hospital, Oxford, UK

J. J. Murray MD FACS
Department of Colon and Rectal Surgery, Lahey Clinic, Burlington, Massachusetts, USA

H. Nelson MD FACS
Consultant, Division of Colon and Rectal Surgery, Mayo Clinic and Mayo Foundation; Associate Professor of Surgery, Mayo Medical School, Rochester, Minnesota, USA

J. R. Oakley MBBS FRACS
Visiting Colorectal Surgeon, Royal Hobart Hospital, Hobart, Tasmania, Australia

Sarah T. P. O'Dwyer BSc MD FRCS
Consultant Colorectal Surgeon, Christie Hospital, Manchester, UK

J. F. C Olliff BMedSci BS MRCP FRCR
Consultant Radiologist, University Hospital Birmingham NHS Trust, Queen Elizabeth Hospital, Birmingham, UK

Colm A. O'Morain MD MSc FRCPI
Professor of Gastroenterology, Academic Head of Department of Medicine, Meath/Adelaide Hospitals, Trinity College, Dublin, Ireland

Tom Öresland MD PhD
Göteborg University, Department of Surgery, Sahlgrenska University Hospital, Göteborg, Sweden

Maria O'Sullivan BSc MINDI
Research Dietitian, Department of Gastroenterology, Meath/Adelaide Hospitals, Trinity College, Dublin, Ireland

J. G. Peiser MD
Senior Lecturer, Ben Gurion University of the Negev, Beer-Sheva; Vice-President of Soroka Medical Center and Director of Operating Theatres, Beer-Sheva, Israel

J. H. Pemberton MD
Professor of Surgery and Consultant in Colon and Rectal Surgery, Mayo Medical School, Mayo Clinic, Rochester, Minnesota, USA

A. S. Peña MD PhD
Professor, Department of Gastroenterology, Free University Hospital, Amsterdam, The Netherlands

A. M. Peters BSc MSc MD MBChB MRCP MRCPath
Consultant in Nuclear Medicine, Hammersmith Hospital, London, UK

Robert E. Petras MD
Chairman, Department of Anatomic Pathology, The Cleveland Clinic Foundation, Cleveland, Ohio, USA

S. F. Phillips MD FRCP FRACP FACP
Professor of Medicine, Mayo Medical School, Rochester, Minnesota, USA; Karl F. and Marjory Hasselmann Professor of Research, Division of Gastroenterology, Mayo Clinic and Foundation, Rochester, Minnesota, USA

Daniel H. Present MD
Clinical Professor of Medicine, Department of Medicine, Mount Sinai School of Medicine, New York, USA

A. B. Price FRCPath
Consultant Histopathologist, Department of Cellular Pathology, Northwick Park and St Mark's Hospitals, Harrow, UK

G. L. Radford-Smith MD MRCP DPhil
Advanced Trainee in Gastroenterology and Hepatology, Department of Gastroenterology and Hepatology, Royal Brisbane Hospital, Brisbane, Australia

D. S. Rampton MA BM BCh DPhil FRCP
Consultant Gastroenterologist, Royal London Hospital, London, UK; Senior Lecturer, St Bartholomew's and Royal London School of Medicine and Dentistry, London, UK

S. S. C. Rao MD MRCP (UK) PhD
Assistant Professor of Medicine, University of Iowa College of Medicine, Iowa, USA

J. M. Rhodes MA MD FRCP
Professor of Medicine (Gastroenterology), Department of Medicine, University of Liverpool, UK

R. H. Riddell MD FRCP(C) FRCPath
Professor of Pathology, McMaster University; Chief of Service, Anatomical Pathology, McMaster University Medical Centre, Hamilton, Ontario, Canada

P. L. Roberts MD
Staff Surgeon, Department of Colon and Rectal Surgery, Lahey Hitchcock Clinic, Burlington, Massachusetts, USA

W. M. C. Rosenberg MA MBBS DPhil MRCP
Clinical Tutor, Nuffield Department of Clinical Medicine, University of Oxford, UK

David A. Rothenberger MD
Clinical Professor and Chief, Division of Colon and Rectal Surgery, Department of Surgery, University of Minnesota, Minneapolis, Minnesota, USA

Peter M. Sagar MD
Division of Colon and Rectal Surgery, Mayo Clinic and Mayo Foundation, Rochester, Minnesota, USA

H. Sandberg-Gertzén MD PhD
Consultant Gastroenterologist, Division of Gastroenterology, Department of Medicine, Örebro Medical Center Hospital, Örebro, Sweden

P. F. Schofield MD FRCS
Consultant Surgeon (Hon.), Christie Hospital, Manchester; Professor of Surgery, Manchester University, UK

N. A. Scott BSc (Hons) MD FRCS
Consultant Colorectal Surgeon, Department of Surgery, Hope Hospital, Salford, UK

E. G. Seidman MDCM FRCP (C) CSPQ
Associate Professor, Departments of Paediatrics and Nutrition, Division of Gastroenterology and Nutrition, Ste Justine Hospital, Faculty of Medicine, University of

Montréal, Canada; Director, Intestinal Immunology Laboratory, Division of Paediatrics and Nutrition, Ste Justine Hospital, Montréal, Canada

John E. Smithson MD MRCP
Senior Registrar (Gastroenterology and General Medicine), Selly Oak Hospital, Birmingham, UK

David Spence BSc (Hons) MRPharmS
Research Fellow, Leicester General Hospital, Leicester, UK

R. C. Spiller MB BChir MSc (London) MD FRCP
Consultant Physician, Division of Gastroenterology, University Hospital, Nottingham, UK

P. J. d'E. Stevens
Chief Professional Nurse, Stomaltherapy Unit, Groote Schuur Hospital, Capetown, South Africa

S. A. Strong MD
Staff Surgeon, Department of Colorectal Surgery, The Cleveland Clinic Foundation, Cleveland, Ohio, USA

Lloyd R. Sutherland MDCM MSc FRCPC FACP
Professor and Head, Department of Community Health Sciences, Faculty of Medicine, University of Calgary, Calgary, Alberta, Canada

Stephan R. Targan MD
Professor, UCLA School of Medicine; Director, Inflammatory Bowel Disease Center; Director, Division of Gastroenterology, Cedars-Sinai Medical Center, Los Angeles, USA

W. R. Thayer, Jr BS MD
Professor of Medicine, Brown University, Providence, Rhode Island, USA; Chief (Emeritus), Gastroenterology Division, Rhode Island Hospital, Providence, Rhode Island, USA

M. G. Thomas BSc MS FRCS FRCS (Gen)
Consultant Senior Lecturer, Department of Surgery, Bristol Royal Infirmary, Bristol, UK

N. P. Thompson MRCP MD
Senior Registrar, Freeman Hospital, Newcastle upon Tyne, UK

J. J. Tjandra MBBS (Melb) MD (Melb) FRACS FRCS FRCPS
Colorectal Surgeon, Royal Melbourne Hospital and University of Melbourne, Australia

H. H. Tsai MD (Hons) MRCP (UK)
Consultant Physician and Gastroenterologist, Castle Hill Hospital, Cottingham, UK

C. Tysk MD PhD
Associate Professor, Consultant Gastroenterologist, Division of Gastroenterology, Department of Medicine, Örebro Medical Center Hospital, Örebro, Sweden

E. P. Variyam MBBS FACP
Chief, Gastroenterology Section, Department of Veterans' Affairs Medical Center; Associate Professor of Medicine, Case Western Reserve University Cleveland, Ohio, USA

Andrew J. Wakefield MBBS FRCS
Senior Lecturer in Medicine and Histopathology and Director of Inflammatory Bowel Disease Study Group, Royal Free Hospital School of Medicine, London, UK

J. A. Walker-Smith MD BS FRACP FRCP (E) (L)
Professor of Paediatric Gastroenterology, University Department of Paediatric Gastroenterology, Royal Free Hospital, London, UK

J. L. Wallace BSc MSc PhD
Professor, Department of Pharmacology and Therapeutics; Director, Intestinal Disease Research Unit, University of Calgary, Alberta, Canada

B. F. Warren MB ChB MRCPath
Consultant Gastrointestinal Pathologist, John Radcliffe Hospital, Oxford, UK

Paul Watkins MA VetMB PhD MRCVS DVR
Veterinary Surgeon, Medical Countermeasures, CBD, Porton Down, Salisbury, UK

Anthony Weiss MD
Clinical Instructor, Burrill Crohn Research Fellow, Department of Medicine, Division of Gastroenterology, Mount Sinai School of Medicine, New York, USA

S. D. Wexner MD FACS FASCRS FACG
Chairman and Residency Program Director, Department of Colorectal Surgery; Vice-Chairman, Division of Surgery; Chairman, Division of Research and Education, Cleveland Clinic Florida, Fort Lauderdale, Florida, USA

G. S. W. Whiteley MS FRCS
Consultant Surgeon, Gwynedd Hospitals NHS Trust, UK

J. G. Williams BSc MCh MBBCh FRCS
Consultant Colo-rectal Surgeon, New Cross Hospital, Wolverhampton, UK

B. G. Wolff MD
Professor of Surgery, Mayo Foundation, Rochester, Minnesota, USA

Cheryl L. Wright MD FRCP (C)
Department of Laboratory Medicine, Chedoke McMaster Hospitals, Hamilton, Ontario, Canada

Matthew J. Zimmerman FRACP
Digestive Disease Center, Medical University of South Carolina, Charleston, South Carolina, USA

Preface

This third edition encompasses the remarkable developments in inflammatory bowel disease that have occurred in this decade. We are delighted to welcome three outstanding members to the Editorial team: Jonathan Rhodes, Stephen Hanauer and Victor Fazio. We have grasped this opportunity to create a new book and enlist the help of a large international group of distinguished contributors. We are grateful that so many experts in the field have contributed their manuscripts to us on time; their remarkable clarity has made editing a pleasure.

Pathogenesis has received particular attention including the new work in basic science which is the key to future advances. The section on diagnosis includes new contributions on CT scanning, ultrasound, MRI and isotope studies. The advances in endoluminal ultrasound have been included in the endoscopy section.

The section concerned with differential diagnosis has been expanded to consider those disorders with which inflammatory bowel disease might be confused.

The natural history of Crohn's disease and ulcerative colitis is followed by a discussion of the therapeutic options and how they can be applied appropriately to specific problems. Special problems receive particular attention including extraintestinal manifestations, the disease in childhood and pregnancy, hepatobiliary disorders and cancer surveillance. The surgical section is completely new. It opens with a discussion of surgical principles and operative technique, including laparoscopy.

The varied approach to the surgical treatment of ulcerative colitis is considered with an expanded section concerned with the role of the ileo-anal pouch. The surgical options for Crohn's disease are then considered followed by specific chapters on the treatment of complications. The volume closes with contributions on stoma management and the social and psychological aspects of the disease.

The project has come to fruition rapidly and we are most grateful to our publishers who have been ever helpful and supportive. If this volume conveys some of the excitement and interest in this rapidly developing and important field then we shall feel the task has been worthwhile.

Birmingham 1997   Robert Allan

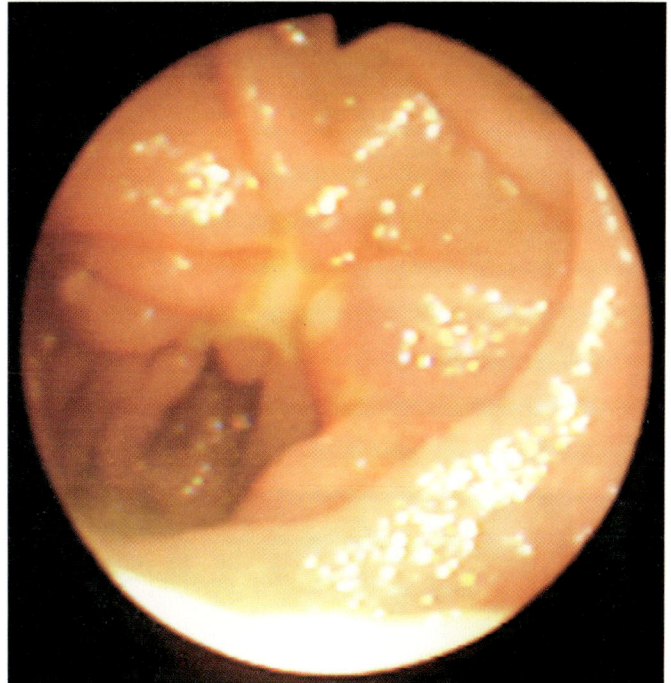

Fig.28.2 See page 271.

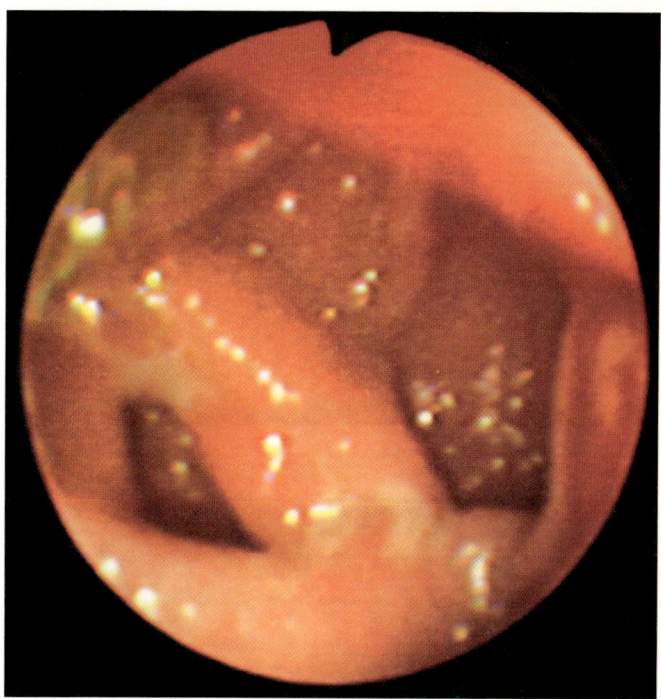

Fig.28.3 See page 272.

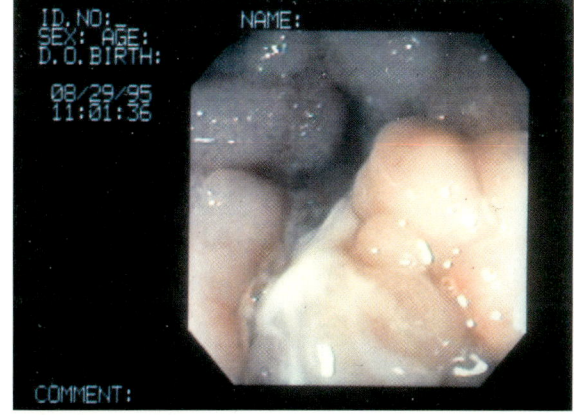

Fig. 29.1 See page 275.

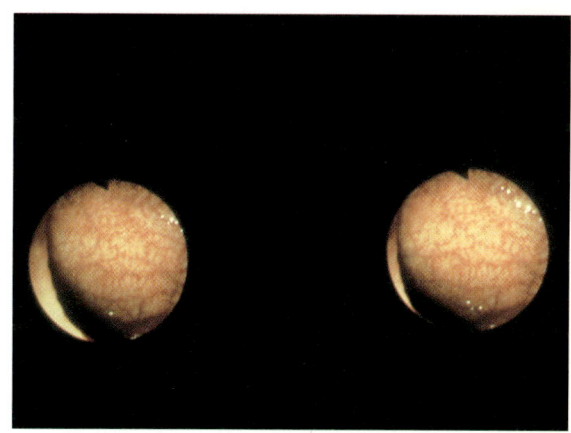

Fig. 29.2 See page 277.

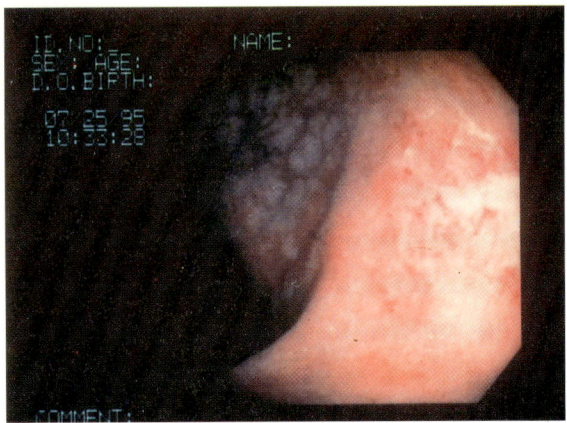

Fig. 29.3 See page 278.

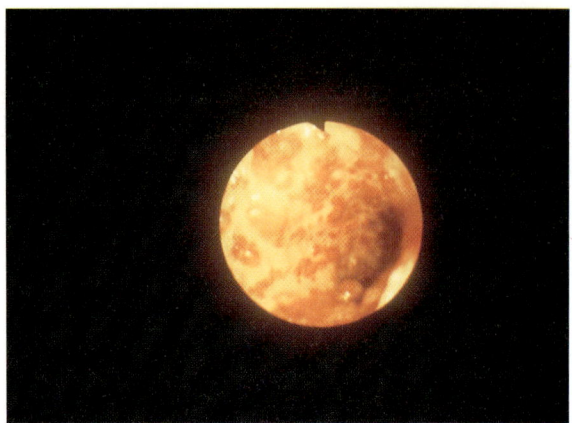

Fig. 29.4 See page 278.

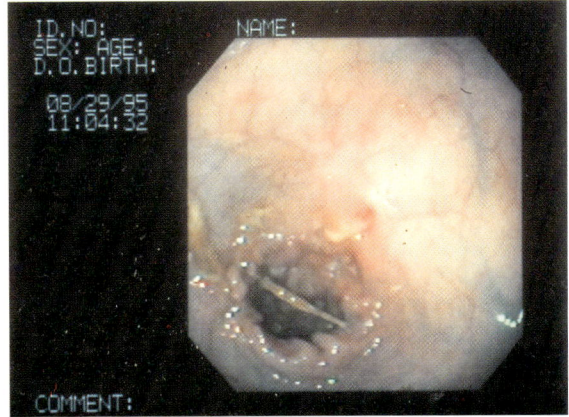

Fig. 29.5 See page 279.

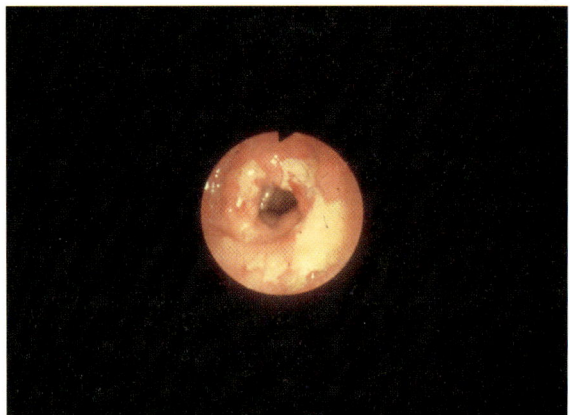

Fig. 29.6 See page 279.

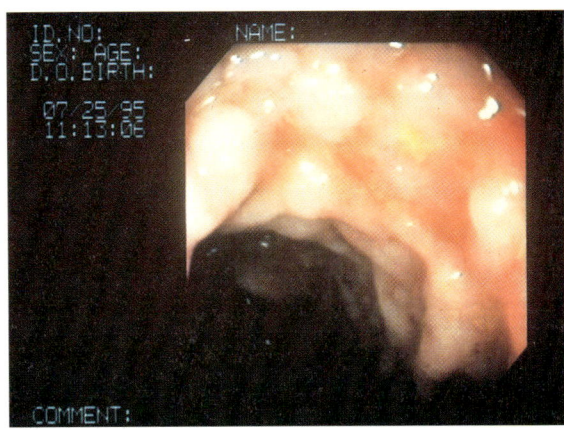

Fig. 29.7 See page 280.

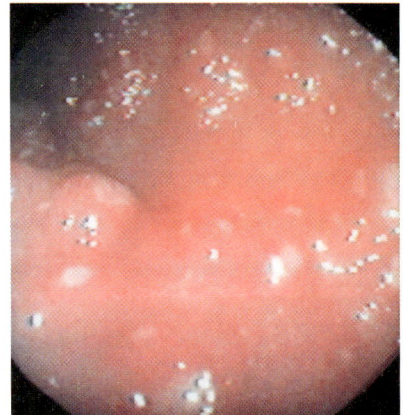

Fig. 42.2 See page 394.

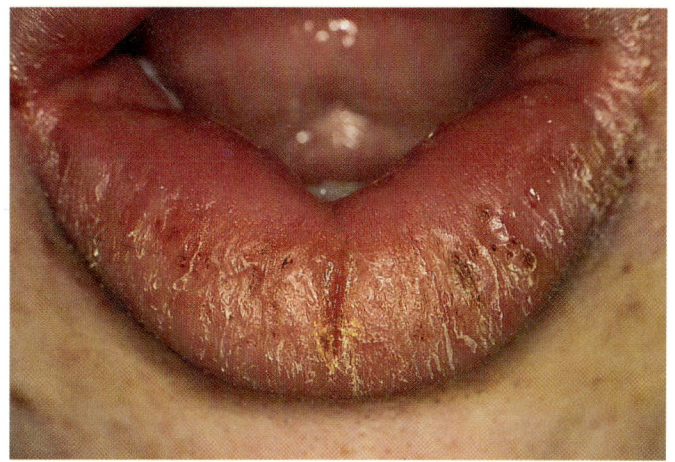

Fig. 70.1

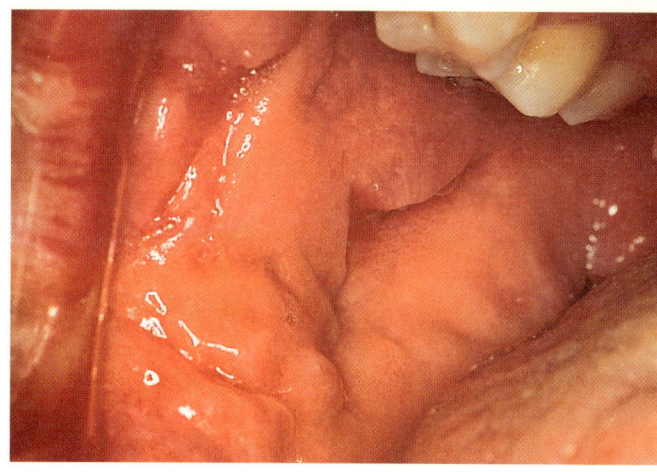

Fig. 70.2

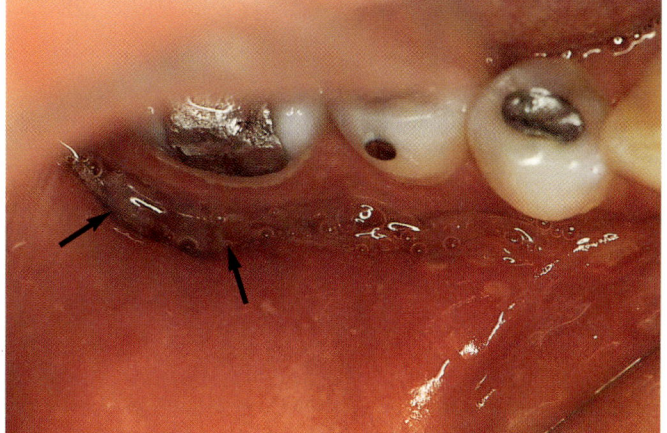

Fig. 70.3

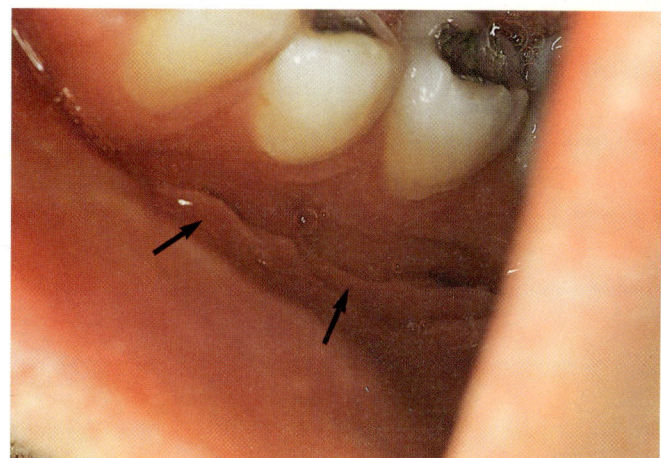

Fig. 70.4

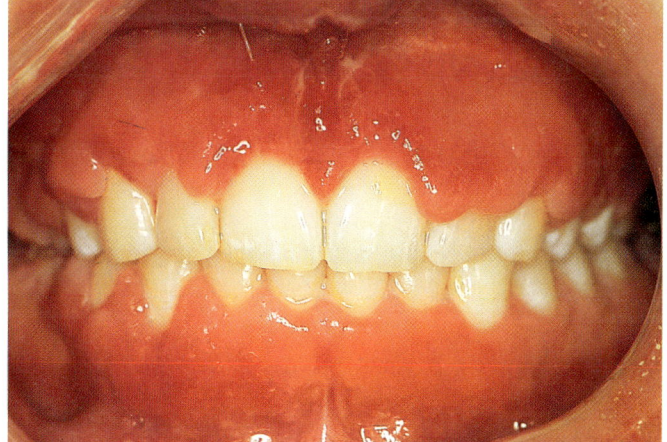

Fig. 70.5

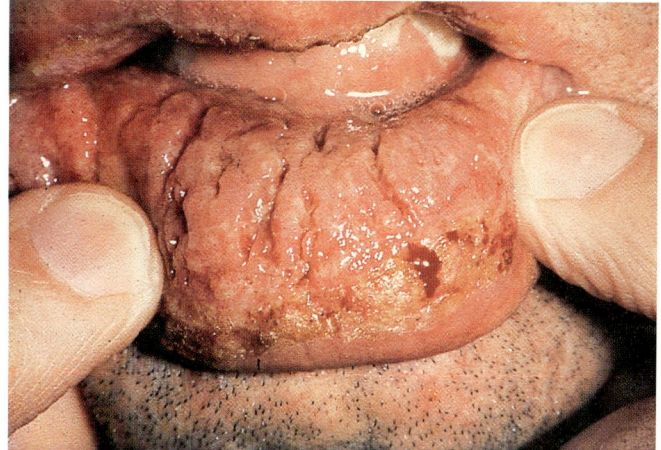

Fig. 70.6

Figs 70.1–70.6 See pages 634–5.

SECTION 1

Historical review

1. Historical review

J. Alexander–Williams

The historian needs to define certain milestones and as a surgeon I am tempted to use as the first the introduction of anesthesia in 1878, when surgeons were first able to contribute to the management of inflammatory bowel disease. The milestone of 1932 was the publication of the first clear description of the disease we now know as Crohn's disease. The history of ulcerative colitis can be divided at 1952, with the simultaneous publication of successful eversion or epithelialized ileostomies by Brooke (1952) and by Crile and Turnbull (1954), giving Brooke precedence because his solution was the more feasible and practical and also because he was my predecessor in Birmingham. I will divide the history of inflammatory bowel disease into AB (ante Brooke) and PB (post Brooke). For more recent milestones I am hard pressed to differentiate between Parks and Nicholls (1978) who recorded their first major successes with continent pouches, or Lee and Papaioannou (1982) with minimal surgery for Crohn's disease. Such is the escalation of the pace of modern change that eras become shorter.

THE HISTORY OF ULCERATIVE COLITIS BEFORE 1952

Historians cannot resist the temptation to attribute to some great historical writer diseases that have been recognized as specific only in modern times. It must have been towards the end of the 19th century, once bacteriology was enough of a science to identify specific causes, that the disease of chronic mucosal ulcerative colitis was able to be differentiated from acute infectious colitis. Nevertheless, in the writings of many early medical heros can be found accounts that would do reasonably well for descriptions of chronic ulcerative colitis. These include Hippocrates of Cos, Aretaeus of Cappadocia and Soranus of Ephesus, who between the years of 640 BC and AD 170 described the clinical details of those who suffered from one or other cause of chronic diarrhea, usually with blood and an ulcerated bowel. Then came the Dark Ages, and it was not until the 17th century that written descriptions of diarrhea or dysenteric diseases were again recorded in graphic detail. It is possible, though never can it be proved, that the 'bloody flux of Sydenham' was the ulcerative colitis that we know today (Kirsner 1988, Hawkins 1990).

The end of the 19th century

Until recently it has been fashionable to attribute the first 'modern' description of ulcerative colitis to Sir Samuel Wilks who, in a letter to the *Medical Times and Gazette* (1859), referred to a death from idiopathic dysentery and suggested that the ulcerated bowel was caused by an abortifacient. This opinion, expressed in the criminal court, almost caused Dr Thomas Smethurst to be hanged for the murder of his mistress, Isabella Banks. However, as Professor John Fielding of Dublin argued so convincingly in the *British Medical Journal* (Fielding 1985), Wilks was almost certainly describing a case of Crohn's disease rather than either ulcerative colitis or homicide. Miss Banks died in early pregnancy after a short illness. Wilks describes the autopsy as follows: 'The intestines lay in a coil adherent by a thin layer of lymph indicative of recent inflammation; the ileum was inflamed for three feet from the ileocaecal valve though otherwise the small intestine looked normal. The large intestine was ulcerated from end to end with ulcers of various sizes mostly *isolated* – though some had run together . . . Inflammation was most marked at the proximal colon and the caecum appeared to be sloughing causing the peritonitis. Tuberculosis was excluded'.

It was Wilks again, writing this time with Walter Moxon (Wilks & Moxon 1875) in lectures on pathological anatomy, who first made the distinction between ulcerative colitis and specific forms of dysentery. His observations are astute and the arguments persuasive, although there are little or no hard data with which could be verified. In those days a doctor's reputation was based more on quality of prose and style rather than on scientific data, and it is easy to see how Wilks attracted the reader's attention when he wrote 'the term colitis is sometimes used as though synonymous with dysentery. Our usual language has indeed been too indefinite, nay, incorrect, in speaking of all affections of the large intestine as dysenteric ... there is quite as much reason to regard febrile epidemic dysentery as a disease distinct from simple ulcerative colitis as there is to regard febrile epidemic diphtheria as a disease distinct from croup ...'. It was perhaps unwise of him to have coined the phrase '*simple* ulcerative colitis', as most of the data were from patients coming to autopsy.

Wilks and Moxon (1875) describe a severe, highly vascular inflammation of the entire colon with scattered minute points of ulceration in a young women who died after experiencing severe bloody and mucoid diarrhea.

Habershon, writing in *Diseases of the Abdomen*, published in London in 1862, was probably the first to describe intestinal pseudopolyps in ulcerative colitis. He wrote: 'in the third stage we find ulceration, sometimes merely as minute circular ulcers but generally of a more extensive character; the ulcers are often oval in form, and based in the transverse axis of the intestine, and their edges are raised and injected, irregular and undermined; and their base is formed by the cellular or muscular coats. These ulcerations gradually extend so as to coalesce till at last nearly the whole of the mucous surface is destroyed, except here and there prominent isolated portions which become intensely congested, and resemble polypoid growths'. Sir William Allchin (1885), from the Westminster Hospital in London, reported on the autopsy of a young woman who died after an acute illness following her fifth confinement: he described gross ulceration of the mucosa of the colon. Allchin comments that the woman experienced relatively little pain, an observation that we can confirm today in patients with fulminant ulcerative colitis. In discussion he states: 'it is to be regretted that the term dysentery is not restricted to the true tropical malady and it should not at once be applied in an adjective form to any diarrhoea dependent upon ulceration of the colon when the factors for the production of the specific disease are, as far as can be recognised, wanting'.

As was so common in the 19th century, serious diseases tended only to be described by pathologists and discussed by physicians. However, at the end of the 19th century we see the first surgical 'breakthrough'. It was probably that great surgical pioneer from Leeds, Mayo-Robson, who performed the first definitive operation for ulceration: in 1893 he created a temporary colostomy. The colitis was then treated, we know not how, and the colostomy later closed (Kirsner 1988).

The first half of the 20th century

With the increasing use of anesthesia, antisepsis and asepsis this century heralded the entry of surgeons into the management of colitis. In 1909 Lockhart-Mummery described the use of sigmoidoscopy in ulcerative colitis and emphasized its value in the detection of large-bowel cancer. In the same year there was a major symposium at the Royal Society of Medicine in London, based on the collected findings of 307 patients observed between 1888 and 1907. Most of the cases were from autopsy reports, with death occurring from colonic perforation, peritonitis, hemorrhage or sepsis. The discussion centered on the value of surgical intervention. Lockhart-Mummery (1909) said that 'the choice of operation lay between caecostomy and appendicostomy', whereas Makins, another contributor to the symposium, expressed a preference for colostomy rather than appendicostomy. In the early 20th century there were no stoma appliances to prevent skin excoriation, which limited all surgical intervention. Nor did doctors appreciate that the exposed serosa of the gut would soon be covered in granulation tissue, which would continue to heal by fibrosis until it produced an unmanageable stenosis.

At the Paris Congress of Medicine in 1913 there was further discussion on ulcerative colitis, although it was largely a regurgitation of the ideas expressed 4 years earlier in London. However, in that same year Brown of the USA proposed the operation of ileostomy 'to rest the bowel' and allow its healing, as had been recommended by the British physicians earlier (Kirsner 1988). This therapeutic approach was adopted briefly in the United States in the 1930s and soon discarded. It is not surprising that in those days surgical intervention had a bad name: it was regarded as 'last-ditch therapy', the effects of the operation usually being considered worse than those of the disease. The first half of the 20th century therefore saw an almost unlimited expansion of ingenious therapeutic regimens, from diet to immune stimulation, with hardly a mention of operation (Kirsner 1988).

The psychogenic basis for ulcerative colitis was proposed (in 1930) by a medical student named Murray. It rapidly gained favour and many patients were subsequently treated by psychotherapy and psychoanalysis. Sadly, the approach was of little therapeutic benefit.

Despite what Brown had written, the early surgical procedures such as appendicostomy, cecostomy and colostomy were performed more to allow proximal instillation of topical antiseptic agents than to 'rest the bowel'. Many liters of antibacterial agents, such as potassium permanganate and hypochloride, were instilled via the stoma, to little effect. In hardly any patient was the success of Mayo-Robson's patient repeated. It was not until Koernig developed an adhesive rubber bag that the era of successful permanent ileostomy arrived. Koernig was a chemistry student who had had an ileostomy for ulcerative colitis under the care of Dr Strauss. Koernig was encouraged to create a rubber bag, cemented to the skin closely around the stoma to prevent contact between the intestinal effluent and the skin. He eventually developed a cement which in most patients was relatively non-irritant.

Largely as a result of this breakthrough, Strauss and Strauss (1944) were able to publish 104 cases of ileostomy. In the following year Clarence Dennis (1945), working in Minneapolis with Wangensteen, emphasized the need for colectomy at the same time as ileostomy.

However, the world was still waiting for the invention of a manageable ileostomy stoma. Stomas at that time were either flush with the skin and leaked constantly, or were brought out as a spout with exposed serosa, with disastrous consequences. At this time Lionel Hardy of Birmingham read of the revolutionary rubber bags from the United States, but despite all his charm and persuasion was unable to obtain them to use on his patients. Therefore, with the help of Dr Clifford Hawkins and the research department at Fort Dunlop in Birmingham, he developed a similar bag which stuck to the skin using a similar latex solution (Hawkins 1990).

THE BROOKE ILEOSTOMY

In the early 1950s conditions were ripe for exploitation by the inventive genius of Bryan Brooke, a young acedemic surgeon working closely with Hardy and Hawkins in Birmingham. He invented what is still known as the 'Brooke ileostomy'.

Brooke's concepts were that if mucocutaneous apposition could be achieved there would be no granulation tissue to contract, and that if the mucosa of the ileum was everted, like a prepuce, there would be a spout of ileum that could fit into the newly developed rubber bag or pouch.

Independently and at the same time, Rupert Turnbull at the Cleveland Clinic in the United States developed the same hypothesis, but he solved it by means of skin grafting the serosal aspect of the ileostomy (Crile & Turnbull 1954). These two surgeons, Brooke and Turnbull, lifelong friends and collaborators, are jointly credited with the birth of the era of successful permanent end ileostomy. It is, however, Brooke's technique of eversion that persists today, hence it is appropriate that it should be termed the 'Brooke ileostomy' (Brooke 1952, 1954).

Since 1950 the history of surgical intervention in ulcerative colitis has developed along three lines:

1. the perfection of the formation of an end ileostomy;
2. the definition of the indications for and limitations of an ileorectal anastomosis;
3. the endeavor to create a continent ileostomy by pouch, by making a small bowel pouch as a neorectum and making it continent with either an inverted nipple valve or anastomosis to the anus, with preservation or recreation of a functioning anal sphincter.

End ileostomy The original Brooke ileostomies were situated just outside the lateral edge of the rectus abdominis muscle, and were sufficiently long to be able to dangle into the large black rubber bags that were then the only relatively odor-free appliances available. It was soon accepted that ileostomy prolapse or retraction was a common complication unless the stoma was brought out through the separated muscle fibers of the rectus abdominis, and that long stomas were both unsightly and easily traumatized. With the development of light odour-proof plastic bags and more effective seals to the skin it was no longer necessary to have a long spout, and this was gradually replaced by the modern 'bud' or 'button', rarely more than 2 cm long. This refinement of the end ileostomy combined with proctocolectomy is arguably the most trouble-free surgical solution to life-threatening or incapacitating chronic mucosal ulcerative colitis.

Ileorectal anastomosis Because ulcerative colitis commonly begins in and predominantly affects the rectum it is rarely possible to salvage a functioning rectum if the colitis is sufficiently severe to warrant colectomy. However, in a few patients (in our series under 10%) there is absolute or relative rectal sparing. Stanley Aylett in the 1950s in Great Britain advocated ileorectal anastomosis (Aylett 1960). He eventually accumulated over 300 cases of diffuse ulcerative colitis treated by total colectomy and ileorectal anastomosis (Aylett 1966, 1971).

Until the recent improvements in function following restorative proctocolectomy, ileorectal anastomosis has had many advocates. It had a number of obvious advantages over the then only alternative of end ileostomy, but there was a risk of anastomotic dehiscence (Veidenheimer et al 1970), postoperative intestinal obstruction (Jones et al 1977) and carcinoma developing in the residual rectal stump (about 5% at 20 years) (Baker et al 1978, Williams and Johnston 1985).

Continent ileostomy with abdominal stoma Nils Kock is acknowledged as the pioneer of the continent abdominal pouch that usually bears his name. His work, pioneered in Gothenburg and developed during a sabbatical year in Zurich, was widely adopted, until it was gradually replaced with restorative proctocolectomy when pouch-to-anus anastomoses were developed (Kock 1969).

The modern era: ileoanal anastomosis Owen Wangensteen of Minneapolis is usually credited with the first ileoanal anastomosis (Wangensteen 1948), although the result was so bad that it was revised to an ileostomy within weeks. Best (1948) and Goligher (1951) tried and abandoned the operation because of the high incidence of frequency, urgency and nocturnal incontinence. Even those advocating the operation reported satisfactory function in less than 50% of patients (Devine & Webb 1951, Schneider 1955).

The first serious attempt to preserve the anal sphincter was made by separating the diseased mucosa from the muscle of the preserved upper anal canal. After successful experiments in dogs, Ravitch (1948) reported two young adults who were said to be continent and able to discriminate flatus from feces. It is only in children and young adults that the operation of 'straight' ileoanal anastomosis has had any success, and even in the young it has now largely been superseded by the pouch.

The total excision of the large-bowel mucosa and the creation of a large reservoir pouch that is anastomosed close to the anal verge, is an operation that evolved rather than was invented. Many names have been associated with its early evolution, names frequently cited and all worthy of recognition, include Ravitch (1948), Valiente and Bacon (1955), Peck and Allenbeck (1964), Glotzer and Phil (1969), Kock (1969), Fonkalsrud and Ament (1978); however, in the United Kingdom the credit is usually attributed to Parks and Nicholls (1978), whereas in Japan Utsunomiya and colleagues (1986) were the first major players in the field. Details of development and operative techniques are to be found in the section on ulcerative colitis.

HISTORY OF CROHN'S DISEASE

Up to 1932

Although the workers from the Mount Sinai Hospital in New York put the disease that we now call Crohn's disease on the medical map, others had clearly recognized its occurrence as a distinct disease entity for at least a century before the most quoted paper of Crohn and colleagues (1932). Historical surveys have revealed descriptions of apparent cases of Crohn's disease as far back as Morgagni in 1769. In 1813 Coombe reported the clinical history and autopsy finding in a young man who died of intestinal obstruction after many years of abdominal pain; the distal ileum was described as thickened and narrowed. In 1828 Abercrombie described a similar case and, according to Kirsner (1988), later in the same century, Moore in 1882 and Fenwick in 1889 produced further single case reports. Fenwick's patient was a young woman who had an intestinal fistula complicating a stenosis. The English speaking world, however, cannot be forgiven for disregarding the paper by Dalziel published in the *British Medical Journal* of 1913. Dalziel described nine cases, of which the first was a doctor who underwent surgery in 1901. Of these nine cases, six almost certainly had what we now call Crohn's disease. In Dalziel's paper the macroscopic appearance of the distal ileum was graphically described as 'an eel in a state of rigor mortis'.

Wilks and Moxon (1875) produced 'Lectures on pathological anatomy' in which they described the case of a young man with a lesion of the ileum that was so narrow that a quill could not be passed through it. In The Netherlands a thesis by De Groot (written in Dutch) described three cases of stenotic lesions of the small intestine in which tubercle bacilli and spirochaetes were excluded (van Coevorden 1989). At operation this patient showed dilatation proximal to two stenotic areas in the terminal ileum. The mesentery was thickened and encroached on the ileal wall. There were nodules like tuberculosis on the serosa, and the ileal wall was rigid and the mucosa ulcerated. Microscopically the inflammation was transmural, with lymphocytes and plasma cells, gross fibrosis and giant cells.

In 1932 there occurred what Janowitz (1985) described as a 'quantum leap', with the presentation of two papers from the group of physicians, surgeons and pathologists from Mount Sinai Hospital. Before this, Janowitz records that the pathologists Willenski and Moschowitz, also of the Mount Sinai Hospital, had reported granulomatous lesions of the small bowel. These had been found in most of the patients who were to make up the series presented to two learned societies in the United States. Ginzburg and Oppenheimer (1933) presented a paper to the American Gastroenterological Association entitled 'non-specific granulomata of the intestines (inflammatory tumor and strictures of the bowel)', which was later published in 1933 in the *Annals of Surgery*. In the same month Crohn presented his paper with Oppenheimer and Ginzburg to the American Medical Association. In its original presentation the paper by Crohn and his colleagues referred only to localized ileitis, which they called 'terminal ileitis'. However, during the discussion Bargen, from the Mayo Clinic, suggested that the term had agonal connotations and that 'regional ileitis' would be more appropriate; such was the title when the classic paper was first published in the same year in the *Journal of the American Medical Association* (Crohn et al 1932).

Before this the Dutch medical literature carried a paper by Nuboer (1932) describing two patients with chronic phlegmonous ileitis, a condition that was obviously the same as that described by Crohn and his colleagues later in the year.

1932 onwards. Which part of the gut is affected?

Although the work of Ginzburg and Oppenheimer (1933) had been concerned with a total of 52 cases presenting with abdominal masses and obstruction, all of which they felt had been described erroneously as tuberculosis or carcinoma, the 1932 paper by Crohn, Oppenheimer and Ginzburg concentrated only on those 14 cases from the same series that affected the terminal ileum. This seminal paper concentrated peoples' minds on the concept of a specific terminal ileal disease.

Ginzburg and Oppenheimer's larger series had included cases of sealed-off perforations of the bowel, strictures secondary to ischemic disease, and hypertrophic ulcerative stenosis with skip lesions. They also described a fourth group of patients with 'localized hypertrophic colitis'. Ginzburg later presented X-ray evidence of films taken in 1925 showing obvious granulomatous disease of the right side of the colon.

Even before the classic 1932 paper, pathologists at the Mount Sinai hospital under Paul Klemperer had recognized that this same non-tuberculous, non-caseating granulomatous disease could affect several parts of the intestine (Janowitz 1985). It is perhaps surprising, therefore, that it took so many years before the disease as we now recognize it was acknowledged as affecting all parts of the alimentary tract.

The chronic granulomatous ulcerative disease of the colon masquerading as carcinoma or tuberculosis, but pathologically distinct from them, was recognized by Moynihan (1907) and Mayo-Robson (1908), both from Leeds. Obviously the Mount Sinai pathologists had recognized the colonic involvement in the 1920s, but it was 1934 before Colp, a surgeon of that institution, described the disease affecting the colon. Harris and colleagues (1933) had described a similar granulomatous disease affecting the duodenum, and had suggested that the name should be changed from regional ileitis to chronic cicatrizing enteritis, but it was soon widely recognized that the disease could occur throughout the alimentary tract. Crohn and Rosenak (1936) described nine cases in which regional enteritis was associated with a chronic granulomatous disease of the colon. They felt that the disease in the colon was a form of ulcerative colitis, and that its association with regional enteritis was interesting and possibly coincidental.

The disease was recognized as affecting the stomach by Bartstra and Kooreman (1939), and as affecting the duodenum by our unit in Birmingham (Fielding et al 1980). In the 1970s many investigators were using the new discovery of the Crosby capsule to obtain mucosal biopsies from throughout the alimentary tract. They used it to investigate the mucosa in patients who apparently had only a localized area affected by Crohn's disease. In these patients some histological abnormality could be detected in the mouth, esophagus, stomach, duodenum and jejunum, and to the rectum and anus. It was recognized that the disease was truly panintestinal in its manifestations; it even occurred in the mouth and pharynx (Croft & Wilkinson 1972, Basu & Asquith 1980, Sculley et al 1982).

Although it is relatively easy to understand the pathology of a disease that affects any part of the alimentary tract, it is difficult to understand when manifestations appear to occur outside the mucous membrane of the alimentary tract. Typical histological manifestations of the disease have been described in the submammary skin (Mountain 1970), the umbilical skin (Phillips & Glazer 1971) and even in the scrotum and prepuce (Atherton et al 1978). These cutaneous and subcutaneous manifestations became known as metastatic Crohn's disease, thereby making it even more difficult to fit the various propounded theories of etiology.

It has been estimated that the overall frequency of extraintestinal manifestations is about 35% (Present 1983), occurring principally in the joints, skin, eye and mouth.

What's in a name?

As we have seen Crohn, Oppenheimer and Ginzburg originally wanted to call the disease they were describing 'terminal ileitis', but this was soon changed to 'regional ileitis', only to be changed to 'regional enteritis' once it was realized that other parts of the small bowel could be affected. It is still known as regional enteritis in much of the United States. Serious problems of nomenclature arose when other parts of the alimentary tract were found to be affected. Initially purely anatomical names were used to describe the depth of penetration of the inflammation, such as 'transmural colitis', or terms that described some of the characteristic histological manifestations, such as 'granulomatous colitis'. As it became clear that these alimentary manifestations, as well as many of the extra-alimentary manifestations, were all part of the same disease, some sort of global terminology was required. In Europe and Scandinavia the term 'Crohn's disease' was readily adopted, as most physicians accepted the 1932 Mount Sinai paper as the classic description of the disease. The physicians in the United States were less ready to accept this eponym, principally because it was realized that the disease was not discovered by Crohn: he was simply first author of a paper about work done, principally, at the Mount Sinai hospital. American physicians in general, and those from Mount Sinai in particular, considered that it would be invidious to single out one name to describe a disease that would perhaps have better been termed 'Berg's disease', 'Klemperer's disease' or 'Mount Sinai disease'.

In the English language we accept what can be termed the law of common usage: whenever a word is commonly used by a body of people communicating in that language and when the word is well understood without ambiguity, then that word becomes accepted. Eventually, after what could be described as a 'decent interval', the word becomes incorporated in the standard dictionaries of the English language. According to the law of common usage, it appears that as 50 years have passed since the classic paper was published, and after the death of Dr Crohn, it would now seem reasonable to accept the term Crohn's disease – at least until such time as the etiology of the disease is known. For this reason in this book, as in most other current English-language contributions, the term Crohn's disease will be used.

MILESTONES IN MEDICAL MANAGEMENT

Medical management is considered in detail in Chapter 2. It is summarized here from a historical perspective seen through surgical eyes. Before and around 1932 the disease was studied rather than treated medically; the only definitive treatment at that time was surgical. Medical management consisted of what was euphemistically called 'general management', which usually consisted of bed rest, nourishing high protein, liquid or semisolid diet, and the replacement of any specific detected deficiencies.

In the early 1940s sulphasalazine began to be used on an entirely empirical basis. In the mid-1970s it was determined that the active ingredient of sulphasalazine was 5-ASA, and at about the same time controlled trials began to be used in the elucidation of its place in the management of Crohn's disease.

Corticosteroids were first used in the management of Crohn's disease in the 1950s, but there are few clinical trials and almost as many people condemned the drug as advocated it. In Birmingham the gastroenterologist W. Trevor Cooke, who was the leading force in the management of inflammatory bowel disease, was an eloquent if dogmatic critic of prolonged steroid therapy. He was responsible for directing many of his patients towards early surgical therapy.

Case reports on the use of immunosuppressive agents such as 5-mercaptopurine and azathioprine appeared in the late 1960s and early 1970s, and by the late 1970s a few controlled clinical trials showed some significant benefit from their use. Since then cyclosporin A and disodium cromoglycate have been introduced, tried and found to be of limited use (Lennard-Jones 1990).

Antibiotics have been used in the management of Crohn's disease from the time of their discovery, particularly to treat the septic complications. Many physicians were using broad-spectrum antibiotics in 1960, and some reported early improvement. However, long-term benefit was not reported until the introduction of metronidazole to the antimicrobial armamentarium (Gitnick 1991).

MILESTONES IN SURGICAL MANAGEMENT

Dalziel (1913) treated chronic inflammatory disease of the terminal ileum by resection, as did Berg, the pioneer surgeon working with the team at Mount Sinai Hospital. It soon became clear that the serious complications of terminal ileal Crohn's disease, such as fistula and abscess, were too complicated to be treated by simple surgical excision, and in the early series of patients from Mount Sinai Hospital a mortality of 16% led to the concept of bypass rather than excision for complicated phlegmonous masses (Garlock & Crohn 1945). The principal advantage of bypass was the lower operative risk; however, after improvements in anesthesia and pre- and postoperative management the surgical mortality was reduced and resection began to regain favour. Resection seems more logical than bypass, particularly because the disease can still progress in the bypassed segment, leading to complications such as fistula, abscess or perforation (Greenstein et al 1974), with the need for frequent reoperation. (Krause et al 1971, Alexander-Williams et al 1972).

In the 1940s the Mount Sinai Hospital surgeons, realizing this, advocated bypass with exclusion, whereby the distal end of the ileum just short of the diseased segment was either brought out as a mucous fistula or closed. The dangers of closing it were that pressure could build up proximal to the remaining obstruction: in some instances perforation occurred. The principal reason for abandoning bypass as a treatment method was the finding of carcinoma by Lightdale et al (1975) and Greenstein et al (1978), who both found a high incidence of terminal ileal carcinoma occurring in bypassed Crohn's disease. Bypass was subsequently used only for the treatment of stenosing duodenal Crohn's disease.

With the return to resection there were many surgeons who took the original advice of Crohn and resected widely, removing all macroscopically diseased tissue with a wide excision of the route of the mesentery and all involved lymph nodes. Many of these surgeons advocated the removal of 20 or 30 cm of normal bowel on either side of the lesion. Later reports showed that there was no great advantage to this and there was always a high risk of recurrence. Surgeons then moved towards minimal excision (see Chapter 80). By the 1980s many stenotic small-bowel lesions were being treated by strictureplasty, and in recent years some of them even by dilatation without excision or operation. The evolution of the surgical treatment of Crohn's disease is not yet complete, although it now has three attainable aims: to be minimal, safe, and therefore able to be used early before complications arise.

REFERENCES

Abercrombie J 1828 Pathological and practical researches on disease of the stomach, the intestinal canal, the liver and other viscera of the abdomen. Waugh and Innes, Edinburgh

Alexander–Williams J 1972 Surgery and the management of Crohn's disease. Clinics in Gastroenterology 1: 469–491

Allchin W H 1885 Case of acute extensive ulceration of the colon. Transactions of the Pathological Society of London 37: 199–202

Atherton D J, Massam M, Wells R S, Harries J T, Pincott T R 1978 Genital Crohn's disease in a 6 year old boy. British Medical Journal 4: 552

Aylett S O 1960 Diffuse ulcerative colitis and its treatment by ileorectal anastomosis. Annals of the Royal College of Surgeons of England 27: 260–265

Aylett S O 1966 Three hundred cases of diffuse ulcerative colitis treatment by total colectomy and ileorectal anastomosis. British Medical Journal 1: 1001–1005

Aylett S O 1971 Ileorectal anastomosis: review 1952–1968. Proceedings of the Royal Society of Medicine 64: 967–971

Baker W N W, Glass R E, Ritchie J K, Aylett S O 1991 Cancer of the rectum following colectomy and ileorectal anastomosis for ulcerative colitis. British Journal of Surgery 65: 862–868

Bartstra D S, Kooreman P J 1939 Peculiar localization of so-called regional ileitis. Clinics in Gastroenterology 9: 307–322

Basu M K, Asquith P 1980 Oral manifestation of inflammatory bowel disease. Clinical Gastroenterology 65: 390–397

Best R R 1948 Anastomosis of the ileum to the lower part of the rectum and anus. A report on experience with ileorectostomy and ileoproctostomy with special reference to polyposis. Archives of Surgery 57: 276–285

Brooke B N 1952 The management of an ileostomy including its complications. Lancet 2: 102–104

Brooke B N 1954 Ulcerative colitis and its surgical treatment. Livingstone, Edinburgh.

Brooke B N, Cave D R, Kind D W 1976 Place of azathioprine for Crohn's disease. Lancet i: 1041–1042

Coombe C, Saunders W 1813 A singular case of stricture and thickening of the ileum. Medical Transactions of the Royal College of Physicians, London 4: 16–18

Crile G Jr, Turnbull R B Jr 1954 The mechanism and prevention of ileostomy dysfunction. Annals of Surgery 140: 459–463

Croft C B, Wilkinson A R 1972 Ulceration of the mouth, pharynx and larynx in Crohn's disease of the intestine. British Journal of Surgery 59: 249–252

Crohn B B, Ginzburg L, Oppenheimer G D 1932 Regional ileitis: a pathologic and clinical entity. Journal of the American Medical Association 99: 1323–1329

Crohn B B, Rosenak B D 1936 A combined form of ileitis and colitis. Journal of the American Medical Association 106: 1

Dalzeil T K 1913 Chronic interstitial enteritis. British Medical Journal 2: 1068–1070

Dennis C 1945 Ileostomy and colectomy in chronic ulcerative colitis Surgery 18: 435–452

Devine J, Webb R 1951 Resection of the rectal mucosa; colectomy and anal ileostomy with normal continence. Surgery, Gynecology and Obstetrics 92: 437–442

Fielding J F 1985 'Inflammatory' bowel disease. British Medical Journal 290: 47–48

Fonkalsrud E W, Ament M E 1978 Endorectal mucosal resection without proctocolectomy as an adjunct for abdominoperineal resection for non-malignant conditions: clinical experience with five patients. Annals of Surgery 188: 245–248

Garlock J H, Crohn B B 1945 An apraisal of the results of surgery in treatment of regional ileitis. Journal of the American Medical Association 127: 205–211

Ginzburg L, Oppenheimer G D 1933 Non-specific granuloma of the intestines. Annals of Surgery 27: 1046–1062

Gitnick G 1991 Inflammatory bowel disease: diagnosis and treatment. Igaku-Shoin, New York

Glotzer P G, Phil B G 1969 Preservation of continence after mucosal graft in the rectum and its feasibility in man. American Journal of Surgery 117: 403–409

Goligher J C 1951 The functional results after sphincter-saving resection of the rectum. Annals of the Royal College of Surgeons of England 8: 421–439

Greenstein A J, Kark A E, Dreiling D A 1974 Crohn's disease of the colon. 1. Fistula in Crohn's disease of the colon, classification presenting features and management in 63 patients. American Journal of Gastroenterology 62: 419–424

Greenstein A J, Sachar D, Pucillo A et al 1978 Cancer in Crohn's disease after diversionary surgery. A report of seven carcinomas occurring excluding bowel. American Journal of Surgery 135: 86–90

Habershon S O 1862 Diseases of the abdomen. J Churchill, London

Harris F I, Bell G H, Brunn H 1933 Chronic cicatrizing enteritis. Surgery, Gynecology and Obstetrics 57: 637–645

Hawkins C F H 1990 Historical review in inflammatory bowel disease. In: Allan R N, Keighley M R B, Alexander–Williams J, Hawkins C F H, (eds) Inflammatory bowel disease. Churchill Livingstone, Edinburgh, pp 3–9

Hawkins H P 1909 Natural history of ulcerative colitis and its bearing on treatment. British Medical Journal I: 765–770

Janowitz H D 1985 Inflammatory bowel disease. A personal view. Field, Rich and Associates, New York

Jones P F, Munro A, Ewen S W B 1977 Colectomy and ileorectal anastomosis for ulcerative colitis: report on a personal series with a critical review. British Journal of Surgery 64: 615–623

Kirsner J B 1988 Historical aspects in inflammatory bowel disease. Journal Clinical Gastroenterology 10: 286–297

Koch N G 1969 Intra-abdominal reservoir in patients with permanent ileostomy. Archives of Surgery 99: 223–231

Krause K U, Bergman L, Norlen B J 1971 Crohn's disease, a clinical study based on 186 patients. Scandinavian Journal of Gastroenterology 6: 97–108

Lee E C G, Papaioannou N 1982 Minimal Surgery for chronic obstruction in patients with extensive and universal Crohn's disease. Annals of the Royal College of Surgery of England 64: 229–233

Lennard-Jones J E 1990 Corticosteroids and immunosuppressive drugs in inflammatory bowel disease. In: Allan R N, Keighley M R B, Alexander–Williams J, Hawkins C (eds) Inflammatory bowel disease. Churchill Livingstone, Edinburgh, pp 373–389

Lightdale C J, Sternberg S S, Psner G, Sherlock P 1975 Carcinoma complicating Crohn's disease. Report of seven cases and review of the literature. American Journal of Medicine 59: 262–268

Lockhart-Mummery J P 1909 In discussion on ulcerative colitis. Proceedings of the Royal Society of Medicine (Medical Section) 2: 92

Morgagni J B 1769 De Sedibu et causis morborum. Remondini, Venice.

Moynihan B G A 1907 The mimicry of malignant disease in the large intestine. Edinburgh Medical Journal 21: 228–233

Mayo-Robson A W 1908 Some abdominal tumours simulating malignant disease and their treatment. British Medical Journal 1: 425–428

Mountain J C 1970 Cutaneous ulceration in Crohn's disease. Gut; 11: 18

Nuboer F J 1932 Chronische phlegnone van hit ileum. Ned T. Geneesk 76: 29–89

Parks A G, Nicholls R J 1978 Proctocolectomy without ileostomy for ulcerative colitis. British Medical Journal; 2: 85–88

Peck P A, Allenbeck G A 1964 Fecal continence in the dog after replacement of rectal mucosa with ileal mucosa. Surgery, Gynecology and Obstetrics 119: 1312–1317

Phillips R K S, Glazer G 1981 Metastatic Crohn's disease of the umbilicus. British Medical Journal 283: 887

Present D H 1983 Crohn's disease: extraintestinal manifestations. Mount Sinai Journal of Medicine 50: 126–132

Ravitch M M 1948 Anal ileostomy with sphincter preservation in patients requiring total colectomy for benign conditions. Surgery 24: 170–187

Royal Society of Medicine Symposium on Ulcerative Colitis 1909 Proceedings of the Royal Society of Medicine 2: 59–156

Schneider S 1955 Anal ileostomy: experiences with a new three-stage procedure. Archives of Surgery 70: 539–544

Sculley C, Cochran K M, Russell R I et al 1982 Crohn's disease of the mouth: an indicator of intestinal involvement. Gut 23: 198–200

Strauss A A, Strauss S F 1944 Surgical treatment of ulcerative colitis. Surgical Clinics of North America 24: 211–224

Utsunomiya J 1986 In: Symposium: Restorative proctocolectomy for ileal reservoir. International Journal of Colorectal Disease 1: 2–19

Valiente M A, Bacon H E 1955 Construction of a pouch using 'pantaloon' technique for pullthrough of ileum following total colectomy. American Journal of Surgery 90: 742–750

van Coevorden F 1989 Surgical aspects of Crohn's disease. Doctoral Thesis, University of Amsterdam

Veidenheimer M C, Dailey T H, Meissner W A 1970 Ileorectal Anastomosis for inflammatory bowel disease of the large bowel. American Journal of Surgery 119: 375–380

Wangensteen O H, Toon R W 1948 Primary resection of the colon and rectum with particular reference to cancer and ulcerative colitis. American Journal of Surgery 75: 384–389

Wilks S, Moxon W 1875 Lectures on pathological anatomy, 2nd edn. Lindsay and Blakiston, Philadelphia, pp 408–409

Williams N S, Johnston D 1985 The current status of mucosal proctectomy and ileoanal anastomosis in the surgical treatment of ulcerative colitis and adenomatous polyposis. British Journal of Surgery 72: 159–168

SECTION 2
Pathogenesis

2. Genetics of inflammatory bowel disease

I. Koutroubakis   A. S. Peña

INTRODUCTION

Genetic studies in inflammatory bowel disease (IBD) can be divided into the following categories:

1. Family studies
2. Twin studies
3. Spouse studies
4. Ethnic studies
5. Associations of IBD with known genetic syndromes
6. Association of IBD with other diseases with known genetic predisposition
7. Association of IBD with autoimmune diseases
8. Genetic marker studies.

Critical analysis of these studies suggests that genetic predisposition is important but not alone sufficient to explain susceptibility to IBD. It is necessary to consider first, that ulcerative colitis and Crohn's disease may not be single entities but rather a group of heterogeneous disorders, and secondly, that these disorders are multi-factorial diseases where both hereditary and environmental factors play a significant part.

FAMILY STUDIES

Familial aggregation of inflammatory bowel disease has long been recognized. First-degree relatives (offspring, siblings and parents) have the greatest risk, particularly the siblings. The first-degree relatives of patients with ulcerative colitis or Crohn's disease have a 10–15-fold increase in the risk of having the same disease as the patient (Monsén et al 1987, Orholm et al 1991). However, the two diseases may also occur in the same family. This discordance of proband/relative pairs was 26% in a recent study (Reed et al 1992).

In the majority of the reports so far, the familial tendency is strongest for Crohn's disease. For example, in a recent study in Leicester (Probert et al 1993) the comparative risk in first-degree relatives of patients with ulcerative colitis to develop ulcerative colitis was 15, but the risk of Crohn's disease was not increased. When the patient had Crohn's disease the comparative risk was increased by up to 35 for Crohn's disease and three for ulcerative colitis. However, in studies from southern Europe (Meucci et al 1992, Manousos et al 1996) the familial prevalence was higher in patients with ulcerative colitis.

Table 2.1 shows the frequency of positive family history among patients with IBD in recent studies. There is a range between 6 and 20%, although some data may be criticized for the inclusion of selected patient groups. Population-based studies in well defined areas and over a long period of time of observation are more likely to give results without bias. These studies have confirmed the increased prevalence of IBD in family members compared to the control population. Age-corrected empirical risk estimates for IBD in the Ashkenazi Jewish population in the United States (Roth et al 1989) demonstrated an increased risk for the offspring, siblings and parents of patients with ulcerative colitis or Crohn's disease.

Bias may result if probands do not have accurate information about the health of all their family members. Patient-controlled studies seem to be more representative than questionnaire-controlled studies. In a recent publication (Reed et al 1992) an effort was made to identify and verify the disease status of first-degree relatives of probands by directly contracting those family members. Although ulcerative colitis probands reported 28.5% and Crohn's disease probands 34.7% of family members with IBD, the real prevalence of family history after confirmation of the diagnosis was only 9.9%.

The age of onset of IBD in some studies was found to be correlated with the familiarity of the disease (Monsén et al 1987, Yang et al 1993a). Patients with a positive family history of IBD had a lower age of onset of the disease. However, in another study (Meucci et al 1992) the mean age at onset of disease was the same in patients with and without a positive family history of IBD. Other clinical characteristics of patients with Crohn's disease, including location, transmural aggressiveness and age of onset have been found to run in families (Tokayer et al 1992). Among

Table 2.1 Incidence of positive family history (first-degree relatives) of inflammatory bowel disease in recent studies

Area	Disease	No. of cases	Positive family history (%)	Reference
Leiden, Netherlands	CD	400	8.0	Weterman & Peña 1984
Stockholm, Sweden	UC	963	7.9	Monsén et al 1987
	CD	1048	13.4	Monsén et al 1991
Liverpool, UK	UC	171	11.7	McConnell et al 1986
	CD	165	18.8	
London, UK	UC	23	8.7	Sanderson et al 1986
	CD	79	8.9	
	IBD	32	6.2	
Oxford, UK	UC	825	12	Satsangi et al 1994
	CD	317	13	
Dublin, Ireland	CD	71	12.7	Fielding 1986
Copenhagen, Denmark	UC	504	11.7*	Orholm et al 1991
	CD	133	8.3*	
Northern Italy	UC	411	6.3	Meucci et al 1992
	CD	241	4.1	
Torino, Italy	CD	125	6.4	Sategna-Guidetti et al 1986
Heraklion, Greece	UC	74	12.2	Manousos et al 1996
	CD	27	7.4	
Israel	IBD	157	6.6	Zlotogora et al 1991
Chicago, USA	IBD	179	22.3	Lashner et al 1986
Cleveland, USA	UC	316	15.8	Farmer & Michener 1986
	CD	522	16.6	
Los Angeles, USA	IBD	188	17.6	Roth et al 1989
Pennsylvania, USA	IBD	352	9.9	Reed et al 1992

UC, ulcerative colitis; CD, Crohn's disease; IBD, inflammatory bowel disease
* First- and second-degree relatives are included

relatives with Crohn's disease, 88% were concordant for location of disease, 67% were concordant for pattern of transmural aggressiveness and 68% were concordant for age of onset. In another study, six cases of parents developing IBD as a later date than their children showed a strong concordance of disease type as well as site of involvement (Burress et al 1994).

The familiality of IBD in different ethnic groups has also been studied. In Israel (Zlotogora et al 1991) the prevalence of first-degree relatives with Crohn's disease was found to be similar in families of both Ashkenazi and non-Ashkenazi origin. However, in the United States it was observed that the lifetime risks for relatives of non-Jewish patients were lower than the corresponding risks of relatives of Jewish patients (Yang et al 1993a). These studies suggest that, in addition to the genetic predisposition, environmental factors are very important in disease manifestation.

TWIN STUDIES

The data derived from studies in twins add strong support to the view that these disorders have a genetic component, since there is a significant increase in the concordance of inflammatory bowel disease in monozygotic twins compared to dizygotic twins.

In a Swedish study (Tysk et al 1988) eight of 18 monozygotic and only one of 26 dizygotic twin pairs were concordant for Crohn's disease. In contrast, in ulcerative colitis cases only one of the 16 monozygotic pairs was concordant for the disease, whereas all the 20 dizygotic or unknown zygosity pairs were discordant. The calculated heritability based on monozygotic pairs was 0.53 for ulcerative colitis and 1.0 for Crohn's disease, suggesting a much larger genetic influence in Crohn's disease than in ulcerative colitis. This was an unbiased study based on the large registry (25 000 pairs) of Swedish twins, although the number of pairs with IBD is still too small to allow definite conclusions to be reached. Other reports consist mainly of case reports, with some bias toward the reporting of concordant pairs. The observation that not all the monozygotic twins are concordant again indicates the importance of environmental factors.

In the Swedish study it was observed that smoking patterns were similar in concordant and discordant twins, implying that the sharing of identical genes and smoking patterns are not enough to develop IBD and that other environmental factors are also important.

There have been no reports of a monozygous twin pair, one with ulcerative colitis and the other with Crohn's disease, and this also supports the concept that the phenotypes of inflammatory bowel disease have a distinct genetic basis.

SPOUSE STUDIES

Indirect evidence supporting the necessity of predisposing genes for the development of the disease in the presence of a common environment is the low prevalence in spouses of patients with IBD. Most reports on IBD in spouses are case reports, and it has been regarded as an unusual occurrence probably no more frequent than would be expected by chance alone (Rhodes et al 1985).

However, Bennett et al (1991) reported 19 cases of couples with IBD among 2500 patients. In five couples both partners had symptoms of IBD before marriage; in seven only one spouse had IBD before marriage and in seven neither spouse had symptoms before marriage. Another interesting observation in the same study is that 36% of the children of these couples developed IBD, with a higher frequency (67%) if both parents had already developed IBD at the time of conception. The high incidence of offspring with IBD when both parents are affected is compatible with a disease of polygenic basis.

In France (Van Kruiningen et al 1993) two families were found, the first with husband, wife and four children, and the second with seven of 11 children with Crohn's disease. There was no history of Crohn's disease in antecedent generations, and the authors suggest that an infectious microorganism might be responsible for these clusterings.

In spite of these unusual reports the incidence of spouse concordance does not seem much increased over population risks, and is dramatically less than the risk to siblings, thus supporting a genetic predisposition.

ETHNIC STUDIES

Several studies have shown that Jews have a two to fourfold higher incidence than other races living in the same area (Table 2.2). Within the Jewish population heterogeneity is found among the different historical ethnic subgroups. American and European Ashkenazi Jews have an increased risk compared to Sephardic or Oriental Jews (Gilat et al 1986, Odes et al 1987). Ashkenazi Jews of middle European origin have an excess risk compared with Jews of Polish/Russian origin (Roth et al 1989, Zlotogora et al 1990).

In the Beer Sheva district of southern Israel the incidence and prevalence of ulcerative colitis and Crohn's disease has been studied in three Jewish populations (Odes et al 1989). Both diseases were more common in European–American-born Jews and in females. The mean annual age-adjusted incidence rates per 100 000 for the period 1979–1987 were 5.4 for ulcerative colitis and 2.1 for Crohn's disease for the total Jewish population of southern Israel, which are lower than those reported in western Europe and North America.

In a prospective epidemiological study in the Bedouin Arabs of southern Israel (Odes et al 1991) a prevalence of 9.8/100 000 for ulcerative colitis and 3.2/100 000 for Crohn's disease as found. These prevalence rates were significantly lower than the corresponding rates in the local Jewish population.

Another ethnic group that has been studied are Asian migrants to the United Kingdom. Studies from London (Chong & Walker-Smith 1986), Bradford (Findlay & Jayarantne 1986), and Leicester (Probert et al 1992, 1993) suggest that Asian immigrants have an increased susceptibility to IBD compared to Asians resident in Asia.

GENETIC SEGREGATION ANALYSIS

The existence of families in which inflammatory bowel disease appears to be inherited has permitted investigators to study the genetics of ulcerative colitis and Crohn's disease. It is apparent that the inheritance of these diseases does not conform to simple Mendelian segregation and more complex patterns of heredity have been investigated. Mathematical modeling of complex patterns of inheritance is dependent upon estimates of candidate gene frequency, gene penetrance and many other factors for which there are few data available in IBD. Different genetic models can be compared to identify the one that most closely approximates the observed patterns of inheritance in IBD families.

A small number of studies have been performed to investigate the mode of inheritance of IBD. The models investigated include simple dominant or recessive heredity, in which IBD is encoded by a single, incompletely penetrant gene which is either dominant or recessive; polygenic inheritance, in which a number of different genes in combination lead to the development of IBD; and multifactorial inheritance, in which genetic and environmental

Table 2.2 Differences in incidence of inflammatory bowel disease between Jewish and non-Jewish populations

Area	Disease	Jewish*	Non-Jewish*	Reference
Baltimore	UC	13.3	3.4	Monk et al 1967
	CD	3.4	1.7	
New York	CD	12.6	5.4	Korelitz 1979
Stockholm	CD	10.0	3.0	Hellers 1979
Malmo	CD	24.0	6.0	Brahme et al 1975
Western Cape (South Africa)	CD	2.8	0.8	Novis et al 1975

UC, ulcerative colitis; CD, Crohn's disease
* Incidence per 100 000 population

factors interact to produce the IBD phenotype. None of these models can be considered to have been absolutely refuted, and it is most likely that differing IBD phenotypes will prove to be inherited in different ways. Evidence has been presented supporting dominant, recessive and polygenic models. In particular there is evidence to support the existence of a recessive gene in about 30% of the members of Crohn's disease families, and a relatively strong additive gene (closer to a dominant than a recessive gene) with low penetrance (22%) in a small proportion (probably less than 10%) of the members of ulcerative colitis families (Monsén et al 1989, Küster et al 1989). A recent study from Copenhagen (Orholm et al 1993) supports the hypothesis that a major dominant gene is present in about 10% of patients with ulcerative colitis, but in patients with Crohn's disease a major recessive gene is present in only 7%.

In ulcerative colitis families the risk of the children acquiring the disease has been calculated as about 11%, a figure similar to that found empirically. The corresponding risk in Crohn's disease families has been estimated as about 20% (Monsén et al 1989). It should be added that hereditary predisposition for disease can be missing in about 70% of patients with Crohn's disease and 90% or more of patients with ulcerative colitis (according to the results of the segregation analysis). This is illustrated by the fact that concordance for disease is low in monozygotic twins with ulcerative colitis, and far from complete in Crohn's disease. This could also explain why first-degree relatives of Ashkenazi Jews have the same risk of acquiring IBD as the first-degree relatives of non-Ashkenazi Jews, in spite of the fact that the prevalence of Crohn's disease is doubled in the non-Ashkenazi Jews (Zlotogora et al 1991). All these findings provide evidence of an important role for environmental factors.

ASSOCIATION OF IBD WITH GENETIC SYNDROMES

Several genetic syndromes have been reported in association with inflammatory bowel disease. However, in only three has the association been consistent and therefore of possible pathogenic importance. These are Turner's syndrome, glycogen storage disease type Ib, and Hermansky–Pudlak syndrome.

Turner's syndrome

The incidence of IBD in Turner's syndrome is significantly higher than in the general population (Price 1979, Kohler & Grant 1981), and this may be the result of an increased genetic predisposition to IBD owing to the abnormal state of the single X chromosome. It is known that chromosomal abnormalities may be associated with a greater liability to autoimmune diseases. Chromosomal studies in both ulcerative colitis and Crohn's disease have shown a significant increase in the number of chromosomal abnormalities: 28.5% and 32.5% respectively, compared to 9.9% of controls (Emerit et al 1972, 1979). In a review of 17 cases of Turner's syndrome and IBD (Manzione et al 1988), in eight of them the chromosomal abnormality was a mosaic pattern where only some of the cell lines have the abnormal X chromosome. Reactivation of at least part of the uniformly sequestered X chromosome could produce autoimmune phenomena.

Glycogen storage disease type Ib

Crohn's disease has recently been reported in association with glycogen storage disease type Ib (Roe et al 1986, Couper et al 1991). This inherited glycogenosis is distinguished clinically from the classic Ia by a predisposition to pyogenic infections caused by neutropenia and neutrophil dysfunction. The association with Crohn's disease is suggested to have possible pathogenetic importance, supporting a role for a neutrophil abnormality in Crohn's disease. Interestingly, oxidative metabolism has been found to be impaired in neutrophils from patients with Crohn's disease, and this could be caused by a reduced content in membrane b-type cytochrome (Solis-Herruzo et al 1993).

Hermansky–Pudlak syndrome

Hermansky and Pudlak (1959) described an inherited syndrome with a triad of albinism, platelet dysfunction and accumulation of a ceroid-like pigment in tissue. In a series of nine patients in two families from Puerto Rico living in New York (Schinella et al 1980), five cases with granulomatous colitis were found. In another series of 37 patients with Hermansky–Pudlak syndrome (Witkop et al 1990), also from Puerto Rico, 12 cases with granulomatous colitis were reported. Two children (one Puerto Rican) with the same combination have been described in New York (Mahadeo et al 1991). The suggestion has been made that the hereditary defect in Hermansky–Pudlak syndrome is an abnormality of lysosomal function, and this abnormality may be involved in the etiology of granulomatous colitis.

ASSOCIATION OF IBD WITH OTHER DISEASES OF KNOWN GENETIC PREDISPOSITION

IBD is associated with various diseases that have known genetic predisposition. These include ankylosing spondylitis, psoriasis, atopy and eczema, celiac disease, cystic fibrosis, primary sclerosing cholangitis, multiple sclerosis and other autoimmune diseases.

Ankylosing spondylitis

Both ulcerative colitis and Crohn's disease are associated with ankylosing spondylitis. It has been estimated that the concurrence of ankylosing spondylitis and IBD is 10–50 times more common than would be expected by chance (Macrae & Wright 1973).

Patients with ankylosing spondylitis are approximately 90% HLA-B27 positive (Feltkamp 1990). Patients with IBD and ankylosing spondylitis are 60–80% HLA-B27 positive (Mallas et al 1976, Dekker-Saeys et al 1978). Studies from Germany showed a special type of genetic heterogeneity of patients with both ankylosing spondylitis and Crohn's disease. The phenotype HLA-B27, -B44 was found to be markedly increased when both diseases coincide. Individuals with this phenotype have a relative risk of 69 for the concurrent manifestation of Crohn's disease and ankylosing spondylitis (Purrmann et al 1988).

Crohn's disease and ankylosing spondylitis in a mother and her son has been described (Czeizel 1992), and the relatives of IBD patients have increased risk for ankylosing spondylitis even when the IBD patient has no evidence of ankylosing spondylitis (Lewkonia & McConnell 1976). On the other hand, endoscopic examination of patients with ankylosing spondylitis (De Vos et al 1989) demonstrated symptomless inflammatory bowel disease in 30% of cases. Ankylosing spondylitis in women with IBD was found to have a significantly younger age of onset compared to other women with ankylosing spondylitis (Kennedy et al 1993).

Inflammatory bowel disease seems to have a facilitating role in those who are genetically predisposed to ankylosing spondylitis. It is still not certain whether the spondylitis is a complication of IBD or an associated disease.

Psoriasis

There is a strong association between psoriasis and inflammatory bowel disease (Table 2.3). In addition there are studies (Yates et al 1982, Lee et al 1990) showing an increased occurrence of psoriasis in first-degree relatives of patients with Crohn's disease, suggesting the possibility of a genetic link.

In a recent study from Germany (Hoffman et al 1991) an increase of HLA B13, Bw58, Cw6 and DR7, which are known to be increased in psoriasis, was found in patients with coexisting Crohn's disease and psoriasis. Intestinal permeability evaluated with ^{51}Cr-labeled EDTA was also found to be increased in patients with psoriasis compared to healthy controls (Humbert et al 1991). This suggests another possible pathogenetic factor to link both disorders. Further investigation is needed to determine the nature of the possible genetic link.

Atopy and eczema

There have been several reports of patients with atopy and eczema, which are known to have a marked hereditary component, also having inflammatory bowel disease. In a series of 200 patients with Crohn's disease (Pugh et al 1979) 36.5% had a positive family history of atopic disease compared to only 10% of controls. In a cooperative study from 14 centres (Gilat et al 1987) eczema was found to occur more frequently in patients with Crohn's disease and their first-degree relatives than in the controls and their families. In ulcerative colitis patients a similar trend was observed but it did not reach statistical significance. There is at present no clear explanation for this association.

Celiac disease

Celiac disease has been associated with more than 20 immunologic disorders. The first report of association with IBD (Salem & Truelove 1965) was followed by several case reports. In a rectal biopsy study of 42 patients with celiac disease (Breen et al 1987) there were three cases with histologic features compatible with ulcerative colitis. In a series of 293 patients with Crohn's disease Cottone and colleagues (1989) found three cases with celiac disease. In a survey of 120 patients with celiac disease (Mayberry et al 1986), their siblings had a twentyfold higher risk of developing celiac disease and fifteenfold higher risk of developing ulcerative colitis than the control groups.

The association may be explained by the influence of HLA-linked genes in both celiac disease and IBD, and/or

Table 2.3 Prevalence of psoriasis that has been reported in patients with inflammatory bowel disease compared to the general population

Area	Disease	No of patients	Prevalence of psoriasis (%)		Reference
			IBD patients*	General population*	
Scotland	UC	88	5.7	1.5	Yates et al 1982
	CD	116	11.2		
Northwest England	CD	128	8.6	1.6	Hughes et al 1983
Blackpool, UK	CD	136	9.6	2.2	Lee et al 1990
Tübingen, Germany	CD	320	4.7	2.0	Hoffmann et al 1991

UC, ulcerative colitis; CD, Crohn's disease
* Prevalence of psoriasis

abnormal permeability of the small intestine, which occurs in celiac disease and has been reported in Crohn's disease.

Cystic fibrosis

There are reports of a possible association of cystic fibrosis with IBD, and especially with Crohn's disease (Ojeda et al 1986, Behrens et al 1989). A recent prospective survey of 11 321 patients with cystic fibrosis from 49 centers (Lloyd-Still 1994) revealed 28 patients with IBD (25 Crohn's disease, 3 ulcerative colitis). The prevalence rate for IBD was seven times higher than the controls and, for Crohn's disease in particular, was 17 times higher.

These data raise the possibility that genes in chromosome 7, where the genetic defect in cystic fibrosis resides, may contribute to the genotype that renders the individual susceptible to Crohn's disease.

Primary sclerosing cholangitis

Primary sclerosing cholangitis (PSC), characterized by chronic inflammation and fibrosis of the intra- and extrahepatic bile ducts, is commonly associated with IBD, especially ulcerative colitis. The prevalence of PSC in ulcerative colitis has been found to be 2–4% (Olsson et al 1991, Wewer et al 1991, Rasmussen et al 1992). Conversely, IBD is present in 50–70% of patients with PSC (Wiesner & La Russo 1980).

Primary sclerosing cholangitis was found to be associated with HLA-DRw52a (Prochazka et al 1990), but other recent studies have not confirmed this (Olerup et al 1991, Zetterquist et al 1992). The haplotype HLA-A1, -B8, -Cw7, DRw17, DQw2, DRw52a appears to confer a special risk of ulcerative colitis complicated by PSC. A dual association of HLA-DR2 and -DR3 with PSC has also been described (Donaldson et al 1991). This observation is of particular interest in view of studies reporting the association of HLA-DR2 with ulcerative colitis.

Multiple sclerosis

A concurrence of multiple sclerosis and IBD has been recognized in families (Minuk & Lewkonia 1986, Sadovnick et al 1989) and in individuals (Rang et al 1982, Kitchin et al 1991, Purrmann et al 1992).

One or more loci contributing specifically to IBD may determine the susceptibility for multiple sclerosis. On the other hand, a common defect in immune regulation may exist in both diseases, and the presence of antilymphocyte antibodies in the serum of patients and their relatives may be a marker for this defect. Multiple sclerosis has also been found to be associated with HLA-DR2.

Other autoimmune diseases

Several other autoimmune diseases have been reported, associated mainly with ulcerative colitis. In a controlled study of 1200 patients with IBD from Oxford (Snook 1990) 'established' autoimmune disorders, including autoimmune thyroid disease and systemic lupus erythematosus, were found in 6.6% of patients with ulcerative colitis, but in only 1.9% of those with Crohn's disease, which is similar to the controls (2%).

Autoimmune hemolytic anemia has been repeatedly reported in association with ulcerative colitis (Batista & Roe 1986). Primary biliary cirrhosis has also been reported in association with ulcerative colitis (Lever et al 1993, Veloso et al 1993). Crohn's disease has been reported in association with myasthenia gravis (Finnie et al 1994) and Cogan's syndrome (Froehlich et al 1994).

Further investigation is needed to determine whether these associations have pathogenetic importance. These studies also point to the possible importance of the regulatory genes of inflammation on the short arm of chromosome 6.

GENETIC MARKER STUDIES

The aim of genetic marker studies is to identify the site of the genes that predispose to inflammatory bowel disease. Early studies of markers, including blood groups, secretor status, α_1-antitrypsin and γ marker genes, have failed to show a consistent association with IBD. At present studies on these markers can be subdivided in those where a genetic element is proved and those subclinical markers where a genetic predisposition may be present. Recent studies have focused on the following genetic markers:

1. HLA antigens
2. Immunoglobulin marker genes
3. Complement haplotypes
4. T-cell receptor genes
5. Cytokine genes.

Genes coded by chromosomes 2, 6 and 7 appear to be important for the susceptibility to suffer from inflammatory bowel disease. Even though not all these associations have been confirmed, interesting results have been published and are worth pursuing.

Histocompatibility antigens (HLA)

The short arm of chromosome 6 is the site of the major histocompatibility complex (MHC) in which the structure of the glycoprotein molecules that make up class I and class II antigens is genetically encoded. A high degree of allelic polymorphism has been established in these genes.

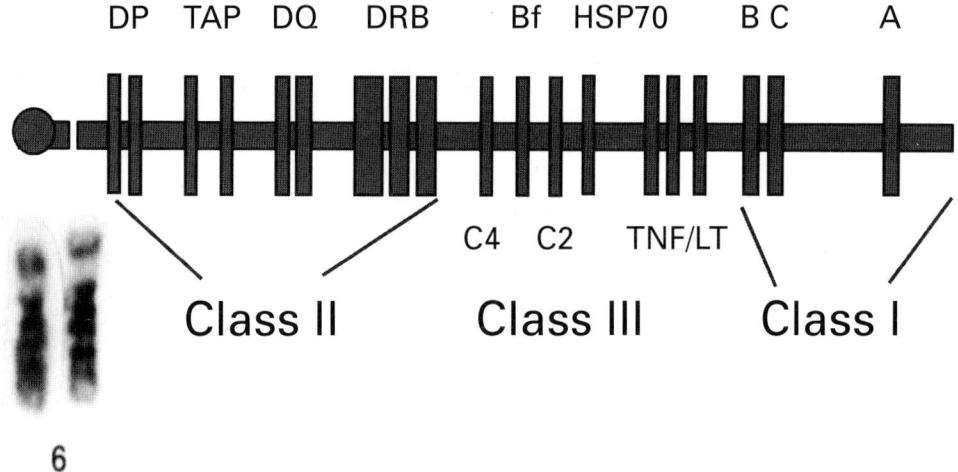

Fig. 2.1 Short arm of human chromosome 6; map of the MHC

Although for a considerable period HLA studies in IBD had been considered inconclusive, recent data, mainly with HLA class II, have increased interest. The frequency of HLA-DR2 in ulcerative colitis has been found to be increased in several studies. Table 2.4 shows the prevalence of HLA-DR2 in ulcerative colitis in different centers compared to healthy controls.

In the initial studies serological techniques were used and only two, from Japan (Asakura et al 1982, Kobayashi et al 1990), reached statistical significance. The association of ulcerative colitis with HLA-DR2 has been confirmed (Sugimura et al 1991) using the polymerase chain reaction. However, their analysis suggested that at least two genetic factors determining susceptibility to ulcerative colitis are located on the HLA-A24, -Bw52, -TNF 10.5kb, DR2, -DQw1, -DPw9 haplotype. More recently, a study from Los Angeles (Toyoda et al 1993), with carefully selected ethnically matched cases and controls and with a combination of molecular and serological techniques, found a significant positive association of ulcerative colitis with the DR2 allele and negative association with DR4 and DRw6 alleles, and a DR-DQ gene combination (DR1-DQw5) which showed a positive association with Crohn's disease. The authors suggest that the genetic susceptibility provided by the HLA class II genes is distinct for each of these forms of IBD, and is not shared between them.

Three recent studies in ulcerative colitis with similar methods also suggest an increased frequency of the HLA-DR2 allele (Farrant et al 1994, Futami et al 1994, Oudkerk Pool et al 1995). However, a study from Pittsburg (Duerr & Neigut 1994) found no association.

It has also been reported that ANCA-positive ulcerative colitis patients had significantly increased levels of DR2 compared to ANCA-negative controls (Yang et al 1993b). In other recent studies, however, HLA-DR2 was not found to be associated with p-ANCA positivity (Duerr & Neigut 1994, Farrant et al 1994, Oudkerk Pool et al 1995).

The association between HLA and IBD so far supports the concept of disease heterogeneity.

Immunoglobulin marker genes

The human immunoglobulin genes encode the immunoglobulin light chains κ and λ and the immunoglobulin heavy chains. Each gene cluster contains genes that encode variable (V), joining (J) and constant (C) elements. The heavy chain constant region genes (C_H) include the $C_\gamma 1$ gene involved in isotype class switching, which may function differently in the ulcerative colitis population.

Table 2.4 Results of studies on HLA-DR2 association with ulcerative colitis

Area	Patients (%)	Controls (%)	Reference
Japan	70	31	Asakura et al 1982
Japan	85	28	Kobayashi et al 1990
Germany	37	20	Smolen et al 1982
United Kingdom	46	30	McConnell 1983
United Kingdom	24	36	Burnham et al 1981
United Kingdom	48	28	Farrant et al 1994
Italy	32	17	Caruso et al 1985
Italy	23	31	Cottone et al 1985
Netherlands	40	28	Oudkerk Pool et al 1995
USA	41	21	Toyoda et al 1993
USA	29	26	Duerr et al 1994

For example, individuals without the G2 marker have lower serum concentrations of IgG2 than carriers of G2m(n) (Rautonen et al 1989). In one study the proportion of IgG1 immunocytes was raised and that of IgG2 decreased in the rectal mucosa of ulcerative colitis twins compared to normal colonic specimens (Helgeland et al 1992). Another mechanism may be that certain V_H genes, directed against antigens which are important to the IgG response in ulcerative colitis, preferentially associate with particular C_H genes in the ulcerative colitis population. A study from Germany showed an association between ulcerative colitis and Gm 1,2,10 (Purrmann et al 1989).

Complement haplotypes

The gene loci coding for the complement components Bf, C3 and C4 are known to be closely linked to the HLA complex. In a study from Denmark (Elmgreen et al 1984) the polymorphism of complement C3 in IBD has been assessed. This found two common alleles for C3, called C3F and C3S, which give rise to the phenotypes F, FS and S. In comparison with healthy controls, the frequency of the C3F allele was significantly increased in patients with Crohn's disease of the small intestine. The frequency of C3F in ulcerative colitis did not differ from that of the controls.

Another study from Germany (Kluge et al 1982) found that the frequency of the Bf-F allotype was significantly higher in patients with Crohn's disease (65.6%) than in controls (28.3%). These observations are highly relevant, since enhanced local production of complement components has been found in the small intestine of these patients (Ahrenstedt et al 1990).

The major role that the complement system plays in the immune response suggests that the observed differences between Crohn's disease and ulcerative colitis (Halstensen et al 1992, 1993) warrant further investigation.

T-cell antigen receptor

The antigen specificity and MHC restriction that are characteristic of all adaptive immune responses are determined by the T-cell antigen receptor (TcR). The repertoire of TcRs expressed by T lymphocytes in the peripheral blood and at specific sites, such as the intestinal mucosa, reflects both the genomically encoded TcR repertoire and the effects of selection due to the interaction between TcRs, self-MHC molecules and self and foreign peptides and proteins. The inheritance of the genetically encoded constituents of these processes may confer disease susceptibility, and thus justifies the study of association and linkage between TcR genes and IBD.

The TcR is a heterodimeric cell surface molecule, non-covalently associated with CD3. The majority of circulating lymphocytes express α and β chains, each of which consists of constant (C), joining (J) and variable (V) elements, with the β chain including a diversity (D) element at the junction of the V and J elements. A minority of TcRs are composed of γ and δ chains, which are assembled in a similar way to α/β heterodimers. Each element in the expressed TcR chain is encoded by a family of genes, approximately 50 V genes, 13–100 J genes and two C genes. During T-cell development the V and (D) J genes encoding α and β chains are rearranged at the genomic level, transcribed and then spliced to a C gene at the RNA level to bring together single V (D) J and C elements as a TcR chain transcript. Diversity among TcRs results from the selection of different representatives of each family of elements, by the random addition and deletion of nucleotides at the V–D–J junctions and the random pairing of α and β chains. This variable recombination process produces a potential diversity of approximately 10^{15} different TcRs. Expressed TcRs undergo a process of selection that leads to the elimination of autoreactive T cells (constituting approximately 90% of all T cells emerging from the bone marrow) and the positive selection of T cells capable of recognizing foreign antigens presented by self-MHC.

Individuals may vary in the numbers and types of TcR element family members that they inherit. Furthermore, a number of TcR element genes have been shown to be allelic. As a result, individuals vary in the genomic TcR repertoire that they inherit. These genomically encoded elements are associated with polymorphisms either within the exons or closely associated introns, and their inheritance can be followed using classic genetic techniques such as restriction fragment polymorphism (RFLP) analysis or tandem repeat analysis. The majority of studies to date have found no association between TcR α and β genes and IBD (Randolph et al 1989, Katakura et al 1989), although one Japanese association study found that a TcR cβ polymorphism was present in all ulcerative colitis patients but no controls (Kobayashi et al 1990).

Although the expressed TcR repertoire formed by gene rearrangement, junctional editing and RNA splicing is based on the genomic repertoire, it may differ in genetically identical individuals. Furthermore, the expressed and selected TcR repertoire, as found in circulating peripheral blood or tissues, will have been subjected to a number of influences that have been shown to induce profound alterations in TcR repertoire, even between identical twins (Loveridge et al 1991). As a result the expressed TcR repertoire cannot be investigated through analysis of DNA but requires the analysis of TCR RNA or, better still, expressed proteins. Several techniques have been developed for the analysis of TcR transcripts, some of which are quantitative and provide interpretable data

(Moss et al 1992). Monoclonal antibodies that recognize specific TcR Vα and Vβ chains are increasingly available but these fail to detect the antigen recognition site of the TcR. Recent studies reporting distortions in TcR repertoire in inflamed Crohn's disease lesions (Gulwani-Akolkar et al 1994, Wong et al 1994) may reflect the influence of environmental agents, such as an infecting organism or superantigen, rather than TcR disease susceptibility genes.

Owing to the differences between genomically encoded and expressed/selected TcR repertoires, the study of TcR at the genomic level may fail to identify association or linkage with IBD, despite TcR playing a major role in the disease. Furthermore, a lack of genetic evidence implicating TcR in disease does not negate the potential of TcR as a target for disease-specific immunotherapies, and this potential justifies the continued investigation of TcR in IBD at the genetic, transcript and protein levels (Loveridge et al 1991).

Cytokine genes

An association of ulcerative colitis with allele 2 of interleukin-1 receptor antagonist (IL-1ra) has been reported (Mansfield et al 1994). Allele 2 of IL-1ra was found in 35% of the ulcerative colitis patients compared to 24% in controls ($P=0.0007$). This IL-1ra locus may represent a marker for a disease-associated gene on chromosome 2. Although in Dutch patients the allele 2 frequency was not significantly different from controls (29% versus 22.6%), the carriers of allele 2 had an increased risk for IBD. No association between IL-1ra, pANCA or HLA-DR2 alleles was found (Bioque et al 1995, 1996).

The location of TNF (tumor necrosis factor) genes within the central region of the major histocompatibility complex (MHC) on the short arm of chromosome 6, the high degree of polymorphism in these genes, and the association between certain HLA alleles and TNF inducibility, has prompted much speculation about the role of TNF in the etiology of IBD. In a recent study the production of biologically active total TNF after T-cell stimulation was found to be decreased in ulcerative colitis patients, and the production of TNFβ found to be significantly increased in those with Crohn's disease (Bouma et al 1995) No significant differences in haplotype frequency were observed when patients with ulcerative colitis and Crohn's disease were compared with normal controls (Bouma et al 1996a, b).

Further investigation is needed to test whether cytokine genes may represent factors for susceptibility to, or severity of, IBD.

SUBCLINICAL MARKERS

Subclinical markers have also been used in genetic studies of IBD to detect the abnormal genotype. These include pANCA, intestinal permeability and, mucin glycoproteins.

Perinuclear antineutrophil cytoplasmic antibodies (pANCA)

In the majority of studies pANCA has been found to be specific for ulcerative colitis rather than Crohn's disease or other forms of colitis. The healthy relatives of patients with ulcerative colitis have been reported to have an increased frequency of positive ANCA compared with environmental controls (Shanahan et al 1992, Seibold et al 1993). However, other studies (Reumaux et al 1992, Lee et al 1994, Monteleone et al 1994) have not confirmed this correlation.

Intestinal permeability

Intestinal permeability to polyethylene glycol was found to be increased in patients with Crohn's disease and their relatives (Hollander et al 1986), but two other studies

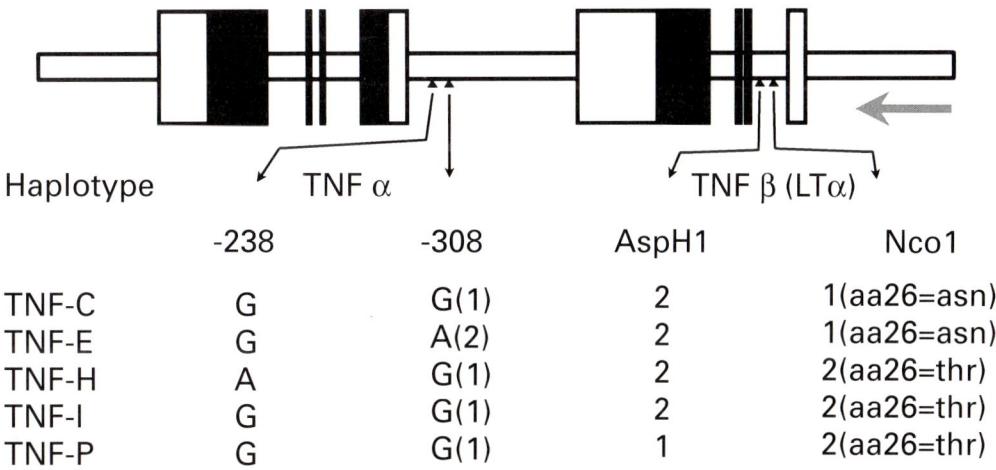

Fig. 2.2 TNF haplotypes; RFLPs in TNFα and TNFβ genes

could not confirm these findings (Theahon et al 1992, Ruttenberg et al 1992). Absorption of the inert sugars lactulose (L), rhamnose (R) and mannitol (M) was also tested, and there are studies which have shown increased L/M ratio in the first-degree healthy relatives of Crohn's disease patients (Pironi et al 1992, May et al 1993). However, in other studies permeability abnormalities could not be found in the relatives but only in patients with IBD (Katz et al 1989, Munkholm et al 1994).

Intestinal mucin glycoproteins

The intestinal mucin glycoproteins have been thought to play an important role in inflammatory bowel disease (Tytgat et al 1993). Deficiency of the subclass IV of mucin glycoproteins in patients with ulcerative colitis has been reported (Podolsky & Isselbacher 1984). In a recent study of monozygotic twins (Tysk et al 1991) reduced mucin subclass IV was found in patients with ulcerative colitis and their healthy identical twin. However, the results of these studies have not been reproduced in other laboratories. Mucin genes have recently been defined and the recognition that they show genetic polymorphism (Gum et al 1989, 1990) offers the opportunity for further investigation. Unpublished preliminary results have shown a lack of association with MUC2 alleles in chromosome 11 (Pladdet et al 1994), and no polymorphism in MUC3 in chromosome 7. Chang et al (1994) have, however, found a defect in the transcription of MUC3. The authors suggested a lack of expression of MUC3 in ulcerative colitis. This observation supports a role for mucin glycoproteins in the pathogenesis of the disease, and should be further studied.

CONCLUSION

Strong evidence for a genetic predisposition towards inflammatory bowel disease is apparent from the data reviewed. Further studies are needed to refine the risks for genetic counseling.

Genetic marker studies have shown a lack of consistent association between these markers and either ulcerative colitis or Crohn's disease. The strongest evidence at present is the association of ulcerative colitis with the HLA-DR2 and interleukin-1 receptor antagonist genes. Thus genes in chromosomes 6 and 2 probably play a part in the predisposition for ulcerative colitis. The association between IBD and several diseases linked with chromosome 6 points to the genes involved in the regulation of inflammation. The association with cystic fibrosis, whose locus is localized in chromosome 7, suggests that genes linked to the T-cell receptor or to MUC3, also localized in chromosome 7, might also be important for another subgroup of patients with IBD (Fig. 2.3).

The recently reported lack of linkage between chromosome 6 and Crohn's disease (Hugot et al 1994, Naom et al 1994) does not exclude the possibility that other genes involved in the regulation of inflammation are important in Crohn's disease susceptibility.

Other markers point to immunological disturbances in ulcerative colitis and Crohn's disease that may not relate to a genetic predisposition. These include pANCA, complement, T-cell receptor and γ marker genes.

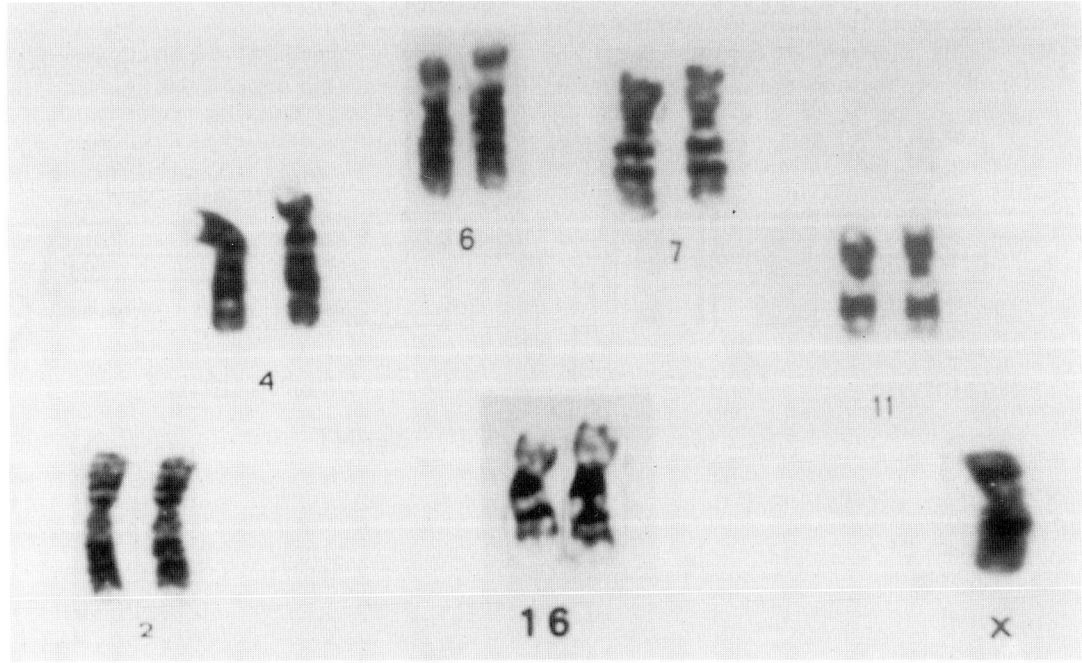

Fig. 2.3 Chromosomes implicated in the susceptibility to IBD

The use of multiply affected families for RFLP linkage studies to identify individual loci that contribute to liability is a promising approach. With this method a locus on the pericentromeric region of chromosome 16 has recently been found to contribute to the increased risk for first-degree relatives of patients with Crohn's disease (Hugot et al 1996). Further investigation of genetic markers may contribute to an understanding of the etiologies of the disease(s) as well as to the development of new therapies.

ACKNOWLEDGEMENTS

I. Koutroubakis is a gastroenterologist of the University Hospital of Heraklion, Greece. For one year he has worked at the Laboratory for Gastrointestinal Immunogenetics, Free University, Amsterdam. We are grateful for the support received from the Greek Society of Gastroenterology.

REFERENCES

Ahrenstedt O, Knutson L, Nilsson-Ekdahl K, Odlind B, Hallgren R 1990 Enhanced local production of complement components in the small intestine of patients with Crohn's disease. New England Journal of Medicine 322: 1345–1349

Asakura H, Tsuchiya M, Aiso S et al 1982 Association of human lymphocyte-DR2 antigens with Japanese ulcerative colitis. Gastroenterology 82: 413–418

Batista M H, Roe D C 1986 A case presentation of hemolytic anemia in ulcerative colitis and review of the literature. American Journal of Gastroenterology 81: 990–992

Behrens R, Segerer H, Bowing B, Bender S W 1989 Crohn's disease in cystic fibrosis. Journal of Pediatric Gastroenterology and Nutrition 9: 528–531

Bennett R A, Rubin P H, Present D H 1991 Frequency of inflammatory bowel disease in offspring of couples both presenting with inflammatory bowel disease. Gastroenterology 100: 1638–1643

Bioque G, Bouma G, Crusius J B A, Koutroubakis I, Kostense P J, Meuwissen S G M, Peña A S 1996 Evidence for genetic heterogenicity in inflammatory bowel disease: the interleukin-1 receptor antagonist in the predisposition to suffer from ulcerative colitis. European Journal of Gastroenterology and Hepatology 8 (2): in press

Bioque G, Crusius J B A, Koutroubakis I, Bouma G, Kostense P J, Meuwissen S G M, Peña A S 1995 Allelic polymorphism in IL-1β and interleukin-1 receptor antagonist (IL-1ra) genes in inflammatory bowel diseases. Clinical and Experimental Immunology 102: 379–383

Bouma G, Oudkerk Pool M, von Blomberg M B E et al 1995 Different spontaneous and stimulated TNF production in patients with Crohn's disease and ulcerative colitis. Gastroenterology 106: A1018

Bouma G, Oudkerk Pool M, Scharenberg J G M et al 1996a Differences in the intrinsic capacity of T cells to produce tumor necrosis alpha and beta in patients with inflammatory bowel disease and healthy controls. Scandinavian Journal of Gastroenterology 30: 1095–1100

Bouma G, Xia B, Crusius J B A, Bioque G et al 1996b Distribution of four polymorphisms in the tumor necrosis factor genes in patients with inflammatory bowel disease. Clinical and Experimental Immunology 103: 391–396

Bouma G, Crusius J B A, Oudkerk Pool M, Kolkman J J et al 1996c Secretion of tumor necrosis factor alpha and lymphotoxin alpha in relation to polymorphisms in the TNF genes and HLA-DR alleles. Relevance for inflammatory bowel disease. Scandinavian Journal of Immunology 43: in press

Brahme, Lindstrom C, Wenckert A 1975 Crohn's disease in a defined population. Gastroenterology 69: 342–352

Breen E G, Coughlan G, Connoly C E, Stevens F M 1987 Coeliac proctitis. Scandinavian Journal of Gastroenterology 22: 471–477

Burnham W R, Gelsthorpe K, Langman M J S 1981 HLA-D related antigens in inflammatory bowel disease. In: Peña A S, Weterman I T, Booth C C, Strober W (eds) Recent advances in Crohn's disease. Martinus Nijhoff, The Hague, pp 192–196

Burress G C, Barclay S K, Kirschner B S 1994 Parents developing IBD after their children. Clincial features and implications for families studies. Gastroenterology 106: A658

Caruso C, Palmeri P, Oliva L, Orlando A, Cottone M 1985 HLA antigens in ulcerative colitis: a study in the Sicilian population. Tissue Antigens 25: 47–49

Chang S K, Park E S, Chung S W et al 1994 Expression of MUC2, MUC3 apomucins and mRNA in ulcerative colitis. Gastroenterology 106: A662

Chong S K F, Walker-Smith J A 1986 Chronic inflammatory bowel disease in immigrants in the United Kingdom. In: McConnell R, Rozen P, Langman M, Gilat T (eds). The genetics of inflammatory bowel disease. Karger, Basel, pp 129–132

Cottone M, Bunce M, Taylor C J, Ting A, Jewell D P 1985 Ulcerative colitis and HLA phenotype. Gut 26: 952–954

Cottone M, Cappello M, Puleo A et al 1989 Familial association of Crohn's disease and coeliac disease. Lancet 2: 338

Couper R, Kapelushnik J, Griffiths A M 1991 Neutrophil dysfunction in glycogen storage disease Ib: association with Crohn's-like colitis. Gastroenterology 100: 549–554

Czeizel A E 1992 Familial aggregation of Crohn's disease and ankylosing spondylitis in a mother and her son. Journal of Clinical Gastroenterology 14: 349–357

Dekker-Saeys B J, Meuwissen S G, van den Berg Loonen E M et al 1978 Ankylosing spondylitis and inflammatory bowel disease. III. Clinical characteristics and results of histocompatibility typing (HLA B27) in 50 patients with both ankylosing spondylitis and inflammatory bowel disease. Annals of Rheumatic Diseases 37: 36–41

De Vos M, Guvelier C, Mielants H et al 1989 Ileocolonoscopy in seronegative spondylarthropathy. Gastroenterology 96: 339–344

Donaldson P T, Farrant J M, Wilkinson M L et al 1991 Dual association of HLA DR2 and DR3 with primary sclerosing cholangitis. Hepatology 13: 129–133

Duerr R H, Neigut D A 1994 HLA DR2 is not associated with ulcerative colitis or perinuclear anti-neutrophil cytoplasmic antibodies. Gastroenterology 106: A674

Elmgreen J, Sorensen H, Berkowicz A 1984 Polymorphism of complement C3 in chronic inflammatory bowel disease. Acta Medica Scandinavica 215: 375–378

Emerit I, Emerit J, Tosoni-Pittoni A et al 1972 Chromosome studies in patients with ulcerative colitis. Human Genetics 16: 313–322

Emerit I, Emerit J, Levy A et al 1979 Chromosomal breakage in Crohn's disease: anticlastogenic effect of D-penicillamine and L-cysteine. Human Genetics 50: 51–57

Farmer R G, Michener W M 1986 Association of inflammatory bowel disease in families. Frontiers of Gastrointestinal Research 11: 17–26

Farrant J M, Bunce M, Artlett C et al 1994 HLA DR2 is a susceptibility marker for ulcerative colitis in British patients irrespective of ANCA positivity. Gastroenterology 106: A679.

Feltkamp T E W, Khan M, López de Castro J 1996 The pathogenetic role of HLA-B27. Immunology Today (in press)

Fielding J F 1986 The relative risk of inflammatory bowel disease among parents and siblings of Crohn's disease patients. Journal of Clinical Gastroenterology 8: 655–657

Findlay J M, Jayarantne S D 1986 Chronic inflammatory bowel disease in immigrants in the United Kingdom. In: McConnell R, Rozen P, Langman M, Gilat T (eds). The genetics of inflammatory bowel disease. Karger, Basel, pp 124–129

Finnie I A, Shields R, Sutton R, Donnelly R, Morris A I 1994 Crohn's disease and myasthenia gravis: a possible role for thymectomy. Gut 35: 278–279

Froehlich F, Friend M, Convers J J, Saraga E, Thorens J, Pecoud A 1994 Association of Crohn's disease and Cogan's syndrome. Digestive Diseases and Sciences 39: 1134–1137

Futami S, Aoyama N, Tamura T et al 1994 HLA-class II β-chain position 86: association with susceptibility to ulcerative colitis. Gastroenterology 106: A684

Gilat T, Grossman A, Fireman Z, Rosen P 1986 Inflammatory bowel disease in Jews. In: McConnell R, Rozen P, Langman M, Gilat T (eds). The genetics of inflammatory bowel disease. Karger, Basel, pp 135–140

Gilat T, Hacohen D, Lilos P, Langman M J S 1987 Childhood factors in ulcerative colitis and Crohn's disease. An international cooperative study. Scandinavian Journal of Gastroenterology 22: 1009–1024

Gulwani-Akolkar B, Akolkar P N, McKinley M, Fisher S E, Silver J 1994 An altered T cell receptor (TCR) repertoire in Crohn's disease (CD). Gastroenterology 106: A695

Gum J R, Byrd J C, Hicks J W, Toribara N W, Lamport D T A, Kim Y S 1989 Molecular cloning of human intestinal mucin cDNAs. Sequence analysis and evidence for genetic polymorphism. Journal of Biological Chemistry 264: 6480–6487

Gum J R, Hicks J W, Swallow D M et al 1990 Molecular cloning of cDNAs derived from a novel human intestinal mucin gene. Biochemistry Biophysics Research Communications 171: 407–415

Halstensen T S, Das K M, Brandtzaeg P 1993 Epithelial deposits of immunoglobulin G1 and activated complement colocalise with the Mr40 kD putative autoantigen in ulcerative colitis. Gut 34: 650–657

Halstensen T S, Mollnes T E, Garred P et al 1992 Surface epithelium related activation of complement differs in Crohn's disease and ulcerative colitis. Gut 33: 902–908

Helgeland L, Tysk C, Järnerot G et al 1992 IgG subclass distribution in serum and rectal mucosa of monozygotic twins with or without inflammatory bowel disease. Gut 33: 1358–1364

Hellers G 1979 Crohn's disease in Stockholm county, 1955–1974: a study of epidemiology, results of surgical treatment and long term prognosis. Acta Chirurgica Scandinavica (Suppl 490): 1–84

Hermansky F, Pudlak P 1959 Albinism associated with hemorrhagic diathesis and unusual pigmented reticular cells in the bone marrow: report of two cases with histochemical studies. Blood 14: 162–169

Hoffmann R, Schieferstein G, Schunter F, Jenss H 1991 Increased occurrence of psoriasis in patients with Crohn's disease and their relatives. American Journal of Gastroenterology 86: 787–788

Hollander D, Vadheim C M, Brettholz E et al 1986 Increased intestinal permeability in patients with Crohn's disease and their relatives. Annals of Internal Medicine 105: 883–885

Hughes S, Williams S E, Turnberg L A 1983 Crohn's disease and psoriasis. New England Journal of Medicine 308: 101

Hugot J P, Laurent-Puig P, Gower-Rousseau C et al 1994 Linkage analyses of chromosome 6 loci, including HLA, in familial aggregations of Crohn's disease. Gastroenterology 106: A703

Hugot J P, Laurent-Puig P, Gower-Rousseau et al 1996 Mapping of a susceptibility locus for Crohn's disease on chromosome 16. Nature 379: 821–823

Humbert P, Bidet A, Treffel P, Drobacheff C, Agache P 1991 Intestinal permeability in patients with psoriasis. Journal of Dermatological Science 2: 324–326

Katakura S, Einarsson L, Hammarström L, Smith C 1989 Restriction fragment length polymorphism analysis of T-cell receptor genes in inflammatory bowel disease. Scandinavian Journal of Gastroenterology 24: 381–384

Katz K D, Hollander D, Vadheim C M et al 1989 Intestinal permeability in patients with Crohn's disease and their healthy relatives. Gastroenterology 97: 927–931

Kennedy L G, Will H, Calin A 1993 Sex ratio in the spondyloarthropathies and its relationship to phenotypic expression, mode of inheritance and age of at onset. Journal of Reumatology 20: 1900–1904

Kitchin L I, Knobler R L, Friedman L S 1991 Crohn's disease in a patient with multiple sclerosis. Journal of Clinical Gastroenterology 13: 331–334

Kluge J, Grosse Wilde H, Kreeb G et al 1982 Association between the HLA-linked complement allotype marker Bf-F and Crohn's disease. Scandinavian Journal of Gastroenterology 17 (Suppl 78): 513

Kobayashi K, Atoh M, Konoeda Y, Yagita A, Inoko H, Sekiguchi S 1990 HLA-DR, DQ and T cell antigen receptor constant beta genes in Japanese patients with ulcerative colitis. Clinical and Experimental Immunology 80: 400–403

Kohler J A, Grant DB 1981 Crohn's disease in Turner's syndrome. British Medical Journal 282: 950

Korelitz B I 1979 From Crohn to Crohn's disease-1979: an epidemiological study in New York City. Mount Sinai Journal of Medicine (NY) 46: 533–540

Küster W, Pascoe L, Purrmann J et al 1989 The genetics of Crohn's disease: complex segregation analysis of a family study with 265 patients with Crohn's disease and 5287 relatives. American Journal of Genetics 32: 105–108

Lashner B A, Evans A A, Kirsner J B, Hanauer S B 1986 Prevalence and incidence of inflammatory bowel disease in family members. Gastroenterology 91: 1395–1400

Lee F I, Bellary S V, Francis C 1990 Increased occurrence of psoriasis in patients with Crohn's disease and their relatives. American Journal of Gastroenterology 85: 962–963

Lee J C W, Cambridge G, Lennard-Jones J E 1994 Prevalence of anti-neutrophil antibodies in familial inflammatory bowel disease: specificity for ulcerative colitis in genetically related individuals. Gastroenterology 106: A718

Lever E, Balasubramanian K, Condon S et al 1993 Primary biliary cirrhosis associated with ulcerative colitis. American Journal of Gastroenterology 88: 945–947

Lewkonia R M, McConnell R B 1976 Familial inflammatory bowel disease – heredity or environment? Gut 17: 235–243

Lloyd-Still J D 1994 Crohn's disease and cystic fibrosis. Digestive Diseases and Sciences 39: 880–885

Loveridge J, Rosenberg W M C, Kirkwood T B L, Bell J I 1991 The genetic contribution to human T cell receptor repertoire. Immunology 74: 246–250

McConnell R B 1983 Ulcerative colitis – genetics feature. Scandinavian Journal of Gastroenterology 18 (Suppl 88): 14–21

McConnell R B, Shaw J M, Whibley E J, McConnell T H 1986 Inflammatory bowel disease: a review of previous genetic studies and the Liverpool Family Data. Frontiers of Gastrointestinal Research 11: 1–11

Macrae I, Wright V 1973 A family study of ulcerative colitis, with particular reference to ankylosing spondylitis and sacroiliitis. Annals of Rheumatic Diseases 32: 16–20

Mahadeo R, Markowitz J, Fisher S, Daum F 1991 Hermansky–Pudlak syndrome with granulomatous colitis in children. Journal of Pediatrics 118: 904–906

Mallas E G, Mackintosh P, Asquith P, Cooke W T 1976 Histocompatiblity antigens in inflammatory bowel disease. Their clinical significance and their association with arthropathy with special reference to HLA-B27(w27). Gut 17: 906–910

Manousos O N, Giannadaki E, Koutroubakis I et al 1996 A prospective epidemiological study of inflammatory bowel disease at Heraklion, Crete, Greece. (Scand J Gastroenterol In press)

Mansfield J C, Holden H, Tarlow J K et al 1994 Novel genetic association between ulcerative colitis and the anti-inflammatory cytokine interleukin-1 receptor antagonist. Gastroenterology 106: 637–642

Manzione N C, Kram M, Kram E, Das K M 1988 Turner's syndrome and inflammatory bowel disease: a case report with immunologic studies 1988. American Journal of Gastroenterology 83: 1294–1297

May G R, Sutherland L R, Meddings J B 1993 Is small intestinal permeability really increased in relatives of patients with Crohn's disease? Gastroenterology 104: 1627–1632

Mayberry J F, Smart H L, Toghill P J 1986 Familial association between coeliac disease and ulcerative colitis. Journal of the Royal Society of Medicine 79: 204–205

Meucci G, Vecchi M, Torgano G et al 1992 Familial aggregation of inflammatory bowel disease in Northern Italy: a multicenter study. Gastroenterology 103: 514–519

Minuk G Y, Lewkonia R M 1986 Possible familial association of multiple sclerosis and inflammatory bowel disease. New England Journal of Medicine 314: 586–587

Monk M, Mendeloff A I, Siegel C I, Lilienfeld A 1967 An epidemiological study of ulcerative colitis and regional enteritis among adults in Baltimore. I. Hospital incidence and prevalence, 1960–1963. Gastroenterology 53: 198–210

Monsén U, Bernell O, Jahansson C, Hellers G 1991 Prevalence of inflammatory bowel disease among relatives of patients with Crohn's disease. Scandinavian Journal of Gastroenterology 26: 302–306

Monsén U, Brostrom O, Nordenvall B et al 1987 Prevalence of inflammatory bowel disease among relatives of patients with ulcerative colitis. Scandinavian Journal of Gastroenterology 22: 214–218

Monsén U, Iselius L, Johansson C, Hellers G 1989 Evidence for a major additive gene in ulcerative colitis. Clinical Genetics 36: 411–414

Monteleone G, Doldo P, Marasco R et al 1994 Perinuclear neutrophil autoantibodies (p-ANCA) in unaffected relatives of patients with ulcerative colitis (UC). Suggestions against familial aggregation. Gut 35 (Suppl 4): A31

Moss P A H, Rosenberg W M C, Bell J I 1992 The human T cell receptor in health and disease. Annual Review of Immunology 10: 71–96

Munkholm P, Langholz E, Hollander D et al 1994 Intestinal permeability in patients with Crohn's disease and ulcerative colitis and their first degree relatives. Gut 35: 68–72

Naom I S, Lee J C W, Ford D, Easton J E, Lennard-Jones J E, Mathew C G 1994 The gene for familial Crohn's disease is not linked to the major histocompatibility complex. Gastroenterology 106: A743

Novis B H, Marks I N, Bank S, Louw J H 1975 Incidence of Crohn's disease at Groote Schuur Hospital during 1970–1974. South African Medical Journal 49: 693–697

Odes H S, Fraser D, Krawiec J 1987 Incidence of idiopathic ulcerative colitis in Jewish population subgroups in the Beer Sheva region of Israel. American Journal of Gastroenterology 82: 854–858

Odes H S, Fraser D, Krawiec J 1989 Inflammatory bowel disease in migrant and native Jewish populations of southern Israel. Scandinavian Journal of Gastroenterology 24 (Suppl 170): 36–38

Odes H S, Fraser D, Krugliak P et al 1991 Inflammatory bowel disease in the Bedouin Arabs of southern Israel: rarity of diagnosis and clinical features. Gut 32: 1024–1026

Ojeda V J, Levitt S, Ryan G, Laurence B H 1986 Cystic fibrosis, Crohn's colitis and adult meconium ileus equivalent. Diseases of the Colon and Rectum 29: 567–571

Olerup O, Broome U, Einarsson K, Zetterquist H 1991 Inability to attribute susceptibility to primary sclerosing cholangitis to specific amino acid positions of the HLA-DRw52a allele. New England Journal of Medicine 325: 1251–1252

Olsson R, Danielsson A, Jarnerot G et al 1991 Prevalence of primary sclerosing cholangitis in ulcerative colitis. Gastroenterology 100: 1319–1323

Orholm M, Iselius L, Sorensen T I A et al 1993 Investigation of inheritance of chronic inflammatory bowel diseases by complex segregation analysis. British Medical Journal 306: 20–24

Orholm M, Munkholm P, Langholz E et al 1991 Familial occurrence of inflammatory bowel disease. New England Journal of Medicine 324: 84–88

Oudkerk Pool M, Bouma G, Crusius J B A et al 1995 Genetic and immunological markers in inflammatory bowel disease. PhD Thesis. Vrije Universitest Amsterdam1995 pp: 134

Pironi L, Miglioni M, Ruggeri E et al 1992 Effect of non-steroidal anti-inflammatory drugs (NSAID) on intestinal permeability in first degree relatives of patients with Crohn's disease. Gastroenterology 102: A697

Pladdct I E, Doekhie F S, Peña A S, Oudejans C B M 1994 Restriction-fragment-length-polymorphism of mucin genes and ulcerative colitis. (submitted)

Podolsky D K, Isselbacher K J 1984 Glycoprotein composition of colonic mucosa. Specific alterations in ulcerative colitis. Gastroenterology 87: 991–998

Price W H 1979 A high incidence of chronic inflammatory bowel disease in patients with Turner's syndrome. Journal of Medical Genetics 16: 263–266

Probert C S J, Jayanthi V, Pinder D et al 1992 Epidemiological study of ulcerative proctocolitis in Indian migrants and the indigenous population of Leicestershire. Gut 33: 687–693

Probert C S J, Jayanthi V, Hughes A O et al 1993 Prevalence and family risk of ulcerative colitis and Crohn's disease: an epidemiological study among Europeans and South Asians in Leicestershire. Gut 34: 1547–1551

Prochazka E J, Terasaki P I, Park M S et al 1990 Association of primary sclerosing cholangitis with HLA-DRw52a. New England Journal of Medicine 322: 1842–1844

Pugh S M, Rhodes J, Mayberry J F, Robers D L, Heatley R V, Newcombe R G 1979 Atopic disease in ulcerative colitis and Crohn's disease. Clinical Allergy 9: 221–223

Purrmann J, Arendt G, Cleveland S et al 1992 Association of Crohn's disease and multiple sclerosis. Is there a common background? Journal of Clinical Gastroenterology 14: 43–46

Purrmann J, Bertrams J, Knapp M et al 1989 Investigation of genetic markers in patients with Crohn's disease and ulcerative colitis. Zeitschrift für Gastroenterologie 27: 366–369

Purrmann J, Zeidler H, Bertrams J et al 1988 HLA antigens in ankylosing spondylitis associated with Crohn's disease. Increased frequency of the HLA phenotype B27, B44. Journal of Reumatology 15: 1658–1661

Randolph L M, Toyoda H, McElree C K, Shanahan F, Targan S P, Rotter J I 1989 Absence of the Eco R V T-cell receptor alpha chain 10-kb RFLP in ulcerative colitis. Gastroenterology 97: 1115–1120

Rang E H, Brooke B N Hermon-Taylor U 1982 Association of ulcerative colitis and multiple sclerosis. Lancet 2: 255

Rasmussen H H, Fallinborg J, Mortesen P B et al 1992 Primary sclerosing cholangitis in patients with ulcerative colitis. Scandinavian Journal of Gastroenterology 27: 732–736

Rautonen N, Sarvas H, Mäkelä O 1989 One allele [G2m(n)] of the human IgG2 locus is more productive than the other. European Journal of Immunology 19: 817–822

Reed J F III, Calkins B M, Rosen L 1992 Concordance of familial characteristics in Crohn's disease and ulcerative colitis. Diseases of the Colon and Rectum 35: 405–410

Reumaux D, Delecourt L, Colombel J F et al 1992 Prevalence of ANCA in first degree relatives of patients with ulcerative colitis. Gastroenterology 102: A683

Rhodes J M, Marshall T, Hamer J D, Allan R N 1985 Case report: Crohn's disease in two married couples. Gut 26: 1086–1087

Roe T F, Thomas D W, Gilsanz V et al 1986 Inflammatory bowel disease in glycogen storage disease type Ib. Journal of Pediatrics 109: 55–59

Roth M P, Petersen G M, McElree C et al 1989 Familial empiric risk estimates of inflammatory bowel disease in Ashkenazi Jews. Gastroenterology 96: 1016–1020

Ruttenberg D, Young G O, Wright J P, Isaacs S 1992 PEG-400 excretion in patients with Crohn's disease, their first degree relatives, and healthy volunteers. Digestive Diseases and Sciences 37: 705–708

Sadovnick A D, Paty D W, Yannakoulias G 1989 Concurrence of multiple sclerosis and inflammatory bowel disease. New England Journal of Medicine 321: 762–763

Salem S N, Truelove S C 1965 Small-intestinal and gastric abnormalities in ulcerative colitis. British Medical Journal 1: 827–831

Sanderson I R, Chong S K F, Walker-Smith J A 1986 Familial occurrence of chronic inflammatory bowel diseases. Frontiers of Gastrointestinal Research 11: 12–16

Sategna-Guidetti C, Bianco L, Bracco E, Marucco E 1986 Familial incidence of Crohn's disease in Italy. Digestive Diseases and Sciences 31: 557–558

Satsangi J, Jewell D P, Rosenberg W M C, Bell J I 1994 Genetics of inflammatory bowel disease. Gut 35: 696–700

Schinella R A, Greco A, Cobert B L et al 1980 Hermansky–Pudlak syndrome with granulomatous colitis. Annals of Internal Medicine 92: 20–23

Seibold F, Klein R, Slametschka D, Weber P, Berg P, Gregor M 1993 p-ANCA in family members of patients with ulcerative colitis and PSC. Gastroenterology 104: A778

Shanahan F, Duerr R, Rotterr J I et al 1992 Neutrophil auto-antibodies in ulcerative colitis: familial aggregation and genetic heterogeneity. Gastroenterology 103: 456–461

Smolen J S, Gangl A, Poltrauer P, Menzel E J, Mayr W R 1982 HLA antigens in inflammatory bowel disease. Gastroenterology 82: 34–38

Snook J 1990 Are the inflammatory bowel diseases autoimmune disorders? Gut 31: 961–963

Solis-Herruzo J A, Fernadez B, Vilalta-Castell E et al 1993 Diminished cytochrome b content and toxic oxygen metabolite production in circulating neutroplils from patients with Crohn's disease. Digestive Diseases and Sciences 38: 1631–1637

Sugimura K, Asakura H, Hibi T, Tsuji T, Inoko H 1991 Molecular analysis of genes responsible for the susceptibility to ulcerative colitis within the HLA region. Gastroenterology 100: A619

Theahon K, Smethurst P, Levi A J et al 1992 Intestinal permeability in patients with Crohn's disease and their first degree relatives. Gut 33: 320–323

Tokayer A Z, Reydel B, Bayless T M 1992 Possible role of heredity in site and transmural aggressiveness of Crohn's disease. Gastroenterology 102: A705

Toyoda H, Wang S-J, Yang H et al 1993 Distinct association of HLA class II genes with inflammatory bowel disease. Gastroenterology 104: 741–748

Tysk C, Lindberg E, Järnerot G, Floderus-Myrhed B 1988 Ulcerative colitis and Crohn's disease in an unselected population of monozygotic and dizygotic twins. A study of heritability and the influence of smoking. Gut 29: 990–996

Tysk C, Riedesel H, Lindberg E, Panzini B, Podolsky D, Järnerot G 1991 Colonic glycoproteins in monozygotic twins with inflammatory bowel disease. Gastroenterology 100: 419–423

Tytgat K M, Dekker J, Büller H A 1993 Mucins in inflammatory bowel disease. European Journal of Gastroenterology and Hepatology 5: 119–127

Van Kruiningen H J, Colombel J F, Cartun R W et al 1993 An in depth study of Crohn's disease in two French families. Gastroenterology 104: 351–360

Veloso F T, Dias L M, Carvalho J et al 1993 Ulcerative colitis, primary biliary cirrhosis, and chronic pancreatitis: Coincident or coexistent? Journal of Clinical Gastroenterology 16: 55–57

Weterman I T, Peña A S 1984 Familial incidence of Crohn's disease in The Netherlands and a review of the literature. Gastroenterology 86: 449–452

Wewer V, Gluud C, Schlicting P, Burchardt F, Binder V 1991 Prevalence of hepatobiliary dysfunction in a regional group of patients with inflammatory bowel disease. Scandinavian Journal of Gastroenterology 26: 97–102

Wiesner R H, La Russo N F 1980 Clinicopathological features of the syndrome of primary sclerosing cholangitis. Gastroenterology 79: 200–206

Witkop C J, Nunez-Babcock M, Rao G H et al 1990 Albinism and Hermansky–Pudlak syndrome in Puerto Rico. Asociacion de Medicina de Puerto Rico 82: 333–339

Wong D K H, Baca-Estrada M E, Croitoru K 1994 Effect of superantigen on the cytolytic function of $V\beta 8$ T cells in Crohn's disease. Gastroenterology 106: A1055

Yang H, McElree C, Roth M-P et al 1993a Familial empiric risks for inflammatory bowel disease: differences between Jews and non-Jews. Gut 34: 517–524

Yang H, Rotter J I, Toyoda H et al 1993b Ulcerative colitis: a genetically heterogeneous disorder defined by genetic (HLA Class II) and subclinical (antineutrophil cytoplasmic antibodies) markers. Journal of Clinical Investigation 92: 1080–1084

Yates V M, Watkinson G, Kelman A 1982 Further evidence of an association between psoriasis, Crohn's disease and ulcerative colitis. British Journal of Dermatology 106: 323–330

Zetterquist H, Broome U, Einarsson K, Olerup O 1992 HLA class II genes in primary sclerosing cholangitis and chronic inflammatory bowel disease: no HLA-DRw52a association in Swedish patients with sclerosing cholangitis. Gut 33: 942–946

Zlotogora J, Zimmerman J, Rachmilewitz D 1990 Crohn's disease in Ashkenazi Jews. Gastroenterology 99: 286–287

Zlotogora J, Zimmerman J, Rachmilewitz D 1991 Prevalence of inflammatory bowel disease in family members of Jewish Crohn's disease patients in Israel. Digestive Diseases and Sciences 36: 471–475

3. Molecular implications of genetic studies
W. M. C. Rosenberg

INTRODUCTION

Familial (Satsangi et al 1994) and twin (Tysk et al 1988) studies of the inheritance of Crohn's disease and ulcerative colitis have provided powerful evidence of a genetic contribution to IBD (inflammatory bowel disease). Identification of the genes that confer susceptibility to ulcerative colitis and Crohn's disease and study of the regulation of genes involved in their pathogenesis will undoubtedly provide powerful tools for diagnosis, insights into etiology and pathobiology, and identify potential targets for therapy. Further study of the regulation of normal genes whose products are involved in the immune responses that contribute to active IBD may also help.

A number of genetic loci have been implicated as conferring susceptibility to IBD. For some highly polymorphic genes, such as those in the HLA class II region, associations between IBD susceptibility and specific alleles have been formally established (Toyoda et al 1993) and the implications of these associations require further consideration. For less polymorphic genes, such as *TNF* (Bouma et al 1994) and the cytokine genes (Gurbindo et al 1993), where the gene products have been characterized in IBD and are clearly implicated in disease pathogenesis, study of the genetic loci may provide important information about the regulation of these genes in disease (Mansfield et al 1994). Disease-associated regulatory polymorphisms may be identified, but information about the normal regulation of these genes in acute and chronic inflammation is likely to identify targets for potential therapy.

The genetic manipulation of laboratory rodents has been used to test hypotheses implicating specific genes in disease causation (Mombaerts et al 1993, Sadlack et al 1993, Strober & Ehrhardt 1993). Although these experiments purport to investigate the role of specific genes in the development of IBD, their interpretation requires an extensive understanding of IBD, the genes studied and the techniques used to investigate them.

MHC GENES AND INFLAMMATORY BOWEL DISEASE

Early studies of HLA association with IBD used serological techniques and failed to detect significant associations. More recently genotyping techniques have been used to identify specific and separate associations for Crohn's disease and ulcerative colitis (Toyoda et al 1993), resolving a long-standing equivocation about the classification of ulcerative colitis and Crohn's disease by establishing that they are separate diseases, ulcerative colitis being associated with *HLA-DR2*, whereas Crohn's disease is associated with *HLA-DR1-DQw5*. Furthermore, subgroup analysis has suggested that different phenotypes within ulcerative colitis may have a genetic basis. The analysis of *HLA-DR2* frequencies in relation to antineutrophil cytoplasmic antibody (ANCA) positivity has suggested that the *HLA-DR2* genotype identifies a distinct phenotype within ulcerative colitis (Yang et al 1993). Apart from establishing a clear disease taxonomy, observations such as these provide important insights into the etiology and pathogenesis of the different subgroups of IBD.

HLA ANTIGENS

Taxonomy and diagnosis

Several groups have found an association between *HLA-DR2* and susceptibility to ulcerative colitis. This association appears to be strongest in Ashkenazi Jews living in North America (Toyoda et al 1993) and in the Japanese (Asakura et al 1982, Sugimura et al 1991). An initial report of *HLA-DR2* being found at increased frequency among English colitics (Farrant et al 1994) has since been refuted (D. P. Jewell, personal communication). Similar HLA, associations have been described in many other immune-mediated disorders (Campbell & Milner 1993), although in most the strength of the associations is much greater than that seen in IBD. The identification of different HLA susceptibility alleles for ulcerative colitis and Crohn's disease represents a major advance in the understanding of the classification of these diseases. HLA typing could now be used as confirmatory evidence of a specific diagnosis, carrying implications for prognosis and therapy. However, the low frequency of the susceptibility alleles in the diseased populations makes HLA typing alone unsuitable as a screening test for diagnosis. Similarly, the identification of different HLA associations for specific disease phenotypes within ulcerative colitis or Crohn's disease will establish discrete diagnostic entities, even if HLA typing will not provide a reliable means of distinguishing the phenotypes. Thus HLA association studies have already contributed major insights into the classification of IBD, and carry some potential for differential diagnosis, if not for screening.

Etiology and pathobiology

In all disorders where HLA alleles are associated with disease susceptibility similar explanations may be invoked to explain the role of HLA molecules in the etiology and pathogenesis.

Antigen presentation

The principal function of the major histocompatibility complex (MHC) class I and class II molecules is to present peptide fragments of antigens to T cells (Townsend & Bodmer 1989, Cresswell 1994). Class I molecules are ubiquitously expressed on nucleated cells and present endogenously processed peptides of approximately eight to nine amino acids in length to cytotoxic T lymphocytes, expressing CD8. The expression of class II molecules is much more restricted, and they present exogenously processed peptides of approximately 12–19 amino acids in length to helper T lymphocytes bearing CD4 (Engelhard 1994). The major sites of genetic variation in these highly polymorphic molecules are clustered in hypervariable regions that encode the walls and pockets of the antigen-binding cleft of the mature protein. Only peptides that can fit into the conformation of the antigen-binding cleft can be bound by the HLA molecule. Thus an HLA molecule of a given specificity can only present a restricted range of peptides to the host's immune system. The principal disease associations for ulcerative colitis are with the class II antigen *HLA-DR2*. It is possible that *HLA-DR2* is directly implicated in presenting an exogenously derived peptide to helper T cells, and that this step is critical in the immune response that lies at the heart of ulcerative colitis. If this explanation is valid then it is the conformation of the *HLA-DR2* antigen-binding cleft that determines peptide binding and permits the development of ulcerative colitis.

The most powerful evidence implicating HLA alleles in disease-specific immune responses arises when polymorphic residues carried by a number of alleles are associated with disease susceptibility or protection. In insulin-dependent diabetes mellitus (Todd et al 1987) and rheumatoid arthritis (Wordsworth et al 1989) specific residues in the antigen-binding cleft of HLA class II molecules have been identified as conferring susceptibility or protection. Similar findings have been described for primary sclerosing cholangitis (Farrant et al 1992), in which leucine at position 38 of the *DR* β chain of *HLA-DR3*0101* or *DRB5*0101* is associated with disease, but *DRB4*0101*, which encodes alanine at position 38, confers protection. Furthermore, these associations appeared to be dose dependent, with leucine 38 homozygosity conferring maximum susceptibility whereas alanine 38 homozygosity confers maximum protection. These findings not only strongly implicate *HLA-DR3* and *DR5* as susceptibility loci, but also imply that it is their function as antigen-presenting molecules that confers disease susceptibility.

The observation of a correlation between *HLA-DR2*, ANCA positivity and ulcerative colitis (Yang et al 1993) suggests that *HLA-DR2* may be involved in a complex network of immunological interactions whereby the presentation of a peptide to helper T cells promotes the production of a pathogenic antibody.

A direct implication of these hypotheses, in which HLA genes are associated with IBD through antigen presentation, is the existence of a specific peptide which, when bound and presented by *HLA-DR2*, can lead to the development of the disease. The identification of this peptide and the protein – or even organism – from which it is derived may now be possible. The elution of peptides from class I and class II molecules has been used to identify the peptides bound by specific MHC alleles (Engelhard 1994). More recently, the genomes of candidate pathogens have been scanned for HLA allele-binding motifs and synthetic peptides used to confirm that a potential epitope can induce the assembly and expression of class I molecules (S. McAdam; manuscript in preparation). 'Reverse genetics' have been applied to the study of the immune response to malaria and have been used to identify peptides critical in disease pathogenesis (Hill et al 1992). The isolation of sufficient quantities of *HLA-DR2* from diseased tissue to permit a similar experiment in active ulcerative colitis remains problematic at present.

T-cell receptor repertoire selection

In addition to presenting immunogenic peptides to mature T cells, MHC molecules have a major functional role in the selection of T-cell receptor repertoire during T-cell maturation. The antigen specificity of T cells is conferred by the T-cell antigen receptor (TcR), a highly polymorphic heterodimeric molecule consisting of α and β or γ and δ chains, each of which is formed by the combination of multiple elements (Moss et al 1992). Each element is encoded by a single representative of families of genes. During T-cell ontogeny the TcR is formed by gene rearrangement, with nucleotide editing at the junctions of the elements increasing the diversity of the expressed TcR. Immature T cells expressing rearranged TcRs migrate from the bone marrow to the thymus, where they undergo a process of selection that results in the deletion of autoreactive T cells and the expansion of T cells capable of recognizing antigens in the context of self-MHC molecules. Both these steps in T-cell selection are dependent upon the interaction of TcR with self-MHC, and thus represent potential sites at which self-MHC molecules may shape the immune response in a way that might influence susceptibility to an environmental disease trigger. In this way, MHC alleles may confer disease susceptibility by shaping the T-cell repertoire.

Recent studies of the immune response to EBV (Epstein–Barr virus) have revealed that combinations of certain HLA molecules can dramatically alter even highly focused T-cell responses (Burrows et al 1994). Moss and colleagues have shown that most *HLA-B8*-positive individuals respond to an immunodominant EBV peptide that has homology with a self-peptide restricted through *HLA-B44*. As a result the majority of *HLA-B8* individuals use T cells expressing a single TcR to control EBV infection, but *HLA-B44* individuals, unable to tolerate the common TcR that would be alloreactive, use a wide variety of TcRs to recognize EBV peptides. Thus HLA molecules may indirectly influence the TcR repertoire by causing the deletion of potentially autoreactive T cells. In this way certain HLA antigens may confer disease protection.

Linked genes

Whereas the HLA association for ulcerative colitis is clearly with a specific HLA allele, that for Crohn's disease is with the *HLA-DR1-DQw5* haplotype. Neither *HLA-DR1* nor *HLA-DQw5* appears to be independently associated with Crohn's disease. This finding is open to a number of interpretations. It is possible that both *HLA-DR1* and *HLA-DQw5* are independently required for the development of Crohn's disease. Association studies are incapable of determining whether the two alleles in a susceptible individual are carried on the same haplotype, or on different haplotypes. This hypothesis could be tested by analyzing the linkage of the two alleles with disease susceptibility in families to determine whether Crohn's disease susceptibility can be conferred by the two alleles on different haplotypes; this is currently being addressed in Oxford.

The alternative interpretation, that Crohn's disease is associated with the *HLA-DR1-DQw5* haplotype, is more likely. Owing to linkage disequilibrium between *HLA-DR* and *HLA-DQ* loci it has proved impossible to distinguish which allele was responsible for Crohn's disease susceptibility in the study by Toyoda et al, in which ethnically similar patients were studied. Similar difficulties arose in studies of celiac disease susceptibility, but were resolved by investigating disease susceptibility alleles in different ethnic groups (Sollid et al 1989). Such a study in Crohn's disease might identify *HLA-DR* or *HLA-DQ* as the major susceptibility locus for Crohn's disease.

A third explanation is that neither locus is responsible for the observed disease susceptibility, but that a third gene, in tight linkage disequilibrium with the *DQw5* haplotype, confers susceptibility to Crohn's disease. This could implicate genes in the MHC class III region, such as those encoding complement and TNF (tumor necrosis factor) (Campbell & Trowsdale 1993). Such an explanation accounts for the observed association between hemochromatosis and *HLA-A3*. For this reason it will be important to define the boundaries of the susceptibility haplotype using markers in the MHC class III region (Mehal et al 1994).

Aberrant expression of HLA molecules has been suggested as a potential trigger for immune-mediated disorders. In active ulcerative colitis *HLA-DR* expression has been described in association with active disease (de Silva et al 1990, Hoang et al 1992, Lowes et al 1992) and is thought to result from immune activation rather than be the trigger. All *HLA* genes are associated with genetically encoded elements that are involved in the control of transcription. These elements are closely linked to the genes that they regulate. It remains possible that *HLA-DR2* in ulcerative colitis-susceptible individuals is linked to an inducible transcription regulation element leading to a primary abnormality of *HLA-DR* expression in response to an environmental trigger. This would explain why few *HLA-DR2*-positive individuals ever develop ulcerative colitis.

Other MHC-encoded genes may confer susceptibility to the inflammatory bowel diseases. The class III region lies between class II and class I on chromosome six, and encodes many genes, only some of which have been fully characterized (Sargent et al 1994). Of those that have been studied, the *TNF-α* and *TNF-β* genes are intimately involved in the immune response. Polymorphisms of *TNF-α* have recently been implicated in susceptibility to malaria (McGuire et al 1994), and it remains possible that the *HLA-DR2* association in ulcerative colitis is merely a marker for a linked susceptibility gene. On the centromeric side of the *HLA-DR* loci lie a number of genes involved in antigen processing and presentation via the endogenous antigen-processing pathway. Although polymorphisms of the *TAP* genes have been associated with immune response phenotypes in rodents, attempts to identify corresponding associations in man have failed (Powis et al 1993, Wordsworth et al 1993).

Ethnic differences

A common characteristic of MHC disease associations is the identification of ethnic differences. Whereas ulcerative colitis appears to be associated with *HLA-DR2* in Ashkenazi Jews, such an association does not appear to exist in northern Europeans. Variations in HLA disease associations in different ethnic groups may arise through a number of mechanisms. In some instances seemingly identical HLA molecules have been found to differ at critical sites in the antigen-binding cleft, which may determine whether variants of an allele confer disease susceptibility or not (Rojo et al 1993). Such confusion may be attributed to the methods used in HLA genotyping. Genetic HLA typing techniques rely on the identification of polymorphism at known sites of variation. However, many of the techniques used, such as sequence-specific oligonucleotide typing and amplification-restricted mutagenesis-PCR, may miss previously unrecognized variants. Genetic HLA variation in ulcerative colitis could only be explored by comparing full-length sequences of the genes encoding *HLA-DR2* in Ashkenazi Jews and northern European caucasoids, but is unlikely to reveal differences. Alternatively, different HLA disease associations may be identified in populations where the common disease allele is only present at a very low frequency; thus among southern Europeans celiac disease is more commonly associated with *HLA-DR5* than with *HLA-DR3*, the common northern European haplotype (Sollid et al 1989).

If the *HLA-DR2* molecules associated with ulcerative colitis in the Ashkenazi Jews do not differ from those not associated with ulcerative colitis in northern Europeans, how can this disparity be explained? The differing patterns of association may either be due to genetically linked genes, or result from the interaction between *HLA-DR2* and other genetically encoded elements.

Therapy

The identification of disease susceptibility HLA alleles raises the potential for a number of new therapies. For class I molecules in-vitro T-cell cytotoxicity assays (Sutton et al 1993) and MHC assembly assays (S. McAdam; manuscript in preparation) have been used to identify peptide epitope motifs for specific HLA alleles. It is now possible to synthesize peptides that are capable of occupying the antigen-binding cleft but which are not recognized by TcR and thus do not trigger activation of the immune response (Sette et al 1994). It is unlikely that synthetic peptides could be delivered in sufficient quantities to compete adequately with pathogenic peptides for the occupancy of MHC antigen-binding clefts.

The recent recognition of the abolition of class II (Ostrov et al 1993) and class I (Klenerman et al 1994, Bertoletti et al 1994) restricted immune responses by 'antagonistic' peptides has raised a new and intriguing therapeutic possibility. These peptides bind to MHC molecules and engage TcR, but their recognition by TcR does not lead to activation of T cells but rather induces anergy in the peptide-specific T cells. The development of specific antagonistic peptides capable of turning off pathogenic T cells is an exciting possibility for the future treatment of immune-mediated disorders, and is dependent on the identification of HLA molecules involved in pathogenesis. These approaches, coupled to the new techniques of peptide vaccination (Cease & Berzofsky 1994) in which peptide epitopes can be delivered to the immune system using genetically engineered constructs, provide exciting potential therapies for IBD.

THE T-CELL RECEPTOR – DIAGNOSIS AND PATHOBIOLOGY

Genomic T-cell receptor repertoire

Selection of T-cell repertoire is shaped by HLA antigens, but the initial potential T-cell repertoire is determined by the genomically encoded TcR repertoire (Moss et al 1992). Some of the TcR V region genes are allelic (Pile et al 1993) and the inheritance of certain alleles has been shown to be associated with autoimmune disorders (Weetman et al 1987, Millward et al 1987, Seboun et al 1989, Oksenberg et al 1988, Heber Katz & Acha-Orbea 1989). In none of these disorders has the association with genetic TcR polymorphism been directly linked to an expressed pathogenic TcR.

Expressed T-cell receptor repertoire

It will be apparent that the inheritance of the genes that encode the elements of the TcR chains, prior to TcR selection, only represents one component of the peripheral blood TcR repertoire which is involved in the immune response. The influence of MHC on TcR repertoire selection has been discussed. Subsequent interaction between TcR and environmentally derived antigens has been shown to exert a major and lasting influence on repertoire, and may contribute to disease susceptibility.

Superantigens (SAg) are complex glycoproteins that bind to MHC class II molecules and stimulate the proliferation of subsets of T cells through their interaction with TcR Vβ elements (Moss et al 1992). They bind both MHC and TcR at sites outside the hypervariable regions involved in classic MHC-restricted peptide antigen recognition. The site on the MHC class II molecule is common to class II molecules, and thus SAgs do not exhibit MHC allele specificity, although the efficiency with which different isotypes and alleles bind SAgs do differ (Scholl et al 1990, Herman et al 1990). Although the TcR SAg binding site is separated from the peptide recognition site, it is encoded within a polymorphic region of the Vβ element and thus SAgs only bind to specific Vβ elements. Two categories of SAg are recognized. Endogenous SAgs, such as murine mammary tumor virus (Choi et al 1991, Marrack et al 1991), have not as yet been found to play a significant role in shaping the TcR repertoire in man. However, for many years it has been recognized that certain bacterial exotoxins are powerful T-cell mitogens (Fleischer & Mittrucker 1991). These are exogenous SAgs and differ from classic T-cell mitogens in that they induce proliferation or T cells bearing specific Vβ elements. SAgs have been shown to be capable of inducing massive expansions of T cells (Hermann et al 1990, Marrack et al 1990) and clonal T-cell anergy (O'Hehir & Lamb 1990, Rellahan et al 1990).

More recently it has become apparent that some viruses may also induce massive clonal expansions of T cells, which in some cases may persist for many years (Carmichael et al 1993). Studies of expressed TcR repertoire in intestinal mucosal cells have described clonal T-cell expansions in healthy individuals (Balk et al 1991). These data suggest that mucosal TcR repertoire differs from peripheral blood, and imply that local mucosal factors may exert major influences an disease susceptibility mediated by TcR. By remodeling the T-cell repertoire SAg and viral effects could have a profound influence on disease susceptibility.

For these reasons it is not sufficient merely to investigate the disease associations of genomically encoded TcR elements to determine the contribution of the TcR to IBD susceptibility. Expressed TcR repertoire must be studied, and tissue-specific TcR repertoire must also be determined. Furthermore, the analysis of appropriate control material is essential. Other cell surface receptors may play a role in conferring specificity on the immune response in IBD. Recent investigation of the expression of the cell surface glycoprotein CD44 has revealed that variants CD44v3 and CD44v6 are selectively overexpressed on colonic crypt epithelial cells in ulcerative colitis but not in other forms of colonic inflammation (Rosenberg et al 1995). CD44 is thought to play a part in lymphocyte homing and adhesion. This finding may prove useful in the differential diagnosis of colonic inflammation and may provide a disease-specific target for immunotherapy.

T-cell receptor and therapy

If it becomes possible to implicate specific TcRs in the pathogenesis of IBD, the TcR will provide a highly specific target for therapy (Wraith et al 1989). In extrinsic allergic encephalomyelitis (EAE) (Acha-Orbea et al 1988, Zamvil et al 1988, Heber Katz & Acha-Orbea 1989), an animal model of multiple sclerosis – Vβ-specific T-cell deletion at different stages of disease induction – has been shown to protect against, abort the development of, or ameliorate the effects of the disease. Currently the reagents and methodologies for investigating TcR repertoire are insufficient to the task. Although it is recognized that animal models such as EAE reveal more about animal immunology than about human disease, the potential use of TcR as a highly specific target for immunotherapy in immune-mediated human disorders remains a sufficiently attractive prospect to encourage further work in this field.

CYTOKINES AND THEIR RECEPTORS

The clinical observation of altered cytokine levels in active IBD is most likely explained as a secondary phenomenon rather than a primary abnormality. Cytokines, their receptors and receptor antagonists are subject to highly complex transcriptional and posttranscriptional regulation (Tanaka & Taniguchi 1992). The genes encoding the major cytokines do not contain sufficient polymorphism to suggest that cytokine polymorphisms will provide a means of diagnosing IBD, or even identifying disease susceptibility. However, polymorphisms have been described in flanking regions that are involved in the regulation of gene transcription. These polymorphisms may lead to over- or underproduction of specific disease-associated cytokines, and this may in turn contribute to the severity or phenotype of IBD. In the future it may be possible to identify specific cytokine-targeted therapy for individuals carrying particular regulatory polymorphisms.

IMPLICATIONS OF TRANSGENIC EXPERIMENTS

The advent of transgenic technology has led to a number of experiments involving the analysis of the phenotype of rodents in which genes have been transfected or disrupted (Strober & Ehrhardt 1993). Transfection of *HLA-B27* (Hammer et al 1990) and disruption of *IL-10* (Kuhn et al 1993), *Il-2* (Sadlack et al 1993) and TcR (Mombaerts et al 1993) have both been associated with enteropathies bearing some superficial similarities to ulcerative colitis or Crohn's disease. However, closer examination of the phenotypes involved has revealed that none of the animal models exactly reflects IBD. The gut can only respond to injury in a finite number of ways, and not all gut inflammation is IBD. Although these experiments may suggest a role for the transgenes in human IBD, they should not be taken to show that the transgenes cause IBD. Transgenic technology is more appropriately used to investigate the function of genes implicated in studies of human diseases.

SUMMARY

Genetic studies of IBD have revealed significant heritable components to Crohn's disease and ulcerative colitis.

Candidate genes have been investigated, and so far the strongest associations have been between HLA alleles and IBD, particularly ulcerative colitis. These studies have clarified the distinction between Crohn's disease and ulcerative colitis, and suggest that there is heterogeneity within Crohn's disease and ulcerative colitis. Already genetic analyses of IBD have improved the accuracy of disease taxonomy, and may in future provide an adjunct to differential diagnosis. These disease associations described so far are open to a number of interpretations. Association with HLA suggests a role for these molecules in antigen presentation or T-cell selection in the pathobiology of IBD. Alternative explanations include the involvement of closely linked MHC genes, such as *TNF*, or genes involved in antigen processing and presentation. Studies of T-cell receptor genes in IBD will have to include the investigation of the expressed and selected TcR repertoire in affected tissues as well as genetically encoded polymorphisms. In addition to yielding important insights into the pathology of IBD, these studies are likely to provide new targets for more specific IBD therapies in the future.

REFERENCES

Acha-Orbea H, Michell D J, Timmerman L et al 1988 Limited heterogeneity of T cell receptors from lymphocytes mediating autoimmune encephalomyelitis allows specific immune intervention. Cell 54: 263–273

Asakura H, Tsuchiya M, Aiso S 1982 Association of human lymphocyte-*DR2* antigens with Japanese ulcerative colitis. Gastroenterology 82: 413–418

Balk S P, Ebert E C, Blumenthal R L et al 1991 Oligoclonal expansion and CD1 recognition by human intestinal intraepithelial lymphocytes. Science 253: 1411–1415

Bertoletti A, Sette A, Chisari F V et al 1994 Natural variants of cytotoxic epitopes are T-cell receptor antagonists for antiviral cytotoxic T cells. Nature 369: 407–410

Bouma G, Oudkerk Pool M, von Bloomberg M B E et al 1994 Different spontaneous and stimulated TNF production in patients with Crohn's disease and ulcerative colitis. Gastroenterology 106: A1018

Burrows S R, Moss D J, Khanna R et al 1994 T-cell receptor repertoire for a viral epitope in humans is diversified by tolerance to a background MHC antigen. Journal of Experimental Medicine (in press)

Campbell R D, Milner C M 1993 M H C genes in autoimmunity. Current Opinion in Immunology 5: 887–893

Campbell R D, Trowsdale J 1993 Map of the human MHC. Immunology Today 14: 349–352

Carmichael A, Jin X, Sissons P, Borysiewicz L 1993 Quantitative analysis of the human immunodeficiency virus type 1 (HIV-1)-specific cytotoxic T-lymphocyte (CTL) response at different stages of HIV-1 infection: differential CTL responses to HIV-1 and Epstein–Barr virus in late disease. Journal of Experimental Medicine 177: 249–256

Cease K B, Berzofsky J A 1994 Toward a vaccine for AIDS: the emergence of immunobiology-based vaccine development. Annual Review of Immunology 12: 923–989

Choi Y, Kappler J W, Marrack P 1991 A superantigen encoded in the open reading frame of the 3' long terminal repeat of mouse mammary tumor virus. Nature 350: 203–207

Cresswell P 1994 Assembly, transport, and function of MHC class II molecules. Annual Review of Immunology 12: 259–294

de Silva H J, Gatter K C, Millard P R et al 1990 Crypt cell proliferation and *HLC-DR* expression in pelvic ileal pouches. Journal of Clinical Pathology 43: 824–828

Engelhard V H 1994 Structure of peptides associated with class I and class II MHC molecules. Annual Review of Immunology 12: 181–208

Farrant J M, Doherty D G, Donaldson P T et al 1992 Amino acid substitutions at position 38 of the DR β polypeptide confer susceptibility to and protection from primary sclerosing cholangitis. Hepatology 16: 390–395

Farrant J M, Bunce M, Artlett C et al 1994 *HLA-DR2* is a susceptibility marker for ulcerative colitis in British patients irrespective of ANCA positivity. Gastroenterology 106: A679

Fleischer B, Mittrucker H 1991 Evidence for T-cell receptor–HLA class II molecule interaction in the response to superantigenic bacterial toxins. European Journal of Immunology 21: 1331–1333

Gurbindo C, Russo P, Sabbah S et al 1993 Interleukin-2 activity of colonic lamina propria mononuclear cells in a rat model of experimental colitis. Gastroenterology 104: 964–972

Hammer R E, Maika S D, Richardson J A et al 1990 Spontaneous inflammatory disease in transgenic rats expressing *HLA-B27* and human-β-*2m*: an animal model of *HLA-B27*-associated human disorders. Cell 63: 1099–1112

Heber Katz E, Acha-Orbea H 1989 V regions disease hypothesis: evidence from autoimmune encephalomyelitis. Immunology Today 10: 164

Herman A, Croteau G, Sekaly R P et al 1990 *HLA-DR* alleles differ in their ability to present staphylococcal enterotoxins to T cells. Journal of Experimental Medicine 172: 709–717

Hermann T, Maryanski J L, Romero P et al 1990 Activation of MHC class I-restricted CD8+ CTL by microbial T-cell mitogens. Journal of Immunology 144: 1181–1186

Hill A V, Elvin J, Willis A C et al 1992 Molecular analysis of the association of *HLA-B35* and resistance to severe malaria. Nature 360: 434–439

Hoang P, Crotty B, Dalton H R, Jewell D P 1992 Epithelial cells bearing class II molecules stimulate allogeneic human colonic intraepithelial lymphocytes. Gut 33: 1089–1093

Klenerman P, Rowland-Jones S, McAdam S et al 1994 Cytotoxic T-cell activity antagonized by naturally occurring *HIV-1 gag* variants. Nature 369: 403–407

Kuhn R, Lohler J, Rennick D et al 1993 Interleukin-10-deficient mice develop chronic enterocolitis. Cell 75: 263–274

Lowes J R, Radwan P, Priddle J D et al 1992 Characterisation and quantification of mucosal cytokine that induces epithelial histocompatibility locus antigen-DR expression in inflammatory bowel disease. Gut 33: 315–319

McGuire W, Hill A V S, Allsop C E M et al 1994 Variation in the TNF-α promoter region associated with susceptibility to cerebral malaria. Nature 371: 508–511

Mansfield J C, Holden H, Tarlow J K 1994 Novel genetic association between ulcerative colitis and the anti-inflammatory cytokine interleukin-1 receptor. Gastroenterology 106: 637–642

Marrack P, Blackman M, Kushnir E, Kappler J 1990 The toxicity of staphylococcal enterotoxin B in mice is mediated by T-cells. Journal of Experimental Medicine 171: 455–464

Marrack P, Kushnir E, Kappler J 1991 A maternally inherited superantigen encoded by a mammary tumour virus. Nature 349: 524–526

Mehal W Z, Gregory W, Cross S J et al 1994 Localisation of the immunogenetic susceptibility to primary biliary cirrhosis. Hepatology 20: 1213–1219

Millward B A, Welsh K I, Leslie R D G et al 1987 T-cell receptor β-chain polymorphisms are associated with insulin-dependent diabetes. Clinical and Experimental Immunology 70: 152–157

Mombaerts P, Mizoguchi E, Grusby M J et al 1993 Spontaneous development of inflammatory bowel disease in T-cell receptor mutant mice. Cell 75: 274–282

Moss P A H, Rosenberg W M C, Bell J I 1992 The human T-cell receptor in health and disease. Annual Review of Immunology 10: 71–96

O'Hehir R E, Lamb J R 1990 Induction of specific clonal anergy in human T lymphocytes by *Staphylococcus aureus* enterotoxins. Proceedings of the National Academy of Sciences USA 87: 1–5

Oksenberg J R, Gaiser C N, Cavalli-Sforza L L et al 1988 Polymorphic markers of human T-cell receptor α and β genes. Family studies and comparison of frequencies in healthy individuals and patients with multiple sclerosis and myasthenia gravis. Human Immunology 22: 111–121

Oksenberg J R, Sherritt M, Begovich A B et al 1989 T-cell receptor Vα and Cα alleles associated with multiple sclerosis and myasthenia gravis. Proceedings of the National Academy of Sciences USA 86: 988–992

Ostrov D, Krieger J, Sidney J et al 1993 T-cell receptor antagonism mediated by interaction between T-cell receptor junctional residues and peptide antigen analogues. Journal of Immunology 150: 4277–4283

Pile K, Wordsworth P, Liote F et al 1993 Analysis of a T-cell receptor Vβ segment implicated in susceptibility to rheumatoid arthritis: Vβ2 germline polymorphism does not encode susceptibility. Annals of Rheumatic Diseases 52: 891–894

Powis S H, Rosenberg W M, Hall M et al 1993 *TAP-1* and *TAP-2* polymorphism in coeliac disease. Immunogenetics 38: 345–350

Rellahan B L, Jones L A, Kruisbeek A M et al 1990 In vivo induction of anergy in peripheral Vβ8 T cells by staphylococcal enterotoxin B. Journal of Experimental Medicine 172: 1091–1100

Rojo S, Garcia F, Villadangos J A et al 1993 Changes in the repertoire of peptides bound to *HLA-B27* subtypes and to site-specific mutants inside and outside pocket B. Journal of Experimental Medicine 177: 613–620

Rosenberg W M C, Prince C, Fox S B et al 1995 Increased expression of CD44v6 and CD44v3 in ulcerative colitis but not Crohn's disease. Lancet 345: 1205–1209

Sadlack B, Merz H, Schorle H et al 1993 Ulcerative colitis-like disease in mice with a disrupted interleukin-2 gene. Cell 75: 253–261

Sargent C A, Anderson M J, Hsieh S L et al 1994 Characterisation of the novel gene *G11* lying adjacent to the complement *C4A* gene in the human major histocompatibility complex. Human Molecular Genetics 3: 481–488

Satsangi J, Jewell D P, Rosenberg W M C, Bell J I 1994 Genetics of inflammatory bowel disease. Gut 35: 696–700

Scholl P R, Diez A, Karr R et al 1990 Effect of isotypes and allelic polymorphism on the binding of staphlococcal exotoxins to MHC class II molecules. Journal of Immunology 144: 226–230

Seboun E, Robinson M A, Doolittle T H et al 1989 A susceptibility locus for multiple sclerosis is linked to the T-cell receptor β-chain complex. Cell 57: 1095–1100

Sette A, Alexander J, Ruppert J et al 1994 Antigen analogs/MHC complexes as specific T-cell receptor antagonists. Annual Review of Immunology 12: 413–431

Sollid L M, Markussen G, Ek J et al 1989 Evidence for a primary association of coeliac disease to a particular *HLA-DQ* α/β heterodimer. Journal of Experimental Medicine 169: 345

Strober W, Ehrhardt R O 1993 Chronic intestinal inflammation: an unexpected outcome in cytokine or T-cell receptor mutant mice. Cell 75: 203–205

Sugimura K, Asakura H, Hibi T et al 1991 Molecular analysis of genes reponsible for susceptibility to ulcerative colitis within the HLA region. Gastroenterology 100: A619

Sutton J, Rowland-Jones S, Rosenberg W et al 1993 A sequence pattern for peptides presented to cytotoxic T lymphocytes by *HLA-B8* revealed by analysis of epitopes and eluted peptides. European Journal of Immunology 23: 447–453

Tanaka N, Taniguchi T 1992 Cytokine gene regulation: regulatory *cis* elements and DNA binding factors involved in the interferon system. Advances in Immunology 52: 263–281

Todd J A, Bell J I, McDevitt H O 1987 *HLA-DQβ* gene contributes to susceptibility and resistance to insulin-dependent diabetes mellitus. Nature 329: 599–604

Townsend A, Bodmer H 1989 Antigen recognition by class I restricted T lymphocytes. Annual Review of Immunology 7: 601–624

Toyoda H, Wang S-J, Yang H et al 1993 Distinct association of HLA class II genes with inflammatory bowel disease. Gastroenterology 104: 741–748

Tysk C, Lindberg E, Järnerot G, Floderus-Myrhed B 1988 Ulcerative colitis and Crohn's disease in an unselected population of monozygotic twins with inflammatory bowel disease. Gut 29: 990–996

Weetman A P, So A K, Roe C et al 1987 T-cell receptor α chain V-region polymorphism linked to primary autoimmune hypothyroidism but not Graves' disease. Human immunology 20: 167–173

Wordsworth B P, Lanchbury J S S, Sakks L I et al 1989 *HLA-DR4* subtype frequencies in rheumatoid arthritis indicate that *DRB1* is the major susceptibility locus within the HLA class II region. Proceedings of the National Academy of Sciences USA 86: 10049–10053

Wordsworth B P, Pile K D, Gibson K et al 1993 Analysis of the MHC-encoded transporters *TAP-1* and *TAP-2* in rheumatoid arthritis: linkage with *DR4* accounts for the association with a minor *TAP-2* allele. Tissue Antigens 42: 153–155

Wraith D C, McDevitt H O, Steinman L, Acha-Orbea H 1989 T-cell recognition as the target for immune intervention in autoimmune disease. Cell 57: 709–715

Yang H, Rotter J I, Toyoda H 1993 Ulcerative colitis: a genetically heterogeneous disorder defined by genetic (HLA class II) and subclinical (antineutrophil cytoplasmic antibodies) markers. Journal of Clinical Investigation 92: 1080–1084

Zamvil S S, Mitchell D J, Lee N E et al 1988 Predominant expression of a T-cell receptor Vβ gene subfamily in autoimmune encephalomyelitis. Journal of Experimental Medicine 167: 1586–1596

4. Epidemiological overview of inflammatory bowel disease

M. J. S. Langman

The study of the epidemiology of inflammatory bowel disease serves three purposes. It allows first, the measurement of the size of the problem that inflammatory bowel disease presents in the community, and secondly the way in which it is changing in frequency, or is associated with specific environmental features. Thirdly, it may provide clues to the etiology of the disease, which is poorly understood.

PROBLEMS IN GATHERING RELIABLE DATA

The prime need is to identify all those who develop the disease under review within a specific population. Non-specific inflammatory bowel disease, with which this chapter is concerned, presents certain analytical difficulties.

Case identification

It is difficult to distinguish between those who clearly have inflammatory bowel disease, those who have symptoms of similar but unrelated disorders, and even those (in a western community where functional disorders are almost the rule) who are disease free.

The vast majority of cases of non-specific inflammatory bowel disease consist of ulcerative colitis or Crohn's disease. In general, ulcerative colitis can be distinguished from Crohn's disease by certain individual features. However, in a minority of affected individuals the patterns cannot reliably be fitted into one or other disease category. Furthermore, detection of disease depends on sophisticated investigative methods being fully available.

Once the nature of the problem is recognized nearly all patients with non-specific inflammatory bowel disease are likely to be referred to hospital, or for a specialist opinion within western communities. Such recognition may be delayed, particularly in Crohn's disease, thus an interval of 2–4 years may occur in the UK or the USA, so that disease frequency may be underestimated if allowance is not made for this interval. Furthermore, in countries with poorly developed healthcare delivery systems, and in which infectious diarrheas present endemic problems, failure to recognize non-specific inflammatory bowel disease can readily occur.

Indices of frequency

Mortality rates

Death from ulcerative colitis or Crohn's disease is uncommon, and measurement of death rates essentially concentrates upon disease complications or complications of surgery. Changing mortality rates may correlate with changing disease incidence rates, but they must also reflect the efficiency of treatment, and even changes in the frequency of associated complications.

Hospital admissions rates

In the past most patients with Crohn's disease were ultimately admitted to hospital; this may no longer be true, and is not true of ulcerative colitis. Many, and probably most, individuals with ulcerative colitis have mild disease limited to the rectum or rectosigmoid area. These, and some with more extensive disease, have intermittent mild symptoms which never occasion hospital admission. Outpatient treatment has probably become more common with improved medical treatment. In consequence, admission rate could remain steady even though the incidence of the disease is increasing.

Where Crohn's disease is concerned a reduction of hospital admission rates during the latter part of a survey period could reflect a true fall in incidence, a lag between outpatient diagnosis and admission to hospital, or improved control with medical treatment.

Repeated admissions pose a further complication. Hospital admission statistics seldom allow distinction between admissions on two or more occasions of a single patient and admissions of different patients. Corrections could be introduced for repeated admissions by reference to the clinical histories of a selected group of patients where the pattern is known, but this may not be representative of the overall picture.

Admission statistics, despite their limitations, can probably be used as a reasonable index for Crohn's disease incidence rates, but they are of little value as indices in ulcerative colitis because only a small proportion of such patients are admitted to hospital.

Outpatient and other diagnostic referral rates

The increasing sophistication of diagnostic indices has resulted in a considerably increased number of studies which have been able to accumulate comprehensive data. In these circumstances there are inevitably problems in interpreting trends. Do they, for example reflect increased diagnostic awareness, new diagnostic techniques, greater intensity of investigation of minor symptoms, or true trends? Conclusive answers may be difficult to obtain, but data sets obtained in defined areas over long periods of time, using largely the same clinics throughout, and which show stability in the frequency of, say, colitis but a rise in that of Crohn's disease, would seem very likely to reflect a true change.

INCIDENCE AND TIME TRENDS

Non-specific inflammatory bowel disease is commonly found in northwestern Europe and North America. The incidence data in Tables 4.1 and 4.2 reflect these patterns. Data sets have been derived in other areas such as Spain (Ruiz & Potel 1986), Italy (Lanfranchi et al 1976), Czechoslovakia (Nedbal & Maratka 1968) as well as New Zealand, Japan, Australia, South Africa and many others. In some of these data based upon hospital recording is likely to be incomplete, but some overall conclusions can be reached.

Table 4.1 Incidence of Crohn's disease. Rates per 100 000 per year in selected populations

Country	Region	Reference	Years	Incidence
United States	Minnesota	Sedlack et al 1980	1968–75	6.6
Sweden	Malmo	Brahme et al 1975	1958–70	6.4
United Kingdom	Blackpool	Lee & Costello 1985	1976–80	6.1
Sweden	Uppsala	Bergman & Krause 1975	1968–73	5.0
France	N. west	Gower-Rousseau et al 1994	1988–90	4.9
United Kingdom	Cardiff	Mayberry & Rhodes 1986	1971–75	4.8
Sweden	Stockholm	Hellers 1979	1970–74	4.5
United States	Minnesota	Gollop et al 1988	1978–82	4.3
Holland	Leiden	Shivananda et al 1987a, b	1979–83	3.9
United Kingdom	Nottingham	Miller et al 1974	1970–72	3.6
Denmark	Copenhagen	Binder et al 1982	1970–78	2.7
Switzerland	Basel	Fahrlander & Baerlocher 1971	1967–69	2.6
United Kingdom	Aberdeen	Kyle & Stark 1980	1973–75	2.6
Faroe Isles		Berner & Kiaer 1986	1964–83	1.7
Israel	Tel Aviv	Rozen et al 1979	1970–78	1.3
Greece	N. west	Tsianos et al 1994	1988–90	0.3

Table 4.2 Incidence of ulcerative colitis. Rates per 100 000 per year in selected populations

Country	Region	Reference	Years	Incidence
United Kingdom	Aberdeen	Sinclair et al 1983	1975	15.8
United Kingdom	Teesside	Devlin et al 1980	1971–77	15.1
United States	Ohmsted	Stonnington et al 1987	1970–79	14.3
Faroe Isles		Berner & Kiaer 1986	1979–83	12.5
Denmark	Copenhagen	Binder et al 1982	1962–78	8.1
United Kingdom	Cardiff	Morris & Rhodes 1984	1968–77	7.2
United Kingdom	Oxford	Evans & Acheson 1965	1951–60	6.5
Sweden	Malmo	Brahme et al 1975	1958–70	6.3
Israel	Jerusalem	Jacobsohn & Levine 1986	1973–78	6.3
Israel	Beersheva	Odes et al 1987	1976–81	5.8
Greece	N. west	Tsianos et al 1994	1988–90	5.1
Sweden	Stockholm	Nordenvall et al 1985	1955–79	4.7
Israel	Tel Aviv	Gilat et al 1974	1961–70	3.6
France	N. west	Gower-Rousseau et al 1994	1988–90	3.2

Areas of proven or probable high incidence

These include Scandinavia, the UK, North America, Australia and much of northwestern Europe in general. Incidence rates are generally higher for ulcerative colitis than for Crohn's disease, although with occasional exceptions such as northwest France (Gower-Rousseau et al 1994). Within Europe incidence rates for ulcerative colitis appear to vary by at least fivefold, although there must inevitably be unevenness in recording the lesser varieties of disease. This may be important because some have noted that the frequency of proctitis in particular, may, be rising (Ekbom et al 1991).

The frequency of Crohn's disease also appears to vary at least sixfold, with the areas of high incidence being the industrialized northwest European and North American countries, as well as Australia and South Africa.

Areas of probable low incidence

There appear to be variations, with some areas, such as Greece, recording a low incidence of Crohn's disease but a distinctly higher frequency of ulcerative colitis. Crohn's disease also seems demonstrably rare in Japan, Israel, Spain and Italy, and in many other areas, although dependence upon hospital databases in case identification makes confident assertions difficult.

Time trends

The incidence of Crohn's disease has increased, whereas no clear trend is identifiable for ulcerative colitis. The figures fit well with the belief that they do not arise from diagnostic transfer from colitis to Crohn's disease. Figures for ulcerative colitis show divergences between those who identify rises in overall frequency (Sinclair et al 1983, Stonnington et al 1987), those who detect little change (Morris & Rhodes 1984) and others who detect change for minor disease only (Ekbom et al 1991).

The incidence of Crohn's disease may now have plateaued (Hellers 1979, Kyle and Stark 1980, Ekbom et al 1991) in the countries of high incidence.

Age and sex incidence

There are considerable variations in patterns. Interpretation is hindered because of recent recognition of the role of smoking in determining the pattern of disease. Age-specific incidence data obtained in one very large study (Ekbom et al 1991) fit with the belief that incidence rates are maximal at the beginning of the third decade of life for both Crohn's disease and colitis. Secondary peaks are described later in life by others, but such findings are, in general, inconsistent.

URBAN/RURAL SOCIOECONOMIC AND ETHNIC FACTORS

Urban/rural differences

A lower incidence of Crohn's disease has been noted in rural populations (Mendeloff et al 1966, Kyle 1971, Ekbom et al 1991, Tsianos et al 1994). Some of the differences are so large and unaccompanied by similar trends for ulcerative colitis (e.g. Tsianos et al) that real differences seem likely. However, where both colitis and Crohn's disease are detected less frequently in rural populations, the possibility of a reduced tendency to present and to be diagnosed in those living outside towns must be remembered.

Socioeconomic factors

Little more than minor variations in incidence have been detected in disease frequency in those of differing socioeconomic groups (Monk et al 1967, 1969, Bonnevie et al 1968, Kyle 1972, Keighley et al 1976).

Examination of factors related to domestic hygiene has shown that Crohn's disease (but not ulcerative colitis) is significantly more common in those who in infancy had separate bathrooms, a hot water tap in the house and mains drainage (Gent et al 1994). Such features are consonant with the raised urban to rural ratio. The cause is unclear, but one possibility is that the hypothesis of delayed exposure to outside sources of infection as a significant factor (Gilat et al 1987) is, in fact, correct.

Ethnic variation

In the USA Crohn's disease and ulcerative colitis have been detected less often in black than in white people. Differences have been of about a third to a fifth in colitis and Crohn's disease, respectively. This marked fluctuation may reflect real differences, although variations in the quality of health care cannot be discounted.

Jews are generally thought to be more susceptible to inflammatory bowel disease than white non-Jewish populations living in the same area (Monk et al 1967, Hellers 1979).

Table 4.3 shows that Jews born in North America or Europe who migrated to Israel were at higher risk of ulcerative colitis than those born in Israel, who were themselves at higher risk than those born in Africa or Asia. These findings suggest the impact of varying environmental influences within the Jewish population.

There are also substantial ethnic minority populations in the UK, and Table 4.3 also shows that the white population living in the middle of England, in Leicestershire, were at increased risk of Crohn's disease compared with south Asians living there. By contrast, south Asians appeared to be at greater risk of ulcerative colitis. It is unclear whether these differences reflect real ethnic variations in susceptibility or differing exposure to risk factors for one or the other disease – notably smoking.

ETIOLOGICAL FACTORS

Interpretation of general epidemiological data

Although general descriptive data have been useful in yielding clues which have allowed the design of case

Table 4.3 Prevalence of inflammatory bowel disease. Comparative data for individuals of different racial origin living in the same area (figures per 100 000 population)

Israel
Age-adjusted prevalence rates of ulcerative colitis according to place of birth (Odes et al 1987)

Place of residence		Place of birth		
		America/Europe	Africa/Asia	Israel
Beersheva	1985	129.3	64.1	97.6
Jerusalem	1978	94.1	24.0	70.2
Tel Aviv	1970	31.3	17.2	23.6

United Kingdom
Age-adjusted prevalence rates of Crohn's disease and ulcerative colitis according to ethnic group of individuals living in Leicestershire (Probert et al 1993)

Disease	European	South Asian		
		Hindu	Sikh	Muslim
Crohn's disease	75.8	31.9	30.8	53.8
Ulcerative colitis	127.8	193.0	207.6	130.6

control, cohort and other investigations of possible causes of colitis and Crohn's disease, the amount of progress has been disappointingly slight. Environmental influences which have been well proven to influence the occurrence of colitis and Crohn's disease are smoking habits: non-smoking in the case of ulcerative colitis, and smoking in the case of Crohn's disease. The strength and consistency of these associations are so great that they cannot be doubted (Harries et al 1982, Logan et al 1984, Somerville et al 1984, Calkins 1989). Without a detailed knowledge of smoking habits it becomes difficult to interpret varying sex ratios for the two diseases in different places. By contrast, the relative weakness of the oral contraceptive–Crohn's disease association (Logan and Kay 1989, Vessey et al 1986, Lesko et al 1988) and its contested nature (Lashner et al 1989) makes it unlikely that increasing oral contraceptive use could account for a rising incidence of Crohn's disease in many areas in the 1970s and early 1980s. None of the above is easily reconciled with possible protection from colitis by appendectomy (Rutgeerts et al 1994).

Some more recent data have tended to indicate that whereas Crohn's disease may be associated with an urban environment, ulcerative colitis may not (Tsianos et al 1994). If Crohn's disease is associated with urbanization, then two possible mechanisms include a greater chance of person-to-person contact, and hence disease transmission, and some other feature of urban domestic life.

Examination of contagion by formal epidemiological study has proved disappointing (Miller et al 1975, 1976). Likewise, an early examination of possible childhood factors has been negative (Gilat et al 1987). The hypothesis then examined was that an overprotective environment against (say) gut pathogens led to later acquisition and a greater likelihood of persistence. However, a more recent study (Gent et al 1994) has shown a highly significant relationship with increased standards of domestic hygiene, thus reviving the protection hypothesis.

Attention given to comparisons of different ethnic populations living in the same area has drawn attention to differences as well as a surprising lack of difference. Thus in the midlands of England ulcerative colitis seems to be at least as common in Asians as in Caucasians, whereas Crohn's disease is not (Probert et al 1993). No obvious reason can be discerned, although there is rough consonance with the urban rural data of Tsianos et al (1994) in Greece, in suggesting that Crohn's disease is an illness developing with urbanization but requiring early life in a western urban environment if it is to occur.

The high prevalence of inflammatory bowel disease in European Jews looks to be at least in part accountable for by environmental factors (nature unknown; see Table 4.3).

Examination of population differences in disease frequency has thrown no light upon the basis for dietary associations, notably the high sucrose intake of Crohn's disease patients (Kaspar and Sommer 1979, Martini and Brandes 1976, Mayberry et al 1980, Järnerot et al 1983).

This disappointing tendency for descriptive studies to fail to bring substantial clues forward – or if there are clues, for recognition to fail – is exemplified by a study of risk factors for extensive ulcerative colitis and ulcerative proctitis (Samuelsson et al 1991). Patients with ulcerative colitis did not differ in most of the socioeconomic, dietary and personal habits compared with the background population.

CONCLUSION

The substantial differences recorded in the frequencies of Crohn's disease and ulcerative colitis remain poorly understood. However, there are indications that Crohn's disease becomes prominent if early life is in an urbanized community, whereas colitis may be more even in its impact, whether life is spent in urban or rural communities. There are also likely substantial differences in disease occurrence in European, particularly north European, populations or those with north European lifestyles and those living in tropical or subtropical areas, but clear confirmatory evidence is lacking, notably because endemic infectious diseases make the confident attribution of non-specific disease difficult.

REFERENCES

Bergman L, Krause U 1975 The incidence of Crohn's disease in central Sweden. Scandinavian Journal of Gastroenterology 10: 725–729

Berner J, Kiaer T 1986 Ulcerative colitis and Crohn's disease on the Faroe islands 1964–83. Scandinavian Journal of Gastroenterology 21: 188–192

Binder V, Both M, Hansen P K, Hendriksen C, Kreiner S, Torp Pedersen K 1982 Incidence and prevalence of ulcerative colitis and Crohn's disease in the County of Copenhagen 1962 to 1978. Gastroenterology 83: 563–568

Bonnevie O, Riis P, Anthoniensen P 1968 An epidemiological study of ulcerative colitis in Copenhagen County. Scandinavian Journal of Gastroenterology 3: 432–438

Brahme F, Lindstrom C, Wenckert A 1975 Crohn's disease in a defined population. An epidemiological study of incidence, prevalence, mortality and secular trends in the city of Malmo. Gastroenterology 69: 342–351

Calkins B M 1989 A meta-analysis of the role of smoking in inflammatory bowel disease. Digestive Diseases and Sciences 34: 1841–1854

Devlin H B, Datta D, Dellipiani A W 1980 The incidence and prevalence of inflammatory bowel disease in North Tees Health District. World Journal of Surgery 4: 133–143

Ekbom A, Helmick C, Zack M, Adami H O 1991 The epidemiology of inflammatory bowel disease: a large population-based study in Sweden. Gastroenterology 100: 350–358

Evans J G, Acheson E C 1965 An epidemiological study of ulcerative colitis and regional enteritis in the Oxford Area. Gut: 311–324

Fahrlander H, Baerlocher C 1971 Clinical features and epidemiological data on Crohn's disease in Basle area. Scandinavian Journal of Gastroenterology 6: 657–662

Gent A E, Hellier M D, Grace R H, Swarbrick E T, Coggon D 1994 Inflammatory bowel disease and domestic hygene in infancy. Lancet 343: 766–767

Gilat T, Hacohen D, Lilos P, Langman M J S 1987 Childhood factors in ulcerative colitis and Crohn's disease. An international co-operative study. Scandinavian Journal of Gastroenterology 22: 1009–1024

Gilat G, Ribak J, Benaroya Y, Zemishlavy Z, Weissman I 1974 Ulcerative colitis in the Jewish population of Tel Aviv–Jafo. Gastroenterology 66: 335–342

Gollop J H, Phillips S F, Melton L J III, Zinsmeister A R 1988 Epidemiological aspects of Crohn's disease; a population-based study in Ohmsted County, Minnesota, 1943–82. Gut 29: 49–56.

Gower-Rousseau C, Salomez J L, Dupas J L et al 1994 Incidence of inflammatory bowel disease in Northern France (1988–1990). Gut 35: 1433–1438

Harries A D, Baird A, Rhodes J 1982 Non-smoking a feature of ulcerative colitis. British Medical Journal 284: 706

Hellers G 1979 Crohn's disease in Stockholm County, 1955–1974. A study of epidemiology, results of surgical treatment and long-term prognosis. Acta Chirurgica Scandinavica Suppl. 490: 1–84

Jacobsohn W Z, Levine Y 1986 Incidence and prevalence of ulcerative colitis in the Jewish population of Jerusalem. Israel Journal of Medical Science 22: 559–563

Järnerot G, Jarnmark I, Nilsson K 1983. Consumption of refined sugar by patients with Crohn's disease. Scandinavian Journal of Gastroenterology 18: 999–1002

Kaspar H, Sommer H 1979 Dietary fibre and nutrient intake in Crohn's disease. American Journal of Clinical Nutrition 32: 898–901

Keighley A, Miller D S, Hughes A O, Langman M J S 1976 The demographic and social characteristics of patients with Crohn's disease in the Nottingham area. Scandinavian Journal of Gastroenterology II: 293–296

Kyle J 1971 An epidemiology study of Crohn's disease in North East Scotland. Gastroenterology 61: 826–833

Kyle J 1972 Crohn's disease. Heinemann Medical, London

Kyle J, Stark J 1980 Fall in the incidence of Crohn's disease. Gut 21: 340–343

Lanfranchi G A, Michelin A, Brignola C 1976 Uno studio epidemiologico sulle malattie inflammatorie intestinali nella provinciade Bologna. Giorno Clinica Medica 57: 235–245

Lashner B A, Kane S V, Hanauer S B 1989 Lack of association between oral contraceptive use and Crohn's disease: a community-based matched case-control study. Gastroenterology 97: 1442–1447

Lee F I, Costello F T 1985 Crohn's disease in Blackpool – incidence and prevalence 1968–80. Gut 26: 274–278

Lesko S M N, Kaufman D W, Rosenberg L et al 1988 Evidence for an increased risk of Crohn's disease in oral contraceptive users. Gastroenterology 89: 1046–1049

Logan R F A, Kay C R 1989 Oral contraception, smoking and inflammatory bowel disease – findings in the Royal College of General Practitioners Oral Contraception Study. International Journal of Epidemiology 18: 105–107

Logan R F A, Edmond M, Somerville K W, Langman M J S 1984 Smoking and ulcerative colitis. British Medical Journal 288: 751–753

Martini G A, Brandes J N 1976 Increased consumption of refined carbohydrates in patients with Crohn's disease. Klinische Wochenschrift 54: 367–371

Mayberry J F, Rhodes J 1986 The changing incidence of Crohn's disease in Wales and the role of heredity in its aetiology. In: McConnell R B, Rozen P, Langman M, Gilat T (eds) The genetics and epidemiology of inflammatory bowel disease. Karger, Basel, pp 114–117

Mayberry J F, Rhodes J, Newcombe R G 1980 Increased consumption of sugar in Crohn's disease. Digestion 20: 323–326

Mendeloff A I, Monk M, Siegal C I, Lilienfeld A 1966 Some epidemiologic features of ulcerative colitis and regional enteritis – a preliminary report. Gastroenterology 51: 748–756

Miller D S, Keighley A C, Langman M J S 1974 Changing patterns in epidemiology of Crohn's disease. Lancet 2: 691–693

Miller D S, Keighley A, Smith P G, Hughes A O, Langman M J S 1975 Crohn's disease in Nottingham: a search for time–space clustering. Gut 16: 454–457

Miller D S, Keighley A, Smith P G, Hughes A O, Langman M J S 1976 A case control method for seeking evidence of contagion in Crohn's disease. Gastroenterology 71: 385–387

Monk M, Mendeloff A I, Siegel C I 1967 An epidemiological study of ulcerative colitis and regional enteritis among adults in Baltimore. Gastroenterology 53: 198–210

Monk M, Mendeloff A I, Siegel C I, Lilienfeld A 1969 An epidemiological study of ulcerative colitis and regional enteritis among adults in Baltimore. Gastroenterology 56: 847–857

Morris T, Rhodes J 1984 Incidence of ulcerative colitis in the Cardiff region 1968–77. Gut 25: 846–848

Nedbal J, Maratka Z 1968 Ulcerative proctocolitis in Czechoslovakia. American Journal of Proctology 19: 106–114

Nordenvall B, Brostrom O, Bergland M 1985 Incidence of ulcerative colitis in Stockholm county 1955–79. Scandinavian Journal of Gastroenterology 20: 783–790

Odes H S, Fraser D, Krawiec J 1987 Ulcerative colitis in the Jewish population of Southern Israel 1961–1985: epidemiological and clinical study. Gut 28: 1630–1636

Probert C S J, Jayanthi V, Hughes A O, Thompson J R, Wicks A C D, Mayberry J 1993 Prevalence and family risk of ulcerative colitis and Crohn's disease: an epidemiological study among Europeans and South Asians in Leicestershire. Gut 34: 154–151

Rozen O, Zonia J, Yekutiel P, Gilat T 1979 Crohn's disease in the Jewish population of Tel-Aviv-Yafo. Gastroenterology 76: 25–30

Ruiz V, Potel J 1986 Crohn's disease in Galicia, Spain, 1968–1982 In: McConnell R, Rozen P, Langman M J S, Gilat T (eds) The genetics and epidemiology of inflammatory bowel disease. Karger, Basel, pp 94–101

Rutgeerts P, D'Haens G, Hiele M, Geboes K, Vantrappen G 1993 Appendectomy protects against ulcerative colitis. Gastroenterology 106: 1251–1253

Samuelsson S M, Ekbom A, Zack M, Helmick C G, Adami H-O 1991 Risk factors for extensive ulcerative colitis and ulcerative proctitis: a population-based case-control study. Gut 32: 1526–1530

Sedlack R E, Whisnant J, Elveback L R, Kurland L T 1980 Incidence of Crohn's disease in Ohmsted County, Minnesota, 1933–1975. American Journal of Epidemiology 112: 759–763

Shivananda S, Pena A S, Mayberry J F, Ruitenberg E J, Hoedemaeker P J 1987a Epidemiology of proctocolitis in the region of Leiden, The Netherlands. Scandinavian Journal of Gastroenterology 22: 993–1002

Shivananda S, Pena A S, Nap M et al 1987b Epidemiology of Crohn's disease the in region of Leiden, The Netherlands. Gastroenterology 93: 966–974

Sinclair J S, Brunt P W, Mowat N A G 1983 Non-specific proctocolitis in north eastern Scotland. Gastroenterology 85: 1–11

Somerville K W, Logan R F A, Edmond M, Langman M J S 1984 Smoking and Crohn's disease. British Medical Journal 289: 954–956

Stonnington C M, Phillips S F, Melton L J III, Zinsmeister A R 1987 Chronic ulcerative colitis: incidence and prevalence in a community. Gut 28: 402–409

Tsianos E V, Masalas C N, Merkouropoulos M, Dalekos G N, Logan R F A 1994 Incidence of inflammatory bowel disease in north west Greece: rarity of Crohn's disease in an area where ulcerative colitis is common. Gut 35: 369–372

Vessey M, Jewell D, Smith A, Yeates D, McPherson K 1986 Chronic inflammatory bowel disease, cigarette smoking and use of oral contraceptives; findings in a large cohort study of women of child-bearing age. British Medical Journal 292: 1101–1103

5. Epidemiology of inflammatory bowel disease

B. Breuer-Katschinski

DIETARY FACTORS

Methodology

Although numerous studies have assessed diet in patients with inflammatory bowel disease, the overall results have been inconclusive. Some of the problems stem from the difficulty of assessing diet. In case control studies dietary habits are usually recalled in prevalent cases either before the onset of the illness or as current habits. Both approaches might not be representative of the pre-illness diet. Although it has been shown that present diet reflects previous diet (Rohan & Potter 1984), there is always a worry that patients with a gastrointestinal disorder might have changed their dietary habits in the past because of gastrointestinal symptoms. Inaccurate reporting of dietary habits in both cases and controls has probably led to an underestimation of the association between diet and disease (Rothman 1986; Table 5.1).

Milk sensitivity

Whether antibodies against dietary antigens play a primary role in inflammatory bowel disease etiology or are secondary to inflammation is not known. There has, however, been a report of a potential relationship between cow's milk sensitivity during infancy and the subsequent development of ulcerative colitis (Glassman et al 1990). Because of the retrospective nature of this study and the difficulty of assessing cow's milk sensitivity, this finding needs to be interpreted with caution.

Breastfeeding

The search for infectious agents, possibly acquired early in life, has stimulated the evaluation of breastfeeding practices in patients with IBD. Although Whorwell et al (1979) found a significant deficiency of breastfeeding in patients with ulcerative colitis compared with controls, no such effect was seen in Crohn's disease. In contrast, Bergstrand and Hellers (1983) reported a significantly shorter breastfeeding period among Crohn's disease patients than in controls. In the latter study information on breastfeeding was checked with the patient's mother or another reliable source. Otherwise the patient was excluded from further analyses. These findings are in accordance with those from Koletzko et al (1989), who found children with Crohn's disease three times less likely to have been breastfed than their unaffected siblings. The same authors reported no protective effect for breastfeeding in children with ulcerative colitis. Two further studies found no association between breastfeeding and IBD (Gilat et al 1987, Ekbom et al 1990). Thus far, the data on breastfeeding in IBD remain inconsistent.

Refined sugar

Considerable interest has been raised by studies on the consumption of refined sugar in Crohn's disease. In 1976, Martini and Brandes reported that the intake of refined sugar was approximately double that of controls. Others have confirmed this observation (Miller et al 1976, Kasper & Sommer 1979, Thornton et al 1979, Silkoff et al 1980, Mayberry et al: 1980, 1981, Penny et al 1983, Järnerot et al 1983). Two studies (Thornton et al 1979, Mayberry et al 1981) examined Crohn's patients with newly diagnosed

Table 5.1 Association between various dietary factors and IBD

Factor	Crohn's disease	Ulcerative colitis
Milk sensitivity	Insufficient data	Insufficient data
Breastfeeding	Inconsistent	Inconsistent
High consumption of refined sugar	Increased risk	No increased risk
Low consumption of fruit and vegetables	Increased risk	Increased risk
Fiber	Inconsistent	Inconsistent
Cereals	Inconsistent	Inconsistent
Fast food	Insufficient data	Insufficient data
Fatty acids	Insufficient data	Insufficient data
Coffee	Insufficient data	Insufficient data
Alcohol	No increased risk	No increased risk
Food additives	Insufficient data	Insufficient data
Food intolerance	Inconsistent	Inconsistent

disease. Both reported a significantly greater intake of sugar in patients compared with controls. Thornton et al (1979) found no difference in the intake of sugar between patients with recent and long-standing symptoms. This finding does not support the suggestion that patients eat more sugar because of disease symptoms. In contrast to these reports, a Swedish study (Järnerot et al 1983) showed that patients with a recent onset of Crohn's disease consumed similar amounts of sugar to controls. An increased taste threshold for sweet foods was postulated to explain the high sugar consumption in patients with Crohn's disease, but three studies (Martini & Brandes 1976, Kasper & Sommer 1980, Thiomny et al 1982) found no evidence for this hypothesis. Thus the question whether high sugar consumption plays an etiological role or is secondary to disease remains unsolved.

When sugar intake was examined in relation to smoking, a higher consumption of refined sugar was only found in non-smokers (Katschinski et al 1988).

If the consumption of refined sugar were a strong determinant for the occurrence of Crohn's disease the per capita consumption of refined sugar in different countries should be related to the incidence of Crohn's disease. According to one study (Sonnenberg 1988), the time trends of Crohn's disease in different countries were not matched by similar time trends of sugar consumption.

The effect of an unrefined diet on the course of Crohn's disease has been examined by means of a controlled multicenter therapeutic trial (Ritchie et al 1987): 352 patients were randomized to two groups; the first group were advised to eat their normal diet, including refined carbohydrate; the second group were advised to eat carbohydrate in its natural unrefined state only. Patients were followed for 2 years. With regard to surgery, hospital admissions and disease deterioration, there were no significant differences between the groups. The results of this trial suggested that the course of mildly active Crohn's disease was unaffected by an unrefined carbohydrate diet. However, this study could not answer the question whether a reduction in sugar intake without a concurrent increase in fiber intake would be beneficial.

Fruit, vegetables and fiber

Several studies reported a decreased consumption of fruit or vegetables among patients with Crohn's disease (Kasper & Sommer 1979, Thornton et al 1979, Bianchi Porro & Panza 1985) and those with ulcerative colitis (Bianchi Porro & Panza 1985, Brandes et al 1979). Whereas Thornton et al (1979) reported a decreased consumption of total dietary fiber in patients with Crohn's disease, the reverse was found in another study (Kasper & Sommer 1979). These studies of dietary fiber intake must be interpreted with caution since it is likely that patients with bowel problems tend to avoid high-fiber foods.

Cereals

An increased consumption of breakfast cereals and bread was reported among patients with ulcerative colitis (Bianchi Porro & Panza 1985, Brandes et al 1979) and Crohn's disease (Bianchi Porro & Panza 1985, Brandes et al 1979, James 1977). These studies were undertaken on the assumption that food eaten on an empty stomach is more likely to reach the areas usually affected by the disease. However, several other studies have not confirmed this association (Martini & Brandes 1976, Thornton et al 1979, Mayberry et al 1980, 1981).

Fast food

In a Swedish case control study by Persson et al (1992) the consumption of fast foods at least twice a week was associated with a three- to fourfold increase in risk for patients with Crohn's disease and ulcerative colitis. Whether the fat composition of these foods plays a role remains speculative.

Fatty acids

Fatty acids of the n-3 type have been shown to alter arachidonic acid metabolism and downregulate the synthesis of leukotriene B4, a potent proinflammatory substance. One study examined dietary intake of essential fatty acids in patients with ulcerative colitis (Katschinski & Goebell 1991), reporting a statistically significant positive association with a high intake of n-3 fatty acids. Further studies are needed to explore the association between fatty acids and IBD.

Coffee and alcohol

In a study by Boyko et al (1989) pre-illness coffee consumption was not significantly altered in patients with ulcerative colitis. In the same study there was an association between alcohol consumption and a decreased risk of ulcerative colitis in those who had never smoked. In another study there was no significant difference in alcohol consumption between patients with Crohn's disease or ulcerative colitis and controls (Katschinski et al 1989). Furthermore, this study showed that in both diseases the relative risk for smoking was not affected by alcohol consumption. Thus it is unlikely that alcohol is an important confounder with regard to the association between smoking and IBD.

Carrageenan

It has been suggested that the increased risk of Crohn's disease associated with high sugar intake might be due to food additives, which may cause local or foreign-body reactions in the intestinal system. Pectin-like polysaccharides such as carrageenan are added to various sweets (Melynk 1975). Carrageenan is a hydrocolloid consisting of a sulfated polysaccharide which is found between and within the cell walls of red seaweeds. In animals such as rabbits, guinea pigs and rats, ulcerative colitis-like lesions developed in the cecum and colon after the ingestion of degraded carrageenan. This observation seems to be limited to certain species of animals. The role of food additives in IBD etiology is still unclear.

Toothpaste

Several authors have speculated that toothpaste may produce a potentially damaging effect to the gut (Chess et al 1950, Sullivan 1990). Most formulations contain abrasives, foaming agents, flavoring mixtures and thickening agents or binders. However, repeated administration of large doses of toothpaste and antacids did not produce changes comparable with those that are characteristic of Crohn's disease (Heatley et al 1980). Epidemiological study shows no convincing correlation between toothpaste consumption and Crohn's incidence or mortality (Ben-Shlomo & Nadanovsky 1990).

Food intolerance

It has been claimed that exclusion of foodstuffs after treatment with elemental diet prolongs remission (Alun Jones et al 1985). These authors reported on the treatment of 77 patients who had achieved full clinical remission by means of parenteral nutrition, enteral nutrition or the use of elimination diets. By excluding suspect foods 64 patients were able subsequently to return to an oral diet. The duration of remission was compared in a controlled trial including 10 patients on an elimination diet and 10 on an unrefined carbohydrate fiber-rich diet. Because of the high relapse rate in the fiber-rich group this study had to end prematurely. More recently, another study has been reported (Pearson et al 1993) in which 20 out of 42 patients identified food sensitivities. When suspect foods were reinvestigated, however, food sensitivity was confirmed in three patients only on double-blind challenge. There was no significant difference in the duration of remission between patients who did or did not identify food sensitivities. These results show that the food sensitivities that can be identified in patients with Crohn's disease tend to be variable and often poorly reproducible.

NUTRITIONAL DEFICIENCIES

Malnutrition is common in patients with inflammatory bowel disease (Table 5.2). There are several mechanisms which are responsible for malnutrition (Harries & Heatley 1983): there may be loss of absorptive surface owing to disease, resection or stagnant loops because of strictures. An enteric loss of nutrients may result from an inflamed intestinal mucosa or an interrupted enterohepatic circulation. Furthermore, medications such as corticosteroids increase nutritional requirements, particularly of protein. Another important cause of malnutrition is reduced food intake as a consequence of anorexia, or fear of eating because of abdominal pain. In patients with Crohn's disease extensive surgical resection of the small intestine often results in short bowel syndrome, which may require artificial feeding. Another consequence of intestinal resection is rapid gastrointestinal transit, which may also cause malnutrition.

Table 5.2 Prevalence of nutritional deficiencies in patients with Crohn's disease

Parameter	Percentage
Weight loss	40–80
Growth failure in children	20–30
Hypoproteinemia	25–76
Anemia	
Iron deficiency	50–70
B_{12} deficiency	10–60
Folate deficiency	30–60
Hyponatremia	10
Hypokalemia	30
Hypomagnesemia	14–88
Vitamin D deficiency	50–75
Steatorrhea	30

Weight and height

Weight and growth retardation are common problems in Crohn's disease; 20–30% of children and adolescents with Crohn's disease develop severe growth retardation as defined by either height below the third percentile for age, or bone age 2 years less than chronological age (Kirschner et al 1978, Gryboski & Spiro 1978). However, most studies reporting weight loss or growth delay did not record the patient's status before the illness. In a study by Kanof et al (1988) the height and weight velocities of 50 children and prepubescent adolescents with Crohn's disease were reviewed. Only patients in whom at least four separate height recordings between the age of 4 years and the onset of symptoms of Crohn's disease existed were included in this study. A significant decrease in height velocity antedated the diagnosis of Crohn's disease in 44 of 50 patients compared with a control population. When height and weight velocities were compared at the time of diagnosis, 17 of 32 children had a decrease in weight velocity before the decrease in height velocity. One of the reasons for delayed linear growth is decreased nutritional intake. Several studies reported that dietary intake is chronically insufficient in the majority of severely growth-retarded children with Crohn's disease (Kelts et al 1979, Kirschner et al 1981,

Motil et al 1982a). When an increased supply of calories was administered intravenously or enterally in some studies (Layden et al 1976, Kirschner et al 1981, Motil et al 1982a) an acceleration in growth velocity was observed.

Although no primary endocrine abnormality has been described in patients with severe growth retardation and Crohn's disease, somatomedin-C levels have been found to be decreased in severely growth-retarded children with Crohn's disease (Kirschner & Sutton 1986). When nutritional status improved, somatomedin-C levels normalized and growth velocity increased (Kirschner & Sutton 1986).

Besides decreased dietary intake, one of the potential causes of weight loss in patients with Crohn's disease is increased energy expenditure. In one study by Chan et al (1986), resting energy expenditure was calculated from oxygen consumption data obtained by indirect calorimetry in 54 patients. There was, however, no evidence of an increased resting energy expenditure in Crohn's disease patients without fever or sepsis.

Protein

Hypoproteinemia in Crohn's disease has been recorded with a frequency between 25% and 76% (Harries & Heatley 1983). Hill et al (1977) studied the incidence of protein malnutrition in 74 patients with established inflammatory bowel disease. Compared with a control group, patients requiring urgent surgery had low values for plasma albumin, transferrin, prealbumin and hemoglobin. These values were even lower in the patients who developed a major complication after surgery. Patients in remission or those with ileostomy showed no evidence of protein malnutrition.

The effect of chronic inflammation, corticosteroid therapy and nutritional supplementation on whole-body protein metabolism and growth was determined in male patients with Crohn's disease (Motil et al 1982a). With regard to nitrogen balance there was no difference between those patients with chronic inflammation, while receiving corticosteroid therapy, and controls. However, lean body mass and muscle mass were, significantly reduced in patients compared to controls. In a further study (Motil et al 1982b) the adaptive response of whole-body leucine metabolism to nutritional supplementation was determined in six adolescents with Crohn's disease and growth failure. During nutritional supplementation given as nocturnal feeding an increase in lean body mass was achieved. The authors stated that this effect was due to increased rates of amino acid incorporation into body protein, and decreased rates of amino acid oxidation.

Anemia

Anemia of varying severity may be found in 50–70% of patients with Crohn's disease who are receiving treatment predominantly in hospital (Beeken 1975). Anemia can result from a deficiency of iron, folic acid or vitamin B_{12}, or may simply be a consequence of chronic inflammation.

A low serum iron may be found in 50–70% of cases. When patients are treated with iron those with true iron deficiency should show a positive response provided the disease is not active, whereas those with chronic inflammation will probably not respond (Harries & Heatley 1983).

The prevalence of vitamin B_{12} malabsorption is variable, with a range of about 10–60% in different series (Harries & Heatley 1983). Vitamin B_{12} deficiency occurs commonly after ileal resection, or may be a result of the inflammation of the terminal ileum (Fausa 1974). Another reason could be bacterial overgrowth (Beeken & Kanich 1973). Substitution of vitamin B_{12} is essential in these cases.

The causes of folate deficiency are undoubtedly often multifactorial. Anorexia, malabsorption, disease activity and low-grade drug-induced hemolysis from sulfasalazine are all important mechanisms (Harries & Heatley 1983). The incidence of folate deficiency varies from 30 to 60% in different series.

Electrolytes

Diarrhea causes electrolyte loss, particularly if water and sodium absorption is impaired in a diseased small intestine. Hyponatremia has been found in only 10% of cases of Crohn's disease (Beeken 1975), whereas hypokalemia is found in about 30% of patients. Hypocalcemia usually occurs in association with hypoalbuminemia.

Hypomagnesemia is common in patients with severe disease or with intestinal resection. Beeken (1975) found hypomagnesemia in only nine of 63 patients, but Main et al (1981) reported that 15 of 17 patients admitted to hospital with severe disease were magnesium deficient.

Carbohydrate and fat absorption

Xylose absorption is usually normal in patients who have not had surgical resections (Heatley 1986). Lactose absorption is also usually normal in Crohn's disease. In contrast, steatorrhea can be found in up to 30% of patients (Heatley 1986). The problem is often masked by the associated anorexia and reduced fat intake.

Vitamins

Deficiencies of the fat-soluble vitamins A, D, E and K are closely related to fat malabsorption. An important problem is the frequency of osteomalacia in patients with Crohn's disease. Compston et al (1978) reported osteomalacia in 22 of 25 patients with small-bowel disease. Harries et al (1982) reported that over 50% of undernourished patients had secondary hyperparathyroidism.

Metals and trace elements

The recognition that zinc may be important for taste, wound healing and growth (Aggett & Harries 1979) has stimulated thought that some problems in Crohn's disease might be due to zinc deficiency. Solomons et al (1976) found evidence of zinc deficiency in five patients with total growth arrest secondary to juvenile Crohn's disease.

The same authors reported that in another group of 12 children with growth retardation none was found with a zinc deficiency syndrome. In a study by Ainley et al (1991) there was no evidence of zinc deficiency in malnourished Crohn's disease patients who presented with depressed non-specific cellular immunity. Information on other metals and trace elements is scarce.

REFERENCES

Aggett P J, Harries J T 1979 Current status of zinc in health and disease states. Archives of Disease in Childhood 54: 909–917

Ainley C, Cason J, Slavin B M, Wolstencroft R A, Thompson R P H 1991 The influence of zinc status and malnutrition on immunological function in Crohn's disease. Gastroenterology 100: 1616–1625

Alun Jones V, Dickinson R J, Workman E, Wilson A J, Freeman A H, Hunter J O 1985 Crohn's disease: maintenance of remission by diet. Lancet 2: 177–180

Beeken W L 1975 Remediable defects in Crohn disease. A prospective study of 63 patients. Archives of Internal Medicine 135: 686–690

Beeken W L, Kanich R E 1973 Microbial flora of the upper small bowel in Crohn's disease. Gastroenterology 65: 390–397

Ben-Shlomo Y, Nadanovsky P 1990 Toothpaste and Crohn's disease. Lancet 336: 1581–1582

Bergstrand O, Hellers G 1983 Breast-feeding during infancy in patients who later develop Crohn's disease. Scandinavian Journal of Gastroenterology 18: 903–906

Bianchi Porro G, Panza E 1985 Smoking, sugar and inflammatory bowel disease. British Medical Journal 291: 971–972

Boyko E J, Perera D R, Koepsell T D, Keane E M, Inui T S 1989 Coffee and alcohol use and the risk of ulcerative colitis. American Journal of Gastroenterology 84: 530–534

Brandes J-W, Stenner A, Martini G A 1979 Ernährungsgewohnheiten der Patienten mit Colitis ulcerosa. Zeitschrift für Gastroenterologie 17: 834–842

Chan A T H, Fleming C R, O'Fallon W M, Huizenga K A 1986 Estimated versus measured basal energy requirements in patients with Crohn's disease. Gastroenterology 91: 75–78

Chess S, Chess D, Olander G, Benner W, Cole W H 1950 Production of chronic enteritis and other systemic lesions by ingestion of finely divided foreign materials. Surgery 27: 221–234

Compston J E, Horton L W L, Ayers A B, Tighe J R, Creamer B 1978 Osteomalacia after small-intestinal resection. Lancet 1: 9–12

Ekbom A, Adami H-O, Helmick C G, Jonzon A, Zack M M 1990 Perinatal risk factors for inflammatory bowel disease: a case-control study. American Journal of Epidemiology 132: 1111–1119

Fausa O 1974 Vitamin B_{12} absorption in intestinal diseases (coeliac disease, dermatitis herpetiformis, ulcerative colitis, Crohn's disease, jejuno-ileal shunting). Scandinavian Journal of Gastroenterology 9 (Suppl 29): 75–79

Gilat T, Hacohen D, Lilos P, Langman M J S 1987 Childhood factors in ulcerative colitis and Crohn's disease. Scandinavian Journal of Gastroenterology 22: 1009–1024

Glassman M S, Newman L J, Berezin S, Gryboski J D 1990 Cow's milk protein sensitivity during infancy in patients with inflammatory bowel disease. American Journal of Gastroenterology 85: 838–840

Gryboski J D, Spiro H M 1978 Prognosis in children with Crohn's disease. Gastroenterology 74: 807–817

Harries A D, Heatley R V 1983 Nutritional disturbances in Crohn's disease. Postgraduate Medical Journal 59: 690–697

Harries A D, Brown R, Heatley R V, Woodhead S, Rhodes J 1982 Vitamin D deficiency in Crohn's disease: an association with undernutrition. Scandinavian Journal of Gastroenterology 17 (Suppl. 78): 151A (abstract)

Heatley R V 1986 Assessing nutritional state in inflammatory bowel disease. Gut 27 (Suppl. 1): 61–66

Heatley R V, Bolton P M, Hughes L E, Owen E W 1980 Mesenteric lymphatic obstruction in Crohn's disease. Digestion 20: 307–313

Hill G L, Blackett R L, Pickford I R, Bradley J A 1977 A survey of protein nutrition in patients with inflammatory bowel disease – a rational basis for nutritional therapy. British Journal of Surgery 64: 894–896

James A H 1977 Breakfast and Crohn's disease. British Medical Journal 1: 943–945

Järnerot G, Järnmark I, Nilsson K 1983 Consumption of refined sugar by patients with Crohn's disease, ulcerative colitis, or irritable bowel syndrome. Scandinavian Journal of Gastroenterology 18: 999–1002

Kanof M E, Lake A M, Bayless T M 1988 Decreased height velocity in children and adolescents before the diagnosis of Crohn's disease. Gastroenterology 95: 1523–1527

Kasper H, Sommer H 1979 Dietary fibre and nutrient intake in Crohn's disease. American Journal of Clinical Nutrition 32: 1898–1901

Kasper H, Sommer H 1980 Taste thresholds in patients with Crohn's disease. Journal of Human Nutrition 34: 455–456

Katschinski B, Goebell H 1991 Dietary essential fatty acids and the risk of ulcerative colitis. Gastroenterology 100: A9

Katschinski B, Logan R F A, Edmond M, Langman M J S 1988 Smoking and sugar intake are separate but interactive risk factors in Crohn's disease. Gut 29: 1202–1206

Katschinski B, Logan R F A, Langman M J S 1989 Rauchen und entzündliche Darmerkrankungen. Zeitschrift für Gastroenterologie 27: 614–618

Kelts D G, Grand R J, Shen G, Watkins J B, Werlin S L, Boehme C 1979 Nutritional basis of growth failure in children and adolescents with Crohn's disease. Gastroenterology 76: 720–727

Kirschner B S, Sutton M M 1986 Somatomedin-C levels in growth-impaired children and adolescents with chronic inflammatory bowel disease. Gastroenterology 91: 830–836

Kirschner B S, Voinchet O, Rosenberg I H 1978 Growth retardation in inflammatory bowel disease. Gastroenterology 75: 504–511

Kirschner B S, Klich J R, Kalman S S, de Favaro M V, Rosenberg I H 1981 Reversal of growth retardation in Crohn's disease with therapy emphasizing oral nutritional restitution. Gastroenterology 80: 10–15

Koletzko S, Griffiths A, Corey M, Smith C, Sherman P 1991 Infant feeding practices and ulcerative colitis in childhood. British Medical Journal 302: 1580–1581

Koletzko S, Sherman P, Corey M, Griffiths A, Smith C 1989 Role of infant feeding practices in development of Crohn's disease in childhood. British Medical Journal 298: 1617–1618

Layden T, Rosenberg J, Nemchausky B, Elson C, Rosenberg I 1976 Reversal of growth arrest in children with Crohn's disease after parenteral alimentation. Gastroenterology 70: 1017–1021

Main A N, Morgan R J, Russell R I et al 1981 Mg deficiency in chronic inflammatory bowel disease and requirements during intravenous nutrition. Journal of Parenteral and Enteral Nutrition 5: 15–19

Martini G A, Brandes J W 1976 Increased consumption of refined carbohydrates in patients with Crohn's disease. Klinische Wochenschrift 54: 367–371

Mayberry J F, Rhodes J, Allan R et al 1981 Diet in Crohn's disease. Two studies of current and previous habits in newly diagnosed patients. Digestive Diseases and Sciences 26: 444–448

Mayberry J F, Rhodes J, Newcombe R G 1980 Increased sugar consumption in Crohn's disease. Digestion 20: 323–326

Melynk C S 1975 Experimental colitis. In: Kirsner J B, Shorter R G (eds) Inflammatory bowel disease. Lea and Febiger, Philadelphia, pp 23–36

Miller B, Fervers F, Rohbeck R, Strohmeyer G 1976 Zuckerkonsum bei Patienten mit Morbus Crohn. Verhandlungen der Deutschen Gesellschaft für Innere Medizin 82: 922–924

Motil K J, Grand R J, Maletskos C J, Young V R 1982a The effect of disease, drugs and diet on whole body protein metabolism in adolescents with Crohn's disease and growth failure. Journal of Pediatrics 101: 345–351

Motil K J, Grand R J, Matthews D E, Bier D M, Maletskos C J, Young V R 1982b Whole body leucine metabolism in adolescents with Crohn's disease and growth failure during nutritional supplementation. Gastroenterology 82: 1359–1368

Pearson M, Teahon K, Levi A J, Bjarnason I 1993 Food intolerance and Crohn's disease. Gut 34: 783–787

Penny W J, Mayberry J F, Aggett P J, Gilbert J O, Newcombe R G, Rhodes J 1983 Relationship between trace elements, sugar consumption, and taste in Crohn's disease. Gut 24: 288–292

Persson P G, Ahlbom A, Hellers G 1992 Diet and inflammatory bowel disease: a case-control study. Epidemiology 3: 47–52

Ritchie J K, Wadsworth J, Lennard-Jones J E, Rogers E 1987 Controlled multicentre therapeutic trial of an unrefined carbohydrate, fibre rich diet in Crohn's disease. British Medical Journal 295: 517–520

Rohan T E, Potter J D 1984 Retrospective assessment of dietary intake. American Journal of Epidemiology 120: 876–887

Rothman K 1986 Modern epidemiology. Little Brown, Boston

Silkoff K, Hallak L, Yegena P et al 1980 Consumption of refined carbohydrate by patients with Crohn's disease in Tel Aviv–Yafo. Postgraduate Medical Journal 56: 842–846

Solomons N W, Rosenfield R L 1976 Growth retardation and zinc nutrition. Pediatric Research 10: 923–927

Sonnenberg A 1988 Geographic and temporal variations of sugar and margarine consumption in relation to Crohn's disease. Digestion 41: 161–171

Sullivan S N 1990 Hypothesis revisited: toothpaste and the cause of Crohn's disease. Lancet 336: 1096–1097

Thiomny E, Horwitz C, Graff E, Rozen P, Gilat T 1982 Serum zinc and taste acuity in Tel Aviv patients with inflammatory bowel disease. American Journal of Gastroenterology 77: 101–104

Thornton J R, Emmett P M, Heaton K W 1979 Diet and Crohn's disease: characteristics of the pre-illness diet. British Medical Journal 2: 762–764

Whorwell P J, Holdstock G, Whorwell G M, Wright R 1979 Bottle feeding, early gastroenteritis, and inflammatory bowel disease. British Medical Journal 1: 382

6. Epidemiology: smoking and oral contraception

R. Logan

After infectious agents and diet, cigarette smoking and oral contraceptive use are the environmental factors that have been most frequently linked to the etiology of inflammatory bowel disease. This is perhaps not surprising, as in many countries the prevalence of smoking and, to a lesser extent, oral contraception has tended to parallel the emergence of inflammatory bowel disease as a serious public health problem. Nevertheless, it is only within the past 10 years that these factors have been studied thoroughly.

SMOKING

In 1982, Harries and others were the first to draw attention to the association of non-smoking with ulcerative colitis, although 6 years earlier Samuelsson had made the same observation (Samuelsson 1976, Harries et al 1982). Since then, more than 20 case control studies have confirmed that, as a group, patients with ulcerative colitis smoke less than their peers of the same age and sex. Any possibility that this surprising finding was due to recall bias (patients tending to underreport smoking) was eliminated when it was shown that, in contrast, Crohn's disease patients tended to be smokers (Somerville et al 1984).

When reviewing the relationship between smoking and the development of inflammatory bowel disease, certain limitations to the data need to be considered. Only two studies have used smoking habit data collected prospectively: data were collected only at recruitment and hence the studies could not allow for any changes in smoking habit (Vessey et al 1986, Logan & Kay 1989). Most studies have been of the case control type, in which data on smoking were obtained some years after the onset of disease, either by questionnaire or by interview, sometimes by physicians. Even in the best designed of these studies the scope for recall bias is considerable, and its effect is difficult to assess.

Ulcerative colitis

Strength, consistency and dose response

Overall, the risk of a smoker developing ulcerative colitis has been around half that of someone who has never smoked, with two meta-analyses estimating relative risks of 0.47 (95% confidence limits 0.4–0.6) and 0.41 (0.3–0.5) (Calkins 1989, Logan 1990). Table 6.1 shows that these summary figures conceal considerable variations in risk estimates between and within different countries (Boyko et al 1987). The 'protective' effect of smoking has generally been similar in both men and women. Some studies have suggested that non-smoking is particularly associated with distal colitis, but this has not been found by others (Tobin et al 1987, Benoni & Nilsson 1987). Whether the risk is lower in pipe or cigar smokers is also not known.

A strong inverse dose–response relationship has been found in several case control studies (Tobin et al 1987, Franceschi et al 1987, Lindberg et al 1988, Nakamura & Labarthe 1994). Although this could be dismissed as being due to patients systematically underreporting amounts smoked, in the prospective cohort studies heavy smokers also had a lower risk of ulcerative colitis than light smokers (Vessey et al 1986, Logan & Kay 1989).

Risk in ex-smokers

One especially striking finding has been the *increased* risk of ulcerative colitis in ex-smokers (Table 6.1). In some studies the risk was particularly increased soon after stopping smoking (Motley et al 1987, Benoni & Nilsson 1987). Although recall bias could be playing a role, it seems likely that there is some further increase in the risk of developing ulcerative colitis within a year of stopping smoking.

Reversibility – effect of restarting smoking

There is evidence that smoking or treatment with nicotine can induce remission in active ulcerative colitis. There have been anecdotal reports of patients whose colitis began after they stopped smoking and improved when they restarted smoking (De Castella 1982, Roberts &

Table 6.1 Inflammatory bowel disease and smoking: relative risks* in smokers and ex-smokers by gender (never smokers RR = 1.0)

Centre (study)	Ulcerative colitis		Crohn's disease	
	Smoking at onset M/F	Ex-smoking M/F	Smoking at onset M/F	Ex-smoking M/F
Nottingham, UK (Logan et al 1986)	0.04/0.15	2.5/1.7	2.1/6.5	1.5/1.3
Liverpool, UK (Tobin et al 1987)	0.15/0.17	0.86/3.0	2.6/3.1	1.4/1.8
Milan, Italy (Franceschi et al 1987)	0.30/1.1	2.1/2.6	4.3/4.8	4.7/3.0
Lund, Sweden (Benoni & Nilsson 1984)	0.36/0.28	1.5/1.8	1.7/2.7	1.1/0.2
Stockholm, Sweden (Persson et al 1990)	0.96/0.72	1.6/1.6	1.3/5.0	1.2/1.0
North Carolina, US (Sandler & Holland 1988)	0.76/0.80	1.2/1.6	1.3/2.6	1.1/2.2
Japan (Nakamura & Labarthe 1994)	0.23/0.41	1.3/2.3	—	—

* Adjusted risks as quoted in papers

Diggle 1982, Jick & Walker 1983). Rudra et al (1989) questioned a group of 30 patients who started or restarted smoking when their colitis was active, and found that 14 thought their symptoms had improved; 13 had noticed no change and three thought they were worse.

These observations are now supported by experimental data from a randomized double-blind trial of transdermal nicotine patches. Pullan and colleagues (1994) found that 49% of patients with active colitis went into complete remission on the equivalent of about 17 cigarettes daily, compared to 24% of those using the placebo patches ($P = 0.03$). Along with symptomatic benefits there were significantly greater improvements in the rectal histology of those using the nicotine patches. In contrast, a randomized trial of transdermal nicotine as maintenance therapy carried out by the same group showed it to be ineffective (Thomas et al 1995).

Smoking and pouchitis

Several observations suggest that 'pouchitis' represents a recurrence of the colitis process in the neorectum. It is of interest, therefore, that smokers appear to be less likely to develop pouchitis or have recurrent pouchitis than non-smokers (Merrett et al 1996).

Crohn's disease

Strength, consistency and dose response

The relationship between smoking and Crohn's disease is almost the exact opposite to that for ulcerative colitis. Overall, the risk of a smoker developing Crohn's disease has been about twice that of a never-smoker, with the two meta-analyses estimating relative risks of 2.4 (95% confidence limit 2.0–2.9) and 2.0 (1.7–2.5) (Calkins 1989, Logan 1990). In contrast to ulcerative colitis, the risk estimates between studies have varied no more than would be expected by chance, and the risk for women has been consistently higher than that for men (Table 6.1). Although some have found smoking to be particularly associated with small-bowel disease, no consistent pattern has emerged.

Light smokers seem to have a risk similar to that for heavier smokers (Tobin et al 1987, Lindberg et al 1988). However, it is possible that in the case control studies recall bias is concealing a dose–response effect, as in the cohort studies heavy smokers had a slightly higher risk of Crohn's disease than light smokers (Vessey et al 1986, Logan & Kay 1989).

Risk in ex-smokers

As shown in Table 6.1, ex-smokers have lower risk of Crohn's disease than smokers, the relative risk estimates from meta-analyses being 1.5 and 1.8. How quickly the risk in ex-smokers falls after stopping is not yet known.

Effect of smoking on prognosis

Several studies have examined the effect of smoking on the course of Crohn's disease, and have invariably found that continued smoking has a powerful adverse effect. Holdstock et al (1984) found that, compared to non-smokers, smokers suffered more relapses, greater diarrhea and needed more hospital admissions. Similarly, in the US Crohn's disease patients in a health maintenance organization who smoked reported an average of 15 days

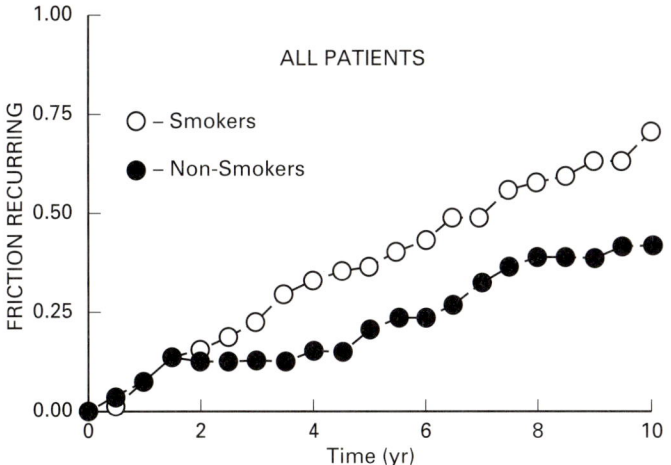

Fig. 6.1 Effect of smoking on prognosis of Crohn's disease: 5- and 10-year cumulative recurrence rate for smokers (36%, 70%) compared with non-smokers (29%, 41%) ($P = 0.0007$). (Reproduced with permission from Sutherland et al 1990)

a month of symptoms compared to 5 days for non-smokers (Kurata et al 1992). Although these studies could not separate cause and effect, Duffy et al (1990) examined relapse rate prospectively and found a 60% increase for smokers. Several groups have assessed smoking habits retrospectively and shown that those smoking at the time of bowel resection or strictureplasty have a twofold increase in risk of needing a second operation (Fig. 6.1, Table 6.2).

Passive smoking and the development of inflammatory bowel disease

Two case control studies have found a higher risk of Crohn's disease in those exposed to passive smoking during childhood. Lashner et al (1993) found that in children with inflammatory bowel disease who did not smoke, the parents were more likely to be smokers than their nominated controls with a fivefold relative risk. There was also an increased but smaller risk for children with ulcerative colitis. In contrast, Persson et al (1990) studied adults and found only a small increased (1.5×) risk of Crohn's disease and no increased risk of ulcerative colitis, whereas Sandler et al (1991) found that passive smoke exposure in childhood was associated with a halving in risk of ulcerative colitis in adults.

Confounding

At present there is no evidence that confounding – the association of smoking with other risk factors – has a significant role. Compared to non-smokers, smokers tend to drink more alcohol, but in two studies of smoking and ulcerative colitis that also assessed alcohol intake the relationship between smoking and colitis was unaffected (Boyko et al 1989, Nakamura & Labarthe 1994).

As a group smokers also consume more refined sugar (sucrose) than non-smokers, often more than twice as much more for heavy smokers (Margetts & Jackson 1993). A high level of refined sugar consumption has also been the only dietary factor consistently associated with Crohn's disease (see Chapter 5). Despite this coincidence, smoking and refined sugar intake appear to be separate risk factors, although they may interact (Thornton et al 1985, Katschinski et al 1988). Similarly, the relationship between ulcerative colitis and smoking is unaffected by adjusting for differences in sugar intake (Katschinski et al 1993b).

Possible mechanisms for the effects of smoking

Taken as a whole, the epidemiological evidence indicates that smoking actively protects against ulcerative colitis, and at the same time promotes the development of Crohn's disease. How smoking has these contrasting effects remains unclear, but several mechanisms have been proposed (Table 6.3). In an ideal world a single mechanism would account for smoking's effect in both diseases, and also for the increased risk of ulcerative colitis in ex-smokers. None of the mechanisms postulated satisfies this criterion.

An alternative possibility is that smoking influences different mechanisms operating in each disease. Thus

Table 6.2 Effect of continued smoking on reoperation rates in Crohn's disease

Centre (study)	n	Patients needing a second operation			
		Time since first operation (years)	Non-smokers (%)	Smokers (%)	Relative risk*
Calgary, Canada (Sutherland et al 1990)	174	5	21	36	2.1
Palermo, Italy (Cottone et al 1994)	182	6	8	24	2.0
Orebro, Sweden (Lindberg et al 1992)	231	10	26	42	1.8

* For heaviest category of smoking

Table 6.3 Some mechanisms by which smoking might promote or protect from inflammatory bowel disease

Immunological
Smokers have reduced IgG, TgH and IgA levels and a reduced ratio of helper to suppressor T cells (Miller et al 1982)

Vascular
Smoking increases procoagulant activity and promotes microvascular thrombosis (Wakefield et al 1991); smoking reduces rectal blood flow (Srivastava et al 1990)

Colonic mucus effects
Smokers with ulcerative colitis have 'normal' colonic mucus compared to non-smokers with colitis (Cope et al 1986) but no abnormality of mucus has been found in Crohn's disease

Intestinal permeability
Permeability reduced in smokers and protects from ulcerative colitis (Prytz et al 1989), but permeability is usually increased in Crohn's disease

Eicosanoid production
Nicotine reduces eicosanoid levels in rectal mucus in animals (Zijlstra et al 1994)

smoking might operate through an adverse vascular effect in Crohn's disease, while affording protection in ulcerative colitis via its effect on colonic mucus. If this were to apply, then the mechanisms affected by smoking would have to be specific to each disease. At present none of the mechanisms postulated has been shown to be specific to Crohn's disease or to ulcerative colitis. The evidence from the trials of nicotine patches or chewing gum suggests that nicotine maybe the mediator in ulcerative colitis. Conceivably, if a vascular mechanism is operating nicotine may also account for the effects of smoking in Crohn's disease.

Conclusion

In the observational studies of smoking and Crohn's disease the recurrence rates for non-smokers were approximately half those of smokers. Assuming that this difference is a consequence of not smoking, then the effect is as large as that obtained in trials of maintenance drug therapy. Therefore physicians should make strenuous efforts to encourage Crohn's disease patients who smoke to stop. Conversely, it may be justifiable to recommend nicotine patches (or even restarting smoking) for patients with severe and intractable ulcerative colitis.

ORAL CONTRACEPTION

The suggestion that the development of inflammatory bowel disease might be related to oral contraception arose from case reports of women developing colitis shortly after starting oral contraceptives and improving after stopping (Kilpatrick et al 1968, Bonfils et al 1977, Heron et al 1981, Tedesco et al 1982). The colitis was frequently atypical, with rectal sparing, segmental inflammation and discrete ulceration suggestive of Crohn's disease, but without granulomas. These reports are difficult to assess, particularly since the use of oral contraceptives is greatest at an age when the incidence of inflammatory bowel disease is also at its highest. Subsequently a range of formal studies have been published including seven case control studies and two cohort studies. The case control studies have generally relied on self-reporting of the timing and duration of pill use, which may be susceptible to bias although less so than for smoking. In contrast, in the cohort studies data on oral contraceptive use were collected on a prospective and continuous basis from the subjects' medical records.

Both case control and cohort studies (Table 6.4) have generally found about a 50% increase in risk of inflammatory bowel disease for current pill users compared to women who have never used the contraceptive pill. The increased risk has been slightly greater for Crohn's disease than for ulcerative colitis, with pill users having a relative risk of Crohn's disease of 1.6 (1.2–2.1) and of ulcerative colitis of 1.4 (1.0–1.9) in a recent meta-analysis (Godet et

Table 6.4 Relative risk of Crohn's disease and ulcerative colitis in oral contraceptive users (never-users RR = 1.0)

Study	Country	Crohn's disease		Ulcerative colitis	
		RR current vs never	(95% cl)	RR current vs never	(95% cl)
Case control studies					
Lesko et al 1985	US	1.7	(1.0–3.2)	–	
Lashner et al* 1989, 1990	US	0.7	(0.3–1.6)	0.7	(0.3–1.8)
Sandler et al* 1992	US	1.3	(0.8–2.0)	1.1	(0.6–1.8)
Persson et al 1993	Sweden	1.9	(0.9–3.9)	1.7	(0.8–3.3)
Katschinski et al 1993a	Germany	2.5	(1.6–6.6)	–	
Boyko et al† 1994	US	2.6	(1.2–5.5)	2.0	(1.2–3.3)
Cohort studies					
Vessey et al 1986	UK	1.5	(0.6–3.8)	2.1	(1.0–4.2)
Logan and Kay 1989	UK	1.5	(0.8–3.1)	1.4	(0.9–2.4)

* Cases asked to nominate friends or neighbors as controls
† Unadjusted for smoking but adjusted risks similar

Table 6.5 Relative risk of Crohn's disease by duration of oral contraception

Study	Country	Never (reference level)	<1 yr	1–5/6 yrs*	>5/6 yrs*
Lesko et al 1985	US	1.0	2.6	4.0	8.0
Boyko et al 1994	US	1.0	1.2	1.7	7.2
				<2/3 yrs†	>2/3 yrs†
Vessey et al 1986	UK	1.0		0.7	2.3
Katschinski et al 1983b	UK	1.0		2.5	4.3

* Lesko et al = 5 yrs, Boyko et al = 6 yrs
† Vessey et al = 2 yrs, Katschinski et al = 3 yrs

al 1995). The significance of this difference is unclear, as oral contraceptive use and smoking are well known to be associated (i.e. women tend to do both), and small differences existing after adjustment for smoking may reflect incomplete statistical adjustment.

If these associations are causal, the risk might be expected to increase with duration of oral contraception. As shown in Table 6.5, the increase in risk of Crohn's disease has been found to be greatest in the women who took the pill for longest. In contrast, in the two studies with data there was no further increase in the risk of ulcerative colitis with long-term use (Vessey et al 1986, Boyko et al 1994). Lesko et al (1985) found that any increased risk seemed to disappear when oral contraceptives were stopped, but no relationship between either disease and former oral contraceptive use was evident in the cohort studies, where the data were most reliable. Demonstration that oral contraception is associated with a particular form of inflammatory bowel disease would support a causal relationship. No data are available for ulcerative colitis, and the evidence for Crohn's disease is conflicting. In an uncontrolled study Rhodes et al (1984) found an association with Crohn's disease that was predominantly accounted for by women with disease confined to the colon, and in Stockholm oral contraception was associated with colonic but not ileal disease (Persson et al 1993). However, in a German study the association was slightly stronger for small-bowel rather than colonic disease (Katschinski et al 1993a).

Although the early reports emphasized that oral contraceptive-associated colitis improved after stopping the pill, the only formal study found that oral contraceptive use had no significant effect on the prognosis of Crohn's disease in terms of need for further surgery (Sutherland et al 1992).

Conclusion

Oral contraception is clearly associated with a small increase in risk of both Crohn's disease and ulcerative colitis. At present it is unclear whether these are directly causal relationships or due to confounding by some factor not yet identified.

An adverse vascular effect, based on analogy with the pill's effects elsewhere, is the mechanism that is most frequently postulated. Wakefield et al (1991) have suggested that Crohn's disease is the result of a chronic mesenteric vasculitis and that oral contraceptives promote a process of multifocal gastrointestinal infarction. Other effects of oral contraceptives have received little consideration; it is notable that use of the oral contraceptive protects against the development of rheumatoid arthritis. There is no evidence that stopping oral contraceptives influences prognosis, although assessment of an effect is clearly difficult. There is therefore no good evidence to suggest that oral contraception should be stopped or avoided by women with either Crohn's disease or ulcerative colitis.

REFERENCES

Benoni C, Nilsson A 1984 Smoking habits in patients with inflammatory bowel disease. Scandinavian Journal of Gastroenterology 19: 824–830

Benoni C, Nilsson A 1987 Smoking habits in patients with inflammatory bowel disease. A case-control study. Scandinavian Journal of Gastroenterology 22: 1130–1136

Bonfils S, Hervior P, Giroder J, Le Quintrec Y, Boucher J P, Gastard J 1977 Acute spontaneously, recovering ulcerative colitis. Digestive Diseases 22: 429–436

Boyko E J, Koepsell T D, Perera D R, Inui T S 1987 Risk of ulcerative colitis among former and current cigarette smokers. New England Journal of Medicine 316: 707–710

Boyko E J, Perero D R, Koepsell T E et al 1989 Coffee and alcohol use and the risk of ulcerative colitis. American Journal of Gastroenterology 84: 530–534

Boyko E J, Theis M K, Vaughan T L, Nicol-Blades B 1994 Increased risk of inflammatory bowel disease associated with oral contraceptive use. Americal Journal of Epidemiology 140: 268–278

Calkins B M 1989 A meta-analysis of the role of smoking in inflammatory bowel disease. Digestive Diseases and Sciences 34: 1841–1854

Cope G F, Heatley R V, Kelleher J 1986 Smoking and colonic mucus in ulcerative colitis. British Medical Journal 293: 481

Cottone M, Rosselli M, Orlando A et al 1994 Smoking habits and recurrence in Crohn's disease. Gastroenterology 106: 643–648

De Castella H 1982 Non-smoking: a feature of ulcerative colitis. (Letter) British Medical Journal 284: 1706

Duffy L C, Zielezny M A, Marshall J R et al 1990 Cigarette smoking and risk of clinical relapse in patients with Crohn's disease. American Journal of Preventive Medicine 6: 161–166

Franceschi S, Panza E, La Vecchia C, Parazzine P, Decarli A, Bianchi Poro G 1987 Non-specific inflammatory bowel disease and smoking.

American Journal of Epidemiology 125: 445–452

Godet P G, May G R, Sutherland L R 1995 A meta-analysis of the role of oral contraceptive agents on inflammatory bowel disease. Gut 1995; 37: 668–673

Harries A D, Baird A, Rhodes J 1982 Non-smoking: a feature of ulcerative colitis. British Medical Journal 284: 706

Heron H C, Khubchandani I T, Trimpi H D, Sheets J A, Stasik J J 1981 Evanescent colitis. Diseases of the Colon and Rectum 24: 555–561

Holdstock G, Savage D, Harman M, Wright R 1984 Should patients with inflammatory bowel disease smoke? British Medical Journal 288: 362

Jick H, Walker A M 1983 Anecdotal accounts of effect of smoking on ulcerative colitis. New England Journal of Medicine 308: 1277–1278

Katschinski B, Logan R F A, Edmond M, Langman M J S 1988 Smoking and sugar intake are separate but interactive risk factors in Crohn's disease. Gut 29: 1202–1206

Katschinski B, Logan R F A, Langman M J S 1989 Rauchen und entzündliche Darmerkrankungen. Zeitschrift fur Gastroenterologie 27: 614–618

Katschinski B, Fingerle D, Scherbaum B, Goebell H 1993a Oral contraceptive use and cigarette smoking in Crohn's disease. Digestive Diseases and Sciences 38: 1596–1600

Katschinski B D, Fisel W, Scjmialek J-P, Bracht J, Goebell H 1993b Smoking and sugar intake in ulcerative colitis: a case-control study. European Journal of Gastroenterology & Hepatology 5: 91–95

Kilpatrick Z M, Silverman J F, Betancourt E, Farman J, Lawson J P 1968 Vascular occlusion of the colon and oral contraceptives. New England Journal of Medicine 278: 438–440

Kurata J H, Kantor-Fish S, Frankl H, Godby P, Vadheim C M 1992 Crohn's disease among ethnic groups in a large health maintenance organization. Gastroenterology 102: 1940–1948

Lashner B A, Kane S V, Hanauer S B 1989 Lack of association between oral contraceptive use and Crohn's disease: a community-based matched case-control study. Gastroenterology 97: 1442–1447

Lashner B A, Kane S V, Hanauer S B 1990 Lack of association between oral contraceptive use and ulcerative colitis. Gastroenterology 99: 1032–1036

Lashner B A, Shaheen N J, Hanauer S B, Kirschner B S 1993 Passive smoking is associated with an increased risk of developing inflammatory bowel disease in children. American Journal of Gastroenterology 88: 356–359

Lesko S M, Kaufman D W, Rosenberg L et al 1985 Evidence for an increased risk of Crohn's disease in oral contraceptive users. Gastroenterology 89: 1046–1049

Lindberg E, Järnerot G, Huitfeldt B 1992 Smoking in Crohn's disease: effect on localisation and clinical course. Gut 33: 779–782

Lindberg E, Tysk C, Andersson K, Järnerot G 1988 Smoking and inflammatory bowel disease. A case control study. Gut 29: 352–357

Logan R F A 1990 Smoking and inflammatory bowel disease. In: Wald N, Baron J (eds) Smoking and hormone-related disorders. Oxford University Press, Oxford, pp 122–134

Logan R F A, Kay C R 1989 Oral contraception, smoking and inflammatory bowel disease. Findings in the Royal College of General Practitioners Oral Contraception Study 18: 105–107

Logan R F A, Katschinski B, Somerville K W, Pearson J C G: 1986 Smoking and inflammatory bowel disease. Gastroenterology 90: 1525

Margetts B M, Jackson A A 1993 Interactions between people's diet and their smoking habits: the dietary and nutritional survey of British adults. British Medical Journal 307: 1381–1384

Merrett M N, Mortensen N, Jewell D P 1996 Smoking may prevent pouchitis in patients with restorative proctocolectomy for ulcerative colitis. Gut 1996; 38: 362–364

Miller L G, Goldstein G, Murphy M, Ginns L C 1982 Reversible alterations in immunoregulatory T cells in smoking. Chest 5: 527–529

Motley R J, Rhodes J, Ford G A et al 1987 Time relationships between cessation of smoking and onset of ulcerative colitis. Digestion 37: 125–127

Nakamura Y, Labarthe D R 1994 A case-control study of ulcerative colitis with relation to smoking habits and alcohol consumption in Japan. American Journal of Epidemiology 140: 902–911

Persson P G, Ahlbom A, Hellers G 1990 Inflammatory bowel disease and tobacco smoke – a case-control study. Gut 31: 1377–1381

Persson P G, Leijonmarck C E, Bernell O, Hellers G, Ahlbom A 1993 Risk indicators for inflammatory bowel disease. International Journal of Epidemiology 22: 268–272

Prytz H, Benoni C, Tagesson C 1989 Does smoking tighten the gut? Scandinavian Journal of Gastroenterology 24: 1084–1088

Pullan R D, Rhodes J, Ganesh S et al 1994 Transdermal nicotine for active ulcerative colitis. New England Journal of Medicine 330: 811–815

Rhodes J M, Cockel R, Allan R N, Hawker P C, Dawson J, Elias E 1984 Colonic Crohn's disease and use of oral contraception. British Medical Journal 288: 595–596

Roberts C J, Diggle R 1982 Non-smoking: a feature of ulcerative colitis. (Letter) British Medical Journal 285: 440

Rudra T, Motley R, Rhodes J 1989 Does smoking improve colitis? Scandinavian Journal of Gastroenterology 24: 61–63

Samuelsson S M 1976 Ulcerative colitis in the county of Uppsala 1945–1964. MD Thesis, Uppsala

Samuelsson S M, Ekbom A, Zack M, Helmick C G, Adami H-O 1991 Risk factors for extensive ulcerative colitis and ulcerative proctitis: a population-based case-control study. Gut 32: 1526–1530

Sandler R S, Holland 1988 Smoking and inflammatory bowel disease. Gastroenterology 94: A398

Sandler R S, Wurzelmann J I, Lyles C M 1992 Oral contraceptive use and the risk of inflammatory bowel disease. Epidemiology 3: 374–378

Sandler R S, Sandler D P, McDonnell C W, Wurzelmann J I 1991 Childhood exposure to environmental tobacco smoke and the risk of ulcerative colitis. Americal Journal of Epidemiology 135: 603–608

Somerville K W, Logan R F A, Edmond M, Langman M J S 1984 Smoking and Crohn's disease. British Medical Journal 289: 954–956

Srivastava E D, Russell M A, Feyerbend C, Rhodes J 1990 Effect of ulcerative colitis and smoking on rectal blood flow. Gut 31: 1021–1024

Sutherland L R, Ramcharan S, Bryant H, Fick G 1990 Effect of cigarette smoking on recurrence of Crohn's disease. Gastroenterology 98: 1123–1128

Sutherland L R, Ramcharan S, Bryant H, Fick G 1992 Effect of contraceptive use on reoperation following surgery for Crohn's disease. Digestive Diseases and Sciences 37: 1377–1382

Tedesco F J, Valpolicelli N A, Moore F S 1982 Oestrogen and progesterone associated colitis: a disorder with clinical and endoscopic features mimicking Crohn's disease. Gastrointestinal Endoscopy 26: 247–249

Thomas G A O, Rhodes J, Mani V et al 1995 Transdermal nicotine as maintenance therapy for ulcerative colitis. New England Journal of Medicine 332: 988–992

Thornton J R, Emmett P M, Heaton K W 1985 Smoking, sugar, and inflammatory bowel disease. British Medical Journal 290: 1786–1787

Tobin M V, Logan R F A, Langman M J, McConnell R B, Gilmore I T 1987 Cigarette smoking and inflammatory bowel disease. Gastroenterology 93: 316–321

Vessey M, Jewell D, Smith A, Yeates D, McPherson K 1986 Chronic inflammatory bowel disease, cigarette smoking, and use of oral contraceptives: findings in a large cohort study of women of childbearing age. British Medical Journal 295: 1101–1103

Wakefield A J, Sawyerr A M, Hudson M, Dhillon A P, Pounder R E 1991 Smoking, the oral contraceptive pill, and Crohn's disease. Digestive Diseases and Sciences 36: 1147–1150

Zijlstra F J, Srivastava E D, Rhodes M et al 1994 Effect of nicotine on rectal mucus and mucosal eicosanoids. Gut 35: 247–251

7. Lymphocytes in inflammatory bowel disease

M. J. Zimmerman   D. P. Jewell

Lymphocytes are a key component of the cellular immune system, and play a major role in amplifying and maintaining the chronic mucosal inflammation seen in inflammatory bowel disease (IBD). In investigating the role of lymphocytes in IBD it is useful to consider the immune system as having separate compartments: systemic – represented by peripheral blood lymphocytes – and gastrointestinal mucosa – lamina propria lymphocytes and intraepithelial lymphocytes. This chapter considers data pertaining to IBD and the phenotypes and functional properties of these separate groups of lymphocytes.

PERIPHERAL BLOOD LYMPHOCYTES

The total numbers of peripheral blood lymphocytes have been found to be within normal limits when patients with IBD are compared with normal controls (Strickland et al 1974, Thayer et al 1976, Auer et al 1979, Richens et al 1980, Victorino & Hodgson 1980, Pepys et al 1982, Davidsen & Kristensen 1987), although some studies have found mild lymphopenia in patients with Crohn's disease (Auer et al 1979, Yuan et al 1983). Peripheral blood B-lymphocyte numbers, and the relative proportions expressing different immunoglobulins, are unchanged in IBD (Strickland et al 1974, Thayer et al 1976, Auer et al 1979). For T lymphocytes, the ratio of CD4 (helper) cells to CD8 (suppressor/cytotoxic) cells is similar to that of normal controls (Selby & Jewell 1983, Learmonth et al 1984, Sieber et al 1984, James et al 1986, Davidsen & Kristensen 1987, Senju et al 1991a), although increased peripheral blood CD4/CD8 ratio has been reported in acute ulcerative colitis (Aiso et al 1982, Godin et al 1984). The mild peripheral lymphopenia noted in some patients is due to reduced T-lymphocyte numbers and has a number of causes, including sequestration of cells within inflamed mucosa, increased cell loss into the gut lumen, and reduced lymphocyte production. Studies of patients with Crohn's disease have shown peripheral blood lymphopenia to be associated with both disease activity and disease chronicity (Auer et al 1979, Yuan et al 1983). Lymphopenia has not been found in patients with recent-onset Crohn's disease (Auer et al 1979), again suggesting that it is associated with disease chronicity rather than acute disease activity.

Although there are no major differences between IBD patients and controls in terms of total lymphocyte numbers, there is evidence that functional differences are present. Peripheral blood lymphocytes in patients with IBD show an increased frequency of cell surface markers, indicating T- and B-cell activation (Raedler et al 1985a, b, Pallone et al 1987). These markers include HLA-DR, interleukin-2 receptor, 4F2 antigen and the transferrin receptor (T9 antigen). Increased expression of peripheral blood lymphocyte surface activation markers is also seen in patients with autoimmune disorders, but not in bacterial or viral colitis (Raedler et al 1985b). In contrast to autoimmune disorders, peripheral blood lymphocytes from patients with IBD also express Fc receptor for IgA, which maybe a more specific lymphocyte activation marker in IBD (Raedler et al 1985b). Other evidence suggesting the increased activation of a subset of peripheral blood lymphocytes in IBD is increased peripheral blood lymphocyte production of soluble interleukin-2 receptor (Crabtree et al 1990, Mahida et al 1990, Mueller et al 1990).

MUCOSAL LYMPHOCYTES

The lamina propria is the major compartment of the mucosal immune system, and contains numerous cell types (Brandtzaeg et al 1989, Beagley & Elson 1992). B lymphocytes constitute 15–40%, with a predominance of IgA-producing cells. T lymphocytes constitute 40–90% and are predominantly CD4+, with a CD4/CD8 ratio similar to peripheral blood. Mucosal lymphocytes differ from peripheral blood lymphocytes in that mucosal lymphocyte surface markers indicate a greater degree of activation and exposure to antigen than peripheral blood lymphocytes (Pallone et al 1987, Allison et al 1990, MacDonald et al 1990, Schreiber et al 1991, Senju et al 1991a). In contrast to peripheral blood cells, the majority of mucosal T cells have the phenotype of memory cells (CD45RO+) rather than naive cells (CD45RA+) (Janossy et al 1989, James 1991). Other cell types within the lamina propria include macrophages (10%), mast cells, granulocytes including eosinophils, and mononuclear cells without T- or B-cell markers but with cytotoxic potential (lymphokine-activated killer (LAK) cells). Few NK (natural killer) cells are present within the intestinal mucosa.

In IBD the total number of lymphoid cells within the intestinal mucosa is increased two to fourfold. Both T- and B-lymphocyte numbers are increased. The ratio of T to B lymphocytes, and the T-cell CD4/CD8 ratio of lamina propria lymphocytes, is similar in both diseased and normal bowel, at approximately 6:1 and 2:1 respectively (Bookman & Bull 1979, Selby et al 1984, James et al 1986, Verspaget et al 1988, Senju et al 1991b). Analysis of immunoglobulin and T-cell receptor gene rearrangements has shown that the T- and B-cell expansion in IBD is polyclonal (Kaulfersch et al 1988, Chao et al 1988). As with peripheral blood lymphocytes, mucosal lymphocytes in IBD show increased expression of surface activation markers compared to mucosal lymphocytes from un-inflamed mucosa (Pallone et al 1987, Allison et al 1990, MacDonald et al 1990, Schreiber et al 1991). Further evidence of increased mucosal lymphocyte activation in IBD includes increased expression of immune activation genes (Matsuura et al 1993) and increased production of T-cell cytokines (Isaacs et al 1992).

Intestinal intraepithelial lymphocytes (IELs) are located at the basolateral aspect of adjacent epithelial cells, and lie on the basement membrane of the epithelial layer. The frequency of IELs in relation to epithelial cell numbers varies throughout the gastrointestinal tract, ranging from 1:6 in the ileum to 1:20 in the colon. Intestinal IELs are a heterogeneous population (Cerf-Bensussan & Guy-Grand 1991). The majority of IELs have the pan-T-cell marker CD3. In contrast to LPL (lamina propria lymphocyte) the majority (75–80%) of IELs are CD8+, and only 5–15% are CD8–. Up to 50% of CD8+ IELs lack CD5, a marker of mature T cells. There is also variation in the type of T-cell receptor (TCR) expressed by IELs. Most (75%) express the $\alpha\beta$ type of TCR. These IELs also express CD2, CD7 and the memory T-cell marker CD45RO. A small proportion (10%) of IELs express the $\gamma\delta$ TCR (Spencer et al 1989). The proportion of $\gamma\delta$ T cells within the intestinal epithelium is much higher than is seen in the lamina propria or peripheral blood. Intraepithelial $\gamma\delta$ T cells use different Vβ genes than do peripheral blood $\gamma\delta$ T cells, and may develop independently of the thymus. Studies of TCR gene rearrangements have shown that IELs are derived from a relatively small number of T-cell clones (Van Kerckhove et al 1992, Blumberg et al 1993). The functional significance of this oligoclonality is unclear. In contrast to the oligoclonality seen in $\alpha\beta$ IELs, there is a greater degree of molecular diversity of the antigen recognition sequences of $\gamma\delta$ IELs (De Libero et al 1993).

The role of $\alpha\beta$ and $\gamma\delta$ T cells in health or disease is uncertain. The heterogeneity of IEL TCR and surface markers probably reflects a diverse range of functional properties. IELs have a variety of effector functions, including cytotoxicity, modulation of epithelial cell function and proliferation, and immunoregulatory roles, including tolerance to dietary antigens and suppressor functions (Cerf-Bensussan & Guy-Grand 1991).

The numbers of IELs in the intact intestinal mucosa of patients with IBD have ben reported as being similar to those in uninflamed mucosa (Ferguson & Murray 1971, Ferguson et al 1975, Selby et al 1984, Hirata et al 1986), although increases have been reported in microscopic colitis (Lazenby et al 1989, Fasoli et al 1992) and in putative early lesions of Crohn's disease (Entrican et al 1987). Hoang et al (1992) examined the phenotypic characteristics of IELs and found no differences between controls and IBD patients. The numbers of $\gamma\delta$ IELs in IBD are no different from those in controls (Trejdosiewicz et al 1991). Although there are no major changes in the total numbers of IELs in IBD, recent evidence suggests that subtle phenotypic differences exist. Culverier et al (1992) found that the expansion of IELs and LPLs in Crohn's disease was due to increases in $\alpha\beta$ T cells, and that the numbers of $\gamma\delta$ T cells were not significantly different between Crohn's disease and controls. Fukushima et al (1991) found a reduced frequency of $\gamma\delta$ IELs in IBD compared to controls. The $\gamma\delta$+ LPLs were CD4+CD8+ in controls and Crohn's disease, but this phenotype was very uncommon in ulcerative colitis. The functional significance of these differences remains unclear.

Before considering the functional properties of isolated lymphocytes, it is important to bear in mind potential limitations imposed by the isolation process. Mucosal lymphocytes are most commonly isolated using enzymatic digestion, in combination with mechanical techniques such as centrifugation. These isolation techniques isolate lamina propria mononuclear cells, which contain a range of cell phenotypes and can include non-lymphocyte mononuclear cells such as macrophages. Although lymphocytes are predominant, the presence of other cell types contaminating the isolates can impart functional properties that may be falsely attributed to lymphocytes. Another limitation of the isolation process is that it may not equally collect the different subsets of lymphocytes. The isolation process may also result in the degradation of labile compounds, with major effects on cell function. Lymphocytes act in complex interrelated networks of different cell types and chemical messengers. Removing elements from these networks may introduce effects that may not be relevant in vivo. Methodological problems are thus likely to be a major source of variability when comparing the results of different studies of lymphocyte function in IBD.

B-LYMPHOCYTE FUNCTION

In IBD the increase in gastrointestinal B lymphocyte numbers is polyclonal, and is associated with an increased number of intestinal plasma cells within the mucosa and through the deeper layers of the bowel wall. The total numbers of intestinal mononuclear cells staining for IgA are increased twofold, whereas staining for IgG is increased 10–30-fold and IgM fivefold (Soltoft et al 1973, Skinner & Whitehead 1974, Baklien & Brandtzaeg 1975, Rosekrans et al 1980, Scott et al 1983, Keren et al 1984). The increase in IgG-staining cells in IBD is much greater than is seen in patients with acute infectious colitis (Van Spreeuwel et al 1985). The pattern of immunoglobulin production is different in IBD. In normal uninflamed intestine, intestinal mononuclear cells spontaneously secrete large amounts of immunoglobulin, predominantly IgA. In IBD there is decreased spontaneous secretion of IgA and upregulation of IgG secretion. Differences also occur in the proportions of immunoglobulin subclasses produced. In uninflamed intestine IgA2 is the predominant form of IgA; however, IgA1 is the most frequent form in IBD (MacDermott et al 1986a). In IBD there is a shift towards increased production of monomeric forms of IgA, and evidence of abnormal IgA production, such as decreased J-chain expression (Kett et al 1988). Differences in immunoglobulin subclasses are also seen in IgG subclasses. In ulcerative colitis intestinal mononuclear cells secrete predominantly IgG1 and IgG3, whereas IgG1 and IgG2 are more common in Crohn's disease (Scott et al 1986). Serum IgG subclasses show similar patterns (MacDermott et al 1988), and the abnormal IgG subclasses in ulcerative colitis persist when the disease is in remission (Ruthlein et al 1992). Twin studies suggest that the differences in IgG subclass production may be determined genetically (Hegeland et al 1992), particularly in ulcerative colitis. As different antigens raise antibody responses restricted to distinct immunoglobulin subclasses, the differences between ulcerative colitis and Crohn's disease may reflect different antigenic stimuli. The abnormalities of immunoglobulin production may also represent abnormal mucosal immune regulation. The pathophysiologic significance of these findings remains undetermined, and it is not clear whether the differences are primary or secondary.

CYTOTOXICITY

A number of different forms of cell-mediated cytotoxicity have been investigated in IBD, including spontaneous (SCMC), antibody-dependent (ADCC), mitogen-induced (MICC), monoclonal antibody-induced ('redirected cytotoxicity') and lymphokine-activated cytotoxicity (LAK). Interpretation of cytotoxicity studies in IBD is difficult owing to the widely varying methodologies. Different studies use a variety of assay systems, with different target cell lines of variable relevance to in-vivo cytotoxicity within the intestinal mucosa. A further limitation of many studies is that it is not clear which cell phenotypes are responsible for the observed cytotoxicity. A further complicating factor is that the phenotype of mucosal cells mediating cytotoxicity may differ from that seen in the peripheral blood (Shanahan et al 1987, Van Tol et al 1992). Cytokines modulate cytolytic function, and probably have a major role in the in-vivo regulation of cytolysis. The absence of cytokines in in-vitro cytotoxicity assay systems may explain the negative results of some studies.

No differences in mitogen-induced cytotoxicity have been found between IBD and controls, and the level of cytotoxicity shown by intestinal lymphocytes is less than that of peripheral lymphocytes (MacDermott et al 1980, Chiba et al 1981, Falchuk et al 1981). General findings have been that intestinal mononuclear cells from IBD and controls are poor mediators of SCMC and ADCC compared to peripheral blood lymphocytes (Fiocchi et al 1985, Bookman & Bull 1979, MacDermott et al 1980, 1981, 1986b). Compared to peripheral blood lymphocytes, mucosal lymphocytes show less induced cytotoxicity when incubated with lectins or interferon (MacDermott et al 1980, 1986b). The relative hyporesponsiveness of intestinal mononuclear cells to lectins or interferon probably reflects the greater degree of activation of intestinal mononuclear cells compared to peripheral blood lymphocytes. The overall cytotoxic capacity of killer (K) cells in the peripheral blood, as assessed by the ability to lyse antibody-coated target cells (ADCC), is normal in IBD (Britton et al 1978, Lyanga et al 1979, Chiba et al 1981, MacDermott et al 1986b). K-cell activity in the lamina propria is poor in both normal tissue and IBD (Bookman & Bull 1979, Chiba et al 1981, MacDermott et al 1986b), though one report suggests increased K-cell activity in mesenteric lymph nodes in Crohn's disease (Britton et al 1978).

Natural killer cells are uncommon in the peripheral blood and intestine of both normal subjects and patients with IBD (Fiocchi et al 1985, Gibson & Jewell 1986, Hirata et al 1986). NK activity, assessed by spontaneous cytotoxicity against certain tumor cell lines, is subnormal in the peripheral blood in IBD (MacDermott et al 1986b, Gibson & Jewell 1986, Manzano et al 1992), particularly in active Crohn's disease (Auer et al 1980, MacDermott et al 1986b, Egawa & Hiwatashi 1986). No difference between IBD and normals has been found in the cytotoxicity of lamina propria lymphocytes (Fiocchi et al 1985, Gibson & Jewell 1986, Macdermott et al 1986b, Gibson et al 1988). A more recent study has suggested subtle differences between Crohn's disease and ulcerative colitis in terms of intestinal mononuclear cell-mediated cytotoxicity. Van Tol et al (1992) showed that intestinal mononuclear cell SCMC was increased in Crohn's disease and reduced in ulcerative colitis. Overall, there is little to suggest a primary abnormality of K or NK function in the pathogenesis of IBD.

Lymphocytes with cytotoxicity against colonic epithelial cell lines have been identified in the peripheral blood of IBD patients (Perlmann & Broberger 1963, Watson et al 1966, Shorter et al 1969b, Stobo et al 1976). These findings suggest that lymphocyte-mediated cytotoxicity resulting in colonic epithelial cell injury may be important to the pathogenesis of IBD. Several lines of evidence argue against a major role for abnormal cytotoxicity in the pathogenesis of IBD. First, specific methodological problems such as a high degree of spontaneous epithelial cell lysis and difficulties in maintaining non-neoplastic colonic epithelial cell lines in culture, make the results of these studies difficult to interpret. Secondly, in contrast to peripheral blood, intestinal mononuclear cells from both inflamed and normal intestine have relatively poor cytotoxicity function in a variety of assay systems. Thirdly, few consistent differences have been shown in lymphocyte-mediated cytotoxicity between IBD patients and controls (Gibson et al 1988). Where such differences are apparent many studies show reduced cytotoxicity function in IBD (Auer & Ziemer 1980, Auer et al 1980, MacDermott et al 1981, 1986b). Fourthly, reduced cytotoxicity function is seen in patients with infectious diarrhea (Auer & Ziemer 1980, Auer et al 1980), suggesting that decreased cytotoxicity is not specific to IBD. Despite these arguments, the concept that lymphocyte-mediated cytotoxicity has a role in epithelial cell injury in IBD remains under investigation. Recently, major histocompatibility antigen-restricted T-cell cytotoxicity against autologous epithelial cells was demonstrated to occur in both Crohn's disease and ulcerative colitis (Okazaki et al 1993). This result is difficult to interpret, as there are no negative disease controls. Intestinal mononuclear cells with cytotoxic activity against cells bearing ileocolonic epithelial antigens have been also been demonstrated in IBD. However, these cells are not found in all patients and there appears to be no correlation between the distribution of disease and the relative response to large- and small-bowel antigens (Roche et al 1985). The general conclusion is that while lymphocyte-mediated cytotoxicity is either normal or non-specifically decreased in IBD, it is unlikely to play a primary role in pathogenesis.

Like lamina propria lymphocytes, intraepithelial lymphocytes have low cytolytic potential against conventional target cell lines. However, lamina propria mononuclear cells and IELs are cytotoxic towards other target cell lines, including epithelial tumour cells. IELs have few Fc receptors for IgG, and do not show ADCC. IEL cytolytic function also differs from peripheral blood lymphocytes in the mechanism of target cell lysis. There are also differences in cytolytic function between IELs and lamina propria mononuclear cells: the latter show both spontaneous and induced cell-mediated cytotoxicity (CMC), whereas IELs only show induced CMC (Ruthlein et al 1993). In inflamed mucosa IELs show reduced induced CMC compared to controls, whereas LPL induced CMC is no different. Furthermore, IELs from patients with IBD or diverticulitis show a similar decrease suggesting that it is non-specific (Ruthlein et al 1993). IELs from human colon, despite their suppressor–cytotoxic phenotype (CD8+), do not exhibit classic MHC class II restricted cytotoxicity (Hoang et al 1995). Further elucidation of the phenotype of IELs and LPLs with cytotoxic function is the focus of current research.

NON-SPECIFIC LYMPHOCYTE FUNCTION

The overall function of T lymphocytes in IBD has been studied by assessment of antigen non-specific responses (in particular, mitogen-induced proliferation in vitro) and of responses to antigens that are not involved in the disease process (delayed-type hypersensitivity (DTH) in vivo, and the mixed lymphocyte reaction (MLR)).

Studies of mitogen-induced in-vitro proliferation of peripheral blood lymphocytes have shown normal (Asquith et al 1973, Bolton et al 1974, Lyanga et al 1979, Fujita et al 1985) or depressed responses (Sachar et al 1973, Rubinstein et al 1978, Victorino & Hodgson 1980, Watanabe et al 1984). No relationship between proliferative response and disease activity has been found (Sachar et al 1973, Lyanga et al 1979, Victorino & Hodgson 1980). The proliferative responses of LPLs to specific antigens has also been assessed in a limited number of studies. In Crohn's disease lamina propria mononuclear cells had an increased proliferative response to *Escherichia coli* lipopolysaccharide and to *Staphylococcus aureus*, but no increased response to *Bacteroides* antigen, lipid A or enterobacterial common antigen (Fiocchi et al 1981). No specific proliferative responses to a variety of mycobacterial and microbial antigens were found in mucosal lymphocytes in IBD (Ibbotson et al 1992). These findings argue against a specific role for any of these antigens in stimulating the mucosal inflammation seen in IBD.

In recent years other mechanisms of lymphocyte activation have been elucidated. A new class of microbial antigens, termed superantigens, have been shown to stimulate activation of peripheral blood and mucosal lymphocytes (Aisenberg et al 1993). Superantigens do not require processing by an antigen-processing cell, and bind (a) to the external domain of class II major histocompatibility molecule rather than the antigen-binding groove, and (b) to a conserved region of the variable region of the β chain (Vβ) of the T-cell receptor rather than to the antigen-binding cleft. In genetically susceptible individuals superantigens stimulate T-cell activation, and have been implicated in the pathogenesis of several chronic inflammatory disorders (Drake & Kotzin 1992). The finding of an increase in Vβ 8+ T cells in mesenteric lymph nodes and peripheral blood in some patients with Crohn's disease suggests a possible role for superantigens in IBD (Posnett et al 1989). As superantigens potentially provide a mechanism by which host genetic factors interact with intestinal microbial flora, investigation of the role of superantigens in IBD will be an area of research in the future.

Impairment of delayed hypersensitivity reactions to a variety of antigens is a consistent finding in patients with IBD. The prevalence of cutaneous anergy is about 50% in ulcerative colitis, and up to 80% in Crohn's disease, compared to 10% in normal controls (Verrier-Jones et al 1969, Bird & Britton 1974, Meuwisen et al 1975, Meyers et al 1976, Sachar et al 1976). Anergy fails to correlate with disease activity (Verrier-Jones et al 1969, Bird & Britton 1974, Meyers et al 1976), although it often resolves after intestinal resection (Heimann et al 1983). As multiple factors affect cutaneous anergy in IBD, including malnutrition and immunosuppressive drug therapy (Forse et al 1981), it is unlikely to reflect an underlying primary defect in cellular immunity.

The proliferative response of peripheral blood lymphocytes in IBD to stimulation in the mixed lymphocyte reaction (MLR) is normal (Auer et al 1978, MacDermott et al 1984) or depressed (Richens et al 1974, Fiske & Falchuk 1980, Ginsberg & Falchuk 1982), and appears to be unrelated to disease activity.

IMMUNOREGULATORY FUNCTIONS

As no single antigen exposure explains the lymphocyte activation in IBD, it is likely that lymphocyte activation reflects abnormal immunoregulation. Particular interest has focused on the investigation of lymphocyte 'suppressor' function. A number of studies, using different assays of suppressor function, have produced confusing results. Although some studies show no difference between IBD patients and controls, the majority show reduced peripheral blood-mediated suppression in IBD (Dalton & Jewell 1992, Dalton et al 1992). LPL-mediated suppression has been found to be decreased in IBD relative to controls (Goodacre & Bienenstock 1982, Dalton et al 1992), no different (Fiocchi et al 1979, Elson et al 1985, James et al 1985, Dalton et al 1992), or increased (Fiocchi et al 1983). Intraepithelial lymphocytes function as suppressor cells (Hoang et al 1991). Normal colonic IELs can suppress the proliferation and spontaneous IgA synthesis of lamina propria and peripheral blood lymphocytes (Hoang et al 1991, Sachdev et al 1993). This function is mediated by CD8+ cells, is γ/δ-independent and is mediated by a soluble factor. IELs from patients with IBD show impaired ability to suppress antigen- and mitogen-induced proliferative responses of lamina propria and peripheral blood lymphocytes (Dalton et al 1993). The significance of suppressor function in IBD remains unclear. Some feel that there is no primary abnormality in suppressor function, and that the alterations observed are probably the result of the inflammatory process.

A recent suggestion has been that reduced suppression may result from abnormal epithelial/lymphocyte interactions (Mayer & Eisenhardt 1990). In-vitro studies have suggested that intestinal epithelial cells can act as antigen-presenting cells to mucosal lymphocytes. Intestinal epithelial cells can activate CD8+ suppressor cells. This is unusual, as CD8+ activation is usually an MHC class 1-related event, whereas intestinal epithelial cells express MHC class II, particularly in IBD. The precise molecular mechanisms by which intestinal epithelial cells activate CD8+ suppressor cells are being defined. Monoclonal antibodies to CD8 block intestinal epithelial cell-mediated CD8+ suppressor activation, whereas monoclonal antibodies to CD4+ and MHC classes I and II are not inhibitory. It is likely that a novel restriction element is involved in cognate intestinal epithelial cell/IEL interactions (Mayer 1994). Recent studies have shown that intestinal epithelial cell/lymphocyte interactions are abnormal in IBD.

In normal intestine, and in non-IBD inflammatory conditions such as diverticulitis, intestinal epithelial cells activate CD8+ suppressor cells. In patients with IBD intestinal epithelial cells activate CD4+ helper cells. Even intestinal epithelial cells from uninflamed areas of bowel activate CD4+ helper cells, suggesting that there is an inherent defect in intestinal epithelial cell/lymphocyte interactions in IBD (Mayer & Eisenhardt 1990, Mayer 1994). This defect may result in inappropriate CD4+ helper activation and failure of CD8+ suppressor mechanisms, and is consistent with other studies showing an increase in 'helper' activity in LPLs from IBD (Elson et al 1985, Kanof et al 1988), due mainly to an increase in CD4+ cells. The finding of abnormal intestinal epithelial cell/lymphocyte interactions as a cause of abnormal mucosal lymphocyte activation is potentially of major significance to the pathogenesis of IBD.

DRUG EFFECTS ON LYMPHOCYTE FUNCTIONS

Many drugs used in the treatment of IBD modulate lymphocyte function. Sulphasalazine inhibits lymphocyte proliferation (Balow et al 1975, Ali et al 1982) and NK activity (MacDermott et al 1986c). Glucocorticoids inhibit T-lymphocyte cytotoxicity (Stavy et al 1973) and inhibit lymphocyte proliferation and cytokine production (Parente & Mugridge 1993). Cyclosporin inhibits T-lymphocyte activation and proliferation (Brynskov 1991, Hodgson 1991), as does azathioprine (Campbell et al 1976). It is likely that these effects contribute to the therapeutic efficacy of these drugs.

CONCLUSION

Overall, there does not appear to be a global defect in lymphocyte function in IBD. Many of the abnormalities are probably secondary to the inflammatory process and reflect an appropriate response to increased antigenic stimulation in the presence of increased mucosal permeability. No one abnormality explains all the aspects of IBD, such as the different clinical phenotypes. Rather, the available evidence illuminates the role of lymphocytes in modulating the inflammatory response that occurs in IBD. There is little evidence to suggest a major role for any lymphocyte abnormality in the primary causation of IBD. The lack of this type of evidence is partially explained by the fact that it is not possible to prospectively identify patients who will develop IBD, and it is thus not possible to follow the serial time course of abnormalities of lymphocyte function. To an extent, the newer animal models of IBD, such as knockout mice (Conner et al 1994), are likely to provide valuable insights; however, one must be cautious in extrapolating the results of these studies to the human disease state. It is possible that the factors involved in the generation of IBD are different from those that sustain the prolonged inflammatory response. Although the 'holy grail' of research into the immunology of IBD is the elucidation of the immunopathogenesis, current research is defining mechanisms by which lymphocytes regulate the inflammatory response and thus provide novel targets for therapeutic intervention (Weldon & Maxwell 1994, Thomson & Forrester 1994).

REFERENCES

Aisenberg J, Ebert E C, Mayer L 1993 T-cell activation in human intestinal mucosa: the role of superantigens. Gastroenterology 105: 1421–1430

Aiso S, Watanabe S, Hibi T, Yoshida T, Tsuchiya M, Tsuru S 1982 Characterisation of immunoregulatory T cells and lymphocytophilic antibodies in ulcerative colitis: analysis with monoclonal antibodies. Journal of Clinical and Laboratory Immunology 9: 109–112

Ali A T M M, Bashan G S, Morley J 1982 Mode of action of sulphasalazine: an alternative view. Lancet 1: 506–507

Allison M C, Poulter L W, Dhillon A P, Pounder R E 1990 Immunohistological studies of surface antigen on colonic lymphoid cells in normal and inflamed mucosa. Gastroenterology 99: 421–430

Asquith P, Kraft S C, Rothberg R M 1973 Lymphocyte responses to non-specific mitogen in inflammatory bowel disease. Gastroenterology 65: 1–7

Auer I O, Ziemer E 1980 Immune status in Crohn's disease. IV In vitro antibody dependent cell mediated cytotoxicity in peripheral blood. Klin Wochensch 58: 779–787

Auer I O, Buschmann C H, Ziemer E 1978 Immune status in Crohn's disease. II Originally unimpaired primary cell mediated immunity in vitro. Gut 19: 618–626

Auer I O, Ziemer E, Sommer H 1980 Immune status in Crohn's disease. V Decreased in vitro natural killer cell activity in Crohn's disease. Clinical and Experimental Immunology 42: 41–49

Auer I O, Gotz S, Ziemer E, Malchow H, Ehms H 1979 Immune status in Crohn's disease. III Peripheral blood lymphocytes, enumerated by means of F(ab)2-antibody fragments, null and T lymphocytes. Gut 20: 261–268

Baklien K, Brandtzaeg P 1975 Comparative mapping of the local distribution of immunoglobulin-containing cells in ulcerative colitis and Crohn's disease of the colon. Clinical and Experimental Immunology 22: 197–209

Balow J E, Hurley D L, Fauci A S 1975 Immunosuppressive effects of glucocorticoids: differential effects of acute vs chronic administration on cell mediated immunity. Journal of Immunology 114: 1072–1076

Beagley K W, Elson C O 1992 Cells and cytokines in mucosal immunity and inflammation. Gastroenterology Clinics of North America 21: 347–366

Bird A G, Britton S 1974 No evidence of decreased lymphocyte reactivity in Crohn's disease. Gastroenterology 67: 926–932

Blumberg R S, Yockey C E, Gross C G, Ebert E C, Balk S P 1993 Human intestinal intraepithelial lymphocytes are derived from a limited number of T cell clones that utilise multiple V beta T cell receptor genes. Journal of Immunology 150: 5144–5153

Bolton P M, James S P, Newcombe R G, WHitehead R H, Hughes L E 1974 The immune competence of patients with inflammatory bowel disease. Gut 15: 213–219

Bookman M A, Bull D M 1979 Characteristics of isolated intestinal mucosal lymphoid cells in inflammatory bowel disease. Gastroenterology 77: 503–510

Brandtzaeg P, Halstensen T S, Kett K et al 1989 Immunobiology and immunopathology of human gut mucosa: humoral immunity and intraepithelial lymphocytes. Gastroenterology 97: 1562–1584

Britton S, Eklund A E, Bird A G 1978 Appearance of killer (K) cells in mesenteric lymph nodes in Crohn's disease. Gastroenterology 75: 218–220

Brynskov J 1991 The role of cyclosporin therapy in Crohn's disease. Digestive Diseases 9: 236–244

Campbell A C, Skinner J M, Hersey P, Waller C A 1976 Immunosuppression in the treatment of inflammatory bowel disease. II The effects of azathioprine on lymphoid cell populations in a double blind trial in ulcerative colitis. Clinical and Experimental Immunology 24: 249–258

Cerf-Bensussan N, Guy-Grand D 1991 Intestinal intraepithelial lymphocytes. Gastroenterology Clinics of North America 20: 549–576

Chao L P, Steele J, Rodrigues C et al 1988 Specificity of antibodies secreted by hybridomas generated from activated B cells in the mesenteric lymph nodes of patients with inflammatory bowel disease. Gut 29: 35–40

Chiba M, Bartnik W, ReMine S G, Thayer W R, Shorter R G 1981 Human colonic intraepithelial and lamina propria lymphocytes: cytotoxicity in vitro and the potential effects of the isolation method on their functional properties. Gut 22: 177–186

Conner E M, Aiko S, Grisham M 1994 Genetically engineered models of inflammatory bowel disease. Current Opinion in Gastroenterology 10: 358–364

Crabtree J E, Juby L D, Heatley R V, Lobo A J, Bullimore D W, Axon A T R 1990 Soluble interleukin-2 receptor in Crohn's disease: relation of serum concentrations to disease activity. Gut 31: 1033–1036

Culvelier C A, De Wever N, Mielants H, De Vos M, Veys E M, Roels H 1992 Expression of T cell receptors à and ë in the ileal mucosa of patients with Crohn's disease and with spondyloarthropathy. Clinical and Experimental Immunology 90: 275–279

Dalton H R, Jewell D P 1992 The immunology of inflammatory bowel disease. In: Jarnerot G, Lennard-Jones J, Truelove S C (eds) Inflammatory bowel disease. Corona Astra, Malmo, Sweden, pp 125–147

Dalton H R, Hoang P, Jewell D P 1992 Antigen induced suppression in peripheral blood and lamina propria mononuclear cells in inflammatory bowel disease. Gut 33: 324–330

Dalton H R, Dipaolo M C, Sachdev G K, Crotty B, Hoang P, Jewell D P 1993 Human colonic intraepithelial cells from patients with inflammatory bowel disease fail to downregulate proliferative responses of primed allogenic peripheral blood mononuclear cells after rechallenge with antigens. Clinical and Experimental Immunology 93: 97–102

Davidsen B, Kristensen E 1987 Lymphocyte subpopulations, lymphoblast transformation activity and concanavalin A induced suppressor activity in patients with ulcerative colitis and Crohn's disease. Scandanavian Journal of Gastroenterology 22: 785–790

De Libero G, Rocci M P, Casorati G et al 1993 T cell receptor heterogeneity in ë T cell clones from intestinal biopsies of patients with celiac disease. European Journal of Immunology 23: 499–504

Drake C G, Kotzin B L 1992 Superantigens: biology, immunology and potential role in disease. Journal of Clinical Immunology 12: 149–162

Egawa S, Hiwatashi N 1986 Natural killer cell activity in patients with inflammatory bowel disease. Journal of Clinical and Laboratory Immunology 20: 187–192

Elson C O, Machelski E, Weiserbs D B 1985 T cell–B cell regulation in the intestinal lamina propria in Crohn's disease. Gastroenterology 89: 321–327

Entrican J H, Busuttil A, Ferguson A 1987 Are the focal microscopic jejunal lesions in Crohn's disease produced by a T-cell mediated response? Scandanavian Journal of Gastroenterology 22: 1071–1075

Falchuk Z M, Barnhard E, Machado I 1981 Human colonic mononuclear cells: studies of cytotoxic function. Gut 22: 290–294

Fasoli R, Talbot I, Reid M, Prince C, Jewell D P 1992 Microscopic colitis: can it be qualitatively and quantitatively characterised? Italian Journal of Gastroenterology 24: 393–396

Ferguson A, Murray D 1971 Quantitation of intraepithelial lymphocytes in human jejunum. Gut 12: 988–994

Ferguson A, Allan R N, Cooke W T 1975 A study of the cellular infiltrate of the proximal jejunal mucosa in ulcerative colitis and Crohn's disease. Gut 16: 205–208

Fiocchi C, Battisto J R, Farmer R G 1981 Studies on gut mucosal lymphocytes in inflammatory bowel disease. Detection of activated T cells and enhanced proliferation to *Staphylococcus aureus* and lipopolysaccharides. Digestive Diseases and Sciences 26: 728–736

Fiocchi C, Battisto J R, Farmer R G 1979 Gut mucosal lymphocytes in inflammatory bowel disease: isolation and preliminary functional characterisation. Digestive Diseases and Sciences 24: 705–717

Fiocchi C, Youngman K R, Farmer R G 1983 Immuno-regulatory function of human intestinal mucosa lymphoid cells: evidence for enhanced suppressor cell activity in inflammatory bowel disease. Gut 24: 692–701

Fiocchi C, Tubbs R R, Youngman K R 1985 Human intestinal mucosal mononuclear cells exhibit lymphokine-activated killer cell activity. Gastroenterology 88: 625–637

Fiske S C, Falchuk Z M 1980 Impaired mixed lymphocyte culture reactions in patients with inflammatory bowel disease. Gastroenterology 79: 682–686

Forse R A, Christou N, Meakins L D, Maclean L D, Shizal H M 1981 Reliability of skin testing as a measure of nutritional state. Archives of Surgery 116: 1284–1288

Fujita K, Okabe N, Yao T 1985 Immunological studies on Crohn's disease. II Lack of evidence for humoral and cellular dysfunction. Journal of Clinical and Laboratory Immunology 16: 155–161

Fukushima K, Masuda T, Ohtani H et al 1991 Immunohistochemical characterisation, distribution and ultrastructure of lymphocytes bearing T cell receptor ë in inflammatory bowel disease. Gastroenterology 101: 670–678

Gibson P R, Jewell D P 1986 Local immune mechanisms in inflammatory bowel disease and colorectal cancer. Gastroenterology 90: 12–19

Gibson P R, Van De Pol E, Pullman W, Doe W F 1988 Lysis of colonic epithelial cells by allogenic mononuclear and lymphokine activated killer cells derived from peripheral blood and intestinal mucosa: evidence against a pathogenic role in inflammatory bowel disease. Gut 29: 1076–1084

Ginsberg C H, Falchuk Z M 1982 Defective autologous mixed lymphocyte reaction and suppressor cell generation in patients with inflammatory bowel disease. Gastroenterology 83: 1–9

Godin N J, Sachar D B, Winchester R, Simon C, Janowitz H D 1984 Loss of suppressor T cells in active inflammatory bowel disease. Gut 25: 743–747

Goodacre R L, Bienenstock J 1982 Reduced suppressed cell activity in intestinal lymphocytes from patients with Crohn's disease. Gastroenterology 82: 653–658

Hegeland L, Tysk C, Jarnerot G et al 1992 IgG subclass distribution in serum and rectal mucosa of monozygotic twins with and without inflammatory bowel disease. Gut 33: 1358–1364

Heimann T, Gelernt I, Schanzer H, Sacher D B, Greenstein A J, Aufses A H 1983 Surgical treatment, skin test reactivity, and lymphocytes in inflammatory bowel disease. American Journal of Surgery 145: 199–201

Hirata I, Berrebi G, Austin L L, Keren D F, Dobbins W O 1986 Immunohistochemical characterisation of intraepithelial and lamina propria lymphocytes in control ileum and colon and in inflammatory bowel disease. Digestive Diseases and Sciences 31: 593–603

Hoang P, Sibille C, Dehennin J P, Vaerman J P, Jewell D P 1995 Cytotoxic activity of human colonic intraepithelial and lamina propria lymphocytes. Gastroenterology 108: A835

Hoang P, Dalton H R, Jewell D P 1991 Human colonic intraepithelial lymphocytes are suppressor cells. Clinical and Experimental Immunology 85: 498–503

Hoang P, Senju M, Lowes J R, Jewell D P 1992 Phenotypic characterisation of isolated intraepithelial lymphocytes in patients with ulcerative colitis and normal controls. Digestive Diseases and Sciences 37: 1725–1728

Hodgson H J F 1991 Cyclosporin in inflammatory bowel disease. Alimentary Pharmacology and Therapeutics 5: 343–350

Ibbotson J P, Lowes J R, Chahal H et al 1992 Mucosal cell-mediated immunity to mycobacterial, enterobacterial and other microbial antigens in inflammatory bowel disease. Clinical and Experimental Immunology 87: 224–230

Isaacs K L, Sartor R B, Haalkill S 1992 Cytokine messenger RNA profiles in inflammatory bowel disease mucosa detected by polymerase chain reaction amplification. Gastroenterology 103: 1587–1595

James S P, Fiocchi C, Graeff A S, Strober W 1985 Immunoregulatory function of lamina propria T cells in Crohn's disease. Gastroenterology 88: 1043–1150

James S P, Fiocchi C, Graeff A S, Strober W 1986 Phenotypic analysis of lamina propria lymphocytes. Gastroenterology 91: 1483–1489

James S P 1991 Mucosal T cell function. Gastroenterology Clinics of North America 20: 597–612

Janossy G, Bofill M, Rowe D, Muir J, Beverley P C L 1989 The tissue distribution of T lymphocytes expressing different CD45 polypeptides. Immunology 66: 517–525

Kanof M E, Strober W, Fiocchi C, Zeitz M, James S P 1988 CD4 positive *leu*-8 negative helper–inducer T cells predominate in the human intestinal lamina propria. Journal of Immunology 141: 3029–3036

Kaulfersch W, Fiocchi C, Waldman T A 1988 Polyclonal nature of the intestinal mucosal lymphocyte population in inflammatory bowel disease. A molecular genetic evaluation of the immunoglobulin and T-cell antigen receptors. Gastroenterology 95: 364–370

Keren D F, Appelman H D, Dobbins W O et al 1984 Correlation of histopathologic evidence of disease activity with the presence of immunoglobulin containing cells in the colon of patients with inflammatory bowel disease. Human Pathology 15: 757–763

Kett K, Brandtzaeg P, Fausa O 1988 J-chain expression is more prominent in immunoglobulin A2 than in immunoglobulin A1 colonic immunocytes and is decreased in both subclasses associated with inflammatory bowel disease. Gastroenterology 94: 1419–1425

Lazenby A J, Yardley J H, Giardiello F M, Jessurun J, Bayless T M 1989 Lymphocytic ('microscopic') colitis: a comparative histopathologic study with particular reference to collagenous colitis. Human Pathology 20: 18–28

Learmonth R P, Phil E, Johnson W R, Barnett M A, McDermott F T, Hughes E R S 1984 Altered blood lymphocyte subclasses in patients with ulcerative colitis. Australia and New Zealand Journal of Surgery 54: 265–269

Lyanga J J, Davis P, Thomson A B R 1979 In vitro testing of immunoresponsiveness in patients with inflammatory bowel disease. Clinical and Experimental Immunology 37: 120–125

MacDermott R P, Bragdon M J, Thurmond R D 1984 Peripheral blood mononuclear cells from patients with inflammatory bowel disease exhibit normal function in the allogeneic and autologous mixed leukocyte reaction and cell-mediated lympholysis. Gastroenterology 86: 476–484

MacDermott R P 1981 Human intestinal mononuclear cells isolated from normal and inflammatory bowel disease specimens are a functionally unique lymphoid population. In: Pea A S, Waterman I T, Booth C C et al (eds) Recent advances in Crohn's disease. The Hague, Martinus Nijhoff, pp 439–444

MacDermott R P, Franklin G O, Jenkins K M et al 1980 Human intestinal mononuclear cells. I Investigation of antibody-dependent lectin-induced and spontaneous cell-mediated cytotoxic capabilities. Gastroenterology 78: 47–56

MacDermott R P, Nash G S, Bertovich M J et al 1986a Evidence for the migration of B cells secreting monomeric IgA and IgA subclass 1

(IgA1) from peripheral compartments into the intestine in inflammatory bowel disease. Gastroenterology 91: 379–385

MacDermott R P, Bragdon M J, Kodner I J, Bertovich K J 1986b Deficient cell-mediated cytotoxicity and hyporesponsiveness to interferon and mitogenic lectin activation by inflammatory bowel disease peripheral blood and intestinal mononuclear intestinal cells. Gastroenterology 90: 6–11

MacDermott R P, Kane M G, Steele L L, Stenson W F 1986c Inhibition of cytotoxicity by sulphasalazine. I Sulphasalazine inhibits spontaneous cell-mediated cytotoxicity by peripheral blood and intestinal mononuclear cells from control and inflammatory bowel disease patients. Immunopharmacology 11: 101–109

MacDermott R P, Nash G S, Auer I O et al 1988 Alterations in serum IgG subclasses in patients with ulcerative colitis and Crohn's disease. Gastroenterology 94: A275

MacDonald T T, Hutchings P, Choy M Y et al 1990 Activated T cells and macrophages in the intestinal mucosa of children with inflammatory bowel disease. In: MacDonald T T, Chalacombe S J, Bland P W et al (eds) Advances in mucosal immunology. Kluwer, Boston, pp 683–690

Mahida Y R, Gallagher A, Kurlak L, Hawkey C J 1990 Plasma and tissue interleukin-2 receptor levels in inflammatory bowel disease. Clinical and Experimental Immunology 82: 75–80

Manzano L, Alvarez-Mon M, Abreu L et al 1992 Functional impairment of natural killer cells in active ulcerative colitis: reversion of the defective natural killer activity by interleukin 2. Gut 33: 246–251

Matsuura T, West G A, Youngman K R, Klein J S, Fiocchi C 1993 Immune activation genes in inflammatory bowel disease. Gastroenterology 104: 448–458

Mayer L 1994 Lymphoepithelial interactions: activation of T-cells by epithelial cells. Mucosal Immunology Update 2. 1, 10–12

Mayer L, Eisenhardt D 1990 Lack of induction of suppressor T cells by intestinal epithelial cells from patients with inflammatory bowel disease. Journal of Clinical Investigation 86: 1255–1260

Meuwisen S G M, Schellekens P T A, Huismans L, Tygat G N 1975 Impaired anamnestic cellular response in patients with Crohn's disease. Gut 16: 854–860

Meyers S, Sachar D B, Taub R N, Janowitz H D 1976 Anergy to dinitrochlorobenzene and depression of T lymphocytes in Crohn's disease and ulcerative colitis. Gut 17: 911–915

Mueller C H, Knoflach P, Zielinski C C 1990 T cell activation in Crohn's disease. Intestinal levels of soluble interleukin-2 receptor in serum and in supernatants of stimulated peripheral blood mononuclear cells. Gastroenterology 98: 639–646

Okazaki K, Morita M, Nishimori I et al 1993 Major histocompatibility antigen restricted cytotoxicity in inflammatory bowel disease. Gastroenterology 104: 384–391

Pallone F, Fais S, Squarcia O, Biancone L, Pozzilli P, Boirivant M 1987 Activation of peripheral blood and intestinal lamina propria lymphocytes in Crohn's disease. Gut 28: 745–753

Parente L, Mugridge M 1993 Glucocorticoids and gastrointestinal inflammation. In: Wallace J L (ed) The handbook of immunopharmacy. Immunopharmacy of the gastrointestinal system. Academic Press, London, pp 169–184

Pepys E O, Fagan E A, Tennent G A, Chadwick V S, Pepys M B 1982 Enumeration of lymphocyte subpopulations defined by surface markers in the whole blood of patients with Crohn's disease. Gut 23: 766–769

Perlmann P, Broberger O 1963 In vitro studies of ulcerative colitis. II Cytotoxic action of white blood cells from patients on human fetal colon cells. Journal of Experimental Medicine 117: 717–733

Posnett D N, Schmelkin I, Burthon D A, August A, McGrath H, Mayer L 1989 T cell antigen receptor V region gene usage: increases in V 8+ T cells in Crohn's disease. Journal of Clinical Investigation 85: 1170–1176

Raedler A, Fraenkel S, Klose G, Seyfarth K, Thiele H G 1985a Involvement of the immune system in the pathogenesis of Crohn's disease: expression of the T9 antigen on peripheral immunocytes correlates with the severity of the disease. Gastroenterology 88: 978–983

Raedler A, Fraenkel S, Klose G, Thiele H G 1985b Increased numbers of peripheral T cells in inflammatory bowel diseases displaying T9 antigen and Fc receptors. Clinical and Experimental Immunology 60: 518–524

Richens E R, Thorpe C M, Field C E 1980 Peripheral blood lymphocytes and mesenteric lymph nodes in Crohn's disease. Gut 21: 507–11

Richens E R, Williams M J, Gough K R, Ancill R J 1974 Mixed lymphocyte reaction as a measure of immunological competence of lymphocytes from patients with Crohn's disease. Gut 15: 24–28

Roche J K, Fiocchi C, Youngman K 1985 Sensitization to epithelial antigens in chronic mucosal inflammatory disease. Characterisation of human intestinal mucosa-derived mononuclear cells reactive with purified epithelial cell-associated components in vitro. Journal of Clinical Investigation 75: 522–530

Rosekrans P C M, Meijer C J L M, Van der Wal A M, Cornelisse C J, Lindeman J 1980 Immunoglobulin containing cells in inflammatory bowel disease of the colon: a morphometric and immunohistochemical study. Gut 21: 941–947

Rubinstein A, Das K M, Melamed J, Murphy R A 1978 Comparative analysis of systemic immunological parameters in ulcerative colitis and idiopathic proctitis: effects of sulphasalazine in vivo and in vitro. Clinical and Experimental Immunology 33: 217–224

Ruthlein J, Heinze G, Auer I O 1993 Anti-CD2 and anti-CD3 induced T cell cytotoxicity of human intraepithelial and lamina propria lymphocytes. Gut 33: 1626–1632

Ruthlein J, Ibe M, Burghardt W, Mossner J, Auer I O 1992 Immunoglobulin G (IgG), IgG1, and IgG2 determinations from endoscopic biopsy specimens in control, Crohn's disease and ulcerative colitis subjects. Gut 33: 507–512

Sachar D B, Taub R N, Brown S M, Present D H, Koerlitz B I, Janowitz H D 1973 Impaired lymphocyte responsiveness in inflammatory bowel disease. Gastroenterology 64: 203–209

Sachar D B, Taub R N, Ramachandar K et al 1976 T and B lymphocytes and cutaneous anergy in inflammatory bowel disease. Annals of the New York Academy of Sciences 278: 565–573

Sachdev G K, Dalton H R, DiPaolo M C, Crotty B, Jewell D P 1993. Human intraepithelial lymphocytes suppress in vitro immunoglobulin synthesis by autologous peripheral blood lymphocytes and lamina propria lymphocytes. Gut 34: 257–263

Schreiber S, MacDermott R P, Raedler A, Pinnau R, Bertovich M J, Nash G S 1991 Increased activation of isolated lamina propria mononuclear cells in inflammatory bowel disease. Gastroenterology 101: 1026–1030

Scott B B, Goodall A, Stephenson P, Jenkins D 1983 Rectal mucosal plasma cells in inflammatory bowel disease. Gut 24: 519–524

Scott M G, Nahm M H, Macke K, Nash G S, Bertovich M J, MacDermott R P 1986 Spontaneous secretion of IgG subclasses by intestinal mononuclear cells: differences between ulcerative colitis, Crohn's disease and controls. Clinical and Experimental Immunology 66: 209–215

Selby W S, Jewell D P 1983 T Lymphocyte subsets in inflammatory bowel disease: peripheral blood. Gut 24: 99–105

Selby W S, Janossy G, Bofill M, Jewell D P 1984 Intestinal lymphocyte subpopulations in inflammatory bowel disease: an analysis by immunohistochemical and cell isolation techniques. Gut 25: 32–40

Senju M, Hulstaert F, Lowder J, Jewell D P 1991a Flow cytometric analysis of peripheral blood lymphocytes in ulcerative colitis and Crohn's disease. Gut 1991a 32: 779–783

Senju M, Wu K C, Mahida Y A, Jewell D P 1991b Two-color immunofluorescence and flow cytometric analysis of lamina propria lymphocyte subsets in ulcerative colitis and Crohn's disease. Digestive Diseases and Sciences 36: 1453–1458

Shanahan F, Brogan M, Targan S 1987 Human mucosal cytotoxic effector cells. Gastroenterology 92: 1951–1957

Shorter R G, Cardoza M, Huizenga K A, ReMine S G, Spencer R J 1969a Further studies of in vitro cytotoxicity of lymphocytes for colonic epithelial cells. Gastroenterology 57: 30–35

Shorter R G, Cardoza M, Spencer R J, Huizenga K A 1969b Further studies of in vitro cytotoxicity of lymphocytes from patients with ulcerative colitis and granulomatous colitis for allogenic colonic epithelial cells. Gastroenterology 56: 304–309

Sieber G, Herrmann F, Zeitz M, Teichmann H, Ruhl H 1984 Abnormalities of B cell activation and immunoregulation in Crohn's disease. Gut 25: 1255–1261

Skinner J M, Whitehead R 1974 The plasma cells in inflammatory disease of the colon: a quantitative study. Journal of Clinical Pathology 27: 643–646

Soltoft J, Binder V, Gudmand-Hoyer E 1973 Intestinal immunoglobulins in ulcerative colitis. Scandanavian Journal of Gastroenterology 8: 293–300

Spencer J, Isaacson P G, Diss T C, MacDonald T T 1989 Expression of disulphide linked and non-disulphide linked forms of the T cell receptor gamma/delta heterodimer in human intestinal intraepithelial lymphocytes. European Journal of Immunology 19: 1335–1339

Stavy L, Cohen I R, Feldman M 1973 The effect of hydrocortisone on lymphocyte mediated cytolysis. Cellular Immunology 7: 302–312

Stobo J D, Tomasi T B, Huizenga K A, Spencer R J, Shorter R G 1976 In vitro studies of inflammatory bowel disease. Surface receptors of the mononuclear cell required to lyse allogeneic colonic epithelial cells. Gastroenterology 70: 71–76

Strickland R G, Korsmeyer S, Soltis R D, Wilson I D, Williams R C 1974 Peripheral blood T and B cells in chronic inflammatory bowel disease. Gastroenterology 67: 569–577

Thayer W R, Charland C, Field C E 1976 The subpopulations of circulating white blood cells in inflammatory bowel disease. Gastroenterology 71: 379–384

Thomson A W, Forrester J V 1994 Therapeutic advances in immunosuppression. Clinical and Experimental Immunology 98: 351–357

Trejdosiewicz L K, Calabrese A, Smart C J et al 1991 Gamma delta T cell receptor positive cells of the human gastrointestinal mucosa: occurrence and V region gene expression in *Helicobacter pylori* associated gastritis, coeliac disease and inflammatory bowel disease. Clinical and Experimental Immunology 84: 440–444

Van Kerckhove C, Russell G J, Deusch K et al 1992 Oligoclonality of human intestinal intraepithelial T cells. Journal of Experimental Medicine 175: 57–63

Van Spreeuwel J P, Lindeman J, Meijer A C J L M 1985 A quantitative study of immunoglobulin-containing cells in the differential diagnosis of acute colitis. Journal of Clinical Pathology 38: 774–777

Van Tol E A, Verspaget H W, Pea A S, Kraemer C V, Lamers C D 1992 The CD56 adhesion molecule is the major determinant for detecting non-major histocompatibility complex restricted cytotoxic mononuclear cells from the intestinal lamina propria. European Journal of Immunology 22: 23–29

Verrier-Jones J, Housley J, Ashurst P M, Hawkins C F 1969 Development of delayed hypersensitivity to dinitrochlorobenzene in patients with Crohn's disease. Gut 10: 52–56

Verspaget H W, Pea A S, Waterman I T, Lamers C B H W 1988 Disordered regulation of in vitro immunoglobulin synthesis by intestinal mononuclear cells in Crohn's disease. Gut 29: 503–510

Victorino R M M, Hodgson H J F 1980 Alteration in T lymphocyte subpopulations in inflammatory bowel disease. Clinical and Experimental Immunology. 41: 156–165

Watanabe M, Tsuru S, Aiso S 1984 Induction of impaired activation of lymphocytes from patients by suppressive factor in Crohn's disease patients. Journal of Clinical and Laboratory Immunology 14: 29–34

Watson D W, Quigley A, Bolt R J 1966 Effect of lymphocytes from patients with ulcerative colitis on human adult colon epithelial cells. Gastroenterology 51: 985–993

Weldon M J, Maxwell J D 1994 Lymphocyte and macrophage interleukin receptors in inflammatory bowel disease: a more selective target for therapy? Gut 35: 867–871

Yuan S, Hanauer S B, Klushens L F, Kraft S C 1983 Circulating lymphocyte subpopulations in Crohn's disease. Gastroenterology 85: 1313–1318

8. Humoral immunity in inflammatory bowel disease

M. T. Abreu-Martin   S. R. Targan

INTRODUCTION

Advances in the field of immunology have changed the way we view syndromes of autoimmunity, including inflammatory bowel diseases. In this chapter we will discuss the normal functions of the humoral immune system, including its specialized role in the gut. We will further highlight changes in the humoral immune system in patients with inflammatory bowel disease, and how they relate to clinical disease. Special attention will be paid to the issue of autoantibodies in inflammatory bowel disease and other autoimmune conditions, specifically as manifestations of immune dysregulation and genetic predisposition to autoimmunity. By examining the delicate balance between a desirable immune response to intestinal pathogens and an excessive immune response to universal intestinal antigens, we hope to shed light on the steps leading to clinical inflammatory bowel disease.

HUMORAL IMMUNITY IN HEALTH

General functions of B lymphocytes

B lymphocytes serve two principal and related functions: antibody production and presentation of antigen to T lymphocytes (Lanzavecchia 1990). When a protein antigen binds to membrane immunoglobulin, it is internalized, processed and presented on the surface of the B lymphocyte in association with a class II MHC molecule. This antigen presentation may have one of two effects, depending on the presence of costimulatory signals: activation of resting T lymphocytes or deletion/anergy of virgin T lymphocytes (Hori et al 1989, Eynon and Parker 1992). This latter function is important in induction of tolerance to self-antigens.

Following the appropriate antigenic challenge, a clone of B lymphocytes proliferates and differentiates into antibody-secreting cells. This process of differentiation includes a switch from the IgM/IgD isotype to another heavy chain isotype: IgA, IgG or IgE, that is both expressed on the cell surface and secreted. The type of immunoglobulin produced by the B cell dictates the effector function of that antibody. For example, the Fc regions of IgM and certain subtypes of IgG can bind and activate the classical complement pathway, while IgE can bind to receptors on mast cells and basophils and cause immediate hypersensitivity. This will be relevant with regard to the immunoglobulin isotype changes seen in inflammatory bowel disease.

B lymphocytes require T-lymphocyte help for full effector function

B lymphocytes present antigen in the context of class II MHC to T-helper lymphocytes, which are then activated to secrete cytokines and express specific membrane receptors. Cytokines produced by T-helper cells, and macrophages, dictate the type of immunoglobulin produced by B cells by specifically promoting the switch to different isotype heavy chains (Rizzo et al 1992; Table 8.1.) The recognition of the importance of cytokines in regulating immunoglobulin production as well as many other immune functions has led to their intensive study in inflammatory bowel disease (Sartor 1994).

Full B-cell differentiation cannot occur, however, in the absence of contact with activated T-helper cells. Many B-cell/T-cell ligand pairs are known to play a part in this contact-dependent help (Parker 1993; Fig. 8.1.) Of the many ligand pairs described, CD40/CD40 (CD40L)

Table 8.1 Cytokine-directed immunoglobulin production. (Reviewed in Parker 1993, *Coffman et al 1989, Tonkonogy et al 1989, Lebman et al 1990a, b)

Predominant source of cytokine(s)	Cytokine(s)	Immunoglobulin type
T-helper 1 and T-helper 2	IL-4, IL-6, IL-2, IFN-γ	IgG
T-helper 2 and T-helper 1	IL-4, IL-6, IL-2, IFN-γ IL-10	IgG1
T-helper 1	IFN-γ	IgG2(a)
T-helper 1	IFN-γ, IL-10	IgG3
T-helper 1 and T-helper 2	IL-4, IL-5, IL-2	IgM
T-helper 2	TGF-β, IL-5, IL-4, IL-6	IgA*
T-helper 2	IL-4	IgE

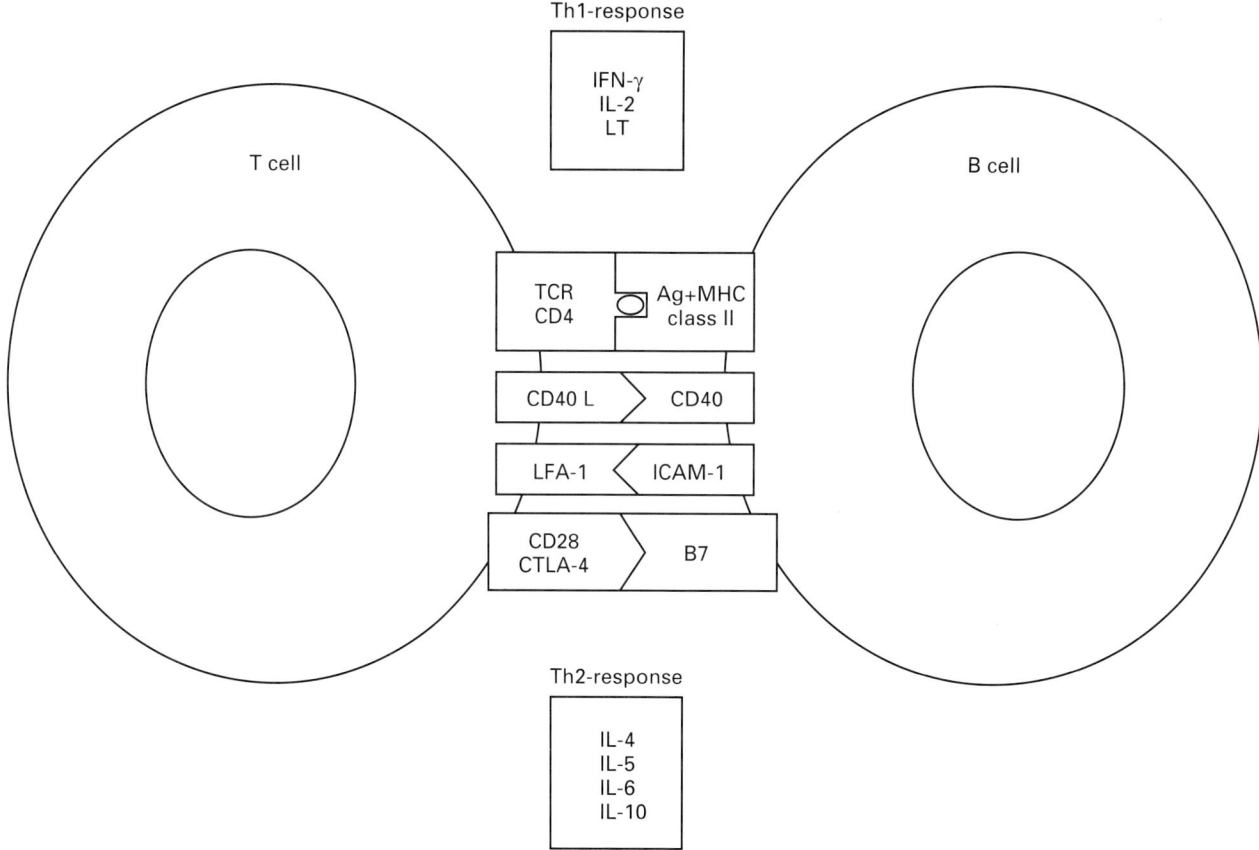

Fig. 8.1 Interactions between T and B cells in the process of isotype switching. Virgin B cells express surface IgM, which captures an antigen, internalizes it and processes the antigen to be re-expressed on the surface of the B cell in the context of a class II MHC molecule. An antigen-specific T cell binds the MHC class II antigen complex through its T-cell receptor and CD4 molecule. This interaction is stabilized by other adhesion molecules, such as LFA-1 and ICAM-1. After activation of the T cell, CD40 ligand (CD40L) is expressed followed by the upregulation B7 on the surface of the B cells. Cytokines produced by the T cell in combination with CD40L then direct the transcription of particular heavy chain isotypes.

appears to be critical in delivering T-cell mediated B-cell help for class switching (Armitage et al 1992, Noelle et al 1992). If the CD40–CD40L interaction is blocked, a peripheral T cell interacting with an appropriate MHC-restricted antigen on the surface of a B cell is rendered anergic (Durie et al 1994). A recent study shows that cyclosporin A inhibits CD40 ligand expression in T lymphocytes (Fuleihan et al 1994). This is of interest in inflammatory bowel disease because of the success in treating ulcerative colitis with cyclosporin A. Based on this work, one of the many mechanisms operative in cyclosporin treatment could be induction of anergy in T cells recognizing particular antigens presented by B cells. This could theoretically prevent inappropriate T-cell activation to intestinal antigens and ameliorate the underlying inflammatory response.

B-lymphocyte function in mucosal immunity

A higher percentage of B lymphocytes from intestinal mucosa express markers of activation than do B lymphocytes from peripheral blood (Peters et al 1989). This is presumably a result of continuous exposure to antigens in the luminal environment. The predominant type of immunoglobulin secreted by the B lymphocytes of the gut is IgA, accounting for 70–90% of all immunoglobulin present in normal intestinal mucosa (Brandtzaeg et al 1991). Secretory IgA produced by B cells from mucosal lymphoid follicles is taken up by the basolateral surface of epithelial cells and released into the bowel lumen, where it prevents invasion of epithelial cells by bacterial, protozoal and viral pathogens (Brandtzaeg 1985). In this way IgA traps potential antigens in the lumen before they elicit an immune response. Unlike other types of immunoglobulin, IgA does not bind complement and is, therefore, well suited to avoid bystander injury of epithelial cells (Imai et al 1988).

Of particular interest is the process leading to preferential differentiation of intestinal B lymphocytes into IgA-secreting cells. Studies using bone marrow-derived pre-B cells show that these cells differentiate into IgA-secreting cells in the presence of dendritic cells and T cells from Peyer's patches, but differentiate into IgG-secreting cells in the presence of dendritic cells and T cells from spleen

(Spalding & Griffin 1986). Thus, cellular and/or soluble signals generated by the combination of dendritic cells and T cells drive the B cell to its tissue-specific immunoglobulin-secreting state. Multiple cytokines are now known to interact to promote the genetic switch to the IgA isotype and the terminal differentiation of an sIgA-positive cell to an IgA-secreting plasma cell.

Transforming growth factor-β (TGF-β), derived from both T cells and non-lymphoid cells, and IL-5, derived from T cells, are involved in enhancing the isotype switch from IgM to IgA in mucosal B lymphocytes (Coffman et al 1989, Lebman et al 1990a, b, Strober & Harriman 1991). From the standpoint of mucosal immune regulation, TGF-β plays additional roles, such as inhibiting T-cell and B-cell activation and promoting wound healing (Snapper & Mond 1993). Terminal differentiation of sIgA-positive B cells to IgA-secreting plasma cells is under the influence of IL-2, IL-4, IL-5 and IL-6 (Harriman et al 1988, Tonkonogy et al 1989, Loughman & Nossal 1989, Beagley et al 1989, Kunimoto et al 1989).

Although cytokines are important in this process of class switching and IgA production by mucosal B lymphocytes, T cells are ultimately responsible for secretion of most of these cytokines. Two general types of T-helper cells are now recognized by the pattern of cytokines they produce. T-helper 1 (Th1) cells secrete IL-2, IFN-γ and lymphotoxin, whereas T-helper 2 (Th2) cells produce IL-4, IL-5, IL-6 and IL-10 (Parker 1993). Thus induction of IgA is largely under the influence of Th2-type responses. In non-human primates, lamina propria lymphocytes express more IFN-γ and IL-2 RNA than do mesenteric lymph node T cells, which express more IL-4 and IL-5 RNA (James et al 1990). Therefore, the inductive site (mesenteric nodes) of the intestinal immune system consists predominantly of Th2-type T cells, whereas the effector compartment (lamina propria) consists predominantly of Th1-type T cells. This point may be relevant in the immunoglobulin shifts that occur in inflammatory bowel disease.

HUMORAL IMMUNITY IN INFLAMMATORY BOWEL DISEASE

In the following sections we will attempt to define the contribution of humoral immunity to clinical inflammatory bowel disease. Alterations in humoral immunity that will be discussed include antibody production by mucosal B cells, complement activation in inflamed mucosa, and serum and mucosal autoantibody production. From the discussion above it is clear that T-cell and B-cell functions are intimately related, and that separation of these two components would be artificial. For this reason, a thorough understanding of the changes in the quantity and type of antibodies predominating in diseased mucosa must encompass what is known about the corresponding T-cell changes in inflammatory bowel disease mucosa. Recently, several animal models of inflammatory bowel disease have been studied. Some models require functional B cells for intestinal inflammation to occur, and others do not. Indeed, patients have been described with common variable immunodeficiency and agammaglobulinemia and inflammatory bowel disease (Ament et al 1973). These observations mean that mucosal destruction cannot always be attributed to changes in mucosal antibody production. The chapter will end with a discussion of the autoantibodies described in inflammatory bowel disease. Although these are not thought to be pathogenic from the standpoint of mucosal inflammation, their presence indicates a fundamental failure of the host immune system to delete B cells expressing high-affinity antibodies to self-antigens. Differences in the type of autoantibodies produced in ulcerative colitis, Crohn's disease and other autoimmune conditions may eventually allow substratification of patients with different natural histories of disease. For the average patient with inflammatory bowel disease, a combination of multiple components of the immune system acts synergistically to cause clinical disease.

Alterations in mucosal and systemic immunoglobulin production

Several lines of evidence indicate that B and T lymphocytes from the mucosa of patients with inflammatory bowel disease express a higher percentage of activation markers than do control mucosa (Schreiber et al 1991, Yacyshyn & Pilarski 1993). Perhaps related to this increased activation of T-helper cells and B cells, there is an increase in the percentage of B lymphocytes producing other types of immunoglobulin in addition to IgA (MacDermott et al 1981, Wu et al 1989; Table 8.2.) Specifically, there is an increase in IgG production by lamina propria mononuclear cells in patients with inflammatory bowel disease compared with healthy controls and patients with acute infectious colitis (Van Spreeuwel et al 1985). This has been demonstrated by both in-vitro cultures of lamina propia B cells and immunohistologic staining of intestinal mucosa (Scott et al 1986, MacDermott & Nahm 1987, Kett et al 1987). Lamina propria mononuclear cells from patients with ulcerative colitis have a shift toward IgG1 and IgG3 production, whereas patients with Crohn's disease have a shift toward IgG1 and IgG2 production (Scott et al 1986). As described above, IgG1 and IgG3 are efficient activators of complement, and therefore this immunoglobulin shift may contribute directly to gut injury. There is also a change in the predominant subtype of IgA produced from IgA2 to IgA1, and a shift towards monomeric IgA instead of dimeric IgA (MacDermott et al 1986, Kett et al 1988). IgA1 is more sensitive to proteolysis, and thus the change in IgA pattern may lead to decreased antigenic exclusion in inflammatory bowel

Table 8.2 Changes in serum and mucosal immunoglobulins in inflammatory bowel disease

Disease type	Serum	Mucosal	References
Crohn's disease	↑total immunoglobulins*	↑IgG2, ↑IgG1§	*MacDermott et al 1981, Beale et al 1982
	↑IgG2†	IgA1>IgA2‡	†MacDermott et al 1989, Gryboski & Buie 1994
Ulcerative colitis	↑total immunoglobulins*	↑IgG1, ↑IgG3§	§MacDermott et al 1981, Wu et al 1989,
	↑IgG1†	IgA1>IgA2‡	Van Spreeuwel et al 1985, Scott et al 1986, ‡MacDermott et al 1986, Kett et al 1988

disease mucosa, perpetuating the inflammatory response. More likely, the change in IgA subtype is a secondary phenomenon related to the changes in T-helper function in inflammatory bowel disease, specifically changes in cytokine profiles (see below).

There are many studies of serum immunoglobulin measurements in patients with inflammatory bowel disease. Gamma globulin levels are elevated in both ulcerative colitis and Crohn's disease. Indeed, the same subtypes that predominate in the lamina propria are represented in sera, which means that patients with ulcerative colitis have elevated IgG1 levels and those with Crohn's disease have elevated IgG2 (MacDermott et al 1989, Gryboski & Buie 1994). In vitro, peripheral blood mononuclear cells from patients with inflammatory bowel disease and other autoimmune conditions, such as systemic lupus erythematosus and Henoch–Schönlein purpura, have an elevated spontaneous production of IgG, IgA and IgM compared to healthy controls (MacDermott et al 1981, Beale et al 1982, Boirivant et al 1990). This probably represents a higher state of lymphocyte activation in vivo and not a primary cause of disease. In general, measurement of serum immunoglobulins in these diseases is not clinically useful because of lack of specificity.

Changes in cytokine patterns in inflammatory bowel disease mucosa lead to shifts in immunoglobulin-secreting cells

B-cell differentiation is greatly dependent on cytokine-mediated class switching and immunoglobulin secretion, therefore changes in the pattern of cytokines present in the lamina propria of patients with ulcerative colitis and Crohn's disease may offer some clues to the increase in IgG synthesis. Several laboratories have described an increase in IL-2 (Mullin et al 1992, Gurbindo et al 1993) and IFN-γ (Breese et al 1993) production by lamina propria mononuclear cells from patients with Crohn's disease but not patients with ulcerative colitis. On this basis, T-helper cells in the lamina propria of Crohn's disease are said to have a Th1 predominance, compared with ulcerative colitis and control lamina propria which have a Th2 predominance. IL-6 mRNA and protein is increased in both active Crohn's disease and ulcerative colitis (Stevens et al 1992, Jones et al 1993). IL-6 can increase the secretion of both IgG1 and IgA. Another interesting observation is the ability of intraepithelial lymphocytes to secrete a soluble factor that suppresses in-vitro IgA production by autologous lamina propria lymphocytes (Sachdev et al 1993). It is hard to know whether intraepithelial lymphocytes can, in vivo, modulate immunoglobulin production by lymphocytes in the lamina propria, but identification of this 'soluble factor' may be useful. At this point, differences in the methodologies used to measure individual mucosal cytokines and the difficulty of many of these assays make them impractical for clinical use, but are provocative with regard to elucidating immunological derangements in inflammatory bowel disease.

Animal models of inflammatory bowel disease: clues to the origins of immune dysregulation

Perhaps the most revealing studies about the potential role of unregulated B-cell function in inflammatory bowel disease come from genetically engineered mouse models. Investigators have developed at least three types of genetically engineered mouse that develop intestinal inflammation when cytokine or T-cell receptor genes are disrupted. Although these models develop chronic enterocolitis or colitis, they do not exactly reproduce human ulcerative colitis or Crohn's disease. Knockout mice with a disruption in the IL-2 gene develop a disease very similar to ulcerative colitis, with colonic bleeding and ulceration (Sadlack et al 1993). These mice have increased numbers of activated B cells, both in peripheral blood and the intestinal mucosa, and increased numbers of IgG1- and IgE-secreting cells. This may occur as a result of a shift to Th2-type cells that produce IL-4. In addition to histologic colitis, these animals produce anticolon antibodies. It is unclear whether these antibodies develop in the late stages of colitis or occur prior to overt disease. The other unexplored possibility is that they cross-react with antigens on luminal bacteria similar to epithelial cell antigens. Thus it seems that in the absence of Th1 activity and IL-2 production B-cell activity is unregulated, leading to the production of autoantibodies.

Mice with mutations in the T-cell receptor (TCR) genes or the class II MHC genes are deficient in both αβ and γδ T cells, and develop a disease like ulcerative colitis. In contrast, mice with mutations in the recombination-activating gene (*RAG-1*), which renders them deficient in mature T and B lymphocytes, do not develop intestinal inflammation (Mombaerts et al 1993). These models imply that in the absence of T-cell help, unregulated B-cell function can lead to intestinal inflammation. The conclusion from these studies is that T-cell functions (both Th1 and Th2) are required to limit excessive B-cell responses to ubiquitous luminal antigens. B cells are necessary in the last mouse model for development of intestinal inflammation; however, SCID mice reconstituted with CD45RB^{high} CD4+ T cells also develop severe colonic inflammation (Powrie et al 1994), indicating that B cells are not always requisite for intestinal inflammation. These animal models highlight the complexity of B-cell/T-cell interactions and the potential for genetic heterogeneity in inflammatory bowel disease, i.e. several genotypes can lead to similar phenotypes. For this reason, measurement of any one cytokine will be insufficient to unravel the essence of chronic intestinal inflammation.

Alterations in complement activation

One consequence of this shift in immunoglobulin type from IgA to IgG is the ability of IgG subtypes to bind and activate complement. Byproducts of the classical complement cascade result in tissue damage through a variety of mechanisms, including neutrophil and macrophage chemotaxis (C5a), opsonization (C3b) and increased vascular permeability (C3a, C5a) (Schreiber et al 1992). Circumstantial evidence that complement is involved in the histologic injury seen in inflammatory bowel disease comes from Halstensen et al (1989, 1990). Using monoclonal antibodies to C3b, these investigators demonstrated the deposition of C3b on the surface of colonic epithelial cells in patients with ulcerative colitis. These C3b deposits were not seen in uninflamed mucosa from the same ulcerative colitis patients or in healthy controls. In these and other studies (Halstensen et al 1993) C3b was found to colocalize with IgG1, supporting the pathogenic role of IgG1 in the epithelial injury seen in inflammatory bowel disease. Unfortunately, it is difficult to prove that IgG1 and complement deposition are causally related to epithelial damage, and not a consequence of epithelial damage followed by an appropriate reaction to bacterial antigens. Ahrenstedt et al (1990) performed in-vivo experiments in patients with Crohn's disease in which they measured jejunal fluid concentrations of C3 and C4. In spite of the fact that the Crohn's disease was thought to be limited to the terminal ileum, investigators found an increase in C3 and C4 in the jejunal fluid of Crohn's disease patients compared with controls. One explanation for these findings is that subclinical disease in patients with Crohn's disease is present in other parts of the small bowel that are not usually accessible to histologic studies. Complement, however, is not integral to the development of inflammatory bowel disease, as evidenced by the fact that patients have been described with both complement deficiency and inflammatory bowel disease (Slade et al 1978). Thus the shift to IgG1 in ulcerative colitis and, to a lesser extent, Crohn's disease leads to complement activation, which may contribute to the inflammatory cascade and mucosal injury, especially in advanced stages of mucosal destruction.

Autoantibodies in inflammatory bowel disease

One of the most intriguing aspects of immunology is the establishment and maintenance of self-tolerance. Analogous to thymic conditioning of T cells, there is evidence that pre-B cells expressing surface IgM with low affinity to autoantigen undergo positive selection (Schwartz & Stollar 1994). This would explain the greater representation of certain V_H segments (variable region of the immunoglobulin heavy chain) in the primary B-cell repertoire than would be expected by chance recombination alone. Based on this reasoning, several laboratories have sought to establish patterns of V_H segment usage in inflammatory bowel disease lamina propria B cells compared with normal ones (McCabe et al 1994). Skewing in the pattern of V_H usage in inflammatory bowel disease might help to predict the nature of the antigenic stimulus driving chronic inflammation and autoantibody production. However, autoantibodies are not necessarily pathogenic – indeed most are not. Autoantibodies are generally considered pathogenic if they are directed towards cell surface targets and not inaccessible intracellular structures (Naparstek & Plotz 1993). More commonly, autoantibodies result from the exposure of antigens due to tissue damage, or as a surrogate marker for immunologic dysfunction.

Investigators have sought the presence of autoantibodies in inflammatory bowel disease both to explain the pathogenesis of the disease and to identify markers to distinguish idiopathic inflammatory bowel disease from other colitides. As early as the 1950s scientists were looking for (and finding) colonic antibodies to explain the inflammation seen in ulcerative colitis (Broberger & Perlmann 1959, Lagercrantz et al 1966, Marcussen 1976, Das et al 1978, Snook et al 1991). Anticolon antibodies are also present in Crohn's disease but are less common. As with most autoantibodies, there is evidence for and against anticolon antibodies having a pathogenic role in inflammatory bowel disease. In vitro, serum antibodies from patients with ulcerative colitis have been shown to direct antibody-dependent cellular cytotoxicity (ADCC) against colon cancer lines (Hibi et al 1993a) and epithelial-cell antigen-coated red blood cells (Fiocchi et al 1989). Arguing against these antibodies having a harmful role in vivo is the inability of some groups to detect anticolon antibodies bound to tissue specimens (Snook et al 1991) and the finding of anticolon antibodies in patients with other non-inflammatory gastrointestinal illnesses (Carlsson et al 1977). Some groups have not even been able to find anticolon antibodies (Cantrell et al 1990). The specific antigens these anticolon antibodies are recognizing have not been absolutely identified, but possible antigens include a 40 kDa colonic protein (Takahasi et al 1990), goblet cells (Harrison 1965, Seibold et al 1991, Hibi et al 1993b), and mucin glycoproteins (Podolsky & Fournier 1988, Hinoda et al 1993). This 40 kDa protein is defined by its ability to react with a monoclonal antibody developed by Das et al (1987). Originally, the 40 kDa protein was felt to be the cytoskeletal protein tropomyosin, but recent data do not concur with this hypothesis and its true nature is yet to be determined (Hamilton et al 1994).

A novel autoantibody to an erythrocyte antigen has recently been identified in the serum of patients with Crohn's disease and ulcerative colitis (Berberian et al 1994). Investigators using anti-idiotypic monoclonal antibodies to specific V_H segments of immunoglobulins have identified V_H3–15-type antibodies bound to erythrocytes in submucosal vessels of biopsies from patients with ulcerative colitis (90%) and Crohn's disease (100%). These antierythrocyte antibodies (AEA) were not found in healthy control subjects but were found in patients with *Campylobacter jejuni* enterocolitis (70%). This study has clinical relevance because it introduces an autoantibody that can be used to distinguish idiopathic inflammatory bowel disease and *C. jejuni* enterocolitis from other colitides. It also supports the theory of molecular mimicry in autoimmunity, and raises the possibility that *C. jejuni* infection serves as a trigger for inflammatory bowel disease in the genetically susceptible host.

Autoantibodies are not only found in patients with inflammatory bowel disease but also in unaffected first-degree relatives. Antibodies directed against epithelial cell components were found in 70% of inflammatory bowel disease patients and 55% of their unaffected relatives, compared to an 8% prevalence in control cases (Fiocchi et al 1989). The high prevalence of these antibodies in first-degree relatives suggests an environmental response, perhaps superimposed on genetic predisposition. This study also supports the idea that anticolon antibodies are not themselves pathogenic, as the relatives did not have clinical disease.

Specific autoantibodies in ulcerative colitis

Antibodies to leukocytes in the sera of patients with inflammatory bowel disease were first described by Korsmeyer et al in 1975. At present, the best-characterized autoantibody in ulcerative colitis is the antineutrophil cytoplasmic antibody (ANCA), which can serve as a paradigm for the study of autoantibodies in inflammatory bowel disease and other autoimmune conditions. ANCA was first described in sera from patients with Wegener's granulomatosis, by Van der Woude et al in 1985. In 1990, Saxon et al described the presence of ANCA in patients with ulcerative colitis. As distinct from Wegener's, the immunofluorescent staining pattern of ANCA in ulcerative colitis is perinuclear, as opposed to cytoplasmic, related to the location of the antigen within the neutrophil. The cytoplasmic ANCA (cANCA) of Wegener's is directed against proteinase-3, a neutrophil granule protein (Gross et al 1993). Still elusive is the antigen being recognized by the pANCA of ulcerative colitis. Many antigens have been implicated, including lactoferrin, proteinase-3, cathepsin G and myeloperoxidase (Peen et al 1993, Broekroelofs et al 1994, Ellerbroek et al 1994). The conventional methodology used to find the antigen recognized by pANCA includes Western blot analysis and ELISAs to the various proteins listed above. The lability of the antigen has, however, made the search for the pANCA antigen difficult. Recent advances in molecular and microscopic technology offer promise in elucidating the antigen and possibly shedding light on immunological abnormalities in ulcerative colitis. Confocal laser microscopy has localized the pANCA reactivity to the inner side of the nuclear membrane, suggesting that chromatin-associated antigens, rather than granule proteins, are being recognized by the pANCA of ulcerative colitis (Tahir et al 1994). Eggena et al (1994) have used phage display technology to clone and characterize pANCA. Using ulcerative colitis lamina propria lymphocytes that spontaneously produced pANCA (Targan et al 1994), a complete IgG1-κ immunoglobulin cDNA library was constructed and expressed in phagemid vectors. This library was enriched for its ability to bind fixed neutrophils, and ultimately a recombinant Fab fragment was purified which could simulate serum pANCA reactivity by ELISA, immunofluorescence and confocal microscopy. Although the antigen has not yet been identified, this technology is very promising for developing highly specific antibodies to unidentified antigens.

There continues to be much debate about the true prevalence of pANCA and its significance in inflammatory bowel disease. There is general agreement in North American and northern European studies that pANCA is present in approximately 60–80% of ulcerative colitis patients and 20–30% of Crohn's disease patients (Cambridge et al 1992, Seibold et al 1992) For this reason, it has become an important serologic marker to distinguish the two diseases. Studies have been carried out around the world to assess the prevalence of pANCA in inflammatory bowel disease (Dalekos et al 1993, Sung et al 1994, Vecchi et al 1994). Many of the reported differences in prevalence can be attributed to the ethnic characteristics of the study populations, as well as the assay methodologies used (Mulder et al 1994). Two principal assays are used: indirect immunofluorescence and fixed-neutrophil ELISA. The former is generally less sensitive than ELISA, but defines the pattern of staining: perinuclear or cytoplasmic. The fixed-neutrophil ELISA can yield different results depending on the laboratory, but in general is more sensitive and less specific than immunofluorescence.

How does one assess the significance of pANCA positivity in patients with inflammatory bowel disease? The presence and titer of pANCA are known not to correlate with disease activity or medical therapy, or to change after colectomy (Cambridge et al 1992, Deusch et al 1993, Oudkerk Pool et al 1993). Family studies in patients with ulcerative colitis or Crohn's disease and their unaffected first-degree relatives show that approximately 70% of ulcerative colitis patients and 15–30% of their relatives are pANCA positive, compared with 27% of Crohn's disease patients and 6% of their relatives (Shanahan et al 1992, Seibold et al 1994). This implies that pANCA is a preclinical marker of disease. More direct evidence of pANCA as a genetic marker of inflammatory bowel disease is data from Yang et al (1993, 1994). ANCA-positive ulcerative colitis patients have a significantly increased frequency of HLA-DR2 positivity compared with pANCA-negative ulcerative colitis patients who have a DR4 association. Because class II MHC molecules dictate the ability of T cells to respond to antigens, the antigen being recognized by pANCA may have steric requirements necessitating certain class II MHC molecules. In addition to HLA associations, pANCA-negative ulcerative colitis patients have an increased frequency of a particular allele for the ICAM-1 gene. This adhesion molecule plays an important role in B-cell/T-cell interactions (Fig. 8.1) and transendothelial migration of leukocytes. Thus, genes coding for immunoregulatory functions may provide the substrate for the pANCA-positive or -negative ulcerative colitis phenotypes.

Although pANCA does not does not change with flares and remissions of ulcerative colitis in a given patient, it may be a marker of treatment-resistant disease (Sandborn et al 1994). This has been defined as lack of response to oral 5-ASA products, topical 5-ASA products or oral steroids within a 4-week period. Compared with treatment-responsive patients, treatment-resistant patients had a significantly higher prevalence of pANCA (87% versus 62%). Interestingly, patients with chronic pouchitis after ileal pouch–anal anastomosis also have an unexpectedly high prevalence of pANCA compared with patients with ileal pouch–anal anastomosis and no pouchitis, (100% versus 50%) (Sandborn et al 1994). Both of these studies support the role of pANCA in defining a subset of ulcerative colitis patients with a different, perhaps more aggressive, natural history.

Specific autoantibodies found in Crohn's disease

In general, autoantibodies are less prevalent in Crohn's disease than in ulcerative colitis. Among the serologic markers thought to be more specific for Crohn's disease than ulcerative colitis are antibodies to pancreatic juice (Stocker et al 1987), cathepsin G (Mayet et al 1992) and cytoskeletal proteins (Mayet et al 1990). Sera from patients with Crohn's disease were analyzed for the presence of antibodies to cathepsin G (cat-G), a myeloid lysosomal enzyme: 74% of patients with Crohn's disease had anti-cat-G antibodies, whereas no ulcerative colitis patients had these antibodies. No healthy control group was studied. Antibodies to pancreatic juice are found in approximately 30% of patients with Crohn's disease, compared with 4% of patients with ulcerative colitis (Stocker et al 1987, Seibold et al 1991). With regard to antibodies against cytoskeletal proteins, the most prevalent are directed against cytokeratin 18, actin and desmin but they are present at relatively low levels (Mayet et al 1990). In an attempt to establish the etiology of Crohn's disease many groups have explored mycobacterial infection. Serum antibodies to mycobacterial antigens do not appear to be overrepresented in patients with Crohn's disease (Kobayashi et al 1988). Unfortunately, although the assays to detect these antibodies may be quite reproducible within a particular laboratory, it is often difficult to duplicate the studies in other laboratories. Moreover, the antibodies described above are present in relatively small percentages of patients with Crohn's disease, or at low titers, and are not very sensitive or specific for the disease. (Table 8.3.)

Table 8.3 Autoantibodies present in inflammatory bowel disease

Autoantibody	Crohn's disease	Ulcerative colitis	References
Antineutrophil cytoplasmic Ab	+low titer (20%)	+high titer (70–80%)	Saxon et al 1990, Seibold et al 1992, Cambridge et al 1992
Antierythrocyte Ab	++high titer (100%)	+low titer (90%)	Eggena et al 1994
Antipancreas	+(30–40%)	(<10%)	Stocker et al 1987, Seibold et al 1991

CONCLUSION

The discussion of humoral immunity in inflammatory bowel disease has evolved from concrete findings of changes in circulating and mucosal immunoglobulins and autoantibodies to the more difficult task of understanding why. We can now correlate particular autoantibodies with genetic markers in inflammatory bowel disease. Whether HLA class II and ICAM-1 are directly related to production of pANCA or linked to other relevant genes is not known. Immunoregulatory genes, such as HLA and ICAM-1, may dictate the potential for antigen recognition. Once a particular intestinal antigen is recognized, another series of poorly defined events results in the production of favorable neutralizing antibodies or the perpetuation of self-reactive antibody-producing cells. Animal models illustrate the important balance between T-helper cell subsets and B cells in dampening the mucosal immune response. The artificial absence of one cytokine, IL-2, leads not only to colitis but also to autoantibody production. Although studies of cytokine production and T-helper subsets in patients with inflammatory bowel disease help to explain certain shifts in immunoglobulin production, they are not explanations for chronic intestinal inflammation. Molecular technology, both in vivo and in vitro, will allow the systematic study of individual populations of cells and their lymphokine products in the hope of answering this question.

Although the causes of chronic inflammatory bowel disease are elusive, our ability to diagnose these diseases correctly continues to improve. Testing patients for the presence of pANCA is already accepted as a way of confirming the diagnosis of ulcerative colitis in clinically equivocal patients, especially prior to surgical therapy. In the future it may be possible to use the autoantibodies present in inflammatory bowel disease patients to predict clinical outcomes, direct therapy, and diagnose genetically susceptible relatives. A panel of tests, including for example pANCA and AEA-15, might be used routinely as a cost-effective way to distinguish inflammatory bowel disease from other causes of colitis or non-inflammatory diarrhea. Autoantibodies present in smaller numbers of patients may also define subsets of patients with distinct natural histories of disease, even if they are not useful for screening purposes. For now, the tests themselves need to be perfected and applied prospectively to studies of clinical outcomes.

REFERENCES

Ament M E, Ochs H D, David S D 1973 Structure and function of the gastrointestinal tract in primary immunodeficiency syndromes: a study of 39 patients. Medicine 52: 227–248

Arhenstedt O, Knutson L, Nillson B, Nilsson-Ekdahl K, Odlind B, Hallgren R 1990 Enhanced local production of complement components in the small intestines of patients with Crohn's disease. New England Journal of Medicine 322: 1345–1349

Armitage R J, Fanslow W C, Strockbine L et al 1992 Molecular and biological characterization of a murine ligand for CD40. Nature 357: 80–82

Beagley K W, Eldridge J H, Lee F et al 1989 Interleukins and IgA synthesis: human and murine interleukin 6 induce high rate IgA secretion in IgA-committed B cells. Journal of Experimental Medicine 169: 2133–2148

Beale M G, Nash G S, Bertovich M J et al 1982 Similar disturbances in B-cell activity and regulatory T-cell function in Henoch–Schönlein purpura and systemic lupus erythematosus. Journal of Immunology 128: 486–491

Berberian L S, Valles-Ayoub Y, Gordon L K, Targan S R, Braun J 1994 Expression of a novel autoantibody defined by the $V_H 3-15$ gene in inflammatory bowel disease and *Campylobacter jejuni* enterocolitis. Journal of Immunology 153: 3756–3763

Boirivant M, Quintieri F, Pugliese O, Famularo G, Fais S, Pallone F 1990 A limited-dilution analysis of activated circulating B cells in Crohn's disease. Journal of Clinical Immunology 19: 128–134

Brandtzaeg P 1985 The role of J chain and secretory component in receptor-mediated glandular and hepatic transport of immunoglobulins in man. Scandinavian Journal of Immunology 22: 111–146

Brandtzaeg P, Nilssen D E, Rognum T O, Thrane P S 1991 Ontogeny of the mucosal immune system and IgA deficiency. Gastroenterology Clinics of North America 20: 397–439

Breese E, Braegger C P, Corrigan C J, Walker-Smith J A, MacDonald T T 1993 Interleukin-2 and interferon-gamma-secreting T cells in normal and diseased human intestinal mucosa. Immunology 78: 127–131

Broberger O, Perlmann P 1959 Autoantibodies in human ulcerative colitis. Journal of Experimental Medicine 110: 657–673

Broekroelofs J, Mulder A H, Nelis G F, Westerveld B D, Tervaert J W, Kallenberg C G 1994 Anti-neutrophil cytoplasmic antibodies (ANCA) in sera from patients with inflammatory bowel disease (IBD). Relation to disease pattern and disease activity. Digestive Diseases and Sciences 39: 545–549

Cambridge G, Rampton D S, Stevens T R, McCarthy D A A, Kamm M, Leaker B 1992 Anti-neutrophil antibodies in inflammatory bowel disease: prevalence and diagnostic role. Gut 33: 668–674

Carlsson H E, Lagercrantz R, Perlmann P 1977 Immunological studies in ulcerative colitis VIII. Antibodies to colon antigen in patients with ulcerative colitis, Crohn's disease and other diseases. Scandinavian Journal of Gastroenterology 12: 707–714

Coffman R L, Lebman D A, Shrader B 1989 Transforming growth factor β specifically enhances IgA production by lipopolysaccharide-stimulated murine B lymphocytes. Journal of Experimental Immunology 170: 1039–1044

Dalekos G N, Manoussakis M N, Goussia A C, Tsianos E V, Moutsopoulos H M 1993 Soluble interleukin-2 receptors, antineutrophil cytoplasmic antibodies, and other autoantibodies in patients with ulcerative colitis. Gut 34: 658–664

Das K M, Dubin R, Nagai T 1978 Isolation and characterization of colonic tissue-bound antibodies from patients with idiopathic ulcerative colitis. Proceedings of the National Academy of Sciences of the United States of America 75: 4528–4532

Das K M, Sakamaki S, Vecchi M, Diamond B 1987 The production and characterization of monoclonal antibodies to a human colonic antigen associated with ulcerative colitis: cellular localization of the antigen by using the monoclonal antibody. Journal of Immunology 139: 77–84

Deusch K, Oberstadt K, Schaedel W, Weber M, Classen M 1993 p-ANCA as a diagnostic marker in ulcerative colitis. Advances in Experimental Medicine and Biology 336: 527–531

Durie F H, Foy T M, Masters S R, Laman J D, Noelle R J 1994 The role of CD40 in the regulation of humoral and cell-mediated immunity. Immunology Today 15: 406–411

Eggena M, Targan S R, Vidrich A, Braun J 1994 Cloning, expression, and characterization of an immunogenetic marker antibody in ulcerative colitis, pANCA. (Submitted)

Ellerbroek P M, Oudkerk Pool M, Ridwan B U et al 1994 Neutrophil cytoplasmic antibodies (p-ANCA) in ulcerative colitis. Journal of Clinical Pathology 47: 257–262

Eynon E E, Parker D C 1992 Small B cells as antigen-presenting cells in the induction of tolerance to soluble protein antigens. Journal of Experimental Medicine 175: 131–138

Fiocchi C, Roche J K, Michener W M 1989 High prevalence of antibodies to intestinal epithelial antigens in patients with inflammatory bowel disease and their relatives. Annals of Internal Medicine 110: 786–794

Fuleihan R, Ramesh N, Horner A et al 1994 Cyclosporin A inhibits CD40 ligand expression in T lymphocytes. Journal of Clinical Investigations 93: 1315–1320

Gross W L, Schmitt W H, Csernok E 1993 ANCA and associated diseases: immunodiagnostic and pathogenetic aspects. Clinical and Experimental Immunology 91: 1–12

Gryboski J D, Buie T 1994 Immunoglobulin studies in children with inflammatory bowel disease. Annals of Allergy 72: 525–527

Gurbindo C, Sabbah S, Menezes J, Justinich C, Marchand R, Seidman E G 1993 Interleukin-2 production in pediatric inflammatory bowel disease: evidence for dissimilar mononuclear cell function in Crohn's disease and ulcerative colitis. Journal of Pediatric Gastroenterology and Nutrition 17: 247–254

Halstensen T S, Mollnes T E, Brandtzaeg P 1989 Persistent complement activation in submucosal vessels of active inflammatory bowel disease: immunohistochemical evidence. Gastroenterology 97: 10–19

Halstensen T S, Mollnes T E, Garred P et al 1990 Epithelial deposition of immunoglobulin G1 and activated complement (C3b and terminal component complex) in ulcerative colitis. Gastroenterology 98: 1264–1271

Halstensen T S, Das K M, Brandtzaeg P 1993 Epithelial deposits of immunoglobulin G1 and activated complement colocalise with the M(r) 40 kD putative autoantigen in ulcerative colitis. Gut 34: 650–657

Hamilton M I, Bradley N J, Thrasivoulou C, Srai S K, Pounder R E, Wakefield A J 1994 Evidence that tropomyosin is not the major antigenic target of the Das antibody 7E12H12 in ulcerative colitis. Annual Meeting of the British Society of Gastroenterology, Abstract T169. Gut 35: S43

Harriman G R, Kunimoto D Y, Elliott J F et al 1988 The role of IL-5 in IgA B cell differentiation. Journal of Immunology 140: 3033–3039

Harrison W J 1965 Autoantibodies against intestinal and gastric mucous cells in ulcerative colitis. Lancet 1: 1346–1350

Hibi T, Ohara M, Watanabe M, Kanai T et al 1993a Interleukin-2 and interferon-gamma augment anticolon antibody dependent cellular cytotoxicity in ulcerative colitis. Gut 34: 788–793

Hibi T, Ohara M, Kobayashi K et al 1993b Enzyme linked immunosorbent assay (ELISA) and immunoprecipitation studies on anti-goblet cell antibody using a mucin producing cell line in patients with inflammatory bowel disease. Gut 35: 224–230

Hinoda Y, Nakagawa N, Nakamura H et al 1993 Detection of a circulating antibody against a peptide epitope on a mucin core protein, MUC1, in ulcerative colitis. Immunology Letters 35: 163–168

Hori S, Sato S, Kitigawa S et al 1989 Tolerance induction of allo-class II H-2 antigen-reactive L3T4$^+$ helper T cells and prolonged survival of the corresponding class II H-2-disparate skin graft. Journal of Immunology 143: 1447–1452

Imai H, Chen A, Wyatt R J, Rifai A 1988 Lack of complement activation by human IgA immune complexes. Clinical and Experimental Immunology 73: 479–483

James S P, Kwan W C, Sneller M C 1990 T cells in inductive and effector compartments of the intestinal mucosal immune system of nonhuman primates differ in lymphokine mRNA expression, lymphokine utilization, and regulatory function. Journal of Immunology 144: 1251–1256

Jarjour W N, Jeffries B D, Davis J S, Welch W J, Mimura T, Winfield J B 1991 Autoantibodies to human stress proteins. A survey of various rheumatic and other inflammatory diseases. Arthritis and Rheumatism 34: 1133–1138

Jones S C, Tejdosiewicz L K, Banks R E et al 1993 Expression of interleukin-6 by intestinal enterocytes. Journal of Clinical Pathology 46: 1097–1100

Kett K, Rognum T O, Brandtzaeg P 1987 Mucosal subclass distribution of immunoglobulin G-producing cells is different in ulcerative colitis and Crohn's disease of the colon. Gastroenterology 93: 919–924

Kett K, Brandtzaeg P, Fausa O 1988 J-chain expression is more prominent in immunoglobulin A2 than in immunoglobulin A1 colonic immunocytes and is decreased in both subclasses associated with inflammatory bowel disease. Gastroenterology 94: 1419–1425

Kobayashi K, Brown W R, Brennan P J, Blaser M J 1988 Serum antibodies to mycobacterial antigens in active Crohn's disease. Gastroenterology 94: 1404–1411

Korsmeyer S J, Williams R C Jr, Wilson I D et al 1975 Lymphocytotoxic antibody in inflammatory bowel disease. A family study. New England Journal of Medicine 293: 1117–1120

Kühn R, Löhler J, Rennick D, Rajewsky K, Müller W 1993 Interleukin-10-deficient mice develop chronic enterocolitis. Cell 75: 263–274

Kunimoto D Y, Nordan R P, Strober W 1988 IL-6 is a potent cofactor of IL-1 in IgM synthesis and of IL-5 in IgA synthesis. Journal of Immunology 143: 2230–2235

Lagercrantz R, Hammarstrom S, Perlmann P, Gustafsson B E 1966 Immunological studies in ulcerative colitis. 3. Incidence of antibodies to colon-antigen in ulcerative colitis and other gastro-intestinal diseases. Clinical and Experimental Immunology 1: 263–276

Lanzavecchia A 1990 Receptor-mediated antigen uptake and its effect on antigen presentation to class II MHC-restricted T lymphocytes. Annual Review of Immunology 8: 773–793

Lebman D A, Lee F D, Coffman R L 1990a Mechanism for transforming growth factor β and IL-2 enhancement of IgA expression in lipopolysaccharide-stimulated B cell cultures. Journal of Immunology 144: 942–959

Lebman D A, Nomura D Y, Coffman R L et al 1990b Molecular characterization of sterile immunoglobulin A transcripts produced during TGF-β induced isotype switching. Proceedings of the National Academy of Sciences of the United States of America 87: 3962–3966

Loughman M S, Nossal G J V 1989 Interleukins 4 and 5 control expression of IL-2 receptor on murine B cells through independent induction of its two chains. Nature 340: 76–79

MacDermott R P, Nahm M H 1987 Expression of human immunoglobulin G subclasses in inflammatory bowel disease. Gastroenterology 91: 379–385

MacDermott R P, Nash G S, Bertovich M J et al 1981 Alterations of IgA, IgM, and IgG by peripheral blood mononuclear cells, and by human bone marrow mononuclear cells from patients with ulcerative colitis and Crohn's disease. Gastroenterology 81: 844–852

MacDermott R P, Bragdon M J, Kodner I J et al 1986 Evidence for the migration of B cells secreting monomeric IgA and IgA subclass I (IgA1) from peripheral compartments into the intestine in inflammatory bowel disease. Gastroenterology 91: 379–385

MacDermott R P, Nash G S, Auer I O et al 1989 Alterations in serum immunoglobulin G subclasses in patients with ulcerative colitis and Crohn's disease. Gastroenterology 96: 764–768

Marcussen H 1976 Anti-colon antibodies in ulcerative colitis. A clinical study. Scandinavian Journal of Gastroenterology 11: 763–767

Mayet W J, Press A G, Hermann E et al 1990 Antibodies to cytoskeletal proteins in patients with Crohn's disease. European Journal of Clinical Investigation 20: 516–524

Mayet W J, Hermann E, Finsterwalder J, Rieder H, Poralla T, Meyer Zum Buschenfelde K H 1992 Antibodies to cathepsin G in Crohn's disease. European Journal of Clinical Investigation 22: 427–433

Mombaerts P, Mizoguchi E, Grusby M J, Glimcher L H, Bhan A K, Tonegawa S 1993 Spontaneous development of inflammatory bowel disease in T cell receptor mutant mice. Cell 75: 275–282

Mulder A H, Broekroelofs J, Horst G, Limburg P C, Nelis G F, Kallenberg C G 1994 Anti-neutrophil cytoplasmic antibodies (ANCA) in inflammatory bowel disease: characterization and clinical correlates. Clinical and Experimental Immunology 95: 490–497

Mullin G E, Lazenby A J, Harris M L, Bayless T M, James S P 1992 Increased interleukin-2 messenger RNA in the intestinal mucosal lesions of Crohn's disease but not ulcerative colitis. Gastroenterology 102: 1620–1627

Naparstek Y, Plotz P H 1993 The role of autoantibodies in autoimmune disease. Annual Review of Immunology 11: 79–104

Noelle R J, Roy M, Shepherd D M, Stamenkovic I, Ledbetter J A, Aruffo A 1992 A novel ligand on activated helper T cells binds CD40 and transduces the signal for cognate activation of B cells. Proceedings of the National Academy of Sciences of the United States of America 89: 6550–6554

Oudkerk Pool M, Ellerbroek P M, Ridwan B U et al 1993 Serum anti-neutrophil cytoplasmic autoantibodies in inflammatory bowel disease are mainly associated with ulcerative colitis. A correlation study between perinuclear antineutrophil cytoplasmic autoantibodies and clinical parameters, medical, and surgical treatment. Gut 34: 46–50

Parker D C 1993 T cell-dependent B cell activation. Annual Review of Immunology 11: 331–360

Peen E, Almer S, Bodemar G et al 1993 Anti-lactoferrin antibodies and other types of ANCA in ulcerative colitis, primary sclerosing cholangitis, and Crohn's disease. Gut 34: 56–62

Peters M G, Secrist H, Anders K A et al 1989 Normal human intestinal B lymphocytes: increased activation compared to peripheral blood. Journal of Clinical Investigation 83: 1827–1833

Podolsky D K, Fournier D A 1988 Emergence of antigenic glycoprotein structures in ulcerative colitis detected through monoclonal antibodies. Gastroenterology 95: 371–378

Powrie F, Correa-Oliveira R, Mauze S, Coffman R L 1994 Regulatory interactions between CD45RB^{high} and CD45RB^{low} CD4+ T cells are important for the balance between protective and pathogenic cell-mediated immunity. Journal of Experimental Medicine 179: 589–600

Reumaux D, Colombel J F, Duclos B et al 1993 Antineutrophil cytoplasmic autoantibodies in sera from patients with ulcerative colitis after proctocolectomy with ileo-anal anastomosis. Advances in Experimental Medicine and Biology 336: 523–525

Rizzo L V, DeKruyff R H, Umetsu D T 1992 Generation of B cell memory and affinity maturation. Induction with Th1 and Th2 cell clones. Journal of Immunology 148: 3733–3739

Sachdev G K, Dalton H R, Hoang P, DiPaolo M C, Crotty B, Jewell D P 1993 Human colonic intraepithelial lymphocytes suppress in vitro immunoglobulin synthesis by autologous peripheral blood lymphocytes and lamina propria lymphocytes. Gut 34: 257–263

Sadlack B, Merz H, Schorle H, Schimpl A, Feller A C, Horak I 1993 Ulcerative colitis-like disease in mice with a disrupted interleukin-2 gene. Cell 75: 253–261

Sandborn W J, Landers C J, Tremaine W J, Targan S R 1994a Unexpectedly high frequency of antineutrophil cytoplasmic antibody in treatment-resistant left-sided ulcerative colitis. (Submitted)

Sandborn W J, Landers C J, Tremaine W J, Targan S R 1994b Antineutrophil cytoplasmic antibody correlates with chronic pouchitis after ileal pouch-anal anastomosis. (Submitted)

Sartor R B 1994 Cytokines in intestinal inflammation: pathophysiological and clinical considerations.

Saxon A, Shanahan F, Landers C, Ganz T, Targan S 1990 A distinct subset of antineutrophil cytoplasmic antibodies is associated with inflammatory bowel disease. Journal of Allergy and Clinical Immunology 86: 202–210

Schreiber S, MacDermott R P, Raedler A et al 1991 Increased activation of isolated intestinal lamina propria mononuclear cells in inflammatory bowel disease. Gastroenterology 101: 1020–1030

Schreiber S, Raedler A, Stenson W F, MacDermott R P 1992 The role of the mucosal immune system in inflammatory bowel disease. Gastroenterology Clinics of North America 21: 451–502

Schwartz R S, Stollar B D 1994 Heavy-chain directed B-cell maturation: continuous clonal selection beginning at the pre-B cell stage. Immunology Today 15: 27–32

Scott M G, Nahm M H, Macke K, Nash G S, Bertovich M J, MacDermott R P 1986 Spontaneous secretion of IgG subclasses by intestinal mononuclear cells: difference between ulcerative colitis, Crohn's disease, and controls. Clinical and Experimental Immunology 66: 209–215

Seibold F, Weber P, Jenss H, Wiedmann K H 1991 Antibodies to a trypsin sensitive pancreatic antigen in chronic inflammatory bowel disease: specific markers for a subgroup of patients with Crohn's disease. Gut 32: 1192–1197

Seibold F, Weber P, Klein R, Berg P A, Wiedmann K H 1992 Clinical significance of antibodies against neutrophils in patients with inflammatory bowel disease and primary sclerosing cholangitis. Gut 33: 657–662

Seibold F, Slametschka D, Gregor M, Weber P 1994 Neutrophil autoantibodies: a genetic marker in primary sclerosing cholangitis and ulcerative colitis. Gastroenterology 107: 532–536

Shanahan F, Duerr R H, Rotter J I et al 1992 Neutrophil autoantibodies in ulcerative colitis: familial aggregation and genetic heterogeneity. Gastroenterology 103: 456–461

Slade J D, Luskin A T, Gewurz H, Kraft S C, Kirsner J B, Zeitz H J 1978 Inherited deficiency of second component of complement and HLA haplotype A10, B18 associated with inflammatory bowel disease. Annals of Internal medicine 88: 796–798

Snapper C M, Mond J J 1993 Towards a comprehensive view of immunoglobulin class switching. Immunology Today 14: 15–17

Snook J A, de Silva H J, Jewell D P The association of autoimmune disorders with inflammatory bowel disease. Quarterly Journal of Medicine 72: 835–840

Snook J A, Lowes J R, Wu K C, Priddle J D, Jewell D P 1991 Serum and tissue autoantibodies to colonic epithelium in ulcerative colitis. Gut 32: 163–166

Spalding D M, Griffin J A 1986 Different pathways of differentiation of pre-B cell lines are induced by dendritic cells and T cells from different lymphoid tissues. Cell 44: 507–515

Stevens C, Walz G, Singaram C et al 1992. Tumor necrosis factor-alpha, interleukin-1 beta, and interleukin-6 expression in inflammatory bowel disease. Digestive Diseases and Sciences 37: 818–826

Stevens T R, Harley S L, Groom J S et al 1993 Anti-endothelial cell antibodies in inflammatory bowel disease. Digestive Diseases and Sciences 38: 426–432

Stocker W, Otte M, Ulrich S et al 1987 Autoimmunity to pancreatic juice in Crohn's disease. Results of an autoantibody screening in patients with chronic inflammatory bowel disease. Scandinavian Journal of Gastroenterology 139 (Suppl): 41–52

Strober W, Harriman G R 1991 The regulation of IgA B-cell differentiation. Gastroenterology Clinics of North America 20: 473–494

Sung J Y, Chan K L, Hsu R, Liew C T, Lawton J W 1993 Ulcerative colitis and antineutrophil cytoplasmic antibodies in Hong Kong Chinese. American Journal of Gastroenterology 88: 864–869

Sung J Y, Chan F K, Lawton J et al 1994 Anti-neutrophil cytoplasmic antibodies (ANCA) and inflammatory bowel diseases in Chinese. Digestive Diseases and Sciences 39: 886–892

Tahir S K, Billing P, Gagne G et al 1994 Nuclear localization of ulcerative colitis specific perinuclear antineutrophil cytoplasmic antibody (pANCA) reactive antigen. American Gastroenterologic Association 1994 Meeting: A2787

Takahasi F, Shah H S, Wise L S, Das K M 1990 Circulating antibodies against human colonic extract enriched with a 40 kDa protein in patients with ulcerative colitis. Gut 31: 1016–1020

Targan S R, Landers C J, MacDermott R P, Vidrich A 1994 Perinuclear antineutrophil cytoplasmic antibodies are spontaneously produced by B-cells from involved and uninvolved mucosa of ulcerative colitis patients. (Submitted)

Tonkonogy S L, McKenzie D T, Swain S L 1989 Regulation of isotype production by IL-4 and IL-5 effects of lymphokines on Ig production depends on the state of activation of the responding B cells. Journal of Immunology 142: 4351–4360

Van der Woude F J, Rasmussen N, Lobatto S et al 1985 Autoantibodies to neutrophils and monocytes: a new tool for diagnosis and a marker of disease activity in Wegener's granulomatosis. Lancet 2: 425–429

Van Spreeuwel J P, Lindeman J, Meijer ACJLM 1985 A quantitative study of immunoglobulin-containing cells in the differential diagnosis of acute colitis. Journal of Clinical Pathology 38: 774–777

Vecchi M, Bianchi M B, Sinico R A et al 1994 Antibodies to neutrophil cytoplasm in Italian patients with ulcerative colitis: sensitivity, specificity and recognition of putative antigens. Digestion 55: 34–39

Wu K C, Mahida Y R, Priddle J D, Jewell D P 1989 Immunoglobulin production by isolated intestinal mononuclear cells from patients with ulcerative colitis and Crohn's disease. Clinical and Experimental Immunology 78: 37–41

Yacyshyn B R, Pilarski L M 1993 Expression of CD45RO on circulating Crohn's disease 19+ B-cells in Crohn's disease. Gut 34: 1698–1704

Yang H, Rotter J I, Toyoda H et al 1993 Ulcerative colitis: a genetically heterogenous disorder defined by genetic (HLA class II) and subclinical (anti-neutrophil cytoplasmic antibodies) markers. Journal of Clinical Investigation 92: 1080–1084

Yang H, Vora D K, Targan S R, Toyoda H, Beaudet A L, Rotter J I 1994 Association of intercellular adhesion molecule-1 (ICAM-1) polymorphisms with subsets of inflammatory bowel disease (IBD) stratified by anti-neutrophil cytoplasmic antibodies (ANCAs) (Submitted)

9. Role of neutrophils in the pathogenesis of inflammatory bowel disease

M. B. Grisham   P. R. Kvietys

INTRODUCTION

Neutrophilic polymorphonuclear leukocytes (neutrophils) are the most prevalent leukocytes in the circulation, comprising approximately 70–80% of the total intravascular pool of leukocytes. The primary function of the neutrophil is to engulf and destroy invading microorganisms. In order to accomplish this task these cells have acquired the ability to synthesize and release large amounts of toxic reactive oxygen metabolites and proteinases. Although this inflammatory response is essential for maintaining normal health, excessive and/or inadvertent recruitment and metabolic activation of neutrophils may result in substantial injury to surrounding tissue (Klebanoff 1992). For example, it is well known that active episodes of inflammatory bowel disease (IBD) are characterized histologically by the extravasation and infiltration of large numbers of neutrophils. This enhanced inflammatory infiltrate is accompanied by extensive mucosal and/or transmural injury, including edema, crypt abscesses, loss of goblet cells, decreased mucus production, erosions and mucosal ulceration. Although it has not been definitively defined whether the neutrophilic infiltrate initiates and/or exacerbates gut injury and dysfunction, there is a growing body of evidence to suggest that pharmacologic or immunologic inhibition of neutrophil function and mediator release attenuates the injury and dysfunction associated with experimental or human IBD (Harris et al 1992, Grisham 1993). Because neutrophils can be observed not only in the gut interstitium but also in the crypt lumen (e.g. crypt abscesses) of the inflamed bowel, it would appear that migration of these cells across the endothelial as well as the epithelial cell barrier is required, and may be important in the development of gut injury and dysfunction.

This chapter describes the molecular interactions between neutrophils and endothelial cells that permit extravasation of neutrophils out of the circulation and into the interstitium; reviews the present state of knowledge regarding the movement of neutrophils within the gut interstitium; characterizes transepithelial migration of neutrophils out of the interstitium and into the crypt lumen; and finally, discusses the biochemical mechanisms by which neutrophils may injure cells and the gut interstitium.

NEUTROPHIL–ENDOTHELIAL CELL INTERACTIONS

One of the cardinal features of acute inflammation is the presence of large numbers of neutrophils in the interstitium of the affected tissue. Neutrophil infiltration of the extravascular space involves a complex sequence of interactions between circulating neutrophils and the vascular endothelium. The initial event is believed to be a weak adhesive interaction which results in neutrophils 'rolling' along the endothelium. Subsequently there is a strengthening of these adhesive forces, such that the neutrophils become attached to the endothelium and remain stationary. Finally, the neutrophils begin to change shape, send out pseudopodia between endothelial cells, and migrate into the interstitium. These adhesive interactions are regulated in an orderly fashion by sequential activation of different families of membrane adherence receptors on neutrophils and endothelial cells (Table 9.1; Fig. 9.1). This section presents a general overview of neutrophil–endothelial cell interactions during acute inflammation. For more comprehensive coverage of specific gastrointestinal inflammatory states the reader is referred to recent reviews (Kvietys & Granger 1993, Granger et al 1993, 1994, Granger & Kubes 1994).

Rolling

In vivo the initial adhesive interaction of neutrophils with vascular endothelium involves the neutrophils moving from the central stream of circulating blood cells toward the vessel wall and subsequent rolling along the endothelium (Schmid-Schönbein et al 1980, Kishimoto 1991). This movement may be due to a hydrodynamic interaction

Table 9.1 Adhesive glycoproteins involved in neutrophil–endothelial cell interactions

Neutrophil adhesion molecules	Family	Surface expression Basal	Stimulated	Stimuli†	Ligand
CD11a/CD18*	β_2 Integrin	Yes	–	a,b,c,k,l,n	ICAM-1, ICAM-2
CD11b/CD18	β_2 Integrin	Yes	↑	a,b,c,d,j,k,l,n	ICAM-1 and others
CD11c/CD18	β_2 Integrin	Yes	↑	a,b,c,d	?
L-selectin	Selectin	Yes	↓	a,c,d,e,f,j	Sialylated moieties (?) P- or E-selectin (?)
PECAM-1	1g supergene	Yes	?	–	PECAM-1
Endothelial cell adhesion molecules					
ICAM-1	1g supergene	Yes	↑	d,e,f,g,k,l,n	CD11a/CD18, CD11b/CD18
ICAM-2	1g supergene	Yes	–	d,e,f,g	CD11a/CD18
E-selectin	Selectin	No	↑	d,e,f	Sialylated Lewis X, L-selectin (?)
P-selectin	Selectin	No	↑	h,i,m	Sialylated Lewis X, L-selectin (?)
PECAM-1	1g supergene	Yes	?	–	PECAM-1

* Alternative designation: CD11a/CD18 (LFA-1), CD11b/CD18 (Mac-1, Mol, CR3, OKM-1), CD11c/CD18 (p150,95,CR4, Lew-M5), L-selectin (LAM-1, LECAM-1, MEL-14, Leu 8, jLHRc, qp100^{MEL}), PECAM-1 (endoCAM, hec7), ICAM-1 (CD54), P-selectin (CD62, PAGEM, GMP-140), E-selectin (ELAM-1).

† a = LTB$_4$; b - fmlp; c = C5a; d = TNF; e = IL-1; f = LPS; g = interferon; h = thrombin; i = histamine; j = PAF; k = anoxia/reoxygenation; l = aspirin; m = H$_2$O$_2$; n = *Helicobacter pylori* extract. (From Andersson 1995, Forrest & Paulson 1995)

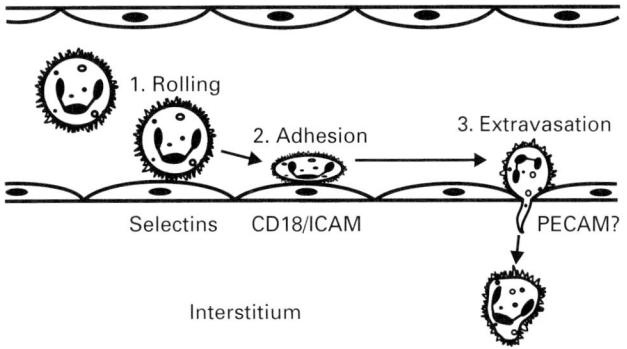

Fig. 9.1 Sequence of events leading to neutrophil rolling, adhesion and extravasation.

between red blood cells and neutrophils as they pass from the smaller-diameter capillaries to the larger-diameter postcapillary venules, i.e. the faster-moving red blood cells displace the neutrophils from the axial stream toward the venular endothelium (Schmid-Schönbein et al 1980). The contribution of red blood cells is underscored by the observation that few neutrophils leave the central stream and approach the venular endothelium when the venules are perfused with leukocyte suspensions devoid of red cells (Bixt et al 1985). The rolling or tumbling of neutrophils along the endothelium is considered to be a result of weak adhesive interactions which are insufficient to overcome the effects of the shear stress along the vessel wall. In-vitro studies indicate that anywhere from 20 to 90% of the neutrophils interacting with endothelial cells are rolling along the monolayer (Smith et al 1990).

The selectins, L-selectin of neutrophils and the P- and E-selectins of endothelial cells, have been implicated in this neutrophils rolling (Lasky 1992, Granger & Kubes 1994). L-selectin is constitutively expressed on quiescent neutrophils, whereas, P- and E-selectins appear on the surface of activated endothelium (McEver 1991a,b). E-selectin mobilization to the surface requires protein synthesis, and maximum surface levels are achieved several hours after activation, with a return to basal levels within 12–24 hours. Very little is known regarding the role of this adhesion molecule in vivo. Koizumi et al (1992) and Nakamura et al (1993) have demonstrated that E-selectin (ELAM-1) is dramatically upregulated on the surface of endothelial cells in mucosa obtained from patients with active but not quiescent ulcerative or Crohn's colitis. Furthermore, Podolsky et al (1993) have shown that two different antibodies to E-selectin did not attenuate the spontaneous colitis that develops in cottontop tamarins. These data suggest that E-selectin-dependent neutrophil adherence is not necessary to sustain the inflammatory response. The authors suggest that if E-selectin is not necessary to promote neutrophil migration into the colonic mucosa, then pathways for neutrophil adhesion must exist in the inflamed colon (Podolsky et al 1993). P-selectin, on the other hand, is rapidly mobilized to the endothelial cell surface, reaching peak levels within 3–10 minutes. The expression of P-selectin is very transient, decreasing to negligible levels within minutes owing to internalization of the selectin via endocytosis. Interestingly, some stimuli (e.g. oxidants) can activate endothelial cells in such a manner that P-selectin expression is prolonged for up to 3 hours (Patel et al 1991). In addition, Nakamura et al (1993) have shown that P-selectin is upregulated in the venules of mucosa obtained from patients with active IBD.

The ligands for the selectins have not been firmly established, but are thought to be sialyl-Lewis x and other fucosylated carbohydrates (Springer & Lasky 1991). A direct interaction between the selectins is also possible, i.e. neutrophil L-selectin with the P- or E-selectin on endothelium (Picker et al 1991). Evidence for the latter contention is provided by in-vitro studies in which neutrophil rolling was studied on artificial lipid membranes (Lawrence & Springer 1991). Neutrophil rolling was observed on membranes containing P-selectin, and the rolling velocity increased with increasing shear stress. For a given shear stress the greater the density of P-selectin in the membranes the lower the velocity of rolling, presumably owing to the greater number of adhesive interactions possible with larger densities. Similar phenomena have been observed using E-selectin-enriched lipid membranes (Kishimoto 1991).

Adhesion

It is believed (Kishimoto 1991) that the rolling of neutrophils keeps them in close apposition to the endothelium, thereby facilitating their activation by inflammatory mediators generated by the endothelium or resident interstitial cells (e.g. mast cells). Activated neutrophils adhere to the venular endothelium (despite the shear stress of flowing blood) by virtue of the strong adhesive interactions between the integrins (CD11/CD18) on neutrophils and ICAM-1 on endothelial cells. Support for this hypothesis is provided by in-vitro observations that neutrophil rolling was negligible on artificial lipid membranes containing only ICAM-1 (Smith 1992). In contrast, on lipid membranes containing both ICAM-1 and P-selectin, neutrophil rolling was observed and ceased within 5 minutes of activation owing to avid adherence of the neutrophils to the membranes. In-vivo studies indicate that neutralization of L-selectin function or removal of L-selectin from the neutrophils prevents firm adhesion to venules exposed to inflammatory mediators (Granger & Kubes 1994). These latter observations support the contention that selectin-mediated rolling is a prerequisite for CD11/CD18-ICAM-1 mediated adhesion.

Upon activation, the neutrophils shed their L-selectin and upregulate and/or activate their integrins (Kishimoto et al 1989). The β_2 integrins on neutrophils are heterodimers consisting of a common β subunit (CD18) non-covalently linked to one of three immunologically distinct α subunits, designated CD11a, CD11b and CD11c (Table 9.1). CD11a/CD18 is basally expressed on the surface of neutrophils and interacts with ICAM-1 and ICAM-2 on endothelial cells to promote adhesive interactions (Marlin & Springer 1987). The addition of unstimulated neutrophils to naive or cytokine-stimulated endothelial cell monolayers in vitro results in neutrophil adherence to the endothelial cells, which is inhibitable by monoclonal antibodies (MAbs) directed against CD11a/CD18 or ICAM-1 (Smith et al 1989). Since CD11a/CD18 is not stored to any appreciable extent in neutrophil granules, there is no reserve from which to mobilize additional CD11a/CD18 to the surface of the neutrophil upon activation. A variety of inflammatory mediators or cytokines are unable to increase the expression of CD11a/CD18 on the surface of neutrophils (Table 9.1). Nakamura et al (1993) have demonstrated that CD11a/CD18 is upregulated in mucosal mononuclear cells in patients with active IBD. In contrast, most of the CD11b/CD18 and CD11c/CD18 adherence glycoproteins are stored in neutrophil granules and can be rapidly (within minutes) mobilized to the surface of neutrophils by fusion of granule membranes with the cell membrane upon stimulation (Carlos & Harlan 1990, Larson & Springer 1990). Stimulation of neutrophils with inflammatory mediators or cytokines results in a three- to tenfold increase in the expression of CD11b/CD18 and CD11c/CD18 on the neutrophil surface. Both anti-CD11a and anti-CD11b MAbs can inhibit the adherence of activated neutrophils to cytokine-stimulated endothelial cell monolayers. When these two MAbs are used simultaneously their inhibitory effects are greater than when either is used alone. Since anti-ICAM-1 MAb is as effective as the combination of anti-CD11a and anti-CD11b MAbs in inhibiting neutrophil adherence, it appears that the CD11b is also using endothelial ICAM-1 as a ligand (Larson & Springer 1990). However, CD11b can also use other ligands to induce adherence to endothelial cells, such as polysaccharide moieties, factor X and other non-specific ligands (as exemplified by the CD11b-dependent adherence of activated neutrophils to inert substrates such as plastic). Although the expression of CD11c is also increased on activated neutrophils, its contribution to neutrophil adhesion to endothelial cells is minimal (Carlos & Harlan 1990). Indeed, in most adhesion assays the inhibitory effect of combinations of anti-CD11a and anti-CD11b MAbs is equivalent to the inhibitory effects of an anti-CD18 MAb (MAb directed against all three of the heterodimers). Taken together, these observations indicate that adhesion of unstimulated neutrophils to endothelium is exclusively dependent on CD11a–ICAM-1 interactions, whereas adhesion of activated neutrophils is dependent on both CD11a and CD11b interactions with ICAM-1.

The avidity with which neutrophils bind to endothelial cells cannot simply be ascribed to changes in surface levels of integrins. For example, under certain conditions neutrophil activators can increase surface levels of CD11b/CD18 on neutrophils without promoting homotypic aggregation (Buyon et al 1990). Alternatively, others have shown that neutrophil activators can increase the avidity of CD11b/CD18 without altering cell surface levels of the glycoprotein (Schwartz & Harlan 1989, Hermanowski-Vosatka et al 1992). These types of observations indicate that neutrophil–endothelial cell interactions involve activation as well as recruitment of neutrophil integrins, and that these two events are independently regulated (Buyon et al 1990). The mechanisms involved in integrin activation are not completely understood, but may involve processes such as conformational changes in the integrins, integrin clustering and/or phosphorylation.

ICAM-1 and ICAM-2 are endothelial cell adhesion molecules which are members of the immunoglobulin supergene family (Carlos & Harlan 1990, Springer 1990, Montefort & Holgate 1991). ICAM-1 contains five Ig-like extracellular domains, of which the first NH_2-terminal Ig-like domain recognizes CD11a/CD18, and the third Ig-like domain recognizes CD11b/CD18 (Diamond et al 1991). ICAM-1 is basally expressed on endothelial cells, and its expression is increased in response to activation of endothelial cells with cytokines (Table 9.1). Maximal expression of ICAM-1 is achieved within 4–8 hours after activating the endothelial cells, and is associated with maximal levels of neutrophil adherence. The mechanism by which ICAM-1 is increased on the cell surface is unclear, but the process involves protein synthesis. ICAM-2 is a truncated form of ICAM-1, containing only two Ig-like extracellular domains (Staunton et al 1989). Like ICAM-1, ICAM-2 is also basally expressed on endothelial cells, but its level of expression is higher (tenfold) than that of ICAM-1 (de Fougerolles et al 1991). In contrast to ICAM-1, ICAM-2 expression is not increased on cytokine-activated endothelial cells (Table 9.1). Malizia et al (1991) and Nakamura et al (1993) have demonstrated enhanced expression of ICAM-1 by mucosal mononuclear cells in biopsies obtained from patients with active ulcerative colitis and Crohn's disease.

Transendothelial migration

After neutrophils have adhered to the endothelium they send pseudopodia between the endothelial cells and migrate into the interstitium. Based on studies using blocking antibodies, neutrophil transmigration across endothelial cell monolayers appears to require CD18–ICAM-1 interactions (Smith 1992). However, it is unclear from these types of studies whether the transmigration process is selectively blocked or whether adhesion of neutrophils, and therefore transmigration, is blocked. Recently, an adhesion molecule, PECAM-1, has been identified which appears to be intimately involved in neutrophil transmigration (Muller et al 1993, Bogen et al 1994). PECAM-1 is preferentially distributed between endothelial cells (intercellular junctions) and the transmigration process appears to involve homotypic adhesive interactions between PECAM-1 on neutrophils and endothelial cells. MAb directed to PECAM-1 blocks neutrophil transmigration without preventing adhesion (Muller et al 1993). Future work should elucidate the precise adhesive interactions involved in the transendothelial migration of neutrophils.

NEUTROPHIL–EPITHELIAL CELL INTERACTIONS

Once extravasated, neutrophils may move through the interstitium in response to certain chemotactic stimuli, including bacterial products and proinflammatory mediators released by the inflamed and/or injured tissue, as well as by bacterial products that have made their way into the interstitium. It is probably this directed migration through the interstitium that ultimately allows the neutrophils to emigrate out of the tissue and into the crypt lumen. Relatively little information is available regarding the movement of neutrophils through the interstitium. The interstitial matrix is composed primarily of a fibrous network of collagen, elastin and glycosaminoglycans. Depending upon the degree of hydration this matrix has been estimated to contain pores with dimensions of 250–1000 Å. These estimates would suggest that neutrophils, even with their ability to readily deform and elongate, would experience significant resistance to movement through the interstitial matrix. A recent study by Bienvenu et al (1994), using intravital microscopic examination of the rat mesentery, has determined that exposure of the mesentery to N-formyl-methionyl-leucyl-phenylalanine (FMLP), leukotriene B_4 (LTB_4), platelet activating factor (PAF) or ischemia and reperfusion, enhanced rates of neutrophil interstitial migration from a mean value of 3.0 μm/min in the unstimulated state to rates of 6–8 μm/min. FMLP-mediated movement of interstitial neutrophils was not inhibited by either elastase or cathepsin G inhibitors, nor by the addition of a monoclonal antibody directed against neutrophil CD11/CD18 (Bienvenu et al 1994). Taken together, these data suggest that interstitial movement of neutrophils activated by various proinflammatory mediators does not require the proteolytic activity of elastase or cathepsin G, nor do the cells require the specific interaction of their adhesion glycoproteins (CD11/CD18) with receptors on the matrix protein.

One of the interesting histologic features of active IBD is the presence of crypt abscesses (Fig. 9.2). In order for neutrophils to be present within the lumen of the crypts, these inflammatory cells must not only have had to extravasate from the circulation and move through the interstitial matrix, but they must also have had to interact with the basement membrane and basolateral surface of the crypt epithelium, and emigrated out of the gut and into the lumen. One would assume that the driving force for this directed migration out of the tissue is provided by the bacterial gradient present in the distal bowel. Indeed, it has been suggested that a major route of elimination of granulocytes (eosinophils, neutrophils) under normal or non-pathological conditions is via diapedesis through the gut epithelial barrier (Teir et al 1963, Arndt et al 1992).

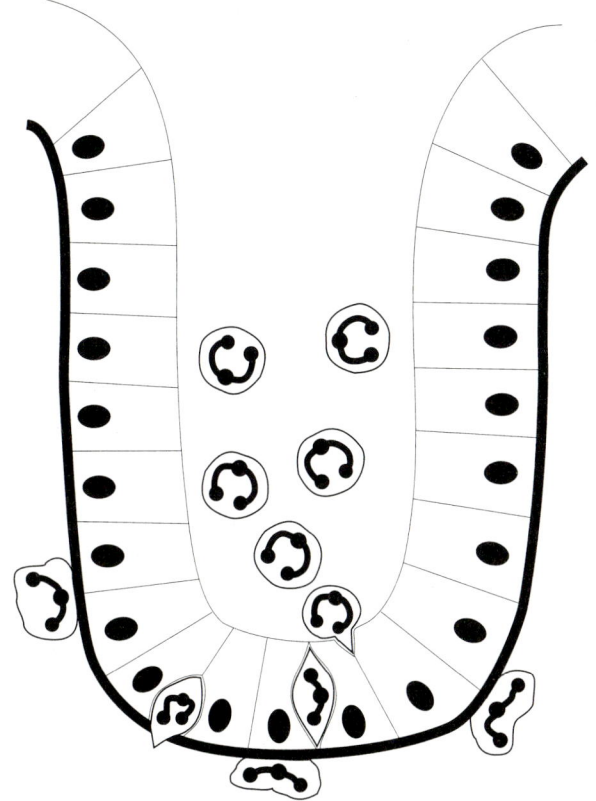

Fig. 9.2 Transepithelial migration of neutrophils and crypt abscess formation.

Active episodes of IBD appear to involve the recruitment of very large numbers of neutrophils out of the circulation and into the interstitium. A chemotactic gradient is apparently established between the interstitium and the crypt lumen, presumably by bacterial products such as FMLP, LPS (lipopolysaccharide) etc. Recent work by Parkos and colleagues (1991) has demonstrated that neutrophil migration across epithelial cells in the basolateral to apical direction (physiological direction of migration) is inhibited 75–85% by antibodies directed against C11b and CD18, but not by antibodies to CD11a or CD11c. Recent antibodies directed against ICAM-1 (known to be the ligand for CD11b/CD18-mediated *transendothelial* migration) did not interfere with the transmigration of neutrophils across epithelial monolayers. Parkos et al concluded that ligands for CD11b/CD18 for neutrophil epithelial interaction are distinct from the CD11b/CD18 ligands for transendothelial cell migration (Parkos et al 1991). These investigators have demonstrated that L-selectin-mediated events do not play a role in neutrophil transmigration (Parkos et al 1991).

Transepithelial migration of neutrophils may account for some of the pathophysiology associated with active episodes of IBD. For example, FMLP-mediated diapedesis of neutrophils across epithelial monolayers in vitro results in a reversible increase in paracellular permeability, as measured by decreased resistance and increased fluxes of small molecular solutes across the monolayer (Parkos et al 1991). During times of intense intestinal inflammation, epithelial cell barrier function may be significantly compromised there, allowing the influx of a variety of pro-inflammatory agents into the interstitium from the lumen. In addition, neutrophils release small molecular weight factors that interact with intestinal epithelial cells to promote Cl^- and water secretion. For example, neutrophil-generated oxidants such as hydrogen peroxide or monochloramine are known to promote Cl^- secretion when applied to the basolateral surface of T_{84} monolayers (Parkos et al 1991, Tamai et al 1992). These data suggest that neutrophils cross the basement membrane and interact with the basolateral aspect of the epithelial plasma membrane. NH_2Cl and possibly other reactive oxygen species may enhance Cl^- secretion and thus may mediate some of the diarrhea known to be associated with active IBD. Nash et al (1991) and Madara et al (1992) have described a low molecular weight factor released by neutrophils which, when applied to the apical but not the basolateral surface of T_{84} cells, induces Cl^- secretion. They have identified this factor as 5'AMP (adenosine monophosphate) (Madara et al 1993). In reality, 5'AMP is metabolized to adenosine by the action of an ectoenzyme located on the apical surface of the endothelial cells. Adenosine is then recognized by specific adenosine receptors located on the apical surface of the epithelial cell, which ultimately induces Cl^- secretion (Thompson et al 1990, Madara et al 1993). Data derived from these studies suggest that the presence of crypt abscesses may not necessarily represent a functionless end-product of neutrophil transepithelial migration. Indeed, neutrophils within the crypt lumen may mediate Cl^- and fluid secretion via the release of 5'AMP.

The neutrophil infiltrate in both ulcerative colitis and Crohn's disease suggests that neutrophils are well capable of migrating through the mucosa; nevertheless, the intriguing resemblance to Crohn's disease of the intestinal manifestations of chronic granulomatous disease, an inherited neutrophil disorder, has prompted several groups to look for defects in neutrophil function. One of the more consistent defects found has been reduced neutrophil chemotaxis into skin window chambers containing patient's serum and placed overlying abraded skin (Segal & Loewi 1976). Further studies suggest that there is no defect in the mobility of the peripheral blood neutrophils in vitro (O'Morain et al 1981, Rhodes & Jewell 1983), but that the sera of patients with Crohn's disease contains inhibitors of chemotaxis (D'Amelio et al 1981, Rhodes et al 1982). A more recent study reports the intriguing findings that Crohn's disease patients are particularly prone to periodontal infection with *Wolinella* spp., and that these bacteria release a potent inhibitor of chemotaxis that is sufficient to alter the serum chemotactic activity (Van Dyke et al 1986).

MECHANISMS OF NEUTROPHIL-MEDIATED TISSUE INJURY

During the course of transendothelial, interstitial and/or transepithelial cell migration of neutrophils, these phagocytes may interact with a variety of proinflammatory agents, such as LTB_4, PAF, immune complexes, complement components or bacterial products (e.g. fMLP, lipopolysaccharide). Interaction of these agents with specific receptors on the neutrophil plasma membrane results in the activation of the latent, plasma membrane-associated NADPH (nicotinamide-adenine-dinucleotide phosphate) oxidase (Klebanoff 1992). Activation of this multicomponent flavoprotein results in the production and release of large amounts of superoxide (O_2^-) and hydrogen peroxide (H_2O_2) as well the myeloperoxidase (MPO)-derived oxidants hypochlorous acid (HOCl) and N-chloramines (RNHCl; Fig. 9.3). In addition to their well characterized cytotoxic properties, H_2O_2, HOCl and certain RNHCls possess several different biological properties. For example, these oxidants are known to promote chloride (Cl^-) secretion, enhance mucosal permeability and increase the resting tension of ileal smooth muscle strips while inhibiting the contractility of electrically stimulated ileal smooth muscle strips (reviewed in Grisham 1994). Furthermore, H_2O_2 and certain RNHCls have been shown to promote mutagenesis in a number of different prokaryotic as well as eukaryotic systems (reviewed in Grisham 1994).

In addition to MPO-generated oxidants, reactive metabolites of oxygen may also be generated by the interaction between H_2O_2 and certain hemoproteins, such as hemoglobin or myoglobin, to yield activated heme plus amino acid radicals, both of which are capable of causing oxidative damage to lipids, protein and carbohydrates (Grisham 1992). Another mechanism by which reactive radicals may be generated at sites of inflammation is by the interaction between O_2^- and the free radical nitric oxide (NO) to produce peroxynitrite (Beckman et al 1990). Several recent studies have demonstrated that active episodes of colonic inflammation in humans or animal models of IBD are associated with enhanced NO production (Boughton-Smith et al 1993, Grisham et al 1994). In fact, NO or NO-derived metabolites may play an important role in mediating some of the pathophysiology associated with some of the models of experimental IBD (Grisham et al 1994). It is known, for example, that NO will rapidly and spontaneously react with molecular oxygen (O_2) to yield a variety of nitrogen oxides:

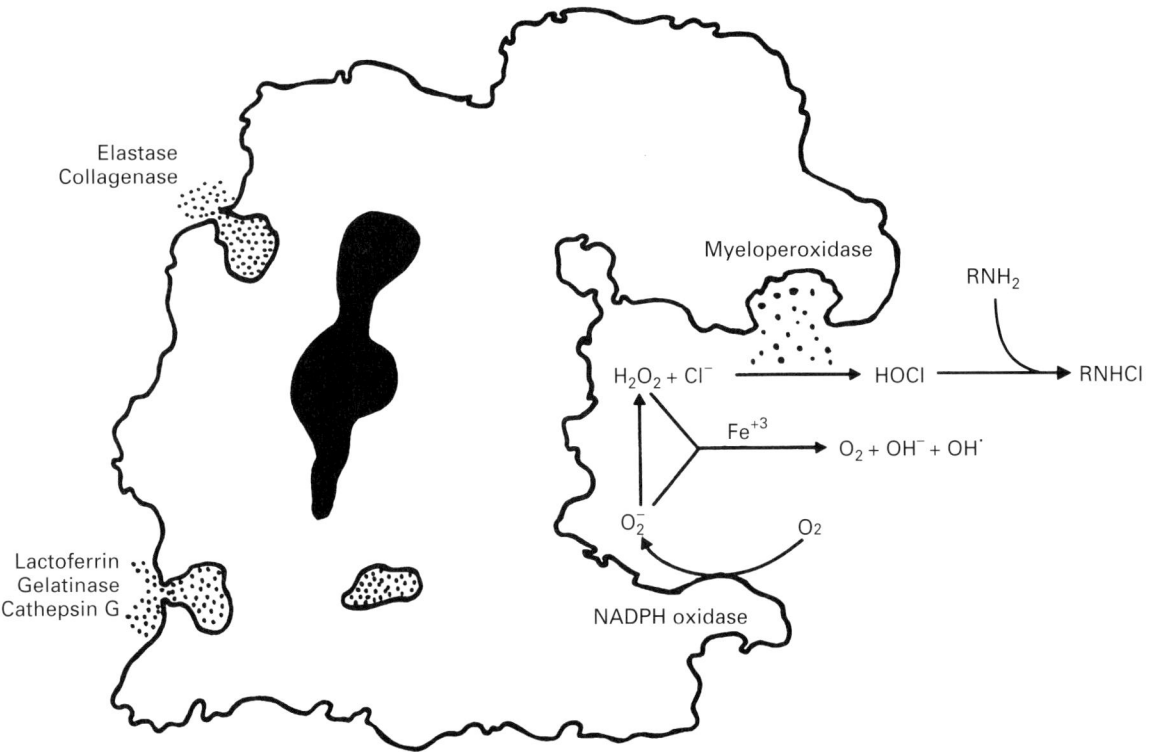

Fig. 9.3 Metabolic activation of neutrophils to produce reactive oxygen metabolites and secrete proteinases. RNH_2 and RNHCl represent primary amines and N-chloramines, respectively.

$$2NO + O_2 \longrightarrow 2NO_2$$
$$2NO + 2NO_2 \longrightarrow 2N_2O_3$$
$$2N_2O_3 + 2H_2O \longrightarrow 4NO_2^- + 4H^+$$

where NO_2, N_2O_3 and NO_2^- represent nitrogen dioxide, dinitrogen trioxide and nitrite, respectively. Dinitrogen trioxide and NO_2 are potent oxidizing and N-nitrosating agents. NO or NO-derived species have been demonstrated to mediate cellular injury and may enhance electrolyte and H_2O secretion (reviewed in Moncada & Higgs 1993). Whether or not NO mediates its pro-inflammatory activity directly or indirectly via its interaction with O_2 or O_2^- remains to be determined.

In addition to direct effects, neutrophil-derived oxidants may damage the epithelium and mucosal interstitium indirectly by altering the proteinase/antiproteinase balance that normally exists within the intestinal interstitium. For example, HOCl (and possibly other lipophilic RNHCls and reactive nitrogen intermediates) may inactivate proteinase inhibitors such as α_1-proteinase inhibitor and α_2 macroglobulin present in the extracellular fluid (plasma, lymph), thus allowing for uncontrolled proteolysis by elastase (reviewed in Weiss 1989). Weiss and colleagues have suggested that the extracellular MPO system (HOCl) may activate the latent collagenase and gelatinase secreted by neutrophils (Weiss 1989). Taken together, these data suggest that oxidative inactivation of important proteinase inhibitors coupled to the oxidant-mediated activation of latent proteases creates an environment favorable for elastase, collagenase and gelatinase-mediated degradation of the mucosal interstitial matrix and epithelial cells.

REFERENCES

Anderson D C 1995 The role of β_2 integrins and intercellular adhesion molecule type 1 in inflammation. In: Granger D N, Schmid-Schönbein G W (eds.) Physiology and pathophysiology of leukocyte adhesion. Oxford Press, NY, pp. 3–42

Arndt H, Kubes P, Grisham M B, Gonzalez E, Granger D N 1992 Granulocyte turnover in the feline intestine. Inflammation 16: 549–559

Beckman J S, Beckman T W, Chen J, Marshall F A, Freeman B A 1990 Apparent hydroxyl radical production by peroxynitrite: implication for endothelial injury from nitric oxide and superoxide. Proceedings of the National Academy of Sciences of the USA 87: 1620–1624

Bienvenu K, Harris N, Granger D N 1994 Modulation of leukocyte migration in mesenteric interstitium. American Journal of Physiology 267: H1573–1577

Bixt A, Johnson P, Braide M, Bagge U 1985 Microscopic studies on the influence of erythrocyte concentration on the postjunctional radial distribution of leukocytes at small venule bifurcations. International Journal of Microcirculation: Clinical and Experimental 4: 141–156

Bogen S, Pak J, Garifallou M, Deng X, Muller W A 1994 Monoclonal antibody to murine PECAM-1 (CD31) blocks acute inflammation in vivo. Journal of Experimental Medicine 179: 1059–1064

Boughton-Smith N K, Evans S M, Hawkey C J et al 1993 Nitric oxide synthase activity in ulcerative colitis and Crohn's disease. Lancet 342: 338–340

Buyon J P, Phillips M R, Abramson S B, Slade S G, Weissman G, Winchester R 1990 Mechanism regulating recruitment of CD11b/CD18 to the cell surface is distinct from that which induces adhesion in homotypic neutrophil aggregation. In: Springer T A, Anderson D C, Rosenthal A S, Rothlein R, (eds) Leukocyte adhesion molecules: structure, function, and regulation. Springer-Verlag, New York, pp 72–83

Carlos T M, Harlan J M 1990 Membrane proteins involved in phagocyte adherence to endothelium. Immunology Review 114: 5–28

D'Amelio R, Rossi P, LeMoli S et al 1981 In vitro studies on cellular and humoral chemotaxis in Crohn's disease using the under agarose technique. Gut 22: 566–570

de Fougerolles A R, Stacker S A, Schwarting R, Springer T A 1991 Characterization of ICAM-2 and evidence for a third counter-receptor for LFA-1. Journal of Experimental Medicine 174: 253–267

Diamond M S, Staunton D E, Marlin S D, Springer T A 1991 Binding of the integrin Mac-1 (CD11b/CD18) to the third immunoglobulin-like domain of ICAM-1 (CD54) and its regulation by glycosylation. Cell 65: 961–971

Forrest M, Paulson J C 1995 Selectin family of adhesion molecules. In: Granger D N, Schmid-Schönbein G W, (eds) Physiology and pathophysiology of leukocyte adhesion. Oxford Press, NY, pp. 43–80

Granger D N, Kubes P 1994 The microcirculation and inflammation: modulation of leukocyte–endothelial cell adhesion. Journal of Leukocyte Biology 55: 662–675

Granger D N, Grisham M B, Kvietys P R 1994 Mechanisms of microvascular injury. In: Johnson L R (ed), Physiology of the gastrointestinal tract. Raven Press, New York, pp 1693–1722

Granger D N, Kvietys P R, Perry M A 1993 Leukocyte–endothelial cell adhesion induced by ischemia and reperfusion. Canadian Journal of Physiology and Pharmacology 71: 67–75

Grisham M B 1992 Reactive metabolites of oxygen and nitrogen in biology and medicine. R G Landes, Austin, Texas

Grisham M B 1993 Role of reactive oxygen metabolites in inflammatory bowel disease. Current Opinion in Gastroenterology 9: 971–980

Grisham M B 1994 Oxidants and free radicals in inflammatory bowel disease. Lancet 344: 859–861

Grisham M B, Specian R D, Zimmerman T E 1994 Effects of nitric oxide synthase inhibition on the pathophysiology observed in a model of chronic granulomatous colitis. Journal of Pharmacology and Experimental Therapeutics 221: 1–8

Harris M L, Schiller H J, Reily P M, Donowitz M, Grisham M B, Bulkley G B 1992 Free radicals and other reactive oxygen metabolites in inflammatory bowel disease. Cause, consequence, or epiphenomenon? Pharmacology and Therapeutics 53: 375–408

Hermanowski-Vosatka A, Van Strijp J A G, Swiggard W J, Wright S D 1992 Integrin modulating factor-1: a lipid that alters the function of leukocyte integrins. Cell 68: 341–352

Kishimoto T K 1991 A dynamic model for neutrophil localization to inflammatory sites. Journal of the National Institutes for Health Research 3: 75–77

Kishimoto T K, Jutila M A, Berg E L, Butcher E C 1989 Neutrophil Mac-1 and MEL-14 adhesion proteins inversely regulated by chemotactic factors. Science 245: 1238–1241

Klebanoff S J 1992 Oxygen metabolites from phagocytes. In: Gallin J I, Goldstein I M, Snyderman R (eds) Inflammation: basic principles and clinical correlates. Raven Press, New York, pp 541–588

Koizumi M, King N, Lobb R, Benjamin C, Podolsky K 1992 Expression of vascular adhesion molecules in inflammatory bowel disease. Gastroenterology 103: 840–847

Kvietys P R, Granger D N 1993 The vascular endothelium in GI inflammation. In: Wallace J (ed) Immunopharmacology of the gastrointestinal system. Academic Press, London, pp 69–103

Larson R S, Springer T A 1990 Structure and function of leukocyte integrins. Immunology Review 114: 181–217

Lasky L A 1992 The homing receptor (LECAM 1/L selectin): a carbohydrate-binding mediator of adhesion in the immune system. In: Harlan J M, Liu D Y, (eds) Adhesion: its role in inflammatory disease. W H Freeman, New York, pp 43–63

Lawrence M B, Springer T A 1991 Leukocytes roll on a selectin at physiologic flow rates: distinction from and prerequisite for adhesion through integrins. Cell 65: 859–873

McEver R P 1991a GMP-140, a receptor that mediates interactions of leukocytes with activated platelets and endothelium. Trends in Cardiovascular Medicine 1: 152–156

McEver R P 1991b Selectins: novel receptors that mediate leukocyte adhesion during inflammation. Thrombosis and Haemostasis 65: 223–228

Madara J L, Parkos C A, Colgan S P et al 1992 Cl^- secretion in a model intestinal epithelium induced by a neutrophil-derived secretagogue. Journal of Clinical Investigation 89: 1938–1944

Madara J L, Patapoff T W, Gillece-Castro B et al 1993 5'AMP is the neutrophil-derived paracrine factor that elicits chloride secretion from T_{84} epithelial monolayers. Journal of Clinical Investigation 91: 2320–2325

Malizia G, Calabrese A, Cottone M et al 1991 Expression of leukocyte adhesion molecules by mucosal mononuclear phagocytes in inflammatory bowel disease. Gastroenterology 100: 150–159

Marlin S D, Springer T A 1987 Purified intercellular adhesion molecule-1 (ICAM-1) is a ligand for lymphocyte function-associated antigen 1 (LFA-1). Cell 51: 813–819

Moncada S, Higgs A 1993 The L-arginine–nitric oxide pathway. New England Journal of Medicine 329: 2002–2012

Montefort S, Holgate S T 1991 Adhesion molecules and their role in inflammation. Respiratory Medicine 85: 91–99

Muller W, Seigl S A, Deng X, Phillips D M 1993 PECAM-1 is required for transendothelial migration of leukocytes. Journal of Experimental Medicine 178: 449–460

Nakamura S, Ohtani H, Watanabe Y et al 1993 In situ cell adhesion molecules in inflammatory bowel disease: evidence of immunologic activation of vascular endothelial cells. Laboratory Investigation 69: 77–85

Nash S, Parkos C A, Nusrat A, Delp C, Madara J L 1991 In vitro model of intestinal crypt abscess: a novel neutrophil-derived secretagogue activity. Journal of Clinical Investigation 87: 1474–1477

O'Morain C O, Segal A A, Walker D, Levi A J 1981 Abnormalities of neutrophil function do not cause the migration defect in Crohn's disease. Gut 22: 817–820

Parkos C A, Delp C, Arnaout M A, Madara J L 1991 Neutrophil migration across a cultured intestinal epithelium: dependence on a CD11b/CD18-mediated event and enhanced efficiency in the physiologic direction. Journal of Clinical Investigation 88: 1605–1612

Patel K D, Zimmerman G A, Prescott S M, McEver R P, McIntyre T M 1991 Oxygen radicals induce human endothelial cells to express GMP-140 and bind neutrophils. Journal of Cell Biology 112: 749–759

Picker L J, Warnock R A, Burns A R, Doerschuk C M, Berg E L, Butcher E C 1991 The neutrophil selectin LECAM-1 presents carbohydrate ligands to the vascular selectins ELAM-1 and GMP-140. Cell 66: 921–933

Podolsky D, Lobb R, King N, Benjamin C, Pepinsky B, Sehgal P, deBeaumont M 1993 Attenuation of colitis in the cotton-top tamarin by anti-α_4 integrin monoclonal antibody. Journal of Clinical Investigation 92: 372–380

Rhodes J M, Potter B J, Brown D J C, Jewell D P 1982 Serum inhibitors of leukocyte chemotaxis in Crohn's disease and ulcerative colitis. Gastroenterology 82: 1327–1384

Rhodes J M, Jewell D P 1983 Motility of neutrophils and monocytes in Crohn's disease and ulcerative colitis

Schmid-Schönbein G W, Usami S, Skalak R, Chien S 1980 The interaction of leukocytes and erythrocytes in capillary and postcapillary vessels. Microvascular Research 19: 45–70

Schwartz B R, Harlan J M 1989 Sulfhydryl reducing agents promote neutrophil adherence without increasing surface expression of CD11b/CD18 (Mac-1, Mo 1). Biochemistry Biophysics Research Communications 165: 51–57

Segal A W, Loewi E 1976 Neutrophil dysfunction in Crohn's disease. Lancet 2: 219–221

Smith C W 1992 Transendothelial migration. In: Harlan J M, Kiu D Y (eds) Adhesion: its role in inflammatory disease. W H Freeman, New York, pp 83–115

Smith C W, Marlin S D, Rothlein R, Toman C, Anderson D C 1989 Cooperative interactions of LFA-1 and Mac-1 with intercellular adhesion molecule-1 in facilitating adherence and transendothelial migration of human neutrophils in vitro. Journal of Clinical Investigation 83: 2008–2017

Smith C W, Marlin S D, Rothlein R, Lawrence M B, McIntire L V, Anderson D C 1990 Role of ICAM-1 in the adherence of human neutrophils to human endothelial cells in vitro. In: Springer T A, Anderson D C, Rosenthal A S, Rothlein R (eds) Leukocyte adhesion molecules: structure, function and regulation. Springer-Verlag, New York, pp 170–189

Springer T A 1990 Adhesion receptors of the immune system. Nature 346: 425–434

Springer T A, Lasky L A 1991 Sticky sugars for selectins. Nature 349: 196–197

Staunton D E, Dustin M L, Springer T A 1989 Functional cloning of ICAM-2, a cell adhesion ligand for LFA-1 homologous to ICAM-1. Nature 339: 61–64

Tamai H, Gaginella T S, Musch M W, Chang E B 1992 Ca-mediated stimulation of Cl^- secretion by reactive oxygen metabolites in human colonic T_{84} cells. Journal of Clinical Investigation 89: 301–307

Teir H, Rytomaa T, Cederberg A, Kiviniemi K 1963 Studies on the elimination of granulocytes in the intestinal tract in the rat. Acta Pathologica Microbiologica Scandinavica 59: 311–324

Thompson L F, Rueoi J M, Glass A et al 1990 Production and characterization of monoclonal antibodies to the glycosyl phosphatidylinositol-anchored lymphocyte differentiation ecto-5'nucleotidase (CD73). Tissue Antigens 35: 9–19

Van Dyke T E, Dowell V R, Offenbacher S, Snyder W, Hersh T 1986 Potential role of microorganisms isolated from periodontal lesions in the pathogenesis of inflammatory bowel disease. Infection and immunity 53: 671–672

Weiss S J 1989 Tissue destruction by neutrophils. New England Journal of Medicine 320: 365–376

10. Monocytes and macrophages in inflammatory bowel disease

Y. R. Mahida

Intestinal inflammation and tissue damage due to migration into the mucosa by circulating monocytes, polymorphonuclear cells and lymphocytes leads to the symptoms associated with active inflammatory bowel disease. During induction of clinical remission, there is resolution of the inflammatory response followed by tissue repair and remodeling, often with a return to a histologically normal intestinal mucosa. The processes of induction, mediation and resolution of inflammatory responses in any tissue require the coordinated actions of many cell types, but the macrophage has a prominent role in all the stages involved. There is a large resident population of macrophages in the human gastrointestinal tract which, together with other cell types (epithelial cells and lymphocytes), are important in host defence against a large array of luminal antigens and microorganisms. In inflammatory bowel disease, penetration by microbes and their products (such as lipopolysaccharide) may exacerbate the mucosal disease via their potent biological effects on macrophages.

There is an increase in the number of intestinal macrophages in active inflammatory bowel disease, and they are especially prominent in the form of granulomata in Crohn's disease. Over the last 20 years there has been an increasing interest in the role of circulating monocytes and intestinal macrophages in the pathogenesis of inflammatory bowel disease. This has coincided with a greater understanding of macrophage cell biology, in particular their capacity to perform a wide range of functions.

GENERAL ASPECTS OF MONOCYTE/MACROPHAGE CELL BIOLOGY

Circulating monocytes and tissue macrophages are heterogeneous cells that are part of the mononuclear phagocyte system (Auger & Ross 1992). They arise from the bone marrow from myeloid-restricted progenitors (which also give rise to granulocytes), which differentiate under the influence of colony-stimulating factors into monocyte-restricted progeny. Monocytes enter the bloodstream after further stages of differentiation and, in humans, circulate for 1–4 days before migrating into tissue to differentiate into macrophages. These resident tissue macrophages assume characteristics normally required for specialized functions in their different microenvironments, such as in the liver (Kupffer cells), lungs (alveolar macrophages), spleen and intestine.

In an inflammatory response large numbers of circulating monocytes migrate preferentially into the injured tissue. The specificity of this response is mediated via interactions between monocytes in circulation and vascular endothelial cells in the injured tissue, and the molecular mechanisms involved in such interactions are being characterized. After stimulation by lipopolysaccharide (which is the outer membrane glycolipid of Gram-negative bacteria) or by cytokines such as interleukin (IL)-1 and tumor necrosis factor-α (TNFα), vascular endothelial cells are induced to express multiple adhesion molecules. These interact with adhesion molecules (designated integrins) expressed on the surface of circulating monocytes to mediate the processes of initial attachment to slow cell transit (cell rolling), followed by stable adhesion, spreading and subsequent diapedesis. Migration of monocytes into the tissues occurs under a chemotactic gradient provided by peptides such as RANTES ('Regulated upon Activation in Normal T cells, Expressed and Secreted') and monocyte chemotactic and activating factor (MCAF).

Monocytes and macrophages are versatile cells with a capacity for carrying out a wide range of functions. Their ability to phagocytose microorganisms has been recognized for over 100 years. Recent studies have shown that in addition to foreign substances, macrophages also phagocytose host cells undergoing programmed cell death (apoptosis), following their specific recognition (Savill et al 1993). The other functions of macrophages can be broadly divided into those maintaining tissue homeostasis and those mediating immunological and inflammatory responses.

Some macrophage functions, such as the induction of immunological responses to foreign antigens, require direct cell–cell interactions. Following its uptake by macrophages, a foreign antigen is processed and presented on the cell surface, in association with MHC class II molecules, to T cells bearing specific receptors.

Direct cell–cell interactions are not required for the many macrophage functions that are mediated via secreted molecules. The cells are capable of secreting over 100 products, including peptide factors (cytokines and growth factors), enzymes, enzyme inhibitors, bioactive lipids and reactive metabolites of oxygen and nitrogen (Nathan 1987).

The macrophage-derived peptide factors mediate not only inflammatory and immunological responses, but also the subsequent process of tissue repair and remodeling. Peptide factors involved in these processes include IL-1, TNFα, basic fibroblast growth factor (bFGF), platelet-derived growth factor (PDGF) and transforming growth factor β (TGFβ). Macrophages can also mediate tissue repair and remodeling via their capacity to change the composition of extracellular matrix, by either synthesizing components of the matrix or by releasing degrading enzymes such as lysosomal acid hydrolases.

Many of the above functions are carried out by activated cells. Activation is a process by which macrophages gain an enhanced capacity for functions such as microbicidal and tumoricidal activities, presentation of antigen to T cells, and secretion of cytokines. Although the process is complex and may not apply to all functions, macrophage activation can be divided into two stages, a state in which the cell is 'primed' and one in which it is 'fully activated' (Hamilton & Adams 1987). Interferon-γ, a product of stimulated T cells, is the best-characterized agent that primes macrophages for activation as characterized by enhanced MHC class II expression, antigen-presenting activity and production of oxygen radicals. Bacterial lipopolysaccharide induces a state of 'full activation' in primed macrophages, when the cells have considerably enhanced microbicidal and tumoricidal activities and increased capacity to produce reactive metabolites of oxygen, nitric oxide and cytokines such as IL-1, IL-6 and TNFα.

MONOCYTES IN INFLAMMATORY BOWEL DISEASE

In patients with active disease there are increased numbers of monocytes in the circulation (Thayer et al 1976, Mee et al 1980a), which would be derived from the increased production of these cells in the bone marrow (Meuret et al 1978). A number of studies have also examined functional activities of circulating monocytes in inflammatory bowel disease. In active disease, the cells have an increased capacity to phagocytose bacteria (Mee et al 1980b, Whorwell et al 1981) and migrate at random in vitro (Rhodes & Jewell 1983). Lysosomal acid hydrolases are intracellular digestive enzymes that can also be released to degrade extracellular molecules (such as extracellular matrix, complement and kinins). The production and release by monocytes of two acid hydrolases, N-acetyl-β-glucosaminidase and β-glucuronidase, have been shown to be markedly elevated in both active ulcerative colitis and Crohn's disease (Ganguly et al 1978, Mee & Jewell 1980). Secretion of the neutral protease, plasminogen activator, is also markedly enhanced in active inflammatory bowel disease (Doe & Dorsman 1982).

Reactive metabolites of oxygen, such as hydrogen peroxide (H_2O_2), superoxide anion (O_2^-), hydroxyl radicals (OH^-) and hypochlorite (OCl^-), mediate microbicidal activity in macrophages but may also induce damage in neighboring cells. A number of studies have shown that peripheral blood monocytes isolated from patients with active inflammatory bowel disease have an enhanced capacity to produce those oxygen radicals (Kitahora et al 1988, Williams et al 1990, Baldassano et al 1993). Increased production of the cytokines IL-1 and IL-6 by monocytes isolated from such patients has also been demonstrated (Satsangi et al 1987, Nakamura et al 1992, Mazlam & Hodgson 1992, Mahida et al 1992).

The increased numbers of circulating monocytes in patients with active inflammatory bowel disease thus have an enhanced capacity to mediate a number of functions that they are likely to perform following migration into the intestinal mucosa.

INTESTINAL MACROPHAGES IN INFLAMMATORY BOWEL DISEASE

Immunohistochemical studies have shown that there are many macrophages in the lamina propria of the normal human small and large intestine (Selby et al 1983, Hume et al 1987, Allison et al 1988, Mahida et al 1989a). A characteristic feature of these cells is their morphological and histochemical heterogeneity. For example, macrophages below the surface epithelium of the normal colon are large, round and strongly express acid phosphatase (ACP) and non-specific esterase (NSE) activities. In contrast, cells in the deeper lamina propria are generally smaller, with many processes, and are negative (or only weakly positive) for these enzymes. Monoclonal antibodies have allowed macrophage heterogeneity in the normal intestine to be studied further, and this is strikingly illustrated in and around Peyer's patches (Mahida et al 1989b).

Intestinal macrophages may have functions common to similar cells in other tissues, but their presence in a site constantly exposed to a large array of luminal antigens and microorganisms suggests that they may also carry out functions unique to this location. It is likely that they play an important role in host defence and interact closely with the large numbers of T and B cells present in the lamina propria, as well as with the surface epithelium.

Functional studies have been performed on macrophages isolated by digestion of the lamina propria with collagenase. Studies on cells isolated from normal mucosa have shown that, despite being constantly exposed to luminal antigens and bacteria, most of the normal colonic and small-intestinal macrophages are downregulated with respect to their capacity to produce oxygen radicals and IL-1 (Mahida et al 1989c, d). This downregulation persists despite stimulation with interferon-γ or lipopolysaccharide (agents known to prime and activate macrophages).

In active ulcerative colitis and Crohn's disease there is an increase in the total macrophage population of the intestinal mucosa, the extent of which is similar to that for other mononuclear cells (Mahida et al 1989a). Studies of these cells in tissue sections (using monoclonal antibodies, histochemical stains and in-situ hybridization) have shown marked heterogeneity, distinct from that seen in the normal mucosa (Gionchetti et al 1988, Allison et al 1988, Mahida et al 1989a, Seldenrijk et al 1989, Allison & Poulter 1991, Cappello et al 1992). Thus macrophages strongly expressing the enzymes acid phosphatase (ACP) and lysozyme (Stamp et al 1992) are present throughout the lamina propria in active inflammatory bowel disease, in contrast to normal colonic and terminal ileal mucosa, where they are only seen below the surface epithelium. ACP is a lysosomal acid hydrolase which, like other acid hydrolases discussed above, degrades molecules intracellularly but can also be secreted in response to cytokines, bacteria or bacterial products. Lysozyme has antibacterial activities and is also found in polymorphonuclear cells.

Using a panel of monoclonal antibodies, subpopulations of macrophages present in the lamina propria of active inflammatory bowel disease mucosa, but absent (or only rarely present) in the normal mucosa, have been identified. In one such subpopulation, the cells express low-affinity IgG receptors as identified with the monoclonal antibody 3G8 (CD16; Mahida et al 1989a), and animal studies suggest that these cells may be involved in clearing immune complexes from the inflamed mucosa. Macrophages labeled with the antibody RFD9 are normally found in germinal centres of lymphoid aggregates, but not in the lamina propria. In active inflammatory bowel disease mucosa, significant numbers of RFD9-positive cells are present in the lamina propria, especially in aggregated clusters in Crohn's disease (Gionchetti et al 1988, Allison et al 1988, Mahida et al 1989a). Some of these clusters may represent microgranulomata, since epithelioid cells in fully developed granulomas are also RFD9 positive and are closely associated with CD4-positive cells (Mahida et al 1988a). Granulomas in Crohn's disease are often found within the walls of blood vessels (Wakefield et al 1991) and the ischemia induced by such lesions may have a role in the pathogenesis of the disease. Interestingly, RFD9-positive cells are also found in the inflamed pouch mucosa of patients with ulcerative colitis who have had a colectomy (de Silva et al 1990). This suggests that immunological mechanisms similar to those in the original ulcerative colitis may be operating in pouchitis. The third subpopulation of macrophages that are found in the mucosa with active ulcerative colitis and Crohn's disease are those expressing IL-2 receptor (Mahida et al 1988b, Choy et al 1990). In contrast to T cells (in which it induces proliferation), IL-2 can induce the production of oxygen radicals in macrophages, and consequently may exacerbate tissue damage.

Functional studies on macrophages isolated from active inflammatory bowel disease mucosa have shown that a majority have an enhanced capacity to produce oxygen radicals (Mahida et al 1989c) and IL-1 (Mahida et al 1989d), and are therefore activated. Despite stimulation, normal intestinal macrophages are downregulated with respect to these functions (see above). This suggests that the activated macrophages in active inflammatory bowel disease are derived from monocytes that have recently migrated into the mucosa. Such recently recruited cells may account for the phenotypically distinct subpopulations of macrophages described above, as well as those found near blood vessels (Rugtveit et al 1994). Such cells may be responsible for perpetuating intestinal inflammation and tissue damage, and studies in an animal model suggest that inhibition of their migration from the circulation could have therapeutic value (Podolsky et al 1993).

As indicated above, macrophages can process and present antigens to T cells. Whereas macrophages may present antigens to primed or sensitized T cells, specialized cells termed dendritic cells (which are the most potent antigen-presenting cells) are required for activation and proliferation of previously resting (unprimed) T cells. Using the allogeneic mixed lymphocyte reaction, cells with potent antigen-presenting activity in the intestine have been shown to have all the characteristics of dendritic cells (Mahida et al 1988c, Pavli et al 1993). In one study these cells were also shown to express markers typically associated with macrophages (Mahida et al 1988c). Isolated cells from active inflammatory bowel disease mucosa have enhanced antigen-presenting activity compared to those from non-inflamed mucosa from the same colon.

Intestinal macrophages are likely to be a major source of the many cytokines (such as IL-1, IL-6, IL-8, IL-10) whose production has been shown to be increased in the mucosa with active ulcerative colitis and Crohn's disease (see Chapter 12). Intestinal macrophages can also influence the functions of B cells (Wu et al 1990) and epithelial cells. For example, a macrophage-derived protein has been shown to act as an intestinal mucin secretagogue (Sperber et al 1993), and alteration in its production could explain the changes in mucin secretion often seen in inflammatory bowel disease.

CONCLUSION

Macrophages are likely to play a major role in the pathogenesis of inflammatory bowel disease, mediating not only intestinal inflammation and tissue damage but also the subsequent process of repair and remodeling. The greatly increased numbers of activated macrophages in the diseased mucosa are capable of performing the functions required for perpetuating intestinal inflammation and tissue damage. These cells are derived predominantly from the circulation following specific interactions with the vascular endothelial cells, and inhibition of this migration could have potential therapeutic value.

REFERENCES

Allison M C, Poulter L W 1991 Changes in phenotypically distinct mucosal macrophage populations may be a prerequisite for the development of inflammatory bowel disease. Clinical and Experimental Immunology 85: 504–509

Allison M C, Cornwall S, Poulter L W, Dhillon A P, Pounder R E 1988 Macrophage heterogeneity in normal colonic mucosa and in inflammatory bowel disease. Gut 28: 1531–1538

Auger M J, Ross J A 1992 The biology of the macrophage. In: Lewis C E, McGee J O'D (eds) The macrophage. Oxford University Press, Oxford, pp 1–74

Baldassano R N, Schreiber S, Johnston R B, Fu R D, Muraki T, MacDermott R P 1993 Crohn's disease monocytes are primed for accentuated release of toxic oxygen metabolites. Gastroenterology 105: 60–66

Cappello M, Keshav S, Prince C, Jewell D P, Gordon S 1992 Detection of mRNAs for macrophage products in inflammatory bowel disease by in situ hybridisation. Gut 33: 1214–1219

Choy M Y, Smith J A W, Williams C B, MacDonald T T 1990 Differential expression of CD25 (interleukin 2 receptor) on lamina propria T cells and macrophages in the intestinal lesions in Crohn's disease and ulcerative colitis. Gut 31: 1365–1370

de Silva H J, Jones M, Prince C, Kettlewell M, Mortensen N J, Jewell D P 1990 Lymphocyte and macrophage subpopulations in pelvic ileal pouches. Gut 32: 1160–1165

Doe W F, Dorsman B 1982 Chronic inflammatory bowel disease: increased plasminogen activator secretion by mononuclear phagocytes. Clinical and Experimental Immunology 48: 256–260

Ganguly N K, Kingham J G C, Lloyd B et al 1978 Acid hydrolases in monocytes from patients with inflammatory bowel disease, chronic liver disease and rheumatoid arthritis. Lancet 1: 1073–1075

Gionchetti P, Mahida Y R, Patel S, Jewell D P 1988 Macrophage and lymphocyte subpopulations in magnifying endoscopic lesions of Crohn's disease. Clinical and Experimental Immunology 72: 373–376

Hamilton T A, Adams D O 1987 Molecular mechanisms of signal transduction in macrophages. Immunology Today 8: 151–158

Hume D A, Allan W, Hogan P G, Doe W F 1987 Immunohistochemical characterisation of macrophages in human liver and gastrointestinal tract: expression of CD4, HLA-DR, OKM1, and the mature macrophage marker 25F9 in normal and diseased tissue. Journal of Leukocyte Biology 42: 474–484

Kitahora T, Suzuki K, Asakura H et al 1988 Active oxygen species generated by monocytes and polymorphonuclear cells in Crohn's disease. Digestive Diseases and Sciences 33: 951–955

Mahida Y R, Patel S, Jewel D P 1988a Macrophage and lymphocyte subpopulations in the granuloma of Crohn's disease. MacDermott R P (ed) Inflammatory bowel disease: current status and future approach. Elsevier Science, pp 137–141

Mahida Y R, Wu K, Patel S, Jewell D P 1988b Interleukin 2 receptor expression by macrophages in inflammatory bowel disease. Clinical and Experimental Immunology 74: 382–386

Mahida Y R, Wu K, Jewell D P 1988c Characterization of antigen presenting activity of mononuclear cells isolated from normal and inflammatory bowel disease colon and ileum. Immunology 65: 543–549

Mahida Y R, Patel S, Gionchetti P, Vaux D, Jewell D P 1989a Macrophage sub-populations in lamina propria of normal and inflamed colon and terminal ileum. Gut 30: 826–834

Mahida Y R, Patel S, Jewell D P 1989b Mononuclear phagocyte system of human Peyer's patches: an immunohistochemical study using monoclonal antibodies. Clinical and Experimental Immunology 75: 82–86

Mahida Y R, Wu K, Jewell D P 1989c Enhanced production of interleukin 1β by mononuclear cells isolated form mucosa with active ulcerative colitis or Crohn's disease. Gut 30: 835–838

Mahida Y R, Wu K, Patel S, Jewell D P 1989d Respiratory burst activity of intestinal macrophages in normal and inflammatory bowel disease. Gut 30: 1362–1370

Mahida Y R, Scott E, Kurlak L, Gallagher A, Hawkey C J 1992 Interleukin 1β, tumour necrosis factor α and interleukin 6 synthesis by circulating mononuclear cells isolated from patients with active ulcerative colitis and Crohn's disease. European Journal of Gastroenterology and Hepatology 4: 501–507

Mazlam M Z, Hodgson H J F 1992 Peripheral blood monocyte cytokine production and acute phase response in inflammatory bowel disease. Gut 33: 773–778

Mee A S, Jewell D P 1980 Monocytes in inflammatory bowel disease: monocyte and serum lysosomal enzyme activity. Clinical Science 58: 295–300

Mee A S, Berney J, Jewell D P 1980a Monocytes in inflammatory bowel disease: absolute monocyte counts. Journal of Clinical Pathology 33: 917–920

Mee A S, Szawatakowski M, Jewell D P 1980b Monocytes in inflammatory bowel disease: phagocytosis and intracellular killing. Journal of Clinical Pathology 33: 921–925

Meuret G A, Bitzi A, Hammer G B 1978 Macrophage turnover in Crohn's disease and ulcerative colitis. Gastroenterology 74: 501–503

Nakamura M, Saito H, Kasanuki J, Tamura Y, Yoshida S 1992 Cytokine production in patients with inflammatory bowel disease. Gut 33: 933–937

Nathan C F 1987 Secretory products of macrophages. Journal of Clinical Investigation 79: 319–326

Pavli P, Hume D A, De Pol E V, Doe W F 1993 Dendritic cells, the major antigen-presenting cells of the human colonic lamina propria. Immunology 78: 132–141

Podolsky, D K, Lobb R, King N et al 1993 Attenuation of colitis in the cotton-top tamarin by anti-α4 integrin monoclonal antibody. Journal of Clinical Investigation 92: 372–380

Rhodes J M, Jewell D P 1983 Motility of neutrophils and monocytes in Crohn's disease and ulcerative colitis. Gut 24: 73–77

Rugtveit J, Brandtzaeg P, Halstensen T S, Fausa O, Scott H 1994 Increased macrophage subset in inflammatory bowel disease: apparent recruitment from peripheral blood monocytes. Gut 35: 669–674

Satsangi J, Wolstencroft R A, Cason J et al 1987 Interleukin 1 in Crohn's disease. Clinical and Experimental Immunology 67: 594–605

Savill J, Fadok V, Henson P, Haslett C 1993 Phagocyte recognition of cells undergoing apoptosis. Immunology Today 14: 131–136

Selby W S, Poulter L W, Hobbs S, Jewell D P, Janossy G 1983 Heterogeneity of HLA-DR positive histiocytes in human intestinal lamina propria: a combined histochemical and immunohistological analysis. Journal of Clinical Pathology 36: 379–384

Seldenrijk C A, Drexhage H A, Menwissen S G M, Palds S T, Meijer J L 1989 Dendritic cells and scavenger macrophages in chronic inflammatory bowel disease. Gut 30: 484–491

Sperber K, Ogata S, Sylvester C et al 1993 A novel human macrophage derived intestinal mucin secretagogue: implications for the pathogenesis of inflammatory bowel disease. Gastroenterology 104: 1302–1309

Stamp G W H, Poulsom R, Chung P et al 1992 Lysozyme gene expression in inflammatory bowel disease. Gastroenterology 103: 532–538

Thayer W R, Charland C, Field C E 1976 The subpopulations of circulating white blood cells in inflammatory bowel disease. Gastroenterology 71: 379–384

Wakefield A J, Sankey E A, Dhillon A P et al 1991 Granulomatous vasculitis in Crohn's disease. Gastroenterology 100: 1279–1287

Whorwell P J, Bennett P, Tanner A R, Wright R 1981 Monocyte function in Crohn's disease and ulcerative colitis. Digestion 22: 271–275

Williams J G, Hughes L E, Hallett M B 1990 Toxic oxygen metabolite production by circulating phagocytic cells in inflammatory bowel disease. Gut 31: 187–193

Wu K C, Mahida Y R, Priddle J D, Jewell D P 1990 Effect of human intestinal macrophages on immunoglobulin production by human intestinal mononuclear cells isolated from patients with inflammatory bowel disease. Clinical and Experimental Immunology 79: 35–40

11. Mast cells and eosinophils in inflammatory bowel disease

S. Bloom

INTRODUCTION

Degranulation of mast cells and eosinophils involves the release of inflammatory mediators that are known to cause mucus secretion, mucosal edema and increased gut permeability; these cells may therefore have a role in the pathogenesis of inflammatory bowel disease (IBD). Mast cell hyperplasia was first reported in ulcerative colitis in 1961 (McAuley & Sommers 1961), although subsequent studies have reported conflicting results. Peripheral blood eosinophilia and raised rectal eosinophil counts have also been reported in IBD. In this chapter mast cell and eosinophil properties and contents will be outlined, together with evidence that these cells are important in the pathogenesis of IBD. This is followed by a consideration of whether the efficacy of therapeutic agents used in IBD may be due to modulation of mast cell and eosinophil function.

MAST CELLS

Mast cells are found throughout the body, but can be classified into several subgroups (Table 11.1). In the human intestinal mucosa mast cells include formaldehyde-sensitive ('mucosal-type') and resistant (connective-tissue type) populations, depending on their abilities to be stained with basic dyes after fixation (Strobel et al 1981, Befus et al 1985). The dominant mast cell of the human intestinal mucosa seems to be the MC_T or formaldehyde-sensitive mast cell (Church et al 1989). For this reason, to visualize mast cells intestinal tissue should be fixed in Carnoys medium and stained with dyes which stain negatively charged proteoglycans in mast cell granules, such as toluidine blue and alcian blue (Enerback 1986, Kitamura 1989). Earlier studies usually failed to address this significant heterogeneity of mast cell populations.

In addition to their traditional role in allergic reactions, activated mast cells are involved in the processes of inflammation, fibrosis and neoplasia (Holgate 1988, Lett-Brown et al 1989) A striking feature of the distribution of mast cells is their close relationship with small vessels and nerves, both in animals (Stead et al 1987) and in man (Stead et al 1989). These data suggest a physiological interaction between mast cells and nerves that may be important in the pathogenesis of mucosal inflammation.

Mast cells share cytochemical and functional characteristics with circulating basophils, but can be distinguished from them electron microscopically (Galli et al

Table 11.1 Heterogeneity among human mast cells

Characteristic	T (mucosal)	TC (connective tissue; submucosal)	Reference
Neutral protease	Tryptase	Tryptase, chymotryptase	(Enerback 1986)
Granule ultrastructure	Scrolls	Gratings/lattices	(Schwartz 1989)
T-cell dependence	+	−	(Irani et al 1987)
Proteoglycans	Chondroitin	Heparin	(Thompson et al 1988)
Eicosanoids	PGD2, LTC4	PDG2, PTC4, D4, E4	
Stimuli for histamine release			
Morphine, vasoactive intestinal peptide, somatostatin, substance P	−	+	(Shanahan et al (1985)
Compound 48/80	−	+	(Befus et al 1987)

1984). Unlike basophils, which circulate as fully differentiated cells that cannot proliferate, mast cells complete their differentiation in tissues and can proliferate extensively (Kitamura & Sonoda 1985, Kitamura et al 1987). Mast cells have high affinity IgE receptors on their surfaces, through which much of their immunological activity is mediated (Metzger et al 1986). Antigen recognition by IgE is followed by cross-linking of receptors and then the release of granules or granule mediators (Ishizaka & Ishizaka 1984).

Table 11.2 Mast cell mediators

Preformed and stored		Newly synthesized
Soluble	Insoluble	
Histamine	Proteoglycans	Prostaglandins
Serotonin	Proteases (e.g. carboxypeptidase)	Leukotrienes
Proteinases (e.g. protease II)	Inflammatory factors	PAF
Chemotactic factors	Peroxidase, superoxide dismutase	Adenosine

Mast cell heterogeneity

Recent reviews of mast cells (Befus et al 1988, Bissonette et al 1989, Kitamura 1989, Schwartz 1989, Benyon et al 1992) have emphasized heterogeneity with regard to morphology, biochemistry, immunology and function. Rodent mast cells can be classified into connective-tissue mast cells and mucosal mast cells based on patterns of dye staining, and these two populations differ extensively in their functional characteristics (Enerback 1986, Befus et al 1988, Kitamura 1989). In humans two mast cell populations can be distinguished on the basis of staining of intracellular tryptase and chymase (Irani et al 1986). Most mast cells in the skin and intestinal submucosa contain tryptase and chymase (TC), whereas lung and intestinal mucosal mast cells usually contain only tryptase (T) (Irani et al 1987, Schwartz et al 1987). The presence of functional differences between these populations (see Table 11.1), makes the classification useful in considering human mast cells, although it does not extend to many other species (Schwartz 1989).

Human mast cells are also heterogeneous in their content of some mediators, such as proteoglycans (Eliakim et al 1986); although overall levels of prostaglandins and leukotrienes have been measured (Fox et al 1985), the technical difficulty in obtaining pure subpopulations of mast cells from human lamina propria means that it is not yet clear whether mast cell subpopulations differ in arachidonic acid metabolism (Befus et al 1987).

Role of mast cell mediators in mucosal inflammation

Mast cell mediators have been reviewed (Schwartz & Austen 1984, Holgate 1988) and are summarized in Table 11.2. These mediators have a variety of actions. Mast cell chemoattractants such as histamine and PGD_2, as well as polypeptide eosinophil and neutrophil chemotactic factors, promote the accumulation of inflammatory leukocytes. Mast cell mediators may increase smooth muscle contractility and affect epithelial cell function (Wallace 1989). Migration is facilitated by mediators having vasodilatory and vascular permeability-enhancing properties. Mast cell mediators have considerable effects on neuronal function (McKay & Bienenstock 1994), which may be relevant considering the close anatomical relation of mast cells to peptidergic nerves (Stead et al 1989). In addition, mast cell protease modulation of neuropeptides may have multiple effects on T and B cells, both of which are sensitive to neuropeptides (McGillis et al 1987).

In view of recent interest in the role of PAF (platelet-activating factor) as a potential mediator in IBD (Wallace et al 1989a, Rachmilewitz et al 1990), it is interesting that studies of mast cell-deficient mice suggest that mast cells are a potential source of PAF (Wallace 1989), whereas in humans synthesis of PAF in intestinal biopsies from patients with ulcerative colitis is enhanced following stimulation with IgE; this is inhibited by sulfasalazine and 5-aminosalicylic acid (5-ASA) (Eliakim et al 1988, Rachmilewitz et al 1992).

Mast cell activation and modulation

As well as the classic IgE-mediated activation pathway, mast cell activating factors have been identified in macrophages, neutrophils, T cells and eosinophils (Lett-Brown et al 1989), although in rodents a number of factors that induce secretion by peritoneal mast cells have no effect on intramucosal mast cells (Benyon et al 1992). Macrophages release a mast cell stimulating factor that is not antigen specific and is IgE dependent (Liu et al 1986). Histamine release from mast cells can be stimulated by cytokines such as IL-1 (Subramanian & Bray 1987) and also by complement components C3a and C5a (Befus et al 1988).

Mast cells in IBD

Morphology

Many published studies report an increase in the number of mast cells in IBD (McAuley & Sommers 1961, Hiatt & Katz 1962, Ranlov et al 1972, Rao 1973, Dvorak et al 1980a, Dvorak & Monahan 1983, Balazs et al 1989, Dvorak et al 1992, King et al 1992). However, there are also reports of mast cells being decreased (Lloyd et al 1975, Sanderson et al 1986) or unchanged (Thompson & Buchmann 1979, Matsueda et al 1982, Sarin et al 1987, Goldsmith et al 1990). There are well known technical difficulties in mast cell quantitation, which may explain some of the discrepancies: traditional fixatives such as formalin may not allow staining of all mast cells, and stains such as toluidine blue used to identify mast cells may stain other cells such as eosinophils and basophils. It has also been suggested (Goldsmith et al 1990) that crypt depletion in ulcerative colitis may make it difficult to distinguish mucosal from submucosal mast cells. Even after excluding those studies done before the instability of mucosal mast cells in formalin was realized, it remains difficult to organize the remaining data into a coherent picture. There is some evidence of different findings in disease subgroups: King et al (1992) reported an increase in mast cells in 80% of ulcerative colitis patients, and suggest that this may correlate with a subgroup of patients who respond to the mast cell stabilizer cromoglycate (Whorwell et al 1981). Increased numbers of mast cells have also been found in other inflammatory bowel diseases (Rao 1973), suggesting that this may be a non-specific finding. Monoclonal antibodies specific for human mast cell tryptase and suitable for use in paraffin-embedded tissue have been developed (Goldsmith et al 1990), but such antibodies may not detect fully degranulated mast cells.

Studies including patients with both ulcerative colitis and Crohn's disease suggest that numbers of mast cells are higher in the former than in the latter (Lloyd et al 1975, Nolte et al 1990); this may be partly explained by difficulties in recognizing degranulated mast cells using light microscopy and conventional staining techniques. However, Sanderson et al (1986) found a significant decrease in mast cell density in Crohn's disease, and also noted that the release of histamine from biopsies of inflamed tissue did not differ greatly from that from normal tissue. In ulcerative colitis and proctitis the mast cells are reported to be increased mainly in the lamina propria, whereas in Crohn's disease there is an increase in submucosal and muscular layer mast cells (Fox et al 1993); mast cells have been reported to be increased in granulomas (Rao 1973). Degranulating mast cells have been observed in active areas of Crohn's disease (Dvorak et al 1978). Mast cells have been found to be increased in cases of pouchitis following colectomy for ulcerative colitis (Dvorak et al 1992).

Functional studies

Several reports describe functional differences in mast cells in IBD, such as increased mediator release (Fox et al 1990, Knutson et al 1990, Nolte et al 1990, Fox et al 1993). Fox et al (1990) showed that mast cells from patients with ulcerative colitis, when stimulated with goat antihuman IgE released more histamine, prostaglandin D_2 and leukotriene C than controls. This group has recently reported that intestinal epithelial cell-associated components (ECAC) can induce a greater release of mast cell mediators in approximately 33% of patients with IBD, compared to normal controls (Fox et al 1993), suggesting that ECAC-induced mast cell reactivity may perpetuate inflammation in a significant number of cases.

Mast cells are closely associated with peptidergic nerves in the gastrointestinal tract (Stead et al 1989). In Crohn's disease, Dvorak and colleagues have shown that mast cells are related to hyperplastic nerves (Dvorak et al 1980b). Human intestinal mast cells contain mostly tryptase, which can inactivate vasoactive intestinal peptide (VIP) while sparing substance P (Caughey 1989). In Crohn's disease, increases in local VIP-containing nerves have been identified (Bishop et al 1980), although there is evidence to suggest that VIP levels are decreased in ulcerative colitis (Watanabe et al 1992).

Effect of therapeutic agents on mast cells in IBD

Salazopyrine

It has been known for some time that sulfasalazine and its active metabolite 5-ASA can block products of the 5-lipoxygenase pathway in neutrophils and inhibit the generation of lipoxygenase and cyclooxygenase products in human colonic biopsies (Stenson & Lobos 1982, Boughton-Smith et al 1983). Recently, an investigation of the modulation of mast cell mediator release by sulfasalazine and 5-ASA (Fox et al 1991) has shown that sulfasalazine significantly enhances goat antihuman IgE-induced histamine release from human intestinal mast cells. This is unlike the situation in the rat, where Barrett et al (1985) have found that sulfasalazine inhibits peritoneal mast cell and mouse bone marrow-derived mast cell histamine release. Sulfasalazine alone did not induce histamine release from mast cells or basophils. The sulfasalazine metabolite 5-ASA effectively inhibits histamine release from basophils and mast cells, and also inhibits the production of prostaglandin D_2 from mast cells. Whether these actions relate to the therapeutic efficacy of 5-ASA in IBD remains unproven.

Steroids

Corticosteroids reduce the number of mast cells within 24 hours in a rodent model (King et al 1985), and have also recently been shown to reduce mast cell numbers in IBD (Goldsmith et al 1990). The mechanism is uncertain, but given that T cells seem to be important for mast cell development (Irani et al 1987) it is interesting that steroids cause reduced production of T cell-derived mast cell growth factors such as IL-3 (Culpepper & Lee 1985). Steroids may also have a direct effect on mast cells to inhibit granule formation (McMenamin et al 1987), and it has been shown that dexamethasone stimulates macrophage engulfment and the destruction of mucosal mast cells (Soda et al 1991).

Immunosuppressants

In mast cells, cyclosporin A and FK506 block degranulation as well as transcriptional activation of several cytokine genes, such as IL-3, IL-5 and the genes involved in leukotriene synthesis (Schreiber & Crabtree 1992). These genes are largely the same as those blocked in T cells, suggesting an effect on a regulatory protein common to mast cells and T cells. In contrast, inhibitors of DNA synthesis such as 6-MP or azathioprine may reduce mastocytosis by a direct effect on mast cell precursors (Butterfield & Weider 1989). Azathioprine, cyclosporin and methotrexate also inhibit PGE_2 production by organ-cultured colonic mucosal biopsies from patients with ulcerative colitis (Eliakim et al 1992).

Effect of experimental and theoretical therapeutic agents on mast cell activators and mediators

Products of lipoxygenase (5-LP) action, such as LTB4, may play a role in IBD and 5-LP inhibitors prevent several of the pathological changes seen in animal models of IBD (Wallace et al 1989b). The 5-LP pathway in mast cells is susceptible to the inhibitor AA-861 (Cohan et al 1989). Some antihistamines inhibit the release of mast cell mediators (Lau & Pearce 1989), as does sodium cromoglycate (Befus et al 1987). There is some evidence that cromoglycate has a differential effect on cutaneous mast cells rather than mucosal mast cells (Clegg et al 1985), and this might account for its disappointing therapeutic effect in IBD. The mast cell stabilizer ketotifen inhibits the release of PGE_2, LTB_4 and LTC_4 (Eliakim et al 1992a), mediators known to be increased in active ulcerative colitis. A recent report (Eliakim et al 1992b) showed that ketotifen can prevent mucosal damage in experimental colitis, and suggests that this agent may be of value in treating IBD. Human mast cells may contain PAF, and PAF antagonists show promise in the therapy of IBD in clinical trials (Rachmilewitz et al 1990).

EOSINOPHILS

Morphology and cell biology

Eosinophils are distinguished by large dense acidophilic cytoplasmic granules, which are membrane bound and morphologically heterogeneous (Egesten et al 1986). Ninety per cent of the granule contents are cationic proteins known to be cytotoxic for mammalian and non-mammalian cells, as well as having other functions (Table 11.3).

Other eosinophil granules secrete arylsulphatase and histamine (Weller & Goetzl 1980). Charcot–Leyden crystals

Table 11.3 Eosinophil granule content and functions

Granule constituent	Function	Reference
Major basic protein (MBP)	Neutralizes heparin or DNA, releases histamine. Also found in basophils and some placental cells	(Venge 1990)
Eosinophil cationic protein (ECP)	Procoagulant, neurotoxic, stimulates fibroblasts to produce hyaluronic acid	(Sarnstrand et al 1988)
Eosinophil peroxidase (EPO)	May cause degranulation of mast cells	(Venge 1990)
Eosinophil-derived neurotoxin (EDN)	Neurotoxic, active ribonuclease	(Venge 1990)

are extracellular deposits of lyophosphatase associated with eosinophil infiltration, and may be important in phospholipid metabolism in the inflammatory process (Ackerman et al 1980, Weller et al 1980). Surface Ig receptors and complement receptors provide recognition sites for cell activation. Variations in eosinophil density exist, with a hypodense activated form often found in inflammation (Prin et al 1983).

The release of major basic protein (MBP), eosinophil cationic protein (ECP) and eosinophil peroxidase (EPO) leads to parasite killing and tissue toxicity. Eosinophils also elaborate arachidonic acid metabolites PGE_2, LTB_4, C_4, D_4 and PAF (Goetzl 1980, Goetzl et al 1980), all of which may be increased in inflamed intestinal mucosa. They release reactive oxygen metabolites and may be more cytotoxic than neutrophils (Bruijnzeel 1989).

Tissue infiltration by eosinophils begins with adherence to the vascular endothelium. Chemotactic factors for eosinophils include complement components, histamine and lipid mediators (Wadee et al 1980, Ogawa et al 1981, Czarnetzki & Rosenbach 1986). Cytokines IL-3 and IL-5 sustain eosinophil viability in culture and are responsible for eosinophil differentiation, maturation and activation (Dvorak et al 1989, Wang et al 1989). IL-5 enhances the eosinophil chemotactic response to PAF (Etienne et al 1989, Wang et al 1989). PAF, which has been shown to be associated with tissue destruction in animal models of IBD (Wallace et al 1989a), also induces eosinophil degranulation (Krogel et al 1989), as do cytokines IL-1a and 1b (Whitcomb et al 1989). The lipid mediator LTB_4 enhances endothelial–eosinophil interaction, and this may explain some of the effect of LTB_4 antagonists in animal models of IBD (Fretland et al 1989).

Eosinophils in IBD

Peripheral blood eosinophilia has been described in ulcerative colitis, and this may vary with ethnic origin (Benfield et al 1990). Eosinophil counts are raised in the rectal mucosa of patients with active ulcerative colitis compared with inactive disease (Wright & Truelove 1966, Sarin et al 1987), although it is uncertain whether the degree of eosinophil infiltrate is related to the severity of inflammation (Willoughby et al 1979, Sarin et al 1987). It has been suggested that because patients with relatively benign disease which responds to treatment have significantly higher eosinophil counts than patients with aggressive disease (Heatley & James 1979), the eosinophil count may be a useful prognostic factor.

Crohn's disease is associated with a prominent eosinophil infiltrate in the lamina propria and the submucosa: eosinophils are reported to lose their crystalline cores (Dvorak 1980), and the contents of the granule matrix are detectable in the lamina propria of intestinal specimens in Crohn's disease, but not in healthy patients (Tai et al 1984, Hallgren et al 1989) or patients with ulcerative colitis (Choy et al 1990). Eosinophils are found close to degranulating mast cells (Dvorak et al 1980a). The release of neurotoxic granule products from eosinophils may explain the alteration in enteric nervous function and the hyperplasia/necrosis of enteric nerves seen in Crohn's disease (Dvorak et al 1980b).

Eosinophils migrate across the colonic epithelium in Crohn's disease (Hallgren et al 1989), and may contribute to crypt abscess formation in IBD. Madara's group has shown that activated eosinophils elicit chloride secretion from intestinal epithelia via the conversion of eosinophil 5' AMP to adenosine (Resnick et al 1993).

SUMMARY

There is considerable evidence that mast cells and eosinophils are involved in the inflammatory process in IBD. The specialization of mucosal-type mast cells and the close relationship between mast cells and enteric nerves are particularly intriguing. This area seems potentially very important and is ripe for further investigation.

REFERENCES

Ackerman S, Loegering D, Gleich G 1980 The human eosinophil Charcot–Leyden crystal protein: biochemical characteristics and measurements by radioimmunoassay. Journal of Immunology 125: 2118–2127

Balazs M, Illyes G, Vadasz G 1989 Mast cells in ulcerative colitis: quantitative and ultrastructural studies. Virchows Archiv B Cell Pathology 57 (6): 353–360

Barrett K, Tashof T, Metcalfe D 1985 Inhibition of IgE-mediated mast cell degranulation by sulfasalazine. European Journal of Pharmacology 107: 279–281

Befus A, Dyck N, Goodacre R, Bienenstock J 1987 Mast cells from human intestinal lamina propria. Isolation, histochemical subtypes, and functional characterisation. Journal of Immunology 138: 2604–2610

Befus F, Fujimaki H, Lee T, Swieter M 1988 Mast cell polymorphisms: present concepts, future directions. Digestive Diseases and Sciences 33: 16S–24S

Befus D, Goodacre R, Dyck N, Bienenstock J 1985 Mast cell heterogeneity in man:1. Histologic studies of the intestine. International Archives of Allergy and Applied Immunology 76: 232–236

Benfield G F, Bryan R, Crocker J 1990 Lamina propria eosinophils and mast cells in ulcerative colitis: comparison between Asians and Caucasians. Journal of Clinical Pathology 43: 27–31

Benyon R, Bissonette E, Befus D 1992 Intestinal mast cells in IBD: pathogenesis and therapeutic implications. In: MacDermott R P, Stenson W F (eds) Inflammatory bowel disease. Elsevier, New York, pp 189–199

Bishop A, Polak J, Bryant M, Bloom S, Hamilton S 1980 Abnormalities of vasoactive intestinal polypeptide containing nerves in Crohn's disease. Gastroenterology 79: 853–860

Bissonette E, Benyon R, Befus A (1989). Mast cells as the targets for the therapy of inflammatory bowel disease. In: Williams C N (ed) Falk Symposium no. 56, Trends in inflammatory bowel disease therapy. Kluwer Academic, pp 41–47

Boughton-Smith N, Hawkey C, Whittle B 1983 Sulfasalazine and the inhibition of thromboxane synthesis in human colonic mucosa. British Journal of Pharacology 80: 604

Bruijnzeel P 1989 Contribution of eosinophil-derived mediators in asthma. International Archives of Allergy and Applied Immunology 90: 57–63

Butterfield J, Weider D 1989 In vitro sensitivity of immature mast cells to chemotherapeutic agents. International Archives of Allergy and Applied Immunology 89: 297–300

Caughey G 1989 Roles of mast cell tryptase and chymase in airway function. American Journal of Physiology 257: L39–L46

Choy M Y, Walker S J, Williams C B, MacDonald T T 1990 Activated eosinophils in chronic inflammatory bowel disease. [Letter] Lancet 336: 126–127

Church M, Benyon R, Rees P 1989 Functional heterogeneity of human mast cells. In: Galli S J, Austen K J (eds) Mast cell and basophil differentiation and function in health and disease. Raven Press, New York, pp 161–170

Clegg L S, Church M K, Holgate S T 1985 Histamine secretion from human skin slices induced by anti-IgE and artificial secretagogues and the effects of sodium cromoglycate and salbutamol. Clinical Allergy 15: 321–328

Cohan V, McKenzie-White J, Triggiani M, Massey W, Kagey-Sobotka A, Lichtenstein L 1989 Heterogeneity of human mast cells and basophils. Effects of a putative 5-lipoxygenase inhibitor. Biochemistry and Pharmacology 38: 4455–4459

Culpepper J, Lee F 1985 Regulation of IL-3 expression by glucocorticoids in cloned murine T-lymphocytes. Journal of Immunology 135: 3191–3197

Czarnetzki B, Rosenbach T 1986 Chemotaxis of human neutrophils and eosinophils towards leukotriene B4 and its 20-w oxidation products in vitro. Prostaglandins 31: 851–858

Dvorak A 1980 Ultrastructural evidence for release of major basic protein-containing crystalline cores of eosinophil granules in vivo: cytotoxic potential in Crohn's disease. Journal of Immunology 125: 460–462

Dvorak A, Monahan R 1983 Crohn's disease: mast cell quantitation using one micron plastic sections for light microscopy. Pathology Annual 18: 181–190

Dvorak A, McLeod R, Onderdonk A et al 1992 Ultrastructural evidence for piecemeal and anaphylactic degranulation of human gut mucosal mast cells in vivo. International Archives of Allergy and Immunology 99: 74–83

Dvorak A, Monahan R, Osage J, Dickersin G 1978 Mast cell degranulation in Crohn's disease. Lancet 1: 498

Dvorak A, Monahan R, Osage J, Dickersin G 1980a Crohn's disease: transmission electron microscopic studies. I. Immunologic inflammatory response. Alterations of mast cells, basophils, eosinophils and the microvasculature. Human Pathology 11: 606–619

Dvorak A M, Osage J E, Monahan R A, Dickersin G R 1980b Crohn's disease: transmission electron microscopic studies. III. Target tissues. Proliferation of and injury to smooth muscle and the autonomic nervous system. Human Pathology 11: 620–634

Dvorak A, Saito H, Hatake K et al 1989 Ultrastructure of eosinophils and basophils stimulated to develop in human cord blood mononuclear cell cultures containing recombinant human IL-5 or IL-3. Laboratory Investigation 61: 116–210

Egesten A, Alumets J, von Mecklenberg C, Palmegren M, Olsen I 1986 Localisation of eosinophil cationic protein, major basic protein, and eosinophil peroxidase in human eosinophils by immunoelectron microscopic technique. Journal of Histochemistry and Cytochemistry 34: 1399–1403

Eliakim R, Gilead L, Ligumsky M, Okon E, Racmilewitz D, Razin E 1986 Histamine and chondroitin sulphate E proteoglycan released by cultured human colonic mucosa: indications for possible presence of E mast cells. Proceedings of the National Academy of Sciences of the USA 83: 461–464

Eliakim R, Karmell F, Razin E, Rachmilewitz D 1988 Role of platelet activating factor in ulcerative colitis. Enhanced production during active disease and inhibition by sulphasalazine and prednisolone. Gastroenterology 95: 1167–1172

Eliakim R, Karmell F, Chorev M, Okon E, Rachmilewitz D 1992a Effect of drugs on colonic eicosanoid accumulation in active ulcerative colitis. Scandinavian Journal of Gastroenterology 27: 968–972

Eliakim R, Karmell F, Okon E, Rachmilewitz D 1992b Ketotifen effectively prevents mucosal damage in experimental colitis. Gut 33: 1498–1503

Enerback L 1986 Mast cell heterogeneity: the evolution of the concept of a specific mucosal mast cell. In: Befus A D, Bienenstock J, Denberg J A (eds) Mast cell differentiation and heterogeneity. Raven, New York, pp 1–26

Etienne A, Soulard C, Thonier F, Braquet P 1989 Modulation by drugs of eosinophil recruitment induced by immune challenge in rats: possible role of IL-5 and PAF. International Archives of Allergy and Applied Immunology 88: 216–221

Fox C C, Lichtenstein L M, Roche J K 1993 Intestinal mast cell responses in idiopathic inflammatory bowel disease. Histamine release from human intestinal mast cells in response to gut epithelial proteins. Digestive Diseases and Sciences 38: 1105–1112

Fox C C, Moore W C, Lichtenstein L M 1991 Modulation of mediator release from human intestinal mast cells by sulfasalazine and 5-aminosalicylic acid. Digestive Diseases and Sciences 36: 179–184

Fox C, Dvorak A, Peters S, Kagey-Sobotka A, Lichtenstein L 1985 Isolation and characterisation of human intestinal mucosal mast cells. Journal of Immunology 135: 483–491

Fox C C, Lazenby A J, Moore W C, Yardley J H, Bayless T M, Lichtenstein L M 1990 Enhancement of human intestinal mast cell mediator release in active ulcerative colitis. Gastroenterology 99: 119–124

Fretland D, Levin S, Tsai B et al 1989 Effect of leukotriene B4 receptor antagonist SC-41930 on acetic acid-induced colon inflammation. Agents and Actions 27: 395–397

Galli S, Dvorak A, Dvorak H 1984 Basophils and mast cells: morphologic insights into their biology, secretory patterns and function. Progress in Allergy 34: 1–141

Goetzl E 1980 Mediators of immune hypersensitivity derived from arachidonic acid. New England Journal of Medicine 303: 822–825

Goetzl E, Weller P, Sunn F 1980 The regulation of human eosinophil function by endogenous monohydroxyeicosatetraenoic acid. Journal of Immunology 124: 926–933

Goldsmith P, McGarity B, Walls A F, Church M K, Millward S G, Robertson D A 1990 Corticosteroid treatment reduces mast cell numbers in inflammatory bowel disease. Digestive Diseases and Sciences 35: 1409–1413

Hallgren R, Colombel J, Dahl R et al 1989 Neutrophil and eosinophil involvement of the small bowel in patients with celiac disease and Crohn's disease: studies on the secretion rate and immunohistochemical localization of granulocyte granule constituents. American Journal of Medicine 86: 56–64

Heatley R V, James P D 1979 Eosinophils in the rectal mucosa. A simple method of predicting the outcome of ulcerative proctocolitis? Gut 20: 787–791

Hiatt R, Katz L 1962 Mast cells in inflammatory lesions of the gastrointestinal tract. American Journal of Gastroenterology 37: 541–545

Holgate S 1988 Mast cells, mediators and disease. Boston, Kluwer Academic

Irani A, Craig S, DeBlois G, Elson C, Schechter N, Schwartz L 1987 Deficiency of the tryptase positive, chymase negative mast cell type in gastrointestinal mucosa of patiens with defective T lymphocyte function. Journal of Immunology 138: 4381–4386

Irani A, Schechter N, Craig S, DeBlois G, Schwartz L 1986 Two types of human mast cells that have subsets with distinct neutral protease compositions. Proceedings of the National Academy of Sciences of the USA 83: 4464–4468

Ishizaka T, Ishizaka K 1984 Activation of mast cells for mediator release through IgE receptors. Progress in Allergy 34: 188–235

King S, Miller H, Newlands G, Woodbury R 1985 Depletion of mucosal mast cell protease by glucocorticoids: effects on intestinal anaphylaxis in the rat. Proceedings of the National Academy of Sciences of the USA 82: 1214–1218

King T, Biddle W, Bhatia P, Moore J, Miner P J 1992 Colonic mucosal mast cell distribution at line of demarcation of active ulcerative colitis. Digestive Diseases and Sciences 37: 490–495

Kitamura Y 1989 Heterogeneity of mast cells and phenotypic change between subpopulations. Annual Review of Immunology 7: 59–76

Kitamura Y, Sonoda T 1985 Differentiation of mast cells and basophils. In: Golde D W (ed) Haemopoietic stem cells. Marcel Dekker, New York, pp 65–80

Kitamura Y, Kanakura Y, Fujita J, Nakano T 1987 Differentiation and transdifferentiation of mast cells: a unique member of the haemopoietic cell family. International Journal of Cell Cloning 5: 108–121

Knutson L, Ahrenstedt O, Odlind B, Hallgren R 1990 The jejunal secretion of histamine is increased in active Crohn's disease. Gastroenterology 98: 849–854

Krogel C, Yukawa T, Dent G, Chung K, Barnes P 1989 Stimulation of degranulation from human eosinophils by platelet activating factor. Journal of Immunology 142: 3519–3526

Lau H, Pearce F 1989 Effects of antihistamines on isolated human lung mast cells, basophils and erythrocytes. Agents and Actions 27: 83–85

Lett-Brown M, Allan R, Grant J 1989 Regulation of human basophils and mast cells. Activation by cytokines. The Year in Immunology 5: 195–204

Liu M, Proud D, Lichtenstein L et al 1986 Human lung macrophage-derived histamine-releasing activity is due to IgE dependent factors. Journal of Immunology 136: 2588–2595

Lloyd G, Green F, Fox H, Mani V, Turnberg L 1975 Mast cells and immunoglobulin E in inflammatory bowel disease. Gut 16: 861–866

McAuley R L, Sommers S C 1961 Mast cells in non-specific ulcerative colitis. American Journal of Digestive Diseases 6: 233–236

McGillis J, Organist M, Payan D 1987 Substance P and immunoregulation. Federal Proceedings 46: 196–199

McKay D, Bienenstock J 1994 The interaction between mast cells and nerves in the gastrointestinal tract. Immunology Today 15: 533–538

McMenamin C, Gault E, Haif D 1987 The effect of dexamethasone on growth and differentiation of bone marrow-derived mucosal mast cells in vitro. Immunology 62: 29–34

Matsueda K, Rimpila J J, Ford J, Levin B, Kraft S 1982 Tissue mast cells in Crohn's disease and ulcerative colitis. In: Peña A S, Weterman I T, Booth C C; Strober W (eds) Recent advances in Crohn's disease. Martinus Nijhoff, The Hague, pp 103–109

Metzger H, Alcaraz G, Hohman R, Kinet J, Pribluda V, Quarto R 1986 The receptor with high affinity for immunoglobulin E. Annual Review of Immunology 4: 419–470

Nolte H, Spjeldnaes N, Kruse A, Windelborg B 1990 Histamine release from gut mast cells from patients with inflammatory bowel diseases. Gut 31: 791–794

Ogawa H, Kunkel S, Fantone J, Ward P 1981 Digestion of the fifth component of complement by eosinophil lysosymal enzymes: production of eosinophil specific chemotactic activity. Virchows Archiv 38: 149–157

Prin L, Capron M, Tonnel A, Bletry O, Capron A 1983 Heterogeneity of human peripheral blood eosinophil; variability in cell density and cytotoxic ability in relation to the level and the origin of hypereosinophilia. International Archives of Allergy and Applied Immunology 72: 336–346

Rachmilewitz D, Eliakim R, Simon P, Ligumsky M, Karmeli F 1992 Cytokines and platelet-activating factor in human inflamed colonic mucosa. Agents and Actions (Spec No.): 32–36

Rachmilewitz D, Karmeli F, Eliakim R 1990 Platelet-activating factor – a possible mediator in the pathogenesis of ulcerative colitis. Scandinavian Journal of Gastroenterology 172 (suppl): 19–21

Ranlov P, Nielson M, Wanstrup J 1972 Ultrastructure of the ileum in Crohn's disease: immune lesions and mastocytosis. Scandinavian Journal of Gastroenterology 7: 471–476

Rao S 1973 Mast cells as a component of the granuloma in Crohn's disease. Journal of Pathology 109: 79–82

Resnick M, Colgan S, Patapoff T et al 1993 Actvated eosinophils evoke chloride secretion in model intestinal epithelia primarily via regulated release of 5'-AMP. Journal of Immunology 151: 5716–5723

Sanderson I, Leung K, Pearce F, Walker-Smith J 1986 Lamina propria mast cells in biopsies from children with Crohn's disease. Journal of Clinical Pathology 39: 279–283

Sarin S, Malhotra V, Sen Gupta S, Karon A, Gaur S, Anand B 1987 Significance of eosinophil and mast cell counts in rectal mucosa in ulcerative colitis: a prospective controlled study. Digestive Diseases and Sciences 32: 363–367

Sarnstrand B, Westegren-Thorsson G, Hernas J, Peterson C, Venge P, Malmstrom A 1988 Eosinophil cationic protein and TGF-alpha stimulate synthesis of hyaluronan and proteoglycan in human lung fibroblast cultures. Fifth International Colloquium on Pulmonary Fibrosis (Abstract)

Schreiber S, Crabtree G 1992 The mechanism of action of cyclosporin A and FK506. Immunology Today 13: 136–142

Schwartz L 1989 Heterogeneity of mast cells in humans. In: Galli S J, Austen K F (eds) Mast cell and basophil differentiation and function in health and disease. Boston, New York, pp 93–105

Schwartz L, Austen K 1984 Structure and function of the chemical mediators of mast cells. Progress in Allergy 34: 271–321

Schwartz L, Irani A, Roller K, Castlls M, Schechter N 1987 Quantitation of histamine, tryptase and chymase in dispersed human T and TC mast cells. Journal of Immunology 138: 2611–2615

Shanahan F, Denburg J, Fox J, Bienenstock J, Befus J 1985. Mast cell heterogeneity: effect of neuroenteric peptides on histamine release. Journal of Immunology 135: 1331–1337

Soda K, Kawabori S, Perdue M, Bienenstock J 1991 Macrophage engulfment of mucosal mast cells in rats treated with dexamethasone. Gastroenterology 100: 929–937

Stead R, Dixon M, Bramwell N, Riddell R, Bienenstock J 1989 Mast cells are closely apposed to nerves in the human gastrointestinal mucosa. Gastroenterology 97: 575–585

Stead R, Tomioka M, Quinonez G, Simon G, Felten S, Bienenstock J 1987 Intestinal mucosal mast cells in normal and nematode-infected rat intestines are in intimate contact with peptidergic nerves. Proceedings of the National Academy of Sciences of the USA 84: 2975–2979

Stenson W, Lobos E 1982 Sulfasalazine inhibits the synthesis of chemotactic lipids by neutrophils. Journal of Clinical Investigation 69: 494–497

Strobel S, Miller H, Ferguson A 1981 Human intestinal mucosal mast cells: evaluation of fixation and staining techniques. Journal of Clinical Pathology 34: 841–858

Subramanian N, Bray M 1987 IL-1 releases histamine from human basophils and mast cells in vitro. Journal of Immunology 138: 271–275

Tai P-C, Spry C, Petersen C, Venge P, Olsson I 1984 Monoclonal antibodies distinguish between storage and secreted forms of eosinophil cationic protein. Nature 309: 182–184

Thompson H, Buchmann P 1979 Mast cell population in rectal biopsies from patients with Crohn's disease. In: Pepys J, Edwards A M (eds) The mast cell: its role in health and disease. Pitman, London, pp 697–701

Thompson H, Schulman E, Metcalfe D 1988 Identification of chondroitin sulphate E in human lung mast cells. Journal of Immunology 140: 2708–2713

Venge P 1990 The human eosinophil in inflammation. Agents and Actions 29: 122–126

Wadee A, Anderson R, Sher R 1980 In vitro effects of histamine on eosinophil migration. International Archives of Allergy and Applied Immunology 63: 322–329

Wallace J 1989 PAF as a mediator of gastrointestinal cell damage. Platelet activating factor and disease. Ed. Kunihiko S, Hanahan D S. Tokyo, International Medical Publishers. 153–186

Wallace J L, Braquet P, Ibbotson G C, MacNaughton W K, Cirino G 1989a Assessment of the role of platelet-activating factor in an animal model of inflammatory bowel disease. Journal of Lipid Mediation 1: 13–23

Wallace J L, MacNaughton W K, Morris G P, Beck P L 1989b Inhibition of leukotriene synthesis markedly accelerates healing in a rat model of inflammatory bowel disease. Gastroenterology 96: 29–36

Wang J, Rambaldi A, Biondi A, Chen Z, Sanderson C, Mantovani A 1989 Recombinant human IL-5 is a selective eosinophil chemoattractant. European Journal of Immunology 19: 701–705

Watanabe T, Kubota Y, Sawada T et al 1992 Neuropeptides and mucosal inflammation in ulcerative colitis. Gastroenterology 102: A710

Weller P, Goetzl E 1980 The regulatory and effector roles of eosinophils Advances in Immunology 27: 339–371

Weller P, Goetzl E, Austen K 1980 Identification of human eosinophil lyophosphatase as the constituent of Charcot–Leyden crystals. Proceedings of the National Academy of Sciences of USA 77: 7440–7443

Whitcomb E, Dinarello C, Pincus S 1989 Differential effects of IL-1 alpha and beta on human peripheral blood eosinophils. Blood 73: 1904–1908

Whorwell P, Whorwell G, Bamforth J et al 1981 A double-blind controlled trial of the effect of sodium cromoglycate in preventing relapse in ulcerative colitis. Postgraduate Medical Journal 57: 436–438

Willoughby C, Piris J, Truelove S 1979 Tissue eosinophils in ulcerative colitis. Scandinavian Journal of Gastroenterology 14: 395–399

Wright R, Truelove S 1966 Circulating and tissue eosinophils. American Journal of Digestive Diseases 11: 831–846

12. Cytokines in inflammatory bowel disease

G. Radford-Smith   D. P. Jewell

INTRODUCTION

Cytokines are small peptide molecules of between 5 and 50 kDa, which can be expressed by a number of different cell lineages but which are most commonly associated with cells of the immune system. The majority of these molecules are released as inactive precursors containing a signal peptide, which is then cleaved to give the mature protein. The active molecules have a vast array of functions, with an enormous amount of redundancy built into the cytokine network (Paul 1989). The reason why certain cytokine functions are unique while others are duplicated has not been established. However, it is likely that those functions which are duplicated do not produce a pathological effect even when in excess, whereas the unique functions 'carry a higher risk' when overexpressed and are therefore more tightly regulated.

The redundancy that is built into the system is generated by several factors, first, by receptor sharing. Interferon-α (IFNα) and interferon-β (IFNβ) bind to a single class of receptor (Uze et al 1990). Interleukin-1α and interleukin-1β can both bind to the type 1 and type 2 IL-1 receptors, whereas the interleukin-1 receptor antagonist (IL-1RA) preferentially binds to the type 1 receptor (Carter et al 1990). Cytokines may also use the same signaling pathways for gene activation. For example, IL-2, IL-3, IL-5 and GM-CSF are all able to activate $p21^{ras}$. However, the extent of overlap after this is as yet unknown (Duronio et al 1992).

Specific functions within this overlapping network are more difficult to explain, but may be due to different combinations of α and β receptor subunits for each cytokine, or different receptors being linked to separate signal transduction pathways, as demonstrated by the two IL-1 receptors (Munoz et al 1991). Different cytokines may also selectively stimulate cells which have achieved responsiveness by previous stimuli.

CLASSIFICATION

There is increasing evidence to suggest that cytokines are fundamentally involved in the control of the immune and inflammatory responses. They enable the cellular components of these responses to communicate with each other and can also determine the nature of the response. Certain molecules, such as IL-1, IL-6, TNFα and the chemokines, are predominantly synthesized and released by activated macrophages. IL-1 and IL-6 have the capacity to stimulate both arms of the immune response by activating T cells to produce IL-2 and express the IL-2 receptor, and also by inducing B-cell proliferation, maturation and increased immunoglobulin synthesis. TNFα similarly has an important and wide-ranging role in the inflammatory response and in host resistance, with its ability to induce or suppress expression of a number of genes. These include genes for growth factors and cytokines, transcription factors, receptors, inflammatory mediators and acute-phase proteins.

The other major cytokines, which include IL-2, IL-4, IL-5, IL-10, IL-13 and γ-interferon (IFN), are predominantly synthesized by activated T lymphocytes. These molecules are now subdivided into the Th1 (IL-2 and IFN) and Th2 (IL-4, IL-5, IL-10 and IL-13) subgroups because of their different actions and effects on the immune response. The Th1 subgroup directs a cell-mediated immune response, whereas the Th2 cytokines generate a humoral response (Mosmann & Coffman 1989, Maggi et al 1992). In view of these properties, several disease states have been assessed on the basis of their Th1/Th2 cytokine profiles to determine which arm of the immune response is predominant. In man, the results of these studies have often been unclear. However, there have been some interesting results obtained from patients with leprosy and leishmaniasis, in which there is a clear spectrum of clinical disease (Yamamura et al 1991, Caceres et al 1993). A Th1 cytokine profile predominates in those patients who successfully eradicate the infection, whereas a Th2 profile is found in those with persistent infection. Similar studies are being carried out for patients with inflammatory bowel disease, and the results are discussed below.

Apart from the molecules described above, which are classically termed cytokines, there are several other peptides which have similar properties but are more closely associated with control of growth, differentiation and repair. These include the transforming growth factors α and β (TGF-α and TGF-β) and the recently described trefoil peptides (Poulsom & Wright 1993). The role of these molecules in the inflammatory process is now being addressed.

CYTOKINE ANALYSIS IN INFLAMMATORY BOWEL DISEASE

The chronic nature of the inflammatory process in Crohn's disease and ulcerative colitis has made cytokines an attractive target for investigation. This has been supported by recent findings in genetically engineered 'knockout' animal models in which a cytokine gene has been deleted. The IL-2 knockout (Sadlack et al 1993) develops an ulcerative colitis-type disease with inflammation limited to the colon, whereas an IL-10 knockout (Kuhn et al 1993) suffers a more widespread enterocolitis. Less specific pathology was found with the TGF-β knockout mouse (Shull et al 1992).

With the dramatic improvement in detection techniques over the last decade, adequate information can now be obtained from a set of 2–4 pinch biopsies rather than having to rely on much larger resection specimens. This provides enough RNA to carry out studies using reverse transcription–PCR (polymerase chain reaction) for analysis of cytokine message. However, the majority of studies which have assessed cytokine protein concentrations have used isolated mucosal cells in culture, with and without stimulation, and either bioassays or ELISA kits.

Monokines

The majority of studies in humans have concentrated on an analysis of the monokines (monocyte/macrophage-derived cytokines), including IL-1, IL-6 and TNF-α. IL-1 and IL-6 are minimally expressed in normal tissue but TNF-α may be expressed at a higher constitutive level. In view of the large amounts of lipopolysaccharide in the intestinal lumen and bathing the mucosa, the resident immune cells, (in particular tissue macrophages) appear to have adapted to their environment and become anergic or tolerant to these stimuli. As may be expected, the concentrations of IL-1β are elevated in both active ulcerative colitis and active Crohn's disease, with the majority of IL-1 activity attributed to mucosal macrophages (Mahida et al 1989). Similar results have been found for both protein and mRNA levels using isolated cells, with all the IL-1 activity present in the mononuclear cell fraction and none in the epithelium (Youngman et al 1993).

The concentrations of IL-6 are similarly elevated in active disease, but some studies have shown a more significant increase in patients with Crohn's disease compared to those with ulcerative colitis (Mitsuyama et al 1991, Lobo et al 1992). However, correlation with other markers of disease activity, such as the ESR, CRP or the Crohn's disease activity index (CDAI), has been poor, and therefore plasma levels of this cytokine have not been further investigated as a potential disease marker. This poor correlation may be explained by its very short half-life (<5 min), the effects of steroids (Woloski et al 1985) and the rapid clearance of mucosally produced IL-6 as it passes through the liver.

Assessment of TNF-α in IBD has given rise to mixed results, with one group reporting elevated serum, stool and lamina propria levels of the protein (Murch et al 1993) while others show no significant difference when looking at mRNA levels alone (Stevens et al 1992, Isaacs et al 1992). A study using isolated cells from the lamina propria supported increased levels of TNF-α protein, but spontaneous secretion was far lower than for IL-1 or IL-6 (Reinecker et al 1993). The presence of membrane-bound TNF or soluble receptors 'mopping' up excess TNF was not addressed in the protocol or in the discussion. The differences between the message and the protein data suggest that TNF expression is controlled at the translational level.

Chemokines

This group of small peptides is predominantly involved in the attraction of effector cells to a site of inflammation or infection. They may display a high degree of specificity in this role: for example, the RANTES (Regulated upon Activation in Normal T cells, Expressed and Secreted) molecule from the β subfamily specifically acts on monocytes and memory (CD45RO+) T cells (Schall et al 1990), whereas macrophage inflammatory protein (MIP)-1β (from the same subfamily) increases binding of CD8+ T cells to VCAM-1 (Tanaka et al 1993). These peptides also play a role in activating specific leukocytes.

The levels of IL-8, GRO (α subfamily) and MCP-1 (β subfamily) have been evaluated in IBD. Although results have suggested that some of these molecules may differentiate between active ulcerative colitis and active Crohn's disease, with increased concentrations above controls only being found in ulcerative colitis (Isaacs et al 1992, Mahida et al 1992), the techniques used have not been truly quantitative. Therefore, all one can say at present is that their expression is elevated in inflammation, as has been elegantly shown for MCP-1 (Reinecker et al 1995).

Immunoregulatory cytokines

Th1: IL-2 and γ-interferon

Investigation of these cytokines has led to conflicting results, which are difficult to resolve solely on the basis of differences in technique. Both IL-2 and IFN have been detected at low concentrations compared to normal controls using isolated lamina propria cells (Fiocchi et al 1984, Lieberman et al 1988). This is in contrast to other data, which have found either no difference (Pullman & Doe 1992) or an increase in Crohn's disease alone (Fais et al 1991, Sasaki et al 1992, Mullin et al 1992, Breese et al 1993). The role of these cytokines therefore still requires clarification, but the most recent evidence favors increased concentrations of IL-2 in Crohn's disease.

Th2: IL-4, IL-10 and IL-13

The limited work that has been done in this area has concentrated on a search for a Th2 defect in IBD. A recent report gives in-vitro evidence to suggest that there is an impaired response to IL-4 by activated mononuclear phagocytes in IBD (Schreiber et al 1995). These experiments indicated that both peripheral blood and intestinal phagocytes from patients with active IBD showed a diminished response to the downregulatory effects of IL-4, such as inhibition of IL-1 and TNF production, superoxide anion generation and elevation of the IL-1RA/IL-1 ratio. The study included both normal controls and disease-specific controls, such as patients with diverticulitis.

Other workers have put forward the hypothesis that Crohn's disease is a Th1-driven disease, whereas ulcerative colitis is Th2 driven (Mullin et al 1993, 1994). Recent work with isolated lamina propria lymphocytes supports this theory. Cells taken from patients with active Crohn's disease spontaneously produce IL-2 and no IL-10, whereas cells from ulcerative colitis patients and controls only produced IL-10 spontaneously. In addition, three out of four normal controls produced IL-13 spontaneously, but this was not detected in any of the IBD patients (Radford-Smith et al 1995). The spontaneous production of IL-2 by T cells in the mucosa implies that they have been released from their state of anergy, which is necessary for maintenance of oral tolerance. This reversal of active suppression in the mucosa, which may normally be maintained by a Th2 cytokine profile (Daynes et al 1990, Santos et al 1993), is a hypothesis which deserves further investigation. The mechanism(s) involved in this reversal also need elucidation.

Detection of IL-4 and IL-13 in vivo using snap-frozen gut biopsies has proved more difficult, even with PCR or nested PCR (Radford-Smith 1994). However, the inflammatory disease seen in IBD does not appear to be associated with a defect or reduction in their synthesis.

CYTOKINE LOCALIZATION AND EFFECTS ON INTESTINAL MUCOSA

Localization

Cytokines may be localized in tissue by in-situ hybridization (for mRNA) or immunohistochemistry (for protein). The majority of this work has been done on the monokines and chemokines, presumably because of their greater abundance in inflamed tissue and because of the availability of monoclonal antibodies to these molecules.

In-situ hybridization has detected IL-1 in subepithelial macrophages, whereas TNF is found deeper in the lamina propria (Cappello et al 1992). As may be expected, the staining for TNF differs between ulcerative colitis and Crohn's disease, with a more superficial distribution in the former and staining throughout the lamina propria in the latter (Murch et al 1993). IL-6 is found in association with T and B cells as well as macrophages (Stevens et al 1992), which correlates with cell depletion studies (Reinecker et al 1993).

The chemokines IL-8 and MCP-1 have been found in macrophages and in the epithelium (Grimm et al 1994, Eckmann et al 1993, Gibson & Rosella 1994). IL-8 is also found in neutrophils (Grumm et al 1994). However, until recently the epithelial findings have only been successful with isolated cells, and this has raised the question as to whether the isolation process itself alters cytokine expression by this group of cells. Very recently, a group have published interesting findings using a polyclonal rabbit antihuman MCP-1 antibody. In the normal colon staining is found in the epithelium, whereas in the inflamed organ staining is widespread (?more non-specific), including spindle cells, mononuclear cells and endothelium (Reinecker et al 1995). The implication from this and previous work on epithelial cells is that they may be capable of engaging in and enhancing a local immune response at a site of injury, thus protecting against potential microbial invasion and further damage.

Localization of immunoregulatory cytokines has not been addressed, although one study (Bromley et al 1994) showed the presence of IL-4 in lamina propria mononuclear cells using digoxigenin-based in situ hybridization in paraffin sections. The scarcity of intestinal IL-4 message detected using PCR, and the relative lack of sensitivity of the techniques used in this study, throws some doubt on the results, and further work by independent investigators in this field is essential.

Pathophysiological effects

Cytokines can work in an autocrine, paracrine or endocrine fashion, and influence not only immune cells but also epithelium, endothelium, mesenchyme and the extracellular matrix. Overproduction can lead to clinical sequelae such as diarrhea and fibrosis, but some of these molecules also have important roles to play in the suppression of both 'physiological' and pathological inflammation, and in healing and repair.

Enhancement of the immune response both locally and systemically is an important feature of most cytokines, but in particular IL-1 and TNF. These induce the synthesis and release of IL-8, which is responsible for further cellular recruitment. IL-1 can also induce IL-2 and IL-2R on T cells. These activated helper cells may then contribute to the cellular (Th1) and humoral (Th2) arms of the immune response. IL-1, IL-6 and TNF all contribute to the hepatic acute-phase response, and other systemic effects such as anorexia, fever, anemia and thrombocytosis.

The Th2 cytokines and TGF-β control the humoral immune response, including the production of mucosal IgA. They have important downregulatory effects on both macrophages and lymphocytes (de Waal Malefyt et al 1991, Oswald et al 1992), and are thought to be an important component of the 'active suppression' mechanism in oral tolerance (Santos et al 1993).

Cytokines produced by local immune cells can induce epithelial cytokine production, as alluded to above. This includes IL-6, IL-8, MCP-1 and TGF-β. IL-8 and MCP-1 act as potent chemoattractants, whereas TGF-β is essential for normal epithelial growth and repair (Barnard et al 1989, Dignass & Podolsky 1993). An excess of TGF may be detrimental, and its role in the development of strictures in Crohn's disease has been evaluated. Fibroblasts taken from Crohn's disease patients produced significantly more type III collagen than controls after exposure to exogenous TGF-β, but excess TGF-β has not as yet been convincingly demonstrated in diseased tissue.

IL-1 may be directly involved in the diarrhea associated with intestinal inflammation. Two mechanisms may be involved: epithelial chloride secretion via increased bradykinin and histamine release; and the effects of prostaglandins released from degranulating mast cells. Both of these can be mediated by IL-1 (Theodorou et al 1994). IFN can increase MHC class II expression on epithelial cells, as exemplified by inflammatory states such as IBD. This may lead to increased antigen presentation, and potentially increased Th1 and Th2 lymphocyte activation. IFN also increases mucosal permeability by damaging epithelial cell tight junctions. This, together with increased adhesion molecule expression, may facilitate neutrophil migration from submucosa to the intestinal lumen or crypt (Colgan et al 1993, Kelly et al 1992). IL-2 is predominantly a T-cell growth factor, but recent studies suggest that it may also be involved in epithelial cell turnover and repair (Ciacci et al 1993).

CYTOKINES AND ANTICYTOKINES AS THERAPEUTIC STRATEGIES

In view of their effects on the immune system several cytokines have already been used in the treatment of various diseases, including IL-2 in renal cell carcinoma and α-interferon in viral hepatitis. The use of cytokines or their antagonists in IBD has only recently been considered. These include the IL-1 receptor antagonist (IL-1 RA), interleukin-10, and humanized antibodies to TNF-α.

The IL-1 RA is a naturally occurring protein that binds to the type 1 and type 2 receptors but has no agonist activity. It therefore acts as an endogenous downregulator of inflammation by blocking the effects of IL-1 (Eisenberg et al 1990). It has been shown to be effective in a rabbit model of colitis (Cominelli et al 1990), and more recently mucosal concentrations were found to be inappropriately low in patients with active IBD compared to non-IBD inflammatory controls. The ratio of IL-1 RA to IL-1 in the IBD group was also much lower, at 5.6 ± 1.8 for Crohn's disease and 6.3 ± 1.5 for ulcerative colitis, compared to 25.2 ± 7.3 for the inflammatory controls (Cominelli et al 1994). A clinical trial of IL-1 RA in IBD is currently in progress.

The use of IL-10 as a therapeutic agent in IBD has been stimulated by its potent downregulatory effects on activated macrophages and the results of the IL-10 knockout model. Human recombinant IL-10 is now available, and a clinical trial using it in the treatment of steroid-resistant Crohn's disease is expected very shortly.

Humanized antibodies to TNF-α have already been assessed in an open-label phase I study in patients with active Crohn's disease. There were no side effects, and in all patients the CDAI dropped to within normal limits in 4 weeks. The average duration of response was 8 weeks after a single infusion (van Dulleman et al 1994). The encouraging early results should stimulate further work in this field, and hopefully provide alternatives to corticosteroids and immunosuppressants in the treatment of these disorders.

CONCLUSIONS AND THE FUTURE

Cytokines contribute to the pathology of IBD by determining the nature of the mucosal immune response. To establish whether they are involved at the etiological level requires further assessment of cytokine gene polymorphisms, in both the diseased and the normal population.

The majority of gene expression studies have established that the monokines are elevated in active disease, but differences between the diseases are less clear and reflect the lack of accuracy and sensitivity in quantification. There is also increasing evidence that Crohn's disease is a Th1-mediated disease, with increased mucosal expression of IL-2 and IFN. The insult or antigen that precipitates this is as yet not established. In contrast, the Th1/Th2 profile in ulcerative colitis is not significantly different from normal controls.

REFERENCES

Barnard J A, Beauchamp R D, Coffey R J, Moses H L 1989 Regulation of intestinal epithelial cell growth by transforming growth factor type beta. Proceedings of the National Academy of Sciences of the USA 86: 1578–1582

Breese E, Braegger C P, Corrigan C J, Walker S J, Mac D T 1993 Interleukin-2- and interferon-gamma-secreting T cells in normal and diseased human intestinal mucosa. Immunology 78: 127–131

Bromley L, McCarthy S P, Stickland J E, Lewis C E, McGee J O 1994 Non-isotopic in situ detection of mRNA for interleukin-4 in archival human tissue. Journal of Immunological Methods 167: 47–54

Caceres D G, Tapia F J, Sanchez M A et al 1993 Determination of the cytokine profile in American cutaneous leishmaniasis using the polymerase chain reaction. Clinical and Experimental Immunology 91: 500–505

Cappello M, Keshav S, Prince C, Jewell D P, Gordon S 1992 Detection of mRNAs for macrophage products in inflammatory bowel disease by in situ hybridisation. Gut 33: 1214–1219

Carter D, Deibel M, Dunn C et al 1990 Purification, cloning, expression and biological characterization of an interleukin-1 receptor antagonist protein. Nature 344: 633–638

Ciacci D, Mahida Y R, Dignass A, Koizumi M, Podolsky D K 1993 Functional interleukin-2 receptors on intestinal epithelial cells. Journal of Clinical Investigation 92: 527–532

Colgan S P, Parkos C A, Delp C, Arnaout M A, Madara J L 1993 Neutrophil migration across cultured intestinal epithelial monolayers is modulated by epithelial exposure to IFN-gamma in a highly polarized fashion. Journal of Cell Biology 120: 785–798

Cominelli F, Nast C C, Clark B D et al 1990 Interleukin 1 (IL-1) gene expression, synthesis, and effect of specific IL-1 receptor blockade in rabbit immune complex colitis. Journal of Clinical Investigation 86: 972–980

Cominelli F, Kam L, Casini-Raggi V et al 1994 Specific mucosal imbalance of IL-1 and IL-1 receptor antagonist (IL-1ra) in IBD: a potential mechanism of chronic inflammation. Gastroenterology 106: A667

Daynes R, Araneo B, Dowell T, Huang K, Dudley D 1990 Regulation of murine lymphokine production in vivo. III. The lymphoid tissue microenvironment exerts regulatory influences over T helper cell function. Journal of Experimental Medicine 171: 979–996

de Waal Malefyt R, Haanen J, Spits H et al 1991 Interleukin 10 (IL-10) and viral IL-10 strongly reduce antigen-specific human T cell proliferation by diminishing the antigen-presenting capacity of monocytes via downregulation of class II major histocompatibility complex expression. Journal of Experimental Medicine 174: 915–924

Dignass A U, Podolsky D K 1993 Cytokine modulation of intestinal epithelial cell restitution: central role of transforming growth factor beta. Gastroenterology 105: 1323–1332

Duronio V, Welham M, Abraham S, Dryden P, Schrader J 1992 $p21^{ras}$ activation via hemopoietin receptors and c-kit requires tyrosine kinase activity but not tyrosine phosphorylation of $p21^{ras}$ GTPase-activating protein. Proceedings of the National Academy of Sciences of the USA 89: 1587–1591

Eckmann L, Jung H C, Schurer M C, Panja A, Morzycka W E, Kagnoff M F 1993 Differential cytokine expression by human intestinal epithelial cell lines: regulated expression of interleukin 8. Gastroenterology 105: 1689–1697

Eisenberg S P, Evans R J, Arend W P et al 1990 Primary structure and functional expression from complementary DNA of a human interleukin-1 receptor antagonist. Nature 343: 341–346

Fais S, Capobianchi M R, Pallone F et al 1991 Spontaneous release of interferon gamma by intestinal lamina propria lymphocytes in Crohn's disease. Kinetics of in vitro response to interferon gamma inducers. Gut 32: 403–407

Fiocchi C, Hilfiker M L, Youngman K R, Doerder N C, Finke J H 1984 Interleukin 2 activity of human intestinal mucosa mononuclear cells. Decreased levels in inflammatory bowel disease. Gastroenterology 86: 734–742

Gibson P, Rosella O 1994 Interleukin-8 secretion by colonic epithelial cells in vitro modulation and effect of disease. Gastroenterlogy 106: A687

Grimm M, Elsbury S, van de Pol E et al 1994 Increased chemokine expression by lamina propria cells in inflammatory bowel disease. Gastroenterology 106: A693

Isaacs K L, Sartor R B, Haskill S 1992 Cytokine messenger RNA profiles in inflammatory bowel disease mucosa detected by polymerase chain reaction amplification. Gastroenterology 103: 1587–1595

Kelly C P, O'Keane J C, Orellana J et al 1992 Human colon cancer cells express ICAM-1 in vivo and support LFA-1-dependent lymphocyte adhesion in vitro. American Journal of Physiology 263: S864–870

Kuhn R, Lohler J, Rennick D, Rajewsky K, Muller W 1993 Interleukin-10-deficient mice develop chronic enterocolitis. Cell 75: 263–274

Lieberman B Y, Fiocchi C, Youngman K R, Sapatnekar W K, Proffitt M R 1988 Interferon γ production by human intestinal mucosal mononuclear cells. Decreased levels in inflammatory bowel disease. Digestive Diseases and Sciences 33: 1297–1304

Lobo A, Evans S, Jones S et al 1992 Plasma interleukin-6 in inflammatory bowel disease. European Journal of Gastionentenology and Hepatology 4: 367–372

Maggi E, Parronchi P, Manetti R et al 1992 Reciprocal regulatory effects of IFN-gamma and IL-4 on the in vitro development of human Th1 and Th2 clones. Journal of Immunology 148: 2142–2147

Mahida Y R, Wu K, Jewell D P 1989 Enhanced production of interleukin 1-beta by mononuclear cells isolated from mucosa with active ulcerative colitis of Crohn's disease. Gut 30: 835–838

Mahida Y R, Ceska M, Effenberger F, Kurlak L, Lindley I, Hawkey C J 1992 Enhanced synthesis of neutrophil-activating peptide-1/interleukin-8 in active ulcerative colitis. Clinical Science 82: 273–275

Mitsuyama K, Sata M, Tanikawa K 1991 Significance of interleukin-6 in patients with inflammatory bowel disease. Gastroenterology Japan 26: 20–28

Mosmann T R, Coffman R L 1989 TH1 and TH2 cells: different patterns of lymphokine secretion lead to different functional properties. Annual Review of Immunology 7: 145–173

Mullin G E, Lazenby A J, Harris M L, Bayless T M, James S P 1992 Increased interleukin-2 messenger RNA in the intestinal mucosal lesions of Crohn's disease but not ulcerative colitis. Gastroenterology 102: 1620–1627

Mullin G, Vezza F, Sampat A et al 1993 Abnormal IL 10 mRNA production in the intestinal mucosal lesions of inflammatory bowel disease. Gastroenterology 104: A751

Mullin G, Maycon Z, Katz R et al 1994 IL-13 in the mucosal lesions of inflammatory bowel disease. Gastroenterology 106: A740

Munoz E, Zubiaga A, Sims J, Huber B 1991 IL-1 signal transduction pathways. I. Two functional IL-1 receptors are expressed in T cells. Journal of Immunology 146: 136–143

Murch S H, Braegger C P, Walker S J, Mac D T 1993 Location of tumour necrosis factor alpha by immunohistochemistry in chronic inflammatory bowel disease. Gut 34: 1705–1709

Oswald I P, Gazzinelli R T, Sher A, James S L 1992 IL-10 synergizes with IL-4 and transforming growth factor-beta to inhibit macrophage cytotoxic activity. Journal of Immunology 148: 3578–3582

Paul W E 1989 Pleiotropy and redundancy: T cell-derived lymphokines in the immune response. Cell 57: 521–524

Poulsom R, Wright N 1993 Trefoil peptides: a newly recognized family of epithelial mucin-associated molecules. American Journal of Physiology 265: G205–G213

Pullman W E, Doe W F 1992 IL-2 production by intestinal lamina propria cells in normal inflamed and cancer-bearing colons. Clinical and Experimental Immunology 88: 132–137

Radford-Smith G L 1994 Cytokine gene expression in inflammatory bowel disease. DPhil Thesis, University of Oxford

Radford-Smith G, McGowan I, Jewell D 1995 Inappropriate spontaneous production of IL-2 mRNA by intestinal lamina propria lymphocytes from patients with Crohn's disease. Evidence for a Th1/Th2 switch. (in preparation)

Reinecker H C, Steffen M, Witthoeft T et al 1993 Enhanced secretion of tumour necrosis factor-alpha, IL-6, and IL-1 beta by isolated lamina propria mononuclear cells from patients with ulcerative colitis and Crohn's disease. Clinical and Experimental Immunology 94: 174–181

Reinecker H-C, Loh E, Ringler D, Mehta A, Rombeau J, MacDermott R 1995 Monocyte-chemoattractant protein 1 gene expression in intestinal epithelial cells and inflammatory bowel disease mucosa. Gastroenterology 108: 40–50

Sadlack B, Merz H, Schorle H, Schimpl A, Feller A C, Horak I 1993 Ulcerative colitis-like disease in mice with a disrupted interleukin-2 gene. Cell 75: 253–261

Santos L, Al-Sabbagh A, Londono A, Weiner H 1993 Oral tolerance to myelin basic protein induces TGF-β secreting T cells in Peyer's patches. Journal of Immunology 150: 115A

Sasaki T, Hiwatashi N, Yamazaki H, Noguchi M, Toyota T 1992 The role of interferon gamma in the pathogenesis of Crohn's disease. Gastroenterology Japan 27: 29–36

Schall T J, Bacon K, Toy K J, Goeddel D V 1990 Selective attraction of monocytes and T lymphocytes of the memory phenotype by cytokine RANTES. Nature 347: 669–671

Schreiber S, Heining T, Panzer U et al 1995 Impaired response of activated mononuclear phagocytes to interleukin 4 in inflammatory bowel disease. Gastroenterology 108: 21–33

Shull M M, Ormsby I, Kier A B et al 1992 Targeted disruption of the mouse transforming growth factor-beta 1 gene results in multifocal inflammatory disease. Nature 359: 693–699

Stevens C, Walz G, Singaram C et al 1992 Tumor necrosis factor-alpha, interleukin-1 beta, and interleukin-6 expression in inflammatory bowel disease. Digestive Diseases and Sciences 37: 818–826

Tanaka Y, Adams D H, Hubscher S, Hirano H, Siebenlist U, Shaw S 1993 T-cell adhesion induced by proteoglycan-immobilized cytokine MIP-1 beta. Nature 361: 79–82

Theodorou V, Eutamene H, Fioramonti J, Junien J, Bueno L 1994 Interleukin 1 induces a neurally mediated colonic secretion in rats: involvement of mast cells and prostaglandins. Gastroenterology 106: 1493–1500

Uze G, Lutfalla G, Gresser G 1990 Genetic transfer of a functional human interferon-α receptor into mouse cells: cloning and expression of its cDNA. Cell 60: 225–234

van Dulleman H, Hommes D, Meenan J et al 1994 Complete remission of steroid-refractory Crohn's disease after administration of monoclonal anti-TNF antibody. Gastroenterology 106: A1054

Woloski B M, Smith E M, Meyer W, Fuller G M, Blalock J E 1985 Corticotropin-releasing activity of monokines. Science 230: 1035–1037

Yamamura M, Uyemura K, Deans R J et al 1991 Defining protective responses to pathogens: cytokine profiles in leprosy lesions. Science 254: 277–279

Youngman K R, Simon P L, West G A et al 1993 Localization of intestinal interleukin 1 activity and protein and gene expression to lamina propria cells. Gastroenterology 104: 749–758

13. Platelets and coagulation
M. Hudson   P. Kesteven

INTRODUCTION

An increased risk of clinical thromboembolic complications is reported to affect 2–6% of patients with inflammatory bowel disease (Bargen & Barker 1936, Ricketts & Palmer 1946, Edwards & Truelove 1954, Talbot et al 1986), rising to an incidence of 39% in some postmortem studies (Graef et al 1966). Elevated levels of plasma fibrinogen, factor V, factor VIII and thrombocytosis may all occur in active ulcerative colitis and Crohn's disease. The thrombotic risk has therefore been attributed to a hypercoagulable state (Lee et al 1968, Morowitz et al 1968, Talstad et al 1970, Lam et al 1975, Lake et al 1978, Talbot et al 1986). However, since most of these proteins may act as acute-phase reactants, elevated blood concentrations of these factors alone may not in themselves constitute a prothrombotic risk.

Thrombosis, vasculitis and tissue infarction have been proposed as contributing factors in Crohn's disease (Wakefield et al 1989). Microvascular thromboses occur in association with granulomatous or lymphocytic inflammation of the affected blood vessels. It has therefore been proposed that activation of the endothelium and the coagulation pathway is central to this enhanced thrombotic tendency. An abnormal tendency to thrombosis may be due to increased activity of procoagulant forces (coagulation cascade, platelet inhibitors, fibrinolytic activators). Under physiological conditions these two forces are kept in homeostatic balance by the vascular endothelium (Fig. 13.1). In 1–2% of the population a specific inherited abnormality in one of the proteins involved in clotting leads to a well defined risk of thrombosis – the thrombophilic syndromes. However, in the majority of cases with thrombosis no such specific abnormality is demonstrable. In such cases the homeostasis is disrupted towards clotting by complex effects on the system and, in particular, by perturbation of the vascular endothelium. Such a tendency towards thrombosis may be demonstrated by decreased concentrations of coagulation proteins or increased levels of markers of activation of coagulation

Procoagulant	Anticoagulant
Coagulation cascade	Antithrombin III Protein C Protein S
Platelet agonists	Prostacyclin
Fibrinolytic inhibitors (PAI-1)	Fibrinolytic activators (tPA)
Perturbed vascular endothelium (tissue factor)	
Thrombosis	**Hemorrhage**

Fig. 13.1 The balance of procoagulant and anticoagulant properties on the endothelial cell surface. PAI-1, plasminogen activator inhibitor; tPA, plasminogen activator.

such as fibrinopeptide-A (FPA) and prothrombin fragments (F1 + 2) (Fig. 13.2). The evidence for systemic and local activation of the coagulation cascade and platelets in inflammatory bowel disease is discussed below.

EVIDENCE OF THROMBOGENESIS

Fibrinopeptide-A (FPA) is a 16-amino acid peptide cleaved from fibrinogen by thrombin. As the half-life of FPA in plasma is <4 minutes, the plasma level of FPA is a sensitive indicator of ongoing in-vivo fibrinogen cleavage and, presumably, fibrin generation. Edwards and colleagues (1987) studied FPA levels in 36 consecutive patients with Crohn's disease. A strong correlation existed between FPA levels and clinical disease activity as determined by the Crohn's disease activity index (CDAI). FPA levels were elevated above the upper limit of normal in 95% of samples from patients with active disease, and 53% of samples from patients with inactive disease. Thus, in-vivo activation of blood coagulation was seen in many patients with inactive disease. These observations were confirmed by Hudson and colleagues (1993a) in 16 patients with Crohn's disease studied serially from relapse through to

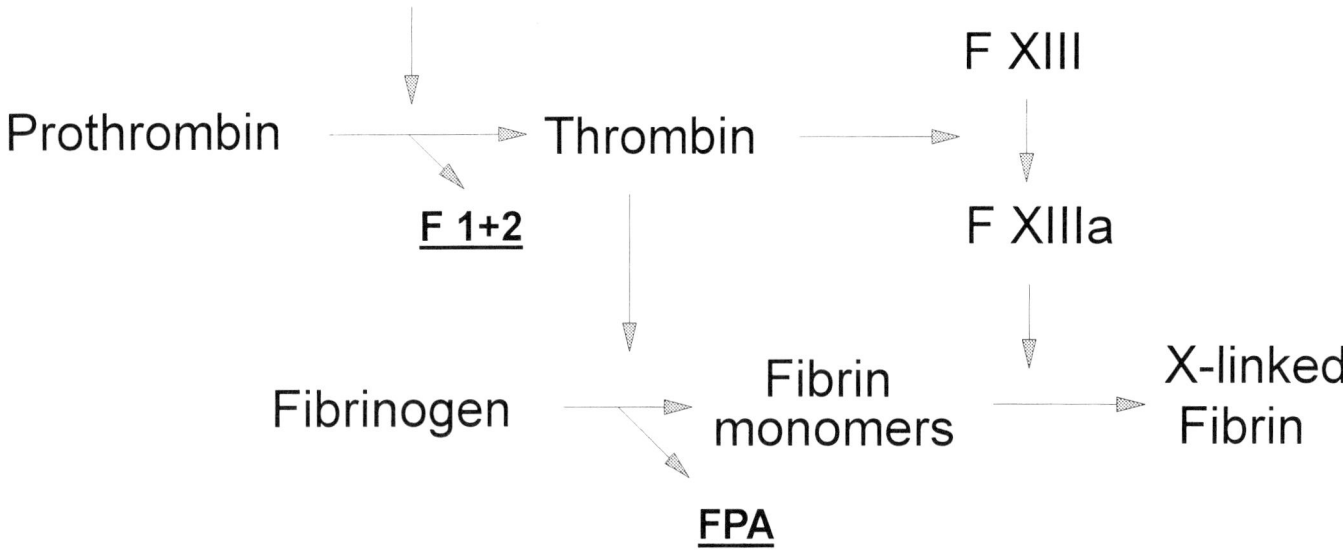

Fig. 13.2 A simplification of the coagulation cascade.

clinical remission, as determined by the Harvey–Bradshaw score. In this study plasma FPA levels and prothrombin fragments F1 + 2 were measured. Elevated concentrations of both were found at times of both active and inactive disease. The majority of samples (35 out of 52: 67%) exhibited evidence of persistent activation of hemostasis (elevated FPA and/or F1 + 2) during phases of apparent clinical remission in Crohn's disease. This was not reflected by clinical activity scores.

In a further study by the same group (Hudson et al 1993b) Factor XIII and its two subunits XIIIA (proenzyme) and XIIIS (carrier protein) were studied. Factor XIII is responsible for cross-linking fibrin into stable adherent clot. Sixteen patients with Crohn's disease were studied prospectively from relapse (CDAI >150) into remission. The plasma Factor XIIIA concentrations were significantly lower in active disease than in remission. In five patients with persistent aggressive disease, the Factor XIIIA concentration remained below the lower range of normal, despite apparent clinical improvement in response to medical treatment (Fig. 13.3). These patients had a poorer outcome in terms of requirements for continued immunosuppression and need for surgery. Tissues from three patients who underwent surgical resection during the study were immunostained for Factor XIIIA. In one patient, capillary thrombi near superficial mucosal erosions immunostained positive for Factor XIIIA in macroscopically normal mucosa. Similar changes were identified in more severely inflamed sections of intestine from the two other patients.

The demonstration of significantly low plasma Factor XIIIA concentrations in active Crohn's disease, and

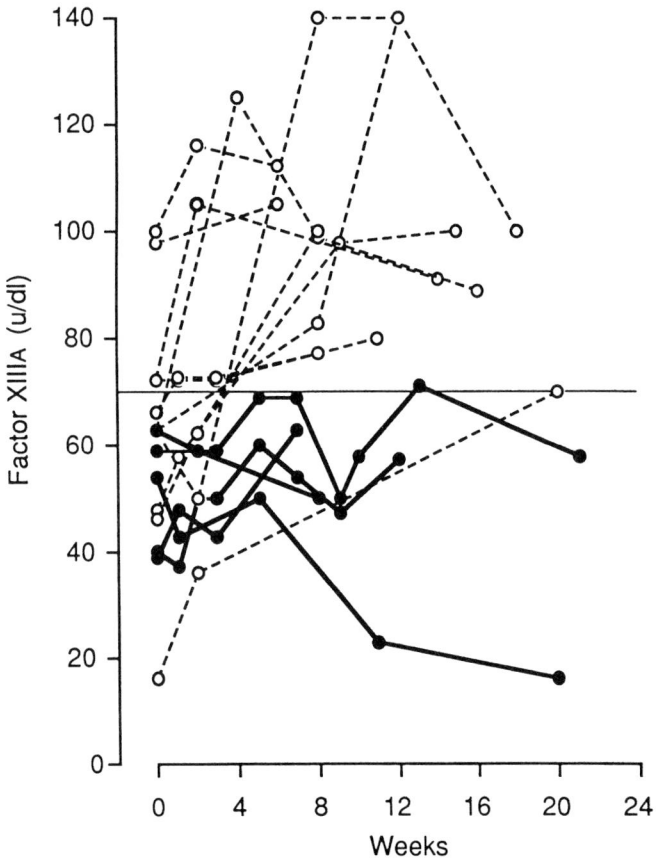

Fig. 13.3 Serum Factors XIIIA in Crohn's disease in response to treatment. ●—● = the five of 16 patients who have a persistently low Factor XIIIA level despite apparent symptomatic response to treatment. (Reproduced with permission of Gut (Hudson et al 1993b)).

immunostaining of Factor XIIIA in capillary thrombi in the bowel wall, suggests that activation of coagulation may be involved in the pathogenesis of Crohn's disease. Similar findings have also been observed in patients with sigmoidoscopically active ulcerative colitis (Hudson, unpublished data).

Activation of the coagulation cascade has long been recognized as an important component of the inflammatory response, and fibrin deposition has been observed in well-characterized delayed hypersensitivity reactions (Colvin et al 1973). Fibrin deposition is implicated in the pathogenesis of a range of inflammatory disorders, including systemic lupus erythematosus (Hardin et al 1978) and renal allograft rejection (Hattler et al 1973). Although the cause of this hypercoagulability has not been fully defined for each of these disorders, the monocyte-derived procoagulant, tissue factor, appears to be central to the activation of coagulation. Monocytes express tissue factor on their surface following in-vitro exposure to immune stimuli (Hattler et al 1973, Edwards & Rickles 1984). This membrane-associated glycoprotein is the cell receptor for Factor VII. Monocyte tissue factor production is regulated by T lymphocytes, cytokines and other immune regulators (Edwards & Rickles 1980, 1984). Edwards and colleagues (1987) studied this further in mononuclear cell suspensions prepared from 18 patients with Crohn's disease and 18 controls. Monocyte procoagulant activity (MPCA) was measured immediately after collection to assess in-vivo MPCA generation. Although patient cells produced twice the MPCA of control cells, the difference was not statistically significant. To assess the potential role of MPCA in the in-vivo activation of coagulation in clinically inactive patients, plasma FPA levels and unstimulated MPCA generation at 24 hours were measured in 15 patients. A strong positive correlation was observed ($r = 0.89$, $P<0.001$), supporting the hypothesis that monocyte activation and increased generation of MPCA may play a role in the activation of blood coagulation in these patients.

Immunohistochemical evidence of tissue factor expression has also been sought in tissue sections. More and colleagues (1993) studied serial cryostat sections of tissue taken from patients with Crohn's disease ($n = 8$), ulcerative colitis ($n = 5$) and from controls ($n = 5$), stained with hematoxylin and eosin and immunostained for tissue factor, collagen type IV, fibrinogen and platelet glycoprotein IIIa. In control tissues, tissue factor was present as a continuous layer along the epithelial basal lamina (as described by Drake and colleagues (1989)), but sections from controls did not immunostain for either fibrinogen or platelets. In non-ulcerated inflamed mucosa, tissue factor staining intensified in cases of Crohn's disease and was associated with fibrin deposition. In ulcerative colitis staining for tissue factor was either patchy or absent, and there was no fibrin deposition. In both diseases tissue factor expression in severely inflamed and ulcerated mucosa was present on lamina propria macrophages and vascular endothelium, and was associated with fibrin or platelet thrombi. In three of eight cases of Crohn's disease tissue factor expression and thrombi were evident in areas of submucosal vasculitis. These were not seen in adjacent normal vessels. These observations are consistent with a tissue factor hemostatic barrier in the intestine: this barrier seems to be incomplete or defective in ulcerative colitis. Tissue factor expression by macrophages and endothelial cells may increase microvascular thrombosis and enhance the prothrombotic environment.

EVIDENCE FOR CHANGES IN ACTIVITY OF THE PHYSIOLOGICAL INHIBITORS OF COAGULATION

Partial deficiencies of antithrombin III to 60% of normal have been described in both active ulcerative colitis and Crohn's disease (Lam et al 1975, Lake et al 1978, Ghosh et al 1983). However, low levels of antithrombin III are not a consistent finding in active Crohn's disease. Hudson and colleagues (1993a) demonstrated no significant difference in antithrombin III levels during active and inactive Crohn's disease in 16 patients followed from relapse into clinical remission. The acquired antithrombin III deficiency is presumed to be due to increased consumption.

There are no reports of reduced protein C activity in inflammatory bowel disease, although reduced protein C antigen levels have been reported in active Crohn's disease (Hudson et al 1993a). This did not reach statistical significance. However, in the same study free protein S (the essential cofactor for protein C) levels were significantly reduced in active disease. Two patients in the study had free protein S levels below the lower limit of normal during both active and inactive disease. This is particularly interesting, as there has been one previous report of a young girl with Crohn's disease and a low free protein S concentration, who experienced nine separate thromboembolic events (Whyshock et al 1988).

EVIDENCE OF IMPAIRED FIBRINOLYSIS

There is evidence for impaired fibrinolysis in inflammatory bowel disease. De Jong and colleagues (1989) demonstrated impaired fibrinolysis in both plasma and colonic mucosa of patients with Crohn's disease and ulcerative colitis when compared to controls. In plasma they demonstrated a small but significant rise in plasminogen activator inhibitor (PAI), with a decrease in tissue plasminogen activator (tPA). Two groups (De Jong et al 1989, de Bruin et al 1988) have demonstrated an increase in mucosal urokinase plasminogen activator (uPA), with a concomitant decrease in tPA. Further evidence of hypofibrinolysis in inflammatory bowel disease has been reported by Conlan and colleagues (1989) in five of eight patients. Four patients had high baseline PAI and in three of these the value rose following venous occlusion. In two patients the euglobulin lysis time remained prolonged (>240 min) following venous occlusion. The fifth patient had low levels of releasable tPA following venous occlusion. These observations are supported by Gris and colleagues (1990). They have demonstrated a defective increase in tPA and residual PAI activity after venous occlusion in 17 patients (7 Crohn's disease, 10 ulcerative colitis). Such changes in fibrinolytic activity would be consistent with perturbation of the vascular endothelium.

PLATELET ABNORMALITIES

A secondary thrombocytosis is not unusual in inflammatory bowel disease, as a response to either chronic inflammation or chronic blood loss. Although qualitative abnormalities (decreased platelet survival) have been demonstrated in a small number of patients with active colitis without thrombosis, these reverted to normal with medical treatment (Morowitz et al 1968). Mori and colleagues (1980) noted accelerated platelet aggregation and retention rates in active Crohn's disease and ulcerative colitis. Webberley and colleagues (1993) investigated platelet function in 104 patients (40 Crohn's disease, 64 ulcerative colitis), of whom eight had previous thromboembolism: 35 had reproducible spontaneous platelet aggregation of more than 30%, which was highly significant when compared to controls. A further 20 patients showed hypersensitivity of platelets to low concentrations of aggregating agents. Plasma thromboxane B_2 and β-thromboglobulin levels were significantly higher than in controls. Platelet survival studies were normal. There was no correlation with disease activity. This suggests that patients with inflammatory bowel disease have abnormal platelet activity, which may contribute to the inflammatory process.

SUMMARY

It is well recognized that a hypercoagulable state exists in patients with inflammatory bowel disease, which involves all components of the clotting system. It is likely that this represents local perturbation of vascular endothelial cell function. Furthermore, such a hypercoagulable state may be closely linked to the pathogenesis of inflammatory bowel disease and may provide a subtle marker of disease activity.

REFERENCES

Bargen J A, Barker N W 1936 Extensive arterial and venous thrombosis complicating chronic ulcerative colitis. Archives of Internal Medicine 58: 17–31

Colvin R B, Johnson R A, Mihm M C, Dvorak H F 1973 Role of clotting system in cell mediated immunity. I. Fibrin deposition in delayed skin reactions in man. Journal of Experimental Medicine 138: 686–698

Conlan M G, Haire W D, Burnett D A 1989 Prothrombotic abnormalities in inflammatory bowel disease. Digestive Diseases and Sciences 34: 1089–1093

de Bruin P A F, Crama-Bohbouth G, Verspaget H W et al 1988 Plasminogen activators in the intestine of patients with inflammatory bowel disease. Thrombosis and Haemostasis 60: 262–266

De Jong E, Porte R J, Knot E A R, Verheijen J H, Dees J 1989 Disturbed fibrinolysis in patients with inflammatory bowel disease. A study in blood plasma, colon mucosa and faeces. Gut 30: 188–194

Drake T A, Morrissey J H, Edgington T S 1989 Selective cellular expression of tissue factor in human tissues. American Journal of Pathology 134: 1087–1097

Edwards R L, Rickles F R 1980 The role of T cells (and T cell products) for monocyte tissue factor generation. Journal of Immunology 125: 606–609

Edwards R L, Rickles F R 1984 Macrophage procoagulants. Progress in Hemostasis Thrombosis 7: 183–209

Edwards F C, Truelove S C 1954 The course and prognosis of ulcerative colitis. Part III: complications. Gut 5: 1–15

Edwards R L, Levine J B, Green R et al 1987 Activation of blood coagulation in Crohn's disease. Gastroenterology 92: 329–337

Ghosh S, Mackie M J, McVerry B A, Galloway M, Ellis A, McKay J 1983 Chronic inflammatory bowel disease, deep-venous thrombosis and antithrombin activity. Acta Haematologica 70: 50–53

Graef V, Baggenstoss A H, Sauer W G, Spittell J A 1966 Venous thrombosis occurring with non-specific ulcerative colitis. Archives of Internal Medicine 117: 277–282

Gris J C, Schved J F, Raffanel C, Dubois A 1990 Impaired fibrinolytic capacity in patients with inflammatory bowel disease. Thrombosis Haemostasis 63: 472–475

Hardin J A, Cronlund M, Haber E, Block K J 1978 Activation of blood clotting in patients with systemic lupus erythematosus. Relationship to disease activity. American Journal of Medicine 65: 430–436

Hattler B G, Rocklin R E, Ward P A, Rickles F R 1973 Functional features of lymphocytes recovered from a human renal allograft. Cellular Immunology 9: 289–295

Hudson M, Hutton R A, Wakefield A J, Sawyerr A M, Pounder R E 1993a Evidence for accelerated thrombogenesis in Crohn's disease. Blood Coagulation and Fibrinolysis 3: 773–778

Hudson M, Wakefield A J, Hutton R A et al 1993b Factor XIIIA subunit and Crohn's disease. Gut 34: 75–79

Lake A M, Stauffer J Q, Stuart M J 1978 Haemostatic alterations in inflammatory bowel disease. American Journal of Digestive Diseases 23: 897–902

Lam A, Borda L T, Inwood M J, Thompson S 1975 Coagulation studies in ulcerative colitis and Crohn's disease. Gastroenterology 68: 245–251

Lee J C L, Spittell J, Sauer W G, Owen C A, Thompson J H 1968 Hypercoagulability associated with chronic ulcerative colitis: changes in blood coagulation factors. Gastroenterology 54: 76–84

More L, Sim R, Hudson M, Dhillon A P, Pounder R E, Wakefield A J 1993 Immunohistochemical study of tissue factor expression in normal intestine and idiopathic inflammatory bowel disease. Journal of Clinical Pathology 46: 703–708

Mori K, Watanabe H, Hiwatashi N, Sugai K, Goto Y 1980 Studies on blood coagulation in ulcerative colitis and Crohn's disease. Tohoku Journal of Experimental Medicine 132: 93–101

Morowitz D A, Allen L W, Kirsner J B 1968 Thrombocytosis in chronic inflammatory bowel disease. Annals of Internal Medicine 68: 1013–1021

Ricketts W E, Palmer W L 1946 Complications of chronic non-specific ulcerative colitis. Gastroenterology 7: 55–56

Talbot R W, Heppell J, Dozois R R, Beart R W 1986 Vascular

complications of inflammatory bowel disease. Mayo Clinic Proceedings 61: 140–145

Talstad I, Rootwelk K, Gjone E 1970 Thrombocytosis in ulcerative colitis and Crohn's disease. Scandinavian Journal of Gastroenterology 8: 135

Wakefield A J, Sawyerr A M, Dhillon A P et al 1989 Pathogenesis of Crohn's disease: multifocal gastrointestinal infarction. Lancet ii: 1057–1062

Webberley M J, Hart M T, Melikian V 1993 Thromboembolism in inflammatory bowel disease: role of platelets. Gut 34: 247–251

Whyshock E, Caldwell M, Crowley J P 1988 Deep venous thrombosis, inflammatory bowel disease and protein S deficiency. American Journal of Clinical Pathology 90: 633–635

14. Inflammatory mediators

D. S. Rampton

INTRODUCTION

Although the etiology of inflammatory bowel disease (IBD) remains obscure, its pathogenesis is gradually being unraveled. In brief, it appears that an initiating factor, for example a microbial or dietary product, triggers an inappropriately severe and prolonged mucosal inflammatory response in genetically predisposed individuals (Fig. 14.1). This response is amplified and perpetuated by recruitment of neutrophils, mononuclear cells and other leukocytes from the intestinal vasculature, with consequent release locally of a variety of inflammatory mediators (Rampton

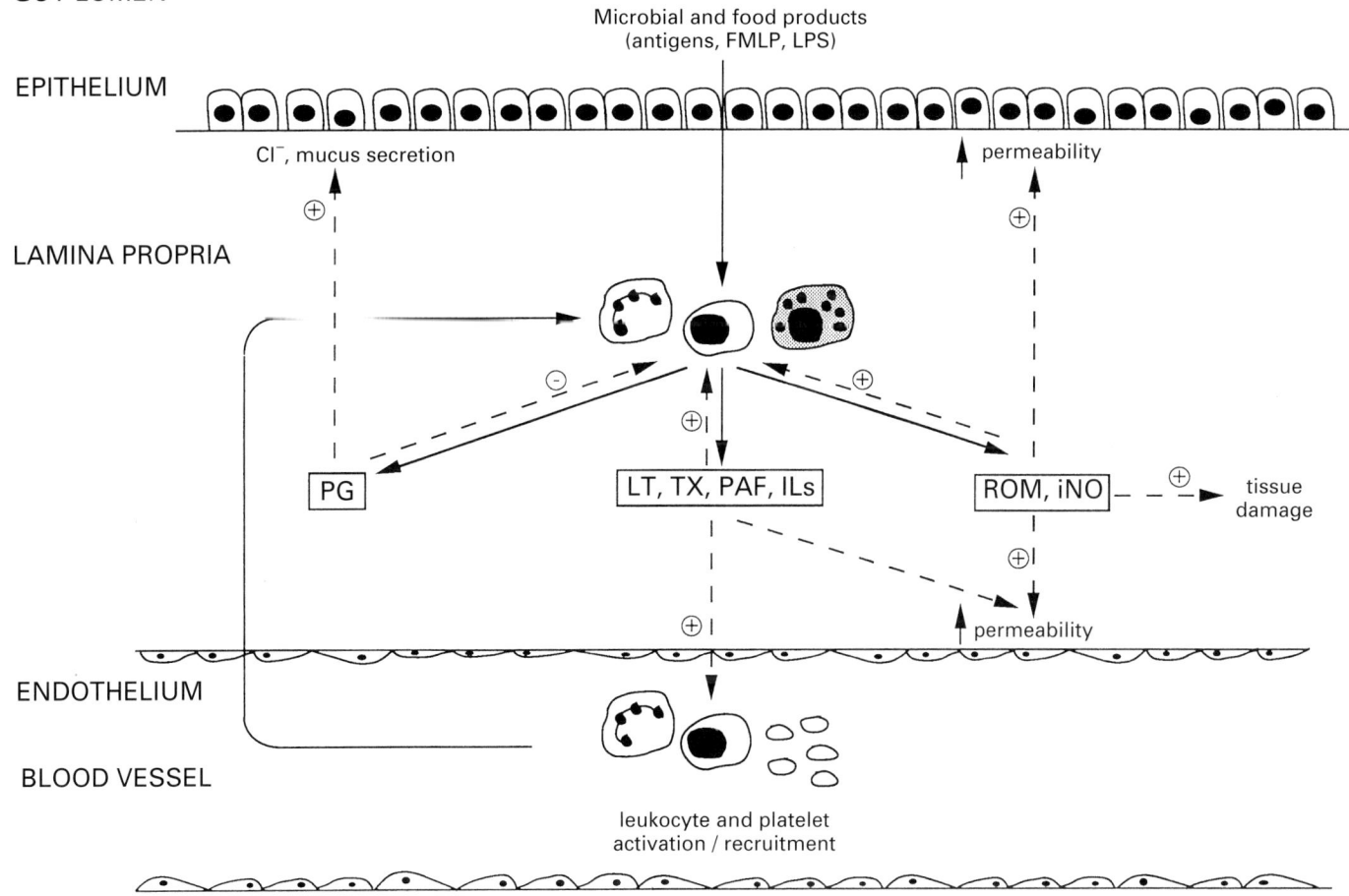

Fig. 14.1 Schematic representation of a cross-section of intestinal mucosa outlining key steps in the pathogenesis of IBD (see text). Dotted arrows denote effects of mediators. FMLP, formylmethionyl-leucyl-phenylalanine; LPS, lipopolysaccharide; ILs, interleukins; PG, prostaglandins; LT, leukotrienes; TX, thromboxanes; PAF, platelet-activating factor; ROM, reactive oxygen metabolites; iNO, nitric oxide synthesized by inducible NO synthase, Cl⁻ chloride.

& Hawkey 1984, Lauritsen et al 1989, Simmonds & Rampton 1993) and cytokines (see Chapter 12). This section reviews the pathophysiological role of lipid mediators (eicosanoids and platelet activating factor (PAF)), reactive metabolites of oxygen (ROMs) and nitrogen (nitric oxide), and kinins.

Criteria for acceptance of a pathophysiological role for a mediator in IBD

To confirm a pathophysiological role for a putative inflammatory mediator in IBD, three major criteria should be fulfilled (Hawkey & Rampton 1985):

1. Changes in IBD: the mediator must be produced in excess in the diseased tissue
2. Potential pathophysiological role: the effects of the mediator must resemble the disordered functions of the diseased organ
3. Effects of inhibitors: specific inhibitors of the synthesis, or receptor antagonists, of the implicated mediator must ameliorate adverse features of the disease.

There are limitations to the application of these criteria. A mediator's bioactivity depends not only on its concentration, but also on the number of receptors, the presence of endogenous inhibitors or receptor antagonists, synergy with other mediators, the site of its production in relation to target cells, and their state of activation and differentiation. Furthermore, a mediator may, as a 'hit-and-run' event, initiate a self-perpetuating inflammatory cascade: subsequent pharmacological inhibition of the initiating mediator may have no effect on ongoing tissue damage. Lastly, few specific potent inhibitors are yet available for use in humans. No conclusions can be drawn, for example, from experiments in which corticosteroids or aminosalicylates are shown to abrogate disease activity in parallel with inhibiting the production of a putative mediator, since the multiple effects of these drugs include inhibition of the mucosal synthesis of both lipid mediators and ROMs (Parente & Mugridge 1993, Gaginella & Walsh 1992). Accordingly, evaluation of the third criterion is often restricted to animal models of IBD, from which extrapolation to the human disease is contentious.

Despite these limitations, the criteria listed above provide a framework for dissecting out the pathophysiological role of individual soluble mediators.

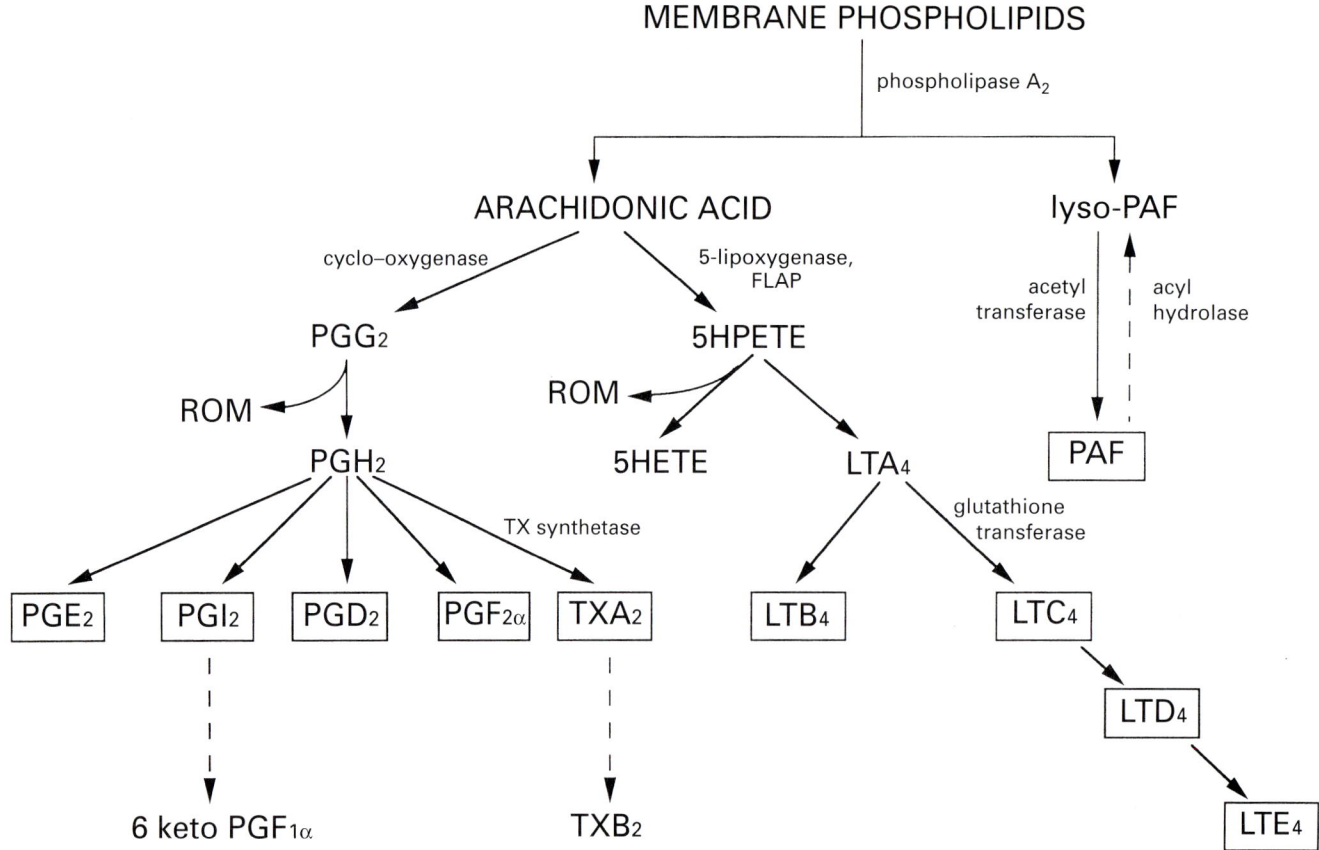

Fig. 14.2 Arachidonic acid metabolism. Abbreviations as in Fig. 14.1; also: HPETE, hydroperoxyeicosatetraenoic acid; HETE, hydroxyeicosatetraenoic acid; FLAP, 5-lipoxygenase activating protein.

EICOSANOIDS

Chemistry

The eicosanoids are hydroxy fatty acids derived from 20-carbon polyunsaturated precursors, in humans predominantly arachidonic acid, released from membrane phospholipids by one or more lipases (Fig. 14.2): the balance of eicosanoids produced depends on cell type. Cyclo-oxygenase activity leads to the formation, via labile cyclic endoperoxides (PGG_2 and PGH_2), of prostaglandins and/or thromboxanes. Synthesis of leukotrienes depends on the actions of 5-lipoxygenase and 5-lipoxygenase activator protein (FLAP), a protein required for the translocation of cytosolic 5-lipoxygenase to the cell membrane and its calcium-dependent activation (Dixon et al 1990). 12- and 15-lipoxygenases produce 12- and 15-hydroperoxy- and hydroxyeicosatetraenoic acids (HPETE and HETE).

Eicosanoids are not stored in cells after synthesis: measurement of their rate of release from tissues, in vitro or in vivo, is more useful than of tissue content (Lauritsen et al 1989). Detection of prostacyclin (PGI_2) and thromboxane A_2 (TXA_2), which are very unstable, is based on assay of their more stable breakdown products (6-keto$PGF_{1\alpha}$ and TXB_2).

Prostaglandins

Changes in IBD

Production of prostaglandins is increased in the intestinal mucosa in IBD, in direct relation to disease activity, whether assessed by in-vitro culture of mucosal biopsies, in-vivo rectal dialysis, or in venous blood, urine or feces (Sharon et al 1978, Rampton et al 1980, Lauritsen et al 1988, Rampton & Hawkey 1984, Lauritsen et al 1989) (Table 14.1). In Crohn's disease, but not ulcerative colitis, prostaglandins are also synthesized in excess by peripheral blood and isolated intestinal mononuclear cells (Rachmilewitz et al 1982, Zifroni et al 1983). Treatment with corticosteroids and aminosalicylates reduces mucosal prostaglandin synthesis but, as for other mediators, it remains uncertain whether this contributes to the achievement of remission or is consequent upon the reduction in tissue inflammation induced by other actions of the drugs (Parente & Mugridge 1993, Gaginella & Walsh 1992).

The cellular sources of mucosal prostaglandin production are diverse. In uninflamed gut, the lamina propria contributes more to PGE_2 production than the epithelium: macrophage recruitment in active IBD probably accentuates this difference (Smith et al 1982, Zifroni et al 1983, Lawson & Powell 1987). PGI_2 is likely to originate mainly from vascular endothelium. Possible stimuli for prostaglandin overproduction in active IBD include bacterial oligopeptides, interleukin-1 and bradykinin (Lawson & Powell 1987, Rampton & Collins 1993).

Potential pathophysiological role

Increased prostaglandin synthesis could contribute to the diarrhea and cramping abdominal pain of active IBD, by inducing mucosal secretion of chloride (and water) and through effects on intestinal smooth muscle (Rampton & Hawkey 1984, Rampton 1989) (Table 14.2). The latter vary with prostaglandin and smooth muscle type: PGE_2, for example, contracts longitudinal but relaxes circular muscle (Rampton & Hawkey 1984). The increased risk of colonic cancer in chronic extensive ulcerative colitis could

Table 14.1 Summary of changes in mediator production in IBD

	PGE_2	TXB_2	LTB_4	LTC_4/D_4	PAF	ROM	NO	Kinins
Ulcerative colitis								
Colorectal mucosa in vitro	+	+	+	+	+	+	+	−
Rectal dialysis in vivo	+	+	+	ND	ND	ND	+†	ND
Isolated intestinal mononuclear cells	+/−	+/−	ND	ND	ND	+	ND	ND
Peripheral blood leukocytes	−	−	+	ND	ND	+/−	ND	ND
Crohn's Disease								
Colorectal mucosa in vitro	+	+*	+	+	+	+	−	+‡
Rectal dialysis in vivo	+	+	+/−	ND	ND	ND	ND	ND
Isolated intestinal mononuclear cells	+	+	ND	ND	ND	+	ND	ND
Peripheral blood leukocytes	+	+	+	ND	ND	+/−	ND	ND

+, increase in comparison with control; −, no change in comparison with control; ND, no data available; * change unrelated to disease activity; † nitric oxide detected as nitrite; ‡ increased kinins inferred from reduced angiotensin-converting enzyme levels
PG, prostaglandin; TX, thromboxane; LT, leukotriene; PAF, platelet-activating factor; ROM, reactive oxygen metabolite; NO, nitric oxide

Table 14.2 The main possible pathophysiological effects of mediators in IBD. The net effects of PGE_2 and constitutively synthesized nitric oxide may be mucoprotective, whereas those of the other mediators are predominantly proinflammatory (see text)

	PGE_2	TXB_2	LTB_4	LTC_4/D_4	PAF	ROM	NO Constitutive	NO Inducible	Kinins
Epithelium									
Cl secretion	↑	↑	–	↑	↑	↑	↓	↑	↑
Mucus	sec	ND	sec	sec	ND	depolym	ND	ND	ND
Inflammatory cell recruitment & activation	↓	↑	↑	↓↑*	↑	↑	↓	↑	↑
Platelet activation	↓	↑	↑	ND	↑	↑	↓	ND	ND
Vasculature									
Tone	↓	↑	–	↑	↑	ND	↓	↓	↓
Permeability	–	–	–	↑	↑	↑	–	↑	↓
Intestinal smooth muscle contraction	↓↑*	ND	–	↑	–	↑↓*	ND	↓	↑↓*
Cell viability	MP	–	–	–	–	CT	MP	CT	–
Carcinogenicity	↑	–	–	–	–	↑	–	↑	–

–, no change in comparison with control; ND, no data available;
*change dependent on experimental conditions
Sec, secretion; depolym, depolymerization; MP, mucoprotection; CT, cytotoxicity.
Other abbreviations as in Table 14.1

conceivably be related to mucosal overproduction of prostaglandins, which has been linked with human and experimental colorectal carcinogenesis (Pugh & Thomas 1994).

In contrast, prostaglandins have well established 'mucoprotective' effects in the upper gastrointestinal tract (Hawkey & Rampton 1985): they could have an anti-inflammatory role in IBD by suppressing neutrophil adherence, diapedesis and activation, macrophage cytokine release and cytotoxicity, T-lymphocyte proliferation and cytotoxicity, mast cell activation and platelet aggregation (Knudson et al 1986, Gryglewski et al 1987, Lauritsen et al 1989). Effects on mucosal blood flow and increased mucus release (Rampton & Hawkey 1984, Lauritsen et al 1989, Rampton 1989) may also be beneficial (Table 14.2).

Effects of inhibitors

At a time when prostaglandins were thought to be proinflammatory in IBD, therapeutic trials with cyclo-oxygenase inhibitors (e.g. indomethacin, flurbiprofen) suggested that patients tended to deteriorate, an impression reinforced by subsequent anecdotes of precipitation of relapse in IBD patients given NSAIDs (Rampton & Hawkey 1984, Rampton 1987 & 1989, Kaufman & Tobin 1987, Lauritsen et al 1989). Indeed, the adverse effects of indomethacin on the small intestine and colon in animals have been advocated as an experimental model of IBD. It is not clear, however, whether the gut toxicity of NSAIDs is due to abrogation of the mucoprotective actions of prostaglandins, diversion of arachidonic acid metabolism to leukotrienes (see Fig. 14.2), or drug effects unrelated to eicosanoid metabolism.

Prostaglandin analogs ameliorate intestinal injury in animal models of IBD (Rampton 1989). In humans, 7 of 12 patients with quiescent ulcerative colitis given 15(R),15-methyl PGE_2 prophylactically developed watery diarrhea (Goldin & Rachmilewitz 1983); studies using a non-diarrheagenic prostaglandin analog are needed to further evaluate the possible mucoprotective role of prostaglandins in IBD.

Thromboxanes

Changes in IBD

Thromboxanes are produced in excess not only in inflamed mucosa, but also in Crohn's disease by uninflamed bowel and by isolated intestinal and peripheral blood mononuclear cells (Rachmilewitz et al 1982, Zifroni et al 1983, Rampton & Collins 1993) (see Table 14.1); furthermore, in one study, a greater excess of TXB_2 than of other eicosanoids was produced by rectal biopsies in Crohn's disease (Hawkey et al 1983). The cellular sources of thromboxanes are likely to include platelets, neutrophils, endothelial cells and epithelial cells, as well as mononuclear cells; soluble stimuli for their synthesis and release include bacterial products (chemotactic peptides, lipopolysaccharide), leukotrienes, PAF, interleukin-1, bradykinin and angiotensin II (Rampton & Collins 1993).

Potential pathophysiological role

The direct proinflammatory effects of thromboxanes

include recruitment and activation of neutrophils, mucosal ulceration and chloride secretion, and reduction of suppressor T-cell activity (Rampton & Collins 1993) (see Table 14.2). Enhanced thromboxane production could also account for increased platelet activation and aggregation in IBD (Collins et al 1994), and multifocal microvascular infarction in Crohn's disease (Wakefield et al 1989). Thromboxanes may thus contribute not only to mucosal disease in IBD, but also, through effects on platelets, to systemic thromboembolism.

Effects of inhibitors

Trials are in progress in IBD using selective thromboxane synthesis inhibitors and receptor antagonists such as ridogrel and picotamide (Casellas et al 1993, Collins et al 1996). Drugs of this type have been shown to suppress endotoxin-, trinitrobenzene sulfonic acid (TNBS)- and NSAID-induced intestinal damage in experimental animals (Boughton-Smith et al 1989, Vilaseca et al 1990, Banerjee & Peters 1990).

Leukotrienes

Changes in IBD

Patients with active IBD have increased mucosal production of LTB_4, LTC_4, LTD_4, 5-, 12- and 15-HETE, the results paralleling those obtained for prostaglandins (Table 14.1) (Rampton & Hawkey 1984, Sharon & Stenson 1984, Peskar et al 1986, Lauritsen et al 1988, Lauritsen et al 1988). 5-lipoxygenation occurs predominantly in neutrophils, eosinophils, mononuclear and mast cells: their recruitment and activation in inflamed mucosa is likely to explain increased leukotriene synthesis in active IBD (Lawson & Powell 1987, Nielsen et al 1987). In contrast, 12-lipoxygenase activity in inflamed IBD tissue has been identified in epithelial cells as well as macrophages, plasma cells and vascular endothelium (Shannon et al 1993).

Potential pathophysiological role

LTB_4 is a potent stimulus of neutrophil adherence, aggregation, chemotaxis and secretion (Rampton & Hawkey 1984, Lauritsen et al 1989) (Table 14.2). Indeed, the demonstration that up to 90% of the chemotactic activity of samples of inflamed intestine is lipid, coelutes with LTB_4 on high-pressure liquid chromatography, and can be removed by incubation with an anti-LTB_4 antibody, suggests that this leukotriene is the principal chemotactic component in IBD tissue (Lobos et al 1987).

LTC_4, LTD_4 and LTE_4, in contrast, are potent constrictors of vascular and intestinal smooth muscle; they also increase vascular permeability, stimulate mucosal secretion of chloride and mucus, inhibit neutrophil migration and stimulate macrophages (Table 14.2) (Fuerstein et al 1981, Smith et al 1988, Thomsen & Ahnfelt-Ronne 1989, Rampton 1989, Smith et al 1990).

12-lipoxygenase products, at least in high concentration, cause degranulation and chemotaxis of neutrophils, and smooth muscle cell migration (Shannon et al 1993).

Effects of inhibitors

Leukotriene synthesis inhibitors and receptor antagonists reduce the severity of experimental animal colitis. In controlled trials in ulcerative colitis, zileuton, a 5-lipoxygenase inhibitor, has proved only modestly efficacious in active disease (Stenson et al 1991, Peppercorn et al 1994) and maintenance of remission (Hawkey et al 1994); in a small open study, SR2640, an LTD_4/LTE_4 antagonist, gave similar results in active ulcerative colitis (Nielsen et al 1991). The pivotal pathophysiological role of neutrophils in active IBD explains the current emphasis on devising more potent LTB_4 inhibitors for the treatment of IBD (Hillingso et al 1994).

PLATELET ACTIVATING FACTOR (PAF)

Chemistry

Like eicosanoids, PAF is not stored in cells. Its immediate precursor, lyso-PAF, is formed in stimulated inflammatory cells, platelets, vascular endothelium and intestinal epithelial cells, by phospholipase A_2-mediated deacylation of membrane phospholipid; lyso-PAF is then acetylated by an acetyltransferase to produce PAF itself (1-O-alkyl-2-O-acetyl-glycero-3-phosphocholine) (see Fig. 14.2).

Changes in IBD

Colorectal synthesis of PAF is increased in active ulcerative colitis, (Eliakim et al 1988), and its ileal, colonic and fecal concentrations are raised in Crohn's disease (Kald et al 1990, Denizot et al 1992) (Table 14.1).

Potential pathophysiological role

The proinflammatory effects of PAF include recruitment and activation of neutrophils, eosinophils, macrophages and platelets (with release of eicosanoids and ROMs), vasoconstriction, and enhancement of transvascular fluid and protein flux (Kubes et al 1990, Buckley & Hoult 1989, Kubes 1993) (Table 14.2).

Effects of inhibitors

A PAF antagonist has been shown to enhance healing in experimental colitis (Wallace 1988) but not, as yet, in human IBD (Malchow et al 1994).

REACTIVE OXYGEN METABOLITES (ROMs)

Chemistry

A free radical is a molecule with one or more unpaired electrons in its outer orbital, and is therefore chemically very reactive: donation of the unpaired electron to, or abstraction of one from, a non-radical produces another radical, and often results in a chain reaction culminating in molecular damage.

ROMs include oxygen-derived true free radicals (e.g. superoxide, hydroxyl ion) as well as other toxic but stable compounds (hydrogen peroxide, hypochlorite) (Fig. 14.3). ROMs are normal byproducts of aerobic metabolism whose potentially adverse effects are usually prevented in vivo by endogenous enzymatic (e.g. mitochondrial cytochrome oxidase, glutathione peroxidase, superoxide dismutase (SOD), catalase) and non-enzymatic (ascorbic acid, β-carotene, α-tocopherol) antioxidants (Fig. 14.3). ROMs are utilized by phagocytes to kill microorganisms. However, excessive ROM generation due to phagocyte activation, ischemia–reperfusion injury, or activation of the arachidonic acid cascade (Fig. 14.2), can overwhelm antioxidant defenses and lead to tissue damage (Fig. 14.3).

The complexity and evanescence of free radical chemistry has made their direct measurement in biological systems difficult. Evidence for ROM activity therefore often requires detection of their 'footprints' (e.g. lipid peroxidation and depletion of endogenous antioxidants).

Changes in IBD

The production of ROMs by inflamed tissue, peripheral blood monocytes and isolated intestinal macrophages is increased in IBD (Mahida et al 1989, Williams et al 1990, Simmonds et al 1992, Simmonds & Rampton 1993) (see Table 14.1); results with peripheral blood neutrophils are conflicting (Williams et al 1990). Reduced levels of endogenous antioxidants, such as SOD, metallothionein and glutathione peroxidase, in both mucosa and blood in IBD (Simmonds & Rampton 1993), are likely to reflect antioxidant consumption by ROMs and, conversely, to

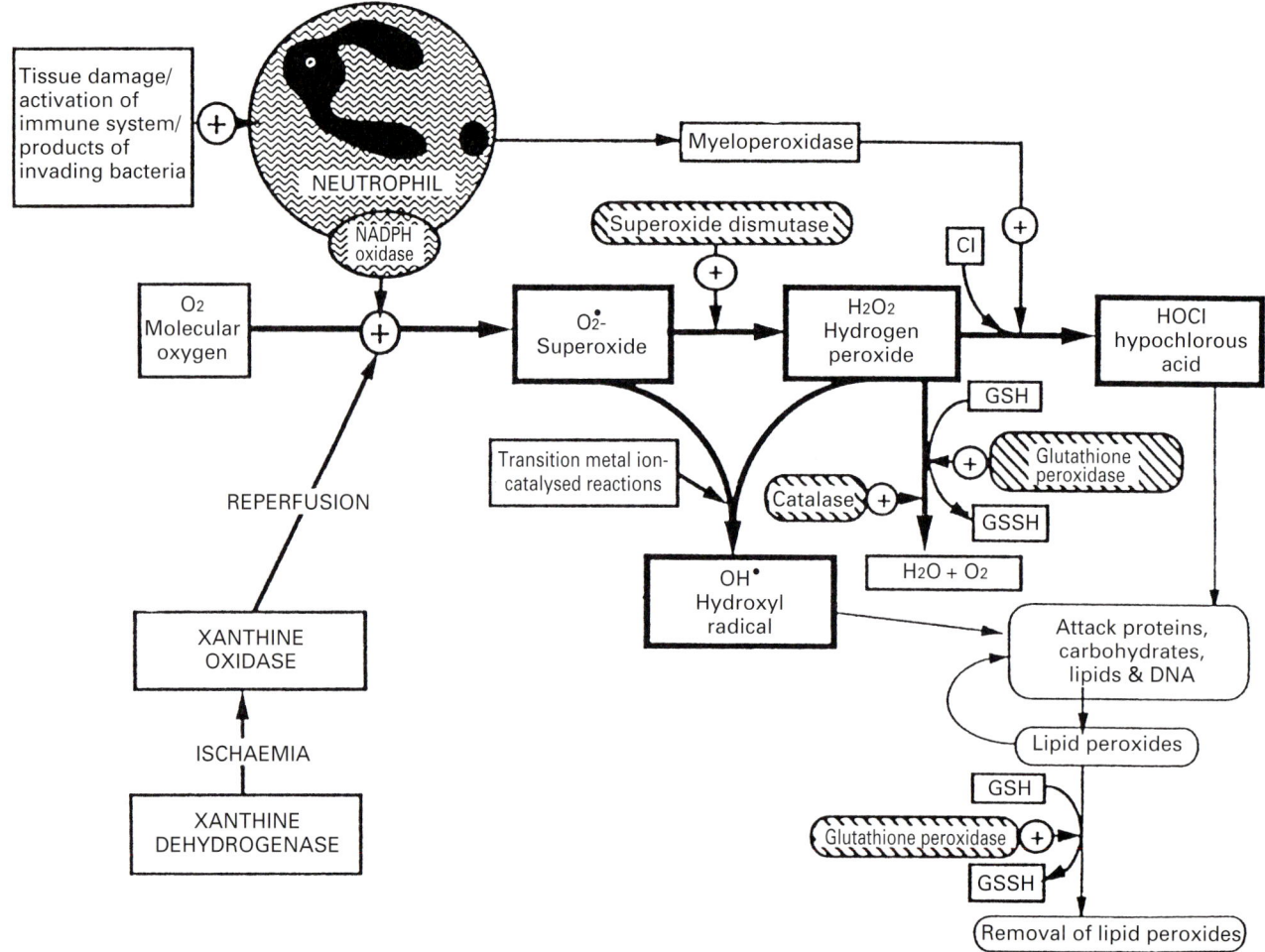

Fig. 14.3 Metabolism of reactive oxygen metabolites (ROMs) of importance in human disease, and sites of action of endogenous antioxidants. NADPH, nicotinamide adenine dinucleotide phosphate; GSH, reduced glutathione; GSSH, oxidized glutathione.

predispose to further oxidative tissue damage. Indeed, normal human colon may be particularly prone to ROM-mediated injury, since it contains very small amounts of SOD and catalase (Grisham et al 1990a). Mucosal lipid peroxidation is increased in active ulcerative colitis (Ahnfelt-Ronne et al 1990); the presence of oxidative products of 5-ASA in the stool also indicates excessive ROM activity in sulfasalazine-treated ulcerative colitis patients (Ahnfelt-Ronne et al 1990).

Potential pathophysiological role

The proinflammatory actions of ROMs (Table 14.2) include recruitment and activation of neutrophils; activation of the arachidonic acid cascade; damage to lipids, DNA, proteins and carbohydrates; direct cytotoxicity; increased epithelial and vascular permeability; mucosal fluid and electrolyte secretion; mucus depolymerization; and alterations in smooth muscle contractility (Grisham et al 1987, 1990b, Bern et al 1989, Moummi et al 1991, Simmonds & Rampton 1993). All these effects could play a role in the pathogenesis of IBD, a conclusion supported by rat studies showing that colitis can be induced by a free radical initiator (Tamai et al 1992), and TNBS-induced colitis may be superoxide-mediated (Grisham et al 1991).

ROMs are mutagenic in vitro (Weitzman & Gordon 1990, Simmonds & Rampton 1993). It is conceivable that prolonged ROM overproduction, for example by causing strand scission or base changes in DNA, contributes to the risk of colonic cancer in chronic extensive ulcerative colitis.

Effects of inhibitors

Antioxidants ameliorate intestinal inflammation in experimental models (Simmonds & Rampton 1993), and the proposal that ROMs contribute to the pathogenesis of human IBD is supported by as yet unconfirmed reports of the beneficial effects of SOD injections with or without desferrioxamine (which, by chelating iron, may reduce hydroxyl ion formation) in steroid-refractory Crohn's disease (Emerit et al 1989), and allopurinol in pouchitis (Levin et al 1992).

NITRIC OXIDE

Chemistry

Nitric oxide, the biologically active component of endothelium-derived relaxing factor (EDRF), is a highly reactive nitrogen metabolite formed from L-arginine by nitric oxide synthase (NOS), with L-citrulline as a by-product (Moncada & Higgs 1993). Its decomposition in the presence of molecular oxygen produces a series of compounds, including nitrite, and the nitrosating compounds N_2O_3 and N_2O_4, which can form carcinogenic nitrosamines from amines (Grisham et al 1992). Furthermore, reaction of nitric oxide with superoxide may generate highly toxic peroxynitrite and hydroxyl ions (Beckman et al 1990).

NOS has three forms, two constitutive, expressed in neurons (NOS 1) and endothelium (NOS 3), and the third inducible (NOS 2); their sites of distribution and stimuli are shown in (Table 14.3) (Moncada & Higgs 1993).

Table 14.3 Comparison of constitutive (NOS 1 and NOS 3) and inducible nitric oxide synthase (NOS 2)

	Constitutive (NOS 1 & 3)	Inducible (NOS 2)
Calcium-dependent	Yes	No
Sites	Neurons (NOS 1), endothelium (NOS 3), platelets	Macrophages, neutrophils, mast cells, endothelium, fibroblasts, smooth muscle cells
Stimuli	Mechanical (shear stress), acetylcholine, ADP, bradykinin	Cytokines (TNFα, IL-1, IFNγ), endotoxin
Corticosteroid sensitive	No	Yes
NO production		
Amounts	Small (picomoles)	Large (nanomoles)
Duration	Short	Longer
Roles	Vascular regulation, neuronal transduction, immune control	Inflammation (Table 14.2), host defence

Changes in IBD

Increased luminal concentrations of nitric oxide in ulcerative colitis (Lundberg et al 1994) and enhanced mucosal activity of inducible NOS in ulcerative colitis, but not in Crohn's disease (Boughton-Smith et al 1993), confirms earlier indirect observations of increased citrulline/arginine ratios in rectal mucosa (Middleton et al 1993a) and nitrite in rectal dialysate in active ulcerative colitis (Roediger et al 1986) (see Table 14.1). Recently, toxic megacolon has been particularly associated with the appearance of inducible NOS in the colonic muscularis propria (Mourelle et al 1995).

Potential pathophysiological role

Excess nitric oxide produced by inducible NOS could exacerbate ulcerative colitis by direct cytotoxicity, activation of neutrophils, vasodilatation, mucosal fluid secretion, reduction of smooth muscle tone, and increased production of carcinogenic nitrosamines (Grisham et al 1992, Moncada & Higgs 1993, Miller et al 1993, 1994, Middleton et al 1993b) (see Table 14.2). Indeed, intrarectally administered peroxynitrite in rats produces a colitis (Rachmilewitz et al 1993). In contrast, constitutive NOS activity may have a protective role through vasodilatation and inhibition of leukocyte–endothelial adherence, platelet aggregation and fluid secretion (Moncada & Higgs 1993, Miller et al 1993) (Table 14.2).

Effects of inhibitors

Although there are no studies to determine which of these actions predominates in human IBD, NOS inhibitors ameliorate experimental colitis in rats (Rachmilewitz et al 1995). The potentially divergent effects of nitric oxide, however, are illustrated by experiments in guinea pigs (Miller et al 1993, 1994): although the NOS inhibitor nitro-L-arginine-methyl ester (L-NAME) caused ileal inflammation and inhibited mucosal fluid absorption in control animals, it reduced inflammation and fluid secretion in those with chronic ileitis induced by TNBS. These results suggest that, when available, a specific inhibitor of inducible (but not constitutive) NOS should be evaluated in human IBD.

KININS

Chemistry

Kinins are unstable peptides formed in blood and tissue by the actions of kallikreins (kininogenases) on kininogens derived from α_2 globulins.

Changes in IBD

Mucosal kallikrein levels are increased in the muscle layer (but not the mucosa) in ulcerative colitis (Zeitlin & Smith 1973), and the activity of angiotensin-converting enzyme, which degrades bradykinin, is reduced in colonic Crohn's disease (Silverstein et al 1981).

Potential pathophysiological role

The effects of kinins, many of which are mediated by eicosanoids (Lawson & Powell 1987, Rampton & Collins 1993), could contribute to vasodilatation, increased vascular permeability, migration of inflammatory cells, motility disturbances and mucosal fluid secretion in IBD (Zeitlin & Smith 1973, Musch et al 1983, Lauritsen et al 1989).

Effects of inhibitors

Kinin inhibitors have not been evaluated in IBD.

CONCLUSION

The net effect of prostaglandins in IBD is probably mucoprotective rather than proinflammatory. Preliminary therapeutic trials using specific inhibitors in humans suggest that leukotrienes and ROMs are of pathophysiological importance, but clarification of the contribution of thromboxanes, PAF, nitric oxide and kinins is still awaited.

However, a clinically important therapeutic advance based on synthesis inhibition or receptor antagonism of a single mediator has not yet occurred. Possible explanations include the non-availability of sufficiently potent, safe, specific inhibitors for use in humans, and, in contrast, the complexity and redundancy of the interactions between different inflammatory pathways: indeed, it is possible that new agents should be broad spectrum, affecting several pathways simultaneously, as do corticosteroids and aminosalicylates.

Increased synthesis of inflammatory mediators is not specific for IBD, and occurs acutely also in infective, pseudomembranous and radiation colitis (Hawkey & Rampton 1985, Lauritsen et al 1988). We remain ignorant of the mechanisms underlying the chronicity of mucosal inflammation in IBD: is this due to persistence of a pathogenic exogenous stimulus, such as an infective agent, to genetically defective downregulation of the inflammatory response after a single infective event, or to an abnormal immune response to normally present (e.g. dietary and microbial) antigenic stimuli?

Answers to these questions must be a priority if we are to make major strides in our understanding of the role of inflammatory mediators in the pathogenesis of IBD, and in its treatment.

REFERENCES

Ahnfelt-Ronne I, Nielsen O H, Christensen A, Langholz E, Binder V, Riis P 1990 Clinical evidence supporting the radical scavenger mechanism of 5-aminosalicylic acid. Gastroenterology 98: 1162–1169

Banerjee A K, Peters T R J 1990 Experimental NSAID-induced enteropathy in the rat: similarities to inflammatory bowel disease and effect of thromboxane synthetase inhibitors. Gut 31: 1358–1363

Beckman J S, Beckman T W, Chen J, Marshall P A 1990 Apparent hydroxyl radical production by peroxynitrite: implications for endothelial injury from nitric oxide and superoxide. Proceedings of the National Academy of Sciences of the USA 87: 1620–1624

Bern M J, Sturbaum C W, Karayalcin S S, Berschneider H M, Wachsman J T, Powell D W 1989 Immune system control of rat and rabbit colonic electrolyte transport. Role of prostaglandins and enteric nervous system. Journal of Clinical Investigation 83: 1810–1820

Boughton-Smith N K, Hutcheson I, Whittle B J R 1989 Relationship between Paf-acether and thromboxane A_2 biosynthesis in endotoxin-induced intestinal damage in the rat. Prostaglandins 38: 319–333

Boughton-Smith N K, Evans S M, Hawkey C J et al 1993 Nitric oxide synthase activity in ulcerative colitis and Crohn's disease. Lancet 342: 338–340

Buckley T L, Hoult J R S 1989 Platelet activating factor is a potent colonic secretagogue with actions independent of specific PAF receptors. European Journal of Pharmacology 163: 275–283

Casellas F, Papo M, Guarner F et al 1993 A selective thromboxane synthetase inhibitor improves chronic ulcerative colitis. Gastroenterology 104: A677

Collins C E, Cahill M, Newland A, Rampton D S 1994 Platelets circulate in an activated state in inflammatory bowel disease. Gastroenterology 106: 840–845

Collins C E, Benson M J, Burnham W R, Rampton D S, 1996 Inhibition of excess in vitro thromboxane B_2 release by colorectal mucosa in inflammatory bowel disease by picotamide. Alimentary Pharmacology and Therapeutics (in press)

Denizot Y, Chaussade S, Nathan N et al 1992 PAF-acether and acetylhydrolase in stool of patients with Crohn's disease. Digestive Diseases and Sciences 37: 432–437

Dixon R A F, Diehl R E, Opas et al 1990 Requirement of a 5-lipoxygenase-activating protein for leucotriene synthesis. Nature 343: 282–284

Eliakim R, Karmeli F, Razin E, Rachmilewitz D 1988 Role of platelet activating factor in ulcerative colitis. Enhanced production during active disease and inhibition by sulfasalazine and prednisolone. Gastroenterology 95: 1167–1172

Emerit J, Pelletier S, Tosoni-Verlignue D, Mollet M 1989 Phase II trial of copper zinc superoxide dismutase (CuZnSOD) in treatment of Crohn's disease. Free Radicals in Biology and Medicine 7: 145–149

Fuerstein N, Foegh M, Ramwell P W 1981 Leucotrienes C4 and D4 induce prostaglandin and thromboxane release from rat peritoneal macrophages. British Journal of Pharmacology 72: 389–391

Gaginella T S, Walsh R E 1992 Sulphasalazine: multiplicity of actions. Digestive Diseases and Sciences 37: 801–812

Goldin E, Rachmilewitz D 1983 Prostanoids cytoprotection for maintaining remission in ulcerative: failure of 15(*R*)-15-methyl prostaglandin E_2. Digestive Diseases and Sciences 28: 807–811

Grisham M B, von Ritter C, Smith B F, LaMont J, Granger D N 1987 Interaction between oxygen radicals and gastric mucin. American Journal of Physiology 253: G93–G96

Grisham M B, MacDermott R P, Deitch E A 1990a Oxidant defence mechanisms in the human colon. Inflammation 14: 669–680

Grisham M B, Gaginella T S, von Ritter C, Tamai H, Be R M, Granger D N 1990b Effects of neutrophil-derived oxidants on intestinal permeability, electrolyte transport and epithelial cell viability. Inflammation 14: 531–542

Grisham M B, Volkmer C, Tso P, Yamada T 1991 Metabolism of trinitrobenzenesulfonic acid by the rat colon produces reactive oxygen species. Gastroenterology 101: 540–547

Grisham M B, Ware K, Gilleland H E, Gilleland L B, Abell C L, Yamada T 1992 Neutrophil-mediated nitrosamine formation: role of nitric oxide in rats. Gastroenterology 103: 1260–1266

Gryglewski R J, Szczeklik A, Wandzilak M 1987 The effect of six prostaglandins, prostacyclin and iloprost on generation of superoxide anions by human polymorphonuclear leucocytes stimulated by zymosan or FMLP. Biochemical Pharmacology 36: 4209–4212

Hawkey C J, Rampton D S 1985 Prostaglandins and the gastrointestinal mucosa: are they important in its function, disease, or treatment? Gastroenterology 89: 1162–1188

Hawkey C J, Karmeli F, Rachmilewitz D 1983 Imbalance of prostacyclin and thromboxane synthesis in Crohn's disease. Gut 24: 881–885

Hawkey C, Gassull M, Lauritsen K et al 1994 Efficacy of zileuton, a 5-lipoxygenase inhibitor, in the maintenance of remission in patients with ulcerative colitis. Gastroenterology 106: A697

Hillingso J, Kjeldsen J, Laursen L S et al 1994 Selective blockade of rectal leucotriene B4 and systemic leucotriene production by a single oral dose of MK591 in patients with active ulcerative colitis: a double-blind, placebo-controlled study. Gastroenterology 106: A698

Kald B, Olaison G, Sjodahl R, Tagesson C 1990 Novel aspects of Crohn's disease: increased content of platelet activating factor in ileal and colonic mucosa. Digestion 46: 199–204

Kaufman H J, Taubin H L 1987 Nonsteroidal antiinflammatory drugs activate quiescent inflammatory bowel disease. Annals of Internal Medicine 107: 513–516

Knudson P J, Dinarello C A, Strom T B 1986 Prostaglandins post-transcriptionally inhibit monocyte expression of interleukin-1 activity by increasing intracellular cyclic adenosine monophosphate. Journal of Immunology 137: 3189–3194

Kubes P 1993 Immunopathophysiology of the gastrointestinal tract: role of platelet activating factor. In: Wallace J L (ed) Immunopharmacology of the gastrointestinal system. Academic Press, London, pp 105–122

Kubes P, Arfors K E, Granger D N 1990 Platelet activating factor-induced mucosal dysfunction: role of oxidants and granulocytes. American Journal of Physiology 260: G965–G971

Lauritsen K, Laursen L S, Bukhave K, Rask-Madsen J 1988 In vivo profiles of eicosanoids in ulcerative colitis, Crohn's colitis and *Cl. difficile* colitis. Gastroenterology 95: 11–17

Lauritsen K, Laursen L S, Bukhave K, Rask-Madsen J 1989 Inflammatory intermediaries in inflammatory bowel disease. International Journal of Colorectal Disease 4: 75–90

Lawson L D, Powell D W 1987 Bradykinin stimulated eicosanoid synthesis and secretion by rabbit ileal components. American Journal of Physiology 252: G783–G790

Levin K E, Pemberton J H, Phillips S F, Zinsmeister A R, Pezim M E 1992 Role of oxygen free radicals in the etiology of pouchitis. Diseases of the Colon and Rectum 35: 452–456

Lobos E A, Sharon P, Stenson W F 1987 Chemotactic activity in inflammatory bowel disease, Role of leucotriene B4. Digestive Diseases and Sciences 32: 1380–1388

Lundberg J O N, Hellström P M, Lundberg J M, Alving K 1994 Greatly increased luminal nitric oxide in ulcerative colitis. Lancet 344: 1673–1674

Mahida Y, Wu K C, Jewell D P 1989 Respiratory burst activity of intestinal macrophages in normal and inflammatory bowel disease. Gut 30: 1362–1370

Malchow H, Ewe K, Goebell H, Wellmann W, Leimer H-G, Kempe R 1994 Failure of the specific PAF-antagonist Apafant in the treatment of ulcerative colitis. Gastroenterology 106: A728

Middleton S J, Shorthouse M, Hunter J O 1993a Increased nitric oxide synthesis in ulcerative colitis. Lancet 341: 465–466

Middleton S J, Shorthouse M, Hunter J O 1993b Relaxation of distal colonic circular smooth muscle by nitric oxide derived from human leucocytes. Gut 34: 814–817

Miller M J S, Sadowska-Krowicka H, Chotinaruemol S, Kakkis J L, Clark D A 1993 Amelioration of chronic ileitis by nitric oxide synthase inhibition. Journal of Pharmacology and Experimental Therapeutics 264: 11–16

Miller M J S, Muashi U K, Sadowska-Kiowicka H et al 1994 Inhibition of calcium-dependent nitric oxide synthase causes ileitis and leucocytosis in guinea pigs. Digestive Diseases and Sciences 39: 1185–1192

Moncada S, Higgs A 1993 The L-arginine–nitric oxide pathway. New England Journal of Medicine 329: 2002–2012

Moummi C, Gullikson G W, Grisham M B, Gaginella T S 1991 Differential effects of reactive oxygen metabolites on neurally stimulated and nonstimulated guinea pig ileum. Journal of Pharmacology and Experimental Therapeutics 256: 266–271

Mouvelle M, Casellas F, Guarner F et al 1995, Induction of nitric oxide synthase in colonic smooth muscle from patients with toxic megacolon. Gastroenterology 109: 1497–1502

Musch M W, Kachur J F, Miller R J, Field M 1983 Bradykinin stimulated electrolyte secretion in rabbit and guinea pig intestine: involvement of arachidonic acid metabolites. Journal of Clinical Investigation 71: 1073–1083

Nielsen O H, Ahnfelt-Ronne I, Elmgreen J 1987 Abnormal metabolism of arachidonic acid in chronic inflammatory bowel disease: enhanced release of leucotriene B4 from activated neutrophils. Gut 28: 181–185

Nielsen O H, Ahnfelt-Ronne I, Thomsen M K, Kissmeyer A-M, Langholz E 1991 Effect of the leucotriene LTD4/LTE4 antagonist, SR2640, in ulcerative colitis: an open clinical study. Prostaglandins Leucotrienes Essential Fatty Acids 42: 181–184

Parente L, Mugridge K G 1993 Glucocorticoids and gastrointestinal inflammation. In: Wallace J L (ed) Immunopharmacology of the gastrointestinal system. Academic Press, London, pp 169–184

Peppercorn M, Das K, Elson E et al 1994 Zileuton, a 5-lipoxygenase inhibitor, in the treatment of active ulcerative colitis: a double-blind, placebo controlled trial. Gastroenterology 106: A751

Peskar B M, Dreyling K W, Peskar B A, May B, Goebell H 1986

Enhanced formation of sulfidopeptide–leucotrienes in ulcerative colitis and Crohn's disease: inhibition by sulfasalazine and 5-aminosalicylic acid. Agents and Actions 18: 381–383

Pugh S, Thomas G A O 1994 Patients with adenomatous polyps and carcinomas have increased colonic mucosal prostaglandin E_2. Gut 35: 675–678

Rachmilewitz D, Ligumsky M, Haimowitz A et al 1982 Prostanoid synthesis by cultured peripheral blood mononuclear cells in inflammatory diseases of the bowel. Gastroenterology 82: 673–679

Rachmilewitz D, Karmeli F, Okun E, Bursztyn M 1995 Experimental colitis is ameliorated by inhibition of nitric oxide synthase activity. Gut 36: 247–255

Rachmilewitz D, Stamler J S, Karmeli F et al 1993 Peroxynitrite-induced rat colitis – a new model of colonic inflammation. Gastroenterology 105: 1681–1688

Rampton D S 1987 Nonsteroidal antiinflammatory drugs and the lower gastrointestinal tract. Scandinavian Journal of Gastroenterology 22: 1–4

Rampton D S 1989 Functional aspects of eicosanoids in inflammatory bowel disease. European Journal of Gastroenterology and Hepatology 1: 145–149

Rampton D S, Collins C E 1993 Thromboxanes in inflammatory bowel disease – pathogenic and therapeutic implications. Alimentary Pharmacology and Therapeutics 7: 357–367

Rampton D S, Hawkey C J 1984 Prostaglandins and ulcerative colitis. Gut 25: 1399–1413

Rampton D S, Sladen G E, Youlten L J 1980 Rectal mucosal prostaglandin E_2 release and its relation to disease activity, electrical potential difference and treatment in ulcerative colitis. Gut 21: 591–596

Roediger W E W, Lawson M J, Nance S H, Radcliffe B C 1986 Detectable colonic nitrite levels in inflammatory bowel disease – mucosal or bacterial malfunction? Digestion 35: 199–204

Shannon V R, Stenson W F, Holtzman M J 1993 Induction of epithelial arachidonate 12-lipoxygenase at active sites of inflammatory bowel disease. American Journal of Physiology 264: G104–G111

Sharon P, Stenson W 1984 Enhanced synthesis of leucotriene B4 by colonic mucosa in inflammatory bowel disease. Gastroenterology 86: 453–460

Sharon P, Ligumsky M, Rachmilewitz D, Zor U 1978 Role of prostaglandins in ulcerative colitis. Enhanced production during active disease and inhibition by sulphasalazine. Gastroenterology 75: 638–640

Silverstein E, Fierst S M, Simon M R, Weinstock J V, Friedland J 1981 Angiotensin-converting enzyme in Crohn's disease and ulcerative colitis. American Journal of Clinical Pathology 75: 175–178

Simmonds N J, Rampton D S 1993 Inflammatory bowel disease – a radical view. Gut 34: 865–868

Simmonds N J, Allen R E, van Someren N V, Blake D R, Rampton D S 1992 Chemiluminescence assay of mucosal reactive oxygen metabolites in inflammatory bowel disease. Gastroenterology 103: 186–196

Smith G S, Warhurst G, Turnberg L A 1982 Synthesis and degradation of prostaglandin E_2 in the epithelium and subepithelial layers of the rat intestine. Biochimica Biophysica Acta 713: 684–687

Smith P L, Montzka D P, McCafferty G P, Wassermann M A, Fondacaro J D 1988 Effect of sulfidopeptide leucotrienes D4 and E4 on ileal ion transport in vitro in the rat and rabbit. American Journal of Physiology 255: G175–G183

Smith P L, Chiossone D C, McCafferty G P 1990 Characterisation of LTC4 effects on rabbit ileal mucosa in vitro. Naunyn Schmiedebergs Archives of Pharmacology 341: 94–100

Stenson W F, Lauritsen K, Laursen J et al 1991 A clinical trial of zileuton, a specific inhibitor of 5-lipoxygenase, in ulcerative colitis. Gastroenterology 100: A253

Tamai H S, Levin S, Gaginella T S 1992 Induction of colitis in rats by 2-2'azobis (2-amidinopropane) dihydrochloride. Inflammation 16: 69–81

Thomsen N K, Ahnfelt-Ronne I 1989 Inhibition by the LTD4 antagonist, SR2640, of effects of LTD4 on canine polymorphonuclear leucocyte functions. Biochemical Pharmacology 38: 2291–2295

Vilaseca J, Sala J, Guarner F, Rodriguez R, Malagelada J-R 1990 Participation of thromboxane and other eicosanoid synthesis in the course of experimental inflammatory colitis. Gastroenterology 98: 269–277

Wakefield A J, Sawyerr A M, Dhillon A P et al 1989 Pathogenesis of Crohn's disease: multifocal gastrointestinal infarction. Lancet 2: 1054–1062

Wallace J L 1988 Release of platelet activating factor (PAF) and accelerated healing induced by a PAF antagonist in an animal model of chronic colitis. Canadian Journal of Physiology and Pharmacology 66: 422–425

Weitzman S A, Gordon L I 1990 Inflammation and cancer: role of phagocyte-derived oxidants in carcinogenesis. Blood 76: 655–663

Williams J G, Hughes L E, Hallett M B 1990 Toxic oxygen metabolite production by circulating phagocytic cells in inflammatory bowel disease. Gut 31: 187–193

Zeitlin I J, Smith A N 1973 Mobilisation of tissue kallikrein in inflammatory disease of the colon. Gut 14: 133–138

Zifroni A, Treves A J, Sachar D B, Rachmilewitz D 1983 Prostanoid synthesis by cultured intestinal epithelial and mononuclear cells in inflammatory bowel disease. Gut 24: 659–664

15. Infective agents – bacterial and viral

S. Mohammed   W. R. Thayer

Major advances in molecular biology have produced innovative techniques for detecting microorganisms present in very low concentrations. This has resulted in the identification of many new bacteria and viruses. As a result, many diseases that were formerly thought to be idiopathic have now been proved to be caused by infectious agents. Examples include the role of *Helicobacter pylori* in peptic ulcer disease and *Escherichia coli* 0157:H7 in hemolytic uremic syndrome. The infectious cause of many diseases was not recognized earlier because of the fastidious growth properties of the causative bacteria, the absence of defined bacterial properties and low bacterial concentrations (Blaser 1994). It was also not recognized that many of these diseases were uncommon sequelae of common diseases. Clinical and epidemiological observations have provided important clues to the causation of many diseases. Techniques such as polymerase chain reaction based on conserved ribosomal sequences have been used to identify the infectious cause of many diseases, for example Whipple's disease (Relman et al 1992). At the same time, developments in molecular immunology have helped us to understand what predisposes an individual to develop disease in response to an infection.

An infectious etiology for inflammatory bowel disease has long been postulated, partly prompted by the similarity of the features of inflammatory bowel disease with classic infectious enteritis. Crohn et al (1932), in their original description of regional ileitis, later called Crohn's disease, were unable to identify a causative agent using cultures and staining techniques. Bargen (1924) and Buie and Bargen (1933) incriminated a diplococcus species in ulcerative colitis. In 1921 Hurst proposed that ulcerative colitis was a sequela of bacillary dysentery. Felsen and Wolarsky (1953) reported that *Shigella dysenteriae* were found in 7% of 994 Crohn's disease and ulcerative colitis stool cultures compared to 0.08% of 6000 controls. A further 11 of 122 proven bacillary dysentery patients studied prospectively developed ulcerative colitis or Crohn's disease within a year. Dach and colleagues (1935) proposed *Bacterium necrophorum*, a Gram-negative bacillus, as the etiologic agent for ulcerative colitis.

The parts of the human body exposed to the largest quantity of infectious agents are the colon and the distal small intestine. Not surprisingly, the largest number of immune cells are also seen in the gastrointestinal tract. Inflammatory bowel disease most commonly involves the parts of the gut with the highest bacterial concentrations, i.e. the terminal ileum and the colon. Some epidemiologic and genetic data also point to an infectious etiology for inflammatory bowel disease. Animal models and clinical observations such as the response to antibiotics, further support this view. This chapter discusses the available data linking infectious agents, specifically bacteria and viruses, to inflammatory bowel disease. The data linking mycobacteria will be discussed in Chapter 16.

EPIDEMIOLOGICAL DATA

Reports of clustering of Crohn's disease have remained unexplained. Mayberry and Hitchens (1978) reported a highly significant concentration of cases of Crohn's disease in Cardiff, South Wales. Allan et al (1986) reported a cluster of Crohn's disease in a small Cotswolds village. Reilly and Robinson (1986) described four Crohn's disease cases developing in adult women who had lived in close contact during their teenage years, and suggested that the illness was caused by an infectious agent with a long latent period. Crohn's disease and ulcerative colitis have been shown to develop in married couples, suggesting an infectious etiology (Lobo et al 1988, Batty et al 1994). Darchis et al (1989) reported the development of Crohn's disease in a married couple and their four children, with three of the cases occurring within 10 months. HLA haplotype linkage analysis of this family (Colombel et al 1989) suggested that this was evidence for an environmental etiology. Bennett et al (1991) reported on the frequency of inflammatory bowel disease in the offspring of couples in which both patients had inflammatory bowel disease. In this study seven couples developed inflammatory bowel disease after marriage. Within this group 17 children were born of whom five have already developed inflammatory bowel disease. Both these studies suggest that even in a genetically predisposed individual exposure to an environmental factor – possibly an infectious agent – is essential to develop the disease. This is further corroborated by an in-depth study of Crohn's disease in two French families (Van Kruiningen et al 1993). In both these families multiple cases occurred among siblings in a 7–13-month period. Radiographs showed a remarkable similarity in the pattern of the disease, which was confined to the distal ileum and cecum. The authors conclude that the circumstances and data point to an infectious microorganism that is responsible for the disease. There is also evidence of a seasonal variation in the incidence of Crohn's disease and ulcerative colitis, suggesting the possibility of an infectious agent (Cave & Freedman 1975). The time of peak incidence of both diseases is different, suggesting that different etiological agents may be involved.

The prevalence of inflammatory bowel disease is highest among whites in North America and northern Europe. It is low among black Americans, native Americans, Asians and Maoris (Mendeloff & Dunn 1971, McConnell & Vadheim 1992). The incidence of inflammatory bowel disease appears to be rising in black Americans in recent years (Calkins et al 1984). Immigrants from Asia in the United Kingdom also have a higher susceptibility to inflammatory bowel disease than Asians resident in Asia (Chong & Walker-Smith 1986, Findlay & Jayarantne 1986). The increasing incidence of inflammatory bowel disease among black Americans and Asians in the UK suggests that exposure to an environmental agent such as an infectious organism may be responsible. The Jewish population has a high risk of developing inflammatory bowel disease (Gilat et al 1986, Mendeloff & Dunn 1991), but prevalence among Jews in Israel is much lower than in Europe or North America (Gilat et al 1986). This suggests that exposure (or lack of it) to an infectious agent may be the reason for the differing prevalence rates.

GENETIC DATA

Considerable amounts of data exist implying a genetic predisposition for the development of inflammatory bowel disease. Critical review of these data suggests that genetic factors interact with environmental factors (Satsangi et al 1994). Studies that report an increased prevalence of inflammatory bowel disease in certain families have shown that first-degree relatives are at a higher risk. Farmer et al (1980) reported that among 522 patients with Crohn's disease, 35.2% had an affected family member (16.7% first degree); among 316 patients with ulcerative colitis, 29.4% had an affected family member (15.8% first degree). McConnell (1990) reported that 31 of 165 patients with Crohn's disease had an affected first-degree relative, including 27 siblings; of 171 patients with ulcerative colitis 20 had an affected relative, including 16 siblings. These studies show a higher risk of developing inflammatory bowel disease among first-degree relatives who share a common environment in the early years of life. This implies that exposure to an infectious agent early in life in the genetically predisposed individual could lead to the development of inflammatory bowel disease.

BOWEL FLORA

The normal human gastrointestinal tract contains a large quantity of bacteria. The primary location of inflammatory bowel disease is in the distal ileum and colon, where there are increased concentrations of both aerobic and anaerobic bacteria, suggesting a role for bowel flora in the pathogenesis of inflammatory bowel disease. Seneca and Henderson (1950) suggested that bacterial flora might be involved in the pathogenesis of ulcerative colitis. The importance of the bowel flora was shown by Harper et al (1985), who introduced ileostomy effluent into colons defunctionalized by Crohn's disease and caused a clinical relapse; a sterile ultrafiltrable fraction did not produce this effect. Initial studies by Cooke (1967) and Gorbach et al (1968) comparing the bowel flora of patients with inflammatory bowel disease with controls, showed minimal or no difference. Subsequent studies by van der Weil-Korstanje and Winkler (1975) showed that ulcerative colitis patients had a hundredfold increase in group-D streptococci, with a reduction of Bifidobacteria, Dickinson et al (1980) reported that coliforms with adhesive properties dominated the fecal flora of ulcerative colitis patients in both active and remission states. Wensinck and Custers-van Lieshaut (1981) showed that the fecal flora of patients with Crohn's disease contained higher number of Gram-positive anaerobic coccoid rods compared to healthy subjects. An *E. coli* strain was isolated from ulcerative colitis patients with increased adhesive properties compared to similar organisms from control subjects (Burke & Axon 1987). Certain strains of *E. coli* (0157:H7) have been responsible for sporadic and epidemic outbreaks of a hemorrhagic colitis (Pai et al 1984, Ryan et al 1986), but these organisms have not been sought in ulcerative colitis.

Crohn's disease patients have a high incidence of agglutinating antibodies against such bowel bacterial strains as *Eubacterium* spp. and *Peptostreptococcus* spp. compared to normal controls (Wensinck and van de Merwr 1981). Antibody titers are also elevated in ulcerative colitis (Auer et al 1983). The higher antibody titers against bowel bacteria in patients with ulcerative colitis and Crohn's disease compared to normal controls may reflect the altered immune response to bowel flora in such patients, or increased absorption of bacterial products.

POSSIBLE ETIOLOGIC AGENTS

Bacteria

Cell-wall defective bacteria

Parent and Mitchell (1976) isolated a cell-wall defective bacterium from Crohn's disease tissue after inoculating homogenized tissue filtrate from patients with Crohn's disease and ulcerative colitis and from controls, into hypertonic media. Following revertance, 11 isolates from eight patients were identified as pseudomonas-like bacteria, most closely resembling group Va; antibodies to these organisms were increased in Crohn's disease sera (Parent & Mitchell 1978). Other studies with enzyme-linked immunosorbent assay (ELISA) and immunofluorescence were unable to confirm these findings (Ibbotson et al 1987). Graham et al (1983) sought bacterial sequences of revertant organisms in inflammatory bowel disease sera by DNA hybridization, with equivocal results. Moreover, immunofluorescence (Whorwell et al 1978) and electron microscopy (Aluwihare 1971) failed to detect such organisms in inflamed tissue. Belsheim et al (1983) and Ibbotson et al (1987) investigated the possible relationship between bacterial cell-wall defective or L-forms and inflammatory bowel disease, and demonstrated a high recovery of bacterial L-forms from intestinal tissue in both Crohn's disease and ulcerative colitis compared to controls. Cell-wall defective mycobacteria have also been considered as possible etiologic agents in Crohn's disease (Chiodini et al 1986). These are discussed in Chapter 16.

Yersinia enterocolitica

Yersinia enterocolitica is a Gram-negative bacillus incriminated in some cases of acute ileitis. The clinical syndrome and postinfectious sequela resembles Crohn's disease, i.e. erythema nodosum and polyarthritis (Alvonen et al 1972, Mygind & Thulin 1970). Radiologically it resembles regional ileitis (van Weichen 1974). Such cases do not usually progress to Crohn's disease (Sjostrom 1971, Persson et al 1976). Specific antibodies to *Yersina* have been observed in ulcerative colitis (Larsen 1980) and Crohn's disease (Cerf et al 1982), but such an association has not been found by others (Swarbrick et al 1979). A recent long-term study from Norway (Saebo & Lassen 1992) suggests an association between yersiniosis and chronic abdominal complaints, including diarrhea and weight loss. Ulcerative colitis is more common in this group than in the usual Scandinavian population. Recently, Heidt et al (1991), using monospecific antibodies, identified plasmid-encoded proteins of *Yersinia enterocolitica* by endoscopic small-bowel biopsy in half of their patients with idiopathic enterocolitis.

Campylobacter

Campylobacter jejuni infections mimic either ulcerative colitis or Crohn's disease. Erythema nodosum and arthritis can occur (Lambert et al 1979, Chandra et al 1982). However, Blaser et al (1984) systematically investigated fecal cultures for *Campylobacter jejuni* in 74 patients with inflammatory bowel disease and healthy controls, with negative results. Campylobacter has, however, been implicated in the exacerbation of inflammatory bowel disease (Goodman et al 1980).

Clostridia

Clostridium difficile has been implicated in the relapse of inflammatory bowel disease (Bolton et al 1980, Lee et al 1986), but other studies could not find an association (Hyams & McLaughlin et al 1985). *Clostridium difficile* toxin could be found either in stool during remission (Dorman et al 1982), or correlated with sulfasalazine or other antibiotic usage (Greenfield et al 1983). Vancomycin therapy was effective in five patients with ulcerative colitis and one patient with Crohn's disease who were *Clostridium difficile* toxin-positive and not responding to standard medical therapy (La Mont & Trnka 1980). At present it appears that *C. difficile* is an unlikely agent for either ulcerative colitis or Crohn's disease, but could possibly exacerbate the illness.

Wolinella

VanDyke et al (1986) suggested that a small motile anaerobic Gram-negative rod (possibly from the genus *Wolinella*) might play a role in the pathogenesis of inflammatory bowel disease. This organism is found in the periodontal flora of inflammatory bowel disease patients with gingival disease, but not in controls. Furthermore, they demonstrated that *Wolinella* extracts and culture supernatants of the isolates inhibited neutrophil chemotaxis in a dose-dependent manner. This defective neutrophil chemotaxis seemed to be serum mediated.

Mycoplasma

Mycoplasma could not be cultured from ulcerative colitis patients in a small study using rectal biopsies and swabs (Jori et al 1968). Antibodies to several mycoplasma species were also not present in sera from patients with inflammatory bowel disease (Beeken 1979).

Chlamydia

Several investigators have suggested that chlamydia might be involved in the pathogenesis of Crohn's disease, using the Frei test (Tomenius et al 1963) and serology (Schuller et al 1978). Such a possibility is unlikely, since electron microscopy would be expected to detect such a large organism. Other investigators, using serology and cultures from rectal biopsies, could not confirm these findings (Taylor-Robinson et al 1979, Elliot et al 1981).

Viruses

Ekbom et al (1990) studied 4000 patients in the Uppsala region of Sweden and showed perinatal virus infection to be a strong risk factor for the subsequent development of inflammatory bowel disease. Kangro et al (1990) investigated 72 children with chronic inflammatory bowel disease for infection with viruses, mycoplasma, chlamydia and coxiella, and observed that viral and respiratory pathogens were temporally associated with exacerbations of inflammatory bowel disease. Thus epidemiological studies have linked viral infections to the development of inflammatory bowel disease.

Von Glahn and Pappenheimer (1925) were the first to implicate viruses after finding intranuclear inclusion bodies in the colonic mucosa of ulcerative colitis patients. Helwig (1959) recognized DNA-containing cytoplasmic inclusion bodies in the colonic mucosa of ulcerative colitis patients, again raising the possibility of a viral etiology. Although the presence of inclusion bodies was confirmed by Monis and Mendeloff (1961), these were interpreted as merely degenerating processes or leukocytes migrating through the intestinal epithelium. Riemann (1977) found virus-like particles with a double membrane and an electron-dense central core, in epithelial cells and macrophages near ulcerative colitis lesions.

Herpes virus

An association between inflammatory bowel disease and herpes viruses (cytomegalovirus and Epstein–Barr virus (EBV)) has been suggested. Cytomegalovirus enterocolitis mimics inflammatory bowel disease (Goodgame 1993), and cytomegalovirus infection can result in a chronic illness similar to ulcerative colitis (Diepersloot et al 1990). Cytomegalic cells have been detected in patients with exacerbation of ulcerative colitis and toxic megacolon (Cooper et al 1977, Berk et al 1985). Cytomegalovirus antibodies were found in one out of four patients with Crohn's disease and three out of six patients with ulcerative colitis (Farmer et al 1973). Patients with exacerbations of ulcerative colitis resistant to steroid therapy, who had cytomegalic inclusions on mucosal biopsy, improved after steroid withdrawal (Berk et al 1985). Wakefield et al (1992) used nested polymerase chain reaction to demonstrate herpes virus DNA in intestinal tissue from patients with Crohn's disease and ulcerative colitis. They found a higher prevalence of both cytomegalovirus DNA and EBV DNA in inflammatory bowel disease than in controls. Using nested polymerase chain reaction and in-situ hybridization, Smith et al (1994) found that intestinal cytomegalovirus and EBV DNA are associated with ulcerative colitis, and intestinal cytomegalovirus DNA was associated with Crohn's disease.

The role of herpes virus in inflammatory bowel disease is still unclear. Cytomegalovirus may be localizing in areas of inflammation, rather than causing the disease. Macrophages form granulomas when presented with antigens which they cannot eliminate. Smith and Wakefield (1993) speculate that if Crohn's disease is caused by a virus, then the granuloma would represent the site of viral antigen presentation. Search of the granuloma and associated vascular structures by immunological, ultrastructural and molecular methods may succeed in finding an infectious agent for Crohn's disease.

Measles virus

Wakefield et al (1993), using transmission electron microscopy, identified paramyxovirus-like particles and inclusions consisting of condensations of nucleocapsid in giant cells and endothelium at foci of vascular injury in nine of nine Crohn's disease patients. Hybridization of measles virus N-protein genomic RNA was identified in all cases of Crohn's disease and localized to the vascular endothelial cells associated with foci of inflammation. In 13 of 15 cases immunohistochemical stains were positive for measles virus nucleocapsid protein. Control tissue was negative. The authors speculate on a possible role for the long persistence of the measles virus in tissue as a pathogenetic factor in Crohn's disease. An epidemiological study from Sweden found a correlation between patients developing Crohn's disease before age 30 and persons who were born up to 3 months after a measles epidemic (Ekbom et al 1994).

Other viruses

Serological methods have been utilized to investigate the presence of viruses in inflammatory bowel disease (Table 15.1). Kyle et al (1963) tested sera from 35 Crohn's disease patients for antibodies to adenovirus and group B Coxsackie virus, but the results did not differ from controls. Antibodies to rotavirus (DeGroote et al 1977) and Norwalk agent (Greenberg et al 1979) were not found to a significant extent in inflammatory bowel disease sera.

TRANSMISSION EXPERIMENTS

Transmission experiments also have supported the role of an infectious agent in causing inflammatory bowel disease. Mitchell and Rees (1970) produced granulomas

Table 15.1 Viral antibody studies in inflammatory bowel disease

RNA viruses
Picorna Virus
   Coxsackie A (1–22, 24) — Beeken 1979
   Coxsackie B (1–66) — Kyle et al 1963
   Polio virus (1–3) — Farmer et al 1973, Beeken 1979
   Echo virus — Farmer et al 1973, Beeken 1979
   (1–7, 9, 11–17, 29–33)

Reoviridae
   Reovirus — Farmer et al 1973, Beeken 1979
   Rota virus — DeGroote et al 1977, Beeken 1979, Greenberg et al 1979

Norwalk virus — Greenberg et al 1979

Paramyxovirus
   Parainfluenza — Farmer et al 1973, Beeken 1979
   Respiratory syncytial virus — Farmer et al 1973, Beeken 1979
   Mumps — Farmer et al 1973, Beeken 1979
   Measles — Beeken 1979

Orthomyxovirus
   Influenza B — Farmer et al 1973, Beeken 1979

Retrovirus
   HIV (Human immunodeficiency virus) — Dourmashkin et al 1986

DNA virus
Adenovirus — Kyle et al 1963, Farmer et al 1973, Beeken 1979

Herpes virus
   Herpes zoster — Farmer et al 1973, Beeken 1979
   Herpes simplex — Farmer et al 1973, Beeken 1979
   Epstein–Barr virus — Grotsky et al 1970, Järnerot & Lantrop 1972, Beeken 1979
   Cytomegalovirus — Swarbrick et al 1979 Farmer et al 1973, Beeken 1979

by inoculating filtrates of intestinal homogenate into the footpad of mice. Taub et al (1974) confirmed this finding, and Simonowitz et al (1979) produced an inflammatory reaction after inoculating Crohn's disease tissue into the bowel wall of rabbits. Cave et al (1975) caused a granulomatous reaction with intraserosal inoculation of Crohn's disease tissue into rabbits. The purported agent could be filtered through a 0.2 μm membrane and inactivated by autoclaving and irradiation (Mitchell & Rees 1976). Similar findings were reported for ulcerative colitis tissue (Taub et al 1974, Cave et al 1976). However, Bolton et al (1973) and Heatley et al (1975) could not detect granulomas after injecting Crohn's disease tissue or homogenate. In order to explain this discrepancy, an independent study was carried out (Thayer 1979) which concluded that many of the granulomas were caused by foreign materials such as pieces of filter.

EXPERIMENTAL MODELS

Animal models of enterocolitis have been designed using transgenic mice. Specific parts of the immune system are disabled using transgenic mice in which specific genes are deleted by gene targeting in the germline. Transgenic mice in which the interleukin-2 (IL-2) gene was disrupted develop inflammatory bowel disease in which the severity of the lesions increases from the cecum to the rectum (Sadlack et al 1993). However, when this strain was bred in a germ-free environment, no disease was seen. An interleukin-10 (IL-10)-defective strain of mice developed chronic enterocolitis involving the entire gastrointestinal tract (Kuhn et al 1993). The enterocolitis was attenuated when the mice were kept in a restricted microbial environment. Similarly, HLA B-27 transgenic rats developed chronic colitis, gastritis and arthritis (Hammer et al 1990). When they were raised in a germ-free state, no colitis was seen (Taurog et al 1993). Colitis does not develop in these experimental models of altered immunity in the absence of the bowel flora, even in the host with an altered immunity; thus the bowel flora are essential to the development of inflammatory bowel disease. Whether the antigenic stimulus is from the bowel flora as a whole or from a specific organism is unclear.

RESPONSE TO ANTIBIOTICS

Antibiotics have been used in inflammatory bowel disease both as primary therapy and also to treat intercurrent infection. Moss et al (1978) found that continuous treatment with broad-spectrum antibiotics such as ampicillin and tetracyclines resulted in symptomatic improvement in 41 of 44 patients with Crohn's disease. Metronidazole has been used as primary therapy for inflammatory bowel disease. In the Swedish Cooperative Crohn's Disease Study (Ursing et al 1982, Rosen et al 1982), metronidazole was compared with sulfasalazine in patients with active Crohn's disease and was found to be just as effective. During the crossover period significant benefit was seen with metronidazole in patients who failed to respond favorably to sulfasalazine. The reverse was not seen, however. A double-blind placebo-controlled trial of metronidazole in Crohn's disease (Sutherland 1991) found that Crohn's disease activity index scores were significantly improved with metronidazole compared to placebo. There were no differences in remission rates.

Ciprofloxacin, a fluoroquinolone, has been used in the treatment of Crohn's disease. Peppercorn (1993) reported resolution of symptoms in four patients with active Crohn's disease after 1 week of ciprofloxacin therapy. Recently, a prospective double-blind placebo-controlled study was performed to assess the effect of ciprofloxacin treatment as an adjunct to conventional treatment in ulcerative colitis (Turunen et al 1994); it was concluded that ciprofloxacin improves the results of long-term therapy. Non-absorbable antibiotics have also been tried in Crohn's disease. In a study of moderately ill hospitalized patients, non-absorbable antibiotics plus an elemental diet were as effective as prednisolone plus a normal diet (Saverymuttu et al 1985). The beneficial role of antibiotics in inflammatory bowel disease is further support for an infectious etiology.

CONCLUSION

Epidemiological and genetic data indicate a role for an infectious agent in the development of inflammatory bowel disease, in addition to a genetic component. Transgenic mice models show that inflammatory bowel disease develops only in the presence of bowel flora. Various infectious agents such as viruses, cell-wall defective bacteria and, more recently, mycobacteria have been suggested as etiologic agents for inflammatory bowel disease. None of these satisfies Koch's postulates.

Transgenic mice models suggest that inflammatory bowel disease can develop in a dysregulated immune state. The gastrointestinal tract contains the largest amount of lymphoid tissue in the body. Progress in molecular immunology has given us a better understanding of the complex interactions that take place between the immune cells of the gastrointestinal system and various antigens in health and disease.

The pathogenesis of inflammatory bowel disease involves an uncontrolled inflammation. This altered immune response may be the result of the genetic make-up of the individual, as well as environmental influences. The immune response may be altered by an infectious agent that involves the immune system, as seen with human immunodeficiency virus infection. The infection may be confined to the immune cells of the gastrointestinal system, or it may be systemic. Long-term exposure to the infectious agent may create a dysregulated immune state, either by a systemic effect or by altering the gastrointestinal mucosal lymphoid cells. Exposure to a specific antigen or multiple antigens from the bowel flora may result in a dysregulated inflammatory state in the bowel, leading to inflammatory bowel disease.

An infectious hypothesis modfied by the host immune and genetic factors provides the best understanding of the pathogenesis of inflammatory bowel disease. The development of sensitive techniques in molecular biology, such as the polymerase chain reaction, may enable us to identify the causative agent(s). Such identification, along with an understanding of the immune interactions, may lead to better understanding, prevention and cure of inflammatory bowel disease.

REFERENCES

Allan R N, Pease P, Ibbotson J P 1986 Clustering of Crohn's disease in a Cotswold village. Quarterly Journal of Medicine 59: 473–478

Aluwihare A P R 1971 Electron microscopy in Crohn's disease. Gut 12: 509–518

Alvonen P, Sievers K, Aho K 1972 Arthritis associated with *Yersinia enterocolitica* infection. Annals of Rheumatic Diseases 31: 34–39

Auer I O, Rhoder A, Wensinck F, van de Merwe J P, Schmidt H 1983 Selected bacterial antibodies in Crohn's disease and ulcerative colitis. Scandinavian Journal of Gastroenterology 18: 217–223

Bargen J A 1924 Experimental studies on the etiology of chronic ulcerative colitis. Journal of the American Medical Association 83: 332

Batty G M, Wilkins W E, Morris J S 1994 Ulcerative colitis in a husband and wife. Gut 35: 562–563

Beeken W 1979 Evidence of virus infection as a cause of Crohn's disease. Zeitschrift für Gastroenterologie 17 (Suppl): 101–104

Belsheim M, Darwisk R, Watson W, Schieven B 1983 Bacterial L-form isolation from inflammatory bowel disease patients. Gastroenterology 85: 364–369

Bennett R A, Rubin P H, Present D H 1991 Frequency of inflammatory bowel disease in offspring of couples both presenting with inflammatory bowel disease. Gastroenterology 100: 1638–1643

Berk T, Gordon S J, Choi H Y, Cooper H S 1985 CMV infecction of the colon: a possible role in exacerbations of inflammatory bowel disease. American Journal of Gastroenterology 80: 355–360

Blaser M J 1994 Bacteria and diseases of unknown cause. Annals of Internal Medicine 121: 144–145

Blaser M J, Hoverson D, Ely I G, Duncan D J, Wang W L, Brown W R 1984 Studies of *Campylobacter jejuni* in patients with inflammatory bowel disease. Gastroenterology 86: 33–38

Bolton P M, Sheriff R, Read A 1980 *Clostridium difficile* associated with diarrhoea: a role in inflammatory bowel disease. Lancet 1: 693–696

Bolton P M, Owen E, Heatley R V, Williams W J, Hughes L E 1973 Negative findings in laboratory animals for a transmissible agent in Crohn's disease. Lancet 2: 1122–1124

Buie L, Bargen J A 1933. Chronic ulcerative colitis. Journal of the American Medical Association 101: 1462

Burke D A, Axon A T 1987 Ulcerative colitis and *E. coli* with adhesive properties. Journal of Clinical Pathology 40: 782–786

Calkins B M, Lilienfeld A M, Garland C F, Mendeloff A I 1984 Trends in the incidence rates of ulcerative colitis and Crohn's disease. Digestive Diseases and Sciences 29: 913

Cave D R, Freedman L S 1975 Seasonal variation in the clinical presentation of Crohn's disease and ulcerative colitis. International Journal of Epidemiology 4: 317–320

Cave D R, Mitchell D N, Brooke B N 1975 Experimental animal studies of the etiology and pathogenesis of Crohn's disease. Gastroenterology 69: 618–624

Cave D R, Mitchell D N, Brooke B N 1976 Evidence of an agent transmissible from ulcerative colitis tissue. Lancet 1: 1311–1315

Cerf M, Mollaret H, Lee A 1982 Peut-on définitivement dissocier maladie de Crohn et infections a Yersinia? Médecine Mal Infectieuse 12: 698

Chandra L, Barrowman J, Kutty K, Bowmer I, Fandy P 1982 Campylobacter infection mimicking a relapse of ulcerative colitis. Canadian Medical Journal 126: 389–390

Chiodini R J, Van Kruiningen H J, Thayer W R, Coutu J A 1986 Spheroplastic phase of mycobacteria isolated from patients with Crohn's disease. Journal of Clinical Microbiology 24: 357–363

Chong S K F, Walker-Smith J A 1986 Chronic inflammatory bowel disease in immigrants in the United Kingdom. In McConnell R, Rozen P, Langman M, Gilat T (eds) The genetics and epidemiology of inflammatory bowel disease. Karger, Basel pp 129–132

Colombel J F, Guillemeo F, VanGossum A et al 1989 Familial Crohn's disease in multiple siblings: no linkage to the HLA system. Gastroenterologie Clinique et Biologique 13: 676–678

Cooke E M 1967 A quantitative comparison of the faecal flora of patients with ulcerative colitis and that of normal persons. Journal of Pathology and Bacteriology 94: 439

Cooper H S, Raffensperger E C, Jonas L, Fitts W T Jr 1977 CMV inclusions in patients with ulcerative colitis and toxic dilatation requiring colon resection. Gastroenterology 72: 1253–1256

Crohn B B, Ginzburg L, Oppenheimer G 1932 Regional ileitis: a pathologic and clinical entity. Journal of the American Medical Association 99: 1323–1329

Dach G M, Heinz T E, Dragstedt L R 1935 Ulcerative colitis: study of bacteria in isolated colons of three patients by cultures and by inoculation of monkeys. Archives of Surgery 31: 225–240

Darchis I, Colombel J F, Cortot A, Devred M, Paris J C 1989 Crohn's disease in a married couple and their four children. (Letter). Lancet: 737

DeGroote G, Desmyter J, Vantrappen G, Philips C A 1977 Rotavirus antibodies in Crohn's disease and ulcerative colitis. Lancet 1: 1263–1264

Dickinson R J, Varian S A, Axon A T, Cooke E M 1980 Increased incidence of faecal coliforms with in vitro adhesive properties in patients with ulcerative colitis. Gut 21: 787–792

Diepersloot R J, Kroes A C, Visser W, Jiwa N M, Rothbarth P H 1990 Acute ulcerative proctocolitis associated with primary CMV infection. Archives of Internal Medicine 150: 1749–1751

Dorman S A, Liggoria E, Winn W C, Beeken W L 1982 Isolation of *Clostridium difficile* from patients with inactive Crohn's disease. Gastroenterology 82: 1348–1351

Dourmashkin R, Sanderson I, Walker-Smith J 1986 Is Crohn's disease caused by a lymphotropic virus? Journal of Pediatric Gastroenterology 5: 334

Ekbom A, Adami H, Helmick C G 1990 Perinatal risk factors for inflammatory bowel disease: a case controlled study. American Journal of Epidemiology 132: 1111–1119

Ekbom A, Wakefield A J, Zaxk M, Adami H O 1994 Perinatal measles infection and subsequent Crohn's disease. Lancet 344: 508–510

Elliott P R, Forsey T, Darougar S, Treharne J D, Lennard-Jones J E 1981 Chlamydia and inflammatory bowel disease. Gut 22: 25–27

Farmer G N, Vincent M M, Vuccilo D A 1973 Viral investigations in ulcerative colitis and regional enteritis. Gastroenterology 65: 8–18

Farmer R G, Michener W M, Mortimer E A 1980 Studies of family history among patients with inflammatory bowel disease. Clinical Gastroenterology 9: 271–277

Findlay J M, Jayarantne S D 1986 Chronic inflammatory bowel disease in immigrants in the United Kingdom. In McConnell R, Rozen P, Langman M, Gilat T (eds) The genetics and epidemiology of inflammatory bowel disease. Karger, Basel, pp 124–129

Felsen J, Wolarsky W 1953 Acute and chronic bacillary dysentery and chronic ulcerative colitis. Journal of the American Medical Association 153: 1069–1072

Gilat T, Grossman A, Fireman Z, Rosen P 1986 Inflammatory bowel disease in Jews. In: McConnell R, Rozen P, Langman M, Gilal T (eds) The genetics and epidemiology of inflammatory bowel disease. Karger, Basel, pp 135–140

Goodgame R W 1993 Gastrointestinal CMV disease. Annals of Internal Medicine 119: 924–935

Goodman M, Pearson K, McGhie D, Dutt S, Deodhar S 1980 Campylobacter and *Giardia lamblia* causing exacerbations of inflammatory bowel disease. Lancet 2: 1247

Gorbach S, Nahas L, Plant A 1968 Studies of intestinal microflora. Fecal microbial ecology in ulcerative colitis and Crohn's disease: its relationship to severity and chemotherapy. Gastroenterology 54: 575

Graham D Y, Yoshimura H H, Estes M 1983 DNA hybridisation studies of the association of *Pseudomonas maltophilia* with inflammatory bowel disease. Journal of Laboratory and Clinical Medicine 101: 940–954

Greenberg H B, Beghard R I, McClain S 1979 Antibodies to viral gastroenteritis viruses in Crohn's disease. Gastroenterology 76: 349–350

Greenfield C, Aguilar R J R, Pounder R E et al 1983 *Clostridium difficile* and inflammatory bowel disease. Gut 24: 713–717

Grotsky H, Glade P R, Hirshaut Y, Sachar D, Janowitz H D 1970 Herpes-like virus and granulomatous colitis. Lancet 2: 1256–1257

Hammer R E, Maika S D, Richardson J A, Tang J P, Taurog J D 1990 Spontaneous inflammatory disease in transgenic rats expressing HLA-B27 and human beta-2 microglobulin: an animal model of HLA-B27 associated human disorders. Cell 63: 1099–1112

Harper P H, Lee E C, Kettlewell M G, Bennet H K, Jewell D P 1985 Role of faecal stream in the maintenance of Crohn's Colitis. Gut 26: 279–284

Heatley R V, Bolto P M, Owen E, Williams W J, Hughes L E 1975 A search for a transmissible agent in Crohn's disease. Gut 16: 528–532

Heidt H, Karch H, Arndt R 1991 Mikrobiologische Befunde bei protrahiert verlaufenden und chronischen Enterocolitiden. Endoscopie Heute 1: 28

Helwig F C 1959 Epithelial cytoplasmic inclusion bodies of possible rival origin in early ulcerative colitis. Diseases of the Colon and Rectum 2: 23–26

Hurst A F 1921 Ulcerative colitis. Guy's Hospital Report 71: 26

Hyams J S, McLaughlin J C 1985 Lack of relationship between *Clostridium difficile* toxin and inflammatory bowel disease in children. Journal of Clinical Gastroenterology 7: 387–390

Ibbotson J P, Pease P E, Allan R N 1987 Serological studies in Crohn's disease. European Journal of Clinical Microbiology 6: 286–290

Jarnerot G, Lantrop K 1972 Antibodies to EB virus in cases of Crohn's disease. New England Journal of Medicine 286: 1215–1216

Jori G P, De Vargas F, Altucci P 1968 Mycoplasmas in chronic ulcerative colitis: a negative study. Pathology and Microbiology (Basel): 31: 209–214

Kangro H, Chang S, Hardiman A 1990 A prospective study of viral and mycoplasma infection in chronic inflammatory bowel disease. Gastroenterology 98: 548

Kuhn R, Lohler J, Rennick D, Rajewsky K, Mullere W 1993 IL-10 deficient mice develop chronic enterocolitis. Cell 75: 263–274

Kyle J, Bell T, Ponteous I, Blair D 1963 Factors in the aetiology of regional enteritis. Bulletin International Surgical Society 22: 575–584

Lambert J, Tischler M, Karmale M, Newman A 1979 Campylobacter ileocolitis: an inflammatory bowel disease. Canadian Medical Journal 121: 1377–1379

LaMont J T, Trnka Y M 1980 Therapeutic implications of *Clostridium difficile* toxin during relapse of chronic inflammatory bowel disease. Lancet 1: 381–383

Larsen J 1980 *Yersinia enterocolitica* infections and rheumatic diseases. Scandinavian Journal of Rheumatology 9: 129

Lee D K, Cooper B T, Barbezat G O 1986 *Clostridium difficile* toxin in chronic idiopathic colitis. New Zealand Medical Journal 27: 620–622

Lobo A J, Foster P N, Sobala G M, Axon A T R 1988 Crohn's disease in married couples. Lancet 1: 704–705

McConnell R B 1990 Genetics of inflammatory bowel disease. In: Allan R N, Keighley M R B, Alexander-Williams J, Hawkins C (eds) Inflammatory bowel disease. Churchill Livingstone, New York, pp 11–23

McConnell R B, Vadheim C M 1992 Inflammatory bowel disease. In: King R A, Rotter J I, Motulsky A O (eds) The genetic basis of common diseases. Oxford University Press, Oxford, pp 326–348

Mayberry J F, Hitchens R A N 1978 Distribution of Crohn's disease in Cardiff. Social Science and Medicine (Oxford) 12: 137–138

Mendcloff A I, Dunn J P 1991 Digestive diseases American Public Health Association Vital and Health Statistics Monograph. Harvard University Press, Cambridge, MA

Mitchell D N, Rees R J W 1970 Agent transmissible from Crohn's disease tissue. Lancet 2: 168–171

Mitchell D N, Rees R J W 1976 Further observations on the transmissibility of Crohn's disease. Annals of the New York Academy of Sciences 178: 546–559

Monis B, Mendeloff A I 1961 Observations on inclusion bodies in normal and pathologic mucosa of the colon in man. Journal of the National Cancer Institute 26: 1429–1443

Moss A A, Carbine J V, Kressel H Y 1978 Radiologic and clinical assessment of broad-spectrum antibiotics in Crohn's disease. American Journal of Radiology 131: 787–790

Mygind N, Thulin H 1970 Yersina enterocolitica: a new cause of erythema nodosum. British Journal of Dermatology 82: 351–354

Pai CH, Gordon R, Sims H V, Bryan L E 1984 Sporadic cases of hemorrhagic colitis associated with *E. coli* 0157: H7. Annals of Internal Medicine 101: 738–742

Parent K, Mitchell P D 1976 Bacterial variants: etiologic agents in Crohn's disease? Gastroenterology 71: 365–372

Parent K, Mitchell P D 1978 Cell wall defective variants of pseudomonas-like (group Va) bacteria in Crohn's disease. Gastroenterology 75: 368–372

Peppercorn M A 1993 Is there a role for antibiotics as primary therapy for Crohn's ileitis? Journal of Clinical Gastroenterology 17: 235–237

Persson S, Danielsson D, Kjellander, Wallenstein S 1976 Studies on Crohn's disease. 1 The relationship between *Yersina enterocolitica* infection and terminal ileitis. Acta Chirurgica Scandinavica 142: 84–90

Reilly R P, Robinson T J 1986 Crohn's disease – is there a long latent period? Postgraduate Medical Journal 62: 353–354
Relman D A, Schmidt T M, MacDermott R P, Falkow S 1992 Identification of the uncultured bacillus of Whipple's disease. New England Journal of Medicine 327: 293–301
Riemann J F 1977 Further electron microscopic evidence of virus-like particles in Crohn's disease. Acta Hepatogastroenterologica 24: 116–118
Rosen A, Ursing B, Alm T 1982 A comparative study of metronidazole and sulfasalazine for active Crohn's disease: the Cooperative Crohn's Disease Study in Sweden. Part I Design and methodologic considerations. Gastroenterology 83: 541–549
Ryan C A, Tauxe R V, Hosek A W et al 1986 E. coli 0157: H7 diarrhea in a nursing home. Journal of Infectious Diseases 154: 631–638
Sadlack B, Merz H, Schorle H, Schimpi A, Feller A C, Horak I 1993 Ulcerative colitis-like disease in mice with a disruptive interleukin-2 gene. Cell 75: 253–261
Saebo A, Lassen J 1992 Acute and chronic gastrointestinal manifestations associated with Yersinia enterocolitica infection. A Norwegian 10-year follow-up study on 458 hospitalised patients. Annals of Surgery 215: 250–255
Satsangi J, Jewell D P, Rosenberg W M C, Bell J I 1994 Genetics of inflammatory bowel disease. Gut 35: 696–700
Saverymuttu S, Hodgson H J F, Chadwick V S 1985 Controlled trial comparing prednisolone with an elemental diet plus non-absorbable antibiotics in active Crohn's disease. Gut 26: 994–998
Schuller J L, Piket-van Ulsen J, Veeken I V D, Michel M F, Stolz E 1978 Antibodies against chlamydia of lymphogranuloma venereum in Crohn's disease. Lancet 2: 19–20
Seneca H, Henderson E 1950 Normal intestinal bacteria in ulcerative colitis. Gastroenterology 15: 34–39
Simonowitz D, Block G E, Riddel R H, Kraft S C, Kirsner J B 1979 Inflammatory tissue reaction in rabbit bowel injected with Crohn's homogenate. American Journal of Surgery 138: 415–417
Sjostrom B 1971 Acute terminal ileitis and its relation to Crohn's disease. In Engel A, Larsson T (eds) Regional enteritis: Crohn's disease. Nordiska Bokhandekins Forlag, Stockholm, pp 73–76
Smith M S H, Wakefield A J 1993 Viral association with Crohn's disease. Annals of Medicine 25: 557–561
Smith M S H, Sawyerr A M, Sim R et al 1994 The distribution of herpes virus DNA within the gastrointestinal tract in inflammatory bowel disease. Gastroenterology 106: 4 Part 2: A775
Sutherland L, Singleton J, Sessions J 1991 Double blind, placebo controlled trial of metronidazole in Crohn's disease. Gut 32: 1071–1075
Swarbrick E, Yungham J, Price H 1979 Chlamydia, cytomegalovirus and yersinia in inflammatory bowel disease. Lancet 2: 11
Taub R N, Sachar D, Siltzbach L, Janowitz 1974 Transmission of ileitis and sarcoid granulomas to mice. Transactions of the Association of American Physicians 87: 219–224
Taurog J D, Hammer R E, Montafiez S et al 1993 Effect of germ free state on the inflammatory disease of HLA-B 27 transgenic rats. Arthritis and Rheumatism 36 (Suppl): S46 (Abstract no 45)
Taylor-Robinson D, O'Morain C A, Thomas B J, Levi A 1979 Low frequency of chlamydial antibodies in patients with Crohn's disease and ulcerative colitis. Lancet 1: 1162–1163
Thayer W R 1979 Executive summary of the AGA-NFIC sponsored workshop on infectious diseases. Digestive Diseases and Sciences 24: 781–784
Tomenius J, Larre E, Lindgren I, Blumenthal B, Lindewall G 1963 Positive Frei test in 7 cases of Morbus Crohn (regional ileitis). Gastroenterologica 99: 368–373
Turunen U, Farkkila M, Vuoristo M et al 1994 A double-blind, placebo controlled six-month ciprofloxacin treatment improves prognosis in ulcerative colitis. Gastroenterology 106: A786 (Abstract)
Ursing B, Alm T, Barany F 1982 A comparative study of metronidazole and sulfasalazine for active Crohn's disease: the Cooperative Crohn's Disease Study in Sweden. Part II Results. Gastroenterology 83: 550–562
van der Weil-Korstanje J A A, Winkler K 1975 The fecal flora of ulcerative colitis. Journal of Medical Microbiology 8: 491–501
Van Dyke T E, Dowell V R, Offenbacher S, Snyder W, Hersh T 1986 Potential role of microorganisms isolated from periodontal lesions in the pathogenesis of inflammatory bowel disease. Infection and Immunity 53: 671–677
van Kruiningen H J, Colombel J F, Cartun R W et al 1993 An in-depth study of Crohn's disease in two French families. Gastroenterology 104: 351–360
van Weichen P 1974 Radiological changes in the distal part of the ileum in association with Yersinia enterocolitica infections. Radiologica Chirurgica Biologica 43: 242–253
Von Glahn W C, Pappenheimer A M 1925 Intranuclear inclusions in visceral disease. American Journal of Pathology 1: 445–466
Wakefield A J, Fox J D, Sawyer A M 1992 Detection of herpes virus DNA in the large intestine of patients with ulcerative colitis and Crohn's disease using nested polymerase chain reaction. Journal of Medical Virology 38: 183–190
Wakefield A J, Pitlilo R, Sim R 1993 Evidence of persistent measles virus infection in Crohn's disease. Journal of Medical Virology 39: 345
Wensinck F, Custers-van Lieshaut L 1981 The fecal flora of patients with Crohn's disease. Journal of Hygiene 87: 1–12
Wensinck F, van de Merwr J P 1981 Serum agglutinins to Eubacterium and Peptostreptococcus species in Crohn's and other diseases. Journal of Hygiene (London) 87: 13–24
Whorwell P J, Davidson I W, Beeken W L, Wright R 1978 Search by immunofluorescence for antigens of rota virus, Pseudomonas maltophilia and Mycobacterium kansasii in Crohn's disease. Lancet 2: 697–698

16. Infective agents – mycobacteria
H. M. Fidler   J. J. McFadden

INTRODUCTION

A link between mycobacterial infection and Crohn's disease was first postulated over 80 years ago, yet despite the application of increasingly sophisticated laboratory techniques the issue remains unresolved. Dalziel (1913) discussed a 'professional colleague' with chronic interstitial enteritis and likened the pathology not only to tuberculous bowel disease, but also to an animal chronic enteric infection termed Johne's disease, caused by *Mycobacterium paratuberculosis*. Crohn himself noted the similarities to ileal tuberculosis when he described 14 cases of a granulomatous disease involving the small intestine (Crohn et al 1932). Many gastroenterologists who have lived with the waxing and waning of research enthusiasm in this field now view the question with some cynicism, but recent work has provided sufficient fresh data and hypotheses to rekindle interest. Obviously the possibility of a role for mycobacteria in Crohn's disease is worth pursuing vigorously, since we may thereby develop a new treatment approach for this increasingly common and disabling disease. Ulcerative colitis presents a clinicopathological syndrome distinct from Crohn's disease, and the likelihood of an etiological mycobacterial role is so remote that it provides a useful experimental control for researchers.

Do mycobacteria cause Crohn's disease? Before reviewing the evidence it is important to consider why this essentially straightforward question has proved so intransigent. First, it is almost certainly incorrect to assume that Crohn's disease has one cause, since most diseases are multifactorial in origin. Many result from a complex interplay of genetic, environmental and infectious elements (McFadden et al 1990), and the episodic nature of Crohn's disease would support this. Even diseases caused by conventional infectious agents, such as enterocolitis, may be associated with a plethora of bacteria, viruses and parasites. Furthermore, disease manifestations may become apparent some time after the acute infection – the 'hit-and-run' mechanism (e.g. reactive arthritis associated with a number of bacterial infections, rheumatic heart disease, or glomerulonephritis associated with group A streptococcal infections).

The anatomical site of possible infection in Crohn's disease, often involving the terminal ileum, makes tissue biopsy difficult and the isolation of possible pathogens from the non-sterile colon requires careful interpretation. If a normal commensal is pathogenic in a given disease, this should ideally be demonstrable by isolation of that organism from a sterile site, such as blood or lung. Since both normal and Crohn's disease-affected gut harbours a host of bacteria, including mycobacteria (Portaels et al 1988), interpretation of any microbiological findings must be cautious, since the mere presence of an organism does not prove causation of disease.

The problem is compounded by the inherent difficulties of studying the *Mycobacterium* genus. The diagnosis of mycobacterial infections has historically been limited by their varied clinical manifestations, low detection rate by microbiological staining, and their slow growth by various culture techniques. Several species of mycobacteria, including *M. tuberculosis* and *M. paratuberculosis*, are thought to be able to survive in a cell-wall deficient form, thereby making themselves undetectable by acid-fast staining (Chiodini et al 1986). In clinical leprosy *Mycobacterium leprae* can still not be cultured; the gold standard for causation, Koch's postulates, cannot be strictly applied.

In such a situation, how can we possibly hope to unravel the probably cofactorial role of mycobacteria in the etiology of Crohn's disease? Fortunately we may not need to analyze all the causative factors involved in this disease, because by isolating a potentially treatable element we may be able to prevent the disease or improve therapy in a recognizable subgroup of sufferers. We will now discuss which mycobacterial organism is the likeliest contender, the detection rates for this organism in Crohn's disease, and whether antimycobacterial chemotherapy has been successful.

MYCOBACTERIUM PARATUBERCULOSIS

M. paratuberculosis has historically been suspected of being

Table 16.1 Distribution and characteristics of *M. avium* complex strains

RFLP type	Human TB	AIDS	Animal TB	Johne's disease	Crohn's disease	Environment	Insertion sequences
M. avium A	+	++	+	–	–	++	–
M. paratb	–	–	–	++	++	–	IS*900*
M. avium A/I	+/–	–	++	+	+	–	IS*901*

++ frequently present
+ rarely present
– absent

involved in Crohn's disease, largely because it has long been recognized to cause an infectious ileitis in ruminants, termed Johne's disease. *M. paratuberculosis* itself belongs to the *Mycobacterium avium* group of mycobacteria, but differs from *M. avium* in being mycobactin-dependent on culture. However, mycobactin-dependent strains of *M. avium* are found, so that mycobactin dependence cannot be used as a taxonomic marker for *M. paratuberculosis* (Collins et al 1983). Members of the *M. avium* group are very closely related, with greater than 95% DNA homology, but can be distinguished by DNA probes which divide the group into three strains/species (McFadden et al 1987b, 1992, Kunze et al. 1991, 1992) which differ in possession of insertion sequences and show marked differences in host range/distribution (Table 16.1). *M. avium* RFLP type A is an environmental opportunist that causes atypical tuberculosis and opportunist infections in immunocompromised patients, particularly AIDS patients. *M. avium* RFLP type A/I is the predominant pathogen causing tuberculosis in animals and birds, but may also occasionally be associated with Johne's disease. *M. paratuberculosis* is the Johne's disease bacillus that has been found only in animals with Johne's disease or in humans with Crohn's disease.

Culture studies

Crohn himself first attempted to culture *M. tuberculosis* from Crohn's disease-affected tissue, and also inoculated such tissue directly into animals (Crohn et al 1932). Neither approach demonstrated mycobacteria in his patients. Perhaps because of the exacting and varied growth requirements of mycobacteria, it was not until 1978 that the first reported culture was made (Burnham et al 1978). Mesenteric lymph nodes from 27 patients with Crohn's disease, 13 with ulcerative colitis and 11 with miscellaneous bowel disorders were cultured for at least 6 months on Lowenstein–Jensen slopes. After 8 months a strain of *Mycobacterium kansasii* grew from one Crohn's disease patient. The first successful cultures of *M. paratuberculosis* from Crohn's disease were reported in a triad of papers by Chiodini in the 1980s. An initially unclassified *Mycobacterium* species, resembling *M. paratuberculosis*, was isolated from the terminal ileum of three patients with Crohn's disease (Chiodini et al 1984b). Remarkably slow growing, it had taken up to 18 months for primary isolation. These three patients formed part of a study group of 14 Crohn's disease patients, six ulcerative colitis patients and seven bowel carcinoma patients. No similar mycobacteria were demonstrated in either control group.

Further work with these cultures employed the rapidly developing DNA technology of the 1980s. A cloned genomic probe derived from the human Crohn's disease isolate of *M. paratuberculosis*, strain Ben, was used to investigate the presence of mycobacterial DNA sequences in Crohn's disease tissues (Butcher et al 1988). DNA was extracted from the colon or terminal ileum of 17 Crohn's disease patients and four controls, and no mycobacterial DNA was detected in any tissue. The sensitivity of this technique was low, being only one organism per 100 human cells for even the bacillary form of *M. paratuberculosis*. DNA extraction methods may have failed to expose spheroplastic DNA. However, restriction fragment-length polymorphism analysis was used to demonstrate that the Crohn's disease-isolated strains of *M. paratuberculosis*, Ben, Linda and Dominic, were identical to each other and the bovine type strain of *M. paratuberculosis* (McFadden et al, 1987a). This was an important finding, since it ruled out the possibility that these strains were in fact isolates of the common environmental opportunist, *M. avium*. Since the initial isolates of Chiodini and co-workers, a number of laboratories around the world have attempted to isolate *M. paratuberculosis* from Crohn's disease tissue. A large number of clinical specimens (more than 200) have been cultured for *M. paratuberculosis* but only six strains of DNA probe-confirmed *M. paratuberculosis* have been successfully isolated from Crohn's disease (Chiodini et al 1984c, Graham et al 1987, Haagsma et al, 1988, Chiodini 1988, McFadden and Seechurn 1992, McFadden et al 1993). *M. avium* RFLP type A/I (which may also cause Johne's disease) has been isolated from two patients in two independent laboratories. A larger number of samples have yielded pleomorphic, spheroplast-like organisms which grow extremely slowly and cannot be identified by conventional means.

Identification of spheroplast-like agents has only become possible with the advent of the polymerase chain reaction (PCR). Thirty of these unidentified spheroplastic organisms grown from 21 patients in Chiodini's laboratory were recently analyzed using PCR: 14 of 25 cultures from

Crohn's disease tissues contained mycobacterial DNA, compared to three of five controls. Six of the Crohn's disease tissue cultures and none of the controls were shown to contain DNA from *M. paratuberculosis* (Wall et al 1993). A similar study on spheroplast-like agents from another laboratory demonstrated *M. paratuberculosis* DNA in spheroplast-like organisms from both Crohn's disease samples and controls (Moss et al 1992). The presence of *M. paratuberculosis* DNA in cultures from control tissue is surprising, since normal control tissues and diseased gut tissues, including ulcerative colitis, have never yielded *M. paratuberculosis* in culture. Immunocompromised AIDS patients have never been found to be colonized with *M. paratuberculosis* (Hampson et al 1988, 1989b), despite the susceptibility of such patients to infection with the very closely related pathogen *M. avium*. When detected in animals *M. paratuberculosis* is always assumed to be pathogenic, and it is reasonable to assume that its presence in Crohn's disease has a similar significance. The detection of *M. paratuberculosis* DNA in cultures from control tissue should therefore be considered in the light of discussion on PCR contamination (see below).

The variability in results from different laboratories should be expected, since *M. paratuberculosis* has exacting and protracted growth requirements and even in multibacillary Johne's disease many laboratories are unable to identify it (Chiodini et al 1984a). If it is present in low numbers, in a vulnerable form with variable biochemical and acid-fast staining, culture alone may always be inadequate for the detection of this organism. More sensitive and specific molecular techniques based on DNA amplification should overcome these inherent problems, and recent PCR work will now be discussed.

DIRECT TISSUE DETECTION OF MYCOBACTERIA AND THE POLYMERASE CHAIN REACTION

Efforts to search directly in Crohn's disease tissue for *M. paratuberculosis* using immunohistochemical techniques have failed to demonstrate any mycobacteria at all (Kobayashi et al 1989). However, the sensitivity of this technique was inadequate to detect paucibacillary disease, and the antibodies used were not derived from spheroplastic forms. Direct detection of DNA within tissues was therefore desirable, yet Butcher et al (1988) failed to identify any mycobacteria by Southern blotting and hybridization alone in Crohn's disease tissue. Doubt remained over the sensitivity of this work, since only one mycobacterial genome per 100 human cells would have been detected. DNA probes were more successful in the diagnosis of Johne's disease from heavily infected fecal material (Vary et al 1990), but the applicability of non-amplification based procedures to Crohn's disease tissue was low.

PCR was designed to increase the efficiency of existing molecular techniques and to provide a sensitive and specific detection mechanism in its own right (Sauki et al 1985). By carrying out repeated cycles of annealing, synthesis and denaturation of nucleic acids in the presence of thermostable DNA polymerase (Taq polymerase) and free nucleic acids, DNA sequences bounded by a pair of sequence-specific primers can be amplified more than a millionfold. PCR product may be detected directly by gel electrophoresis and ethidium bromide staining if more than 10 ng of DNA is produced. When combined with Southern transfer of the product on to membrane and hybridization with labeled probe, the sensitivity is increased by a further factor of 10. This technique has already been used in the diagnosis of tuberculosis and leprosy (Hermans et al 1990, Brisson-Noel et al 1991, De Wit et al 1993, Noordhoek et al 1994).

Before the PCR can be used, species-specific primer sequences must first be identified. With respect to *M. paratuberculosis*, some groups have used the single-copy 16S rRNA sequences and the conserved *groEl* gene (Wu et al 1991). However, the use of species-specific insertion sequences allows greater sensitivity and specificity. Insertion sequences are small, mobile genetic elements containing genes related only to their mobility. They are typically 0.8–1.8 kilobase pairs long, and one genome may contain several copies of these identical sequences as potential PCR targets. Two of these are relevant to the study of Crohn's disease (Table 16.1). IS*900* is specific to *M. paratuberculosis* and present in multiple copies of 15–20 per genome (Green et al 1989). When validated for PCR with cultures, it had a sensitivity of 10 fg DNA, the equivalent of two *M. paratuberculosis* genomes (Vary et al 1990). IS*900* has been applied in PCR to Johne's disease fecal material, but cattle feces inhibited the PCR and a drop in sensitivity was seen (Vary et al 1990). With purified fecal DNA, an IS*900*-based PCR had a sensitivity of 100% for detection of *M. paratuberculosis* organisms in Johne's disease (Vary et al 1990). *M. avium* RFLP type A/I, also implicated in Crohn's and Johne's disease (McFadden et al 1993), also contains an insertion sequence, termed IS*901* (Kunze et al 1991, 1992). IS*901* is absent in the other closely related organism, including *M. avium* RFLP type A, which affects AIDS patients. Thus these closely related strains within the *M. avium* complex can be sensitively and specifically detected by PCR using IS*900* and IS*901*, despite a sequence homology of approximately 98% in their chromosomal DNA (Kunze et al 1992).

A summary of the results obtained by different laboratories in detecting *M. paratuberculosis* infection in Crohn's disease tissue by PCR, can be seen in Table 16.2 (Quirke et al 1991, Wu et al 1991, Cellier et al 1993, Rowotham et al 1993, Dell'Isola et al 1994, Fidler et al 1994). Unfortunately, many of the results are published only in abstract form, and so full details of experimental

Table 16.2 Detection of *M. paratuberculosis* DNA in Crohn's disease tissue by PCR

Reference	Tissue	Crohn's disease	Ulcerative colitis	Controls	Phenol used	Granulomas assessed	Southern hybridization
Quirke et al 1991	gut	2/5	1/5	–		no	yes
Wu et al 1991	gut	0/20	–	0/10	–	yes	no
Rosenberg et al 1991	mln, gut	0/21	–	0/6		no	yes
Sanderson et al 1992	gut	26/40	1/23	5/40	yes	no	yes
Cellier et al 1993	gut	0/45	0/24	0/18		no	no
Koltun et al 1993	gut	5/16	1/7	3/13		no	yes
Fidler et al 1993	mln	0/30	0/2	0/13	no	no	yes
Fidler et al 1994	gut	4/31	0/10	0/20	no	yes	yes
Rowbotham et al 1993	gut	0/57	0/45	0/9		no	no
Dell'Isola et al 1994	gut	13/18	7/24	7/24	yes	no	yes

mln, mesenteric lymphnode

protocols are not available. However, the table makes grim reading for those who had hoped that PCR would resolve the question of mycobacterial infection in Crohn's disease. A number of features are immediately apparent.

1. In contrast to culture results, *M. paratuberculosis* DNA was detected in control specimens in three out of nine of the studies.
2. *M. paratuberculosis* DNA was detected in Crohn's disease tissue in five out of nine of the studies, but the frequency of detection ranged from 13% to 72% of specimens examined. However, it should be noted that in the study in which 65% of Crohn's disease specimens were positive, samples were examined in triplicate and were scored positive if *M. paratuberculosis* DNA could be detected in only one of the triplicate samples (Sanderson et al 1992).
3. *M. paratuberculosis* DNA could not be detected in Crohn's disease tissue in three out of nine of the studies.

Before analyzing these results in detail, it is instructive to compare them with results obtained from a study sponsored by the World Health Organization, evaluating the potential use of PCR for the diagnosis of tuberculosis (Noordhoek et al 1994). Pooled sputum was spiked with various numbers of BCG (*Mycobacterium bovis* strain BCG) cells and sent with control uninfected sputum (randomized and blinded) to seven research laboratories for PCR detection of BCG DNA. The results obtained for part of this study, in which 0.2 ml sputum samples were spiked with 10^3 and 10^4 BCG cells, are summarized in Table 16.3. As can be seen, the results bear some similarities to the Crohn's disease studies. Each of the laboratories was experienced in PCR and each included negative controls. Yet over the whole study, 19% of the negative samples were reported to be positive! Of the samples containing 10^3 BCG cells in 0.2 ml (the sensitivity of microscopy for comparison is 10^3–10^4/ml) the percentage of samples that were found to be positive ranged from 0 to 90% in different laboratories.

This study illustrated the difficulties of PCR tests for detection of mycobacterial DNA. The sensitivity of PCR

Table 16.3 Sensitivity and specificity of PCR for the detection of BCG in sputum by PCR: results of a blinded trial involving seven independent laboratories. (Data from Noordhoek et al 1994)

Laboratory	10^3 BCG in sputum (25 samples)	10^4 BCG in sputum (10 samples)	0 BCG in sputum (20 samples)
1	5	7	11
2	3	2	3
3	1	3	6
4	15	9	4
5	12	8	0
6	20	10	3
7	13	10	0

can be its own downfall, and its ability to produce large numbers of copies of a sequence from minute quantities of DNA is likely to generate false positive results. Although these can result from sample-to-sample contamination, a more serious source of false positives is the carryover of DNA from a previous amplification of the same target, termed 'amplicon carryover'. Even minute quantities of a PCR sample can lead to serious contamination problems. Since these can exist in aerosol form, or on hair and skin, simple sterile techniques may not remove them.

The problems of PCR are not, however, insurmountable. Two of the laboratories engaged in the tuberculosis study reported zero false positives (Table 16.3). Both these laboratories used guanidinium thiocyanate for pretreatment and lysis of the samples, and silica particles to purify the DNA. With 10^4 BCG cells these two laboratories reported 80% and 100% sensitivity, although with only 10^3 BCG cells the sensitivities dropped to 60 and 70% detection. Two laboratories (1 and 4) used phenol extraction to purify the DNA and had false positive rates of 44% and 16% respectively. Phenol extraction produces a fine aerosol of tiny particles that may contain thousands of PCR amplicons – sufficient to contaminate many PCR tubes.

Of the Crohn's disease studies (Table 16.2) that reported detection of *M. paratuberculosis* DNA in ulcerative colitis or control tissue, two used phenol extraction to purify DNA. Details are not available on the third. Only the studies described by Fidler et al (1993, 1994) used guanidinium thiocyanate for sample pretreatment and

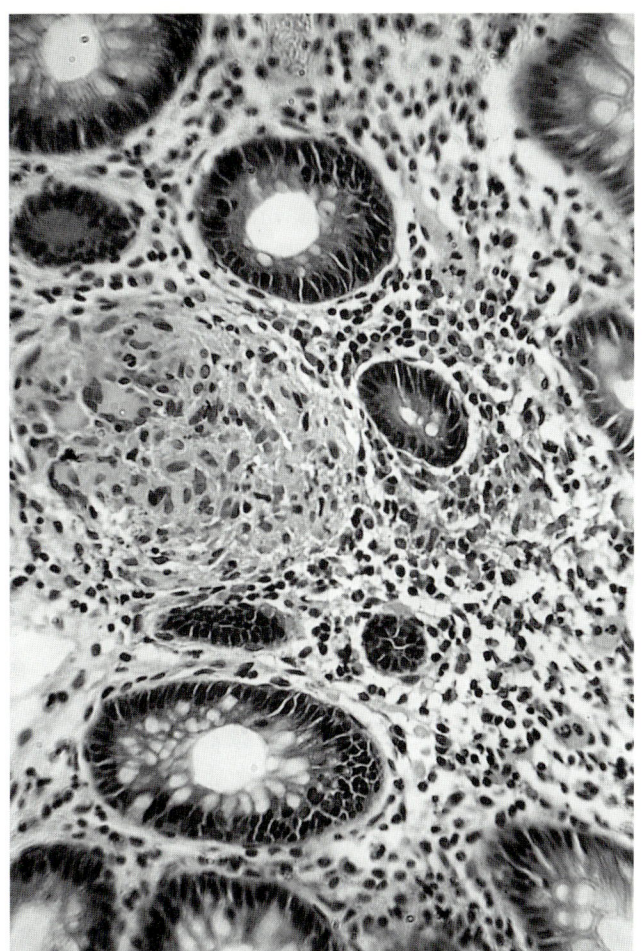

Fig. 16.1 Photomicrograph of Crohn's rectal tissue section containing a granuloma. A parallel section was investigated by PCR and contained more than 2000 genomes of *M. paratuberculosis* DNA. (Hematoxylin and eosin stain, ×250)

Crohn's disease tissues contained granulomata, and Crohn's disease tissues containing granulomata were significantly more likely to amplify IS*900* than the non-Crohn's disease tissues ($P = 0.02$). One of these specimens, from a rectal biopsy, contained up to 2000 genomes when assessed by serial dilution (Fig. 16.1), but no acid-fast bacilli were visible on Ziehl–Neelsen staining. These PCR results suggest that *M. paratuberculosis* is present in concentrated foci within some granulomata of Crohn's disease.

ANTIMYCOBACTERIAL THERAPY IN CROHN'S DISEASE

The myriad difficulties of research in this area are nowhere more apparent than when designing a trial of antimycobacterial chemotherapy in Crohn's disease. *M. paratuberculosis* cultured from primates has a wide range of sensitivities (McClure et al 1987). One early report of the use of quadruple therapy in Crohn's disease was encouraging (Hampson et al 1989a). Further small studies did not support these findings, and a recent large well-controlled 2-year treatment trial of rifampicin, isoniazid and ethambutol likewise provided no evidence of any tangible benefit (Swift et al 1994). Negative results for antimycobacterial regimens in Crohn's disease may be interpreted in a number of ways. First, mycobacteria may not be involved in the pathology. Secondly, the effectiveness of drugs assessed in vitro may not be appropriate to all *M. paratuberculosis* organisms in vivo. The differences between the sensitivity of this organism in vitro and in vivo, and between drug sensitivities of the three Crohn's disease isolates examined in detail so far, would support this (Marsheck et al 1972). The failure of antimycobacterial chemotherapy in Johne's disease (Chiodini et al 1984a) and the problems of treating atypical mycobacterial disease in humans (Horsburg et al 1991, Young et al 1991) are indicative that much longer and multidrug treatment regimens may be necessary.

It is probable that we do not yet possess an appropriate antimicrobial agent to tackle an organism that may lack a cell wall, be exceptionally slow growing, have great biochemical heterogeneity and live within parasitized host cells. Finally, and probably most importantly, both culture- and PCR-based work suggests that *M. paratuberculosis* may be involved in only a proportion of patients with Crohn's disease. Future trails should therefore target this group specifically if we hope to detect a clinical response.

WHERE NEXT FOR MYCOBACTERIA AND CROHN'S DISEASE?

The use of molecular techniques has not resolved the issue of mycobacterial involvement in Crohn's disease. There have been too many poorly conducted and improperly controlled studies that have effectively 'muddied the

lysis, and silica beads for the purification of DNA. Neither of these studies detected *M. paratuberculosis* DNA in control specimens, a result entirely in accordance with culture results.

However, perhaps the most important conclusion to be drawn from the tuberculosis study is that there is no substitute for a properly conducted blinded trial with appropriate positive and negative controls. Most of the participating laboratories had previously reported successful results with their own in-house PCRs, yet when examined by the ultimate test of a fully blinded trail most tests yielded low sensitivities and specificities. Of the studies described in Table 16.1, only those by Fidler et al (1993, 1994) were reported to have been performed blinded, with appropriate positive and negative controls.

In one of the Crohn's disease studies (Fidler et al 1994) in which fixed tissue sections were examined, histopathological examination of adjacent tissue sections was also performed. Twenty of the 31 Crohn's disease tissues contained granulomata. Interestingly, all four positive waters' for any proper evaluation of the role of the likely presence of mycobacterial DNA in Crohn's disease. Further in-house studies will only add to the confusion. We propose that the following studies should be performed to resolve the issue:

1. A bank of Crohn's disease and control (positive and negative) tissue specimens should be collected. Specimens should be coded and identical samples sent to a number of laboratories for a fully blinded multicenter trial of detection of mycobacterial DNA in Crohn's disease tissue by PCR.

2. Serum samples from the same patients should be examined for the presence of antibody to mycobacterial antigens.
3. Any reproducibly positive specimens should be examined by either in-situ PCR or immunohistochemistry to attempt to determine the localization of mycobacteria within the tissue and their association with lesions.
4. A trial of antimycobacterial therapy in Crohn's disease. should be performed with patients reproducibly demonstrated to be infected with *Mycobacterium paratuberculosis*.

REFERENCES

Brisson-Noel A, Aznar C, Chureau C et al 1991 Diagnosis of tuberculosis by DNA amplification in clinical practice evaluation. Lancet 338: 364–366

Burnham W R, Lennard-Jones J E, Stanford J L, Bird R G 1978. Mycobacteria as a possible cause of inflammatory bowel disease. Lancet 2: 693–696

Butcher P D, McFadden J J, Hermon-Taylor J 1988. Investigation of mycobacteria in Crohn's disease tissue by Southern blotting and DNA hybridisation with cloned mycobacterial genomic DNA probes from a Crohn's disease isolated mycobacteria. Gut 29: 1222–1228

Cellier C, De Benhouwer H, Faucheron J L et al 1993. *Mycobacterium paratuberculosis* and *avium silvaticum* DNA cannot be detected in Crohn's disease tissues. Gastroenterology 140: A678

Chiodini R J 1988 Identification of mycobacteria from Crohn's disease by restriction polymorphism of the 5S ribosomal DNA genes. In: MacDermott R P (ed) Inflammatory bowel disease. Elsevier Science Publications, Amsterdam, pp 509–514

Chiodini R J, van Kruiningen H J, Merkal R S 1984a Ruminant paratuberculosis (Johne's disease). The current status and future prospects. The Cornell Veterinarium 74: 218–262

Chiodini R J, van Kruiningen H J, Merkal R S, Thayer W R, Coutu J A 1984b Characteristics of an unclassified *Mycobacterium* species isolated from patients with Crohn's disease. Journal of Clinical Microbiology 20: 966–971

Chiodini R J, van Kruiningen H J, Thayer W R, Merkal R S, Coutu J A 1984c Possible role of mycobacteria in inflammatory bowel disease. I. An unclassified *Mycobacterium* species isolated from patients with Crohn's disease. Digestive Diseases and Sciences 29: 1073–1079

Chiodini R J, van Kruiningen H J, Thayer W R, Coutu J A 1986 Spheroplastic phase of mycobacteria isolated from patients with Crohn's disease. Journal of Clinical Microbiology 24: 357–363

Collins P, Mathews P R J, McDiarmid A, Brown A 1983 The pathogenicity of *Mycobacterium avium* and related mycobacteria for experimental animals. Journal of Medical Microbiology 16: 27–35

Crohn B Ginzberg L Oppenheimer G 1932 Regional ileitis, a pathological and clinical entity. Journal of the American Medicial Association 99: 1323–1329

Dalziel T K 1913 Chronic interstitial enteritis. British Medical Journal ii: 1068–1070

Dell'Isola B, Poyart C, Goulet O et al 1994 Detection of *Mycobacterium paratuberculosis* by polymerase chain reaction in children with Crohn's disease. Journal of Infectious Diseases 169: 449–451

De Wit M Y, Douglas J T, McFadden J, Klatser P R 1993 Polymerase chain reaction for detection of *Mycobacterium leprae* in nasal swab specimens. Journal of Clinical Microbiology 31: 502–506

Fidler H M, Ibbotson J, Chahal H et al 1993 Abdominal lymph-node granulomas and *Helicobacter pylori*. Lancet 342: 299–300

Fidler H M, Thurrell W, Rook G A, Johnson N M, McFadden J J 1994 Specific detection of *Mycobacterium paratuberculosis* DNA associated with granulomatous tissue in Crohn's disease. Gut 35: 506–510

Graham D Y, Markesich D C, Yoshimura H H 1987 Mycobacteria and inflammatory bowel disease. Results of culture. Gastroenterology 92: 436–442

Green E P, Tizard M L V, Moss M T et al, 1989 Sequence and characteristics of IS900, and insertion element identified in a human Crohn's disease isolate of *Mycobacterium paratuberculosis*. Nucleic Acids Research 17: 9063–9073

Haagsma J, Mulder C, Eger A, Bruins J, Ketel J, Tytgat G 1988 *Mycobacterium* species isolated from patients with Crohn's disease. In: MacDermott R P (ed) Inflamatory bowel disease: current status and future approaches. Elsevier, Amsterdam, pp 535–537

Hampson S J, McFadden J J, Hermon-Taylor J 1988 Mycobacteria and Crohn's disease. Gut 29: 1017–1019

Hampson S, Parker M, Saverymuttu S, Joseph A E J, McFadden J J, Hermon-Taylor J J 1989a Quadruple antimicrobial therapy in Crohn's disease: results at 9 months of a pilot study in 20 patients. Alimentary Pharmacology and Therapeutics 3: 343–352

Hampson S J Portaels F, Thompson J et al, 1989b DNA probes demonstrate a single highly conserved strain of *Mycobacterium avium* infecting AIDS patients. Lancet i: 65–68

Hermans P W M, Van Soolingen D, Dale J W et al 1990 Insertion element IS986 from *Mycobacterium tuberculosis*: a useful tool for diagnosis and epidemiology of tuberculosis. Journal of Clinical Microbiology 28: 2051–2058

Horsburgh C R, Havlik J A, Ellis D A et al 1991 Survival of patients with acquired immune deficiency syndrome and disseminated *Mycobacterium avium* complex infection with and without antimycobacterial chemotherapy. American Review of Respiratory Disease 144: 557–559

Kobayashi K, Blaser M J, Brown W R 1989 Immunohistochemical examination for mycobacteria in intestinal tissues from patients with Crohn's disease. Gastroenterology 96: 1009–1015

Koltun W A, Bloomer M M, Kauffman G L et al 1993 Mycobacteria other than paratuberculosis may play a role in Crohn's disease. Gastroenterology 104: A726

Kunze Z M, Portaels F, McFadden J J 1992 Biologically distinct subtypes of *Mycobacterium avium* differ in possession of insertion sequence IS901. Journal of Clinical Microbiology (30(9): 2366–2372

Kunze Z M, Wall S, Appelberg R, Silva M T, Portaels F, McFadden J J 1991 IS901, a new member of a widespread class of atypical insertion sequences, is associated with pathogenicity in *Mycobacterium avium*. Molecular Microbiology 5: 2265–2272

McClure H M, Chiodini R J, Anderson D C, Swenson B, Thayer W R, Coutu J A 1987 *Mycobacterium paratuberculosis* infection in a colony of stumptail macaques *Macaca artoides*. Journal of Infectious Diseases 155: 1011–1018

McFadden J J, Seechurn P 1992 Mycobacteria and Crohn's disease. Molecular approaches. In: Macdermott R, Stenson W (eds) Inflammatory bowel disease. Elsevier, New York, pp 259–271

McFadden J J, Kunze Z, Seechurn P 1990 DNA probes for detection and identification. In: McFadden J J (ed) Molecular biology of the mycobacteria. Surrey University Press, Guildford, pp. 139–172

McFadden J J, Butcher P D, Chiodini R J, Hermon-Taylor J J 1987a Crohn's disease-isolated mycobacteria are identical to *Mycobacterium paratuberculosis*, as determined by DNA probes that distinguish between mycobacterial species. Journal of Clinical Microbiology 25: 796–801

McFadden J J, Butcher P D, Thompson J, Chiodini R J, Hermon-Taylor J 1987b The use of DNA probes identifying restriction-fragment-length polymorphisms to examine the *Mycobacterium avium* complex. Molecular Microbiology 1: 283–291

McFadden J, Collins J, Beaman B, Arthur M, Gitnick G 1993 Mycobacteria in Crohn's disease: DNA probes identify the wood-pigeon strain of *Mycobacterium avium*. Journal of Clinical Microbiology 30: 3070–3073

McFadden J J, Kunze Z M, Portaels F, Labrousse V, Rastogi N 1992 Epidemiological and genetic markers, virulence factors and intracellular growth of *Mycobacterium avium* in AIDS. Research Microbiology 143: 423–436

Marsheck W J, Kraychy S, Muir R D 1972 Microbial degradation of sterols. Applied Microbiology 23: 72–77

Moss M T, Sanderson J D, Tizard M L V et al 1992 Polymerase chain reaction detection of *Mycobacterium paratuberculosis* and *Mycobacterium avium* subsp. *silvaticum* in long term cultures from Crohn's disease and control tissues. Gut 33: 1209–1213

Noordhoek G T, Kolk A H, Bjune G et al 1994 Sensitivity and specificity of PCR for detection of *Mycobacterium tuberculosis*: a blind comparison study among seven laboratories. Journal of Clinical Microbiology 32: 277–284

Portaels F, Larsson L, Smeets P 1988 Isolation of mycobacteria from healthy persons' stools. International Journal of Leprosy 56: 469–471

Quirke P, Dockey D, Taylor G R, Lewis, F A, Hawkey P, Graham D 1991 Detection of *Mycobacterium paratuberculosis* in Crohn's disease. Gut 32: A572

Rosenberg W M C, Bell J L, Jewel D P 1991 *Mycobacterium paratuberculosis* DNA cannot be detected in Crohn's disease. Gastroenterology 100: A611

Rowbotham D S, Mapstone N P, Trejdosiewicz L K, Howdle P D, Quirke P 1993 *Mycobacterium paratuberculosis* DNA is not detected by the polymerase chain reaction in Crohn's disease. Gut A228.

Sanderson, J D, Moss, M T, Tizard M L V, Hermon-Taylor J 1992 *Mycobacterium paratuberculosis* in Crohn's disease tissue. Gut 33: 890–896

Sauki R K, Scharf S, Faloona F et al 1985 Enzymic amplification of the β-globin genomic sequences and restriction site analysis for diagnosis of sickle cell anemia. Science 230: 1350–1354

Swift G L, Srivastava E D, Stone R et al 1994 Controlled trail of anti-tuberculous chemotherapy for two years in Crohn's disease. Gut 35: 363–368

Vary P H, Andersen P R, Green E, Hermon-Taylor J, McFadden J J 1990 Use of highly specific DNA probes and the polymerase chain reaction to detect *Mycobacterium paratuberculosis* in Johne's disease. Journal of Clinical Microbiology 28: 933–937

Wall S, Kunze Z M, Saboor, S et al 1993 Identification of spheroplast-like agents isolated from tissues of patients with Crohn's disease and control tissues by polymerase chain reaction. Journal of Clinical Microbiology 31: 1241–1245

Wu S W P, Pao C C, Chan J 1991 Lack of mycobacterial DNA in Crohn's disease tissue. Lancet 337: 174–175

Young L S, Wiviot L, Wu M, Kolonoski P, Bolan R, Inderlied C B 1991 Azithromycin for treatment of *Mycobacterium avium–intracellulare* complex infection in patients with AIDS. Lancet 338: 1107–1109

17. Infective agents – vascular factors

N. P. Thompson   A. J. Wakefield

INTRODUCTION

Using standard histological techniques, vascular abnormalities have been noted, particularly in specimens of Crohn's disease, for many years, although these have been thought to be of secondary importance. More recently, with perfusion–fixation, the microvasculature has been examined more precisely and additional immunohistochemical studies have given insights into significant endothelial changes and vascular abnormalities in both active and quiescent disease states.

HISTOLOGICAL VASCULAR CHANGES

Knutson and Lunderquist, in 1968, described characteristic vascular abnormalities in Crohn's disease: arterial and venous mural thickening was usual, with inflammatory lesions of 'endovasculitis' and 'perivasculitis' seen less often. Cases of ulcerative colitis revealed hyperemia only, with no evidence of vasculitis. In Crohn's disease the presence of arterial mural thickening, predominantly due to medial hypertrophy, has been confirmed in Japanese (Funayama et al 1987), German (Furst et al 1992) and French (Roussel 1993) series: histological evidence of vasculitis with damage to the endothelium was supported by ultrastructural studies (Dvorak et al 1980).

In 1989 a series of studies was undertaken by the authors' group to investigate in detail the microvasculature in inflammatory bowel disease, based upon the hypothesis that Crohn's disease is primarily a granulomatous vasculopathy. Initially, perfusion–fixation at mean arterial pressure with glutaraldehyde was used, with subsequent histological and ultrastructural analysis. This revealed intraluminal fibrin and inflammatory cells in direct contact with arterial, as well as venous, endothelium (Fig. 17.1a, b). These inflammatory cells appeared not only to produce intravascular aggregates, but also to migrate through to the subendothelial space, with associated destruction of the vessel wall architecture.

The relationship of granulomas – one of the characteristic lesions of Crohn's disease – to blood vessels was examined further using perfusion–fixation of resected specimens with formalin. The relationship of blood vessels, stained with collagen type-IV antibodies, and macrophages (KPI) was studied: of 485 granulomas from 15 specimens, 85% were identified as arising in association with blood vessels (Wakefield et al 1991; Fig. 17.2). Undoubtedly a number of granulomas also involve lymphatics, although perfusion–fixation and vascular immunostaining helped to resolve the vessel origin of the majority of these lesions.

It has been assumed by most authors (Knutson & Lunderquist 1968, Roussel 1993) that the vascular abnormalities seen in Crohn's disease are secondary, non-specific lesions. To detect whether vascular changes occurred at an early stage non-inflamed, apparently normal mucosa was examined (Sankey et al 1993). Specimens from 35 patients with Crohn's disease were examined using immunostaining to identify small mucosal capillaries. Mucosal capillary damage and rupture was seen in those with Crohn's disease but not in inflammatory or normal controls, suggesting that vascular damage was an early and potentially important event (Fig. 17.3).

Histological vascular changes in ulcerative colitis have attracted less attention than those in Crohn's disease, as they are less dramatic. Knutson and Lunderquist (1968) noted only hyperemia, which was related to the degree of inflammation. Subsequent immunohistochemical studies reported mucosal microvascular thrombi in colonic resections (Shubnich et al 1976), and more recently in rectal biopsies, using monoclonal antibody against Factor XIIIA, to identify thrombi in eight and of 13 cases (Dhillon et al 1992; Fig. 17.4).

IMMUNOHISTOCHEMICAL STUDIES

Although morphological, resin-casting and angiographic studies of the vasculature (see below) have provided an impression of the frequency and significance of vascular changes, immunohistochemistry has been increasingly used to investigate the microvasculature in inflammatory bowel disease. This has provided information on the function of

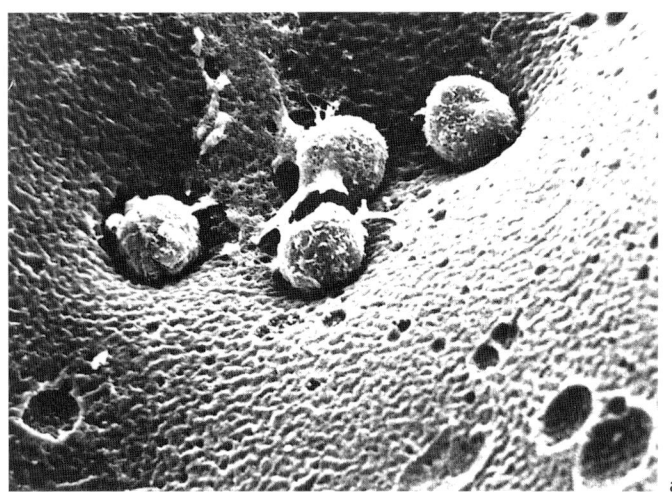

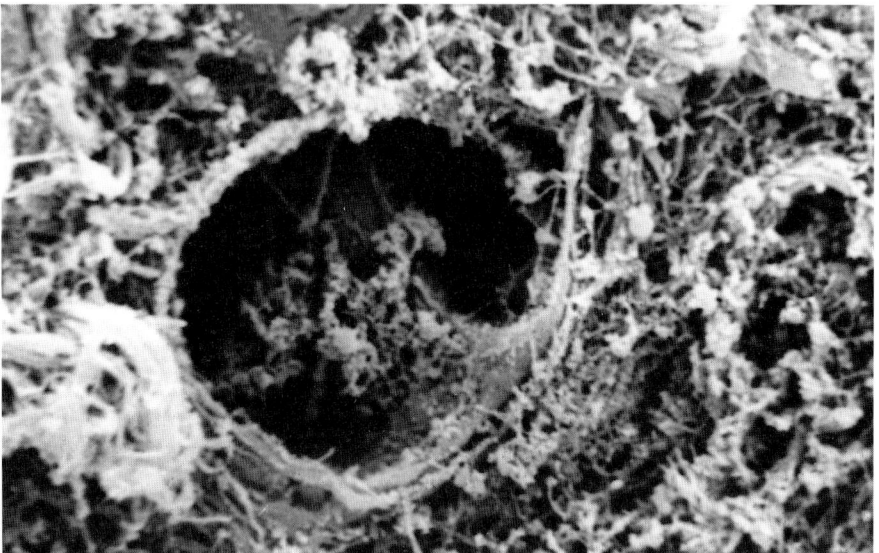

Fig. 17.1a Freeze–fracture scanning electron micrograph of arterial resin cast in terminal ileal Crohn's disease. Craters on the resin cast are produced by inflammatory cells adherent to the arterial endothelium in macroscopically normal, non-ulcerated Crohn's disease. Magnification × 1950. **b** Freeze–fracture scanning electron micrograph of a perfusion-fixed vessel in the lamina propria of Crohn's disease, showing intravascular thrombus formation occluding the vessel lumen. Magnification × 1250

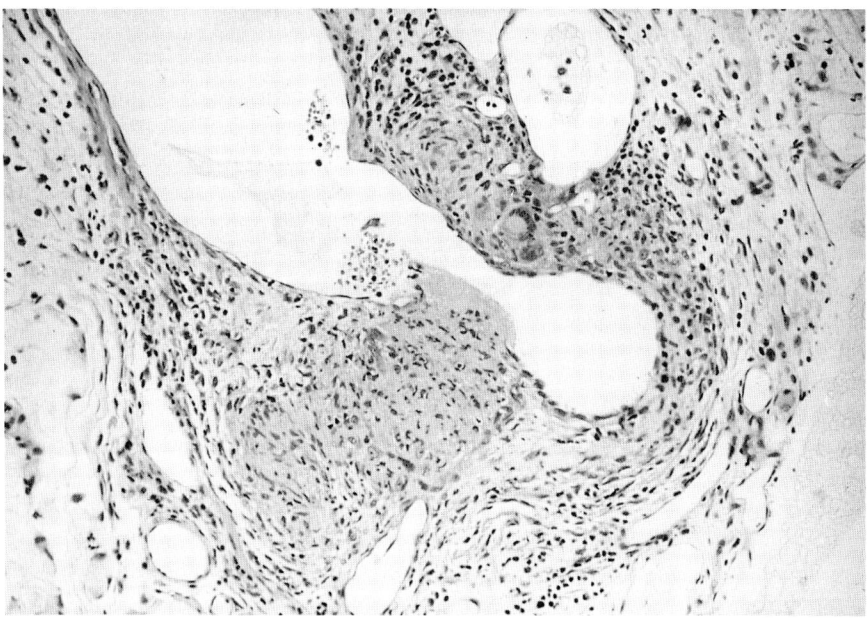

Fig. 17.2 Photomicrograph of arterial perfusion-fixed specimen of Crohn's disease. There is granulomatous destruction of the vessel wall which is focal and associated with rupture of the intima and thrombus deposition. The thrombus has propagated in the direction of blood flow, confirming the arterial origin of this lesion. Magnification × 284

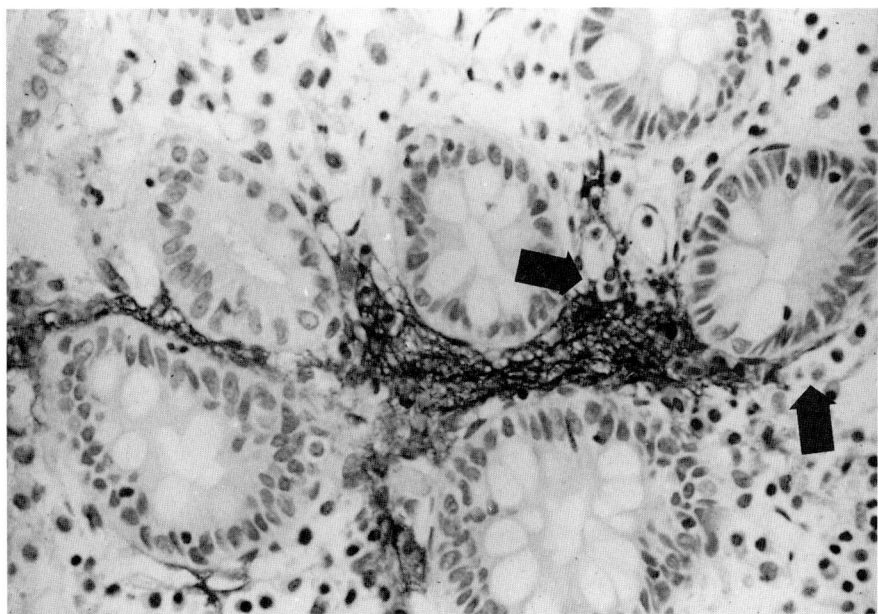

Fig. 17.3 Photomicrograph showing fibrillary trail of fibrin immunostained with polyclonal antibody against fibrinogen. The fibrin emanates from two vessels (arrowed), identified in serial section by vascular immunostaining for collagen type IV (not shown). These features precede evidence of mucosal inflammation. Original magnification × 426

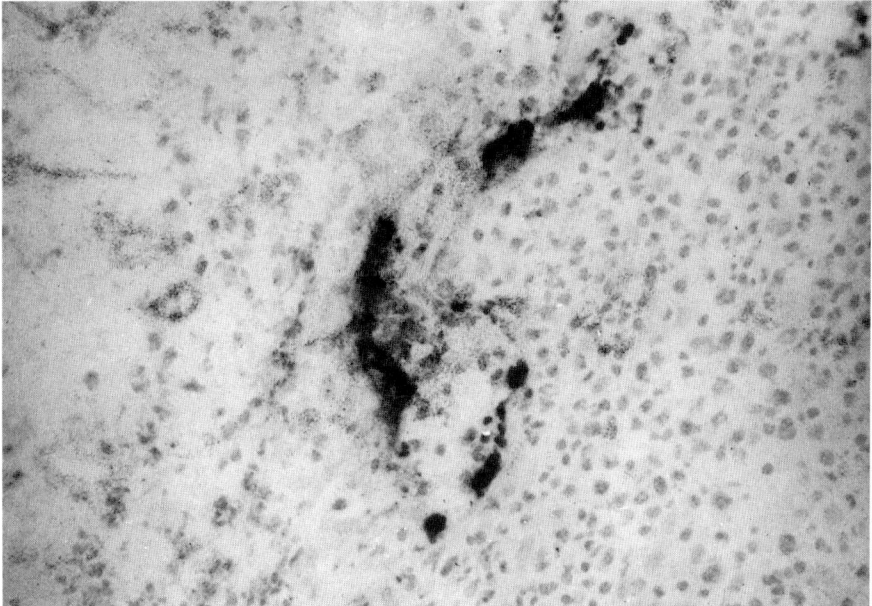

Fig. 17.4 Photomicrograph of the mucosa in ulcerative colitis immunostained with platelet glycoprotein IIIa, showing a microthrombus formation. Magnification × 426

endothelial cells and their possible role in the pathophysiological processes taking place.

There is evidence that endothelial cells actively participate in the inflammatory process: in patients with ulcerative colitis mesenteric endothelial cells have been shown to express interleukin-1 (IL-1) (Matsumoto et al 1989). Endothelial cells in both Crohn's disease (Momburg et al 1988) and ulcerative colitis (Matsumoto et al 1989) have been shown to express HLA class II antigens, suggesting that they might be actively involved in antigen presentation; similar changes were not seen in healthy controls.

There has recently been considerable interest in the expression of adhesion molecules by the vascular endothelium in those with inflammatory bowel disease compared with healthy controls. The differential expression of these

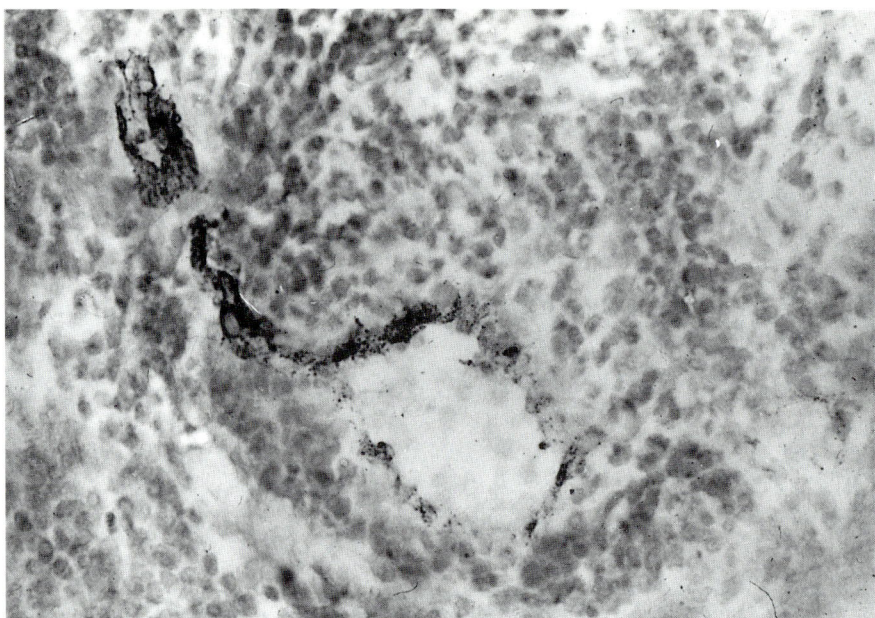

Fig. 17.5 Focus of granulomatous vasculitis in Crohn's disease immunostained for E-selectin, showing expression along the endothelial cell surface. Magnification × 461

molecules between those with active and quiescent disease has also been studied. Selectins are thought to be involved in the initial phases of cell adhesion to capture leukocytes, and expression of both E-selectin and P-selectin is increased in active disease (Koizumi et al 1992, Ohtani et al 1992, Nakamura et al 1993; Fig. 17.5) Interestingly, E-selectin expression, which was raised in active ulcerative colitis, did not return to control levels even during remission of the disease (Cellier et al 1994).

The immunoglobulin superfamily adhesins, such as ICAM-1, VCAM-1 and PECAM, are involved in producing firm adhesion and migration of leukocytes. ICAM-1, but not VCAM-1, expression has been shown to be increased in active inflammatory bowel disease (Nakamura et al 1993). Less is known about the expression of endothelial adhesion molecules in inactive disease. One study suggested that the patterns of expression differ among healthy controls, those with Crohn's disease and those with ulcerative colitis (Schuerman et al 1993). Specifically, there was increased expression of PECAM in inactive ulcerative colitis and decreased expression of ICAM-1 in Crohn's disease, compared with controls.

Endothelial cells not only interact with other cell types involved in the inflammatory process but also are influenced by cytokines produced by them. Macrophages positively staining for tumor necrosis factor-α (TNF-α) cluster around arterioles and venules in Crohn's disease but not ulcerative colitis, potentially impairing endothelial integrity and increasing inflammatory cell recruitment (Murch et al 1993a). Local TNF-α synthesis may then contribute to prothrombotic events at the endothelial cell surface. Expression of tissue factor, a potent procoagulant, was observed in foci of vasculitis in non-ulcerated Crohn's disease, but not in uninflamed vessels either in Crohn's disease or in moderate ulcerative colitis (More et al 1993; Fig. 17.6). In severe ulcerative colitis, as well as in Crohn's disease, tissue factor expression by both macrophages and endothelial cells was associated with thrombus formation, particularly at the base of ulcers. This finding contrasts with the increased mucosal levels of tissue-type plasminogen activator (t-PA) found in those with ulcerative colitis compared with controls (Kurose et al 1992). The control of hemostasis depends on multiple factors, and it is the local balance of these factors that determines microvascular thrombus formation.

OTHER EFFECTOR MECHANISMS IN VASCULAR EVENTS

Endothelin-1 (ET-1) is a potent vasoconstrictor and both its expression and tissue concentration in Crohn's disease and ulcerative colitis are increased over healthy controls (Murch et al 1992). Although the cellular origins of ET-1 have not been clearly defined, local synthesis may represent an effector mechanism that contributes to tissue ischemia. That ET-1 is acting on the microvasculature was further suggested by the recent observation that ET-1 receptors were increased in mucosal and submucosal vessels in active inflammatory bowel disease (Hudson et al 1994; Fig. 17.7).

It has been suggested that in patients with active ulcerative colitis endothelial cells and infiltrating mononuclear cells produce increased amounts of nitric oxide compared with controls (Oshitani et al 1993). The

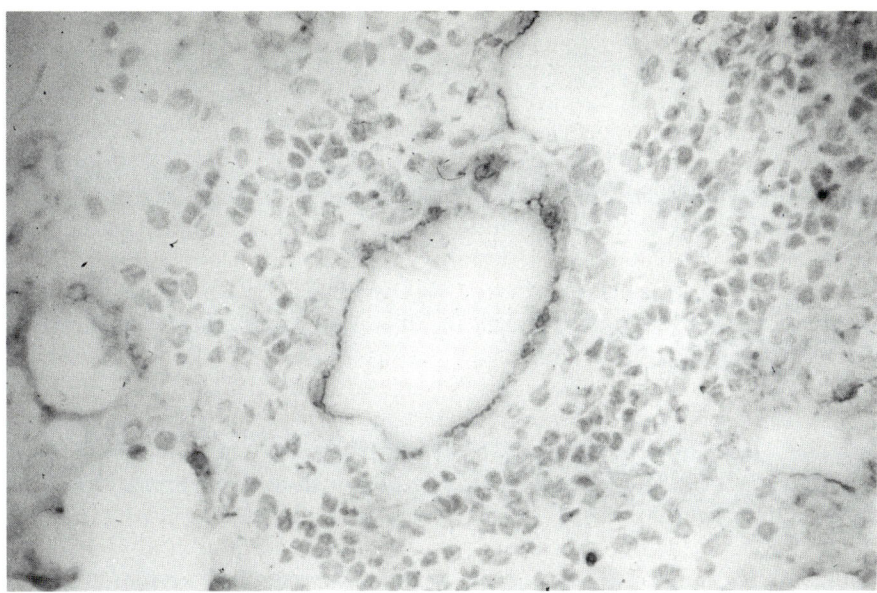

Fig. 17.6 Focus of vasculitis in Crohn's disease immunostained for tissue factor, showing endothelial expression which is not seen in normal vessels. Magnification × 426

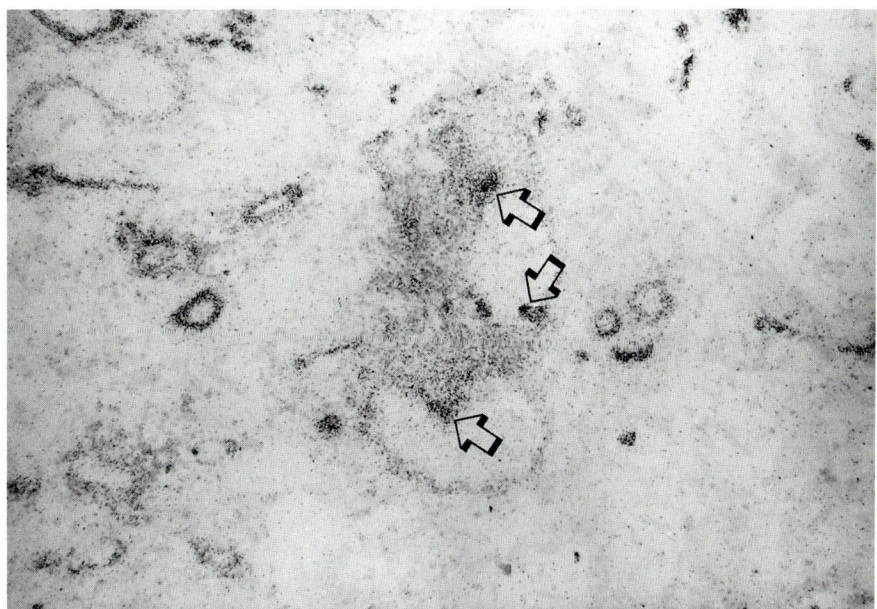

Fig. 17.7 Autoradiograph of endothelin receptor expression in Crohn's disease. Constitutive endothelin receptor expression is seen on submucosal arteries: a vein in the centre of the picture also shows increased expression of endothelin receptors, specifically in foci of inflammation (arrowed). Magnification × 177

vasodilator action of this agent may be related to the hyperemia that has been noted in both histological studies (Knutson & Lunderquist 1968) and angiographic studies (see below). Again, the balance between vasoconstriction and vasodilatation presumably depends on the local balance of multiple agents, some of which (for example ET-1 and nitric oxide) may exert antagonistic effects.

Sulphated glycosaminoglycans (GACs) are negatively charged polysaccharides which both regulate the ability of albumin to leave the vasculature and inhibit thrombosis. The distribution of these molecules in inflammatory bowel disease has been studied using gold-labeled probes. In inflammatory bowel disease there is extensive loss of GAGs from the vascular endothelium, which is particularly marked in the submucosa in Crohn's disease (Murch et al 1993b).

SEROLOGICAL AND HEMATOLOGICAL EVIDENCE OF VASCULAR DAMAGE

Humoral changes in inflammatory bowel disease are described in full in Chapter 8, and changes in platelets and coagulation in Chapter 13. With specific reference to vascular injury, antiendothelial antibodies have been studied in patients with inflammatory bowel disease and healthy controls (Stevens et al 1993). Titers were noted to be raised in both those with Crohn's disease and those with ulcerative colitis; in the latter, levels were related to disease activity. In-vitro studies, however, suggested that the antibodies were not directly cytotoxic to endothelial cells.

There is evidence of vascular complement activation in active inflammatory bowel disease (Halstensen & Brandtzaeg 1991, Halstensen et al 1989a, Halstensen et al 1989b). As well as contributing to thrombus formation, local complement activation may be one of the mechanisms involved in direct endothelial cell damage (Sankey et al 1993, Murch et al 1993b).

Circulating von Willebrand's factor is a marker of vascular damage and concentrations have been found to be raised in patients with both active and quiescent inflammatory bowel disease. The observation that concentrations are raised in inactive disease might suggest that ongoing vascular injury is a fundamental abnormality in these diseases (Stevens et al 1992). However, the same study also found elevated concentrations of von Willebrand's factor in those with acute bacterial diarrhea, suggesting that elevated concentrations might be a result of nonspecific intestinal inflammation.

ANIMAL MODELS

The vascular changes that occur in boxer dogs with canine histiocytic ulcerative colitis have been studied and are similar to those found in patients with ulcerative colitis (Lawson et al 1975). Diseased segments showed vascular dilatation and hypervascularity; more severely diseased areas showed arteriolar attenuation. Ulcerated areas demonstrated complete disruption of the microvasculature.

In order to determine whether the phenotypic idiosyncrasies of Crohn's disease, including 'skip' lesions and transmural inflammation, could be explained by a submucosal vascular insult, an animal (ferret) model was developed (Hudson et al 1992). Styrene microspheres of varying sizes injected into the ferret midgut microvasculature produced acute focal and transmural inflammation and mucosal ulceration. Mucosal integrity to this single insult was restored within 72 hours. A similar model, using hamsters and degradable starch microspheres, also produced inflammation, with complete healing within 2 weeks (Boyd et al 1994).

The well known clinical entity of anastomotic recurrence of Crohn's disease was also investigated using the ferret model (Osbourne et al 1993). Styrene microspheres were

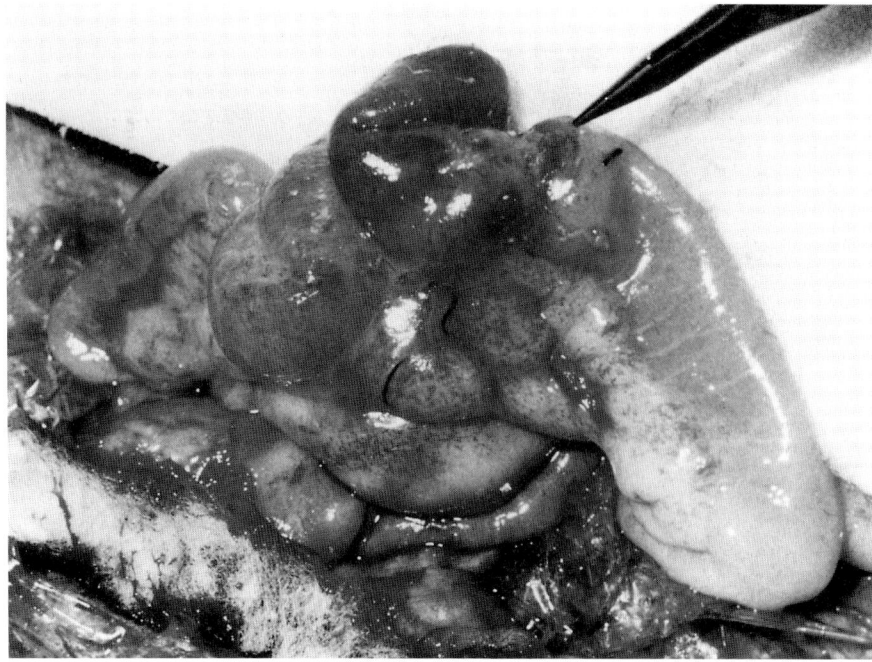

Fig. 17.8 Chronic inflammation at the anastomosis in a ferret model of submucosal microvascular occlusion. Forceps indicate the site of anastomosis; to the right the bowel is uninflamed, to the left it is grossly inflamed. The bowel to the left had been injected 2 weeks prior to anastomosis with microspheres, followed 72 hours later by division of the intestine and anastomosis to a normal, non-embolized loop.

injected intra-arterially into isolated intestinal loops, and after 72 hours interloop anastomoses were formed. Two weeks later chronic transmural inflammation, ulceration and granulomas were found in those loops injected with microspheres, but not in control loops (Fig. 17.8). The combination of two ischemic insults resulted in chronic inflammation and pathological appearances which were similar to Crohn's disease. This work has received support from recent clinical observations in Crohn's disease using Doppler flowmetry – see below (Angerson et al 1993).

ANGIOGRAPHIC AND RESIN-CASTING STUDIES

There have been several angiographic studies of the mesenteric vasculature in inflammatory bowel disease; reported abnormalities have been largely ascribed to changes of generalized inflammation. Kalima et al (1975) noted increased numbers of small, narrow vasa recta vessels in inflamed sections of Crohn's bowel on angiography. Vascular abnormalities have been misinterpreted as vascular malformations or neoplastic lesions (DeNardi et al 1989). A further angiographic study confirmed the destruction of the primary mesenteric vasculature, with replacement by bizarre ectatic neovasculature (Schafer et al 1992). In ulcerative colitis changes observed in a series of 25 patients were more prominent in the microvasculature, with findings of either capillary blush or loss of normal tapering of the vasa recta (Tsuchiya et al 1980).

Resin-casting studies revealed very similar patterns to angiographic studies, with stenosis or destruction of the vasa recta in affected Crohn's bowel (Wakefield et al 1989; Fig. 17.9). These changes were also seen in macroscopically normal bowel, suggesting that vascular changes may be early and pathogenetically important. Abnormalities of the intestinal vasculature, detected by resin-casting studies, in bowel which was unapparently affected by Crohn's disease, have been interpreted as revealing coexistent angiodysplasia (Arenas et al 1990).

Estimates of vascular volume in resected specimens using barium concentrations suggest that this is reduced in segmental Crohn's disease but not in ulcerative colitis (Carr et al 1986). Radioisotope washout studies have also suggested that blood flow is decreased in Crohn's disease-affected bowel but increased in active colitis; inactive colitis has normal flow (Hulten et al 1977). It is notable that in active colitis a rapid venous phase suggested shunting of blood across a potentially ischemic mucosa. These findings are consistent both with the earlier finding of decreased rectal vascular resistance compared with controls, in those with ulcerative colitis, particularly those with active disease (Binder 1968), and with the hyperemia noted histologically (Knutson & Lunderquist 1968). Significantly decreased blood flow at the site of anastomotic recurrence of Crohn's disease was also detected using Doppler flowmetry (Angerson et al 1993).

INTERVENTION TRIALS

There has been a single, open-labeled trial of intravenous heparin in acute ulcerative colitis (Gaffney et al 1993). This was conducted after the observation of dramatic clinical improvement in two patients treated with heparin after developing deep-vein thromboses during relapse of their colitis. An improvement was seen in all 10 patients studied. This interesting observation requires proper evaluation in a randomized controlled trial.

EXTRAINTESTINAL ASSOCIATIONS OF INFLAMMATORY BOWEL DISEASE

The extraintestinal associations of inflammatory bowel disease are discussed in detail elsewhere (Chapter 69). However, there are numerous case reports which suggest that these associated conditions frequently have a vasculitis basis, particularly those associated with Crohn's disease. Pyoderma gangrenosa is one of the more common dermatological associations of inflammatory bowel disease, and is typified histologically by a lymphocytic vasculitis (Powell et al 1985); other forms of cutaneous vasculitis have also been described in Crohn's disease (Humbert et al 1989, Shum & Guenther 1990).

Retinal vasculitis occurring with Crohn's disease has been reported (Duker et al 1987, Ruby & Jampol 1990), and central nervous system vasculitis has been reported in both Crohn's disease and ulcerative colitis (Nelson et al 1986, Adamek et al 1993). Pulmonary vasculitis has been described in association with exacerbations of ulcerative colitis (Collins et al 1979, Sargent et al 1985).

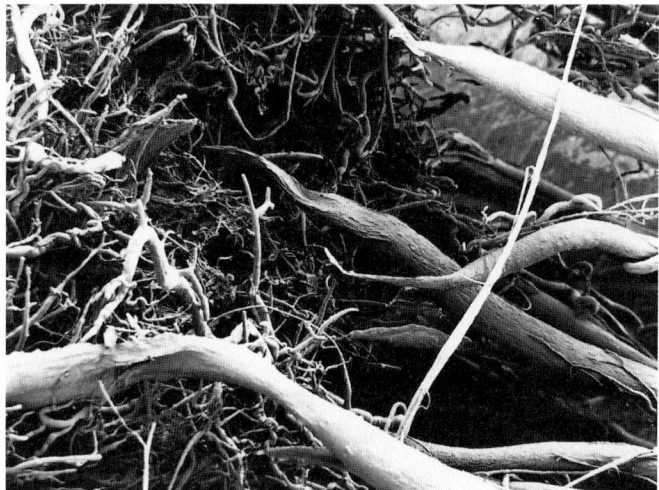

Fig. 17.9 Arterial resin-cast specimen of perfusion-fixed Crohn's disease. Vasa recta passing through the intestinal wall become stenosed and occluded within the diseased submucosa. Beyond is an intense neovascularization, presumably consequent upon the ischemic process. Magnification × 12.5

The increased risk of thromboembolic disease in association with inflammatory bowel disease is discussed fully elsewhere (Chapter 78). The clinical manifestations of this increased risk include arterial and venous occlusion, in the absence of the usual risk factors for thromboembolic disease (Schneiderman et al 1979, Talbot et al 1986, Halliday & Farthing 1988). A recent case report of a patient with recurrent venous thrombosis in association with Crohn's disease also reported an underlying vasculitis as the cause for the extraintestinal thrombosis (Motte et al 1992).

ASSOCIATIONS WITH OTHER DISEASES

There are numerous case reports describing the coexistence of Crohn's disease with other vasculitic diseases, such as Takayasu's disease (Van Elburg et al 1992), Cogan's disease (Froehlich et al 1994) and polyarteritis nodosa (Kahn et al 1980, Gudbjornsson & Hallgren 1990). These suggest a possible common pathogenesis and provide further circumstantial evidence that Crohn's disease may have a vasculitic pathogenesis. Nailbed capillaroscopic findings in a series of seven patients with Crohn's disease were similar to those found in other systemic vasculitidies (Jouanny et al 1991).

A possible protective effect against the development of inflammatory bowel disease of hemophilia and von Willebrand's disease was suggested by the apparent paucity of cases among the UK population of those with inherited coagulopathies (Thompson et al 1994). This provided epidemiological evidence that intravascular thrombotic events might be important in the development of both ulcerative colitis and Crohn's disease.

POSSIBLE ETIOLOGICAL AGENTS

Infectious agents which have a possible role in the etiology of inflammatory bowel disease are discussed elsewhere, but there has been relatively little research into how these agents might cause the vascular and hemostatic

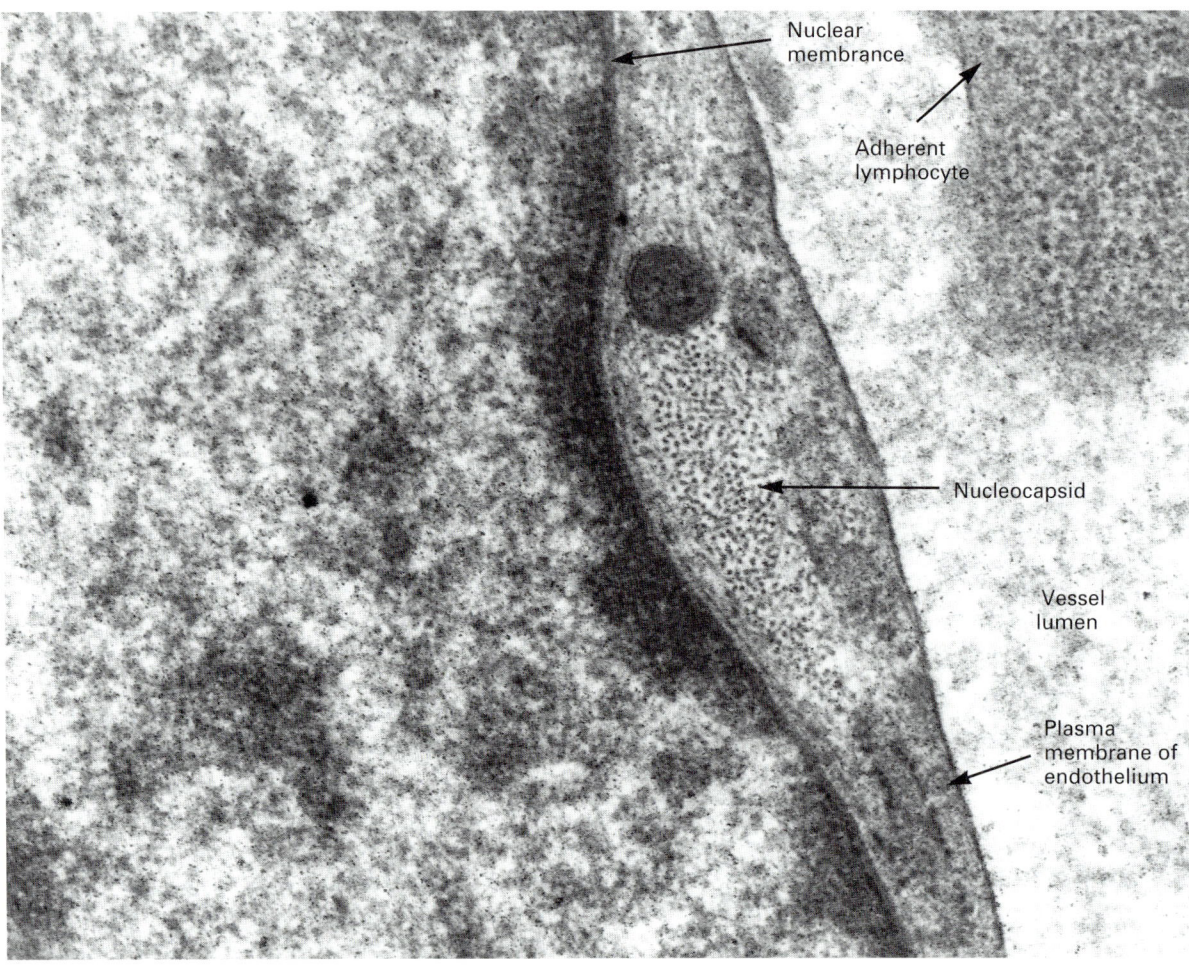

Fig. 17.10 An endothelial cell in Crohn's disease showing 17 nm intracytoplasmic fibrillary arrays consistent with paramyxovirus nucleocapsids. There is a lymphocyte adherent to the endothelium in this focus of vasculitis in a perfusion-fixed specimen of Crohn's disease. Magnification × 52 080

changes described earlier in this chapter. Mycobacteria have long been postulated as being involved in the etiology of Crohn's disease, and it is interesting that granulomatous vasculitis has been described as occurring in ileocecal tuberculosis (Mapstone & Dixon 1992).

Measles virus persistence in Crohn's disease has been described using techniques of transmission electron microscopy, immunohistochemistry and RNA in-situ hybridization. In all those with Crohn's disease measles localized to foci of granulomatous vasculitis (ultrastructurally to both endothelial cells and macrophages), whereas measles virus was only identified in a minority of controls or those with ulcerative colitis (Wakefield et al 1993; Fig. 17.10). Vasculitis associated with endothelial cell infection is an important component of measles virus pathology, and may be relevant to Crohn's disease (Jirapinyo et al 1990, Norrby & Oxman 1990). Other viruses, such as cytomegalovirus, have been shown to be capable of producing a vasculitis affecting the gastrointestinal tract (Roberts et al 1989), though whether or not this is of significance to the development of inflammatory bowel disease is unknown.

SUMMARY

There is histological and ultrastructural evidence of frequent vasculitis and endothelial damage in Crohn's disease. Angiographic, resin-casting and blood-flow studies all suggest that mucosal ischemia occurs, particularly in Crohn's disease, and animal models suggest that ischemia can result in multifocal inflammation and ulceration. That extraintestinal manifestations of both Crohn's disease and ulcerative colitis frequently have a vasculitic basis is further supportive evidence of an important role for vascular injury in these conditions. In ulcerative colitis mucosal microthrombi appear to be an early feature of the disease. Endothelial cells appear to have important roles as both affector and effector cells in the pathogenesis of these diseases. The further elucidation of the role of endothelial injury in both conditions is likely to be a fruitful line of research.

REFERENCES

Adamek R J, Wegener M, Wedmann B, Buttner T, Ricken D 1993 Cerebral vasculitis in Crohn's disease. Leber, Magen, Darm 23: 91–93

Angerson W J, Allison M C, Baxter J N, Russell R I 1993 Neoterminal ileal blood flow after ileocolonic resection for Crohn's disease. Gut 34: 1513–1514

Arenas R J, Cremades M A, Almenar del Poyo L et al 1990 Angiodysplasia of the colon and Crohn's disease. A study with vascular resin casts. Revista Espanola de Enfermedades Digestivas 78: 171–174

Binder V 1968 Rectal vascular resistance in ulcerative colitis. Scandinavian Journal of Gastroenterology 3: 36–42

Boyd A J, Sherman I A, Huang S N, Saibi F G 1994 Differences in intestinal inflammation induced by mesenteric intravascular administration of hapten or degradable starch microspheres. Gastroenterology 106: A1019

Carr N D, Pullan B R, Schofield P F 1986 Microvascular studies in non-specific inflammatory bowel disease. Gut 27: 542–549

Cellier C, Fromont-Hankard G, Leborgne M, Chaussade S, Land B 1994 Variations of in situ expression of vascular adhesion molecules in ulcerative colitis. Gastroenterology 106: A662

Collins W J, Bendig D W, Taylor W F 1979 Pulmonary vasculitis complicating childhood ulcerative colitis. Gastroenterology 77: 1091–1093

DeNardi F, Burns K, Peterson R A, Barron P T, Patel D G, Chambers R J 1989 Crohn's disease angiographically mimicking vascular malformation or neoplasm. Canadian Association of Radiologists Journal 40: 279–282

Dhillon A P, Anthony A, Sim R et al 1992 Mucosal capillary thrombi in rectal biopsies. Histopathology 21: 127–133

Duker J S, Brown G C, Brooks L 1987 Retinal vasculitis in Crohn's disease. American Journal of Ophthalmology 103: 664–668

Dvorak A M, Monahan R A, Osage J E, Dickersin G R 1980 Crohn's disease: transmission electron microscopic studies. II. Immunologic inflammatory response. Alterations of mast cells, basophils, eosinophils, and the microvasculature. Human Pathology 11: 606–619

Froehlich F, Fried M, Gonvers J J, Saraga E, Thorens J, Pecoud A 1994 Association of Crohn's disease and Cogan's syndrome. Digestive Diseases and Sciences 39: 1134–1137

Funayama Y, Sasaki I, Imamura M, Naito H, Sato T 1987 The analysis of intestinal microcirculation by histometrical studies of arterial media in Crohn's disease. Journal of the Japanese Surgical Society 88: 1695–704

Furst H, Storck M, Jauch K W, Scheurlen C, Kaltenecker A, Wiebecke B 1992 Crohn's disease in advanced age. Chirurgie 63: 26–30

Gaffney P R, Doyle C T, Hogan J, Gaffney A 1993 Paradoxical response to heparin in 10 patients with ulcerative colitis. Gastroenterology 104: A703

Gudbjornsson B, Hallgren R 1990 Cutaneous polyarteritis nodosa associated with Crohn's disease. Report and review of the literature. Journal of Rheumatology 17: 386–390

Halliday C E, Farthing M J 1988 Arterial thrombosis in Crohn's disease. Medical Journal of Australia 149: 559–560

Halstensen T S, Brandtzaeg P 1991 Local complement activation in inflammatory bowel disease. Immunologic Research 10: 485–492

Halstensen T S, Mollnes T E, Brandtzaeg P 1989a Persistent complement activation in submucosal blood vessels of active inflammatory bowel disease: immunohistochemical evidence. Gastroenterology 97: 10–19

Halstensen T S, Mollnes T E, Fausa O, Brandtzaeg P 1989b Deposits of terminal complement complex (TCC) in muscularis mucosae and submucosal vessels in ulcerative colitis and Crohn's disease of the colon. Gut 30: 361–366

Hudson M, Dashwood M R, Pounder R E, Wakefield A J 1994 ^{125}I endothelin-1 binding in normal human intestine and inflammatory bowel disease. Gastroenterology 106: A239

Hudson M, Piasecki C, Sankey E A et al 1992 A ferret model of acute multifocal gastrointestinal infarction. Gastroenterology 102: 1591–1596

Hulten L, Lindhagen J, Lundgren O, Fasth S, Ahren C 1977 Regional intestinal blood flow in ulcerative colitis and Crohn's disease. Gastroenterology 72: 388–396

Humbert P, Monnier G, Billerey C, Birgen C, Dupond J L 1989 Polyneuropathy: an unusual extraintestinal manifestation of Crohn's disease. Acta Neurologica Scandinavica 80: 301–306

Jirapinyo P, Thakerngpol K, Chaichanwatanakul K 1990 Cytopathologic effects of measles virus on the human intestinal mucosa. Journal of Paediatric Gastroenterology 10: 550–554

Jouanny P, Schmidt C, Wahl D, De Korwin J D, Schmitt J 1991 Nailbed capillaroscopy in Crohn's disease. Revue de Médecine Interne 12: 377–379

Kahn E I, Daum F, Aiges H W, Silverberg M 1980 Cutaneous polyarteritis nodosa associated with Crohn's disease. Diseases of the Colon and Rectum 23: 258–262

Kalima T V, Peltokallio P, Myllarniemi H 1975 Vascular patter in ileal Crohn's disease. Annals of Clinical Research 7: 23–31

Knutson H, Lunderquist A 1968 Vascular changes in Crohn's disease. American Journal of Roentgenology, Radium Therapy and Nuclear Medicine 103: 380–385

Koizumi M, King N, Lobb R, Benjamin C, Podolsky D K 1992 Expression of vascular adhesion molecules in inflammatory bowel disease. Gastroenterology 103: 840–847

Kurose I, Miura S, Suematsu M et al 1992 Tissue-type plasminogen activator of colonic mucosa in ulcerative colitis. Evidence of endothelium-derived fibrinolytic activation. Digestive Diseases and Sciences 37: 307–311

Lawson T L, Gomez J A, Margulis A R 1975 Vascula alterations in canine histiocytic ulcerative colitis. Investigative Radiology 10: 212–242

Mapstone N P, Dixon M F 1992 Vasculitis in ileocaecal tuberculosis: similarities to Crohn's disease. Histopathology 21: 477–479

Matsumoto T, Kitano A, Nakamura S et al 1989 Possible role of vascular endothelial cells in immune responses in colonic mucosa examined immunocytochemically in subjects with and without ulcerative colitis. Clinical and Experimental Immunology 78: 424–430

Momburg F, Koretz K, Von Herbay A, Moller P 1988 Nonimmune human cells can express MHC class II antigens in the absence of invariant chain – an immunohistological study on normal and chronically inflamed small intestine. Clinical and Experimental Immunology 72: 367–372

More L, Sim R, Hudson M, Dhillon A P, Pounder R, Wakefield A J 1993 Immunohistochemical study of tissue factor expression in normal intestine and idiopathic inflammatory bowel disease. Journal of Clinical Pathology 46: 703–708

Motte S, Flamme F, Depierreux M, Wautrecht J C, Van Gossum A, Dereume J P 1992 Venous thromboangiitis associated with regional enteritis. International Angiology 11: 237–240

Murch S H, Braegger C P, Sessa W C, MacDonald T T 1992 High endothelin-1 immunoreactivity in Crohn's disease and ulcerative colitis. Lancet 339: 381–385

Murch S H, Braegger C P, Walker-Smith J A, MacDonald T T 1993a Location of tumour necrosis factor alpha by immunohistochemistry in chronic inflammatory bowel disease. Gut 34: 1705–1709

Murch S H, MacDonald T T, Walker-Smith J A, Levin M, Lionetti P, Klein N J 1993b Disruption of sulphated glycosaminoglycans in intestinal inflammation. Lancet 341: 711–714

Nakamura S, Ohtani H, Watanabe Y et al 1993 In situ expression of the cell adhesion molecules in inflammatory bowel disease. Evidence of immunologic activation of vascular endothelial cells. Laboratory Investigation 69: 77–85

Nelson J, Barron M M, Riggs J E, Gutmann L, Schochet S S Jr 1986 Cerebral vasculitis and ulcerative colitis. Neurology 36: 719–721

Norrby E, Oxman N 1990 Measles virus. In: Fields B N, Kripe D (eds) Virology, 2nd edn. Raven Press, New York, pp 1013–1044

Ohtani H, Nakamura S, Watanabe Y et al 1992 Light and electron microscopic immunolocalization of endothelial leucocyte adhesion molecule-1 in inflammatory bowel disease. Morphological evidence of active synthesis and secretion into vascular lumen. Virchows Archiv A, Pathological Anatomy and Histopathology 420: 403–409

Osbourne M J, Hudson M, Piasecki C et al 1993 Crohn's disease and anastomotic recurrence: microvascular ischaemia and anastomotic healing in an animal model. British Journal of Surgery 80: 226–229

Oshitani N, Kitano A, Okabe H, Nakamura S, Matsumoto T, Kobayashi K 1993 Location of superoxide anion generation in human colonic mucosa obtained by biopsy. Gut 34: 936–938

Powell F C, Schroeter A L, Su W P, Perry H O 1985 Pyoderma gangrenosum: a review of 86 patients. Quarterly Journal of Medicine 55: 173–186

Roberts W H, Sneddon J M, Waldman J, Stephens R E 1989 Cytomegalovirus infection of gastrointestinal endothelium demonstrated by simultaneous nucleic acid hybridization and immunohistochemistry. Archives of Pathology and Laboratory Medicine 113: 461–464

Roussel F 1993 Vascular lesions in Crohn's disease. Histopathology 23: 394–396

Ruby A J, Jampol L M 1990 Crohn's disease and retinal vascular disease. American Journal of Ophthalmology 110: 349–353

Sankey E A, Dhillon A P, Anthony A et al 1993 Early mucosal changes in Crohn's disease. Gut 34: 375–381

Sargent D, Sessions J T, Fairman R P 1985 Pulmonary vasculitis complicating ulcerative colitis. Southern Medical Journal 78: 624–625

Schafer K, Tiedjen K U, Bohm E, Ernst R 1992 Angioarchitecture of the ileum and colon in Crohn disease. Zentralblatt für Chirurgie 117: 417–422

Schneiderman J H, Sharpe J A, Sutton D M 1979 Cerebral and retinal vascular complications of inflammatory bowel disease. Annals of Neurology 5: 331–337

Schuermann G M, Aber-Bishop A E, Facer P, Lee J C, Rampton D S, Dore C J 1993 Altered expression of cell adhesion molecules in uninvolved gut in inflammatory bowel disease. Clinical and Experimental Immunology 94: 341–347

Shubnich M G, Lopunova Zhk., Karbovnitskaia L P, Litvinenko M D 1976 Histochemical properties of the heparin–protein complex of mast cells and the state of the blood coagulating system in a primary lesion focus of non-specific ulcerative colitis. Arkhiv Patologii 38: 60–65

Shum D T, Guenther L 1990 Metastatic Crohn's disease. Case report and review of the literature. Archives of Dermatology 126: 645–648

Stevens T R, Harley S L, Groom J S, Cambridge G, Leaker B, Blake D R 1993 Anti-endothelial cell antibodies in inflammatory bowel disease. Digestive Diseases and Sciences 38: 426–432

Stevens T R, James J P, Simmonds N J, McCarthy D A, Laurenson I F, Rampton D S 1992 Circulating von Willebrand factor in inflammatory bowel disease. Gut 33: 502–506

Talbot R W, Heppell J, Dozois R R, Beart R W Jr 1986 Vascular complications of inflammatory bowel disease. Mayo Clinic Proceedings 61: 140–145

Thompson N P, Wakefield A J, Pounder R E 1994 Inherited disorders of coagulation appear to protect against inflammatory bowel disease. Gut 35 (Supplement 5): T111

Tsuchiya M, Miura S, Asakura H et al 1980. Angiographic evaluation of vascular changes in ulcerative colitis. Angiology 31: 147–153

Van Elburg R M, Henar E L, Bijleveld C M, Prins T R, Heymans H S 1992 Vascular compromise prior to intestinal manifestations of Crohn's disease in a 14-year-old girl. Journal of Pediatric Gastroenterology and Nutrition 14: 97–100

Wakefield A J, Pittilo R M, Sim R, Cosby S L, Stephenson J R, Dhillon A P 1993 Evidence of persistent measles virus infection in Crohn's disease. Journal of Medical Virology 39: 345–353

Wakefield A J, Sankey E A, Dhillon A P et al 1991 Granulomatous vasculitis in Crohn's disease. Gastroenterology 100: 1279–1287

Wakefield A J, Sawyerr A M, Dhillon A P et al 1989 Pathogenesis of Crohn's disease: multifocal gastrointestinal infarction. Lancet 2: 1057–1062

18. Mucosal defenses

J. M. Rhodes   B. J. Campbell   R. C. Evans

This chapter will focus on the mucus barrier and its role in protecting the intestinal mucosa from physical damage and from penetration by toxins or allergens.

NORMAL STRUCTURE AND PHYSIOLOGY OF MUCUS GLYCOPROTEINS

Mucus composition

The gel-forming properties of mucus are a function of its important glycoprotein (mucin) component. Mucins are high $M(r)$ glycoproteins (range $1–20 \times 10^6$ Da) whose linear protein core is highly glycosylated by O-linked oligosaccharide chains which account for 50–80% of the dry weight. The 'bottle brush' arrangement of oligosaccharides around the core (Lamont 1992) allows the mucin to bind large quantities of water, resulting in a gel that expands rapidly following secretion into the intestinal lumen. This gel not only constitutes a physical barrier and lubricant, but also generates a protective diffusion barrier for the underlying epithelium, with this latter effect being particularly important in the stomach, where the low pH also increases mucus viscosity at the luminal surface (Bhaskar et al 1991). Mucus can also function as a free radical scavenger, partly as a consequence of its ability to bind lipids (Gong et al 1991).

Other constituents of mucus include secretory IgA, α_1-antitrypsin, lysozyme and lactoferrin (both of the latter having significant bactericidal properties), shed cell membrane glycoproteins, glycolipids and dialysable salts. Growth factors are secreted in mucus, for example epidermal growth factor (EGF) and trefoil peptides (Wright et al 1990, 1993), which are secreted by the specialized goblet cells found as an adaptive phenomenon adjacent to areas of ulceration. A 60 kDa stress (heat shock) protein, localized in normal colorectal epithelial cells, is also secreted with mucus, where it functions as a chaperone molecule associating with colonic mucin and possibly aiding in its synthesis and/or secretion (Winrow et al 1993). These stress proteins are markedly induced in vivo in ulcerative colitis, but no change is seen in Crohn's disease. In addition, a mucin-associated protease inhibitor has been described and sequenced (Van-Seuningen et al 1989), and this may well have an important role in protecting the epithelium.

The recent application of molecular cloning techniques to the study of mucins has increased our understanding of their polypeptide backbones. Currently, at least seven different apomucin core sequences have been identified, and these are differentially expressed in different tissues and in different disease states (see below). Although all these gene products contain large numbers of tandem repeat sequences which are rich in the amino acids serine and/or threonine, their sequences are dissimilar. It is not yet known whether this heterogeneity results in the different patterns of glycosylation found in various organs. Each mucin chain contains a small number of N-linked oligosaccharides, which are added before O-glycosylation can proceed (Strous & Dekker 1992), particularly in the cysteine-rich N- and C-terminal unique regions (Gum et al 1992, Bobek et al 1993), but they are greatly outnumbered by O-linked oligosaccharide side-chains, which are usually in excess of 150 per molecule. These O-linked side-chains are always initiated by N-acetylgalactosamine, α-linked on to either serine or threonine, but further extension of the oligosaccharide chain (up to 15 or more monosaccharides) is characterized by enormous variation in branching, linkage, substitution by ester sulphate or sialic acid (N-acetylneuraminic acid), or O-acetylation of the sialic acids themselves. Consequently, this leads to a much higher degree of polydiversity than would be achievable with similar numbers of amino acid residues.

Most of the mucin protein core is so protected by glycosylation that it is resistant to protease attack, but mucins also have relatively non-glycosylated regions which are susceptible to protease attack, which degrades the mucin to non gel-forming subunits of variable length, according to their protein core type. Physical and electron-microscopic evidence suggests that these glycopeptide subunits are linked end-to-end via disulfide (S–S) bonds,

Table 18.1 Human mucin cDNA

Mucin	Origin	Chromosome	Tandem repeat (a/a)		Reference
MUC1 (PEM)	Mammary carcinoma Pancreatic carcinoma	1q21–24	20	Thr/Ser rich	Swallow et al 1987 Gendler et al 1990 Lan et al 1990
MUC2	Intestine	11p15.5	23	Thr/Pro/Cys rich	Gum et al 1989, 1994 Griffiths et al 1990 Toribara et al 1991
MUC3	Intestine	7q22	17	Thr/Ser rich	Gum et al 1990 Fox et al 1992
MUC4	Tracheobronchial	3q29	16	Thr/Ser rich	Porchet et al 1991 Gross et al 1992
MUC5a/c	Tracheobronchial Stomach	11p15	8	Thr/Ser rich	Nguyen et al 1990 Aubert et al 1991
MUC5b	Tracheobronchial Stomach	11p15	29	Alternating hydrophilic/ hydrophobic peptide domains	Dufosse et al 1993 Toribara et al 1993
MUC6	Stomach	11p15	169	Thr/Ser/Pro rich	Toribara et al 1993
MUC7	Salivary gland	4	23	Pro/Ala/Thr/Ser rich	Bobek et al 1993

forming an elongated thread structure, although the precise orientation of the monomers (i.e. N- and C-terminus positions) within the polymer has yet to be established (Sheehan et al 1986). In contrast, however, the membrane-bound epithelial mucin MUC1 (Table 18.1) does not possess a high cysteine content and does not form these characteristic disulfide-dependent polymers (Gendler et al 1991).

Mucin core-protein genes

In humans seven mucin genes (MUC1–7) have so far been identified, of which only MUC2 and MUC3 have been cloned from small-intestinal cDNA libraries, both encoding for secreted intestinal mucins (Gum et al 1989, 1990, Griffiths et al 1990, Fox et al 1992). All MUC genes encode for the mucin core polypeptide, and possess distinct tandem repeat sequences, lengths and chromosomal locations (Table 18.1). MUC2 both exhibits a high degree of length and sequence polymorphisms, and has different ethnic distributions (Toribara et al 1991). It also possesses unique cysteine-rich subdomains upstream and downstream of its central repetitive region, and these are likely to be involved in the polymerization of MUC2 into biopolymers via intramolecular disulphide bonds, as well as the expected linear end-to-end biopolymers (Gum et al 1992). Recent evidence has also shown MUC2 to contain a repetitive element of approximately 350 amino acids, with sequence similarity to the four D domains of prepro-von Willebrand factor (vWf) (Gum et al 1994). In addition, the MUC2 N-terminal region also contains another sequence similar to that of a 741 residue proprotein contained within prepro-vWf, which has been implicated in disulphide-linked oligomerization and packaging of vWf into secretory vacuoles, hence suggesting that parallel mechanisms may also exist for MUC2 (Gum et al 1994). MUC2 is thought to be the major secreted mucin type in the normal colon (Tytgat et al 1994).

Of the other mucin genes, MUC1 (cloned from mammary epithelium, and later from pancreas) is the best characterized, coding for membrane-bound polymorphic epithelial mucin (PEM) (Swallow et al 1987, Gendler et al 1990, Lan et al 1990). Four tracheobronchial mucin cDNAs have been cloned and are derived from two different human genes, MUC4 and MUC5 (Porchet et al 1991, Gross et al 1992). MUC5 cDNAs can be divided into two distinct groups of non-overlapping clones, MUC5a/c and MUC5b (Nguyen et al 1990, Aubert et al 1991, Dufosse et al 1993); one of the bronchial mucins is homologous with MUC2 (Jany et al 1991). MUC6 is one of two described gastric mucin cDNAs (Toribara et al 1993), the other gene being MUC5. The location of both these genes and that of intestinal MUC2 to chromosome 11p15 suggests a functional clustering of secretory mucin genes. Recently, the protein core of a low molecular weight human salivary mucin MUC 7 (M52) has been cloned, sequenced and located to chromosome 4 (Bobek et al 1993).

Polymorphism of mucins at the level of both DNA and mRNA is a common phenomenon and consistent with the size heterogeneity of mucins observed during purification. This polydispersity may well reflect rapid turnover, instability, partial degradation, or even incomplete or alternative splicing of mucin genes.

Normal intestinal mucin gene expression

MUC2 is highly expressed in the jejunum, duodenum, ileum and colon, and to a lesser extent in the gallbladder and bronchus (Ho et al 1993b, Gambús et al 1993).

MUC3 is expressed in the jejunum, ileum, colon and gallbladder (Gambús et al 1993, Audie et al 1993). The lack of MUC2 and MUC3 seen in the stomach may indicate that the major secreted gastric mucin is structurally adapted for resistance against acid, whereas the presence of high levels of MUC3 in the gallbladder and intestinal epithelium perhaps indicates that this mucin is more protective against bile salts. A recent study demonstrated that MUC2 and MUC3 show differences in their intracellular localization (MUC2 in intestinal goblet cells and MUC3 both in goblets and absorptive cells lacking secretory granules) and provides evidence for the existence of a maturational gradient for MUC3 but not MUC2, reflecting possible functional differences between the two (Chang et al 1994a).

MUC1, highly expressed on apical membranes of many epithelial tissues (e.g. breast, pancreas, bronchus etc.) is only sparsely expressed in small-intestinal and colonic epithelium. Higher MUC1 expression in the colon can be detected by immunohistochemistry after periodate or α-fucosidase treatment has revealed the antibody epitope (Ho et al 1993b, Bara et al 1993). Furthermore, a recent study has demonstrated MUC1 mRNA as well as MUC4 in the normal colonic mucosa (Ogata et al 1992). MUC6, a gastrointestinal tract-specific mucin core, highly expressed in the stomach and gallbladder, shows weak expression in both ileum and colon (Toribara et al 1993).

Although the synthesis and structure of the mucin core proteins is becoming much better understood as a result of these molecular studies, there is still very little known about the factors that regulate the synthesis and structure of the O-linked oligosaccharide chains, which give the mucins most of their important biological properties. This lack of knowledge is still at a fundamental level. In particular, it is not known whether the structure of the oligosaccharides is determined by the mucin core sequence or alternatively by differential expression of the relevant glycosyltransferases. Furthermore, although the structures of the major neutral O-linked oligosaccharides of normal colonic mucus have been carefully documented by Podolsky (1985a, b) the structure of the acid (sialylated and/or sulfated) oligosaccharides is unknown, yet these are probably more numerous and potentially more important.

MUCIN ABNORMALITIES IN COLORECTAL DISEASE

In both inflammatory and neoplastic colonic diseases disorders in mucin biosynthesis are observed which result either from differences in the relative expression of the different apomucins (Table 18.2) or from changes in the synthesis of the oligosaccharide side-chains, each of which may affect the physical properties of the viscous mucus gel.

Ulcerative colitis is associated with both qualitative and quantitative alterations in mucin glycoproteins. In 1983, Podolsky and Isselbacher reported a selective reduction in a mucin subclass (IV) defined by discontinuous gradient anion-exchange gel chromatography. However, this may chiefly reflect mucus depletion, as it has been notoriously difficult to obtain pure mucin preparations free from contamination by tissue glycoproteins, and in the authors' laboratory pure mucins from normal colon subjected to linear salt-gradient ion-exchange chromatography were mostly eluted with a similar salt concentration to the fraction that was apparently deficient (Raouf et al 1991). It is intriguing, though, that Podolsky's group have also been able to find a similar defect in apparently unaffected twins, perhaps implying that these individuals had a

Table 18.2 Mucin core alterations in colonic disease

		Colonic carcinoma		Ulcerative colitis	
MUC1	mRNA	↔	Ogata et al 1992 Ho et al 1993c	?	
	apomucin epitopes	↑	Ho et al 1993c Nakamori et al 1994	?	
MUC2	mRNA	↑ ↔/↓ ↔/↓	Ho et al 1993b Chang et al 1994a Ogata et al 1992	↑	Chang et al 1994b
	apomucin epitopes	↑ ↔/↓ ↔/↓	Ho et al 1993b Gambus et al 1993 Chang et al 1994a	↑	Chang et al 1994b
MUC3	mRNA	↑ ↓ ↓	Ho et al 1993b Chang et al 1994a Ogata et al 1992	↓	Chang et al 1994b
	apomucin epitopes	↑ ↓	Ho et al 1993b Chang et al 1994a	↓	Chang et al 1994b
MUC4	mRNA	↑	Ogata et al 1992	?	
	apomucin epitopes	?		?	

latent form of the disease. There certainly are alterations in the oligosaccharide chains in inflammatory bowel disease, but anion-exchange gel chromatography of intact mucins is probably too insensitive a technique for their detection. Changes in mucin oligosaccharide structure have been demonstrated, however, by alteration in the binding of anticarbohydrate antibodies and lectins (see below).

Altered mucin gene expression

In severe ulcerative colitis increased expression of MUC2 mRNA has been seen in the epithelial goblet cells, particularly in the crypt base; in mild colitis MUC2 showed even globlet cell expression throughout the crypt (Chang et al 1994b). In contrast, MUC3 was markedly decreased or absent in the glands of severely inflamed colitic epithelium (Chang et al 1994b), and this lack of MUC3 expression could potentially have an important role in the pathogenesis of ulcerative colitis. Increased expression of MUC1, 2 and 3 epitopes has been found in colonic adenocarcinoma of all histological subtypes, but the highest expression of MUC2 epitopes and MUC2 mRNA is observed in mucinous (colloid) cancers (Ho et al 1993b), correlating with decreased patient survival (Ho et al 1993c). In contrast, decreased MUC2 and 3 apomucin levels and mRNA expression have been reported in well-differentiated colonic cancers (Ogata et al 1992, Chang et al 1994a). Increased MUC4 mRNA has also been seen in colonic cancer tissue (Ogata et al 1992).

Altered glycosylation and expression of glycosyltransferases

There is good evidence of a general reduction in O-glycosylation in human colonic adenocarcinoma (Boland & Deshmukh 1990, Campbell et al 1995). Similar decreased oligosaccharide side-chain length is seen in both active ulcerative colitis and Crohn's disease (Clamp et al 1981), and oligosaccharide changes have also been demonstrated by alteration in the binding of anticarbohydrate antibodies and lectins (Jacobs & Huber 1985, Yuan et al 1986, Rhodes et al 1988, Podolsky & Fournier 1988).

In many cases blood group carbohydrate antigens expressed during fetal development, but absent in adult epithelium, return as oncofetal antigens during carcinogenesis (Yuan et al 1985). Some of these cancer-associated blood group antigens, such as sialyl-Le^x, are present not only on secreted mucus but also on the cell surface. They may also serve as ligands for endothelial cell adhesion molecules such as E-selectin (ELAM1) (Berg et al 1991), and may play an important role in the adhesion of cancer cells to vascular endothelium (Takada et al 1993). Advanced primary colorectal carcinomas show loss of sulfomucin, increased sialomucin expression, and increased sialyl-dimeric-Le^x antigen expression. This extended Le^x antigen seems to function as an ectopic adhesion ligand which promotes metastatic tumor cell implantation, and its high expression is correlated with a poor prognosis (Hoff et al 1989, Matsushita et al 1991). Le^x and Le^y antigens (positional isomers of Le^a and Le^b), minimally expressed in normal colonic epithelia, are both increased in colonic cancer and adenomatous polyps (Kim et al 1986, Itzkowitz et al 1986).

The extended type-2 chain, polylactosamine backbone structure (blood group I antigen) is also synthesized preferentially by premalignant and malignant colonocytes (Miyake et al 1989), a consequence of increased $\beta1{\rightarrow}3$GlcNAc-transferase activity (Holmes et al 1987).

Mucin core-region carbohydrate changes include the appearance of Tn, sialyl-Tn and TF(T/core 1) antigens in colonic and other epithelial carcinomas (e.g. pancreatic and cholangiocarcinoma) (Itzkowitz et al 1989, Osata et al 1993, Yamashita et al 1993). Sialyl-Tn antigen (SAα2-6GalNAcα-O-Ser/Thr), increasingly expressed during the dysplasia–carcinoma sequence, has been associated with a poor prognosis (Itzkowitz et al 1990) and immunotherapy with tumor antigens (such as sialyl-Tn), in order to enhance immune recognition, is being explored as an approach to cancer treatment (O'Boyle et al 1992, Ho et al 1993a).

Many of the same alterations in glycosylation have also been demonstrated in inflammatory bowel disease: indeed, no alteration has so far been shown in inflammatory bowel disease that has not also been found in colon cancer. Increased expression of the Thomsen–Friedenreich antigen (TFα; galactose $\beta1{\rightarrow}3$ N-acetylgalactosamine $\alpha1{\rightarrow}O$-Ser/Thr) for example, is seen in ulcerative colitis and Crohn's disease, adenomatous polyps and colorectal cancer (Rhodes et al 1986, 1988, Itzkowitz et al 1989). In the past there has been some discrepancy over the presence of TFα antigen, since most evidence for its existence in malignant tissue comes from either binding with the peanut lectin (PNA), which is not totally specific for TFα antigen possessing some affinity for both TFβ antigen (Galβ1-3GalNAcβ-, on glycolipids) and type 1 (Galβ1-3GlcNAcβ1-3)$_n$ chains, or using an indirect D-galactose oxidase/Schiff's reagent detection method (Xu et al 1992). The uncertainty has been further increased by studies which have failed to demonstrate TFα in malignant tissue using specific monoclonal antibodies (Longenecker et al 1987, Orntoft et al 1990). However, a recent study in our own laboratory, using oligosaccharide analysis by high-performance liquid chromatography (HPLC) combined with specific enzymatic release of TFα antigen, demonstrated increased expression of TFα antigen in both ulcerative colitis and colonic adenocarcinoma mucin, and its concealment in normal mucin (Campbell et al 1995).

The mechanism of increased TF, Tn and sTn expression in malignancy and in colitis may be due to altered glycosyltransferase expression. The increased expression of Galβ1-3GalNAc could be explained by either reduced sialylation (Springer 1984, Lance & Lev 1991) or reduced fucosylation (Okada et al 1994), or by a loss of the more common core 3 structure GlcNAcβ1-3GalNAc (Podolsky 1985a, b), allowing preferential synthesis of core 1 Galβ1-3GalNAc. Evidence that mild acid hydrolysis reveals TF antigen in normal mucin would suggest reduced sialylation or fucosylation as the mechanism (Campbell et al 1995), but a recent study has reported reduced activity of GlcNAc→GalNAc transferase in human colorectal carcinoma cells, but unchanged β1-3Gal→GalNAc transferase (King et al 1994), and this would be an alternative explanation for the increased expression of both TF and Tn antigens. A loss of the GlcNAc-GalNAc transferase has also been reported in cultured human colorectal adenoma and adenocarcinoma cell lines (Vavasseur et al 1994). Little is currently known about the mechanisms that regulate the relevant glycosyltransferases, but ras oncogene transformation has been shown to result in decreased α2-3→Galβ1-3GalNAc sialyltransferase activity (Delannoy et al 1993). Overall, however, mucus sialylation is increased in inflammatory bowel disease (Parker et al 1995), as in colorectal cancer.

It has recently been reported that Galβ1-3GalNAc is a major site for sulfation in the colon (Kuhns et al 1995, Vavasseur et al 1994) and this provides an alternative explanation which could clarify the situation considerably. If Galβ1-3GalNAc is usually sulfated, this would explain why Podolsky (1995a, b) did not find it among the neutral oligosaccharide structures. Moreover, the increased expression of Galβ1-3GalNAc (TF) in cancer and inflammatory bowel disease could be the direct result of the reduced sulfation that has also been demonstrated (see below).

It has been proposed that increased TF expression, which is present not only on intestinal mucins but also on O-linked epithelial cell surface glycoproteins, may allow interaction with dietary lectins such as PNA. This lectin, like many others, is highly resistant to cooking or digestion, and is present in active form in the colonic lumen after ingestion. Interaction with such lectins has the potential to cause marked stimulation (Ryder et al 1992, 1994a, b) or inhibition (Yu et al 1993) of proliferation, which may be quantitatively as important as interaction with growth factors in determining the increased proliferation that occurs in hyperplasia and as a prelude to malignant change. It follows that it is reasonable to hypothesize that the altered glycosylation found in ulcerative colitis and Crohn's disease may be a major factor determining increased proliferation, and hence the increased risk for colon cancer in these conditions.

The most obvious histochemical feature that distinguishes normal colonic mucus from small-intestinal mucus is its high degree of sulfation. Altered sulfation of epithelial glycoconjugates may play an important pathophysiological role by altering mucus function, cell–cell interactions and cell–pathogen interactions. Whereas mucins of the colorectal mucosa are normally rich in carbohydrate O-sulphate esters, in ulcerative colitis most (Corfield et al 1992a, b, Raouf et al 1992) but not all studies (Morita et al 1993) have shown a decrease in sulfation. Lower activity of the relevant sulfotransferase has also been demonstrated in human colon cancer (Vavasseur et al 1994, Kuhns et al 1995).

It is unclear whether the colonic sulfomucin has MUC2, MUC3 or any other specific apomucin core type, or whether mucins based on any core type may become sulfated in the presence of the appropriate sulfotransferase. Sulfation is potentially particularly important, since it greatly increases the resistance of mucus glycoproteins to further degradation by glycosidases (Tsai et al 1992). Increased sulfation (correlated with the presence of bacteria) occurs in gastric intestinal metaplasia (Jass & Filipe 1981), and in the neocolonic epithelium that forms after surgical pouch reconstruction (O'Connell et al 1986; Shepherd et al 1987) and this all lends indirect support to the hypothesis that sulfation may be an important defense against bacterial breakdown of the secreted mucus.

Loss of O-acetylation of sialomucin, usually at the C8 site in normal colonic mucin, has been demonstrated in ulcerative colitis, familial polyposis coli, and in colonic adenomas and carcinomas (Jass & Smith 1992, Muto et al 1985, Milton et al 1993). Furthermore, studies have also demonstrated an interesting genetic inheritance of O-acetylation (Sugihara & Jass 1986, Fuller et al 1990). The use of mild periodic acid–Schiff staining to identify sialomucins with non-O-acetylated sialic acid residues has revealed that 9% of normal individuals are homozygous for lack of C8 O-acetylation throughout their colonic goblet cells, whereas in about 25% of normal adults (but not normal children) there are occasional non-O-acetylated crypts. This phenomenon increases with age, and has been interpreted as evidence of clonal mutation (Fuller et al 1990). Similar changes have been observed in adenomatous crypts in the colons of people whose other crypts are normally O-acetylated (Jass & Smith 1992); the same crypts also express cryptic TF activity. The functional importance of these changes is at present uncertain, but at least some quantification of clonal mutation may be made which may prove very useful in the experimental assessment of carcinogens. Loss of O-acetylation makes the sialic acids much more susceptible to enzymatic cleavage; however, there appears to be no increased risk for ulcerative colitis in individuals who are homozygous for non-O-acetylated sialomucins (Jass et al 1988).

It is interesting that so far no change in mucin structure has been found in inflammatory bowel disease that has not also been found in colon cancer and in hyperplastic or adenomatous colonic polyps. The changes seen in carbohydrate expression seem likely to be secondary to the disease process, and may reflect incomplete glycosylation by a hyperplastic mucosa rather than any disease-specific change. Nevertheless, they are likely to have important functional consequences for mucosal protection (Rhodes 1989), perhaps making the mucus more susceptible to degradation by bacterial mucus-degrading glycosidases which are secreted into the colonic lumen (Hoskins & Boulding 1981), and provide a good explanation for the marked thinning of the surface mucus layer seen in ulcerative colitis (Pullan et al 1994). It should be also noted that the changes in O-linked oligosaccharide structure of intestinal mucins tend to be mirrored by similar changes in cell-surface oligosaccharides, which could also have considerable functional importance.

MUCIN SYNTHESIS AND SECRETION

Mucin synthesis

Mucin protein cores typically have a high proline content, which is thought to prevent α-helix formation, thus leaving the molecule in an expanded conformation which facilitates the high degree of glycosylation (Allen 1978). Following synthesis of the protein core in the ribosomes and subsequent leading sequence cleavage and translocation into the lumen of the endoplasmic reticulum, post-translational modifications of mucin (including glycosylation) take place, and continue as the molecule migrates from the *cis* to the *trans* side of the Golgi apparatus (Roth 1987).

O-glycosylation is initiated in the *cis* Golgi by binding of N-acetyl galactosamine (GalNAc) as its uridine diphosphate (UDP) nucleotide derivative to the oxygen of the serine (Ser) and threonine (Thr) residues (i.e. an O-glycosidic bond) by the action of UDP-GalNAcα→Ser/Thr transferase (Babczinski 1980). One transferase can form both GalNAc-O-Ser and GalNAc-O-Thr, although the amino acid sequence adjacent to the serine and threonine markedly influences their formation (Wang et al 1993). The oligosaccharide chain can then be terminated by the addition of sialic acid (forming the tumor-associated sialyl-Tn antigen) or more typically can be progressively elongated by further addition of alternating N-acetylglucosamine (GlcNAc) and galactose (Gal). Elongation is probably controlled at least to some extent by the structure and glycosylation of the peptide core of glycoproteins, for example Galβ1→3GalNAc glycoprotein transferase, active in O-glycan core 1 synthesis, shows a preference for GalNAc-Thr over GalNAc-Ser, but the presence of Galβ1-3GalNAcα side-chains adjacent to GalNAc-Thr reduces its activity (Granovsky et al 1994).

The oligosaccharide chains can be considered as comprising core, backbone and peripheral regions. Glycosylation is mediated by glycosyltransferases specific not only for the donor molecule but also for the oligosaccharide acceptor. Core formation and elongation occur in the *cis* Golgi, and terminal residues (e.g. fucose, sialic acid and sulfate) are added in the *trans* Golgi. At least six types of mucin oligosaccharide core region have been identified (Table 18.3), with core 3 most commonly found in neutral colonic mucins (GlcNAcβ1→3GalNAc) (Podolsky 1985a, b). These core structures are usually elongated by major backbone chains (Table 18.3), and can be branched in a β1,6 configuration, usually using galactose as a branching point. The oligosaccharide chains are terminated or terminally branched by an α-linked residue, either sialic acid, N-acetyl galactosamine (blood group A) or galactose (blood group B), in association with focuse (blood group H(O)) on the subterminal galactose (depending on the presence or absence of the fucosyltransferases that are encoded by the secretor gene (*Se*) and *H* genes) (Hounsell & Feizi 1982, Mollicone et al 1985, Torrado et al 1989). Most – arguably all – of the mucin oligosaccharide structures are blood group antigens, with Lewis, I, TF, Tn and Forssman, as well as ABO, antigens being commonly expressed. Addition of ester sulfate to N-acetylglucosamine and/or galactose occurs, particularly in colonic mucin.

Each mucin in the human intestine probably contains 30–40 different oligosaccharide structures, but it is not yet clear what determines their sequence. At present it seems more likely to depend on the relative proportions of the different glycosyltransferases, rather than on the type of mucin core protein sequence.

Table 18.3 Mucin O-linked oligosaccharide regions

Peripheral region	Backbone region	Core region
[A] GalNAcα1-3→R	Type 1 Galβ1-3GlcNAcβ1-3Galβ→R	Galβ1-3GalNAcα-O-Ser/Thr Type 1
[B] Galα1-3→R	Type 2 Galβ1-4GlcNAcβ1-3Galβ→R	Galβ1-3[GlcNAcβ1-6]GalNAcα-O-Ser/Thr Type 2
[H] Fucα1-2Galβ1-4/3GlcNAcβ→R		GlcNAcβ1-3GalNAcα-O-Ser/Thr Type 3
[Le^a] Galβ1-3[Fucα1-4]GlcNAcβ→R		GlcNAcβ1-3[GlcNAcβ1-6]GalNAcα-O-Ser/Thr Type 4
[Le^x] Galβ1-4[Fucα1-3]GlcNAcβ→R		Galα1-3GalNAcα-O-Ser/Thr Type 5
[Le^b] Fucα1-2Galβ1-3[Fucα1-4]GlcNAcβ→R		Galβ1-3[Galβ1-6]GalNAcα-O-Ser/Thr Type 6
[Le^y] Fucα1-2Galβ1-4[Fucα1-3]GlcNAcβ→R		

Normal colonic mucin synthesis, generally measured in vitro by incorporation of radiolabeled *N*-acetylglucosamine or gluosamine, can be increased by butyrate (Finnie et al 1995) and has recently has been shown to be enhanced by carbenoxolone, corticosteroids (prednisolone and hydrocortisone) and nicotine (Finnie et al 1994).

Goblet cell depletion of the mucus is a characteristic histological feature of ulcerative colitis (McCormick et al 1990), and previous studies of mucin synthesis by colitic biopsy specimens cultured *in vitro* have had conflicting conclusions, with reduced synthesis in inactive colitis in one study (Cope et al 1988) but normal synthesis in another (Smith & Podolsky 1987). The consensus is that there is probably a slight reduction in inactive disease, which may be accounted for at least partly by sparsity of crypts, but that synthesis increases to normal levels in active disease (Ryder et al 1995). Synthesis is generally increased in Crohn's disease (Ryder et al 1995), in keeping with the increased thickness of the mucus layer (Pullan et al 1994). A recent study has demonstrated that the lectin PNA increases mucus synthesis in cultured colonic explants from patients with normal and diseased colonic epithelium (Ryder et al 1994a).

Mucus secretion

The intestinal mucosa consists of absorptive epithelial cells and specialized mucus-secreting goblet cells. Both secrete mucus, but the goblet cell provides the main source of mucus to protect and lubricate the epithelial surface. Goblet cells can arise from either multipotent basal crypt stem cells or poorly differentiated lower crypt oligomucous cells. Following oligosaccharide synthesis, the mature mucins and other mucus constituents are packaged and stored in secretory granules as a compact mass at the apical membrane, and await secretion. The signal for storage is generally contained within the primary structure of secretory proteins such as renin and growth hormone (Trahair et al 1989, Chu et al 1990). It is likely that the primary sequence of mucins also contains a signal that directs them to storage granules and mutation, or alternative splicing of mucins presumably could result in the redirection of the secretory product into the non-storage pathway, providing one possible mechanism for the relative absence of goblet cells in ulcerative colitis. The stored mucins are then condensed in the storage granules, as is seen from their increased electron density (Sandoz et al 1985). Condensing granules are most numerous near the *trans* Golgi, and are not found near the plasma membrane or in the main granule mass of the goblet cell. Condensation is associated with an increase in intragranular Ca^{2+}, which probably acts via 'charge shielding', enhancing apolar interactions and mucin compaction, whereas Ca^{2+} in association with other granule factors perhaps aids mucin polymer–polymer affinity (Verdugo 1990). Upon maturation they migrate up the villus, where they are sloughed into the lumen over 2–3 days (Merzel & Leblond 1969). As they migrate they undergo morphological change, acquiring an organized array of microtubules and intermediate filaments (theca) which separate granule from cytoplasm and give the goblet cell its typical shape (Radwan et al 1990). In addition, they undergo changes in mucin type, with distal colonic lower crypt goblet cells containing predominantly sulfated mucins, whereas upper crypt goblets contain fewer sulfated mucins (Lapertosa et al 1984).

Two types of goblet cell mucus secretion have been described.

Slow baseline secretion involves continual secretion of single secretory granules via conventional but immediate exocytosis, i.e. the intermittent fusion of a single mucous granule membrane and the apical plasma membrane. Exocytosis is non-regulated, although one study has shown arachidonic acid partially to inhibit baseline secretion (Yedger et al 1992), and this probably ensures continual replenishment of the mucosal surface mucus coat. Granule translocation from the supranuclear region to luminal cell surface is inhibited by nocadazole, suggesting involvement of microtubules in baseline secretion (Olivier & Specian 1991). Actin filaments at the cell apex act as a functional barrier to secretion, and depolymerization of actin by cytochalasin accelerates baseline secretion (Specian & Neutra 1980, Olivier & Specian 1990).

Rapid mucus secretion occurring in response to stimuli and providing protection to a threatened epithelial surface, involves fusion of multiple storage granules and the apical membrane, resulting in secretion of the granule cluster/mass together with cytoplasm and excess apical membrane, i.e. regulated exocytosis. Rapid expansion of mucin molecules takes place on exposure to the extracellular fluid, and may be a phenomenon of charge repulsion of the polyanionic chains once the intragranule Ca^{2+} charge shielding is negated (Verdugo 1990). The empty or near-empty goblet then gradually refills over a period of 1–2 hours. This process is not inhibited by drugs interfering with the cellular cytoskeleton (actin), but may be mediated by an alteration in the concentration of intracellular calcium (Olivier & Specian 1990). Rapid secretion seems to be independent of changes in the concentration of cyclic nucleotides (Neutra et al 1982).

Our own group has preliminary evidence that there may be a third type of mucus secretion in inflamed tissue. This involves the expulsion of entire goblets from the goblet cells, leaving behind apparently healthy non-goblet cells (Sadek et al 1994). This is in keeping with the observation (Kaftan & Wright, 1989) that there is an apparent selective loss of goblet cells relative to non-goblet epithelial cells in experimental colitis. The mechanism for this type of goblet expulsion is unknown, but its probable specificity for inflamed tissue suggests that it might involve leukocyte components as secretagogues.

Mucus secretagogues

Intestinal studies have tended to use mucin-secreting cell lines derived from colonic adenocarcinomas which produce mucins, resemble goblet cells and grow in monolayers. Cholinergic agonists (e.g. acetylcholine) and cholinomimetic drugs (such as pilocarpine and carbachol, stimulate mucin secretion in small-intestine mucin-producing cells (Phillips 1992) and in colonic adenocarcinoma cells (Phillips et al 1988, McCool et al 1990). Muscarinic receptors have been identified by ^{3}H-QNB binding on both villus and crypt cells of the small intestine and colon (Rimele et al 1981, Wahawaisan et al 1983). Goblet cell discharge by electric field stimulation in vitro is only partially blocked by atropine, indicating the presence of a non-cholinergic secretagogue as part of the enteric nervous system (Phillips et al 1984).

Vasoactive intestinal polypeptide (VIP) stimulated secretion of mucin in the T84 colonic cells (McCool et al 1990) but not in colonic goblet cell line CL.16E (HT29-derived cells), even though VIP receptors were present (Laberthe et al 1989). However, carbachol-induced secretion in CL.16E cells was strongly potentiated by VIP, proving these receptors to be functionally active in the control of mucin secretion (Laberthe et al 1989). 'Cross-talk' probably occurs between the cAMP (cyclic adenosine monophosphate) pathway stimulated by VIP and the Ca^{2+} pathway stimulated by neurotensin or carbachol. The combined action of carbachol and VIP requires extracellular calcium (Bou-Hanna et al 1994). In addition to VIP, other neuropeptides such as neurotensin and neuromedin N have also been shown to stimulate secretion in colonic cells, both via the same shared receptor (Augeron et al 1992). Neurotensin stimulation was proceeded by a rise in intracellular Ca^{2+} without an increase in cAMP, suggesting that receptor binding may activate phospholipase C.

Agents which elevate intracellular calcium (ionophores), activate protein kinase C (diacylglycerol, phorbol esters) and elevate intracellular cAMP (forskolin, IBMX), all stimulate mucin secretion in various colonic adenocarcinoma cell lines (Yedger et al 1992, McCool et al 1990). A number of other agents have also been shown to stimulate mucin secretion in intestinal cells and explants, including adenosine triphosphate (ATP) (Merlin et al 1994), immunoglobulins and interleukin-1 (Cohan et al 1991). Secretion with interleukin-1 and a recently described macrophage-derived secretagogue (Sperber et al 1993) suggests a link between the immune response and mucus hypersecretion, which may explain the mucus depletion that is a feature of most forms of mucosal inflammation.

Induction of rapid mucus secretion has been demonstrated in response to anaphylaxis (Lake et al 1980), mucosal irritants (e.g. mustard oil, alcohol, hypertonic saline, triglycerides and bile acids), mechanical trauma and histamine (Neutra et al 1982). Mucin secretion can also be activated by bacterial enterotoxins released by *Vibrio cholera* and *Escherichia coli* from the small intestine (Moon et al 1971, Forstner et al 1981) and colon (Chadee et al 1991). The release of mucin from human colonic cells LS174T induced by *Entamoeba histolytica* is dependent on contact and protein kinase C activation (Keller et al 1992).

Enzymatic breakdown of secreted mucus

Secreted colonic mucus undergoes continual degradation, mainly as a result of attack by bacterial enzymes (Hoskins & Zamcheck 1968, Forstner 1978). It seems likely that only a small proportion of normal colonic bacteria have the ability to secrete all the enzymes necessary for mucin degradation (Miller & Hoskins 1981); however, many bacteria produce some of the relevant enzymes and it is probable that a symbiotic relationship exists between them. In-vitro studies have shown that many of these bacterial enzymes are inducible in the presence of mucus (Macfarlane et al 1989). In these studies the addition of mucus to the culture medium resulted in a marked increase in the secretion of proteases and glycosidases relevant to mucus degradation, whereas the proteases in particular were largely cell-bound in the absence of mucin.

The fact that colonic bacteria are able to secrete mucin-degrading enzymes (Hoskins & Boulding 1981, Variyam & Hoskins 1981, Hoskins et al 1985) implies that the concentration of these enzymes is likely to rise progressively from the proximal to the distal colon. This allows the hypothesis to be proposed that ulcerative colitis could be the result of increased susceptibility of the colonic mucus layer to breakdown by bacterial enzymes, thus exposing the mucosa to penetration by toxins or allergens (Rhodes 1989). The progressive rise in concentration of the mucus-degrading enzymes in the distal colon would then explain the characteristic distribution of ulcerative colitis.

In theory, bacterial degradation of secreted mucus could occur either by stepwise breakdown of the oligosaccharide side-chains or by a more direct attack on the relatively non-glycosylated regions of the mucin protein core. Protease digestion of mucins certainly results in the formation of subunits which have lost their ability to form gels (Sellers et al 1988), but it is unclear which of these mechanisms predominates in vivo. Histochemical studies have shown that fecal extracts can desulfate and desialylate colonic mucins in tissue sections, leaving behind apparently intact goblets filled with neutral mucin (Rhodes et al 1985a), but these studies were performed on fixed tissue, where the response to proteases may be very different. Disappointingly, these studies failed to show any increased susceptibility of ulcerative colitis mucus to desialylation or desulfation. Fecal extracts have been shown to contain protease activity which is capable of degrading mucin polymers to their subunits, has a broad pH range (4.5–11.0) and, perhaps surprisingly, is 100% inhibitable by soybean trypsin inhibitor (Hutton et al 1990). At least some of this activity is likely to be of pancreatic rather than bacterial origin (Scawen & Allen 1977). Protease activity has been shown to be increased in fecal samples from patients with ulcerative colitis (Samson et al 1993). One possibility which has yet to be excluded is that some of these abnormalities might result from altered secretion of mucus-associated protease inhibitors (Van-Seuningen et al 1989).

Human feces usually also contain all the enzymes necessary for breakdown of the mucin oligosaccharides. Endoglycosidases capable of breaking off the entire oligosaccharide chain seem to be rare or non-existent, however, so breakdown proceeds in a stepwise fashion from the tip of the chain. O-acyl esterases are needed to remove the O-acyl residues from the sialic acids before the sialidases themselves can act, and the sialic acids then have to be removed before other specific glycosidases can further degrade the oligosaccharide. All the relevant enzymes seem to be present in human feces (Corfield et al 1992c), and there is increased fecal activity of O-acyl esterase in ulcerative colitis (Corfield et al 1988, 1993). Colonic mucins are distinguished by their marked sulfation and the presence of ester sulfate also renders the oligosaccharide chains resistant to glycosidase attack (Tsai et al 1992). Human feces have also been shown to contain mucin sulfatases (Tsai et al 1991, 1992, Corfield et al 1993, Roberton et al 1993) and increased activity of these enzymes has been demonstrated in active ulcerative colitis (Corfield et al 1993, Tsai et al 1995).

Because of the difficulty in assessing the relative roles of proteases, glycosidases, sulfatases, O-acyl esterases and sialidases in the degradation of secreted mucus, a subsequent study has used ^{14}C-threonine labeled mucin as a substrate for a 'total mucinase' assay (Dwarakanath et al 1995). Gel filtration was then used to assess the proportion of label released into lower molecular weight fragments. Fecal mucinase activity assessed by this assay was again shown to have a wide pH range (4.5–9.5), suggesting multiple enzymes, but was 83% inhibitable by the chymotrypsin inhibitor chymostatin. Mucinase activity was increased by >50% in fecal samples from patients with ulcerative colitis, irrespective of disease activity, providing another possible explanation for the thin mucus layer in this condition.

Most of the evidence suggests that alterations in fecal mucus-degrading activity in ulcerative colitis are likely to be secondary to the disease rather than a primary event, possibly as a result of increased substrate availability if mucus is shed more rapidly. Nevertheless, any process that reduces the effect of the protective mucus layer is likely to be harmful, and so inhibition of this process represents a potentially useful therapeutic target. Agents so far shown to inhibit the relevant enzymes include bismuth salts (Tsai et al 1995, Dwarakanath et al 1995) and polyacrylates (Hutton et al 1990). Other agents, such as the sialic acid analogs that inhibit sialidases (von Itztein et al 1993) are also worthy of study.

Studies of mucus degradation in Crohn's disease show intriguing differences from those in ulcerative colitis. The intramucosal mucus in tissue sections is relatively resistant to fecal sialidase activity (Rhodes et al 1985a) and fecal sulfatase (Tsai et al 1992) and mucinase activity (Dwarakanath et al 1995) is not increased. Furthermore, some (Mizon et al 1991, El Yamani et al 1992) but not all (Rhodes et al 1985b, Ruseler-van Embden & van Lieshout 1987) studies have also shown reduced fecal glycosidase activity in Crohn's disease. These findings would all help to explain the relatively thick mucus layer that is found in Crohn's disease (Pullan et al 1994).

SUMMARY

In ulcerative colitis the surface mucus layer is thin and the mucosa is depleted of goblet cells, whereas in Crohn's disease the mucus layer is thick and goblet cells are retained, even in the presence of inflammation. There are no changes in mucin synthesis sufficient to account for these differences, which seem more likely to be due either to differences in mucus secretion or differences in the rate at which mucus is degraded after secretion. Although much is known about secretion of mucus from normal mucosa, there is currently no clear understanding of how this process is altered in the presence of inflammation. Preliminary evidence suggests that the goblet cell depletion seen in ulcerative colitis may be the result of expulsion of goblets from the cells, rather than shedding of the goblet cells themselves. Once mucus has been secreted, increased activity of the fecal mucus-degrading enzymes in ulcerative colitis are likely to hasten its breakdown.

Alterations in glycosylation and sulfation in inflammatory bowel disease are similar to those found in colorectal cancer, and affect not only mucin but also glycosylation of the cell surface glycoproteins. These changes result in changes in lectin binding which allow interaction with dietary lectins, which may be important in determining the hyperproliferation which is thought to precede colonic cancer. The same changes may also result in altered binding of bacterial lectins, and hence in an altered mucosal flora, but further studies are required to assess this. The shortening and reduced sulfation of oligosaccharide chains in inflammatory bowel disease are likely to reduce the efficacy of the mucus layer as a barrier.

It is not yet clear to what extent the changes in glycosylation might be primary rather than secondary events, nor is it clear whether they are the result of altered glycosyltransferase activity or altered MUC core protein expression. The hypothesis that inherited alterations in mucus formation or secretion underlie the pathogenesis of colitis remains viable (Rhodes 1996) and has the attraction that it can explain many of the clinical features of the disease, including its anatomical distribution.

REFERENCES

Allen A 1978 Structure of gastrointestinal mucus glycoproteins and the viscous and gel-forming properties of mucus. British Medical Bulletin 34: 28–33

Aubert J P, Porchet N, Crepin M et al 1991 Evidence for different human tracheobronchial mucin peptides deduced from nucleotide cDNA sequences. American Journal of Respiratory Cellular and Molecular Biology, 5: 178–185

Audie J P, Janin A, Porchet N, Copin M C, Gosselin B, Aubert J P 1993 Expression of human mucin genes in respiratory, digestive and reproductive tracts ascertained by in situ hybridisation. Journal of Histochemistry and Cytochemistry 41: 1479–1485

Augeron C, Voisin T, Laboisse C L 1992 Neurotensin and neuromedin N stimulate mucin output from human goblet cells (C1.16E) via neurotensin receptors. American Journal of Physiology 262: G470–G476

Babczinski P 1980 Evidence against the participation of lipid intermediates in the in vitro biosynthesis of serine (threonine) N-acetyl D-galactosamine linkages in sub-maxillary mucin. FEBS Letters 117: 207–211

Bara J, Imberty A, Perez S, Imai K, Yachi A, Oriol R 1993 A fucose residue can mask the MUC1 epitopes in normal and cancerous gastric mucosae. International Journal of Cancer 54: 607–613

Berg E L, Robinson M K, Mansson O, Butcher E C, Magnani J L 1991 A carbohydrate domain common to both sialyl Le^a and sialyl Le^x is recognised by the endothelial cell leukocyte adhesion molecule ELAM-1. Journal of Biological Chemistry 266: 14869–14872

Bhaskar K R, Gong D H, Bansil R et al 1991 Profound increase in viscosity and aggregation of pig gastric mucin at low pH. American Journal of Physiology 261: G827–G832

Bobek L A, Tsai H, Biesbrock A R, Levine M J 1993 Molecular cloning, sequence, and specificity of expression of the gene encoding the low molecular weight human salivary mucin (MUC7). Journal of Biological Chemistry 268: 20563–20569

Boland C R, Deshmukh S T 1990 The carbohydrate composition of mucin colon cancer. Gastroenterology 98: 1170–1177

Bou-Hanna C, Berthon B, Combettes L, Claret M, Laboisse C L 1994 Role of calcium in carbachol- and neurotensin-induced mucin exocytosis in a human colonic goblet cell line and cross talk with the cAMP pathway. Biochemical Journal 299: 579–585

Campbell B J, Finnie I A, Hounsell E F, Rhodes J M 1995 Direct demonstration of increased expression of Thomsen–Friedenreich (TF) antigen in colonic adenocarcinoma and ulcerative colitis mucin and its concealment in normal mucin. Journal of Clinical Investigation 95: 571–576

Chadee K, Keller K, Forstner J, Innes D J, Ravdin J I 1991 Mucin and non-mucin secretagogue activity of *Entamoeba histolytica* and cholera toxin in rat colon. Gastroenterology 100: 986–997

Chang S K, Dohrman A F, Basbaum C B et al 1994a Localisation of mucin (MUC2 & MUC3) mRNA and peptide expression in human normal intestine and colon cancer. Gastroenterology 107: 28–36

Chang S K, Park E S, Chung W S et al 1994b Expression of MUC2, MUC3 apomucins and mRNA in ulcerative colitis. Gastroenterology 106: 662

Chu W N, Baxter J D, Reudelhuber T L 1990 A targeting sequence for dense secretory granules resides in the active renin protein moiety of human preprorenin. Molecular Endocrinology 90: 1905–1913

Clamp J R, Fraser G, Read A E 1981 Study of the carbohydrate content to mucus glycoproteins from normal and diseased colons. Clinical Science 61: 229–234

Cohan V L, Scott A L, Dinarello C A, Prendergast R A 1991 Interleukin-1 is a mucus secretagogue. Cellular Immunology 136: 425–434

Cope G F, Heatley R V, Kelleher J, Axon A T R 1988 *In vitro* mucus glycoprotein production by colonic tissue from patients with ulcerative colitis. Gut 29: 229–243

Corfield A P, Williams A J K, Clamp J R, Wagner S A, Mountford R A 1988 Degradation by bacterial enzymes of colonic mucus from normal subjects and patients with inflammatory bowel disease: the role of sialic acid metabolism and the detection of a novel esterase. Clinical Science 74: 71–78

Corfield A P, Do Amaral-Corfield C, Wagner S A, Warren B, Mountford R A, Bartolo D C C, Clamp J R 1992a Loss of sulphate in human colonic mucins during ulcerative colitis. Biochemical Society Transactions 20: 95S

Corfield A P, Warren B, Bartolo D C C, Wagner S A, Clamp J R 1992b Mucin changes in ileoanal pouches monitored by metabolic labelling and histochemistry. British Journal of Surgery 79: 1209–1212

Corfield A P, Wagner S A, Clamp J R, Kriaris M S, Hoskins L C 1992c Mucin degradation in the human colon: production of sialidase, sialate *O*-acetylesterase. *N*-acetylneuraminate lyase, arylesterase, and glycosulfatase activities by strains of fecal bacteria. Infection and Immunity 60: 3971–3978

Corfield A P, Wagner S A, O'Donnell L J D, Durdey P, Mountford R A, Clamp J R 1993 The roles of enteric bacterial sialidase, sialate *O*-acetyl esterase and glycosulfatase in the degradation of human colonic mucin. Glycoconjugate Journal 10: 72–81

Delannoy P, Pelczar H, Vandamme V, Verbert A 1993 Sialyltransferase activity in FR3T3 cells transformed with *ras* oncogene: decreased CMP-NeuAc:Galβ1-3GalNAc alpha-2,3-sialyltransferase. Glycoconjugate Journal 10: 91–98

Dufosse J, Porchet N, Audie J P et al 1993 Degenerate 87 base pair tandem repeats create hydrophilic/hydrophobic alternating domains in human peptide mucins mapped to 11p15. Biochemical Journal 293: 329–337

Dwarakanath A D, Campbell B J, Tsai H H, Sunderland D, Hart C A, Rhodes J M 1995 Faecal mucinase activity assessed in inflammatory bowel disease using 14C-threonine labelled mucin substrate. Gut 37: 58–62

El Yamani J, Mizon C, Capon C et al 1992 Decreased faecal exoglycosidase activities identify a subset of patients with active Crohn's disease. Clinical Science 83: 409–415

Finnie I A, Campbell B J, Dwarakanath A D, Taylor B A, Rhodes J M 1994 Nicotine, corticosteroids and sodium butyrate increase mucin synthesis by human colonic epithelium. Gastroenterology 106: A680

Finnie I A, Dwarakanath A D, Taylor B A, Rhodes J M 1995 Colonic mucin synthesis is increased by sodium butyrate. Gut 36: 93–99

Forstner J F 1978 Intestinal mucins in health and disease. Digestion 17: 234–263

Forstner J F, Roomi N W, Fahim R E F, Forstner G G 1981 Cholera toxin stimulates secretion of immunoreactive intestinal mucin. American Journal of Physiology 240: G10–G16

Fox M F, Lahbib F, Pratt W et al 1992 Regional localisation of the intestinal mucin gene MUC3 to chromosome 7q22. Annals of Human Genetics 56: 281

Fuller C E, Davies R P, Williams G T, Williams E D 1990 Crypt restricted heterogeneity of goblet cell mucus glycoprotein in histologically normal human colonic mucosa: a potential marker of somatic mutation. British Journal of Cancer 61: 382–384

Gambús G, De Bolos C, Andreu D, Franci C, Egea G, Real F X 1993 Detection of the MUC2 apomucin tandem repeat with a mouse monoclonal antibody. Gastroenterology 104: 93–102

Gendler S J, Lancaster C A, Taylor-Papadimitriou J et al 1990 Molecular cloning and expression of the human tumour-associated polymorphic epithelial mucin (PEM). Journal of Biological Chemistry 265: 15286–15293

Gendler S J, Spicer A P, Lalani E N et al 1991 Structure and biology of a carcinoma-associated mucin, MUC1. American Review of

Respiratory Diseases 144: S42–47

Gong D H, Turner B, Bhaskar K R, Lamont J T 1991 Lipid binding to gastric mucin: protective effect against oxygen free radicals. American Journal of Physiology 259: G681–686

Granovsky M, Bielfeldt T, Peters S et al 1994 UDP galactose: glycoprotein-N-acetylgalactosamine 3-beta-D-galactosyltransferase activity synthesising O-glycan core 1 is controlled by the amino acid sequence and glycosylation of glycopeptide substrates. European Journal of Biochemistry 221: 1039–1046

Griffiths B, Matthews D J, West L et al 1990 Assignment of the polymorphic intestinal mucin gene (MUC2) to chromosome 11p15. Annals of Human Genetics 54: 277–285

Gross M S, Guyonnet-Duperat V, Porchet N, Bernheim A, Aubert J P, Nguyen V C 1992 Mucin 4 (MUC4) gene: regional assignment (3q29) and RFLP analysis. Annals of Genetics 35: 21–26

Gum J R, Byrd J C, Hicks J W et al 1989 Molecular cloning of human intestinal cDNAs. Sequence analysis and evidence for genetic polymorphism. Journal of Biological Chemistry 264: 6480–6487

Gum J R, Hicks J W, Swallow D M et al 1990 Molecular cloning of cDNAs derived from a novel human intestinal mucin gene. Biochemistry and Biophysics Research Communications 171: 407–415

Gum J R, Hicks J W, Toribara N W, Rothe E M, Lagace R E, Kim Y S 1992 The human MUC2 intestinal mucin has cysteine-rich subdomains located both upstream and downstream of its central repetitive region. Journal of Biological Chemistry 267: 21375–21383

Gum J R, Hicks J W, Toribara N W, Siddiki B, Kim Y S 1994 Molecular cloning of human intestinal mucin (MUC2) cDNA. Identification of the amino-terminus and overall sequence similarity of prepro-von Willebrand factor. Journal of Biological Chemistry 269: 2440–2446

Halvorsen T B, Sein E 1988 Influence of mucinous components on survival in colorectal adenocarcinomas. A multivariate analysis. Journal of Clinical Pathology 41: 1068–1072

Ho I, Ogata S, Chen A, Makalansky J, Werther J L, Itzkowitz S H 1993a Establishment of a rat colon cancer model for immunotherapy based on sialosyl-Tn antigen. Gastroenterology 104 (4): A410

Ho S B, Chandler D J, Logan G, Toribara N W, Kim Y S, Ewing S L 1993b Intestinal and gastric mucin core peptide expression in colon cancer: correlation with histology, stage and survival. Gastroenterology 104 (4), A410

Ho S B, Neihans G A, Lyftogt C et al 1993c Heterogeneity of mucin gene expression in normal and neoplastic tissues. Cancer Research 53: 641–651

Hoff S D, Matsushita Y, Ota D M et al 1989 Increased expression of sialyl-dimeric Le^x antigen in advanced primary colorectal carcinomas and liver metastases. Cancer Research 49: 6883–6888

Holmes E H, Hakamori S, Ostander G K 1987 Synthesis of type 1 & 2 lacto series glycolipid antigens in human colonic adenocarcinoma and derived cell lines due to activation of a normally unexpressed β1-3N-acetyl glucosaminyltransferase. Journal of Biological Chemistry 262: 15649–15658

Hoskins L C, Boulding E T 1981 Mucin degradation in human colon ecosystems. Evidence for the existence and role of bacterial subpopulations producing glycosidases as extracellular enzymes. Journal of Clinical Investigation 67: 163–172

Hoskins L C, Zamcheck N 1968 Bacterial degradation of gastrointestinal mucins. I. Comparison of mucus constituents in the stools of germ-free and conventional rats. Gastroenterology 54: 210–217

Hoskins L C, Agustines M, McKee W B, Boulding E T, Kriaris M, Niedermeyer G 1985 Mucin degradation in human colon ecosystems. Isolation and properties of fecal strains that degrade ABH blood group antigens and oligosaccharides from mucin glycoproteins. Journal of Clinical Investigation 75: 944–953

Hounsell E F, Feizi T 1982 Gastrointestinal mucins, structures and antigenicities of their carbohydrate chains in health and disease. Medical Biology 60: 227–236

Hutton D A, Pearson J P, Allen A, Foster S N E 1990 Mucolysis of the colonic mucus barrier by faecal proteinases inhibition by interacting polyacrylate. Clinical Science 78: 265–271

Itzkowitz S H, Bloom E J, Kokal W A, Modin G, Hakamori S, Kim Y S 1990 Sialosyl Tn: a novel mucin antigen associated with poor prognosis in colorectal cancer patients. Cancer 66: 1960–1966

Itzkowitz S H, Yuan M, Fukushi Y et al 1986 Lewis x and sialylated Lewis x-related antigen expression in human malignant and non-malignant colonic tissues. Cancer Research 46: 2627–2632

Itzkowitz S H, Yuan M, Montgomery C K et al 1989 Expression of Tn, sialosyl Tn and T antigens in human colon cancer. Cancer Research 49: 197–204

Jacobs L R, Huber P W 1985 Regional distribution and alterations of lectin binding to colorectal mucin in mucosal biopsies from controls and subjects with inflammatory bowel disease. Journal of Clinical Investigation 75: 112–118

Jany B H, Gallup M W, Yan P S, Gum J R, Kim Y S, Basbaum C B 1991 Human bronchus and intestine express the same mucin gene. Journal of Clinical Investigation 87: 77–82

Jass J R, Filipe M I 1981 The mucin profile of normal gastric mucosa, intestinal metaplasia and its variants and gastric carcinoma. Histochemical Journal 13: 931–939

Jass J R, Smith M 1992 Sialic acid and epithelial differentiation in colorectal polyps and cancer; a morphological, mucin and lectin histochemical study. Pathology 24: 233–242

Jass J R, Sugihara K, Love S B 1988 Basis of sialic acid heterogenity in ulcerative colitis. Journal of Clinical Pathology 41: 388–392

Kaftan S M, Wright N A (1989). Studies on the mechanisms of mucous cell depletion in experimental colitis. Journal of Pathology 159: 75–85

Keller K, Olivier M, Chadee K 1992 The fast release of mucin secretion from human colonic cells induced by *Entamoeba histolytica* is dependent on contact and protein kinase C activation. Archives of Medical Research 23: 217–221

Kim Y S, Yuan M, Itzkovitz S H et al 1986 Expression of Le^y and extended Le^y blood group-related antigens in human malignant, premalignant and non-malignant colonic tissues. Cancer Research 46: 5985–5992

King M-J, Chan A, Roe R et al 1994 Two different glycosyltransferase defects that result in GalNAcα-O-peptide (Tn) expression. Glycobiology 4: 267–279

Kuhns W, Jain R K, Matta K L et al 1995 Characterisation of a novel mucin sulphotransferase activity synthesising sulphated O-glycan core 1, 3-sulphate- Galβ1-3GalNAcα-R. Glycobiology 5: 689–697

Laberthe M A, Augeron C, Rouyer-Fessard C et al 1989 Functional VIP receptors in the human mucin-secreting colonic epithelial cell line CL.16E. American Journal of Physiology 256: G443–G450

Lake A M, Bloch K J, Sinclair K J, Walker W 1980 Anaphylactic release of intestinal goblet cell mucus. Immunology 39: 173–178

Lamont J T 1992 Mucus: the front line of intestinal mucosal defence Annals of the New York Academy of Sciences 664: 190–201

Lan M S, Batra S K, Qi W N, Metzar R S, Hollingsworth M A 1990 Cloning and sequencing of a human pancreatic tumor mucin cDNA. Journal of Biological Chemistry 265: 15294–15299

Lance P, Lev R 1991 Colonic oligosaccharide structures deduced from lectin-binding studies before and after desialylation. Human Pathology 22: 307–312

Lapertosa G, Fulcheri E, Acquarone M, Filipe M I 1984 Mucin profiles in the mucosa adjacent to large bowel non-adenocarcinoma neoplasias. Histopathology 8: 805–811

Longenecker B M, Willans D J, MacLean G D, Selvaraj S, Suresh M R, Noujaim A A 1987 Monoclonal antibodies and synthetic tumour-associated glycoconjugates in the study of the expression of Thomsen–Friedenreich-like and Tn-like antigens on human cancers. Journal of the National Cancer Institute 78: 489–492

McCool D J, Marcon M A, Forstner J F, Forstner G G 1990 The T84 human adenocarcinoma cell line produces mucin in culture and releases it in response to various secretagogues. Biochemical Journal 267: 491–500

McCormick D A, Horton L W, Mee A S 1990 Mucin depletion in inflammatory bowel disease. Journal of Clinical Pathology 43: 143–146

Macfarlane G T, Hay S, Gibson G R 1989 Influence of mucin on glycosidase, protease and arylamidase activities of human gut bacteria grown in a 3-stage continuous culture system. Journal of Applied Bacteriology 66: 407–417

Matsushita Y, Nakamori S, Seftor E A, Hendrix M J, Irimura T 1991 Human colon carcinoma cells with invasive capacity obtained by selection for sialyl-dimeric Le x antigen. Experimental Cell Research 196: 20–25

Merlin D, Augeron C, Tien X Y, Guo X, Laboisse C L, Hopfer U 1994 ATP-stimulated electrolyte and mucin secretion in the human intestinal goblet cell line HT29-Cl.16E Journal of Membrane Biology 137: 137–149

Merzel J, Leblond C P 1969 Origin and renewal of goblet cells in the epithelium of the mouse small intestine. American Journal of Anatomy 124: 281–306

Miller R S, Hoskins L C 1981 Mucin degradation in human colon ecosystems. Fecal population densities of mucin-degrading bacteria estimated by a 'most probable number' method. Gastroenterology; 81: 759–765

Milton J D, Eccleston D, Parker N et al 1993 Distribution of O-acetylated sialomucin in the normal and diseased gastrointestinal tract shown by a new monoclonal antibody. Journal of Clinical Pathology 46: 323–329

Miyake M, Kohno N, Nudelman E D, Hakomori S I 1989 Human IgG3 monoclonal antibody directed to an unbranched repeated type 2 chain Galβ1-4GlcNAcβ1-3Galβ1-4GlcNAcβ1-3Galβ-R which is highly expressed in colonic and hepatocellular carcinoma. Cancer Research 49: 5689–5695

Mizon C, el Yamani J, Colombel J F et al 1991 Deglycosylation of α1-proteinase inhibitor is impaired in the faeces of patients with active inflammatory bowel disease (Crohn's disease). Clinical Science 80: 517–523

Mollicone R, Bara J, Le Pendu J, Oriol R 1985 Immunological pattern of type 1 (Le[a], Le[b]) and type 2 (X,Y,H) blood group-related antigens in the human pyloric and duodenal mucosae. Laboratory Investigation 53: 219

Moon H W, Whipp D C, Baetz A L 1971 The comparative effects of enterotoxins from *Escherichia coli* and *Vibrio cholerae* on rabbit and swine small intestine. Laboratory Investigation 25: 133–140

Morita H, Kettlewell M G, Jewell D P, Kent P W 1993 Glycosylation and sulphation of colonic glycoproteins in patients with ulcerative colitis and in healthy subjects. Gut 34: 926–932

Muto T, Kamiya J, Sawada T, Agawa S, Morioka Y, Utsunomiya J 1985 Mucin abnormality of colonic mucosa in patients with familial polyposis coli: a new tool for early detection of the carrier? Diseases of the Colon and Rectum 28: 147–148

Nakamori S, Ota D M, Cleary K R, Shirotani, Inmura T, 1994 MUC1 mucin expression as a marker of progression and metastasis of human colorectal carcinoma. Gastroenterology 106: 353–361

Neutra M R, O'Malley L J, Special R D 1982 Regulation of intestinal goblet cell secretion. II. A survey of potential secretagogues. American Journal of Physiology 242: G380–387

Nguyen V C, Aubert J P, Gross M S, Porchet N, Degand P, Frezal J 1990 Assignment of human tracheobronchial mucin gene(s) to 11p15 and a tracheobronchial mucin-related sequence to chromosome 13. Human Genetics 86: 167–172

O'Boyle K P, Zamore R, Adluri S et al 1992 Immunisation of colorectal cancer patients with modified ovine submaxillary gland mucin and adjuvants induces IgM and IgG antibodies to sialylated Tn. Cancer Research 52: 5663–5667

O'Connell P R, Rankin D R, Weiland L H, Kelly K A 1986 Enteric bacteriology, absorption, morphology and emptying after ileal pouch–anal anastomosis. British Journal of Surgery 73: 909–914

Ogata S, Uehara H, Chen A, Itzkowitz S H 1992 Mucin gene expression in colonic tissues and cell lines. Cancer Research 52: 5971–5978

Okada Y, Sotozono M A, Sakai N, Yonei S, Nakanishi S, Tsuji T 1994 Fucosylated Thomsen–Friedenreich antigen in α-anomeric configuration in human gastric surface epithelia: an allogenic carbohydrate antigen possibly controlled by the Se gene. Journal of Histochemistry and Cytochemistry 42: 371–376

Olivier M G, Special R D 1990 Cytoskeleton of intestinal goblet cells: role of actin filaments in baseline secretion. American Journal of Physiology 259: G991–G997

Olivier M G, Special R D 1991 Cytoskeleton of intestinal goblets cells: role of microtubules in baseilne secretion. American Journal of Physiology 260: G850–G857

Orntoft T F, Harving N, Langkilde N C 1990 O-linked mucin type glycoproteins in normal and malignant colon mucosa: lack of T antigen and accumulation of Tn and sialosyl Tn antigens in carcinomas. International Journal of Cancer 45: 666–672

Osata M, Yonezawa S, Siddiki B et al 1993 Immunohistochemical study of mucin carbohydrates and core proteins in human pancreatic tumors. Cancer 71: 2191–2199

Parker N, Tsai H H, Ryder S D, Raouf A H, Rhodes J M 1995 Increased rate of sialylation of colonic mucin by cultured ulcerative colitis mucosal explants. Digestion 56: 52–56

Phillips T E 1992 Both crypt and villus intestinal goblet cells secrete mucin in response to cholinergic stimulation. American Journal of Physiology 262: G327–G331

Phillips T E, Phillips T H, Neutra M R 1984 Regulation of intestinal goblet cell secretion. IV. Electric field stimulation in vitro. American Journal of Physiology 247: G682–G687

Phillips T E, Huet C, Bilbo P R, Podolsky D K, Louvard D, Neutra M R 1988 Human intestinal globlet cells in monolayer culture: characterisation of a mucus-secreting subclone derived from HT29 colonic adenocarcinoma cell-line. Gastroenterology 94: 1390–1403

Podolsky D K 1985a Oligosaccharide structures of human colonic mucin. Journal of Biological Chemistry 260: 8262–8271

Podolsky D K 1985b Oligosaccharide structures of isolated human colonic mucin species. Journal of Biological Chemistry 260: 15510–15515

Podolsky D K, Fournier D A 1988 Alterations in mucosal content of colonic glycoconjugates in inflammatory bowel disease defined by monoclonal antibodies. Gastroenterology 95: 371–378

Podolsky D K, Isselbacher K J 1983 Composition of human colonic mucin. Selective alteration in inflammatory bowel disease. Journal of Clinical Investigation 72: 142–153

Porchet N, Cong N V, Dufosse J et al 1991 Molecular cloning and chromosomal localisation of a novel human tracheo-bronchial mucin cDNA containing tandemly repeated sequences of 48 base pairs. Biochemistry and Biophysics Research Communications 175: 414–422

Pullan R D, Thomas G A O, Rhodes M et al 1994 Thickness of adherent mucus gel on colonic mucosa in humans and its relevance to colitis. Gut 35: 353–359

Radwan K A, Oliver M G, Special R D 1990 Cytoarchitectural reorganisation of rabbit colonic goblet cells during baseline secretion. Anatomical Record 189: 365–376

Raouf A H, Parker N, Iddon D et al 1991 Ion-exchange chromatography of purified mucus glycoproteins in inflammatory bowel disease: absence of a selective subclass defect. Gut 32: 1139–1145

Raouf A H, Tsai H H, Parker N, Hoffman J, Walker R J, Rhodes J M 1992 Sulphation of colonic mucin in ulcerative colitis and Crohn's disease. Clinical Science 83: 623–626

Rhodes J M 1989 Colonic mucus and mucosal glycoproteins: the key to colitis and cancer? Gut 30: 1660–1666

Rhodes J M 1996. Unifying hypothesis for inflammatory bowel disease and related colon cancer: sticking the pieces together with sugar. Lancet 347: 40–44

Rhodes J M, Black R R, Savage A 1988 Altered lectin binding by colonic epithelial glycoconjugates in ulcerative colitis and Crohn's disease. Digestive Diseases and Sciences 33: 1359–1363

Rhodes J M, Black R R, Gallimore R, Savage R 1985a Histochemical demonstration of desialylation and desulphation of normal and inflammatory bowel disease rectal mucus by faecal extracts. Gut 26: 1312–1318

Rhodes J M, Gallimore R, Elias E, Allan R N, Kennedy J F 1985b Faecal mucus degrading glycosidases in ulcerative colitis and Crohn's disease. Gut 26: 761–765

Rhodes J M, Black R R, Savage A 1986 Glycoprotein abnormalities in colonic carcinoma, adenoma and hyperplastic polyps shown by lectin peroxidase histochemistry. Journal of Clinical Pathology 39: 1331–1334

Rimele T J, O'Doriso M S, Gaginella T 1981 Evidence of muscarinic receptors on rat colonic epithelial cells: binding of ^{3}H-quinuclidinyl benzilate. Journal of Pharmacology and Experimental Therapy 218: 426–434

Roberton A M, McKenzie C G, Sharfe N, Stubbs L B 1993 A glycosulphatase that removes sulphate from mucus glycoprotein. Biochemical Journal 293: 683–689

Roth J 1987 Subcellular organisation of glycosylation in mammalian cells. Biochimica Biophysica Acta 7: 405–436

Ruseler-van Embden J G H, van Leishout L M C 1987 Increased faecal glycosidases in patients with Crohn's disease. Digestion 37: 43–50

Ryder S D, Smith J A, Rhodes J M 1992 Peanut lectin is a mitogen for normal human colonic epithelium and HT colorectal cancer cells. Journal National Cancer Institute 84: 1410–1416

Ryder S D, Smith J A, Rhodes E G H, Rhodes J M 1994a Proliferative response of HT29 and Caco2 human colorectal cancer cells to a panel of lectins. Gastroenterology 106: 85–93

Ryder S D, Parker N, Eccleston D, Haqqani M T, Rhodes J M 1994b Peanut lectin stimulates proliferation in colonic explants from patients with ulcerative colitis and colonic polyps. Gastroenterology 106: 117–124

Ryder S D, Raouf A H, Parker N, Walker R J, Rhodes J M 1995 Abnormal mucosal glycoprotein synthesis in inflammatory bowel diseases is not related to cigarette smoking. Digestion 56: 370–376

Sadek S K, Finnie I A, O'Dowd G M, Rhodes J M 1994 Effect of formyl- methionyl-leucyl-phenylalanine on mucus secretion in the normal human colon: a novel mechanism of mucus secretion. Clinical Science 86: 33 (Abstract)

Samson H J, Pearson J R, Allen A, Srivastava E D, Record C O 1993 Significant increase in negatively charged serine dependent proteases in ulcerative colitis. Gut 34: W39 (Abstract)

Sandoz D, Nicolas G, Laine M 1985 Two mucous cell types revisited after quick-freezing and cryosubstitution. Biological Chemistry 54: 79–88

Scawen M, Allen A 1977 The action of proteolytic enzymes on the glycoprotein from pig gastric mucus. Biochemical Journal 163: 363–368

Sellers L A, Allen A, Morris E R, Ross-Murphy S B 1988 Mucus glycoprotein gels: role of glycoprotein polymeric structure and carbohydrate side-chains in gel formation. Carbohydrate Research 178: 93–110

Sheehan J, Oates K, Carlstedt I 1986 Electron microscopy of cervical, gastric and bronchial glycoproteins. Biochemical Journal 239: 147

Shepherd N A, Jass J R, Duval I, Moskowitz R L, Nicholls R J, Morson B C 1987 Restorative protocolectomy with ileal reservoir: pathological and histochemical study of mucosal biopsy specimens. Journal of Clinical Pathology 40: 601–607

Smith A C, Podolsky D K 1987 Biosynthesis and secretion of human colonic mucin glycoproteins. Journal of Clinical Investigation 80: 300–307

Specian R D, Neutra M R 1980 Mucous granule transport and secretion: effects of colchicine and cytochalasin. British Journal of Cell Biology 87: 300a

Sperber K, Ogata S, Sylvester C et al 1993 A novel human macrophage-derived intestinal mucin secretagogue: implications for the pathogenesis of inflammatory bowel disease. Gastroenterology 104: 1302–1309

Springer G F 1984 T and Tn: general carcinoma autoantigens. Science 224: 1198–1206

Strous G J, Dekker J 1992 Mucin type glycoproteins. Critical Reviews in Biochemistry and Molecular Biology 27: 57–92

Sugihara K, Jass J R 1986 Colorectal goblet cell sialomucin heterogeneity: its relation to malignant disease. Journal of Clinical Pathology 39: 1088–1095

Swallow D B, Gendler S, Griffiths B et al 1987 The hypervariable gene locus PUM, which codes for the tumour associated epithelial mucins is located on chromosome 1, within the region 1q21–24. Annals of Human Genetics 51: 289–294

Takada A, Ohmori K, Yoneda T et al 1993 Contribution of carbohydrate antigens sialyl Lewis a and sialyl Lewis x to adhesion of human cancer cells to vascular endothelium. Cancer Research 53: 354–361

Toribara N W, Gum J R, Culhane P J et al 1991 MUC2 human small intestinal mucin gene structure: repeated arrays and polymorphism. Journal of Clinical Investigation 88: 1005–1013

Toribara N W, Roberton A M, Ho S B et al 1993 Human gastric mucin: identification of a unique species by expression cloning. Journal of Biological Chemistry 268: 5879–5885

Torrado J, Blasco E, Cosme A, Gutierrez-Hoyos A, Arenas J I 1989 Expression of type 1 and type 2 blood group-related antigens in normal and neoplastic gastric mucosa. American Journal of Pathology 91: 249

Trahair J F, Neutra M R, Gordon J 1989 Use of transgenic mice to study routing of secretory proteins in intestinal epithelial cells. Analysis of human growth hormone compartmentalisation as a function of cell type and differentiation. Journal of Cell Biology 109: 3231–3242

Tsai H H, Hart C A, Rhodes J M 1991 Production of mucin degrading sulphatase and glycosidases by *Bacteroides thetaiotaomicron*. Letters in Applied Microbiology 13: 97–101

Tsai H H, Sunderland D, Gibson G, Hart C A, Rhodes J M 1992 A novel mucin sulphatase from human faeces: its identification, purification and characterisation. Clinical Science 82: 447–454

Tsai H H, Dwarakanath A D, Hart C A, Milton J D, Rhodes J M 1995 Increased faecal mucin sulphatase activity in ulcerative colitis: a potential target for treatment. Gut 36: 570–576

Tytgat K M A J, Buller H A, Opdam F J M, Kim Y S, Linerhand Auk, Dekker J 1994 Biosynthesis of human colonic mucin – MUC2 is the prominent secretory mucin. Gastroenterology 107(5): 1352–1363

Van-Seuningen I, Davril M, Hayem A 1989 Evidence for the tight binding of human mucus proteinase inhibitor to highly glycosylated macromolecules in sputum. Biological Chemistry Hoppe-Seyler; 370: 749–755

Variyam E P, Hoskins L C 1981 Mucin degradation in human colon ecosystems. Gastroenteroloogy 8: 751–758

Vavasseur F, Dole K, Yang J et al 1994 O-glycan biosynthesis in human colorectal adenoma cells during progression to cancer. European Journal of Biochemistry 222: 415–424

Verdugo P 1990 Goblet cell secretion and mucogenesis. Annual Review of Physiology 52: 157–176

von Itzstein M, Wu W-Y, Kok G B et al 1993 Rational design of potent sialidase-based inhibitors of influenza virus replication. Nature 363: 418–423

Wahawaisan R, Wallace L J, Gaginella T S 1983 Muscarinic receptors exist on ileal crypt and villus cells of the rat. Federal Proceedings 42: 761

Wang Y, Agrwal N, Eckhardt A E, Stevens R D, Hill R L 1993 The acceptor specificity of porcine submaxillary UDP-GalNAc:polypeptide N-acetylgalactosaminyltransferase is dependent on the amino acid sequence adjacent to serine and threonine residues. Journal of Biological Chemistry 268: 22979–22983

Winrow V R, Mojdehi G M, Ryder S D, Rhodes J M, Blake D R, Rampton D S 1993 Stress proteins in colorectal mucosa: enhanced expression in ulcerative colitis. Digestive Diseases and Sciences 38: 1994–2000

Wright N A, Pike C, Elia G 1990 Induction of a novel epidermal growth factor-secreting cell lineage by mucosal ulceration in human gastrointestinal stem cells. Nature 343: 82–85

Wright N A, Poulson R, Stamp G W H et al 1993 Trefoil peptide expression in gastrointestinal cells in inflammatory bowel disease. Gastroenterology 104: 12–20

Xu H, Sakamoto K, Shamsuddin A M 1992 Detection of the tumour marker D-galactose β1-3N-acetylgalactosamine in colonic cancer and precancer. Archives of Pathology Laboratory Medicine 116: 1234–1238

Yamashita K, Yonezawa S, Tanaka S et al 1993 Immunohistochemical study of mucin carbohydrates and core proteins in hepatolithiasis and cholangiocarcinoma. International Journal of Cancer 55: 82–91

Yedger S, Eidelman O, Malden E et al 1992 Cyclic AMP-independent secretion of mucin by SW 1116 human colon carcinoma cells. Biochemical Journal 283: 421–426

Yu L, Fernig D G, Smith J A, Milton J D, Rhodes J M 1993 Reversible inhibition of proliferation of epithelial cell lines by *Agaricus bisporus* (edible mushroom) lectin. Cancer Research 53: 4627–4632

Yuan M, Itzkowitz S H, Boland C R et al 1986 Comparison of T-antigen expression in normal, premalignant and malignant human colonic tissue using lectin and antibody immunohistochemistry. Cancer 46: 4841–4847

Yuan M, Itzkowitz S H, Palekar A et al 1985 Distribution of blood group antigens A B H Lewis a and Lewis b in human normal, fetal and malignant colonic tissue. Cancer Research 45: 4499–4511

19. Animal models – naturally occurring

B. F. Warren   P. Watkins

INTRODUCTION

Naturally occurring animal models of chronic inflammatory bowel disease (IBD), both Crohn's disease and ulcerative colitis, may help to fill some of the gaps in our knowledge of these ill-understood conditions. However, before we can extrapolate from such animal models to human disease they need careful evaluation, clinically, endoscopically, histologically, in their response to treatment, and in their development of complications within and outside the gastrointestinal tract. This chapter deals entirely with proposed models of IBD that occur naturally. It does not include any models induced experimentally, whether by chemical instillation or by genetic manipulation, as in the case of the IL-2 and IL-10 knockout mice (Sadlach et al 1993, Kuhn et al 1993). These experimentally induced models can be useful in identifying specific parts of the inflammatory process in IBD, such as cell movement, neutrophil–epithelial cell interactions, or mucin depletion, but many of them should be regarded as useful models of intestinal inflammation or ulceration rather than true models of IBD (Warren & Watkins 1993).

NATURALLY OCCURRING MODELS OF CROHN'S DISEASE

Johne's disease

The best-known spontaneously occurring model of Crohn's disease is Johne's disease of ruminants, which is caused by *Mycobacterium paratuberculosis*. This is a wasting disease of cattle with diarrhea. It causes intestinal strictures, which histologically have transmural inflammation with wall thickening and granulomas, and a profound histiocytic infiltrate in the lamina propria. In Johne's disease tissue mycobacteria can be found using special stains. Mycobacteria and mycobacteria-like organisms have never been easy to find in cases of Crohn's disease, but the similarity to Johne's disease has led to an extensive search by some workers for a mycobacterial cause of Crohn's disease (Chiodini et al 1984, McFadden et al 1987).

In 1984, Chiodini et al isolated *Mycobacterium "linda"* from two Crohn's patients: this organism was not pathogenic to rats, rabbits, guinea pigs or chickens, but following injection into an infant goat a granulomatous ileocolitis developed within 10 months. The organism bore close resemblance to *Mycobacterium paratuberculosis*, and has since been isolated by others from Crohn's patients and from stump-tailed macaques (*Macaca arctoides*) with a spontaneously occurring epidemic form of granulomatous ileocolitis which bears some pathological resemblance to Crohn's disease.

Johne's disease has been the main stimulus for studies of the role of mycobacteria in Crohn's disease (Yoshimura et al 1987) and is an important spontaneously occurring model. However, the two diseases are really quite different, in particular the frequency of finding mycobacteria is dramatically greater in Johne's disease, and the lack of metastatic spread in human Crohn's disease treated with long-term immunosuppression is also different from the expected course in a primarily infective disease treated in this way. Johne's disease is not associated with any extra intestinal manifestations of disease. Fat wrapping, an important feature of Crohn's disease in humans (Sheehan et al 1992), has not been seen in any spontaneous model of Crohn's disease, but has been seen in one induced model (Sartor et al 1995).

Ferrets

Ferrets develop a proliferative colitis associated with diarrhea, often progressing to rectal prolapse. The colon appears thickened at postmortem and there is proliferation of the colonic mucosa, with a mixed inflammatory cell infiltrate (Fox et al 1982). Intracytoplasmic campylobacter-like organisms have been demonstrated in such cases, and *Campylobacter fetus* subspecies *jejuni* has been isolated (Fox & Lawson 1988).

Pigs

Ileitis is not uncommon in pigs. Adsersen (1931) found small-bowel inflammation in 378 of 4097 animals examined at an abattoir. Pigs suffer from more than one form of ileitis, collectively referred to as the intestinal adenomatosis complex (Jubb et al 1993). The fundamental lesion is a proliferation of epithelial cells which are infected by campylobacter-like organisms (McOrist et al 1989). The lesions may progress to one of several conditions:

1. Necrotizing enteritis
2. Regional ileitis with ulceration and connective tissue changes, which result in severe thickening of the wall and stricture formation. Cases with hyperplastic changes have grown *Campylobacter sputa* subspecies *mucosalis* (Lawson & Roland 1974)
3. Proliferative hemorrhagic enteropathy, with acute or subacute intestinal haemorrhage (Emsbo 1951).

Hamsters

A terminal ileitis is seen in the Syrian hamster which has a 90% mortality and causes wall thickening and inflammation, with granuloma formation. This seems to be caused by a rod-shaped bacillus, and its histological appearance in some cases is more like yersinia than Crohn's disease (Booth & Cheveral 1967, Jackson & Wagner 1970, Amend et al 1972, Johnson & Jacoby 1978). Hamsters with chronic diarrhea often suffer from rectal bleeding due to mucosal prolapse, which is frequently fatal.

Hamsters also suffer from an enterocecocolitis caused by a campylobacter-like organism which has been demonstrated in epithelial cells (McOrist et al 1989, Schoeb & Fox 1989). Most recently it has been suggested that there is a synergistic effect between *Escherichia coli* and campylobacter, the former allowing the latter to invade enterocytes (Dillehay et al 1994).

Horses

Cimprich (1974) has described a granulomatous ileal disease of horses with associated linear ulceration and submucosal granuloma formation (Merritt et al 1976). The cause of this condition has not yet been identified.

Sheep

Sheep occasionally suffer from a terminal ileitis with linear ulceration. This usually occurs in a variety known as Texel sheep (Wensvoort 1962).

Birds

Fatal hemorrhagic ulceration of the small intestine and right colon may occur in the quail and is due to a Gram-positive anerobic rod (Berkhoff et al 1974, Berkhoff & Campbell 1974). A granulomatous small-bowel disease occurs in free-range chickens infected by mucoid-encapsulated *Escherichia coli* (Hamilton & Conrad 1958), and coccidial infection also gives rise to ileocaecal inflammation (Reid 1978).

NATURALLY OCCURRING MODELS OF ULCERATIVE COLITIS

Rodent models

The spontaneous colitis which arises in genetically manipulated rodents, such as the HLA B27 rat or the IL-2 and IL-10 knockout mice mentioned earlier, are not included here because of their previous genetic manipulation, which consigns them to the category of 'induced' models of colitis.

Spontaneous mouse models are readily available from a variety of sources. They do, however, have several disadvantages as models of human IBD. They frequently turn out to be due to an infection, and bear little clinical or histopathological resemblance to human disease. The other obvious disadvantage of small rodent models is the technical problem of repeated endoscopy and biopsy. This is usually not possible in small rodents, and therefore precludes any meaningful follow-up study of either the progress of the disease with time, or the effects of drugs on the disease.

Japanese waltzing mice suffer from a spontaneous colitis which affects predominantly the ascending colon and cecum (Tyzzer 1917). The disease has also been found to affect rats, rabbits and horses, and, as is the case with most other forms of spontaneous animal colitis, was found to be due to infection, this time by a spore-bearing bacterium, *Bacillus pyliformis* (Allen et al 1965, Mayberry et al 1984). Infectious colitis is also seen in Swiss–Webster mice infected with *Citrobacter freundii*. The mice have a distal colitis affecting the descending colon, with mucosal hyperplasia followed by diffuse mucosal inflammation, crypt abscess formation and ulceration (Barthold et al 1976). A large outbreak of colitis in mice caused by this organism was reported by Ediger et al (1974). There was increased mortality coupled with a high incidence of rectal prolapse.

Dogs

Boxer dogs are prone to develop a total colitis which is usually histiocytic, whereas other dogs may develop a lymphocytic and plasmacytic colitis.

Kennedy and Cello (1966) first described this colitis in Boxer dogs. The affected animals have bloody diarrhea, the disease is characterized by relapses and remissions, and there is usually a response to treatment with sulfasalazine.

The histopathology is somewhat different from human IBD: although granulomata are seen in the mucosa and submucosa, the overwhelming microscopic feature of this condition is the presence of large numbers of histiocytes in the lamina propria, which contain granules that stain with the periodic acid–Schiff reagent, rather like Whipple's disease in humans. Electron microscopic studies have shown chlamydia-like organisms within phagocytic vacuoles (Van Kruiningen 1967). In a subsequent study Van Kruiningen (1972) pointed out that there are several distinguishable forms of colitis in dogs, apart from the histiocytic colitis of boxers. Some examples, such as the lymphocytic plasmacytic colitis (Bush 1985) that affects many different species, resemble human ulcerative colitis clinically, and a variable response to sulfasalazine (van Meeuwisen, personal communication) and to corticosteroids has been reported. Histiocytic colitis of boxer dogs often does not respond to standard human IBD therapy, and has a much worse prognosis than other cases of idiopathic canine colitis (Bush 1992, Hall et al 1994). The boxer dog colitis does, however, seem to have a genetic component in that it is not seen in other species of dog, but plans to breed out the disease have so far been unsuccessful (Hall et al 1994).

Cats

In Germany cats have been recently observed to develop a steroid-responsive colitis, making infection an unlikely cause (Ghermai 1989).

Horses

In the horse acute colitis with severe diarrhea is often life-threatening. There are several recognized causes of this, including salmonellosis (Roberts & O'Boyle 1982), *Ehrlichia risticii* (causing Potomac horse fever) (Whitlock 1986), and enterotoxemia produced by *Clostridium perfringens* type A. Histology of the large intestine usually shows edema, hyperaemia and hemorrhage, sometimes with frank infarction.

'Colitis X' is a severe but fortunately rare disease of horses (Rooney et al 1963). This is an acute sporadic illness characterized by sudden onset of severe diarrhea without blood, which is often fatal. Histology of the large intestine shows edema, hyperemia and petechial hemorrhage, and sometimes frank infarction. In some cases *Clostridium difficile* has been implicated (Onderdonk 1985). This is an acute ischemic colitis, presumably mediated via *Clostridium difficile* toxin, which is clinically and histologically quite different from human chronic inflammatory bowel disease.

Pigs

Pigs are susceptible to an acute diarrheal illness known as swine dysentery, thought to be caused by *Spirulina hyodysenteriae* acting in synergy with other enteric bacteria such as *Bacteroides vulgatus*, *Fusobacterium necrophorum*, and *Campylobacter* species (Onderdonk 1985). Histologically there is an acute colitis and the response to antibiotic therapy is good.

More recently, *Yersinia pseudotuberculosis* has also been implicated as a cause of infective ulcerative typhylocolitis in pigs (Neef & Lysons 1994). This disease is characterized by microabscesses of the lamina propria with ulceration of the overlying epithelium. This was discovered in a 7-week-old pig with ulcerative typhylocolitis. The organism (serotype IIa) was inoculated orally into 16 growing pigs. When autopsies were performed at 10 days, typhylocolitis was present in 10 cases (Neef & Lysons 1994). The histological appearance in the published pictures is more like that of an infective colitis than human inflammatory bowel disease.

Primates

Spontaneous colitis in primates offers most hope in providing a useful model of human IBD. Colitis of varying types has been reported in several primate species over the years, but until recently very little attention has been paid to their validity as models of human disease. Primate models are usually spontaneous and require careful characterization before they can be used. They need to be similar to human disease clinically, endoscopically, histologically, and in their response to treatment – in particular to steroid therapy. The histological subclassification of human colitides is a relatively recent refinement (Day et al 1978), which is often ignored when evaluating animal models (Warren & Watkins 1994). This has allowed many infective colitides in primates, and other animals, to pass as models of human IBD.

Lowland gorilla colitis is extremely rare and not particularly useful as a model, since endoscopy presents distinct handling difficulties. Also, histologically this condition has more features resembling low-grade chronic ischemic colitis than chronic idiopathic ulcerative colitis.

Stress-induced fatal acute dysentery has been reported in four Siamang gibbons (Stout & Snyder 1969). This was ascribed to 'socioenvironmental upheaval', since no bacterial pathogen was detected. A similar colitis has been observed in orangutans (Scott & Keymer 1974), which also occurred in sporadic and unpredictable episodes.

Rhesus macaques develop a spontaneous colitis in which nitric oxide synthase induction is thought to be important in the pathogenesis (Ribbons et al 1995). The authors stress the importance of finding a spontaneous model of human IBD which is comparable to that in the cotton-top tamarin, but present in an animal which is more readily available for study. However, they go on to state that although there are similarities to the human condition the amount of ulceration and acute inflammation is much less. This model may provide a further way of studying the role of nitric oxide in IBD, although this can also be studied in humans (Boughton Smith et al 1993) and in mice (Rachmilewitz et al 1994).

Many New World monkeys develop a colitis which bears very close resemblance to human ulcerative colitis, clinically, endoscopically, histologically and in its response to treatment. *Saguinus fuscicollis illigeri* (the white-lipped tamarin) and *Callithrix jacchus* (the common marmoset) develop such a colitis (Chalmers et al 1983), but without an increased risk for complications, including colorectal carcinoma (Boland & Clapp 1987).

The cotton-top tamarin (*Saguinus oedipus oedipus*) (Fig. 19.1) is unique among New World monkeys, and indeed all spontaneous models of ulcerative colitis, in that it also develops some of the intra- and extraintestinal complications seen in humans (Kirkwood et al 1986, Warren et al 1993). The cotton-top tamarin not only quite predictably develops a colitis resembling human ulcerative colitis, but according to some reports also has a 25–40% risk for developing colonic cancer after 2–5 years in captivity (Lushbaug et al 1978, Chalifoux & Bronson 1981, Chalifoux et al 1982, Kirkwood et al 1986).

In the literature on human IBD and colorectal cancer tamarins are frequently confused with their more common relatives marmosets, another variety of New World monkey. It is therefore worth spending some time here explaining the taxonomy and characteristic features of the cotton-top tamarin. The cotton-top tamarin was first identified by Linnaeus in 1758 (Mast et al 1993) as a monkey with a striking mane of white hair. It is a New World monkey whose entire natural distribution is now in a small area of rainforest in northwest Colombia; it is an endangered species which has been listed under the highest conservation rating by CITES (Convention on International Trade in Endangered Species of Flora and Fauna). The cotton-top belongs to the family Callitrichidae, which includes 32 species in total. These comprise 15 species of Callithrix (including the common marmoset *Callithrix jacchus*), Cebuella, four lion tamarins of the genus Leontopithecus, and 12 tamarins within the species *Saguinus* (including the cotton-top tamarin, *Saguinus oedipus oedipus*).

Tamarins have been further subdivided into Amazonean and extra Amazonean, which include three taxa found in Colombia. These are *Saguinus geoffroyi*, *Saguinus oedipus* and *Saguinus leucopus*. This family provides the smallest examples of New World monkeys: they have non-prehensile tails, claws, and they move as quadrupeds. Consequently they have been referred to as 'little squirrel-like monkeys with claws' (Kavanagh 1983). All Callitrids lack the set of paired molars seen in all other New World monkeys. The teeth are an important difference between marmosets and tamarins, and reflect their different feeding habits. Marmosets have short, chisel-shaped lower incisors, which are well suited to perforating the bark of trees to extract sap and gum, on which these animals feed. The cotton-top tamarin, however, has long canines, reflecting its hunting habit for live first-class animal protein, in the form of grubs and small rodents. Apart from the constant incorrect referral in the literature to the cotton-top tamarin as a marmoset, the cotton-top goes under several alternative names. In Germany it is referred to as the 'Franz Liszt' monkey, because of the composer's equally prolific white hair. Nomenclature is even confused in southwest Colombia, its country of origin, where it is often called by the same name as *S. geoffroyi*, – bichichi – whereas in the north, titi, titis, or titi pielroja are all used synonymously for the cotton-top tamarin alone (Mast 1993).

A register of all captive cotton-top tamarins (the International Stud Book) was established in 1987 (Tardiff & Colley 1990).

The cotton-top's suitability as a model has been under discussion for some time. One of the problems has been that organisms (usually *Campylobacter jejuni*) have been isolated from some cases and not others. Some animals have responded to 5-ASA compounds whereas others have not. Recent work has helped to clarify this situation. From clinical, bacteriological, endoscopic, histologic and therapeutic studies, the cotton-top seems to develop not one but five types of colitis. One is an obvious infective colitis due to *Campylobacter jejuni*; another is a rare infection due to *Klebsiella pneumoniae*; a third resembles human pseudomembranous colitis, and the majority are

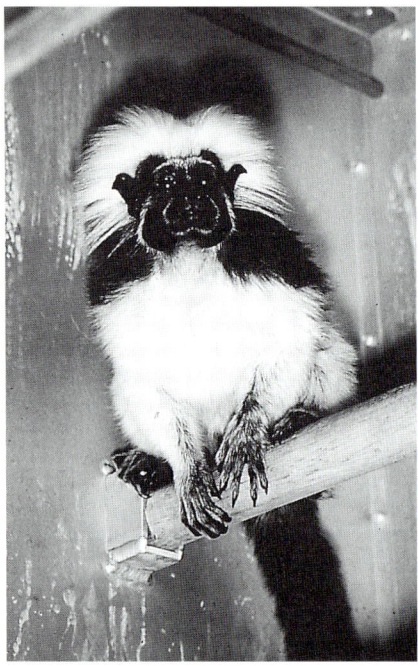

Fig. 19.1 The cotton-top tamarin (*Saguinus oedipus oedipus*).

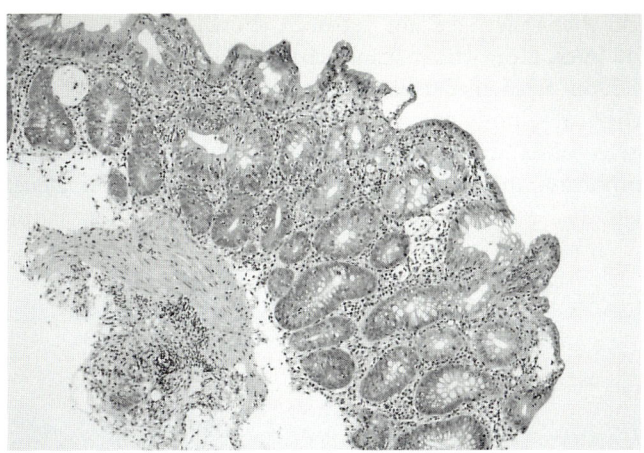

Fig. 19.2 Campylobacter colitis in the cotton-top tamarin. There is little crypt distortion, and predominantly acute inflammation with eccentric, superficial crypt abscesses.

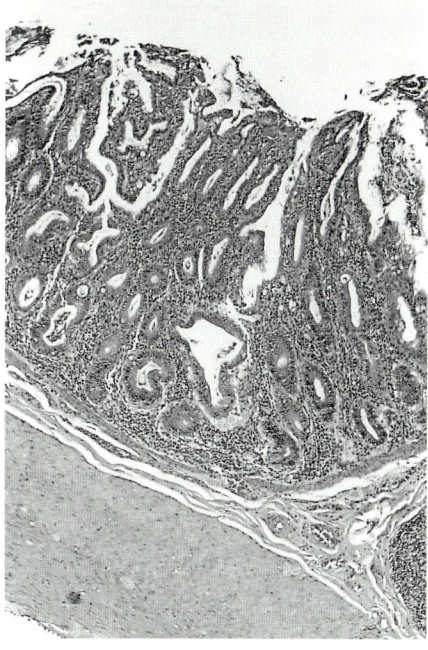

Fig. 19.3 Ulcerative colitis in the cotton-top tamarin. Here there is crypt distortion and branching. The lamina propria contains a diffuse chronic inflammatory cell infiltrate and collections of neutrophils with cryptitis and central, deep, crypt abscess formation.

like human IBD, a very small fraction of which bear some similarity to Crohn's disease.

Cotton-tops with Campylobacter colitis have offensive stools, a high peripheral blood white cell count, a total or patchy colitis endoscopically and histological appearances identical to those seen in infective colitis in humans (Day et al 1978). In this condition there is little crypt distortion and superficial, predominantly acute, inflammation with the formation of neutrophil polymorph collections in the lamina propria and superficial and eccentric crypt abscesses. Failure to recognize and treat this condition results in the rapid death of the animal. However, early treatment with erythromycin brings about rapid resolution of the colitis.

Klebsiella pneumoniae colitis is a very rare disorder of neonatal cotton-top tamarins and is the only colitis in the cotton-top which does not have a direct human counterpart. The histological appearance is of gross mucosal edema, in which many organisms may be seen.

As in humans, treatment with antibiotics in the cotton-top tamarin is not without hazard. Pseudomembranous colitis follows antibiotic therapy and is endoscopically patchy with a histological appearance of intercrypt erosions, with volcano-like eruptions of neutrophils and fibrin on the surface – a picture identical to human pseudomembranous colitis (Price & Davies 1977). This is a frequently fatal condition in the cotton-top. This is no longer seen in the Bristol colony now that antibiotics are no longer the first-line therapy for all cotton-tops with diarrhea.

We have seen only four cases that resemble Crohn's disease more closely than ulcerative colitis. Here the endoscopic inflammation and the histological inflammation were patchy, and mucosal microgranulomas were seen in two cases. These responded to the same treatment as cotton-top tamarin ulcerative colitis.

Fortunately for researchers the great majority of cases of cotton-top tamarin colitis resemble human ulcerative colitis, and the infective cases described above are quite rare. As in humans, this disease is of unknown cause but affects about 40% of captive cotton-tops at any point in time.

In some animals the disease is chronic and persisting, but in most it follows a pattern of relapse and remission. Histologically there is crypt distortion and mucin depletion. The lamina propria contains a diffuse chronic inflammatory cell infiltrate and varying amounts of acute inflammatory cells, depending on disease activity. When the disease is active crypt abscesses form, just as in humans (Madara et al 1985, Clapp et al 1988, Warren & Watkins 1994). Staining for mucin with high iron diamine/alcian blue (Spicer 1964) shows a change from normal colonic-type sulfated sialomucin to small-bowel type non-sulfated sialomucin with the development of colitis, as is seen in humans (Makwakwa et al 1992). This can be confirmed by biochemical analysis using a dual labeling technique with ^{35}S sulfate and ^{3}H glucosamine (Corfield, personal communication). There is an altered pattern of lectin binding by mucin similar to that seen in human colitis. The lectin peanut agglutinin, which binds to the mucin core disaccharide galactose β1-3-N-acetylgalactosamine, has been shown to bind to colonic goblet cell mucin in 65% of cases (Boland & Clapp 1987). Selective depletion of a mucin subclass definable by ion-exchange chromatography similar to that reported in ulcerative colitis has also been observed (Podolsky et al 1985). Active colitis is associated with elevated eicosanoid levels (leukotrienes and prostaglandins), as seen in human ulcerative colitis (Madara et al 1985, Panzini et al 1990).

The response of this condition to therapy with 5-ASA compounds and steroids is an important indicator of its non-infective nature. There has been a report of successful treatment with sulfasalazine in one colony (Madara et al 1985). In our colony the cotton-top tamarins found sulfasalazine unpalatable, no matter how well it was disguised by food. Problems of administration also occurred with enteric-coated 5-ASA compounds owing to the large size of the tablets. Fortunately, the powdered form of 5-ASA linked to another 5-ASA molecule by diazo bonds (olsalazine) has been found to be both palatable and successful in the Bristol cotton-top colony. If the colitis is mild this is the only treatment needed. However, if it is more severe (judged endoscopically), treatment with prednisolone and olsalazine is instituted, provided the stool culture is negative.

The complications of cotton-top tamarin colitis make it unique among models of human IBD (Warren & Watkins 1994). Cotton-top tamarins have for some time been known to develop colorectal carcinoma (Kirkwood et al 1986), but this has not been reported in the absence of ulcerative colitis. Like the carcinomas complicating human ulcerative colitis, these tumors are predominantly right-sided, flat and multiple; 65% are in the right side of the colon (Clapp & Henke 1993). The only two differences between cotton-top and human colonic carcinomas are that the cotton-top tumors are invariably mucinous and that they have not yet been shown to metastasize to the liver. Coexistent dysplasia (Riddell et al 1993) is rare (Clapp & Henke 1993, Warren & Watkins 1994), but when mucinous carcinomas are seen complicating ulcerative colitis in humans, dysplasia is also uncommon. It is important to realize that the cotton-top tamarin closely

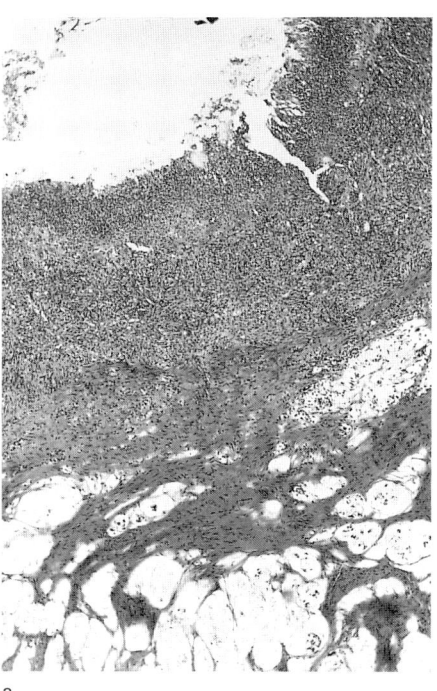

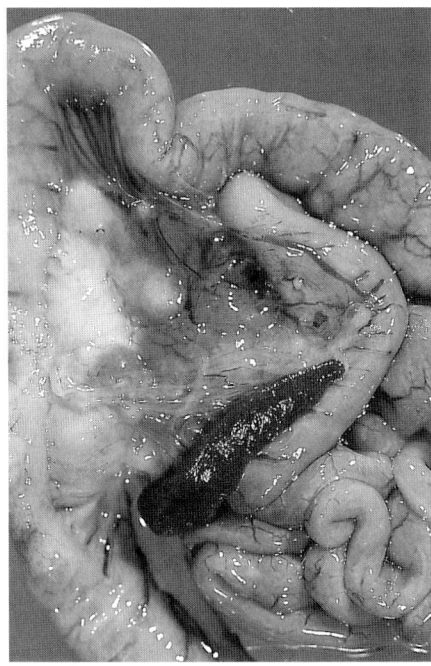

Fig. 19.4 Cotton-top tamarin colon with total ulcerative colitis and locally invasive mucinous carcinoma, with local lymph node involvement.

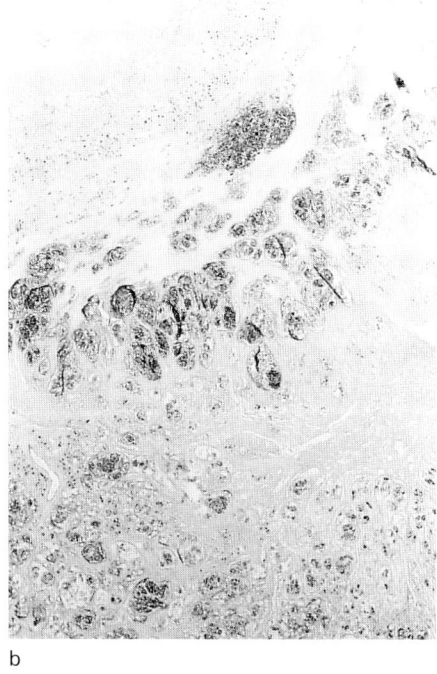

Fig. 19.5 Mucinous carcinoma invading through the full thickness of the bowel wall in the cotton-top tamarin colon. Large lakes of mucin are seen containing clumps of adenocarcinoma cells within the external muscle coat. a. HPE stained b. Alian blue/PAS stained.

parallels the non-polypoid route to carcinogenesis seen in human ulcerative colitis. In particular, this is not a model of the adenoma carcinoma sequence as seen in people without colitis. This has been a point of confusion in older publications. The lack of liver metastasis is fascinating. There is no apparent anatomical reason for this, but careful histological examination (Clapp et al 1985, Clapp & Henke 1993) has revealed a lack of angioinvasion, whereas intralymphatic and lymph node deposits are extremely common early in the course of the disease. Metastasis to sites other than lymph nodes occurs only very late in the disease process. A possible explanation for the lack of hepatic metastases and late extralymphatic spread may be that the tumors elicit a strong host response to tumor antigens, which confines them within the lymphatics until immune surveillance is eventually overwhelmed by tumor (Clapp & Henke 1993).

Another interesting similarity is the fact that cotton-top tamarin colitis is complicated by colorectal carcinoma at a specific age (usually 4–6 years) rather than after a certain duration of disease (Clapp & Henke 1993, Warren & Watkins 1994). This parallels the important three-centre study by Gyde et al (1988) in which it was proposed that some of the patients who have a genetic susceptibility to total ulcerative colitis also have a genetic susceptibility to multiple, flat, right-sided colon cancer.

More recently, liver disease has been recognized at postmortem in cotton-tops with ulcerative colitis (Warren et al 1993). The histological features seen in the liver include periportal chronic inflammation and a histological appearance wich resembles human sclerosing cholangitis, in a small number of animals dying from severe total colitis.

The cause of cotton-top tamarin colitis remains unknown. The role of any genetic susceptibility is yet to be established, although the colon cancer complicating the colitis tends to run in families (Clapp & Henke 1993, Warren & Watkins 1994). The possibility that a particular MHC class I allele may be important has been revived by demonstration that HLA B27 transgenic rats develop an ulcerative colitis-like illness (Hammer et al 1990). The cotton-top tamarin's MHC class I genes are unique, with different antigen recognition sites from any other primate (Watkins et al 1991). They are also very limited in their variation and polymorphisms compared to other species, whereas the MHC class III molecules in the cotton-top are polymorphic. It may be that one of the conserved MHC class I molecules expressed by tamarins may be similar to human HLA B27. Selective environmental pressure for a limited number of MHC class I alleles may have rendered the tamarin extremely susceptible to environmental factors not encountered in its natural habitat, which may turn out to be the cause of ulcerative colitis.

The possibility that this may be an autoimmune disorder has gained some support from the finding of an autoantibody in the cotton-top tamarin which will cross-react with colonic antigens shared by both humans and cotton-tops (Das et al 1990).

Captivity, stresss and low environmental temperature have also been suggested as possible causes (Wood et al 1993), but the true prevalence of this condition in the wild remains unknown.

Infective causes of cotton-top tamarin ulcerative colitis have been sought for many years without success. Coronavirus-like particles have been found in the feces of cotton-tops with colitis, but their significance is unknown (Brian and Shockley 1993).

CONCLUSION

The only disadvantage of cotton-top tamarin colitis as a model of human disease is the rarity of the species. This animal has a unique and important place as a model of human ulcerative colitis once it is realized that it may suffer from either infective colitis or ulcerative colitis of unknown cause, which resembles human chronic ulcerative colitis. This model may provide many of the answers concerning the pathogenesis of ulcerative colitis, the development of its complications, and meaningful studies of its therapy.

REFERENCES

Adsersen V 1931 Fortsatte undersogelser vedrorende forebyggelse of anaemi hos pattergrise. Maandschr Drylaeger 44: 465–495

Allen A M, Ganaway J R, Moore T D, Kinard R F 1965 Tyzzer's disease syndrome in laboratory rabbits. American Journal of Pathology 46: 859–882

Amend N K, Loeffler D G, Ward B C, Van Hoosier G L 1972 Transmission of enteritis in the Syrian hamster. Laboratory Animal Science 26: 566–572

Barthold S W, Coleman G L, Bhatt P N, Osbaldiston G M, Jonas A M 1976 The aetiology of transmissible murine colonic hyperplasia. Laboratory Animal Science 26: 889–894

Berkhoff G A, Campbell S G 1974 Etiology and pathogenesis of ulcerative enteritis ('quail disease'). Experimental Disease 18: 205–212

Berkhoff G A, Campbell S G, Naylor H B 1974 Etiology and pathogenesis of ulcerative enteritis ('quail disease') Characterisation of the causative anaerobe. Avian Disease 18: 195–204

Boland C R, Clapp N K 1987 Glycoconjugates in the colons of new world monkeys with spontaneous colitis. Association between inflammation and neoplasia. Gastroenterology 92: 625–634

Booth A D, Cheveral N F 1967 The pathology of proliferative ileitis of the golden hamster. Pathologia Veterinaria (Basel) 4: 31–44

Boughton-Smith N K, Evans S M, Hawkey C J et al 1993 Nitric oxide synthetase activity in ulcerative colitis. Lancet 341: 338–340

Brian D A, Shockley L J 1993 Coronavirus in tamarin and marmoset colitis. In: Clapp NK (ed) A primate mode for the study of colitis and colonic carcinoma. CRC Press, Boca Raton, pp 145–159

Bush B M 1985 Colitis in the dog. Veterinary Annual 25: 337–347

Bush B M 1992 Boxer colitis. Veterinary Record 130: 191

Chalifoux F V, Bronson R T 1981 Colonic adenocarcinoma associated with chronic colitis in cotton top marmosets, *Saguinus oedipus*. Gastroenterology 80: 942–946

Chalifoux L V, Bronson R T, Escajadillo A, McKenna S 1982 An analysis of the association of gastroenteric lesions with chronic wasting syndrome of marmosets. Veterinary Pathology 19 (Suppl 7): 141–162

Chalmers D T, Murgatroyd L B, Wadsworth P F 1983 A survey of the pathology of marmosets (*Callithrix jacchus*) derived from a marmoset breeding unit. Laboratory Animals 17: 270–279

Chiodini R J, Van Kruiningen H J, Thayer W R, Merkal R S, Coutu J 1984 A possible role of mycobacteria in inflammatory bowel disease. I An unclassified mycobacterium species isolated from patients wih Crohn's disease. Digestive Diseases and Sciences 29: 1073–1079

Cimprich R E 1974 Equine granulomatous enteritis. Veterinary Pathology I: 535–547

Clapp N K, Henke M A 1993 Spontaneous colonic carcinoma. Observations in the Oak Ridge Associated Universities' 26 year old cotton top tamarin (*Saguinus oedipus*) colony. In: Clapp N K (ed) A primate model for the study of colitis and colonic carcinoma. CRC Press, Boca Raton, pp 171–185

Clapp N K, Henke M L, Lushbaugh C, Humason G L, Gangaware B L 1988 Effect of various biological factors on spontaneous marmoset and tamarin colitis. A retrospective histopathologic study. Digestive Diseases and Sciences 33: 1013–1019

Clapp N K, Henke M A, Hansard R M, Carson R L, Adams L J Nardi R V 1993 Natural history, time course, and pathogenesis of idiopathic colitis in the cotton top tamarin (*Saguinus oedipus oedipus*). In: Clapp N K (ed) A primate model for the study of colitis and colonic carcinoma. CRC Press, Boca Raton, pp 83–89

Clapp N K, Lushbaugh C, Humason G L, Gangaware B L, Henke M A 1985 Natural history and pathology of colon cancer in *Saguinus oedipus oedipus*. Digestive Diseases and Sciences 30: 1075–1135

Das K M, Squillante L, Henke M A, Clapp N K 1990 The presence of circulating antibodies in cotton top tamarins (CTT) with spontaneous colitis against an epitope on MR 40 000 protein shared by human and CT colon epithelial cells. Gastroenterology 98: A444

Day D W, Mandal B K, Morson B C 1978 The rectal biopsy appearances in Salmonella colitis. Histopathology 2: 117–131

Dillehay D L, Paul K S, Boosinger T R, Fox J G 1994 Enterocecocolitis associated with *E. coli* and Campylobacter-like organisms in a hamster (*Mesocretus auratus*) colony. Laboratory Animal Science 44: 12–16

Ediger R D, Kovatch R M, Rabstein M M 1974 Colitis in mice with a high incidence of rectal prolapse. Laboratory Animal Science 24: 488–494

Emsbo P 1951 Terminal or regional ileitis in swine. Scandinavian Journal of Veterinary Science 3: 1–28

Fox J G, Lawson G H K 1988 Campylobacter-like omega intracellular antigen in proliferative colitis in ferrets. Laboratory Animal Science 38: 34–36

Fox J G, Murphy J C, Ackerman, Prostack K S, Gallagher C A, Rainbow V J 1982 Proliferative colitis in ferrets. American Journal of Veterinary Research 43: 858–864

Ghermai A K 1989 Chronic inflammatory bowel disease in cats. Tiermarztl-Prax 17: 195–199

Gyde S N, Prior P, Stevens A et al 1988 Colorectal carcinoma in ulcerative colitis: a cohort study of primary referrals from three centres. Gut 29: 206–217

Hall E J, Rutgers H C, Scholes S E F et al 1994 Journal of Small Animal Practice. 35: 509–515

Hamilton C M, Conrad C D 1958 Extreme mortality in Hjarre's disease (coligranuloma in chickens). Journal of the American Veterinary Medical Association 132: 84–85

Hammer R E, Maika S D, Richardson J A, Tang J P, Taurog J D 1990 Spontaneous inflammatory disease in transgenic rats expressing HLA B27 and human beta 2m: an animal model of HLA associated human disorders. Cell 63: 1099–1112

Jackson S T, Wagner J E 1970 Proliferative ileitis in Syrian hamsters (*Mesocricetus auratus*). Laboratory Animal Science 6: 12–15

Johnson E A, Jacoby R O 1978 Transmissible ileal hyperplasia of hamster. II Ultrastructure. American Journal of Pathology 91: 451–468

Jubb K V F, Kennedy P C, Palmer N 1993 Pathology of domestic animals, 4th edn. Academic Press, San Diego

Kavanagh M 1983 A complete guide to monkeys, apes, and other primates. Viking Press, New York

Kennedy P C, Cello R M 1966 Colitis of boxer dogs. Gastroenterology 51: 926–931

Kirkwood J K, Pearson G R, Epstein M A 1986 Adenocarcinoma of the large bowel and colitis in captive cotton-top tamarins *Saguinus o. oedipus*. Journal of Comparative Pathology 96: 507–515

Kuhn R, Lohler J, Rennick D, Rajewsky K, Muller W 1993 Interleukin-10-deficient mice develop chronic enterocolitis. Cell 75: 263–274

Lawson G H K, Rowland A C 1974 Intestinal adenomatosis in the pig: a bacteriological study. Research in Veterinary Science 17: 331–336

Lushbaug C C, Humason G L, Swatzendruber D C, Richter C B, Gengozian N 1978 Spontaneous colonic adenocarcinoma in marmosets. Primates in Medicine 10: 119–134

McFadden J J, Butcher P D, Chiodini R, Hermon-Taylor J 1987 Crohn's disease – isolated mycobacteria are identical to *Mycobacterium paratuberculosis* as determined by DNA probes that distinguish between mycobacterial species. Journal of Clinical Microbiology 25: 796–801

McOrist S M, Lawson G H K, Rowland A C, MacIntyre N 1989 Early lesions of proliferative enteritis in pigs and hamsters. Veterinary Pathology 26: 260–264

Madara J L, Podolsky D K, King N W, Sehgal P K, Moore R, Winter H S 1985 Characterisation of spontaneous colitis in cotton-top tamarins (*Saguinus oedipus*) and its response to sulfasalazine. Gastroenterology 88: 13–19

Makwakwa K, Warren B F, Watkins P E, Bradfield J W B 1992 Mucins in cotton top tamarin colitis. Journal of Pathology 168: 144A

Mast R B, Rodriguez J V, Mittermeier R A 1993 The Colombian cotton top tamarin in the wild. In: Clapp N K (ed) A primate model for the study of colitis and colonic carcinoma. CRC Press, Boca Raton, pp 3–43

Mayberry J F, Rhodes J, Heatley R V 1984 Infections which cause ileocolic disease in animals: are they relevant to Crohn's disease? Gastroenterology 78: 1080–1084

Merritt A M, Cimprich R E, Beech J 1976 Granulomatous enteritis in nine horses. Journal of the American Veterinary Medical Association 169: 603–609

Neef N A, Lysons R J 1994 Pathogenicity of a strain of *Yersinia pseudotuberculosis* isolated from a pig with porcine colitis syndrome. Veterinary Record 135: 58–63

Onderdonk A B 1985 Experimental models for ulcerative colitis. Digestive Diseases and Sciences 30: 405–455

Panzini B, King N, Seghal P, Podolsky D K 1990 Role of leukotrienes in the colitis of the cotton top tamarin: effect of a 5-lipoxygenase inhibitor. Gastroenterology 98: A468

Podolsky d K, Madara J L, King N, Sehgal P, Moore R, Winter H S 1985 Colonic mucin composition in primates. Selective alterations associated with spontaneous colitis in the cotton-top tamarin. Gastroenterology 88: 20–25

Price A B, Davies D R 1977 Pseudomembranous colitis. Journal of Clinical Pathology 30: 1–12

Rachmilewitz D, Stamler J S, Karmeli F, Loscalzo J, Xavier R J, Podolsky D K 1994 Role of nitric oxide in the pathogenesis of IBD. In: Rachmilewitz D (ed) Inflammatory bowel diseases. Kluwer Academic Press, Lancaster, pp 82–90

Reid W M 1978 Coccidiosis. In: Hofstad M S, Calnek B W Hambolett C F, Reid W M, Yoder H W (eds) Diseases of poultry. Iowa State University Press, Ames, Iowa, pp 784–815

Ribbons K A, Zhang X-J, Thompson J H et al 1995 Potential role of nitric oxide in a model of chronic colitis in Rhesus macaques. Gastroenterology 108: 705–711

Riddell R H, Goldman H, Ransohoff D F et al 1983 Dysplasia in inflammatory bowel disease: standardised classification with provisional clinical applications. Human Pathology 14: 931–948

Roberts M C, O'Boyle D A 1982 Experimental *Salmonella anatum* infection in horses. Australian Veterinary Journal 58: 232–240

Rooney J R, Brayans J T, Poll E R 1963 Colitis 'X' of horses. Journal of the American Veterinary Medical Association 142: 510–511

Sadlach B, Merz H, Schorle H, Schimpl A, Feller A C, Horak I 1993 Ulcerative colitis-like disease in mice with disrupted interleukin 2 gene. Cell 75: 253–261

Sartor R B, Cromarties W J, Powell D W, Schwab J H 1985 Granulomatous enterocolitis induced in rats by purified bacterial cell wall fragments. Gastroenterology 89: 587–595

Schoeb T R, Fox J G 1989 Enterocecocolitis associated with intraepithelial Campylobacter-like bacteria in rabbits. Veterinary Pathology 26: 260–264

Scott G B D, Keymer I F 1974 Ulcerative colitis in apes: comparison with the human disease. Journal of Pathology 115: 241–244

Sheehan A L, Warren B F, Shepherd N A, Gear M W L 1992 Fat wrapping in Crohn's disease. British Journal of Surgery 79: 955–958

Spicer S S 1964 Diamine methods for differentiating mucosubstances histochemically. Journal of Histochemistry and Cytochemistry 13: 211–233

Stout C, Snyder R L 1969 Ulcerative colitis-like lesion in siamang gibbons. Gastroenterology 57: 256–260

Tardiff S D, Colley R. International cotton top tamarin stud book, 3rd edn. Oak Ridge Association University, Oak Ridge T N 1990

Tyzzer E 1917 A fatal disease of the Japanese waltzing mouse characterised by a spore-bearing bacillus. Journal of Medical Research 37: 307–338

Van Kruiningen H J 1967 Granulomatous colitis of boxer dogs: comparative aspects. Gastroenterology 53: 114–122

Van Kruiningen H J 1972 Canine colitis comparable to regional enteritis and mucosal colitis of man. Gastroenterology 62: 1128–1142

Warren B F, Watkins P E 1993 Animal models. In: Scholmerich J, Kruis W, Goebel H, Hohenberger W, Gross V (eds) Inflammatory bowel diseases. Kluwer Academic Press, London, pp 3–7

Warren B F, Watkins P E 1994 Animal models of inflammatory bowel disease. Journal of Pathology 172: 313–316

Warren B F, Henke M, Clapp N K 1993 Extraintestinal manifestations. In: Clapp N K (ed) A primate model for the study of colitis and colonic carcinoma. CRC Press, Boca Raton, pp 127–132

Watkins D I, Chen Z W, Toukatly G, Hughes A L, Letvin N L 1991 Unusually limited nucleotide sequence variation of the expressed major histocompatibility complex class I genes for a New World primate species (*Saguinus oedipus oedipus*). Immunogenetics 33: 79

Watkins P E, Foulkes R, Stephens S, Ward P, Warren B F 1993 Faecal tumour necrosis factor alpha in cotton top tamarin colitis. Journal of Pathology 170: 364A

Wensvoort P 1962 Rekkers of strekkers een aandoening bij lammeren. Tijdschr Diergeneesk 87: 841–884

Whitlock R H 1986 Colitis: differential diagnosis and treatment. Equine Veterinary Journal 18: 278–283

Wood J D, Peck O C, Sharma H M et al 1993 Stress induced inflammatory changes in the cotton top tamarin model for spontaneous colitis and colon cancer. Gastroenterology 104: A803

Yoshimura H H, Graham D Y, Estes M K, Merkal R S 1987 Investigation of association of mycobacteria with inflammatory bowel disease by nucleic acid hybridisation. Journal of Clinical Microbiology 25: 45–51

20. Animal models of inflammatory bowel disease – experimental

J. L. Wallace   C. M. Hogaboam

INTRODUCTION

An ideal animal model of inflammatory bowel disease (IBD) is one that exhibits the entire spectrum of clinical and pathological manifestations of the human condition (MacPherson & Pfeiffer 1976). In addition, for an animal model to be a practical investigational tool it should be inexpensive, easy to reproduce, and therapeutically manipulated with the same agents that are used to treat the human counterpart. For many applications it is also desirable that the animal model has a predictable clinical course. For this reason, and because of their cost, some of the 'spontaneous' models of colitis are less attractive for some applications, and efforts have been made to develop simple, inexpensive and reproducible models of IBD that involve induction of intestinal inflammation, usually via administration of a chemical irritant or by elicitation of a mucosal immune response.

The various strategies taken to develop models are based on the following premises regarding the etiology of inflammatory bowel disease:

1. IBD is most likely triggered by a luminal agent such as a microbe, a microbial byproduct, a dietary antigen or other environmental factors.
2. An inappropriate response of the mucosal immune system to the triggering event may produce an inflammatory reaction that is self-amplifying.
3. The impaired mucosal immune response may be a consequence of an inheritable defect.

Thus experimental models have been developed that involve the administration of an antigen (or hapten), other forms of stimulation of the mucosal immune system, administration of bacterial products into the lamina propria, or dietary manipulation that gives rise to intestinal inflammation. In some cases the genetic component of chronic inflammation has been probed by eliciting intestinal inflammation in a variety of inbred strains of rodents.

INFECTIOUS AGENTS

Many models of IBD are the products of early experiments in which patient tissue or potential causative factors of IBD were introduced into animals. For example, Crohn et al (1932) originally described what is now called 'Crohn's disease' as histologically resembling intestinal tuberculosis. Many years later, Mitchell and Rees (1970) demonstrated that filtered tissue homogenates from Crohn's disease patients injected into the footpads of mice induced local and ileal granulomatous inflammation. Similarly, Cave et al (1975) found that intestinal tissue homogenates from Crohn's disease patients injected into the ileal wall of the rabbit induced granulomatous inflammation and mucosal ulceration. Das et al (1980) observed that athymic mice developed lymphomas following the injection of homogenates of lymph nodes from Crohn's disease patients, providing further support for the proposal that some transmissible 'biological factor' induced Crohn's disease. However, these studies have proved difficult to reproduce (Cohen et al 1981), and the transmissible factor capable of inducing intestinal inflammation in these animal models has never been identified, despite repeated attempts (Phillpotts et al 1980).

Intestinal inflammation can also be produced by administering various strains of bacteria or bacterial components to animals. For example, Chiodini et al (1984) isolated *Mycobacterium paratuberculosis* from resected Crohn's disease tissue by prolonged in-vitro culturing techniques and demonstrated that this organism could induce ileal granulomatous lesions when administered to young goats and mice.

Another 'infectious' model of IBD is that described by Sartor et al (1985), who demonstrated that the injection of streptococcal cell wall fragments (a peptidoglycan–polysaccharide complex) into the cecal wall of inbred rats produced a chronic granulomatous inflammation. Granulomatous inflammation could also be produced by injecting the peptidoglycan–polysaccharide complex into the wall of the rat colon (Yamada et al 1993a). Interestingly, some of the rats treated with peptidoglycan–polysaccharide developed extraintestinal inflammation similar to that seen in human Crohn's disease, including arthritis and biliary tract inflammation. McCall et al (1994) have also used this model to probe the genetic component of intestinal inflammation, and have identified some strains of inbred rats which are resistant to both the intestinal and extraintestinal inflammation following peptidoglycan–polysaccharide complex administration.

Infection of rodents with intestinal parasites has provided valuable models of intestinal inflammation that have been extensively studied (Moqbel 1986). Although these are not purported to be models of IBD per se, they are reliable and predictable models of intestinal inflammation. Two helminths that are commonly used to induce intestinal inflammation in the rat and other species are *Nippostrongylus brasiliensis* and *Trichinella spiralis*. In both of these infections the inflammatory response has been shown to be T-lymphocyte dependent. Both models are characterized by significant increases in the numbers of eosinophils and mast cells in the small intestine. This is significant, since the numbers of both of these cell types are elevated in affected tissues in IBD (Dvorak et al 1980, King et al 1992). These models are also characterized by profound changes in epithelial secretion (Perdue et al 1984, Russell & Castro 1985), smooth muscle structure and function (Diamant et al 1989, Muller et al 1989) and inflammatory mediator production (Perdue et al 1989, Hogaboam et al 1991).

CHEMICAL- AND HAPTEN-INDUCED COLITIS

Experimental intestinal inflammation can be produced using a single agent or a mixture of agents, administered directly into the lumen of the intestine or injected into the lamina propria. Typically, the luminally applied agents destroy the epithelial barrier and/or activate resident mucosal inflammatory cells, and either directly or indirectly promote the influx of granulocytes into the mucosa. Although many caustic agents can induce an acute inflammatory response in the intestine, the development of chronic inflammation usually involves the persistent presence of a foreign material or antigen, or an alteration in the quantity or composition of enteric flora.

Acetic acid

Perhaps the most widely used of the 'caustic' models of colitis is that induced by intraluminal administration of acetic acid, usually in concentrations in the range of 4–10%. This solution produces widespread epithelial injury to the tissue with which it has direct contact. Within 24–48 hours after its application, a considerable infiltration of granulocytes into the affected area can be detected. Ulceration is evident during the first few days after acetic acid administration, but heals rapidly. This simple model has been used in rats, rabbits and guinea pigs (Krawisz et al 1984, Fretland et al 1990). Many drugs which accelerate healing in IBD also reduce the severity of injury in this model (Conzentino et al 1986, Fedorak et al 1990). The major drawback of this model is the relatively short period of active inflammation, thereby preventing its being used for studies of repeated drug administration or dietary manipulation. Moreover, from a histological standpoint the injury induced by acetic acid more closely resembles ischemic colitis than IBD.

Trinitrobenzene sulfonic acid

A major disadvantage of most of the models of IBD that employ a caustic agent is the lack of chronicity of the inflammatory response. The colitis induced by intracolonic administration of trinitrobenzene sulfonic acid (TNBS) has become a widely used model (Kim & Berstad 1992) because the inflammation persists for several months. Furthermore, the model has been reproduced in numerous laboratory animal species (including rat, mouse, rabbit, cat and guinea pig), is relatively inexpensive, shares many histological similarities with IBD, and is characterized by augmented inflammatory mediator synthesis similar to IBD. The development of this model by Morris and colleagues (1989) was based on the hypothesis of Ward (1977) that IBD develops because an abnormally permeable mucosal barrier allows the entry of a luminal antigen into the lamina propria, which is poorly cleared by the mucosal immune system (Morris et al 1989). Although a single antigen responsible for initiating IBD has never been identified, there is considerable evidence that altered mucosal permeability may play an important role (Hollander et al 1986, May et al 1993). A single instillation into the rat colon of TNBS dissolved in ethanol produces chronic ulceration and inflammation, which persists for more than 8 weeks. Ethanol acts as a barrier breaker, allowing the hapten, TNBS, access to the lamina propria. TNBS covalently binds to cell surface proteins, and thereafter behaves as an antigen. If the animal has previously been sensitized to this antigen, T lymphocytes will subsequently lyse these cells (Teh et al 1978). However, this model also works in animals that have not been presensitized, since macrophages will also destroy the TNBS-binding cells. Furthermore, it has been shown that TNBS can undergo metabolism in the colon to yield various reactive oxygen metabolites, which are cytotoxic (Grisham et al 1991). In support of the hypothesis that TNBS acts through these immune mechanisms, rather than purely as a caustic agent, are the observations that prior sensitization or tolerization of animals to TNBS results in an increase or decrease, respectively, in the severity of colitis (Beck et al 1988). Systemic re-exposure to TNBS many weeks after the initial intracolonic administration results in a 'reactivation' of the colitis (Appleyard & Wallace 1995). Furthermore, the severity of colonic epithelial injury can be significantly attenuated through treatment with an immunosuppressant (Higa et al 1993).

A substantial portion of the mucosal injury associated with TNBS-induced colitis is attributable to infiltration granulocytes. The increases in colonic epithelial permeability associated with TNBS colitis in the rabbit were prevented or reversed by treating the animals with monoclonal antibodies directed against CD18, a leukocyte adhesion glycoprotein that mediates leukocyte adherence to and migration across the vascular endothelium (Wallace et al 1992b).

Dinitrochlorobenzene

Another hapten that has been utilized to elicit experimental colitis is dinitrobenzenesulfonic acid (DNCB). Rosenberg and Fischer (1964) demonstrated that painting a solution of this hapten on the skin of guinea pigs, and intrarectal administration of the hapten 7 days later, resulted in colonic edema, vasodilation and significant inflammatory cell infiltration. This inflammatory response was transient, however, with the colon appearing histologically normal within 3 days (Glick & Falchuk 1981). This model is believed to represent delayed-type hypersensitivity, with an involvement of T lymphocytes supported by the observation that sensitivity to the hapten could be passively transferred by T cells (Bicks et al 1965).

Sulfated polysaccharides

Marcus and Watt (1969) demonstrated that the addition of degraded carrageenan (a sulfated polysaccharide from red seaweed) to the drinking water of guinea pigs and rabbits produced large mucosal lesions in the cecum and colon of these animals. The lesions typically appeared within 7–14 days in the cecum, and 30 days later in the colon and rectum. In other studies it was shown that carrageenan promoted cecal and colonic damage through mechanisms that involved the activation of resident macrophages (Abraham et al 1974) and alteration of the cecal microflora to specifically promote the overgrowth of *Bacteroides vulgatus* (Onderdonk et al 1983). Carrageenan did not induce ulcers in germ-free rats, and antimicrobials were only effective when administered before the carrageenan (Onderdonk et al 1978). Although the lesions induced by carrageenan are histologically similar to those seen in IBD, the utility of this model is limited by the damage being predominantly localized to the cecum, as well as the considerable amount of time required for the development of the lesions. Maintenance of inflammation depends upon continued administration of carrageenan (Watt & Marcus 1973).

The importance of bacterial overgrowth in the development of animal colitis has also been demonstrated using a model in which dextran sulfate sodium (DSS) was administered orally to mice (Okayasu et al 1990). DSS administration for 8 days produced an overgrowth of anerobic microbes, including *Bacteroides* and *Clostridium* species and, similarly to carrageenan-induced colitis, augmented macrophage function was apparent. This model is unique, however, in that DSS induced mucosal erosions and inflammation only in the colon and rectum. Furthermore, a chronic intestinal inflammatory response was produced if the mice received a cycled regimen of oral DSS in distilled water for 7 days followed by distilled water alone for 10 days. After four or five cycles, chronic intestinal inflammation was apparent which did not require further administration of DSS.

Non-steroidal anti-inflammatory drugs

Ingestion of non-steroidal anti-inflammatory drugs (NSAIDs) has been associated with exacerbation of pre-existing or reactivation of quiescent IBD (Kauffman & Taubin 1987), and has also been shown to exacerbate experimental colitis (Woolverton et al 1989, Wallace et al 1992b). Bjarnason and Peters (1989) suggested that NSAIDs may play a role in the etiology of IBD, particularly Crohn's disease, since these drugs were found to cause a profound and long-lasting increase in intestinal permeability which could lead to enhanced translocation of bacterial and/or antigen. Data from animal studies support this hypothesis. Stewart et al (1980) reported that dogs given indomethacin or cincophen for up to 1 month developed colitis, which was characterized by patchy ulceration of the mucosa, predominantly around lymphoid follicles, and granulomatous inflammation in the mucosa and mesenteric lymph nodes. Inflammation of the jejunum and ileum resembling that in Crohn's disease can be induced in rats within 24 hours of oral administration of indomethacin or other NSAIDs. Lesions were substantially less severe when indomethacin was administered to germ-free rats (Robert 1975), and can be prevented by treatment with some antimicrobials (Kent et al 1969, Bjarnason et al 1992, Yamada et al 1993b), supporting a role for enteric bacteria in their pathogenesis. This is further supported by the observation that luminal bacterial counts increased markedly after administration of NSAIDs to rats (Kent et al 1969, Yamada et al 1993b), although it is not yet clear if this occurs before or purely as a consequence of the onset of damage.

VASCULAR OCCLUSION

Attempts have been made to develop animal models of colitis through the occlusion of mesenteric microvessels. For example, Hudson et al (1992) ligated as many as 30 adjacent vasae rectae in the ferret, but found that this produced no evidence of ischemic damage. On the other hand, this group (using ferrets) and Boley et al (1965) (using dogs) produced colitis by administering microspheres into the mesenteric circulation. Hudson et al (1992) reported that a combination of 27 and 90 μm microspheres, injected into the submucosal collateral plexus, resulted in focal mucosal inflammation, necrosis and ulceration. Lesions were observed 48 hours after microsphere administration, and by 72 hours there was evidence of regeneration of the mucosa. The inflammatory infiltrate at 24 hours post injection was primarily neutrophilic, and by 48 hours there was a predominance of lymphocytes in the infiltrate. The authors conclude that their study provides evidence that focal gastrointestinal infarct leading to mucosal inflammation can be elicited by this method, with adjacent regions of mucosa appearing normal.

IMMUNE COMPLEX-INDUCED COLITIS

Kraft et al (1963) first demonstrated that colonic inflammation could be induced using the 'Auer' procedure. This involved immunization of rabbits with egg albumin to induce a generalized antibody response, followed 10–14 days later by the intracolonic injection of 1% formalin. Colitis was subsequently induced by intravenous injection of egg albumin, or by its local injection into the wall of the intestine. In this manner, circulating immune complexes entered the intestinal mucosa at the areas where formalin had damaged the vasculature (Lowes & Jewell 1990), thus evoking a local inflammatory response. Hodgson et al (1978) simplified this model by directly infusing immune complexes into non-sensitized rabbits subsequent to a formalin enema. They also noted that an acute colitis developed that was self-limiting and healed rapidly if the formalin or egg albumin was not constantly reapplied (Lowes & Jewell 1990). This technique was modified further by Mee et al (1979) to obtain a chronic model of intestinal damage. In this study, animals were immunized with an *Escherichia coli* antigen prior to the formalin enema, and then rechallenged with the same antigen. They found that severe intestinal damage was still apparent 6 months after its initiation. These results suggest that hypersensitivity to native bacterial antigens in the intestine may be one mechanism through which acute colitis develops into more chronic inflammation (Kim & Berstad 1992).

SUMMARY

Although experimental models of intestinal inflammation cannot provide a complete representation of all of the clinical features of a complex disease such as IBD, they are nevertheless valuable tools for studying the pathogenesis of intestinal inflammation and for assessing novel anti-inflammatory regimens. Each model has a number of advantages and disadvantages, and the relative value of each depends primarily on the question or hypothesis that is to be addressed. For example, if a model is being used as a primary screen for the efficacy of a novel anti-inflammatory drug, some of the simple chemical models may be the most suitable. On the other hand, if an investigator is interested in studying the factors affecting the progression from acute to chronic inflammation, or the role of enteric bacteria in chronic inflammation, some of the immune-mediated models may be more suitable.

This chapter has reviewed the experimental models of colitis that are most suitable for the testing of therapeutic agents. Recent gene knock-out animals have given us considerable information about the complex relationship between the immune system and the colonic flora but are as yet less available and arguably less suitable for testing therapy. They are discussed in Chapter 15 and well reviewed by Elson et al (1995).

REFERENCES

Abraham R, Fabian R J, Goldberg L, Coulston F 1974 Role of lysosomes in carrageenan-induced cecal ulceration. Gastroenterology 67: 1169–1181

Appleyard C B, Wallace J L 1995 Reactivation of hapten-induced colitis and its prevention by anti-inflammatory drugs. American Journal of Physiology 269: G119–G125

Beck P L, Morris G P, Wade A W, Szewczuk M, Wallace J L 1988 Immunological manipulation of disease progression in a rat model of chronic inflammatory disease of the colon. In MacDermott R P (ed) Inflammatory bowel disease: current status and future approach. Elsevier Science Publishers, Amsterdam, pp 201–206

Bicks R O, Brown G, Hicky D, Rosenberg E W 1965 Further observations on a delayed hypersensitivity reaction in guinea pig colon. Gastroenterology 48: 425–429

Bjarnason I, Peters T J 1989 Intestinal permeability, non-steroidal anti-inflammatory drug enteropathy and inflammatory bowel disease: an overview. Gut 30 (Suppl): 22–28

Bjarnason I, Hayllar J, Smethurst P, Price A, Gumpel M J 1992 Metronidazole reduces intestinal inflammation and blood loss in non-steroidal anti-inflammatory drug induced enteropathy. Gut 33: 1204–1208

Boley S J, Krieger H, Schultz L et al 1965 Experimental aspects of peripheral vascular occlusion of the intestine. Surgery Gynecology and Obstetrics 789–794

Cave D R, Mitchell D N, Brooke B N 1975 Experimental animal studies of the etiology and pathogenesis of Crohn's disease. Gastroenterology 69: 618–624

Chiodini R J, Van Kruiningen H J, Thayer W R Jr, Merkal R S, Contu J A 1984 Possible role of mycobacteria in inflammatory bowel disease. I. An unclassified mycobacterium species isolated from patients with Crohn's disease. Digestive Diseases and Sciences 29: 1073–1079

Cohen Z, Leung M K, Jirsch D, Archibald S, Cullen J, Gardner J 1981 Transmission of IBD homogenates in inbred mice and rabbits. In Pena A S (ed) Recent advances in Crohn's disease. Martinus Nijhoff, Boston, pp 259–265

Conzentino P, Will P C, Lin A, Gaginella T S 1986 Effect of 5-lipoxygenase inhibitors on acetic acid colitis in the rat. Pharmacologist 28: 163

Crohn B B, Ginzburg L, Oppenheimer G D 1932 Regional ileitis: a pathological and clinical entity. Journal of the American Medical Association 99: 1323–1328

Das K M, Valenzuela I, Morecki P 1980 Crohn's disease lymph node homogenates produce murine lymphoma in athymic mice.

Proceedings of the National Academy of Sciences of the USA 77: 588–592

Diamant S C, Gall D G, Scott R B 1989 The effect of intestinal anaphylaxis on postprandial motility in the rat. Canadian Journal of Physiology and Pharmacology 67: 1326–1330

Dvorak A M, Monahan R A, Osage J E, Dickerson G R 1980 Crohn's disease: transmission electron microscope studies. II. Immunologic inflammatory response. Alterations of mast cell, basophils and eosinophils, and the microvasculature. Human Pathology 11: 606–619

Elson C O, Sartor R B, Tennyson G S, Riddell R H 1995 Experimental models of inflammatory bowel disease. Gastroenterology 109: 1344–1367

Fedorak R N, Empey L R, MacArthur C, Jewell L D 1990 Misoprostol provides a colonic mucosal protective effect during acetic acid-induced colitis in rats. Gastroenterology 98: 615–622

Fretland D J, Widomski D L, Tsai B S 1990 Effect of leukotriene B4 receptor antagonist SC-41930 on colonic inflammation in rat, guinea pig and rabbit. Journal of Pharmacology and Experimental Therapeutics 255: 572–576

Glick M E, Falchuk Z M 1981 Dinitrochlorobenzene-induced colitis in the guinea pig: studies of colonic lamina propria lymphocytes. Gut 22: 120–125

Grisham M B, Volkmer C, Tso P, Yamada T 1991 Metabolism of trinitrobenzene sulfonic acid by the rat colon produces reactive oxygen species. Gastroenterology 101: 540–547

Higa A, McKnight G W, Wallace J L 1993 Attenuation of epithelial injury in acute experimental colitis by immunomodulators. European Journal of Pharmacology 239: 171–176

Hodgson H J F, Potter B J, Skinner J, Jewell D P 1978 Immune-complex mediated colitis in rabbits. Gut 19: 225–232

Hogaboam C M, Befus A D, Wallace J L 1991 Intestinal platelet-activating factor synthesis during Nippostrongylus brasiliensis infection in the rat. Journal of Lipid Mediators 4: 211–224

Hollander D, Vadheim C M, Brettholz E, Peterson G M, Delahunty T, Rotter J I 1986 Increased intestinal permeability in patients with Crohn's disease and their relatives. Annals of Internal Medicine 105: 883–885

Hudson M, Piasecki C, Sankey E A et al 1992 A ferret model of acute multifocal gastrointestinal infarction. Gastroenterology 102: 1591–1596

Kaufmann H J, Taubin H L 1987 Nonsteroidal anti-inflammatory drugs activate quiescent inflammatory bowel disease. Annals of Internal Medicine 107: 513–516

Kent T H, Cardelli R M, Stamler F W 1969 Small intestinal ulcers and intestinal flora in rats given indomethacin. American Journal of Pathology 54: 237–249

Kim H-S, Berstad A 1992 Experimental colitis in animal models. Scandinavian Journal of Gastroenterology 27: 529–537

King T, Biddle W, Bhatia P, Moore J, Miner P B 1992 Colonic mucosal mast cell distribution at line of demarcation of active ulcerative colitis. Digestive Diseases and Sciences 37: 490–495

Kraft S C, Fitch F W, Kirsner J B 1963 Histologic and immunohistochemical features of Auer 'colitis' in rabbits. American Journal of Pathology 43: 913–923

Krawisz J E, Sharon P, Stenson W F 1984 Quantitative assay for acute intestinal inflammation based on myeloperoxidase activity. Gastroenterology 87: 1344–1350

Lowes J R, Jewell D P 1990 The immunology of inflammatory bowel disease. Springer Seminars in Immunopathology 12: 251–268

McCall R D, Haskill S, Zimmerman E M, Lund P K, Thompson R C, Sartor R B 1994 Tissue interleukin-1 and interleukin-1 receptor antagonist expression in enterocolitis in resistant and susceptible rats. Gastroenterology 106: 960–972

MacPherson B, Pfeiffer C J 1976 Experimental colitis. Digestion 14: 424–452

Marcus R, Watt J 1969 Seaweeds and ulcerative colitis in laboratory animals. Lancet 2: 489–490

May G R, Sutherland L R, Meddings J B 1993 Is small intestinal permeability really increased in relatives of patients with Crohn's disease? Gastroenterology 104: 1627–1632

Mee A S, McLaughlin J E, Hodgson H J F, Jewell D P 1979 Chronic immune colitis in rabbits. Gut 20: 1–5

Mitchell D N, Rees R J W 1970 Agent transmissible from Crohn's disease tissue. Lancet 2: 168–171

Moqbel R 1986 Helminth-induced intestinal inflammation. Transactions of the Royal Society of Tropical Medicine and Hygiene 80: 719–727

Morris G P, Beck P L, Herridge M S, Depew W T, Szewczuk M R, Wallace J L 1989 Hapten-induced model of chronic inflammation and ulceration in the rat colon. Gastroenterology 96: 795–803

Muller M J, Huizinga J D, Collins S M 1989 Altered smooth muscle contraction and sodium pump activity in the inflamed rat intestine. American Journal of Physiology 257: G570–G577

Okayasu I, Hatakeyama S, Yamada M, Ohkusa T, Inagaki Y, Nakaya R 1990 A novel method in the induction of reliable experimental acute and chronic ulcerative colitis in mice. Gastroenterology 98: 694–702

Onderdonk A B, Cisneros R L, Bronson R T 1983 Enhancement of experimental ulcerative colitis by immunization with Bacteroides vulgatus. Infection and Immunity 42: 783–788

Onderdonk A B, Hermos J A, Dzink J L, Bartlett J G 1978 Protective effect of metronidazole in experimental ulcerative colitis. Gastroenterology 74: 521–526

Perdue M H, Chung M, Gall D G 1984 Effect of intestinal anaphylaxis on gut function in the rat. Gastroenterology 86: 391–397

Perdue M H, Ramage J K, Burget D, Marshall J, Masson S 1989 Intestinal mucosal injury is associated with mast cell activation and leukotriene generation during Nippostrongylus-induced inflammation in the rat. Digestive Diseases and Sciences 34: 724–731

Phillpotts R J, Hermon-Taylor J, Teich N M, Brooke B N 1980 A search for persistent virus infection in Crohn's disease. Gut 21: 202–207

Robert A 1975 An intestinal disease produced experimentally by a prostaglandin deficiency. Gastroenterology 69: 1045–1047

Rosenberg E W, Fischer R W 1964 DNCB allergy in the guinea pig colon. Archives of Dermatology 89: 99–103

Russell D A, Castro G A 1985 Anaphylactic-like reaction of small intestinal epithelium in parasitized guinea-pigs. Immunology 54: 573–579

Sartor R B, Cromartie W J, Powell D W, Schwab J H 1985 Granulomatous enterocolitis induced in rats by purified bacterial cell wall fragments. Gastroenterology 89: 587–595

Stewart T H M, Hetenyi C, Rowsell H, Orizaga M 1980 Ulcerative colitis in dogs induced by drugs. Journal of Pathology 131: 363–378

Teh H S, Phillips R A, Miller R G 1978 Quantitative studies on the precursors of cytotoxic lymphocytes. The cellular basis of the cross-reactivity of TNP-specific clones. Journal of Immunology 121: 1711–1718

Wallace J L, Keenan C M, Gale D, Shoupe T S 1992 Exacerbation of experimental colitis by nonsteroidal anti-inflammatory drugs is not related to elevated leukotriene B_4 synthesis. Gastroenterology 101: 18–27

Wallace J L, Higa A, McKnight G W, McIntyre D E 1992 Prevention and reversal of experimental colitis by a monoclonal antibody which inhibits leukocyte adherence. Inflammation 16: 343–354

Ward M 1977 The pathogenesis of Crohn's disease. Lancet 1: 903–905

Watt J, Marcus R 1973 Experimental ulcerative disease of the colon in animals. Gut 14: 506–510

Woolverton C J, White J J, Sartor R B 1989 Eicosanoid regulation of acute intestinal vascular permeability induced by intravenous peptidoglycan–polysaccharide polymers. Agents and Actions 26: 301–309

Yamada T, Sartor R B, Marshall S, Specian R D, Grisham M B 1993a Mucosal injury and inflammation in a model of chronic granulomatous colitis in rats. Gastroenterology 104: 759–771

Yamada T, Deitch E, Specian R D, Perry M A, Sartor R D, Grisham M B 1993b Mechanisms of acute and chronic intestinal inflammation induced by indomethacin. Inflammation 17: 641–662

21. Pathophysiology of small-intestinal dysfunction in Crohn's disease

R. C. Spiller

The impact of Crohn's disease on small-bowel function is very variable, depending on the distribution and severity of the disease. This is often underestimated radiologically, panendoscopy revealing unsuspected aphthous ulcers, mucosal edema and radiologically occult stenoses (Fitzgerald et al 1992, Lescut et al 1993). This may explain why abnormalities of small-bowel function are frequently reported in Crohn's colitis in spite of normal radiology. Although the brunt of Crohn's disease is usually born by the ileum, the jejunum and the duodenum are often occultly involved, especially where anorexia and nausea are prominent symptoms (Lenaerts et al 1989), when gastric emptying is often delayed.

The effect of radiologically occult disease is relatively subtle compared with the severe, often debilitating, malabsorptive syndromes that develop following repeated surgical resection, which usually includes the terminal ileum. The functions served by this region are those most often affected (Fig. 21.1), including most importantly salt and water absorption, vitamin B_{12} and bile salt absorption. The loss of the ileocecal valve which frequently accompanies ileal resection may also lead to small-bowel contamination, with consequent malabsorption of fat, B_{12} and other nutrients.

WATER AND ELECTROLYTE ABSORPTION

Although a normal homogenized diet has a relatively low sodium concentration (35 mmol/l), after the addition of sodium-rich pancreatic and biliary secretions there is a rapid equilibration with extracellular fluid across the relatively permeable jejunum, which usually means a further influx of sodium, yielding a luminal concentration of 120–140 mmol per liter (Fig. 21.2). This means that sodium is the dominant electrolyte, whose absorption largely determines water absorption and hence fluid fluxes through the small bowel (Spiller et al 1986a). Inflamed small (Allan et al 1975) and large (Head et al 1969) bowel affected by Crohn's disease has been shown to demonstrate impaired net absorption of sodium and water, due mainly to decreased mucosa→serosa, as well as a small increase in serosa→mucosa, fluxes (Atwell & Duthie 1964). Increased permeability and decreased absorption appears to be a generalized feature of intestinal inflammation (Hawker et al 1980).

Numerous inflammatory mediators have been shown to stimulate secretion, including histamine, bradykinin,

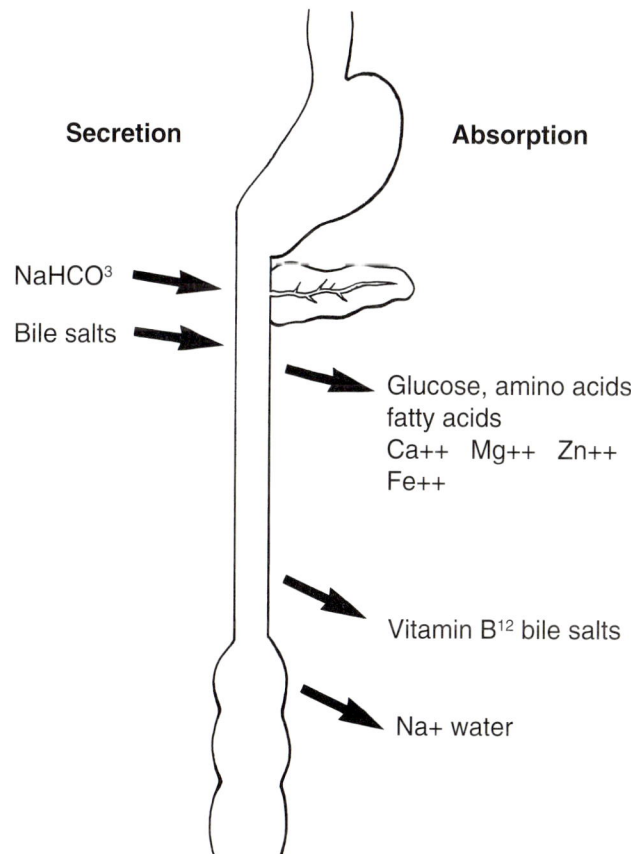

Fig. 21.1 Regional variations in absorption and secretion. After a substantial initial secretion of facilitators of digestion and absorption, namely sodium, water, bile and pancreatic enzymes, most nutrients and minerals are absorbed proximally. This leaves the bulk of the sodium and water to be absorbed distally, together with bile acids and vitamin B_{12}.

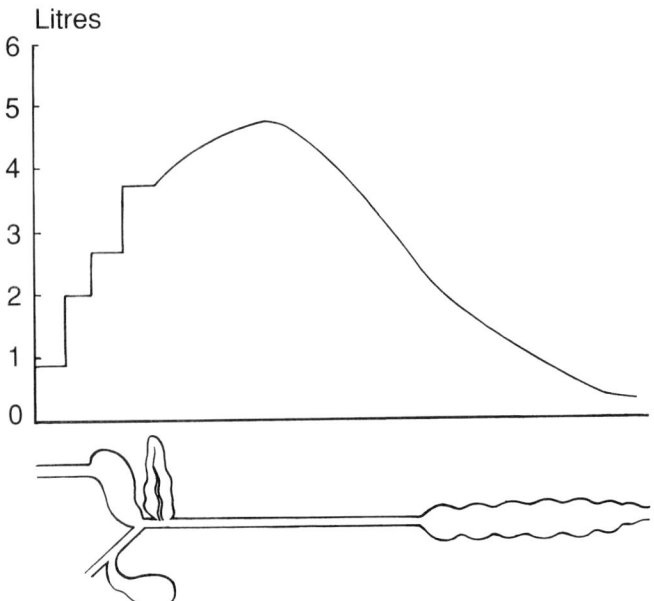

Fig. 21.2 24-hour fluid flow through the gut. Normal intake approximates to 1 l, to which is added 1 l saliva, 1–2 l gastric juice, 1–2 l pancreaticobiliary secretions and 1–2 l of intestinal secretions, resulting in a flow which increases until the midjejunum. Absorption predominates thereafter, but flow is still 1–2 l at the ileocecal valve. The colon normally absorbs 90% of ileocolonic inflow; however, resection of the ileum markedly increases this to 3–4 l, which can overwhelm the colon's absorptive capacity.

Table 21.1 Fecal electrolyte loss in Crohn's disease compared with normal subjects and those with secretory diarrhea due to enterotoxigenic *E. coli* (ETEC)

	Control	Small-bowel Crohn's	Crohn's enterocolitis	ETEC
n	29	18	11	38
Stool/24h	149±101 g	325±139 g	397±164 g	117±66 ml/kg
Na^+ mmol/l	18±17	29±19	41±19*	54±28
K^+ mmol/l	61±25	49±19	52±34	38±22
Cl^- mmol/l	14±11	17±11	28±19*	24

* Significantly different from controls $P < 0.05$
Control data, Crohn's small-bowel and enterocolitis from Caprilli et al 1985, and data from diarrhea due to enterotoxigenic *E. coli* (ETEC) from Molla et al 1981

platelet-activating factor, adenosine and prostaglandin-D_2. Serotonin, like several other mediators such as bradykinin, appears to act via neurally mediated prostaglandin release, since its secretory effects are blocked by both prostaglandin synthetase inhibitors and blockade of the enteric nervous system (for review see Sartor & Powell 1991).

The patchy nature of Crohn's disease means that the resulting increased stool output is modest compared with the secretory diarrheas observed in cholera or enterotoxigenic *Escherichia coli*, where the entire small bowel is affected (Table 21.1). Compensatory absorption by the colon in small-bowel Crohn's disease may be impaired by excessive bile salts and accelerated colonic transit.

Compared with ulcerative colitis, Crohn's disease of the colon is associated with a lower fecal sodium and a higher osmotic gap, 271 ± 98 versus 140 ± 56 mmol/l (calculated as stool osmolality $-2(\{Na^+\}+\{K^+\})$) (Schilli et al 1982). This is most likely due to the fermentation products of malabsorbed carbohydrate caused by occult small bowel disease.

Effect of right hemicolectomy

Fecal sodium loss is much increased after right hemicolectomy, the effect being mainly determined by the amount of colon remaining (Cummings et al 1973; Fig. 21.3), rather than the amount of terminal ileum resected. As can be seen from Figure 21.2, loss of the distal small bowel results in greatly increased colonic inflows, which may reach 4–5 litres per 24 hours. This exceeds the normally very adequate colonic absorptive reserve of up to 6ml per minute (Palma et al 1981). After a right hemicolectomy there is a 20–30% reduction in capacity to absorb sodium and water, as assessed by whole-gut perfusion with saline (Arrambide et al 1989). This effect is in addition to any further inhibitory effect of malabsorbed bile acids, and explains the often modest effect of bile acid-binding agents on the resulting diarrhea. Opioid drugs such as loperamide or codeine, which delay small-bowel transit, are often more effective in such cases.

CARBOHYDRATE ABSORPTION

Monosaccharides

Since most carbohydrate is absorbed in the first 100 cm of the small bowel, one would predict that a predominantly distal small-bowel disease such as Crohn's would not

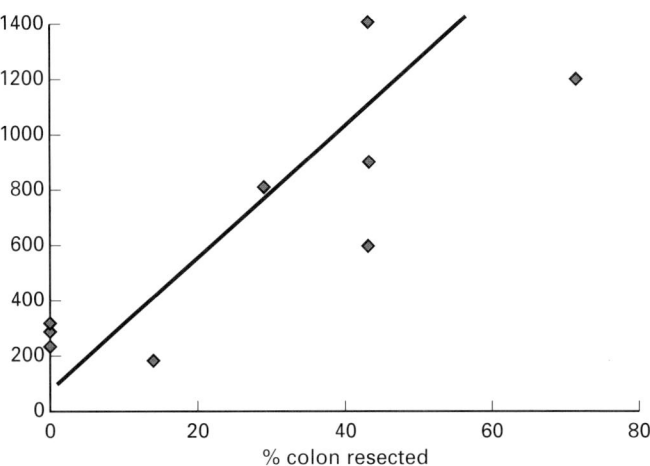

Fig. 21.3 Relationship between stool weight and percentage of colon resected in patients undergoing ileal and colonic resection for Crohn's disease and following trauma (Cummings et al 1973).

substantially alter absorption. Indeed, using xylose as a model monosaccharide it is apparent that significant malabsorption only occurs when more than 100 cm of bowel has either been resected or is diseased (Gerson et al 1973). The exception to this is when small-bowel contamination occurs, which markedly increases the frequency of xylose malabsorption (see below; Beeken & Kanich 1973).

Disaccharides

Disaccharide malabsorption due to diminished brush border enzyme activity is most likely to be a problem with lactose, the disaccharide with the lowest brush border hydrolase activity. When detailed morphometry and enzymatic analysis has been done in patients with disease apparently confined radiologically to the ileum and colon, reduced mucosal surface area and disaccharidase activity have been demonstrated (Dunne et al 1977). About one in 10 of Crohn's disease patients in the UK experience an exacerbation of symptoms with milk (Pearson et al 1993), an incidence similar to that in the adult population at large. Lactose malabsorption is more common in the USA, and was demonstrated in nearly one-third of pediatric patients with inflammatory bowel disease in Chicago, the incidence largely in keeping with the ethnic background of the subjects and not significantly different from controls. However, in those with extensive small-bowel disease the incidence increased to 66%, compared with only 25% of those with terminal ileitis alone, suggesting that the disease does significantly impair lactose absorption in these cases (Kirschner et al 1980).

NITROGEN ABSORPTION

Excessive protein loss is one of the most common abnormalities in small-bowel Crohn's disease, with a negative nitrogen balance and increased fecal output of nitrogen in about 50% of cases (Beeken 1975). This is more likely to be due to increased loss of plasma proteins than impaired protein digestion and absorption, since it does not correlate well with other indices of malabsorption (Beeken 1975). Increased gut clearance of ^{51}Cr-labeled plasma proteins does, however, correlate well with the extent of small-bowel disease and, in the absence of sepsis, with a lowering of serum albumin (Nordgren et al 1990). Other probe proteins, such as ^{59}Fe-iron-dextran and α_1-antitrypsin (Karbach et al 1985), can also be used to show increased loss of plasma proteins in stool.

FAT ABSORPTION

Although most fat absorption takes place in the jejunum, the normal ileum provides an important functional reserve. Disease or resection of the ileum results in the loss of this reserve, accelerated small-bowel transit, and also, by inter-

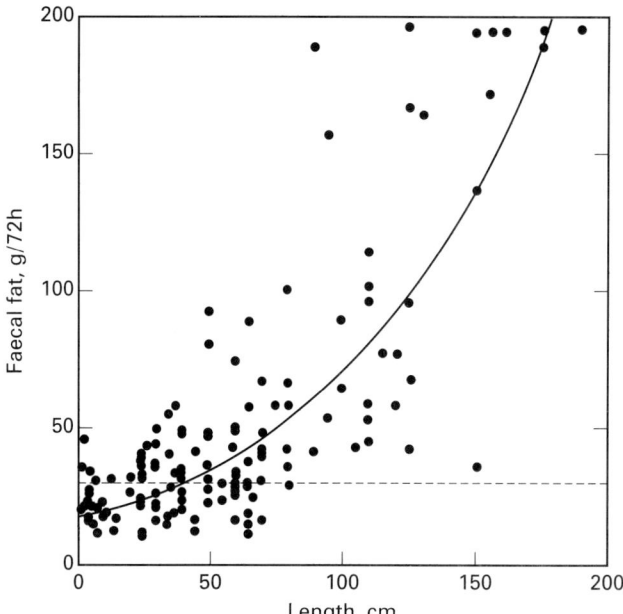

Fig. 21.4 Correlation between 72 hour fecal fat excretion and length of small bowel resected for Crohn's disease (Filipsson et al 1978).

rupting bile salt recirculation, impairment of duodenal fat emulsification and micelle formation (see below under bile acids). Furthermore, severe small-bowel disease is associated with impaired pancreatic secretions (Hegnhoj et al 1990). Finally, bacterial overgrowth deranges fat digestion, both by deconjugating bile acids and also by toxic effects on the mucosa by bacterial products, increasing the incidence of steatorrhea from 28% to 57% (Beeken 1975).

Some or all of these mechanisms variably contribute to a correlation between the length of small bowel affected by, or resected because of, Crohn's disease and fecal fat excretion, which rises above the normal limits when 50–100 cm of bowel are involved. Although inflammation of the small bowel contributes to fat malabsorption, surgical resection has a much greater effect (Filipsson et al 1978). These authors found a poor correlation of fecal fat excretion with extent of ileal disease, but a highly significant correlation with length of small-bowel resection (Fig. 21.4). Serial measurements clearly showed that 60% of patients experienced an increase in fecal fat after resection, resulting in 20% excreting more than 10 g per 24 hours (Filipsson et al 1978).

The malabsorbed fat makes an important contribution to symptoms, as can be seen by the improvement when fat intake is reduced from 100 g to 40 g daily (Andersson et al 1974). The benefits of a low-fat diet include reduced fecal fat, a reduction in stool sodium and water content, and diminished colonic oxalate absorption (Andersson & Jagenburg 1974). On the higher-fat diet unabsorbed free fatty acid may well inhibit water and electrolyte absorption, both directly as well as indirectly through acceleration of transit (Spiller et al 1986b).

Hyperoxaluria, which may result in renal calculus formation, appears to be due to increased absorption (Chadwick et al 1973), probably from the colon. There has been much interest in mechanisms (Harper & Mansell 1991), and it has been shown that both unabsorbed free fatty acids and excess bile salts can increase colonic permeability to oxalate (Saunders et al 1975, Dobbins & Binder 1976). Furthermore, by precipitating calcium as soaps, unabsorbed long-chain fatty acids increase oxalate solubility, which may also enhance absorption. Within the small bowel these fatty acids also significantly impair mineral absorption (see below).

SMALL-BOWEL BACTERIAL OVERGROWTH

Small-bowel bacterial overgrowth, defined as a colony count of 1×10^5/ml or greater in jejunal aspirates, was reported in six out of 36 patients with Crohn's disease (Beeken & Kanich 1973). The organisms isolated included *E. coli*, *Bacteroides* species, *proprioni bacterium* and *enterobacter*. Patients with small-bowel contamination were significantly more likely to have experienced weight loss, anemia, vitamin B_{12} malabsorption, xylose malabsorption and fat malabsorption, and also had evidence of increased protein loss from the gut. High counts are associated with jejunal disease and enteroenteric fistulae, and hence are more likely to be seen in patients with severe disease. This makes it somewhat difficult to disentangle the effects of such overgrowth. Bacteria ferment carbohydrate, generating short-chain fatty acids which in themselves have a cathartic effect, inducing propulsive ileal activity (Kamath & Phillips 1988). In addition, such bacteria deconjugate bile acids and consume vitamin B_{12} (Simon & Corbach 1984).

In the case of coloileal and colojejunal fistulae the seeding of sterile small-bowel contents with colonic bacteria is the obvious mechanism. Where no such fistulae exist intermittent subacute intestinal obstruction may be the mechanism, since anything which interferes with the normal clearance mechanism of the small bowel tends to lead to bacterial overgrowth (Vantrappen et al 1977b).

Both jejunal aspiration and ^{14}C-d-xylose breath test are necessary to reliably diagnose bacterial overgrowth in patients in whom there is a strong clinical suspicion of this problem, since false negatives may occur with both tests (Rumessen et al 1985).

MINERAL ABSORPTION

Calcium, magnesium, zinc and iron

Negative balances for calcium, magnesium and zinc are relatively common in Crohn's disease (Hessov et al 1983a, b). Like magnesium, zinc and iron, calcium is largely absorbed in the upper small intestine, with appreciable excretion in gut secretions. Balance studies are difficult, since one is measuring the difference between two substantial fluxes. In an extensive study of calcium absorption in Crohn's disease a negative balance was found in only four of 31 patients (Krawitt et al 1976). Although no association was noted between fat and xylose malabsorption, there was a correlation between calcium balance and enteric protein loss, which was markedly increased in those with extensive ileal disease. In spite of the apparently normal calcium balance results, bone disease in Crohn's disease is in fact quite common (Pigot et al 1992). This is undoubtedly multifactorial, with cortico-steroids and the non-specific effects of disease and anorexia being important, as well as the frequent occurrence of low serum levels of 25-hydroxy vitamin D (Vogelsang et al 1989). There is a poor relationship between the extent of small-bowel resection and calcium balance, the only exception here being those who have had an ileostomy formed (Hylander et al 1980), suggesting that after small-bowel resection the colon can exert some compensatory effect.

Significant magnesium depletion, as evidenced by diminished urinary magnesium excretion and low muscle biopsy magnesium content, relates well with the extent of small-bowel resection in Crohn's disease. Significant magnesium depletion has been reported in about 50% of subjects with more than 100 cm resected, in spite of a finding of normal serum magnesium in all but 6% of patients (Hessov et al 1983).

Zinc absorption is often impaired in patients with small-bowel Crohn's disease, with slower absorption (Sturniolo et al 1980) and, in a smaller number of cases, increased excretion compared with controls (Nakamura et al 1988). This increased loss of zinc may well be due to excessive loss of zinc-containing intestinal mucosal cells. Not surprisingly, symptomatic zinc deficiency is most often found in patients with massive small-bowel resection (McClain et al 1980).

Iron deficiency is common, caused by both impaired absorption (De Vizia et al 1992) and increased excretion in desquamated cells and occult blood loss.

FOLATE AND B_{12} ABSORPTION

Anemia is common, owing to the effects of chronic inflammation and increased gastrointestinal blood loss, as well as impaired absorption of specific hematinics.

Folate

Patients with anorexia and postprandial abdominal pain often have a poor dietary intake of fresh fruit and vegetables, which are the most important source of dietary folate. The low serum folate commonly seen in Crohn's disease is undoubtedly partially due to this. However, about 25% of patients also appear to have impaired absorption of folate (Hoffbrand et al 1968) without any obvious relationship to their intake of salazopyrin, which is known to impair folic acid absorption (Franklin & Rosenberg 1973, Elsborg & Larsen 1979). Folic acid is predominantly actively absorbed in the proximal small intestine, with little absorption in the ileum (Hepner et al 1968). This impaired absorption may be due to subtle changes in the jejunum, with impairment of the acid microclimate which facilitates folate absorption (Lucas et al 1978), or to loss of absorptive surface area (Dunne et al 1977). Supplementation with oral folate can usually easily overcome this defect.

Vitamin B_{12}

Absorption of vitamin B_{12} has traditionally been used as a measure of ileal disease. There is a close relationship between B_{12} malabsorption and the length of bowel affected by the Crohn's disease, which is of course usually ileum.

Surgical resection is associated with an impairment of B_{12} absorption in about half of patients, with absorption falling below normal once more than 50 cm has been resected (Gerson et al 1973, Filipsson et al 1978). Small-bowel contamination with bacterial degradation of B_{12} is also a possible mechanism. It is therefore apparent that increasing dietary B_{12} is of little use, and that parenteral B_{12} is necessary in most cases once B_{12} malabsorption develops.

BILE ACID ABSORPTION

As shown in Figure 21.1, bile acids are predominantly absorbed in the distal ileum, and impaired bile acid absorption has been used as a simple test of ileal dysfunction for some years (Fagan et al 1983). This impairment is associated with a decrease in bile acid pool size (Vantrappen et al 1977a) and an increased fecal excretion of bile acids (Kruis et al 1986). In addition, although fasting duodenal contents are normal, after a meal, especially the second meal of the day, duodenal bile acid concentrations are reduced below the critical micellar concentration, owing to failure of the normal enterohepatic recirculation (Mansbach et al 1972, Poley & Hofmann 1976, Van Deest et al 1986)

Impairment of the enterohepatic circulation can be demonstrated in patients with ileitis or ileal resection, but not in those with colitis, by a reduction in the postprandial rise in serum choleglycine (Suchy & Balistreri 1981).

The resulting increased delivery of bile acids to the colon has a number of important effects, including accelerated colonic transit with increased stool water, the so-called 'bile acid catharsis' (Hofmann & Poley 1969), as well as a qualitative change in bile salt pool composition. The proportion of deoxycholic acid falls, whereas that of ursodeoxycholate rises, reflecting changes in colonic bacterial metabolism (Rutgeerts et al 1986, Lapidus & Einarsson 1991). The decrease in bile acid pool size may well contribute to the increased incidence of gallstones in Crohn's disease following ileal resection. Bile acid catharsis is most obvious in those with a limited (<50 cm) resection of the terminal ileum, who respond well to cholestyramine (Jacobsen et al 1985). Where larger resections are involved bile acid catharsis is only a small part of the problem, which relates more to sodium and water malabsorption, and cholestyramine has a correspondingly smaller effect (Arrambide et al 1989).

INTESTINAL PERMEABILITY

Impaired 'barrier' function of the small-bowel epithelium has been demonstrated in Crohn's disease using a range of 'permeability probes', which have demonstrated increased permeation of probe molecules such as lactulose (Pearson et al 1982) and ^{51}Cr EDTA (ethylene diamine tetra-acetic acid) (O'Morain et al 1986). There has been some confusion in the literature owing to the different behaviours of various types of permeability probes (Table 21.2).

In disordered permeability there is the paradox of an increased permeation of the high molecular weight species and a decreased permeation of the lower molecular weights. This is usually expressed as a ratio of urinary excretions of the two species, thereby controlling for other variables that affect permeation, including gastric emptying, tonicity of the test meal and small-intestinal transit. In normal subjects permeability rapidly decreases as the molecular radius increases from less than 0.4 nm to 04–0.8 nm. This has been explained by hypothesizing that there is a large population of small pores 0.4–0.7 nm in diameter, and a much smaller population of larger pores of 6.5 nm diameter. Transmembrane pores and intercellular tight junctions may provide the anatomical counterpart of these two components. The tight junction space is about 20 nm, criss-crossed by strands of proteins attached to the cytoskeleton. The tightness of the junction can be altered by changes in intracellular mediators, including cyclic adenosine monophosphate (cAMP) and calcium (for review see Travis & Menzies 1992).

Permeation of these various probes depends on their route of administration and the degree of inflammation of the mucosa. Direct installation of the probes into inflamed segments of terminal ileum in Crohn's disease shows an

Table 21.2 Absorption and renal clearance of various probes used to assess permeability

Probe	Mol wt. (Da)	Diameter (nm)	% urinary excretion in 5 h	% urinary excretion after i.v. dose
PEG-400	194–502	0.53	18–20	41
Mannitol	182	0.67	17–21	79
Rhamnose	164	0.83	10–12	72
Lactulose	342	0.95	0.25–0.41	97
^{51}Cr-EDTA	359	1.05	0.64–0.70*	96

* 12 h collection, 2–3× greater at 24 h owing to colonic absorption

increased permeability of this area to a range of polyethylene glycols, molecular weights 590–1042 Da (Olaison et al 1988). This increase in absorption is non-specific with respect to molecular size. By comparison, when low molecular weight polyethylene glycols are given by mouth to patients with terminal ileal disease, their absorption is diminished (Olaison et al 1989). Numerous subsequent studies have confirmed this trend (for review see Olaison et al 1990). Diminished absorption of the smaller probes reflects the greater contribution of reduced surface area and accelerated transit in reducing absorption from the numerous smaller pores. By contrast, the erosions, epithelial disruptions and fissures seen in areas of active Crohn's ileitis provide routes of access for the larger molecular weight probes, whose absorption is correspondingly increased.

The most widely used probe, ^{51}Cr EDTA, is assessed by excretion over 24 hours following an oral test dose, which has consistently been reported as higher in patients with Crohn's disease but not their healthy relatives, indicating that it is a reflection of inflammation rather than a feature predisposing to Crohn's disease (Bjarnason et al 1983, Ainsworth et al 1989). In normal controls and patients with ulcerative colitis less than 2.6% of the test dose is excreted while in small bowel Crohn's disease excretions of 3.3–14% have been reported (Bjarnason et al 1983). Although one study has suggested increased permeability to PEG (polyethylene glycol) 400 in patients with Crohn's disease and their healthy first-degree relatives, these findings do not appear to have been confirmed by others, for reasons which are not yet quite clear (Travis & Menzies 1992, Wyatt et al 1993).

Wyatt's suggestion that the increased permeability demonstrated by the lactulose/mannitol test predicts frequency of relapse is interesting, but still needs to be confirmed. Although permeability tests have been available for nearly 15 years they have not been widely used in clinical practice as they lack specificity. However, they may be useful for following responses to treatment (Sanderson et al 1987). If such tests are to be used it is important to control for the test conditions, since the luminal contents at the time the probe is administered do appear to make a difference, with least permeability being found when the probes are given with 250 ml of a mixed nutrient polymeric diet (Peeters et al 1994). Subjects should avoid alcohol the night before, as this has been shown to alter permeability. The test otherwise seems fairly robust with respect to variations in body size, creatinine clearance, urinary volume and small-bowel transit time (Aabakken 1989).

Mechanisms of increased permeability

Many factors are likely to be responsible for increased permeability in Crohn's disease. Inflammatory mediators such as α-interferon, platelet activating factor (PAF) and tumor necrosis factor have all been shown to alter permeability in various cultured monolayers, although of these only PAF has so far been demonstrated to be increased in Crohn's disease (Cominelli & Kam 1993). In-vivo evidence is sparse, but during acute inflammatory responses to nematode worms villous atrophy is common, and the resulting relative immaturity of the epithelial barrier may contribute, among other factors, to the increase permeability noted (Ramage et al 1988). Whether this increase in permeability is merely an epiphenomenon or contributes causally to inflammation by allowing certain antigens to breach the mucosa, is as yet unknown.

SUMMARY

1. Crohn's disease of the small bowel is often underestimated by radiology.
2. Impaired absorption of sodium and water leads to increased ileocolonic inflow.
3. Increased ileal protein loss is associated with negative balance of calcium, magnesium and zinc.
4. Malabsorption of nutrients is usually relatively modest, unless there has been small-bowel resection or bacterial overgrowth.
5. Loss of >50 cm of ileum is associated with vitamin B_{12} malabsorption, >100 cm with malabsorption of bile acids and fat.
6. Increased permeability is common and appears to mirror the severity of mucosal inflammation.

REFERENCES

Aabakken L 1989 ^{51}Cr-ethylenediaminetetraacetic acid absorption test. Methodologic aspects. Scandinavian Journal of Gastroenterology 24: 351–358

Ainsworth M, Eriksen J, Waever Rasmussen J, Schaffalitzky De Muckadell O B 1989 Intestinal permeability of ^{51}Cr-labelled ethylenediaminetetraacetic acid in patients with Crohn's disease and their healthy relatives. Scandinavian Journal of Gastroenterology 24: 993–998

Allan R, Steinberg D M, Dixon K, Cooke W T 1975 Changes in the bidirectional sodium flux across the intestinal mucosa in Crohn's disease. Gut 16: 201–204

Andersson H, Jagenburg R 1974 Fat-reduced diet in the treatment of hyperoxaluria in patients with ileopathy. Gut 15: 360–366

Andersson H, Isaksson B, Sjogren B 1974 Fat-reduced diet in the symptomatic treatment of small bowel disease. Gut 15: 351–359

Arrambide K A, Santa Ana C A, Schiller L R, Little K H, Santangelo W C, Fordtran J S 1989 Loss of absorptive capacity for sodium chloride as a cause of diarrhea following partial ileal and right colon resection. Digestive Diseases and Sciences 34: 193–201

Atwell J D, Duthie H L 1964 The absorption of water, sodium, and potassium from the ileum of humans showing the effects of regional enteritis. Gastroenterology 46: 16–22

Beeken W L 1975 Remediable defects in Crohn's disease. Archives of Internal Medicine 135: 686–690

Beeken W L, Kanich R E 1973 Microbial flora of the upper small bowel in Crohn's disease. Gastroenterology 65: 390–397

Bjarnason I, O'Morain C, Levi A J, Peters T J 1983 Absorption of ^{51}chromium-labeled ethylenediaminetetraacetate in inflammatory

bowel disease. Gastroenterology 85: 318–322
Caprilli R, Vernia P, Latella, G, Frieri G 1985 Consequence of colonic involvement on electrolyte and acid–base homeostasis in Crohn's disease. American Journal of Gastroenterology 80: 509–512
Chadwick V S, Modha K, Dowling R H 1973 Mechanism for hyperoxaluria in patients with ileal dysfunction. New England Journal of Medicine 289: 172–176
Cominelli F, Kam L 1993 Inflammatory mediators of inflammatory bowel disease. Current Opinion in Gastroenterology 9: 534–543
Cummings J H, James W P T, Wiggins H S 1973 Role of the colon in ileal-resection diarrhoea. Lancet 17: 344–347
De Vizia B, Poggi V, Conenna R, Fiorillo A, Scippa L 1992 Iron absorption and iron deficiency in infants and children with gastrointestinal diseases. Journal of Pediatric Gastroenterology and Nutrition 14: 21–26
Dobbins J W, Binder H J 1976 Effect of bile salts and fatty acids on the colonic absorption of oxalate. Gastroenterology 70: 1096–1100
Dunne W T, Cooke W T, Allan R N 1977 Enzymatic and morphometric evidence for Crohn's disease as a diffuse lesion of the gastrointestinal tract. Gut 18: 290–294
Elsborg L, Larsen L 1979 Folate deficiency in chronic inflammatory bowel diseases. Scandinavian Journal of Gastroenterology 14: 1019–1024
Fagan E A, Chadwick V S, McLean Baird I 1983 SeHCAT absorption: a simple test of ileal dysfunction. Digestion 26: 159–165
Filipsson S, Hulten L, Lindstedt G 1978 Malabsorption of fat and vitamin B_{12} before and after intestinal resection for Crohn's disease. Scandinavian Journal of Gastroenterology 13: 529–536
Fitzgerald P G, Topp TJ, Walton J M, Jackson J R, Gillis D A 1992 The use of indium-111 leukocyte scans in children with inflammatory bowel disease. Journal of Pediatric Surgery 27: 1298–1300
Franklin J L, Rosenberg I H 1973 Impaired folic acid absorption in inflammatory bowel disease: effect of salicylazosulphapyridine (Azulfidine). Gastroenterology 64: 517–525
Gerson C D, Cohen N, Janowitz H D 1973 Small intestinal absorptive function in regional enteritis. Gastroenterology 64: 907–912
Harper J, Mansell M A 1991 Treatment of enteric hyperoxaluria. Postgraduate Medical Journal 67: 219–222
Hawker P C, McKay J S, Turnberg L A 1980 Electrolyte transport across colonic mucosa from patients with inflammatory bowel disease. Gastroenterology 79: 508–511
Head L H, Heaton J W, Kivel R M 1969 Absorption of water and electrolytes in Crohn's disease of the colon. Gastroenterology 56: 571–579
Hegnhoj J, Hansen C P, Rannem T, Sobirk H, Andersen L B, Andersen J R 1990 Pancreatic function in Crohn's disease. Gut 31: 1076–1079
Hepner G W, Booth C C, Cowan J, Hoffbrand A V, Mollin D L 1968 Absorption of crystalline folic acid in man. Lancet ii: 302–306
Hessov I, Andersson H, Isaksson B 1983a Effects of a low-fat diet on mineral absorption in small-bowel disease. Scandinavian Journal of Gastroenterology 18: 551–554
Hessov I, Hasselblad C, Fasth S, Hulten L 1983b Magnesium deficiency after ileal resections for Crohn's disease. Scandinavian Journal of Gastroenterology 18: 643–649
Hoffbrand A V, Stewart J S, Booth C C, Mollins D L 1968 Folate deficiency in Crohn's disease: incidence, pathogenesis, and treatment. British Medical Journal 2: 71–75
Hofmann A F, Poley R J 1969 Cholestyramine treatment of diarrhea associated with ileal resection. New England Journal of Medicine 281: 398–401
Hylander E, Ladefoged K, Jarnum S 1980 The importance of the colon in calcium absorption following small-intestinal resection. Scandinavaian Journal of Gastroenterology 15: 55–60
Jacobsen O, Hojgaard L, Moller E H et al 1985 Effect of enterocoated cholestyramine on bowel habit after ileal resection: double blind crossover study. British Medical Journal 290: 1315–1318
Kamath P S, Phillips S F 1988 Initiation of motility in canine ileum by short chain fatty acids and inhibition by pharmacological agents. Gut 29: 941–948
Karbach U, Ewe K, Dehos H 1985 Antiinflammatory treatment and intestinal alpha-1-antitrypsin clearance in active Crohn's disease. Digestive Diseases and Sciences 30: 229–235
Kirschner B S, DeFavaro M, Jensen W 1980 Lactose malabsorption in children and adolescents with chronic inflammatory bowel disease (IBD). Gastroenterology 78: 1195
Krawitt E L, Beeken W L, Janney C D 1976 Calcium absorption in Crohn's disease. Gastroenterology 71: 251–254
Kruis W, Kalek H D, Stellaard F, Paumgartner G 1986 Altered fecal bile acid pattern in patients with inflammatory bowel disease. Digestion 35: 189–198
Lapidus A, Einarsson K 1991 Effects of ileal resection on biliary lipids and bile acid composition in patients with Crohn's disease. Gut 32: 1488–1491
Lenaerts C, Roy CC, Vaillancourt M, Weber A M, Morin C L, Seidman E 1989 High incidence of upper gastrointestinal tract involvement in children with Crohn's disease. Pediatrics 83: 777–781
Lescut D, Vanco D, Bonniere P et al 1993 Perioperative endoscopy of the whole small bowel in Crohn's disease. Gut 34: 647–649
Lucas M L, Cooper B T, Lei F H et al 1978 Acid microclimate in coeliac and Crohn's disease: a model for folate malabsorption. Gut 19: 735–742
McClain C, Soutor C, Zieve L 1980 Zinc deficiency: a complication of Crohn's disease. Gastroenterology 78: 272–279
Mansbach C M, Garbutt J T, Tyor M P 1972 Bile salt and lipid metabolism in patients with ileal disease with and without steatorrhea. Digestive Diseases 17: 1089–1099
Molla A M, Rahman M, Sarker S A et al 1981 Stool electrolyte content and purging rates in diarrhea caused by rotavirus, enterotoxigenic E. coli, and V. cholerae in children. Journal of Pediatrics 98: 835–838
Nakamura T, Higashi A, Takano S, Akagi M, Matsuda I 1988 Zinc clearance correlates with clinical severity of Crohn's disease. A kinetic study. Digestive Diseases and Sciences 33: 1520–1524
Nordgren S, Hellberg R, Cederblad A, Fasth S, Lindstedt G, Hulten L 1990 Fecal excretion of radiolabeled ($^{51}CrCl^{3}$) proteins in patients with Crohn's disease. Scandinavian Journal of Gastroenterology 25: 345–351
Olaison G, Leandersson P, Sjodahl R, Tagesson C 1988 Intestinal permeability to polyethyleneglycol 600 in Crohn's disease. Peroperative determination in a defined segment of the small intestine. Gut 29: 196–199
Olaison G, Sjodahl R, Leandersson P, Tagesson C 1989 Abnormal intestinal permeability pattern in colonic Crohn's disease. Absorption of low molecular weight polyethylene glycols after oral or colonic load. Scandinavian Journal of Gastroenterology 24: 571–576
Olaison G, Sjodahl R, Tagesson C 1990 Abnormal intestinal permeability in Crohn's disease. A possible pathogenic factor. Scandinavian Journal of Gastroenterology 25: 321–328
O'Morain C A, Abelow A C, Chervu L R, Fleischner G M, Das K M 1986 Chromium 51-ethylenediaminetetraacetate test: useful test in the assessment of inflammatory bowel disease. Journal of Laboratory and Clinical Medicine 108: 430–435
Palma R, Vidon N, Bernier J J 1981 Maximal capacity for fluid absorption in human bowel. Digestive Diseases and Sciences 26: 929–934
Pearson A D J, Eastham E J, Laker M F et al 1982 Intestinal permeability in children with Crohn's disease and coeliac disease. British Medical Journal 285: 20–21
Pearson M, Teahon K, Levi A J, Bjarnason I 1993 Food intolerance and Crohn's disease. Gut 34: 783–787
Peeters M, Hiele M, Ghoos Y et al 1994 Test conditions greatly influence permeation of water soluble molecules through the intestinal mucosa: need for standardisation. Gut 35: 1404–1408
Pigot F, Roux C, Chaussade S et al 1992 Low bone mineral density in patients with inflammatory bowel disease. Digestive Diseases and Sciences 37: 1396–1403
Poley R J, Hofmann A F 1976 Fat digestion after two sequential test meals with and without cholestyramine. Gastroenterology 71: 38–44
Ramage J K, Hunt R H, Perdue M H 1988 Changes in intestinal permeability and epithelial differentiation during inflammation in the rat. Gut 29: 57–61
Rumessen J J, Gudmand-Hoyer E, Bachmann E, Justesen T 1985 Diagnosis of bacterial overgrowth of the small intestine. Scandinavian Journal of Gastroenterology 20: 1267–1275
Rutgeerts P, Ghoos Y, Vantrappen G, Fevery J 1986 Biliary lipid composition in patients with nonoperated Crohn's disease. Digestive Diseases and Sciences 31: 27–32

Sanderson I R, Boulton P, Menzies I, Walker Smith J A 1987 Improvement of abnormal lactulose/rhamnose permeability in active Crohn's disease of the small bowel by an elemental diet. Gut 28: 1073–1076

Sartor R B, Powell D W 1991 Mechanisms of diarrhea in intestinal inflammation and hypersensitivity: immune system modulation of intestinal transport. Current Topics in Gastroenterology 75–113

Saunders D R, Sillery J, McDonald G B 1975 Regional differences in oxalate absorption by rat intestine: evidence for excessive absorption by the colon in steatorrhoea. Gut 16: 543–554

Schilli R, Breuer R I, Klein F et al 1982 Comparison of the composition of faecal fluid in Crohn's disease and ulcerative colitis. Gut 23: 326–332

Simon G L, Gorbach S L 1984 Intestinal flora in health and disease. Gastroenterology 86: 174–193

Spiller R C, Jones B J M, Silk D B A 1986a Jejunal water and electrolyte absorption from two proprietary enteral feeds in man: importance of sodium content. Gut 28: 681–687

Spiller R C, Brown M L, Phillips S F 1986b Decreased fluid tolerance, accelerated transit, and abnormal motility of the human colon induced by oleic acid. Gastroenterology 91: 100–107

Sturniolo G C, Molokhia M M, Shields R, Turnberg L A 1980 Zinc absorption in Crohn's disease. Gut 21: 387–391

Suchy F S, Balistreri W F 1981 Ileal dysfunction in Crohn's disease assessed by the postprandial serum bile acid response. Gut 22: 948–952

Travis S, Menzies I 1992 Intestinal permeability: functional assessment and significance. Clinical Science 82: 471–488

Van Deest B W, Fordtran J S, Morawski S G, Wilson J D 1986 Bile salt and micellar fat concentration in proximal small bowel contents of ileectomy patients. Journal of Clinical Investigation 47: 1314–1324

Vantrappen G, Ghoos Y, Rutgeerts P, Janssens J 1977a Bile acid studies in uncomplicated Crohn's disease. Gut 18: 730–735

Vantrappen G, Janssens J, Hellemans J, Ghoos Y 1977b The interdigestive motor complex of normal subjects and patients with bacterial overgrowth of the small intestine. Journal of Clinical Investigation 59: 1158–1163

Vogelsang H, Ferenci P, Woloszczuk W et al 1989 Bone disease in vitamin D-deficient patients with Crohn's disease. Digestive Diseases and Sciences 34: 1094–1099

Wyatt J, Vogelsang H, Hubl W, Waldhoer T, Lochs H 1993 Intestinal permeability and the prediction of relapse in Crohn's disease. Lancet 341: 1437–1439

22. Absorption of fluids and electrolytes by the colon – relevance to inflammatory bowel disease

A. M. Levy   S. F. Phillips

INTRODUCTION

In health, the colon conserves the electrolytes and water in chyme so effectively that desiccated stools can be stored and eliminated later, at a socially convenient time. Frequent, uncontrolled evacuation of blood, mucus and liquid feces by patients with inflammatory bowel disease (IBD) represents a dramatic change from this orderly function, and indicates a major disturbance of colonic function. Study of the normal function of the colon in humans is complicated by regional differences in absorption, a complex and poorly understood pattern of motility, and the largely unexplored relationships between the host and the resident bacterial flora. With such an incomplete understanding of normal physiology it is not surprising that the pathophysiology of IBD is largely unknown. Moreover, clinical factors, such as the severity of inflammation and the anatomical sites of involvement, are variables which are difficult to quantify and which may vary with time in any individual.

Current hypotheses of colonic absorption, motility and metabolism are based on results from in-vitro and in-vivo approaches which are best viewed as complementary. This chapter aims to integrate these results and relate them to the clinical problems of IBD.

PARTICULAR PROPERTIES OF THE COLON AS AN ABSORBING ORGAN

Colonic mucosa as a 'tight' epithelium

The functions of the colonic epithelium largely reflect its structure as a bilayer phospholipid membrane, which readily allows diffusion of lipophilic solutes across it while restricting the movement of water and hydrophilic molecules. These probably require specific carrier proteins for active transport, or water-filled 'pores' if they are to cross the membrane. The pores are probably located in the tight junction region between epithelial cells, and these have, indeed, been classified as 'tight' or 'leaky' (Diamond 1974). The colon, unlike the small intestine, normally has a 'tight' mucosa that restricts the passive fluxes of ions and thereby minimizes water and electrolyte loss in the stool. The basic research that established knowledge of these features of the colon was accomplished years ago, and focused on three concepts: pore size, mucosal permeability and transepithelial potential difference. Effective pore size in the colon has been estimated to be less than 23 nm (2.3 Å) (smaller than the urea molecule) by the demonstration that water flow into the lumen in response to perfusion with equimolar solutions of mannitol and urea was equal (Billich & Levitan 1969). Comparable values for the jejunum and ileum are 8 Å and 4 Å, respectively (Fordtran et al 1965). Permeability studies have demonstrated that the human colon can absorb water even in the face of a large osmotic gradient (Billich & Levitan 1969), whereas transport in the small bowel is isotonic (Fordtran et al 1965). In addition, the colon restricts the movement of molecules such as polyethylene glycol more so than does the ileum or jejunum, as evidenced by studies of urinary excretion of these substances after their colonic instillation (Chadwick et al 1977). This limited permeability of water and non-charged solutes also applies to ions. A functional consequence of these membrane properties, when combined with active sodium absorption, is the spontaneous generation of a large transepithelial potential difference, which has been localized to the mucosa (Edmonds 1975). This results in the mucosa being 30–40 mV negative compared to the serosa, but the actual potential difference in vivo is variable, being increased by mineralocorticoids (endogenous or exogenous) and decreased when mucosal disease is present (Edmonds & Pilcher 1973, Rask-Madsen & Dalmark 1973).

Regional differences

Another important point relates to the variable absorptive function found in different anatomical regions. The most persuasive data comes from animal models, which indicate that there is regional variability in the major mechanisms of sodium absorption; this material is well reviewed in detail elsewhere (Binder et al 1991). It remains to be seen whether or not these regional differences are as important in humans. Regional differences in chloride absorption have also been reported (Hubel et al 1987).

ABSORPTION AND SECRETION

Absorption of inorganic ions and water

In most mammalian species the colonic mucosa actively absorbs sodium (Na) and chloride (Cl), whereas bicarbonate (HCO_3) accumulates on the mucosal side (Schultz 1980, Chang & Rao 1994). Net movements of ions follow the same general principles in humans, but the major mechanisms for ionic transport vary in relative importance from the proximal to the distal colon (Sellin & DeSoignie 1987). Sodium absorption is active and occurs against electrical and concentration gradients, such that a linear relationship is maintained between the rate of Na absorption and luminal concentrations of Na from 25 to 150 mmol/l (Billich & Levitan 1969, Devroede & Phillips 1969). Both active electrogenic (i.e. giving rise to a potential difference) and electroneutral processes transport Na out of the colon, but mechanisms accounting for all of Na transport across the colonic mucosa have not yet been described (Donowitz 1987).

Three types of membrane pump are important. The first is an ouabain-sensitive sodium–potassium (Na–K) ATPase (adenosine triphosphatase) located at the basal surface of colonic epithelial cells that actively extrudes Na^+ into the extracellular fluid, thereby lowering the intracellular Na concentration. The second pump operates at the apical surface, is electrogenic, and can be blocked by amiloride. This pump is more important in the distal colon. Electrogenic Na absorption thus exhibits a gradient from proximal to distal bowel, and contributes most to Na absorption in distal segments. The third pump accomplishes electroneutral Na and Cl absorption by parallel Na–H and Cl–HCO_3 exchange, and has been localized to the brush border of colonocytes (Binder et al 1986, Foster et al 1986a). Exchangers of sodium and hydrogen are not unique to the colon: they are found in almost all cells and are probably driven by sodium gradients established by Na–K ATP-ase (VanDyke & Ives 1988). In contrast to findings in the small bowel, the addition of glucose or amino acids to solutions in contact with colonic mucosa does not augment sodium uptake (Grady et al 1970, Hawker et al 1978).

Like Na, chloride, is actively absorbed against large concentration gradients, and absorption continues even when the flow of water is into the lumen. At equal concentrations Cl absorption exceeds that of Na, the difference being accounted for by HCO_3 secretion. Cl–HCO_3 exchange has been estimated to provide for approximately 25% of total Cl absorption in the human colon (Davis et al 1983). Carbonic anhydrase is involved, since Cl absorption and HCO_3 secretion are abolished by acetazolamide (Phillips & Schmalz 1970). Failure of Cl–HCO_3 exchange has been demonstrated in the dramatic diarrheal syndrome of infants, congenital chloridorrhea (Holmberg et al 1975).

Several mechanisms regulate the movement of K in and out of the colon. Both luminal concentrations of K and the total body K load appear to influence the balance between absorption and secretion. Potassium accumulates in the lumen when the luminal fluid contains less than 15 mmol/l, but is absorbed when greater concentrations are present (Devroede & Phillips 1969, Giller & Phillips 1972). These findings are consistent with passive K movement along electrochemical gradients. However, other mechanisms also operate, including a secretion of K that is dependent on luminal Na (Edmonds & Nielsen 1968, Hawker et al 1978).

Calcium (Ca), magnesium (Mg) and zinc (Zn) are largely absorbed in the small intestine and there is very little information on the role of the colon in their homeostasis. Hypermagnesaemia has been described after administration of enemas that contain magnesium sulphate (Wacker & Parisi 1968), and during colonic perfusion magnesium was absorbed and calcium secreted (Phillips & Giller 1973). Radioactive Mg and Ca were absorbed and readily detectable in the blood of healthy volunteers after rectal instillation (Gooptu et al 1969). These ions are relevant clinically, since excessive loss of Mg and Ca may occur in severe IBD (Posey & Bargen 1950, Thoren 1962). Nevertheless, absorption of these cations has been said to be enhanced in inflammatory bowel disease (Gooptu et al 1969). Zinc deficiency may also occur with prolonged parenteral nutrition, but its handling by the human colon is as yet unexplored.

Short-chain fatty acids

Short-chain fatty acids (SCFA) constitute the major fecal anion of all herbivores and omnivores (Dawson et al 1964, Rubinstein et al 1969, Bjork et al 1976). The three principal SCFAs are acetic, propionic and butyric acid. SCFAs are produced by anerobic fermentation of undigested carbohydrate by colonic bacteria, and they are present in the colon almost completely in the form of anions (pK_a 4.8). SCFAs are the preferred energy source for colonocytes (Roediger 1980, 1982), and have been shown to increase luminal bacterial mass (Stephen & Cummings 1979); they also affect colonic epithelial cell proliferation, and deficiencies of SCFAs have been implicated in the pathogenesis of ulcerative colitis (Roediger 1980). Indeed, local treatment with enemas of SCFAs can reduce the inflammation of ulcerative (Breuer et al 1991) and diversion (Harig et al 1989) colitis. Although it has long been known that absorption of sodium and water is augmented by the absorption of SCFA (Ruppin et al 1980, Roediger & Moore 1981), the mechanisms of SCFA absorption was controversial until recently. Previously two theories garnered support: non-ionic diffusion and anion exchange systems. It is now clear that non-ionic diffusion accounts for a significant proportion of SCFA absorption, and is dependent upon hydrogen ion availability for protonation of SCFA ions to their non-ionic forms (von Engelhardt et al 1993). In the cecum and proximal colon non-ionic diffusion is responsible for 35% and 40–50% of SCFA absorption, respectively. In these areas of the colon non-ionic diffusion is dependent upon apical membrane exchange of Na^+–H^+. In contrast, distal colonic absorption by non-ionic diffusion accounts for >80% of SCFA absorption, and requires an apical K^+–H^+ ATPase for H^+ ions to protonate the SCFA anions (von Engelhardt et al 1993). This means that another mechanism must account for the remainder of SCFA absorption, and the most likely one is transport mediated by an anion carrier. Also being pursued is an understanding of the mechanism by which SCFAs enhance Na^+ and Cl^- absorption in the colon. There is evidence that the electroneutral NaCl absorption that results from Na–H exchange allows butyrate to be protonated, followed by non-ionic diffusion of the SCFA into the colonocyte (Binder & Mehta 1989). H^+-butyrate then dissociates and butyrate anion is exchanged for luminal Cl. The question of whether SCFAs cross the basolateral membrane of the colonic epithelial cell or are used exclusively as a fuel source by the cell is not resolved.

Secretion of ions and water

A net accumulation of fluid in the intestine could result from inhibition of absorption, especially if a basal state of secretion was thereby unmasked. Conversely, fluid would also accumulate in the lumen if ions and water were actively secreted. The relative contribution of either mechanism is not clear. Active secretion requires that ions move from serosal to mucosal fluids against electrochemical gradients. The phenomenon fundamental to intestinal secretion is an active secretion of chloride ions; thus, basic studies now focus on the control of chloride channels. Chloride secretion can be stimulated in colonic mucosa by the phosphodiesterase inhibitor theophylline, thus implicating cyclic nucleotides. Secretion can be inhibited by both serosal ouabain and furosemide. Presumably by blocking Na–K ATP-ase, ouabain interferes with sodium-chloride (NaCl) exchange at the basolateral membrane, thus making chloride unavailable for apical secretion (Frizzell & Heintze 1979).

Control of secretion is discussed below, but among the stimuli that elicit net secretion in the intact colon a number are of particular clinical relevance. These include the laxatives ricinoleic acid (Ammon & Phillips 1973, Bright-Asare & Binder 1973, Racusen & Binder 1979), bisacodyl (Ewe & Holker 1974), dicotyl sodium sulfosuccinate (Saunders et al 1975), dihydroxy bile acids (Mekhjian et al 1971, Binder & Rawlins 1973) and prostaglandins (Frizzell & Heintze 1979, Racusen & Binder 1980). Most of these compounds have also been shown to stimulate secretion in vitro.

Cholera toxin (CT) binds predominantly to villous (as opposed to crypt) epithelial cells of the small intestine (Weiser & Quill 1975), but evokes secretion from crypt cells through nervous mechanisms mediated by the enteric nervous system (Jodal 1990, Tantisera et al 1990). Previously it had been thought that the secretory effect induced by CT was merely local, within the segment in which the toxin was placed (Hubel et al 1991), but recent evidence demonstrates that CT in the small intestine can, in fact, induce colonic secretion of electrolytes and water, and that this effect is abolished by neural disconnection of the large from the small intestine (Nocerino et al 1995). Thus the pathophysiology of cholera diarrhea includes a secretory response of the colon. The neural pathways that propagate this effect are unknown, but vasoactive intestinal polypeptide (VIP)-containing neurons are a likely effector candidate (Jiang et al 1993, Cassuto et al 1981). The role of this new pathophysiological mechanism in other human diseases affecting the small and large bowel remains to be explored.

Modulation of absorption and secretion

Neurohumoral and extracellular control

Both mineralocorticoids and glucocorticoids affect electrolyte transport in the mammalian colon. It is of note that these changes the produced by aldosterone and by glucocorticoids considered to have little or no mineralocorticoid activity. These crossover effects may result from specific ligand–receptor interaction, or may be produced by partial binding of one ligand to the other ligand's receptor if the interaction is less restricted (Sandle & Binder 1987). In addition, ligand–receptor binding may augment an existing membrane transport process, or induce new processes. For example, aldosterone, which has only modest effects in the small intestine, increases electrogenic Na^+ transport in the distal colon of the rabbit, where this mechanism of amiloride-sensitive absorption exists under baseline conditions (Frizzell & Schultz 1978). In contrast, the rat distal colon does not possess electrogenic Na^+ transport at baseline, but rather absorbs Na^+ and Cl^- by electroneutral NaCl absorption. Thus, in the rat aldosterone apparently induces a new Na^+ transport mechanism and inhibits the existing NaCl absorption pathway (Foster et al 1983). Further complexity is added because the physiological responses vary with the segment of the colon being studied. Unlike its effects in the distal colon, aldosterone in the rat proximal colon increases electroneutral absorption of NaCl, and does not induce a new amiloride-sensitive process of electrogenic Na^+ transport (Foster et al 1986b). In sum, aldosterone increases NaCl absorption in the colon. Pure glucocorticoids also augment NaCl absorption, by both electrogenic and electroneutral mechanisms. Interestingly, it has been shown that this increase by glucocorticoids of electrogenic Na^+ absorption is mediated by binding of the glucocorticoid to the aldosterone receptor, and is thus an example of overlap of gluco- into mineralocorticoid activity (Binder et al 1991). On the other hand, the increase in electroneutral NaCl absorption is mediated by the glucocorticoid receptor (Bastl 1987). It is not known whether the increase in electroneutral NaCl transport described for aldosterone above is mediated through interaction with the glucocorticoid receptor, or whether another aldosterone-specific receptor exists for this purpose.

The net effect of aldosterone on K^+ transport is secretion, but this is achieved by a combination of increased absorption and secretion of K^+, the latter effect being the greater. These changes are mediated by binding to the aldosterone receptor. Similarly, glucocorticoids enhance net K^+ secretion by partial binding to the aldosterone receptor (Binder et al 1991).

The gastrointestinal tract contains abundant neurons, estimated to be as many as in the spinal cord; indeed, the enteric nervous system (ENS) has been termed a 'minibrain in the gut'. The ENS is composed of the myenteric, submucosal and mucosal subdivisions. Most neurons of the myenteric plexus project to smooth muscle in the tunica muscularis, whereas most submucosal plexus neurons project to the epithelium, where they probably serve to modulate ion transport (Furness & Costa 1980, Furness et al 1985, Carey et al 1985, Hubel et al 1987). Neuropeptides may be the shared intermediates, participating in both humoral and neural regulation. Thus, most submucosal neurons contain several neuropeptides, including VIP, galanin, neuropeptide Y, somatostatin and others. Although most of the experimental observations have been gathered from the small bowel, comparable principles must apply to the colon and some investigators have studied colonic tissues specifically. Thus, in the guinea pig colon electrical stimulation of submucosal neurons evoked a serosal-to-mucosal flux of Cl (Kuwahara et al 1987). In comparable experiments with human tissue, cecal mucosa responded by Cl secretion and reduced Na absorption, the transverse colon did not respond, and the sigmoid colon showed reduced Cl absorption only (Hubel et al 1987). Additional observations on colonic tissue also support this key concept (Bridges et al 1986). It is clear that mucosal transport can be modulated – and may be ultimately controlled – by the ENS, a system of nervous mediation that also orchestrates motility and blood flow. In cholera, the ENS also mediates interactions between the small and large intestines, relationships that could be relevant to other human diseases.

Eicosanoids. Prostaglandins and leukotrienes are derived from long-chain unsaturated fatty acids present in the plasma membrane of all cells. In parallel with the growing understanding that the healthy gastrointestinal tract exists in a dynamic state of balanced inflammation (Chang & Rao 1994), it is clear that there exists a baseline level of prostaglandin and leukotriene production throughout the intestine. Thus even the healthy intestine may have a subclinical, secretory state. There is much overlap in the functions of these inflammatory–secretory molecules, which makes their study in vivo difficult. It is clear, however, that leukotrienes such as LTB4 amplify the inflammatory response by stimulating and recruiting PMN (polymorph neutrophils), which in turn impair the barrier function of the colonic epithelium and facilitate net secretion. In addition, prostaglandins exert a mucosal protective effect, to varying degrees, in different regions (Hawkey & Rampton 1985). Yet another layer of complexity has been discerned with the expanding knowledge of the connections between prostaglandins and other systems that mediate inflammation, such as the mast cells and the cytokine network. Thus, it is now apparent that the increase in prostaglandins when fluid is secreted into the colon in anaphylaxis depends on the degranulation of mast cells, and is expressed via interleukin-1 (IL-1), a potent cellular stimulator of prostaglandin secretion (Theodorou et al 1994). The complexity of the cascade is revealed by the observation that agents that stabilize mast cells or neutralize IL-1 completely abolish the hypersecretion induced by antigen challenge in sensitized animals, whereas prostaglandin inhibitors only partially reduce this response (Theodorou et al 1994).

Intracellular mechanisms. Regulatory mechanisms alter cellular function by changing the function of cell membranes and by stimulating intracellular second-messenger systems. Mechanisms generating intracellular cyclic adenosine monophosphate (cAMP) are involved in the response to secretagogues such as prostaglandins (PG) and theophylline (Frizzell et al 1976, Simon et al 1978), although the more fundamental interaction is with systems depending on the release of calcium ions (Warhurst et al 1988). Intracellular Ca release is linked with two major pathways, the Ca–calmodulin complex and the protein kinase C cascade. These pathways act on the state of phosphorylation of intracellular proteins. Sodium chloride and water absorption are increased in epithelial cells exposed to low Ca concentrations and after administration of the calcium-channel blocker verapamil (Donowitz 1985). Serotonin acts on cells through a Ca-dependent mechanism which stimulates active Cl secretion and reduces NaCl absorption (Zimmerman & Binder 1984). Protein kinase C is activated by diacylglycerol and phorbol esters (diacylglycerol analogs) released from cell membranes.

Animal experiments in vitro have shown that phorbol esters inhibit NaCl absorption, may inhibit apical membrane Na–H exchange and attenuate PGE_2-mediated secretion (Ahn et al 1985, Warhurst et al 1988).

Colonic absorptive capacity

Colonic function can be assessed in humans by comparing the composition of stools and the ileal input to the colon. Indirect assessments of the volume and composition of ileal flow were based on the volumes (400–600 ml/day) collected from well established ileostomies (Hill 1976). However, intestinal absorption after colectomy may be influenced by many factors, including the extent of ileal resection or residual ileal disease, and any intestinal adaptation that may occur after colectomy. An alternative approach was a direct measurement of flow in the terminal ileum by applying dye-dilution techniques (Phillips & Giller 1973). These studies concluded that the fasting ileal flow in healthy humans is 0.1–0.7 ml/min, with peaks of 5 ml/min 1–2 hours after a meal (Phillips & Giller 1973). By integrating such data over 24 hours, about 1500 ml is estimated to enter the colon each day: this volume contains 200 mmol Na, 100 mmol Cl and 10 mmol K. By comparison, normal stools contain up to 100–150 ml of water, 1–5 mmol Na, 1–2 mmol Cl and 5–15 mmol K per day. Thus, the healthy colon absorbs more than 90% of what it receives.

Colonic reserve

A logical extension of the above observations is to ask what the colon can accomplish under stress? An exogenous load of isotonic fluid was delivered into the cecum, to augment the endogenous flow; thus, the threshold at which the fecal volume increases was determined (Debongnie & Phillips 1978). A load of 2 l per day did not produce diarrhea, whereas 4 l per day increased the fecal output. When these exogenous and endogenous loads were combined, almost 5 l of a 6 l load was absorbed from the healthy human colon (Debongnie & Phillips 1978). Moreover, the size of a single fluid bolus delivered to the colon also influenced absorption. Thus, a 250 ml bolus of fluid did not influence fecal output, whereas 500 ml delivered at the same rate overwhelmed the absorptive capacity of the colon and produced loose stools (Debongnie & Phillips 1978). Palma et al (1981) confirmed that a sudden increase in the rate of ileal discharge into the cecum could overcome the ability of the colon to handle fluids, producing diarrhea. Thus, the colon has major reserves to handle a fluid overload but this is only effective if the excess is presented to it at a rate less than some critical value.

Relationships with motility

The proximal colon has been postulated to possess the major reservoir functions by which increased volumes of ileal effluent are accommodated (Phillips 1988). Thus, with proximal accommodation sufficient time would be available for slow transit to facilitate absorption, and Na, Cl and water conservation to be maximized. The system was disturbed pharmacologically when the cecum and ascending colon were perfused with diarrheogenic long-chain fatty acids (Spiller et al 1986). The proximal colon constricted and distal flow was increased, resulting in diarrhea. The effect of these fatty acids on cecal accommodation and colonic transit was countered by morphine, which also controlled the diarrhea (Kamath et al 1990). The concept that the proximal colon was the reservoir was further tested by the scintigraphic studies of Hammer and Phillips (1993). A healthy human colon was loaded with increasing volumes of saline, labeled for scintigraphic imaging. The entire proximal colon (cecum, ascending and transverse colons) stored liquids and solids; residence time was particularly important in the transverse colon. However, in response to the fastest infusions (500 ml in 30 minutes) fluid reached the rectum quickly; nevertheless, this segment was also able to store fluids and solids and therefore to provide impressive compensating potential. Thus it appears that reservoir function of the rectum has been underestimated, and is deserving of more scrutiny. In this regard, the reduced compliance and increased sensitivity of the inflamed rectum are thought to contribute importantly to the symptoms of IBD.

It is not possible to state a simple relationship between motility, transit and absorption. Colonic motility is more complex than the patterns seen in the upper gut: for instance, it shows diurnal variations, with maximum activity occurring after waking in the morning and following meals (Narducci et al 1987). Increased non-propulsive or segmenting contractions probably promote contact between the mucosa and luminal contents, and facilitate NaCl and water absorption. On the other hand, strongly propulsive, high-amplitude distally propagated contractions emptied the colon very rapidly when a mucosal irritant (oleic acid) was present (Spiller et al 1986, Kamath 1990). Ileal effluents will contain excess fat in any state of malabsorption. Similar waves of pressure were recorded from the colon in ulcerative colitis (Spriggs et al 1951). Rapid transit of colonic contents predisposes to diarrhea and increased fecal salt and water losses from the body.

PATHOPHYSIOLOGICAL CHANGES IN DISEASE

Chronic ulcerative colitis and Crohn's disease

The pathophysiology of IBD and its effects on colonic function are still obscure. The uncertain effects of mucosal inflammation cannot be ignored. Thus, in addition to deranged absorption, IBD might be anticipated to provoke exudation and possibly other mechanisms of fluid secretion. Inflammatory disease may therefore lead to diarrhea by several mechanisms. Blood, serum and mucus may exude from sites of ulceration or inflammation. When exudation is prominent, as in distal proctitis, rectal bleeding and diarrhea (with frequent, small, sometimes hard stools) may be a feature even though the fecal excretion of water is normal (Lennard-Jones et al 1962). Another mechanism of diarrhea is the accumulation of fluid in the lumen, as a result of active secretion by the diseased colon (Hawker et al 1980). Alternatively, the capacity of even a normal colon to handle an excess of fluid and electrolytes arriving from the ileum might be overwhelmed, as in Crohn's disease of the small bowel. Another mechanism is due to malabsorbed bile acids or dietary fat, which act as endogenous secretagogues. It is probable that combinations of these mechanisms are present in many patients with IBD.

Fluid and electrolytes losses in severe colitis

Disturbances of base and electrolyte homeostasis only occur when the disease is severe and acute. Losses of fluid and electrolytes from the inflamed colon range from 100 to 1500 ml, 10–170 mmol Na and 20–50 mmol K per day (Smiddy et al 1960). Corticosteroid therapy may intensify potassium loss. In severe ulcerative colitis and toxic megacolon a metabolic or mixed alkalosis may occur; this contrasts with the metabolic acidosis encountered in severe diarrhea from many other causes. Excessive chloride is lost in the stools, suggesting a defect in $Cl-HCO_3$ exchange. A rising arterial blood pH has been suggested by one group as an index of severity of proctocolitis (Caprilli et al 1976).

Pore size, permeability and PD

Transmucosal PD has been assessed in IBD by direct mucosal contact, and was found to be depressed in active colitis (Edmonds & Pilcher 1973, Rask-Madsen & Dalmark 1973); the PD returned to normal with resolution of the proctitis. It is suggested that the PD decreases as a consequence of impaired Na absorption. The alternative theory is of a back diffusion of Na ions into the lumen, with ions leaking freely back to the lumen owing to enhanced mucosal permeability (Levitan et al 1963, Rask-Madsen et al 1973).

Absorption in vitro

Mucosal transport in vitro in the sigmoid and descending colons has been studied in material removed by colectomy (Hawker et al 1980). Sodium absorption was impaired associated with a low PD and I_{sc} (short-circuit current) in the diseased mucosa, primarily due to a decreased flux of Na from mucosa to serosa. Secretion of Na, from serosal to mucosal fluids, was unaltered. Net fluxes of Cl and K were normal. However, Na fluxes and other indices of transport were normal in patients who received preoperative corticosteroids. There is some variance between these results and an earlier study (Archampong et al 1972) which demonstrated secretion of Na, Cl and K by the mucosa in IBD.

Absorption in vivo

In vivo studies have utilized a variety of techniques, including absorptive capacity of an intestinal loop isolated during colonic resection; total colonic perfusion; rectal instillation of test solutions; and dialysis bags inserted into the rectum.

Absorption of Na and water appears to be impaired in ulcerative colitis and Crohn's colitis (Duthie et al 1964, Harris and Shields 1970, Rask-Madsen et al 1973), and similar findings apply for Cl (Duthie et al 1964, Head et al 1969, Harris & Shields 1970). Potassium absorption is also impaired, and active secretion has even been suggested (Harris & Shields 1970).

Collagenous and microscopic colitis

Collagenous colitis causes a secretory diarrhea characterized by marked secretion of Na, Cl and water (Rask-Madsen et al 1983). Although normal on gross inspection, the histology of the colonic mucosa exhibits a subepithelial collagenous layer throughout. This collagen layer may be important in the pathogenesis of diarrhea, by acting as a simple physical barrier to absorption. Indeed, perfusion studies have demonstrated that Na and Cl fluxes from the colonic lumen to the bloodstream are decreased, and sodium movement in the opposite direction is increased in this illness. In contrast, Cl secretion is unchanged.

Another diarrhea of unknown origin was first identified by Fordtran's group as being due to non-specific inflammation of the colon (Read et al 1980). This entity was called microscopic colitis, because endoscopic and radiographic studies demonstrated the colonic mucosa to be grossly normal. A subsequent study (Bo-Linn et al 1985) showed that the histology could be easily differentiated from healthy tissue and some other forms of chronic diarrhea (without colonic inflammation). In most of the patients biopsy specimens from throughout the colon were abnormal, with similar severity, implicating a diffuse process. The main histologic findings consisted of acute inflammatory cells in the lamina propria, cryptitis, reactive changes in the surface epithelium (decreased mucus, loss of cellular polarity, and nuclear irregularity), mitotic figures, and goblet cell depletion. The investigators also performed colonic perfusion studies to determine fluid absorption, electrolyte flux and transmucosal potential difference. These showed decreased net absorption of water, Na and Cl by the colon, normal K secretion, and decreased HCO_3 secretion. The potential difference was not altered. Thus a histological abnormality with an associated defect in colonic water and electrolyte absorption was demonstrated, although a causal relationship could not be inferred. The etiology of the inflammation remains unknown, but the possibility that it represents a variant or early non-progressive form of inflammatory bowel disease has been raised.

Diarrhea following ileal resection

Bile acid and fat malabsorption

Disease or resection of the ileum in Crohn's disease impairs active absorption of bile acids, and can also cause fat malabsorption. Hofmann and Poley (1972) hypothesized that the diarrhea of limited ileal resections (<100 cm) is due to increased colonic secretion induced by bile acids, and that their sequestration with cholestyramine would be effective treatment. Conversely, 'fatty acid diarrhea' should occur after resections of more than 100 cm; fat is then the primary secretagogue, and reduction of dietary fat should be an effective treatment. Colonic secretion therefore appears to be the major physiological mechanism for diarrhea after ileal resection. It is also well established that bile acids and fatty acids reduce colonic absorption and can evoke a net secretion of fluid (Mekhjian et al 1971, Ammon & Phillips 1973, 1974, Bright-Asare & Binder 1973, Binder & Rawlins 1973). Mucosal inflammation in the proximal colon will also increase exposure of the remaining colonic mucosa to bile acids by further reducing bile acid absorption from the colon (Holmquist et al 1986, Mekhjian et al 1979).

The essential features of bile acid catharsis are that it is (a) dose-related, (b) rapidly reversible, and (c) highly stereospecific (Chadwick et al 1979, Gordon et al 1979). Bile acids with two hydroxy groups in the steroid nucleus, in the positions 3,7; 3,12; or 7,12, are the most potent. Similar comments apply to long-chain fatty acids. Ricinoleic acid, the active principle of castor oil, has been utilized as a model of endogenous overload of the colon by fatty acids. Ricinoleate is a C18 monohydroxy fatty acid which inhibits net absorption of water and electrolytes by the colon, and induces net fluid secretion at higher doses (Ammon & Phillips 1973, Bright-Asare & Binder 1973, Gaginella et al 1977). Dietary fatty acids have a similar effect, and their hydroxylation by intestinal bacteria enhances their secretory potency (Ammon & Phillips 1973). Thus, oleic acid is a less potent secretagogue than its bacterial hydration product, 10-OH stearic acid (Ammon & Phillips 1973). These differences may be explained in part by the fact that hydroxylated fatty acids are absorbed more slowly than their more hydrophobic, non-hydroxylated cogenors (Ammon & Phillips 1974).

The mechanism by which bile acids and fatty acids induce secretion is uncertain. Both classes of secretagogue stimulate adenylate cyclase activity, with a resultant increase in mucosal cAMP (Coyne et al 1977, Binder et al 1978). Thus, active secretion of Cl, an established property of cAMP, has been proposed as a mechanism for the action of bile acids and fatty acids on human colonic tissue (Coyne et al 1977). Pretreatment with propranolol prevented stimulation of adenylate cyclase, implicating β-adrenergic pathways (Coyne et al 1977); however, β-blockade failed to ameliorate bile acid diarrhea in one clinical report (Donowitz & Charney 1979).

Bile acid diarrhea is accompanied by increased bidirectional fluxes of small molecular weight hydrophilic probes, reflecting a generalized increase in mucosal permeability (Bright-Asare & Binder 1973, Gaginella et al 1977). However, a primary role for altered permeability is doubted, because although pretreatment with propranolol blocked the secretory response to bile acids, it did not prevent the increase in permeability (Binder et al 1978). A further potential mechanism for secretory diarrhea is mucosal damage, since both bile acids and fatty acids are potent cytotoxins and their perfusion through the colon produces epitheliolysis (Gaginella & Phillips 1976, Gaginella et al 1977). Another possible mechanism involves increased transit through the colon, since bile acids stimulate colonic motility (Snape et al 1980).

Associated partial resection of the colon

Less attention has been directed to the influence of concurrent resection of the colon. However, it is not surprising that the severity of diarrhea following ileal resection is modified by the extent of colonic resection (Cummings et al 1973, Mitchell et al 1980). The observations of Cummings et al (1973) are particularly cogent: not only was the loss of colonic absorbing surface incriminated, but reduced bacterial production of SCFA in the shortened colon might also lead to a reduction in Na absorption. Adaptive changes in the colonic mucosa which reduce the effects of resection have been observed in rats following cecectomy and partial jejunoilectomy (Fabritius et al 1986).

Kock and ileal pouches

After proctocolectomy surgical construction of a reservoir for ileal chyme maintains continence, with planned intermittent evacuation through an ileostomy (Kock pouch) or transanally (ileal pouch) being possible. These pouches have improved patient lifestyle following colonic resection; indeed, construction of an ileal pouch after proctocolectomy is standard in many major centers. After a period of adaptation the frequency of stooling is 5–7 per day, and fecal weight is approximately that of discharge from an ileostomy. The absorptive function of Kock pouch mucosa was similar to that of normal healthy ileum (Gadacz et al 1977), but comparable studies have not been performed with ileal pouches. Pouch function is perturbed in 10–30% of otherwise successful outcomes by the development of non-specific inflammation (pouchitis), which can be accompanied by diarrhea and increased fecal weight (Sandborn 1994). Although pouch absorptive function is presumed to be altered by the inflammation of pouchitis, no experimental data are available (Kelly et al 1980, 1983). The etiology is unknown, but may relate to abnormal proliferation of anerobic bacteria in the small intestine.

Enteric hyperoxaluria

Renal oxalate stones are common after ileal resection and in other forms of steatorrhea. Hyperoxaluria is due to increased absorption of dietary oxalate in the colon (Dobbins & Binder 1977), and is one of the few examples of pathological hyperabsorption. Increased mucosal permeability to oxalate is produced by the action of bile acids or fat on colonic epithelium; this is aggravated by high dietary intakes of oxalate and intraluminal binding of calcium ions by fatty acid anions as a result of steatorrhea (Dobbins & Binder 1977). Contributing factors to stone formation include oliguria and a low total ionic strength of urine (Smith 1980); these in turn are aggravated by intestinal loss of water and salts.

REFERENCES

Ahn J, Chang E B, Field M 1985 Phorbol ester inhibition of Na–H exchange in rabbit proximal colon. American Journal of Physiology 249: C527–C530

Ammon H V, Phillips S F 1973 Inhibition of colonic water and electrolyte absorption by fatty acids in man. Gastroenterology 65: 744–749

Ammon H V, Phillips S F 1974 Inhibition of ileal water absorption by intraluminal fatty acids. Journal of Clinical Investigation 53: 205–210

Archampong E Q, Harris J, Clark C G 1972 The absorption and secretion of water and electrolytes across the healthy and the diseased human colonic mucosa measured in vitro. Gut 13: 880–886

Bastl C P 1987 Regulation of cation transport by low doses of glucorticoids in *in vivo* adrenalectomized rat colon. Journal of Clinical Investigation 80: 748–756

Billich C O, Levitan R 1969 Effect of sodium concentration and osmolality on water and electrolyte absorption from the intact human colon. Journal of Clinical Investigation 48: 1336–1347

Binder H J, Mehta P 1989 Short-chain fatty acids stimulate active Na and Cl absorption *in vitro* in the rat distal colon. Gastroenterology 96: 989–996

Binder H J, Rawlins C L 1973 Effect of conjugated dihydroxy bile salts on electrolyte transport in rat colon. Journal of Clinical Investigation 52: 1460–1466

Binder H J, Dobbins J W, Racusen L C, Whiting D S 1978 Effect of propranolol on ricinoleic acid and deoxycholic acid induced changes of intestinal electrolyte movement and mucosal permeability. Gastroenterology 75: 668–673

Binder H J, Sandle G I, Rajendrum V M 1991 Colonic fluid and electrolyte transport in health and disease. In: Phillips S F, Pemberton J H, Shorter R G (eds) The large intestine: physiology, pathophysiology and disease. Raven Press, New York, pp 141–168

Binder H J, Stange G, Murer H, Stieger B, Hauri H 1986 Sodium–proton exchange in colon brush-border membranes. American Journal of Physiology 251: G382–G390

Bjork J T, Soergel K H, Wood C M 1976 The composition of 'free' stool water. Gastroenterology 70: 864 (Abstract)

Bo-Linn G W, Vendrell D D, Lee E, Fordtran J S 1985 An evaluation of the significance of microscopic colitis in patients with chronic diarrhea. Journal of Clinical Investigation 75: 1559–1569

Breuer R I, Buto S K, Christ M L et al 1991 Rectal irrigation with short-chain fatty acids for distal ulcerative colitis. Preliminary report. Digestive Diseases and Sciences 36: 185–187

Bridges R J, Rack M, Rummel W, Schreiner J 1986 Mucosal plexus and electrolyte transport across the rat colonic mucosa. Journal of Physiology (London) 376: 531–542

Bright-Asare P, Binder H J 1973 Stimulation of colonic secretion of water and electrolytes by hydroxy fatty acids. Gastroenterology 64: 81–88

Caprilli R, Vernia P, Colaneri O, Torsoli A 1976 Blood pH: a test for assessment of severity in proctocolitis. Gut 17: 763–769

Carey H V, Cooke H J, Zafirova M 1985 Mucosal responses evoked by stimulation of ganglion cell somas in the submucosal plexus of the guinea pig ileum. Journal of Physiology (London) 364: 69–79

Cassuto J, Ahrenkrug J, Jodal M, Tuttle R, Lundgren O 1981 Release of vasoactive intestinal polypeptide from the cat small intestine exposed to cholera toxin. Gut 22: 958–963

Chadwick V S, Phillips S F, Hofmann A F 1977 Measurements of intestinal permeability using low molecular weight polyethylene glycols (PEG 400). II. Application to normal and abnormal permeability states in man and animals. Gastroenterology 73: 247–251

Chadwick V S, Gaginella T S, Carlson G L, Debongnie J C, Phillips S F 1979 Effects of molecular structure on bile acid induced alterations in absorptive function, permeability, and morphology in perfused rabbit colon. Journal of Laboratory and Clinical Medicine 94: 661–674

Chang E B, Rao M C 1994 Intestinal water and electrolyte transport: mechanisms of physiological and adaptive responses, In: Johnson L R (ed) Physiology of the gasrointestinal tract, 3rd edn. Raven Press, New York, pp 2022–2087

Coyne M J, Bonorris G G, Chung A, Conley D, Schoenfield L J 1977 Propranolol inhibits bile acid and fatty acid stimulation of cyclic AMP in human colon. Gastroenterology 73: 971–974

Cummings J H, James W P T, Wiggins H S 1973 Role of the colon in ileal resection diarrhea. Lancet 1: 344–347

Davis G R, Morawski S G, Santa Ana C A, Fordtran J S 1983 Evaluation of chloride/bicarbonate exchange in the human colon *in vivo*. Journal of Clinical Investigation 71: 201–207

Dawson A M, Holdsworth C D, Webb J 1964 Absorption of short chain fatty acids in man. Proceedings of the Society for Experimental Biology and Medicine 117: 97–100

Debongnie J C, Phillips S F 1978 Capacity of the human colon to absorb fluid. Gastroenterology 74: 698–703

Devroede G J, Phillips S F 1969 Conservation of sodium, chloride, and water by the human colon. Gastroenterology 56: 101–109

Diamond J M 1974 Tight and leaky junctions of epithelia: a perspective on kisses in the dark. Federation Proceedings 33: 2220–2224

Dobbins J W, Binder H J 1977 Importance of the colon in enteric hyperoxaluria. New England Journal of Medicine 296: 298–301

Donowitz M 1987 Small intestinal and colonic linked sodium chloride absorption. New understanding of distribution and regulation. Gastroenterology 93: 640–651

Donowitz M, Charney A N 1979 No effect of propranolol in chronic diarrhea. (Correspondence) New England Journal of Medicine 300: 201

Duthie H L, Watts J M, De Dombal F T, Goligher J C 1964 Serum electrolytes and colonic transfer of water and electrolytes in chronic ulcerative colitis. Gastroenterology 47: 525–530

Edmonds C J 1975 Electrical potential difference of colonic mucosa. Gut 16: 315–318

Edmonds C J, Nielsen O E 1968 Transmembrane electrical potential differences and ionic composition of mucosal cells of rat colon. Acta Physiologica Scandinavica 72: 338–349

Edmonds C J, Pilcher D 1973 Electrical potential difference and sodium and potassium fluxes across rectal mucosa in ulcerative colitis. Gut 14: 784–789

Ewe K, Holker B 1974 Einfluss eines diphenolischer Laxars Bisacodyl auf den Wasser-und Elektrolyttransport im menschlichen Colon. Klinische Wochenschrift 52: 827–833

Fabritius J, Nell G, Loeschke K 1986 Adaptation of electrolyte transport in rat large intestine after proximal resection. II. Colon after 50% jejunoilectomy combined with cecectomy. Pflügers Archiv 406: 328–332

Fordtran J S, Rector F C, Ewton M F, Soter N, Kinney J 1965 Permeability characteristics of the human small intestine. Journal of Clinical Investigation 44: 1935–1944

Foster E S, Dudeja P K, Brasitus T A 1986a $Na^+–H^+$ exchange in rat colonic brush-border membrane vesicles. American Journal of Physiology 250: G781–G787

Foster E S, Budinger M E, Hayslet J P, Binder H J 1986b Ion transport in proximal colon of the rat: sodium depletion stimulates neutral sodium chloride absorption. Journal of Clinical Investigation 77: 228–235

Foster E S, Zimmerman T W, Hayslett J P, Binder H J 1983 Corticosteroid alteration of active electrolyte transport in rat distal colon. American Journal of Physiology 245: G668–G675

Frizzell R A, Heintze K 1979 Electrogenic chloride secretion by mammalian colon. In: Binder H J (ed) Mechanisms of intestinal secretion. Alan R. Liss, New York, pp 101–110

Frizzell R A, Schultz S G 1978 Effects of aldosterone on ion transport by rabbit colon in vitro. Journal of Membrane Biology 39: 1–26

Frizzell R A, Koch M J, Schultz S G 1976 Ion transport by rabbit colon. 1: Active and passive components. Journal of Membrane Biology 27: 297–316

Furness J B, Costa M 1980 Types of nerves in the enteric nervous system. Neuroscience 5: 1–20

Furness J B, Costa M, Gibbins I L, Llewellyn-Smith I J, Oliver J R 1985 Neurochemically similar myenteric and submucous neurons directly traced to the mucosa of the small intestine. Cell and Tissue Research 241: 155–163

Gadacz T R, Kelly K A, Phillips S F 1977 The continent ileal pouch: absorptive and motor features. Gastroenterology 72: 1287–1291

Gaginella T S, Phillips S F 1976 Ricinoleic acid (castor oil) alters intestinal surface structure: a scanning electron microscopic study. Mayo Clinic Proceedings 51: 6–12

Gaginella T S, Chadwick V S, Debongnie J C, Lewis J C, Phillips S F 1977 Perfusion of rabbit colon with ricinoleic acid: dose-related mucosal injury, fluid secretion, and increased permeability. Gastroenterology 73: 95–101

Giller J, Phillips S F 1972 Electrolyte absorption and secretion in the human colon. American Journal of Digestive Diseases 17: 1003–1011

Gooptu D, Truelove S C, Warner G T 1969 Absorption of electrolytes from the colon in cases of ulcerative colitis and in control subjects. Gut 10: 555–561

Gordon S J, Kinsey M D, Magen J S, Joseph R E, Kowlessar O D 1979 Structure of bile acids associated with secretion in the rat cecum. Gastroenterology 77: 38–44

Grady G F, Duhamel R C, Moore E W 1970 Active transport of sodium by human colon in vitro. Gastroenterology 59: 583–588

Hammer J, Phillips S F 1993 Fluid loading of the human colon: effects of segmental transit and stool composition. Gastroenterology 105: 988–998

Harig J M, Soergel K H, Komorowski R A, Wood C M 1989 Treatment of diversion colitis with short-chain-fatty acid irrigation. New England Journal of Medicine 320: 23–28

Harris J, Shields R 1970 Absorption and secretion of water and electrolytes by the intact human colon in diffuse untreated proctocolitis. Gut 11: 27–33

Hawker P C, Mashiter K E, Turnberg L A 1978 Mechanisms of transport of Na, Cl, and K in the human colon. Gastroenterology 74: 1241–1247

Hawker P C, McKay J S, Turnberg L A 1980 Electrolyte transport across colonic mucosa from patients with inflammatory bowel disease. Gastroenterology 79: 508–511

Hawkey C J, Rampton D S 1985 Prostaglandins and the gastrointestinal mucosa: are they important in its function, disease or treatment? Gastroenterology 89: 1162–1188

Head L H, Heaton J W, Kivel R M 1969 Absorption of water and electrolytes in Crohn's disease of the colon. Gastroenterology 56: 571–579

Hill G 1976 Ileostomy: surgery, physiology and management. Grune and Stratton, New York

Hofmann A F, Poley J R 1972 Role of bile acid malabsorption in pathogenesis of diarrhea and steatorrhea in patients with ileal resection. I. Response to cholestyramine or replacement of dietary long-chain triglyceride by medium-chain triglyceride. Gastroenterology 62: 918–934

Holmberg C, Perheentupa J, Launiala K 1975 Colonic electrolyte transport in health and in congenital chloride diarrhea. Journal of Clinical Investigation 56: 302–310

Holmquist L, Andersson H, Rudic N, Ahren C, Fallstrom S P 1986 Bile acid malabsorption in children and adolescents with chronic colitis. Scandanavian Journal of Gastroenterology 21: 87–92

Hubel K A, Renquist K, Shirazi S 1987 Ion transport in human cecum, transverse colon, and sigmoid colon in vitro. Baseline and response to electrical stimulation of intrinsic nerves. Gastroenterology 92: 501–507

Hubel K A, Renquist K S, Varley G 1991 Secretory reflexes in ileum and jejunum: absence of remote effects. Journal of the Autonomic Nervous System 35: 53–62

Jiang M M, Kirchgessner A, Gershon M D, Surprenant A 1993 Cholera toxin-sensitive neurons in guinea pig submucosal plexus. American Journal of Physiology 264: G86–G94

Jodal M 1990 Neuronal influence on intestinal transport. Journal of Internal Medicine 228(Suppl 732): 125–132

Kamath P S, Phillips S F, O'Connor M K, Brown M L, Zinsmeister A R 1990 Colonic capacitance and transit in man: modulation by luminal contents and drugs. Gut 31: 443–449

Kelly D G, Branon M E, Phillips S F, Kelly K A 1980 Diarrhea after continent ileostomy. Gut 21: 711–716

Kelly D G, Phillips S F, Kelly K A, Weinstein W M, Gilchrist M J 1983 Dysfunction of the continent ileostomy: clinical features and bacteriology. Gut 24: 193–201

Kuwahara A, Bowen S, Wang J, Condon C, Cooke H 1987 Epithelial responses evoked by stimulation of submucosal neurons in guinea pig distal colon. American Journal of Physiology 252: G667–G674

Lennard-Jones J E, Cooper G W, Newell A C, Wilson C W E, Jones F A 1962 Observations on idiopathic proctitis. Gut 3: 201–206

Levitan R, Bikerman V, Burrows B A, Ingelfinger F J 1963 Rectosigmoidal absorption of phenolsulfonphthalein (PSP), sulfisoxazole diethanolamine (Gantrisin), and radioiodine (^{131}I) in normal subjects and patients with idiopathic ulcerative colitis. Journal of Laboratory and Clinical Medicine 62: 639–645

Mekhjian H S, Phillips S F, Hofmann A F 1971 Colonic secretion of water and electrolytes induced by bile acids: perfusion studies in man. Journal of Clinical Investigation 50: 1569–1577

Mekhjian H S, Phillips S F, Hofmann A F 1979 Colonic absorption of unconjugated bile acids: perfusion studies in man. Digestive Diseases and Sciences 24: 545–550

Mitchell J E, Breuer R I, Zuckerman L, Berlin J, Schilli R, Dunn J K 1980 The colon influences ileal resection diarrhea. Digestive Diseases and Sciences 25: 33–41

Narducci F, Bassotti G, Gaburri M, Morelli A 1987 Twenty-four hour manometric recording of colonic motor activity in healthy man. Gut 28: 17–25

Nocerino A, Iafusco M, Guandalini S 1995 Cholera toxin-induced small intestinal secretion has a secretory effect on the colon of the rat. Gastroenterology 108: 34–39

Palma R, Vidon N, Bernier J 1981 Maximal capacity for fluid absorption in human bowel. Digestive Diseases and Sciences 26: 929–934

Phillips S F 1988 Physiology and pathophysiology of the large intestine and anal canal. In: Kirsner J B, Shorter R G (eds) Diseases of the colon, rectum and anal canal. Williams & Wilkins, Baltimore, pp 23–46

Phillips S F, Giller J 1973 The contribution of the colon to electrolyte and water conservation in man. Journal of Laboratory and Clinical Medicine 81: 733–746

Phillips S F, Schmalz P F 1970 Bicarbonate secretion by the rat colon:

effect of intraluminal chloride and acetazolamide. Proceedings of the Society for Experimental Biology and Medicine 135: 116–122

Posey E L, Bargen J A 1950 Metabolic derangements in chronic ulcerative colitis. Gastroenterology 16: 39–50

Racusen L C, Binder H J 1979 Ricinoleic acid stimulation of active anion secretion in colonic mucosa of the rat. Journal of Clinical Investigation 63:743–749

Racusen L C, Binder H J 1980 Effect of prostaglandin on ion transport across isolated colonic mucosa. Digestive Diseases and Sciences 25: 900–904

Rask-Madsen J, Dalmark M 1973 Decreased transmucosal potential difference across the human rectum in ulcerative colitis. Scandinavian Journal of Gastroenterology 8: 321–326

Rask-Madsen J, Hammersgaard E A, Knudsen E 1973 Rectal electrolyte transport and mucosal permeability in ulcerative colitis and Crohn's disease. Journal of Laboratory and Clinical Medicine 81: 342–353

Read N W, Krejs G J, Read M G, Santa Ana C A, Morawski S G, Fordtran J S 1980 Chronic diarrhea of unknown origin. Gastroenterology 78: 264–271

Roediger W E 1980 The role of anaerobic bacteria in the metabolic welfare of the colonic mucosa in man. Gut 21: 793–798

Roediger W E 1982 Utilization of nutrients by isolated epithelial cells of the rat colon. Gastroenterology 83: 424–429

Roediger W E W, Moore A 1981 Effect of short-chain fatty acid on sodium absorption in isolated human colon perfused through the vascular bed. Digestive Diseases and Sciences 26: 100–106

Rubinstein R, Howard A V, Wrong O M 1969 In vivo dialysis of faeces as a method of stool analysis. IV. The organic anion component. Clinical Science 37: 549–564

Ruppin H, Bar-Meir S, Soergel K H, Wood C M, Schmitt M G 1980 Absorption of short-chain fatty acids by the colon. Gastroenterology 78: 1500–1507

Sandborn W J 1994 Pouchitis following ileal pouch–anal anastomosis: definition, pathogenesis and treatment. Gastroenterology 107: 1848–1855

Sandle G I, Binder H J 1987 Corticosteroids and intestinal ion transport. Gastroenterology 93: 188–196

Saunders D R, Sillery J, Rachmilewitz D 1975 Effect of dioctylsodium sulfosuccinate on structure and function of rodent and human intestine. Gastroenterology 69: 380–386

Schultz S G 1980 Cellular models of sodium and chloride absorption by mammalian small and large intestine. In: Field M, Fordtran J S, Schultz S G (eds) Secretory diarrhea. American Physiological Society, Bethesda, Maryland, pp 1–9

Sellin J H, DeSoignie R 1987 Ion transport in human colon *in vitro*. Gastroenterology 93: 441–448

Simon B, Czygan P, Spaan G, Dittrich J, Kather H 1978 Hormone-sensitive adenylate cyclase in human colonic tissue. Digestion 17: 229–233

Smiddy F G, Gregory S D, Smith I B, Goligher J C 1960 Faecal loss of fluid, electrolytes, and nitrogen in colitis before and after ileostomy. Lancet 1: 14–19

Smith L H 1980 Enteric hyperoxaluria and other hyperoxaluric states. In: Coe F L (guest ed.), Brenner B N, Stein J H (eds) Contemporary issues in nephrology, Vol 5. Churchill Livingstone, New York, pp 136–164

Snape W J, Schiff S, Cohen S 1980 Effect of deoxycholic acid on colonic motility in the rabbit. American Journal of Physiology 238: G321–G325

Spiller R C, Brown M L, Phillips S F 1986 Decreased fluid tolerance, accelerated transit and abnormal motility of the human colon induced by oleic acid. Gastroenterology 91: 100–107

Spriggs E A, Code C F, Bargen J A, Curtis R K, Hightower N C 1951 Motility of the pelvic colon and rectum of normal persons and patients with ulcerative colitis. Gastroenterology 19: 480–491

Stephen A M, Cummings J H 1979 Effects of dietary fibre on fecal bacterial mass. Gut 20: A457–A458 (Abstract)

Tantisira M H, Fändriks L, Jönsson C, Jodal M, Lundgren O 1990 Studies on cholera toxin-induced changes of alkaline secretion and transmural potential difference in the rat small intestine *in vivo*. Acta Physiologica Scandinavica 138: 75–84

Theodorou V, Fioramonti J, Junien J L, Bueno L 1994 Anaphylactic colonic hypersecretion in cow's milk sensitized guinea-pigs depends upon release of interleukin-1, prostaglandins and mast cell degranulation. Alimentary Pharmacology and Therapeutics 8: 301–307

Thoren L 1962 Magnesium deficiency: studied in two cases of acute fulminant ulcerative colitis treated by colectomy. Acta Chirurgica Scandinavica 124: 134–143

Van Dyke R W, Ives H E 1988 Na^+/H^+ exchange: what, where and why? Hepatology 8: 960–965

von Engelhardt W, Burmester M, Hansen K, Becker G, Rechkemmer G 1993 Effects of amiloride and ouabain on short-chain fatty acid transport in guinea-pig large intestine. Journal of Physiology 460: 455–466

Wacker W E C, Parisi A F 1968 Magnesium metabolism. New England Journal of Medicine 278: 658–663

Warhurst G, Higgs N B, Lees M, Tonge A, Turnberg L A 1988 Activation of protein kinase C attenuates prostaglandin E_2 responses in a colonic cell line. American Journal of Physiology 255: G27–G32

Weiser M M, Quill H 1975 Intestinal villus and crypt cell responses to cholera toxin. Gastroenterology 69: 479–482

Zimmerman T W, Binder H J 1984 Serotonin induced alteration of colonic electrolyte transport in the rat. Gastroenterology 86: 310–317

23. Pathophysiology of gastrointestinal motor disturbances in inflammatory bowel disease

S. S. C. Rao

INTRODUCTION

The tonic and phasic contractions of the intestinal smooth muscle control the rate at which material travels along the gut before it is finally expelled through the anus. In theory, excessive propulsive motor activity would accelerate the transit of material, producing diarrhea, whereas a preponderance of mixing or segmental contractions could result in delayed transit and constipation.

The mechanisms responsible for the bowel disturbance in inflammatory bowel disease are presumably caused by interactions of abnormal motor activity (Read & Johnson 1983) and epithelial transport (Steadman & Phillips 1990). Impaired colonic absorption of sodium and chloride (Duthie et al 1964, Harris & Shields 1970, Rask-Madsen et al 1973, Hawker et al 1980) and excessive secretion of fluid and electrolytes (Archampong et al 1972, Edmonds & Pilcher 1973) are thought to be responsible for the liquid diarrhea observed in patients with active colitis. Failure of the diseased colon to salvage unabsorbable carbohydrate may also contribute to the diarrhea in some patients (Montgomery et al 1968, Read 1982, Rao et al 1987a). Until recently, disturbances of intestinal motor activity in ulcerative colitis and Crohn's disease were less well understood. These motor abnormalities may not only affect the colon but may also involve the small intestine and the stomach. This chapter provides an understanding of the role of motor activity in the pathophysiology of inflammatory bowel disease.

DISTURBANCES OF INTESTINAL MOTOR ACTIVITY IN ULCERATIVE COLITIS

Nature of bowel disturbance

For a condition in which change of bowel habit is a major manifestation, there is only limited information regarding objective data on bowel symptoms. In a recent study (Rao et al 1988a) the prevalence of symptom and stool patterns was assessed prospectively in 96 patients with colitis (Table 23.1). Increased frequency of defecation, urgency, a feeling

Table 23.1 The prevalence of stool patterns and bowel symptoms in patients with ulcerative colitis, subdivided according to the extent and activity of disease

	Total colitis		Distal colitis	
	Active	Quiescent	Active	Quiescent
No. studied	26	19	34	31
Symptoms				
Urgency	24 (92%)*	2 (11%)	27 (79%)†	5 (16%)
Incomplete evacuation	20 (77%)*	3 (16%)	27 (79%)†	6 (19%)
Tenesmus	18 (69%)*	2 (11%)	20 (59%)†	3 (10%)
Pain	12 (46%)*	2 (11%)	18 (53%)†	5 (16%)
Anal soreness	13 (50%)*	2 (11%)	11 (32%)†	2 (6%)
Incontinence	8 (31%)*	0	6 (18%)†	0
Nocturnal defecation	21 (81%)*	0	19 (56%)†	0
Predominant stool consistency				
Unformed	17 (65%)*	3 (16%)	15 (44%)†	2 (7%)
Formed	4 (15%)*	15 (79%)	8 (23%)†	26 (84%)
Hard	5 (19%)	1 (5%) NS	11 (33%)‡	3 (9%)

Data expressed as the proportion of patients in each group who reported the symptom
*, significantly different from quiescent total colitis ($P < 0.01$)
†, significantly different from quiescent total colitis ($P < 0.01$)
‡, significantly different from quiescent total colitis ($P < 0.05$)
NS, not significant

of incomplete evacuation and tenesmus were the most frequent symptoms experienced by patients with active colitis. The occurrence of nocturnal defecation and fecal incontinence invariably suggested active disease. The prevalence of these symptoms was similar in patients with total and distal colitis, suggesting that they are related to an inflamed and irritable distal colon. Although most patients with active colitis had increased stool frequency and were voiding blood and mucus in their stools, the results of stool consistency tests were surprising: 27% of all patients with active colitis voided hard pellet-like stools indicative of constipation. This feature was more common in patients with active rather than quiescent colitis. Another 20% of patients passed formed stools; thus approximately 50% of patients with active disease did not have diarrhea.

Analysis of stool output demonstrated that patients with active colitis had increased stool weight and frequency

Table 23.2 Measurements of stool output in normal controls and in patients with ulcerative colitis, subdivided according to disease extent and activity

	Control $n = 20$	Ulcerative colitis			
		Total		Distal	
		Active $n = 15$	Quiescent $n = 15$	Active $n = 23$	Quiescent $n = 23$
Mean daily stool frequency	1.1 ± 0.5	$4.6 \pm 1.3^{*\dagger}$	$1.9 \pm 0.9^{*}$	$2.7 \pm 0.9^{*\dagger}$	1.3 ± 0.6
Mean daily stool weight (g)	152 ± 61	$296 \pm 98^{*\dagger}$	161 ± 53	$203 \pm 94^{*}$	162 ± 73
Mean weight of each bowel movement (g)	136 ± 72	$64 \pm 19^{*\dagger}$	99 ± 38	$73 \pm 32^{*\dagger}$	139 ± 46
Percentage stools unformed	—	$80^{\dagger}$	18	$57^{\dagger}$	24
Percentage stools with blood	—	$71^{\dagger}$	9	$59^{\dagger}$	5
Percentage stools with mucus	—	$56^{\dagger}$	10	$68^{\dagger}$	15

Results are expressed as mean ± SD
*, significantly different from controls
†, significantly different from quiescent disease

compared to patients with quiescent colitis (Rao et al 1987b; Table 23.2). Patients with active disease also passed smaller amounts of stool during each bowel movement, indicating that these patients defecate at lower rectal volumes (Rao et al 1987b); thus, the colitic rectum appears to be more irritable than normal.

Disturbances in gastric and small-intestinal transit

Gastric stasis and small-intestinal pseudo-obstruction have been described in patients with colitis (Manousos & Salem 1965), although some of these cases may be explained by hypokalemia. Duodenal and jejunal motor activity recorded during resting conditions and in response to various stimuli indicate that the intraluminal pressures are lower and the rate of intestinal propulsion slower in patients with colitis than in controls (Ritchie & Salem 1965). In another study, delay in the clearance of barium from the small intestine was observed in nine of 16 patients with ulcerative colitis (Manousos & Salem 1965). Mouth-to-cecum transit was also estimated using radiotelemetric capsules in eight patients with colitis, and a delay in gastric emptying and small-bowel transit time was reported (Rosswick et al 1967).

In a more recent study the small-bowel transit time of a solid meal was delayed in all patients irrespective of the extent or activity of colitis (Table 23.3). All groups of colitics except those with quiescent distal colitis had normal gastric emptying (Rao et al 1987b). Since gastric emptying was normal, this delay in mouth-to-cecum transit must represent a slowing of small-bowel transit time. Moreover, the small-bowel transit time in the same individuals did not change during active and quiescent phases of the disease (Rao et al 1987b; Table 23.4). The reason for this delayed transit is not known, but suppression of small-bowel contractile activity and delayed small-bowel transit can be induced by prolonged rectal stimulation (Youle & Read 1984, Kellow et al 1986).

Disturbances in colonic transit

Nearly all the measurements of colonic motor activity in colitic patients have been carried out in the distal colon, but this may not represent changes in motor function along the whole length of the colon. The only available

Table 23.3 Measurements of gastrointestinal transit and breath concentration in normal controls and in patients with ulcerative colitis subdivided according to disease extent and activity

	Control $n = 20$	Ulcerative Colitis			
		Total		Distal	
		Active $n = 15$	Quiescent $n = 15$	Active $n = 23$	Quiescent $n = 23$
Half time for gastric emptying (min)	52 ± 22	48 ± 19	53 ± 31	57 ± 27	$67 \pm 27^{*}$
Breath H$_2$ concentration (ppm)					
Basal value	10 ± 4	9 ± 6	12 ± 8	14 ± 10	17 ± 12
1 hour after rise	18 ± 7	27 ± 21	28 ± 12	27 ± 14	31 ± 16
Mouth to cecum transit time (min)	229 ± 65	$296 \pm 57^{\dagger}$	$317 \pm 80^{\dagger}$	$327 \pm 77^{\dagger}$	$314 \pm 88^{\dagger}$
Whole-gut transit time (h)					
1st marker	32 ± 13	28 ± 12	36 ± 19	42 ± 32	44 ± 36
50% markers	48 ± 22	55 ± 22	53 ± 33	55 ± 22	60 ± 42

Results are expressed as mean ± SD
*, significantly different from controls $P < 0.05$
†, significantly different from controls $P < 0.001$

Table 23.4 Transit measurements and stool output during active and quiescent disease (paired data)

	Total colitis ($n = 6$)			Distal colitis ($n = 8$)		
	Active	Quiescent	P	Active	Quiescent	P
Gastric emptying ($t\frac{1}{2}$) (min)	46 ± 22	41 ± 6	NS	51 ± 23	78 ± 33	<0.05
Mouth to cecum transit (min)	298 ± 62	310 ± 60	NS	313 ± 87	293 ± 82	NS
Whole gut transit (h)	63.8 ± 22.2	55.7 ± 29.3	NS	68.1 ± 49.4	78.3 ± 55.1	NS
Mean daily stool weight (g)	253 ± 72	159 ± 62	<0.02	192 ± 99	144 ± 79	<0.05
Mean daily stool frequency	4.1 ± 1.0	1.9 ± 1.0	<0.002	3.0 ± 0.8	1.2 ± 0.7	<0.001

Results are expressed as mean ± SD
NS, not significant

information regarding proximal colonic motility in colitis is from measurements of colonic transit. Although it is widely assumed that ulcerative colitis is associated with rapid colonic transit (Van Hees et al 1979), recent studies have indicated that the whole-gut transit time of solid and liquid markers is not accelerated in either active or quiescent colitics, compared to normal subjects (Rao et al 1987b; Table 23.4).

There are, however, significant differences in segmental colonic transit. A plain abdominal X-ray taken 48 hours after ingestion of the test meal indicated that transit through the proximal colon is slowed in patients with active colitis, whereas distal colonic transit is accelerated. This effect is independent of the extent of the colitis (Rao et al 1987b; Fig. 23.1). Hence, in contrast to the concept of rapid colonic transit, there is proximal colonic stasis in patients with active colitis. This has been commented upon previously, but has been largely ignored. Mackie (1938) reported that there was a considerable delay in the transit of barium through the proximal colon in 50% of patients with active colitis. Lennard-Jones et al (1962a, b) reported that 33% of patients with proctitis and six other cases of more extensive disease exhibited proximal colonic stasis. Impaired propulsive activity in the proximal colon was also observed when intraluminal pressures were recorded using a radiotelemetric capsule (Jalan et al 1970). A recent study investigated the mouth-to-anus transit of a blue dye in patients with proctitis, and reported that the dye appeared

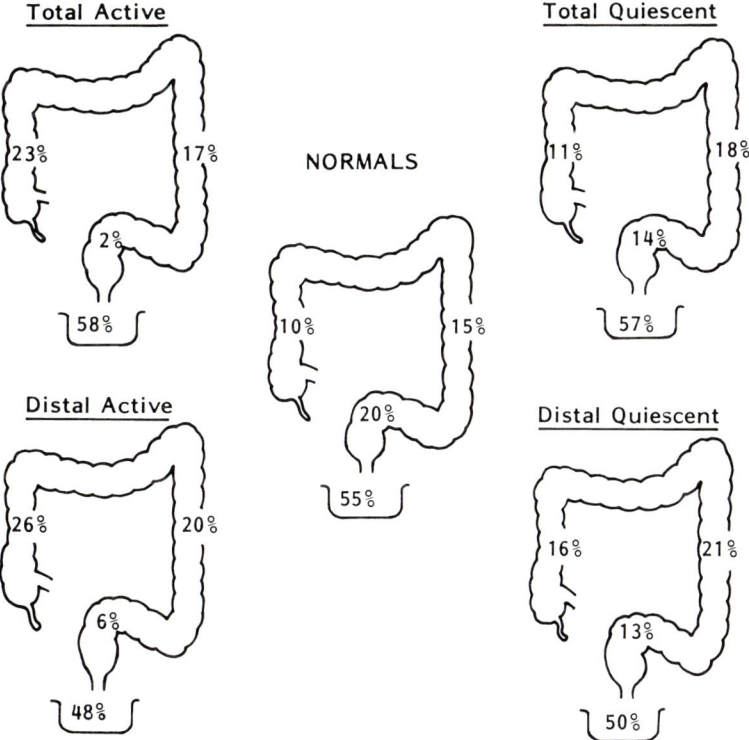

Fig. 23.1 Segmental distribution of the mean percentage of the number of markers in the colon in patients with colitis and normal subjects. (from Rao et al 1987b)

in the stool at the same time as in control subjects but took a significantly longer time to disappear from stool (Black et al 1987), further supporting the hypothesis of fecal stasis. A retrospective radiological survey showed that 6% of patients with total colitis and 30% of patients with distal colitis had evidence of proximal colonic stasis (Jalan et al 1970). These clinical accounts may have underestimated the true incidence, since many patients with colitis are unaware that they are constipated as they are distracted by the passage of blood and mucus (Engel 1954a, b).

Previous studies have shown that the proximal and the distal colon react differently when stimulated by the same pharmacological agent: for example, opiates cause proximal colonic stasis and distal colonic hyperactivity (Garrett et al 1967, Spiller et al 1985), whereas serotonin has an opposite effect (Fink & Friedman 1960). Another study demonstrated marked differences in the electrophysiological and mechanical properties of smooth muscle from the two regions (Gill et al 1986). Hence, although the large intestine is considered as a single organ, the functional characteristics of the proximal and the distal colon appear to be different, and consequently their responses to inflammation may also differ. Furthermore, stimulation of the distal colon may produce changes in the proximal colon, either through neurohormonal mechanisms or via an extrinsic reflex (Youle & Read 1984, Kellow et al 1986).

Proximal colonic stasis may enhance the tendency for patients with severe colitis to develop toxic megacolon. The exact mechanisms responsible for this are unknown, but one explanation is that a transmural inflammatory response may affect the ganglion cells, causing inhibition of the tonic contraction of the intestinal smooth muscle (Read & Johnson 1983, Youle & Read 1984). This loss of resting tone may lead to luminal dilation. Factors which predispose the inflamed colon to become dilated include administration of opiates and belladonna alkaloids to control diarrhea, barium studies and electrolyte disturbances, particularly hypokalemia (Smith et al 1962, Jalan et al 1969, Norland & Kirsner 1969, Binder et al 1974, Truelove & Marks 1981). Opiates relax the proximal colon and induce increased segmental contractions of the distal colon (Garrett et al 1967, Spiller et al 1985). Since colitics with active disease have a slower transit through the proximal colon (Rao et al 1987b), opiates could only worsen this inherent tendency for colonic inertia and can lead to toxic dilatation.

Colonic motility in ulcerative colitis

Since the colon is not easily accessible, early observations of colonic motor patterns were based on measurements of rectosigmoid contractility, which have shown conflicting results. In 1951, Posey and Bargen recorded intraluminal pressures in the rectosigmoid region with a tandem balloon system, and concluded that diarrhea in colitis was caused by an excessive propulsive activity of the colon. Using a similar system, two other groups (Kern et al 1951, Spriggs et al 1951) found that active colitics have a diminished total activity but an increased incidence of large propulsive waves. Similar phenomena have been noted in myoelectrical recordings from patients with painless diarrhea, but without colonic inflammation (Frexinos et al 1987). Davidson et al (1957a, b) described similar propulsive waves from the rectosigmoid region of children with colitis, but they interpreted these as a feature of the diarrheal state and not of ulcerative colitis per se. Direct observations on the exteriorized colon in two patients with colitis also suggested the occurrence of increased propulsive activity (Grace et al 1951). In contrast, Connell (1962), using miniature balloons, found that sigmoid motility was diminished during active colitis but reverted to a normal pattern once the inflammation improved. He suggested that diarrhea in colitis could result from a failure of segmental contractile activity in the sigmoid colon, which normally delays the distal flow of fecal matter.

The discrepancies in the results from different studies reflect differences in the design of the pressure sensors, in the recording sites, and in the selection of patients (Chaudhary & Truelove 1961a, Rao et al 1988b). Intraluminal pressures at different sites in the colon show a considerable variation in the pattern, frequency and amplitude of contractions, both within and between subjects (Chaudhary & Truelove 1961a, Ritchie & Tuckey 1969, Dinoso et al 1983, Rao et al 1988b), and recordings may need to be made at multiple sites to gain a clear impression of rectosigmoid contractility.

In one study which investigated the integrated pressure activity of the sigmoid colon, rectum and anal canal using open-tip perfused catheters, patients with active colitis showed a relative lack of spontaneous rectal contractions, with 40% showing total quiescence throughout the recording period (Rao et al 1988b; Fig. 23.2). These findings have since been further confirmed (Loening-Baucke et al 1989a, Reddy et al 1991). It is possible that the occurrence of propulsive waves (reported in previous studies) was related to the use of large balloons as pressure sensors in the rectum. A tandem balloon system is not only more likely than open-tip perfused catheters to detect propagating contractions and to exaggerate their duration and amplitude, but may also induce large-amplitude rectal contractions in a tense rectum. This hypothesis is supported by the results of balloon distension of the rectum (Rao et al 1987c) and rapid infusion of fluid into the rectum (Rao et al 1988b).

When a large volume of saline was infused the inflamed rectum generated abnormally strong contractions that challenged the continence mechanism and caused early leakage of saline, which occurred in spurts when the intrarectal pressures exceeded the anal relaxation pressures

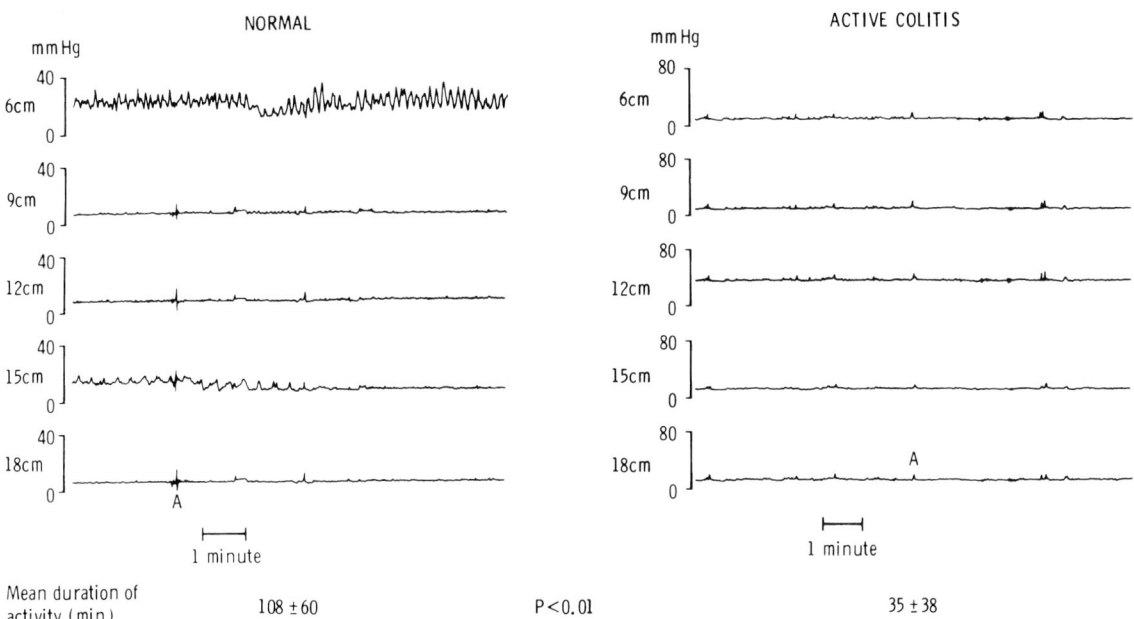

Fig. 23.2 Typical patterns of the resting pressure activity in the rectosigmoid channels at different distances from the anal verge in a normal subject and in a patient with active colitis. 'A' represents artefacts.

(Rao et al 1988b; Fig. 23.3). The total volume of saline retained was lower in patients with active colitis than in those with quiescent colitis and normal controls (Rao et al 1988b). Continence to rectal infusion of saline was also influenced by the severity of inflammation, since patients with mild colitis retained more saline than those with moderately severe colitis (Rao et al 1988b). Putting all these results together, it seems that the distal colon in active colitis is programmed to react to relatively small volumes of distension with the generation of large-amplitude propagative contractions.

Some workers have suggested that increased colonic motility in ulcerative colitis could result in mucosal ischemia, which may be primarily responsible for mucosal damage (Fairburn 1973, Hiatt 1984). Lium and Porter (1939) showed that spastic contractions of colonic explants in dogs resulted in ulceration and ischemic mucosal damage. Furthermore, administration of mecholyl caused sustained contractions and mucosal erosions similar to those seen in colitis (Wener et al 1949, Rostad 1973). A similar pattern of hypermotility has been induced experimentally by administering cholinergic agents (Moeller & Kirsner 1954, Almy 1961) during stimulation of the pelvic nerves (Rostad 1973) and after postganglionic sympathectomy (Berger & Lium 1960). These changes revert to a more normal pattern after the administration of anticholinergic or ganglion-blocking drugs (Kern et al 1951, Almy 1961). These observations led to the suggestion that in patients with colitis the colon is in a state of continued readiness for defecation (Almy 1961), and that this is a result of excessive parasympathetic tone brought about by continued emotional stress (Wener & Polonsky 1950, Davidson et al 1957a, b, Almy 1961). However, it is unlikely that emotional stress is solely responsible for these changes, as the same proportion of normal subjects and colitics exhibited hyperactivity when intraluminal pressures were recorded during an interview on a wide range of emotive topics (Chaudhary & Truelove 1961b).

Anorectal function in colitis

Lium (1939) reported that the rectal wall in patients with colitis exhibited a greater tone in response to balloon distension than in normal subjects, and Farthing and colleagues showed that the maximum volume of air that could be tolerated in the rectum is reduced in patients with active colitis (Farthing & Lennard-Jones 1978).

These findings were confirmed and extended by a more recent and integrated assessment of the motor activity of the anorectum (Rao et al 1987c). During serial distension of a balloon in the rectum, patients with active colitis perceived the balloon and experienced an urgent desire to defecate at under 50% of the rectal volume required to elicit these sensations in normal subjects, or in patients with quiescent colitis (Rao et al 1987c; Table 23.5). The perception of a desire to defecate at an abnormally low rectal volume could explain symptoms of urgency, and the passage of small, frequent stools (Rao et al 1987b).

The increased rectal sensitivity in active colitis was associated with a marked decrease in rectal compliance

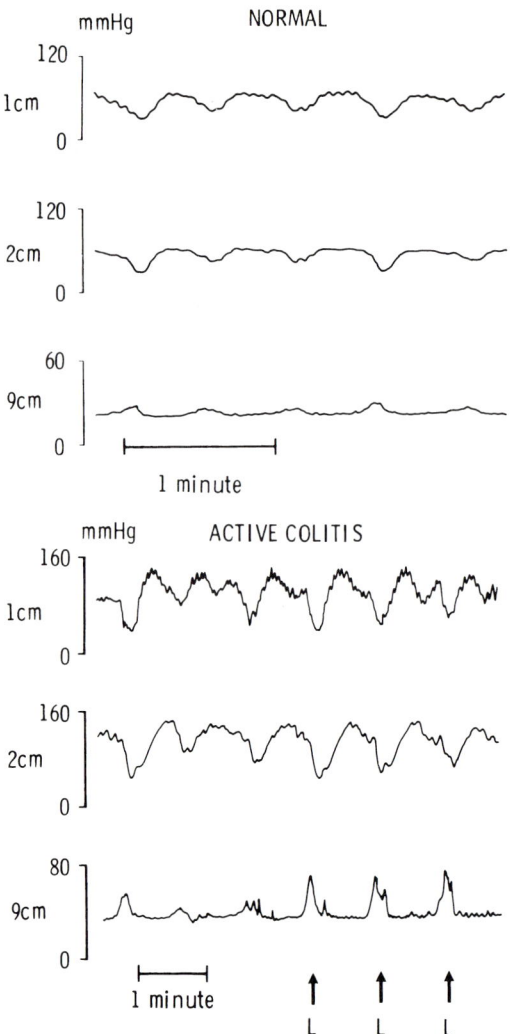

Fig. 23.3 Typical patterns of the pressure activity during the last 5 minutes of saline infusion in a normal subject and a patient with active colitis showing the large amplitude rectal contractions associated with anal relaxations. L – indicates leakage of saline.

Table 23.5 Results of anal sphincter pressure and anal and rectal responses to balloon distension in normal subjects and in patients with ulcerative colitis

	Normal subjects ($n = 12$)	Active colitis ($n = 18$)	Quiescent colitis ($n = 17$)
Maximum basal sphincter pressure (mmHg)	68 ± 20	63 ± 24	69 ± 22
Maximum squeeze sphincter pressure (mmHg)	199 ± 39	156 ± 74	165 ± 67
Rectal volume required for perception of balloon (ml)	38 ± 15	13 ± 5^{ox}	51 ± 38
Rectal volume required for a desire to defecate (ml)	73 ± 29	35 ± 21^{ox}	91 ± 59
Rectal volume required for an urgent desire to defecate (ml)	167 ± 39	75 ± 34^{ox}	169 ± 74
Maximum tolerable volume (ml)	229 ± 45	98 ± 41^{ox}	$178 \pm 74*$
Rectal volume required to cause anal relaxation (ml)	18 ± 12	12 ± 5	17 ± 14
Rectal volume required to cause sustained anal relaxation (ml)	75 ± 45	$43 \pm 30*†$	65 ± 32
Rectal compliance (dv/dp) ml/mmHg	12 ± 5	3 ± 2^{ox}	8 ± 4

Results are expressed as mean $\pm$ SD
^{ox}, significantly different from normal controls ^{ox}, $P < 0.001$, ^{ox}, $P < 0.05$
$*†$, significantly different from quiescent colitis, $*$, $P < 0.001$, $†$, $P < 0.05$

(Rao et al 1987c, Loening-Baucke et al 1989b) and an increase in the initial reactivity to rectal distension (Rao et al 1987c). When Denis et al (1979) measured the viscoelastic properties of the rectal wall with a spherical balloon, they found that the rectal intraluminal pressures and the rectal elasticity coefficient (after accommodation to balloon distension) were higher in patients with active colitis than those with quiescent colitis and controls. This suggested that the reduced rectal size observed in colitics (Farthing & Lennard-Jones 1977) is due to a loss of rectal distensibility. However, rectal compliance in patients with quiescent colitis was not significantly reduced compared to normal subjects, and paired studies indicated that increased rectal sensitivity and reactivity was related to the presence of active inflammation (Rao et al 1987c; Table 23.4). Thus the decrease in rectal compliance in active colitis appears to be caused by an increase in smooth muscle tone rather than intramural fibrosis. It is possible that both the sensory changes and the increased rectal contractile responses could be caused by sensitization of intramural receptors by the inflammatory changes (Rao et al 1987c). This mechanism could also account for the prolonged anal sphincter relaxation in response to small volumes of rectal distension in active colitis (Rao et al 1987c). This could lead to incontinence unless the external anal sphincter is able to contract with sufficient strength and rapidity. Patients with active colitis who are incontinent have abnormally low sphincter pressures (Rao et al 1987c), although the weak sphincter is related in most instances to pudendal neuropathy and obstetric trauma, and not to the effects of colitis.

Effect of food on colonic and anorectal activity

Patients with active colitis often complain of an increased urge to defecate after eating a meal. Spriggs (1951) recorded intraluminal pressures before and after a meal in patients with active colitis and normal subjects, and concluded that although there was an overall increase in the rectosigmoid activity, no differences were seen between the two groups. Another study, however, indicated that in patients with colitis the maximal colonic myoelectrical response to a meal is decreased and the duration of activity is shorter than in normal subjects (Snape et al 1980a).

Moreover, unlike normal subjects, there was no simultaneous increase in colonic contractility. The authors of this study suggested that the electrical activity of muscle function is preserved but diminished in colitics, whereas the contractile response to eating is impaired (Snape et al 1980a). This reduction in sigmoid contractility may allow unimpeded flow of fecal matter to the rectum (Connell 1962). These findings were further confirmed by measuring intraluminal pressures in the rectosigmoid region after a meal (Loening-Baucke et al 1989b). More recently, combined recording of intraluminal pressure with scintigraphic transit also showed that preprandially, patients with colitis have decreased contractile activity of the distal colon, but after a meal there was more irregular movement of tracer and a greater number of propagating contractions than in normal subjects (Reddy et al 1991). Since the normal motor response following a meal consists of an increased number of segmental contractions (Reddy et al 1991), in patients with active colitis, the reduced frequency of these contractions together with the occurrence of more frequent and low-amplitude propulsive contractions, could give rise to a greater urge to defecate.

Motor activity of the anorectum and the ileoanal pouch

Restorative proctocolectomy with an ileal reservoir (pouch), or a mucosal proctectomy with an ileoanal anastomosis, have been recently introduced as options for patients with severe colitis requiring colectomy. Although useful, they are associated with functional disturbances of the neorectum. Mucosal proctectomy causes significant reduction of the resting anal tone, as well as impairment of rectal and anal sensation. These changes are believed to be responsible for a higher incidence of fecal incontinence in these patients (Johnston et al 1987, Nicholls et al 1981). On the other hand, if the anal canal is left undisturbed, sphincteric tone and anal sensation appear to be better preserved (Johnston et al 1987, Holdsworth & Johnson 1988). In a study of ambulatory manometry of the anal canal and the terminal ileum in patients who underwent restorative proctocolectomy, the resting activity of the internal anal sphincter, consisting of ultraslow waves and slow waves, was absent in 62% of patients with mucosal proctectomy (Holdsworth et al 1994). Furthermore, the number of isolated rectal contractions with anal relaxation (sampling reflex) was also reduced, suggesting significant disruption of the normal anorectal function. In contrast, all patients who had an ileal reservoir (pouch) exhibited normal anal sphincter activity as well as the anal sampling reflex. In another study the myoelectrical activity of the terminal ileum was normal in patients with an ileal pouch, but the motor activity of the pouch itself was reduced, suggesting that the latter may serve as a useful reservoir (Pescatori 1985). Furthermore, in response to a meal, neostigmine or balloon distension of the pouch, the anal sphincter appeared to contract appropriately, suggesting that proctocolectomy with an ileal reservoir may better preserve continence. However, when compared with healthy subjects, patients with an ileal pouch exhibited reduced rectal sensation for flatus and for perceiving the sampling reflex, as well as diminished motor activity (Miller et al 1990). Recently, it has also been suggested that the J pouch with a smaller capacity may show more activity prior to defecation (Stryker et al 1986) than the W pouch (Miller et al 1990).

Another study examined the relationship of small-bowel motility to ileoanal reservoir function, and found that patients with a higher defecation frequency tended to have a greater number of migrating motor complexes (MMC) in the small bowel (although they were not propagated to the reservoir), and a lower threshold for the maximum tolerable volume of the reservoir (Groom et al 1994). This study suggested that changes in small-bowel motor activity may influence pouch function and stool frequency. These observations indicate that surgical reconstruction induces important changes in anorectal and bowel function. However, in order to establish the beneficial effects of these procedures, further studies comparing the motor activity in different types of pouches, together with an assessment of the defecatory function in these patients, are desirable. Pouchitis has been described as a complication in 25–50% of patients (Pemberton et al 1987, Michelassi et al 1993). Whether this problem is related to abnormal motor function of the pouch together with small-bowel dysfunction remains to be explored.

Conclusions

Increased propulsive activity of the small bowel and proximal colon is not the cause of diarrhea in patients with active colitis. The increase in stool weight in active colitics is probably related to the secretion of mucus from the inflamed epithelium, and reduced absorption of fluid and electrolytes. Paradoxical slowing of proximal colonic and small-bowel transit is consistent with the finding of fecal stasis and the passage of hard, pellety stools in some patients. The combination of quiescent basal pressure recordings, increased rectal tone, increased rectal sensitivity, increased phasic pressure response to distension, and reduced rectal capacitance suggests that the distal colon in patients with active colitis appears to be programmed to react to intraluminal contents by generating strong contractions that challenge the continence barrier and cause frequent, urgent and often painful defecation.

DISTURBANCES OF INTESTINAL MOTOR ACTIVITY IN CROHN'S DISEASE

Although Crohn's disease is not primarily a motility disorder, the accompanying inflammation, tissue swelling and intestinal obstruction may have a profound effect on intestinal motor activity, leading to the symptoms observed in many of these patients.

The pathological abnormality in Crohn's disease is a patchy inflammatory change, which commences in the submucosa and can spread to involve all layers of the gut. This causes thickening of the bowel wall and leads to progressive stasis and distension proximal to the area, and eventually obstruction. Involvement of the muscle layers and myenteric plexus by the inflammatory process results in a rigid aperistaltic segment of bowel, which acts as a passive conduit relying on pressure differences caused by proximal contractions for the propulsion of food through the segment. Very few direct recordings of gastrointestinal motor activity have been made in patients with Crohn's disease. Thus, our knowledge of the motor disturbances is largely based on observations during radiological studies and transit measurements, and from inferences based on pathology.

Stomach

Crohn's disease of the stomach is rare but predominantly affects the antral region, causing weakness or absence of antral peristalsis and a rigid tubular appearance on barium meal. In some cases the pylorus may become obstructed; in others it may be dilated. Impairment of gastric emptying occurs in up to 70% of cases (Fielding et al 1970), and is much worse for solids than for liquids. Liquid emptying of a meal in patients with small-bowel Crohn's disease was similar to healthy controls, but solid emptying was delayed in all seven patients who had Crohn's disease with malnutrition, whereas Crohn's patients without growth retardation had normal emptying (Grill et al 1985). Moreover, 80% of patients with radiological and endoscopic evidence of non-constrictive Crohn's lesions in the duodenum had delayed gastric emptying; surprisingly, 57% of patients without such involvement also had delayed emptying. These results suggest that delayed gastric emptying occurs in patients with active disease even in the absence of luminal obstruction, and could lead to reduced caloric intake and malnutrition. Whether this is a specific effect of the disease process on gut motor function, or a result of generalized debility and esthenia is, however, unclear. Reflex inhibition of gastric emptying can be induced by distension of the small or large intestine, such as occurs proximal to an obstruction (Loew & Patterson 1935, Youmans & Meek 1937). It is also possible that the inflammation of the bowel itself may slow gastric emptying, possibly by stimulating pain receptors.

Small intestine

Crohn's disease of the small intestine obstructs the passage of food, causing distension of the bowel proximally. This may stimulate sensory stretch receptors in the bowel wall, inducing abdominal pain, vomiting, and possibly also intestinal secretion via local nervous reflex (Caren et al 1974).

Recordings of intestinal motility proximal to an experimental obstruction (Dahlgren & Thoren 1967) have shown that the bowel is very active and generates strong peristaltic contractions to overcome the obstruction. Summers et al (1983) found that Crohn's patients with partial small-bowel obstruction had repetitive contractions interspersed with periods of quiescence lasting at least a minute. This pattern is highly propulsive and may represent an adaptation to luminal obstruction. It was present throughout the small intestine and was exacerbated by food (Foulk et al 1954).

A recent study reported that the orocecal transit time was slower in younger patients (<20 years of age) with small-bowel Crohn's disease (Gotze & Ptok 1993). In less than half of these patients normalization of small-bowel transit time was associated with an improvement in disease activity. Although 50% of patients in this study had large-bowel Crohn's disease, the orocecal transit time of this subgroup was not stated. Furthermore, it was unclear what proportion of patients with small-bowel disease had intestinal stricture, which may have contributed to the motor abnormalities.

Stasis of food proximal to a Crohn's stricture may not only be associated with impaired transit, but may also lead to an overgrowth of bacteria. This can lead to diarrhea, because bacteria degrade bile acids and fatty acids to unconjugated dihydroxy bile acids and hydroxy fatty acids, which are poorly absorbed in the small intestine and enter the colon, where they stimulate secretion and propulsive motor activity (Binder 1980, Snape et al 1980a, b, Vantrappen et al 1981, Spiller et al 1985). Furthermore, bacterial overgrowth of the small intestine may be associated with absence of the normal fasting motor activity (Vantrappen et al 1977).

Colon

Crohn's colitis frequently presents with diarrhea, which may be caused by the presence of unabsorbed bile acids or fat (Binder 1980, Snape et al 1980b, Vantrappen et al 1981). The release of prostaglandins and other transmitter substances by the inflamed tissue may also stimulate colonic propulsive activity (Bennet 1975). There is no information regarding disturbances in colonic motor function in Crohn's disease, but a recent study (Kangas et al 1992) examined anorectal function and found that sphincter pressure, rectal sensation and rectal compliance were similar in normal subjects and those patients with Crohn's disease who did not have anorectal disease. However, patients with Crohn's disease affecting the anorectal segment showed low sphincter pressures and reduced rectal capacity, and these changes predisposed many of these patients to fecal incontinence. Interestingly, several patients without anal disease but who had had previous surgery also had fecal incontinence (Kangas et al 1992). This suggests that factors other than anal dysfunction may also lead to incontinence in some of these patients.

These limited studies have shed new light on the motor disturbances in Crohn's disease, but clearly further studies are required to better define the pathophysiological abnormalities in such patients and the effect of disease on symptoms and nutritional status.

REFERENCES

Almy T P 1961 Observations on the pathologic physiology of ulcerative colitis. Gastroenterology 40: 299–306

Archampong E Q, Harris J, Clark C G 1972 Absorption and secretion of water and electrolytes across the healthy and the diseased human colonic mucosa measured in-vitro. Gut 13: 880–886

Bennett A 1975 Pharmacology of colonic muscle. Gut 16: 307–311

Berger R L, Lium R 1960 Abdominal postganglionic sympathectomy. A method for production of an ulcerative colitis-like state in dogs. Annals of Surgery 152: 266–273

Binder H J 1980 Pathophysiology of bile acid and fatty acid induced diarrhoea. In: Field M, Fordtran J S, Schultz S G (eds) Secretory diarrhea. American Physiology Society, Washington DC, pp 159–178

Binder S C, Patterson J F, Glotzer D J 1974 Toxic megacolon in ulcerative colitis. Gastroenterology 66: 909–915

Black D A, Ainley C C, Senapati A, Thompson R P H 1987 Transit time in ulcerative proctitis. Scandinavian Journal of Gastroenterology 22: 872–876

Caren J F, Meyer J H, Grossman M I 1974 Canine intestinal secretion during and after rapid distension of the small bowel. America Journal of Physiology 227: 183–188

Chaudhary N A, Truelove S C 1961a Colonic motility. A critical review of methods and results. American Journal of Medicine 31: 86–106

Chaudhary N A, Truelove S C 1961b Human colonic motility: a comparative study of normal subjects, patients with ulcerative colitis and patients with the irritable colon syndrome. III. Effects of emotions. Gastroenterology 40: 27–36

Connell A M 1962 The motility of the pelvic colon. II. Paradoxical motility in diarrhoea and constipation. Gut 3: 342–348

Dahlgren S, Thoren L 1967 Intestinal motility in low small bowel obstruction. Acta Chirurgica Scandinavica 133: 417–421

Davidson M, Sleisenger M H, Almy P T, Levine S Z 1957a Studies in distal colon motility in child. II. Propulsive activity in diarrhoeal states. Paediatrics 17: 820–832

Davidson M, Sleisenger M H, Almy P T, Levine S Z 1957b Studies in distal colon motility in child. I. Non-propulsive patterns in normal children. Paediatrics 17: 807–819

Denis Ph, Colin R, Galmiche J P 1979 Elastic properties of the rectal wall in normal adults and in patients with ulcerative colitis. Gastroenterology 77: 45–48

Dinoso V P, Murthy S N S, Goldstein J, Rosner B 1983 Basal motor activity of the distal colon: a reappraisal. Gastroenterology 85: 637–642

Duthie H L, Watts J M, De Dombal F T, Golligher J C 1964 Serum electrolytes and colonic transfer of water and electrolytes in chronic ulcerative colitis. Gastroenterology 47: 525–530

Edmonds C J, Pilcher D 1973 Electrical potential differences and sodium and potassium fluxes across rectal mucosa in ulcerative colitis. Gut 14: 784–789

Engel G L 1954a Studies of ulcerative colitis. I. Clinical data bearing on the nature of the somatic process. Psychosomatic Medicine 16: 496

Engel G L 1954b Studies of ulcerative colitis. I. The nature of the somatic process and the adequacy of psychosomatic hypotheses. American Journal of Medicine 16: 416–426

Fairburn R A 1973 On the aetiology of ulcerative colitis. A vascular hypothesis. Lancet i: 697–699

Farthing M J G, Lennard-Jones J E 1977 Rectosacral distance and rectal size in ulcerative colitis. British Medical Journal 2: 1266

Farthing M J G, Lennard-Jones J E 1978 Sensibility of the rectum to distension and the anorectal distension reflex in ulcerative colitis. Gut 19: 64–69

Fielding J, Toye D, Beton D, Cooke W 1970 Crohn's disease of the stomach and duodenum. Gut 11: 1001–1006

Fink S, Friedman G 1960 The differential effect of drugs on the proximal and distal colon. American Journal of Medicine 28: 534–540

Foulk W T, Code C F, Morlock C G, Bargen J A 1954 A study of the motility patterns and basal rhythm in the duodenum and upper part of the jejunum in human beings. Gastroenterology 26: 601–611

Frexinos J, Fioramonti J, Bueno L 1987 Colonic myoelectrical activity in IBS painless diarrhoea. Gut 28: 1613–1618

Garrett J M, Sauer W G, Moertel C B 1967 Colonic motility in ulcerative colitis after opiate administration. Gastroenterology 53: 93–100

Gill R C, Cote K R, Bowes K L, Kingma Y J 1986 Human colonic smooth muscle: spontaneous contractile activity and response to stretch. Gut 27: 1006–1013

Gotze H, Ptok A 1993 Orocaecal transit time in patients with Crohn's disease. European Journal of Pediatrics 152: 193–196

Grace W J, Wolf S, Wolff H G 1951 The human colon. Paul B. Hoeber, New York

Grill B B, Lange R, Markowitz R, Hillemeier A C, McCallum R W, Gryboski J D 1985 Delayed gastric emptying in children with Crohn's disease. Journal of Clinical Gastroenterology 7: 216–226

Groom J S, Kamm M A, Nicholls R J 1994 Relationship of small bowel motility to ileoanal reservoir function. Gut 35: 523–529

Harris J, Shields R 1970 Absorption and secretion of water and electrolytes by the intact human colon in diffuse untreated proctocolitis. Gut 11: 27–33

Hawker P C, McKay J S, Turnberg L A 1980 Electrolyte transport across colonic mucosa form patients with inflammatory bowel disease. Gastroenterology 79: 508–511

Hiatt R B 1984 Abnormal intestinal motility as an etiological factor in inflammatory bowel disease. Journal of Clinical Gastroenterology 6: 201–203

Holdsworth P J, Johnston D 1988 Anal sensation after restorative proctocolectomy for ulcerative colitis. British Journal of Surgery 75: 993–996

Holdsworth P J, Sagar P M, Lewis W G, Williamson M, Johnston D 1994 Internal anal sphincter activity after restorative proctocolectomy for ulcerative colitis: a study using continuous ambulatory manometry. Diseases of the Colon and Rectum 37: 32–36

Jalan K N, Sircus W, Card W I et al 1969 An experience of ulcerative colitis. I. Toxic dilation in 55 cases. Gastroenterology 55: 68–82

Jalan K N, Walker R J, Prescott R J, Butterworth S T G, Smith A N, Sircus W 1970 Fecal stasis and diverticular disease in ulcerative colitis. Gut 11: 688–696

Johnston D, Holdsworth P J, Nasmyth D G et al 1987 Preservation of the entire anal canal in conservative proctocolectomy for ulcerative colitis: a pilot study comparing end-to-end ileoanal anastomosis without mucosal resection with mucosal proctectomy. British Journal of Surgery 74: 940–944

Kangas E, Hiltunen K M, Matikainen M 1992 Anorectal function in Crohn's disease. Annales Chirugiae et Gynaecologiae 81: 43–47

Kellow J E, Gill R C, Joene De M, Parnell N, Wingate D L 1986 Rectal distension modifies upper gastrointestinal (GI) motor activity. Gut 27: A1252

Kern F Jr, Almy T P, Abbott F K, Bondanoff M D 1951 The motility of the distal colon in non-specific ulcerative colitis. Gastroenterology 19: 493–503

Lennard-Jones J E, Langman M J S, Jones F A 1962a Faecal stasis in proctocolitis. Gut 3: 301–305

Lennard-Jones J E, Cooper G W, Newell A C, Wilson C W E, Avery Jones F 1962b Observations of idiopathic proctitis. Gut 3: 201–206

Lium R 1939 Observations on the etiology of ulcerative colitis. IV. The rectometrogram and the rectal reactions of 8 normal subjects and 1 patient with ulcerative colitis (before and after spinal anaesthesia). American Journal of Medical Science 197: 841–846

Lium R, Porter J 1939 Etiology of ulcerative colitis. II. Effects of induced muscular spasm on colonic explants in dogs with comments on the relation of muscular spasm to ulcerative colitis. Archives of Internal Medicine 63: 210–225

Loening-Baucke V, Metcalf A M, Shirazi S 1989a Anorectal manometry in active and quiescent ulcerative colitis. American Journal of Gastroenterology 84: 892–897

Loening-Baucke V, Metcalf A M, Shirazi S 1989b Rectosigmoid motility in patients with quiescent and active ulcerative colitis. American Journal of Gastroenterology 84: 34–39

Loew E R, Patterson T L 1935 The reflex influence of the lower portion of the large gut on tonus and movement of the empty stomach in dogs. American Journal of Physiology 113: 89–90

Mackie T T 1938 The medical management of chronic ulcerative colitis. Journal of the American Medical Association 111: 2071–2076

Manousos O N, Salem S N 1965 Abnormal motility of the small intestine in ulcerative colitis. Gastroenterologia 104: 249–257

Michelassi F, Stella M, Block G E 1993 Prospective assessment of functional results after ileal J pouch–anal restorative proctocolectomy. Archives of Surgery 128: 889–895

Miller R, Orrom W J, Duthie G, Bartolo D C C, Mortensen N J McC 1990 Ambulatory anorectal physiology in patients following restorative proctocolectomy for ulcerative colitis: comparison with normal controls. British Journal of Surgery 77: 895–897

Moeller H C, Kirsner J B 1954 The effect of drug induced hypermotility on the intestinal tract of dogs. Gastroenterology 26: 303–311

Montgomery R D, Frazer A C, Hood C, Goodhart J M, Holland M R, Schneider R 1968 Studies of intestinal fermentation in ulcerative colitis. Gut 9: 521–526

Nicholls R J, Belliveam P, Neill M, Wilks M, Tabaqohali S 1981 Restorative proctocolectomy with ileal reservoir: a pathophysiological assessment. Gut 22: 462–468

Norland C C, Kirsner J B 1969 Toxic dilatation of colon (toxic megacolon): etiology, treatment and prognosis in 42 patients. Medicine 48: 229–250

Pemberton J H, Kelly K A, Beart R W, Dozois R R, Wolff B G, Ilstrup D M 1987 Ileal pouch–anal anastomosis for chronic ulcerative colitis. Annals of Surgery 206: 504–513

Pescatori M 1985 Myoelectric and motor activity of the terminal ileum after pelvic pouch for ulcerative colitis. Diseases of the Colon and Rectum 28: 246–253

Posey E L, Bargen J A 1951 Observations of normal and abnormal human intestinal motor function. American Journal of Medical Science 221: 10–20

Rao S S C, Read N W, Holdsworth C D 1987a Is the diarrhoea in ulcerative colitis related to a failure of colonic salvage of carbohydrate? Gut 28: 1090–1094

Rao S S C, Read N W, Brown C, Bruce C, Holdsworth C D 1987b Studies on the mechanism of bowel disturbance in ulcerative colitis. Gastroenterology 93: 934–940

Rao S S C, Read N W, Davidson P A, Bannister J J, Holdsworth C D 1987c Anorectal sensitivity and responses to rectal distension in patients with ulcerative colitis. Gastroenterology 93: 1270–1275

Rao S S C, Holdsworth C D, Read N W 1988a Symptoms and stool patterns in patients with ulcerative colitis. Gut 29: 342–345

Rao S S C, Read N W, Stobhart J A H, Haynes W G, Benjamin S, Holdsworth C D 1988b Anorectal contractility under basal conditions and during rectal infusion of saline in ulcerative colitis. Gut 29: 769–777

Rask-Madsen J, Hammersgaard E A, Knudsen E 1973 Rectal electrolyte transport and mucosal permeability in ulcerative colitis and Crohn's disease. Journal of Laboratory and Clinical Medicine 81: 342–353

Read N W 1982 Diarrhoea. The failure of colonic salvage. Lancet ii: 481–483

Read N W, Johnson A J 1983 Disturbance of intestinal motor activity. In: Allan R N, Keighley M R B, Alexander-Williams J, Hawkins C (eds) Inflammatory bowel disease. Churchill Livingstone, Edinburgh, pp 54–62

Reddy S N, Bazzocchi G, Chan S et al 1991 Colonic motility and transit in health and ulcerative colitis. Gastroenterology 101: 1289–1297

Ritchie J A, Salem S N 1965 Upper intestinal motility in ulcerative colitis, idiopathic steatorrhoea and the irritable bowel syndrome. Gut 6: 325–337

Ritchie J A, Tuckey N S 1969 Intraluminal pressure studies at different distances from the anus in normal subjects and in patients with the irritable colon syndrome. American Journal of Digestive Diseases 14: 96–106

Rosswick R P, Stedeford R D, Brooke B N 1967 New methods of studying intestinal transit times. Gut 8: 195–196

Rostad H 1973 Colonic motility in the cat. II. Extrinsic nerve control. Acta Physiologica Scandinavica 89: 91–103

Smith F W, Law D H, Nickel Jr W F, Sleisenger M H 1962 Fulminant ulcerative colitis with toxic dilatation of the colon: medical and surgical management of eleven cases with observations regarding etiology. Gastroenterology 42: 233–243

Snape W J, Matarazzo S A, Cohen S 1980a Abnormal gastrocolonic response in patients with ulcerative colitis. Gut 21: 392–396

Snape W J, Shiff S, Cohen S 1980b Effect of deoxycholic acid on colonic motility in the rabbit. American Journal of Physiology 23: G321–G325

Spiller R C, Brown M L, Phillips S F 1985 Segmental colonic function in experimental steatorrhoea – decreased capacitance of the proximal colon. Gut 26: A1136–1137

Spriggs E A 1951 The motility of the human pelvic colon and rectum in health and in certain abnormal conditions. DM Thesis, University of Cambridge

Spriggs E A, Code C F, Bargen J A, Curtiss R K, Hightower N C 1951 Motility of the pelvic colon and rectum of normal persons and patients with ulcerative colitis. Gastroenterology 19: 480–491

Steadman C, Phillips S F 1990 Absorption of fluids and electrolytes by the colon: relevance to inflammatory bowel disease. In: Allan R N, Keighley M R B, Alexander-Williams J, Hawkins C (eds) Inflammatory bowel disease. Churchill Livingstone, Edinburgh, pp 55–70

Stryker S J, Phillips S F, Dozois R R, Kelly K A, Beart R W 1986 Anal and neorectal function after ileal pouch–anal anastomosis. Annals of Surgery 203: 55–61

Summers R W, Anuras S, Green J 1983 Jejunal manometry pattern in health, partial intestinal obstruction and pseudo-obstruction. Gastroenterology 85: 1290–1300

Truelove S C, Marks C G 1981 Toxic megacolon. Part I: Pathogenesis, diagnosis and treatment. Clinics in Gastroenterology 10: 107–117

Van Hees P A M, Tuinte J H M, Van Rossum J M, Van Tongeren J H M 1979 Influence of intestinal transit time on azo-reduction of salicylazosulphapyridine (salazopyrin). Gut 20: 300–304

Vantrappen G, Janssens J, Hellemans J, Ghoos Y 1977 The interdigestive motor complex of normal subjects and patients with bacterial overgrowth of the small intestine. Journal of Clinical Investigation 9: 1158–1166

Vantrappen G, Janssens J, Rolemberg S, Hellemans J 1981 Intestinal motility and diarrhoea. In: Read N W (ed) Diarrhoea. New insights. Clinical & Research Reviews 1 (Suppl. 1): pp 83–90

Wener J, Polonsky A 1950 The reaction of the human colon to naturally occurring and experimentally induced emotional states; observation through a transverse colostomy on a patient with ulcerative colitis. Gastroenterology 15: 84–94

Wener J, Hoff H E, Simon M A 1949 Production of ulcerative colitis in dogs by the prolonged administration of mecholyl. Gastroenterology 12: 637–644

Youle M S, Read N W 1984 Effect of painless rectal distension on gastrointestinal transit of a solid meal. Digestive Diseases and Sciences 29: 902–906

Youmans W B, Meek W J 1937 Gastrointestinal inhibition in unanaesthetised dogs during rectal stimulation. American Journal of Physiology 120: 750–760

24. Mucosal metabolism and proliferation

P. R. Gibson   D. H. Barkla

The efficient and effective function of intestinal epithelium as a barrier between luminal macromolecules and microorganisms on the one hand, and the internal milieu on the other, is central to the health of the intestines and of the organism as a whole. Failure to achieve an effective barrier has several deleterious consequences: for example, the lamina propria may be exposed to luminal macromolecules, many of which are potent inducers of immunoinflammatory events; the epithelium may have a reduced capacity to perform its absorptive/secretory roles; and tissue fluid and cells may cross the epithelium and be lost to the lumen. An understanding of the biology, pathobiology and modulation of injury to, and maintenance and repair of, the epithelial barrier may offer insight into pathogenic mechanisms and potential therapeutic strategies in inflammatory bowel disease (IBD). This chapter addresses issues of epithelial turnover, metabolic activity and repair that have particular relevance to barrier function in relation to both health and IBD.

NUTRITIONAL REQUIREMENTS OF INTESTINAL EPITHELIAL CELLS

The nutrition of the intestinal mucosa is of particular importance to maintenance of health of the organism (Table 24.1). Adequate delivery of oxygen to the mucosa is also essential for tissue viability for a wide variety of reasons, ranging from cellular energy supply to maintenance of the structure of connective tissue, but will not be further addressed here (see Chapter 17). The intestinal mucosa is a high consumer of energy and other nutrients because of the need to support high proliferative rates and considerable synthetic, secretory and other active processes of mucosal cells, especially in the epithelial and immunological compartments. Deficiencies can result from quantitative or qualitative inadequacies of diet, and may be aggravated by the route of delivery of nutrients (Table 24.1). Although much of our understanding of mucosal nutritional requirements and the consequences of deficiencies have come from studies in experimental animals, the findings in general appear to apply to humans.

Table 24.1 Causes and consequences of nutritionally deficient intestinal mucosa

Nutritional substrate deficiency
Quantitative deficiencies (*protein, protein-energy*)
Qualitative deficiencies (*glutamine, non-starch polysaccharides and/or resistant starch, nucleotides*)
Route of delivery of nutrients (*total parenteral nutrition*)

Impairment of intestinal mucosal
growth (atrophy)
protein synthesis
immune competence
barrier function
healing/repair
resistance to injury

Small-intestinal epithelium

The major energy substrates for small-intestinal epithelium are glutamine and, to a lesser extent, ketone bodies, in preference to glucose (Windmueller & Spaeth 1978, Watford et al 1979, Newsholme & Carrié 1994). Atrophy is observed during glutamine-deficient total parenteral nutrition (TPN) and this can be reversed by the addition of glutamine to the intravenous feeding solution (Hwang et al 1986, Grant 1988) or, more effectively, by its use orally (Salloum et al 1989). Glutamine is actively transported into enterocytes via both the basolateral and the apical membranes, and then metabolized by glutaminase, which has a very high substrate affinity (Souba et al 1990a). Enterally delivered glutamine stimulates both brush border uptake and glutaminase activity (Salloum et al 1990), whereas fasting has the opposite effect, even when plasma glutamine levels are maintained.

Glutamine feeding accelerates mucosal healing following methotrexate therapy (Jacobs et al 1987, Fox et al 1988) or irradiation (Klimberg et al 1989, Souba et al 1990b), and attenuates mucosal injury induced by irradiation (Klimberg et al 1990), indicating the importance of glutamine to the maintenance of the epithelial barrier. However, oral glutamine did not reduce the proportion of elemental diet-fed rats exhibiting bacterial translocation (as a measure of mucosal barrier function) (Xu et al 1993), although it did attenuate translocation associated with TPN (Burke et al 1989).

Other nutritional substrates may also be important. Nucleotides administered either enterally or parenterally can improve gut morphology and promote mucosal healing (Grimble 1994). Arginine and ornithine, as precursors of nitric oxide and polyamines, may be important (Cynober 1994), especially given the key roles of nitric oxide and polyamines in many intestinal functions. Short-chain fatty acids (SCFAs) given intravenously (Koruda et al 1988) or intraluminally in the large bowel (Kripke et al 1989) are also trophic for small-bowel mucosa. The mechanism for this effect is unclear, but hepatic metabolism of SCFAs results in the production of ketone bodies and glutamine (Desmoulin et al 1985, Cross et al 1984) which, by themselves, are trophic for small-bowel mucosa (Windmueller & Spaeth 1978, Kripke et al 1988).

Large-bowel (colonic) epithelium

The major energy source for colonic epithelial cells is of luminal origin and comprises SCFAs, of which butyrate is the most important (Roediger 1980a, 1982). Of circulating substrates, ketone bodies are preferred to glutamine or glucose. High luminal concentrations of SCFAs are generated by bacterial fermentation of carbohydrates, principally non-starch polysaccharide (fiber) and resistant starch of dietary origin (Cummings 1994). SCFAs are rapidly absorbed by colonic epithelium but are handled differently: butyrate is largely metabolized by the epithelium, whereas the major proportion of propionate and acetate passes to the liver via the portal blood (Cummings 1994). In isolated colonocytes butyrate oxidation has a sparing effect on oxidation of glutamine or glucose, but the reverse does not occur (Roediger 1980a). This preference for butyrate may be more marked in the distal than the proximal large bowel (Roediger 1980a), although this has not been a consistent observation (Finnie et al 1993, Chapman et al 1994).

The level of butyrate in the colon is reduced following starvation, consumption of a no/minimal residue diet, diversion of the fecal stream away from the colonic lumen, or TPN. In all of these situations the colonic mucosa atrophies, even when the protein and energy requirements of the organism as a whole are met. The atrophy is reversed by reintroducing non-starch polysaccharide into the diet (Hosoda et al 1989), or by direct instillation of SCFAs or butyrate alone into the colonic lumen (Sakata & Englehardt 1983, Kripke et al 1989, Edwards 1993), but not by intravenous SCFAs (Koruda et al 1988) or intraluminal instillation of glucose (Edwards 1993).

In-vitro studies of colonic and non-colonic cell lines have shown that butyrate variably arrests cell growth, modulates the synthesis of many proteins, predominantly

Table 24.2 Direct effects of butyrate on normal colonic epithelium

	Human	Animal	In vitro	In vivo	References
Certain or probable effects					
Major supply of energy and acetyl CoA	+	+	+	+	Roediger 1980a, Roediger et al 1984, Ardawi & Newsholme 1985
Promotion of sodium and water absorption	+	+	+	+	Argenzio et al 1975, Bond & Levitt 1976, Ruppin et al 1980
Aid in lipogenesis and lipid assembly	+	+	+		Caamano et al 1988, Roediger et al 1992
Necessary for metabolism of xenobiotics	+		+		Ireland et al 1990, Roediger et al 1989
Inhibition of cell-associated urokinase activity	+	+	+	+	Gibson et al 1994c, 1995a
Inhibition of interleukin-8 secretion	+		+		Gibson & Rosella 1994
Possible effects					
Stimulation of transglutaminase production		+		+	D'Argenio et al 1994
Variable effects					
Proliferation					
inhibits in active ulcerative colitis	+			+	Scheppach et al 1992
stimulates in SCFA deficiency	+	+		+	Sakata & Engelhardt 1983, Kripke et al 1989, Edwards 1993
no effect on normal mucosa	+		+		Gibson et al 1991, Gibson et al 1995b
No effects					
Differentiation	+	+	+	+	Gibson et al 1991, Gibson et al 1995a Gibson et al 1995b
Unknown effects					
Barrier function					
Restitution					

via alteration of transcription, and modifies cell morphology, cytoskeletal organization and phenotypic differentiation (reviewed by Kruh et al 1994). However, colonic epithelial cells in vivo are unique in that they are *normally* exposed to high concentrations of butyrate, and many of the effects of butyrate observed in other cell types do not occur. Thus, any putative cellular effects of butyrate cannot be assumed to occur in normal colonic epithelium. Some of the effects of butyrate on normal colonic epithelial cells are shown in Table 24.2

There is only limited information available on the functional effects of luminal butyrate in the colon. Its deficiency results in mucosal atrophy, which reduces sodium and water absorption. Bacterial translocation, as a measure of mucosal barrier function, can be reduced by the addition of fiber to the diet in experimental animals, but poorly fermented fibers seem to be more effective than highly fermented ones (Spaeth et al 1990, Alverdy et al 1990, Barber et al 1990). Thus, the role of butyrate in the improvement seen in these animals is questionable. There are no data more directly examining the relationship between butyrate and barrier function, except that butyrate reduces paracellular permeability in the Caco-2 model of intestinal epithelium (Mariadason & Gibson 1994). Luminal butyrate deficiency in humans, best observed following diversion of the fecal stream from a segment of colon, is often associated with the development of colitis in that segment (Glotzer et al 1981). Whether diversion colitis is a manifestation of reduced barrier function of the colonic epithelium has not been directly studied, but instillation of luminal SCFAs has therapeutic benefit in many such patients (Harig et al 1989). The bursting pressure of a colonic anastomosis was enhanced by luminal instillation of butyrate in an animal model (Rolandelli et al 1986), indicating a positive effect of butyrate on the healing process and subsequent strength of the extracellular matrix, possibly via stimulation of blood flow (Kvietys & Granger 1981) and/or transglutaminase activity (D'Argenio et al 1994). Re-epithelialization was also accelerated. However, the effect of butyrate specifically on the epithelial restitution is unknown.

Implications for IBD

Crohn's disease and small-intestinal mucosa

Problems of glutamine supply may occur in patients with Crohn's disease owing to poor intake of nutrients and/or the use of glutamine-deficient TPN. The effect of Crohn's disease on glutamine uptake and utilization by enterocytes is not known. In experimental animals surgical stress is associated with reduced brush border uptake of glutamine but enhanced glutaminase activity and uptake via the basolateral membrane (Souba et al 1990a). Exogenously administered corticosteroids mimic this response (Souba et al 1985). In contrast, endotoxemia or sepsis are associated with reduction of uptake and metabolism of glutamine, mimicking the fasting state. The possible enhancement of glutamine utilization by corticosteroid therapy might contribute to its efficacy. The promotion of epithelial regeneration by EGF (epidermal growth factor) (see below) may be due in part to stimulation of glutamine uptake by enterocytes (Salloum et al 1993). However, the efficacy of elemental diets in ileal Crohn's disease (O'Morain et al 1980) cannot be attributed to improved glutamine delivery, since those preparations used in clinical trials are deficient in glutamine. The effect on Crohn's disease activity of adding glutamine and/or nucleotides to elemental/polymeric diets or to TPN is worthy of further investigation.

Ulcerative colitis and colonic epithelium

Roediger first proposed that the primary problem in ulcerative colitis was energy deficiency of the colonic epithelium, based upon the observation that isolated colonocytes from patients with ulcerative colitis had diminished ability to oxidize butyrate (Roediger 1980b). Furthermore, inhibition of butyrate oxidation in rats by the rectal administration of 2-bromo-octanoate leads to a diffuse colitis (Roediger & Nance 1986). Since substrate (butyrate) supply is unlikely to be significantly diminished except in more severe disease (Vernia et al 1988), the critical point of this hypothesis is whether the oxidation of butyrate is indeed abnormal in the epithelium of patients with ulcerative colitis. Several groups have addressed this issue, and the results are summarized in Table 24.3. Three conclusions can be drawn from the sometimes conflicting data about colonic epithelium in ulcerative colitis:

1. Impaired butyrate oxidation is evident when concentrations used are high (5 mM or greater) and generally toxic to cells (normal or transformed) in culture. This effect is not secondary to the presence of mucosal inflammation per se.
2. Normal butyrate oxidation is observed when lower, non-toxic concentrations are used.
3. Glutamine utilization, at least in distal colonic epithelium, is probably increased, indicating stimulation of glutaminase activity and/or glutamine uptake, possibly as a compensatory response to reduced utilization of other substrates.

Thus the critical issue remains unresolved. More information on intracellular butyrate concentrations in both experimental situations and in vivo, and substrate utilization experiments over a wide range of butyrate concentrations in the presence and absence of glutamine, are required.

Table 24.3 Butyrate and glutamine utilization by the colonic epithelium in ulcerative colitis

Cell system	Reference	Butyrate oxidation	Butyrate concentration	Glutamine oxidation	Comments
Isolated colonocytes	Roediger 1980b	Reduced Rectum Active/quiescent	10 mM	Increased	Minimal contamination with non-epithelial cells Uncertain effects of cell injury during isolation
	Ireland & Jewell 1990	Reduced Proximal/distal Active/quiescent Non-inflamed	?	Not studied	No disease controls Only surgically resected bowel studied
	Clausen et al 1994	Normal	0.125–2 mM	Not studied	Normal oxidation of acetate/proprionate
Colonoscopic biopsies	Finnie et al 1993	Normal Proximal/distal Quiescent	1 mM	Increased Distal only	Minimal contribution by leukocytes Butyrate > 2 mM inhibited oxidation
	Chapman et al 1994	Reduced Proximal/distal Quiescent	5 mM	Normal	Low levels of substrate utilization
Bicarbonate output *in vivo*	Roediger et al 1984	Reduced (active) Normal (quiescent)	40 mM	Not studied	Indirect measure only Disease specificity

A parallel approach to studying colonic epithelial butyrate utilization in ulcerative colitis is to examine factors that might modulate its oxidation. Sulfides, which are normally produced by bacteria in the colonic lumen, selectively inhibit butyrate oxidation in isolated colonocytes (Roediger et al 1993a,b). Excessive exposure to sulfides may occur owing to excessive production, as is suggested occurs in ulcerative colitis (Florin et al 1990, G F Gibson et al 1991), or to reduced detoxification. In contrast, nitrites, which may be of dietary or of inflammatory cell origin, stimulate butyrate oxidation (Roediger et al 1986, Ireland & Jewell 1990). Of the drugs used to treat ulcerative colitis, corticosteroids and immune-modulating agents are unlikely to directly influence butyrate oxidation. Mesalazine has no effect on isolated colonocytes (Ireland & Jewell 1990) but may inhibit nitrite-induced stimulation of butyrate oxidation (Roediger et al 1989), although this effect has not been confirmed (Ireland & Jewell 1990). Non-steroidal anti-inflammatory drugs, which may worsen ulcerative colitis, inhibit butyrate oxidation in isolated cells (Roediger 1994).

Butyrate delivered alone, or together with other SCFAs, twice daily as enemas to patients with active distal ulcerative colitis is effective therapy (Breuer et al 1991, Scheppach et al 1992). The mechanism by which butyrate might act is not established, but may involve the improvement of energy substrate supply (a problem in severe colitis), 'stabilization' of the colonic epithelium on its basement membrane by reducing cell surface urokinase activity (see below) (Gibson et al 1994c), elevation of transglutaminase activity (D'Argenio et al 1994), reduction of cytokine secretion (Gibson et al 1994c), or improvement of blood flow and oxygen uptake (Kvietys & Granger 1981).

Ileal mucosa and the ileoanal reservoir

Ileal reservoir surgery for ulcerative colitis leads to changes in epithelial morphology (more colon-like) in the pouch after establishment of the fecal stream through it. This is likely to be a response to changes in exposure to luminal molecules associated with stasis of contents and with bacterial fermentation within the pouch, but which molecules are responsible has not been determined. Substrate utilization experiments have shown ileal epithelium to be just as capable as colonic epithelium of oxidizing butyrate (Finnie et al 1993), but whether butyrate becomes the 'preferred' energy substrate is not known. When the pouch becomes inflamed (pouchitis) the use of SCFA enemas has produced disappointing results, but glutamine enemas appear more promising (Wischmeyer et al 1993). This preliminary observation suggests that pouchitis may be associated with nutritional depletion, and that glutamine remains the preferred energy substrate.

XENOBIOTIC METABOLISM

The colonic mucosa is exposed to a range of foreign compounds of dietary, microbial and pharmacological origin. Information on the capabilities of colonic epithelium to metabolize xenobiotics is, however, limited. Studies in experimental animals and humans have demonstrated colonic mucosa to be capable of acetylation (Ireland et al 1990), sulfation of phenols (Sund & Lauterbach 1986, Bostrom et al 1968, Ramakrishna et al 1991), hydroxylation (Oshinsky & Strobel 1897) and S-methylation (Weisiger et al 1980), but not of glucuronidation (Hackford et al 1988).

Xenobiotic metabolism by colonic epithelial cells is of particular interest in ulcerative colitis for three reasons:

1. Failure to detoxify molecules may lead to mucosal injury. For example, impaired sulfation of phenols (specifically paracetamol) by colonic mucosa has been demonstrated in vivo in patients with ulcerative colitis (Ramakrishna et al 1991). Since colonic mucosa is continuously exposed to phenols (Murray & Adams 1988), and since phenols may have adverse effects on cells, their impaired detoxification may injure colonic epithelium and play a role in the pathogenesis of ulcerative colitis.
2. Drugs administered topically in the therapy of ulcerative colitis depend upon their local metabolism to ensure restriction of their pharmacological action to the mucosa. For example, the rapid acetylation of mesalazine by colonic epithelial cells (Ireland et al 1990) limits its systemic absorption.
3. Butyrate appears to be necessary for the adequate supply of cofactors in xenobiotic metabolism. For example, in the acetylation of mesalazine, acetyl groups are donated by acetyl CoA, of which about 70% has been predicted to derive from butyrate oxidation (Roediger 1994). If butyrate oxidation is indeed impaired in ulcerative colitis, then the efficiency of such detoxification processes may also be impaired.

HIERARCHICAL ORGANIZATION OF INTESTINAL EPITHELIUM

The topographical organization of the small and large intestine is basically similar, comprising three overlapping zones: a proliferative zone in the lower third of the crypt, a functional compartment on the surface of the colon or on the upper parts of the villi of the small intestine, and a zone of differentiation lying between them. The proliferative zone contains stem cells, which are believed to divide relatively constantly and slowly and to comprise only a small proportion of the total population of crypt cells (4–5 per crypt in the small intestine and one per crypt in the colon) (Jankowski et al 1994). Stem cells give rise to progenitor cells, which undergo clonogenic and rapid expansion to produce a population of functional end-cells. All differentiated cell types (absorptive, goblet, enteroendocrine and, in the small intestine, paneth cells) arise from a common precursor stem cell, and differentiated progeny migrate towards the surface/villus, except for enteroendocrine and paneth cells, which may migrate towards the base of the crypt.

The functional zone comprises cells that are mature and are principally responsible for the digestive and absorptive functions of the intestines. This is also the zone where most cells die. Cell death is best defined as occurring when cells leave the hierarchical organization, and this may occur by one of three mechanisms:

1. By *apoptosis* (programmed cell death), in which a series of events culminate in rapid condensation and breaking up of the cell into membrane-bound apoptotic bodies, which are phagocytosed either by macrophages (Walker et al 1988, Iwanaga et al 1993, Barkla et al 1994) or by adjacent cells. This occurs predominantly in the surface epithelium or villus tip, but may occur anywhere along the length of the crypt.
2. By *cell shedding* (suicide) into the lumen. These cells often display features of commitment to the apoptotic pathway (such as DNA fragmentation) (Gavrieli et al 1992) but are shed before apoptosis is completed. This process may also occur in sheets of cells (Barkla et al 1994), and is restricted to surface cells which are only loosely attached to the basement membrane and easily dislodged (Buck 1986).
3. By *necrosis* (cell lysis), which may occur as a result of cell injury by cellular and/or soluble factors.

The proportion of cells dying by each of these mechanisms is not known. The traditional view is that cell shedding predominates, but this is being challenged (Iwanaga et al 1993, Barkla et al 1994).

The number and arrangement of each cell type in each region of the intestine are 'pre set' within certain limits. Clearly there are mechanisms for maintaining this system, but their nature remains unexplained.

Factors influencing epithelial turnover

Isolated colonic crypt cells continue to synthesize DNA at a relatively constant rate in the absence of both a mesenchymal association and extraneous growth factors, even when protein synthesis is markedly suppressed (Gibson et al 1994d). Thus, unlike lymphocytes, their proliferation is not driven by exogenous mitogens but is, at least in part, constitutive. Under these conditions control of cell proliferation may occur via local tissue-specific inhibitors (Bullough 1952) such as TGFβ (tumour growth factor β) (Barnard et al 1989). However, many mitogens have been described and these are outlined in Table 24.4 Factors that specifically modulate crypt fission or budding are unknown, but may be similar to those modulating cell proliferation listed in Table 24.4.

There is increasing interest in factors that might influence the rate of cell death in the intestine, especially since controlling cell death may be a useful means to control cell proliferation. Apart from the identification of cells early in the process of apoptosis (Gavrieli et al 1992), little is known of the control of apoptosis in the gut. Cell shedding occurs owing to mechanical forces separating cells that are loosely adherent to their basement membrane in the surface/villus compartment, but why the cells are loosely attached at those sites is uncertain. One factor of potential importance is the

Table 24.4 Some 'mitogenic' factors for the intestinal epithelium

Setting	Factors stimulating epithelial proliferation and/or growth	Postulated mechanisms
'Starved' intestine	Butyrate (colon) [1,2] Glutamine (small intestine) [3–5]	Improved energy supply Improved oxygen supply

Accelerated cell death	High-fat diet [6, 7]
	Irradiation
	Cytotoxic drugs
	Dimethylhydrazine (rats)
		Suppression of
		  diamine oxidase activity [8,9]
		  chalones
		  other inhibitory factors [10,11]
		cell migration per se [12]

Regeneration following injury	EGF, TGFα, TGFβ, PDGF [13,14] IGF-1 [15]	Direct mitogenic effect Promotion of migration Enhanced glutamine uptake [16]
Mucosal inflammation	T-cell mediated immune reactions [17]	Cytokines secreted from T- cells and/or macrophages → cell injury and/or mitogenic
Normal energy-replete epithelium	IGF-1 [18] Peanut lectin [19,20]	Direct mitogenic effect General stimulation of metabolic activity

1, Sakata & Engelhardt 1983; 2, Kripke et al 1989; 3, Hwang et al 1986; 4, Grant 1988; 5, Salloum et al 1989; 6, Lapre et al 1993; 7, Govers et al 1994; 8, Mennigen et al 1987; 9, Erdman et al 1989; 10, Barnard et al 1989; 11, May et al 1981; 12, Winkle 1968; 13, Thompson et al 1989; 14, Mustoe et al 1990; 15, Huang et al 1993; 16 Salloum et al 1993; 17, Castro 1982; 18, Steeb et al 1994; 19, Ryder et al 1992; 20, Ryder et al 1994

activity of cell surface proteases, especially urokinase and its major activation product plasmin, which has a wide spectrum of proteolytic substrates, including most components of the basement membrane. Urokinase is secreted by colonic epithelial cells (Gibson et al 1994d) and can be identified immunohistologically on the basolateral membrane of surface epithelial cells (P R Gibson, unpublished observations), and in the small intestine its activity is predominantly associated with cells from the villus tip (Gibson et al 1994a). The localization of maximal urokinase expression/activity to areas where cell shedding predominates suggests that urokinase may be related to cell shedding.

Factors affecting cell differentiation and maturation

In vitro, colonic epithelial cells increase their expression of markers of differentiation during culture and further enhance their expression when serum-starved, despite a reduction in the rate of protein synthesis (Gibson et al 1994d). These observations suggest that adverse conditions may accelerate the rate of differentiation, perhaps via induction of a stimulating factor (such as TGFβ) or suppression of an inhibitory factor. Although basement membrane components and soluble factors produced by mesenchymal cells may play an important role in promoting the differentiation of fetal epithelial cells (Hahn et al 1990), a role in regulating differentiation in adult intestinal epithelium remains unexplored. Colonic epithelial cells undergo a remarkable change as they move from the mouth of the crypt to the surface compartment immediately adjacent: an increase in the density and length of microvilli, and in the expression of brush border enzymes (Young et al 1992), suggesting regulation by microenvironmental influences.

Implications for IBD

In the rectum of patients with active or quiescent ulcerative colitis the proliferative rate of colonic epithelial cells is elevated (Bleiberg et al 1970, Eastwood & Trier 1973, Serafini et al 1981, Allan et al 1985) and the crypts are usually shorter, indicating increased cell turnover. In addition, branching and budding of crypts is commonly observed (Cheng et al 1986). This increased rate of cell production may be a response to an increase in the rate of cell death. All types of cell death may be involved: cells die in association with crypt abscesses (by necrosis); apoptotic bodies are found with increased frequency in crypt and surface compartments (Lee 1993); and mucosal urokinase activity is increased (De Bruin et al 1986, Elliott et al 1987), raising the likelihood of increased susceptibility to cell loss to the lumen. Several factors are likely to contribute to an increased rate of cell death, and these include exposure to reactive oxygen metabolites, cytokines (such as TNFα – tumor necrosis factor-α), hypoxia and proteases; regenerative responses or putative mitogenic effects of T-cell products may also be driving proliferation. Branching of crypts is a regenerative response to crypt destruction, but the reduced crypt density (mucosal atrophy) seen in some patients may be a long-term consequence of destruction of crypt stem cells, estimated by some to be as few as one cell per crypt (Ponder et al 1985).

Despite the shortened lifespan of colonic epithelial cells, the expression of some markers associated with a differentiated phenotype are paradoxically normal or increased in association with mucosal inflammation (Cooper & Steplewski 1988, Wolf et al 1989). However, cells lacking the hallmarks of maturation have been reported in the surface epithelium of patients with ulcerative colitis (Donnellan 1966).

Table 24.5 Diffuse abnormalities of colonic epithelium occurring specifically in ulcerative colitis, independently of the presence of mucosal inflammation

Plasma membrane	Focal diminution and shortening of microvilli	Delpre et al 1989
	Reduced ability to retain intracellular proteins	Gibson et al 1988
Phenotype	Reduced mucin chromatographic fraction IV	Podolsky & Isselbacher 1984, Tysk et al 1991
	Reduced mucin glycosylation and sulfation	Morita et al 1993
	Expression of novel glycoprotein epitopes	Podolsky & Fournier 1988a
		Podolsky & Fournier 1988b
	Abnormal response of alkaline phosphatase to butyrate	Gibson et al 1994c
Metabolism	Reduced butyrate oxidation	Roediger 1980b, Chapman et al 1994
	Reduced sulfation of phenols	Ramakrishna et al 1991
Secretory products	Abnormal suppression of interleukin-8 by TNFα	Gibson & Rosella 1994
	Abnormalities in urokinase system	Gibson & Rosella 1996

Increasing evidence (Table 24.5) indicates that colonic epithelial cells are diffusely abnormal in ulcerative colitis, even those in apparently non-involved proximal segments. Whether some or all of these findings are secondary to subclinical mucosal inflammation, drugs used in treatment, or other ill-defined effects of inflammation, has not been determined, with one exception: in monozygotic twins mucin abnormalities are also present in the mucosa of the unaffected twin (Tysk et al 1991), pointing to a major genetic contribution. Their disease specificity and apparent independence of mucosal inflammation, however, do suggest that they reflect early changes in disease pathogenesis (Gibson 1994).

MUCOSAL INJURY AND REPAIR

Injury that involves only the mucosa heals without marked inflammatory/repair responses and is not associated with fibrosis. Physical or chemical insults that cause local denuding of the surface epithelium trigger a rapid response. Epithelial cells from adjacent undamaged sites flatten and rapidly migrate over the basal lamina to cover the exposed site, a process termed restitution. This response begins within minutes of the injury, is complete within hours (Buck 1986, Feil et al 1989), and is independent of cell proliferation. On completion of the 'sealing' process, re-establishment of the colonic crypts occurs in a similar way to that seen in the embryo, where single crypts become larger and then bifurcate from the base upwards. This process occurs more slowly than restitution and is dependent upon increased cell proliferation. Lateral 'budding' of crypts at higher levels may also occur. Deeper injuries into the submucosa/muscularis layers invokes an inflammatory response and repair processes that take days to weeks to complete, depending upon the penetration of the injury to the gut wall.

Regulation of restitution

EGF and motility-stimulating proteins appear to promote epithelial cell migration in intestinal wound healing (Rosen & Goldberg 1989). 'Restitution' of wounded IEC-6 cell monolayers (a poorly differentiated intestinal epithelial cell line) over a plastic substratum is promoted by TGFβ (Ciacci et al 1993), by several other soluble factors – EGF, TGFα, IL-1β and interferon-γ – via a TGFβ-dependent pathway (Dignass & Podolsky 1993), and by trefoil peptides independently of TGFβ (Dignass et al 1994). Studies in differentiated cell lines have shown hepatocyte growth factor to promote restitution (T84 cells) (Nusrat et al 1994), but have also indicated the importance of cell substratum in the modulation of responses (Caco-2 cells) (Basson et al 1992). Restitution assays using whole mucosa in vitro have also indicated the importance of the substrate over which the epithelial cells migrate; restitution is faster when the basement membrane remains intact (Feil et al 1989), and is promoted by collagens in the small intestine (Moore et al 1992) and by laminin in the colon (Feil et al 1992).

Regulation of regeneration

Epithelial proliferation and regeneration associated with surgical wounds or other intestinal injury is stimulated by systemic and – for some – enteral administration of several growth factors, such as EGF, TGFα, TGFβ, PDGF (plateler-derived growth factor) (Thompson et al 1989, Mustoe et al 1990) or IGF-1 (insulin-like growth factor-1) (Huang et al 1993) in experimental animals, and EGF in children with enterocolitis (Sullivan et al 1991). Epithelial cell differentiation is also altered in regenerating mucosa: cells with a novel phenotype and the ability to secrete EGF appear to develop in association with budding crypts (Wright et al 1990). Factors that improve the energy substrate supply to the cells also promote regeneration and healing in animal models following injury induced by surgery, drugs or irradiation.

Susceptibility to injury

Epithelia have the ability to adapt to adverse conditions so that susceptibility to injury is reduced. Stress (heat shock) proteins appear to be important in this response. Factors such as heat, hypoxia and reactive oxygen metabolites induce the synthesis of stress proteins, and these subsequently render the cells more resistant to injury by those stimuli (Lindquist 1986). Colonic mucosal stress protein expression is elevated in ulcerative colitis but not in Crohn's disease (Winrow et al 1993), but little else is known of their expression or modulation in intestinal epithelium. Exogenous growth factors may also be cytoprotective: for example, EGF protects against chemically induced colitis in the rat (Luck & Bass 1993). Luminal glutamine or butyrate also modulate mucosal susceptibility to injury (see above).

Implications for IBD

Efficient repair of breaches in the intestinal epithelium is of obvious importance for the maintenance of barrier function in patients with inflammatory bowel disease. Any intervention that can promote restitution and/or stimulate regeneration may have therapeutic efficacy in healing, in prevention of relapse, or in the minimization of atrophy from loss of crypt numbers. Likewise, 'cytoprotection' may have therapeutic advantage. In effect, however, few if any current therapies are known to act via such mechanisms. Corticosteroids inhibit wound healing, but the effects of mesalazine-delivering drugs on epithelial restitution and regeneration are unknown. The systemic infusions of growth factors such as EGF or IGF-1 may indeed be efficacious, but their high cost precludes their serious consideration at the present time. Since peanut lectin stimulates proliferation of colonic epithelial cells in ulcerative colitis (Ryder et al 1994), its therapeutic use in promoting regeneration is worthy of study.

CONCLUSION

A better understanding of mucosal metabolism and of epithelial turnover and repair mechanisms would offer potential insights into the pathogenic mechanisms in ulcerative colitis and Crohn's disease, and might lead to the design of better therapeutic strategies. Relevant information in some areas is already forthcoming, but has yet to be translated into practical therapy and evaluated in patients. The best example is the considerable amount of data underlining the importance of mucosal nutrition to the function, repair and susceptibility to injury of intestinal mucosa, and of the notion that the specific metabolic needs of the mucosa should be addressed in addition to the general nutritional needs of the whole patient. Although these approaches may not in themselves offer great therapeutic benefit, they may play key adjunctive roles in improving responses to drug therapy aimed principally at immunoinflammatory events.

REFERENCES

Allan A, Bristol J B, Williamson R C N 1985 Crypt cell production rate in ulcerative proctocolitis: differential increments in remission and relapse. Gut 26: 999–1003

Alverdy J C, Aoys E, Moss G S 1990 Effect of commercially available chemically defined liquid diets on the intestinal microflora and bacterial translocation from the gut. Journal of Parenteral and Enteral Nutrition 14: 1–6

Ardawi M S M, Newsholme E A 1985 Fuel utilisation in colonocytes of the rat. Biochemical Journal 231: 713–719

Argeugio R A, Miller N, von Engelhardt W 1975 Effect of volatile fatty acids on water and ion absorption from the goat colon. American Journal of Physiology 229: 997–1002

Barber A E, Jones W G, Minei J P et al 1990 Glutamine or fiber supplementation of a defined formula diet: impact on bacterial translocation, tissue composition, and response to endotoxin. Journal of Parenteral and Enteral Nutrition 14: 335

Barkla D H, Gibson P R, Nov R 1994 Cell death in human colonic epithelium. Journal of Gastroenterology and Hepatology 9: A77 (Abstract)

Barnard J A, Beauchamp R D, Coffey R J, Moses H L 1989 Regulation of intestinal epithelial cell growth by transforming growth factor type beta. Proceedings of the National Academy of Science, USA 86: 1578–1582

Basson M D, Modlin I M, Madri J A 1992 Human enterocyte (Caco-2) migration is modulated in vitro by extracellular matrix composition and epidermal growth factor. Journal of Clinical Investigation 90: 15–23

Bleiberg H, Mainguet P, Galand P, Chreien J, Dupont-Mariesse N 1970 Cell renewal in the human rectum. In vivo autoradiographic study on active ulcerative colitis. Gastroenterology 58: 851–855

Bond J H, Levitt M D 1976 Fate of soluble carbohydrate in the colon of rats and man. Journal of Clinical Investigation 57: 1158–1164

Bostrom H, Bromster D, Nordenstam H, Wengle B 1968 On the occurrence of phenol and steroid sulphokinases in the human gastrointestinal tract. Scandinavian Journal of Gastroenterology 3: 369–375

Breuer R I, Buto S K, Christ M L et al 1991 Rectal irrigation with short-chain fatty acids for distal ulcerative colitis: preliminary report. Digestive Diseases and Sciences 36: 185–187

Buck R 1986 Ultrastructural features of rectal epithelium of the mouse during the early phases of migration to repair a defect. Virchows Archiv [Cell Pathology] 51: 331–340

Bullough W S 1952 Stress and epidermal mitotic activity. I. The effects of adrenal hormones. Journal of Endocrinology 8: 265–270

Burke D, Alverdy J C, Aoys E, Moss G S 1989 Glutamine-supplemented total parenteral nutrition improves gut immune function. Archives of Surgery 124: 1300–1396

Camaño G J, Iglesias J, Marco C, Limares A 1988 In vivo utilization of [3–14c] acetoacetate for lipid and amino acid synthesis in the 15-day-old chick. Comparative Biochemistry and Physiology 91: 1–5

Castro G A 1982 Immunological regulation of epithelial function. American Journal of Physiology 243: G321–G329

Chapman M A S, Grahn M F, Boyle M A, Hutton M, Rogers J, Williams N S 1994 Butyrate oxidation is impaired in the colonic mucosa of sufferers of quiescent ulcerative colitis. Gut 35: 73–76

Cheng H, Bjerknes M, Amar J, Gardiner G 1986 Crypt prodcution in normal and diseased human colonic epithelium. Anatomical Record 216: 44–48

Ciacci C, Lind S E, Podolsky D K 1993 Transforming growth factor β regulation of migration in wounded rat intestinal epithelial monolayers. Gastroenterology 105: 93–101

Clausen M R, Nortensen P B, Holtug K, Nordgaard I, Hove P B 1994 Kinetic studies on colonocyte metabolism of short-chain fatty acids and glucose in patients with ulcerative colitis. Gastroenterology 106: A666 (Abstract)

Cooper H S, Steplewski Z 1988 Immunohistologic study of ulcerative colitis with monoclonal antibodies against tumour-associated and/or differentiation antigens. Gastroenterology 95: 686–693

Cross T A, Pahl C, Oberhansli R, Aue W P, Keller V, Seilig J 1984 Ketogenesis in the living rat followed by ^{13}C NMR spectroscopy. Biochemistry 23: 6398–6402

Cummings J H 1994 Quantitating short chain fatty acid production in humans. In: Binder H J, Cummings J, Soergel K H (eds) Short chain fatty acids. Kluwer, Dordrecht, pp 11–19

Cynober L 1994 Can arginine and ornithine support gut functions? Gut 35 (Suppl 1): S42–S45

D'Argenio G, Cosenza V, Sorrentini I et al 1994 Butyrate, mesalamine, and factor XIII in experimental colitis in the rat: effects on transglutaminase activity. Gastroenterology 106: 399–404

De Bruin P A F, Crama-Bohbouth G, Verspaget H W et al 1986 Plasminogen activators in the intestine of patients with inflammatory bowel disease. Thrombosis and Haemostasis 60: 262–266

Delpre G, Avidor I, Steinherz R, Kadish U, Ben-Bassat M 1989 Ultrastructural abnormalities in endoscopically and histologically normal and involved colon in ulcerative colitis. American Journal of Gastroenterology 84: 1038–1046

Desmoulin F, Canioni P, Cozzone P J 1985 Glutamate–glutamine metabolism in the perfused rat liver. ^{13}C NMR study using 2-^{13}C-enriched acetate. FEBS Letters 185: 29–32

Dignass A U, Podolsky D K 1993 Cytokine modulation of intestinal epithelial cell restitution: central role of transforming growth factor β. Gastroenterology 105: 1323–1332

Dignass A, Lynch-Devaney K, Kindon H, Thim L, Podolsky D K 1994 Trefoil peptides promote epithelial migration through a transforming growth factor β-independent pathway. Journal of Clinical Investigation 94: 376–383

Donnellan W L 1966 Early histological changes in ulcerative colitis. Gastroenterology 50: 519–540

Eastwood G L, Trier J S 1973 Epithelial cell renewal in cultured rectal biopsies in ulcerative colitis. Gastroenterology 64: 383–390

Edwards W H B 1993 Growth factors and colonic mucosa. MS Dissertation, University of Melbourne

Elliott R, Stephens R W, Doe W F 1987 Expression of urokinase-type plasminogen activator in the mucosal lesions of inflammatory bowel disease. Journal of Gastroenterology and Hepatology 2: 517–523

Erdman S H, Jung H, Park Y et al 1989 Suppression of diamine oxidase activity enhances postresection ileal proliferation in the rat. Gastroenterology 96: 1533–1536

Feil W, Lacy E R, Wong Y-M M et al 1989 Rapid epithelial restitution of human and rabbit colonic mucosa. Gastroenterology 97: 685–701

Feil W, Riegler T, Sogukuglu T et al 1992 Laminin stimulates rapid epithelial restitution of the human colon in vitro. Gastroenterology 102: A67 (Abstract)

Finnie I A, Taylor B A, Rhodes J M 1993 Ileal and colonic epithelial metabolism in quiescent ulcerative colitis: increased glutamine metabolism in distal colon but no defect in butyrate metabolism. Gut 34: 1552–1558

Florin T H J, Gibson G R, Neale G, Cummings J H 1990 A role for sulfate reducing bacteria in ulcerative colitis. Gastroenterology 98: A170 (Abstract)

Fox A D, Kripke S A, DePaula J, Berman J M, Settle R G, Rombeau J L 1988 Effect of a glutamine-supplemented enteral diet on methotrexate-induced enterocolitis. Journal of Parenteral and Enteral Nutrition 12: 325–331

Gavrieli Y, Sherman Y, Ben-Sasson S A 1992 Identification of programmed cell death in situ via specific labeling of nuclear DNA fragmentation. Journal of Cell Biology 119: 493–501

Gibson G R, Cummings J H, Macfarlane G T 1991 Growth and activities of sulfate-reducing bacteria in gut contents of healthy subjects and patients with ulcerative colitis. FEMA Microbiological Ecology 86: 103–112

Gibson P R 1994 Current concepts in the pathogenesis and therapy of inflammatory bowel disease. Clinical Immunotherapeutics 2: 134–160

Gibson P R, Rosella O 1994 Interleukin-8 secretion by colonic epithelial cell in vitro, response to injury suppressed by butyrate and enhanced in inflammatory bowel disease. Gut 37: 536–545

Gibson P R, van de Pol E, Barratt P J, Doe W F 1988 Ulcerative colitis – a disease characterized by the abnormal colonic epithelial cell? Gut 29: 516–521

Gibson P R, Moeller I, Kagelari O, Folino M, Young G P 1991 Contrasting effects of butyrate on expression of phenotypic markers of differentiation in neoplastic and non-neoplastic colonic epithelial cells in vitro. Journal of Gastroenterology and Hepatology 7: 165–172

Gibson P R, Albert V, Nov R, Rosella O, Young G P 1994a The relation of enterocyte-associated urokinase activity to position on the crypt–villus axis in rats. Journal of Gastroenterology and Hepatology 9: A108 (Abstract)

Gibson P R, Folino M, Rosella O, McIntyre A, Finch C, Young G P 1995a Dietary modulation of colonic mucosal urokinase activity in rats. Journal of Gastroenterology and Hepatology 10: 324–330

Gibson P R, Rosella R, Nov R, Young G 1995b Colonic epithelium is diffusely abnormal in ulcerative colitis and colorectal carcinoma. Gut 36: 857–863

Gibson P R, Rosella O, Rosella G, Young G P 1994b Constitutive secretion by colonic epithelium of urokinase-type plasminogen activator and plasminogen activator inhibitor-1. Gut 35: 969–975

Gibson P R, Rosella O, Rosella G, Young G P 1994c Butyrate is a potent inhibitor of urokinase secretion by normal colonic epithelium in vitro. Gastroenterology 107: 410–419

Gibson P R, Rosella O, Young G P 1994d Serum-free medium increases the expression of markers of differentiation of human colonic crypt cells in vitro. Gut 35: 791–797

Gibson P R, Rosella O 1996 Abnormalities of the urokinase system in colonic crypt cells from patients with ulcerative colitis. Inflammatory Bowel Diseases (in press)

Glotzer D J, Glick M E, Goldman H 1981 Proctitis and colitis following diversion of the faecal stream. Gastroenterology 80: 438–441

Govers M J A P, Termont D S M L, Van der Meer R 1994 The mechanism of the antiproliferative effect of milk mineral and other calcium supplements on colonic epithelium. Cancer Research 54: 95–100

Grant J 1988 Use of L-glutamine in total parenteral nutrition. Journal of Clinical Research 44: 506–513

Grimble G K 1994 Dietary nucleotides and gut mucosal defence. Gut 35 (Suppl 1): S46–S51

Hackford A W, Mayhew J W, Goldin B R 1988 An isolated perfused model for the study of colonic metabolism and transport. Journal of Surgical Research 44: 14–25

Hahn U, Stallmach A, Hahn E G, Riecken E O 1990 Basement membrane components are potent promoters of rat intestinal epithelial cell differentiation in vitro. Gastroenterology 98: 322–335

Harig J M, Soergel K H, Komorowski R A, Wood C M 1989 Treatment of diversion colitis with short-chain fatty acid irrigation. New England Journal of Medicine 320: 23–28

Hosoda N, Nisht M, Nakagawa M, Hiramatsu Y, Hioki K, Yamamoto M 1989 Structural and functional alterations in the gut of parenterally or enterally fed rats. Journal of Surgical Research 47: 129–133

Huang K F, Chung D H, Herndon D N 1993 Insulin-like growth factor 1 (IGF-1) reduces gut atrophy and bacterial translocation after severe burn injury. Archives of Surgery 128: 47–54

Hwang T L, O'Dwyer S T, Smith R J, Wilmore D W 1986 Preservation of small bowel mucosa using glutamine-enriched parenteral nutrition. Surgical Forum 37: 56–58

Ireland A, Jewell D P 1990 5-Aminosalicylic acid (5-ASA) has no effect on butyrate metabolism in human colonic epithelial cells. Gastroenterology 98: A176 (Abstract)

Ireland A, Priddle J D, Jewell D P 1990 Acetylation of 5-aminosalicylic acid by isolated human colonic epithelial cells. Clinical Science 78: 105–111

Iwanaga Y, Han H, Adachi K, Fujita T 1993 A novel mechanism for disposing of effete epithelial cells in the small intestine of guinea pigs. Gastroenterology 105: 1089–1097

Jacobs D O, Evans D A, O'Dwyer S T, Smith R J, Wilmore D W 1987 Disparate effects of 5-fluorouracil on the ileum and colon of enterally fed rats with protection by dietary glutamine. Surgical Forum 38: 45–49

Jankowski J A, Goodlad R A, Wright N A 1994 Maintenance of normal intestinal mucosa function, structure and adaptation. Gut 35 (Suppl 1): S1–S4

Klimberg V S, Souba W W, Dolson D J et al 1989 Oral glutamine supports crypt cell turnover and accelerates intestinal healing following abdominal radiation. Journal of Parenteral and Enteral Nutrition 13: 35

Klimberg V S, Salloum R M, Kasper M et al 1990 Oral glutamine accelerates healing of the small intestine and improves outcome after whole abdominal radiation. Archives of Surgery 125: 1040–1045

Koruda M J, Rolandelli R H, Settle R G, Zimmano D M, Rombeau J L 1988 Effect of parenteral nutrition supplemented with short-chain fatty acids on adaptation of massive small bowel resection. Gastroenterology 95: 715–720

Kripke S A, Fox A D, Berman J M, De Paula J A, Rombeau J L, Settle R G 1988 Inhibition of TPN-associated colonic atrophy with β-hydroxybutyrate. Surgical Forum 39: 48–50

Kripke S A, Fox A D, Berman J L, Settle R G, Rombeau J L 1989 Stimulation of intestinal mucosal growth with intracolonic infusion of short chain fatty acids. Journal of Parenteral and Enteral Nutrition 13: 109–116

Kruh J, Tichonicky L, Defer N 1994 Effect of butyrate on gene expression. In: Binder H J, Cummings J, Soergel K H (eds) Short chain fatty acids. Kluwer, Dordrecht, pp 135–147

Kvietys P R, Granger D N 1981 Effects of volatile fatty acids on blood flow and oxygen uptake by the dog colon. Gastroenterology 80: 962

Lapre J A, De Vries H T, Koeman J H, Van der Meer R 1993 The antiproliferative effect of dietary calcium on colonic epithelium is mediated by luminal surfactants on the type of dietary fat. Cancer Research 53: 784–789

Lee F D 1993 Importance of apoptosis in the histopathology of drug related lesions in large intestine. Journal of Clinical Pathology 46: 118–122

Lindquist S 1986 The heat shock response. Annual Review of Biochemistry 55: 1151–1191

Luck M S, Bass P 1993 Effect of epidermal growth factor on experimental colitis in the rat. Journal of Pharmacological and Experimental Therapeutics 264: 984–990

Mariadasan J M, Gibson P R 1994 The effect of butyrate on paracellular permeability in the Caco-2 model of colonic epithelium. Gastroenterology 106: A729 (Abstract)

May R J, Quaroni A, Kirsch K, Isselbacher K J 1981 A villous cell-derived inhibitor of intestinal cell proliferation. American Journal of Physiology 241: G520–G527

Mennigen R, Kusche J, Leisten L, Erpenbach K 1987 Diamine oxidase (DAO) activity and intestinal mucosa integrity: influence of suture techniques. Agents and Actions 20: 277–280

Moore R, Madri J, Carbro S, Madara J L 1992 Collagens facilitate epithelial migration in restitution of native guinea pig intestinal epithelium. Gastroenterology 102: 119–130

Morita H, Kettlewell M G, Jewell D P, Kent P W 1993 Glycosylation and sulphation of colonic mucus glycoproteins in patients with ulcerative colitis and in healthy subjects. Gut 34: 926–932

Murray K E, Adams R F 1988 Determination of simple phenols in faeces and urine by high performance liquid chromatography. Journal of Chromatography 431: 143–149

Mustoe T A, Landes A, Cormak D T 1990 Differential acceleration of healing of surgical incisions in the rabbit gastrointestinal tract by platelet-derived growth factor and transforming growth factor, type beta. Surgery 108: 324–330

Newsholme E A, Carrié A-L 1994 Quantitative aspects of glucose and glutamine metabolism by intestinal cells. Gut 35 (Suppl 1): S13–S17

Nusrat A, Parkos C A, Godowski P J, Delp-Archer C, Rosen E M, Madara J L 1994 Hepatocyte growth factor/scatter effects on epithelia. Journal of Clinical Investigation 91: 2056–2065

O'Morain C, Segal A W, Levi A J 1980 Elemental diets in the treatment of acute Crohn's disease. British Medical Journal 281: 1173–1175

Oshinsky R J, Strobel H W 1987 Drug metabolism in rat colon: resolution of enzymatic constituents and characterization of activity. Molecular and Cellular Biochemistry 75: 51–60

Podolsky D K, Fournier D A 1988a Emergence of antigenic glycoprotein structures in ulcerative colitis detected through monoclonal antibodies. Gastroenterology 95: 371–378

Podolsky D K, Fournier D A 1988b Alterations in mucosal content of colonic glycoconjugates in inflammatory bowel disease defined by monoclonal antibodies. Gastroenterology 95: 379–381

Podolsky D K, Isselbacher K J 1984 Glycoprotein composition of colonic mucosa: specific alterations in ulcerative colitis. Gastroenterology 87: 991–998

Ponder B A J, Schmidt G H, Wilkinson M M, Wood M J, Monk M, Reid A 1985 A derivation of mouse intestinal crypts from single progenitor cells. Nature 313: 689–691

Ramakrishna B S, Roberts-Thompson J C, Pannall P R, Roediger W E W 1991 Impaired sulphation of phenol by the colonic mucosa in quiescent and active ulcerative colitis. Gut 32: 46–49

Roediger W E W 1980a Role of anaerobic bacteria in the metabolic welfare of the colonic mucosa in man. Gut 21: 793–798

Roediger W E W 1980b The colonic epithelium in ulcerative colitis – an energy deficiency disease? Lancet 2: 712–715

Roediger W E W 1982 Utilization of nutrients by isolated epithelial cells of the rat colon. Gastroenterology 83: 424–429

Roediger W E W 1994 The imprint of disease on short chain fatty acid metabolism by colonocytes. In: Binder H J, Cummings J, Soergel K H (eds) Short chain fatty acids. Kluwer, Dordrecht, pp 195–205

Roediger W E W, Nance S 1986 Metabolic induction of experimental ulcerative colitis by inhibition of fatty acid oxidation. British Journal of Experimental Pathology 67: 773–782

Roediger W E W, Lawson M J, Kwok V, Kerr Grant A, Pannal P R 1984 Colonic bicarbonate output as a test of disease activity in ulcerative colitis. Journal of Clinical Pathology 37: 704–707

Roediger W E W, Radcliffe B C, Deakin E J, Nance S H 1986 Specific metabolic effect of sodium nitrite on fat metabolism by mucosal cells of the colon. Digestive Diseases and Sciences 31: 535–539

Roediger W E W, Deakin E J, Walker G, Nance S H 1989 Assessment of salicylate derivatives for potential use in ulcerative colitis: proposal for a new action of 5-aminosalicylic acid? Pharmacology 39: 39–45

Roediger W E, Kapaniris O, Millard S 1992 Lipogenesis from n-butyrate in colonocytes. Action of reducing agent and 5-aminosalicylic acid with relevance to ulcerative colitis. Molecular and Cellular Biochemistry 118: 113–118

Roediger W E W, Duncan A, Kapaniris O, Millard S 1993a Reducing sulfur compounds of the colon impairs colonocyte nutrition: implications for ulcerative colitis. Gastroenterology 104: 802–809

Roediger W E W, Duncan A, Kapaniris O, Millard S 1993b Sulphide impairment of substrate oxidation in rat colonocytes: a biochemical basis for ulcerative colitis? Clinical Science 85: 623–627

Rolandelli R H, Koruda M J, Settle R G 1986 Effects of intraluminal infusion of short chain fatty acids on the healing of colonic anastomosis in the rat. Surgery 100: 198–203

Rosen E N, Goldberg I D 1989 Protein factors which regulate cell motility. In Vitro Cellular and Developmental Biology 25: 1079–1087

Ruppin H, Bar-Meir S, Saergel K H et al 1980 Absorption of short chain fatty acids by the colon. Gastroenterology 78: 1500–1507

Ryder S D, Smith J A, Rhodes J M 1992 Peanut lectin is a mitogen for normal human colonic epithelium and for HT29 human colorectal cancer cells. Journal of the National Cancer Institute 84: 1410–1416

Ryder S D, Parker N, Ecclestone D, Haqqani M T, Rhodes J M 1994 Peanut lectin stimulates proliferation in colonic explants from patients with inflammatory bowel disease and colon polyps. Gastroenterology 106: 117–124

Sakata T, Engelhardt W V 1983 Stimulating effect of short chain fatty acids on the epithelial cell proliferation in the rat large intestine. Comparative Biochemistry and Physiology 74A: 459–462

Salloum R M, Souba W W, Klimberg V S et al 1989 Glutamine is superior to glutamate in supporting gut metabolism, stimulating intestinal glutaminase activity, and preventing bacterial translocation. Surgical Forum 40: 6–8

Salloum R M, Souba W W, Fernandez A, Stevens B R 1990 Dietary modulation of intestinal glutamine transport in intestinal brush border membrane vesicles of rats. Journal of Surgical Research 48: 635–638

Salloum R M, Stevens B R, Schultz G S, Souba W W 1993 Regulation of small intestinal glutamine transport by epidermal growth factor. Surgery 113: 552–559

Scheppach W, Sommer H, Kirchner T et al 1992 Effect of butyrate enemas on the colonic mucosa in distal ulcerative colitis. Gastroenterology 103: 51–56

Serafini E P, Kirk A P, Chambers T J 1981 Rate and pattern of epithelial cell proliferation in ulcerative colitis. Gut 22: 648–652

Souba W W, Smith R J, Wilmore D W 1985 Effect of glucocorticoids on glutamine metabolism in visceral organs. Metabolism 34: 450–456

Souba W W, Herskowitz K, Salloum R M, Chen M K, Austgen T R 1990a Gut glutamine metabolism. Journal of Parenteral and Enteral Nutrition 14 (Suppl 4): 45S–50S

Souba W W, Klimberg V S, Hautamaki R D et al 1990b Oral glutamine reduces bacterial translocation following abdominal radiation. Journal of Surgical Research 48: 1–5

Spaeth G, Specian R D, Berg R D 1990 Bulk prevents bacterial translocation induced by the oral administration of total parenteral nutrition solution. Journal of Parenteral and Enteral Nutrition 14: 442–447

Steeb C B, Trahair J F, Tomas F M, Read L C 1994 Prolonged administration of IGF peptides enhances growth of gastrointestinal tissues in normal rats. American Journal of Physiology 266: G1090–G1098

Sullivan P B, Brueton M J, Tabara Z B, Goodlad R A, Lee C Y, Wright N A 1991 Epidermal growth factor in necrotising enteritis. Lancet 338: 53–54

Sund R B, Lauterbach F 1986 Drug metabolism and metabolite transport in the small and large intestine: experiments with 1-naphthol and phenolphthalein by luminal and contra-luminal administration in the isolate guinea pig mucosa. Acta Pharmacologica Toxocologica 58: 74–83

Thompson J S, Saxena S K, Greaton C, Shultz G, Sharp J G 1989 The effect of route of delivery of urogastrone on intestinal regeneration. Surgery 106: 45–51

Tysk C, Riedesel H, Lindberg E, Panzini B, Podolsky D, Jarnerot G 1991 Colonic glycoproteins in monozygotic twins with inflammatory bowel disease. Gastroenterology 100: 419–423

Vernia P, Gnaedinger A, Hauck W, Breuer R I 1988 Organic anions and the diarrhea of inflammatory bowel disease. Digestive Diseases and Sciences 33: 1353–1358

Walker N I, Bennett R E, Axelsen R A 1988 Melanosis coli: a consequence of anthraquinone-induced apoptosis of colonic epithelial cells. American Journal of Pathology 131: 465–476

Watford M, Lund P, Krebs H A 1979 Isolation and metabolic characteristics of rat and chicken enterocytes. Biochemical Journal 178: 589–596

Weisiger R A, Pinkus L M, Jakoby W B 1980 Thiol 5-methyltransferase: suggested role in detoxication of intestinal hydrogen sulfide. Biochemical Pharmacology 29: 2885–2887

Windmueller H G, Spaeth A E 1978 Identification of ketone bodies and glutamine as the major respiratory fuels in vivo for postabsorptive rat small intestine. Journal of Biological Chemistry 253: 69–76

Winkle W V 1968 The epithelium in wound healing. Surgery Gynecology and Obstetrics 314: 1089–1115

Winrow V R, Mojdehi G M, Ryder S D et al 1993 Stress proteins in colorectal mucosa: enhanced expression in ulcerative colitis. Digestive Diseases and Science 38: 1994–2000

Wischmeyer P, Pemberton J H, Phillips S F 1993 Chronic pouchitis after ileal pouch–anal anastomosis: responses to butyrate and glutamine suppositories in a pilot study. Mayo Clinic Proceedings 68: 978

Wolf B C, D'Emilia J C, Salem R R et al 1989 Detection of the tumor-associated glycoprotein antigen (TAG-72) in premalignant lesions of the colon. Journal of the National Cancer Institute 81: 1913–1917

Wright N A, Pike C, Elia G 1990 Induction of a novel epidermal growth factor-secreting cell lineage by mucosal ulceration in human gastrointestinal stem cells. Nature 343: 82–85

Xu D, Qi L, Thirstrup C, Berg R, Deitch E A 1993 Elemental diet-induced bacterial translocation and immunosuppression is not reversed by glutamine. Journal of Trauma 35: 821–824

Young G P, Macrae F A, Gibson P R, Alexeyeff M, Whitehead R H 1992 Brush border hydrolases in normal and neoplastic colonic epithelium. Journal of Gastroenterology and Hepatology 7: 347–354

//
SECTION 3

Clinical diagnosis

25. Radiology – contrast studies

J. R. Lee

INTRODUCTION

Despite the advent of cross-sectional imaging systems such as ultrasound, computerized tomography (CT) and magnetic resonance (MRI), bowel inflammation is usually more satisfactorily demonstrated by contrast radiography. The extraluminal effects of bowel inflammation, such as abscess formation, lymph node enlargement and fibrofatty proliferation are, however, best examined by cross-sectional imaging (Gore 1987).

Contrast imaging is cheap compared to other forms of imaging and is generally extremely safe. A further advantage is that a permanent record of the examination is made and can be kept for future reference and comparison, which is not commonly the case with endoscopy, which is increasingly being used as an alternative.

AIR CONTRAST STUDIES

As the bowel may contain little natural gas, air can be added as a supplement. This is most widely used as an 'air enema' in the assessment of acute colitis (Bartram et al 1983). This is a comfortable examination for patients, especially if a smooth muscle relaxant such as buscopan (hyoscine *N*-butylbromide) or glucagon is used as an adjunct. Some practitioners prefer the use of carbon dioxide gas instead of air as this is more readily absorbed and is said to cause less patient discomfort. With such an examination, the extent, and occasionally the severity of, ulcerative colitis can be determined (Fig. 25.1). With Crohn's colitis this examination is not so useful as the disease process is usually patchy in distribution.

POSITIVE CONTRAST MEDIA STUDIES

Water soluble

Solutions of organic iodine ions similar to the parenterally administered media used to diagnose vascular and urinary tract disease are used. They are not absorbed to any significant extent by an intact gastrointestinal mucosa, and therefore do not give rise to contrast reactions. However, they do not adhere well to mucosal surfaces and mucosal detail is poor. Their main use is where there is suspicion of an intestinal leak. One further advantage is that, if required, CT examination can be performed soon afterwards.

Barium sulfate

Barium sulfate is virtually insoluble and its suspension is therefore generally hazard free, provided it is confined within the intestinal lumen. However, all modern commercial barium sulfate preparations contain small amounts of organic substances which improve the stability of the suspensions. These organic compounds may very rarely cause an allergic response, especially if the mucosal surface is ulcerated or breached. The main danger from barium is spill into the peritoneal cavity or, rarely, intravasation from a severely ulcerated mucosa.

Barium air 'double contrast' examinations give the best mucosal detail and are usually routine in the examination of the esophagus, stomach, duodenum and large bowel. These examinations can be improved by the use of short-acting smooth muscle relaxants, which allow greater distension of the bowel wall as well as preventing bowel movement. There is still a place for single contrast studies provided they are aided by careful palpation with fluoroscopy by dedicated examiners (Carlson 1986), particularly in patients with severe colitis, where air insufflation may increase the risk of perforation or toxic dilatation.

EXAMINATION TECHNIQUES FOR SPECIFIC AREAS

The esophagus, stomach and duodenum are conventionally examined with a double contrast barium meal examination (DCBM) following a 6-hour fast. Water-soluble contrast should be used if there is any suspicion of intestinal perforation.

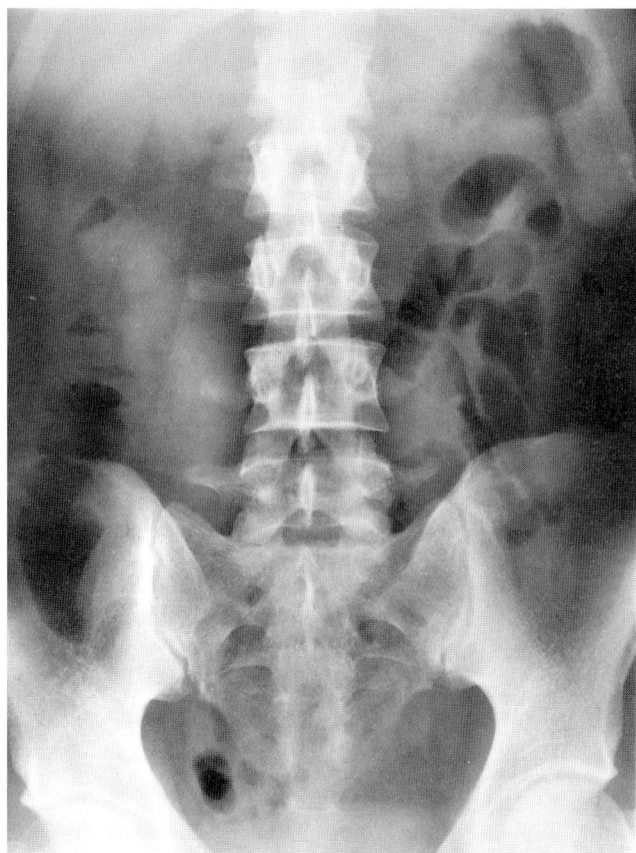 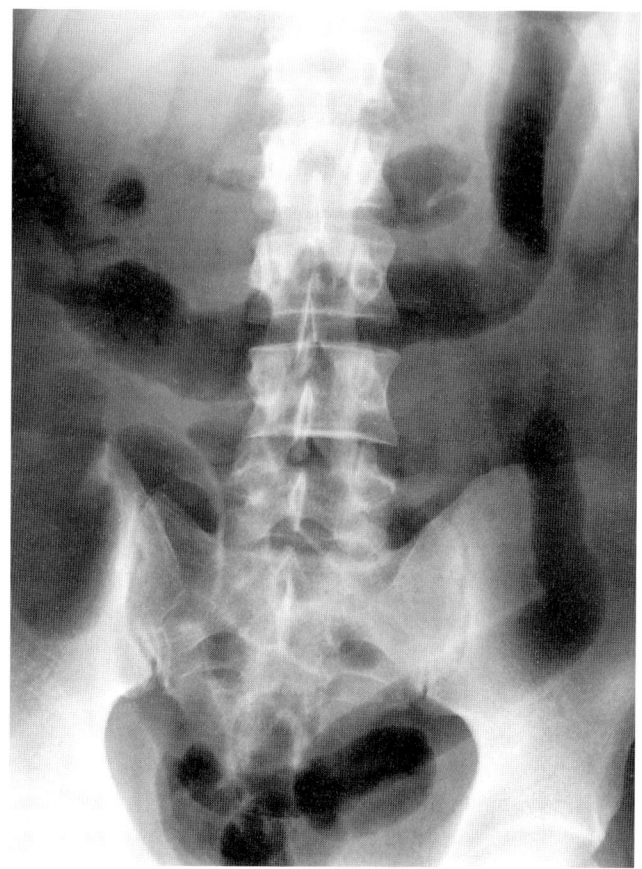

Fig. 25.1 Air enema in chronic ulcerative colitis. **a** Preliminary and **b** following insufflation of air per rectal catheter. The colon is narrowed from the proximal transverse colon to the rectum.

Small-bowel barium meal

The question of the best method of examining the small intestine still causes controversy among radiologists (Maglinte et al 1987). For many years the traditional 'barium meal and follow-through' examination was used almost exclusively (Marshak 1975). This involved the patient drinking a large volume of a dilute barium suspension and radiographs of the abdomen were taken at intervals until the barium reached the colon, when the terminal ileum was examined with fluoroscopy. The examination is often poorly performed, with too little barium being given and infrequent radiographs taken, with too-long intervals between. This, together with the fact that barium may take several hours – perhaps most of the day – to traverse the small bowel, leads to a degradation of the barium column and poor anatomical demonstration. The examination can be improved by giving further barium drinks and taking frequent (10–15 min intervals) radiographs in the initial stages. The radiologist must see each film and be prepared to examine the bowel with fluoroscopy at any moment. Further refinements can be achieved by giving the patient drugs such as metoclopramide to promote intestinal hurry. The addition of a small amount of a water-soluble iodide contrast agent to the barium mixture also gives the same effect (Fraser & Adam 1988). These refinements result in a more predictable and quicker examination: all of the small bowel can be examined within $1-1\frac{1}{2}$ hours in 95% of patients (Howarth et al 1969). Fraser and Preston (1983) have described a simple technique of examining the small bowel with barium and gas to obtain a double contrast examination (Fig. 25.2).

Small-bowel enema (enteroclysis)

Despite these refinements, many radiologists claim that the 'follow-through' is inaccurate and will fail to demonstrate small lesions and short strictures, and will underestimate the extent of diseased segments, because of failure of distension of the intestine which is necessary to attain an optimum morphological examination, as it is in radiography of the stomach and large bowel (Maglinte et al 1992). Many authorities believe this is best achieved by intubating the proximal jejunum and infusing barium at a constant rate – 'enteroclysis' (Sellink 1976). This technique can be single contrast using dilute barium (Nolan & Gourtsoyiannis 1980) (Fig. 25.3), or double contrast by

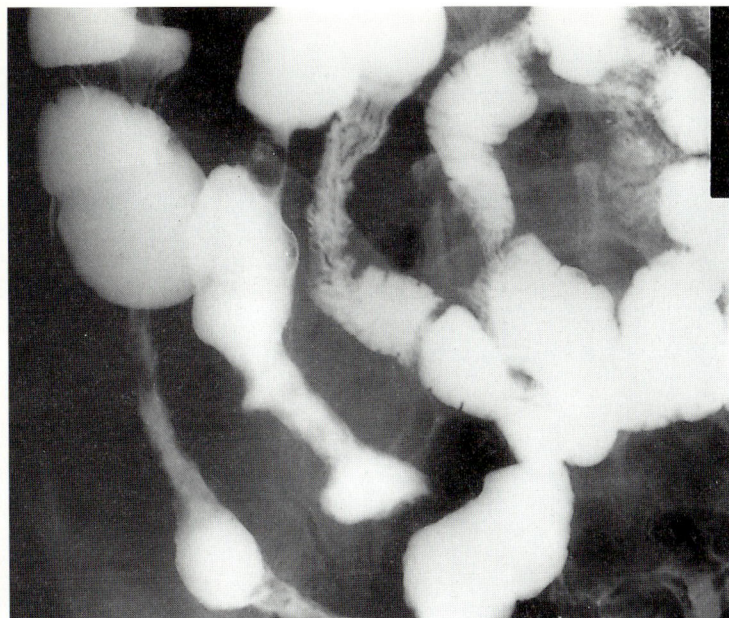

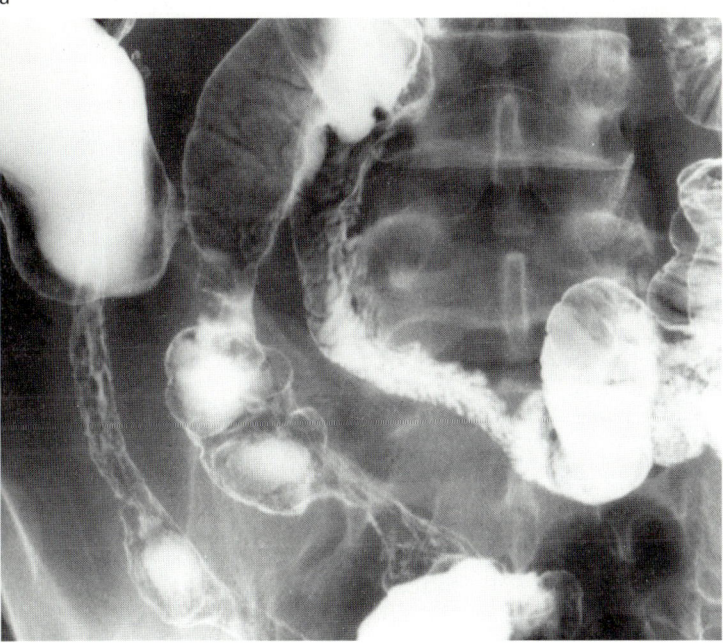

Fig. 25.2 Example of a 'gas-enhanced barium follow-through'. **a** Shows barium in the neoterminal ileum and **b** shortly after the passage of carbon dioxide through the small bowel. Note how the full extent of the several strictures is now demonstrated.

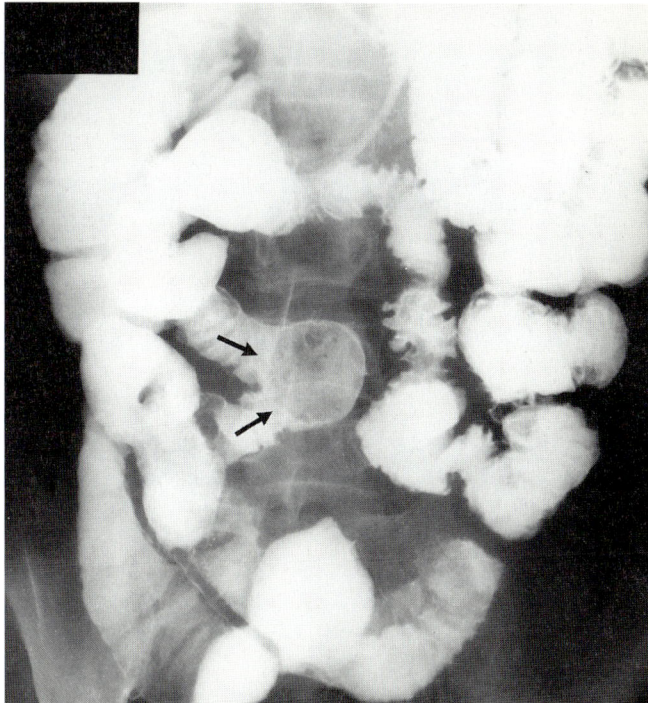

Fig. 25.3 Enteroclysis with dilute barium. Several short strictures are shown, some of which have been treated with a strictureplasty (arrows).

following the barium with air or a dilute methylcellulose mixture (Ekberg 1977, Herlinger 1978). Using such techniques the whole small bowel can be examined within 10–20 minutes. However, it is not possible to examine the stomach and duodenum at the same time.

Retrograde imaging of small intestine

A rarely used method of examining the small bowel is by the retrograde infusion of large quantities of dilute barium via the rectum (Miller 1965), sometimes also using paralysing agents such as glucagon. In patients with an ileostomy the small intestine may be examined easily with a retrograde ileogram. This involves infusing barium via a cannula inserted into the ileostomy (Fig. 25.4). Using this method it is possible to demonstrate the whole small bowel within 10–20 minutes. A further method of examining the distal ileum is the 'oral pneumocolon', whereby air is introduced into the large bowel via a rectal tube when barium has reached the ileum in the orthograde manner in a conventional 'follow-through' examination (Kellet et al 1977). Reflux of air into the barium-filled terminal ileum gives double contrast detail of this commonly affected segment of the bowel (Fig. 25.5).

The best anatomical demonstration of the distal ileum is obtained by a double contrast barium enema (DCBE) (Fig. 25.6), but reflux into the terminal ileum only occurs in about 60% of patients (Lee & Ferrando unpublished data). If there has been an ileocecal resection for Crohn's disease a DCBE is the preferred examination to assess recurrent disease (see Fig. 25.43b).

Barium enema

The large intestine is most accurately examined by DCBE, which can give excellent demonstration of the mucosa including the fine mucosal grooves (innominate folds)

218 INFLAMMATORY BOWEL DISEASES

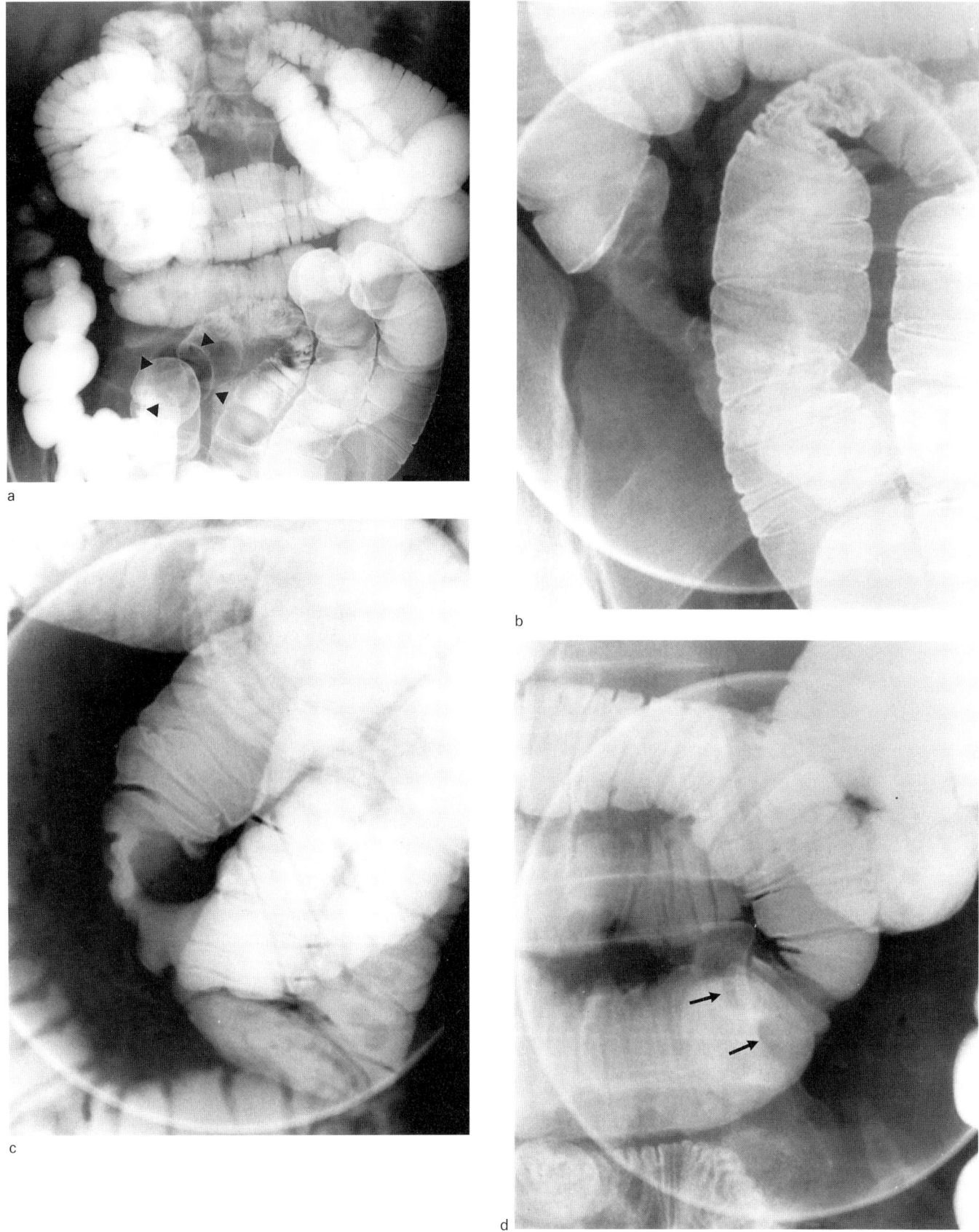

Fig. 25.4 **a** Retrograde ileogram with Foley catheter (balloon arrowed) in ileostomy. At first glance the bowel may appear normal, but careful compression **b, c, d** reveals three isolated short strictures. Note scattered aphthous ulceration near short stricture **d**.

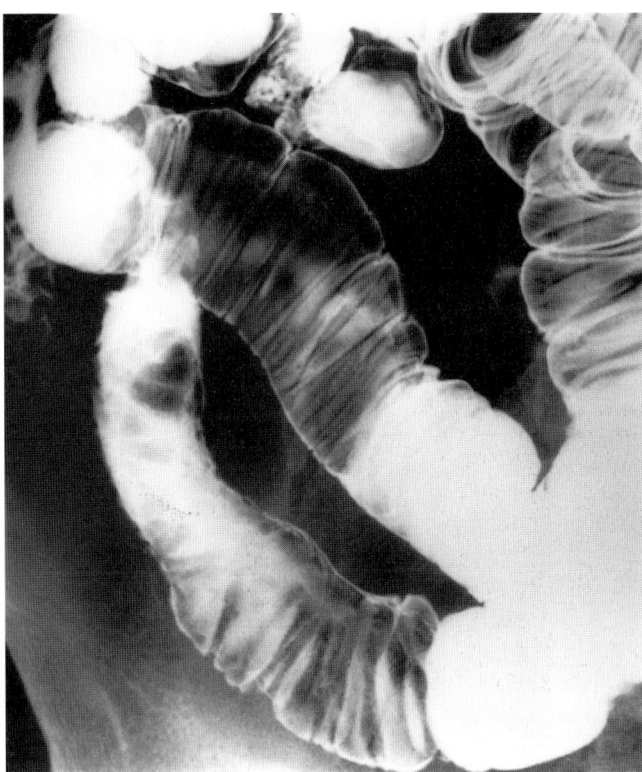

Fig. 25.5 An example of an oral pneumocolon – air insufflated per rectum after oral ingestion of barium. There is Crohn's ulceration in the terminal ileum, maximal on the mesenteric border.

(Williams 1975) (Fig. 25.7). The examination is dependent upon good bowel cleansing, which can be easily achieved following a 30–40 hour period of solid food restriction and ingestion of saline laxatives (Lee & Ferrando 1984). Some clinicians and radiologists are apprehensive about the potential risks of bowel preparation in patients with inflammatory bowel disease. However, in the author's experience all patients, except those bordering on a toxic colon, can safely undergo full bowel preparation and few are too ill to be examined by DCBE. A simplified barium enema without prior bowel preparation, the 'instant barium enema', can be used with advantage, in some patients or situations (Thomas 1979). This can give a quick evaluation of the extent of ulcerative colitis and is particularly useful in conjunction with an outpatient clinic. It is dependent upon an inflamed colon being empty of feces so as not to obscure mucosal detail. This examination is not so accurate in the assessment of Crohn's colitis, which tends to have patchy distribution, but may still be useful (Patel & Bartram 1993).

DIAGNOSTIC FEATURES

Ulcerative colitis

Ulcerative colitis is an inflammatory process of the mucosa which usually heals without fibrosis. The rectum is nearly

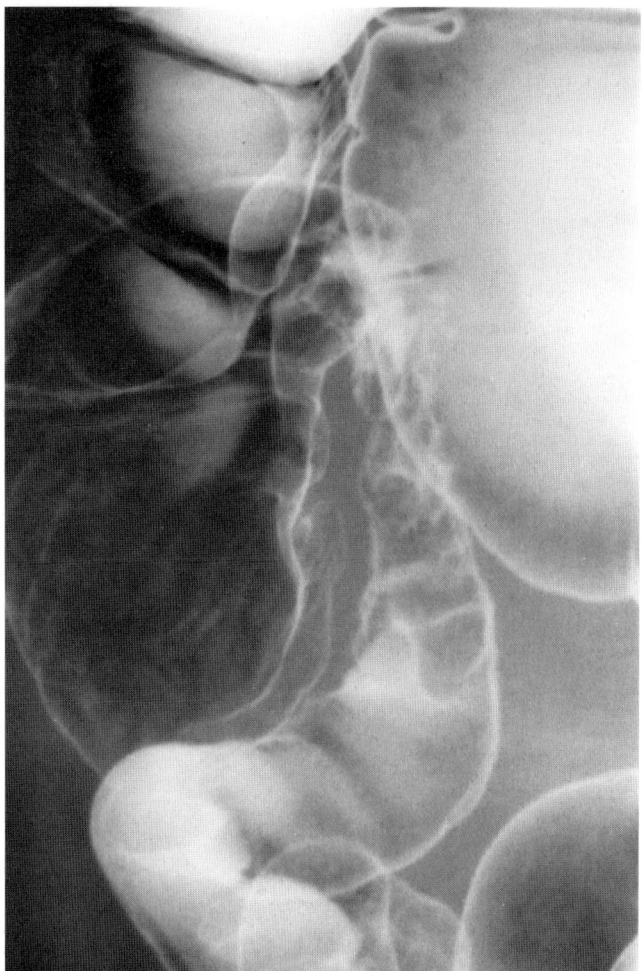

Fig. 25.6 An example of how the distal ileum can be well demonstrated in approximately 60% of patients by means of a DCBE. The terminal few centimeters are affected by early nodular Crohn's disease, with an apparent sharp demarcation from normal mucosa.

always affected, but the proximal progression is variable and in many patients may be always confined to the rectum and sigmoid. Characteristically the inflammation affects the large bowel in a continuous and symmetrical fashion, in contrast to colonic Crohn's disease (Morson et al 1990)

RADIOLOGICAL FEATURES

Ulceration

On a DCBE the normal rectal and colonic mucosa is smooth and featureless, with a fine even line of the bowel wall (Fig. 25.7a). Occasionally the fine mucosal innominate grooves can be seen both 'en face' and tangentially (Fig. 25.7b), but with the more frequent use of high-dose laxatives these are not so often seen. The earliest inflammatory change seen radiographically is an even granularity of the mucosa 'en face' and a thickening of the

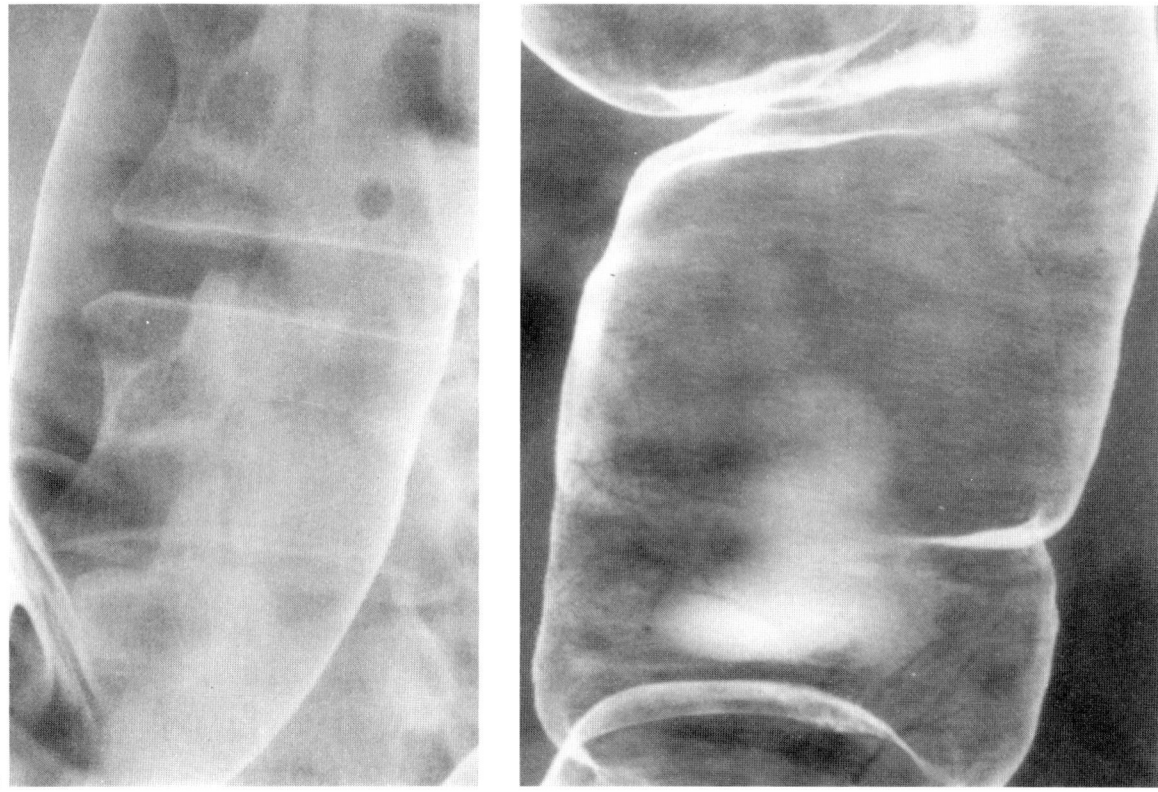

Fig. 25.7 **a** Smooth, featureless appearance of mucosa on DCBE. **b** Fine shallow transverse grooves in colonic mucosa shown on DCBE. Both **a** and **b** are normal appearances.

bowel margin tangentially (Fig. 25.8a). This represents hyperemic friable mucosa. With increasing disease severity the granular pattern becomes coarsened and uneven (Fig. 25.8b).

In its earliest form ulceration is a superficial erosion of the mucosa (Morson et al 1990). This may be seen as larger accumulations of barium superimposed upon the granular background 'en face', but in coarsened granular pattern these superficial ulcerations may not be identified on tangential outline. With deeper ulceration the granular pattern becomes more uneven 'en face', and in profile the outline is more irregular with more clearly defined projections (Fig. 25.8c).

With deeper undermining ulceration 'collar-stud' ulceration may occasionally be seen and may become confluent, giving rise to a parallel tracking of the bowel wall. Although the ulceration may be focal, there is usually a background granularity with no intervening or background normal mucosa. In some patients the rectum may be radiographically normal, owing to the effect of local steroid application (Fig. 25.9) (Morson et al 1990).

Fibrosis

Histologically there is little evidence of fibrosis but in patients with severe or long-standing disease abnormal tone of the bowel wall smooth muscle can cause radiological evidence of bowel shortening and narrowing (Fig. 25.9) (Morson et al 1990). The most commonly seen effect is a shortening of the bowel, which is more severe distally, in keeping with the disease distribution. An earlier manifestation of shortening is seen as blunting and widening of the haustral outlines, leading to complete loss in severe cases. However, the observer must be aware that the haustral pattern may be poor or completely absent in the left colon in normal patients, particularly when viewed with a well distended colon. The change in muscle tone appears to run parallel with the severity of the mucosal inflammation, and in patients in remission the shortening and haustral change may revert to normal.

In patients with severe rectal disease the rectum can become very narrow, giving rise to an apparent widening of the presacral or postrectal space when viewed on a lateral projection. This severe narrowing does not appear to revert to normal and the majority of these patients eventually proceed to proctocolectomy. Concentric strictures, which are usually short and tapering in appearance (Fig. 25.10), are uncommon but may be seen in patients with long-standing disease. Colonoscopy is then essential to exclude malignant change.

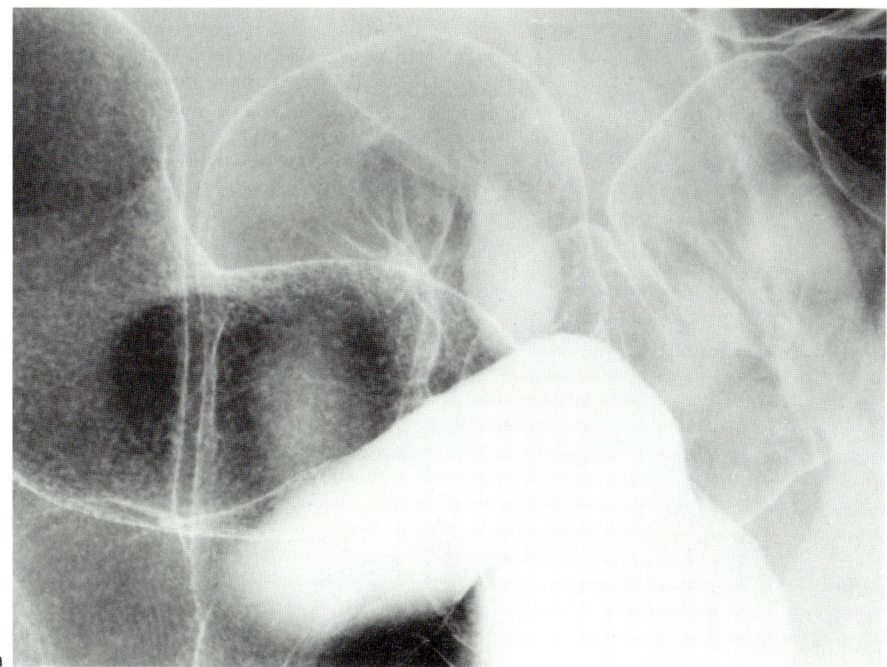

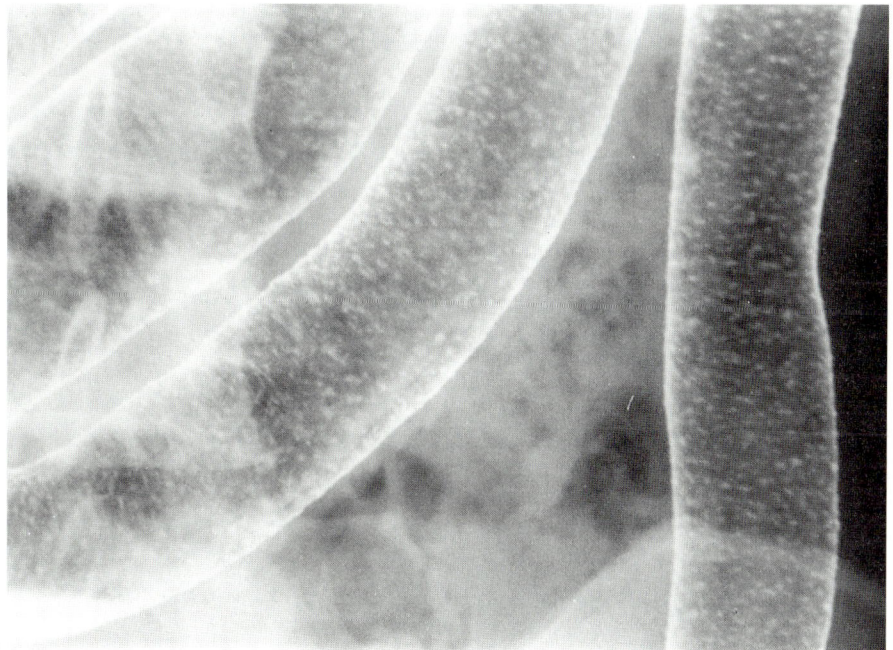

Fig. 25.8 Mucosal ulceration in ulcerative colitis. **a** Fine even granulation of mucosa of the distal sigmoid colon with normal featureless mucosa of proximal sigmoid colon above. **b** Coarse but even granular mucosa. There is shallow ulceration, as shown by fine stippling of the bowel margins.

222 INFLAMMATORY BOWEL DISEASES

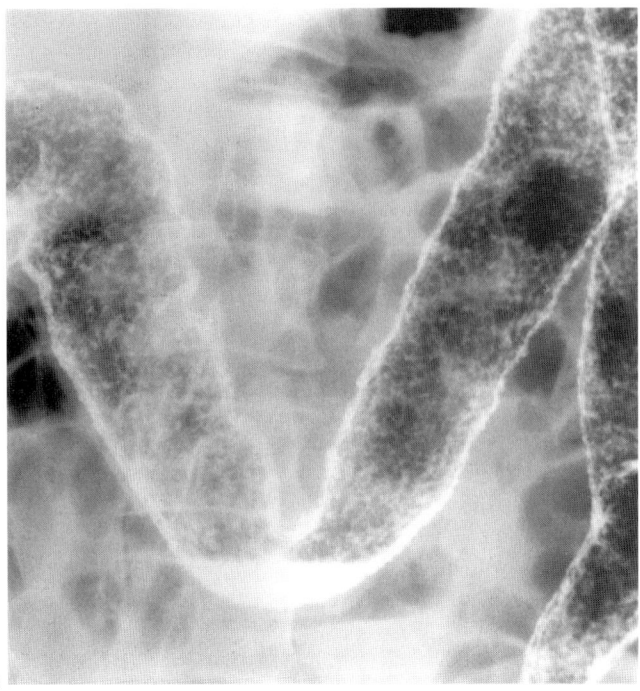

Fig. 25.8 *(Cont'd)* **c** More severe ulceration, as shown by a coarse uneven mucosal surface both 'en face' and tangentially. The haustral pattern is lost. Note how in all affected areas the ulceration is continuous and symmetrical.

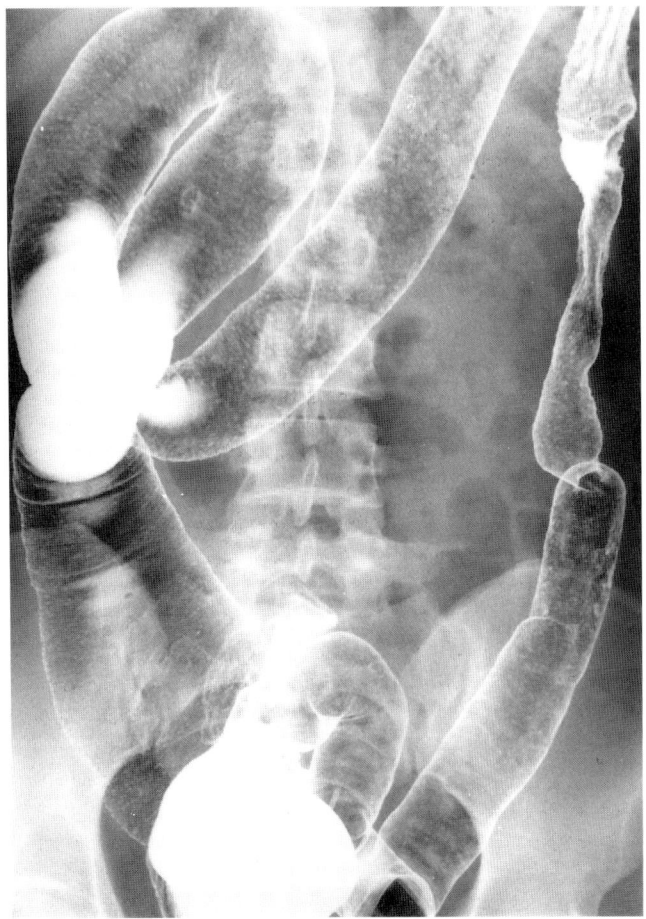

Fig. 25.9 Complete involvement of the colon with ulcerative colitis: demonstration of continual, symmetrical ulceration and loss of haustration. The cecum and ascending colon show a lesser degree of ulceration than the transverse colon. The sigmoid is virtually normal, having been treated with topical steroid enemas.

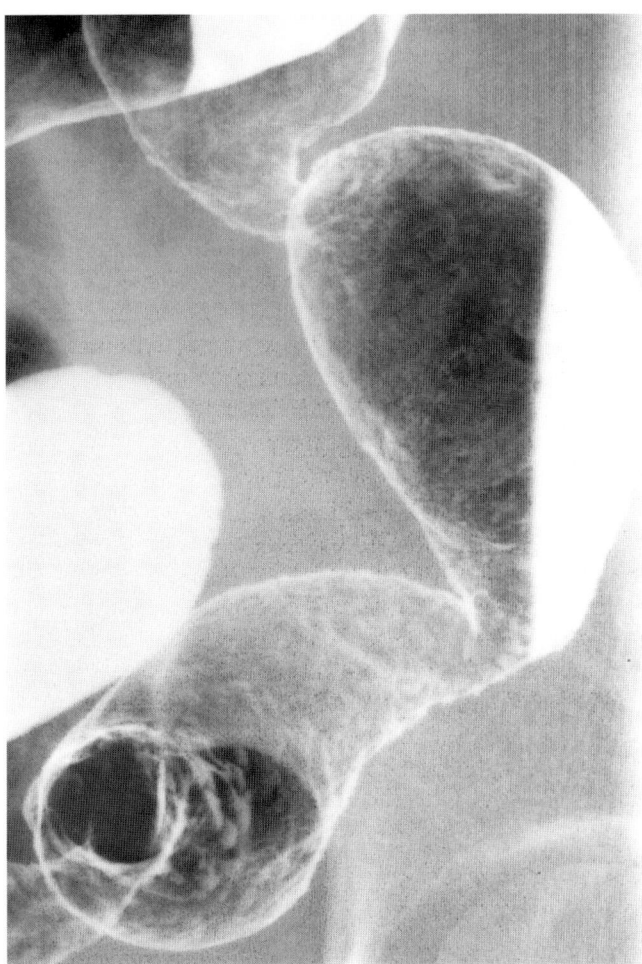

Fig. 25.10 Short tapering strictures in chronic ulcerative colitis.

Fistulae

Fistulae are not a common feature of ulcerative colitis, although simple perianal fistulae may occasionally occur.

Polyps

Irregular severity of mucosal ulceration can lead to relative elevation of islands of inflamed mucosa, causing an uneven polypoid appearance. These are pseudopolyps (Fig. 25.11), and lead to a coarsely nodular appearance of the mucosa both 'en face' and in profile. Occasionally, localized areas of inflamed mucosa may be hypertrophic and appear as a granular sessile protuberance surrounded by granular mucosa. These are sometimes separately categorized as inflammatory polyps (Fig. 25.12). More commonly, in patients with quiescent disease multiple small, usually filiform excrescences are seen against a smooth mucosal background. These are post inflammatory pseudopolyps (Fig. 25.13), and represent previously severe ulceration which has healed. This latter appearance may be seen in all forms of inflammatory bowel disease, including Crohn's disease, and is not specific for ulcerative colitis (Zegal & Laufer 1978). All these polyps are benign and do not herald malignant change. Multiple frondlike postinflammatory polyps do not usually cause any problems in diagnosis. Inflammatory polyps, when surrounded with a smooth mucosa, may cause confusion with neoplastic change and should be biopsied.

Neoplasia

The risk of colon cancer is increased approximately 11-fold in patients with long-standing extensive colitis (Fig. 25.14). (Lennard-Jones et al 1990, Sugita et al 1991). Tumors may be annular or polypoidal in appearance, and may occur anywhere in the colon. Studies have differingly reported an excess cancer rate in either the cecum or the distal colon (Gyde et al 1988) Epithelial dysplasia is common, but unfortunately is not readily distinguishable radiographically, even with good-quality DCBE. However, Frank et al (1978) and Hooyman et al (1987) have reported radiological features of dysplasia.

Terminal ileum

In most patients with ulcerative colitis the terminal ileum is normal, but in some patients who have a total colitis, usually of long-standing low-grade severity, the distal ileum may be dilated, with a granular appearance. There is no focal ulceration. The ileocecal valve is patulous and allows free retrograde reflux (Fig. 25.15). This appearance is termed 'backwash ileitis'.

PLAIN FILM EXAMINATIONS

An important feature of inflammatory bowel disease is that the inflamed bowel segment does not usually contain feces. As ulcerative colitis is a continuous disease, commencing distally, a plain abdominal film will usually show little air and no feces in the affected segment, and the extent of the disease can often be gauged by noting where feces are present in the colon. In acute severe disease fecal stasis may be prominent proximal to the diseased area, and this in itself may cause clinical symptoms. If there is sufficient gas in the bowel the edematous mucosa will be shown with an abnormal contour and loss of haustral pattern, and in severe inflammation swollen mucosa will show a nodular pattern. This becomes extreme in patients with fulminating disease, where the colon often becomes dilated and markedly nodular, caused by islands of edematous mucosa surrounded by severe deep ulceration (Fig. 25.16b). This appearance is usually termed 'toxic megacolon' (Fazio 1980). In supine patients the bowel gas will be maximally situated in the transverse colon

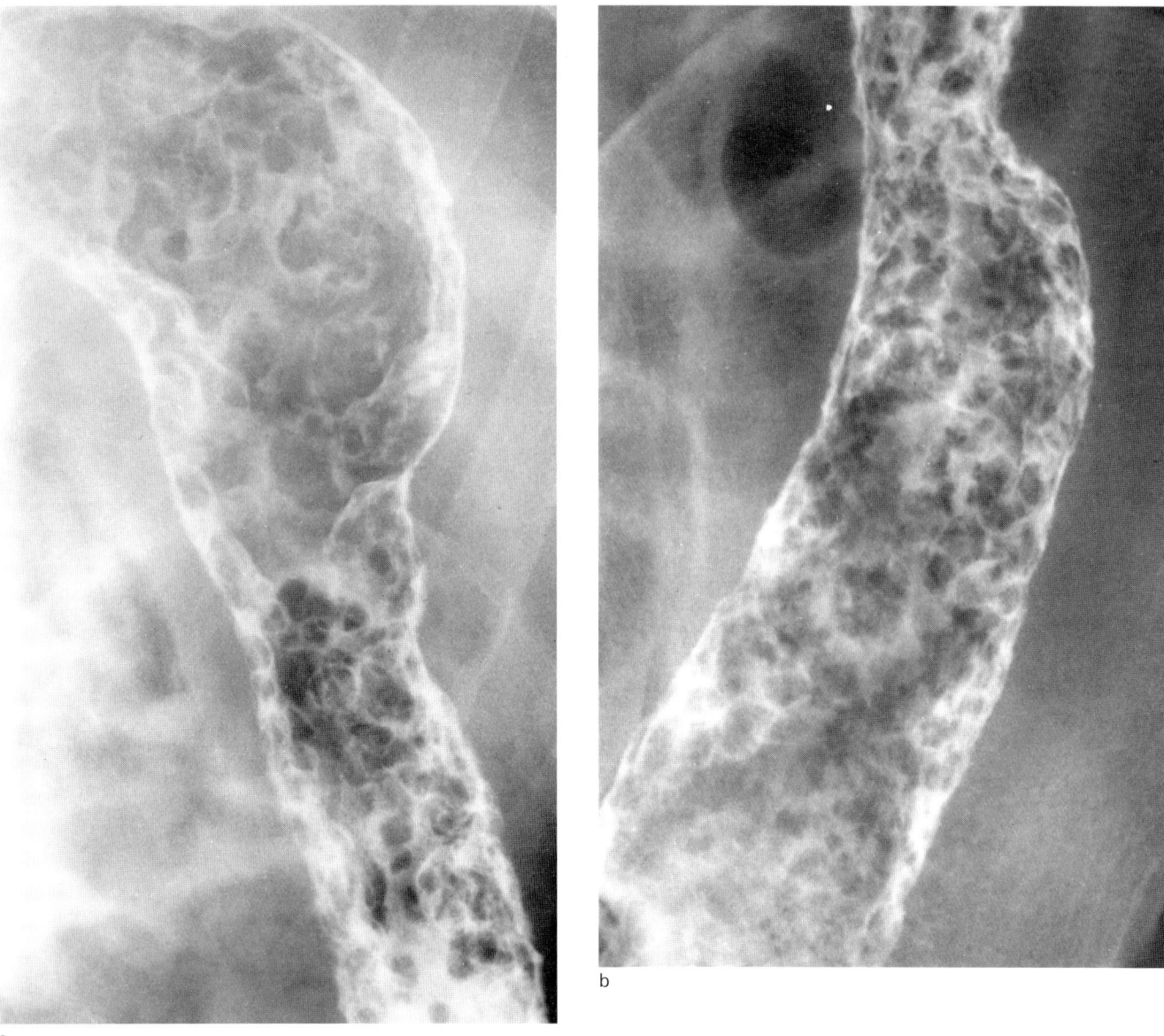

Fig. 25.11 Two examples **a** and **b**, showing severe ulcerative colitis with irregular mucosal islands – pseudopolyps.

(Fig. 25.16a). Observers often place stress upon the maximum width of the dilated colon, which should be less than 5 cm (Fazio 1980) or 6 cm (Halpert 1987). The important feature in the diagnosis of toxic megacolon is the presence of mucosal nodularity (Fig. 25.16a). Not all cases of toxic colon are dilated (Halpert 1987). In patients with acute disease, but not those with fulminating colitis, extra air can be inserted per rectum to give a better assessment of the inflamed bowel (Lindstrom & Noren 1992) (Fig. 25.1).

DIFFERENTIAL DIAGNOSIS

The main difficulty is in separating ulcerative from Crohn's colitis (see pp. 237–239). Other forms of colitis may occasionally cause problems. Patients taking long-term non-steroidal anti-inflammatory drugs may develop a continuous symmetrical colitis similar to ulcerative colitis, and may also develop web-like bowel strictures (Bjarnason et al 1993). Linear ulceration is common in Crohn's colitis, but may also occasionally be seen in ulcerative colitis (Suekane et al 1990).

Crohn's Disease

Crohn's disease affects all parts of the gastrointestinal tract, although the distal small bowel and the large bowel are most commonly involved. The inflammation is transmural and features include edema, ulceration and fibrosis of all layers of the bowel wall, and complications such as

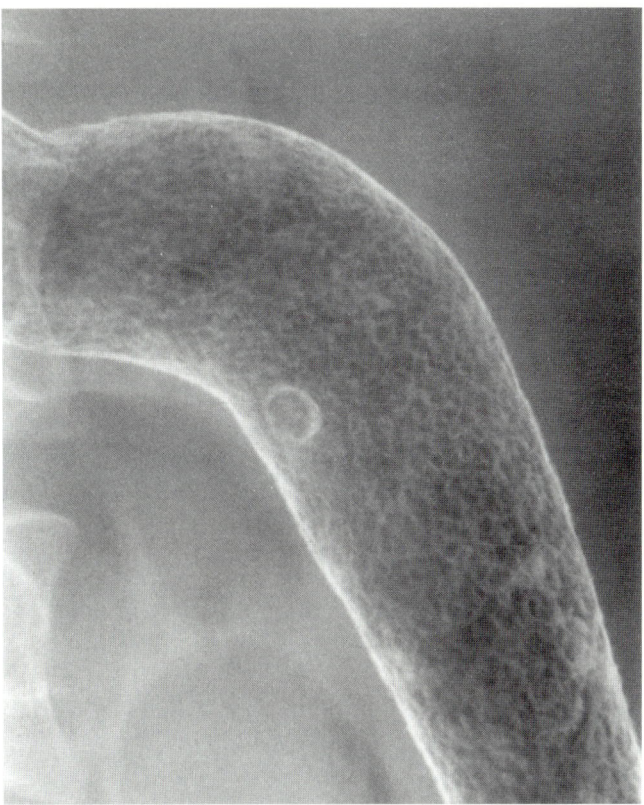

Fig. 25.12 An inflammatory polyp shown against a background of granular mucosa in long-standing ulcerative colitis.

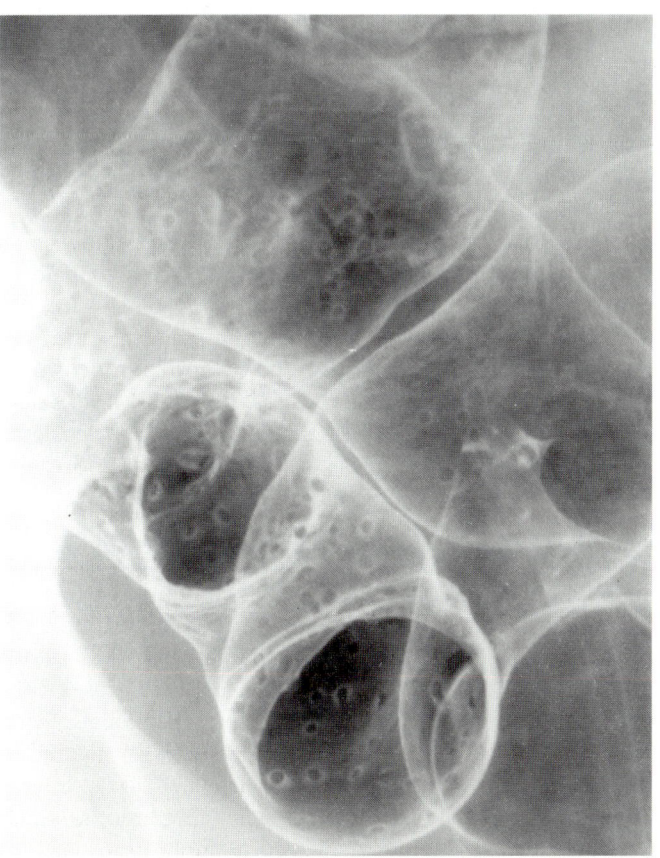

Fig. 25.13 Postinflammatory polyps. Small smooth filiform excrescences shown against a smooth colonic mucosa – long-standing but quiescent ulcerative colitis.

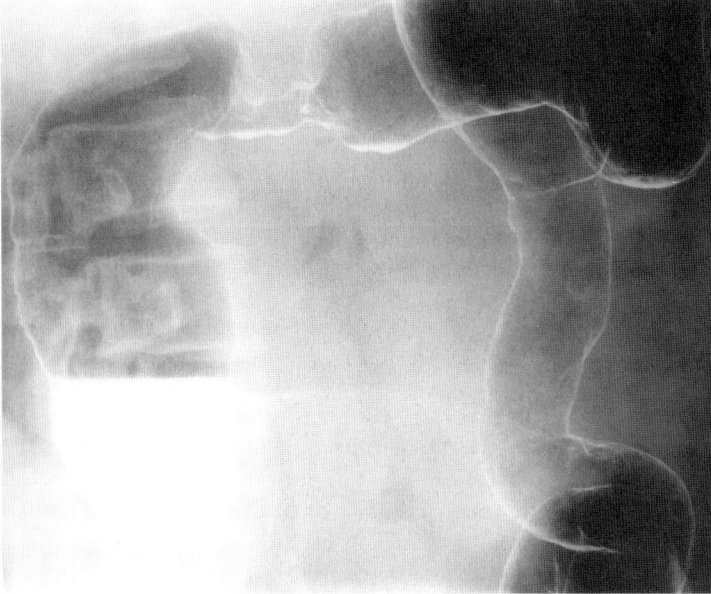

Fig. 25.14 An example of an annular carcinoma developing in a patient with long-standing quiescent inflammatory bowel disease.

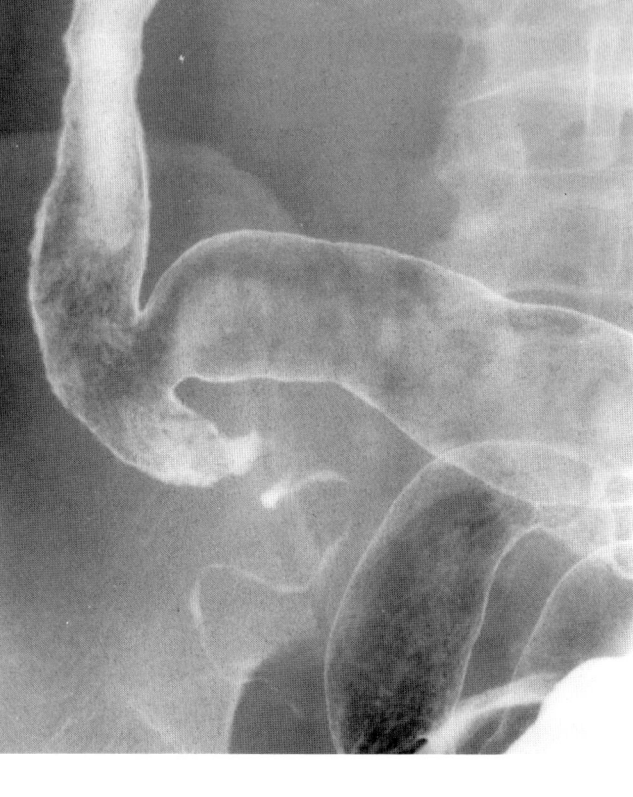

Fig. 25.15 'Backwash ileitis'. The whole colon is affected by long-standing ulcerative colitis. The ileocecal valve is patulous, allowing free reflux into the terminal ileum, which is dilated and featureless.

fistula. The radiological hallmark of Crohn's disease is its discontinuity: there are 'skip' areas of disease, with normal bowel intervening (Fig. 25.17). It is also asymmetrical, with one side of the bowel wall being affected to a different degree from the other.

Radiological features

Edema. Initially, mucosal edema is seen as alteration of the fine mucosal detail. More edema will cause the mucosa to be altered. In the stomach, thickening of folds usually occurs in the antrum. The valvulae conniventes of the small intestine may show varying patterns, including diffuse granularity (Glick & Teplick 1985), thickening, straightening, blunting and distortion. All these abnormal appearances may be present at the same time within the same area. Sometimes nodularity is due to a combination of linear and transverse ulceration, but it may also be due to localized areas of mucosal edema not associated with ulceration (Fig. 25.18). Edema of the deeper layers of the bowel wall may lead to an increase of the whole bowel thickness – 'hosepipe thickening' and is shown by separation of barium-filled bowel loops (Fig. 25.19). Fibrofatty invasion of the mesentery is another cause of separation of barium-filled bowel loops. This cause is not apparent on barium radiology, but is readily seen on CT scanning.

Ulceration. The earliest manifestation is the aphthous or aphthoid ulcer (Morson et al 1990). This is a shallow intramucosal lesion and is seen 'en face' as a small speck of retained barium surrounded by a translucent halo of mucosal edema (Fig. 25.20). Aphthous ulcers are too shallow to be seen in profile. In the initial stages they are seen as discrete lesions surrounded by normal mucosa. As the disease progresses larger ulcers of variable size, shape and depth occur (Figs. 25.21, 25.22). Ulcers may coalesce to form large denuded areas, often both linear and transverse, leading to a cobblestone appearance (Fig. 25.18). Deep penetrating ulcers often have a spike or a 'rosethorn' appearance (Fig. 25.23) which is characteristic, but not pathognomic, of Crohn's disease (Stanley et al 1971). Deep ulcers may undermine the mucosa, leading to a 'collar-stud' lesion (Fig. 25.24) (Lichtenstein et al 1979). These may be discrete or multiple, appearing as a continuous track in the submucosal layers. This is also seen in ulcerative colitis. The progressive stages of ulceration are often seen within the same localized area. Severe ulceration is usually surrounded by smaller lesions, which gradually merge into normal mucosa.

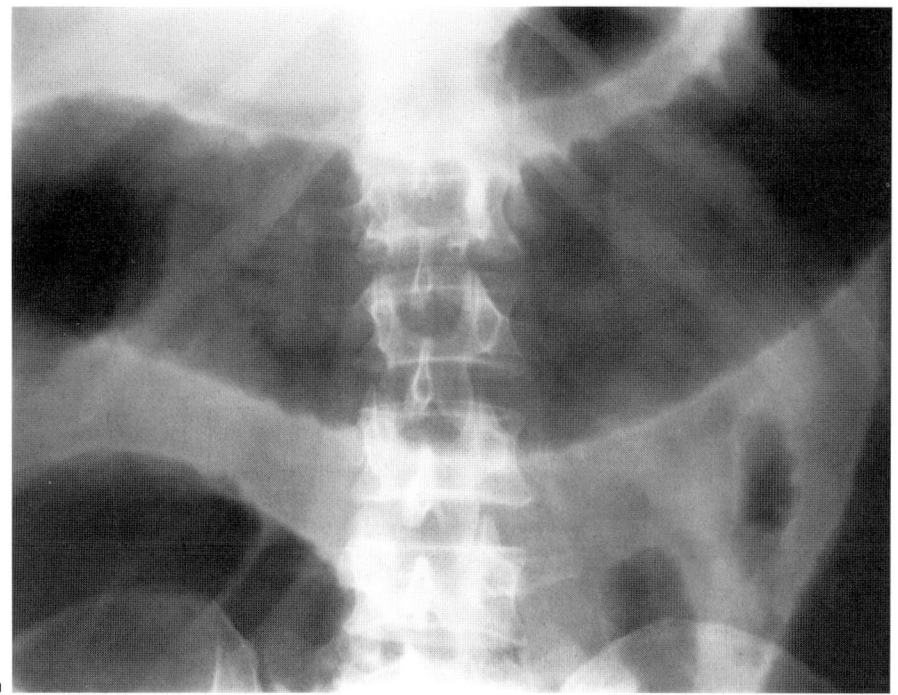

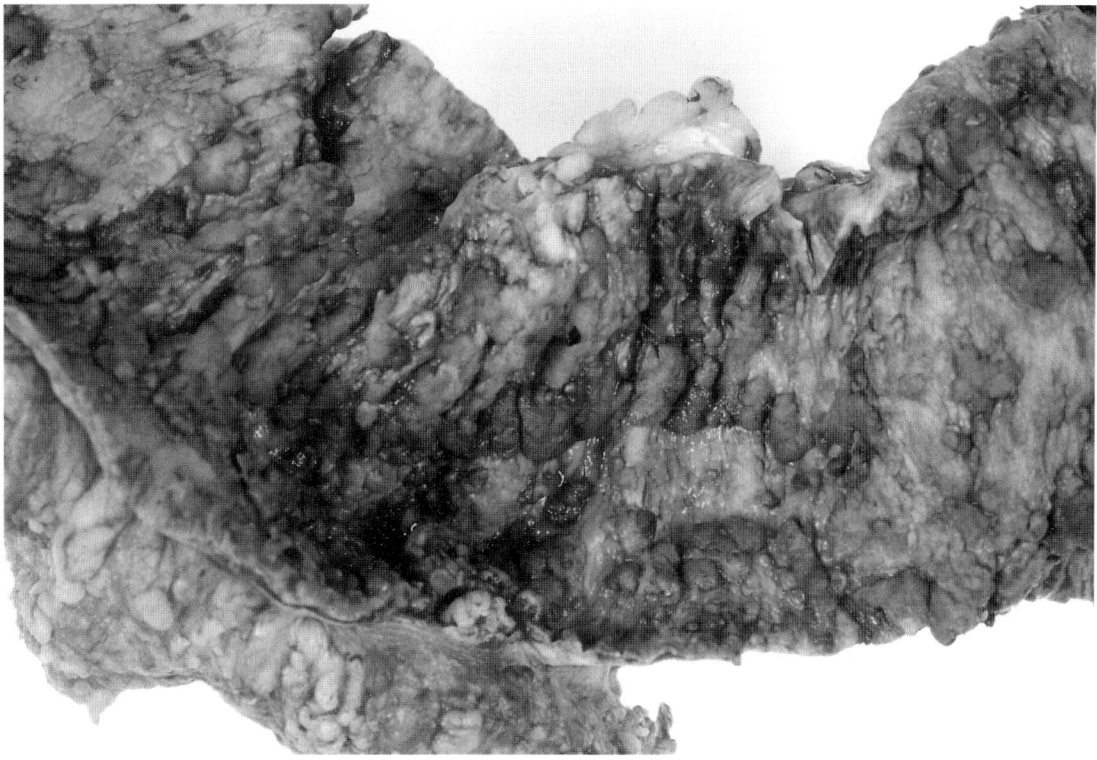

Fig. 25.16 Toxic (mega) colon. **a** Plain abdominal radiograph showing a dilated gas-filled colon. The essential feature is that the outline of the colon is irregular, with mucosal islands projecting into the lumen. These can also be seen 'en face'. **b** Colonic specimen of toxic colon, showing deep confluent ulceration with isolated mucosal islands.

228 INFLAMMATORY BOWEL DISEASES

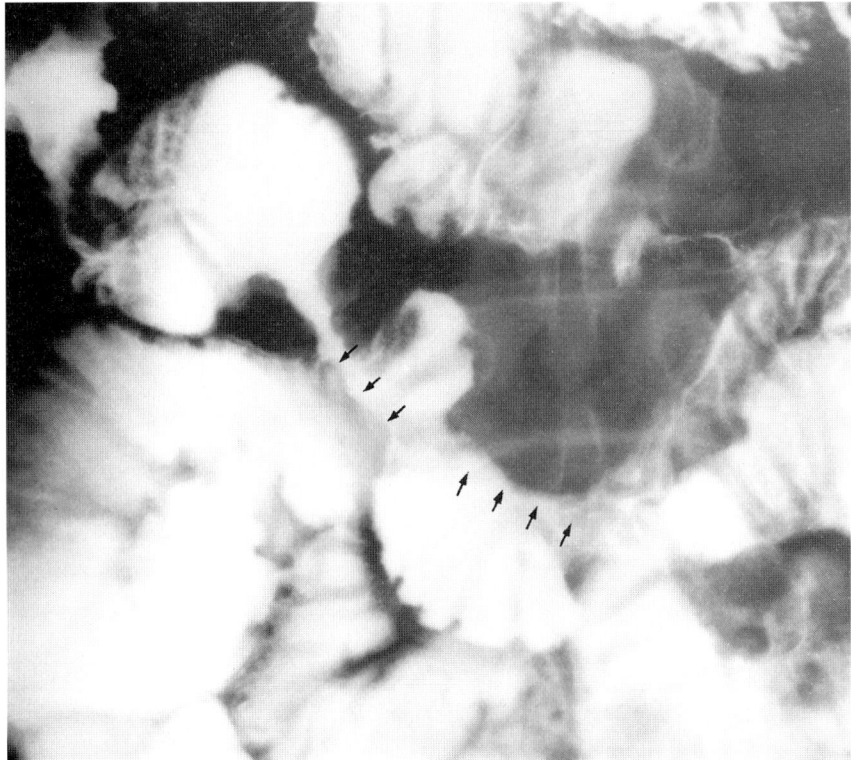

Fig. 25.17 Crohn's disease of the small bowel, showing several ulcerated segments with intervening normal small bowel. The ulceration is also asymmetrical, with apparent normal mucosa opposite ulcerated segments (arrows).

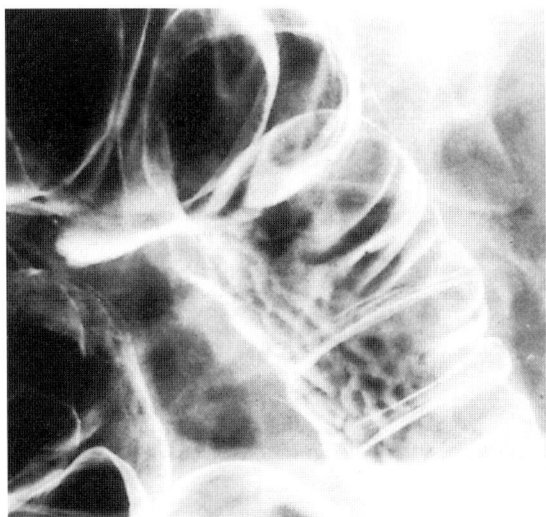

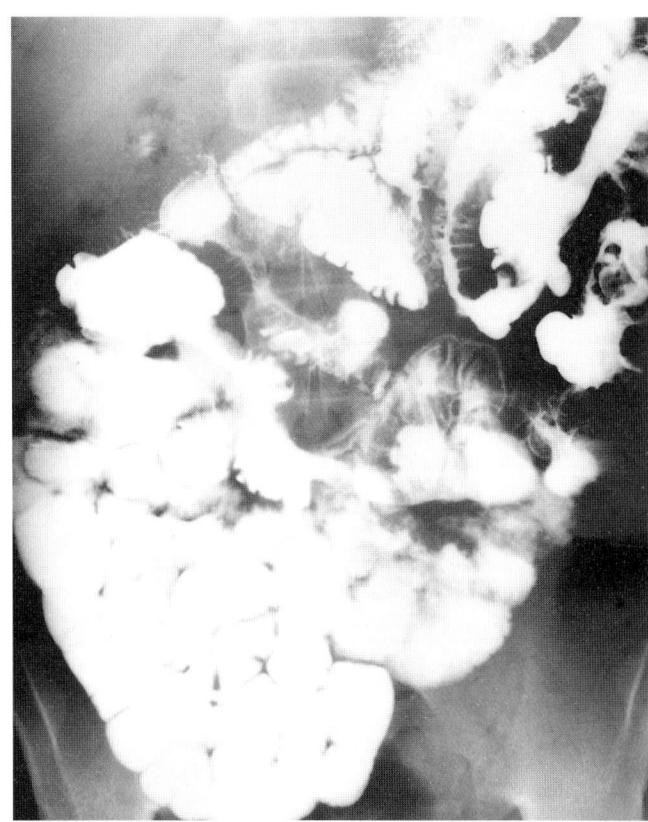

Fig. 25.18 'Cobblestone' mucosa seen on the mesenteric border of the colon on double contrast barium enema. Note the asymmetrical distribution with the opposite wall of the colon apparently normal.

Fig. 25.19 Barium follow-through showing severe Crohn's disease in the jejunum with a normal ileum. Note how the barium-filled loops are separated in the jejunum owing to marked bowel wall 'hosepipe' thickening, whereas in the ileum the bowel loops are closely adjacent.

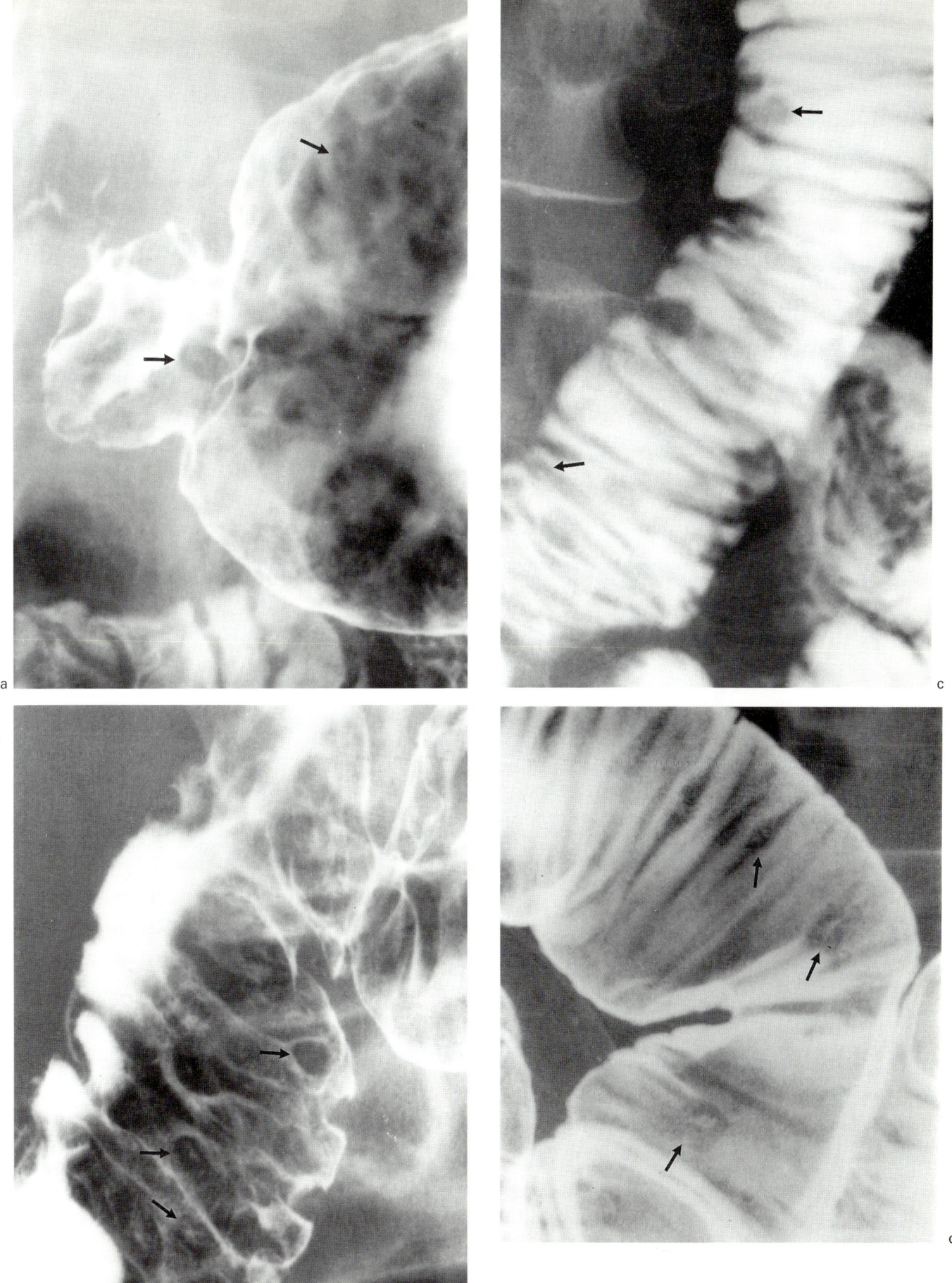

Fig. 25.20 Aphthous ulceration in **a** stomach antrum, **b** descending duodenum, **c** jejunum, **d** ileum.

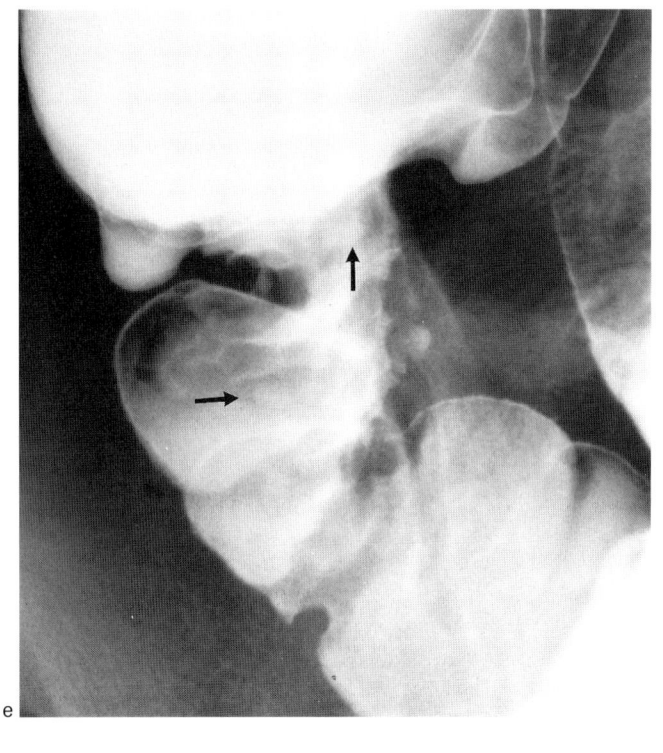

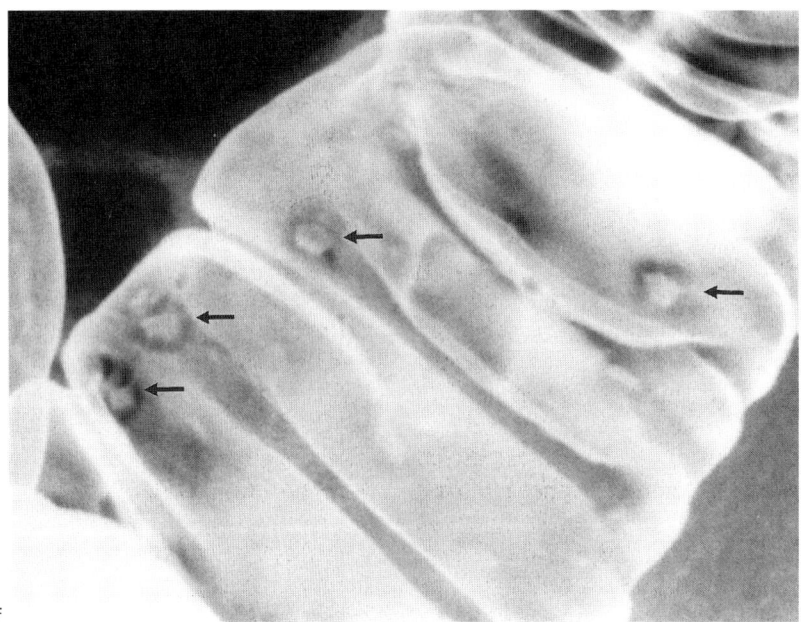

Fig. 25.20 (*Cont'd*) **e** neo-terminal ileum and **f** colon.

Fibrosis. As the disease heals, fibrosis leads to contraction. If fibrosis occurs circumferentially, narrowing and obstruction will result. Often, however, much of the apparent bowel narrowing is due to spasm rather than fibrosis (Fig. 25.25). The differentiation can be made by using smooth muscle relaxants. As much of the disease is asymmetric and involves predominantly the mesenteric border (Meyers 1976), shortening occurring in the long axis of the bowel leads to pseudosacculation. If the disease extends through the bowel wall and adjacent loops become adherent, fibrosis will cause angulation and kinking. It may be difficult to differentiate quiescent adherent fibrotic bowel from active disease segments, as the obstructed bowel may show secondary mucosal edema, but in practice the distinction is rarely in doubt (Bartram 1980).

RADIOLOGY – CONTRAST STUDIES   231

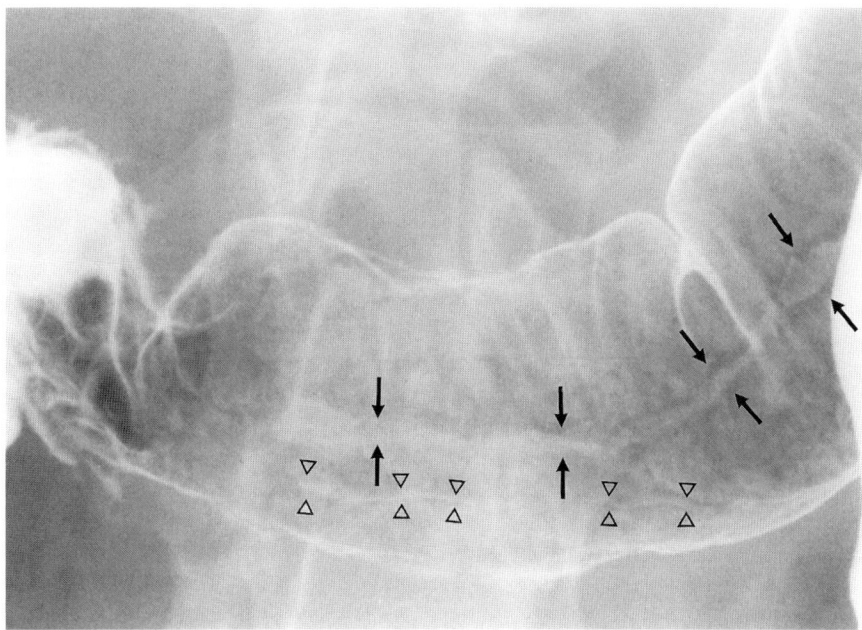

Fig. 25.21 Long linear ulceration in the colon (arrows), with a further, narrower, linear ulcer adjacent (arrowheads).

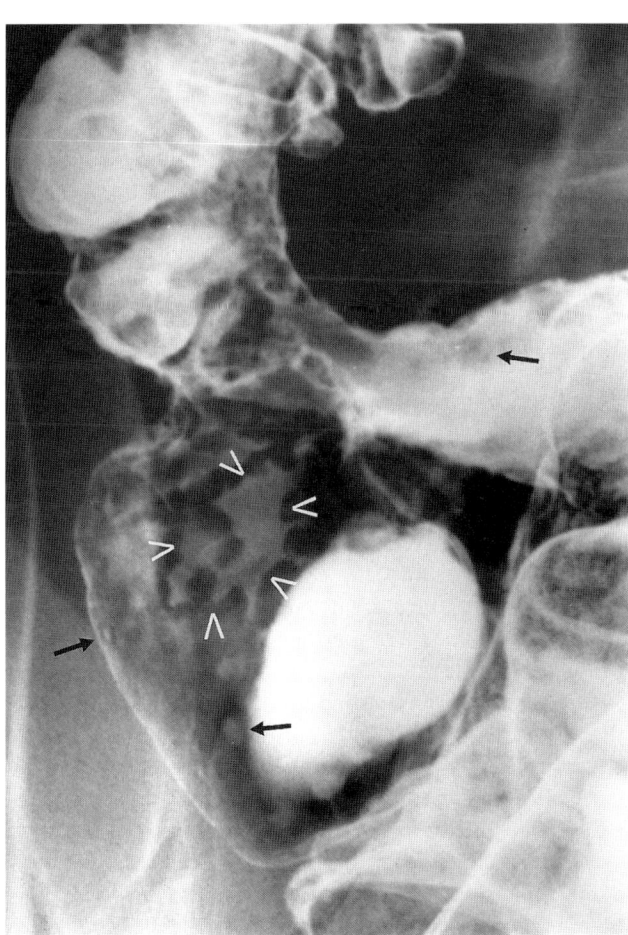

Fig. 25.22 Confluent irregular shallow ulcer in the cecum (open arrowheads), with smaller aphthous ulceration in cecum and terminal ileum (arrows).

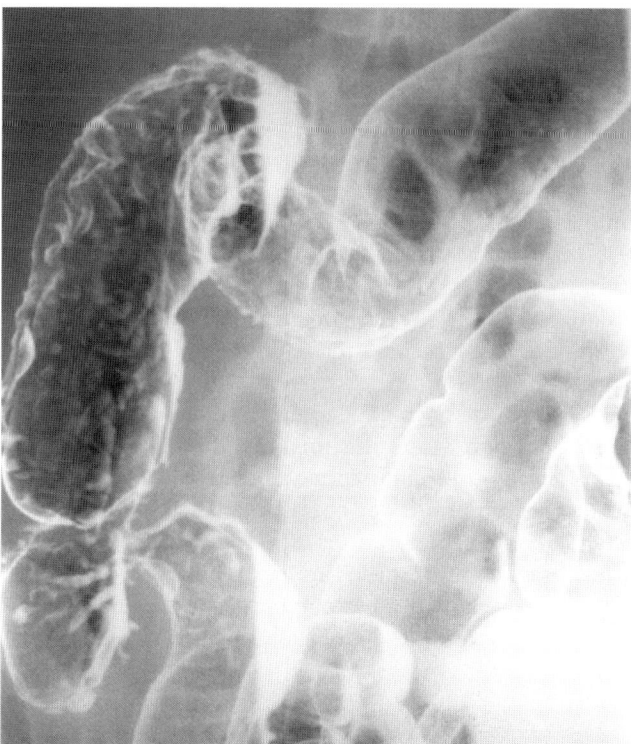

Fig. 25.23 Severe ulceration in the right colon and adjacent terminal ileum. There are penetrating ulcers/sinuses projecting out from the bowel margin.

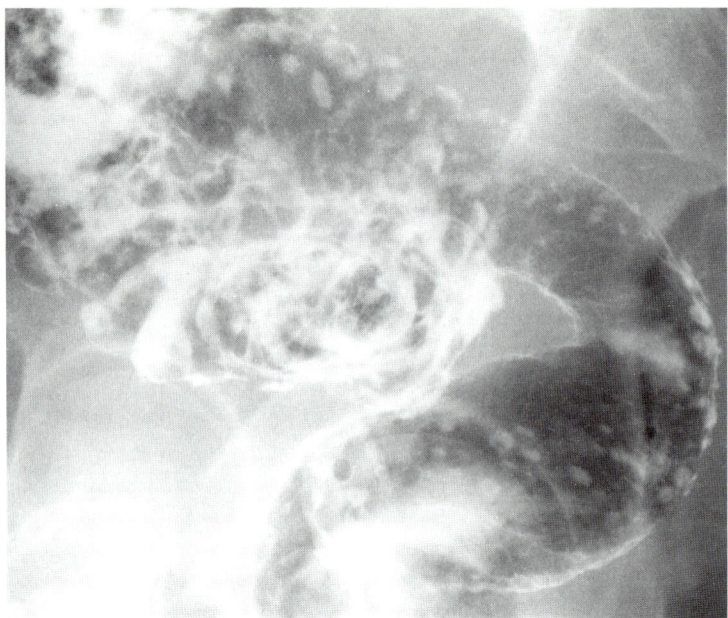

Fig. 25.24 Deep, punched-out 'collar-stud' ulceration in Crohn's disease of the rectum.

Fistulae. Fistulae result from the transmural ulcers penetrating into adjacent structures. Ulcers between adjacent small bowel loops result in enteroenteric fistulae, whereas involvement of the parietal peritoneum lead to enterocutaneous fistulae. Less commonly, fistulae occur between the bowel and the bladder or vagina. The majority of enteroenteric fistulae are short and occur within a few centimeters of the ileocecal valve (Fig. 25.26). As the amount of short circuit is small, many are not apparent clinically. Enterocolic fistulae may lead to a significant short circuit, as between ileum and sigmoid loop, and cause sudden worsening of symptoms such as diarrhea. Some fistulae are simple single tracks but others are complex, resulting from abscesses perforating via numerous pathways (Fig. 25.27).

Sinuses are often seen, probably caused by the progression of deep penetrating ulcers (Fig. 25.28). Many are intra-abdominal in association with abscesses, especially around the terminal ileum. Another common site of sinus formation is in the anal region. These may be shown on barium examination, especially if the anal canal and lower rectum are not obscured by an over-distended rectal balloon catheter. It is now recognized that perirectal abscesses and sinuses are best demonstrated by CT or MRI scanning. In most patients with perianal inflammation the rectum is radiologically normal.

Radiological features at specific sites

Esophagus, stomach and duodenum. Crohn's disease of the esophagus is uncommon. The few reports of the radiological appearances in proven esophageal Crohn's disease describe ulceration, fibrosis, stricture, inflammatory polyps and, occasionally, fistulae (Dyer et al 1969, Cynn et al 1975, Cockey et al 1985, Tishler & Helman 1984). As it is difficult to obtain reliable mucosal detail in the lower esophagus radiologically, often owing to movement blurring from adjacent cardiac pulsation, endoscopic examination is more rewarding.

In the stomach and duodenum the disease usually affects both the gastric antrum and the duodenum continuously, although single contrast barium studies have shown a higher (2–7%) incidence of duodenal involvement (Nugent et al 1977, Ariyama et al 1980) than stomach at 1–4% (Fielding et al 1970). However, the use of double contrast barium studies has shown mucosal abnormalities in the stomach and duodenum in 20–40% of patients with Crohn's disease elsewhere in the intestinal tract (Stevenson 1978, Bartram & Laufer 1979). It is extremely rare for the esophagus, stomach and/or duodenum to be affected without other parts of the bowel also being involved. The earliest sign is aphthous ulceration, best seen in the stomach antrum (Fig. 25.20a), but less often in the descending duodenum (Fig. 25.20b). This may be associated with spasm and, later, with more fixed fibrosis and deformity (Fig. 25.29). This may become extreme, leading to a narrow antrum and obliteration of the duodenal bulb – the 'ramshorn' deformity – (Farman et al 1975). In long-standing cases the mucosa may become effaced and replaced with a mosaic appearance. Mucosal edema may occasionally be seen in the stomach in the form of discrete nodules along the line of rugal folds or around the cardia, without the presence of ulceration. Uncommonly, the distal duodenum may be affected by

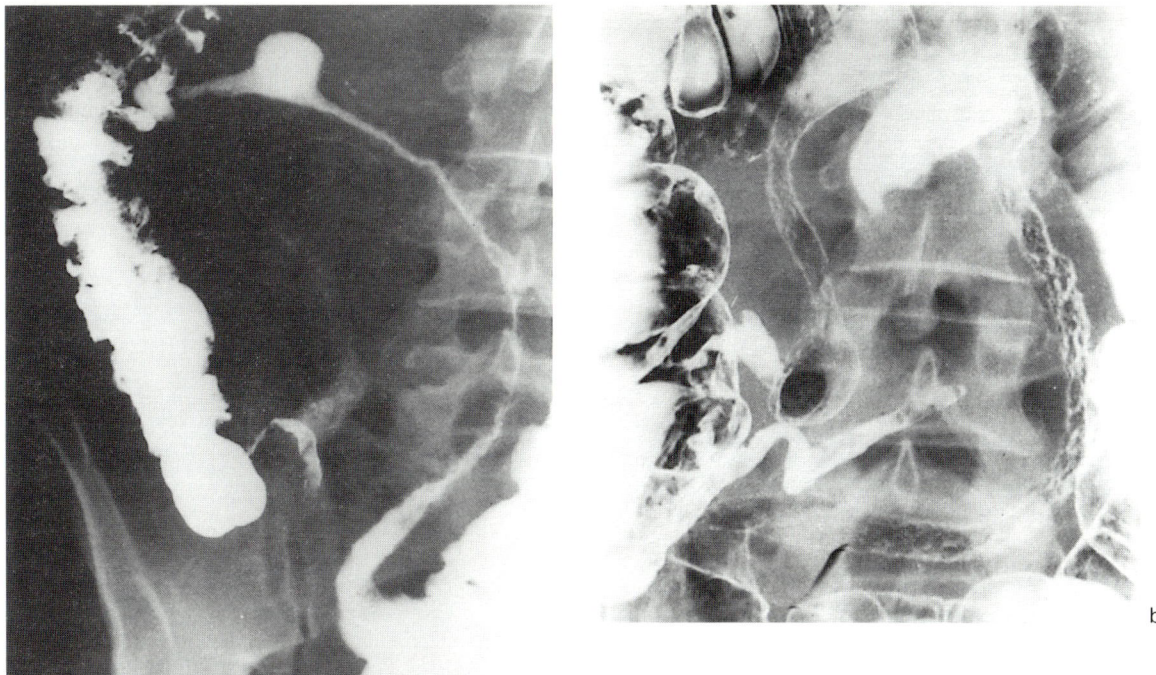

Fig. 25.25 **a**, Severe ulceration of the distal ileum with marked narrowing of the bowel. **b**, Insufflation of air per rectum causes some dilation of the ileum, showing that the narrowing is not entirely due to fibrosis. The mucosal ulceration is better shown in the air contrast film.

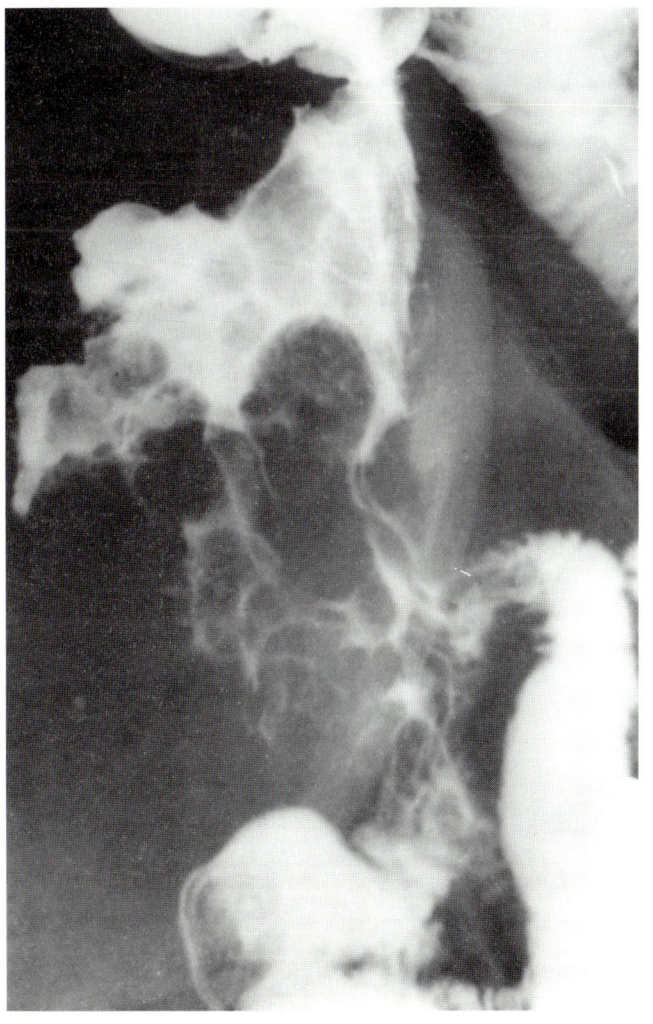

Fig. 25.26 Short internal fistulae between the cecum and terminal small bowel.

short lengths of ulceration and stricture formation without associated involvement of the antroduodenum. Fistulae involving the stomach and duodenum are rare, and are thought to be secondarily involved by concurrent disease in the adjacent small or large bowel (Jacobsen et al 1985).

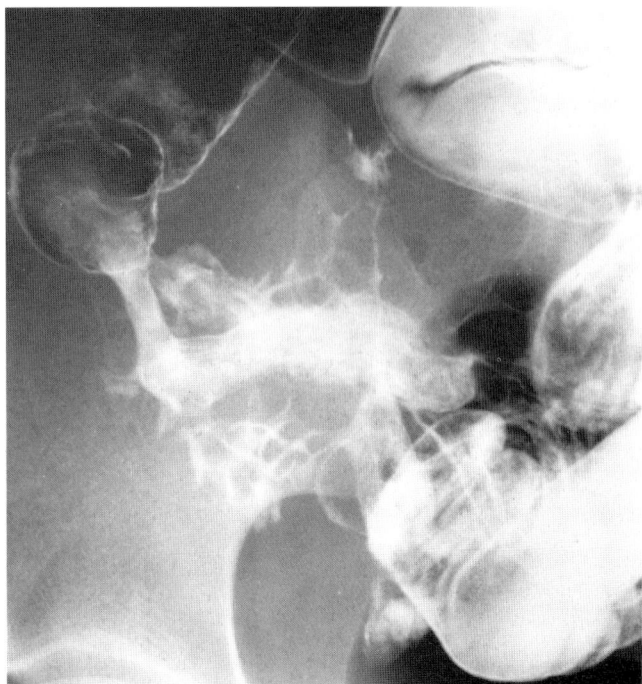

Fig. 25.27 More complex internal fistulation between cecum, terminal ileum and abscess cavity.

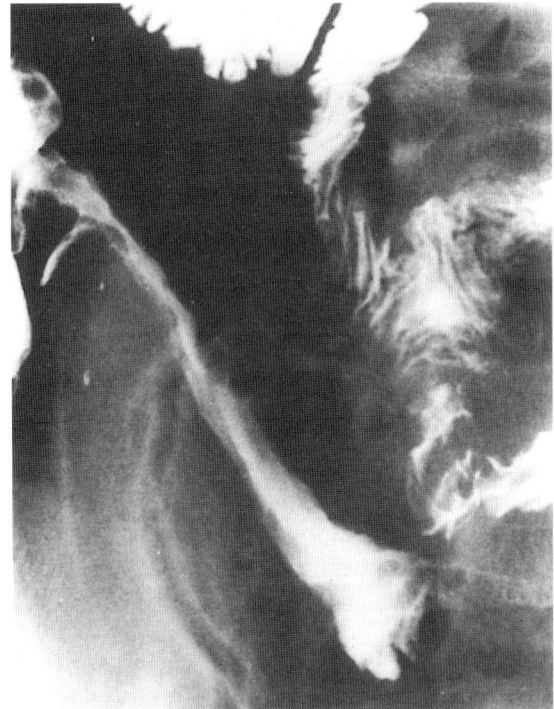

Fig. 25.28 Acutely inflammed terminal ileum with spasm and marked bowel thickening. A deep penetrating sinus is apparent within a centimeter of the ileo-caecal valve. This type of lesion is the likely precursor to the type of fistula seen in Fig. 25.26.

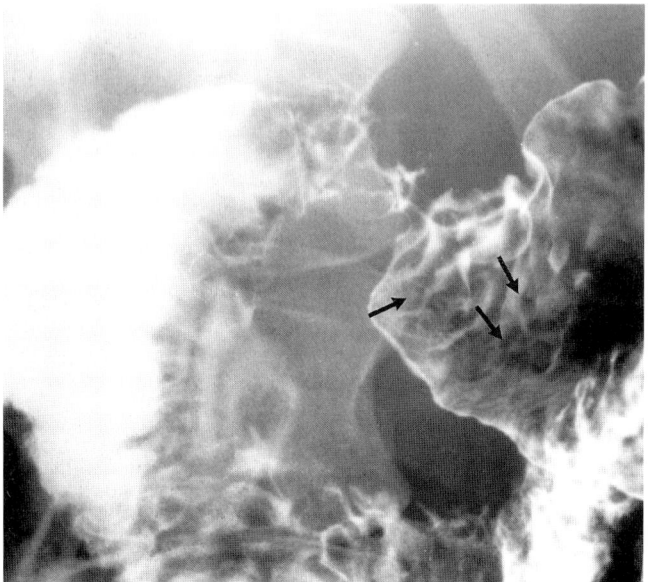

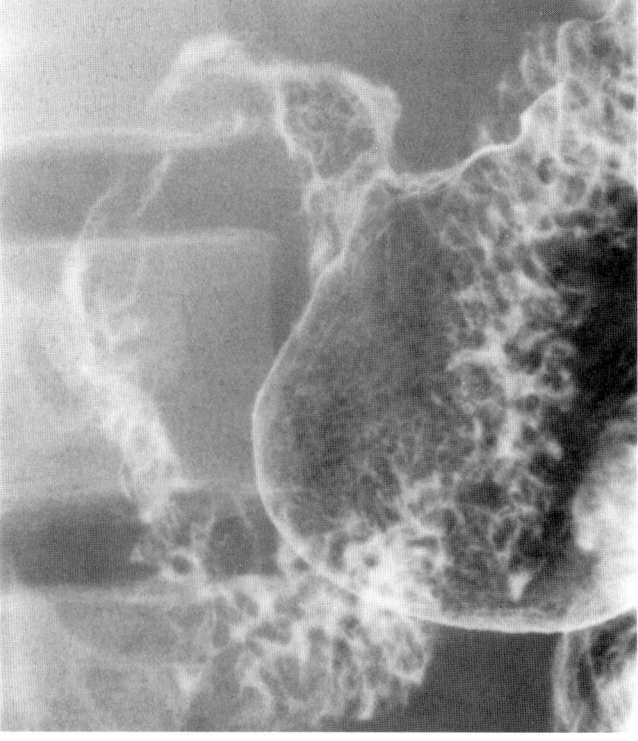

Fig. 25.29 Contiguous Crohn's disease of the stomach, antrum and duodenum. **a** The duodenum is still recognizable. There are aphthous ulcers in the antrum (arrows). **b** Severe antroduodenal narrowing with complete loss of duodenal bulb and descending duodenal mucosa.

Differential diagnosis

Erosive peptic ulcer disease, which commonly affects the lower esophagus, distal stomach and proximal duodenum, causes spasm, edema and aphthous and linear ulceration, and may be difficult or impossible to differentiate from Crohn's disease without histology. Unfortunately, deep diagnostic biopsies may be difficult to obtain with fiber optic endoscopes, and large surgical biopsies or resections are rarely performed. Postinflammatory polyps have been described in the esophagus and stomach in Crohn's disease (Cockey et al 1985). In more severe disease distinction from carcinoma, lymphoma, sarcoid and tuberculosis may be difficult (Farman et al 1975, Thompson et al 1975, Huchzermeyer et al 1976).

Small intestine

Terminal ileum. The terminal ileum is the part of the bowel most commonly affected by Crohn's disease. It is also the area most difficult to examine by double contrast radiography. This may be one of the reasons why the disease is often well advanced before being diagnosed. An early finding in Crohn's disease is irritability of the terminal ileum, with spasm and nodularity (Fig. 25.6). Thickening of the valvulae conniventes may appear sometimes, with the classic signs of aphthous ulceration. In the later stages ulceration may penetrate deeply into the submucosa. Edema of the bowel wall causes separation from adjacent loops. (Figs. 25.19, 25.30, 25.31). In the terminal ileum Crohn' disease often shows as a long, continuous symmetrical diseased segment, extending back from the ileocecal valve, sometimes for 30 cm or more (Fig. 25.30). The classic narrow, long terminal ileal segment – the 'string sign' – is more often due to spasm and edema of the acutely inflamed bowel than to a permanent fibrotic narrowing. Careful fluoroscopy, aided by antispasmodic drugs and air insufflation, will often demonstrate temporary relaxation of the narrowing (Fig. 25.25).

Involvement of the ileum is often continuous with the cecum and ascending colon (Figs 25.23 and 25.32) (Nelson et al 1973). Occasionally narrowing of the cecum is caused by extrinsic pressure on the medial wall by an edematous thickened terminal ileal loop (Berridge 1971). This is best demonstrated by a barium enema examination, and will be seen even if no reflux occurs into the terminal ileum.

Jejunoileum. In a few patients the terminal ileum is not involved when other parts of the small intestine show evidence of the disease. Disease in the proximal small intestine is usually either multiple or diffuse. In the first type there are scattered areas of disease showing the usual characteristics of discontinuous, asymmetric segments with nodular mucosa and ulceration, sometimes leading to isolated strictures, which may be short (Fig. 25.33). In diffuse jejunoileitis most of the small-intestinal mucosa shows generalized edema, thickening of the valvulae conniventes, nodularity and discrete superficial ulceration (Fig. 25.31). Diffuse disease can heal, giving a virtually normal appearance on subsequent barium examination, even when the whole small gut appears involved initially. Occasionally the diffuse form of the disease leads to enormous dilation of the bowel segments between

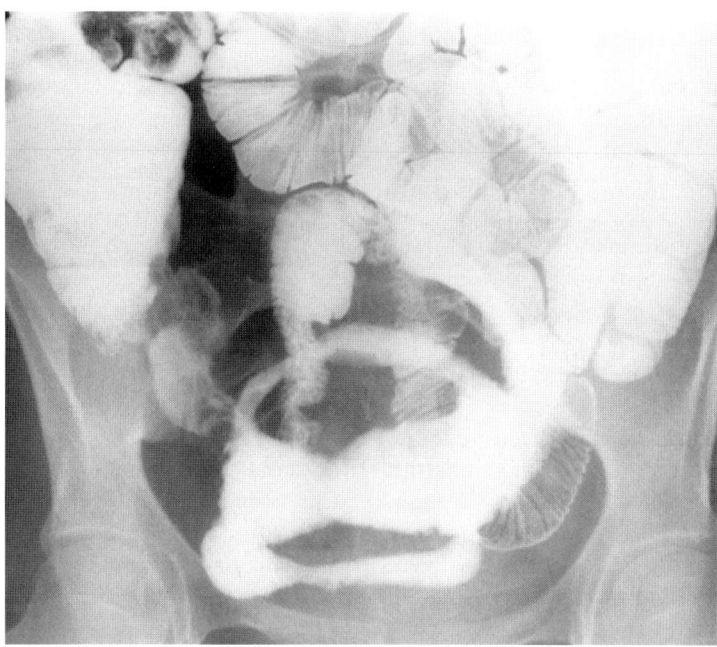

Fig. 25.30 Severe continuous ulceration of the distal ileum, with separation of the bowel lumina caused by marked 'hosepipe' thickening of the bowel wall.

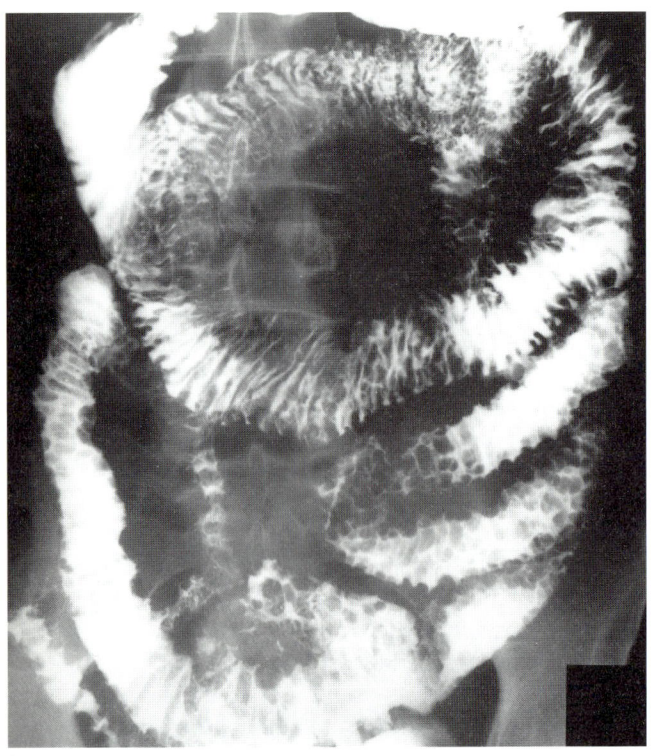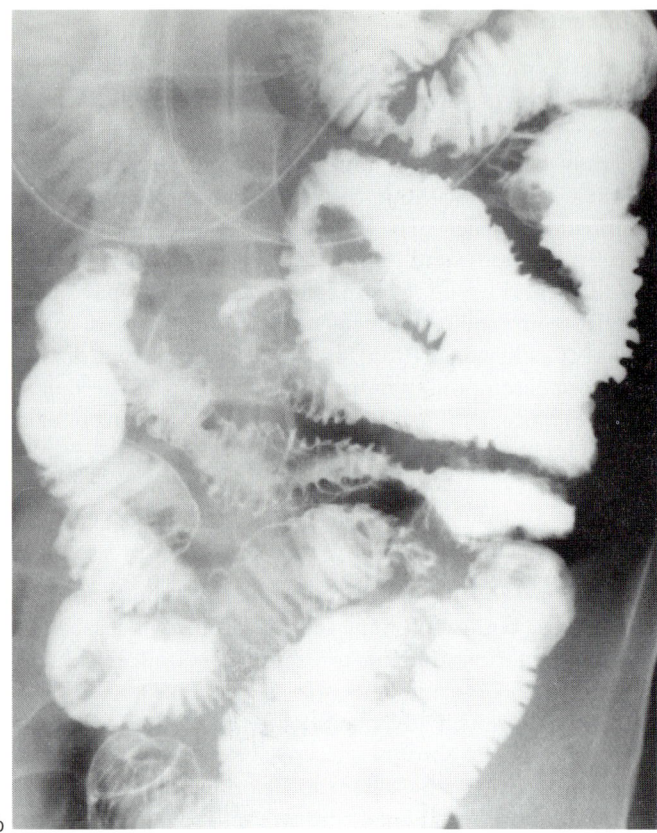

Fig. 25.31 **a** Diffuse mucosal thickening and nodularity with loop separation due to diffuse small bowel Crohn's disease. **b** Diffuse small-bowel disease with stricture formation.

strictures (Fig. 25.34). These patients are difficult to examine radiologically: the dilated loops retain secretions and food residues, which prevent adequate demonstration of the anatomy.

Fistulae in Crohn's disease are most commonly seen when the small bowel is affected. The most common fistulae are situated near to the ileocecal valve and occur between ileum and ileum, or ileum and cecum (Fig. 25.26). They may be single or multiple, and most are short. Another common fistula is between terminal ileum and an adherent sigmoid colon (Simpkins 1976). Enterovaginal and enterovesical fistulae are relatively uncommon, and are usually the sequel of a pelvic abscess.

Differential diagnosis

In the terminal ileum early disease with mucosal edema, nodularity and spasm can be simulated by infection with *Yersinia enterocolitica* (Ekberg et al 1977). It is a benign, short-lived disease and, unlike in Crohn's enteritis, the mucosal abnormality always reverts to a normal pattern. It never leads to stricture or fistula (Vantrappen et al 1977).

Tuberculosis is difficult to differentiate from terminal ileal Crohn's disease. Both often also affect the cecum and ascending colon. The two diseases are virtually impossible to separate radiologically, although there have been reports suggesting that longitudinal ulceration is an important finding in Crohn's disease, which differentiates it from intestinal tuberculosis (Tsukasa et al 1978).

Patients receiving long-term non-steroidal anti-inflammatory drugs may develop ulceration and strictures in the terminal ileum which are radiologically indistinguishable from Crohn's disease (Bjarnason et al 1987).

Gross nodularity, ulceration and strictures may occur in lymphoma, which may also be difficult to differentiate from Crohn's disease. Cross-sectional imaging may, however, be helpful in detecting extraluminal and lymphnodal masses. Imaging techniques may also be useful in diagnosing primary carcinoma or neoplastic change in long-standing or bypassed Crohn's segments. Carcinoid tumors of the ileocecal area have a propensity for fibrosis and may cause nodularity, distortion and tethering of the terminal small bowel, and may simulate Crohn's disease in which the bowel loops have become adherent and fibrotic around an abscess (Chang et al 1978). Ischemia will produce mucosal thickening, but this usually assumes a gross appearance, described as 'picket fence', which can normally be differentiated from Crohn's disease.

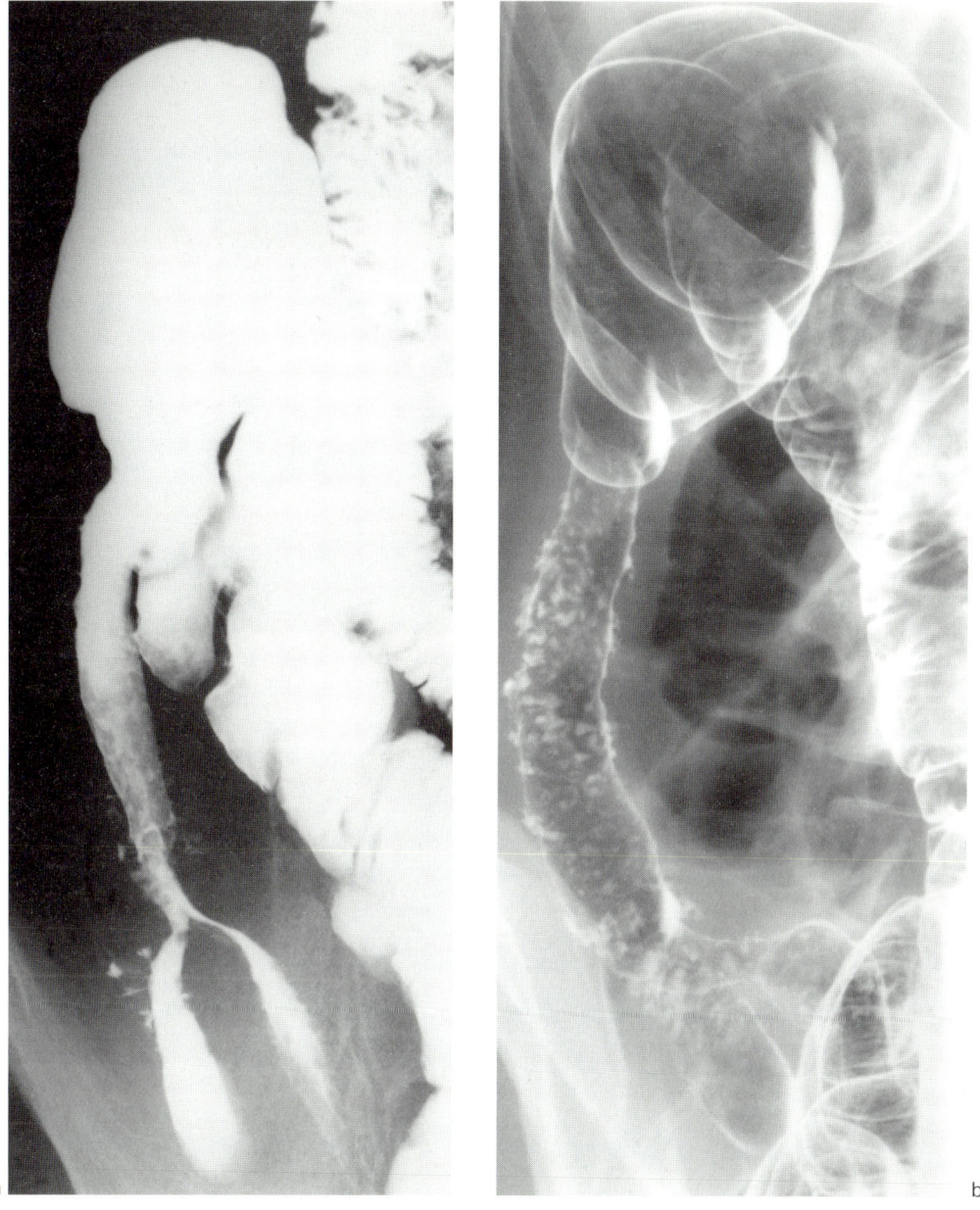

Fig. 25.32 Severe ileocolonic Crohn's disease. **a** In a barium follow-through examination the bowel appears to be extremely narrow, but a DCBE later **b** shows that the narrowing is in part due to spasm.

Large bowel. The incidence of Crohn's colitis appears to be increasing, possibly owing to improved diagnostic methods of endoscopy and double contrast barium radiography, which allow better visualization of the mucosal anatomy than do the earlier methods of single contrast barium enema. These methods show earlier and smaller mucosal abnormalities, such as shallow aphthous ulceration (Figs 25.20f, 25.22), and allow a definitive diagnosis of Crohn's colitis, which can be differentiated from specific and ulcerative colitis, which characteristically has a diffuse granular appearance. Patients previously thought to have ulcerative colitis, including some who were so labeled for many years, are now classified as having Crohn's disease. In our experience, patients in whom the initial radiological diagnosis was in some doubt, or was classified as 'intermediate colitis', usually have Crohn's disease.

Classically, colonic Crohn's disease affects the proximal colon, usually with associated disease in the terminal ileum (Nelson et al 1973) (Figs 25.23, 25.32). The disease is patchy and the rectum is often spared, in contrast to ulcerative colitis, in which the rectum is almost invariably involved (Morson et al 1990). However, some report that about 50% of patients with Crohn's colitis have rectal disease (Simpkins 1976, Margulis et al 1971) (Fig. 25.35). There are reports of patients with continuous total Crohn's

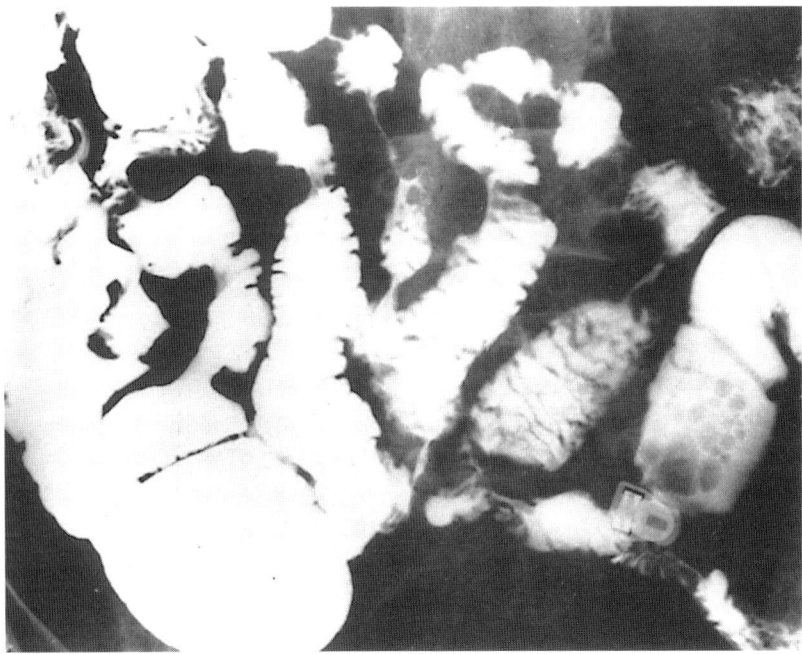

Fig. 25.33 Multiple short stricture in the small bowel. Some are typically asymmetrical but others are symmetrical. Between the strictures the mucosa is normal.

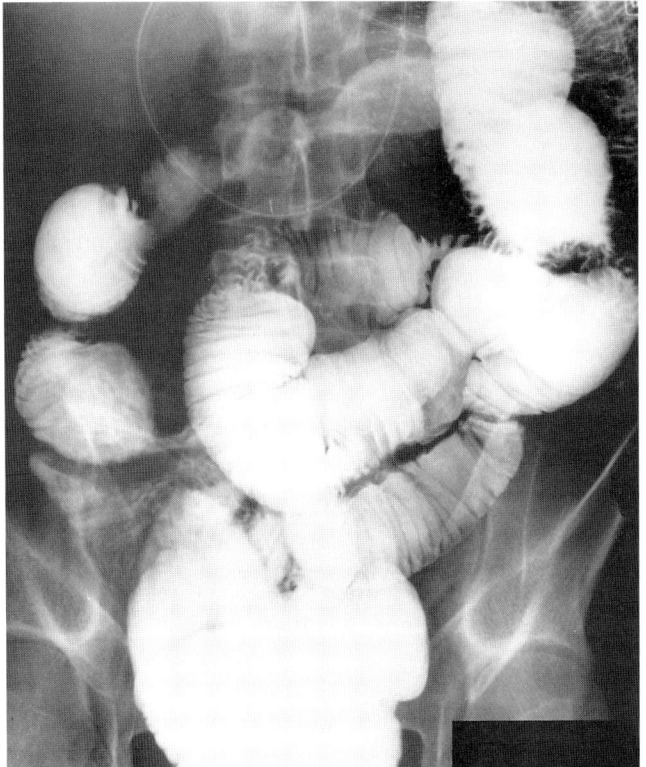

Fig. 25.34 Small-bowel enema showing dilated segment of small bowel and strictures. The strictures will often be shown more clearly with careful palpation and compression with fluoroscopy (see also Fig. 25.4).

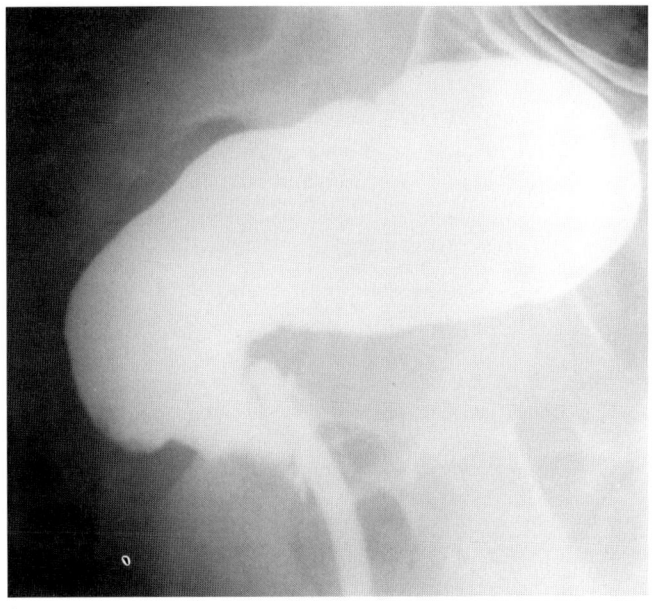 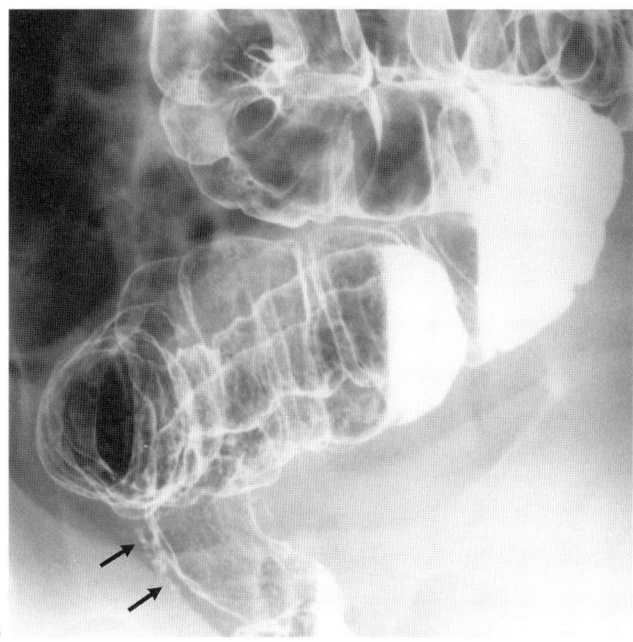

Fig. 25.35 Rectal Crohn's disease. **a** Irregular narrowing of distal rectum and **b** more extensive ulceration of rectum and sigmoid. There is a penetrating sinus (arrows).

colitis that is difficult to differentiate from the classic appearance of ulcerative colitis (Joffe 1981).

Radiological features

The earliest radiological changes are scattered discrete aphthous ulcers (Fig. 25.20). The areas of abnormality are usually discontinuous, surrounded by areas of normal mucosa, and are commonly on the mesenteric margin. As the disease progresses larger deeper ulcers form. The coalescence of transverse and linear ulceration leads to the classic 'cobblestone' configuration. In a remission aphthous ulceration may regress but rarely disappears completely (Ni & Goldberg 1986). Occasionally the ulceration remains shallow but enlarges in area, often causing curiously irregular (Fig. 25.22), sometimes linear (Fig. 25.21), completely isolated ulcers within normal mucosa. Areas of ulceration may gradually progress to normal mucosa (see Fig. 25.39), or the change may be acute, abrupt and clearly delineated (Fig. 25.36).

The appearance of the terminal ileum is said to be important in the differentiation between Crohn's colitis and ulcerative colitis. In Crohn's disease the ileum is either normal or narrowed and ulcerated by disease. The narrow ulcerated areas can be distinguished from the 'backwash ileitis' (Fig. 25.15) that can occur in total ulcerative colitis, in which strictures and frank ulceration are not seen. The terminal ileum is involved in about 50–70% of patients with Crohn's colitis, and there is usually contiguous disease of the cecum and ascending colon (Nelson et al 1973, Simpkins 1976) (Figs 25.23,

25.32). During remission the ulcerated mucosa may heal to produce postinflammatory polyps (Fig. 25.37). These are simply a sign of quiescence and occur with other types of inflammatory bowel disease (Zegal & Laufer 1978). Rarely, they may be large and proliferative (Bernstein et al 1978, Kelly et al 1986) and simulate localized neoplasia (Jones & Abbruzzese 1978). Rarely also, Crohn's colitis may progress to toxic megacolon, giving an appearance similar to that seen in ulcerative colitis. In later stages of the disease fibrosis causes shortening of the bowel (Fig. 25.38). In the long axis fibrosis will lead to pseudosacculation, especially when this occurs on the mesenteric border, whereas circumferential fibrosis will lead to a stricture, which may be difficult to differentiate from a neoplastic narrowing. Strictures are seen in about a quarter of examinations on patients with Crohn's colitis (Fig. 25.39), and half of these tend to be multiple (Simpkins & Young 1971). Colonoscopy may be necessary to exclude malignancy.

Fistulae from the colon are not common. Most are associated with involvement of the adjacent inflamed terminal ileum, but occasionally direct communication is seen between the vaginal vault and the rectum or sigmoid colon. Duodenal–colic fistulae are rare (Laufer et al 1977) and are due to colonic disease (Jacobsen et al 1985).

Differential diagnosis of Crohn's disease of the large bowel

The differential diagnosis from ulcerative colitis has already been discussed. Colonic tuberculosis can appear

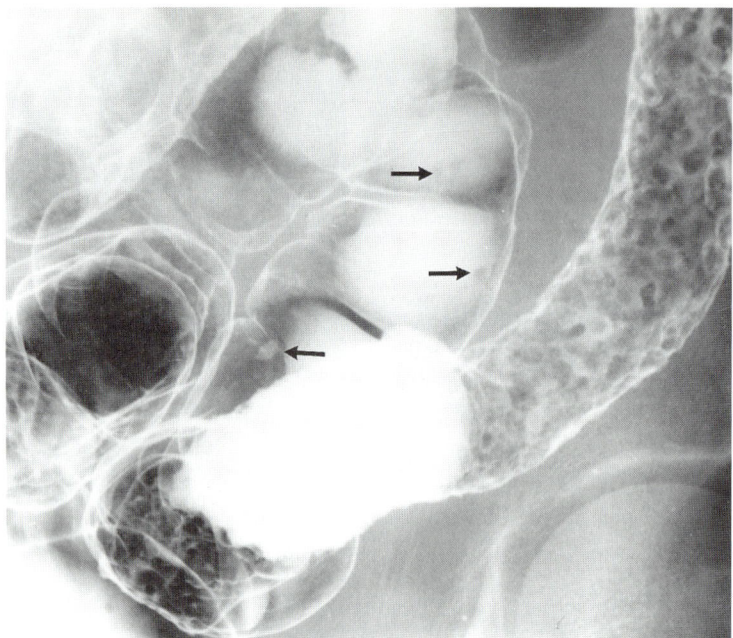

Fig. 25.36 Continuous symmetrical involvement of the descending colon with Crohn's disease having a marked resemblance to ulcerative colitis (see also Fig. 25.11). Note, however, the relative normality of the sigmoid colon, with scattered aphthous ulceration (arrows), which makes the differentiation easy.

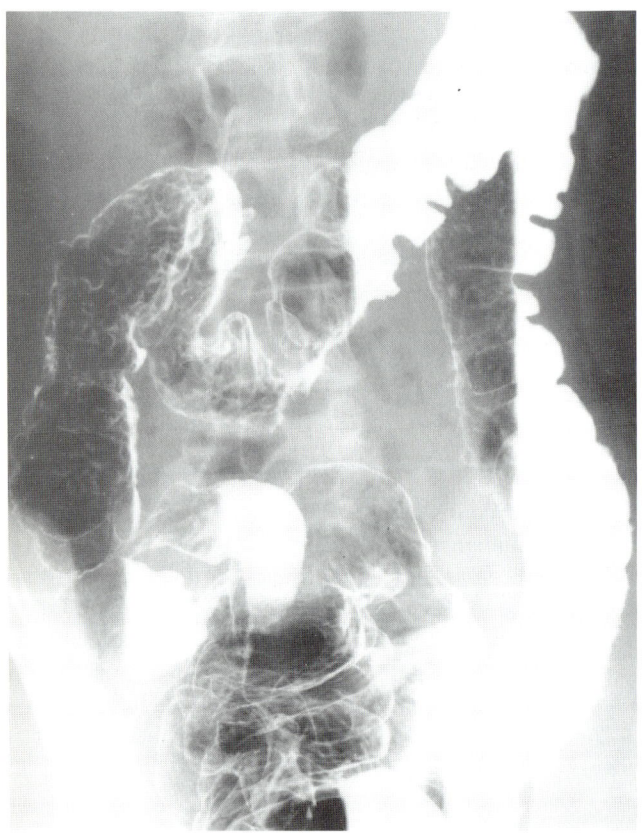

Fig. 25.37 Almost complete involvement of the large bowel by Crohn's disease. Around the hepatic flexure there are postinflammatory polyps. In the descending colon both aphthous and deep ulceration is present.

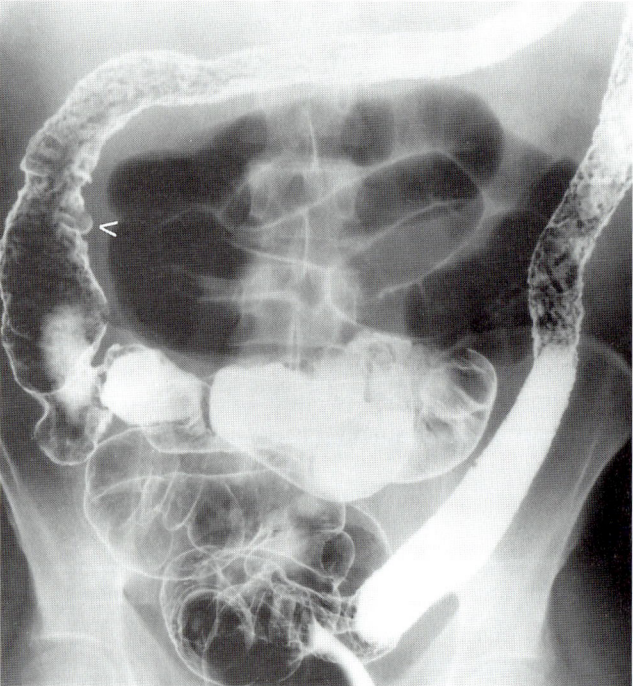

Fig. 25.38 Marked shortening of the large bowel caused by long-standing Crohn's disease. Appearances are similar to those seen in chronic ulcerative colitis, but the small area of normal mucosa in the ascending colon (arrowhead) and relative normality of the sigmoid confirm that this is Crohn's disease.

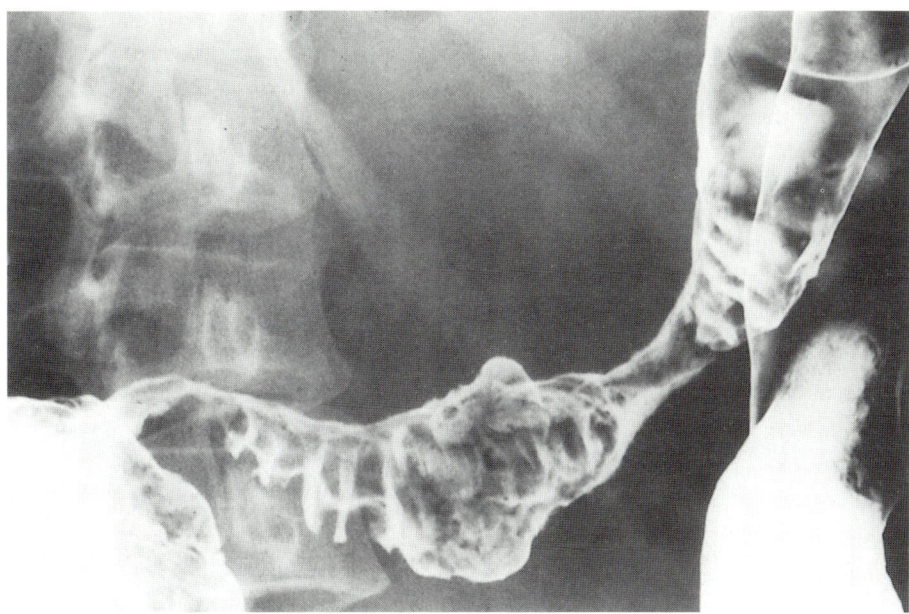

Fig. 25.39 Double contrast barium enema examination showing a long asymmetrical stricture with tapering margins in the transverse colon. On the distal side of the stricture near the splenic flexure are aphthous ulcers.

identical to Crohn's colitis (Healy et al 1992) (Fig. 25.40). In patients from western European countries both conditions are prone to affect the terminal ileum and ascending colon, but isolated segments of tuberculosis may occur in the colon (Balthazar & Bryk 1980). Filiform polyposis may occur in both (Peh 1988). The diagnosis of tuberculosis is not usually made until the colon has been examined histologically.

The strictures of Crohn's disease may be confused with neoplasia and ischemia. Neoplastic strictures are usually single and have a shouldered margin with an abrupt transition (Simpkins & Young 1971). However, sometimes they mimic tapered benign inflammatory strictures. Ischemic disease of the colon usually occurs in the elderly and is predominantly left-sided. Crohn's colitis may easily be confused with ischemic colitis (British Medical Journal 1973) as both can present with areas of mucosal edema, thumbprinting and ulceration (Iida et al 1986, Reeders & Tygat 1987), which is often linear and occasionally aphthous and sharply demarcated from adjacent normal mucosa. Ischemic colitis often settles clinically within a few weeks and the radiological abnormalities then usually disappear, making differentiation easier. However, linear ulceration and permanent fibrous strictures may remain, which are impossible to differentiate from Crohn's disease (Fig. 25.41).

In elderly patients diverticular disease may also be difficult to differentiate from Crohn's disease. In both conditions there may be mucosal thickening with associated spasm and narrowing. Longitudinal submucosal sinuses and tracks (Fig. 25.42) may be seen in both

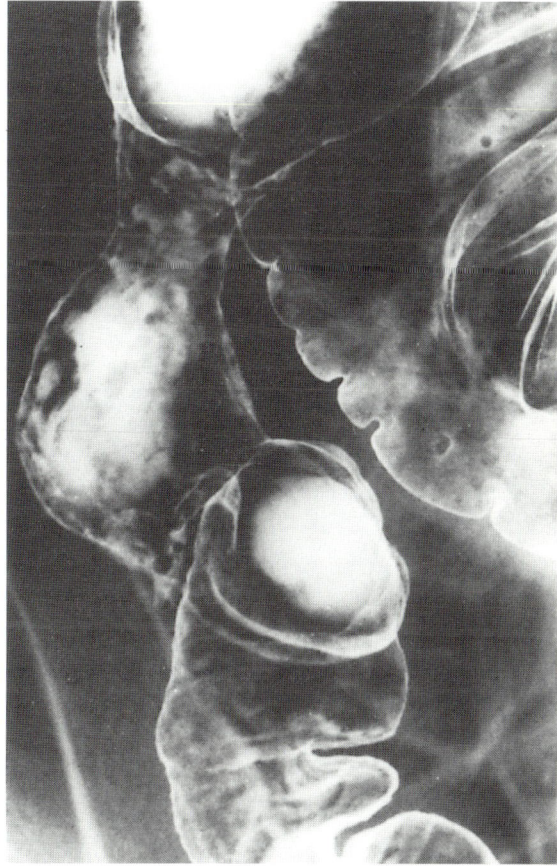

Fig. 25.40 Distortion and contraction of the ileocecal region with shallow ulceration. Appearances indicated Crohn's disease but pathological examination of the resected specimen revealed tuberculosis.

Crohn's colitis and in severe diverticular disease of the sigmoid colon (Marshak 1975), and cutaneous fistulae develop. Crohn's and diverticular disease may coexist (Berman et al 1979), as may either or both with ischemic colitis.

In the early stages of Crohn's colitis, when there is only mucosal edema and aphthous ulceration, the appearances may resemble those seen in Behçet's disease (O'Connell et al 1980) or amoebic colitis (Cardoso et al 1977, Max & Kelvin 1980). Behçet's disease is rare and amoebic colitis is not common in western Europe, but may be seen in visitors from Africa and Asia. For practical purposes, in patients from western countries the demonstration of aphthous ulceration justifies the diagnosis of Crohn's colitis (Simpkins 1977).

Rectal sparing may occur in pseudomembranous colitis (Rubesin et al 1989).

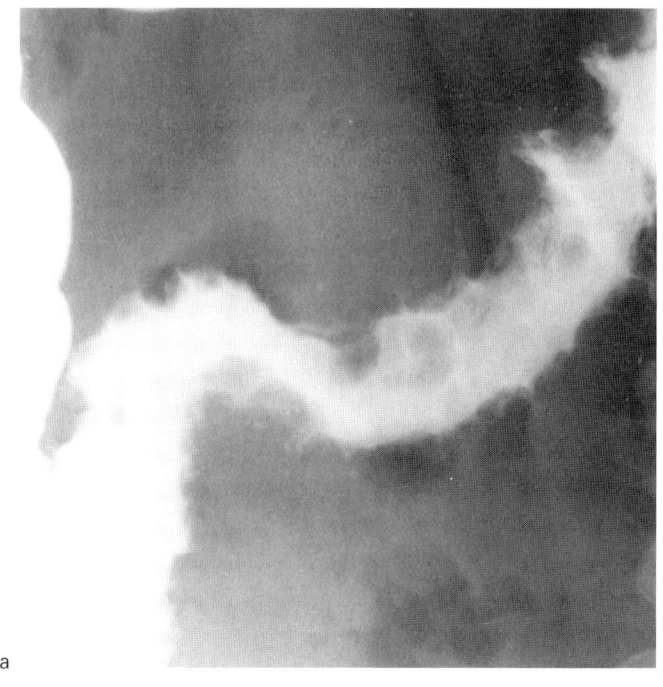

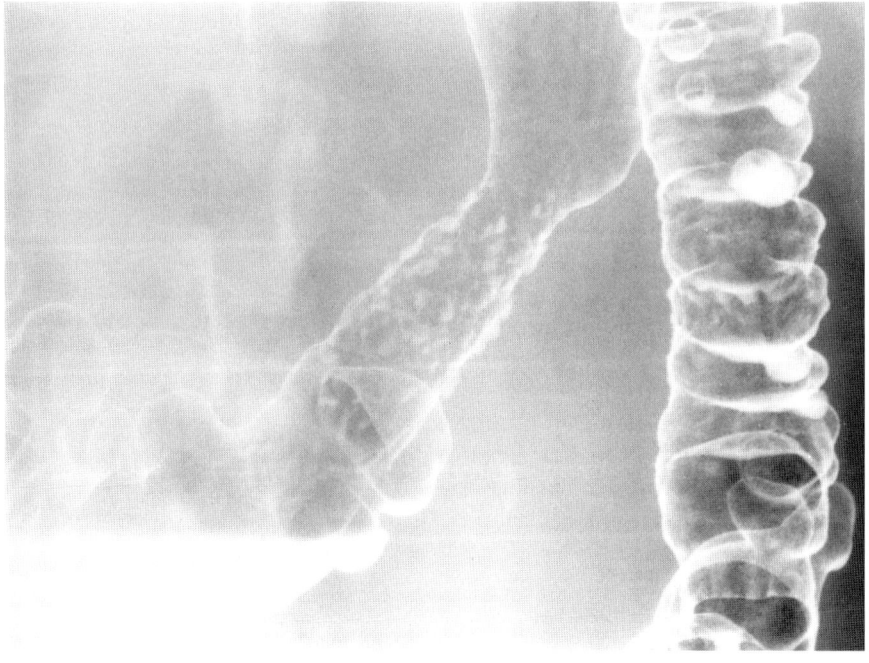

Fig. 25.41 Ischemic colitis. **a** Acute phase. **b** Weeks later, showing stricturing with asymmetric sacculation. Without the early phase appearances in **b** could be confused with Crohn's disease.

Diagnostic pitfalls

Plain films. The extent of colitis can easily be underestimated from plain films. 'Thumbprinting' as an indication of colitis may easily be overdiagnosed. In both situations, the use of an 'air enema' will be helpful. Gaseous distension of the transverse colon greater than 5 or 6 cm is commonly seen in ileus, colonic obstruction, pseudo-obstruction and following a barium enema or colonoscopy, and the colon diameter in itself should not compel the diagnosis of toxic dilatation. Irregularity of the colon margin by mucosal islands is the important feature.

Contrast examinations. Fine adherent fecal residue in the colon and flocculation of the barium layer can often cause difficulty in differentiation from mucosal ulceration and granularity. Careful inspection of all films may be helpful, but further examinations, either radiological or endoscopic, may be required. Lymphoid hyperplasia in the small bowel and colon may cause problems, particularly if it is confined to the terminal ileum and the patient has symptoms in that area. Lymphoid hyperplasia has been associated with bowel inflammation and neoplasia (Kenney et al 1982, Bronen et al 1984), but it is most commonly a normal feature, especially in children and young adults (Laufer & de Sa 1978, Kelvin et al 1979). 'Rosethorn' ulceration is often quoted as being pathognomonic of Crohn's disease. This feature is greatly overdiagnosed on barium examinations and the appearance is frequently due to underdistension of the bowel, with barium pooled between swollen mucosal folds. Occasionally, tiny diverticula in the sigmoid colon may simulate aphthous ulcers when viewed 'en face'. If the observer is aware of this, a search for diverticula projecting outwards from the bowel margins tangentially and the absence of other evidence of disease will be helpful.

A tubular colon, with lack of haustration and a normal mucosal surface, is not an uncommon finding and is usually a normal variant. The normal left colon, in particular, may lack a haustral contour.

Use in monitoring. Because of the theoretical dangers of radiation, the use of X-ray imaging in the follow-up of inflammatory bowel disease requires thought. It should be used sparingly, and simpler, quicker examinations such as the 'air' and 'instant' enemas given more precedence. Fiber optic endoscopy can usually be used as an alternative.

Disease extent

The full extent of disease and the number and length of strictures, in particular, may not be so accurately demonstrated in the small bowel. In the proximal small intestine more information may be obtained by enteroscopy, but in the distal small bowel additional lesions may only be found if laparotomy is performed. If laparotomy is

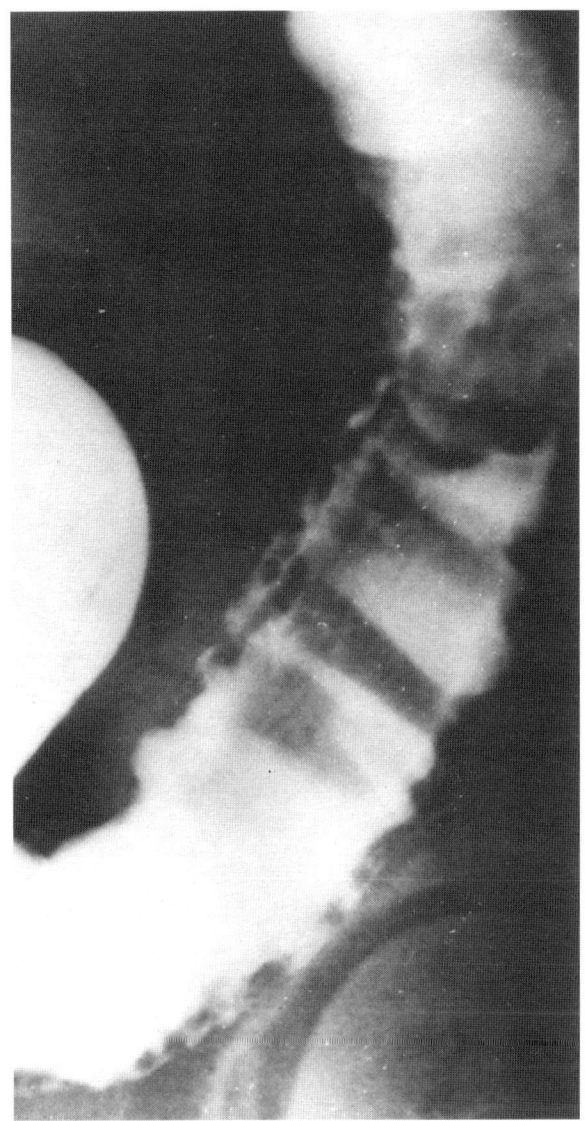

Fig. 25.42 Barium enema examination showing intramural ulceration in the sigmoid colon which connected to give parallel submucosal tracks. Note the irregularly thickened colonic mucosa adjacent to the track. The smooth appearance of the rectum is not involved.

Recurrent Crohn's disease

Recurrent disease after resection is not uncommon and has the same radiological features as the primary disease (Rutgeerts et al 1990). The operation most often performed for Crohn's disease is resection of the terminal ileum, usually with removal of the cecum and a portion of the ascending colon. When Crohn's disease recurs, the area affected is invariably the 'new' terminal ileum (Fig. 25.43). This happens whether the ileal anastomosis is to the ascending, transverse or the sigmoid colon (Rutgeerts et al 1990). For gastric or duodenal Crohn's disease the usual operation is a bypass gastroenterostomy. After this operation we have seen florid disease in the stomach and adjacent jejunal loops, occasionally requiring a further bypass.

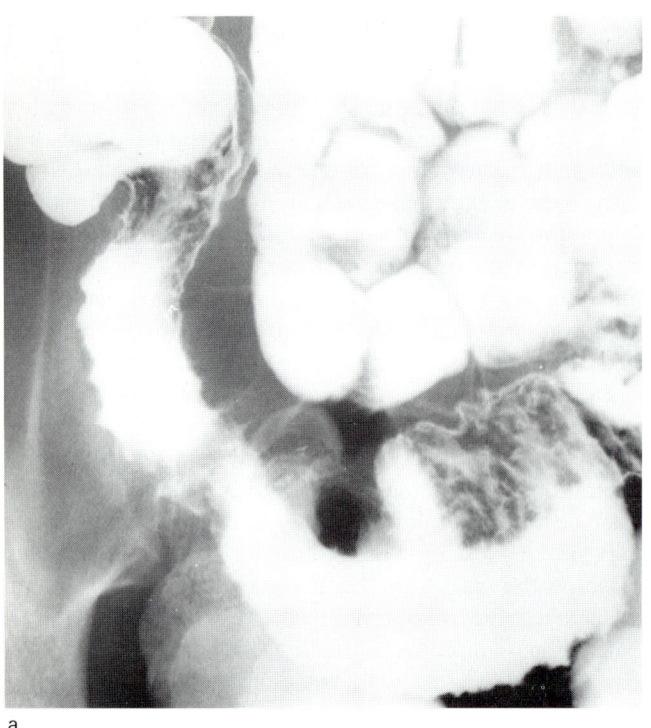
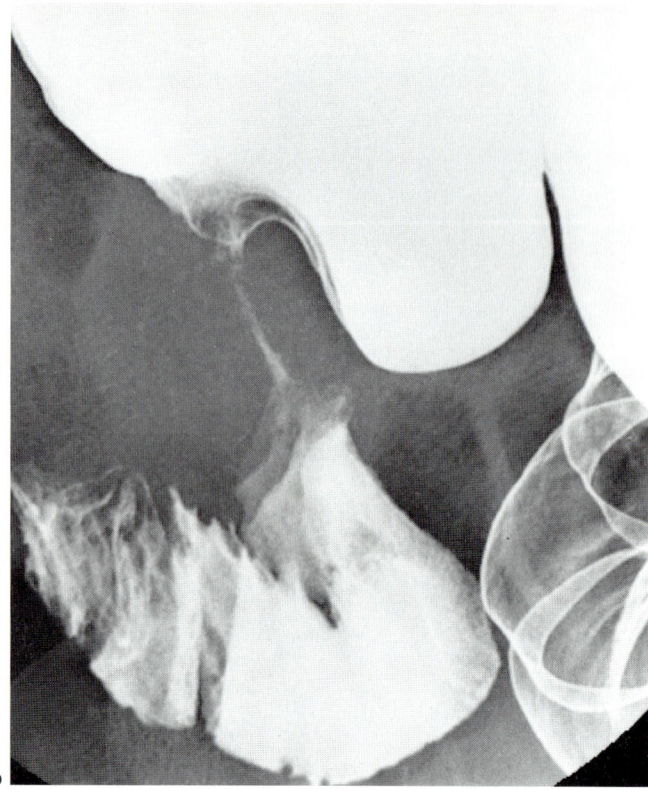

Fig. 25.43 Recurrent disease in the ileum following ileocecal resection. **a** Long-segment ulcerative disease. **b** Short-segment fibrotic disease.

performed for strictures the whole small bowel may be assessed better by pullthrough using a distensible balloon (Alexander-Williams 1994, personal communication)

Assessment of fistulae

Clinicians require not only demonstration of the fistula tract(s) and a communication with the bowel, but to show the bowel adjacent to the fistula and, if possible, an assessment of the nature of the underlying disease: how extensive it is and what is the condition of the adjacent bowel (Alexander-Williams & Irving 1982). It is particularly important to demonstrate whether there is any degree of distal obstruction, as this will almost certainly delay or prevent spontaneous closure of the fistula and may determine the choice of treatment. Some fistulae may be shown quite satisfactorily as part of the routine barium contrast assessment of the bowel (Figs 25.26, 25.27). This particularly applies to short internal fistulae, such as are commonly seen around the terminal ileum and adjacent cecum/right colon. The most difficult fistulae to assess are those with cutaneous connections, particularly if these are multiple. In general these are best assessed by instilling a water-soluble iodide-based contrast agent down the track. If the fistula is a single direct tract from the skin to the bowel this is usually a simple examination. Unfortunately, many fistulas are multitracked, often with multiple skin openings and bowel connections. If contrast media is injected down a track in this situation it usually leaks from other skin openings or formal stomas, leading to obscuration of the anatomy, failing to enter adjacent bowel or all fistulous and sinus tracks, and giving rise to an incomplete and unsatisfactory examination. These problems can be overcome by the use of soft rubber balloon catheters, which should be inserted into all skin openings, including any mucosal stomas, and the rectum prior to any contrast instillation (Fig. 25.44). With the use of selective catheter occlusion and injection, the procedure can be controlled and the anatomy demonstrated (Fig. 25.45). Often this can be achieved in a single examination, but occasionally two or more examinations on separate days will be required to obtain the required results.

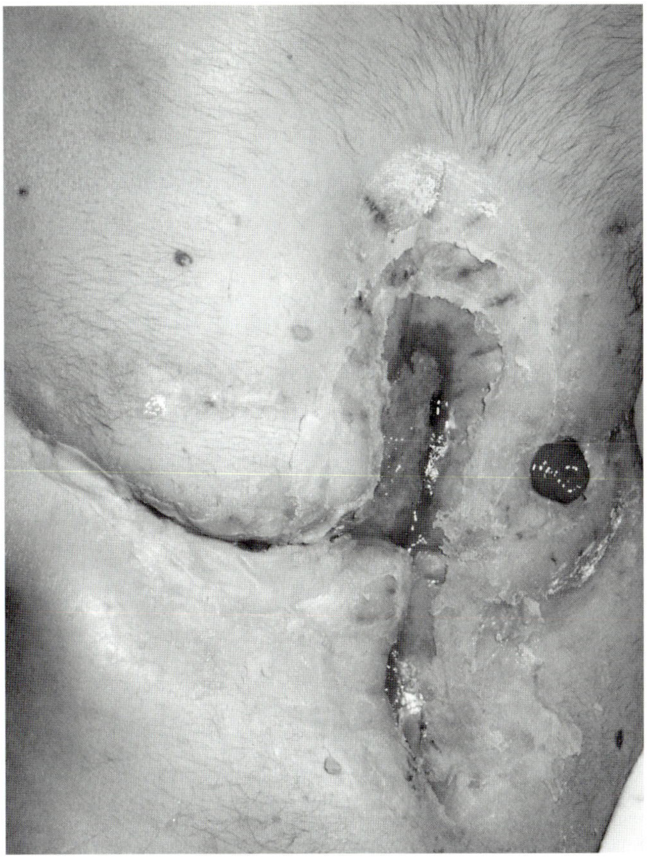

Fig. 25.44 Fistulography for extensive enterocutaneous fistulation of anterior abdominal wall. **a** Appearance before and **b** following insertion of soft rubber balloon catheters into fistulae and ileostomy.

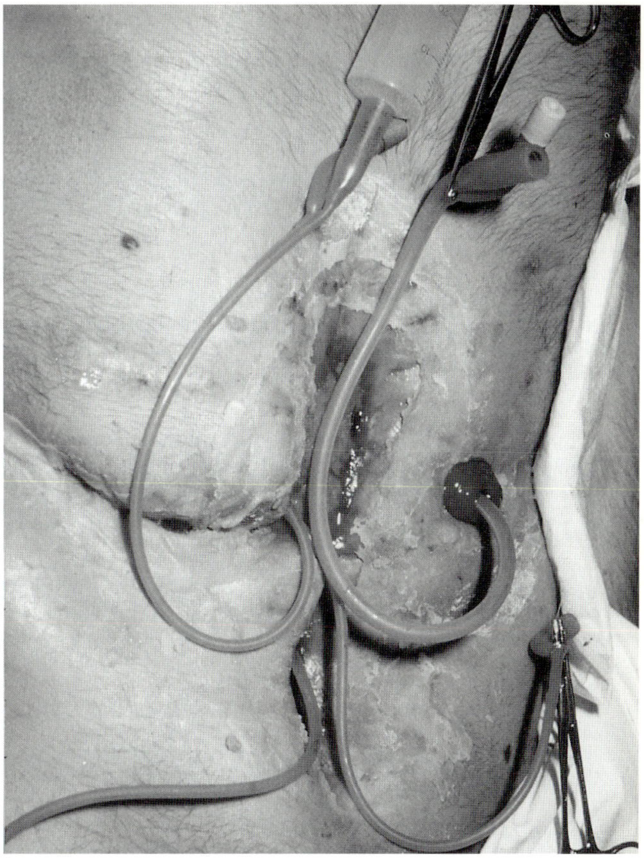

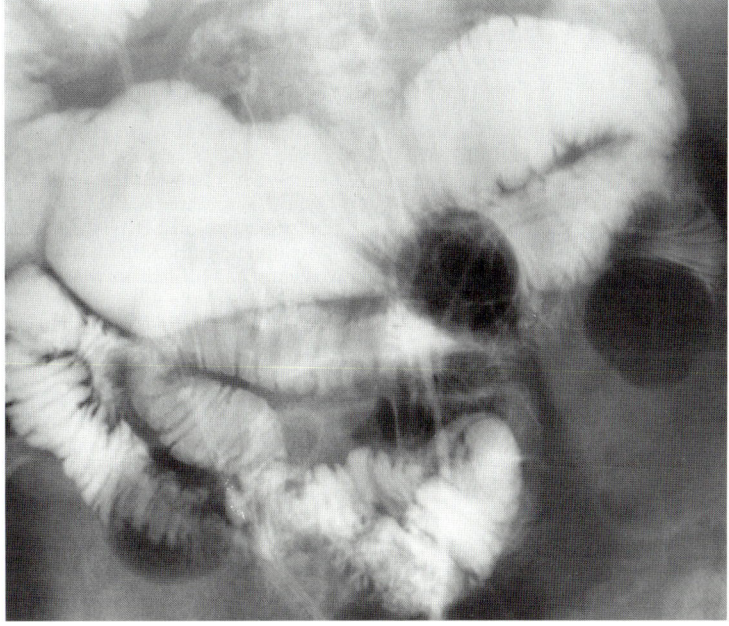

Fig. 25.45 Example of fistulogram. The balloons are airfilled and show as black circles.

REFERENCES

Alexander-Williams J, Irving M 1982 Investigation of the patient with an intestinal fistula. In: Intestinal fistulas. Wright, Bristol, pp 54–68

Ariyama J, Wehlin L, Lindstrom C G, Wenkert A, Roberts G M 1980 Gastroduodenal erosions in Crohn's disease. Gastrointestinal Radiology 5: 121–125

Balthazar E J, Bryk D 1980 Segmental tuberculosis of the distal colon: radiographic features in seven cases. Gastrointestinal Radiology 5: 75–80

Bartram C I 1980 The radiological demonstration of adhesions following surgery for inflammatory bowel disease. British Journal of Radiology 53: 650–653

Bartram C I, Laufer I 1979 Inflammatory bowel disease In: Laufer I (ed) Double contrast gastrointestinal radiology with endoscopic correlation. Saunders, Philadelphia, pp. 601–688

Bartram C, Preston D, Lennard-Jones J 1983 The 'air enema' in acute colitis. Gastrointestinal Radiology 8: 61–65

Berman I R, Corman M L, Coller J A, Veidenheimer M C 1979 Late onset Crohn's disease in patients with colonic diverticulitis. Diseases of the Colon and Rectum 22: 524–529

Bernstein J R, Ghahremani G G, Paige M L, Rosenberg J L 1978 Localised giant psuedopolyposis of the colon in ulcerative and granulomatous colitis. Gastrointestinal Radiology 3: 431–435

Berridge F R 1971 Two unusual radiological signs of Crohn's disease of the colon. Clinical Radiology 32: 443–448

Bjarnason I, Hallyar J, Macpherson A J, Russell A J 1993 Side effects of nonsteroidal anti-inflammatory drugs on the small and large intestines in humans. Gastroenterology 104: 1832–1847

Bjarnason I, Zanelli G, Smith T et al 1987 Nonsteroidal anti-inflammatory drug-induced intestinal inflammation in humans. Gastroenterology 93: 480–489

British Medical Journal 1973 Crohn's disease in the elderly: a diagnostic problem. British Medical Journal 3: 188–189

Bronen R A, Glick S N, Teplick S K 1984 Diffuse lymphoid follicle of the colon associated with colonic carcinoma. American Journal of Roentgenology 142: 105–109

Cardoso J M, Kimura K, Stoopen M et al 1977 Radiology of invasive amebiasis of the colon. American Journal of Roentgenology 128: 935–941

Carlson H C 1986 Perspective. The small bowel examination in the diagnosis of Crohn's disease. American Journal of Roentgenology 147: 63–65

Chang S F, Burrell M I, Belleza N A, Spiro H M 1978 Borderlands with diagnosis of regional enteritis? Trends in overdiagnosis and value of a therapeutic trial. Gastrointestinal Radiology 3: 67–72

Cockey B M, Jones B, Bayless T M, Shauer A B 1985 Filiform polyps of the esophagus with inflammatory bowel disease. American Journal of Roentgenology 144: 1207–1208

Cynn W-S, Chon H, Gureghian R A, Levin B L 1975 Crohn's disease of the esophagus. American Journal of Roentgenology 125: 359–364

Dyer N H, Cook P L, Kempharper R A 1969 Oesophageal stricture associated with Crohn's disease. Gut 10: 549–554

Ekberg O 1977 Double contrast examination of the small bowel. Gastrointestinal Radiology 1: 349–353

Ekberg O, Sjostrom B, Brahme F 1977 Radiological findings in Yersinia ileitis. Radiology 123: 15–19

Farman J, Faegenberg D, Dallemand S, Chen C-K 1975 Crohn's disease of the stomach. The 'ram's horn' sign. American Journal of Roentgenology 123: 242–251

Fazio V W 1980 Toxic megacolon in ulcerative colitis and Crohn's disease. Clinical Gastroenterology 9: 389–407

Fielding J F, Toye D K M, Beton D C, Cooke W T 1970. Crohn's disease of the stomach and duodenum. Gut 11: 1001–1006

Frank P H, Riddell R H, Feczko P J, Levin B 1978 Radiological detection of colonic dysplasia (precarcinoma) in chronic ulcerative colitis. Gastrointestinal Radiology 3: 209–219

Fraser G M, Adam R D 1988 Modifications of the gas enhanced small bowel barium follow-through using gastrografin and compression. Clinical Radiology 39: 537–541

Fraser G M, Preston P G 1983 The small bowel barium follow-through enhanced with an oral effervescent agent. Clinical Radiology 34: 673–679

Glick S N, Teplick S K 1985 Crohn's disease of the small intestine. Diffuse mucosal granularity. Radiology 154: 313–317

Gore R M 1987 Cross-section imaging of inflammatory bowel disease. Radiologic Clinics of North America 25: 115–131

Gyde S N, Prior P, Allan R N et al 1988 Colorectal cancer in ulcerative colitis: a cohort study of primary referrals from three centers. Gut 29: 206–217

Halpert R D 1987 Toxic dilatation of the colon. Radiologic Clinics of North America 25: 147–155

Healy J C, Gorman S, Kumar P J 1992 Case report: tuberculous colitis mimicking Crohn's disease. Clinical Radiology 46: 131–132

Herlinger H 1978 A modified technique for the double contrast small bowel enema. Gastrointestinal Radiology 3: 201–207

Hooyman J R, MacCarty R L, Carpenter H A, Schroeder K W, Carlson H C 1987 Radiographic appearance of mucosal dysplasia associated with ulcerative colitis. American Journal of Roentgenology 149: 47–51

Howarth F H, Cockel R, Roper B H, Hawkins C F 1969 The effect of metoclopramide upon gastric motility and its value in barium progress meals. Clinical Radiology 20: 294–300

Huchzermeyer H, Paul F, Seifert E, Frohilch H, Rasmussen Ch W 1976. Endoscopic results in five patients with Crohn's disease of the oesophagus. Endoscopy 8: 75–81

Iida M, Matsu T, Fuchigami T, Iwashita A, Yao T, Fujishima M 1986 Ischaemic colitis: serial changes in DCBE. Radiology 159: 327–341

Jacobsen I M, Schapiro R H, Warshaw A L 1985 Gastric and duodenal fistulas in Crohn's disease. Gastroenterology 89: 1347–1352

Joffe N 1981 Diffuse mucosal granularity in double contrast studies of Crohn's disease of the colon. Clinical Radiology 32: 85–90

Jones B, Abbruzzese A A 1978 Obstruction giant pseudopolyps in granulomatous colitis. Gastrointestinal Radiology 3: 437–438

Kellett M J, Zboralske F F, Margulis A R 1977 Per oral pneumocolon examination of the ileo-cecal region. Gastrointestinal Radiology 1: 361–365

Kelly J K, Langevin J M, Price L M 1986 Giant and symptomatic inflammatory polyps of the colon in ideopathic inflammatory bowel disease. American Journal of Surgical Pathology 10: 420–428

Kelvin F M, Max R J, Norton G A et al 1979 Lymphoid follicular pattern of the colon in adults. American Journal of Roentgenology 133: 821–825

Kenney P J, Koehler R E, Shackelford G D 1982 The clinical significance of large lymphoid follicles in the colon. Radiology 142: 41–46

Laufer I, de Sa D 1978 Lymphoid follicular pattern: a normal feature of the paediatric colon. American Journal of Roentgenology 130: 51–55

Laufer I, Joffe N, Stolberg H 1977 Unusual causes of gastrocolic fistula. Gastrointestinal Radiology 2: 21–25

Lee J R, Ferrando J R 1984 Variables in the preparation of the large intestine for DCBE. Gut 25: 69–72

Lennard-Jones J E, Melville D M, Morson B C, Ritchie J K, Williams C B 1990 Precancer and cancer in extensive colitis: findings among 401 patients over 22 years. Gut 31: 800–806

Lichtenstein J E, Madewell J E, Feigin D S 1979 The collar button ulcer. Gastrointestinal Radiology 4: 79–84

Lindstrom E, Noren G 1992 Air enema revisited in assessment of colitis. Acta Radiologica 33: 360–364

Maglinte D D J, Chernish S M, Kelvin F M, O'Connor K W, Hage J P 1992 Crohn's disease of the small intestine. Accuracy and relevance of enteroclysis. Radiology 184: 541–554

Maglinte D D J, Lappas J C, Kelvin F M, Rex D, Chermish S M 1987 Small bowel radiography: how, when and why? Radiology 163: 297–305

Margulis A R, Goldberg H I, Lawson T L et al 1971 The overlapping spectrum of ulcerative and granulomatous colitis: a roentgenographic–pathologic study. American Journal of Roentgenology 113: 325–334

Marshak R H 1975 Granulomatous disease of the intestinal tract (Crohn's disease). Radiology 114: 3–22

Max R J, Kelvin F M 1980 Non-specificity of discrete colonic ulceration on double contrast barium enema study. American Journal of Roentgenology 134: 1265–1267

Meyers M A 1976 Clinical involvement of mesenteric and antimesenteric borders of small bowel loops. Radiologic interpretation of pathologic alterations. Gastrointestinal Radiology 1: 49–58

Miller R E 1965 Complete reflux small bowel examination. Radiology 84: 457–462

Morson B C, Dawson M P, Way D W, Jass J R, Price A B, Williams G T 1990 (eds) Morson and Dawson's Gastrointestinal Pathology 3rd edn. Blackwell Scientific, Oxford

Nelson J A, Margulis A R, Goldberg H I, Lawson T L 1973 Granulomatous colitis: significance of involvement of the terminal ileum. Gastroenterology 64: 1071–1076

Ni X-Y, Goldberg H I 1986 Aphthous ulcers in Crohn's disease. Radiographic course and relationship to bowel appearance. Radiology 158: 589–596

Nolan D J, Gourtsoyiannis N C 1980 Crohn's disease of the small intestine: a review of the radiological appearances in 100 consecutive patients examined by a barium infusion technique. Clinical Radiology 31: 597–603

Nugent F W, Richmond M, Park S K 1977 Crohn's disease of the duodenum. Gut 18: 115–120

O'Connell D S, Courtney J V, Riddell R H 1980 Colitis of Behçet's syndrome – radiological and pathologic features. Gastrointestinal Radiology 5: 173–179

Patel U, Bartram C 1993 Utility of the instant (unprepared) enema in Crohn's colitis. Clinical Radiology 47: 351–354

Peh W C G 1988 Filiform polyposis in tuberculosis of the colon. Clinical Radiology 39: 534–536

Reeders J W A J, Tytgat G N J 1987 Ischaemic colitis. Serial changes in DCBE. Radiology 162: 583

Rubesin S E, Levine M S, Glick S N, Hellinger H, Laufer I 1989 Pseudomembranous colitis with rectosigmoid sparing on barium studies. Radiology 170: 811–813

Rutgeerts P, Geboes K, Vantrappen G, Beyus J, Kerremans R, Hiele M 1990 Predictability of postoperative course of Crohn's disease. Gastroenterology 99: 956–963

Sellink J L 1976 Radiological atlas of common disease of the small intestine. H E Stenfert, Kroese B V, Leiden

Simpkins K C 1976 The barium enema in Crohn's colitis In: Waterman I T, Pena A S, Booth C C (eds) The management of Crohn's disease. Excerpta Medica, Amsterdam, pp 62–67

Simpkins K C 1977 Aphthoid ulcers in Crohn's colitis. Clinical Radiology 28: 601–608

Simpkins K C, Young A C 1971 The differential diagnosis of large bowel strictures. Clinical Radiology 22: 449–457

Stanley P, Kelsey Fry I, Dawson A M, Dyer N 1971 Radiological signs of ulcerative colitis and Crohn's disease of the colon. Clinical Radiology 22: 434–442

Stevenson G W 1978 Gastroduodenal lesions in Crohn's disease. Gut 19: 962–963

Suekane H, Iida M, Matsui T, Yao T, Fujishima M 1990 Radiographic demonstration of longitudinal ulcers in patients with ulcerative colitis. Gastrointestinal Radiology 15: 333–337

Sugita A, Sachar D B, Bodian C, Ribeiro M B, Aufses A H, Greenstein A J 1991 Colorectal cancer in ulcerative colitis. Influence of anatomical extent and age at onset or colitis–cancer interval. Gut 32: 167–169

Thomas B M 1979 The instant enema in inflammatory disease of the colon. Clinical Radiology 30: 165–173

Thompson W M, Cockrill H, Rice R P 1975 Regional enteritis of the duodenum. American Journal of Roentgenology 123: 252–261

Tishler J M A, Helman C A 1984 Crohn's disease of the oesophagus. Journal of the Canadian Association of Radiology 35: 28–30

Tsukasa S, Tokjdome K, Irisa T, Nishimata Y, Hashimoto S, Shirakabe H 1978 Roentgenographic diagnosis of Crohn's disease of the small intestine. Stomach and Intestine 13: 335–349

Vantrappen G, Agg H O, Ponette E, Geboes K, Bertrand P H 1977 Yersinia enteritis and entero-colitis: gastroenterological aspects. Gastroenterology 72: 220–227

Williams I 1975 Innominate grooves in the surface of the mucosa. Radiology 84: 877

Zegel H G, Laufer I 1978 Filiform polyposis. Radiology 127: 615–619

26. Radiology – CT, ultrasound and MRI

J. F. C. Olliff

Barium examination remains the imaging modality of choice in the diagnosis of inflammatory bowel disease (IBD), whether it involves large or small bowel. It can demonstrate good mucosal detail and allow determination of the length involved and whether the involvement is continuous or discontinuous. Cross-sectional imaging (scanning) has a complementary role, demonstrating the mucosa poorly but showing adjacent mesentery and other abdominal and pelvic contents well.

GENERAL ASPECTS OF ULTRASOUND, CT AND MRI SCANNING OF THE INTESTINE

Ultrasound is readily available and cheaper than MRI (magnetic resonance imaging) or CT (computed tomography). It is possible to scan very ill patients on the ward. Ultrasound can identify bowel wall thickening and show abscesses or collections within the abdomen or pelvis which are not obscured by bowel gas, but it may not demonstrate interloop abscesses and does not give good mesenteric detail. It can be impossible to obtain a diagnostic scan in the obese patient. CT gives excellent soft tissue contrast and abnormal soft tissue is readily shown within mesenteric fat. It will show interloop abscesses if there has been good bowel opacification with oral contrast medium. It can also be used to examine solid organs within the abdomen and pelvis. MRI also gives excellent soft tissue contrast but suffers from the lack of a good bowel contrast agent to delineate small- and large-bowel loops. MRI can image in any plane and this is particularly useful in the pelvis, where it can be used to examine the pelvic floor. It will also show abnormalities within solid organs and is the best imaging modality to demonstrate marrow abnormality.

ULTRASOUND

Transabdominal ultrasound may be used to detect bowel wall thickening (Fig. 26.1). However, many different

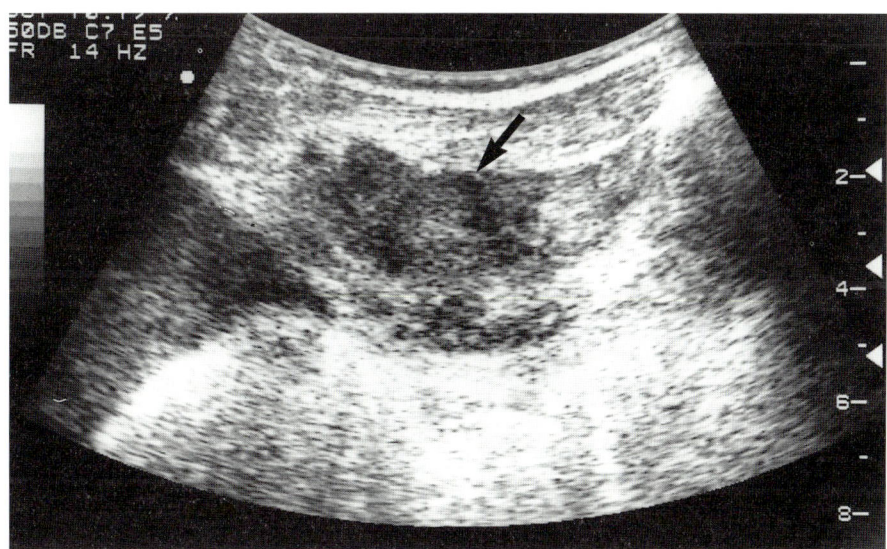

Fig. 26.1 Transabdominal ultrasound of the right iliac fossa demonstrating an abdominal bowel loop, with bowel wall thickening and an inflammatory mass.

processes produce bowel wall thickening and distinction between the differing pathologies may not be possible with ultrasound. Some authors have attempted to distinguish between Crohn's disease and ulcerative colitis on the basis of different degrees of bowel wall thickening (Dubbins 1984, Kimi, et al 1990). Others have attempted to distinguish between the different conditions using specific ultrasound appearances and patterns of bowel involvement. These have been described as 'Crohn's pattern' or 'ulcerative colitic pattern' (Khaw et al 1991). It was found that the Crohn's pattern reflected mural thickening, with inflammation, edema and fibrosis, and produced a typical target lesion. The ulcerative colitis pattern gave rise to a poorly defined inhomogeneous wall and lumen, with irregular air trapping between mucosal folds and ulcers. These two patterns were found to be of significant value in the differentiation between causes of inflammatory bowel pathology. No cases of ulcerative colitis produced a Crohn's-type pattern, and infective causes of bowel inflammation showed more typically an ulcerative colitic pattern.

COMPUTED TOMOGRAPHY (CT)

On CT the normal wall thickness of the small bowel and colon is 2–3 mm and it is homogeneous in attenuation. The bowel wall thickness will be artificially increased if the gut is scanned obliquely. The normal mesenteric fat has an attenuation value of –75 to –125 Hounsfield units, and should thus appear black on 'standard' window width and level settings. The normal mesentery contains blood vessels, seen either end-on as small rounded soft tissue dots, or seen along their length. Normal mesenteric lymph nodes measure less than 5 mm in size (Gore 1989).

CROHN'S DISEASE

CT can appear normal in early disease when only mucosal abnormality is present (Fig. 26.2). The bowel wall then becomes thickened, with a homogeneous appearance caused by edema, inflammation and fibrosis (Fig. 26.3). Occasionally an inhomogeneous appearance is seen, with a double halo (Fig. 26.4) due to an inner low-density ring corresponding to severe mucosal edema or to submucosal fat accumulation (Frager et al 1983, Jones et al 1986). Abnormality is most frequently seen in the terminal ileum, and is often discontinuous. Thickened bowel wall can be seen on CT when the mucosa appears normal in patients with quiescent disease (Gore 1989). Bowel dilatation will be evident proximal to an obstructing diseased segment.

CT is very useful for the assessment of mesenteric disease. Bowel loop separation seen on barium study may be due to bowel wall thickening, fibrofatty proliferation (Fig. 26.5), enlarged lymph nodes, phlegmon (Fig. 26.6) or abscess. Fibrofatty proliferation results in streaky densities within the mesenteric fat, and the mesenteric fat will have an increased attenuation value (increased by 20–60 Hounsfield units) (Fig 26.7) (Gore 1989). Lymphadenopathy can be marked in patients with Crohn's disease (Fig. 26.8), but if it exceeds 8 mm in diameter small-bowel lymphoma or carcinoma should be considered as an underlying cause (Gore 1989). Mesenteric abscesses are a common complication of Crohn's disease (Goldberg et al 1983). In this series 25% of patients being investigated further following suspicious barium study had evidence on CT of mesenteric abscesses. These appear as well circumscribed fluid densities, which may have a thick wall and often contain gas (Fig. 26.9). Contrast medium within a collection indicates fistulous communication.

Abscesses occur in 12–25% of patients with Crohn's disease at some time. Although most of these patients have had surgery the abscesses are not usually related to this (i.e. anastomotic breakdown) but are related to other diseased segments of bowel (Alexander-Williams 1982).

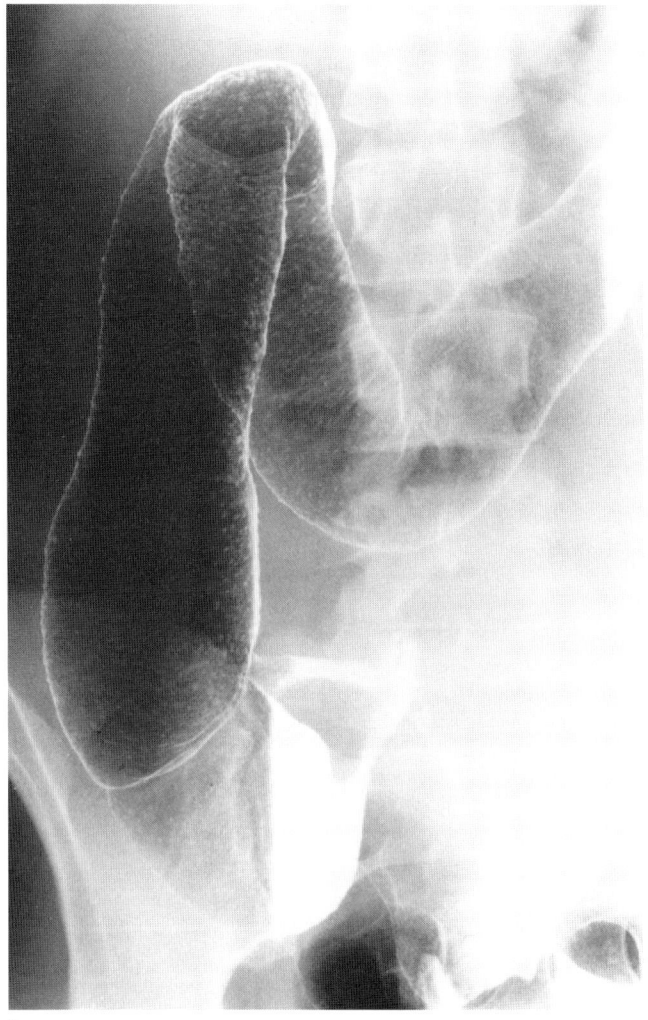

Fig. 26.2a Barium enema demonstrating extensive Crohn's colitis and terminal ileal involvement.

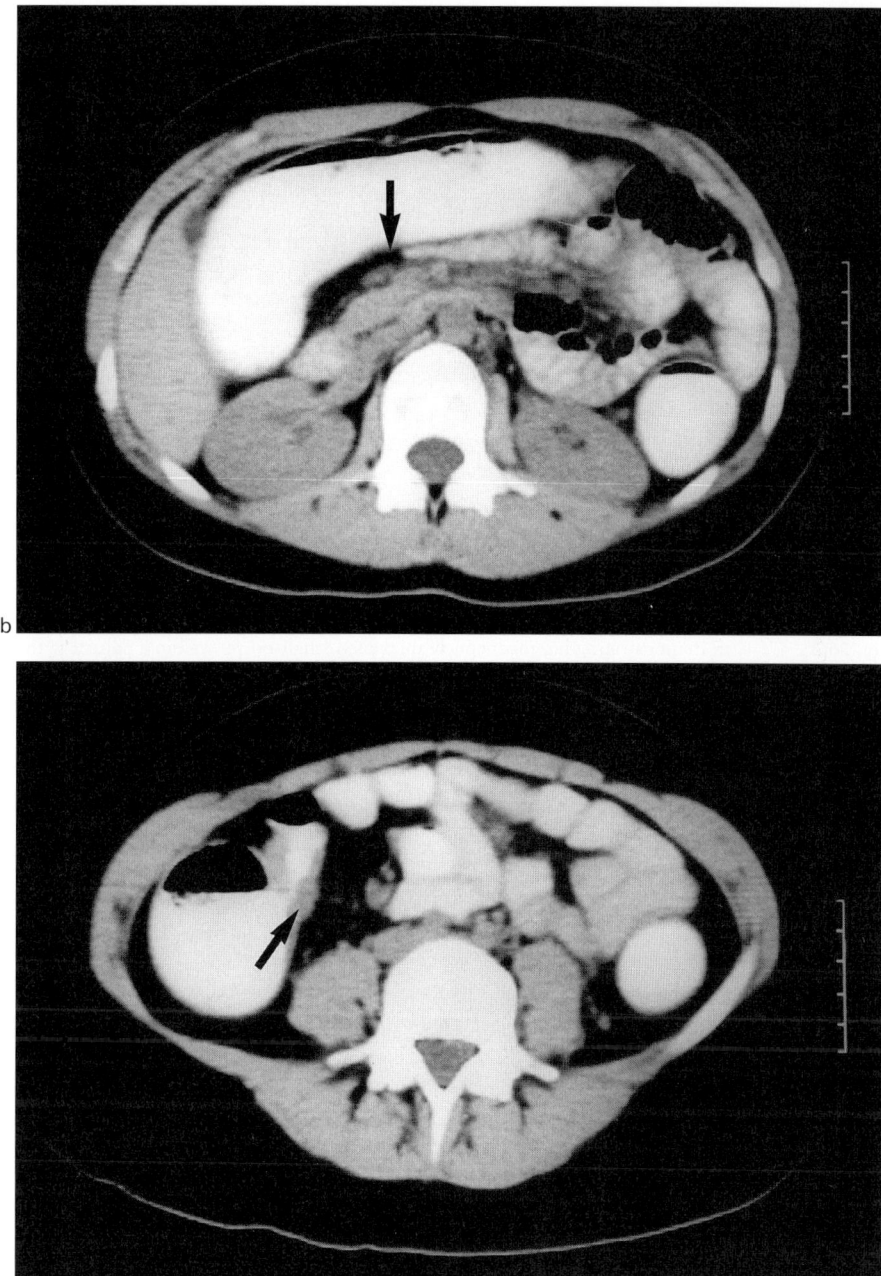

Fig. 26.2 *(Cont'd)* **b** CT scan of the same patient, demonstrating very little abnormality of the transverse, descending or ascending colon. **c** The involvement of the terminal ileum with wall thickening is clearly seen (arrow): note adjacent fibrofatty proliferation.

Percutaneous drainage can be performed using ultrasound or CT guidance. This is unlikely to result in healing if there is evidence of enteric communication, but can be used to tide the patient over until they are well enough for definitive surgery (Lambiase et al 1988). Abscess formation may also occur in the liver and retroperitoneum, including the psoas muscles (Kerber et al 1984). CT is very useful in diagnosing pyogenic liver abscesses, with a reported sensitivity of 95–98% (Halvorsen et al 1984, Mathieu et al 1985).

CT will frequently demonstrate abnormality in the perirectal and perianal region in patients with Crohn's disease (Yousmen et al 1988). These authors found abnormalities in 82% of 200 patients scanned. The most commonest was inflammatory streaking of fat in the perirectal region and ischiorectal fossa, often associated with thickening of the perirectal fascia. Rectal wall thickening occurred in 30% of their patients (Fig. 26.10), and 22% were found to have perirectal or perianal fistulae or sinus tracts. It can be difficult on CT to distinguish between

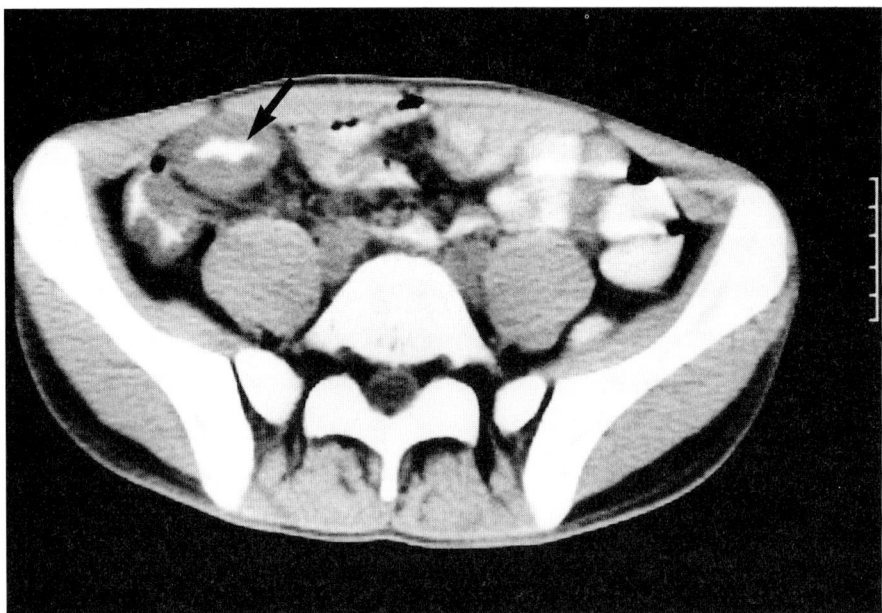

Fig. 26.3 CT scan demonstrating homogeneously thickened small-bowel wall in a patient with Crohn's disease.

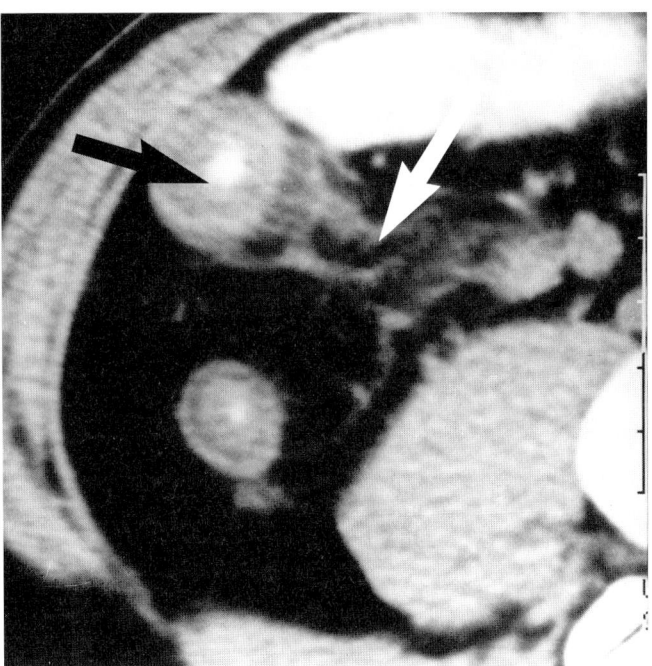

Fig. 26.4 CT scan showing inhomogeneous wall thickening with a halo in a patient with severe active Crohn's disease (black arrow). There is also inflammatory streaking of the mesenteric fat (white arrow).

inflammatory streaking and tract formation when air or contrast material is not present in the sinus tract. The presence of a double wall thickness and origin from inflamed bowel wall may allow this diagnosis to be made. Abscess was found in 14% of Yousmen's study group, associated either with adjacent rectosigmoid colon or in the perirectal fat, most frequently at the level of the acetabula. These authors found that disease was present below the symphysis pubis in more than one-third of patients, and this fact should be borne in mind when CT scans are being performed in patients with Crohn's disease so that scans are obtained below the level of the external anal sphincter.

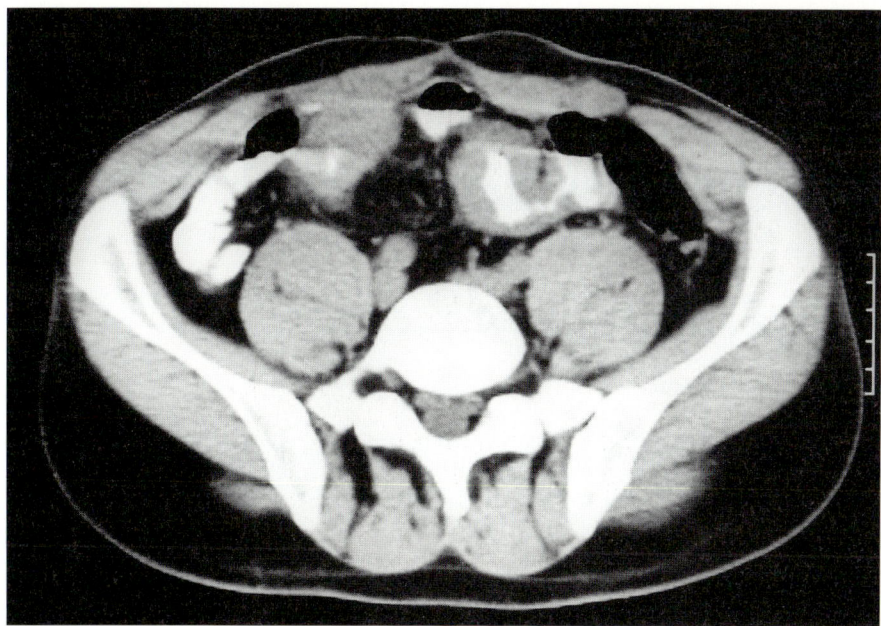

Fig. 26.5 In this patient CT demonstrates that bowel loop separation is due to a combination of bowel wall thickening and fibrofatty proliferation.

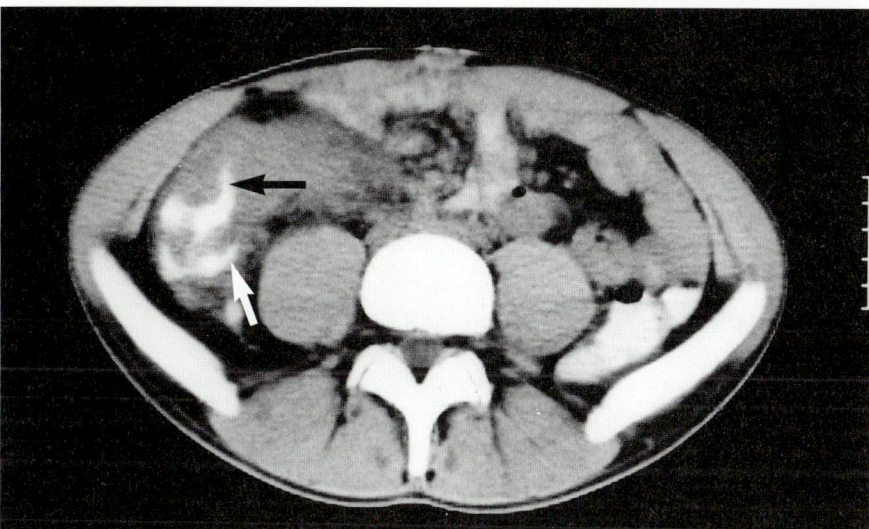

Fig. 26.6 CT scan demonstrating an inflammatory mass extending into the mesentery from a very abnormal bowel loop with short contrast-filled tracks within it (arrow).

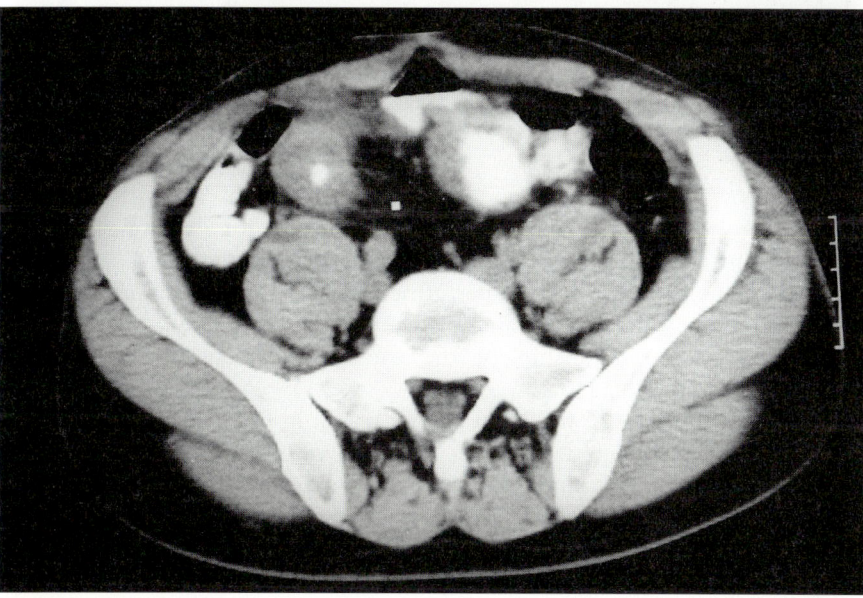

Fig. 26.7a The cursor reported a reading of −50 Hounsfield units from the mesenteric fat in this patient.

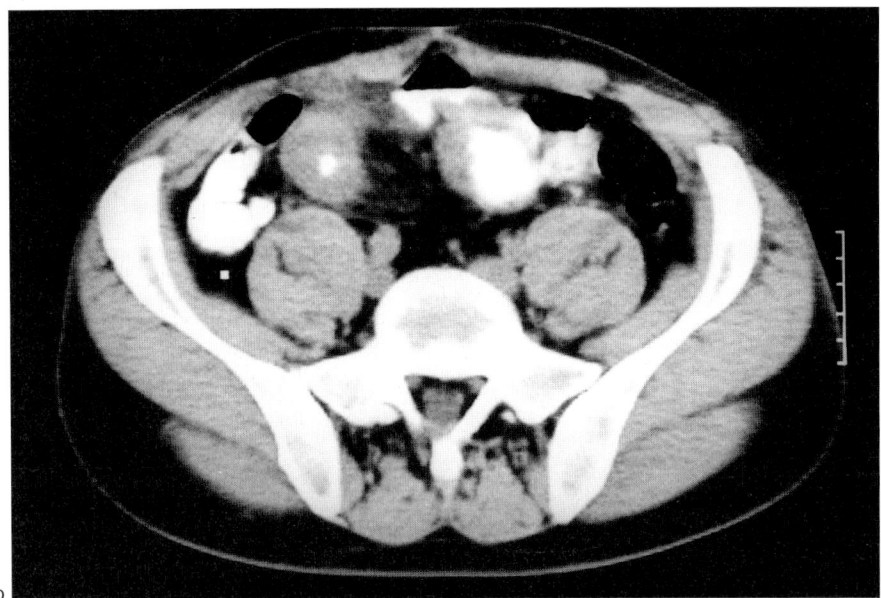

Fig. 26.7 (Cont'd) **b** The retroperitoneal fat measured −100 Hounsfield units.

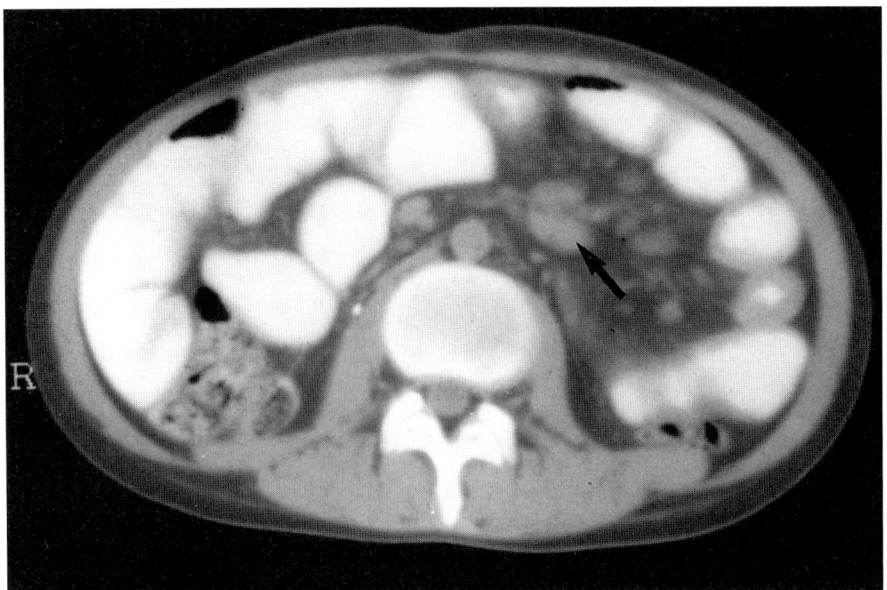

Fig. 26.8 Quite marked mesenteric lymphadenopathy is seen in this patient with Crohn's disease (arrow). There was no evidence of underlying lymphoma.

CT may be used in the detection and evaluation of bladder involvement by Crohn's disease, which can cause focal wall thickening adjacent to an extravesical soft tissue mass and/or focal bowel wall thickening. CT may demonstrate fistula formation with intravesical air (Merine et al 1989).

There is an increased incidence of adenocarcinoma of the colon and small bowel in patients with long-standing Crohn's disease: 31% of these lesions occur in bypassed segments of gut (Shorter 1985). These segments are not amenable to examination by conventional barium studies and CT can therefore be useful for detecting a tumor mass and staging local and distant disease.

CT can be performed following conventional sinogram or, if the opening cannot be cannulated, to show the relationship of the tract to adjacent structures (Fig. 26.11).

CT has been proved useful in the investigative workup of patients with Crohn's disease. In a study of 80 consecutive patients with clinically symptomatic disease (Fishman et al 1987), CT scanning provided information that altered the medical or surgical management of 28%

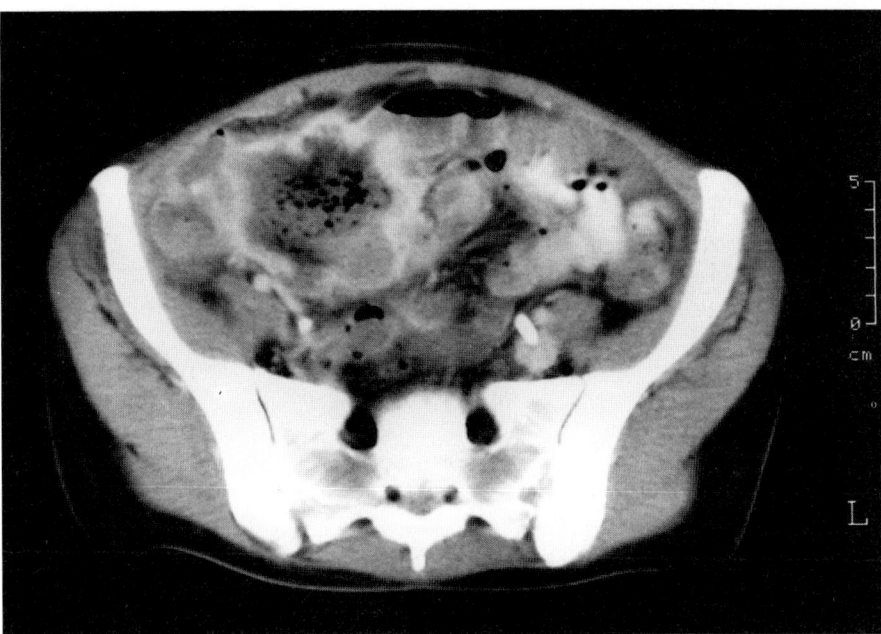

Fig. 26.9 This mesenteric abscess has a strongly enhancing capsule and contains gas.

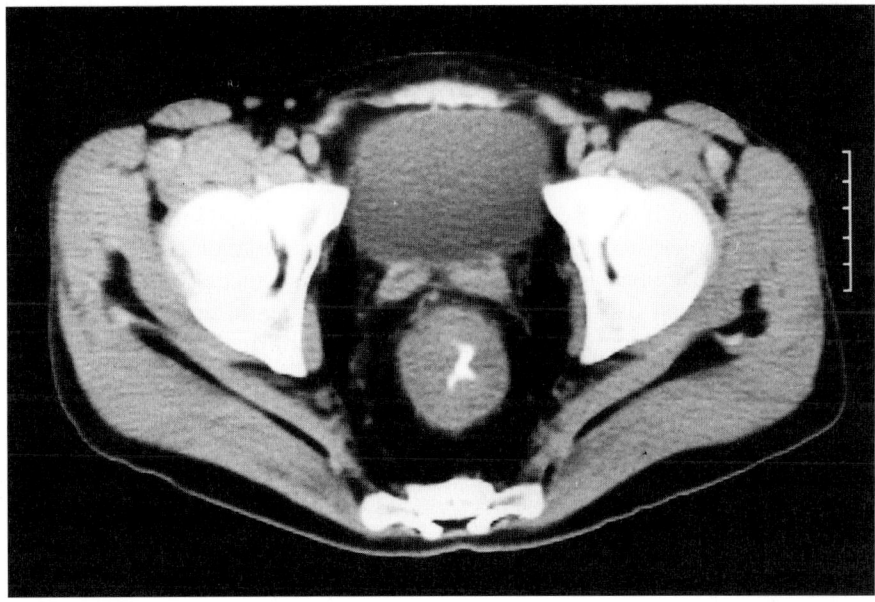

Fig. 26.10 Marked rectal wall thickening with some perirectal steaking is shown in this patient with severe perianal and rectal Crohn's disease.

of cases. These patients had fistulae, abscesses, avascular necrosis of the femoral head, sacral osteomyelitis, pelvic inflammatory disease and femoral vein thrombosis.

CT can be used to determine the cause of bowel loop separation or luminal narrowing, and to investigate patients with suspected sepsis. Some authors suggest that it should be the initial investigation in children known to have Crohn's disease, who have a changing pattern of clinical symptoms (Jabra et al 1991). It has also been suggested that it may be used to follow clinical activity. Both CT and small-bowel meal/enema use ionizing radiation. A recent paper from Hart et al (1994) estimated a mean effective dose to the patient for enteroclysis of 1.5 mSv. This study was performed in a teaching hospital by a radiologist with an interest in small-bowel examination. Doses received for small-bowel enema in several hospitals within the West Midlands region ranged from 6.2 to 13 mSv (Elizabeth McNeil, personal communication) – a routine CT scan of the abdomen has been said to give a mean effective dose of 7.16 mSv (Shrimpton et al 1991).

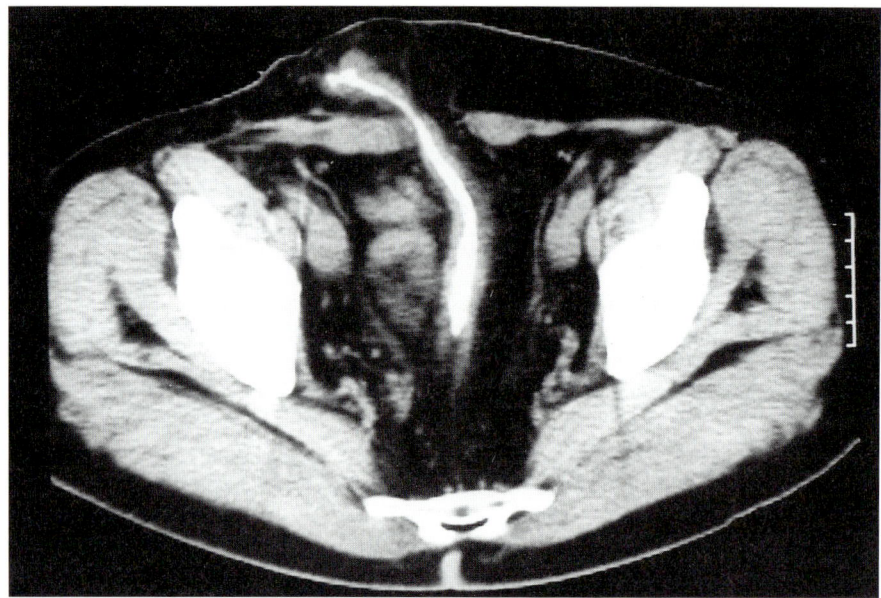

Fig. 26.11 The length of a sinus tract and its relationship to adjacent structures can be demonstrated by CT following a conventional sinogram.

CT examination may, however, be tailored to examine abnormal areas only, and thus this dose can be reduced.

CT scanning in ulcerative colitis

CT scanning is used less often in the investigation of patients with ulcerative colitis. Again barium and endoscopy will show early mucosal changes not appreciated on CT. In chronic ulcerative colitis wall thickening and lumen narrowing occur, and these changes can be appreciated. The degree of thickening is usually less than that seen in Crohn's disease. Unlike Crohn's disease the walls often have an inhomogeneous attenuation. Fatty infiltration of the mucosa can be found, with corresponding regions of low density on CT scans. Again, severe wall edema can cause reduction of wall attenuation (Fig. 26.12).

The colonic wall may be thinned in toxic megacolon, although CT should not routinely be used in this situation.

The accumulation of fat in the presacral space in patients with chronic ulcerative colitis will increase the diameter of the space, and this will be appreciated on CT. This fat appears abnormal on CT, with added streaky soft tissue

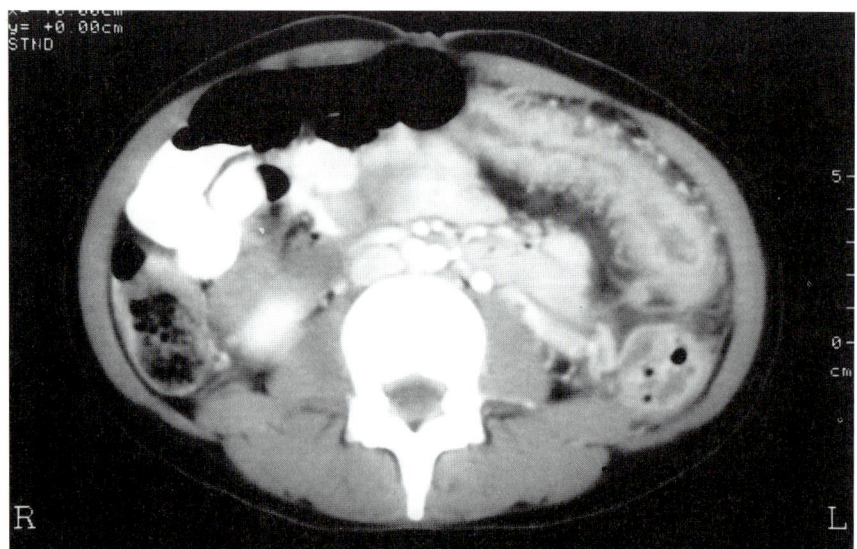

Fig. 26.12 CT demonstrating severely inflamed transverse and descending colon in a patient with ulcerative colitis. The ascending colon appears normal.

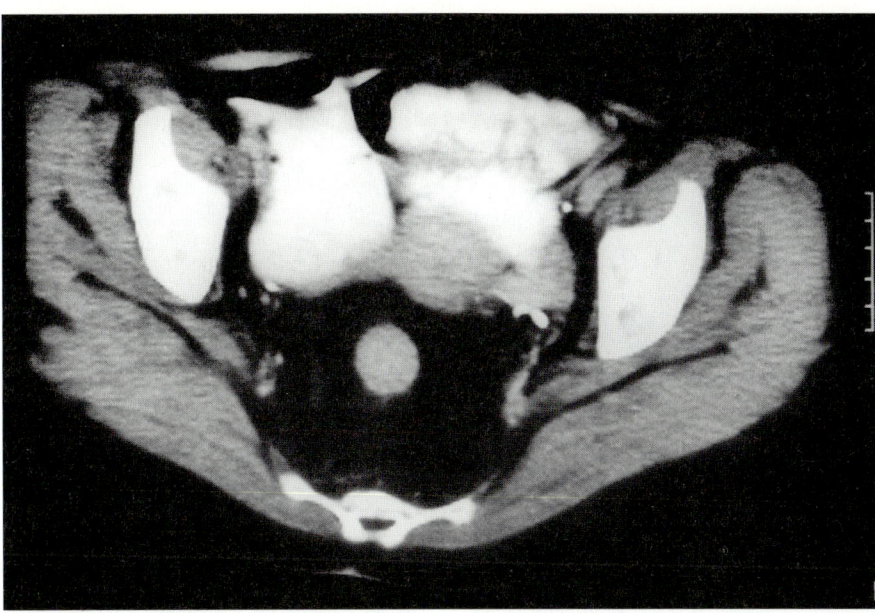

Fig. 26.13 There is a marked increase in the diameter of the presacral fat in this patient with long-standing ulcerative colitis, and streaking densities are seen within it.

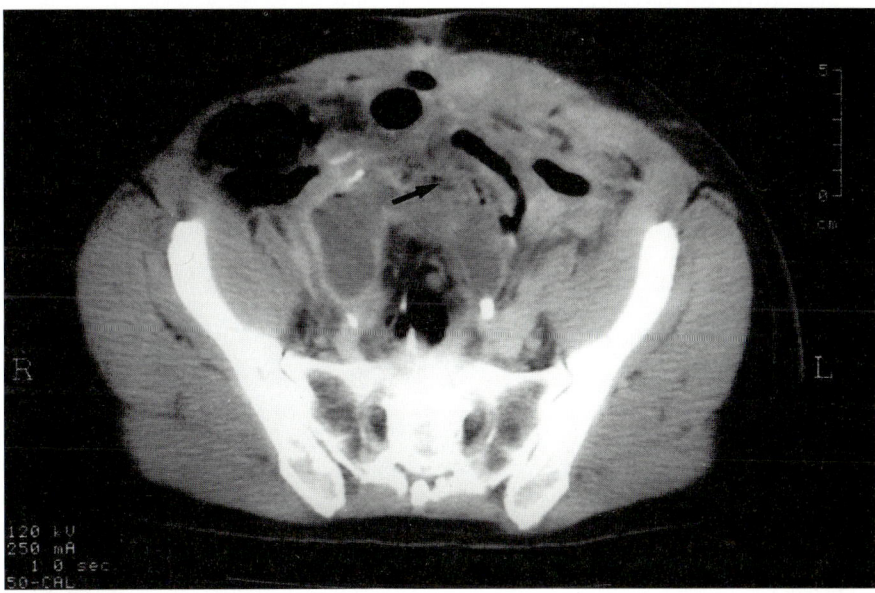

Fig. 26.14 CT scan showing the upper portion of an ileoanal reservoir. There is an abnormal collection of gas anteriorly (arrow). Several abscesses were found at surgery.

densities within it (Fig. 26.13). Enlarged lymph nodes can again be seen in patients with ulcerative colitis, especially in the perirectal region and also within the mesentery.

In patients with an ileoanal reservoir (pouch) contrast may be instilled into the pouch at the time of CT scanning to demonstrate postoperative complications such as leak or pelvic abscess. CT will show a healthy reservoir close to the sacrum, but following surgery fibrosis can occur. The pouch usually has well defined margins and its afferent and efferent limbs can be traced (Fig. 26.14).

MRI in Crohn's disease

MRI is becoming the imaging modality of choice for the investigation of perianal and perirectal fistulae (Koelber et al 1989). Its ability to image in the sagittal, coronal and axial planes, and its excellent soft tissue contrast, allows delineation of the fistulous tracts and demonstration of their relationship to the pelvic floor muscles, with determination of the internal opening and the relationship of the tract to the external and internal sphincters (Fig. 26.15).

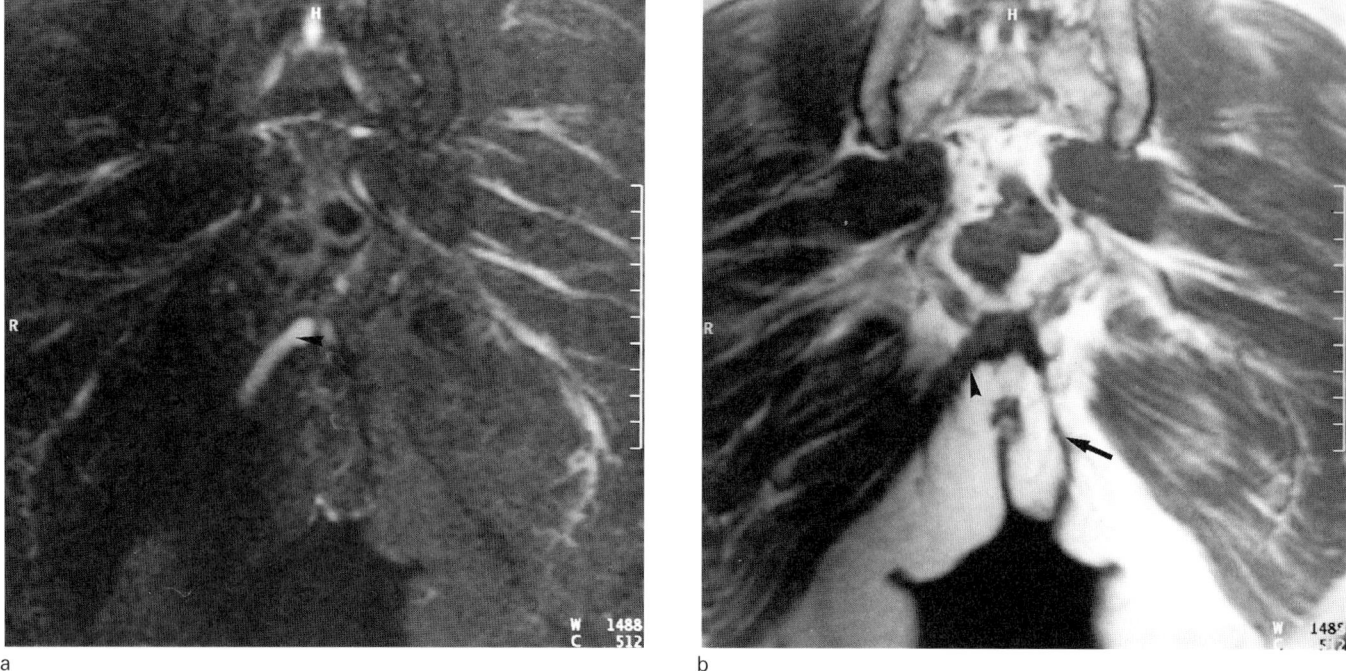

Fig. 26.15a Coronal MRI scan, the STIR sequence suppresses signal from fat. There is a transsphincteric tract on the right which is of high signal (arrow) and consistent with inflammation. **b** The corresponding T_1-weighted spin echo coronal image demonstrates another left-sided tract (arrow), which is of low signal on both sequences and is therefore fibrotic. The right-sided tract is also seen (arrowhead).

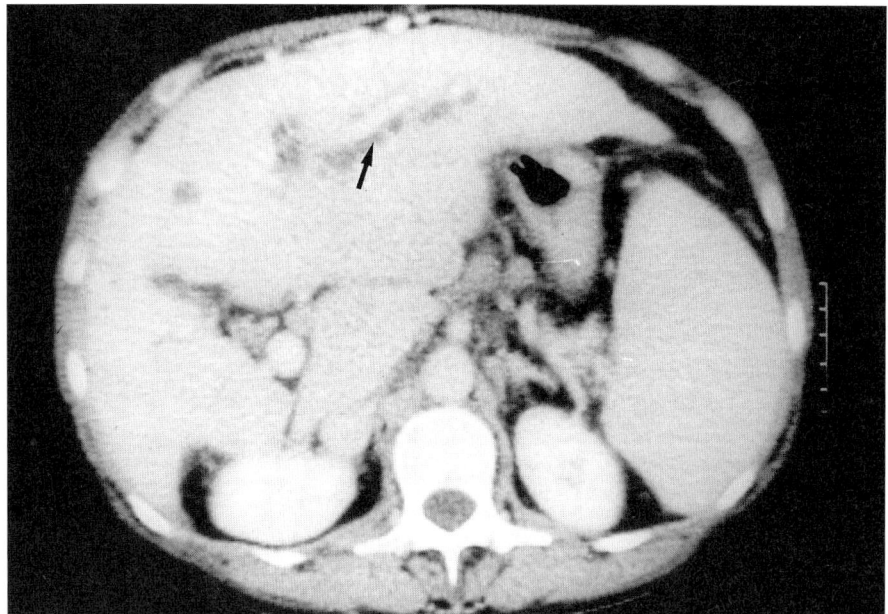

Fig. 26.16 CT scan of the liver in a patient with sclerosing cholangitis, demonstrating irregular duct dilation in the left lobe (arrow) and an atrophic right lobe.

Although endoanal ultrasound has also established a role, its limited field of view is its major disadvantage here. A recent study (Barker et al 1994) showed concordance rates between MRI and operative findings of 86% for the presence and course of the primary tract, 91% for the presence and site of secondary extensions or abscesses, and 97% for the presence of horseshoeing.

EXTRAINTESTINAL FEATURES OF INFLAMMATORY BOWEL DISEASE

Hepatobiliary complications

Fatty infiltration of the liver is a common finding in patients with Crohn's disease and can be diffuse or focal. On CT scanning this results in reduced attenuation of the liver, and vessels running through these regions have a higher attenuation than surrounding fatty liver. The incidence of gallstones is also increased in patients with Crohn's disease. Ultrasound is the imaging modality of choice for the diagnosis of cholelithiasis and possible biliary obstruction. Sclerosing cholangitis is seen more commonly in patients with ulcerative colitis, but can occur in patients with Crohn's disease. Irregular dilatation of the intrahepatic ducts can be appreciated (Rahn et al 1983) on CT, ultrasound and MRI, but endoscopic cholangiography (ERCP) remains the best imaging modality. The right lobe of the liver is often atrophic compared to the left (Fig. 26.16). Patients with sclerosing cholangitis develop portal hypertension, and features consistent with this can be seen on all scanning modalities, e.g. collateral vessels and splenomegaly. There is an increased incidence of cholangiocarcinoma in these patients. These tumors can be very difficult to diagnose with any cross-sectional imaging modality and are better detected by a combination of cholangiography and guided cytology or biopsy. This is because the tumors often invade along the ductal walls and large masses may not be visible. If a large mass is present this may be seen on CT as an area of low attenuation following a dynamic contrast-enhanced scan of the liver, and on ultrasound it may be recognized as a hypoechoic mass. It has been suggested that cholangiocarcinoma will retain contrast and appear as areas of increased attenuation if delayed scans are obtained following i.v. contrast-enhanced CT (Takayasu et al 1990).

REFERENCES

Alexander-Williams J 1982 Surgical management. In: Rachmilewitz D (ed) Inflammatory bowel disease. Nijhoff, Boston, pp 269–291

Barker P G Lunniss P J, Armstrong P, Reznek R H, Cottam K, Phillips R K 1994 Magnetic resonance imaging of fistula in ano: technique, interpretation and accuracy. Clinical Radiology 49: 7–13

Dubbins P A 1984 Ultrasound demonstration of bowel wall thickness in inflammatory bowel disease. Clinical Radiology 35: 227

Fishman E K, Wolf E J, Jones B et al 1987 CT evaluation of Crohn's disease: effect on patient management. American Journal of Roentgenology 148: 537–549

Frager D H, Goldman M, Beneventano T C 1983 Computed tomography in Crohn's disease. Journal of Computerised Assisted Tomography 7: 819–824

Goldberg H T, Gore R M, Margulis A R et al 1983 Computed tomography in the evaluation of Crohn's disease. American Journal of Roentgenology 140: 277–282

Gore R M 1989 CT of inflammatory bowel disease. Radiologic Clinics of North America 27: 717–729

Halvorsen R A, Korobkin M, Foster W L, Silverman P M, Thompson W M 1984 The variable CT appearance of hepatic abscesses. American Journal of Roentgenology 142: 941–946

Hart D, Haggett P J, Borderman P, Nolan D J, Wall B F 1994 Patient radiation doses from enteroclysis examinations. British Journal of Radiology 67: 997–1000

Jabra A, Fishman E K, Taylor G A 1991 Crohn's disease in the pediatric patient: CT evaluation. Radiology 179: 495–498

Jones B, Fishman E K, Hamilton S R et al 1986 Submucosal accumulation of fat in inflammatory bowel disease: CT/pathologic correlation. Journal of Computerised Assisted Tomography 10: 759–763

Kerber G W, Greenberg M, Rubin J M 1984 Computed tomography evaluation of local extra-intestinal complications of Crohn's disease. Gastrointestinal Radiology 9: 143–148

Khaw K T, Yeoman L J, Saverymutu S H et al 1991 Ultrasonic patterns in inflammatory bowel disease. Clinical Radiology 43: 171

Kimi M B, Wang K Y, Huggett R C et al 1990 Diagnosis of inflammatory bowel disease with ultrasound: an in-vitro study. Investigative Radiology 25: 1085

Koelber G, Schmiedl G, Majer M C et al 1989 Diagnosis of fistulae and sinus tracts in patients with Crohn's disease: value of MR imaging. American Journal of Roentgenology 152: 999–1003

Lambiase R A, Cronan J J, Dorfman G F et al 1988 Percutaneous drainage of abscesses in patients with Crohn's disease. American Journal of Roentgenology 150: 1043–1046

Mathieu D, Zasile N, Grenier P 1985 Portal thrombosis: dynamic CT features and course. Radiology 154: 737–741

Merine D, Fishman E K, Kuhlman J G, Jones B, Bayless T M, Siegelmarc S 1989 Bladder involvement in Crohn's disease: role of CT in detection and evaluation. Journal of Computer Assisted Tomography 13: 90–93

Rahn N H, Koehler R E, Weyman P J et al 1983 CT appearance of sclerosing cholangitis. American Journal of Roentgenology 141: 549–552

Shorter R G 1985 Risks of intestinal cancer in Crohn's disease: Diseases of the Colon and Rectum 26: 686–689

Shrimpton P C, Jones D G, Hiller M C et al 1991 Survey of CT practice in the UK, Part II: Dosimetric aspects. National Radiological Protection Board

Takayasu K et al 1990 CT of hilar cholangiocarcinoma: late contrast enhancement in six patients. American Journal of Roentgenology 154: 1203–1206

Yousmen D M, Fishman E K, Jones B 1988 Crohn's disease: perirectal and perianal findings at CT. Radiology 167: 331–334

27. Radiology – isotope scanning

A. M. Peters   J. P. Lavender

INTRODUCTION

There are several agents available for radionuclide imaging of inflammatory bowel disease (IBD), including radiolabeled autologous leukocytes, polyclonal immunoglobulin, antigranulocyte monoclonal antibodies and, more recently, monoclonal antibodies which recognize activated endothelial adhesion molecules. The most important and widely used are labeled leukocytes.

LABELED WHITE CELLS

Radiolabeled leukocytes or granulocytes have become established as a routine means of localizing various forms of inflammatory disease and infections, including IBD and intra-abdominal and soft tissue sepsis associated with IBD (Thakur et al 1977, Peters et al 1983, 1986, Roddie et al 1988). Leukocytes can be labeled with ^{111}In (Thakur et al 1977, Peters et al 1983) (physical half-life 28 days) or ^{99m}Tc (Peters et al 1986, Roddie et al 1988) (half-life 6 hours). ^{99m}Tc offers several advantages in respect of cost, convenience, image resolution and radiation dosimetry (Peters 1994).

Cell labeling

The principle of cell labeling is that when blood cells are exposed to a radioactive lipophilic metal–chelate complex, they are indiscriminately labeled as a result of nonspecific penetration of the cell membrane by the lipophilic complex (McAfee & Thakur 1976). The cells to be labeled have to be first separated from the other blood cell types. ^{111}In is firmly retained within the cell, although the precise intracellular binding sites are not clearly known. Because of competition between intracellular and plasma proteins for the available ^{111}In, the labeling efficiency, i.e. the percentage of the available ^{111}In taken up by the cell during labeling, is higher when the cells are labeled in saline. ^{111}In oxine and ^{111}In tropolonate are the most widely used complexes: the latter has the advantage of a higher labeling efficiency in plasma-enriched medium (Peters et al 1983). This is important with respect to the ultimate viability and behavior of the cells, which is impaired if the cells are comletely deprived of plasma in the suspending medium (Saverymuttu et al 1983a).

^{99m}Tc-hexamethyleneamine oxime (HMPAO) (Peters et al 1986, Roddie et al 1988) is also a lipophilic complex and readily penetrates blood cells. After entering the cell it becomes hydrophilic and is trapped inside. Its profile of labeling efficiencies across different blood cell types is similar to ^{111}In tropolonate, with some degree of selectivity for granulocytes. It is not as stably bound by blood cells as ^{111}In (Peters et al 1988).

For some clinical indications 'pure' granulocytes are preferable to so-called 'mixed' leukocytes, which contain contaminating red cells and platelets. Because of their radiosensitivity, lymphocytes probably fail to survive after being labeled with ^{111}In. Isolation of 'pure' granulocytes is achieved by centrifugation on a density-gradient, which consists of a dense material, such as metrizamide or Percoll, mixed with saline, or preferably autologous plasma, in varying ratios. The less dense mixtures are layered on top of the more dense to produce a discontinuous gradient. The mixed leukocyte preparation is placed at the top and, after centrifugation, the different blood cells, depending on their size and density, sediment to different gradient interfaces. Labeled granulocytes should be used for kinetic or quantitative studies, or when the patient has a low peripheral granulocyte count. Otherwise, mixed leukocytes are adequate for routine imaging.

Cell labeling with ^{99m}Tc offers the advantage of convenience because ^{99m}Tc is eluted from a 'generator', whereas ^{111}In is delivered on a weekly basis. Furthermore, because of its shorter half-life, ^{99m}Tc-labeled cells give a lower radiation dose than ^{111}In.

Kinetics of labeled leukocytes and normal distribution

The early normal distribution of radiolabeled leukocytes or granulocytes (1–3 h after injection) reflects the distribution of the marginated granulocyte pool, which in normal humans accounts for about half of the total blood granulocyte pool (Athens et al 1961) and is mostly in the liver, lungs, bone marrow, and especially the spleen (Peters et al 1985). The circulating granulocyte pool (i.e. the difference between the marginated pool and the total blood granulocyte pool) can be seen on early images as blood pool radioactivity in the cardiac chambers and major vessels. In-vitro manipulation, particularly separation on density-gradient columns, exposes granulocytes to damage or activation, which may lead to premature removal from the blood. The most sensitive criterion of granulocyte integrity following labeling is therefore the 'recovery', which is the fraction of injected labeled cells present in the circulating granulocyte pool at about 45 minutes after injection, when they have equilibrated throughout their marginated pools (Peters et al 1988). ^{99m}Tc and ^{111}In labeled leukocytes show similar kinetics and give similar recoveries in blood (Peters et al 1988).

^{111}In granulocytes circulate in blood with a half-life of about 6 hours. In the absence of inflammatory disease they are destroyed in the reticuloendothelial system at random, thereby giving an exponential blood disappearance curve (Saverymuttu et al 1985b). The half-life of ^{99m}Tc-labeled granulocytes is shorter, at about 4 hours. This is the result of ^{99m}Tc elution rather than a manifestation of cell damage; correction of elution, based on in-vitro data, gives a half-life of about 6 hours. Images taken 24 hours after injection, when the circulating cell-bound activity has been cleared, show an image of the reticuloendothelial system (Saverymuttu et al 1985b). Stability of the label in 'targeted' tissue, whether normal or abnormal, is obviously important, and it is less for ^{99m}Tc than for ^{111}In (Peters et al 1988).

^{99m}Tc-labeled leukocytes show additional normal features not seen on ^{111}In scans. These include non-specific bowel activity, seen from about 3 hours after injection, urinary activity, and occasionally gallbladder activity, all of which are the result of the excretion of secondary hydrophilic complexes of ^{99m}Tc HMPAO (Roddie et al 1988). Gallbladder activity suggests that biliary excretion of these complexes is the basis for the non-specific bowel activity, although whereas colonic activity is seen in virtually all patients by 24 hours, gallbladder activity is seen in less than 10% of patients at any time.

The non-specific bowel activity is a problem with ^{99m}Tc HMPAO-labeled leukocytes, particularly in the imaging of IBD and abdominal collections. Since it does not appear for at least 3 hours after injection, it can be circumvented by early imaging. The resolution and count density offered by ^{99m}Tc compensate for this need to image early, when the majority of the injected labeled cells are still present in the circulation. Renal and urinary activity can almost always be identified as such, although bladder activity may interfere with rectal imaging. Their clear separation requires an outlet view, in which the pelvis is imaged with the patient sitting on the camera face (see below).

Applications in IBD

Labeled leukocytes and/or granulocytes have several applications in IBD, including localization of segments of active inflammation, identification of complications such as intra-abdominal sepsis, quantification of disease activity, imaging the extra-abdominal manifestations of IBD, and assessment of new forms of treatment.

The basis for disease localization and quantification is early migration of labeled granulocytes into segments of inflamed bowel, rapidly followed by migration into the bowel lumen and distal intraluminal transit (Fig. 27.1). The label itself is ultimately excreted in the feces. Imaging must therefore be early (within 3 h) in order to identify the sites within the gastrointestinal tract where the cells

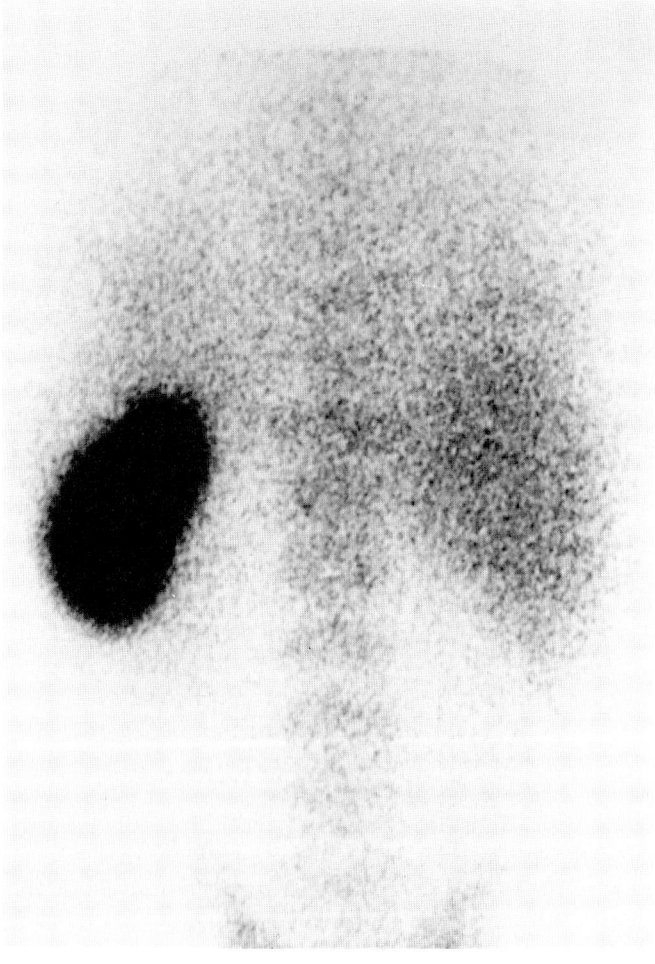

Fig. 27.1 Distribution of ^{99m}Tc-labeled leukocytes (posterior view) in a patient with inactive inflammatory bowel disease 1 hour after injection. Note prominent splenic, hepatic and bone marrow activity representing physiological leukocyte distribution. The lungs are also prominent, slightly more so than in the normal subject.

are migrating. Late images simply demonstrate distal intraluminal transit of labeled cells that have migrated more proximally. In this respect, leukocyte scanning in IBD is analogous to ^{99m}Tc-labeled red cell imaging for the localization of gastrointestinal bleeding.

Imaging for identification of diseased segments

Imaging may help to diagnose and localize IBD in patients presenting with chronic diarrhea who do not have a diagnosis, or to assess recurrence in patients with known chronic disease in whom other radiological studies may be difficult to interpret. ^{99m}Tc-labeled cells have now essentially replaced ^{111}In for this purpose, because of their superiority in localizing disease to specific bowel segments, particularly small bowel (Arndt et al 1993, Scholmerich et al 1988, Allen et al 1993, Lantto et al 1991) (Fig. 27.2). ^{111}In leukocytes, although giving reliable images of the colon (Saverymuttu et al 1982), may miss small-bowel disease. This is not only because of inferior image resolution, but also because the small bowel is mobile and its contents are in rapid transit. The shorter imaging time with ^{99m}Tc minimizes movement artefacts during image acquisition. The localization of ^{99m}Tc-labeled leukocytes in inflamed bowel is extremely rapid: Lantto et al (1991) have claimed to obtain clearly abnormal images as early as 2 minutes after injection, although others have made more modest claims (Weldon et al 1993).

Crohn's disease and ulcerative colitis can usually be distinguished from each other from the distribution of disease activity (Saverymuttu et al 1988). Thus, rectal sparing, small-bowel involvement and skip areas suggest Crohn's disease (Fig. 27.3), whereas continuous involvement from the rectum, without small-bowel involvement, suggests ulcerative colitis (Fig. 27.4). In Crohn's disease, fistulae involving the urinary tract may be difficult to assess with ^{99m}Tc because of urinary activity, and therefore have to be imaged early in order to avoid confusion with non-specific bowel activity. ^{111}In-labeled cells may be preferable in this setting.

IBD, especially Crohn's disease, may be associated with intra-abdominal sepsis. In Crohn's disease, abdominal abscesses not infrequently communicate with the bowel lumen, and cells migrating into the abscess may gain access to the bowel lumen and pass distally in the feces. Because they arrive in the lumen later than cells migrating directly into the abscess, the typical appearance of a communicating abscess is early discrete localization in the abdomen, followed several hours later by activity in the bowel lumen (Saverymuttu et al 1985a) (Fig. 27.5). Delayed imaging at 48 hours may be useful in order to demonstrate persistence of activity at the site of the abscess. Because of its physiological excretion in bowel and the short physical half-life, ^{99m}Tc-labeled cells are not suitable in patients with suspected communicating abscess, and ^{111}In is preferable.

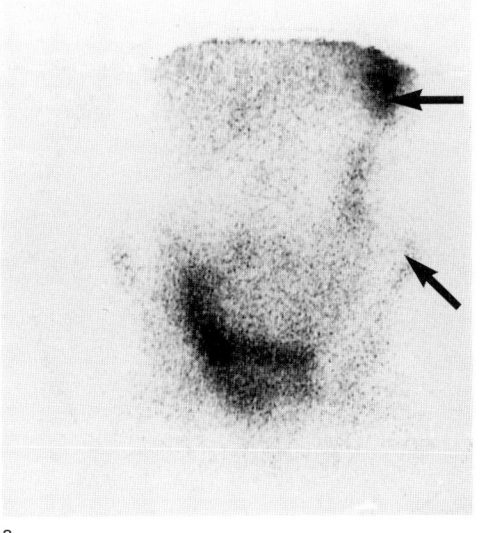 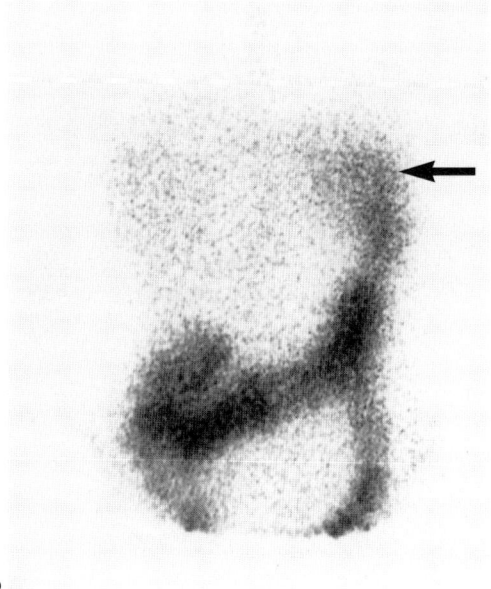

a

b

Fig. 27.2 Abnormal anterior abdominal ^{111}In-labeled granulocyte scan in a young adult with Crohn's disease. **a** The 3-hour image shows evidence of active distal small bowel disease and colitis involving the proximal descending colon. **b** The 24-hour image shows abnormal activity throughout the colon. This is due to distal intraluminal transit of migrated labeled cells, which are all ultimately excreted in the feces and quantification of which, in a 4-day fecal collection, allows assessment of overall disease activity. Note the decrease in prominence of splenic and marrow activities (arrows) between the images, reflecting recruitment of cells from splenic and marrow pools for migration between 3 and 24 hours.

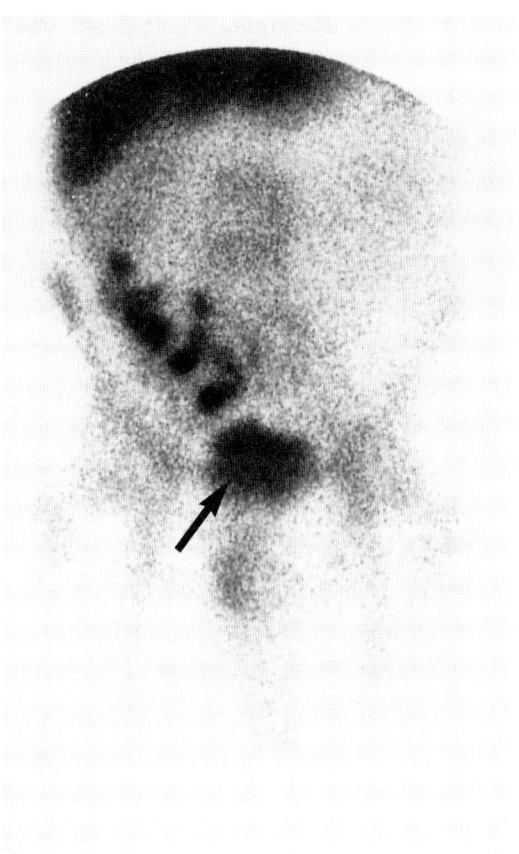

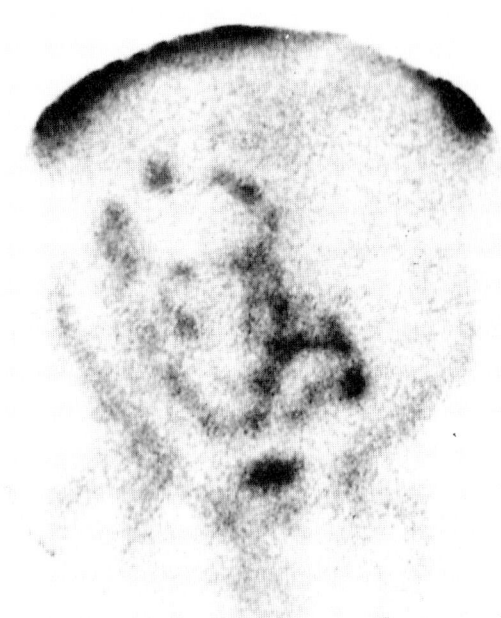

Fig. 27.4 Small-bowel Crohn's disease imaged with ^{99m}Tc-HMPAO-labeled leukocytes and showing clear evidence of skip lesions.

Fig. 27.3 Abnormal ^{99m}Tc-HMPAO leukocyte scan (2-hour image) in a young patient with Crohn's disease involving loops of distal small bowel. Urinary activity in the bladder (arrow) is normal. Note the improved resolution compared with Figure 27.2**a**.

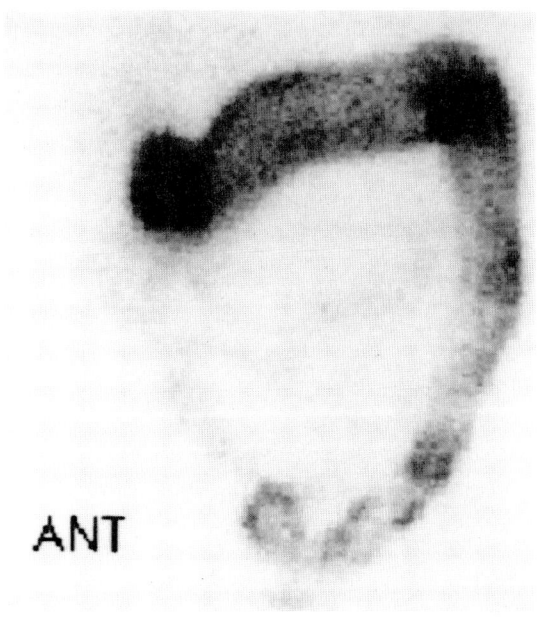

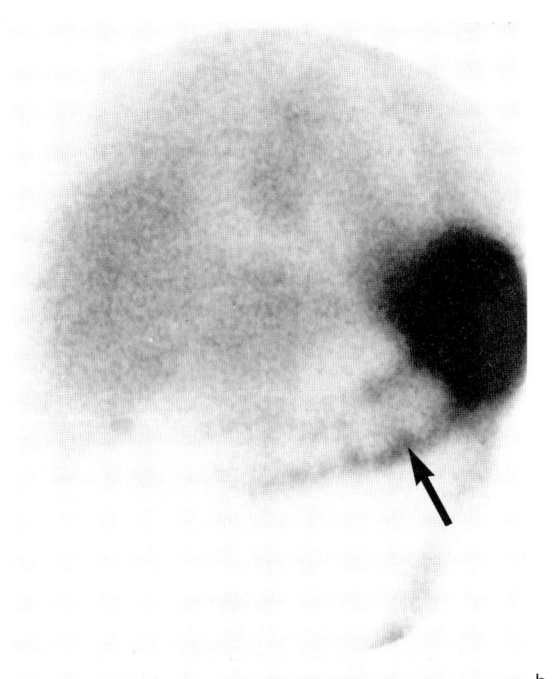

Fig. 27.5 ^{99m}Tc-HMPAO leukocyte scans in two patients with toxic megacolon complicating ulcerative colitis. In **a** the colon is continuously involved from rectum to hepatic flexure, whereas, in **b** the disease involves up to mid-transverse colon. Note the extensive dilatation in **a** and the localized dilatation (arrow) in **b**.

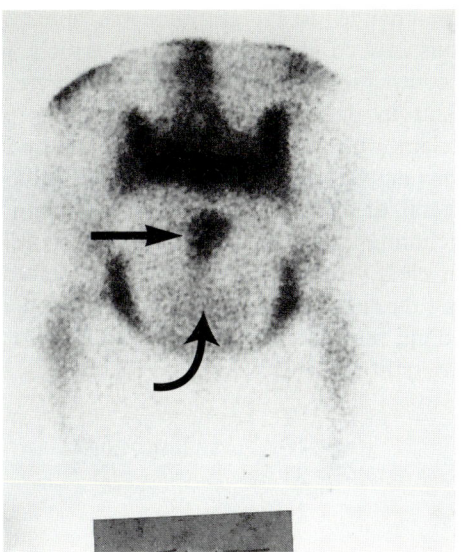

Fig. 27.6 Pelvic outlet view (^{99m}Tc-HMPAO) showing abnormal rectal uptake (straight arrow) behind the bladder (curved arrow), indicative of proctitis.

Because of non-specific bowel activity, sequential imaging with ^{99m}Tc-labeled leukocytes is obviously important in IBD. It also modifies the accuracy of the technique. Thus, as Almer et al (1992) have shown, segments positive at 1 hour and showing increased positivity at 4 hours have a high positive predictive value (97% versus endoscopy and 80% versus histology), in contrast to segments which are negative at 1 hour and become positive at 4 hours (positive predictive value of 73% versus endoscopy and 53% versus histology) or equally positive at both times (96% versus endoscopy and 70% versus histology). In addition to non-specific bowel activity, urinary activity may obscure pathological uptake of ^{99m}Tc-labeled leukocytes in the bowel, although this problem can usually be circumvented by a pelvic outlet view, obtained with the patient sitting on the camera face (Fig. 27.6).

Uptake of labeled leukocytes in segments of bowel is not specific for Crohn's disease and ulcerative colitis, but is also seen in a variety of other gastrointestinal inflammatory conditions, including gastritis, acute infections, vasculitis (Jonker et al 1992a), radiation enteritis, graft versus host disease (Saverymuttu et al 1986), pseudo-membranous colitis, and after excessive use of non-steroidal analgesics. Causes of false positive leukocyte scans for inflamed bowel include recent anastomosis and gastrointestinal bleeding, in which the circulating labeled cells behave as if they were labeled red cells. Copious radioactivity may also be seen in the bowel in patients with intrathoracic sepsis, who may cough up and swallow labeled cells (Currie et al 1987). Swallowed activity is not usually seen in the abdomen until several hours after injection of the cells, and so this is more a problem with ^{111}In-labeled cells. Communicating abscess and sepsis within the biliary tree are other potential causes of a false positive scan for IBD.

Quantification of disease activity

The gold standard for quantification of disease activity is measurement of the total ^{111}In excreted in a 4-day fecal collection (Saverymuttu et al 1983b). This provides an accurate assessment of disease extent and activity because all the granulocytes migrating into the bowel wall in IBD continue to migrate into the bowel lumen and are excreted in the stools. This test should be performed with ^{111}In labeled 'pure' granulocytes, since the fecal ^{111}In is expressed in relation to the injected dose; any activity on formed elements other than granulocytes will lead to underestimation of the disease activity. Alternatively, the fraction of the ^{111}In associated with granulocytes in the injected dose can be measured from a small aliquot of the injectate, after cell separation, on a suitable density-gradient column. Patients with active IBD may lose up to 80% of their injected granulocyte-associated ^{111}In; patients with IBD in remission usually have a marginally abnormal ^{111}In excretion, but patients with irritable bowel syndrome or non-inflammatory forms of bowel disease such as colonic carcinoma excrete less than 2%. These low values are important, since they offer no support for the view that granulocytes normally leave the circulation in a scavenging role in the tissues, including the gastro-intestinal tract.

As an esthetically preferable alternative, fecal excretion can be calculated from whole-body ^{111}In counting (Carpani de Kaski et al 1992). This is feasible because in normal individuals $95 \pm 5\%$ of injected ^{111}In is retained at 5 days (Currie et al 1987). Using an imaging dose of ^{111}In-labeled granulocytes, a conventional gamma camera, with its collimator removed, can be used to count the whole-body radioactivity. The erect patient is counted from a distance of 4 m for a period of 2 minutes from both anterior and posterior projections. This is performed at about 3 hours after injection, before any activity has been lost, and again at 4 days. A standard is counted at the same time from the same distance. The percentage loss of ^{111}In is calculated from the decrease in the geometric mean of anterior and posterior counts, corrected for physical decay of the radionuclide, between the first and second measurements, or by comparison with the standard, assuming that no ^{111}In has been lost at the time of the first measurement. Whole-body counting can be performed on outpatients, an advantage over a 4-day fecal collection, which has been shown to be reliable only in supervised patients (Carpani de Kaski et al 1992). Whole-body counting slightly overestimates fecal ^{111}In excretion because of losses in other body fluids, although these only amount to about 5% (Saverymuttu et al 1985b).

Fecal counting cannot be applied to ^{99m}Tc-labeled leukocytes because of the short physical half-life of the radionuclide and the non-specific fecal ^{99m}Tc excretion. Several alternative approaches have been applied which generally depend on quantifying the intensity of abnormal uptake on early gamma camera images (Giaffer et al 1993, Tindale et al 1992). The main disadvantage of these approaches is that they are critically dependent on the time after injection, and therefore on rates of granulocyte localization, extent of intraluminal transit of radioactivity, and size of the marginating pools, particularly the spleen. Accordingly, Almer et al have recently demonstrated no superiority of these computerized quantification techniques over subjective visual assessment against the gold standards of endoscopy and histology (Almer et al, in press).

The radiation dose from any radionuclide investigation is conventionally expressed in terms of the effective dose equivalent (EDE), which takes into account the target organs and their susceptibility to radiation, as well as the amount of radioactivity administered. For the usual imaging doses, about 200 MBq for ^{99m}Tc and 15 MBq for ^{111}In-labeled cells, the respective EDEs are 3 mSv and 9 mSv. These compare with about 4 ± 2 mSv for a barium meal and 8 ± 4 mSv for a barium enema, although doses from such radiological procedures are less precise because of variations in the number of exposures. Because of the relatively high EDE of ^{111}In, ^{99m}Tc HMPAO is generally preferred for pediatric studies. The dose, especially from ^{99m}Tc, should not, however, deter regular follow-up with white cell scanning if there is a genuine clinical need; a barium study gives at least as high a dose and is likely to be performed as an alternative. Other than at presentation, there is little justification for performing a white cell scan *and* a barium study. For the assessment of disease activity, a white cell scan is generally preferred.

Extraintestinal manifestations in IBD

Imaging of the lung with labeled granulocytes has turned out to be of interest in IBD because of recent evidence of abnormalities of granulocyte traffic in the lungs of patients with IBD, and of subtle degrees of lung injury as shown by pulmonary ^{99m}Tc-DTPA aerosol clearance (Lecouffe et al 1990).

In patients with IBD the early lung signal is frequently increased, although this is not accompanied by a reduced recovery or abnormal cell biodistribution, and therefore represents a real abnormality of pulmonary granulocyte traffic (Jonker et al 1992b, Ussov et al 1994, in press). This elevated lung activity decreases broadly in proportion to the decreasing blood activity, implying reversible pooling in the lung. The mechanism of the increased pooling is uncertain, although, as can be shown by a shape-change assay, granulocytes show increased spontaneous in-vivo activation in IBD, which, insofar as this is accompanied by increased granulocyte stiffness, would result in delayed pulmonary vascular transit. A close correlation has recently been demonstrated between spontaneous activation and pulmonary granulocyte pooling in several diseases associated with systemic inflammation, including IBD (Ussov et al, submitted) (Fig. 27.7).

It is not clearly known whether this increased pooling causes lung damage. Nevertheless, comparison of granulocyte pooling and granulocyte migration into the pulmonary interstitium with ^{99m}Tc-DTPA aerosol clearance

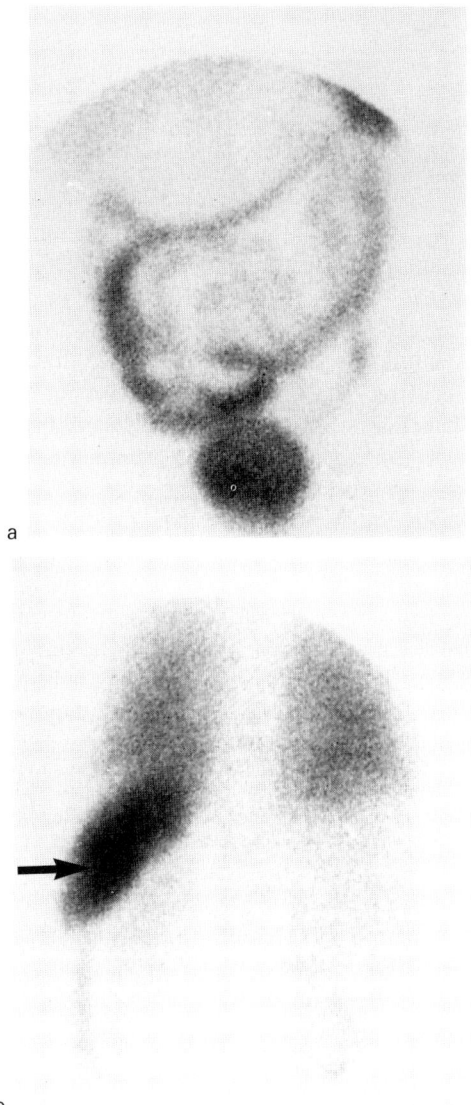

Fig. 27.7 ^{99m}Tc-HMPAO leukocyte scan (2 h) in a patient with severe enteric graft-versus-host disease. Extensive abnormal bowel uptake can be seen in **a**, an anterior view over the abdomen. Diffuse increased pulmonary can also be seen **b** (posterior view) associated with a normal distribution of activity between liver and spleen (arrowed). The patient had no overt respiratory difficulties. A very similar picture is not infrequently seen in inflammatory bowel disease.

as a sensitive index of lung damage, suggests that if the cells migrate lung injury may result (Ussov et al, submitted). Although not on the same scale as in acute lung injury, such as adult respiratory distress syndrome, there is a low level of pulmonary granulocyte migration in IBD (Ussov et al 1994 & submitted), and this may account for the pulmonary abnormalities occasionally encountered in this condition (Eade et al 1980, Camus et al 1993).

OTHER AGENTS AND FUTURE DIRECTIONS

Radiolabeled human immunoglobulin (HIG) (Datz et al 1994) and antigranulocyte monoclonal antibodies (Segarra et al 1991) have been claimed to give good results in IBD, but they are not yet established as routine diagnostic agents. Uptake of HIG is probably non-specific via a compromised vascular endothelium, although if labeled with ^{111}In the label appears to be retained in the extravascular space. Antigranulocyte monoclonal antibodies target the bone marrow because of its enormous number of myeloid cells; there is very little labeling of circulating granulocytes, so the mechanism of uptake in inflamed tissue is not clear. Radioactivity localizing in inflamed bowel remains extraluminal, thereby facilitating localization of disease. Phagocytic labeling of leukocytes, in which the cells are labeled by offering them labeled colloid for phagocytosis (Pullman et al 1988), was briefly popular, although since the recovery of intact labeled granulocytes is so low, the mechanism of uptake in inflammation is obscure. A novel technique is the targeting of activated endothelial molecules with specific radiolabeled monoclonal antibodies (Jamar et al, submitted). ^{111}In-labeled anti-E-selectin, for example, has recently been successfully used to image inflamed bowel and synovitis. The antibody is internalized, so that the radioactivity remains at the site of inflammation.

CONCLUSION

With the increasing refinement of conventional radiological techniques for imaging IBD, such as small bowel enema (Dixon et al 1993), ultrasonography (Holt 1992) and air enema (Lindstroma Noren 1992), as well as non-radiological techniques such as gut lavage (Choudari et al 1993), the precise role of leukocyte scintigraphy in the clinical management of IBD needs to be clearly defined, especially with respect to the most appropriate investigation for exclusion of IBD in the patient with chronic diarrhea, follow-up of the patient with known disease, and the value of quantitative assessment of disease activity in the individual patient.

The use made of leukocyte scintigraphy within a gastroenterology unit will depend on the availability of the technique. It will nevertheless be seen to allow imaging of the entire gastrointestinal tract, as well as extra-intestinal manifestations of IBD, in one procedure, unlike radiology or endoscopy, and with a high diagnostic accuracy. Its most useful clinical role is probably in the assessment of recurrence and activity in known disease, and it is therefore a valuable tool in planning therapy. A major drawback of white cell scintigraphy is the time-consuming requirement for cell isolation in vitro. Recent developments outlined above may result in more direct and simpler imaging of inflammatory disease.

REFERENCES

Allan R A, Sladen G E, Bassingham S, Clarke S E M, Fogelman I 1993 Comparison of simultaneous ^{99m}Tc HMPAO and ^{111}In oxine labelled white cell scans in the assessment of inflammatory bowel disease. European Journal of Nuclear Medicine 20: 195–200

Almer S, Franzen L, Peters A M et al 1992 Do technetium-99m hexamethyleneamine oxime (HMPAO) labelled leukocytes truly reflect the mucosal inflammation in patients with ulcerative colitis? Scandinavian Journal of Gastroenterology 27: 1031–1038

Almer S, Peters A M, Ekberg S, Franzen L, Granerus G, Strom M. Do computer-aided interpretations of technetium-99m HMPAO leukocyte scans add anything to interpretation by naked eye? (submitted)

Arndt J-W, Van der Sluys Veer A, Blok D et al 1993 Prospective comparative study of technetium-99m WBCs and indium-111 granulocytes for the examination of patients with inflammatory bowel disease. Journal of Nuclear Medicine 34: 1052–1057

Athens J W, Mauer A M, Ashenbrucker H, Cartwright G E, Wintrobe M M 1961 Leukokinetic studies III. The distribution of granulocytes in the blood of normal subjects. Journal of Clinical Investigation 40: 159–164

Camus P, Piard F, Ashcroft T, Gal A A, Colby T V 1993 The lung in inflammatory bowel disease. Medicine 72: 151–183

Carpani de Kaski M, Peters A M, Knight D, Stuttle A W J, Lavender J P, Hodgson H J 1992 ^{111}In whole body retention: a new method for quantification of disease activity in inflammatory bowel disease. Journal of Nuclear Medicine 33: 756–762

Choudari C P, O'Mahony S, Brydon G et al 1993 Gut lavage fluid protein concentrations: objective measures of disease activity in inflammatory bowel disease. Gastroenterology 104: 1064–1071

Currie D C, Saverymuttu S H, Peters A M et al 1987 Indium-111 labelled granulocyte accumulation in the respiratory tracts of patients with bronchiectasis. Lancet 1: 1335–1339

Datz F L, Anderson C E, Ahluwalia R et al 1994 The efficacy of indium-111-polyclonal IgG for the detection of infection and inflammation. Journal of Nuclear Medicine 35: 74–83

Dixon P M, Roulston M E, Nolan D J 1993 The small bowel enema: a ten year review. Clinical Radiology 47: 46–48

Eade O E, Smith C L, Alexander J R, Whorwell P J 1980 Pulmonary function in patients with inflammatory bowel disease. American Journal of Gastroenterology 73: 154–156

Giaffer M H, Tindale W, Senior S, Barber D C, Holdsworth C D 1993 Quantification of disease activity in Crohn's disease by computerised analysis of ^{99m}Tc hexamethylpropylineamine oxime (HMPAO) labelled leucocyte images. Gut 34: 68–74

Holt S 1992 Ultrasonic assessment of inflammatory bowel disease. American Journal of Gastroenterology 87: 1889–1890

Jamar F, Chapman P, Keelan E T M, Peters A M, Haskard D O. Targeting endothelial activation using radiolabelled monoclonal antibody against E-selectin. (submitted)

Jonker N, Peters A M, Gaskin G, Pusey C D, Lavender J P 1992a A retrospective study of granulocyte kinetics in patients with systemic vasculitis. Journal of Nuclear Medicine 33: 491–497

Jonker N D, Peters A M, Carpani de Kaski M, Hodgson H J, Lavender J P 1992b Pulmonary granulocyte margination is increased in patients

with inflammatory bowel disease. Nuclear Medicine Communications 13: 806–810
Lantto E H, Lantto T J, Vorne M 1991 Fast diagnosis of abdominal infections and inflammation with ^{99m}Tc HMPAO labelled leucocytes. Journal of Nuclear Medicine 32: 2029–2034
Lecouffe P, Vendel H, Huglo D, Colombel J-F, Wallaert B, Marchandise X 1990 Pulmonary and intestinal permeabilities in Crohn's disease. European Journal of Nuclear Medicine 16: S180
Lindstrom E, Noren B 1992 Air enema revisited in assessment of colitis. Acta Radiologica 33: 360–364
McAfee J G, Thakur M L 1976 Survey of radioactive agents for in vitro labelling of phagocytic leukocytes. I Soluble agents. Journal of Nuclear Medicine 17: 480–487
Peters A M 1994 The utility of ^{99m}Tc HMPAO labeled leukocytes for imaging infection. Seminars in Nuclear Medicine 24: 110–127
Peters A M, Danpure H J, Osman S et al 1986 Preliminary clinical experience with ^{99m}Tc HMPAO for labelling leucocytes and imaging inflammation. Lancet 2: 946–949
Peters A M, Roddie M E, Danpure H J et al 1988 ^{99m}Tc HMPAO labelled leucocytes: comparison with ^{111}In-tropolonate labelled granulocytes. Nuclear Medicine Communications 9: 449–463
Peters A M, Saverymuttu S H, Reavy H J, Danpure H J, Osman S, Lavender J P 1983 Imaging inflammation with ^{111}In tropolonate labeled leukocytes. Journal of Nuclear Medicine 24: 39–44
Peters A M, Saverymuttu S H, Keshavarzian A, Bell R N, Lavender J P 1985 Splenic pooling of granulocytes. Clinical Science 68: 283–289
Pullman W, Sullivan P, Barratt P J, Lising J, Booth J A, Doe W F 1988 Assessment of inflammatory bowel disease activity by technetium-99m phagocyte scanning: a new imaging technique. Gastroenterology 95: 989–996
Roddie M E, Peters A M, Danpure H J et al 1988 Imaging inflammation with ^{99m}Tc hexamethyl propylene amine oxime (HMPAO) labeled leukocytes. Radiology 166: 767–772
Saverymuttu S H, Chadwick V S, Joseph A E A, Northfield T C, Maxwell J D, Hodgson H J F 1988 Distinction between Chrohn's colitis and ulcerative colitis by indium-111 granulocyte scanning. Gut 29: A707
Saverymuttu S H, Peters A M, Hodgson H J, Chadwick V S, Lavender J P 1982 Indium-111 autologous leucocyte scanning: comparison with radiology for imaging the colon in inflammatory bowel disease. British Medical Journal 285: 255–257
Saverymuttu S H, Peters A M, Danpure H J, Reavy H J, Osman S, Lavender J P 1983a Lung transit of ^{111}In-labelled granulocytes. Relationship to labelling techniques. Scandinavian Journal of Haematology 30: 151–160
Saverymuttu S H, Peters A M, Hodgson H J, Chadwick V S, Lavender J P 1983b Quantitative fecal ^{111}In-leukocyte excretion in the assessment of disease activity in Crohn's disease. Gastroenterology 85: 1333–1339
Saverymuttu S H, Peters A M, Lavender J P 1985a Clinical importance of enteric communication with abdominal abscesses. British Medical Journal 290: 23–27
Saverymuttu S H, Peters A M, Keshavarzian A, Reavy H J, Lavender J P 1985b The kinetics of 111-indium distribution following injection of 111-indium labelled autologous granulocytes in man. British Journal of Haematology 61: 675–685
Saverymuttu S H, Peters A M, O'Brien C et al 1986 Indium-111 labelled autologous leucocyte scanning in gastrointestinal graft versus host disease. Digestive Diseases and Sciences 31: 829–832
Scholmerich J, Schmidt E, Shumichen C, Billmann P, Schmidt H, Gerok W 1988 Scintigraphic assessment of bowel involvement and disease activity in Crohn's disease using ^{99m}Tc hexamethylpropyleneamine oxime as a leucocyte label. Gastroenterology 95: 1287–1293
Segarra I, Rocha M, Balleillas C et al 1991 Granulocyte specific monoclonal antibody ^{99m}Tc BW 250/183 and ^{111}In-oxine labelled leukocyte scintigraphy in inflammatory bowel disease. European Journal of Nuclear Medicine 18: 715–719
Thakur M L, Lavender J P, Arnot R N, Silvester D J, Segal A W 1977 Indium-111 labeled autologous leukocytes in man. Journal of Nuclear Medicine 18: 1014–1021
Tindale W B, Barber D C, Giaffer M H, Senior S, Holdsworth C D 1992 ^{99m}Tc HMPAO labelled leucocyte imaging in Crohn's disease: a subtraction technique for the quantification of disease activity. Clinical Physics and Physiological Measurements 13: 37–50
Ussov W Yu, Peters A M, Hodgson H J, Hughes J M B 1994 Quantification of pulmonary uptake of indium-111 labelled granulocytes in inflammatory bowel disease. European Journal of Nuclear Medicine 21: 6–11
Ussov W, Peters A M, Glass D, Gunasekera R D, Hughes J M B. Measurement of the pulmonary vascular granulocyte pool. Validation of technique and initial results in inflammatory conditions. Journal of Applied Physiology (in press).
Ussov W Yu, Peters A M, Savill J, Hughes J M B. Relationship between granulocyte activation, pulmonary granulocyte kinetics and alveolocapillary barrier integrity in extrapulmonary inflammatory disease. (submitted)
Weldon M, Saverymuttu S, Findlayson C, Joseph A, Maxwell J 1993 Accurate assessment of colonic inflammatory bowel disease (IBD) using early (1 hr) technetium (^{99m}Tc) HMPAO white cell scanning. Gut 34: S62

28. Endoscopy – upper gastrointestinal tract
A. I. Morris

INTRODUCTION

Since the development of flexible fiberoptic endoscopy in the 1960s the progress and sophistication of instrument design has permitted gastroenterologists to reach progressively further into the gastrointestinal (GI) tract. Not only can most of the GI tract be directly visualized and biopsied, but in addition therapy can be delivered to stop bleeding, dilate strictures, remove foreign bodies and ablate tumors.

With a standard forward-viewing upper gastrointestinal endoscope, lesions down to the junction of the second and third parts of the duodenum can be reached. Before the era of small-bowel enteroscopy attempts to visualize below this level were usually carried out with either a standard or a pediatric colonoscope. These instruments, not being specifically designed for this purpose, had inappropriate handling and stiffness characteristics that limited their use and depth of penetration down the GI tract.

In the last 10 years small-bowel enteroscopes have been designed to enable better visualization of the small bowel, which may have particular importance in the assessment of small-bowel Crohn's disease.

SMALL-BOWEL ENTEROSCOPY

Three basic types of small-bowel enteroscope have been developed, but only two have gone into commercial production. The three types are the push enteroscope, the sonde enteroscope and the 'rope-way'. The latter has not been widely used; it involved the patient swallowing a weighted thread which was allowed to pass through the entire GI tract until it emerged through the anus. A very flexible, narrow non-steerable scope was attached to the upper end of the thread and was slowly pulled through

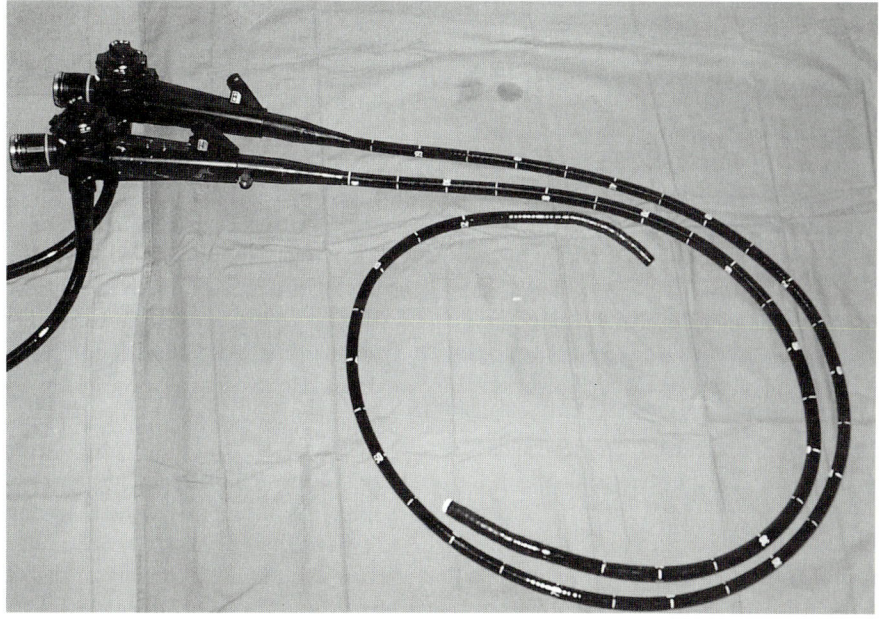

Fig. 28.1 Small-bowel push enteroscope alongside standard-length gastroscope (Olympus).

the patient, from mouth to anus. Hardly surprisingly, this technique never achieved popularity.

The current models of sonde scope are very thin (about 6 mm in diameter) but have no biopsy channel and are not steerable. They are passed transnasally into the GI tract and, once positioned in the duodenum, are propelled further down the small bowel with the aid of a balloon at the tip which, when inflated, stimulates peristalsis as the motive force. These endoscopes can intubate the entire small bowel and views of the mucosa are obtained on extubation by gentle traction. Because of folds and the concertina effect of the bowel on the scope, the entire mucosal surface cannot be inspected and it is estimated that between 30 and 50% of the surface may not be visualized. The other frustration with this instrument is the inability to reposition the scope should a lesion be seen transiently, the inability to biopsy or treat lesions, and the prolonged nature of the examination, which may take up to 6 hours.

The push-type enteroscope, now available from several manufacturers, either in the form of a fiberoptic instrument or as a videoendoscope, can generally only reach to the mid or lower jejunum. The advantage of this type of scope is that it can be reinserted and steered, as well as permitting targeted biopsies and the delivery of therapy. Laser therapy, injection therapy, polypectomy and balloon dilatation accessories can all be passed through the standard biopsy channel (usually 2.8 mm diameter). These endoscopes are very floppy by comparison with gastroduodenoscopes and colonoscopes, and thus although they can pass down the small bowel, looping in the stomach can be a problem, which some endoscopists overcome by using overtubes down to the duodenum.

USE OF ENDOSCOPY IN DIFFERENTIAL DIAGNOSIS

The main use for endoscopy is in the diagnosis of Crohn's disease of the upper GI tract and in determining its severity and extent. It is uncommon for Crohn's disease to present with upper GI symptoms, but when it does it has to be distinguished from other inflammatory or ulcerative diseases of the esophagus, stomach and duodenum.

In the esophagus the principal differential diagnosis is from gastroesophageal reflux disease. The endoscopic appearance of mucosal edema, hyperemia or ulceration is not specific and is subjective. Even strictures in the esophagus cannot be confidently diagnosed on the basis of their appearance, as they may be peptic, malignant, or due to Crohn's diseases. Biopsies can help in distinguishing between these conditions, but often if Crohn's is considered it is because of pre-existing knowledge of Crohn's elsewhere in the GI tract. Similarly, the diagnosis of the cause of gastritis, duodenitis and ulceration in both these sites has to be based on the macroscopic, microscopic and other associated features and history from the patient. Failure of peptic ulceration to heal with acid suppressant therapy and/or *Helicobacter pylori* eradication may alert the endoscopist to the possibility that the lesion is not simply peptic. The ingestion of NSAIDs can give similar findings, with erosions being a common endoscopic finding in addition to gastritis, duodenitis and more marked ulceration. The usual hallmark taken as being diagnostic of Crohn's disease in the upper GI tract is the presence of non-caseating granulomas. It must not be forgotten that there are many causes of granulomas, and that sarcoid and tuberculosis must be thought of in the appropriate patient.

Endoscopy of the small bowel is a relatively new development, and currently complements the use of contrast radiology. In the upper GI tract, however, endoscopy has replaced radiology in many centres as the first method of assessment.

UPPER GI ENDOSCOPY AND THE ESOPHAGUS

There are few if any specific endoscopic appearances of IBD in the esophagus. During treatment with immunosuppressive drugs patients might acquire monilial esophagitis or, very occasionally, a viral esophagitis. Beck et al (1994) reported a case of aphthous ulceration as the presenting feature of Crohn's disease, which settled with steroids but not a proton pump inhibitor. Similar aphthoid ulcers in the esophagus have been reported by Hizawa et al (1994). In a pediatric series of Crohn's patients studied prospectively, 16% had abnormal endoscopic esophageal biopsies without abnormal endoscopic appearances (Cameron 1991).

Very occasionally Crohn's disease may present with a stricture or fistula. Few prospective surveys of the extent of involvement of the esophagus in Crohn's disease have been published. In one study (Schmitz-Moormann et al 1985) 225 patients with Crohn's disease affecting the large and/or small bowel were endoscoped. Endoscopic lesions were found in the esophagus in 15%, of which only 57% revealed histological alterations. Geboes et al (1986) found histological proof of esophageal disease in seven or nine patients with esophageal involvement in a cohort of 500 Crohn's patients followed for 4 years. The clinical presentation was usually with painful dysphagia, and large aphthoid lesions were the most common endoscopic finding.

Because of the high prevalence of gastroesophageal reflux disease in the general population, the finding of esophagitis in a patient with Crohn's disease should not automatically be taken to indicate Crohn's involvement of the esophagus. The finding of discrete aphthoid ulcers, or the histological confirmation of granulomas in biopsies from inflamed mucosa, is more suggestive.

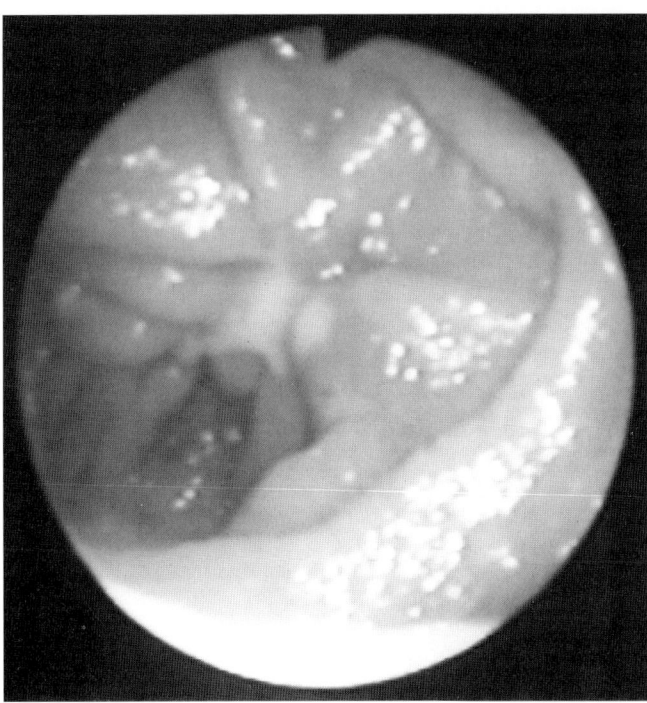

Fig. 28.2 Small-bowel endoscopic photograph of jejunal ulceration due to Crohn's disease, with stellate radiating folds centered on ulcerated area. Small erosion adjacent to larger ulcer. (See page xix.)

Stricture dilatation for dysphagia has been reported (Rowe et al 1987), although most cases with fistulation seem to have been treated surgically.

UPPER GI ENDOSCOPY AND THE STOMACH AND DUODENUM

As in the esophagus, there are no specific endoscopic findings that are pathognomonic of Crohn's disease. A variety of macroscopic lesions have been reported, including aphthoid erosions, ulcers, fold thickening, nodules, erythema and areas of stenosis (Alcantara et al 1993), with granularity and cobblestoning also being noted (Sukhabote & Freeman 1993).

In Cameron's (1991) prospective series of endoscopy in 56 children and adolescents with Crohn's disease, 46% had involvement of the body of the stomach and 36% antral involvement. Duodenal involvement occurred in only 21%. These results are not very different from those of Schmitz-Moorman et al (1985), where endoscopic lesions were seen in the stomach in 49% of 221 patients. Only 60% revealed histological changes, with confirmation of Crohn's disease based on non-caseating granulomas in 29.4%. These authors comment that the only predictive lesions for the presence of granulomas in the stomach were chronic erosions. Mucosal edema and redness were not specific and, interestingly, less predictive of granulomas than their presence in the duodenum. Thirty-four percent of the patients had duodenal abnormalities.

Fistulation from the stomach to the colon, small bowel or bronchial tree has been reported, but there are no specific endoscopic reports of its diagnosis or treatment. Fistulation from the duodenum into the small and large bowel, pancreas and biliary tree has also been reported, but in most cases radiology has been the predominant diagnostic mode. Pancreatitis and cholangitis have both been described secondary to duodenal obstruction caused by Crohn's stricturing of the infra-ampullary region of the second part of the duodenum (Kato et al 1992). As yet endoscopic management of such cases has not been published, although duodenal stenoses alone have been dilated by through-the-scope balloon dilators. Even a persimmon bezoar has given rise to pancreatitis when it caused ampullary obstruction by becoming lodged in an area of duodenal Crohn's (Eliakim et al 1987).

Although there are only reports of endosonographic differentiation of mucosal from transmucosal IBD in the colon using an endoscopic ultrasound colonoscope (Hildebrandt et al 1992), with the increasing availability of gastric and duodenal endoscopic ultrasound scopes it may be anticipated that this might enhance the endoscopist's ability to diagnose Crohn's disease.

ENDOSCOPY OF THE UPPER SMALL INTESTINE

The main use of small-bowel enteroscopy has been in the investigation of obscure GI bleeding and the effects of NSAIDs on the small intestine. Increasing use is now being made of enteroscopy to search for evidence of Crohn's disease in the upper small intestine. Inspection and biopsy of strictures shown on contrast radiographic studies and the biopsy of abnormal mucosa seen on X-rays is another increasing use. The availability of specially designed small-bowel enteroscopes will to a great extent replace the need for intraoperative endoscopy. Similar lesions to those found in the stomach and duodenum have been described (Lescut et al 1993).

THERAPEUTIC POTENTIAL

Currently only the push enteroscope allows the gastroenterologist to delivery therapy into the small bowel. Laser, bicap diathermy, heater probe and injection of adrenaline or sclerosants can all be safely used down a push enteroscope to stop bleeding. The author has removed multiple polyps from the entire small bowel in a patient with Peutz–Jeghers syndrome by this means, and the dilatation of small-bowel strictures with through-the-scope balloon dilators is already being undertaken. This technique for the dilatation of anastomotic colonic strictures, and for strictures due to Crohn's, is already well described and must surely be the main therapeutic potential for enteroscopes in IBD. The placement of fine-

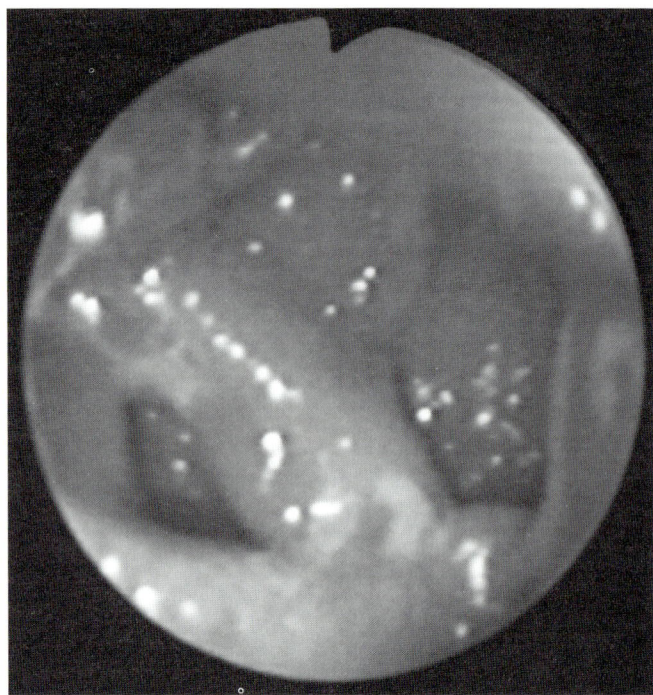

Fig. 28.3 Further enteroscopic picture of several small ulcers on distorted, thickened and inflamed jejunal fold. (See page xix.)

bore feeding tubes by endoscopy and the insertion of percutaneous endoscopic gastrotomy and jejunostomy feeding tubes is another developing area. Few gastroenterologists are willing to consider such tubes in patients with Crohn's disease for fear of fistulation, but nutritional support might be offered to ulcerative colitis patients during an exacerbation, or following colectomy if oral feeding is difficult to re-establish early.

REFERENCES

Alcantara M, Rodriguez R, Potenciano J L, Carrobles J L, Munoz C, Gomez R 1993 Endoscopic and bioptic findings in the upper gastrointestinal tract in patients with Crohn's disease. Endoscopy 25: 282–286

Beck P L, Blustein P K, Andersen M A 1994 Aphthous esophageal ulceration. A novel presentation of Crohn's disease? Canadian Journal of Gastroenterology 8: 101–104

Cameron D J 1991 Upper and lower gastrointestinal endoscopy in children and adolescents with Crohn's disease: a prospective study. Journal of Gastroenterology and Hepatology 6: 355–358

Eliakim R, Fich A, Libson E, Katz E, Rachmilewitz D 1987 Crohn's disease of the duodenum presented as pancreatitis due to persimmon bezoar. Journal of Clinical Gastroenterology 9: 553–555

Geboes K, Jannssens J, Rutgeerts P, Vantrappen G 1986 Crohn's disease of the oesophagus. Journal of Clinical Gastroenterology 8: 31–37

Hildebrandt U, Kraus J, Ecker K W, Schmid T, Schuder G, Feifel G 1992 Endosonographic differentiation of musocal and transmural nonspecific inflammatory bowel disease. Endoscopy 24 (Suppl 1); 359–363

Hizawa K, Iida M, Kohrogi N, Yao T, Sakamoto K, Fujishima M 1994 Crohn's disease: early recognition and progress of aphthous lesions. Radiology 190: 451–454

Kato M, Ninomiya M, Sugiura J et al 1992 A case of duodenal Crohn's disease associated with ampullary insufficiency and cholangitis. Dig. Endosc. 1992, 4: 159–164

Lescut D, Vanco D, Bonniere P et al 1993 Perioperative endoscopy of the whole small bowel in Crohn's disease. Gut 34: 647–649

Rowe P H, Taylor P R, Sladen G E, Owen W J 1987 Cricopharyngeal Crohn's disease. Postgraduate Medical Journal 63: 1101–1102

Schmitz-Moorman P, Malchow H, Pittner P M 1985 Endoscopic and bioptic study of the upper gastrointestinal tract in Crohn's disease patients. Pathol. Res. Pract. 179: 377–387

Sukhabote J, Freeman H J 1993 Granulomatous (Crohn's) disease of the upper gastrointestinal tract: a study of 22 patients with mucosal granulomas. Canadian Journal of Gastroenterology 7: 605–609

29. Endoscopy – lower intestinal tract

E. J. Irvine   R. H. Hunt

ROLE OF ENDOSCOPY IN INFLAMMATORY BOWEL DISEASE

Fiberoptic endoscopy is well established, safe and accurate for the diagnosis and management of inflammatory bowel disease (IBD). Direct visualization of the mucosa and biopsy of suspected abnormalities are possible. The principal applications of endoscopy in IBD include discrimination of Crohn's disease from ulcerative colitis or other inflammatory conditions, delineation of the sites of disease or extent, grading of endoscopic disease severity, and confirmation of complications such as stricture, fistula or mass. Finally, diagnosis of pouchitis, surveillance to detect precancer, or therapeutic interventions such as dilatation of strictures or electrocautery of bleeding sites are also important endoscopic applications.

Standard lavage bowel preparations (Ernstoff et al 1983, Pockros et al 1985) and oral sodium phosphate do not significantly alter the mucosal endoscopic or histological appearance. The normal colonic mucosa is smooth, pale, glistening and transparent, varying from grey to pink (Hunt 1986), with a blue tone at the splenic and hepatic flexures where the spleen or liver impress on the colonic wall. The vascular pattern, a branching network of superficial vessels which increase in diameter distally, is most prominent in the rectum. The colonic haustra are also prominent in the left colon, while in the transverse colon the lumen has a triangular appearance due to mesenteric suspension. In the terminal ileum a carpet of finger-like villi may be seen, particularly after instillation of water and air insufflation. Submucosal nodules of up to 2 mm in diameter represent benign lymphoid hyperplasia, which may occur in patients well into the fourth and fifth decades.

Specific indications

Colonoscopy, although not critical for initiation of therapy, is important in making a definitive diagnosis of IBD and to differentiate Crohn's disease from ulcerative colitis (Waye 1992). It is essential for defining the extent and severity of colonic or ileal inflammation. Specific drug therapies or formulations may then be selected for disease severity or site of maximum inflammation. Endoscopy also provides the opportunity to take random as well as targeted biopsies, which are vital for confirming a presumptive diagnosis or differentiating difficult disease. Subsequent endoscopy may be necessary to document changes in disease extent or severity, for example to determine eligibility or to monitor response to therapy in clinical trials, particularly in patients with ulcerative colitis. An additional advantage of endoscopy is the ability to take photographs or video recordings for objective or subsequent evaluation.

Outside clinical trials, evidence does not support the use of colonoscopy to monitor the disease's clinical course, except for cancer surveillance in extensive or pancolitis (Gyde 1990). Indeed, in severe or fulminant disease colonoscopy is contraindicated. Although a careful flexible sigmoidoscopy may carry less risk in a severe first attack of IBD, it still has a limited role, as the rectum is often spared and histologic features can only be used confidently to differentiate Crohn's disease from ulcerative colitis in the 15–20% of cases with granulomas. A recent review has reported a perforation rate for colonoscopy of between 0.09% and 0.36%, (0.2–0.5% after therapeutic and 0.1–0.3% after diagnostic colonoscopy), with an attendant mortality rate of 0.02% (Hall et al 1991). Data pertinent to a selected population of IBD patients are not available.

When the clinical course of the disease is more severe than anticipated, or in the presence of specific complications, such as a mass, stricture or hemorrhage, colonoscopy is mandatory to obtain biopsies or to execute therapeutic interventions. Performing colonoscopy preoperatively is also strongly advised in patients who are having (semi-)elective surgery, to define clearly the type of IBD and its extent and severity. These parameters can then be weighed to minimize the risk of undertaking inappropriate surgery. Some surgeons still favor a barium enema to provide the 'road map' for surgery, since estimates of disease extent at colonoscopy may be less accurate owing to the variability in location of important

Table 29.1 Indications for endoscopy in inflammatory bowel disease

Differential diagnosis (according to symptoms suggestive of upper gut, small bowel, biliary tract or colon)
Disease
    Extent (ulcerative colitis)
    Site (Crohn's disease)
Disease severity (entry/exit clinical trials; postoperative recurrence)
Intractability of symptoms
Complication (fistula, hemorrhage, anemia)
Visualization and biopsy (mass or stricture)
Therapeutic intervention (dilatation of stricture, electrocautery of hemorrhage)
Peri- or intraoperative assessment
Examination of stoma, Kock or pelvic pouch
Surveillance for dysplasia

Table 29.2 Differential diagnosis of IBD by site of involvement

Terminal ileum
Crohn's disease
Lymphoid nodular hyperplasia
NSAID injury
Lymphoma
Carcinoid
Ischemia
Tuberculosis
Histoplasmosis
Yersinia
Anisakiasis

Colon
Inflammatory
    Ulcerative colitis
    Crohn's disease
    Collagenous colitis
    Microscopic colitis
    Radiation-induced colitis
    Diverticular disease
    Behçet's syndrome
    Cediua
    Pneumatosis coli
    NSAID colitis
    Chronic granulomatous disease
    Malakoplakia
Infectious
    Antibiotic-associated colitis
    Yersinia enterocolitica
    Tuberculosis
    Amebiasis
    Endolimax nana
    Schistosomiasis
    Entameba histolytica
    Syphilis
    Lymphogranuloma venereum
    Cytomegalovirus
    Spirochetosis
    Chlamydia
    Gonorrhea

HIV-associated
Infection
    Giardiasis
    Candidiasis
    Herpes simplex
    CMV colitis
    Cryptosporidiosis
    Kaposi's sarcoma
    Entameba coli
    Histoplasmosis

landmarks. Table 29.1 lists the various indications for endoscopy in IBD.

Differential diagnosis

The etiology of mucosal inflammation is often difficult to ascertain because of the lack of specific endoscopic features. In attempting a definitive diagnosis, clinicians must consider the clinical findings, the patient's age, the presence of risk factors for IBD or other inflammatory conditions (including infection), family history, smoking status, the duration of intestinal or extraintestinal symptoms, and prior medication use.

A diagnosis of IBD is anticipated only after infection and acute self-limiting colitis have been excluded. Several studies have shown that 22–38% of patients suspected of having IBD will be found to have infection (Tedesco et al 1983, Bayerdorffer et al 1986, Lumb and Hunt 1987, Waye 1992). Infectious and acute self-limited colitis are usually short-lived, lasting less than 2 weeks, but may have associated systemic symptoms such as fever. Features such as rectal bleeding, frequent or loose stools, abdominal pain, urgency and tenesmus are non-specific, whereas a history of travel or clustering of cases is more suggestive of infection.

In making a diagnosis of Crohn's disease or ulcerative colitis, the stool should be cultured for bacterial pathogens, including *Clostridium difficile* and its toxin, and a microscopic examination performed to look for parasites and red or white blood cells. Although the differential diagnosis of IBD is extensive, as shown in Table 29.2, the most common entities to consider are *Campylobacter jejuni*, *Yersinia enterocolitica*, *Clostridium difficile*, venereal diseases, tuberculosis, drug-induced colitis, graft-versus-host disease, obstruction, ischemia, solitary rectal ulcer, and collagenous and lymphocytic colitis (Rutgeerts et al 1992). In patients with significant risk factors or known HIV infection, rarer opportunistic infections should also be considered.

Macroscopic lesions should generally be biopsied, taking two additional biopsies per 10 cm of bowel for histological assessment to facilitate diagnosis (Waye 1990) while culture of ileal biopsies if inflammation is present may confirm Yersinia or Chlamydia infection (Bayerdorffer et al 1986). If opportunistic infections such as cytomegalovirus (Mentec et al 1994) or *Mycobacterium avium* complex are a possibility, biopsies and brushings should also be sent for the appropriate culture and cytological examination.

Acute infectious colitis

Colonoscopy is not recommended when infectious colitis is suspected, although rigid or flexible sigmoidoscopy may be appropriate if bloody diarrhea is present. In the presence of *Escherichia coli* or *Campylobacter jejuni*, patchy erythema or mucosal edema may be the only abnormality (Cooper et al 1992), but Campylobacter, Salmonella or Shigella may also be indistinguishable endoscopically from ulcerative colitis (Waye 1992). Yersinia can produce microscopic ulceration throughout the colon or terminal ileum. Biopsies will show the acute polymorphonuclear inflammatory infiltrate in the lamina propria with normal architecture which is also observed in acute self-limited colitis, when no pathogen is identified (Surawicz and Belic 1984).

Antibiotic associated colitis due to *Clostridium difficile* infection, although typically portrayed as having pale yellow or white plaques overlying a hemorrhagic inflamed rectal mucosa, may also have a segmental distribution, occurring in the sigmoid or ascending colon, with rectal sparing (Lumb & Hunt 1987). Kishida et al (1992) have described less obvious features, such as erosions and aphthoid and linear ulcers. Histology showing the typical 'volcano lesion', together with a mucous exudate, may suggest antibiotic-associated colitis or demonstrate the presence of a specific pathogen. Occasionally elderly or debilitated patients may present with a fulminant colitis mimicking an acute abdomen (Triadafilopoulos & Hallstone 1991). A history of prior antibiotics is usually present in such cases, and the diagnosis may be confirmed by the presence of toxin in the stool or by culture. However, empirical treatment with metronidazole or vancomycin may be appropriate if a strong suspicion exists, since false negative results may delay the diagnosis.

The endoscopic appearance of acute amebic colitis is similar to that of ulcerative colitis, with diffuse friability, granularity and erythema (Crowson & Hines 1978, Larsson et al 1991). In chronic amebic colitis, discrete or localized ulcers with a rolled edge, giving the ulcers a punched-out appearance, may help distinguish it from Crohn's disease. A history of foreign travel or exposure in an endemic area should suggest this diagnosis. Biopsies of inflamed mucosa should be taken from the edge of ulcerated areas: trophozoites may be detected in the mucosa (Prathap & Gilman 1970). The presence of an inflammatory mass in the cecum may also be confused with Crohn's disease or carcinoma. Consideration should be given to empirical treatment in patients from endemic areas.

Chronic infections

With the increased migration of patients from less developed countries, tuberculosis should be considered (Palmer et al 1985). In intestinal tuberculosis the ileocecal region is frequently involved, but diffuse aphthous ulcers, cobblestoning or skip lesions, polypoid folds and strictures may also occur in the colon, simulating Crohn's disease (Shah et al 1992). Radiologically detectable lung disease is present in only about 50% of patients (Carr-Locke & Finlay 1983). A high index of suspicion by the clinician, endoscopist and pathologist is essential to prevent this treatable condition being overlooked. Langhans' giant cells and agglomerations of epithelioid cells in biopsies,

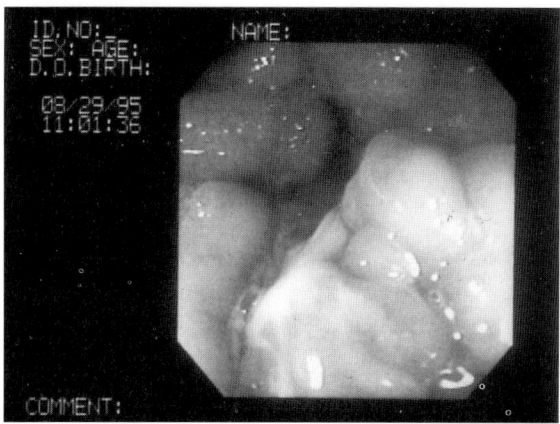

Fig. 29.1 Tuberculosis of the colon, shown here, may mimic the cobblestoned appearance of Crohn's disease with thickened edematous folds in areas of healed ulceration. (See page xix.)

plus cultures, will provide a diagnosis in over 75% of subjects (Bhargava et al 1992, Shah et al 1992).

Less commonly, but also in Asian, African or Middle Eastern immigrants, long-standing schistosomiasis infection may cause a severe extensive colitis or segmental lesions, ranging from small mucosal excrescences to multiple large proliferative polyps (Nebel et al 1974, Mohamed et al 1990). The diagnosis should be considered in patients from endemic areas, and although it may be confirmed by demonstrating viable Schistosoma ova in the stools (11%) (Mohamed et al 1990), the colonoscopic appearance and biopsy demonstration of organisms are most useful.

In immunocompromized patients with diarrhea, particularly those rendered neutropenic during chemotherapy (Prescott et al 1992) and who have received prolonged antibiotics, endoscopic ulceration, ulcerated sloughed mucosa, polyps or segmental lesions have been noted. Fungal stains may demonstrate mucosal candida or aspergillus in the submucosa and these infections are associated with a high mortality, even after treatment with systemic antifungal agents.

Microscopic colitis

Collagenous and lymphocytic colitis are often discussed together, as these conditions are both associated with chronic watery diarrhea and may have a normal mucosal appearance, or subtle changes such as patchy erythema, alterations in vascular pattern or mucosal edema (Zeroogian & Chopra 1994). A diagnosis is made in the absence of infection, primarily by histology, and biopsies must be taken from multiple colonic segments, since the histologic features are frequently focal (Tanaka et al 1992). Both collagenous and lymphocytic colitis have increased numbers of intraepithelial lymphocytes in the colonic epthelium, with a chronic inflammatory infiltrate in the lamina propria. In collagenous colitis, which occurs predominantly in middle-aged and older women, possibly in those with a prior history of NSAID use (Riddell et al 1992), there is also a widened focal subepithelial collagen band (Widgren et al 1988). Both of these forms of colitis have been reported to respond to therapy with binding resins, such as cholestyramine, or anti-inflammatory drugs such as 5-ASA or corticosteroids (Rokkas et al 1988). However, the natural history of these entities and their outcomes have not been well described. In our own series of consecutive patients with irritable bowel syndrome, five of 30 patients were ultimately diagnosed to have lymphocytic or collagenous colitis, suggesting that routine biopsy of the colon is useful in patients with diarrhea-predominant irritable bowel syndrome (Irvine et al 1995, unpublished data).

Ischemic/radiation colitis

Patients with colonic ischemia may complain of overt rectal bleeding, with or without abdominal pain, but diarrhea is not a usual feature. A history of cardiovascular disease or the use of oral contraceptives should be also ascertained. Colonoscopic findings are commonly segmental, involving the splenic flexure and the descending or sigmoid colon (Hunt & Buchanan 1979). The affected segment may initially show petechiae in a pale mucosa, superficial ulceration, or a hemorrhagic friable ulcerated mucosa with a pseudomembrane (Snowcroft et al 1981, Seow-Chen et al 1993). A sharp line of demarcation may or may not be present. Radiation colitis in women who have undergone radiation for pelvic malignancy may show a similar appearance, with thinning of the mucosa or acute hemorrhagic ulceration, usually in the upper rectum or sigmoid (Anseline et al 1981). After healing, mucosal telangiectasia is common and may be a source of bleeding. Loss of haustra or strictures may occur after healing of acute ischemia or radiation. Biopsy of strictured areas should be performed to rule out malignancy, and may demonstrate hemosiderin within macrophages, fibrosis, a paucity of vessels or the typical telangiectasias (Hunt & Buchanan 1979).

Segmental or isolated ulceration

Solitary rectal ulcer syndrome, thought to be due to intussusception and ischemia of the anterior rectal mucosa, may be confused with Crohn's disease in patients with rectal bleeding and localized ulceration in the rectum (Madigan & Morson 1969, Hizawa et al 1994). The area may be edematous, cystic, ulcerated or have a polypoid appearance. However, the histology demonstrating fibrosis, hyperplasia of the muscularis mucosa and the presence of colitis cystica profunda will identify the true diagnosis (Rutter & Riddell 1975).

A segmental colitis has also been described in middle-aged or elderly patients with rectal bleeding and diverticular disease (Gore et al 1992, Peppercorn 1992). In a series of 2380 colonoscopies, 1.42% had 'crescentic fold disease of the sigmoid colon', and of those 82% had diverticular disease. Half were treated with anti-inflammatory drugs such as 5-ASA or sulfasalazine, with a positive response, while two of 34 required resection. Endoscopically there was localized mucosal edema, erythema, hemorrhage and exudate, with sparing of the diverticular orifices. Biopsies demonstrated chronic inflammatory infiltration of the lamina propria and crypt microabscesses.

NSAIDs and chronic systemic disease

Certain multi-organ systemic diseases involving the gastrointestinal tract may cause diarrhea, abdominal pain or rectal bleeding. Specific forms of arthritis, collagen vascular diseases or vasculitis may have associated intestinal inflammation which can be confused with IBD.

Several studies have observed an increased relative risk for Crohn's disease in HLA B27-positive patients with ankylosing spondylitis (Macrae & Wright 1973, Costello et al 1980) and patients with B27 and B44 may be at very high risk for both diseases (Purrmann et al 1988). Ulcerating or stricturing lesions occurring throughout the intestine have also been described in patients taking NSAIDs (Bjarnasson et al 1993), making it difficult to discern whether this association is genetic or secondary to the treatment. A case control study of 118 patients with various inflammatory arthritides and 24 patients with acute bacterial gastroenteritis, reported ileocolonic lesions in over 80% of the latter (Leirisalo-Repo et al 1994). The acute findings included mucus, mucosal edema, a change in vascularity, small ulcers or hemorrhage. Chronic changes, primarily large ulcers, were found in the ileum of 20% or descending colon of 30% of those with sacroiliitis or ankylosing spondylitis, and were thought to be typical or diagnostic of Crohn's disease in 26%. Patients with seronegative oligoarthropathy who were taking NSAIDs had no chronic changes. These findings suggested that the NSAIDs were not playing a significant role in the etiology of the chronic gut inflammation.

A chronic colitis, endoscopically indistinguishable from ulcerative colitis and with histology showing a chronic inflammatory infiltrate in the lamina propria, has been shown in some patients with portal hypertension and rectal bleeding (Kozarek et al 1991). In a small series of patients with diarrhea, normal colonoscopy and mixed connective tissue diseases, eosinophils were noted deep in the pericrypt area. These patients improved after treatment with corticosteroids or azathioprine (Clouse et al 1992).

Diversion colitis

Diversion colitis, a chronic mucosal inflammation occurring in the excluded bowel of patients who have undergone a subtotal colectomy or split ileostomy (Glotzer et al 1981), is endoscopically and microscopically indistinguishable from ulcerative colitis (Harig et al 1989). The postulated etiology, a deficiency of short-chain fatty acids, the primary nutrient for colonocytes (Roediger 1980), was initially thought to permit discrimination of the two entities. However, both forms of colitis have now been treated successfully using daily butyrate enemas (Harig et al 1989, Steinhart et al 1994). A recent study of 37 children who underwent colostomy plus a Hartmann procedure or mucous fistula for Hirschsprung's disease demonstrated that 70% had histological evidence of diversion colitis at the time of reanastomosis 6–12 months later (Haque & West 1992). Histologically, diversion colitis in the non-IBD population may show normal architecture without crypt abscesses accompanying chronic inflammation in the lamina propria (Roe et al 1993). In the presence of prior IBD, however, the two entities remain difficult to separate.

Pediatric patients

The differential diagnosis of IBD in children and adolescents differs somewhat from that in adults. Allergic proctocolitis in the first year of life in children ingesting formula, cow's or soya milk may be associated with the typical endoscopic features of ulcerative colitis. Taking at least three biopsies has been suggested to identify focal eosinophilic infiltration in all mucosal compartments, which will assist in the diagnosis (Odze et al 1993). Despite a conservative approach to diagnosis in the pediatric population, Lipson et al (1990) have suggested that colonoscopy is the investigation of choice to diagnose colonic and terminal ileal inflammation in children with chronic diarrhea and/or rectal bleeding. As in adults, biopsies are essential to discriminate between ulcerative colitis and Crohn's disease or other conditions (Chong et al 1985, Bertele-Harms et al 1986). Benign lymphoid nodular hyperplasia is common, and occurred in 18% of the children who underwent ileoscopy to rule out inflammatory bowel disease (Lipson et al 1990).

CROHN'S DISEASE AND ULCERATIVE COLITIS

Endoscopic lesions, even in patients with known IBD, may be worsened by a superimposed infection or drug therapies, such as NSAIDs. Other lesions, such as diverticular disease, adenomas or hemorrhoids, may occur independently of the IBD.

Discriminating ulcerative colitis from Crohn's disease may be helped by the history, when rectal bleeding is not a significant symptom or if there is concomitant small-bowel or perianal disease. However, about two-thirds of those with Crohn's colitis will have rectal disease, rendering standard rigid sigmoidoscopy inadequate to provide a definitive diagnosis in over 80% of cases. Clinicians with access to immediate flexible sigmoidoscopy are more likely to discriminate successfully between the two initially. Colonoscopy of the colon and terminal ileum, combined with multiple biopsies and histologic assessment, is the most efficient and accurate diagnostic investigation, once IBD is considered to be present.

Comparison of colonoscopy with other imaging techniques

There are very few studies comparing the accuracy of diagnosis of different imaging techniques in IBD. One review (Freeny 1986) has shown that 18–20% of patients with endoscopically detectable Crohn's disease had normal X-rays. The authors' own prospective study reported the sensitivity of colonoscopy for detecting IBD to be 83%, but 100% if biopsies were included (Irvine et al 1988). In studies determining the extent of disease in ulcerative colitis, those patients with a false negative barium enema appeared to have endoscopically mild disease. Although barium studies appear to be less sensitive than endoscopy for diagnosis, the ability to discriminate between Crohn's disease and ulcerative colitis has been comparable, with an accuracy of between 95% and 98% (Freeny 1986).

Ulcerative colitis

Disease severity

A standardized endoscopic description of ulcerative colitis was undertaken by Baron and colleagues in the mid-1960s (Baron et al 1964). This index, shown in Table 29.3, is still utilized by clinicians and investigators for scoring disease severity. Until now, many clinical trials have relied primarily on symptomatic improvement to demonstrate therapeutic efficacy in ulcerative colitis (Irvine 1993). In a recent meta analysis of rectal 5-ASA therapies we have shown that symptomatic improvement and remission rates are greater than the corresponding endoscopic improvement, which in turn are also greater than histologic improvement (Marshall & Irvine 1995). Carbonnel et al (1994) demonstrated in 51 patients who required colectomy for a severe attack, that deep and extensive ulcerations, mucosal detatchment, well-like ulcerations or total mucosal abrasion were highly correlated with histological findings of severe disease in 96% of cases.

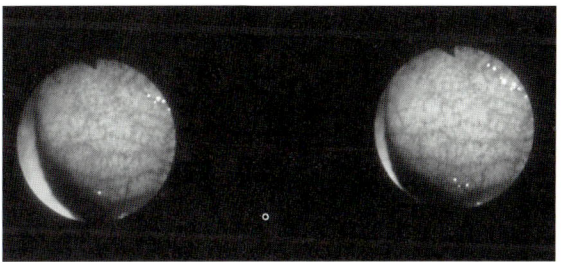

Fig. 29.2 Inactive or mild ulcerative colitis in which the vascular pattern is altered with tortuous vessels and pseudoaneurysms. (See page xix.)

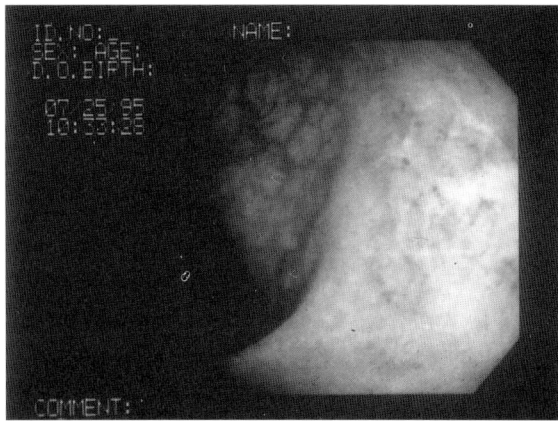

Fig. 29.3 Moderately active ulcerative proctitis with a normal vascular pattern proximal to the inflamed mucosa which is granular, edematous and friable with visible petechial hemorrhages. (See page xx.)

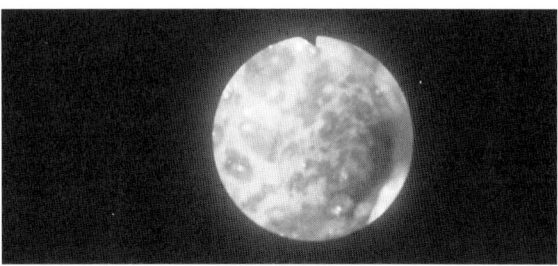

Fig. 29.4 In more severe ulcerative colitis, there is diffuse superficial ulceration of the mucosa with the islands of non-ulcerated mucosa giving the appearance of pseudo-polyps. (See page xx.)

Table 29.3 Ulcerative colitis severity

Graded endoscopic severity

0 Normal (normal, uninflamed)
1 Mild (mucosal edema, erythema, absent vascular pattern, granularity)
2 Moderate (friability, petechiae, presence of pus or mucopus)
3 Severe (spontaneous bleeding, erosions, ulceration)

Adapted from Baron et al (1964)

Thus clinical, endoscopic and histological assessments are complementary in the assessment of disease severity.

Predicting relapse

Meyers and Janowitz (1989) first suggested that incomplete endoscopic healing at sigmoidoscopy was a predictor of an increased likelihood of relapse. Riley et al (1991) prospectively evaluated this question in 82 patients with endoscopically quiescent ulcerative colitis over 12 months. Baseline rectal biopsies demonstrated chronic inflammation in the lamina propria of all biopsies, while 58% showed architectural irregularities. Predictors of relapse, which occurred in 27 patients (33%), included epithelial ulceration (present in 75% who relapsed versus 31% who did not relapse), crypt abscess (78% versus 27%), acute inflammatory cell infiltrate (52% versus 25%), and mucin depletion (56% versus 26%), but chronic inflammatory cell infiltrate or crypt architectural distortion were not predictive. Another study, which assessed endoscopic and histologic criteria predicting disease exacerbation in 82 patients, found an increased frequency of relapses in patients who had endoscopic mucosal edema or erythema (Courtney et al 1991), but no relationship to the histology. These results suggest that a biopsy is an indispensable adjunct to endoscopy to quantify improvement, and both criteria should be considered for stratifying patients at entry to trials assessing maintenance therapy. Perhaps those at high risk of relapse also should be targeted for higher-dose maintenance 5-ASA.

Disease extent

Based on barium enema studies, Farmer (1979) suggested that patients initially diagnosed to have proctitis or limited colitis had a low risk (10%) of developing extensive colitis within the first few years of diagnosis. Later, using colonoscopy, disease extent varied depending on the activity at the time of colonoscopy, with less active disease appearing to regress (Niv et al 1987). In a follow-up of 828 patients at the Cleveland Clinic (Farmer et al 1993), 34% of those with proctitis and 70% with left-sided colitis progressed to pancolitis, with 58.1% requiring surgery. Risk factors associated with extension of disease included toxic or fulminant colitis early in the clinical course, association of joint symptoms, and younger age at diagnosis. In 1161 patients in Copenhagen County (Langholz et al 1995), 53% who had left-sided disease at diagnosis progressed to pancolitis endoscopically or radiologically over 25 years, whereas 76% of those with extensive colitis had regression of disease over a similar period.

Several studies have shown that some patients with ulcerative colitis may have patchy inflammation. In a retrospective review of 12 children with surgically proven ulcerative colitis (Markowitz et al 1993), three had patchy inflammation or a normal rectum endoscopically and six had patchy rectal or sigmoid inflammation or a normal biopsy histologically. Two other series have suggested that untreated patients (Spiliadis and Lennard-Jones 1987) or younger adults (Bernstein et al 1995) were more likely to have patchy disease. In these studies a good correlation was demonstrated between endoscopic and histologic appearance. Indeed, with the development of more sophisticated high-resolution endoscopes, such variability in disease severity and extent may be reported more frequently.

Several groups have also reported subsets of patients with ulcerative colitis in which the initial diagnosis was later changed to Crohn's disease (Langevin et al 1992). In our own series of such patients (Irvine et al 1990), changes in diagnosis were due to variable endoscopic or histologic appearances over time, or to endoscopist or histologist observer errors, but not to treatment with rectal therapy.

Table 29.4 Endoscopic appearance of inflammatory bowel disease

Ulcerative colitis (colon only)	Crohn's disease (any part of the gut)
Rectum involved	Rectum may be spared
Diffuse/continuous disease	Focal/asymmetric disease
Loss of vascular pattern	Loss of vascular pattern
Erythema/mucus/hemorrhage	Erythema/mucus/hemorrhage
Friability/granularity	Friability/granularity
Microulceration	Discrete (aphthous) ulceration
	Linear/serpiginous ulcers
	Discoid ulcers amid normal mucosa
	Poor distensibility
	Cobblestoning
	Fistula
	Perianal disease
Stricture	Stricture
Pseudopolyp	Pseudopolyp
Mucosal bridge	Mucosal bridge
Inflammatory mass	Inflammatory mass

Adapted from Pera et al (1987)

The first large study to critically evaluate the endoscopic features that discriminate Crohn's disease from ulcerative colitis was performed by Pera et al (1987). They assessed 357 patients with colitis during 606 colonoscopies over 22 months, and compared the endoscopic scores to an independent diagnosis by histology, surgery or autopsy. Colonoscopy made an accurate diagnosis in 89%, errors occurred in 4%, and 7% were diagnosed to have indeterminate colitis, predominantly in the presence of severe inflammation. Discontinuous disease, anal lesions and cobblestoning were the best predictors of Crohn's disease; those for ulcerative colitis were erosions, microulcers and granularity. Additional features are also summarized in Table 29.4.

Crohn's disease

Mary and Modigliani (1989) further standardized an endoscopic scoring system for Crohn's disease of the colon, part of which is shown in Table 29.5. In a study assessing observer agreement using this scale (Modigliani et al 1987), 112 colonoscopies were carried out by 18

Table 29.5 Crohn's disease endoscopic index of severity (CDEIS)

Check all findings that are present	
Rectum	[ ] Normal or
	[ ] Pseudopolyps
	[ ] Healed ulceration
	[ ] Erythema
	[ ] Edema
	[ ] Aphthous ulcers
	[ ] Superficial or shallow ulcers
	[ ] Deep ulcers
	[ ] Non-ulcerated stenosis
	[ ] Ulcerated stenosis
Place an X on the line to represent the	
% surface area involved by disease	|-------------------|
% surface area involved by ulceration	|-------------------|

Adapted from Mary and Modigliani (1989)

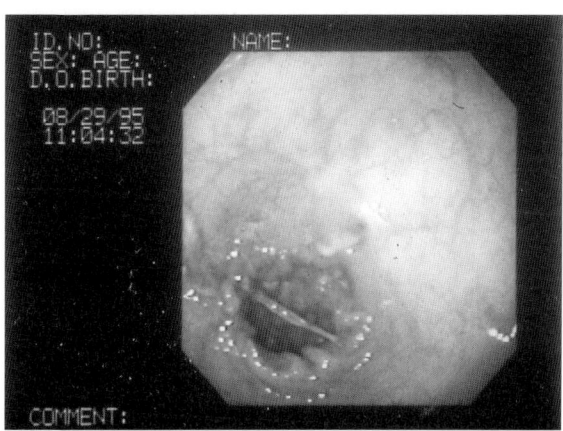

Fig. 29.5 An apthous ulcer, a small raised edematous lesion with a central erosion and surrounding erythema is the earliest typical lesion of Crohn's disease but may also occur in infections such as Yersinia, amebiasis or tuberculosis. (See page xx.)

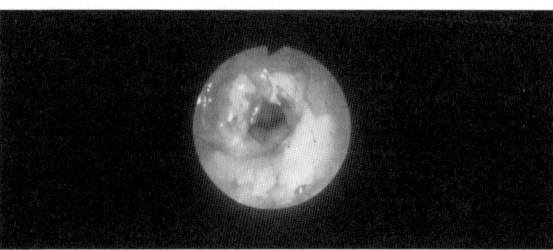

Fig. 29.6 Larger confluent ulcers occur in more severe Crohn's disease in association with rigidity and narrowing of the colonic lumen. (See page xx.)

paired endoscopists. The agreement on estimating diseased and ulcerated surfaces was good, with intraclass correlation coefficients of >0.85, and was similar for the presence or absence of ulcerated or non-ulcerated stenosis, deep ulcers, shallow ulcers and pseudopolyps. Reliability for aphthous ulcers was slightly less (70% agreement) and was poor for edema, erythema and healed ulceration. Consistency was also poorer when endoscopists were from different centers. This suggested that prior training would be required in clinical trials to ensure observer agreement, and that a simplified index might gain wider acceptance for application by clinicians.

In contrast to the findings in ulcerative colitis, several European studies on Crohn's disease have reported a lack of correlation between endoscopic and symptom severity (Modigliani et al 1990, Cellier et al 1994). In one study 92% of patients experiencing an acute attack of ileocolonic Crohn's disease achieved remission after treatment with prednisolone 1 mg/kg/day. However, 71% failed to achieve endoscopic remission (Modigliani et al 1990). Landi et al (1992) subsequently demonstrated, in a randomized clinical trial of 147 patients with ileocolonic or colonic Crohn's disease, that the presence of endoscopic lesions after induction of remission with corticosteroids did not predict those who would relapse over an 18-month follow-up period; 78% of the initial cohort experienced a relapse

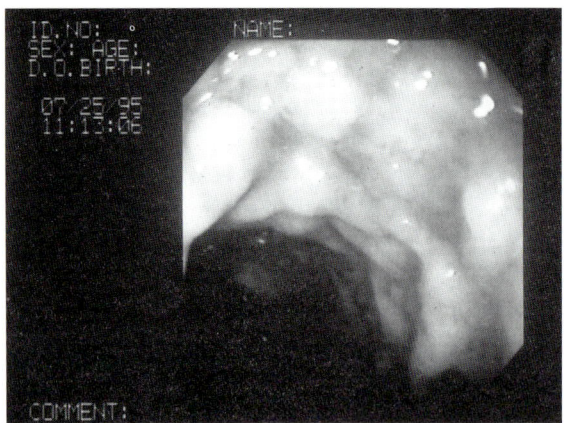

Fig. 29.7 Lymphoid nodular hyperplasia may be seen in the terminal ileum of normal subjects or patients with inflammatory bowel disease. Biopsies of this area will be normal. (See page xx.)

over the 18-month study. The authors concluded that ritual colonoscopy was not beneficial in determining therapy, but would add risk and costs to patient management.

Ileoscopy

The value of intubation of the terminal ileum during colonoscopy is increasingly being demonstrated. Kundrotas et al (1994) reported successful ileal intubation in over 90% of 295 consecutive unselected colonoscopies, requiring less than 10 minutes to examine an average of 10 cm of terminal ileum. In their series lesions were found in 2% of patients. Rokkas et al (1992) performed retrograde ileography by introducing barium through a catheter after intubation of the ileum, and obtained good visualization of 20–40 cm of ileum in patients with possible IBD. Concordance of diagnosis by ileoscopy and small-bowel meal in a retrospective series of 46 children with suspected Crohn's disease was 91% (Lipson et al 1990). They reported 100% sensitivity for detecting ileal Crohn's disease by ileoscopy and biopsy, although the gold standard of diagnosis was colonoscopy alone. Hewak et al (1995), using all available radiology, endoscopy and histology and follow-up for diagnosis in 48 patients, observed that ileoscopy detected ileal Crohn's disease accurately in 20 of 21 patients, but five with benign lymphoid nodular hyperplasia were overdiagnosed to have Crohn's disease by small-bowel meal with pneumocolon. Another small series of seven patients with iron deficiency, pain or diarrhea and a normal small-bowel meal all had Crohn's disease detected by ileoscopy (Zwas et al 1993). Ileoscopy should thus be attempted at the time of colonoscopy in patients with possible IBD, and this approach is likely to be more accurate for diagnosing ileal disease. Colonoscopy should be used to confirm isolated mild ileal disease before initiating therapy, and retrograde ileography may be useful in selected patients.

Perioperative endoscopy

Colonoscopy before surgery is most useful in patients with Crohn's disease to determine the extent of disease involvement prior to laparotomy and segmental resection. Postoperatively, colonoscopy is generally undertaken because of recurrence of symptoms, such as diarrhea, and to evaluate the anastomosis.

Rutgeerts et al (1990), in a follow-up study of patients who underwent segmental ileal resection, showed a 73% recurrence in the neoterminal ileum of 98 patients within 1 year, with 20% of patients having symptoms (Rutgeerts et al 1990). A 3-year follow-up showed 85% endoscopic recurrence and symptomatic recurrence in 34%. The likelihood of developing symptoms was related to the endoscopic severity of recurrent lesions. In a clinical trial to prevent postoperative disease recurrence, the recurrence rate in controls was observed to be only 22% at 1 year and 79% at 4 years, with only one-third of patients being symptomatic (McLeod et al 1995). However, not all the evaluations in this study were undertaken endoscopically. They confirmed that patients with aphthous ulcers were less likely to become symptomatic than those with larger ulcerations. The results of these studies contrast with those of clinical trials in patients with well established endoscopic disease, and suggest that there is indeed a correlation between lesion severity and symptoms.

An ileostomy, colostomy, Kock or pelvic pouch also may be intubated with a colonoscope or upper GI endoscope, and may be useful in patients with anemia, bleeding, high-output diarrhea or obstruction. Careful inspection should be made for adhesions, stricture, recurrent Crohn's disease or pouchitis. In patients with a Koch or pelvic pouch after total colectomy for ulcerative colitis (Kock et al 1977), pouchitis looks similar endoscopically to ulcerative colitis. The etiology may be multifactorial, relating to the underlying disease, an altered bacterial profile or underlying immune factors (Nicholls 1994). Refractory pouchitis with endoscopic features closely resembling Crohn's disease has been described in 24 patients, who had a greater prevalence of extraintestinal disease manifestations than did 21 controls (38% versus 5%) (Subramani et al 1993). Biopsies to confirm microscopic inflammation should always be obtained (Knobler et al 1986) to demonstrate a mixed acute epithelial inflammation with crypt abscesses and lymphocytic and plasma cell infiltrate in the lamina propria. Villous atrophy or colonic metaplasia may also be present (Nicholls 1994). Causes other than pouchitis, such as a fistula or loss of the nipple, should also be sought in cases of incontinence of a Kock pouch, and these can be readily visualized at endoscopy, as can recurrence of Crohn's disease (Waye 1988). A pediatric gastroscope, with its shorter bending section and acute angulation, is especially useful to obtain full visualization of the pouch.

The use of intraoperative enteroscopy is seldom required and not widely recommended (Lescut et al 1993, Smedh et al 1993). In these two modest series, scattered lesions varying from aphthous to larger ulcers were noted throughout the small bowel. External findings tended to underestimate the disease. In one study surgery was modified by the endoscopic findings, often resulting in a more limited resection. Biopsies of early lesions were noted to have increased eosinophils in the inflammatory infiltrate (Lescut et al 1993).

COMPLICATIONS OF INFLAMMATORY BOWEL DISEASE

Complications of inflammatory bowel disease may be a further indication for an endoscopic examination. Although toxic megacolon has generally been a definitive contraindication to colonoscopy, it has been successfully treated by endoscopic decompression in several case reports (Hoashi et al 1991, Riedler et al 1989), similar to that used in the treatment of Ogilvie's syndrome. However, given the potentially high risk, this should not yet be generally recommended.

Hemorrhage

Robert et al (1991) reported 21 of 1526 patients with Crohn's disease over 26 years who presented with severe gastrointestinal hemorrhage. Bleeding occurred more frequently in patients with colonic involvement (1.9%) than in those with small-bowel disease alone (0.7%) ($P < 0.001$). The mean age of the patients at the time of first hemorrhage was 28 years, and more than half required surgical resection; 3–9% of the series of patients with rectal bleeding who have undergone colonoscopy have been found to have IBD (Irvine et al 1988, Rossini et al 1989), and bleeding may be the presenting feature, especially in elderly patients with right-sided Crohn's disease. Persistent hemorrhage is more likely to be due to ulcerative colitis and, if massive, merits urgent colectomy (Rossini et al 1989). Colonoscopy can be useful to determine the site of bleeding, whether from small aphthous ulcers or a visible vessel, or to estimate the extent of resection required. Injection with epinephrine, ethanol or a sclerosing agent can be attempted. However, more experience will be needed to define clearly the role of these interventions in patients with inflammatory bowel disease.

Strictures

Strictures in ulcerative colitis are not uncommon and should always suggest the possibility of malignancy. In one series (Gumaste et al 1992) strictures occurred in 5% of 1156 patients. Of 70 stenoses in 59 patients, 17 (24%) were found to be malignant. Features associated with malignancy included occurrence after 20 years of disease; site proximal to the splenic flexure; and the presence of obstructive symptoms. Inflammatory strictures are often friable and may be ulcerated, whereas fibrotic strictures appear short and are often weblike. About 10% of strictures cannot be intubated with the adult colonoscope and an attempt with a smaller diameter pediatric instrument should be made to obtain biopsies and cytologic brushings. The presence of an abrupt or shelflike margin should also raise the suspicion of malignancy (Waye 1978). Since carcinoma in colitis can extend submucosally, giving negative superficial biopsies (Crowson et al 1976), lesions which appear endoscopically to be malignant should always be considered for resection. Those that are confidently confirmed to be benign may then be dilated endoscopically.

Yamazaki and colleagues (1991) examined strictures in 980 hospitalized patients with Crohn's disease during a 26-year period. Approximately 20% had colonic strictures, with about one-fifth having more than one stricture. Strictures were more common in colitis (19%) than ileocolitis (11%), and 10 malignant strictures were identified in nine patients (three ileocolitis, six colitis). Although malignancy was more common in a strictured than nonstrictured bowel segment, there were no clinical features, other than longer duration of disease which suggested a microscopic diagnosis of malignancy.

Benign terminal ileal, colonic and postsurgical anastomotic strictures in Crohn's disease, or benign strictures in ulcerative colitis, may be managed effectively by balloon dilatation, although the measurement tools to assess the effectiveness of such interventions have not been defined (Blomberg et al 1991, Bell et al 1991). Blomberg and colleagues (1991) reported their experience in 27 patients with Crohn's disease using hydrostatic balloon dilators with a built-in guide wire (Microvasive Rigiflex TTS). The procedure was performed through the endoscope under direct vision using balloons from 3 to 8 cm in length. Balloons were inflated for between 30 seconds and 5 minutes one to four times per session to achieve a postdilatation diameter of 10–15 mm. In this and other series, several dilatations were often necessary (Blomberg et al 1991, Bell et al 1991, Williams and Palmer 1991, Breysem et al 1992), and features which suggested that dilatation may be ineffective included stricture length (average 12 cm) or the presence of active disease. Perforation or bleeding are potential complications of dilatation and in one series were each reported in 4% of patients (Blomberg et al 1991). Recently combined injection of triamcinolone with balloon dilatation has been performed in at least one case report (Lavy 1994). Critical evaluation of the follow-up, and other techniques such as electrocautery or laser incision and dilatation, will be needed before they can be recommended.

OTHER ENDOSCOPIC TECHNIQUES

Ultrasonography

Anorectal pathology is common in Crohn's disease and occurs in approximately 22–85% of cases. Hypertrophic skin tags, anal fissures or ulceration, fistulae, abscesses and strictures of the anal canal have been reported (Wijers et al 1992, Schratter-Sehn et al 1993). Transrectal ultrasonography, when available, is easy to perform and well tolerated by patients, and provides useful information about the rectal wall and pararectal tissues. Van Outryve and colleagues (1991) described the use of this technique in 40 healthy individuals and 40 patients with Crohn's disease. In healthy subjects ultrasound of the rectal wall demonstrated five distinct layers, with clear visualization of the anal sphincter and no pararectal pathology. In the Crohn's patients, thickening of the rectal wall was seen in 16 cases and heterogeneity at the anal sphincter in 19. This technique detected a number of lesions missed by the routine proctoscopy: four pararectal abscesses, two pararectal fistulae, two para-anal abscesses and one para-anal fistula. Abscesses were echopoor areas, whereas fistulae appeared to be echopoor areas with a ductlike appearance. Transrectal ultrasound has also been useful in diagnosing solitary rectal ulcers, in which the five rectal layers are preserved (Hizawa et al 1994), and in evaluating anal sphincter abnormalities such as fissures, ulcers or destruction secondary to trauma during vaginal delivery. Future applications, such as preoperative assessment in female patients who require colectomy and pelvic pouch construction, may be useful.

Dye-spraying techniques

Japanese investigators have been instrumental in developing dye-spraying techniques and the use of magnifying endoscopes to detect dysplastic or malignant mucosa in the gastrointestinal tract. These same techniques may also be adapted to detect subtle inflammation in inflammatory bowel disease. Okada and colleagues (1991) sprayed 0.1% indigo carmine through a sigmoidoscope on to the macroscopically normal rectum and sigmoid colon of 20 patients with Crohn's disease and ten age-matched healthy volunteers. Minute lesions such as aphthoid ulcers, erythema or small ulcers, were observed in 90% of the Crohn's patients and no healthy volunteers. Histologically granulomas were found in 15% of patients with Crohn's disease. Makiyama et al (1989) assessed 27 patients with Crohn's disease (37 occasions) by incorporating methylene blue into the colonic lavage solution. They described a worm-eaten appearance with endoscopic magnification, and biopsies of these areas also had a high incidence of granulomata. Application of dyes has not been well evaluated for the detection of dysplasia or cancer.

MASS LESIONS

Inflammatory polyps

Mass lesions detected by barium enema may represent carcinoma, adenomatous polyp or non-neoplastic pseudopolyp, and all require full evaluation by colonoscopy and biopsy. Inflammatory or pseudopolyps are generally multiple and small, with a surface mucosal appearance similar to that of the surrounding mucosa. They may occur in both ulcerative colitis and Crohn's disease, usually in areas of healed prior ulceration, and although they have no malignant potential (Jalan et al 1969, Teague & Waye 1981), may be confused with a dysplasia-associated lesion or mass (Blackstone et al 1981). When solitary or large, the appearance may be more suggestive of carcinoma. Inflammatory polyps also may consist of granulation tissue, which rarely can bleed, occlude the colonic lumen or cause intussusception (Forde et al 1978). Filiform inflammatory polyps are usually multiple, long and slender, and are covered by normal non-dysplastic epithelium (Rozenbajgier et al 1992). Biopsy or removal of solitary lesions, large lesions (>1 cm) or those with an appearance distinct from the surrounding mucosa should be performed to permit histological appraisal.

Adenomatous polyps

Adenomatous polyps, although uncommon in inflammatory bowel disease, may be difficult to distinguish from inflammatory polyps. In one series of 150 patients with ulcerative colitis, 3% had adenomatous polyps, of which three were solitary (Teague & Read 1975) Thus, removal of singular or large polyps by the usual snare polypectomy technique is recommended; follow-up is similar to that for non-IBD related adenomas. The dysplasia-associated lesion or mass, which may be poorly circumscribed, can appear as a slightly raised velvety plaque or an irregular area of nodularity or ulceration, and is not usually confused with an adenoma (Blackstone et al 1981).

REFERENCES

Anseline P F, Laver I C, Fazio V W et al 1981 Radiation injury of the rectum: evaluation of surgical treatment. Annals of Surgery 194: 716–724

Baron J H, Connell A M, Lennard-Jones J E 1964 Variation between observers in describing mucosal appearances in proctocolitis. British Medical Journal 1: 89–92

Bayerdorffer E, Hochter W, Schwarzkopf-Steinhauser G et al 1986 Bioptic microbiology in the differential diagnosis of enterocolitis. Endoscopy 18: 177–181

Bell N J V, Rademaker J W, Hunt R H 1991 Through-the-scope (TTS) balloon dilation of ileocolonic and colonic anastomotic strictures. Gastrointestinal Endoscopy 37: A272 (Abstract)

Bernstein C N, Shanahan F, Anton P A, Weinstein W A 1995 Patchiness of mucosal inflammation in treated ulcerative colitis: a prospective study. Gastrointestinal Endoscopy 42: 232–237

Bertele-Harms R M, Harms H K, Schmitz-Moormann P 1986 Significance of endoscopy in influencing bowel disease in childhood. Wien Klin Ische Wochenschrift 98: 540–543

Bhargava D K, Shriniwas M D, Chopra P et al 1992 Peritoneal tuberculosis: laparoscopic patterns and its diagnostic accuracy. American Journal of Gastroenterology 87: 109–112

Bjarnason I, Hayllar J, Macpherson A J, Russell A S 1983 Side effects of non-steroidal anti-inflammatory drugs on the small and large intestine in humans. Gastroenterology 104: 1832–1847

Blackstone M O, Riddell R H, Rogers B H G 1981 Dysplasia-associated lesion or mass (DALM) detected by colonoscopy in longstanding ulcerative colitis; an indication for colectomy. Gastroenterology 80: 366–374

Blomberg B, Rolny P, Jarnerot G 1991 Endoscopic treatment of anastomotic strictures. Endoscopy 23: 195–198

Breysem Y, Janssens J F, Coremans G et al 1992 Endoscopic balloon dilation of colonic and ileo-colonic Crohn's strictures: long term results. Gastrointestinal Endoscopy 38: 142–147

Carbonnel F, Lavergne A, Lemann M et al 1994 Colonoscopy of acute colitis. A safe and reliable tool for assessment of severity. Digestive Diseases and Sciences 39: 1550–1557

Carr-Locke D L, Finlay D B L 1983 Radiological demonstration of colonic aphthoid ulcers in patients with intestinal tuberculosis. Gut 24: 453–455

Cellier C, Sahmoud T, Froguel E et al 1994 Correlation between clinical activity, endoscopic severity and biological parameters in colonic or ileocolonic Crohn's disease. Gut 35: 231–235

Chong S K, Blackshaw A J, Boyle S et al 1985 Histological diagnosis of chronic inflammatory bowel in childhood. Digestive Diseases and Sciences 29: 731–734

Clouse R E, Alpers D H, Hockenbery D M, DeSchryver-Kecskemeti K 1992 Pericrypt eosinophilic enterocolitis and chronic diarrhea. Gastroenterology 103: 168–176

Cooper R, Murphy S, Midlick D 1992 *Campylobacter jejuni* enteritis mistaken for ulcerative colitis. Journal of Family Practice 34: 357–362

Costello P B, Alea J A, Kennedy A C et al 1980 Prevalence of occult inflammatory bowel disease in ankylosing spondylitis. Annals of Rheumatic Disease 39: 453–446

Crowson T D, Hines C 1978 Amebiasis diagnosed by colonoscopy. Gastrointestinal Endoscopy 24: 254–255

Crowson T D, Ferrante W F, Gathright J B 1976 Colonoscopy: inefficacy for early carcinoma detection in patients with ulcerative colitis. Journal of the American Medical Association 236: 2651–2652

Ernstoff J J, Howard D A, Marshall J B et al 1983 A randomized blinded clinical trial of rapid colonic lavage solution (Golytely) compared with standard preparation for colonoscopy and barium enema. Gastroenterology 84: 512–516

Farmer R G 1979 Longterm prognosis for patients with ulcerative proctosigmoiditis. Journal of Clinical Gastroenterology 8: 47–50

Farmer R G, Easley K A, Rankin G B 1993 Clinical patterns, natural history and progression of ulcerative colitis: a long term follow-up of 1116 patients. Digestive Diseases and Sciences 38: 1137–1146

Forde K, Gold R P, Halck S et al 1978 Giant pseudopolyposis in colitis with colonic intussusception. Gastroenterology 75: 1142–1146

Freeny P C 1986 Crohn's disease and ulcerative colitis. Evaluation with double contrast barium enema examination and endoscopy. Postgraduate Medicine 80: 139–156

Glotzer D J, Glick M E, Goldman H 1981 Proctitis and colitis following diversion of the fecal stream. Gastroenterology 80: 438–441

Gore S, Shepherd N A, Wilkinson S P 1992 Endoscopic crescentic fold disease of the sigmoid colon: the clinical and histopathological spectrum of a distinctive endoscopic appearance. International Journal of Colorectal Disease 7: 76–81

Gumaste W, Sachar D B, Greenstein A J et al 1992 Benign and malignant stenoses in ulcerative colitis. Gut 33: 938–941

Gyde S 1990 Screening for colorectal cancer in ulcerative colitis: dubious benefits and high costs. Gut 31: 1089–1092

Hall C, Dorricott N J, Donovan I A, Neoptolemos J P 1991 Colon perforation during colonoscopy: surgical versus conservative management. British Journal of Surgery 78: 542–544

Haque S, West A B 1992 Editorial: Diversion colitis – 20 years a-growing. Journal of Clinical Gastroenterology 15: 281–283

Harig J M, Soergel K H, Komorowski et al 1989 Treatment of diversion colitis with short chain fatty acid irrigation. New England Journal of Medicine 320: 23–28

Hewak J, Farrow R, Wright C et al 1995 Diagnosis of ileal Crohn's disease: a comparative study of ileoscopy versus small bowel meal with pneumocolon. Gastroenterology 108: A834 (Abstract)

Hizawa K, Iida M, Suekane H et al 1994 Mucosal prolapse syndrome: diagnosis with endoscopic ultrasound. Radiology 191: 527–530

Hoashi T, Tsuda S, Yao T et al 1991 A case of ulcerative colitis with toxic megacolon, successfully treated with colonoscopic decompression. Nippon Shokakibyo Gakkai Zasshi 88: 91–95

Hunt R H 1986 Lower gastrointestinal tract. In: Schiller K F R, Cockel R, Hunt R H (eds) Atlas of gastrointestinal endoscopy. Chapman & Hall, London pp 177–228

Hunt R H, Buchanan J K 1979 Transient ischemic colitis – colonoscopy and biopsy in diagnosis. Journal of the Royal Naval Medical Service 65: 15–19

Hunt R H, Teague R H, Swarbrick E T, Williams C B 1975 Colonoscopy in the management of colonic strictures. British Medical Journal ii: 360–361

Irvine E J 1993 Assessing outcome in randomized clinical trials: inflammatory bowel disease. Canadian Journal of Gastroenterology 7: 561–567

Irvine E J, O'Connor, Frost R A et al 1988 A prospective comparison of double contrast barium enema plus flexible sigmoidoscopy versus colonoscopy in rectal bleeding. Gut 29: 1188–1193

Irvine E J, Somers S, Seaton T, Riddell R H 1990 Reasons for change in diagnosis from ulcerative colitis to Crohn's disease. World Congress of Gastroenterology Abstracts

Jalan K N, Sircus W, Walker R J et al 1969 Pseudopolyposis in ulcerative colitis. Lancet 2: 555–559

Kishida T, Sato J, Fujimori S et al 1992 An endoscopic study of antibiotic associated colitis. Journal of Nippon Medical School 59: 450–456

Knobler H, Ligumsky M, Okon E et al 1986 Pouch ileitis – recurrence of inflammatory bowel disease in the ileal reservoir. American Journal of Gastroenterology 81: 199–201

Kock N G, Darle N, Hulton L et al 1977 Ileostomy. Current Problems in Surgery 14: 36–38

Kozarek R A, Botoman V A, Bredfeldt J E et al 1991 Portal colopathy: prospective study of colonoscopy in patients with portal hypertension. Gastroenterology 101: 1192–1197

Kundrotas L W, Clement D J, Crain M et al 1994 A prospective evaluation of successful terminal ileum intubation during routine colonoscopy. Gastrointestinal Endoscopy 40: 544–546

Landi B, N'Guyen A N H T, Cortot A et al 1992 Endoscopic monitoring of Crohn's disease treatment: a prospective, randomized clinical trial. Gastroenterology 102: 1647–1653

Langevin S, Menard D, Haddad H et al 1992 Idiopathic ulcerative colitis may be the initial manifestation of Crohn's disease. Journal of Clinical Gastroenterology 15: 199–204

Langholz E, Nielsen O H, Munkholm et al 1995 Course and prognostic factors influencing changes in the anatomical extent of ulcerative colitis. Gastroenterology 108: A857 (Abstract)

Larsson P A, Olling S, Darle N 1991 Amebic colitis presenting as acute inflammatory bowel disease. European Journal of Surgery 157: 553–555

Lavy A 1994 Steroid injection improves outcome in Crohn's disease strictures. Endoscopy 26: 366

Leirisalo-Repo M, Turunen U, Stenman et al 1994 High frequency of silent inflammatory bowel disease in spondyloarthopathy. Arthritis and Rheumatism 37: 23–31

Lescut D, Vanco D, Bonniere P et al 1993 Perioperative endoscopy of the whole small bowel in Crohn's disease. Gut 34: 647–649

Lipson A, Bartram C I, Williams C B et al 1990 Barium studies and ileoscopy compared in children with suspected Crohn's disease. Clinical Radiology 41: 5–8

Lumb B J, Hunt R H 1987 Miscellaneous disorders of the colon. In: Sivak M (ed) Gastroenterologic endoscopy. WB Saunders Company, Philadelphia, pp 946–959

McLeod R S, Wolff B G, Steinhart A H et al 1995 Risk and significance of endoscopic and radiological recurrence of Crohn's disease post operatively. Gastroenterology 108: A874 (Abstract)

Macrae I, Wright V 1973 A family study of ulcerative colitis with particular reference to ankylosing spondylitis and sacroiliitis. Annals of Rheumatic Diseases 32: 16–20

Madigan M R, Morson B C 1969 Solitary ulcer of the rectum. Gut 10: 871–881

Makiyama K, Tanaka T, Senju M et al 1989 Clinical course and magnifying endoscopic findings of fine lesions of the large intestinal mucosa in Crohn's disease. Gastroenterology (Japan) 24: 120–126

Markowitz J, Kahn E, Grancer K et al 1993 Atypical rectosigmoid histology in children with newly diagnosed ulcerative colitis. American Journal of Gastroenterology 88: 2034–2037

Marshall J K, Irvine E J 1995 Rectal aminosalicylate therapy in distal ulcerative colitis: a meta-analysis. Aliment Pharmacol Therapeut 9: 293–300

Mary J Y, Modigliani R for Groupe d'Etudes Thérapeutiques des Affections Inflammatoires du Tube Digestif (GETAID) 1989 Development and validation of an endoscopic index of the severity of Crohn's disease: a prospective multicentre study. Gut 30: 983–989

Mentec H, Leport C, Leport J et al 1994 Cytomegalovirus in HIV-1 infected patients: a prospective research in 55 patients. AIDS 8: 461–467

Meyers S, Janowitz H D 1989 The natural history of ulcerative colitis: an analysis of the placebo response. Journal of Clinical Gastroenterology 11: 33–37

Modigliani R, Mary J Y, Simon J F et al 1990 Clinical biological and endoscopic picture of attacks of Crohn's disease: evolution on prednisolone. Gastroenterology 98: 811–818

Modigliani R, Mary J Y and the Groupe d'Etudes Thérapeutiques des Affections Inflammatoroires du Tube Digestif 1987 Reproducibility of colonoscopic findings in Crohn's disease. Digestive Diseases and Sciences 32: 1370–1379

Mohamed A R, al Karawi M, Yasawy M I 1990 Schistosomal colonic disease. Gut 31: 439–442

Nebel O T, El-Masry N A, Castell D O et al 1974 Schistosomal colonic polyposis: endoscopic and histological characteristics. Gastrointestinal Endoscopy 20: 99–101

Nicholls R J 1994 Pouchitis – what's new in etiology and management? In: Sutherland L R, Collins S M, Martin F et al (eds) Inflammatory bowel disease: basic research, clinical implications and trends in therapy. Kluwer Academic Publishers, Lancaster, pp 303–312

Niv Y, Bat L, Ron E, Theodor E 1987 Change in the extent of colonic involvement in ulcerative colitis: a colonoscopic study. American Journal of Gastroenterology 82: 1046–1051

Odze R, Bines J, Leightner A et al 1993 Allergic proctocolitis in infants: a prospective clinicopathogic biopsy study. Human Pathology 24: 668–674

Okada M, Maeda K, Yao T, Iwashita A, Nomiyama Y, Kitahara K 1991 Minute lesions of the rectum and sigmoid colon in patients with Crohn's disease. Gastrointestinal Endoscopy 37: 319–324

Palmer K R, Patil D H, Basran G S et al 1985 Abdominal tuberculosis in urban Britain – a common disease. Gut 26: 1296–1305

Peppercorn M 1992 Drug-responsive chronic segmental colitis associated with diverticula: a clinical syndrome in the elderly. American Journal of Gastroenterology 87: 609–612

Pera A, Bellardo P, Caldera D et al 1987 Colonoscopy in inflammatory bowel disease. Diagnostic accuracy and proposal of endoscopic score. Gastroenterology 92: 181–185

Pockros P J, Foroozan P 1985 Golytely lavage versus a standard colonoscopy preparation: effect on normal mucosal histology. Gastroenterology 88: 545–548

Prathap K, Gilman R 1970 The histopathology of acute intestinal amebiasis: a rectal biopsy study. American Journal of Pathology 60: 229–246

Prescott R J, Harris M, Banerjee S S 1992 Fungal infections of the small and large intestine. Journal of Clinical Pathology 45: 806–811

Purrmann J, Zeidler H, Bertrams J et al 1988 HLA antigens in ankylosing spondylitis associated with Crohn's disease. Increased frequency of HLA phenotype B27, B44. Journal of Rheumatology 15: 1658–1661

Riddell R H, Tanaka M, Mazzoleni G 1992 Non-steroidal anti-inflammatory drugs as a possible cause of collagenous colitis. Gut 33: 683–686

Riedler L, Wohlgenannt D, Stoss F et al 1989 Endoscopic decompression in toxic megacolon. Surgical Endoscopy 13: 190–192

Riley S A, Mani V, Goodman M J, Dutt S, Herd M E 1991 Microscopic activity in ulcerative colitis: what does it mean? Gut 32: 174–178

Robert J R, Sachar D B, Greenstein A J 1991 Severe gastrointestinal hemorrhage in Crohn's disease. Annals of Surgery 213: 207–211

Roe A M, Warren B F, Brodribb A J M, Brown C 1993 Diversion colitis and involution of the defunctioned anorectum. Gut 34: 382–385

Roediger W E W 1980 The colonic epithelium in ulcerative colitis: an energy deficient disease. Lancet ii: 712–715

Rokkas T, Filipe M I, Sladen G E 1988 Collagenous colitis with rapid response to sulfasalazine. Postgraduate Medical Journal 64: 74–76

Rokkas T, Psaras P, Niotos E et al 1992 Endoscopic retrograde ileography. Gastrointestinal Endoscopy 38: 375–376

Rossini F P, Ferrari A, Spandre M et al 1989 Emergency colonoscopy. World Journal of Surgery 13: 190–192

Rozenbajgier C, Puck R, Jenss H, Kaiserling E 1992 Filiform polyposis: a case report describing clinical, morphological and immunohistochemical findings. Clinical Investigation 70: 520–528

Rutgeerts P, Geboes K, Vantrappen G et al 1990 Predictability of the postoperative course of Crohn's disease. Gastroenterology 99: 956–962

Rutgeerts P, Peeters M, Geboes K, Vantrappen G 1992 Infectious agents in inflammatory bowel disease. Endoscopy 26: 565–567

Rutter K R P, Riddell R H 1975 The solitary ulcer syndrome of the rectum. Clinical Gastroenterology 4: 505–530

Schratter-Sehn A U, Lochs H, Vogelsang H et al 1993 Endoscopic ultrasonography versus computed tomography in the differential diagnosis of perianorectal complication in Crohn's disease. Endoscopy 25: 582–586

Seow-Chen F, Chua T L, Goh H S 1993 Ischemic colitis and colorectal cancer: some problems and pitfalls. International Journal of Colorectal Diseases 8: 210–212

Shah K S, Thomas V, Mathan M et al 1992 Colonoscopic study of 50 patients with colonic tuberculosis. Gut 33: 337–351

Smedh K, Olaison G, Nystrom P O, Sjodahl R 1993 Intraoperative enteroscopy in Crohn's disease. British Journal of Surgery 80: 897–900

Snowcroft C W, Sanowski R A, Kozarek R A 1981 Colonoscopy in ischemic colitis. Gastrointestinal Endoscopy 27: 156–161

Spiliadis C A, Lennard-Jones J E 1987 Ulcerative colitis with relative sparing of the rectum. Clinical features, histology and prognosis. Diseases of the Colon and Rectum 30: 334–336

Steinhart A H, Brzezinski A, Baker J P 1994 Treatment of refractory ulcerative proctosigmoiditis with butyrate enemas. American Journal of Gastroenterology 89: 179–183

Subramani K, Harpaz N, Bilotta J et al 1993 Refractory pouchitis: does it reflect underlying Crohn's disease? Gut 34: 1539–1542

Surawicz C M, Belic L 1984 Rectal biopsy helps to distinguish acute self-limited colitis from idiopathic inflammatory bowel disease. Gastroenterology 86: 104–113

Tanaka M, Mazzoleni G, Riddell R H 1992 Distribution of collagenous colitis: utility of flexible sigmoidoscopy. Gut 33: 65–70

Teague R H, Read A E 1975 Polyposis in ulcerative colitis. Gut 16: 792–792

Teague R H, Waye J D 1981 Endoscopy in inflammatory bowel disease. In: Hunt R H, Waye J D (eds) Colonoscopy: techniques clinical practice and colour atlas. Chapman & Hall, London, pp 343–362

Tedesco F J, Hardin R D, Harper R N et al 1983 Infectious colitis endoscopically simulating inflammatory bowel disease: a prospective evaluation. Gastrointestinal Endoscopy 29: 195–197

Triadafilopoulos G, Hallstone A 1991 Acute abdomen as the first presentation of pseudomembranous colitis. Gastroenterology 101: 685–691

Van Outryve M J, Pelckmans P A, Michielsen P P, Van Maercke Y M 1991 Value of transrectal ultrasonography in Crohn's disease. Gastroenterology 101: 1171–1177

Waye J D 1978 Colitis, cancer and colonoscopy. Medical Clinics of North America 62: 211–224

Waye J D 1988 Endoscopy in idiopathic inflammatory bowel disease. In: Kirsner J B, Shorter R G (eds) Inflammatory bowel disease. Lea and Febiger, Philadelphia, pp 353–376

Waye J D 1990 Endoscopy in inflammatory bowel disease: indications and differential diagnosis. Medical Clinics of North American 74: 51–65

Waye J D 1992 Differentiation of inflammatory bowel conditions. Endoscopy 24: 551–554

Wijers O B, Tio T L, Tytgat G N J 1992 Ultrasonography and endosonography in the diagnosis and management of inflammatory bowel disease. Endoscopy 24: 559–564

Widgren S, Jlidi R, Cox N 1988 Collagenous colitis: histologic, morphometric and ultrastructural studies. Report of 21 cases. Virchows Archiv 413: 287–296

Williams A J, Palmer K R 1991 Endoscopic balloon dilatation as a therapeutic option in the management of intestinal strictures resulting from Crohn's disease. British Journal of Surgery 78: 453–454

Yamazaki Y, Ribeiro M B, Sachar D B, Aufses A H, Greenstein A J 1991 Malignant colorectal strictures in Crohn's disease. American Journal of Gastroenterology 86: 882–885

Zeroogian J M, Chopra S 1994 Collangenous colitis and lymphocytic colitis. Annual Review of Medicine 45a: 105–118

Zwas F, Bonheim N A, Berken C A, Gray S 1993 Ileoscopy as an important tool for the diagnosis of Crohn's disease: a report of seven cases. Gastrointestinal Endoscopy 40: 89–91

30. Endoluminal ultrasound

M. S. Bhutani   R. H. Hawes

INTRODUCTION

Endoluminal ultrasound was first developed in the 1950s (Wild & Reid 1956), when the probe was positioned in the rectum and used to image the prostate. In the late 1970s ultrasound transducers were mounted on the end of flexible endoscopes, initially to improve ultrasound imaging of the pancreas. It was quickly realized, however, that using high-frequency transducers within the gut lumen produced exquisitely detailed images of the gastrointestinal tract wall, and that correlates existed between the echo layers and the histologic layers. This technology has become widely utilized in Europe and Japan, and is being increasingly accepted in the United States. Its principal role to date has been to stage gastrointestinal cancers (Hawes 1993), but with more widespread availability new applications have been discovered. This chapter will focus on the utility of endoscopic ultrasound in inflammatory bowel disease.

INSTRUMENTATION

Both rigid and flexible echoendoscopes are available for colorectal imaging. Rigid probes do not incorporate optics and their use is confined to the rectum. Flexible echoendoscopes have incorporated fiberoptic bundles and can be passed into the more proximal colon. The most commonly used rectal probe is manufactured by Bruel and Kjaer (Naerum, Denmark; Marlborough, MA) (Fig. 30.1). It uses a single-element transducer which operates at 7.5 MHz. The transducer is mechanically rotated, providing a 360° radial image perpendicular to the axis of the probe. A balloon is fitted around the transducer to provide acoustic coupling with the gut wall. Rigid probes are also manufactured which incorporate linear array transducers (Hitachi, Tarry Town, NY, and Acuson, Mountainview, CA). The linear array systems have the advantage of ultrasound-directed needle puncture, but their use to date has been almost exclusively in prostate imaging.

Two flexible endoscopic systems are available which can perform colorectal endosonography. One incorporates a linear array transducer (Pentax FG-32UA, Orangeburg, NY). This echoendoscope connects to a Hitachi console (model 515, Hitachi, Conshohocken, PA). The most commonly used flexible echoendoscope is manufactured by Olympus (Olympus Optical, Tokyo; Olympus America, Lake Success, NY). The upper gastrointestinal echoendoscope (GF-UM20) (Fig. 30.2) incorporates oblique viewing optics and can often be passed into the distal sigmoid colon. It can image at 7.5 and 12 MHz, and scans by mechanically rotating the transducer 360° around the axis of the endoscope. Olympus also makes an echocolonoscope (CF-UM20) (Fig. 30.3). This instrument has a mechanically rotating single-element transducer (7.5 MHz), but the light and image bundles run alongside the transducer to provide endviewing optics. This allows the instrument to be passed into the more proximal colon, and in most cases to the cecum (80%). This system provides the only mechanism for endoluminal ultrasound of the entire colon.

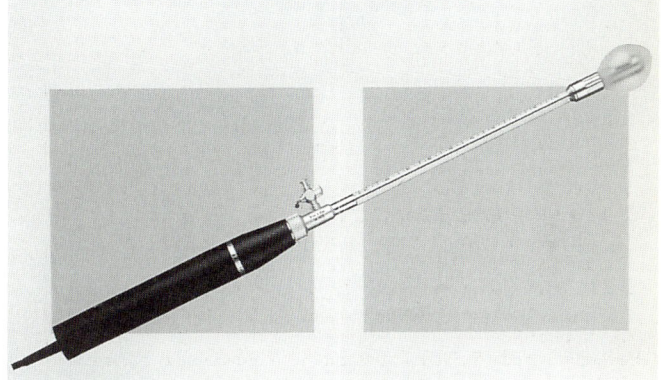

Fig. 30.1 Bruel and Kjaer rectal ultrasound probe.

ROLE IN THE DIFFERENTIAL DIAGNOSIS OF INFLAMMATORY BOWEL DISEASE

Five echolayers of the gastrointestinal wall are identified sonographically (Figs 30.4, 30.5). The first (closest to the

286 INFLAMMATORY BOWEL DISEASES

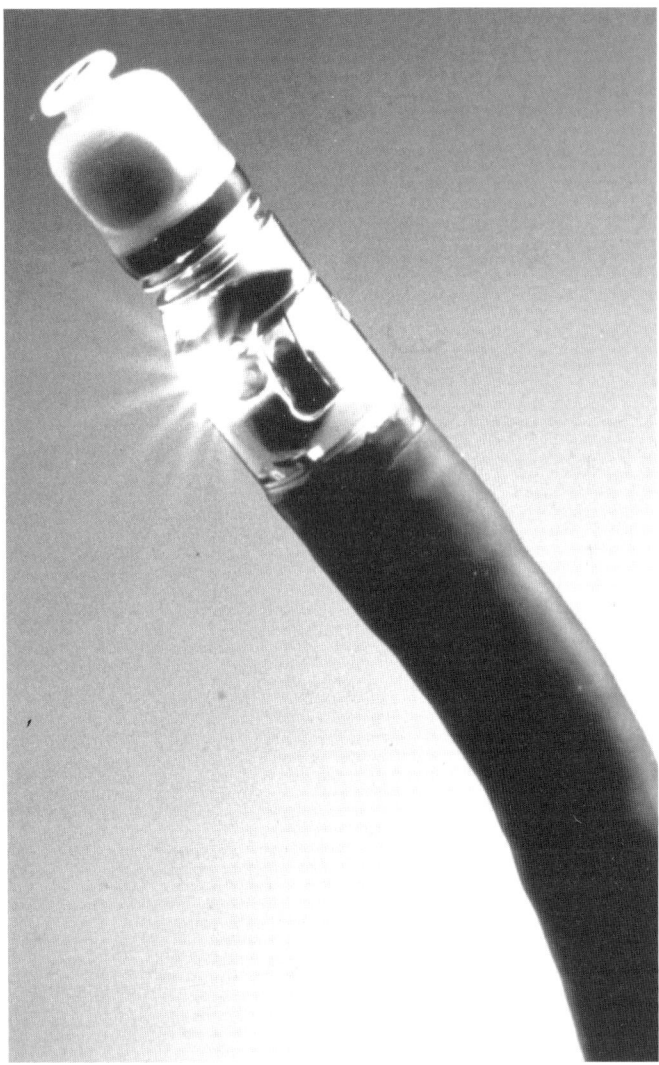

Fig. 30.2 Olympus GF-UM20 radial scanning flexible fiberoptic echoendoscope.

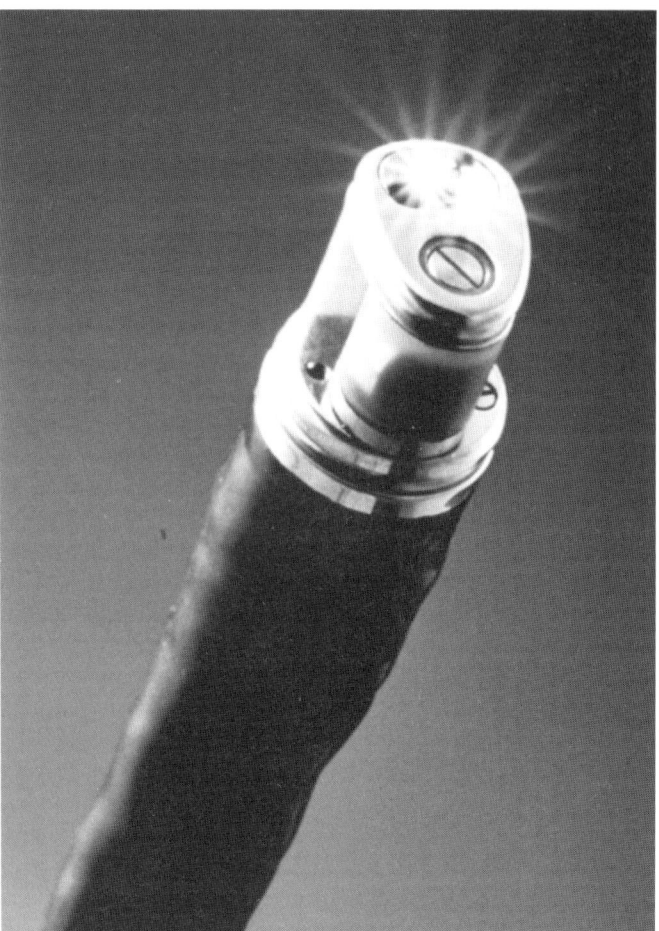

Fig. 30.3 Distal end of the Olympus CF-UM20 echocolonscope with end-viewing optics.

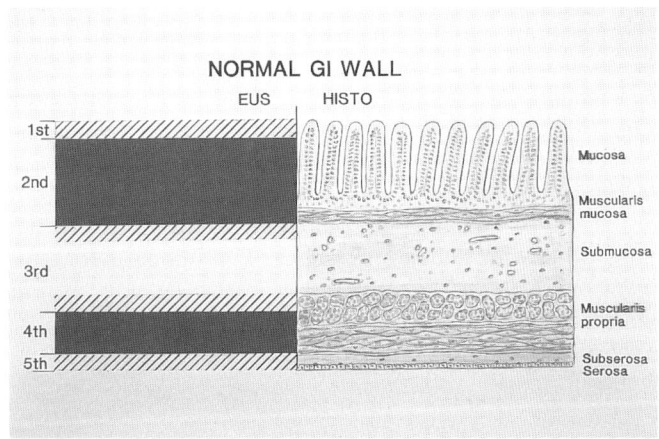

Fig. 30.4 Schematic representation of endosonographic appearance of the gastrointestinal wall layers, with histologic correlates.

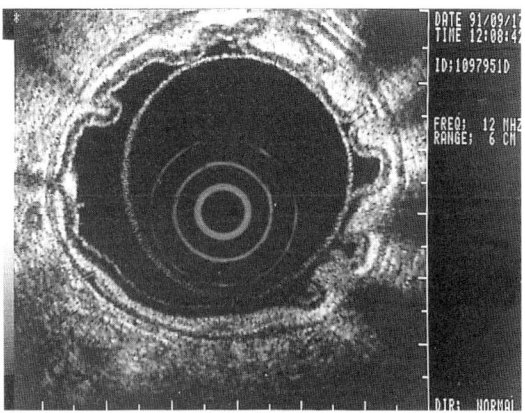

Fig. 30.5 Endoscopic ultrasound image demonstrating the five echolayers of the stomach wall imaged with the radial scanning echoendoscope at a frequency of 12 MHz.

transducer), hyperechoic layer represents a mucosal interface echo. The second layer is hypoechoic and roughly correlates with the mucosa. The third layer is hyperechoic and corresponds to the submucosa. The fourth layer, which is hypoechoic, represents the muscularis propria. The fifth layer is hyperechoic and results from an acoustic interface with the serosa/subserosa or surrounding fat.

Transabdominal ultrasonography has been studied as a diagnostic modality for inflammatory bowel disease (Bozkurt et al 1994). It is performed after retrograde instillation of water into the colon, and has been used to image the colonic wall in an effort to define criteria which might differentiate ulcerative colitis from Crohn's disease (Fig. 30.6). Thickened, echopoor bowel wall with loss of the typical five-layer wall stratification has been found to be a sonographic feature of Crohn's colitis. Ulcerative colitis, on the other hand, while revealing a thickened echopoor bowel wall, maintained the integrity of the echolayers without disruption (Limberg 1989) (Fig. 30.7). The in-vivo data from Limberg, however, have not been confirmed in an in-vitro model. Kimmey et al (1990) looked at normal colons as well as those resected in patients with inflammatory bowel disease. The normal colonic wall thickness is less than 3 mm. This in-vitro analysis did show thickening of the bowel wall and loss of the five-layer stratification in some cases, and although normal colon could be distinguished from inflamed colon, a differentiation between Crohn's colitis and ulcerative colitis could not be made with accuracy.

The findings reported with extracorporeal ultrasound should be applicable to endoluminal ultrasound, but greater detail of the bowel wall structure should be achievable with the higher-frequency transducers. Experience with this application is limited, but Shimizu et al (1992) performed endosonography in patients with ulcerative colitis and demonstrated varying degrees of gastrointestinal wall abnormalities in 47%. As the severity of disease increased, progressively deeper layers of the gut wall became thickened (third and fourth layers, representing submucosa and muscularis propria respectively). Related applications for endosonography in the future may include:

1. Endosonography in combination with endoscopy may provide information about the extent and degree of inflammation – information that could improve therapy (Cho et al 1990).
2. It may also be possible that endosonography will aid in evaluating patients who achieve an endoscopic remission but who are still experiencing symptoms (possibly representing residual submucosal inflammation).
3. Endosonography may also play a role in the small subset of patients in whom there are mixed characteristics of Crohn's disease and ulcerative colitis. Visualization of the entire gut wall may add information to help discriminate between the two diseases.

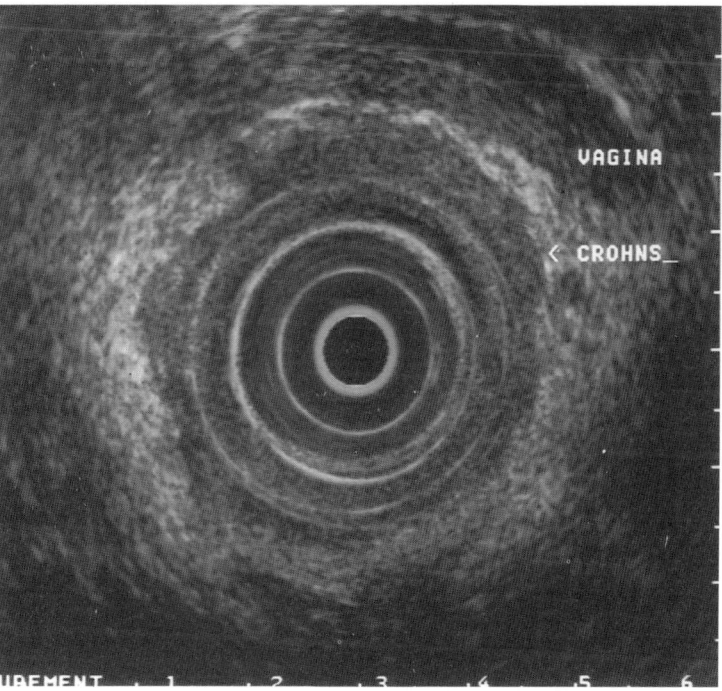

Fig. 30.6 Thickening of the rectal wall in a patient with Crohn's disease. Note the loss of echolayers, the irregular outer (deep) contour of the bowel wall and the close proximity to the vagina. No fistula was identified.

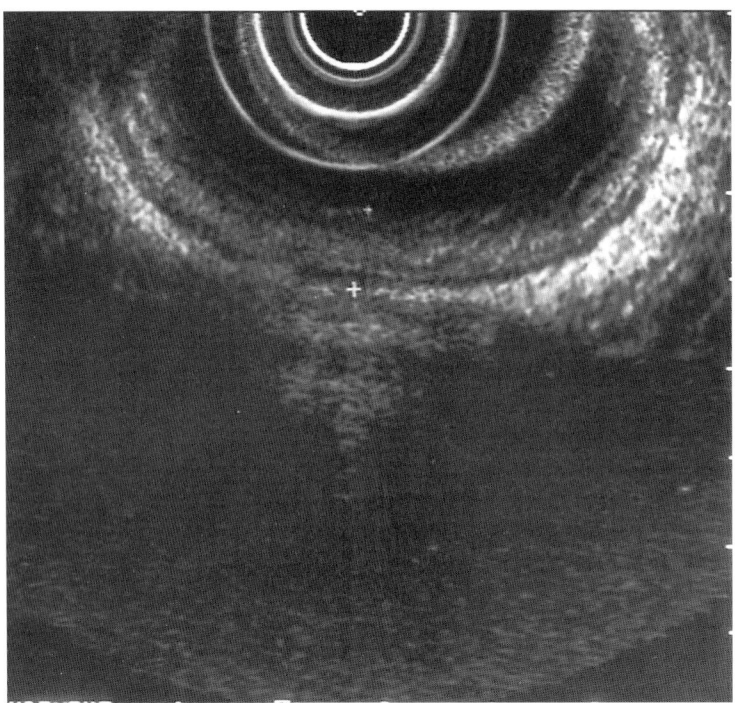

Fig. 30.7 Thickening of the mucosa and submucosa in a patient with ulcerative colitis without disruption of the echolayers.

Patients with Crohn's disease are generally excluded from surgical procedures that involve an ileal reservoir, such as an ileal pouch–anal anastomosis or Kock's continent ileostomy, because of the risk of recurrence (Dozois et al 1980, Pezim et al 1989). Approximately 5% of patients undergoing total colectomy for presumed ulcerative colitis will in fact have gross and/or microscopic features which overlap with Crohn's colitis. In such cases of 'indeterminate colitis' it is difficult to decide whether an ileal pouch–anal anastomosis should be performed (Pezim et al 1989). Hildebrandt et al (1992) have used endoluminal ultrasound to study this group of patients and found that it was helpful in preoperative evaluation because it can determine whether the inflammation is mucosal or transmural. They hypothesized that finding transmural inflammation would reflect a disease spectrum more consistent with Crohn's, and excluded these patients from surgical procedures requiring an ileal reservoir. Using this information resulted in improved long-term outcome for surgery in patients with indeterminate colitis.

ROLE IN EVALUATING FISTULA AND ABSCESS IN CROHN'S DISEASE

Perianal complications occur in 22–54% of patients with Crohn's disease, and may be the first manifestation of the disease in some patients (Rankin et al 1979, Williams et al 1981). These include abscesses, strictures, fistulae and anal fissures. Fistulography, endoscopy, barium studies and computed tomography (CT) have traditionally been the methods used to evaluate for these lesions. Problems with these examinations include incomplete definition of the lesion(s) (barium studies, CT, endoscopy) and pain and dissemination of infection (fistulography). Endoluminal ultrasound is a less invasive and less painful alternative and provides high-resolution images (Tio et al 1990). A fistula appears on ultrasound as a hypoechoic or anechoic serpiginous-like structure localized within the perianorectal area. Reverberation echoes from air bubbles within the fistulous track can provide a clue to its presence. An abscess appears as a hypoechoic or anechoic cavity with irregular borders (Fig. 30.8), which may contain material of increased echogenicity representing necrotic debris (Tio et al 1990, Wiersema & Hawes 1992). Tio et al (1990) performed endoscopic ultrasound in 36 patients with Crohn's disease suspected of having a fistula or an abscess. The exams were performed primarily with rigid probes operating at frequencies of 5 and 7.5 MHz. A perirectal structure compatible with a fistula was found in 32 patients. In all of these a communication between the fistulous tract and an adjacent structure (skin, anal canal or vagina) was detected. Abscesses associated with the fistula were seen in 29 of the 32 patients. Seventeen of the 32 patients subsequently underwent surgery and the endosonography finding of an abscess or a fistula was confirmed in all 17.

Positioning the ultrasound probe in the anal canal is a reliable and safe method to detect and define perianal

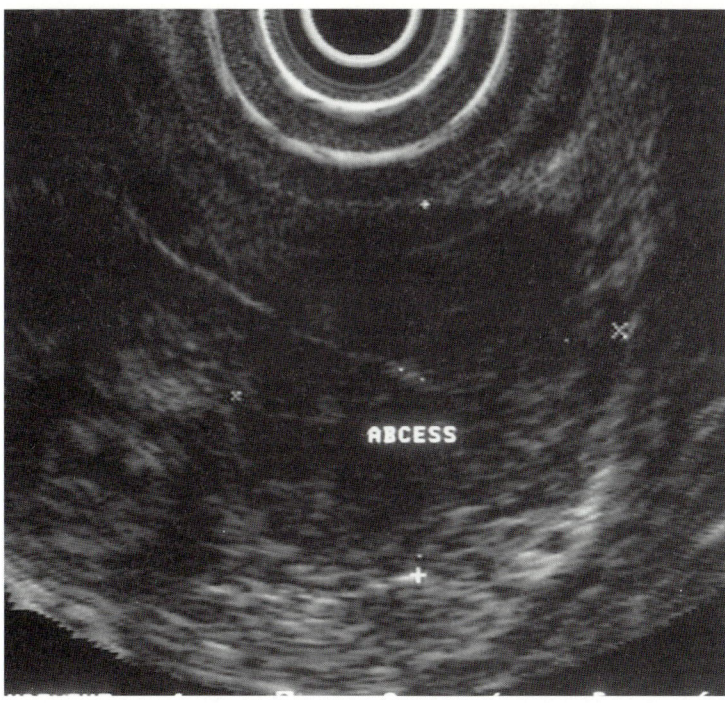

Fig. 30.8 A 2 cm perirectal abscess in a patient with Crohn's disease imaged with the radial scanning flexible echoendoscope.

fistulae. Endoluminal ultrasound can define the course of the fistula, identify unusual patterns (horseshoe-track fistulae) and define complicated fistulae preoperatively (Law et al 1989, Deen et al 1994). It can also be helpful in following the response to therapy and documenting closure in patients treated medically. Rectovaginal fistulas are more clearly imaged using a transvaginal approach (Tio et al 1990), and this provides an alternative route to image female patients who have rectal stenosis, severe rectal pain or have undergone a proctectomy (Wijers et al 1992).

Conventional imaging procedures probably underreport perineal complications in Crohn's disease patients. When 40 unselected patients with Crohn's disease underwent transrectal ultrasound, 75% (30 patients) were found to have perineal complications but only 30% were detected by endoscopy and proctography combined (Van Outryve et al 1991). The abnormalities detected by ultrasound included abscesses, fistulae, a thickened rectal wall and an abnormal anal sphincter. The normal ultrasound appearance of the anal sphincter is an echopoor, homogeneous structure. A striking heterogeneity of the anal sphincter was noted in 47% of the patients with Crohn's disease. This finding has been suggested as a possible predictor of the development of anal canal stenosis (Van Outryve et al 1991).

Comparison has been made between transanal endosconography and digital examination in the detection of anal fistulae (Choen et al 1991). Ultrasound and digital examination were comparable in identifying intersphincteric and transphincteric tracts. In this study a rigid, non-optical rectal probe fitted with a hard sonolucent cone was used. This hard cone was especially designed for imaging the anal canal. When used for rectal imaging, however, it may not provide sufficient contact with the rectal wall, resulting in loss of acoustic coupling and poor image quality. The drawback of digital examination is that it is unable to delineate the course of a fistula, or whether it communicates with an abscess or an adjacent organ.

CT has been used to evaluate the perineum in patients with inflammatory bowel disease, and in a prospective trial transrectal ultrasound was compared to CT in 25 patients with Crohn's disease (Schratter-Sehn et al 1993). Surgical findings were used as the standard with which both CT and ultrasound were compared. Fistulae were found in 17 of the 25 patients. Ultrasound detected the fistula in 14 (82%), whereas CT visualized only four (24%). Endosonography and CT had equivalent accuracy in detecting abscesses.

The advantages of endoluminal ultrasound in rectal and perirectal disease appear to be its efficacy, safety, simplicity, low cost and lack of irradiation. More studies are needed comparing the utility of ultrasound versus other imaging devices. A likely future application of endoluminal ultrasound will be in drainage of perineal abscesses. Linear array echoendoscopes can accurately detect abscess cavities and can effectively place a needle catheter into the target. This would permit acute aspiration (for culture and drainage) and could potentially be followed with the passage of a guide wire through the needle and a drainage tube over the wire. The combination of effective drainage, appropriate antibiotics and systemic Crohn's disease treatment (steroids/imuran) may serve as an effective treatment for some of these difficult patients.

SUMMARY

Endoluminal ultrasound is likely to see wider application in the future in patients with inflammatory bowel disease. Its use in evaluating patients with perineal Crohn's disease is well established. Endosonography may have a role in patients who exhibit characteristics of both Crohn's and ulcerative colitis, especially if surgical treatment involving an ileoanal anastomosis is contemplated. Future research should focus on determining the relationship between the endoscopic and endosonographic appearance of the colon, and whether or not endosonographic information concerning the extent and thickness of bowel wall inflammation could influence treatment.

REFERENCES

Bozkurt T, Richter F, Lux G 1994 Ultrasonography as a primary diagnostic tool in patients with inflammatory disease and tumors of the small intestine and large bowel. Journal of Clinical Ultrasound 22: 85–91

Cho E, Yasuda K, Nakajima M 1990 Endoscopic ultrasonography (EUS) in the diagnosis of ulcerative colitis. Gastroenterology 98 (Part 2): A164

Choen S, Burnett S, Bartram C I, Nicholls R J 1991 Comparison between anal endosonography and digital examination in the evaluation of anal fistulae. British Journal of Surgery 78: 445–447

Deen K I, Williams J G, Hutchinson R, Keighley M R B, Kumar D 1994 Fistulas in ano: endoanal ultrasonographic assessment assists decision making for surgery. Gut 35: 391–394

Dozois R R, Kelly K A, Beart Jr R W, Beahrs O H 1980 Improved results with continent ileostomy. Annals of Surgery 192: 319–324

Hawes R H 1993 New staging techniques. Endoscopic ultrasound. Cancer 71: 4207–4213

Hildebrandt U, Kraus J, Ecker K W, Schmid T, Schuder G, Feifel G 1992 Endosonographic differentiation of mucosal and transmural nonspecific inflammatory bowel disease. Endoscopy 24 (Suppl 1): 359–363

Kimmey M B, Wang K Y, Haggit R C, Mack L A, Silverstein F 1990 Diagnosis of inflammatory bowel disease with ultrasound. Investigative Radiology 25: 1085–1090

Law P J, Talbot R W, Bartram C I, Northover J M A 1989 Anal endosonography in the evaluation of peri-anal sepsis and fistula in ano. British Journal of Surgery 76: 752–755

Limberg B 1989 Diagnosis of acute ulcerative colitis and colonic Crohn's disease by colonic sonography. Journal of Clinical Ultrasound 17: 25–31

Pezim M E, Pemberton J H, Beart R W Jr et al 1989 Outcome of 'indeterminate colitis' following ileal-pouch anal anastomosis. Diseases of the Colon and Rectum 31: 653–658

Rankin G B, Watts H D, Melnyk C S, Kelley M L Jr 1979 National cooperative Crohn's disease study: extraintestinal manifestations and peri-anal complications. Gastroenterology 77: 914–920

Schratter-Sehn A U, Lochs H, Vogelsang H, Schurawitzki H, Herold C, Schratter M 1993 Endoscopic ultrasonography versus computed tomography in the differential diagnosis of perianorectal complications in Crohn's disease. Endoscopy 25: 582–586

Shimizu S, Tada M, Kawai K 1992 Value of endoscopic ultrasonography in the assessment of inflammatory bowel diseases Endoscopy 24 (Suppl 1): 354–358

Tio T L, Mulder C J J, Wijers O B, Sars P R A, Tytgat G N J 1990 Endosonography of peri-anal and peri-colorectal fistula and/or abscess in Crohn's disease. Gastrointestinal Endoscopy 36: 331–336

Van Outryve M J, Pelckmans P A, Michielsen P P, Van Maercke Y M 1991 Value of transrectal ultrasonography in Crohn's disease. Gastroenterology 101: 1171–1177

Wiersema M J, Hawes R H 1992 Normal colorectal anatomy and benign colon conditions. Gastrointestinal Endoscopy Clinics of North American 77: 914–920

Wijers O B, Tio T L, Tytgat G N J 1992 Ultrasonography and endosonography in the diagnosis and management of inflammatory bowel disease. Endoscopy 24: 559–564

Wild J J, Reid J M 1956 Diagnostic use of ultrasound. British Journal of Physiology 19: 248–254

Williams D R, Coller J A, Corman M L, Nugent W, Veidenheimer M C 1981 Anal complications in Crohn's disease. Diseases of the Colon and Rectum 24: 22–24

PART THREE   HISTOPATHOLOGY

31. Histopathology of ulcerative colitis

R. H. Riddell

Ulcerative colitis is a chronic disease of unknown cause characterized by exacerbations and remissions of bloody diarrhea, usually beginning in the rectum and extending proximally in continuity to involve all or part of the remaining colon, and affecting almost exclusively the mucosa of the large bowel. Although there is some overlap in the gross and histopathological features of many colonic inflammatory conditions and few of the specific findings are diagnostic, some patterns are sufficiently characteristic to permit a diagnosis that is both accurate and clinically useful. The biopsy features may require augmentation by careful consideration of a constellation of features, including clinical, endoscopic and radiological findings. Biopsies can distinguish active ulcerative colitis from infections in the acute phase, but culture and stool examinations for ova, parasites and toxins often provide the diagnosis of infection. Ulcerative colitis must be distinguished from Crohn's disease, the other major form of idiopathic chronic inflammatory bowel disease (IBD). In most western countries this differentiation is the most frequent diagnostic dilemma in the clinical and histopathological diagnosis of IBD.

From the clinical viewpoint questions include the problems in an initial presentation, and those in patients with known IBD. In a fisrt presentation the major questions include the following:

1. In a patient with diarrhea or bloody diarrhea, what is the underlying disease? The differential diagnosis here is primarily between ulcerative colitis and acute infectious colitis sometimes called acute self-limited colitis. However, in bloody diarrhea other diseases requiring consideration are many, but include Crohn's disease and acute ischemia.
2. In patients with non-bloody diarrhea, both ulcerative colitis and Crohn's disease require consideration, but the emphasis shifts more to Crohn's disease, particularly if abdominal pain, mass or fistula is present, and symptoms are long-standing. Watery diarrhea raises the question of infection, particularly if symptoms are of recent onset, but if symptoms are more chronic microscopic colitis, which includes lymphocytic colitis, or collagenous colitis enters into the differential diagnosis.

In patients known to have IBD the questions include:

1. In patients not responding to therapy is there anything to explain this, such as the wrong diagnosis, underestimated extent or activity, or superimposed infection?
2. Does the patient have dysplasia or cancer?

HISTOPATHOLOGICAL CRITERIA FOR ULCERATIVE PROCTOCOLITIS

There is a gulf between current morphological criteria for IBD available in the literature and the criteria actually used in practice, many of which have never been formally tested. The major reasons for this are:

1. Original criteria for IBD were based on pathology findings in surgical resections carried out primarily for complications, including intractable disease and on rectal biopsies. These were therefore largely personal experience and subject to considerable referral and selection biases.
2. Studies in the literature are based almost entirely on rectal biopsies, primarily in the first attack of the disease.
3. Neither of these reflect current clinical practice, in which the first investigation is increasingly flexible sigmoidoscopy rather than rigid proctoscopy or sigmoidoscopy, which allows evaluation and biopsy of considerably more bowel, and multiple biopsies from several regions, including biopsy above an upper margin in ulcerative proctitis or proctosigmoiditis to confirm that this is the case.
4. In current practice interpretation is the result of examining patterns of inflammation and architecture in mutiple biopsies, and the distribution of the disease throughout the terminal ileum, large bowel, and

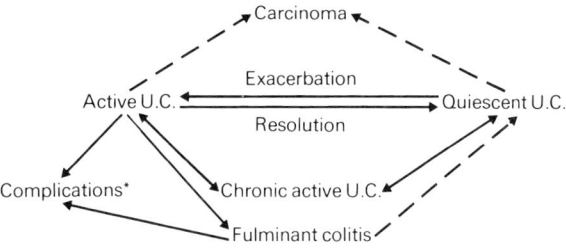

Fig. 31.1 The interrelationships of recognizable clinicopathological patterns of disease in ulcerative colitis.
* Complications include inflammatory polyps, hemorrhage, toxic dilatation, perforation and stricture.

sometimes the upper gastrointestinal tract in addition. For over two decades colonoscopy with multiple biopsies has been used to define the extent and distribution of activity of ulcerative colitis, and to a large extent the different distribution of Crohn's disease, but these have never really been extended to diagnostic criteria or found their way into the literature.

5. The effects of therapy and how it may modify biopsy appearances remains poorly understood. Furthermore, with the advent of 'designer drugs' which are activated in the large bowel, the possibility that unusual patterns of disease may be the result of delayed or inappropriate drug release, and the effect this may have on morphology remains anecdotal.

Despite these disclaimers, the appearances of biopsies obtained at full colonoscopy are widely acknowledged and taught, which has resulted in an oral tradition of ulcerative colitis that is not reflected by data in the literature. The reason for this is not difficult to see, for the design of a study to determine the predictive value of each histological feature would be extraordinarily complex, with numerous variables. This chapter is therefore based on a combination of what is in the literature and personal experience, but I shall try to distinguish which is which.

The pathology of ulcerative colitis often parallels the variability in the clinical course of the disease, as illustrated by Figure 31.1. The important topics of dysplasia and cancer in ulcerative colitis, as well as extraintestinal manifestations of ulcerative colitis, are discussed elsewhere.

ACTIVE ULCERATIVE COLITIS

Ulcerative colitis is characteristically a mucosal disease, usually beginning in the rectum and extending proximally in continuity to involve all or part of the remaining colon. Other than in fulminant colitis, focal disease or skip areas are not part of the picture and should strongly suggest that the underlying disease is another entity, particularly Crohn's disease. In some patients, particularly the young, ulcerative colitis may be extensive or involve the entire colon from the beginning. In many patients the disease begins in the rectum and remains limited to that site (ulcerative proctitis) or the rectosigmoid region (ulcerative proctosigmoiditis) for its entire course.

Colonoscopically there may be mucosal hyperemia, granularity, friability, erosions, ulceration and bleeding, variable in degree depending on the severity of the attack. Mucosal vascular congestion with edema and focal hemorrhage is often present, and tends to be more prominent in severe cases. Shallow ulcers are frequent in active disease, but deeper ulcers penetrating the muscularis mucosa into the superficial submucosa are less common, and are seen principally in severe cases. Most of the histopathological findings in ulcerative colitis are limited to the mucosa and superficial submucosa, with the deeper layers unaffected except in fulminant disease. Therefore, most of the diagnostic features of ulcerative colitis can be seen in mucosal biopsies. In distal disease normal mucosa may be found proximally. Macroscopic examination of the colon is almost entirely a function of the colonoscopist, and the material submitted to the pathologist is limited to mucosal biopsies. The training of colonoscopists regarding sites to be biopsied is far from uniform, resulting in little uniformity as to the number or sites of biopsies taken.

The histopathological findings in biopsies taken from patients with acute active ulcerative colitis correlate reasonably well with the endoscopic appearance; however, this is a broad correlation and in any individual patient correlation between clinical activity, colonoscopic appearances and histology may be far from perfect.

The distinction between ulcerative colitis in particular and infections colitis can be impossible to make endoscopically, hence the notion of 'non-specific' ulcerative colitis, despite the fact that in active disease the histologic changes of ulcerative colitis in their fully developed form are highly specific. Major criteria separating IBD (i.e. ulcerative colitis or Crohn's disease) from normal and from acute infectious colitis (Dickinson et al 1979, Kumar et al 1982, Surawicz & Belic 1984, Lazenby et al 1989, McCormick et al 1990, Seldenrijk et al 1991, Schumacher 1993, Surawicz et al 1994, Theodossi et al 1994) are discussed in more detail in Chapter 38, but are primarily as follows.

Epithelium: architectural changes – crypt branching and distortion in which the normal crypt parallelism is lost, this being replaced by irregular, distorted or branched crypts, frequently failing to reach the muscularis mucosa and the number of crypts may also be reduced (this indicates previous crypt destruction of any cause); a villous surface (a feature primarily of active disease); mucin depletion (usually seen in association with crypt abscesses and therefore not specific or sensitive); and crypt dilatation.

Inflammation: lymphoplasmacytic infiltrate with plasma cells down to the muscularis mucosae, and with an excess of lymphoid aggregates and basal giant cells, granulomas (see later for criteria for distinguishing ulcerative colitis and Crohn's disease). Excessive mononuclear cells and the presence of neutrophils distinguish the inflamed from the normal colon. The second major feature is diffuse inflammation, in which chronic inflammation, both plasma cells and lymphoid tissue, is invariably present immediately above the muscularis mucosae, either as multiple nodules (occasional nodules are normal), or as a distinct band (Fig. 31.2); occasionally both the band and nodules are present. These two features indicate the presence of IBD as opposed to an acute infection.

Although these two features indicate IBD more detailed examination of the mucosa is needed to confirm ulcerative colitis. I find that in active ulcerative colitis neutrophils show a characteristic attraction to crypt epithelium, which they infiltrate. This constellation of histological features is so characteristic that there is virtually no differential diagnosis if they are all present: they are certainly not 'non-specific' (as in non-specific ulcerative colitis).

Crypt abscess. Aggregates of neutrophils near and invading the crypt epithelium form crypt abscesses which, when numerous, are a characteristic and reliable indicator of activity (Fig. 31.3). Crypt abscesses range from small accumulations of neutrophils within crypt lumina and epithelium to large intramucosal abscesses which completely destroy the crypt epithelium and extend into the surrounding lamina propria. Most crypts in a diseased segment show some degree of involvement and, when the mid and deeper parts of the crypt are the worst affected, the diagnosis of ulcerative colitis can be made with confidence. This contrasts with the appearances in infective and toxic colitis, where there is a distinct tendency for the acute inflammation to affect primarily the luminal epithelium and the superficial portion of the crypts. Isolated crypt abscesses, particularly intermixed with completely uninvolved crypts when associated with focal chronic inflammation are more typical of Crohn's disease than of ulcerative colitis. The epithelial invasion characterized by the polymorphonuclear infiltrate and resulting crypt abscesses is an important characteristic of ulcerative colitis, although not completely specific. In contrast,

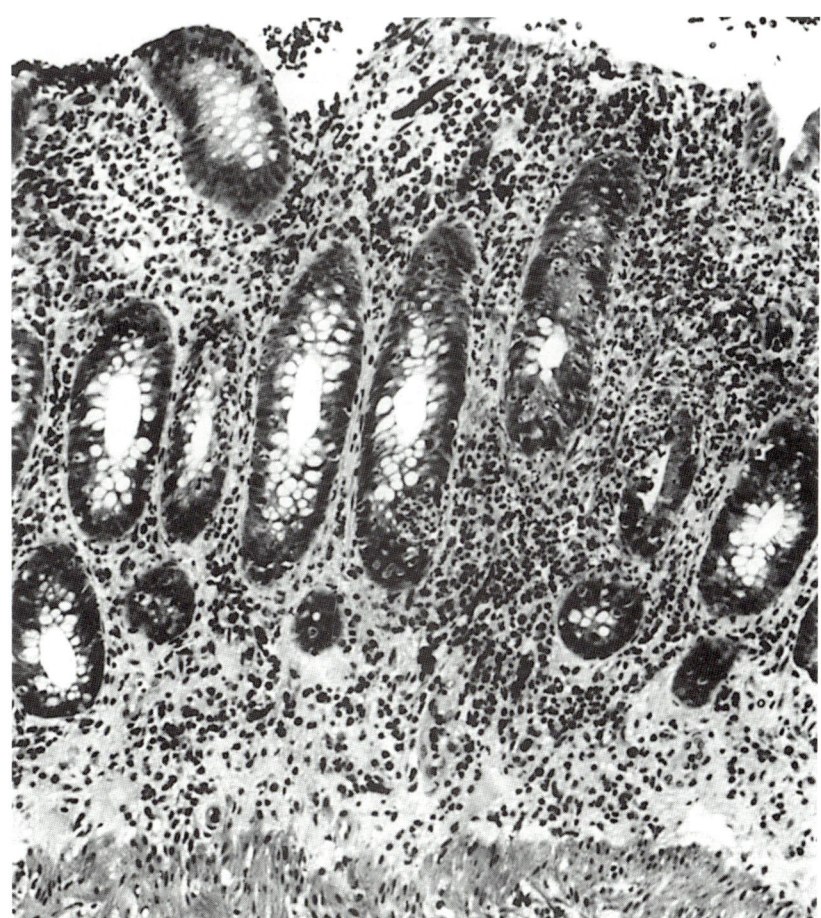

Fig. 31.2 Inflammatory bowel disease in a rectal biopsy showing a diffuse transmucosal inflammation and crypts that fail to reach the muscularis mucosae, and mild reduction in epithelial mucin that is usually associated with acute inflammation.

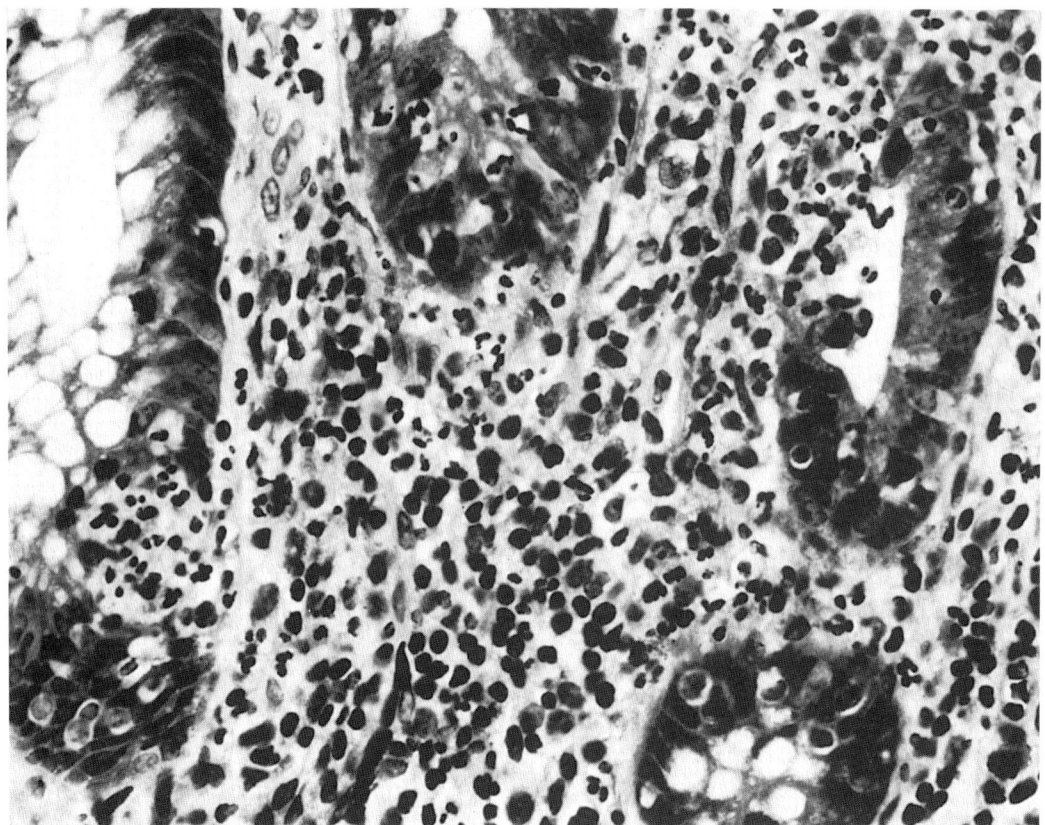

Fig. 31.3 Detail of Figure 31.2. Neutrophils are invading all of the crypts to form early crypt abscesses. In the presence of the other changes of IBD seen in Fig. 31.2, this change is highly characteristic of ulcerative colitis, and highly unusual in other diseases.

ulcerative colitis is unlikely if there is absent or minimal epithelial invasion by polymorphonuclear infiltrate.

It is important to realize that crypt abscesses are also a feature of acute colitis from many other causes. They will sometimes indicate more about the activity of the acute inflammatory process than the underlying etiology. Numerous free neutrophils in the lamina propria with crypt sparing seems rare in ulcerative colitis, to the point that I usually raise the question of whether there are other features present clinically or endoscopically that might suggest that the underlying disease is Crohn's disease rather than ulcerative colitis, or whether, if the patient really has ulcerative colitis, whether the current exacerbation may be related to a superimposed infection, in which lamina propria neutrophils are also the rule. In addition, crypts are frequently depleted of mucin; although mucin depletion is usually associated with cryptitis, the two may be dissociated. Thus, acute inflammation of crypts may occur in the absence of mucin depletion, whereas marked mucin depletion may occur in the absence of acute cryptitis.

Ulceration is quite uncommon in biopsies, but the luminal epithelium is frequently attenuated and cuboidal rather than tall and columnar, suggesting restitution of the epithelium. Clearly, the distinguishing nature of the cryptitis cannot be used if disease is quiescent; similarly, the deep plasma cell and lymphocytic infiltrate cannot be used if disease has been in remission and these changes have resolved.

Chronic inflammatory infiltrate. Typically, in ulcerative colitis a chronic inflammatory infiltrate, mostly of lymphocytes and plasma cells, accompanied by variable numbers of eosinophils, extends diffusely throughout the lamina propria (Figs 31.2, 31.3). Variability in intensity of inflammation in ulcerative colitis may result in a somewhat patchy distribution, but a clearly focal distribution is more suggestive of Crohn's disease (Haggitt 1983). The chronic inflammatory infiltrate does not show the epithelial trophism that is typical of the acute inflammatory infiltrate. Mast cells may also be increased, but these are not readily appreciated in hematoxylin and eosin sections. Some functional characteristics of the chronic inflammatory infiltrate are now being described using both immunological and immunohistochemical methods. However, the results of all studies have not been in complete agreement and the significance of the findings is not clear. Some studies have reported an increase in both numbers and proportions of IgG-producing cells (Brandtzaeg et al 1974, Bookman et al 1979), but this has not been a universal conclusion (O'Donoghue & Kumar

1979). Eosinophils may form such a large part of the infiltrate, particularly when the disease is quiescent, that the possibility of an eosinophilic colitis may be entertained. However, eosinophilic colitis is a poorly described entity and far less common than is ulcerative colitis, with numerous eosinophils in the infiltrate.

Lymphoid follicles. In the normal colonic mucosa one finds lymphoid follicles adjacent to the muscularis mucosa. In some subjects the follicles may become especially large and numerous in the rectum, and less common in the colon. This finding has been termed by some 'follicular proctitis or colitis' and is often accompanied by epithelium showing regenerative features. Although usually regarded primarily as a variant of ulcerative colitis, there has been a suggestion that follicular proctitis behaves like ulcerative colitis only in the presence of architectural distortion (Fig. 31.4), and that in its absence there is no response to therapy (Flejou et al 1988).

Mucin depletion. Depletion of goblet cell mucin is a characteristic and fairly consistent finding in ulcerative colitis and, except where dysplasia is present, is another reliable indicator of activity. Mucin depletion tends to affect all crypts and to be pronounced when there is an intense inflammatory infiltrate. Restoration of normal mucin content, usually beginning in the most superficial portion of the crypts, occurs with resolution and returns to normal levels in the state of quiescence. An increased rate of epithelial cell proliferation may be reflected by increased numbers of mitotic figures, from the usual of about one per three crypts to one or more per crypt. Other, not so prominent, features of epithelial regeneration may also be seen in active disease. When the acute attack is resolving and the patient's symptoms have diminished, epithelial regeneration becomes a prominent histological feature (Fig. 31.5).

The distribution of mucosal lesions in ulcerative colitis usually begins distally in the rectosigmoid area and spreads proximally in continuity (Fig. 31.6). This is a useful diagnostic feature for both endoscopist and pathologist, especially when the pathologist is provided with multiple separately identified biopsies. The rectum is usually involved, but the extent of the proximal spread is variable. Some patients, particularly the young, have disease which appears to involve much or all of the colon from the onset. Some patients have disease limited to the rectum which, although it is proctoscopically and histologically indistinguishable from the local findings in ulcerative colitis, rarely extends distally and is sometimes referred to as idiopathic proctitis (Farmer 1979, 1989). The degree of inflammation in these patients may be much more marked than in those with more extensive disease (Jenkins et al 1990). In cases with limited colonic involvement the transition from diseased to normal mucosa is usually gradual, but is occasionally abrupt. Proximal spread is in continuity without intervening areas of uninvolved mucosa. This is an important feature of ulcerative colitis which contrasts with the discontinuous pattern of involvement often seen in Crohn's colitis. Variation in macroscopic activity and severity may falsely suggest that there are skip areas. However, biopsies from such apparent skip areas always confirm that there is involvement. Likewise, sigmoidoscopically uninvolved rectal mucosa is occasionally observed but almost always found to be diseased when examined histologically (Odze et al, 1993). This emphasizes

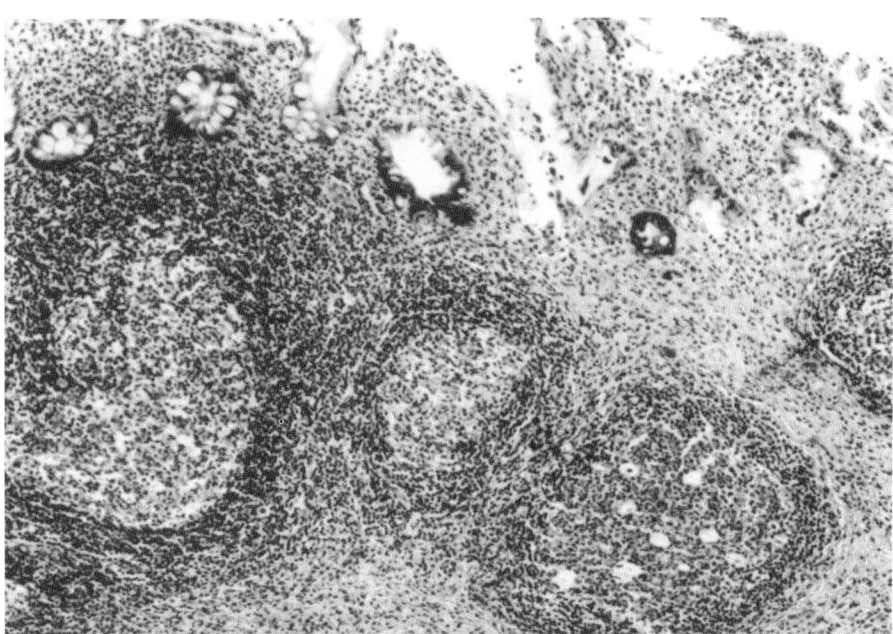

Fig. 31.4 Follicular proctitis with prominent lymphoid follicles containing germinal centers.

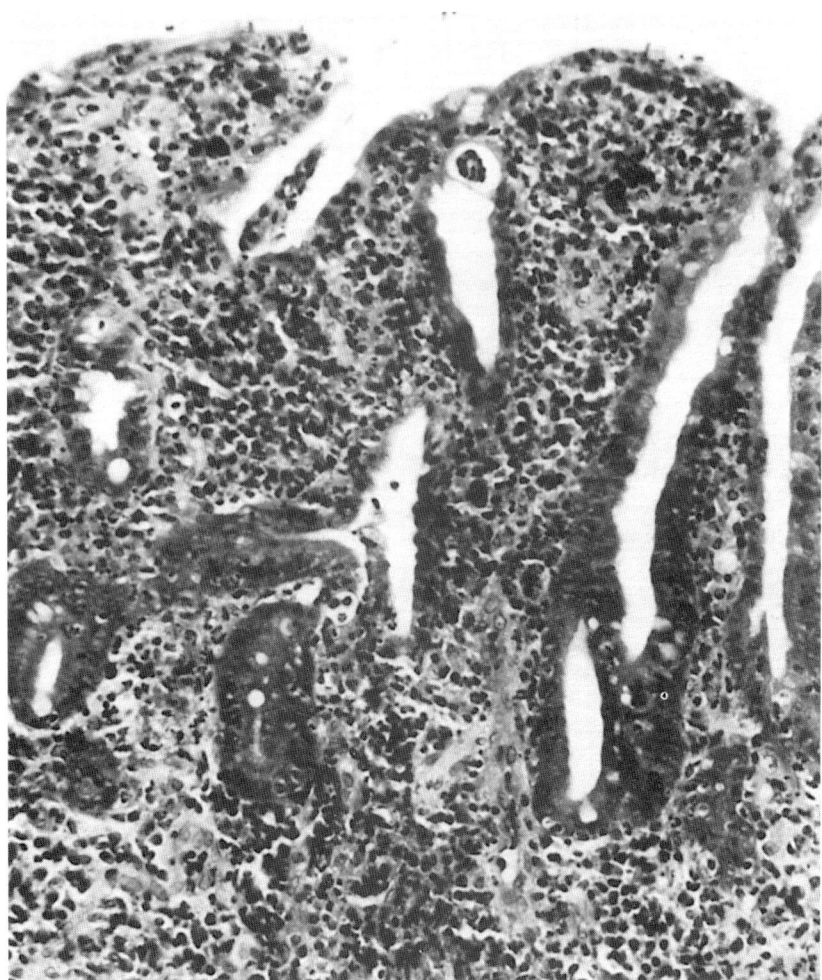

Fig. 31.5 Early resolving colitis in musocal biopsy. Attenuated mucin-depleted regenerating epithelium covering a previously ulcerated surface is seen particularly in the upper mucosa, and is the predominant feature of restituting epithelium, although acute and chronic inflammation is still present.

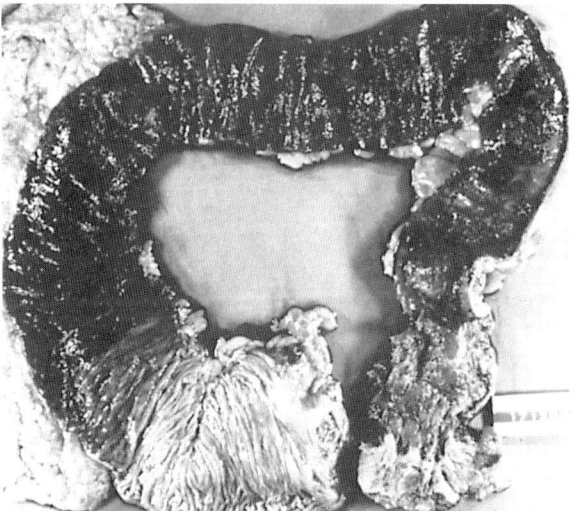

Fig. 31.6 Severe active ulcerative colitis showing continuity of active disease from rectum to mid-ascending colon. The proximal segment of the ascending colon and the cecum are not involved.

the importance of always obtaining a biopsy from apparently uninvolved mucosa.

Backwash ileitis. Total colonic involvement is accompanied by extension of mucosal inflammation into the distal terminal ileum in between 10 and 20% of patients. It is usually associated with a dilated patulous ileocecal valve. Whether this lesion represents a reaction to regurgitation of colonic content into the terminal ileum (Morson & Dawson 1979) or primary ileal involvement (Saltzstein & Rosenberg 1963) is not yet established. Morphologically the ileitis looks almost identical to colonic disease (Saltzstein & Rosenberg 1963). Therefore the commonly used term 'backwash ileitis' should not be given too much pathological significance, nor does it have any prognostic significance, and it usually resolves following colectomy. Despite rare reported cases of ileal perforation in ulcerative colitis (Markowitz 1960) the affected ileum can even be utilized for anastomosis or ileostomy formation without appreciable hazard.

RESOLUTION OF ACTIVE DISEASE FOLLOWING THERAPY

As a patient recovers from an acute attack the signs of clinical resolution often precede those of histological resolution. As activity begins to subside, regenerative features become prominent as epithelial continuity is restored (Fig. 31.5). The epithelium is at first attenuated as it stretches over recently ulcerated surfaces, then it gradually becomes columnar. It is important to distinguish the nuclear changes characteristic of regenerating epithelia (Fig. 31.7) from those of true dysplasia. During the early stages of regeneration, when the epithelium appears flattened, the nuclei may also be attenuated. However, they may also be large with prominent nucleoli and an open chromatin pattern, but are widely separated. As the cells become cuboidal to low columnar, the nuclei appear closer together, sometimes overlapping, but do not show polarity. Basal polarity appears after the epithelium has become columnar, but varying degrees of stratification may be seen while columnar differentiation is in progress. At this stage, when the nuclei are stratified, the chromatin tends to be diffuse with loss of nuclear detail, nucleoli are less conspicuous, and overlapping nuclear boundaries are difficult to define. This change is in marked contrast to the findings in true dysplasia, where the nuclei, although often stratified, have easily defined

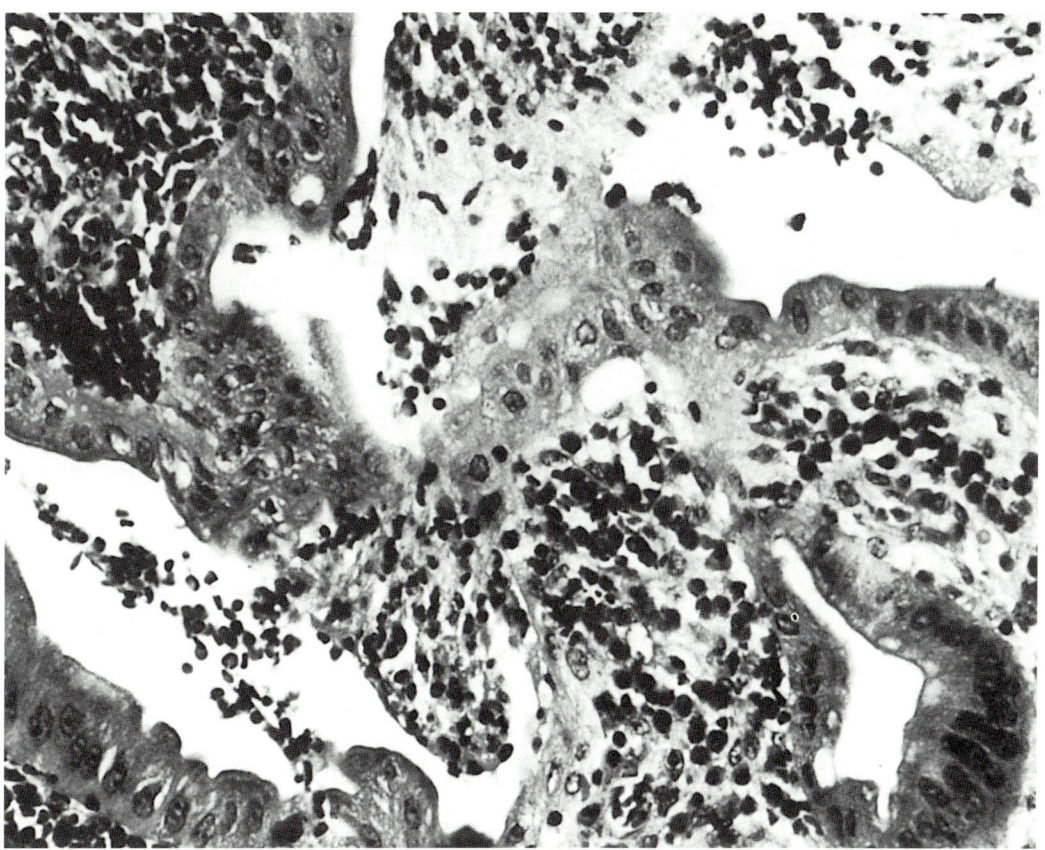

Fig. 31.7 Detail of regenerating restituting epithelium in which there is a decreased number of cells, as indicated by the increased separation between nuclei in cells of reduced height, showing variation in cell height. Basal polarity is developing in some columnar cells but stratification and loss of polarity is indicated by nuclei not localized to the bases of the cells.

boundaries with deposits of chromatin at the periphery. It can be said that 'epithelium may be judged by the company it keeps', so that obviously regenerating epithelium in the same or adjacent crypts is strong evidence against true dysplasia. However, it should be remembered that dysplastic epithelium may also be involved in an acute exacerbation and undergo regeneration. It is usually necessary for resolution to be well advanced before the diagnosis of underlying dysplasia can be made with confidence.

Neutrophils disappear as the acute inflammation subsides, but may still be seen in and around the crypts in the early stages of resolution (Fig. 31.5). As the epithelium matures the goblet cell population is restored and mitotic figures decrease. The final feature of the resolution is the gradual decline in the diffuse infiltrate of lymphocytes and plasma cells. Uneven resolution of the chronic inflammation may produce a patchy infiltrate which could be misdiagnosed as Crohn's disease. However, in ulcerative colitis it is uncommon to see the marked focal change with parts of the mucosa heavily inflamed while the adjacent mucosa appears virtually normal that is so typical of some forms of Crohn's disease. Complete histological resolution may take several months after the symptoms have resolved and the endoscopic appearances returned to normal. In patients with quiescent disease who have no histological abnormality it may be impossible to make or exclude a diagnosis of ulcerative colitis (Odze et al 1993).

QUIESCENT ULCERATIVE COLITIS

When the disease is quiescent an intact but architecturally abnormal mucosa usually persists as an indication of previous mucosal injury. The degree of architectural change may vary from none (Odze et al 1993) to slight abnormalities to marked mucosal atrophy, and is related to the severity, duration and frequency of the previous active disease. Macroscopically the mucosa may appear normal, or be smooth and atrophic. Careful attention must be given to any small nodules, villous foci or flat plaque-like areas, which should raise suspicion that there could be a small carcinoma or dysplasia (Riddell 1977). In general, endoscopic appearances of ulcerative colitis during the resolving or quiescent stages do not correlate as well with the histological findings as they do in the acute phase.

Some shortening and reduction in the diameter of the bowel, which is usually most apparent distally, is often present and may be severe. Such shortening in ulcerative colitis is attributed to muscular contraction and thickening, and is usually not accompanied by fibrosis (Morson & Dawson 1979). Shortening is usually more pronounced in long-standing colitis than in early attacks and, when present in colectomy specimens, even those resected with active disease, is usually an indication of prolonged disease.

A total lack of haustra may ultimately give rise to a tube-like appearance, but these radiological findings may occasionally revert to normal if the disease remains quiescent for a long period (Kirsner et al 1951).

Microscopically, the normal parallel arrangement of closely packed crypts is usually lost. The crypts are reduced in number, more widely separated and often branched (Fig. 31.8). Shortening of crypts may leave a prominent gap between the crypt bases and the muscularis mucosae. Shortening and branching of crypts is particularly useful in differential diagnosis, as it is frequent in ulcerative colitis but less common in Crohn's disease and rare in infective colitis. In the quiescent state the goblet cell population is restored to normal. Inflammatory cell infiltrates are resolved and other features of active disease are absent. Paneth cells, almost never found in the normal colon except in the vicinity of the ileocecal valve, may appear in any region of the colon or rectum. They are usually located at the base of crypts and are occasionally numerous. Argentaffin cells may also be increased.

Characteristically there is hypertrophy of the muscularis mucosae, accompanied by some separation of fibers. It is generally most prominent in the rectum, where the muscularis mucosae is normally thickest. Repeated episodes of activity may cause a multilayered muscularis mucosae, which may be a major factor in the benign strictures sometimes observed in ulcerative colitis (Goulston & McGovern 1969). Similar thickening of the muscularis mucosae is observed in chronic colitides of other etiologies, and thus represents a non-specific feature of chronic inflammation of the colon. All of these findings can be expected in patients with long-standing ulcerative colitis, particularly those associated with repeated episodes of exacerbation. Mild cases may show only minimal loss of parallelism, slightly increased separation and occasional branching of crypts. These findings, especially shortening and branching of crypts, are most suggestive of ulcerative colitis when found diffusely or in multiple biopsies. In other forms of colitis, including Crohn's disease, they may be found focally. Rarely, the mucosa in ulcerative colitis may regenerate so well that it is virtually indistinguishable from normal mucosa, both clinically (Spiliadis & Lennard-Jones 1987) and histologically.

CHRONIC ACTIVE AND INTRACTABLE ULCERATIVE COLITIS

Some patients have disease with evidence of persistent histopathological change, although the symptoms can vary from minimal to severe. The term 'chronic active ulcerative colitis' seems appropriate here. The mucosa, whether examined endoscopically or grossly in resected specimens, may vary in appearance from almost normal to severely inflamed. The involved mucosa in such patients is often difficult to classify histologically into the classic three

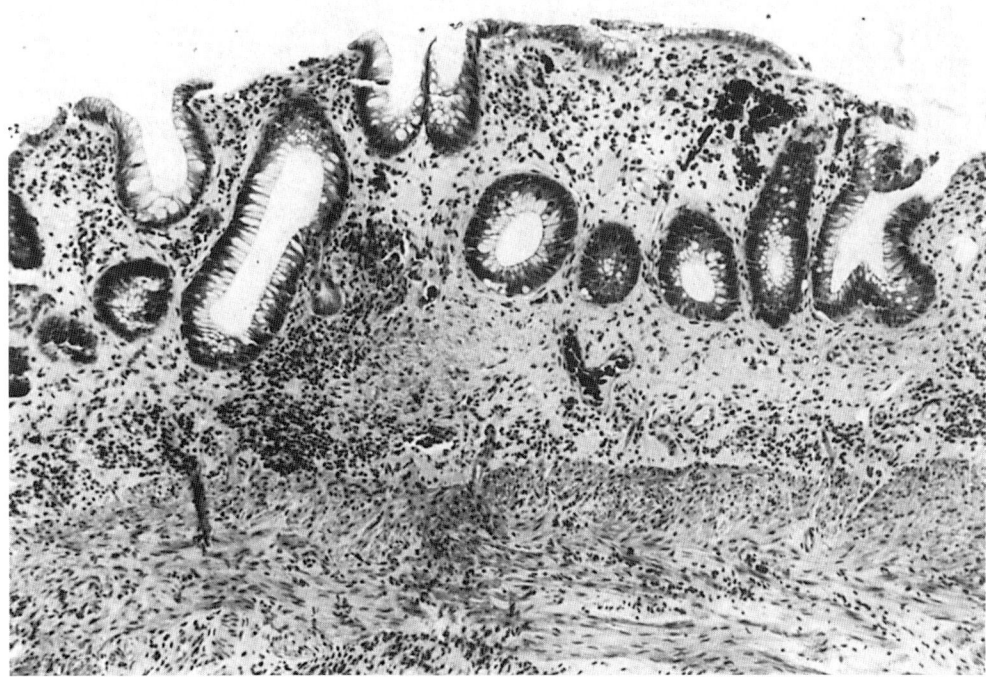

Fig. 31.8 Quiescent IBD, that is a picture of chronic injury although usually associated with ulcerative colitis in rectal biopsy showing loss of parallelism, shortening and branching of crypts, near normal goblet cell population, and thickened muscularis mucosae.

stages of active, resolving or quiescent colitis. Generally the mucosa shows partially developed features of activity combined with findings more typical of resolving disease, although invariably there is a dense chronic inflammatory infiltrate and a variable amount of acute inflammation. Crypt distortion and atrophy are invariably present. Muscular abnormalities may result in shortening, reduction in diameter and loss of the normal haustral pattern.

SEVERE ACTIVE ULCERATIVE COLITIS

About 15% of patients with ulcerative colitis experience a particularly severe or fulminant episode which is unresponsive to intensive medical therapy or accompanied by massive uncontrollable hemorrhage and requires urgent colectomy. These fulminating attacks tend to occur early in the course of the disease, but may be seen in patients with a history of long-standing disease. Most are not complicated by toxic dilatation, but the colectomy specimens from these patients who do not resolve show the characteristic features of ulcerative colitis. Such cases form the basis of most of the macroscopic descriptions of ulcerative colitis. The distribution of lesions in these severe cases usually shows rectosigmoid involvement with variable degrees of proximal extension in continuity, similar to that seen in the more common pattern of mild or moderately severe disease. External examination of such specimens usually shows only minimal external changes, as might be expected in a disease predominantly affecting the mucosa.

The serosal surfaces are generally free of inflammatory change. They are smooth, often glistening and free of adhesions or exudate, but may be hyperemic owing to dilatation of subserosal vessels. The wall is characteristically soft and pliable and lacks fibrosis. In contrast to the minimal change observed on the serosal surface, the mucosal changes are usually dramatic (Fig. 31.6). The most severely involved mucosa is dark red or purple, hemorrhagic and friable with extensive ulceration. It is covered by a mixture of blood, mucus, pus, necrotic debris and liquid stool. Extensive and deep ulceration, which exposes the underlying submucosa or muscularis propria, is common. The described changes are very florid because disease entirely confined to the mucosa rarely, if ever, causes illness sufficiently severe to require urgent colectomy (Buckell et al 1980).

Confluence of ulcers often leaves isolated polypoid islands of mucosa (Fig. 31.9) and may produce longitudinal furrows. This is possibly the only time when the term 'pseudopolyp' is appropriate. However, because of the ambiguity of the term 'polyp' we prefer the term 'mucosal islands'. Deep fissuring, which is characteristic of Crohn's disease, is seen rarely except in toxic dilatation. Even in severe cases where ulcers extend into the submucosa or muscularis propria, the inflammatory infiltrate is restricted to the immediate vicinity of the ulcer

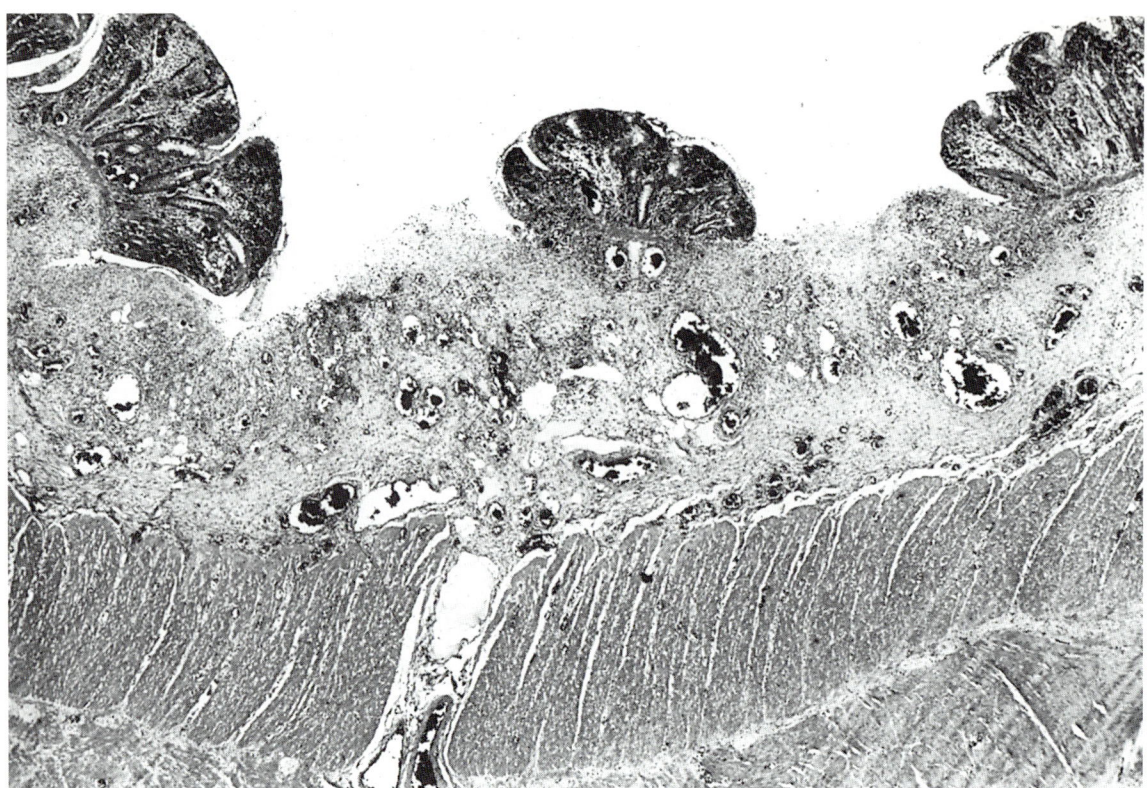

Fig. 31.9 Severe active ulcerative colitis with deep ulcers extending into the submucosa and musocal islands. The muscularis propria is virtually unaffected.

(Fig. 31.9). Changes in the remainder of the submucosa are limited to vascular dilatation and edema. Fibrosis, granulomas or lymphocytic aggregates in the submucosa, muscularis or serosal layers away from areas of ulceration are absent. Occasional foreign-body granulomas are sometimes found adjacent to deep ulcers which extend into the submucosa. These should not be confused with the sarcoid-like granulomas seen in Crohn's disease, which are independent of overlying ulcers. The foreign-body granulomas that occur in ulcerative colitis are usually associated with foreign material, the identification of which may be facilitated by the use of polarized light. Our experience does not include the diffuse submucosal periarteritis-like vasculitis described by Warren and Sommers (1949). The St Mark's experience appears similar to ours (Morson & Dawson 1979), as does that of Lumb and Protheroe (1955).

In a few patients with ulcerative colitis the characteristic features of the disease are obscured or absent during fulminant attacks (Markowitz 1960, Price 1978, Lee et al 1979). The rectum, although usually involved, may be relatively spared, with the brunt of the disease falling on the mucosa proximal to the rectum. The role of steroid enemas as a cause of apparent rectal sparing is unclear, but is sometimes evoked as an explanation. Before the advent of steroid therapy rectal sparing was often attributed to the effect of cod liver oil enemas or other typical therapy that was in vogue at the time (Kirsner, personal communication). In such cases careful sigmoidoscopy often reveals relatively normal-appearing rectum and above that scattered ulcers, before the more proximal diffusely affected mucosa is seen. Biopsies show focal disease and can be misinterpreted as Crohn's disease because of its focality. The mucosa between ulcers may appear surprisingly normal, both grossly and histologically, in marked contrast to the normal continuity of musocal disease seen in ulcerative colitis. In the severely diseased areas fissure ulcers extend into the muscularis propria as V-shaped clefts, and are frequently accompanied by some degree of dilatation of the colon. These cleft-like fissures in ulcerative colitis are always found in areas of extensive ulceration and are accompanied by signs of myocytolysis and vascular dilatation in the adjacent tissue. They differ from the typical fissures of Crohn's disease, which have a more prominent inflammatory cell component, show less myocytolysis in adjacent muscle, and are not limited to areas of extensive overlying musocal ulceration. Such cases represent some of the 10% of colectomy specimens that cannot be confidently identified as either ulcerative colitis or Crohn's disease (Price 1978, Lee et al 1979). The term 'indeterminate colitis' has been proposed as an appropriate diagnostic term for these cases, which represent the area of maximal overlap of pathologic features of ulcerative colitis and

Crohn's disease. Unfortunately, this term is now frequently used as a synonym for idiopathic IBD of uncertain type. A firm diagnosis of either ulcerative colitis or Crohn's disease may depend on the review of previous material, or have to await the evidence from subsequent follow-up.

LOCAL COMPLICATIONS

The most serious complication of acute ulcerative colitis is colonic perforation, which may occur in either toxic megacolon or severe active colitis without dilatation. Toxic megacolon is reported to occur in 2–4% of all patients with ulcerative colitis (Edwards & Truelove 1964, Gilat et al 1976), and in up to 13% of hospital patients (Jalan et al 1969a). It may develop at any time but is most commonly seen early in the course of the disease; it may be the presenting manifestation. Dilatation is most often greatest in the transverse colon, but may involve only the sigmoid colon and occasionally almost the entire colon. In some areas, and sometimes over long segments of bowel, it involves all layers, including the muscularis propria and serosa. The serosa is congested, dull, opaque and often covered by a fibrinous or fibrinopurulent exudate. The thin friable wall, which has been likened to wet tissue paper, is easily ruptured and perforation may occur spontaneously or with even the most gentle surgical handling. In the affected area musocal ulceration is severe, with frequent cleft-like extensions into the muscularis propria accompanied by extensive myocytolysis (Figs 31.10, 31.11). Vascular dilatation and engorgement is often present and may be a more prominent feature than the inflammatory cell infiltrate.

Although no definite explanation is yet available for the state of toxic megacolon, of the specific factors studied the muscular lesions and depth of ulceration have the strongest correlation with the area of dilatation (Norland & Kirsner 1969, Buckell et al 1980). It is presumed that all patients with toxic dilatation, even those who respond to intensive medical therapy, have similar pathological features during the acute episode. This is because the extension of regenerated mucosa into the muscularis propria is found also in colectomy specimens from patients who are successfully brought through an episode of toxic dilatation, but in whom colectomy is performed subsequently (Fig. 31.12). No consistent neurological abnormality has been reported and obvious obstructive lesions are absent. Hypokalemia and drugs such as narcotics and anticholinergics, which decrease motility, are recognized as aggravating factors but not as primary etiological agents (Norland & Kirsner 1969).

Occasionally patients with severe active ulcerative colitis without toxic dilatation are unresponsive to medical therapy; they may also be complicated by colonic perforation. These cases also show focal cleft-like extension of the mucosal ulcers into the muscularis propria which create potential sites of perforation. The penetration of the muscularis propria is usually less extensive than that in toxic megacolon, and myocytolysis and muscular inflammation are more closely confined to the immediate

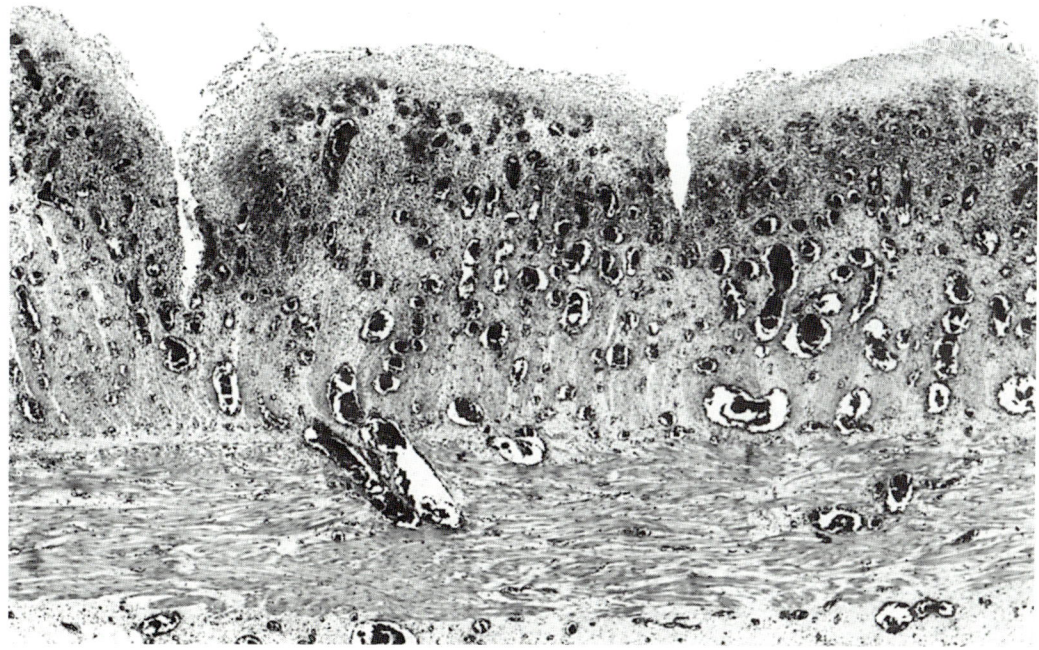

Fig. 31.10 Toxic dilatation with extensive mucosal loss and ulcers extending into the muscularis propria as cleft-like extensions. Vascular dilatation and engorgement are prominent in comparison to the degree of inflammation.

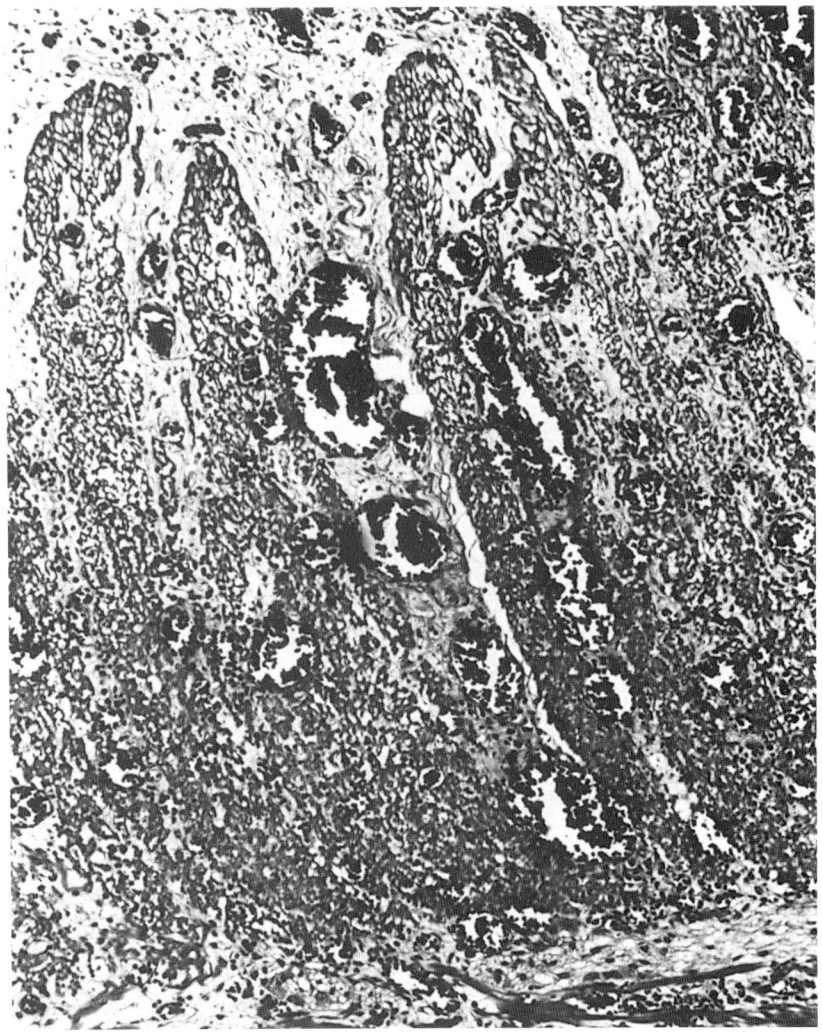

Fig. 31.11 Same case as Figure 31.10. Myocytolysis of the circular layer is apparent and not confined to the immediate vicinity of the deep ulcers, which extend into the muscularis propria.

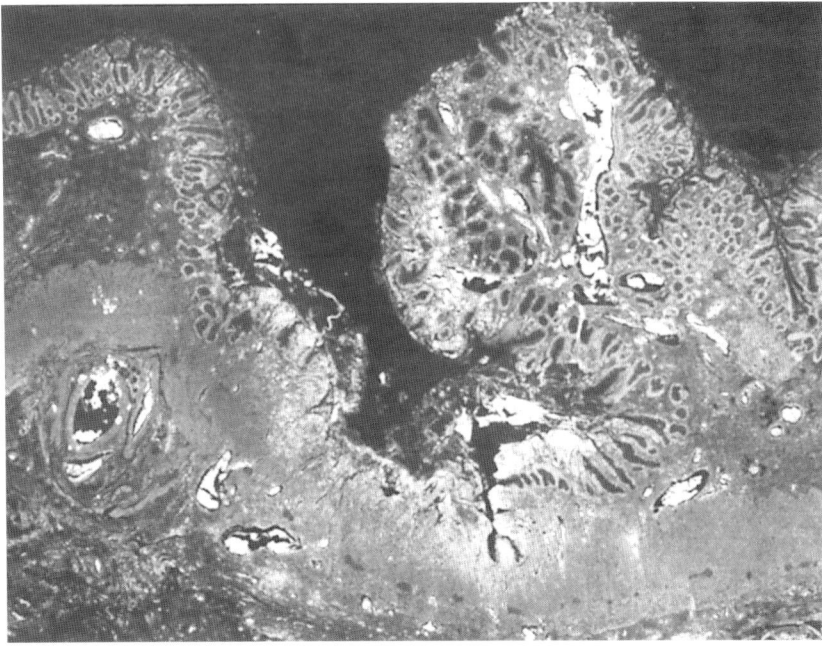

Fig. 31.12 Colon from a patient who had fulminant ulcerative colitis managed medically, resulting in regenerated mucosa extending over the base of deep ulcers into the muscularis propria.

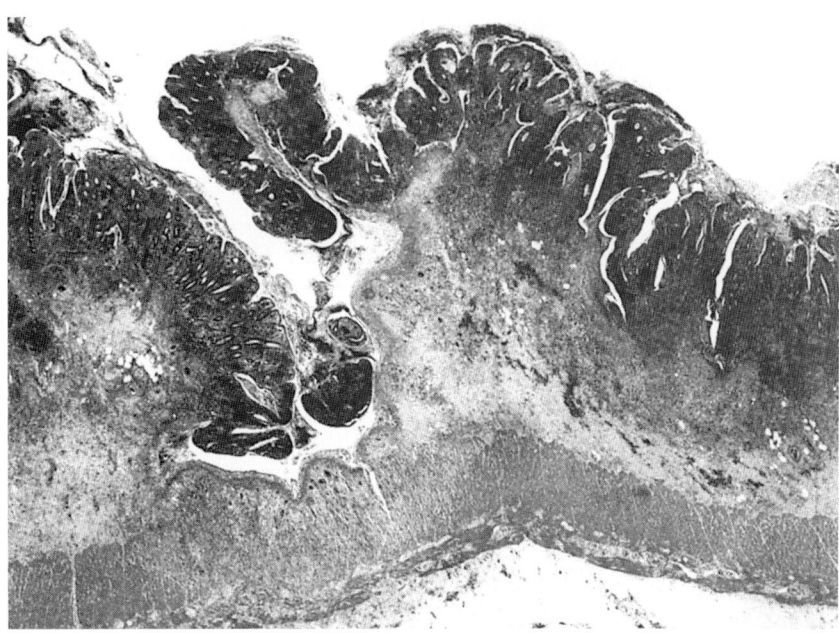

Fig. 31.13 Impending perforation in severe active ulcerative colitis without dilatation. A deep ulcer extends into the muscularis propria. Myocytolysis is confined to the immediate vicinity of the ulcer.

vicinity of the deep ulcers (Fig. 31.13). They also differ from patients with toxic megacolon in that the inflammatory infiltrate tends to be more prominent relative to the degree of vascular dilatation.

Benign strictures and inflammatory polyps are local sequelae of ulcerative colitis which are usually of little consequence to the patient and not an indication for colectomy. However, colectomy is sometimes considered if there is doubt as to their underlying pathology, or if they prevent the colonoscopist from reaching the proximal colon in cancer surveillance programs. Benign strictures attributed to hypertrophy of the muscularis mucosae (Goulston & McGovern 1969) have been described radiologically and are sometimes seen in resected specimens. They are usually smooth, may be multiple, are sometimes reversible and are rarely sufficiently narrow to cause obstruction. Strictures that are not reversible may include some due to fibrosis of the submucosa or muscularis propria as a result of previous severe ulcerative disease which did not remain confined to the mucosa. Benign strictures are most commonly seen in patients with long-standing disease, although they are occasionally observed at the time of presentation (deDombal et al 1966, Goulston & McGovern 1969).

Polypoid mucosal tags are a relatively common benign sequela of active ulceration colitis. The term 'pseudopolyp' is commonly used also for these mucosal projections, to avoid confusion with adenomas. These mucosal tags, unlike those seen as 'mucosal islands' in acute disease, clearly fit the definition of polyp and so the alternative term 'inflammatory polyp' is preferred (Morson & Dawson 1979). When they occur in active disease before there is re-epithelialization they consist of isolated edematous and congested mucosal remnants rising above the surrounding ulcerated surface (Figs 31.9, 31.13). Another mechanism of inflammatory polyp formation is the exuberant proliferation of granulation tissue to form the polypoid nodules that are later covered with regenerated mucosa. The histological appearance of inflammatory polyps shows some variability, depending on whether the mucosa originated from a mucosal island or from regenerated mucosa, and depending on the degree of inflammation and the amount of intermixed granulation tissue. Some polyps with pronounced inflammation and cystic dilated crypts may resemble juvenile polyps histologically.

Inflammatory polyps assume many shapes and occasionally form mucosal bridges, but usually they lack the distinct lobulated head typical of pedunculated adenomas. Most inflammatory polyps are less than 1.5 cm long, although they do show considerable variation in size and occasionally may reach several centimeters in length or diameter. They persist in the quiescent stage after re-epithelialization, and often remain as a constant monument to the severity of the preceding ulceration. When especially numerous they can form a forest of polyps, for which the term 'colitis polyposa' has been used. Although in the past there has been controversy concerning the precancerous potential of inflammatory polyps (Dawson & Pryse-Davies 1959), they are now considered benign (deDombal et al 1966, Hinrichs & Goldman 1968, Jalan et al 1969b). Occasionally they may become large and create a suspicion of carcinoma or cause obstruction (Hinrichs & Goldman 1968, Joffe 1977). Most commonly they occur in patients with severe disease, especially those with total colonic involvement (deDombal et al 1966, Jalan et al 1969b). This is the probable basis for the reported positive association of inflammatory polyps with toxic megacolon and the arthropathy of ulcerative colitis (Jalan et al 1969b), for both tend to occur with severe total colitis. Patients with mild disease, as judged by clinical criteria, rarely have inflammatory polyposis.

Inflammatory polyps are generally distributed in a diffuse or irregular fashion throughout the colon, but they are relatively uncommon in the rectum, especially close to the anal verge (deDombal et al 1966). Inflammatory polyps are not exclusive to ulcerative colitis and may be found following ulceration or inflammatory bowel disease of other etiologies. True adenomatous polyps may occur as coincidental finding in patients with ulcerative colitis, although their incidence is low.

Anal lesions occur in a minority of patients with ulcerative colitis and are thought to be secondary to the diarrhea. These include anal fissure, rectal prolapse, hemorrhoids and perianal excoriations and perirectal abscesses. In ulcerative colitis the anal complications are considerably less frequent and less severe than in Crohn's disease. Rectovaginal fistulae are rare in ulcerative colitis and should always raise the suspicion of a diagnosis of Crohn's disease.

DIFFERENTIAL DIAGNOSIS

Acute infectious colitis

The main changes in infectious colitis which help to distinguish it from normal and from IBD are the epithelium, where the architecture is preserved, with occasional mucin depletion, and inflammation, with neutrophils or both acute and chronic inflammation in the lamina propria and superficial crypt abscesses. In one report of infectious colitis neutrophils were most marked in the first few days after the onset of bloody diarrhea along with edema, the neutrophils becoming focal a week after the onset of diarrhea (Kumar et al 1982). Unlike active ulcerative colitis in which, if neutrophils are present they are invariably found in the crypt epithelium in at least the same density as found in the lamina propria, in infection (like Crohn's disease) they predominate in the lamina propria, to the point that the lamina propria may be purulent.

These criteria seem relatively straightforward, but in practice they are not so easy to utilize. In an interobserver study of 60 rectal biopsies from patients with bloody diarrhea, 41 had IBD but only a mean of 33 of these (about 80%) were correctly identified; the figure for infectious colitis was even less (Lessells et al 1994). There are several reasons why problems in diagnosis occur:

1. Ulcerative colitis in the first 2 weeks or so may not have architectural distortion, and if treated promptly the architecture may return quickly to normal and architectural distortion and basal plasmacytosis may not be found until considerably later than the initial presentation (Schumacher 1993, Odze et al 1993).
2. The basal plasmacytosis that is so useful in the diagnosis of IBD may be focal and not always present, whereas a few deep plasma cells may apparently sometimes be found in infective colitis (Schumacher 1993).
3. Infective colitis can cause focal changes endoscopically (Rutgeerts et al 1982).
4. Although most infections do not cause architectural distortion, the most severe diseases causing ulceration, such as shigella (Anand et al 1986), pseudomembranous colitis, and occasionally salmonella, may result in architectural distortion (Lewin et al 1992).
5. Selection bias plays a major role in the morphological descriptions of infective colitis, for these are selected on the basis of patients with recognized pathogens, or those with bloody diarrhea; they also have to be patients with sufficient concern to seek a physician; as such they represent a highly select subgroup of those with infective colitis, albeit probably the most severe.
6. In practice, the spectrum of appearances caused by infective colitis varies from virtually a normal mucosa for enteric organisms such as *Vibrio* and rotavirus (not associated with blood), to the typical biopsy appearances of infective colitis as cited in the literature.

Although the clinical picture and microbiological studies of the stool usually establish the correct diagnosis, several points are worth remembering. Standard microbiological methods may be inadequate and special methods are necessary to isolate some organisms, such as Campylobacter. Furthermore, a predisposition for salmonella infection has been reported in patients with ulcerative colitis and Crohn's disease (Lindeman et al 1967, Dronfield et al 1974), although this has been challenged (Szilagyi 1985). In some patients exacerbations of ulcerative colitis occur with stools that contain Campylobacter (Newman & Lambert 1980) or *Clostridium difficile* toxin (Bolton et al 1980, LaMont & Trnka 1980). It is not clear whether the apparent predisposition to infection with these organisms is peculiar to ulcerative colitis or a consequence of antibiotics or steroid therapy.

In infective colitis the crypt abscesses tend to be superficial, in contrast to ulcerative colitis in which they are usually prominently basal. In infective colitis mucin depletion and accompanying chronic inflammatory cell infiltration is often less than is expected in ulcerative colitis. Recovery from infective colitis is usually followed by restoration of histologically normal mucosa. The diffuse mucosal atrophy and crypt distortion indicative of previous active disease, which typify quiescent ulcerative colitis, are notably absent, unless infection is superimposed on underlying ulcerative colitis or unless the infection has been so severe that musocal destruction has occurred. This may be seen in infections such as pseudomembranous colitis and Shigella (Anand et al 1986) and rarely in Campylobacter, syphilis and herpes virus infection (Surawicz et al 1986, Allison et al 1987, Surawicz 1988). Conversely, some patients without architectural distortion may ultimately prove to have inflammatory bowel disease (Therkildsen et al 1989). Gram stains are rarely successful in demonstrating the infecting organisms and therefore usually of little value in differential diagnosis. Pseudomembranous colitis due to *Cl. difficile* toxin in patients without underlying ulcerative colitis has histological features which distinguish it from those of patients with ulcerative colitis whose exacerbation is associated with *Cl. difficile* toxin. Therefore there should be no confusion with ulcerative colitis except when it is complicated by toxic dilatation, when differentiation may be difficult.

Criteria for the distinction of Crohn's disease from ulcerative colitis (see also Chapter 32)

Histologic criteria for Crohn's disease in the literature are still largely based on the finding of granulomas, in addition to the presence of criteria for IBD (Cook et al 1973, Schmitz-Moormann & Himmelmann 1988, Theodossi et al 1994). In one recent interobserver variability study by ten pathologists examining numerous defined features, some were consistently identified in patients with Crohn's disease, including granulomas and Langhan's giant cells; focal inflammation was seen more frequently in Crohn's disease than ulcerative colitis, but was also seen in normals. Crypt architecture and distortion, branching and Paneth cell metaplasia did not distinguish but were seen more frequently in ulcerative colitis. Other features were of little value (Theodossi et al 1994). This latter study differed from most previous ones by examining two biopsies from each patient, although their sites are not stated. Note that no study examining full colonoscopic series of biopsies has yet reached the literature. Some features which one would normally consider to be reproducible, such as the presence of neutrophils, were surprisingly variably reported, and this has also been found in other studies (Seldenrijk et al 1991).

In Crohn's disease, and also some patients with fulminant colitis of any (or undetermined) cause, aphthoid ulcers, serpiginous or bear-claw ulcers, longitudinal and transverse ulcers with intervening mucosa that is edematous and therefore may be endoscopically cobblestoned, may all be present. Yet the biopsy appearances of these 'specific' endoscopic lesions have received very little attention (Tanaka & Riddell 1990). In practice, biopsies of aphthoid ulcers are usually reflected by focal erosion or ulceration, on a background of a largely normal mucosa or one in which the inflammation reduces dramatically over the extent of the biopsy. Typically, one side of a biopsy may be ulcerated and the other have either a minimal increase in chronic inflammation or even be normal, and contain few or no neutrophils away from the ulcer. Given an endoscopic appearance of this type, it will be appreciated that the colonoscopist can under these circumstances completely bias any morphological diagnosis based on these features, since the colonoscopist will deliberately take biopsies to demonstrate the presence of focal ulceration on the background of a relatively normal mucosa.

A second untested feature of Crohn's disease is that, unlike ulcerative colitis, where if neutrophils are present they usually attack most of the crypts in their immediate neighbourhood, in Crohn's disease this seems to be much less frequent and neutrophils are therefore largely confined to the lamina propria with relative crypt sparing, a feature shared with infective colitis (so much so that the question of an infection-driven exacerbation of IBD may come to mind). Involvement of crypts and surface epithelium, or villi in the terminal ileum, may be exquisitely focal.

Using these criteria, the hallmark of Crohn's disease is the presence of focal inflammation within and between biopsies, especially with focal ulceration at one end of the biopsy and relatively uninvolved mucosa at the other. Granulomas are a bonus, but terminal ileal inflammation, and occasionally pyloric metaplasia, may also be found and are extremely helpful when present. Fulminant colitis of any cause can result in an identical morphological appearance. If neutrophils are found in the lamina propria they usually extend up to the crypt epithelium but not into it; however, focal infiltration particularly into the surface epithelium may occur. Although ischemia can produce similar changes, these are usually associated with mucosal fibrosis and sometimes with a pseudomembrane. Conversely, the hallmark of ulcerative colitis is architectural distortion in association with chronic and acute inflammation, all of which tend to increase distally, although all may extend proximally and maximally to the cecum in a small group of patients with active total disease. More typically, proximal biopsies may be normal and, passing distally, architectural changes then creep in, and at some point a cryptophilic neutrophilic infiltrate. Sometimes these may be condensed, with a transition from active to normal over a few centimeters. Relative rectal sparing may exist but it is rare for rectal mucosa to be absolutely normal in the presence of more proximal active disease.

In mucosal biopsy specimens a diagnosis of either ulcerative colitis or Crohn's disease can be made in the majority of cases, but with somewhat less reliability than in resected specimens. Histological distinction between these two diseases is generally easier in the acute stage than during the resolving phase, when definitive diagnosis may be more difficult or impossible. Increasing the mucosal area sampled with multiple biopsies improves the chances of reliable histological diagnosis. This is especially true with multiple colonoscopic biopsies, when focal inflammation within and between biopsies is typical of Crohn's disease, even in the absence of granulomas (inflammatory polyps must be excluded as these are often inflamed). However, the term indeterminate colitis has also been used clinically for patients in whom the underlying disease is unclear in the absence of the severely active disease for which this term was originally coined.

In a few patients the subsequent evolution of disease may necessitate a change in diagnosis – it is invariably from ulcerative colitis to Crohn's disease rather than the other way round. In some of these patients careful review of previous material may then reveal either marked focality or 'missed' granulomas. It should be remembered that Crohn's colitis passed unrecognized as a clinical entity until the early 1960s. Patients undergoing proctocolectomy and ileostomy before that time were virtually all called ulcerative colitis. Some of them returned much later with evidence of ileostomy dysfunction or further disease in the small bowel. Review of resected material from these patients often reveals that the underlying disease was indeed Crohn's disease and, presumably, always had been.

Finally, a question asked with increasing frequency is whether ulcerative colitis can coexist with Crohn's disease in the same patient. Suggestions that this might occur have appeared in the literature following the recognition of Crohn's disease of the colon and its distinction from ulcerative colitis (Edwards & Truelove 1964, Voitk et al 1976, Eyer et al 1980). Clearly, if both diseases ultimately prove to have different etiologies there is no reason, statistically, why this should not occur. Indeed, given the prevalence of ulcerative colitis as approximately 40–80 per 100 000, and that of Crohn's disease as approximately 15 per 100 000, this coexistence would be expected to occur in 6–12 per 100 000 000 of the population, or 20–40 cases in the USA. Conversely, if they prove to be different manifestations of the same etiological agent it might not happen at all. We are currently sceptical about reports of both diseases occurring in the same patient, probably because we have yet to be convinced of an acceptable example. Nevertheless, it is possible that our underlying bias in trying to make most diseases fit one or other category might prevent us from recognizing such cases should they occur. Thus, any patient with typical ulcerative colitis in whom biopsy or resected material shows a typical granuloma or other features of Crohn's disease is immediately classified as having Crohn's disease. This approach is of course pragmatic, as most of such patients ultimately appear to be have as Crohn's disease, with the risk of any of its complications and, if follow-up is sufficiently long, most are not 'cured' by proctocolectomy.

Indeterminate colitis

Most cases of idiopathic IBD can be readily identified as either ulcerative colitis or Crohn's disease, and pose little diagnostic problem. This distinction is most easily made in resected specimens, where extensive gross and histological examination is possible and confident diagnosis can be expected in about 90% of cases. Reliable classification may not be possible in the remaining specimens, which almost always represent severe active disease, often with some degree of dilatation, and where transmural inflammation is invariably present. For them, the term 'indeterminate colitis' has been proposed (Price 1978, Lee et al 1979). These cases represent the area of maximal overlap of pathological features of Crohn's disease and ulcerative colitis. Under these circumstances a firm diagnosis of Crohn's disease depends on the histological demonstration of additional features such as non-caseating sarcoid-like granulomas that are not due to foreign material, typical lymphoid aggregates away from areas of ulceration, and typical fistula tracts.

In patients with indeterminate colitis coming to resection there is increasing evidence that, compared to patients with ulcerative colitis, those undergoing restorative proctocolectomy have a greater number of complications, including the need to remove the pouch (McIntyre et al 1995, Luukkonen et al 1994, Grobler et al 1993, Koltun et al 1991, Atkinson et al 1994).

Ischemic colitis

In the elderly and arteriopathic patient it may be difficult to differentiate histologically between acute ulcerative colitis and acute ischemic colitis. The subsequent clinical course provides better differentiation than does the evolution of the histological changes. Although hemosiderin deposition is the distinguishing feature of the later stages of ischemic colitis, it may also be found following hemorrhage into the lamina propria in both ulcerative colitis and Crohn's disease.

Taking biopsies in the absence of endoscopic disease

The last decade has seen increasing acknowledgement of the presence of chronic colitis that can cause symptoms not apparent endoscopically. In the presence of a thickened subepithelial collagen band this is collagenous colitis, but both inflammation and a thickened collagen band are required for the diagnosis. The collagen band may be focal and the inflammation may be rectal sparing (Lazenby et al 1990, Tanaka et al 1992). In the absence of a collagen band the diagnosis is commuted to microscopic colitis or, in the presence of an excess of intraepithelial lymphocytes, to lymphocytic colitis.

Importantly, although the morphology of IBD is distinguishable from microscopic/lymphocytic colitis (Lazenby et al 1989, Fasoli et al 1992), the typical biopsy of microscopic colitis can be seen in patients with both ulcerative colitis and Crohn's disease under appropriate circumstances. For example, a patient with distal active ulcerative colitis can have a more proximal biopsy in which the architecture has returned to normal but an excess of plasma cells exists, reaching the lamina propria. Random biopsies from Crohn's disease may be identical, but in both circumstances there is sufficient gross disease that microscopic colitis is not a consideration.

In patients with diarrhea in whom no or minimal endoscopic abnormality is found, a small number of biopsies are required to exclude microscopic abnormalities, particularly collagenous or microscopic/lymphocytic colitis. At flexible sigmoidoscopy, normal biopsies from the sigmoid, descending colon and rectum are an excellent indicator that significant disease will not be present proximal to this (Tanaka et al 1992). At full colonoscopy additional biopsies from the cecum and transverse colon are useful for detecting collagenous colitis in patients apparently having microscopic colitis, because the thickened subepithelial collagen band can be extremely focal (Lazenby et al 1990, Tanaka et al 1992). Under these circumstances it should be recalled that data are accumulating suggesting that the mucosa in ulcerative colitis may return to normal in some patients (Kirsner et al 1951, Odze et al 1993).

Changing patterns of disease as the result of therapy

Although it is generally accepted that a variety of medications modify inflammation and symptoms, this is very poorly documented in the literature. Patients are treated primarily for symptomatic relief, but this shows only a poor correlation with inflammation in individual patients, although a reasonable overall correlation. Drugs with a therapeutic effect include steroids given either systemically or in enemas, immunosuppressives, and numerous salicylate preparations, many of which have been designed to be released into specific parts of the small or large intestine. Failure of drugs to be released into the required segment of bowel, for example because of rapid transit through that segment prior to release, or conditions dissimilar to those at which release occurs physiologically, may result in areas of bowel that remain inflamed, with subsequent unusual or even new patterns of disease. It is therefore necessary to be alert to the possibility that new distributions of disease may be iatrogenic and the result of new 'designer drugs' that may not work, or be released, precisely as or where planned. Also, even diffuse disease such as typical ulcerative colitis may not resolve diffusely, but rather with a degree of focality that may cause the possibility of underlying Crohn's disease to be raised. Similarly, the effect of enemas on causing distal healing is well known, but what if these changes are present without enema use? Is this acceptable for ulcerative colitis, or does ulcerative colitis by definition always have to involve the rectum? Two studies, currently in abstract form only, suggest that the colitis associated with diverticulitis, and limited to that segment of bowel, may be morphologically indistinguishable from ulcerative colitis, and may recur as typical ulcerative colitis, raising the possibility that ulcerative colitis may not necessarily always involve the rectum from the beginning (Makapugay & Dean 1995, Hart et al 1995).

VARIATION BETWEEN COLONOSCOPISTS, AND IMPLICATIONS FOR PATHOLOGY

There is a perception among gastroenterologists that some pathologists are more able to render an accurate interpretation than others. One reason why this might be true is that there may also be considerable variability between colonoscopists as to how many biopsies are taken, given identical clinical circumstances. Interestingly, almost 30% of gastroenterologists believe that their pathologists are unable reliably to distinguish ulcerative colitis from infective colitis (which may be true) (Riddell et al 1995). A 'catch-22' situation exists in that if the pathology response is perceived as being inadequate or suboptimal then fewer biopsies will be taken.

These problems are compounded by interobserver variation among colonoscopists. For example, there is considerable variation in the endoscopist's definition of an aphthoid ulcer; this in turn affects first the sensitivity and specificity of aphthoid ulcers, particularly in separating ulcerative colitis from Crohn's disease; and secondly whether some gastroenterologists accept aphthoid ulcers as part of the endoscopic spectrum of ulcerative colitis, and whether they are correct in doing this. There are also variations in the amount of emphasis put on continuity of disease and location, particularly if this is rectal. These problems are further compounded by variations in the endoscopic accuracy of terms such as erosions or ulcers, and the modifying effect of therapy on all of these features. It is surely time for studies to clarify these issues.

REFERENCES

Allison M C, Hamilton-Dhillon A P, Pounder R E 1987 The value of rectal biopsy in distinguishing self-limited colitis from early inflammatory bowel disease. Quarterly Journal of Medicine 65: 985–995

Anand B S, Malhotra V, Bhattacharya S K et al 1986a Rectal histology in acute bacillary dysentery. Gastroenterology 90: 654–660

Atkinson K G, Owen D A, Wankling G 1994 Restorative proctocolectomy and indeterminate colitis. American Journal of Surgery 167: 516–518

Bolton R P, Sheriff R J, Read A D 1980 *Clostridium difficile* associated diarrhoea: a role in inflammatory bowel disease. Lancet 1: 383–384

Bookman M A, Bull D M 1979 Characteristics of isolated intestinal musocal lymphoid cells in inflammatory bowel disease. Gastroenterology 77: 503–510

Brandtzaeg P, Baklien K, Fauso O, Hoel P S 1974 Immunohistochemical characterization of local immunoglobulin formation in ulcerative colitis. Gastroenterology 66: 1123–1136

Buckell N A, Williams G T, Bartram C I, Lennard-Jones J E 1980 Depth of ulceration in acute ulcerative colitis. Gastroenterology 79: 19–25

Cook M G, Dixon M F 1973 An analysis of the reliability of detection and diagnostic value of various pathological features in Crohn's disease and ulcerative colitis. Gut 14: 255–262

Dawson I M P, Pryse-Davies J 1959 The development of carcinoma of the large intestine in ulcerative colitis. British Journal of Surgery 47: 113–128

deDombal F T, Watts J McK, Watkinson G, Goligher J C 1966 Local complications of ulcerative colitis: stricture, pseudopoliposis, and carcinoma of colon and rectum. British Medical Journal 1: 1442–1447

Dickinson R J, Gilmour H M, McClelland B L 1979 Rectal biopsy in patients admitted to an infectious disease unit with diarrhoeal disease. Gut 20: 141–148

Dronfield M W, Fletcher J, Langman M J S 1974 Coincident Salmonella infection and ulcerative colitis: problems of recognition and management. British Medical Journal 1: 99–100

Edwards F C, Truelove S C 1964 The course and prognosis of ulcerative colitis. Gut 5: 1–22

Eyer S, Spadaccini C, Walker P, Ansel H, Schwartz M, Sumner H W 1980 Simultaneous ulcerative colitis and Crohn's disease. American Journal of Gastroenterology 73: 345–349

Farmer R G 1979 Long-term prognosis for patients with ulcerative proctosigmoiditis (ulcerative colitis confined to the rectum and sigmoid colon). Journal of Clinical Gastroenterology 1: 47–50

Farmer R G 1989 Ulcerative proctitis: tractable or intractable. In: Barkin J S, Rogers A L (eds) Difficult decisions in digestive disease Year Book Medical Publishers, Chicago, pp 368–379

Fasoli R, Talbot I, Reid M, Prince C, Jewell D P 1992 Microscopic colitis: can it be qualitatively and quantitatively characterized? Italian Journal of Gastroenterology 24: 393–396

Flejou J F, Potet F, Bogomoletz W V et al 1988 Lymphoid follicular proctitis. A condition different from ulcerative proctitis? Digestive Diseases and Sciences 33: 314–320

Gilat T, Lilas P, Zemishany Z, Ribak J, Benroya Y 1976 Ulcerative colitis in the Jewish population of Tel-Aviv Yafo: clinical course. Gastroenterology 70: 14–19

Goulston S J M, McGovern V J 1969 The nature of benign strictures in ulcerative colitis. New England Journal of Medicine 281: 3290–3295

Grobler S P, Hosie K B, Affie E, Thompson H, Keighley M R 1993 Outcome of restorative proctocolectomy when the diagnosis is suggestive of Crohn's disease. Gut 34: 1384–1388

Haggitt R C 1983 The differential diagnosis of inflammatory bowel disease. In: Norris H T (ed) Pathology of the colon, small intestine and anus. Churchill Livingstone, New York, pp 21–60

Hart J, Baert F, Hanauer S 1995 Sigmoiditis: a clinical syndrome with a spectrum of pathologic features, including a distinctive form of IBD. Laboratory Investigation (in press)

Hinrichs R H, Goldman H 1968 Localized giant pseudopoliposis of the colon. Journal of the American Medical Association 205: 108–109

Jalan K N, Sircus W, Card W I et al 1969a An experience in ulcerative colitis. I. Toxic dilatation in 55 cases. Gastroenterology 57: 68–82

Jalan K N, Walker R J, Sircus W, McManus J P A, Prescott R J, Card W I 1969b Pseudopoliposis in ulcerative colitis. Lancet 2: 555–559

Jenkins D, Goodall A, Scott B B 1990 Ulcerative colitis: one disease or two? (Quantitative histological differences between distal and extensive disease). Gut 31: 426–430

Joffe N 1977 Localized giant pseudopoliposis secondary to ulcerative or granulomatous colitis. Clinical Radiology 28: 609–616

Kirsner J B, Palmer W L, Klotz A P 1951 Reversibility in ulcerative colitis: clinical and radiological observations. Radiology 57: 1–14

Koltun W A, Schoetz Jr D J, Roberts P L, Murray J J, Collen J A, Veidenheimer M C 1991 Indeterminate colitis predisposes to perineal complications after ileal pouch–anal anastomosis. Diseases of the Colon and Rectum 34: 857–860

Kumar N B, Nostrant T T, Appelman H D 1982 This histopathologic spectrum of acute self-limited colitis. American Journal of Surgical Pathology 6: 523–529

LaMont J T, Trnka Y M 1980 Therapeutic implications of *Clostridium difficile* toxin during relapse of chronic inflammatory bowel disease. Lancet 1: 381–383

Lazenby A J, Yardley J H, Giardiello F M, Jessurun J, Bayless T M 1989 Lymphocytic ('microscopic') colitis: a comparative histologic study with particular reference to collagenous colitis. Human Pathology 20: 18–28

Lazenby A J, Yardley J H, Giardiello F M, Bayless T M 1990 Pitfalls in the diagnosis of collagenous colitis: experience with 75 cases from a registry of collagenous colitis at the Johns Hopkins Hospital. Human Pathology 21: 905–910

Lee K S, Medline A, Shockey S 1979 Indeterminate colitis in the spectrum of inflammatory bowel disease. Archives of Pathology and Laboratory Medicine 103: 173–176

Lessells A M, Beck J S, Burnett R A et al 1994 Observer variability in the histopathological reporting of abnormal rectal biopsy specimens. Journal of Clinical Pathology 47: 48–52

Lewin K J, Riddell R H, Weinstein W M 1992 Gastrointestinal pathology and its clinical implications. Igaku-Shoin, New York

Lindeman R J, Weinstein L, Levitan R, Patterson J F 1967 Ulcerative colitis and intestinal salmonellosis. American Journal of Medical Science 254: 855–861

Lumb G, Protheroe R H B 1955 Biopsy of the rectum in ulcerative colitis. Lancet 2: 1208–1215

Luukkonen P, Jarvinen H, Tanskanen M, Kahri A 1994 Pouchitis – recurrence of the inflammatory bowel disease? Gut 35: 243–246

McCormick D A, Horton L W, Mee A S 1990 Mucin depletion in inflammatory bowel disease. Journal of Clinical Pathology 43: 143–146

McIntyre P B, Pemberton J H, Wolff B G, Dozois R R, Beart Jr R W 1995 Indeterminate colitis: long-term outcome in patients after ileal pouch–anal anastomosis. Diseases of the Colon and Rectum 38: 51–54

Makapugay L M, Dean P J 1995 Diverticular disease-associated colitis. A study of 23 cases. American Journal of Surgical Pathology (in press)

Morson B C, Dawson I M P 1979 Gastrointestinal pathology. Blackwell, Oxford

Newman A, Lambert J R 1980 *Campylobacter jejuni* causing flare-up of inflammatory bowel disease. Lancet 2: 919

Norland C C, Kirsner J B 1969 Toxic dilatation of colon (toxin megacolon): etiology, treatment and prognosis in 42 patients. Medicine 48: 229–250

O'Donoghue D P, Kumar P 1979 Rectal IgE cells in inflammatory bowel disease. Gut 20: 149–153

Odze R, Antonioli D, Peppercorn M, Goldman H 1993 Effects of topical 5-aminosalicylic acid (5-ASA) therapy on rectal mucosal biopsy morphology in chronic ulcerative colitis. American Journal of Surgical Pathology 17: 869–875

Price A B 1978 Overlap in the spectrum of non-specific inflammatory bowel disease: colitis indeterminate. Journal of Clinical Pathology 31: 567–577

Riddell R H 1977 The precancerous lesion of ulcerative colitis. In: Yardley J H, Morson B C (eds) The gastrointestinal tract. Williams and Wilkins, Baltimore, pp 109–123

Riddell R H, Geboes K, Meuwissen S G M 1995 Are gastroenterologists uniform in their response to specific clinical problems? Implications for pathologists. (in preparation)

Rutgeerts P, Geboes K, Ponette E, Coremans G, Vantrappen G 1982 Acute infective colitis caused by endemic pathogens in western Europe: endoscopic features. Endoscopy 14: 212–219

Saltzstein S I, Rosenberg B F 1963 Ulcerative colitis of the ileum and regional enteritis of the colon, a comparative histologic study. American Journal of Clinical Pathology 40: 610–623

Schmitz-Moormann P, Himmelmann G W 1988 Does quantitative histology of rectal biopsy improve the differential diagnosis of Crohn's disease and ulcerative colitis in adults? Pathology Research and Practice 183: 481–488

Schumacher G 1993 First attack of inflammatory bowel disease and infectious colitis. A clinical histological and microbiological study with special reference to early diagnosis. Scandinavian Journal of Gastroenterology 198: (Suppl.) 1–24

Seldenrijk C A, Morson B C, Meuwissen S G, Schipper N W, Lindeman J, Meijer C J 1991 Histopathological evaluation of colonic mucosal biopsy specimens in chronic inflammatory bowel disease: diagnostic implications. Gut 32: 1514–1520

Spiliadis C A, Lennard-Jones J E 1987 Ulcerative colitis with relative sparing of the rectum. Clinical features, histology and prognosis. Diseases of the Colon and Rectum 30: 334–336

Surawicz C M 1988 The role of rectal biopsy in infectious colitis. American Journal of Surgical Pathology 12: 82–88

Surawicz C M, Belic L 1984 Rectal biopsy helps to distinguish acute self-limited colitis from idiopathic inflammatory bowel disease. Gastroenterology 86: 104–113

Surawicz C M, Goodell S E, Quinn T C et al 1986 Spectrum of rectal biopsy abnormalities in homosexual men with intestinal symptoms. Gastroenterology 91: 645–649

Surawicz C M, Haggitt R C, Husseman M, McFarland L V 1994 Mucosal biopsy diagnosis of colitis: acute self-limited colitis and idiopathic inflammatory bowel disease. Gastroenterology 107: 755–763

Szilagyi A, Gerson M, Mendolson J, Yusuf N. A 1985 Salmonella infections complicating inflammatory bowel disease. Journal of Clinical Gastroenterology 7: 251–255

Tanaka M, Riddell R H 1990 The pathological diagnosis and differential diagnosis of Crohn's disease. Hepatogastroenterology 37: 18–31

Tanaka M, Mazzoleni G, Riddell R H 1992 Distribution of collagenous colitis: utility of flexible sigmoidoscopy. Gut 33: 65–70

Theodossi A, Spiegelhalter D J, Jass J et al 1994 Observer variation and discriminatory value of biopsy features in inflammatory bowel disease. Gut 35: 961–968

Therkildsen M H, Jensen B Y, Teglbjaerg P S, Rasmussen N 1989 The final outcome of patients presenting with their first episode of acute diarrhea and an inflamed rectal mucosa with preserved crypt architecture. A clinicopathologic study. Scandinavian Journal of Gastroenterology 24: 158–164

Voitk A J, Owen D R, Lough J 1976 Coexistent regional enteritis and ulcerative colitis. International Surgery 61: 535–571

Warren S, Sommers S C 1949 Pathogenesis of ulcerative colitis. American Journal of Pathology 25: 657–679

32. Histopathology of Crohn's disease

J. R. Goldblum   R. E. Petras

GENERAL ASPECTS

Crohn's disease is an idiopathic chronic inflammatory disorder which may affect any portion of the gastrointestinal tract, but most commonly the small intestine, particularly the distal terminal ileum, and the right colon. Crohn's disease has also been referred to as regional enterocolitis or regional enteritis/ileitis because of the frequent involvement of these sites. The differential diagnosis of Crohn's disease depends upon the site of involvement within the gastrointestinal tract. To the pathologist the diagnosis of Crohn's disease usually requires a combination of both gross and microscopic features, particularly with respect to the distribution of the disease.

MACROSCOPIC FEATURES

In the authors' experience, approximately 70% of patients with Crohn's disease will have involvement of the small bowel, either alone or together with the colon (Farmer et al 1985). Grossly, the first evident lesion of Crohn's disease is a small, well-demarcated mucosal ulcer referred to as an aphthous ulcer. These are often multiple and are typically separated by grossly unremarkable intervening mucosa. As these ulcers grow they coalesce to form continuous areas of ulceration of the intestinal mucosa. Thus the mucosal aspect of the opened specimen can reveal ulcers which are discrete, linear, serpiginous or diffuse. Given the presence of normal mucosa between these ulcers, a cobblestone-like appearance may be present. Ulcers may be superficial or can extend well into the muscularis propria, with the occasional formation of fissures and sinus tracts which are apparent on the gross specimen (Kelly & Siu 1986).

Fistulae and sinus tracts can be found near areas of stenosis. On cross-section one can often appreciate marked submucosal fibrosis and hypertrophy of the muscularis mucosae and propria, resulting in stricture formation, particularly in the terminal ileum (Kelly & Sutherland 1988). Characteristically the serosal fat wraps itself around the external surface, often obscuring most of the serosal surface, a process referred to as 'fat-wrapping'. The extension of sinus tracts through the bowel wall can result in perforation and the formation of external abscesses, which tend to remain localized in the area of the perforation. If the inflammatory reaction involves adjacent tissues, including other portions of the bowel, urinary bladder, vagina and abdominal skin, fistulous connections may result. Mesenteric lymph nodes are often enlarged as a result of reactive follicular hyperplasia or granulomatous inflammation.

In classic cases of Crohn's colitis, the colectomy specimen is typically of normal length. The mucosa shows variable ulceration and edema, with patterns that are indistinguishable from those seen in the small intestine (Fig. 32.1). In addition, the intersection of linear ulcers with small horizontal crevices results in isolated small islands of normal or edematous mucosa, resulting in a cobblestone-like pattern. Deep fissuring ulcers, with the formation of longitudinal sinus tracts and fistulous connections, may also occur in Crohn's colitis. Inflammatory polyps can be seen, but their presence or absence is not particularly useful in distinguishing Crohn's from ulcerative colitis. The bowel wall is usually irregularly thickened, most prominently in areas of stricture. Evidence of patchy serositis, with encroachment of the mesenteric fat on to the serosal aspect of the colon, is occasionally prominent. Sometimes the peri-intestinal fat and serosa show extensive fibrosis, with areas of adhesion. As with the mucosal involvement, the serosal and peri-intestinal involvement is typically patchy.

Of all the gross features stated above, the most important information that one can obtain from the surgically resected specimen is the precise location, extent and distribution of disease. In most cases, evaluation of these features will allow for an accurate gross diagnosis. However, some cases of diffuse ulcerative or fulminant Crohn's colitis may be difficult or impossible to distinguish from ulcerative colitis, both grossly and microscopically. Although controversial, some investigators believe that

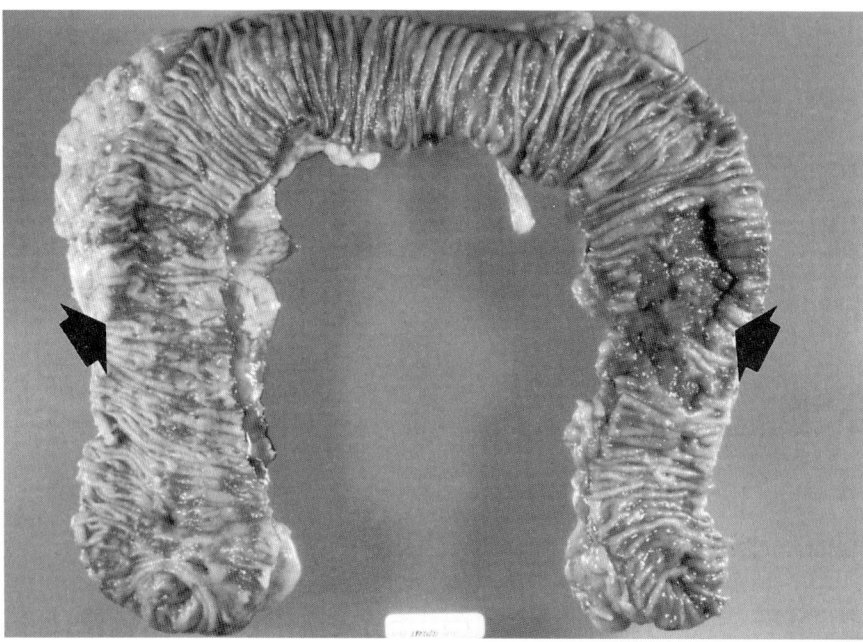

Fig. 32.1 Gross specimen of total proctocolectomy for Crohn's disease. The arrows note areas of ulceration in both the left and right colon, in between which there is normal-appearing mucosa.

the presence of gross ulceration at the surgical margins is a strong indicator that the disease will clinically recur and/or progress (Pennington et al 1980).

MICROSCOPIC FEATURES OF SMALL-INTESTINAL CROHN'S DISEASE

The earliest gross and histologic lesion of Crohn's disease is the aphthous ulcer, in which there is a discrete area of mucosal ulceration often overlying a lymphoid follicle. The mucosa between the ulcers is typically normal. As these ulcers grow in size and number they coalesce to form more diffuse areas of mucosal ulceration. Some ulcers become slitlike and deep, forming fissures which may extend into the deep submucosa, muscularis propria or beyond. When cut in cross-section these fissures appear as submucosal abscesses. The walls of the fissures are lined by granulation tissue and histiocytes, and are rich in lymphoid tissue. The surrounding mucosa which is non-ulcerated often shows variable villous blunting, with an expansion of the lamina propria by plasma cells and neutrophil- or eosinophil-mediated epithelial injury (cryptitis and crypt abscesses). Very importantly, there are typically areas of normal mucosa which intervene between areas of obvious active mucosal inflammation.

A major histologic feature of Crohn's disease is the presence of transmural inflammation, which takes the form of lymphoid aggregates that show a propensity to form around lymphatic and small blood vessels. These lymphoid aggregates may be seen anywhere within the intestinal wall, but are often most pronounced in the submucosa. On occasion the inflammation can spill over into the vascular walls, resulting in a 'Crohn's vasculitis.' This is thought to be a secondary phenomenon and not an etiologic factor in Crohn's disease (Geller & Cohen 1983).

The other major histologic feature of Crohn's disease is the presence of non-necrotizing granulomas (Fig. 32.2). These are typically few in number, scattered and not well formed, and have been estimated to be present in approximately 50–70% of cases (Chambers & Morson 1979, Kuramoto et al 1987). They may be seen in any portion of the bowel wall, as well as within regional lymph nodes. They closely resemble those granulomas seen in sarcoidosis, and consist of a collection of epithelioid histiocytes with occasional giant cells and a variable admixture of other inflammatory cells, including lymphocytes and eosinophils. Necrosis is characteristically not present. Although granulomas may be present in markedly inflamed mucosa, diagnostic granulomas are more frequently seen in histologically normal mucosa. It is important to exclude a granulomatous response to extravasated mucin from an injured crypt (so-called 'crypt rupture granuloma') from a true Crohn's-like granuloma. Occasionally small aggregates of epithelioid histiocytes are present, forming less well-formed granulomas or 'microgranulomas' (Rotterdam et al 1977).

A variety of other histologic features are characteristically seen in Crohn's disease, but are not diagnostic. These include submucosal fibrosis, neuronal hyperplasia, particularly of the myenteric plexus, hypertrophy of both the muscularis mucosae and propria, and pyloric gland

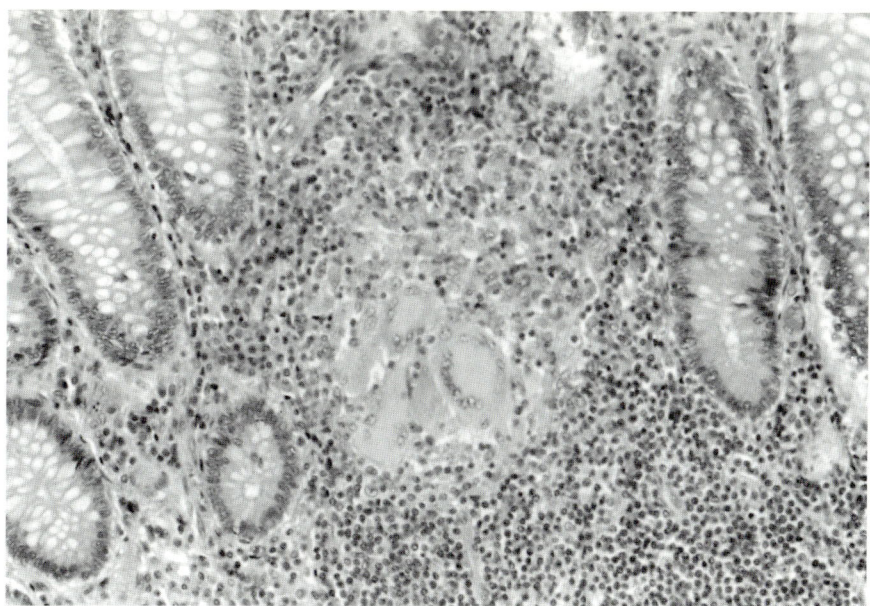

Fig. 32.2 Typical granuloma seen between mucosal crypts in a case of Crohn's disease. Several giant cells are surrounded by groups of epithelioid histiocytes, forming a sarcoid-like granuloma. There is an absence of active inflammation in the vicinity.

metaplasia. As mentioned below, these features may be seen in a variety of entities which enter the differential diagnosis of small-intestinal Crohn's disease.

The major indication for surgery in Crohn's disease is intestinal obstruction (Mekhjian et al 1979, Lee & Papaioannou 1982). Resection of the stenosed segment remains the standard therapy, but even with patients with localized disease that has been totally excised, approximately two-thirds will suffer anastomotic recurrence (Bergman & Krause 1977, Nygaard & Fousa 1977, Kotanagi et al 1991). This has prompted some surgeons to remove more bowel and even to advocate frozen-section analysis of the surgical margins (Ihasz et al 1975, Bergman & Krause 1977, Nygaard & Fousa 1977). We believe that it has been established that the histologic status of the resection margins in Crohn's disease is not associated with anastomotic recurrence (Pennington et al 1980, Hamilton et al 1985, Kotanagi et al 1991). Therefore, frozen-section analysis of a margin is never justified and the routine histologic examination of resection margins is of doubtful clinical relevance (Petras & Oakley 1992).

Differential diagnosis of small-intestinal Crohn's disease

The principal differential diagnostic considerations in Crohn's enteritis and ileocolitis are ischemic bowel disease and tuberculosis, as well as other chronic granulomatous infections with a predilection for the ileocecal region, including yersiniosis and histoplasmosis.

Ischemic bowel disease can closely mimic Crohn's disease because the bowel involvement is typically patchy, ulcers may be discrete or serpiginous, and healing may result in strictures. Acute ischemic enteritis may be focal or diffuse. There is typically superficial epithelial necrosis, with sparing of the deep portion of the crypt compartment (Whitehead 1972), as well as hemorrhage into the lamina propria, which is typically hypocellular. Occasionally the formation of pseudomembranes on the mucosal surface may closely mimic an infectious process. Depending upon the severity and duration of the ischemia, these changes may involve the entire mucosal thickness or, when severe, result in transmural ischemic necrosis (Robinson et al 1981). Although this early phase of ischemia is histologically characteristic, in its organizing phase ischemic damage becomes somewhat non-specific in appearance. However, an ischemic etiology should be suspected when an ulcer and organizing inflammation appear bland and unassociated with the marked chronic inflammation and lymphoid aggregates typical of Crohn's disease. In the healing phase the mucosa may become architecturally distorted, with villous blunting and even pyloric gland metaplasia (Petras 1994). Healed phases of ischemia are often accompanied by stricture formation, including fibrosis of the muscularis propria, an uncommon feature in primary inflammatory bowel disease (Petras 1994). Finally, granulomatous inflammation is not seen in ischemic bowel disease.

Grossly, intestinal tuberculosis may be indistinguishable from Crohn's disease (Tandon & Prakash 1972), as strictures of the ileum and cecum are common.

Histologically, although the granulomas may be non-necrotizing, many will show prominent caseous necrosis, a feature which is typically absent in granulomas related to Crohn's disease. There are often numerous granulomas present, and coalescence may result in grossly identifiable nodules. Although there may be discrete ulcers present in the mucosa, longitudinally running ulcers with the formation of a cobblestone-like appearance are absent. The diagnosis is confirmed by special stains for acid-fast bacilli, and by cultures.

Yersiniosis, caused by *Yersinia pseudotuberculosis* or *Yersinia enterocolitica*, may cause a fatal systemic illness or a self-limited enteritis which can closely mimic Crohn's disease. Both organisms are small Gram-negative pleomorphic coccobacilli, and may cause mesenteric adenitis with or without involvement of the terminal ileum, appendix or cecum. Most patients are young and present with fever and colicky abdominal pain (El-Miraghi & Mair 1979). Histologically there is typically lymphofollicular hyperplasia with prominent germinal center formation and suppurative granulomas, often in the germinal centers (Bradford et al 1974). Palisading histiocytes are found around a necrotic center, often with microabscesses (Gleason & Patterson 1982). Careful histologic examination, serologic tests and microbial cultures aid in this distinction from Crohn's disease.

Histoplasmosis may also be centered around the ileocecal area, and is characterized by the presence of both non-necrotizing and necrotizing granulomatous inflammation (Miller & Everett 1979). The mucosal changes and transmural lymphoid inflammation characteristic of Crohn's disease are typically absent in histoplasmosis, and this diagnosis can be confirmed with special stains and cultures.

MICROSCOPIC FEATURES OF COLONIC CROHN'S DISEASE

The most characteristic pattern of injury seen on mucosal biopsy in Crohn's disease is a focal active colitis, in which there is a patchy distribution of both architectural and inflammatory changes (Fig. 32.3). At low magnification there is typically a patchy expansion of the lamina propria, primarily by plasma cells coupled with focal architecture distortion, which is often minor. Characteristically some areas of the mucosa maintain an essentially normal appearance (Petras 1994). Ulcers, including fissural ulcers, may be present. Although granulomas may be present in Crohn's colitis, they are less frequent and often less well formed than the granulomas seen in Crohn's enteritis or ileocolitis. Active inflammation with crypt rupture and mucin extravasation may elicit a granulomatous response. Thus, if a granuloma is present in an area which is not actively inflamed, this feature strongly suggests a diagnosis of Crohn's disease. As in the small intestine, transmural lymphoid aggregates are characteristically present and have a propensity to form around blood vessels and lymphatics. Minor histologic features often seen in Crohn's colitis are neuronal hyperplasia, pyloric gland metaplasia (more often seen in small-intestinal Crohn's disease), inflammatory polyps, and patchy muscularis propria fibrosis.

On occasion Crohn's disease may result in a fulminant colitis, requiring urgent or emergent colectomy (Price

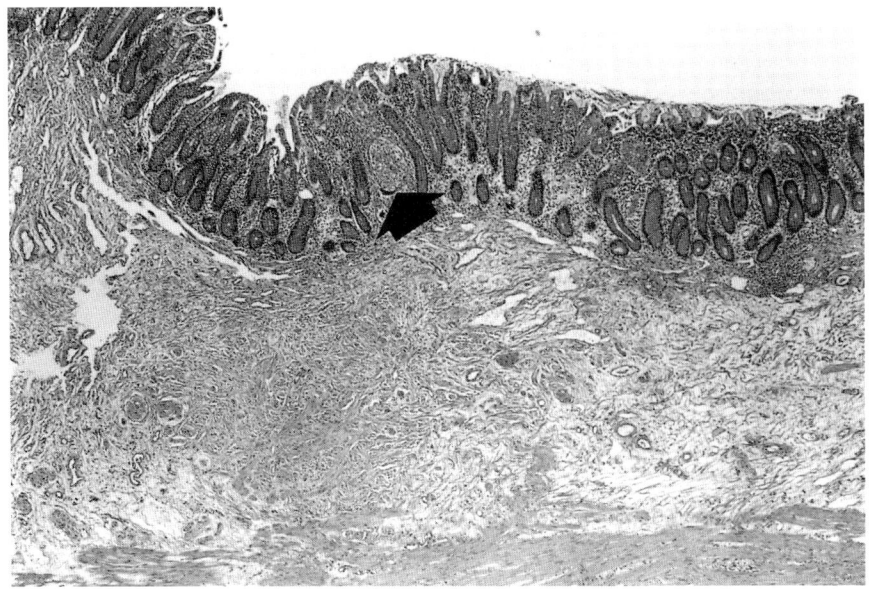

Fig. 32.3 Low-magnification view of colonic mucosa and submucosa in Crohn's disease. The arrow denotes an area of crypt injury. This is a focal active colitis pattern, given the normal surrounding mucosa.

1978). In these cases careful examination of the gross specimen with thorough sampling is critical in arriving at a diagnosis of Crohn's disease as the etiology of the fulminant colitis. Skip lesions, found either grossly or microscopically, suggest Crohn's disease. If the mucosa adjacent to a deep ulcer is almost completely normal, then this is suggestive of Crohn's disease. In contrast to active ulcerative colitis, in fulminant Crohn's disease the submucosa tends to be expanded and edematous, with prominent lymphangiectasia. Deep lymphoid aggregates are characteristically present in areas not involved by deep fissuring ulcers. In some cases a diagnosis of Crohn's disease can only be suggested based upon the gross and microscopic features of the specimen, and the designation 'fulminant colitis, indeterminate type, possibly/probably Crohn's disease' is appropriate.

Differential diagnosis of Crohn's colitis

The differential diagnosis of Crohn's colitis is wide, and depends to a large degree upon the type of specimen available for evaluation (endoscopic biopsy or colonic resection specimen). On mucosal biopsy, although a pattern of focal active colitis is characteristic of Crohn's disease, this pattern may be seen in infectious colitis (acute self-limited colitis) or in some cases of ulcerative colitis resolving under medical treatment (Odze et al 1993). Although the presence of granulomas strongly suggests Crohn's disease, they are commonly not present. In addition, germinal centers, tangential cuts of blood vessels or of the pericryptal fibroblastic sheath may be misinterpreted as the granulomas of Crohn's disease. Although the mucosal biopsy features of infectious colitis may be indistinguishable from those of Crohn's disease in the absence of granulomas, there is typically a predominance of neutrophils in the lamina propria in cases of infectious colitis, whereas in Crohn's disease the neutrophils tend to predominate within the crypt epithelium (Surawicz & Belic 1984, Schumacher 1993). On rare occasions a diffuse active colitis pattern of injury may also be seen in some examples of Crohn's colitis (Schumacher 1993), and in some cases of documented infectious colitis (Anand et al 1986).

Numerous other conditions may be associated with mucosal ulceration which, particularly on mucosal biopsy, may cause some difficulty in differentiation from Crohn's colitis. Behçet's disease, a rare disorder which involves the gastrointestinal tract in up to 50% of cases, is characterized by ulcers which are concentrated in the distal terminal ileum and right colon (Johnson & Everhart 1986, Lee 1986). The ulcers are typically superficial and well defined, but may form fissures and rarely cause perforation. However, large serpiginous ulcers are typically not present. In addition, granulomas and transmural lymphoid aggregates are not present. Perivascular inflammation and necrotizing vasculitis may be seen.

Non-specific ulcers of the colon may also be caused by a variety of drugs, including non-steroidal anti-inflammatory agents (NSAIDs) and oral contraceptives. NSAIDs, can result in changes which are indistinguishable from ischemic enteritis or colitis, with superficial epithelial necrosis and preservation of the deep crypts (Huber et al 1991, Haque et al 1992, Monahan et al 1992). The lamina propria is not expanded by inflammatory cells, but rather is replaced by granulation tissue. Eosinophils may be prominent. Subsequent fibrosis may result in broad-based strictures. These changes are most often localized to the right side of the colon, particularly the cecum (Uribe et al 1986). Similarly, patients treated with oral contraceptive pills may develop discrete colonic ulcers, again primarily localized to the right colon (Tedesco et al 1982, Schneiderman & Cello 1986). The estrogenic component may result in subendothelial intimal proliferation of mesenteric arteries and subsequent ischemic enteritis or colitis. Thus, on endoscopy either of these conditions could be confused with Crohn's colitis, given their propensity to involve the right colon in a patchy manner. However, histologic examination of biopsy specimens will allow for distinction.

Diverticular disease may appear grossly similar to Crohn's disease. Given that inflammatory bowel disease and diverticular disease are both rather common, it is not unusual to see both disease processes affecting the colon at the same time. Not infrequently, pathologists attribute all the changes to one disease (usually diverticular disease) and overlook the coexisting Crohn's colitis. Features which should suggest that Crohn's disease is complicating diverticular disease include the presence of fissuring ulcers, ulcers outside areas with active diverticulitis, and internal fistulae other than colovesical or vaginal fistulae (Schmidt et al 1968).

As mentioned previously, on rare occasions Crohn's disease can result in a fulminant colitis, and in this situation it may be difficult or impossible to differentiate Crohn's disease from ulcerative colitis. Since both deep fissuring ulcers and transmural inflammation in the area of deep ulceration may be seen in cases of fulminant ulcerative colitis, these major histologic criteria for the diagnosis of Crohn's disease are no longer reliable. In fulminant colitis which is due to ulcerative colitis one should not encounter skip lesions, either grossly or microscopically. Although transmural inflammation may be seen, this should be confined to areas of deep ulceration (Petras 1994). The status of the intervening mucosa between the deep ulcers is critical to assess. In ulcerative colitis the intervening mucosa, although relatively less inflamed, should still show changes of active ulcerative colitis. On the other hand, if skip lesions are found this strongly suggests Crohn's disease. In addition, transmural lymphoid aggregates in areas without deep ulceration also suggest Crohn's disease. Even in closely examined and well-sectioned cases of fulminant colitis, some cases can still not be placed into one of these categories. In these cases the designation of 'colitis, type indeterminate' is appropriate, but this should be considered as a temporary designation, since additional clinical information or the subsequent clinical course may allow for discrimination between ulcerative colitis and Crohn's disease (Pezin et al 1989).

REFERENCES

Anand B S, Malhotra V, Bhattacharya S K et al 1986 Rectal histology in acute bacillary dysentery. Gastroenterology 90: 654–660

Bergman L, Krause U 1977 Crohn's disease: a long-term study of the clinical course in 186 patients. Scandinavian Journal of Gastroenterology 12: 937–944

Bradford W D, Norce P S, Gutman L T et al 1974 Pathologic features of enteric infection with *Yersinia entercolitica*. Archives of Pathology 98: 17–22

Chambers T J, Morson B C 1979 The granuloma in Crohn's disease. Gut 20: 269–274

El-Miraghi N R H, Mair N S 1979 The histopathology of enteric infection with *Yersinia pseudotuberculosis*. American Journal of Clinical Pathology 71: 631–639

Farmer R G, Whelan G, Fazio V W 1985 Long-term follow-up of patients with Crohn's disease. Relationship between the clinical pattern and prognosis. Gastroenterology 88: 1818–1825

Geller S A, Cohen A 1983 Arterial inflammatory cell infiltrates in Crohn's disease. Archives of Pathology and Laboratory Medicine 107: 473–475

Gleason T H, Patterson S D 1982 The pathology of *Yersinia enterocolitica* ileocolitis. American Journal of Surgical Pathology 6: 347–355

Hamilton S R, Reese J, Pennington L et al 1985 The role of resection margin frozen section in the surgical management of Crohn's disease. Surgery Gynecology and Obstetrics 160: 57–62

Haque S, Haswell J E, Dreznick J T, West A B 1992 A cecal diaphragm associated with the use of nonsteroidal anti-inflammatory drugs. Journal of Clinical Gastroenterology 15: 332–335

Huber T, Ruchti C, Halter F 1991 Nonsteroidal anti-inflammatory drug-induced colonic strictures: a case report. Gastroenterology 100: 1119–1122

Ihasz M, Mester E, Refi M 1975 Experience in surgical management of Crohn's disease. American Journal of Proctology 26: 47–62

Johnson D A, Everhart C V 1986 Colitis in Behçet's syndrome. Gastrointestinal Endoscopy 32: 58–59

Kelly J K, Siu T O 1986 The strictures, sinus, and fissures of Crohn's disease. Journal of Clinical Gastroenterology 8: 594–598

Kelly J K, Sutherland L R 1988 The chronological sequence in the pathology of Crohn's disease. Journal of Clinical Gastroenterology 10: 28–33

Kotanagi H, Kramer K, Fazio V W et al 1991 Do microscopic abnormalities at resection margins correlate with increased anastomotic recurrence in Crohn's disease? Retrospective analysis of 100 cases. Diseases of the Colon and Rectum 34: 909–916

Kuramoto S, Oohara T, Ihara O et al 1987 Granulomas of the gut in Crohn's disease. A step sectioning study. Diseases of the Colon and Rectum 30: 6–11

Lee E C G, Papaioannou N 1982 Minimal surgery for chronic obstruction in patients with extensive or universal Crohn's disease. Annals of Colonic Surgery of England 64: 229–233

Lee R G 1986 The colitis of Behçet's syndrome. American Journal of Surgical Pathology 10: 888–893

Mekhjian H S, Switz D M, Watts H D et al 1979 National cooperative Crohn's disease study: factors determining recurrence of Crohn's disease after surgery. Gastroenterology 77: 907–913

Miller D P, Everett E D 1979 Gastrointestinal histoplasmosis. Journal of Clinical Gastroenterology 1: 233–236

Monahan D W, Sarnes E C, Parker A C 1992 Colonic strictures in a patient on long-term nonsteroidal anti-inflammatory drugs. Gastrointestinal Endoscopy 38: 385–388

Nygaar D K, Fousa O 1977 Crohn's disease: recurrence after surgical treatment. Scandinavian Journal of Gastroenterology 12: 577–584

Odze R, Antonioli D, Peppercorn M, Goldman H 1993 Effect of topical 5-aminosalicylic acid (5-ASA) therapy in rectal mucosal biopsy morphology in chronic ulcerative colitis. American Journal of Surgical Pathology 17: 869–875

Pennington L, Hamilton S R, Bayless T R et al 1980 Surgical management of Crohn's disease: influence of disease at margin of resection. Annals of Surgery 192: 311–318

Petras R E 1994 Non-neoplastic intestinal diseases. In: Sternberg S, Antonioli D, Carter D, Mills S E, Oberman H A (eds) Diagnostic surgical pathology, 2nd edn. Raven Press, New York, pp 1346–1348

Petras R E, Oakley J R 1992 Intestinal complications of inflammatory bowel disease: pathologic aspects. Seminars in Colon and Rectal Surgery 3: 160–172

Pezin M E, Pemberton S H, Beart R W et al 1989 Outcome of 'indeterminate' colitis following ileal pouch–anal anastomosis. Diseases of the Colon and Rectum 32: 653–658

Price A B 1978 Overlap in the spectrum of non-specific inflammatory bowel disease – 'colitis indeterminate'. Journal of Clinical Pathology 31: 567–577

Robinson J W L, Mirkovitch V, Winistorfer B, Saegesser F 1981 Response of the intestinal mucosa to ischaemia. Gut 22: 512–527

Rotterdam H, Korelitz B I, Sommers S C 1977 Microgranulomas in grossly normal rectal mucosa in Crohn's disease. American Journal of Clinical Pathology 67: 550–554

Schmidt G T, Lennard-Jones J E, Morson B C, Young A C 1968 Crohn's disease of the colon and its distinction from diverticulitis. Gut 9: 7–16

Schneiderman D J, Cello J P 1986 Intestinal ischemia and infarction associated with oral contraceptives. Western Journal of Medicine 145: 350

Schumacher G 1993 First attack of inflammatory bowel disease and infectious colitis. Scandinavian Journal of Gastroenterology 28: 1–24

Surawicz C M, Belic L 1984 Rectal biopsy helps to distinguish acute self-limited colitis from idiopathic inflammatory bowel disease. Gastroenterology 86: 104–113

Tandon H D, Prakash A 1972 Pathology of intestinal tuberculosis and its distinction from Crohn's disease. Gut 13: 260–269

Tedesco F J, Volpicelli N A, Moore F S 1982 Estrogen and progesterone-associated colitis: a disorder with clinical and endoscopic features mimicking Crohn's disease. Gastrointestinal Endoscopy 28: 247–249

Uribe A, Johansson C, Sczezak P, Rubio C 1986 Ulceration of the colon associated with naproxen and acetylsalicylic acid therapy. Gastrointestinal Endoscopy 32: 242–244

Whitehead R 1972 The pathology of intestinal ischemia. Clinical Gastroenterology 1: 613–637

33. Histopathology – dysplasia and cancer
J. R. Jass

NATURE OF DYSPLASIA

In the context of the gastrointestinal tract dysplasia has come to signify a precancerous lesion, synonymous with intraepithelial neoplasia. Neoplasia, in turn, is understood to be a clonal, proliferative disorder governed by mutation or loss of genes (oncogenes and oncosuppressor genes) implicated in the control of growth and differentiation. New and fundamental insights into the molecular genetics of gastrointestinal dysplasia, including dysplasia in inflammatory bowel disease, are being gained at a rapid pace. Although dysplasia may certainly complicate Crohn's disease, most of the clinical–pathological–molecular correlations to date have applied to dysplasia in ulcerative colitis. Accordingly, this chapter will focus on the pathobiology of dysplasia in ulcerative colitis.

MICROSCOPIC APPEARANCES OF DYSPLASIA

Dysplasia is characterized by a combination of cytological atypia, abnormal differentiation and disordered architecture. Cytological atypia may occur on a reactive and reversible basis during phases of acute inflammation in ulcerative colitis. It is inadvisable to diagnose dysplasia in the presence of acute inflammation. Dysplasia often adopts a villous configuration (Fig. 33.1), with the cytological changes occurring mainly in the basally located epithelium (Rubio et al 1984). More superficially, the villi are covered with mucous cells showing little or no atypia. Regenerative mucosa may also assume a villous configuration (Fig. 33.2) (Rubio et al 1982, Lee 1987). Features that aid the recognition of villous dysplasia are abnormal cytology, the presence of a single population of tall mucous cells, and the tendency for villi to be pointed rather than blunt-ended.

Dysplasia in ulcerative colitis may be similar to adenomatous epithelium, with characteristic enlarged, elongated, crowded and pseudostratified nuclei (Fig. 33.3). Criteria for grading adenomatous dysplasia (as mild, moderate and severe) are well established (Figs 33.4, 33.5).

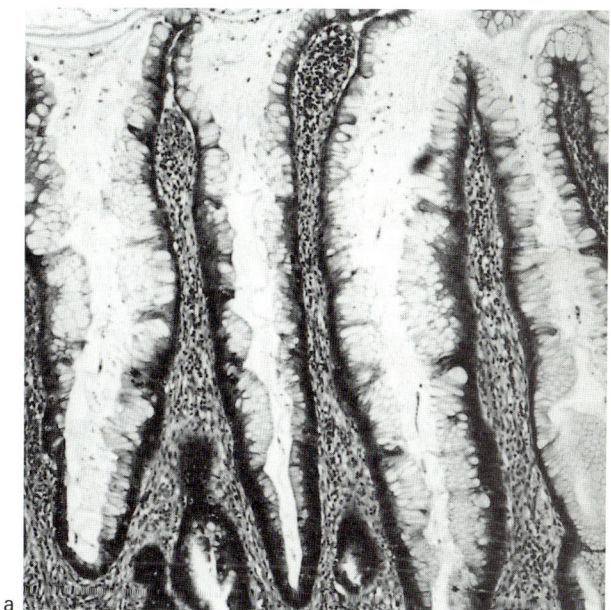
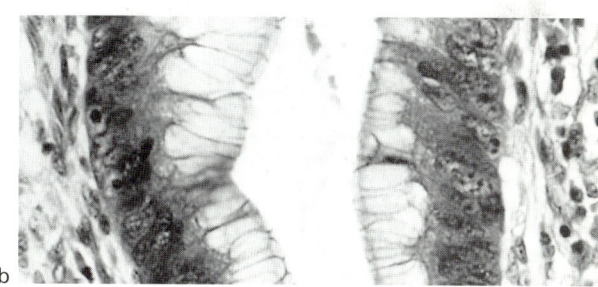

Fig. 33.1 Epithelial dysplasia with a villous architecture. **a** At low magnification villi show pointed tips and are covered by tall, columnar mucus cells. **b** High magnification shows nuclear enlargement, elongation and crowding. This is most apparent within the lower third of the mucosa. (Hematoxylin & eosin)

Dysplasia in flat mucosa may assume a variety of alternative patterns, characterized mainly by nuclear and cytoplasmic abnormalities and less by architectural changes such as villosity or tubular branching and budding. The nuclei are typically enlarged, round and intensely hyper-

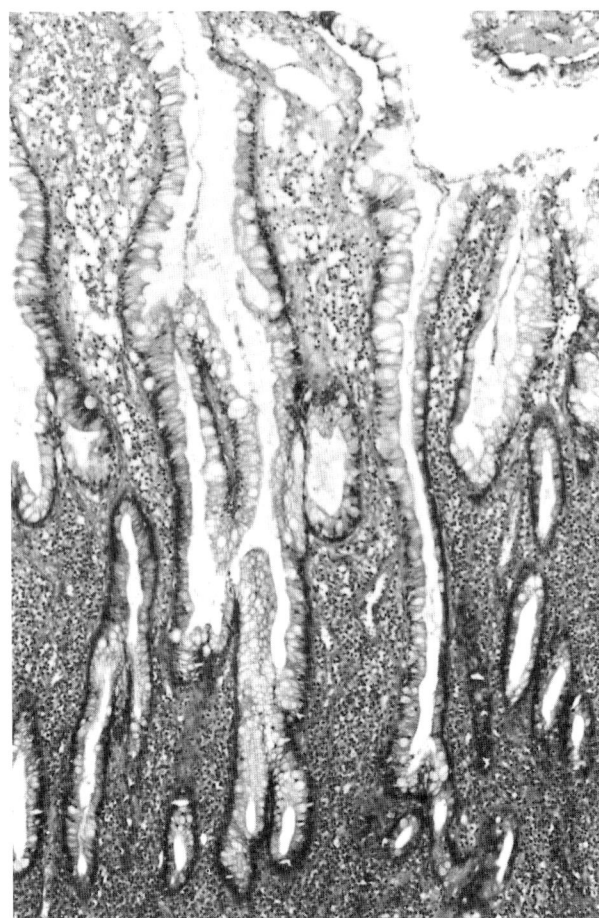

Fig. 33.2 Villous change within non-dysplastic regenerative mucosa. The villi are blunt-ended and are covered by goblet cells that differ little from their normal counterparts. (Hematoxylin & eosin)

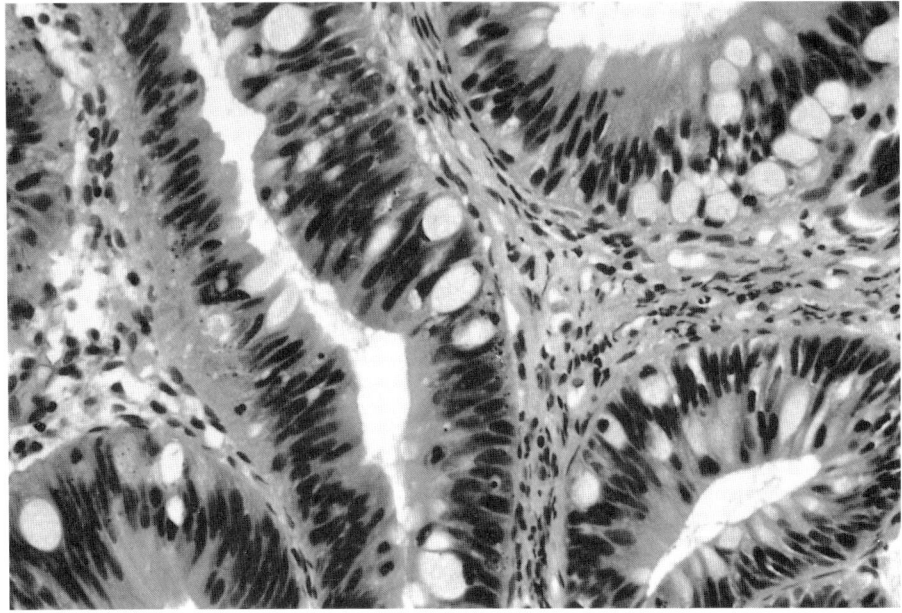

Fig. 33.3 High magnification showing adenomatous dysplasia (low grade) with crowded, elongated nuclei. Inverted or 'upside-down' goblet cells are conspicuous (among or below nuclei). These are a frequent hallmark of dysplasia in ulcerative colitis. (Hematoxylin & eosin)

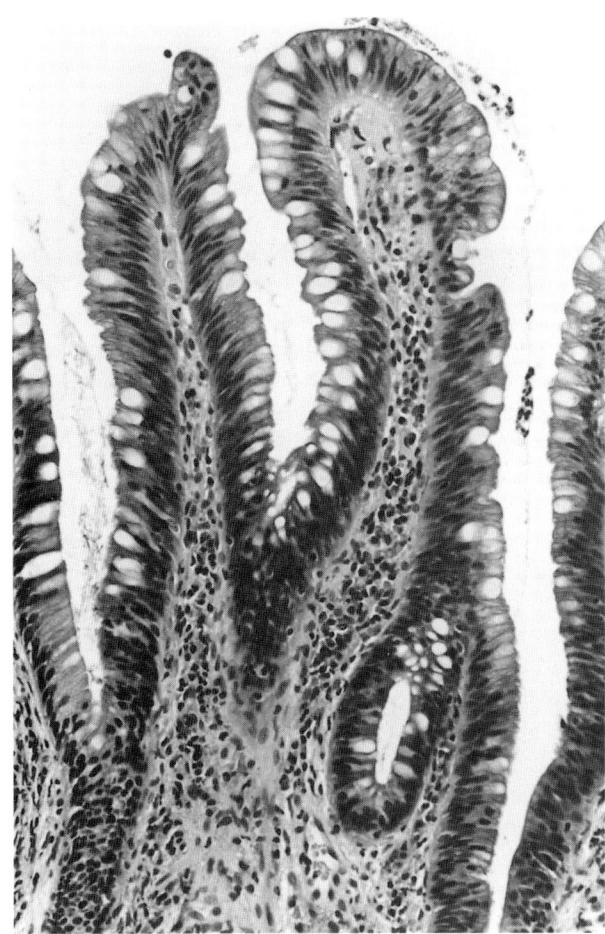

Fig. 33.4 Low-grade dysplasia within flat mucosa. Nuclear enlargement and stratification is most obvious in the lower right-hand portion of the field. (Hematoxylin & eosin)

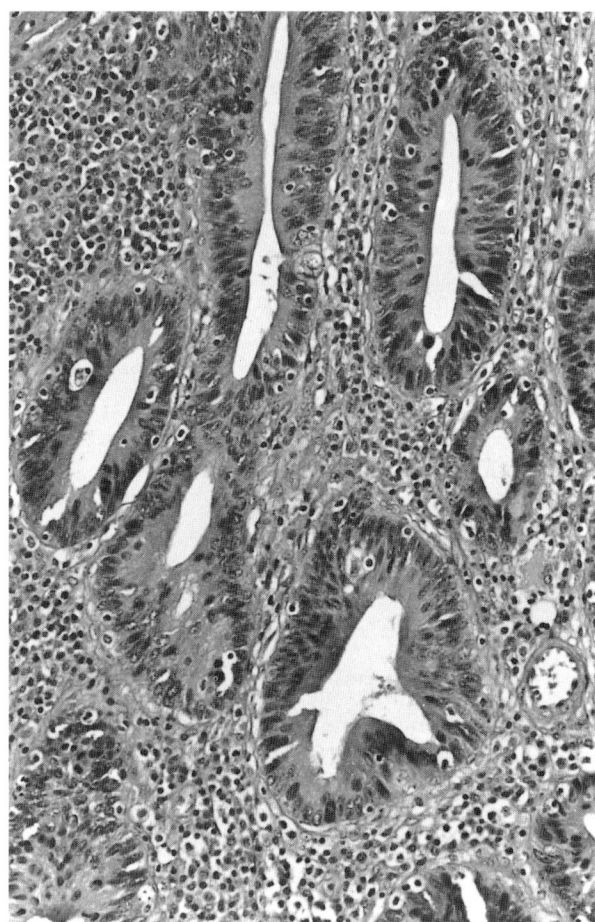

Fig. 33.5 High-grade dysplasia within an elevated lesion (dysplasia-associated lesion or mass). Nuclei are enlarged and pleomorphic. (Hematoxylin & eosin)

chromatic, but show little evidence of pseudostratification, and cytoplasm is usually eosinophilic. Criteria for grading non-adenomatous forms of dysplasia are less well established (Riddell 1976).

A useful working classification of dysplasia in ulcerative colitis was developed in recognition of the tendency for reactive or regenerative changes to mimic dysplasia, the existence of epithelial patterns of unknown portent, and the subjectivity of grading dysplasia as mild, moderate and severe. It was recommended that biopsies should be classified as negative, indefinite or positive for dysplasia (Table 33.1). The indefinite category was expanded further as probably negative, unknown, or probably positive for dysplasia. Biopsies positive for dysplasia were subdivided as low-grade or high-grade (Figs 33.4, 33.5) (Riddell et al 1983). Interobserver studies have demonstrated acceptable levels of agreement for biopsies that are either negative for dysplasia or show high-grade dysplasia. In contrast, marked disagreement arises in relation to intermediate grades (Melville et al 1989). In practice, the somewhat artificial results of interobserver studies were eclipsed by the successful outcome of the associated cancer prevention programme (Melville et al 1989). This is explained by the fact that patients are managed on the basis of multiple observations over time, and placed in clinical context.

MACROSCOPIC APPEARANCES OF DYSPLASIA

Dysplasia in ulcerative colitis may be invisible macroscopically or may present as either a well-circumscribed

Table 33.1 Classification of dysplasia in ulcerative colitis (Riddell et al 1983)

Negative	Normal mucosa
	Inactive (quiescent) colitis
	Active colitis
Indefinite	Probably negative (probably inflammatory)
	Unknown
	Probably positive/probably dysplastic
Positive	Low-grade dysplasia
	High-grade dysplasia

polypoid mass with the morphology of a tubular, tubulovillous or villous adenoma, or as an ill-defined elevated lesion with a nodular and/or velvety mucosal appearance. The visible forms of dysplasia have been described as 'dysplasia-associated lesion or mass' (DALM) (Blackstone et al 1981). There is evidence of a progression in time from dysplasia in flat mucosa through DALM to invasive adenocarcinoma. The incidence of cancer in specimens with visible dysplastic lesions was 58%, compared to 4% in specimens with flat dysplasia only. No elevated lesions were found in four colectomy specimens with low-grade dysplasia only, but were present in 83% of colectomy specimens with high-grade dysplasia (Butt et al 1983). Elevated lesions were larger and more numerous in patients with cancer, and 50% of cancers were shown to arise in either elevated or polypoid lesions (Butt et al 1983).

HISTOCHEMISTRY AND BIOCHEMISTRY

Alterations to epithelial mucin

Structural differences exist between epithelial mucin expressed by normal versus neoplastic epithelium of the colorectum.

Sialic acid and sulfate

A relative increase in the ratio of sialic acid to sulfate may be demonstrated by the high iron diamine/Alcian blue technique through a brown to blue color change; this alteration is frequently seen in dysplasia in ulcerative colitis (Ehsanullah et al 1985, Jass et al 1986). However, a similar switch may be observed in non-dysplastic colitic mucosa. Although the change in non-dysplastic mucosal biopsies has been found by some to be a reasonably sensitive marker for dysplasia or cancer elsewhere in the bowel (Ehsanullah et al 1985, Fozard et al 1987), others report a similar incidence of mucin change in biopsies from subjects with no concurrent neoplasia (Jass et al 1986, Ahnen et al 1987).

O-acetyl to non-O-acetyl sialic acid

A switch from O-acetyl to non-O-acetyl sialic acid has been described in dysplasia in ulcerative colitis using a modification of the periodic acid–Schiff technique (Agawa et al 1988). This is, however, a non-specific change that occurs in regenerative mucosa in ulcerative colitis (Jass et al 1986). Such regenerative mucosa shows a characteristic morphology, evidenced by crypt serration, mucin secretion by columnar cells, reduction in goblet cell numbers, and prominent peanut agglutinin binding within the Golgi zone. These lesions, similar structurally and histochemically to the hyperplastic polyp, were found to be more frequent in colitis with cancer than matched colitics with no cancer (Jass et al 1986).

Peanut agglutinin (PNA) reactivity

This lectin binds to oligosaccharides lacking a terminally substituted sialic acid (polylactosamine, i.e. nGalβ1→3GlcNAc→ and Galβ1→3GalNAc or T antigen) (Jass & Roberton 1994). Galβ1-3 GalNAc has been directly quantified in mucus extracted from colon cancers and shown to be increased in ulcerative colitis compared to normal colonic mucus (Campbell et al 1995). However, in histochemical studies PNA shows only a limited propensity to bind to mucinous material, indicating that there is relatively little T expression, even within malignant epithelial mucins (Jass & Smith 1992). In regenerative (hyperplastic) mucosa in ulcerative colitis, increased PNA reactivity is generally limited to the Golgi zone. Dysplastic epithelium may include columnar cells showing cytoplasmic binding, and occasional focally positive goblet cells (Jass et al 1986, Ahnen et al 1987). In actively inflamed epithelium the pattern of PNA binding approximates to that of dysplasia (Cooper et al 1987). Increased PNA reactivity within non-neoplastic colitic mucosa has been stated to herald the subsequent development of dysplasia (Boland et al 1984). This observation has not been extended, and subsequent studies have not shown PNA to be diagnostically useful (Jass et al 1986, Ahnen et al 1987, Cooper et al 1987).

Ulex europaeus agglutinin (UEA-1) reactivity

As with PNA there is increased expression, limited not only to dysplasia but occurring also in specimens of active and inactive ulcerative colitis. UEA-1 binding was not found to be diagnostically useful (Ahnen et al 1987).

Carcinoembryonic antigen (CEA) and secretory component (SC)

Preliminary work indicated that regenerative change and dysplasia in ulcerative colitis could be distinguished by their contrasting patterns of immunoreactivity in relation to CEA and SC (Isaacson 1976, 1982). Subsequently, neither CEA neoexpression nor loss of SC immunoreactivity has been shown to be specific for epithelial dysplasia (Rognum et al 1982, Allen et al 1985b). High-grade epithelial dysplasia did not show loss of polarity (apical expression) of CEA, which has been shown to accompany loss of differentiation in colorectal cancer (Ahnen et al 1987).

Enzymology

Enzymatic analyses of biopsies showing epithelial dysplasia reveal altered lactic dehydrogenase (LDH) isoenzyme patterns (Lewis et al 1970), increased activities of lactate dehydrogenase and glucose-6 phosphate dehydrogenase (Vatn et al 1984), and increased activity of N-acetyl-β-D-glucosaminidase (Borkje et al 1987). These changes, consistent with a switch to anerobic respiration, are typical of neoplastic epithelium but have not been used in routine diagnosis.

CELL CYCLE STUDIES IN ULCERATIVE COLITIS

Cell kinetics

There is a report describing increased rectal cell proliferation in colitics with dysplasia (Biasco et al 1990). This has not been confirmed and is unlikely to be sufficiently specific for diagnostic purposes.

DNA aneuploidy

Clones with an abnormal chromosomal constitution are described as aneuploid and may be identified by their increased DNA content. DNA aneuploidy can be measured by microdensitometry or flow cytometry (FCM). In the normal–adenoma–carcinoma sequence of the colorectum, the frequency of aneuploidy increases from 0 in samples of normal mucosa through 4%, 18%, 36% and 63% in samples obtained from adenomas showing mild, moderate and severe dysplasia and adenocarcinomas respectively (Goh & Jass 1986). In serving as a prerequisite for *p53* allele loss (Burmer et al 1992), aneuploidy is clearly a fundamental event in the process of neoplastic evolution and not merely an epiphenomenon. Given the problems of recognizing and grading dysplasia in ulcerative colitis, the assessment of DNA content offers promise of a technique which is both objective and reproducible. However, the relationship between aneuploidy and the normal–dysplasia–carcinoma sequence in ulcerative colitis is not straightforward. Some studies have reported an increasing frequency of aneuploidy in step with histopathological progression (Hammarberg et al 1984, Melville et al 1988, Suzuki et al 1990), whereas others have reported a relatively high frequency of aneuploidy in non-dysplastic mucosa (Fozard et al 1986, Rutegard et al 1989). The reasons for these conflicting data include the following:

1. Differing patient selection, notably biopsies from patients in surveillance programs versus samples from surgical specimens with established neoplasia
2. Problems of histopathological interpretation, particularly the distinction between negative for dysplasia, indefinite for dysplasia, and low-grade dysplasia
3. The use of paraffin-embedded tissue versus fresh tissue
4. Variation in frequency of near-diploid (potentially false) aneuploidy.

Although it can no longer be doubted that a clear relationship exists between aneuploidy and neoplastic progression in ulcerative colitis, it is evident that samples that are either negative or indefinite for dysplasia may occasionally be aneuploid (Ahnen et al 1990, Burmer et al 1992). In other words, aneuploidy occurs earlier in the evolution of cancer in ulcerative colitis than in the sporadic adenoma–carcinoma sequence. To what extent can this knowledge be exploited in cancer prevention? Aneuploidy was seen in one out of 33 (3%) high-risk patients who were negative for dysplasia, and in four out of 13 (30%) patients with changes indefinite for dysplasia. All of the five patients with aneuploidy developed dysplasia within 30 months (Rubin et al 1992). Nineteen patients without aneuploidy were followed for at least 2 years and none developed either aneuploidy or dysplasia (Rubin et al 1992). It should be appreciated, however, that an average of 40 biopsy samples was obtained from each patient, using a technique that ensured that each sample was at least 5 mm in diameter. The analysis was performed on fresh tissue. It was estimated that in order to achieve 95% confidence in detecting dysplasia or aneuploidy, 56 histological and 30 FCM samples respectively would be required. This enormous investment in time and technology could be justified only if it was shown that the high-risk colitics without aneuploidy never went on to develop dysplasia or carcinoma (at least within a particular timeframe). A lesser strategy, namely the demonstration of the absence or presence of aneuploidy within indefinite biopsies, could be useful in refining a purely histopathological approach. However, microdensitometry rather than FCM would probably be the technique of choice for the retrospective analysis of small, formalin-fixed tissue samples.

MOLECULAR BIOLOGY

p53 and oncosuppressor genes

p53 is implicated in the pathogenesis of a wide range of tumors, including colorectal neoplasms. The full oncogenic effect is seen when both copies of the gene are inactivated, the first by mutation and the second generally by loss of the wild-type allele, as demonstrated through loss of heterozygosity (LOH). The frequency of *p53* LOH in samples obtained from surgical specimens was shown to be closely related to neoplastic progression: negative for dysplasia (6%); indefinite for dysplasia (9%); low-grade dysplasia (33%); high-grade dysplasia (63%); and cancer (85%). Interestingly, *p53* LOH was detected only in aneuploid populations, though not all aneuploid populations showed *p53* LOH (Burmer et al 1992). LOH implicating the oncosuppressor genes *p53*, *Rb* and *MCC/APC* was noted to occur more frequently in dysplasia in cancer originating in the distal as opposed to the proximal colon (Greenwald et al 1992). This is also the pattern recorded in sporadic neoplasia (Delattre et al 1989, Scott et al 1991).

Like DNA aneuploidy, *p53* LOH appears to occur earlier in ulcerative colitis than in sporadic neoplasia. Mutations in *p53* may also occur at a relatively early stage in colitic neoplasia (Yin 1993). In fact, such studies underestimate the frequency of *p53* mutations, because of the enormous investment of resources that would be required to cover the entire *p53* mutational hotspot region. *p53* mutations occur not only in dysplastic mucosa but also in diploid, non-dysplastic mucosa adjacent to dysplasia (Crispin et al 1993). This would fit with the requirement for *p53* mutation to precede loss of the second, normal allele at the somatic level.

A number of monoclonal antibodies have been raised to the *p53* protein. These react with the mutated and/or wild-type *p53* protein according to the antibody clone and conditions of staining. At the time of writing it seems prudent to review only the more reliable molecular findings; further research is required before the immunohistochemical approach can be evaluated critically.

Ki-*ras* mutations

Ki-*ras* mutations occur early in the evolution of sporadic adenoma and are present in the majority of sporadic colorectal cancers. However, these mutations occur less frequently in colitic cancers, and are not identified in the early stages of neoplastic evolution in ulcerative colitis (Bell et al 1991, Burmer et al 1992, Chen et al 1992, Chaubert et al 1994). Thus, in sporadic neoplasia Ki-*ras* and *p53* are implicated at early and late stages of neoplastic progression respectively, whereas the converse applies in ulcerative colitis. There is a report of a Ki-*ras* mutation in regenerative mucosa showing villous change (Chaubert et al 1994).

Clonal expansion and field change

Dysplasia in ulcerative colitis may occupy a large area and is often multifocal. To what extent can such an extensive change be traced back to a single cell? Specific molecular events such as Ki-*ras* mutations or *p53* allele loss can be shown to occur throughout large plaques of dysplasia, indicating their clonal nature (Burmer et al 1992). However, the multistep process of neoplasia requires the successive development of subclones, in turn arising through increasing genetic instability (Nowell 1976). In ulcerative colitis the last is evidenced by the early onset of aneuploidy. The selection and expansion of subclones with a growth advantage underlies the process of neoplastic progression.

The demonstration of a specific *p53* mutation within non-dysplastic mucosa would be indicative of clonal expansion, since limitation of the mutation to a single clonal unit (crypt) would preclude its detection through a dilutional effect. Such clonal expansion would presumably have occurred through regenerative crypt division following ulceration (Ahnen et al 1990). Separate foci of dysplasia probably arise as independent events, and have been shown to differ in their molecular constitution (Burmer et al 1992). Conceivably, neoplastic cells could exfoliate and reimplant within ulcerated areas, thereby producing spatially separated lesions that are clonally related.

CLINICAL SIGNIFICANCE AND CANCER PREVENTION

The success of cancer prevention programs for ulcerative colitis will be influenced by the number and size of dysplastic lesions and the proportion of cancers that arise therefrom. Although the majority of cancers in ulcerative colitis are associated with extensive epithelial dysplasia (Riddell & Morson 1979), dysplasia may be limited to a focus away from the cancer (Riddell & Morson 1979, Kewenter et al 1982, Allen et al 1985a) or may be absent altogether in approximately 20% of colectomies for cancer (Ransohoff et al 1985, Riddell 1976). These cancers have presumably destroyed a small area of dysplasia in the course of their evolution. In such cases, cancers may yet be detected at an early stage because the majority present as lesions visible to the endoscopist (Butt et al 1983). New insights into the molecular biology of dysplasia may allow early detection of such cases in the future (see above).

Endoscopic biopsies should be taken from both macroscopically visible lesions and flat mucosa. Elevated lesions will often turn out to be regenerative polypoid mucosa. Conversely, dysplasia may be detected in flat mucosa. Severe dysplasia in flat mucosa is an indication for colectomy, whereas biopsies showing changes indefinite for dysplasia or low-grade dysplasia are an indication for more frequent surveillance. DALM is often associated with an underlying cancer and colectomy is indicated for either low or high-grade dysplasia occurring in the context of a macroscopically visible lesion (Blackstone et al 1981).

FUTURE PROSPECTS FOR DYSPLASIA

Over the last 20 years successive generations of special techniques have been hailed as diagnostic advances in the management of cancer risk in ulcerative colitis, but have subsequently failed to live up to their early promise. Now that neoplasia is understood to be a multistep process implicating specific cancer genes, molecular biology offers the main diagnostic challenge to the current mainstay of routine light macroscopic examination. Within a few years molecular diagnosis should provide both sensitivity and specificity, and may be applied not only to biopsy specimens but to stool samples, thereby obviating the requirement for regular endoscopy. It is hoped that molecular technology will be particularly helpful in identifying the subset of patients who develop cancer without producing extensive epithelial dysplasia.

INCIDENCE OF CANCER IN ULCERATIVE COLITIS

Colorectal cancer is a relatively uncommon complication of ulcerative colitis, accounting for no more than 1% of large-bowel cancer occurring in the general population (Butt et al 1980). However, the magnitude of the clinical problem posed by colitis-associated colorectal cancer is appreciated when the young age of onset of malignancy is noted. Using standardized mortality ratios, the relative cancer risk was increased (compared to the general population) eightfold for subjects with ulcerative colitis (Gyde et al 1988).

The risk of cancer in ulcerative colitis is influenced by the extent of the disease and the duration of symptoms. Extensive ulcerative colitis may be defined as radiological evidence of extension of the disease at least as far as the hepatic flexure (Butt et al 1980). Although this definition is arbitrary, may underestimate the extent of mild disease and will be influenced by observer variation, it has nonetheless helped to identify an important high-risk subgroup. Within this subgroup, however, early estimates of the incidence of cancer were inflated (de Dombal et al 1966, Devroede & Taylor 1976, Lennard-Jones et al 1977, Greenstein et al 1979). Lower estimates of risk could reflect the low background risk of sporadic colorectal cancer in particular populations (Maratka et al 1985). More important, though, will be the various types of selection bias associated with hospital series (Gyde et al 1988). Population studies (in which all subjects with ulcerative colitis in a defined geographical area are followed up) would provide the ideal method for determining cancer incidence. Two such studies had a short median follow-up and estimates of long-term cancer incidence were associated with wide confidence limits (Kewenter et al 1978, Hendriksen et al 1985). The most reliable guide to colorectal cancer incidence in extensive ulcerative colitis is provided by a retrospective cohort study of primary referrals at three centres (Gyde et al 1988) (Table 33.2).

If repeated cycles of injury and regeneration were important in the pathogenesis of cancer in colitis, one would expect malignant change to occur with increased frequency in subjects with less extensive disease, albeit limited to the affected segments of bowel. In fact, there is a small excess of colorectal cancer in subjects with left-sided colitis, estimated as fourfold as compared with 19-fold in subjects with extensive colitis (Gyde et al 1988). Of 100 cases of colitis-associated colorectal cancer, 15 occurred in patients with left-sided colitis (Sugita et al 1991). In those with left-sided colitis the age of onset of cancer was a decade later than in subjects with extensive disease. Interestingly, the onset of left-sided colitis was also delayed by a decade relative to extensive colitis. In both groups there was a correlation between age at onset of ulcerative colitis and age at diagnosis of cancer (Sugita et al 1991). Gyde et al (1988) found that cancers presented around the age of 50 years, and that this was independent of disease duration. This observation was based on only 29 subjects developing colorectal cancer against a background of extensive ulcerative colitis. In addition, attempts to pinpoint the date of onset of ulcerative colitis are unlikely to be reliable.

Table 33.2 Cumulative frequency of colorectal cancer based on a retrospective cohort of 823 patients residing in three areas (Gyde et al 1988)

Years from onset	Patients (no.)	Colorectal cancers (no.)	Cumulative frequency (%)	95% CI
5	308	2	0.0	
10	244	6	0.7	0–1.1
15	195	7	3.4	1.0–5.8
20	132	5	7.2	3.6–10.8
25	73	3	11.6	6.4–16.8
30	36	6	16.5	9.0–24.0
35	12	0	33.4	19.3–47.6

PATHOLOGY OF CANCER IN ULCERATIVE COLITIS

Site

Attempts to compare sites of colitis associated with sporadic bowel cancer have produced conflicting data (Slaney & Brooke 1959, Edling & Eklof 1961, Goldgraber & Kirsner 1964, Riddell 1976). This may be due in part to the fact that the anatomical distribution of sporadic bowel cancer varies with age and gender. In addition, several studies have shown an increasing predilection of sporadic colorectal cancer for the proximal colon with time (Jass 1991). Comparison is also complicated by the fact that cancer in colitis is more likely to be multiple (Butt et al 1983, Mir-Madjlessi et al 1986). It is probable that the site distribution of colitis-associated cancer does not differ to any great extent from that of sporadic bowel cancer (Slater et al 1985). Anatomical distribution of cancer by gender is similar in colitis-associated versus sporadic bowel cancer, with males in both groups showing an increased proportion of rectal cancers (Riddell 1976).

Macroscopic appearances

The gross appearance of colitis-associated cancer has been described as nodular, plaque-like, polypoid, ulcerated and stricturing (Dawson & Pryse-Davies 1959, Cook & Goligher 1975) (Fig. 33.6). The terms nodular and plaque-like probably apply to macroscopically visible forms of dysplasia rather than to cancer (Fig. 33.1). Thus the major macroscopic differences between sporadic and colitis-associated neoplasms may relate to precancerous lesions as opposed to established cancers. Within an endoscopically detected DALM may be an incidental microscopic focus of early cancer. It is important to note that the great majority of colitis-associated cancers present either as gross lesions or in association with a macroscopically visible form of dysplasia (or both) (Butt et al 1983).

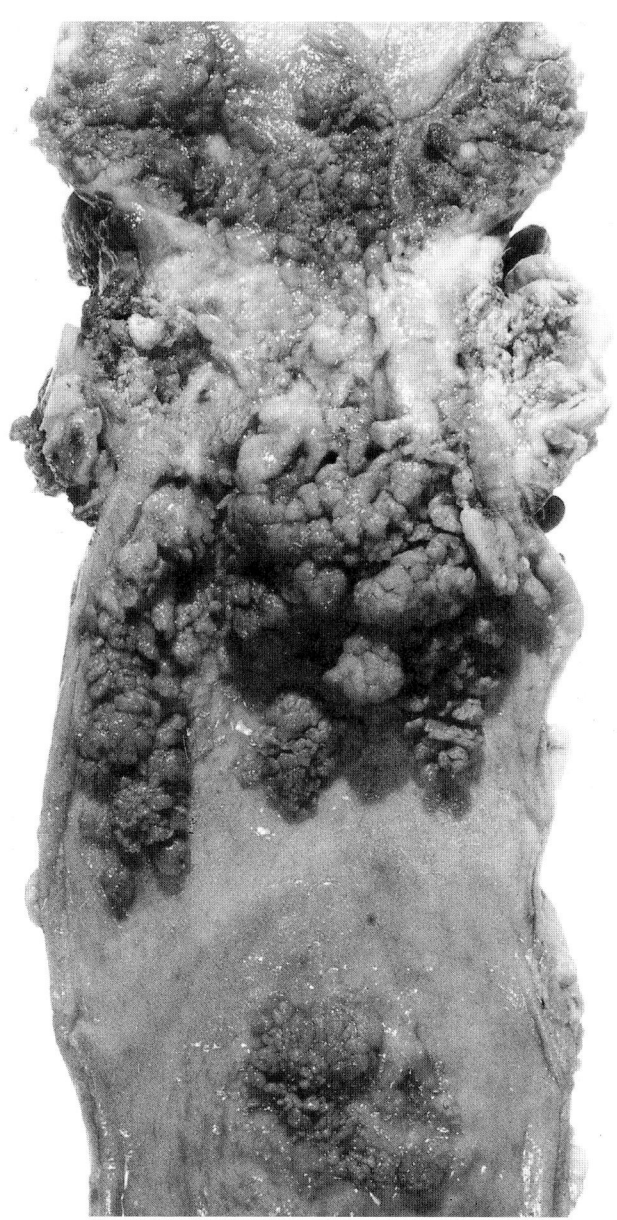

Fig. 33.6 Stricturing cancer arising within mass of polypoid dysplasia (dysplasia-associated lesion or mass) in a patient with ulcerative colitis. There is a small focus of DALM below the main mass.

Microscopic appearances

A relatively high proportion of cancers complicating ulcerative colitis are poorly differentiated and/or mucinous (Riddell 1976, Ritchie et al 1981, Mir-Madjlessi et al 1986), yet the overall prognosis of cancer in colitis is similar to that of sporadic bowel cancer. The worse prognosis associated with poorly differentiated tumors may be balanced by the higher proportion of early cancers detected by screening. Most cancers are adenocarcinomas, but colorectal lymphoma may complicate ulcerative colitis and Crohn's disease (Shepherd et al 1989).

SPORADIC VERSUS ULCERATIVE COLITIS-ASSOCIATED CANCER

A number of fundamental differences between sporadic and colitis-associated colorectal neoplasia have been highlighted: incidence, age at onset, pathogenesis, gross and microscopic appearances, and molecular biology. It is likely that the background activity of cyclical inflammation, injury and regeneration occurring in ulcerative colitis accounts for many of these differences. The increased incidence of cancer in ulcerative colitis could be due to increased cellular turnover or (more likely) to increased periods of exposure of target cells to potential environmental mutagens as a result of breakdown of normal mucosal defence mechanisms. Cycles of regeneration will be associated with crypt division, leading to horizontal mucosal expansion of clones and subclones of cells in various stages of neoplastic progression (Ahnen et al 1990). This would account for the development of large areas of epithelial dysplasia. Differences between sporadic and colitis-associated cancer are not marked, however. This may be explained by the fact that although the timing and order of the steps leading to cancer may differ, the endpoint is the same.

CANCER IN CROHN'S DISEASE

Cancer is an uncommon complication of Crohn's disease. Relatively recent reviews of the world literature documented only 61 case reports of small-bowel cancer (Hawker et al 1982) and 44 cases of large-bowel cancer (Zinkin & Brandwein 1980). Various clinical factors will influence the incidence of cancer in Crohn's disease. Unlike ulcerative colitis, the disease affects the entire gastrointestinal tract. Surgical excision of macroscopic disease will prevent the onset of cancer within the affected segment, whereas bypass procedures (Greenstein et al 1978) and strictureplasty that leave the diseased segment in situ will increase the risk. Estimating the true incidence of cancer in colonic Crohn's disease is complicated by the relatively recent recognition of Crohn's colitis, and the difficulties of distinguishing Crohn's from ulcerative colitis.

SMALL-BOWEL CANCER IN CROHN'S DISEASE

The fact that small-bowel cancer is extremely rare, whereas the terminal ileum is the most frequent site of Crohn's disease, should render the ileum the most obvious location for demonstrating an increased relative risk of malignancy. Greenstein et al (1980) observed four small-bowel cancers in 579 subjects with Crohn's disease diagnosed between 1960 and 1976, giving a relative risk of 86-fold compared with the general population. Small-bowel cancers are described in other hospital series that would again indicate a high relative risk, despite the low number of cases (Darke et al 1973, Weedon et al 1973, Gyde et al 1980, Cooke et al 1980, Harper et al 1987, Petras et al 1987). One population study based in the Copenhagen area (population 500 000) observed one case of small-bowel cancer among 185 patients with Crohn's disease reviewed over a period of 18 years (Binder et al 1985).

The majority of small-bowel cancers (67%) occur in the ileum (Hawker et al 1982), whereas the periampullary region is the site of predilection for small-bowel cancer in the general population. Most cancers occur at the site of macroscopic disease (Darke et al 1973, Frank & Shorey 1973, Valdes-Dapena et al 1976, Greenstein et al 1980), including in association with fistulae (Fleming & Pollock 1975, Burbige et al 1977, Greenstein et al 1980, Traube et al 1980) and bypassed loops of bowel. There is a long latent period between onset of disease and cancer, but cancers still occur at a relatively young age. Most are adenocarcinomas but carcinoid tumors and non-Hodgkin's lymphomas have been described.

COLORECTAL CANCER IN CROHN'S DISEASE

The incidence of colorectal cancer in Crohn's disease has been published in a number of hospital series without providing the relative risk as compared with the general population (Darke et al 1973, Truelove & Pena 1976, Cooke et at 1980, Harper et al 1987, Petras et al 1987). Weedon et al (1973) found a 26-fold relative risk for colorectal cancer in a selected series of young patients with onset of disease before the age of 21 years. Where age of onset was not restricted, Gyde et al (1980) found a fourfold increased relative risk and Greenstein et al (1978, 1980) sevenfold, as compared with the general population. A population study is the ideal epidemiological method for defining cancer incidence in a disease. In practice, because of the rarity of Crohn's disease such studies are rendered difficult through the long period of time required to accrue relatively small numbers of patients. Five such studies failed to show an increase in the incidence of colorectal cancer (Brahme et al 1975, Binder et al 1985, Kvist et al 1986, Gollop et al 1988, Fireman et al 1989). A sixth population study based in the Uppsala healthcare region followed up a cohort of 1655 patients with Crohn's disease (Ekbom et al 1990). Twelve colorectal cancers were diagnosed, giving an overall increased risk of 2.5. The risk was higher for individuals with colonic involvement alone (5.6) and highest of all for subjects diagnosed as having Crohn's disease with colonic involvement below 30 years of age (20.9). A recent hospital series removed all inherent selection biases to derive an accurate estimate of overall relative risk of 3.4 in a cohort of 281 patients (Gillen et al 1994a). However, a further study by the same group has shown a much higher relative risk (18-fold) in patients with extensive colonic Crohn's disease similar to the relative risk for colon cancer found in ulcerative colitis in the same center (Gillen et al 1994b).

A detailed account of the pathology of colorectal cancer in Crohn's disease was based upon 11 specimens (two occurring in the same patient) seen at Johns Hopkins Hospital, Baltimore, between 1949 and 1983 (Hamilton 1985). The anatomical distribution was similar to that of sporadic bowel cancer. Seven cancers arose in grossly affected segments and three in microscopically affected areas with gross disease elsewhere. Two occurred in bypassed rectum. Patients were relatively young (mean age 55 years).

Cancers are more likely to be mucinous and/or poorly differentiated, as in ulcerative colitis (Hamilton 1985, Petras et al 1987, Richards et al 1989, Choi & Zelig 1994). Epithelial dysplasia (Fig. 33.7) is frequently found adjacent to cancer, and has also been noted to occur at a distance from tumors (Hamilton 1985, Petras et al 1987, Richards et al 1989). Given the contrasting clinical and pathological features of Crohn's colitis cancer versus sporadic colorectal cancer, the usual origin of Crohn's colitis cancer within a diseased segment of bowel, the similar pathological findings in cancers occurring in Crohn's disease and ulcerative colitis, as well as the epidemiological data relating to cancer incidence, there can be little doubt that an association exists between Crohn's disease and cancer of the large bowel. Nonetheless, colorectal cancer remains as an uncommon complication of Crohn's disease.

CANCER OF THE ANORECTAL REGION IN CROHN'S DISEASE

A study based at St Mark's Hospital, London, collated 32 case reports of cancers arising in the lower rectum and anal canal, or in association with anal or rectal fistulae (Connell et al 1994). Twelve of these patients were treated at St Mark's Hospital; the relatively high incidence of anorectal cancers seen at this institution reflects the selected nature of its patient population. The 32 cancers included 18 adenocarcinomas, 13 squamous cell carcinomas (two in situ) and one undifferentiated carcinoma.

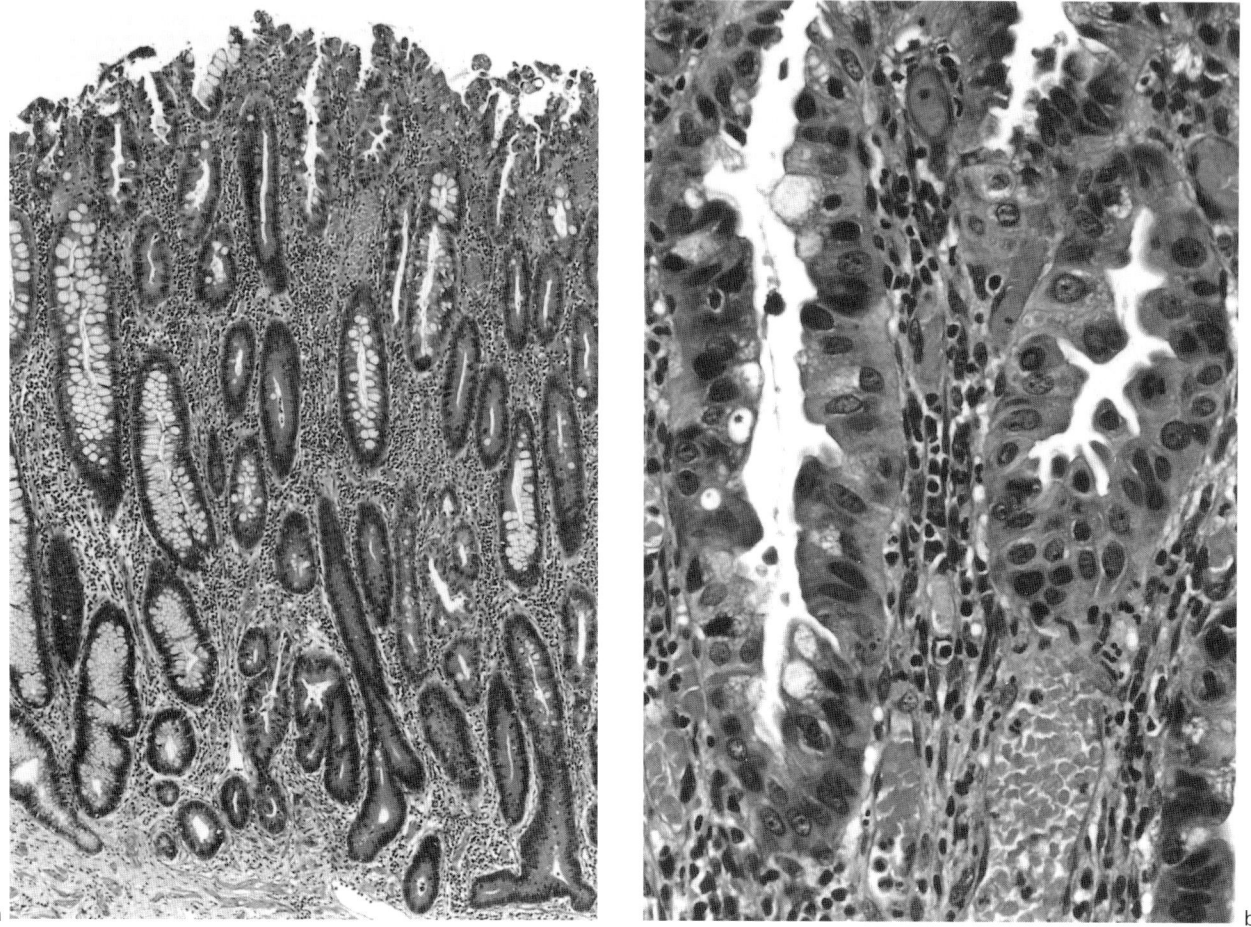

Fig. 33.7 Epithelial dysplasia in a patient with Crohn's colitis. **a** Low magnification shows the change to be intramucosal, although there was a contiguous Dukes B carcinoma (not shown). **b** High magnification shows areas of high-grade dysplasia. (Hematoxylin & eosin)

In addition to the involvement of chronic inflammation and long-standing fistulae (Buchmann et al 1980, Chaikhouni et al 1981, Church et al 1985), the use of immunosuppressive drugs in the treatment of Crohn's disease has been offered as an additional factor in the etiology of anorectal cancer (Ball et al 1988). No evidence of human papilloma virus (type 16) was found in eight patients who were tested (Gilbert et al 1991).

REFERENCES

Agawa S, Muto T, Morioka Y 1988 Mucin abnormality of colonic mucosa in ulcerative colitis associated with carcinoma and/or dysplasia. Diseases of the Colon and Rectum 31: 387–389

Ahnen D J, McHugh J B, Bozdeck J M, Warren G H 1990 Carcinogenesis in chronic ulcerative colitis: flow cytometry. Canadian Journal of Gastroenterology 4: 390–396

Ahnen D J, Warren G H, Greene L J, Singleton J W, Brown W R 1987 Search for a specific marker of mucosal dysplasia in chronic ulcerative colitis. Gastroenterology 93: 1346–1355

Allen D C, Biggart J D, Pyper P C 1985a Large bowel mucosal dysplasia and carcinoma in ulcerative colitis. Journal of Clinical Pathology 38: 30–43

Allen D C, Biggart J D, Orchin J C 1985b An immunoperoxidase study of epithelial marker antigens in ulcerative colitis with dysplasia and carcinoma. Journal of Clinical Pathology 38: 18–29

Ball C S, Wujanto R, Haboubi N Y, Schofield P S 1988 Carcinoma in anal Crohn's disease: discussion paper. Journal of the Royal Society of Medicine 81: 217–219

Bell S M, Kelly S A, Hoyle J A et al 1991 c-Ki-*ras* gene mutations in dysplasia and carcinomas complicating ulcerative colitis. British Journal of Cancer 64: 174–178

Biasco G, Lipkin M, Minarini A, Higgins P, Miglioli M, Barbara L 1990 Proliferative and antigenic properties of rectal cells in patients with chronic ulcerative colitis. Cancer Research 44: 5450–5454

Binder V, Hendriksen C, Kreiner S 1985 Prognosis in Crohn's disease based on results from a regional patient group from the County of Copenhagen. Gut 26: 146–150

Blackstone M O, Riddell R H, Rogers B H G, Levin B 1981 Dysplasia-associated lesion or mass (DALM) detected by colonoscopy in long-standing ulcerative colitis: an indication for colectomy. Gastroenterology 80: 366–374

Boland C R, Lance P, Levin B et al 1984 Abnormal goblet cell glycoconjugates in rectal biopsies associated with an increased risk of neoplasia in patients with ulcerative colitis: early results of a prospective study. Gut 25: 1364–1371

Borkje B, Laerum O D, Schrumpf E 1987 Enzyme activities in biopsy specimens from large bowel mucosa in ulcerative colitis. Scandinavian Journal of Gastroenterology 22: 443–448

Brahme F, Lindstrom C, Wenekert A 1975 Crohn's disease in a defined population. An epidemiological study of incidence, prevalence, mortality and secular trends in the City of Malmo, Sweden. Gastroenterology 69: 342–351

Buchmann P, Allan R B, Thompson H, Alexander-Williams J 1980 Carcinoma in a rectovaginal fistula in a patient with Crohn's disease. American Journal of Surgery 140: 462–463

Burbige E J, Bedine M S, Handelsman J C 1977 Adenocarcinoma of the small intestine in Crohn's disease involving the small bowel. Western Journal of Medicine 127: 43–45

Burmer G C, Rabinovitch P S, Haggitt R C et al 1992 Neoplastic progression in ulcerative colitis: histology, DNA content and loss of a p53 allele. Gastroenterology 103: 1602–1610

Butt J H, Lennard-Jones J E, Ritchie J K 1980 A practical approach to the cancer risk in inflammatory bowel disease. Medical Clinics of North America 4: 1203–1220

Butt J H, Konishi F, Morson B C, Lennard-Jones J E, Ritchie J K 1983 Macroscopic lesions in dysplasia and carcinoma complicating ulcerative colitis. Digestive Diseases and Sciences 28: 18–26

Campbell B J, Finnie I A, Hounsell E F, Rhodes J M 1995 Direct demonstration of increased expression of Thomson–Friedenreich (TF) antigen in colonic adenocarcinoma and ulcerative colitis mucin and its concealment in normal mucin. Journal of Clinical Investigation 95: 571–576

Chaikhouni A, Regueyra F T, Stevens J R 1981 Adenocarcinoma in perineal fistulas of Crohn's disease. Diseases of the Colon and Rectum 24: 639–643

Chaubert P, Benhattar J, Saraga, Costa J 1994 K-ras mutations and p53 alterations in neoplastic and non-neoplastic lesions associated with longstanding ulcerative colitis. American Journal of Pathology 144: 767–775

Chen J, Compton C, Cheng E, Fromowitz F, Viola M V 1992 c-Ki-ras mutations in dysplastic fields and cancers in ulcerative colitis. Gastroenterology 102: 1983–1987

Choi P M, Zelig M P 1994 Similarity of colorectal cancer in Crohn's disease and ulcerative colitis: implications for carcinogenesis and prevention. Gut 35: 950–954

Church J M, Weakley F L, Fazio V W, Sebek B A, Achkar E, Carwell M 1985 The relationship between fistulas in Crohn's disease and associated carcinoma. Diseases of the Colon and Rectum 26: 361–366

Connell W R, Sheffield J P, Kamm M A, Ritchie J K, Hawley P R, Lennard-Jones J E 1994 Lower gastrointestinal malignancy in Crohn's disease. Gut 35: 347–352

Cook M G, Goligher J C 1975 Carcinoma and epithelial dysplasia complicating ulcerative colitis. Gastroenterology 68: 1127–1136

Cooke W T, Mallas E, Prior P, Allen R N 1980 Crohn's disease: course treatment and long term prognosis. Quarterly Journal of Medicine 49: 363–384

Cooper H S, Farano P, Coapman R A 1987 Peanut lectin binding sites in colons of patients with ulcertive colitis. Archives of Pathology and Laboratory Medicine 111: 270–275

Crispin D, Brentnall T, Haggitt R et al 1993 p53 mutations can be an early event in ulcerative colitis with dysplasia or cancer. Gastroenterology 104: A395

Darke S G, Parks A G, Grogono J I, Pollock D J 1973 Adenocarcinoma and Crohn's disease: a report of two cases and analysis of the literature. British Journal of Surgery 60: 169–175

Dawson I M P, Pryse-Davies J 1959 The development of the carcinoma of the large intestine in ulcerative colitis. British Journal of Surgery 47: 113–128

de Dombal F T, Watts J M, Watkinson G, Goligher J C 1966 Local complications of ulcerative colitis: stricture, pseudopolyposis and carcinoma of colon and rectum. British Medical Journal 1: 1442–1447

Delattre O, Law D J, Remvikos Y et al 1989 Multiple genetic alterations in distal and proximal colorectal cancer. Lancet 2: 353–356

Devroede G J, Taylor W F 1976 On calculating cancer risk and survival of ulcerative colitis patients with the life table method. Gastroenterology 71: 505–509

Edling N P G, Eklof O 1961 Distribution of malignancy in ulcerative colitis. Gastroenterology 41: 465–466

Ehsanullah M, Naunton-Morgan M, Filipe M I, Gazzard B 1985 Sialomucins in the assessment of dysplasia and cancer risk patients with ulcerative colitis treated with colectomy and ileorectal anastomosis. Histopathology 9: 223–236

Ekbom A, Helmick C, Zack M, Adami H O 1990 Increased risk of large-bowel cancer in Crohn's disease with colonic involvement. Lancet 336: 357–359

Fireman Z, Grossman A, Lilos P, Hacohen D, Bar Meir S, Rozen P et al 1989 Intestinal cancer in patients with Crohn's disease: a population study in central Israel. Scandinavian Journal of Gastroenterology 24: 346–350

Fleming K A, Pollock A C 1975 A case of Crohn's carcinoma. Gut 16: 533–537

Fozard J B J, Dixon M F, Axon A T R, Giles G R 1987 Lectin and mucin histochemistry as an aid to cancer surveillance in ulcerative colitis. Histopathology 11: 385–394

Fozard J B J, Quirke P, Dixon M F, Giles G R, Bird C C 1986 DNA aneuploidy in ulcerative colitis. Gut 27: 1414–1418

Frank J D, Shorey B A 1973 Adenocarcinoma of the small bowel as a complication of Crohn's disease. Gut 14: 120–124

Gallop J H, Phillips S F, Melton L J, Zinsmeister A R 1988 Epidemiological aspects of Crohn's disease: a population based study in Ohmsted County, Minnesota. Gut 29: 49–56

Gilbert J M, Mann C V, Scholefield J, Domizio P 1991 The aetiology and surgery of carcinoma of the anus, rectum and sigmoid colon in Crohn's disease. Negative correlation with human papillomavirus type 16 (HPV-16). European Journal of Surgical Oncology 17: 507–513

Gillen C D, Andrews H A, Prior P, Allan R N 1994a Crohn's disease and colorectal cancer. Gut 35: 651–655

Gillen C D, Walmsley R S, Prior P, Andrews H A, Allen R N 1994b Ulcerative colitis and Crohn's disease: a comparison of the colorectal cancer risk in extensive colitis. Gut 35: 1590–1592

Goh H S, Jass J R 1986 DNA content and the adenoma–carcinoma sequence in the colorectum. Journal of Clinical Pathology 39: 387–392

Goldgraber M B, Kirsner J B 1964 Carcinoma of the colon in ulcerative colitis. Cancer 17: 657–665

Greenstein A J, Sachar D B, Smith H 1979 Cancer in universal and left-sided ulcerative colitis: factors determining risk. Gastroenterology 77: 290–294

Greenstein A J, Sachar D B, Pucillo A, Kreel I, Geller S, Janowitz H D et al 1978. Cancer in Crohn's disease after diversionary surgery. American Journal of Surgery 135: 86–90

Greenstein A J, Sachar D B, Smith H, Janowitz H D, Aufses A H Jr 1980 Patterns of neoplasia in Crohn's disease and ulcerative colitis. Cancer 46: 403–407

Greenwald B D, Harpaz N, Yin J et al 1992 Loss of heterozygosity affecting the p53, Rb, and mcc/apc tumour suppressor gene loci in dysplastic and cancerous ulcerative colitis. Cancer Research 52: 741–745

Gyde S N, Prior P, Allan R N et al 1988 Colorectal cancer in ulcerative colitis: a cohort study of primary referrals from three centres. Gut 29: 206–217

Gyde S N, Prior P, Macartney J C, Thompson H, Waterhouse J A, Allan R N 1980 Malignancy in Crohn's disease. Gut 21: 1024–1029

Hamilton S R 1985 Colorectal carcinoma in patients with Crohn's disease. Gastroenterology 89: 398–407

Hammarberg C, Slezak P, Tribukait B 1984 Early detection of malignancy in ulcerative colitis. A flow-cytometric study. Cancer 53: 291–295

Harper P H, Fazio V W, Lavery L C et al The long-term outcome in Crohn's disease. Diseases of the Colon and Rectum 30: 174–179

Hawker P C, Gyde S N, Thompson H, Allan R N 1982 Adenocarcinoma of the small intestine complicating Crohn's disease. Gut 23: 188–193

Hendriksen C, Kreiner S, Binder V 1985 Long term prognosis in ulcerative colitis – based on results of a regional patient group from the country of Copenhagen. Gut 26: 158–163

Isaacson P 1976 Tissue demonstration of carcinoembryonic antigen (CEA) in ulcerative colitis. Gut 17: 561–567

Isaacson P 1982 Immunoperoxidase study of the secretory immunoglobulin system in colonic neoplasia. Journal of Clinical Pathology 34: 14–25

Jass J R 1991 Subsite distribution and incidence of colorectal cancer in New Zealand 1974–1983. Diseases of the Colon and Rectum 34: 56–59

Jass J R, Roberton A M 1994 Colorectal mucin histochemistry in health and disease: A critical review. Pathology International 44: 487–504

Jass J R, Smith M 1992 Sialic acid and epithelial differentiation in colorectal polyps and cancer – a morphological mucin and lectin histochemical study. Pathology 24: 233–242

Jass J R, England J, Miller K 1986 Value of mucin histochemistry in follow up surveillance of patients with long-standing ulcerative colitis. Journal of Clinical Pathology 39: 393–398

Kewenter J, Ahlman H, Hulten L 1978 Cancer risk in extensive ulcerative colitis. Annals of Surgery 188: 824–828

Kewenter J, Hulten L, Ahren C 1982 The occurrence of severe epithelial dysplasia and its bearing on treatment of long-standing ulcerative colitis. Annals of Surgery 195: 209–213

Kvist N, Jacobsen O, Norgaard P, Ockelmann H H, Kvist H K, Schou G et al 1986 Malignancy in Crohn's disease. Scandinavian Journal of Gastroenterology 21: 82–86

Lee R G 1987 Villous regeneration in ulcerative colitis. Archives of Pathology and Laboratory Medicine 111: 276–278

Lennard-Jones J E, Morson B C, Ritchie J K, Shove D C, Williams C B 1977 Cancer in colitis: assessment of the individual risk by clinical and histological criteria. Gastroenterology 73: 1280–1289

Lewis B, Morson B C, February A W, Hywel Jones J, Misiewics J J 1970 Abnormal lactic dehydrogenase isoenzyme patterns in ulcerative colitis with precancerous change. Gut 12: 16–19

Maratka Z, Nedbal J, Kocianova J, Havelka J, Kudrmann J, Hendl J 1985 Incidence of colorectal cancer in proctocolitis: a retrospective study of 959 cases over 40 years. Gut 26: 43–49

Melville D M, Jass J R, Morson B C et al 1989 Observer study of the grading of dysplasia in ulcerative colitis: comparison with clinical outcome. Human Pathology 20: 1008–1014

Melville D M, Jass J R, Shepherd N A et al 1988 Dysplasia and deoxyribonucleic acid aneuploidy in the assessment of precancerous changes in chronic ulcerative colitis. Gastroenterology 95: 668–675

Mir-Madjlessi S H, Farmer R G, Easley K A, Beck G J 1986 Colorectal and extracolonic malignancy in ulcerative colitis. Cancer 58: 1569–1574

Nowell 1976 The clonal evolution of tumour cell populations. Science 194: 23–28

Petras R E, Mir-Madjlessi S H, Farmer R G 1987 Crohn's disease and intestinal carcinoma: a report of 11 cases with emphasis on associated epithelial dysplasia. Gastroenterology 93: 1307–1314

Ransohoff D F, Riddell R H, Levin B 1985 Ulcerative colitis and colonic cancer. Problems in assessing the diagnostic usefulness of mucosal dysplasia. Diseases of the Colon and Rectum 28: 383–388

Richards M E, Rickert R R, Nance F C 1989 Crohn's disease associated carcinoma. Annals of Surgery 209: 764–773

Riddell R H 1976 The precarcinomatous phase of ulcerative colitis. In: Morsan B C (ed) Current topics in pathology: pathology of the gastrointestinal tract. Springer-Verlag, Berlin, pp 179–219

Riddell R H, Morson B C 1979 Value of sigmoidoscopy and biopsy in detection of carcinoma and premalignant change in ulcerative colitis. Gut 20: 575–580

Riddell R H, Goldman H, Ransohoff et al 1983 Dysplasia in inflammatory bowel disease: standardized classification with provisional clinical applications. Human Pathology 14: 931–968

Ritchie J K, Hawley P R, Lennard-Jones J E 1981 Prognosis of carcinoma in ulcerative colitis. Gut 22: 752–755

Rognum T O, Elgjo K, Fausa O, Brandtzaeg P 1982 Immunohistochemical evaluation of carcinoembryonic antigen, secretory component, and epithelial IgA in ulcerative colitis with dysplasia. Gut 23: 123–133

Rubin C E, Haggitt R C, Burmer G C, Brentnall T A et al 1992 DNA aneuploidy in colonic biopsies predicts future development of dysplasia in ulcerative colitis. Gastroenterology 103: 1611–1620

Rubio C A, Johansson C, Slezak P, Ohman U, Hammarberg C 1984 Villous dysplasia: an ominous histologic sign in colitic patients. Diseases of the Colon and Rectum 27: 283–287

Rubio C A, Nylander G, Johansson C, Slezak P 1982 Non-dysplastic villous changes in endoscopic biopsies in ulcerative colitis with carcinoma. Acta Pathologica Microbiologica Immunologica Scandinavica A, 90: 277–282

Rutegard J, Ahsgren L, Stenling R, Roos G 1989 DNA content and mucosal dysplasia in ulcerative colitis: flow cytometric analysis in patients with dysplastic or indefinite morphologic changes in the colorectal mucosa. Diseases of the Colon and Rectum 32: 1055–1059

Scott N, Sagar P, Stewart J, Blaire G E, Dixon M F, Quirke P 1991 p53 in colorectal cancer. Clinicopathological correlation and prognostic significance. British Journal of Cancer 63: 317–319

Shepherd N A, Hall P A, Williams G T et al 1989 Primary malignant lymphoma of the large intestine complicating chronic inflammatory bowel disease. Histopathology 15: 325–337

Slaney G, Brooke B N 1959 Cancer in ulcertive colitis. Lancet 2: 694–698

Slater G, Greenstein A J, Gelernt I, Kreel I, Bauer J, Aufses A H 1985 Distribution of colorectal cancer in patients with and without ulcerative colitis. American Journal of Surgery 149: 780–782

Sugita A, Sachar D B, Bodian C, Ribeiro M B, Aufses Jr A H, Greenstein A J 1991 Colorectal cancer in ulcerative colitis. Influence of anatomical extent and age at onset on colitis–cancer interval. Gut 32: 167–169

Suzuki K, Muto T, Masaki T, Morioka Y 1990 Microspectrophotometric DNA analysis in ulcerative colitis with special referenc to its application in diagnosis of carcinoma and dysplasia. Gut 31: 1266–1270

Traube J, Simpson S, Riddell R H, Levin B, Kirsner J B 1980 Crohn's disease and adenocarcinoma of the bowel. Digestive Diseases and Sciences 25: 939–944

Truelove S C, Pena A S 1976 Course and prognosis of Crohn's disease. Gut 17: 192–201

Valdes-Dapena A, Rudolph I, Hidayat A et al 1976 Adenocarcinoma of the small bowel in association with regional enteritis. Four new cases. Cancer 37: 2938–2947

Van M H, Elgjo K, Norheim A, Bergan A 1984 Measurement of enzyme activity in colonic biopsies: a test for premalignancy in ulcerative colitis? Scandinavian Journal of Gastroenterology 19: 889–892

Weedon D D, Shorter R G, Ilstrup D M et al 1973 Crohn's disease and cancer. New England Journal of Medicine 289: 1099–1103

Yin J, Harpaz N, Tong Y et al 1993 p53 point mutations in dysplasia and cancerous ulcerative colitis lesions. Gastroenterology 104: 1633–1639

Zinkin L D, Brandwein C 1980 Adenocarcinoma in Crohn's colitis. Diseases of the Colon and Rectum 23: 115–117

34. Laboratory markers of inflammatory bowel disease

H. J. F. Hodgson

Ideally, laboratory markers – in the sense of readily available biochemical, hematological or serological tests – in idiopathic inflammatory bowel disease would distinguish patients with these conditions from other individuals, both when the disease was active and when quiescent, would distinguish ulcerative colitis from Crohn's disease, would define and quantify inflammatory activity, and would indicate remission and give early warning of relapse. Clearly, we have no single laboratory marker to do this; even using a panel of markers these aims cannot be achieved. The laboratory markers in regular use are, even at their best, not specific in reflecting the presence of inflammation in the gut: their value is as part of total assessment of the patient, and they need to be taken in conjunction with history, examination and radiological, endoscopic and other information.

This chapter will survey individually both commonly and less frequently used laboratory markers in inflammatory bowel disease, and then discuss their use in the management of these conditions.

THE ACUTE-PHASE RESPONSE

The acute-phase response in its full form is *illness* – fever, malaise, anorexia, leukocytosis and negative nitrogen balance – a cardinal response of the body to many kinds of infection or trauma, including inflammatory bowel disease. The response involves many immunological and inflammatory processes, and changes in function in many organs. Many of the changes in the blood are due to alterations in the rate of synthesis of proteins by the liver (Trautwein et al 1994). There are small increases in the plasma concentration of weak acute-phase proteins such as complement C_3 two- to fourfold rises in proteins such as α_1 acid glycoprotein fibrinogen and α_1-antitrypsin, and spectacular rises up to 100-fold or more in the concentration of C-reactive protein (CRP) and amyloid A-associated protein (SAA). The increased hepatic synthesis of these proteins during the acute-phase response is accompanied by transient reduction in the rate of synthesis of negative acute-phase proteins, of which albumin and transferrin are typical examples. The production of acute-phase proteins is regulated by proinflammatory cytokines, such as interleukins IL-1 and IL-6, produced in sites of inflammation, altering gene expression by hepatocytes. The majority of the laboratory markers that are used to reflect acute inflammation in inflammatory bowel disease reflect some part of the acute-phase response; abnormalities in these tests are not specific for either ulcerative colitis or Crohn's disease.

ERYTHROCYTE SEDIMENTATION RATE (ESR)

The ESR is the traditional approach to quantifying the acute-phase response. ESR varies with plasma protein concentration, particularly alphaglobulins, fibrinogen and gammaglobulins, and hematocrit. Few clinicians bother with the correction for the latter, but severe anemia can elevate the ESR. Hyperglobulinemia in many individuals does not reflect acute inflammation (e.g. patients with paraproteinemia), although it raises the ESR. In the context of inflammatory bowel disease, however, the ESR provides a crude and rapid approach to the labile plasma protein alterations of the acute-phase response. As there are alterations in the serum levels of many proteins, some of which have long half-lives, the ESR is slow to alter when there are major changes in clinical state. The use of the ESR in inflammatory bowel disease is, however, time-honoured and cost-effective.

In ulcerative colitis, where clinical, endoscopic and histological grading of disease severity is a straightforward means of providing a clinical assessment of disease activity, there is a good overall correlation between ESR and disease activity. For example, mean ESR (mm/h) was 18 mm/h in a group of patients with quiescent disease, 43 mm/h in mildly active disease, 62 mm/h in moderately active disease and 83 mm/h in severely active disease (Dearing et al 1969). However, the scatter was great, with considerable overlap between groups, and among the severe group with bloody diarrhea, weight loss, anemia and fever, the range was 3–120. ESR also reflects disease extent, to some degree. Among patients with comparable disease activity the ESR is similar in both universal and left-sided colitis, but low in patients with limited proctitis, even if that is quite severe. Reflecting the long half-life of the various contributory proteins, the ESR may take several days to fall even when clinical improvement is rapid.

In Crohn's disease, assessing the extent to which a laboratory parameter reflects disease activity is more complicated than in ulcerative colitis, as discussed later. In particular, clinical activity may not always parallel the inflammatory activity. Using clinical indices of activity, the ESR is higher in active disease than in remission, but there is considerable overlap between groups (e.g. median ESR was 18 in 36 mildly active patients, and 17 in 40 moderately active patients (Fagan et al 1982). Disease site is also relevant. The ESR emerges as a better correlate of clinical activity in predominantly colonic Crohn's disease than in localized small-bowel disease. Sachar et al (1986, 1990) combined observations in ulcerative colitis and Crohn's disease to demonstrate that, over most ranges of activity, the order of mean ESR was proctitis and proctosigmoiditis < ileiitis and ileojejunitis < left-sided ulcerative colitis < ileocolitis < universal ulcerative colitis < Crohn's colitis.

C-REACTIVE PROTEIN

C-reactive protein (CRP) is a single protein, one component of the acute-phase response, with the major advantage as a laboratory marker that it responds very rapidly to the onset and disappearance of inflammation, with up to 1000-fold changes in its concentration (Mazlam & Hodgson 1994). The protein itself (MW 105 000 Da) is selectively deposited on damaged cell membranes, and complexes with free DNA. CRP is released from the liver into the circulation within 6 hours of tissue injury, reaching peak level after 24–48 hours. The short half-life (19 hours) explains the rapid falls that occur in serum concentration after reduction in inflammation. IL-1β, IL-6, tumor necrosis factor-α (TNFα) and transforming growth factor-β (TGF-β) can all enchance CRP production by liver cells (Trautwein et al 1994). CRP rises in both ulcerative colitis and Crohn's disease activity, but this is more marked in Crohn's disease than ulcerative colitis (Fagan et al 1982). In ulcerative colitis CRP correlates with extent in active disease, and in severe colitis, when urgent medical treatment is undertaken and the risk of colectomy high, persisting elevation of the CRP during treatment was associated with a failure to respond to corticosteroids and, therefore, recourse to surgery (Prantera et al 1988).

CRP is more generally used in assessing Crohn's disease. In part this reflects the greater need for such assessments in Crohn's disease rather than ulcerative colitis, as the clinical criteria are more likely to be ambiguous (Hodgson & Mazlam 1991). In addition, CRP tends to rise to higher levels in active Crohn's disease than in active ulcerative colitis (Saverymuttu et al 1986) – perhaps reflecting differences in cytokines produced in these two conditions (Mazlam & Hodgson 1992). CRP (normal <1 mg/ml) had a median value of 4 in mild, 15 in moderate, and 85 in severe Crohn's disease, although there was considerable overlap, and successful therapy led to a fall in levels over the first 24–48 hours (Fagan et al 1982). Helpfully, clinically unsuccessful corticosteroid treatment does not lower CRP. In an extensive series of reported studies, CRP has correlated well with other assessments, including colonoscopic appearance, disease extent and leukocyte excretion (Fagan et al 1982, André et al 1980, 1981, Saverymuttu et al 1983, Prantera et al 1985). It is important to recognize, however, that a lack of anticipated concordance between different assessments may in fact be valuable when individual patients are considered. Thus, patients with high symptomatic scores due to a fibrous stricture causing obstruction will probably have a low CRP, reflecting the fixed rather than inflammatory nature of the obstruction. Patients with diffuse low-grade disease restricted to the small intestine may have low CRP levels. Unsuspected abscesses may be associated with CRP elevations. In a longitudinal study in Crohn's disease, Boirivant et al (1988) showed that if clinical remission was achieved but an elevated CRP persisted, the chances of subsequent clinical relapse were greater than if the CRP normalized.

One particular usage of CRP is in the differential diagnosis of mild symptomatology, where a normal CRP will favor functional bowel disorder rather than Crohn's disease (Shine et al 1985).

SERUM AMYLOID A (SAA)

Normal individuals produce SAA from the liver in response to inflammation; persistent unregulated production leads to amyloidosis. SAA, a protein with structural similarities to CRP, responds in the same way during active inflammation in inflammatory bowel disease, with higher levels in Crohn's disease than in ulcerative colitis (Chambers et al 1987). This probably explains why there is a much stronger association of amyloidosis with Crohn's disease than ulcerative colitis. As a routine assay, serum SAA seems to have no advantage over CRP.

α_1-ACID GLYCOPROTEIN

Seromucoids (a group of α_1-glycoproteins first analysed as perchloric acid-soluble, phosphotungstic acid-insoluble material (Cooke et al 1958) contribute to the acute-phase response. Current assays measure orosomucoid–α_1-acid glycoprotein (Thaw & Albutt, 1980). In ulcerative colitis serum levels correlate well with clinical disease activity, with less overlap between groups than with ESR (Dearing et al 1969), and one study reported a good correlation of serum α_1-acid glycoprotein with protein loss into the gut (Jensen et al 1976). The half-life is 5 days, so the speed of response is no better than with ESR. In Crohn's disease good correlations between orosomucoid and the clinical Crohn's disease activity index (CDAI) were reported (André et al 1980, 1981).

α_1-ANTITRYPSIN

The serum level of the acute-phase response α_1-antitrypsin is also a correlate of disease activity (Meryn et al 1985). The fact that this protein is highly protease resistant means that fecal measurement of α_1-antitrypsin can be used as a measure of protein-losing enteropathy, and it is this feature that has attracted most attention in inflammatory bowel disease (Karbach et al 1983, Meyers et al 1988a, b).

OTHER ACUTE-PHASE PROTEINS

Despite the fact that other acute-phase proteins also alter in active disease, little attention has been paid to using the elevations of, for example, fibrinogen, α_2-macroglobulin, or a variety of other proteins, as routine laboratory parameters. Serum albumin falls in active disease, as a negative acute-phase reactant, although other factors such as protein loss into the gut (Bendixen et al 1970) and malnutrition also affect albumin levels.

OTHER SERUM PROTEIN MEASUREMENTS

Immunoglobulins. Immunoglobulins G, A and M are all slightly elevated in ulcerative colitis and Crohn's disease compared with controls – notably IgA reflecting the recruitment of the gut mucosal immune system. However, the increase is relatively small, the range of normality wide, and the precise relationship with clinical activity inexact (Weeke & Jarnum, 1971, Hodgson & Jewell 1978). Patients with associated liver disease may have striking Ig elevations.

Neutrophil elastase. The serum level of elastase, one of the proteolytic enzymes released from polymorphonuclear leukocyte granules in inflammatory reactions, rises during acute inflammation – more prominently in Crohn's disease than in ulcerative colitis – and good correlations with clinical activity indices and the CRP level have been reported (Adeyemi et al 1985). Serum lactoferrin, another neutrophil granule constituent, is also elevated in active disease of either type (Adeyemi & Hodgson 1991).

Neopterin; soluble IL-2 receptor. Serum neopterin levels rise in conditions associated with the activation of T cells and macrophages; elevated serum levels thus occur in a variety of conditions associated with activated cellular immunity, including viral infections; serum (and urinary) neopterin levels correlate with disease activity in Crohn's disease (Niederwieser et al 1985, Prior et al 1986). T-cell activation and expansion of T-cell clones involves IL-2 generation by T cells themselves, and consequent receptor shedding into the circulation elevates IL-2 receptor levels in Crohn's disease, in parallel with other parameters of activity such as α_1-antitrypsin levels, CRP and clinical activity indices (Crabtree et al, 1990, Mahida et al 1990). These two assays have not proved more valuable than simpler assays such as the CRP, and are not in general clinical use.

HEMATOLOGICAL PARAMETERS

Hemoglobin. Although a vital clinical measurement, hemoglobin level is a poor correlate of contemporary inflammatory or clinical activity. Current or previous hemorrhage, iron and other hematinic deficiencies, and depression of hemopoiesis as a direct correlate of inflammation (anemia of chronic disease) all contribute to anemia.

White cell count. Mild elevations of white cell count, predominantly polymorphonuclear neutrophil leukocytes, occur in active disease; systemic corticosteroids also elevate the granulocyte count. Conversely, immunosuppressants may lower the lymphocyte count. In Crohn's disease complicating abscesses may lead to high neutrophil counts, and complicating lymphangiectasia to lymphocyte loss within the gut and reduced circulating T-cell numbers. In ulcerative colitis a few patients have a distinct eosinophilia, and at a tissue level this has been thought to be associated with the healing phase.

Platelet count. In both ulcerative colitis and Crohn's disease the platelet count rises during relapse. Thrombocytosis of >400 000/µl is more common in severe than in mild or moderate ulcerative colitis, and in large groups of patients with Crohn's disease the platelet count correlates well with the CDAI (Talstad et al 1973, Harris et al 1983, Phillips & Dronfield 1983). However, the fairly wide range of normality, the fairly small range of abnormality (rarely to >2 × upper limit of normal), and other compounding factors (acute hemorrhage of any sort can raise the platelet count) mean that, although readily available, this parameter is not widely utilized.

Hematinic levels. Parameters of iron status are often abnormal in inflammatory bowel disease, but again are complex. Iron deficiency raises transferrin levels, but inflammation lowers the rate of transferrin synthesis by the liver. Serum B_{12} levels may fall in Crohn's disease, but slowly as a consequence of malabsorption, and generally after ileal resection rather than merely ileal disease. Serum and red cell folate levels are often low in active Crohn's disease, reflecting both anorexia (the body stores of folate can be depleted in weeks) and a diffuse reduction in small-intestinal absorptive capacity (even in disease apparently limited to the colon).

MEASUREMENT OF OTHER CIRCULATING SUBSTANCES

In experimental studies many other substances circulate at higher than normal levels in the blood during active disease. These include IL-1, IL-6, TNF-α soluble TNF receptors, complement breakdown products, etc. (Satsangi et al 1987, Miura & Hiwatashi 1985, Mahida et al 1990). Some observations suggest differences between the inflammatory process in ulcerative colitis and Crohn's disease, for example greater levels of IL-6 and IL-1 are often – although not invariably – reported in Crohn's disease than in ulcerative colitis (Mazlam & Hodgson 1992). Most of these measurements have not been translated into routine clinical use.

OTHER LABORATORY ASSESSMENTS OF DISEASE ACTIVITY

As already discussed, all these readily measured markers correlate with inflammation, but an elevated level in a patient with a diagnosis of inflammatory bowel disease does not confirm that the gut is actively inflamed. Other inflammatory processes – pneumonia, bronchiectasis, or often an associated inflammatory process such as arthritis or spondylitis, may confuse the issue. Therefore, laboratory assessments that directly reflect gastrointestinal inflammation have been explored. These include (1) detection of increased intestinal permeability, in general by detecting increased urinary excretion of ingested probe molecules (PEG, ^{51}Cr–EDTA, non-metabolized sugars); (2) detection of protein-losing enteropathy by stool measurement using exogenously administered markers (^{111}In- or ^{51}Cr-labeled protein (Nordgren et al 1990)) or the endogenous protein α_1-antitrypsin; (3) detection of inflammatory mediators or cells in the feces (fecal elastase (Adeyemi & Hodgson 1988), ^{111}In-labeled leukocyte excretion (Saverymuttu et al 1982), assessment of stool prostanoids or leukotrienes by rectal dialysis (Lauritsen et al 1987)). None of these have been generally accepted for routine use, though as research tools they may be useful owing to their specificity for gut disease.

THE USE OF LABORATORY ASSESSMENTS OF DISEASE ACTIVITY

In ulcerative colitis, the relationship between symptomatology and the presence of active inflammation, and the ready accessibility of rectal mucosa to endoscopic assessment, means that laboratory markers of activity are ancillary rather than critical aids to clinical management.

In defining severe disease, and thus the need for hospitalization and urgent treatment, an ESR of >30 mm/h and Hb of <11 were the laboratory markers that contributed to the six features (otherwise stool frequency, bleeding, temperature and tachycardia) identified by Truelove and Witts (1955). A low albumin level has also been defined as an association of severe disease and the potential necessity for colectomy. In practice, however, the clinical features are far more relevant.

In Crohn's disease, however, the heterogeneity of the disease and the poor correlation between symptomatology and the presence of active inflammation has rendered laboratory markers of inflammation much more interesting and potentially more useful. The simplest example of this is the observation that subacute obstruction plus a high ESR means active inflammation; subacute obstruction plus a normal ESR probably means a fibrous stricture. It is of little surprise that there are often discrepancies between the clinical indices of activity and the results of laboratory indices in individual patients, even if the two correlate well overall, and it is precisely because these discrepancies arise that both sets of assessments are needed. As mentioned, high symptomatic scores but low indices often reflect non-inflammatory complications, such as strictures or the consequences of bowel resection; low clinical scores with high laboratory indices may reflect other causes of inflammation than gut disease; the euphoriant effect of corticosteroids; or the presence of gut inflammation at a subsymptomatic level.

This last possibility has led a number of workers to investigate whether laboratory markers can be used to identify patients at risk of relapse. Brignola et al (1986), Boirivant et al (1988) and Wright et al (1987) have all performed serial studies and demonstrated that elevations of acute-phase reactants identify a subgroup at greater risk of clinical relapse. It is likely that these exercises identify patients who currently have inflammation which is not yet clinically apparent, rather than those in whom a relapse has not yet started. Whether clinically well patients with abnormal laboratory markers merit treatment is an open question, which will need to be reassessed at intervals as more acceptable medications such as non-systemically active corticosteroids become available.

The final – but perhaps most general – use of laboratory studies is to discriminate normality from disease, particularly in the assessment of patients with mild intermittent diarrhea – ? irritable bowel ? inflammatory bowel disease. In clinical remission all the laboratory parameters referred to thus far can be normal, and a clean return of laboratory assessments is thus not conclusive evidence of the absence of inflammatory bowel disease. ANCA, antineutrophil cytoplasmic antibodies, are found in 60–70% of patients with ulcerative colitis, and persist in remission (Snook et al 1989), but their role in diagnosing colitis during remission has not been formally assessed. In any case, the ? IBS ? IBD problem is much more characteristic of possible Crohn's disease than ulcerative colitis, and ANCA are only found in a minority of patients with Crohn's disease. The finding of abnormal laboratory markers is very useful in encouraging further investigation to identify the presence of inflammation; normal results are reassuring, but unfortunately not conclusive evidence of the absence of inflammatory bowel disease.

REFERENCES

Adeyemi E O, Hodgson H J F 1988 Faecal elastase in inflammatory bowel disease. Gut 29: A1474
Adeyemi E O, Hodgson H J F 1991 Lactoferrin: a correlate of disease activity in inflammatory bowel disease. European Journal of Gastroenterology and Hepatology 3: 51–56
Adeyemi E O, Neumann S, Chadwick V S, Hodgson H J F, Pepys M B 1985 Circulating human leucocyte elastase in patients with inflammatory bowel disease. Gut 26: 1306–1311
André C, Descos L, Landais P, Fermanian J 1980 Laboratory supplementation of Crohn's disease activity index. Lancet ii: 594–595
André C, Descos L, Landais P, Fermanian J 1981 Assessment of appropriate laboratory measurements to supplement the Crohn's disease activity index. Gut 22: 571–574
Bendixen G, Goltermann N, Jarnum S 1970 Immunoglobulin and albumin turnover in ulcerative colitis. Scandavanian Journal of Gastroenterology 5: 441–443
Boirivant M, Leoni M, Tariciotti D, Fais S, Squarcia O, Pallone F 1988 The clinical significance of serum C-reactive protein levels in Crohn's disease. Journal of Clinical Gastroenterology 10: 401–405
Brignola C, Campieri M, Bazzocchi G, Farruggia P, Tragnone A, Lanfranchi G A 1986 A laboratory index for predicting relapse in asymptomatic patients with Crohn's disease. Gastroenterology 91: 1490–1494
Chambers R E, Stross P, Barry R E, Whicher J T 1987 Serum amyloid A protein compared with C-reactive protein, alpha$_1$-antichymotrypsin and alpha$_1$-acid glycoprotein as a monitor of inflammatory bowel disease. European Journal of Clinical Investigation 17: 460–467
Cooke W T, Fowler D C, Cox E V 1958 The clinical significances of seromucoids in regional ileitis and ulcerative colitis. Gastroenterology 34: 910–919
Crabtree J E, Juby L D, Heatley R V, Lobo A J, Bullimore D W, Axon A T R 1990 Soluble interleukin-2 receptor in Crohn's disease: relation of serum concentrations to disease activity. Gut 31: 1033–1036
Dearing W H, McGuckin W H, Elveback L R 1969 Serum alpha$_1$-acid glycoprotein in chronic ulcerative colitis. Gastroenterology 56: 295–303
Fagan E A, Dyck R F, Maton P N, Hodgson H J F, Chadwick V S, Pepys M B 1982 Serum levels of C-reactive protein in Crohn's disease and ulcerative colitis. European Journal of Clinical Investigation 12: 351–360
Harris A D, Fitzsimons E, Fifield R et al 1983 Platelet count: a simple measure of activity in Crohn's disease. British Medical Journal 286: 1476
Hodgson H J F, Jewell D P 1978 The humoral immune system in inflammatory bowel disease. 2. Immunoglobulin levels. American Journal of Digestive Diseases 23: 123–128
Hodgson H J F, Mazlam M Z 1991 Assessment of disease activity in inflammatory bowel disease. Alimentary Pharmacology and Therapeutics 5: 555–584
Jensen K B, Jarnum S, Koudhal G, Kristensen M 1976 Serum orosomucoid ulcerative colitis. Its relation to clinical activity, protein loss and turnover of albumin and IgG. Scandinavian Journal of Gastroenterology 11: 177–193
Karbach U, Ewe K, Bodenstein H 1983 Alpha-1-antitrypsin, a reliable endogenous marker for intestinal protein loss and its application in patients with Crohn's disease. Gut 24: 718–723
Lauritsen K, Laursen L S, Bukhave K, Rask-Madsen J 1987 Intraluminal colonic levels of arachidonic acid metabolites in ulcerative colitis. Advances in Prostaglandin, Thromboxane, Leukotriene Research 17: 347–352
Mahida Y R, Gallagher A, Kurlak L, Hawkey C J 1990 Plasma and tissue interleukin-2 receptor level in IBD. Clinical Experimental Immunology 82: 75–80
Mazlam M Z, Hodgson H J F 1992 Peripheral blood monocyte cytokine production and acute phase response in inflammatory bowel disease. Gut 33: 773–778
Mazlam M Z, Hodgson H J F 1994 Why measure C reactive protein? Gut 35: 5–7
Meyers S, Lichtiger S, Feuer E J, Lahman E A, Janowitz H D 1988a Fecal alpha$_1$-antitrypsin as a measure of Crohn's disease activity. Journal of Clinical Gastroenterology 10: 491–497
Meyers S, Wolke A, Field S P, Feuer E J, Johnson J W, Janowitz H D 1988b Fecal alpha$_1$-antitrypsin measurement: an indicator of Crohn's disease activity. Gastroenterology 89: 13–18
Meryn S, Lochs H, Bettelheim P, Sertl K, Mulak K 1985 Serumproteinkonzentrationen – parameter für die krankheitsaktivitt bei morbus Crohn? Leber Magen Darm 15: 160–164
Miura M, Hiwatashi N 1985 Cytokine production in inflammatory bowel disease. Clinical and laboratory Immunology 18: 81–86
Niederwieser D, Fuchs D, Hausen A, Judmaier G, Reibnegger G, Wachter H 1985 Neopterin as a new biochemical marker in the clinical assessment of ulcerative colitis. Immunobiology 170: 320–326
Nordgren S, Hellberg R, Cederblad A, Fasth S, Lindstedt G, Hulten L 1990 Fecal excretion of radiolabelled (^{51}CrCl$_3$) proteins in patients with Crohn's disease. Journal of Gastroenterology 25: 345–351
Phillips M S, Dronfield M W 1983 Platelet count in patients with Crohn's disease. British Medical Journal 286: 1895
Prantera C, Davoli M, Lorenzetti F et al 1988 Clinical and laboratory indicators of extent of ulcerative colitis. Serum C-reactive protein helps the most. Journal of Clinical Gastroenterology 10: 41–45
Prantera C, Luzi C, Olivotto P, Levenstein S, Cerro P, Frances A 1985 Relationship between clinical and laboratory parameters and length of lesions in Crohn's disease of the small bowel. Digestive Diseases and Sciences 29: 1093–1097
Prior C, Bollbach R, Fuchs D et al 1986 Urinary neopterin, a marker of clinical activity in patients with Crohn's disease. Clinica Chimica Acta 155: 11–22
Sachar D B, Luppescu N E, Bodian C, Shlien R D, Fabry T L, Gumaste V V 1990 Erythrocyte sedimentation as a measure of Crohn's disease activity: opposite trends in ileitis versus colitis. Journal of Clinical Gastroenterology 12: 643–646
Sachar D B, Smith H, Chan S, Cohen L B, Lichtiger S, Messer J 1986 Erythrocytic sedimentation rate as a measure of clinical activity in inflammatory bowel disease. Journal of Clinical Gastroenterology 8: 647–650
Satsangi J, Wolstencroft R A, Cason J, Ainley C C, Dumonde D C, Thompson R P H 1987 Interleukin 1 in Crohn's disease. Clinical Experimental Immunology 67: 594–605
Saverymuttu S H, Hodgson H J F, Chadwick V S, Pepys M B 1986 Differing acute phase responses in Crohn's disease and ulcerative colitis. Gut 27: 809–813
Saverymuttu S H, Peters A M, Lavender J P, Hodgson H J F, Chadwick V S 1982 ^{111}Indium-labelled leucocytes – a new method of imaging the colon in inflammatory bowel disease. British Medical Journal 285: 225–257
Saverymuttu S H, Peters A M, Hodgson H J F, Chadwick V S 1983 Assessment of disease activity in ulcerative colitis using ^{111}Indium labelled faecal leucocyte excretion. Scandinavian Journal of Gastroenterology 18: 907–912
Shine B, Berghouse L, Lennard-Jones J E, Landon J 1985 C-Reactive protein as an aid in the differentiation of functional and inflammatory bowel disorders. Clinica Chimica Acta 148: 105–109
Snook J A, Chapman R W, Fleming K et al 1989 Anti-neutrophil nuclear antibody in ulcerative colitis, Crohn's disease and primary sclerosing cholangitis. Clinical Experimental Immunology 76: 30–33
Talstad I, Rootwelt K, Gjone E 1973 Thrombocytosis in ulcerative colitis and Crohn's disease. Scandinavian Journal of Gastroenterology 8: 135–138
Thaw P A, Albutt E C 1980 A critical evaluation of a serum seromucoid

assay and its replacement by a serum alpha$_1$-acid glycoprotein assay. Annals of Clinical Biochemistry 17: 140–143

Trautwein C, Böker K, Manns M O 1994 Hepatocyte and immune system: acute phase reaction as a contribution to early defence mechanisms. Gut 35: 1163–1166

Truelove S C, Witts L J 1955 Cortisone in ulcerative colitis: final report of a therapeutic trial. British Medical Journal 2: 1041–1044

Weeke B, Jarnum S 1971 Serum concentrations of 19 serum proteins in Crohn's disease and ulcerative colitis. Gut 12: 297–302

Wright J P, Alp M N, Young G O, Tigler-Wybrandi N 1987 Predictors of acute relapse of Crohn's disease. Digestive Diseases and Sciences 32: 164–170

35. Clinical indices in inflammatory bowel disease

D. T. Spence   J. F. Mayberry

INTRODUCTION

The use of clinical indices in inflammatory bowel disease (IBD) began in the early 1950s and has enabled clinicians to improve patient management and to monitor the effects of therapeutic interventions. Almost all activity indices in inflammatory bowel disease have been developed because of the need to quantify disease activity in clinical trials. One of the first indices was formulated by Truelove and Witts (1955), who needed to measure the severity of illness in patients with ulcerative colitis who were participating in a trial of cortisone. Their observation that the severity of illness could be measured using predefined criteria set a precedent for disease activity measurement in IBD.

Considerable controversy surrounds the use of disease activity indices. Most combine varying degrees of objective and subjective measurements in order to derive a single figure or set of figures which best describe the level of disease in a given individual. Such measurements may include symptomatology, laboratory tests, histology, radiology and endoscopic appearances (Fig. 35.1). There is an ever growing number of indices, each of which places emphasis on different aspects of disease, and there is a clear need for consensus on this issue. Moreover, the wider issue of health status measurement in IBD proposed by Garrett and Drossman (1990) deserves attention. Such measurements should encompass psychosocial aspects as well as disease activity. This chapter will examine some of the disease activity indices used in IBD and issues which surround their use in both clinical trials and clinical practice.

TERMINOLOGY

Terms such as disease activity, disease severity, degree of illness and, more recently, health status have all been used in the assessment of IBD. Singleton (1987) has discussed the problems in defining terms which may encompass both subjective feelings of illness and objective measures of the extent or degree of inflammation. Highly subjective measurements are often regarded as measuring the degree of illness rather than disease activity (Singleton 1987). Objective measures can describe 'actual disease severity', but they may or may not agree with the patient's current subjective measures. It is important, however, that both subjective and objective measures are used to determine disease activity, as knowledge of both is needed to make clinical decisions (Talsted and Gjone 1976; Gomes et al 1986, Singleton 1987). Thus the severity index for ulcerative colitis proposed by Truelove and Witts (1955) incorporates objective elements of disease activity (laboratory tests) and subjective elements or degree of illness (physical symptoms).

CLINICAL INDICES IN ULCERATIVE COLITIS

The extent and degree of ulceration in ulcerative colitis was first described by Stierlin (1912) using radiological studies. Since the disease is localized to the colon and rectum, and primarily involves the mucosa, the severity of disease (grade of inflammation) can also be reasonably assessed using endoscopy with biopsy (Singleton 1987, Beck 1987). This makes the assessment of ulcerative colitis relatively easy compared to Crohn's disease, and the complexity of disease activity indices in the latter condition reflect this.

The index described by Truelove and Witts (1955) defines three levels of severity: severe, moderately severe and mild. The components of the index are shown in

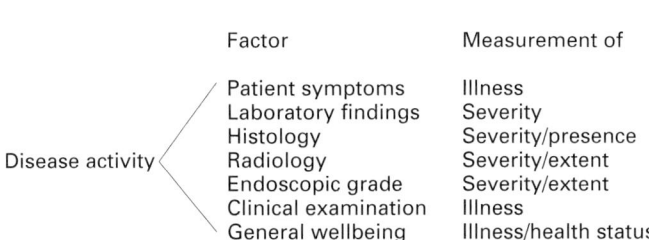

Fig. 35.1 Factors contributing to disease activity

Table 35.1 Truelove and Witts' disease severity index

Severe	Diarrhea > 6 times per day
	Macroscopic blood in stool
	Temperature >37.5° or >37.8°C on 2 out of 4 days
	Pulse >90 bpm
	Anemia (Hb <75% normal)
	ESR raised (>30 mm/h)
Mild	Diarrhea <4 times per day
	Small amounts of macroscopic blood
	Apyrexial
	Normal pulse
	No severe anemia
	ESR not raised (<30 mm/h)

Moderately severe is defined as intermediate between severe and mild

Table 35.1; each was equally weighted and the score has been used widely to determine disease activity in ulcerative colitis. Its two main disadvantages are the lack of sensitivity that results from having only three levels of severity (Singleton 1987) and a relative inability to predict short-term prognosis in response to treatment, or to predict the need for surgery (de Dombal 1986, Garrett and Drossman 1990). Garrett and Drossman (1990) further criticized the lack of attention paid to the patient's experience of illness, and this is their basis for arguing the use of health status measures. Endoscopy and biopsy evaluation have been shown to correlate poorly with a slightly modified form of Truelove and Witts' index, which might be construed as evidence that disease activity indices are poor indicators of macroscopic disease severity (Gomes et al 1986).

Early work with these indices in ulcerative colitis looked not only at the patient's response to treatment but also at their value as predictors of outcome (Edwards & Truelove 1963, Lennard-Jones et al 1975). The higher the stool frequency and body temperature the less likely the patient would be to respond to treatment, suggesting that early surgical intervention would be required.

In 1978 Powell-Tuck et al produced an activity index which placed more emphasis on the quantitative assessment of disease, for the first time including weighting of endoscopic appearance and extraintestinal complications of disease. This index was used in a study of prednisolone in active proctocolitis, and was later recommended by Singleton (1987) for monitoring patients in both research and clinical practice. The Organisation Mondiale de Gastroenterologie (OMGE) survey report (Myren et al 1979) discussed the use of Truelove and Witts' index in clinical practice and produced a consensus view which removed rectal bleeding, anemia and ESR from the index, but added weight loss, distension and pain. A series of studies in the mid-1970s included the use of diary cards, where the degree of urgency and level of incontinence were also recorded (Hodgson 1982) together with related criteria such as general wellbeing and ability to work (Heatley et al 1975, Bucknell et al 1978, Hodgson 1982).

Talsted and Gjone (1976) devised a disease activity index consisting of 18 parameters, many of which were laboratory tests which were difficult to carry out routinely; as a result the index has been regarded as impractical for everyday use (Seo et al 1992).

Table 35.2 shows the content of three indices used in clinical trials of 5-aminosalycylic acid (5-ASA) therapy in the late 1980s and early 1990s (Schroeder et al 1987, Rachmilewitz 1989, Sninsky et al 1991). Two of the studies used essentially the same index, albeit in modified form. This was based on a physician's global assessment and scores for stool frequency, rectal bleeding and endoscopic findings, and in one study included the patient's functional assessment of general wellbeing and ability to perform tasks. A third study (Rachmilewitz 1989) used an assessment similar to the St Marks Ulcerative Colitis Index (Powell-Tuck et al 1978) but included an investigator's global assessment of the patient's symptomatic state. These studies reflect a shift in emphasis towards the inclusion of subjective measures of health or degree of illness, as proposed by Garrett and Drossman in the 1980s, thus including the effect of disease on the patient's daily life.

In 1992 Seo et al performed multiple regression analysis in a similar way to that used by Best et al (1976) and Van Hees et al (1980) in developing Crohn's disease indices, using 18 clinical, laboratory and endoscopic parameters to produce a 'definitive' activity index for ulcerative colitis. Their index consists of an equation containing clinical and laboratory data multiplied by prederived constants, and claimed to improve upon the index produced by Truelove and Witts, but it has not yet been widely adopted.

Unfortunately, no consensus exists for which index best determines disease activity in ulcerative colitis. Truelove and Witts' (1955) index has been used widely, whereas a number of reviews have mentioned the merits of the index derived by Powell-Tuck et al (1978). With the advent of health status and quality of life measures in IBD it is preferable that future measurement of disease activity should include not only an accurate description of disease severity but also an assessment of the effects the disease has on the patient's quality of life.

CLINICAL INDICES IN CROHN'S DISEASE

Disease activity indices for Crohn's disease are more numerous and more complicated than those used in ulcerative colitis. Crohn's disease has a variable clinical picture, and in some individuals inflammatory activity and symptomatology do not correlate well (Hodgson 1982). Recent studies have demonstrated problems with scoring systems, whether they are based on symptomatology, endoscopic findings as laboratory measurement (Oliason et al 1990). The assessment of Crohn's disease is com-

Table 35.2 Disease indices in ulcerative colitis

Reference	Truelove & Witts 1955	Lennard-Jones et al 1975	Talsted & Gjone 1976	Powell-Tuck et al 1978	Myren et al 1979/84	Schroeder et al 1987	Rachmilewitz 1989	Sninsky et al 1991	Seo et al 1992
Setting	CT	CP	CP	CT	CT	CT	CT	CT	CP/CT
Features									
Diarrhea/bowel habit	✓	✓	✓	✓	✓	✓	✓	✓	✓
Rectal bleeding	✓			✓		✓	✓	✓	✓
Temperature	✓	✓	✓	✓	✓		✓		
Stool consistency				✓					
Pulse	✓		✓	✓					
Abdominal pain/tenderness		✓		✓	✓				
Abdominal mass									
Weight loss				✓	✓				
Nausea & vomiting				✓					
Extraintestinal manifestations		✓		✓			✓		
General health				✓					
ESR	✓		✓				✓		✓
Hemoglobin	✓		✓				✓		✓
Albumin		✓	✓						
Other lab tests			✓						
Sigmoidoscopy			✓	✓		✓	✓	✓	
Radiological		✓	✓						
Functional assessment						✓	✓	✓	

CP, developed for use in clinical practice
CT, part of clinical trial

plicated by symptoms that result from previous surgical resections and the difficulty of scoring for complications such as strictures and fistulae.

One of the earliest British activity measures in Crohn's disease was the St Marks Crohn's Disease Index (Willoughby et al 1971, Burnham et al 1979). It has been used in clinical trials and includes clinical and laboratory criteria (Table 35.3). Burnham et al (1979) added the functional concepts of sense of wellbeing and limitations on activity, and discussed the similarity between this index and the Crohn's Disease Activity Index (CDAI, Best et al 1976) (see later).

In 1974 de Domball et al modified the Truelove and Witts' ulcerative colitis index in a study of the short-term course and prognosis of Crohn's disease in the OMGE trial. Hodgson (1982) considered this index suitable for colonic disease, but unlikely to be of value in severe small-bowel disease. Talsted and Gjone (1976) devised an activity index for Crohn's disease which identified mild, moderate and severe disease using a combination of symptoms and laboratory data (Table 35.3). These were weighted to give a figure which described the disease activity as a percentage. As with their 1976 ulcerative colitis activity index, the parameters used in the calculation were so numerous that use of this index in practice is difficult. Garrett and Drossman (1990) highlighted the fact that none of the newer indices had been validated against existing ones. This may well have been because existing indices were felt to be so flawed as to make any correlation relatively meaningless.

The Crohn's Disease Activity Index (CDAI) developed by Best et al (1976) for the United States National Cooperative Crohn's Disease Study and later modified (Best et al 1979), is perhaps the most widely used disease activity index for Crohn's disease. It was developed in a preliminary study to ensure a uniform approach to the measurement of disease activity in a number of centers participating in therapeutic clinical trials. Eighteen predictors of disease activity were selected by participating clinicians, together with a physician-based global assessment score consisting of four categories from very well to very poor. Multiple regression and stepwise deletion analyses were applied to derive an equation and weightings that could be used to measure Crohn's disease activity.

The CDAI requires completion of a patient diary card over 7 days, and computation on the eight variables that were finally selected from the original 18. Total CDAI scores range from negative to over 600, and the index has been validated against the physician's global score. In 1979, Best et al rederived the weightings for each of the weight parameters used in the original CDAI, using a larger patient group. As little difference was found between the original and new values, they suggested that there was no advantage in using the rederived values in place of the original.

A number of clinicians found the CDAI difficult to use and this has been a major criticism (Mee et al 1978, Singleton 1987, Hyams et al 1991). Best and Becktel (1981) suggested a simplified version using diarrhea, pain and wellbeing assessed on 1 rather than 7 days, and deleted

Table 35.3 Disease indices in Crohn's disease

Reference	Willoughby et al 1971	De Dombal et al 1974	Talsted & Gjone 1976	Best et al 1976	Harvey & Bradshaw 1980	Van Hees et al 1980	Myren et al 1984	Wright et al 1985	Sandler et al 1988
Index name	St Marks CD	De Dombal	Talsted	CDAI	Harvey–Bradshaw	DUTCHAI	IOIBD Oxford	Cape Town index	
Setting	CT	CP	CP	CT	CP	CP	CT	CP	CT
Features									
Bowel habit	✓	✓	✓	✓	✓		✓	✓	✓
Rectal bleeding	✓	✓		✓					
Stool consistency				✓		✓			
Abdominal tenderness/pain	✓	✓	✓	✓	✓		✓	✓	✓
Abdominal mass	✓			✓			✓	✓	
Weight loss/gain	✓	✓	✓	✓				✓	
Temperature	✓	✓	✓	✓		✓	✓	✓	
Pulse		✓	✓						
Nausea & vomiting				✓					
General health	✓			✓	✓			✓	✓
Surgery						✓			
Perianal complication	✓			✓			✓		
Fistula	✓		✓	✓			✓	✓	
Extraintestinal complications	✓			✓	✓		✓	✓	
Laboratory tests				✓					
ESR	✓		✓			✓			
Hemoglobin	✓		✓						
Albumin	✓		✓			✓			
Other lab tests	✓		✓						
Endoscopy			✓						
Quetelet (body weight/height)						✓			
Drug therapy for diarrhea				✓					
Weighting	variable	1–3	variable	variable	0–5	variable	equal	0–3	variable

CP, developed for use in clinical practice
CT, part of clinical trial

opiate use, hematocrit and weight. This simplifed version has not been widely used by other investigators, many of whom have chosen to derive their own indices. More fundamental to the accuracy of the CDAI in measuring disease activity is the subjective aspect of the index, which has a high impact on the final score (Hodgson 1982, Singleton 1987). In addition, the inclusion of hematocrit has been criticized as it is not the most accurate laboratory determinant of disease activity (Andre et al 1981, Beck 1987). In 1980 Harvey and Bradshaw proposed a simplified activity index using five variables, which correlated well with the CDAI ($r = 0.9$); this index has subsequently seen widespread use in clinical studies but suffers from the same subjectivity as the CDAI. In particular, Myren et al (1984) highlighted the effect that the number of loose motions had on the score, and proposed an amended version for which the score for the number of bowel motions per day ranged from 0 to 5 maximum. In addition, Brooke (1980) suggested that the Harvey–Bradshaw score was inappropriate for patients who had undergone resection of diseased bowel.

In order to increase the objectivity of assessment of disease severity Van Hees et al (1980) proposed an activity index using laboratory tests and clinical findings. Like the Talsted and Gjone activity index (1976) before it, the Van Hees index is quite lengthy and may be too time-consuming for routine clinical practice. Its objective nature means that it correlates poorly with other more subjective indices (Myren et al 1984). Nevertheless, it has been used in a number of studies and is less prone to interobserver variation (de Dombal and Softley 1987). In an attempt to clarify some of these issues the OMGE and the International Organization for the study of Inflammatory Bowel Disease (IOIBD) conducted a study comparing various indices, including the IOIBD index (Oxford index). These indices showed poor correlation with the Van Hees index and the other more subjective indices leading to the conclusion that the Van Hees index was measuring inherently different values from most other assessments. By way of contrast, Crama-Bohbouth et al (1989) felt that many activity indices were poor indicators of inflammation compared to specific laboratory tests. However, laboratory tests did correlate with the Van Hees index, presumably because this index itself contains laboratory parameters.

Studies by Myren et al (1984) and Reed et al (1991), which used predefined objectives, have shown that subjective indices such as the CDAI, Harvey–Bradshaw and Oxford index tend to correlate well with each other, with physician scores and with patient wellbeing scores (Myren et al 1984). Conversely, Reed et al (1991) found that physician scores correlated best with the Van Hees index. In addition, Goebell et al (1990) reported a better correlation between the CDAI and a clinical rating scale than was the case for the Van Hees index, which correlated best with a laboratory rating. Wright et al (1985) produced a modified version of the IOIBD (Oxford) index in which 10 parameters were scored from 0 to 3; this version is also known as the Capetown Index, and correlated better than seven other indices, including the CDAI, Harvey–Bradshaw and Van Hees, with patient assessment of wellbeing (Reed et al 1991).

OTHER CLINICAL INDICES

A number of disease indices have been suggested for use in children with Crohn's disease. These take account of the effects of the disease on growth rate, and pay particular attention to height and weight (Lloyd-Still and Green 1979, Hyams et al 1991). Both indices have been validated against the CDAI and a modified Harvey–Bradshaw index (Myrens et al 1984) respectively.

Relatively little attention has been given to clinical indices in patients who have undergone surgery, or who have specific complications such as perianal bleeding. Allan et al (1992) developed a specific index to measure anal disease activity for use in therapeutic trials and clinical management consisting of three parameters, namely spontaneous anal pain, pain on defecation and inhibition of locomotion. Morowitz and Kirsner (1981) discussed the functional impairment of ileostomy patients before and after surgery using parameters such as general health, medical therapy, duration of illness and patient outcomes. This study showed that most patients with an ileostomy have an active and productive life. Likewise, Kennedy et al (1982) found that the general health of such patients, when measured using clinical and laboratory tests, was good. The health-related quality of life improved after surgery in a group of ulcerative colitis patients studied by Mcleod et al (1991).

In an alternative approach to the measurement of Crohn's diseases activity, Present et al (1980) used individual goal setting for patients. They scored improvements or deterioration in their condition based on specific problems that individuals experienced. This approach would be difficult to implement in clinical trials, but does provide a means of focusing and individualizing patient treatment in clinical practice.

ENDOSCOPIC INDICES IN IBD

Table 35.2 and 35.3 indicate some of the clinical activity indices that have utilized endoscopic appearance. Baron et al (1964) proposed grading system (I–IV) for endoscopic appearance in order to reduce interobserver variation. This has been widely used in research and clinical practice. Hodgson (1982) highlighted some of the problems with relating endoscopic appearance to clinical assessment, citing Truelove and Witts (1955) as an example in which patients in clinical remission still showed active endoscopic appearances. Subsequently, Modigliani et al (1990) found that only 38 of 131 patients with Crohn's disease in clinical remission demonstrated endoscopic remission, and Cellier et al (1994) have also concluded that clinical activity in Crohn's disease seems to be independent of mucosal lesion severity. In 1989 Rachmilewitz proposed an endoscopic index which was used in a multicenter study of 5-aminosalicylic acid versus sulfasalazine. This index included four categories, with severity weighting in each category; the authors do not comment on whether this increased the sensitivity of their index. Mary and Modigliani (1989) have also described an endoscopic index which correlated with global assessment of endoscopic disease severity.

HEALTH STATUS MEASURES IN IBD

There has recently been interest in the impact of IBD on the everyday lives of patients, including their worries and fears about present and future health (Drossman et al 1989). Garrett and Drossman (1990) have suggested that assessment of health status should include psychological status, culture, coping strategies, stressful life events and level of social support. They argue that disease activity alone is insufficient to measure a patient's illness experience. Drossman et al (1989) suggested that clinical evaluation should include assessment of physical, psychological and social functioning. They also used the Sickness Impact Profile, which is a general measure of quality of life, to show that IBD patients experience moderate social and psychological functional impairment. Patients with Crohn's disease also appeared to have more impairment than those with ulcerative colitis. Later workers found that although patients with IBD had both physical symptoms and impaired psychosocial functioning, their health status was still generally good (Drossman et al 1991). These findings agree with Mitchell et al (1988), who developed the McMaster Inflammatory Bowel Disease Quality of Life Index. This is one of the most commonly used indices in IBD (Guyatt et al 1989). Arguably these quality of life indices have become the IBD activity indices of the 1990s, since the use of clinical activity indices alone, has poor sensitivity to changes in health status (Garrett and Drossman 1990).

In a review of quality of life assessment in IBD Moody and Mayberry (1992) commented on the current view that quality of life is impaired at numerous levels. They suggested that a uniformly agreed, reliable and valid measure of quality of life was required, and later developed a disease-specific index of the quality of life in Crohn's and ulcerative colitis (QuICC), which has since been validated (Moody & Mayberry 1993). Irvine (1993) and Irvine et al (1994) have discussed the validity and reliability of the use of the McMaster quality of life index in therapeutic trials, recognizing that newer indices are required for specific patient subgroups. The development and use of quality of life indices is discussed in more depth elsewhere in this book.

CONCLUSION

The application of clinical indices in IBD is complex, with no real consensus as to which parameters should be used. Some features, however, are common to most of the indices used today. In ulcerative colitis these include bowel habit, rectal blood loss and endoscopic grading, together with hemoglobin, albumin and ESR, whereas in Crohn's disease they include bowel habit, abdominal tenderness or pain, abdominal mass, extraintestinal complications, and laboratory tests consisting of orosomucoid, ESR and C-reactive protein. An increase in the number of parameters included in an index seems to reduce 'user friendliness' and compliance in practice. The increasing use of health status and quality of life measures shows that investigators are beginning to place appropriate emphasis on the 'illness experience', which is rightly used to determine clinical decisions and predict outcome.

REFERENCES

Allan A, Linares M D, Spooner H A, Alexander-Williams J 1992 Clinical index to quantitate symptoms of perianal Crohn's disease. Diseases of the Colon and Rectum 35: 656–661

Andre C, Descos L, Landais P, Fermanian J 1981 Assessment of appropriate laboratory measurements to supplement the Crohn's Disease Activity Index. Gut 22: 571–574

Baron J H, Connell A M, Lennard-Jones J E 1964 Variations between answers in describing mucosal appearances in protocolitis. British Medical Journal 1: 89–92

Beck I T 1987 Laboratory assessment of inflammatory bowel disease. Digestive Diseases and Sciences 32: 26s–41s

Best W R, Becktel J M 1981 Crohn's disease activity index as a clinical instrument. In: Recent advances in Crohn's disease. Nijhoff, Amsterdam, pp 7–11

Best W R, Becktel J M, Singleton J W 1979 Rederived values of the eight coefficients of the Crohn's Disease Activity Index. Gastroenterology 77: 843–846

Best W R, Becktel J M, Singleton J W, Kern F Jr 1976 Development of a Crohn's disease activity index. Gastroenterology 70: 439–444

Brooke B N 1980 Index of Crohn's disease activity. Lancet 1: 711

Bucknell N A, Gould S R, Day D W, Lennard-Jones J E, Edwards A M 1978 Controlled trial of disodium cromoglycate in chronic persistent ulcerative colitis. Gut 19: 1140–1143

Burnham W R, Lennard-Jones J E, Heckesweiller P, Colin R, Geffroy Y 1979 Oral BCG vaccine in Crohn's disease. Gut 20: p 229–233

Cellier C, Sahmond T, Froguel E et al 1994 Correlations between clinical activity, endoscopic severity and biological parameters in colonic or ileocolonic Crohn's disease. A prospective multicentre study of 121 cases. Gut 35: 231–235

Crama-Bohbouth G, Pena A S, Biemond I et al 1989 Are activity indices helpful in assessing active intestinal inflammation in Crohn's disease? Gut 30: 1236–1240

De Dombal F T 1986 Measuring and quantifying the status of patients with inflammatory bowel disease: some international data and reflections. Oxford University Press, New York

De Dombal F T, Softley A 1987 IOIBD report No. 1: observer variation in calculating indices of severity and activity in Crohn's disease. Gut 28: 474–481

De Dombal F T, Burton I L, Clamp S E, Goligher J C 1974, Short term prognosis of Crohn's disease. Gut 15: 435–443

Drossman D A, Leserman J, Mitchell C M, Li Z, Zagami E A, Patrick D L 1991 Health status and health care use in persons with inflammatory bowel disease. A national sample. Digestive Diseases and Sciences 36: 1746–1755

Drossman D A, Patrick D L, Mitchell C M, Zagami E A, Appelbaum M I 1989 Health related quality of life in inflammatory bowel disease functional status and patient worries and concerns. Digestive Diseases and Sciences 34: 1379–1386

Edwards F C, Truelove S C 1963 The course and prognosis of ulcerative colitis. Gut 4: 299–315

Garrett J W, Drossman D A 1990 Health status in inflammatory bowel disease: biological and behavioural considerations. Gastroenterology 99: 90–96

Goebell H, Wienbeck M, Schomerus H, Malchow H 1990 Evaluation of Crohn's disease activity index and the Dutch index for severity and activity of Crohn's disease. An analysis of the data from the European Cooperative Crohn's disease study. Medizinische Klinik 85: 573–576

Gomes P, Du Boulay C, Smith C, Holdstock G 1986 Relationship between disease activity indices and colonscopic findings in patients with colonic IBD. Gut 27: 92–95

Guyatt G, Mitchell A, Irvine E J 1989 A new measure of health status for clinical trials in inflammatory bowel disease. Gastroenterology 96: 804–810

Harvey R F, Bradshaw J M 1980 A simple index of Crohn's disease activity. Lancet 1: 514

Heatley R V, Calcraft B J, Rhodes J, Owen E, Evans B K 1975 Disodium cromoglycate in treatment of chronic proctitis. Gut 16: 559–563

Hodgson H J F 1982 Assessment of drug therapy in inflammatory bowel disease. British Journal of Clinical Pharmacology 14: 159–170

Hyams J S, Ferry G D, Mandell F S et al 1991 Development and validation of a pediatric Crohn's disease activity index. Journal of Pediatric Gastroenterology and Nutrition 12: 439–447

Irvine E J 1993 Quality of life – measurement in inflammatory bowel disease. Scandinavian Journal of Gastroenterology 28: 36s–39s

Irvine E J, Feagan B, Rochon J et al 1994 Quality of life: a valid and reliable measure of therapeutic efficacy in the treatment of inflammatory bowel disease. Gastroenterology 106: 287–296

Kennedy H K, Lee E C, Claridge G, Truelove S C 1982 The health of subjects living with a permanent ileostomy. Quarterly Journal of Medicine 203: 341–357

Lennard-Jones J E, Ritchie J K, Hilder W, Spicer C C 1975 Assessment of severity of colitis. Gut 16: 579–584

Lloyd-Still J D, Green O C 1979 A clinical scoring system for chronic inflammatory bowel disease in children. Digestive Diseases and Sciences 24: 620–624

McLeod R S, Churchill D N, Lock A M, Vanderburch S, Cohen Z 1991 Quality of life of patients with ulcerative colitis preoperatively and postoperatively. Gastroenterology 101: 1307–1313

Mary J F, Modigliani R 1989 Development and validation of an endoscopic index of severity for Crohn's disease: a prospective multicentre study. Gut 30: 983–989

Mee A S, Brown D J, Pewell D P 1978 Crohn's disease activity index is it useful? Gut 19: A990

Mitchell A, Guyatt G, Singer J et al 1988 Quality of life in patients with inflammatory bowel disease. Journal of Clinical Gastroenterology 10: 306–310

Modigliani R, Mary J Y, Simon J et al 1990 Clinical, biological and endoscopic picture of attacks on Crohn's disease. Gastroenterology 98: 811–818

Moody G A, Mayberry J F 1992 Quality of life: its assessment in gastroenterology. European Journal of Gastroenterology and Hepatology 4: 1025–1030

Moody G A, Mayberry J F 1993 Quality index in Crohn's and colitis. Gastrointestinal Research Unit, Leicester

Morowitz D A, Kirsner J B 1981 Ileostomy in ulcerative colitis. American Journal of Surgery 141: 370–375

Myren J, Boucher I A D, Watkinson G, De Dombal F T 1979 Inflammatory bowel disease – an OMGE survey. Scandinavian Journal of Gastroenterology 14 (Suppl 56): 1–27

Myren J, Boucher I A D, Watkinson G, Softley A, Clamp S E, De Dombal F 1984 The OMGE multinational inflammatory bowel disease survey 1976–1982: a further report on 2657 cases. Scandinavian Journal of Gastroenterology 19 (Suppl 95): 1–27

Oliason G, Sjodahl R, Tagesson C 1990 Glucocorticoid treatment in Ileal Crohn's disease: relief of symptoms but not of endoscopically viewed inflammation. Gut 31: 325–328

Powell-Tuck J, Brown R L, Lennard-Jones J E 1978 A comparison of oral prednisolone given as single or multiple daily doses. Scandinavian Journal of Gastroenterology 13: 833–837

Present D H, Korelitz B I, Wisch N, Glass J L, Sachar D B, Pasternack B S 1980 Treatment of Crohn's disease with 6-mercaptopurine. New England Journal of Medicine 302: 981–987

Rachmilewitz D 1989 Coated mesalazine 5-amino salicylic acid versus sulphasalazine in the treatment of active ulcerative colitis: a randomised trial. British Medical Journal 298: 82–86

Reed J F, Faust L A, Rosen L 1991 Assessment of disease activity in a registry of Crohn's disease in Eastern Pennsylvania. Gastroenterology 29: 378–382

Sandler R S, Matthew C J, Kupper L L 1988 Development of a Crohn's disease index for survey research. Journal of Clinical Epidemiology 41: 451–458

Schroeder K W, Tremaine W J, Ilstrup D M 1987 Coated oral 5-amino salicyclic acid therapy for mildly to moderately active ulcerative colitis. New England Journal of Medicine 317: 1625–1629

Seo M, Okada M, Yao T, Ueki M, Arima S, Okumura M 1992 An index of disease activity in patients with ulcerative colitis. American Journal of Gastroenterology 87: 971–976

Singleton J W 1987 Clinical activity assessment in inflammatory bowel disease. Digestive Diseases and Sciences 32: 42s–45s

Sninsky C A, Cort D H, Shanahan F 1991 Oral mesalamine (Asacol) for mildly to moderately active ulcerative colitis. Annals of Internal Medicine 115: 350–355

Stierlin E 1912 Zur rontgendiagnostic der colitis ulcerosa. Zeitschrift für Klinische Medizin 75: 486–493

Talsted I, Gjone E 1976 The disease activity of ulcerative colitis and Crohn's disease. Scandinavian Journal of Gastroenterology 11: 403–408

Truelove S C, Witts L J 1955 Cortisone in ulcerative colitis. British Medical Journal 1: 1041–1048

Van Hees P, Van Elteren P H, Van Lier H J J, Van Tongren J H M 1980 An index of inflammatory activity in patients with Crohn's disease. Gut 21: 279–286

Willoughby J M T, Kumar A M, Beckett J, Dawson A M 1971 Controlled trial of azathioprine in Crohn's disease. Lancet 2: 944–946

Wright J P, Marks I N, Parfitt A 1985 A simple index of Crohn's disease activity. The Cape Town index. South African Medical Journal 68: 502–503

36. Ulcerative colitis versus Crohn's disease – one disease or two?

H. J. F. Hodgson

When all the clinical, radiological, endoscopic and histopathological data have been collated, 85–90% patients with inflammatory bowel disease can be classified with confidence as suffering from either ulcerative colitis or Crohn's disease. It is important to bear in mind that, in the absence of firm evidence as to the etiology of these conditions, the criteria on which the assignment to ulcerative colitis or Crohn's disease is made are purely descriptive. Among patients thought to have idiopathic inflammatory bowel disease, 15% or so remain unclassified between these two diagnoses. Some of these will fit the histological criteria that have been put forward for a diagnosis of 'indeterminate colitis'. However, clinicians often use this term on more general grounds, meaning merely that the available information does not at the moment allow a distinction to be drawn between ulcerative colitis and Crohn's disease.

Clearly, making a clinical distinction between ulcerative colitis and Crohn's disease is worthwhile, because experience demonstrates that clinical course, response to treatment, recurrence rate after colectomy and the propensity to develop various complications differ significantly between the two clinical groups. The first section of this chapter will therefore describe the clinical, pathological, radiological, endoscopic and other distinctions of these two conditions (recalling that these distinctions are descriptive). However, the existence of the 10–15% of patients with unclassified colonic inflammation raises the questions: are the two clinically distinct forms, ulcerative colitis and Crohn's disease, truly distinct, or are they the well defined poles of a continuous spectrum of inflammatory bowel disease? Indeterminate colitis, and the arguments concerning 'inflammatory bowel disease – one disease or two?' – will be covered in the latter half of the chapter.

ULCERATIVE COLITIS VERSUS CROHN'S DISEASE – DISTINGUISHING FEATURES

If a patient with inflammatory bowel disease has significant small-intestinal disease, or inflammation which extends proximal to the colon with more than just a few inches of contiguous backwash ileitis, the diagnosis of ulcerative colitis will immediately be dismissed; the difficulties of diagnosis arise when inflammation is apparently confined to the colon.

Clinical

Local symptoms

Classically ulcerative colitis is episodic, often with quite prolonged periods of remission of symptoms, whereas Crohn's disease is more likely to follow a chronic continuous course. Frank rectal bleeding and tenesmus are more suggestive of ulcerative colitis, whereas many patients with Crohn's colitis may have active disease with neither symptom. The distinction reflects largely the disease distribution, with rectal involvement being characteristic of ulcerative colitis but often absent in Crohn's disease. Pain in ulcerative colitis is characteristically hypogastric and tends to occur just before defecation; Crohn's colitis can give similar colicky spasms but (if the left side of the colon/rectum is spared) not closely associated with defecation. Among these clinical features only persistent severe diarrhea without bleeding is really helpful in making a clinical distinction, pushing the classification towards Crohn's disease.

Associated conditions

Perianal disease, either concurrently or historically, is a strong clinical association of Crohn's disease. Features include anal fissures, perianal fistulae – particularly if complicated and extending to above the intestinal sphincter – and fleshy skin tags with dusky cyanotic skin colour, which are often surprisingly painless. Anal stenosis can also occur, but is seen also in ulcerative colitis, and anal fissures and low fistulae may also occur in ulcerative colitis as they do in the general population. Other fistulae – coloenteric, colovesical or colocutaneous – are all strongly suggestive of Crohn's disease, but rectovaginal fistulae are reported in up to 4% of patients with ulcerative colitis.

The extraintestinal manifestations of ulcerative colitis and Crohn's disease are not identical, but the differences are largely in the frequency with which they occur. Erythema nodosum is more common in Crohn's disease than in ulcerative colitis (Samitz 1973), whereas pyoderma gangrenosum is more common in ulcerative colitis (Shatin 1971). Aphthous mouth ulcers are more common in Crohn's disease. Ulcerative colitis and Crohn's disease have a similar incidence of ankylosing spondylitis: the peripheral joint manifestations tend to be more episodic in ulcerative colitis, reflecting the easily recognized acute relapses characteristic of that condition; small joint arthralgias may be more common and less episodic in Crohn's disease, probably reflecting a response to clinically inapparent gut inflammation (Palumbo et al 1973). Finger clubbing is more common in Crohn's disease (Perry et al 1972). Eye complications are common in both, although both episcleritis and iritis are probably more common in Crohn's disease (Greenstein et al 1976).

There are some systemic associations which do occur with marked differences in frequency between the two types of disease. In some cases the difference reflects the presence of small-intestinal disease (hyperoxaluria and renal stones in extensive Crohn's disease, ureteric obstruction and a high incidence of biliary stones in terminal ileal disease), and there are straightforward physiological reasons for these complications. It is intriguing, however, that there are two significant associated systemic diseases whose incidence varies strikingly between ulcerative colitis and Crohn's disease. Systemic amyloidosis is well recognized in Crohn's disease – clinically apparent in 1% or so (Greenstein et al 1976) and a reported incidence of up to 25% of amyloid deposits at autopsy; it is very rare indeed in ulcerative colitis (Shorvon 1977, Rand et al 1980). Conversely, the hepatic complication of sclerosing cholangitis is in general much more commonly associated with ulcerative colitis than Crohn's disease (Chapman et al 1983).

Endoscopic appearances

Unless local therapy with corticosteroid or 5-aminosalicylate preparations has led to rectal improvement while the more proximal bowel is still inflamed, proctoscopic examination in active ulcerative colitis will reveal inflammation, with diffusely erythematous friable mucosa extending for a variable length proximally. The concept that ulcerative colitis can spare the rectum still has some adherents, but is certainly unfashionable (Spiliadis & Lennard-Jones 1987), and rectal sparing will usually lead to classification as indeterminate colitis. The continuous diffuse involvement of ulcerative colitis usually clearly differs from that of Crohn's, which is generally segmental, although some patients with Crohn's disease may have a proctitis very similar to that of ulcerative colitis. In active Crohn's colitis the features include rectal sparing in 50%, and positive colonoscopic features of superficial ulceration (93%), deep ulceration (49%), erythema (44%), aphthous ulceration (35%) and ulcerated stenosis (10%) (Modigliani et al 1990). Pseudopolyps, often thought of as associated predominantly with severe ulcerative colitis, were reported in 41% of patients with active Crohn's colitis at colonoscopy. Pera et al (1987) prospectively studied over 250 patients with inflammatory bowel disease by colonoscopy, and in comparison with a final overall diagnosis reported that endoscopy allowed correct classification in 89%. In 7% diagnosis was indeterminate, and either this diagnosis or a misassignment with respect to the final agreed diagnosis was more common when inflammation was severe. Continuous symmetrical granularity and erosions were the most diagnostically helpful features for ulcerative colitis, and discontinuous involvement, cobblestoning, rectal sparing and discrete ulcers were most helpful for classification as Crohn's colitis.

Radiology

The impact of radiology in differentiating ulcerative colitis and Crohn's disease is broadly similar to that of colonoscopy, although since even double contrast barium enema examination underestimates disease extent compared to endoscopic and histological examination, it is probably less sensitive (Geboes & Vantrappen 1975). Fine continuous granularity of the mucosal wall, with symmetrical involvement extending for a varying distance proximally, characterizes mild ulcerative colitis; as already referred to above, rectal sparing is rare and probably generally secondary to treatment. With more severe disease, haustrae disappear and ulcerations become more prominent, and may give rise to 'collar-stud'-like abscesses. Inflammatory polyps, or surviving mucosa standing proud above adjacent denuded areas of mucosa, are found in severe disease and regenerative polyps may persist after healing. In severe pancolitis there may be an associated patulous ileocecal valve and a short symmetrically inflamed but non-stenosed segment of terminal ileum. Benign strictures may occur (in less than 10% of patients): these are generally smooth and tapered, and are more common in pancolitis.

Radiologically Crohn's disease is generally patchy, more likely to be proximal than distal, often spares the rectum, and the tendency for submucosal fibrosis to occur characteristically leads to asymmetry of the colonic wall. Aphthoid ulcers may be clearly seen in good-quality examinations, but ulceration can also be diffusely granular, as in ulcerative colitis. Pseudopolyps and strictures and occur, although the latter are generally not smooth and symmetrical as in ulcerative colitis. Transmural fissures give rise to 'rosethorn' ulcers, and sometimes to fistulae, but collar-stud-like ulcers similar to those in ulcerative colitis may occur. The terminal ileal involvement of Crohn's generally differs strikingly from the backwash ileitis of ulcerative colitis – usually with narrowing and edematous cobblestoning.

Other diagnostic approaches

More recent diagnostic approaches – ultrasound, CT (computed tomography) and magnetic resonance imaging – have contributed to distinguishing ulcerative colitis from colonic Crohn's disease by identifying the thicker wall of the colon affected with Crohn's disease, and allowing the identification of fistulae and abscesses, each suggesting Crohn's disease. Leukocyte scanning techniques show active inflammation of both types, and help clinical distinction between ulcerative colitis and colonic Crohn's disease by the evidence they give of disease distribution in the colon, by the identification of abscesses, and by the simultaneous identification of inflamed small intestine.

Laboratory parameters

Blood tests

The laboratory parameters relevant to assessing inflammatory bowel disease are discussed in Chapter 34. There are measurements that vary between ulcerative colitis and Crohn's disease, although they often reflect disease site (e.g. low B_{12} and folate in Crohn's disease reflecting small-intestinal involvement). However, the higher levels of the acute-phase reactants, C-reactive protein and serum amyloid A, probably reflect differences in the cytokines generated in the tissues and present in the circulation (e.g. higher IL-1 and IL-6 levels), and may be diagnostically helpful (though not definitive). Circulating ANCA (antineutrophil cytoplasmic antibodies) are much more common in ulcerative colitis.

Histological examination

The characteristic features of active ulcerative colitis – a mixed pleomorphic inflammatory cell infiltrate in the lamina propria, flattening and, in severe cases, ulceration of the surface epithelium, distortion of crypts, with loss of mucus from goblet cells, cryptitis and crypt abscesses – should all be readily appreciable from mucosal biopsy specimens (Morson et al 1990). In contrast, some of the features that argue most strongly for the diagnosis of Crohn's disease – transmural inflammation, submucosal fibrosis, fissures and fistulae – are not appreciable without full-thickness specimens (Cook & Dixon 1973, Price 1978). Patchiness of inflammation, prominent lymphoid follicles and mucus retention, in rectal or colonoscopic biopsies, will favor Crohn's disease, but the 'hallmark', the granuloma, is often not found in such specimens. Geboes and Vantrappen (1975) made 'definitive' diagnoses of Crohn's disease in colonic biopsies, on the basis of granulomas, in 24% of cases.

OVERALL PICTURE

The author's estimate is that 20% of patients with inflammation confined to the colon present a diagnostic problem between ulcerative colitis and Crohn's disease. With time, these clinically indeterminate cases often become clearer and are more likely to develop features that favor a diagnosis of Crohn's disease rather than ulcerative colitis. Mild proctitis, for example, may turn out in time to be associated with terminal ileal Crohn's disease or Crohn's disease elsewhere in the colon. Surgical practice generally admits of less doubt, but even here there are patients in whom reclassification takes place. Certain surgical procedures are conventionally limited to patients with ulcerative colitis, notably ileal pouch anastomosis. Despite a preoperative diagnosis of ulcerative colitis in 100%, subsequent events have led to reclassification as Crohn's disease in 1–7% in different series (Pemberton 1987, Hyman et al 1991). It is less common for Crohn's disease to be reclassified as ulcerative colitis, although interestingly in a group of over 100 patients submitted to split ileostomy under the impression that Crohn's disease was present, at least 10 eventually were diagnosed as having ulcerative colitis (Harper et al 1983).

INDETERMINATE COLITIS

The term indeterminate colitis is used loosely. The clinician's usage has been referred to above, and might be better as 'inflammatory bowel disease, type uncertain'. Adopting this phrase would leave the term indeterminate colitis to describe that group of patients whom – even though a colectomy specimen has become available – histopathological examination cannot assign to either ulcerative colitis or Crohn's disease. Price (1978) described the histological features characteristic of this group, which constitute 10–15% of colectomy specimens, and commented that this histological diagnosis is more likely to be assigned when the colectomy was performed as an emergency. The growing popularity of restorative surgery, performing ileal pouch anastomosis, makes this group significant; the majority of surgeons regard the operation as the gold standard in ulcerative colitis, but fraught with hazard in Crohn's disease, and thus the postcolectomy patient with indeterminate colitis prevents a particular problem for future management. Recent data demonstrate that perhaps half or more cases of histologically indeterminate colitis can be assigned to either ulcerative colitis or Crohn's disease if all clinical features are taken into account, and that the patient whose colitis is still indeterminate after review of the histology of the resected colon does *not* develop Crohn's disease in the long term (Wells et al 1991). In conclusion, the patient with true, histologically defined 'indeterminate colitis' is a suitable candidate for restorative surgery (Pezim et al 1989). In contrast, the patient with clinically defined 'inflammatory bowel disease, type uncertain' may well turn out to have Crohn's disease.

ONE DISEASE OR TWO?

As already mentioned, in the absence of etiological information the definitions of ulcerative colitis and Crohn's disease are descriptive. It is possible that recognition of an etiological agent, such as an infectious agent in one and not the other condition, will short-circuit debate on the relationship of these two conditions in the future. It is interesting to reflect, however, that a single agent can give very different patterns of disease, reflecting either evolution over time (consider the evolution of primary chance, secondary syphilis and a gumma in syphilis) or differences in immune response (the granulomatous, paucibacillary lesions of tuberculoid leprosy contrast with the bacteria-loaded, non-granulomatous diffuse inflammation of lepromatous leprosy).

There is no doubt that most patients can be clinically assigned to a diagnosis of one or other condition. The first part of this chapter surveyed this with respect to colonic disease, and clearly patients with involvement of the small intestine in addition are not perceived as diagnostic problems. However, there are issues which arise because our definitions are descriptive. *If* ulcerative colitis does not affect the small intestine (except for backwash ileitis), a patient with small intestinal involvement *cannot* have ulcerative colitis. *If* granulomas are taken as the hallmark of Crohn's disease, a patient with ulcerative colitis *cannot* have granulomas.

These tenets are easily accepted because they are clinically helpful (at least in 90% of cases). However, meticulous reading of the descriptive literature shows that many of the 'certainties' are either misremembered or incorrect. Granulomas, for example – anyway detected in only 60–70% of tissues from Crohn's disease (Holdstock et al 1982) – are found in 4% of patients who in all other criteria have ulcerative colitis (Schachter et al 1970). Severe ulcerative colitis can spread transmurally. Up to 20% of ulcerative colitis patients have some perianal problems. The pouchitis that occurs in the small intestine of ulcerative colitis patients after ileal pouch procedures demonstrates the tendency of these patients to develop small-intestinal inflammation (this very rarely occurs when the same procedure is performed for familial polyposis). Crypt abscesses occur in Crohn's disease as well as ulcerative colitis (Morson et al 1990).

I believe it is now possible to link current concepts of the pathogenesis of these diseases with our knowledge of their genetic, geographic and environmental background, and support the hypothesis that these diseases form a spectrum. Although we have as yet no definitive evidence for a single infectious agent, we have overwhelming evidence that the tissue damage in inflammatory bowel disease is mediated by the expression of immune pro-inflammatory processes, of many different kinds, in the mucosa. Activated T cells, increased B-cell numbers, recruited macrophages, activated polymorphonuclear leukocytes, synthesized and released proinflammatory cytokines and eicosanoids, and perhaps dysregulation of anti-inflammatory cytokines, are all implicated. We are now aware that the immune responses demonstrated by an individual – in the case of inflammatory bowel disease perhaps only to the constituents of the gut lumen – are not solely driven by the antigenic challenge. They reflect perhaps equally the genetic constitution of the individual. We already have some clear clues that some of the manifestations in ulcerative colitis and Crohn's disease can be related to genetic makeup. Although there is no overall strong HLA association with either type of inflammatory bowel disease, certain manifestations are more likely to occur when inflammatory bowel disease affects patients with a given HLA haplotype. Among those with Crohn's disease, HLA B8-positive individuals have less tendency to develop granulomas (Holdstock et al 1982). Patients with ulcerative colitis who are HLA B8 and DR3 positive have a tenfold increase in their risk of developing sclerosing cholangitis (Chapman et al 1983). Increasing knowledge of inflammatory processes shows that genetics and inflammation are closely linked. Ulcerative colitis patients, and not those with Crohn's, have an increased frequency of a particular polymorphism of the IL-1 receptor antagonist gene, which may indicate to different ability, control endogenous IL-1 mediated inflammation (Mansfield et al 1994). Another example is the evidence concerning TNF-α (tumor necrosis factor-α). The tendency to produce TNF-α, a major proinflammatory cytokine, is linked to polymorphisms of the TNF-α gene. At the phenotypic level TNF-α is generated more readily from monocytes in Crohn's disease than in ulcerative colitis (Mazlam & Hodgson 1992), and preliminary evidence implicates TNF-α as a major contributor to the inflammatory process in Crohn's disease, with apparently good responses to therapy with anti-TNF-α antibodies (Van Dullemen et al 1994).

There is strong genetic evidence of a predisposition to inflammatory bowel disease. Within many affected families, however, both ulcerative colitis and Crohn's disease are found (Mons'en et al 1987), indicating perhaps that in such families the common genetic factor is a tendency to develop inflammation in the bowel. Coinheritance of one set of genes might push this inflammatory process along a pathway leading to diffuse mucosal inflammation; another set might predispose to produce cytokines which lead to granulomatous inflammation. Those genes predisposing to diffuse mucosal inflammation might be associated with a greater tendency to mount an immune response to ANCA, and to affect the biliary tract (Snook et al 1989); those associated with the granulomatous inflammatory tendency might segregate with a greater tendency to produce cytokines generating C-reactive protein and serum amyloid A (Chambers et al 1987). Environmental factors are also relevant. Smoking, for example, predisposing to Crohn's disease in most but not all populations studied, might exert its effects by enhancing the production of those cytokines leading to granulomatous inflammation. In most instances the combination of the variety of genetic factors and environmental factors leads to a pattern clearly describable as ulcerative colitis or Crohn's disease. Clearly, however, in such a complex situation individuals will emerge whose condition cannot be clearly categorized, and who lie at varying points along a continuous spectrum.

REFERENCES

Chambers R E, Stross P, Barry R E, Whicher J T 1987 Serum amyloid A protein compared with C-reactive protein, alpha 1-antichymotrypsin and alpha 1-acid glycoprotein as a monitor of inflammatory bowel disease. European Journal of Clinical Investigation 17: 460–467

Chapman R W, Barghese Z, Gaul R, Patel G, Kokinon N, Sherlock S 1983 Association of primary sclerosing cholangitis with HLA-B8. Gut 24: 38–41

Cooke E M, Dixon M F 1973 An analysis of the reliability of detection and diagnostic value of various pathological features in Crohn's disease and ulcerative colitis. Gut 14: 255–262

Geboes K, Vantrappen G 1975 The value of colonoscopy in the diagnosis of Crohn's disease. Gastrointestinal Endoscopy 22: 18–23

Greenstein A J, Janowitz H D, Sachar B D 1976 The extraintestinal complication of Crohn's disease and ulcerative colitis: a study of 700 patients. Medicine 55: 401–412

Harper P H, Truelove S C, Lee E C G, Kettlewell M G W, Jewell D P 1983 Split ileostomy and ileocolostomy for Crohn's disease of the colon and ulcerative colitis: a 20 year survey. Gut 24: 106–113

Holdstock G, MacPherson B, Beeken W L 1982 HLA B8 and granuloma formation in Crohn's disease. Gut 23: 600–602

Hyman N H, Fazio W, Tukson W B, Lavery I C 1991 The consequences of an ileal pouch–anal anastomosis for Crohn's colitis. Diseases of the Colon and Rectum 34: 653–657

Mansfield J C, Holden H, Tarlow J K et al 1994 Novel genetic association between ulcerative colitis and the anti-inflammatory cytokine interleukin-1 receptor antagonist. Gastroenterology 106: 637–642

Mazlam M Z, Hodgson H J F 1992 Peripheral blood monocyte cytokine production and acute phase response in inflammatory bowel disease. Gut 33: 773–778

Modigliani R, Mary J Y, Simon J F et al 1990 Clinical, biological, and endoscopic picture of attacks of Crohn's disease. Evolution on prednisolone. Gastroenterology 98: 811–818

Mons'en V, Bromstrom O, Nordenrall B, Sorstad J, Hellers G 1987 Prevalence of inflammatory bowel disease among relatives of patients with ulcerative colitis. Scandinavian Journal of Gastroenterology 22: 214–218

Morson B C, Dawson I M P, Day D W et al 1990 Inflammatory disorders. In: Morson B C, Dawson I M P, Day D W, Jass J R, Price A B, Williams G T (eds) Morson and Dawson's gastrointestinal pathology, 3rd edn. Blackwell Scientific, Oxford, pp 477–549

Palumbo P J, Ward L E, Sauer W G, Scudamore H H 1973 Musculoskeletal manifestations of inflammatory bowel disease – ulcerative and granulomatous colitis and ulcerative proctitis. Mayo Clinic Proceedings 48: 411–416

Pemberton J H 1987 Surgery for ulcerative colitis. Surgical Clinics of North America 67: 633–673

Pera A, Bellando P, Caldera V et al 1987 Colonoscopy in inflammatory bowel disease. Diagnosis accuracy and proposal of an endoscopic score. Gastroenterology 92: 181–185

Perry P M, Evans G A, Davies J D 1972 Regional ileitis, ulcerative colitis and clubbed colitis. Gastroenterologica 107: 272–282

Pezim M E, Pemberto J H, Beart R W et al 1989 Outcome of indeterminate colitis following ileal pouch and anastomosis. Diseases of the Colon and Rectum 32: 653–658

Price A B 1978 Overlap in the spectrum of non-specific inflammatory bowel disease – 'colitis indeterminate'. Journal of Clinical Pathology 31: 567–577

Rand J A, Brandt L J, Baker N H, Lynch J 1980 Ulcerative colitis complicated by amyloid. American Journal of Gastroenterology 74: 185–188

Samitz M H 1973 Skin complications of ulcerative colitis and Crohn's disease. Cutis 16: 533–537

Schachter H, Goldstein M J, Rappaport H, Fennessy M B, Kirsner J B 1970 Ulcerative and granulomatous colitis: validity of different diagnostic criteria. Annals of Internal Medicine 72: 841–851

Shatin H 1971 How I treat pyoderma gangrenosum. Postgraduate Medical Journal 49: 251–253

Shorvon P J 1977 Amyloidosis and inflammatory bowel disease. American Journal of Digestive Disease 22: 209–213

Snook J A, Champan R W, Fleming K et al 1989 Anti-neutrophil nuclear antibody in ulcerative colitis, Crohn's disease and primary sclerosing cholangitis. Clinical Experimental Immunology 76: 30–33

Spiliadis C A, Lennard-Jones J E 1987 Ulcerative colitis with relative sparing of the rectum. Diseases of the Colon and Rectum 30: 354–356

van Dullemen H M, Hommes D W, Meenan J et al 1994 Complete remissions of steroid-refractory Crohn's disease after administration of monoclonal anti-TNF antibody cA2. Gastroenterology 107: A576

Wells A D, McMillan I, Price A B et al 1991 Natural history of indeterminate colitis. British Journal of Surgery 78: 179–181

37. Infective colitis

C. A. Hart

INTRODUCTION

As a cause of death worldwide, diarrheal diseases are second only to cardiovascular disease (Hibbs 1993), and in infancy they are the most common cause of death (Walsh & Warren 1979, Synder & Merson 1982).

It is estimated that in developing countries each child experiences three to eight episodes of diarrheal disease per year (Mata et al 1983, WHO 1984). In Asia, Africa and Latin America this results in 4.6–6 million deaths each year, the majority of which are in children (Snyder & Merson 1982). In contrast, in the USA the attack rates of diarrheal disease in children is two episodes per year (Glass et al 1991). The overall estimated mortality rate is 3000–4000 per year and the majority of deaths occur in the elderly (>74 years) (Lew et al 1991). In the UK the numbers of cases of diarrheal disease reported to the Public Health Laboratory continues to rise each year. For example, since 1980 reported cases of campylobacteriosis have increased by 450%, salmonellosis by 250%, and shigellosis by 200% (Davies et al 1995).

There are approximately 35 different microorganisms capable of causing diarrheal disease. Although it is not possible to diagnose clinically the etiological agents causing diarrheal disease, it is possible to assign them to two groups: those causing inflammatory and those causing non-inflammatory diarrhea (Table 37.1). Under normal circumstances the two may be differentiated on clinical grounds and by examination of a wet or stained preparation of feces for pus cells. The presence of five or more pus cells per high-power field indicates an inflammatory diarrhea. This is of course less useful in patients with coexistent active inflammatory bowel disease, when pus cells would be excreted as part of the disease. Nevertheless, this classification does provide a useful method for discussing causes of acute colitis (Table 37.2).

CAMPYLOBACTER spp.

Only as recently as 1977 was campylobacter finally recognized as an important cause of diarrheal disease

Table 37.1 Inflammatory and non-inflammatory diarrhea

	Inflammatory	Non-inflammatory
Symptoms	Fever, abdominal pain tenesmus	Nausea, vomiting abdominal pain and fever not prominent
Stool	Frequent, small to moderate volume. Mucus, bloodstained, pus cells present	Voluminous, watery, pus cells absent
Site	Distal ileum and colon	Proximal small intestine
Mechanisms	Death of enterocytes due to toxin or invasion. Loss of mucosa initiating inflammatory response	Osmotic or secretory

(Skirrow 1977). It is now the most common cause of diarrheal disease in adults and a not insignificant cause in children.

Microbiology

Campylobacter is a curved or spiral Gram-negative rod varying in length from 1.5 to 3.5 μm and in diameter from 0.2 to 0.4 μm. It is motile by means of one or more flagella. There are 15 species in the genus, but only four, *C. jejuni*, *C. coli*, *C. upsaliensis* and *C. lari*, are important in human diarrheal disease. Each is thermophilic (optimally at 42–43°C and not at 25°C) and microaerophilic.

Epidemiology

In the UK and USA the estimated incidence of infection is between 68 and 1100 infections per 100 000 population per year (Pearson & Healing 1992, Allos & Blaser 1995). The highest rates of infection are in young adults, and males in the age ranges 15–24 years and 45–54 years are at the greatest risk. In UK campylobacteriosis peaks in late May or early June, but infections occur throughout the year. *C. jejuni* is associated with the majority of infections. It is part of the normal enteric flora of cattle, poultry, sheep, domestic pets, wild animals and birds, and

Table 37.2 Pathogens in inflammatory and non-inflammatory diarrhea

	Inflammatory	Non-inflammatory
Viruses	Human immunodeficiency virus* Cytomegalovirus*	Rotavirus Adenovirus 40/41 Astrovirus Calicivirus Norwalk Agent Small round structureless viruses Coronavirus Torovirus Bredavirus Pestivirus
Bacteria	Enteroinvasive *E. coli* (EIEC) Enterohemorrhagic *E. coli* (EHEC) Enteroaggregative *E. coli* (EAggEc) *Aeromonas hydrophila* *Plesiomonas shigelloides* *Campylobacter* spp. *Salmonella* spp. *Shigella* spp. *Yersinia enterocolitica* *Clostridium difficile* *Myobacterium avium/intracellulare**	Enterotoxigenic *E. coli* (ETEC) Enteropathogenic *E. coli* (EPEC) *Vibrio cholerae* *Vibrio parahaemolyticus* *Plesiomonas shigelloides* *Campylobacter* spp. *Salmonella* spp. *Bacillus cereus* *Clostridium perfringens*
Protozoa	*Entamoeba histolytica*	*Cryptosporidium parvum* *Giardia lamblia* *Blastocystis hominis* *Cyclospora cayetanensis* *Isospora belli** *Enterocytozoon bieneusi**

* In immunocompromised patients

can be acquired from them directly or indirectly in water. Person-to-person transmission occurs rarely, primarily in young children. The reservoir of *C. coli* is the intestinal flora of pigs and poultry, that of *C. upsaliensis* dogs and cats and that of *C. lari* is the intestines of seagulls, dogs and horses. In outbreaks milk, water and poultry are the most common sources. A mode of acquisition which is perhaps unique to the UK is by bird attack on bottled milk delivered to the doorstep (Southern et al 1990). When jackdaws and magpies, in particular, peck through foil milk bottle tops they also defecate, leaving *C. jejuni* in the milk. Campylobacter can survive for 2–5 weeks in milk at 4°C, but do not multiply. Approximately 10% of reported cases of campylobacteriosis are associated with foreign travel.

Pathogenesis

The infective dose can be as low as 500 organisms and as high as 10^6 organisms, with an incubation period of 2–5 days. Campylobacter can produce either inflammatory or non-inflammatory diarrhea. Examination of colonic biopsies shows a neutrophil inflammatory infiltrate with ulcerated epithelium, glandular atrophy, loss of mucus production and crypt abscesses. This histopathology may thus easily be confused with Crohn's disease or ulcerative colitis. The precise pathogenic mechanisms are unclear, but it does appear that the organisms can elaborate an enterotoxin with a mode of action similar to cholera toxin (Ruiz-Palacios et al 1985) and a cytotoxin (Yeen et al 1983), but the clinical significance of the latter is unclear (Everest et al 1992). Campylobacters are also able to invade intestinal cells in vitro (Everest et al 1992) and in animal models (Caldwell et al 1983). How they invade or induce intestinal cell death and inflammation is not known. However, non-motile mutants of *C. jejuni* lacking flagella are much less pathogenic.

Diagnosis

Campylobacteriosis cannot be diagnosed clinically. Specific diagnosis is by culture of feces on appropriate selective media (e.g. Skirrow's medium) at 42°C under microaerophilic conditions. Direct Gram stain of feces can be of value.

Clinical features

In outbreaks, approximately 20% of patients are asymptomatic. Diarrhea is the prominent feature and can be severe (20% of patients have more than 14 stools per day). Most patients will also have fever, abdominal pain, malaise and nausea. On average diarrhea persists for 6–7 days. Campylobacter can also cause bacteremia (in about 1% of cases of diarrheal disease). This generally occurs in older patients (>65 years) and those with immune deficit (e.g. hypogammaglobulinemia, AIDS or malnutrition). The mortality rate is 2.4 per 1000 infections (Smith & Blaser 1986).

Other complications include reactive arthritis in patients with the HLA-B27 phenotype, encephalopathy and carditis. Symptomatic or asymptomatic *C. jejuni* infection is also associated with Guillain–Barré syndrome (GBS), and it is estimated that it is responsible for 20–40% of cases of GBS.

Treatment and prevention

Most patients require no specific antimicrobial chemotherapy and oral rehydration is sufficient. However, this may not be the case for patients with bacteremia, those with immune deficit, and pregnant women. Macrolides such as erythromycin or clindamycin are the treatment of choice. Although fluoroquinolones such as ciprofloxacin or ofloxacin might be effective, increasing resistance is being reported.

There is no vaccine available, so prevention of infection is by avoiding ingestion of the bacteria. This requires education of the public about potential reservoirs and improved food and kitchen hygiene.

SALMONELLA spp.

There are over 2250 serovars of Salmonellae. *S. typhi*, which causes typhoid fever, and *S. paratyphi* A, B and C, which cause paratyphoid fever, rarely cause simple diarrheal disease and therefore will not be considered further. The remainder are able to infect a wide variety of animals, reptiles and birds, either symptomatically or asymptomatically. Infections in humans are termed salmonelloses.

Microbiology

Salmonellae are Gram-negative rods (0.6 μm × 2–3 μm) that are motile by virtue of peritrichate flagella. They grow aerobically and anerobically from 7°C to 48°C (optimally at 37°C). They are killed by heat (e.g. 72°C for 15 seconds or 65.6°C for 12 minutes), but are resistant to freezing and drying (Baird-Parker 1990). The serovars are defined by the possession of O or somatic antigens (on lipopolysaccharides) and H or flagellar antigens in the Kauffman–White scheme. With so many serovars and the development of new DNA typing methods the wisdom of such a scheme has been challenged, but to change nomenclature would introduce too many problems (Old 1992).

Epidemiology

In the UK the reported incidence of salmonellosis is 50 per 100 000 per year (Baird-Parker 1990) and in the USA between 40 and 50 thousand cases are reported each year (CDC 1993). These figures are thought to underestimate the problems by 20 to 100-fold. Recently the number of reported cases of salmonellosis has plateaued, or even declined slightly. In the UK, salmonellosis peaks in summer and in the USA in late summer and autumn. Most infections in the UK are due to *S. enteritidis* (50–60% of cases), *S. typhimurium* (20–25%), and *S. virchow* (5%). Most cases are acquired by ingesting food or water contaminated by Salmonellae, although secondary person-to-person spread may also occur. Unlike *Campylobacter* spp. Salmonellae can and do multiply on food. Certain animal species tend to be associated with different Salmonellae. For example *S. typhimurium* is associated with cattle and *S. enteritidis* with poultry. The remarkable increase in the incidence of salmonellosis over the past 20 years has been a result of changes in eating habits (e.g. fast-food restaurants and deep-frozen poultry) and intensive farming techniques (e.g. battery hens, minimal-graze cattle). The latter has resulted in Salmonellae becoming established as part of the normal flora of cattle and poultry (between 1970 and 1980, 80% of frozen chickens were contaminated by Salmonellae) and the former has resulted in incomplete cooking and thus incomplete killing of the Salmonellae. A recent trend has been the colonization of chickens' egg-laying apparatus by *S. enteritidis* phage type 4, which has resulted in outbreaks of diarrhea following ingestion of uncooked (e.g. in mayonnaise) or partially cooked eggs. Infection may also occur when animal feces contaminate fruit and vegetables that are eaten uncooked. There has even been an outbreak in the USA following contamination of a marijuana crop.

Pathogenesis

Generally the infective dose is high ($>10^6$ organisms) but in certain patients (young children, the elderly), with certain serovars (e.g. *S. enteritidis*) and when ingested in high-fat foods (e.g. chocolate or salami) the infective dose can be much lower (10^1–10^4 organisms). The incubation period is 12–48 hours (but can rarely be up to 7 days). Salmonellae induce an inflammatory diarrhea by binding to and penetrating enterocytes. This leads to a neutrophil infiltration and eventual enterocyte death. There is evidence of upregulation of Salmonella pathogenicity genes once at the site of infection (Macbeth & Lee 1993, Mahan et al 1993). This results in the expression of surface appendages on the bacteria that are necessary for entry into epithelial cells (Ginocchio et al 1994). The bacteria bind to an unknown receptor on the enterocyte and induce its membrane to form ruffles (Francis et al 1993). The bacteria are then taken into the cell by pinocytosis into membrane-bound vacuoles. This results in disruption of epithelial barrier function (Jepson et al 1995) and release of interleukin (IL)-8 (Eckmann et al 1993, MacCormick et al 1993), which is a neutrophil chemoattractant. Salmonellae are also able to survive within macrophages, which is important in the pathogenesis of disseminated Salmonella infection. Genes present on cryptic (virulence) plasmids (Gulig & Doyle 1993) as well as on the bacterial chromosome are necessary for full expression of disease. A cluster of 12 chromosomal genes are involved in attachment and entry into epithelial cells and survival in phagosomes (Groisman & Ochman 1993). Some share homology with *Shigella flexneri* virulence plasmid genes and some are upregulated in the acid environment of phagocytic vacuoles (Alpuche-Aranda et al 1994).

Clinical features

Salmonella infection may result in diarrheal disease, enteric fever, bacteremia with or without localization, or asymptomatic carriage. Gastroenteritis is the most common presentation and does not differ greatly from that due to *Campylobacter* spp., and may also present as 'pseudo-appendicitis'. Illness lasts from 2 to 7 days. Enteric fever is rarely due to the food-poisoning Salmonellae. Certain serovars (*S. typhimurium*, *S. choleraesuis* and *S. dublin*) are more likely to result in bacteremic spread. Bacteremia occurs more frequently in those under 5, the elderly and those with immune deficit. Intact humoral and cell-mediated immunity is necessary for recovery from and defense against salmonellosis. In mice a gene encoding a macrophage membrane transporter protein is linked to protection from bacteremic illness (Vidal et al 1993). A similar gene has been described in humans (Levin et al 1995). Salmonella bacteremia is a feature in HIV-infected patients prior to the development of AIDS (Gilks et al 1990).

Localization of bacteremic infection occurs particularly in cardiovascular lesions, bones and meninges, although infections have been reported from most sites in the body. Between 0.2 and 0.6% of patients with salmonellosis become chronic intestinal carriers. Finally, salmonelloses are associated with reactive arthritis in susceptible individuals (HLA-B27).

Diagnosis

Specific diagnosis is by isolation of Salmonellae from feces, blood or other infected sites. Isolation from feces requires liquid (e.g. selenite) or solid (e.g. DCA or SS agar) selective media. Methods involving various DNA technologies are under investigation, but no one method is universally accepted.

Treatment and prevention

Fluid and electrolyte replacement is the most important therapy. Previously antibiotic therapy was avoided because of concerns about the development of resistance and induction of the carrier state. Some now recommend treatment of traveller's diarrhea with fluoroquinolones such as ciprofloxacin, but quinolone resistance in enteric pathogens is on the increase (Keystone 1994). Antibiotic therapy should be given to the febrile toxic patient with salmonellosis. There is as yet no vaccine available, and prevention is as for Campylobacter infection.

SHIGELLA spp.

Shigellae are the cause of bacillary dysentery and the genus is named after Shiga, who first demonstrated the bacteria in 1898. Dysentery has been a disease of poor and crowded communities throughout history, and is a major cause of morbidity and mortality in developing countries. After over 25 years of decline the incidence of shigellosis has recently greatly increased in the UK (Newman 1993).

Microbiology

Shigellae are Gram-negative bacilli which differ from Salmonellae in being aflagellate and thus non-motile. There are four species. *Sh. dysenteriae* (ten serotypes), *Sh. flexneri* (six serotypes), *Sh. boydii* (15 serotypes) and *Sh. sonnei* (one serotype). All will grow on simple media under aerobic and anerobic conditions.

Epidemiology

Sh. dysenteriae is rarely encountered outside the tropics, where it causes epidemics of bacillary dysentery with mortality rates up to 20%. In the UK 90% of cases are due to *Sh. sonnei*, and most of the rest are caused by *Sh. flexneri*. Outbreaks of *Sh. sonnei* infection tend to occur in nurseries and primary schools. Shigellae are solely human pathogens and infection is spread feco-orally, directly or in food and water. They are maintained in the community by asymptomatic carriers. Over 50% of cases in the UK are in children under 10. However, up to 50% of household contacts of a case of shigellosis will also become infected (Davies 1952).

Pathogenesis

The infective dose of Shigellae is low (10–100 organisms). All pathogenic Shigellae carry a large (c. 220 kb) plasmid which is essential for pathogenicity (Sansonetti 1991). It carries pathogenicity genes clustered in two loci, which are transcribed in opposite directions. One cluster of genes encodes invasion plasmid antigens (ipa) A–D. These gene products, together with some in the other cluster, mediate attachment to and entry into colonic enterocytes. Bacteria are taken up by a process of endocytosis (Fig. 37.1). They lyse the endocytoxic vesicle and escape into the cytoplasm, where they multiply (Sansonetti et al 1986). In the colonocyte cytoplasm they attach to microfilaments and stress fibers, and move to the periphery of the cell in a manner similar to the movement of intracellular organelles (Vasselon et al 1991). They then penetrate into adjacent colonocytes, thus moving from cell to cell without re-entering the gut lumen. Colonocyte death is induced by apoptosis (Zychlinsky et al 1992) rather than necrosis. Invasion of epithelial cells by Shigellae also results in the release of IL-8 and other cytokines, which attract neutrophils (Raqib et al 1995) and result in the inflammatory diarrhea. *Sh. dysenteriae* in particular, but probably other species also, secrete shiga toxin and shiga-like toxins (or verocytotoxins) 1 and 2. These inhibit protein synthesis and lead to cell death. Their production is related to development of the hemolytic uremic syndrome (HUS) and possibly encephalopathy.

Clinical features

Sh. sonnei infection in the UK and the USA tends to be mild and seldom results in fulminant dysentery. *Sh. flexneri*, and especially *Sh. dysenteriae*, are more likely to produce

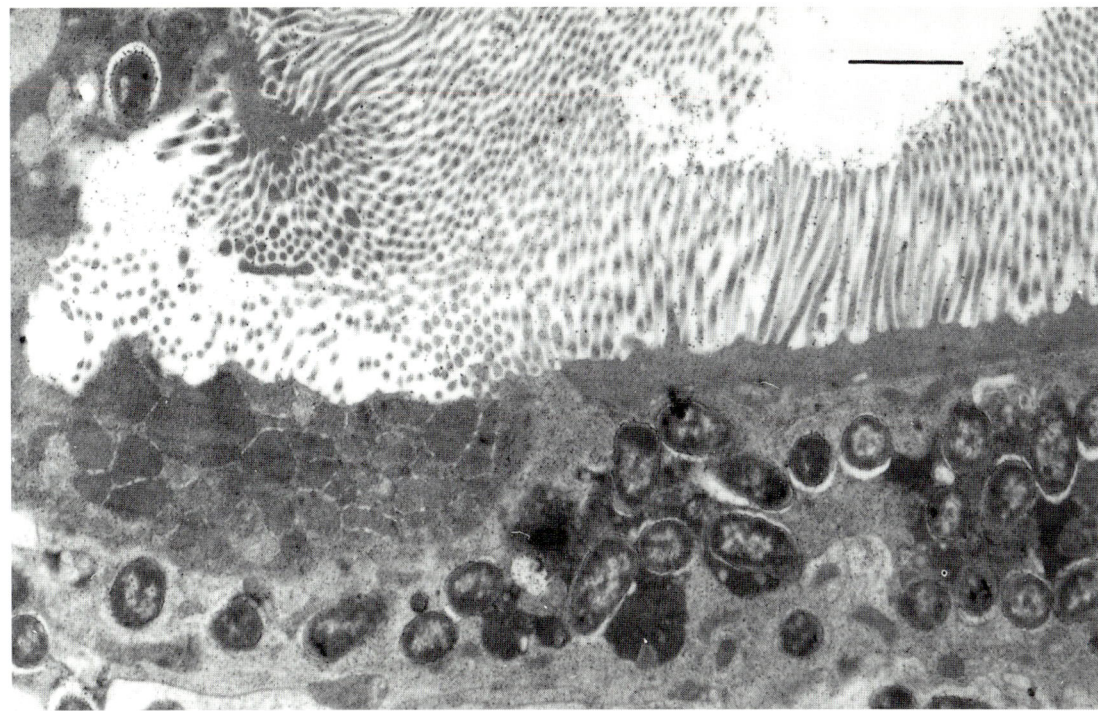

Fig. 37.1 Thin-section electron micrograph of colonic epithelium infected with *Shigella sonnei*. The bacteria are present within the cytoplasm and most have been released from their endocytotic vesicles. (bar = 2 μm).

severe disease. Mild infection, which often has features of a secretory diarrhea, lasts from 5 to 7 days. Prolonged carriage seldom extends beyond 2 months. Local complications, such as toxic megacolon, perforation and rectal prolapse, are common in younger patients infected with *Sh. dysenteriae*. HUS is seen almost exclusively with *Sh. dysenteriae* 1 infection, but reactive arthritis can occur with any of the Shigellae in susceptible individuals.

Treatment and prevention

Severe shigellosis, and especially that due to *Sh. dysenteriae*, requires antimicrobial chemotherapy. Multidrug resistance in Shigellae is problematic, but most are still susceptible to fluoroquinolones. These are not currently licenced for use in children because of the possibility of cartilage damage (seen in young beagle dogs). There is no vaccine for Shigellae and prevention must rely on appropriate hygienic precautions (PHLS 1993).

ESCHERICHIA COLI

There are at least five different pathogenic strategies used by *E. coli* to cause diarrheal disease (Hart et al 1993). Of these, three (enteroinvasive *E. coli*, enterohemorrhagic *E. coli* and enteroaggregative *E. coli*) cause colitis.

Enterohemorrhagic *E. coli* (EHEC)

This is an increasingly important cause of food poisoning.

Microbiology

E. coli is a motile Gram-negative rod indistinguishable from Salmonellae and Shigellae microscopically. It grows readily on most media aerobically or anerobically. It is part of the normal intestinal flora (c. 10^7 organisms/g). The enteropathic strains of *E. coli*, however, are not normal flora but to distinguish them from the normally excreted *E. coli* can be difficult. *E. coli* strains can be serotyped by possession of different O- or somatic antigens present on lipopolysaccharide molecules in the outer leaflet of their outer membrane. Certain O- serogroups are linked to the different enteropathic strains. For example, one of the major EHEC strains is O157:H7; however, other serogroups such as O26, O103, O111, O113, as well as some 50 other serogroups, have been implicated. Unfortunately, serogrouping is insufficiently sensitive or specific for absolute delineation of EHECs. This is done by detection of EHEC pathogenicity genes or gene products.

Epidemiology

EHEC can be part of the normal flora of cattle and pigs; in addition, some outbreaks of infection have been associated with contact with chicken coops (Tozzi et al 1994). Most information has come from studies of outbreaks of hemorrhagic colitis and/or HUS. Such outbreaks have been associated with the consumption of minced beef, luncheon meat, potatoes, unpasteurized cider and milk, mayonnaise and drinking water, and contact with swimming-pool water or cow manure (Tarr 1995). Direct person-to-person spread has also been described. Most outbreaks have been due to 0157:H9, and the role of other EHEC serogroups is unclear. However, there have been few surveys of sporadic EHEC infection.

Pathogenesis

The infective dose of EHEC is low. EHEC adhere to the intestinal mucosa using a fimbrial adhesin encoded on a large (>80 kb) plasmid. They produce characteristic ultrastructural lesions confined to the terminal ileum and colon, termed attaching/effacement (Fig. 37.2). These are the same as those induced by enteropathogenic *E. coli*, but their effect is greater on the proximal small intestine (Embaye et al 1989). Indeed, both EHEC and EPEC chromosomes encode the *eae* (EPEC attachment/ effacement) gene which expresses a transmembrane protein, intimin, that results in F-actin accumulation and the subsequent development of ultrastructural lesions. In addition, EHEC express one or both of the toxins, verotoxin (VT) 1 and 2 (in American literature termed shiga-like toxins (SLT) 1 and 2). The VT1 and VT2 genes are present on bacteriophages rather than plasmids. The toxins are composed of five B subunits (the toxophore) and one A subunit (the toxin). The B subunits bind the VT to target cells. The receptor is the glycolipid, globotriasylceramide (Gb3 or gal (α) 1-4gal (β) 1–4 glucosylceramide). This is also the blood group antigen Pk or CD77, and it is believed that the tissue distribution of this antigen is related to disease manifestations (Taylor 1995). After attachment of the B subunit the whole molecule is internalized via clathrin-coated pits, the A subunit is cleaved by proteolysis and the 27 kDa A_1 subunit cleaves an adenine residue in 28S rRNA, thus terminating protein synthesis. This, it is presumed, leads to colonocyte death, perhaps by apoptosis (Inward et al 1995), and the resultant widespread inflammation causes the bloody diarrhea. HUS occurs in a proportion (*c.* 10%) of those with EHEC infection but is predominantly found in children under 10yr. It is presumed that VT enters the circulation and binds to renal glomerular endothelium, causing a thrombotic microangiopathy perhaps mediated by tumor necrosis factor release (Harel et al 1993). This resuls in intravascular hemolysis and renal failure. VT is also a neurotoxin, which might explain the encephalopathy occurring in some patients with hemorrhagic colitis.

Clinical features

In outbreaks approximately 10% of patients have a watery diarrhea alone, 90% have hemorrhagic colitis, and 10%

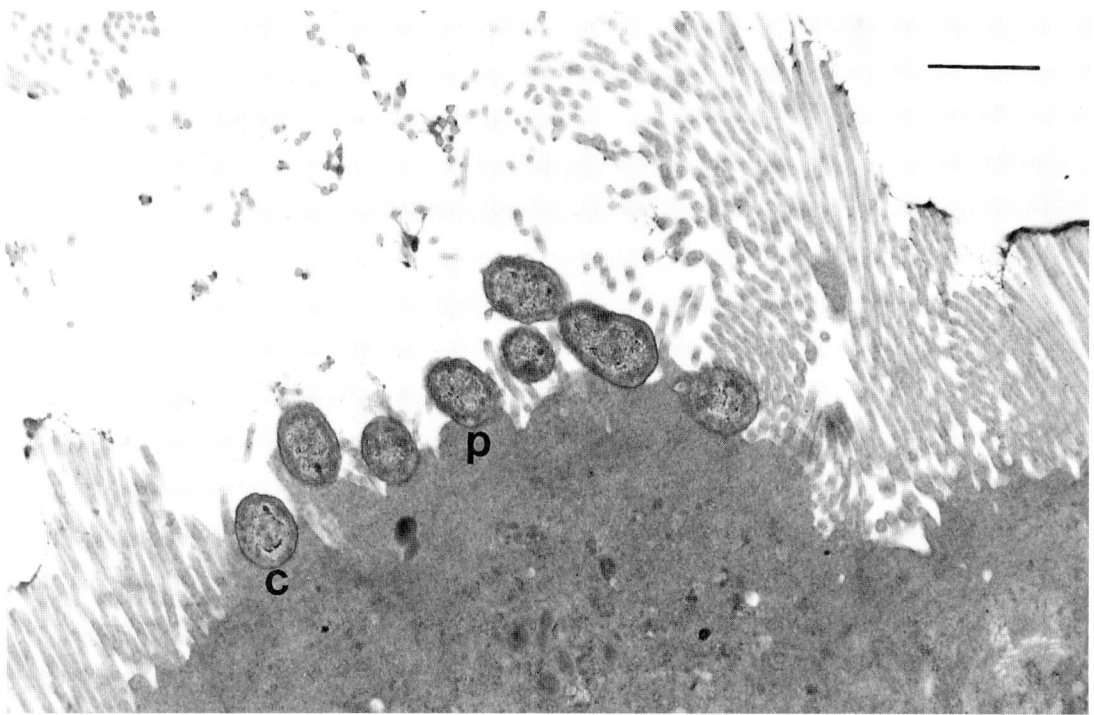

Fig. 37.2 Thin-section electron micrograph of ileal epithelium infected with an enterohemorrhagic *Escherichia coli* O157:H9. The ultrastructural damage, which involves intimate adherence of the bacteria and loss of microvilli, is termed attaching-effacement. The bacteria cause disruption of the terminal web, which results in a very plastic cell membrane and cup (c) and pedestal (p) formation is seen at sites of bacterial attachment. The enterocytes are subsequently killed by verotoxins. (bar = 2 μm).

also develop HUS. After an incubation period of 3–4 days a prodrome of cramping abdominal pain and transient pyrexia is often reported. Within 2 days this progresses to a non-bloody secretory-like diarrhea with or without vomiting. Then 1–2 days later in this progresses to a bloody diarrhea with abdominal tenderness. HUS develops, predominantly in children, and on average presents 1 week after onset of diarrhea. Diarrhea lasts from 4 to 10 days.

Diagnosis

E. coli O157:H7 can be detected by culture on sorbitol–MacConkey agar (it is sorbitol non-fermenting) and serogrouping. The other EHECs are more difficult and precise diagnosis depends upon detection of pathogenicity genes (*eae*, EHEC, VT1 and 2) or gene products (VT). Retrospective diagnosis can be by detection of antibodies to VT or O157 lipopolysaccharide.

Treatment and prevention

Treatment is by replacing fluid and electrolytes. Antibiotics are not indicated. No vaccine is available.

Enteroinvasive E. coli (EIEC)

These carry a virulence plasmid (*c*. 200 kb) and virulence genes that are almost identical to those of Shigellae, and produce colitis in the same way. They are of minor importance (<5% of cases) as a cause of diarrheal disease in the tropics, and are rarely encountered in developed countries. The diarrheal disease caused by EIEC is less severe than that of Shigellae.

Enteroaggregative E. coli (EAggEC)

EAggEc are a recently described cause of diarrheal disease and are so called because of their ability to form brick-like aggregates on cultured cells. They are associated with acute and persistent bloody diarrhea in children in the tropics (Bhan et al 1989). Little information is available on their role in developed countries. They adhere to colonic mucosa via bundle-forming fimbriae (Knutton et al 1993), and some strains elaborate a heat-stable toxin (Savarino et al 1993).

YERSINIA ENTEROCOLITICA

The frequency of isolation of *Y. enterocolitica* has increased in recent years, perhaps owing to increased awareness (Cover & Aber 1989). Nevertheless, it is still of minor importance (<3% of cases). It is a Gram-negative coccobacillus which is motile at lower temperatures (<25°C). Yersiniosis is more prevalent in the cooler parts of the northern hemisphere and most cases occur in autumn and winter (Doyle 1990). Infection is usually acquired as food poisoning, and the pig is the main reservoir of the major serovars (03 and 09). Infection can occur from eating improperly cooked pork, or indirectly via water. *Y. enterocolitica* can grow at temperatures as low as 0–2°C. Bacteria invade the ileal enterocytes, causing thickening and inflammation of the mucosa. Pathogenic strains carry a virulence plasmid (*c*. 60 kb) and its expression is temperature dependent. They also possess chromosomal *eae*-like genes. Diarrheal disease due to *Y. enterocolitica* is most common in young children. It does not differ greatly from other inflammatory diarrheas but persists for longer than most (about 2 weeks). *Y. enterocolitica* may also cause mesenteric adentitis, terminal ileitis (in children less than 5yr) and 'pseudoappendicitis'. Infection is also linked with reactive arthritis in HLA-B27-positive patients, erythema nodosum predominantly in women, and may cause bacteremia and metastatic infection. Treatment should be directed to managing dehydration. Extraintestinal infection is treated with aminoglycosides.

CLOSTRIDIUM DIFFICILE

Clostridium difficile was first recognized as an enteric pathogen in 1978 (Bartlett et al 1978), although a toxin associated with pseudomembranous colitis (PMC) was described a year earlier (Larson et al 1977).

Microbiology

Cl. difficile is a spore-bearing Gram-positive anerobic bacillus.

Epidemiology

Cl. difficile is part of the normal flora of from 3 to 15% of adults, but increases to over 45% in volunteers given antibiotics. Up to two-thirds of neonates carry toxigenic *Cl. difficile* with no ill effect. Development of PMC is usually related to administration of antibiotics that alter intestinal flora, such as macrolides, β-lactams, tetracyclines, trimethoprim, sulfonamides and quinolones. Recently some antineoplastic agents have also been associated with PMC. Most cases of PMC occur in elderly susceptible patients in hospital, or who have been recently discharged from hospital. Nosocomial spread of infection can cause major problems (Anglim & Farr 1994).

Pathogenesis

The acquisition rate of *Cl. difficile* depends upon environmental contamination by spores. For example, patients on leukemia wards have an acquisition rate of 2.5%, which rises to 21.5% in an outbreak (Tabaqchali & Jumaa

1995). Treatment with broad-spectrum antibiotics that are re-excreted into the intestine allows overgrowth of *Cl. difficile*. Two different toxins, A (308 kDa; enterotoxin) and B (250–270 kDa; cytotoxin), are elaborated by *Cl. difficile*. Toxin A causes fluid secretion and is a neutrophil chemoattractant. Toxin B is a potent cytotoxin. Both stimulate cytokine release from colonocytes. This results in the spectrum of changes including erythema, edema, severe inflammation and pseudomembrane formation, seen on colonoscopy. Early lesions are punctate but can coalesce with time to produce large areas of damage. The histopathological appearances are of acute and chronic inflammation in the lamina propria. The pseudomembranes are composed of fibrin, mucin, inflammatory cells and necrotic mucosal cells.

Diagnosis

This is by detection of *Cl. difficile* and/or its toxins by culture, antigen detection (for toxin), cytotoxicity assays or detection of genome by polymerase chain reaction.

Clinical features

Diarrhea varies in severity from a self-limiting change in bowel habit to severe copious (up to 30 stools per day) watery diarrhea. Other features include abdominal cramps, pyrexia (up to 105°F) and leukocytosis. There can be hypoalbuminemia, and it may be necessary to resect part of the bowel in severe disease.

Treatment and prevention

Metronidazole (400 mg every 8 hours orally for 7–10 days) is the treatment of choice. An alternative therapy is vancomycin (125 mg every 6 hours orally for 7–10 days). Approximately 20% of patients have relapse, when the diagnosis should be reconfirmed. Most relapses will respond to further courses of vancomycin or metronidazole. Prevention is aimed at stopping cross-infection and inappropriate use of antibiotics in hospitals.

ENTAMOEBA HISTOLYTICA

It is estimated that there are about 50 million cases of amebiasis, resulting in 100 000 deaths each year (Walsh & Warren 1979). The prevalence of infection can be up to 50% of populations in developing countries (Ravdin 1995).

Microbiology

Ent. histolytica is a protozoan parasite. The cyst (*c.* 12 μm in diameter) is the infective form and has a chitinous wall which allows it to remain viable for weeks under appropriate environmental conditions. Following ingestion they excyst in the small intestine to produce four trophozoites (*c.* 25 μm) per cyst. The cysts move to the large intestine where they feed on exfoliated cells and bacteria. The recently described *Ent. dispar* is morphologically indistinguishable from *Ent. histolytica*, but is non-pathogenic (Tannich et al 1989). All *Ent. dispar* and approximately 90% of *Ent. histolytica* infections are asymptomatic.

Epidemiology

High rates of amebiasis are found in Latin America, India, southern and western Africa and the Far East. High prevalence is related to poor socioeconomic and hygienic conditions, communal living, and being institutionalized. In developed countries amebiasis is found primarily in immigrants from endemic areas and in promiscuous male homosexuals. It is a very uncommon cause of travellers' diarrhea.

Pathogenesis

Trophozoites have a surface adherence lectin. This brings the trophozoite into close apposition to mucus, colonocytes and phagocytic cells by binding to galactose receptors. The trophozoites kill target cells on direct contact, perhaps by utilizing a saponin-like ionophore, by hemolysins or by proteolytic activity. This galactose-inhibitable lectin appears to function as an inhibitor of C8 and C9, thus avoiding the lytic activity of complement.

Diagnosis

Examination of fresh stool or material from ulcers or abscess to demonstrate motile amebae containing ingested erythrocytes is the most sensitive diagnostic tool. Serological assays using recombinant antigens are useful adjuncts. Detection of the galactose-inhibitable lectin in stool is currently under evaluation.

Clinical features

Amebic colitis presents with abdominal pain, tenesmus and frequent watery stools which contain blood and mucus. There may also be abdominal tenderness. Endoscopy will reveal characteristic hemorrhagic ulcers. Fulminant progressive colitis presents with severe bloody diarrhea and children under 2 are at particular risk. Chronic amebic colitis is clinically indistinguishable from idiopathic inflammatory bowel disease. Other local complications exclude ameboma, strictures of the anus, rectum or sigmoid colon, and perianal ulceration.

Extraintestinal amebiasis centers on hepatic amebic abscesses, which may extend to the pleura, lungs, pericardium, peritoneum, or even the brain.

Treatment and prevention

Invasive colitis and liver abscess are treated with metronidazole (750 mg orally 8-hourly for 10 days). For intraluminal infection diloxanide furoate or paromomycin are recommended. Prevention relies on public health measures, including improved sanitation and identifying and treating carriers (intraluminal infection). No vaccine is available, but a recombinant protein comprising part of the galactose-inhibitable lectin prevents amebic liver abscesses in gerbils (Soong et al 1995).

REFERENCES

Allos B M, Blaser M J 1995 *Campylobacter jejuni* and the expanding spectrum of related infections. Clinical Infectious Diseases 20: 1092–1101

Alpuche-Aranda C M, Racoosin E L, Swanson J A, Miller S I 1994 *Salmonella* stimulate macrophage micropinocytosis and persist within spacious phagosomes. Journal of Experimental Medicine 179: 601–608

Anglim A M, Farr B M 1994 Nosocomial diarrhea due to *Clostridium difficile*. Current Opinion in Infectious Diseases 7: 602–608

Baird-Parker A L 1990 Foodborne salmonellosis. Lancet 336: 1231–1235

Bartlett J G, Chang T W, Gurwith M, Gorbach S L, Onderdonk A B 1978 Antibiotic-associated pseudomembranous colitis due to toxin producing clostridia. New England Journal of Medicine 298: 531–534

Bhan M K, Raj P, Levine M M et al 1989 Enteroaggregative *Escherichia coli* associated with persistent diarrhoea in a cohort of rural children in India. Journal of Infectious Diseases 159: 1061–1064

Caldwell M B, Walker R I, Stewart S D, Rogers J E 1983 Simple adult model for *C. jejuni* enteritis. Infection and Immunity 42: 1176–1182

CDC 1993 Summary of notifiable diseases: United States 1992. Morbidity and Mortality Weekly Report 41: 3

Cover T L, Aber R C 1989 *Yersinia enterocolitica*. New England Journal of Medicine 321: 16–24

Davies E G, Elliman D A C, Hart C A, Nicoll A, Rudd P T 1995 Manual of childhood infections. WB Saunders, London, pp 328–329

Davies J B M 1952 Symptomless carriers in home contacts in Sonne dysentery. British Medical Journal 2: 191–192

Doyle M P 1990 Pathogenic *Escherichia coli*, *Yersinia enterocolitica* and *Vibrio parahaemolyticus*. Lancet 336: 1111–1115

Eckmann L, Kagnoff M F, Fierer J 1993 Epithelial cells secrete the chemokine interleukin-8 in response to bacterial entry. Infection and Immunity 61: 4569–4574

Embaye H, Batt R M, Saunders J R, Getty B, Hart C A 1989 Interaction of enteropathogenic *Escherichia coli* O111 with rabbit intestinal mucosa in vitro. Gastroenterology 96: 1079–1086

Everest P H, Goosens H, Butzler J-P et al 1992 Differentiated Caco-2 cells as a model for enteric invasion by *Campylobacter jejuni* and *C. coli*. Journal of Medical Microbiology 37: 319–325

Francis C L, Ryan T A, Jones B D, Smith S J, Falkow S 1993 Ruffles induced by *Salmonella* and other stimuli direct macropinocytosis of bacteria. Nature 364: 639–642

Gilks C F, Brindle R J, Otieno L S et al 1990 Life threatening bacteraemia in HIV-1 seropositive adults admitted to hospital in Nairobi, Kenya. Lancet 336: 545–549

Ginocchio C C, Olmstead S B, Wells C L, Galan J E 1994 Contact with epithelial cells induces the formation of surface appendages on *Salmonella typhimurium*. Cell 76: 717–724

Glass R I, Lew J F, Gangarosa R E, Le Baron C W, Ho M 1991 Estimates of morbidity and mortality rates for diarrheal disease in American children. Journal of Pediatrics 118: S27–S33

Groisman E A, Ochman H 1993 Cognate gene clusters govern invasion of host epithelial cells by *Salmonella typhimurium* and *Shigella flexneri*. EMBO Journal 12: 3779–3787

Gulig P A, Doyle T J 1993 The *Salmonella typhimurium* virulence plasmid increases the growth rate of *Salmonellae* in mice. Infection and Immunity 61: 504–511

Harel Y, Silva M, Giroir B, Weinberg A, Clearey T B, Beutler B 1993 A reporter transgene indicates renal-specific induction of tumor necrosis factor (TNF) by shiga-like toxin. Journal of Clinical Investigation 92: 2110–2116

Hart C A, Batt R M, Saunders J R 1993 Diarrhoea caused by *Escherichia coli*. Annals of Tropical Paediatrics 13: 121–131

Hibbs R G 1993 Diarrhoeal disease: current concepts and future challenges. Transactions of the Royal Society of Tropical Medicine and Hygiene (Suppl 3) 87: 1–2

Inward C D, Williams J, Chant I et al 1995 Verocytotoxin-1 induces apoptosis in vero cells. Journal of Infection 30: 213–218

Jepson M A, Collares-Buzato C B, Clark A, Hirst B H, Simmons N L 1995 Rapid disrupton of epithelial barrier function by *Salmonella typhimurium* is associated with structural modification of intercellular junctions. Infection and Immunity 63: 356–359

Keystone J S 1994 Single-dose antibiotic treatment for travellers' diarrhoea. Lancet 344: 1520–1521

Knutton S, Shaw R K, Bhan M K et al 1993 Ability of enteroaggregative *Escherichia coli* strains to adhere in vitro to human intestinal mucosa. Infection and Immunity 60: 2083–2091

Larson H E, Parry J V, Price A B et al 1977 Undescribed toxin in pseudomembranous colitis. British Medical Journal 1: 1246–1248

Levin M, Newport M J, D'Souza S et al 1995 Familial disseminated atypical mycobacterial infection in childhood: a human mycobacterial susceptibility gene. Lancet 345: 79–83

Lew J F, Glass R I, Gangarosa R E, Cohen I P, Bern C, Moe C L 1991 Diarrheal deaths in the United States, 1979 through 1987: a special problem for the elderly. Journal of the American Medical Association 265: 3280–3284

MacBeth K J, Lee C A 1993 Prolonged inhibition of bacterial protein synthesis abolishes *Salmonella* invasion. Infection and Immunity 61: 1544–1546

MacCormick B A, Colgan S P, Delp-Archer C, Miller S I, Madara J L 1993 *Salmonella typhimurium* attachment to human intestinal epithelial monolayers: transcellular signalling to subepthelial neutrophils. Journal of Cell Biology 123: 895–907

Mahan M J, Slauch J M, MeKalanos J J 1993 Selection of bacterial virulence genes that are specifically induced in host tissue. Science 259: 666–668

Mata L, Simhon A, Urrutia J, Kronmal R, Fernandez R, Crareia B 1983 Epidemiology of rotavirus in a cohort of 45 Guatemalan Mayan Indian children from birth to age 3 years. Journal of Infectious Diseases 148: 452–461

Newman C P S 1993 Surveillance and control of *Shigella sonnei* infection. Communicable Disease Report Review 3: 63–68

Old D C 1992 Nomenclature of *Salmonella*. Journal of Medical Microbiology 37: 361–363

Pearson A D, Healing T D 1992 The surveillance and control of campylobacter infection. Communicable Disease Report Review 2: 133–139

PHLS Working Group 1993 Revised guidelines for the control of *Shigella sonnei* infection and other infective diarrhoeas. Communicable Disease Report Review 3: 69–70

Raqib R, Wretlind B, Anderson J, Lindberg A A 1995 Cytokine secretion in acute shigellosis is correlated to disease activity and directed more to stool than plasma. Journal of Infectious Diseases 171: 376–384

Ravdin J I 1995 Amebiasis. Clinical Infectious Diseases 20: 1453–1466

Ruiz-Palacios G M, Lopez-Vidal Y, Torres J, Torres N 1985 Serum antibodies to heat labile enterotoxin of *Campylobacter jejuni*. Journal of Infectious Diseases 152: 413–416

Sansonetti P J 1991 Genetic and molecular basis of cell invasion by *Shigella* spp. Reviews of Infectious Diseases 13 (Suppl 4): 285–292

Sansonetti P J, Ryter A, Clerc P et al 1986 Multiplication of *Shigella flexneri* within HeLa cells: lysis of the phagocytic vacuole and plasmid mediated contact haemolysis. Infection and Immunity 51: 461–469

Savarino S J, Fasano A, Watson J et al 1993 Enteroaggregative *Escherichia coli* heat-stable enterotoxin 1 represents another family of *E. coli* heat-stable toxin. Proceedings of the National Academy of Science USA 90: 3093–3097

Skirrow M 1977 Campylobacter enteritis a 'new' disease. British Medical Journal 2: 9–11
Smith G S, Blaser M J 1986 Fatalities associated with *Campylobacter jejuni* infections. Journal of the American Medical Association 253: 2873–2875
Snyder J D, Merson M H 1982 The magnitude of the global problem of acute diarrhoeal disease: a review of active surveillance. Bulletin of the World Health Organization 60: 605–613
Soong C-J G, Kain K C, Abd-Alla M, Jackson T F H G, Ravdin J I 1995 A recombinant cysteine-rich section of the *Entamoeba histolytica* galactose-inhibitable lectin is efficacious as a subunit vaccine in the gerbil model of amebic liver abscess. Journal of Infectious Diseases 171: 645–651
Southern J P, Smith R M M, Palmer S R 1990 Bird attack on milk bottles: possible mode of transmission of *Campylobacter jejuni* to man. Lancet 336: 1425–1427
Tabaqchali S, Jumaa P 1995 Diagnosis and management of *Clostridium difficile* infection. British Medical Journal 310: 1375–1380
Tannich E, Horstmann R D, Knobloch J et al 1989 Genomic DNA differences between pathogenic and non-pathogenic *Entamoeba histolytica*. Proceedings of the National Academy of Sciences USA 86: 5118–5122
Tarr P I 1995 *Escherichia coli* O157: H7: clinical, diagnostic and epidemiological aspects of human infection. Clinical Infectious Diseases 20: 1–10
Taylor C M 1995 Verotoxin-producing *Escherichia coli* and the haemolytic uraemic syndrome. Journal of Infection 30: 189–192
Tozzi A E, Niccolini A, Caprioti A et al 1994 A community outbreak of haemolytic uraemic syndrome in children occurring in a large area of Northern Italy over a period of several months. Epidemiology and Infection 113: 209–219
Vasselon T, Mounier J, Prevost M-C, Hellio R, Sansonetti P J 1991 Stress fiber-based movement of *Shigella flexneri* within cells. Infection and Immunity 59: 1723–1732
Vidal S M, Malo D, Vogan K, Skamene E, Gros P 1993 Natural resistance to infection with intracellular parasites: isolation of candidate for *Bcg*. Cell 73: 469–485
Walsh J A, Warren K S 1979 Selective primary health care: an interim strategy for disease control in developing countries. New England Journal of Medicine 301: 967–974
WHO/CDD/VID/84.4 Diarrhoeal Disease Control Programme 1984 Report of the Third Meeting of the Scientific Working Group on Viral Diarrhoeas. Microbiology, epidemiology and vaccine development, WHO, Geneva, pp 8–14
Yeen W P, Puthuchearly S D, Pang T 1983 Demonstration of a cytotoxin from *Campylobacter jejuni*. Journal of Clinical Pathology 36: 1237–1240
Zychlinsky A, Precost M C, Sansonetti P 1992 *Shigella flexneri* induces apoptosis in infected macrophages. Nature 358: 167–169

38. Acute infectious colitis – diagnostic dilemmas

C. L. Wright   R. H. Riddell

Bloody diarrhea is generally only found in more severe cases of infective colitis, but these constitute a higher proportion of those referring themselves for medical attention (Nostrant et al 1987, Lewin et al 1992). There may be a proven infectious etiology, but many have no identifiable infectious organism, or do not resolve without antibiotics. These have been referred to as 'infectious-type colitis' (Lewin et al 1992) or 'non-relapsing colitis' (Janda et al 1991). Since some of these cases are not self-limiting, and an offending pathogen cannot always be isolated (Schumacher et al 1991), we prefer the term 'acute infectious-type colitis' (AIC).

The major problems faced in diagnosis occur in the selected group of patients with symptoms severe enough to come to medical attention. These are as follows:

1. Atypical clinical features raising suspicions of inflammatory bowel disease (IBD)
2. Failure to identify a pathogen
3. Organisms of uncertain pathogenicity isolated
4. Evolution of AIC into IBD.

ATYPICAL CLINICAL FEATURES RAISING SUSPICIONS OF IBD

The typical presentation of AIC is of a sudden onset of diarrhea that is often initially watery but which may become bloody. It is usually accompanied by fever and abdominal pain. The underlying diagnosis of AIC may be obscured by atypical or non-classical clinical features, causing the physician to consider IBD as a possible etiology. The enteroinvasive organisms produce bloody diarrhea, may have a prolonged course, and may thus cause a clinical picture similar to IBD, especially ulcerative colitis. A further endoscopic twist is that although ulcerative colitis may be suspected clinically, the endoscopic and histologic appearances of AIC may mimic Crohn's disease.

AIC must be distinguished from an initial attack of IBD, since management differs. Rapid steroid treatment may be immensely beneficial in severe ulcerative colitis, but is inappropriate in infectious colitis, and may result in dissemination of the infection and possibly toxic megacolon or fulminant disease. An incorrect diagnosis of IBD can result in inappropriate therapy, long-term cancer surveillance, and possible colectomy (Nostrant et al 1987).

Features favoring infectious colitis include acute onset of diarrhea (within 24 hours), fever within 1 week of onset of disease, severe abdominal pain, vomiting, and more than 12 bowel movements per 24 hours at the onset (Table 38.1) (Vinje et al 1995). In comparison, inflammatory bowel disease usually has a more insidious onset, is more protracted, and has remissions and exacerbations (Farmer 1990). However, the clinical features of AIC and IBD, especially ulcerative colitis, frequently overlap. Ulcerative colitis has an acute or abrupt onset in 36–62% of cases (Edwards & Truelove 1964, Evans et al 1965) and 10% of cases of AIC may have an insidious onset (Janda et al 1991). Although most patients with infectious colitis presented within 1 week of onset of symptoms, those with *Salmonella* or *Cl. difficile* infection had symptoms of longer duration. *Cl. difficile* has a high incidence of recurrence, even after stopping the inciting antibiotics. *C. jejuni* infections may also relapse (Farmer 1990). *Yersinia* infections may last for several months before spontaneously resolving (Jewell 1993). A subacute presentation (rapidly increasing diarrhea during a period of more than 24 hours) was common in both the AIC and IBD groups.

Recovery from AIC is usually complete within 10–14 days (Nostrant et al 1987; Vinje et al 1995) but the duration of the active phase is not diagnostic since infectious colitis can occasionally last longer than 6 weeks (Blaser 1986, Nostrant et al 1987, Janda et al 1991, Vinje et al 1995). An outbreak of a chronic diarrheal syndrome in Henderson County, Illinois, in the United States, was attributed to an unidentified infection arising from contaminated water. Symptoms persisted for up to 2 years (Schumacher et al 1991). The endoscopic appearance is not always helpful in distinguishing AIC from IBD. AIC

Table 38.1 Clinical features at first visit in IBD and infectious colitis

Clinical feature	Infectious colitis	Inflammatory bowel disease
Onset	Acute	Insidious
Fever	Early (within 1st week)	No fever
		Late (after 1st week)
Bowel movements	>12/24 h at onset	<4/24 h at onset
Other symptoms	Severe abdominal pain	Acute deterioration, previous slight symptoms
	Vomiting	

may have diffuse uniform fine mucosal friability, with touch bleeding, features which mimic ulcerative colitis (hence the outdated notion of 'non-specific ulcerative colitis') (Nostrant et al 1987, Farmer 1990).

Tissue biopsy of the colon is usually able to distinguish AIC from IBD. Some have suggested that AIC has specific histologic characteristics if biopsied within the first several days (Nostrant et al 1987), but other studies contradict this (Surawicz & Belic 1984, Therkildsen et al 1989, Schumacher et al 1994). The diagnosis of AIC in patients with active disease is best based upon the absence of histologic criteria favoring IBD (Surawicz & Belic 1984, Schumacher et al 1994), and the presence of other combinations that are usually only found in infection. There is a spectrum of changes found in AIC that may depend on the timing of the biopsy and the organism involved.

There are several strong histologic predictors of IBD (Table 38.2). A key feature is basal plasmacytosis (Kumar et al 1982, Nostrant et al 1987, Surawicz et al 1994, Schumacher et al 1994). Although plasma cells are a normal constituent of the colonic lamina propria, they are usually confined to the upper two-thirds of the mucosa. The presence of more than rare plasma cells at the base of the mucosa usually indicates a long-standing chronic inflammatory process, such as IBD, microscopic/lymphocytic colitis, or collagenous colitis. It is often present early in IBD, and is rarely seen in AIC (Fig. 38.1). Basal plasmacytosis in IBD is present focally within the first 2 weeks from onset of symptoms, and eventually becomes more diffuse (Schumacher et al 1994). Over one-third of IBD patients presenting within 2 weeks had only this and no other feature of IBD. Within 3–5 weeks from onset of symptoms, 85% of the

Table 38.2 Histopathology in IBD and AIC

Features favoring IBD	Features favoring AIC
Inflammation	Acute inflammation only
basal plasmacytosis	None to minimal architectural distortion,
basal lymphoid aggregates	fewer than two crypt branches
granulomas	*No* basal plasmacytosis
Paneth cell metaplasia	Absence of villiform surface
Architecture	
two or more crypt branches	
villiform surface	
crypt atrophy	

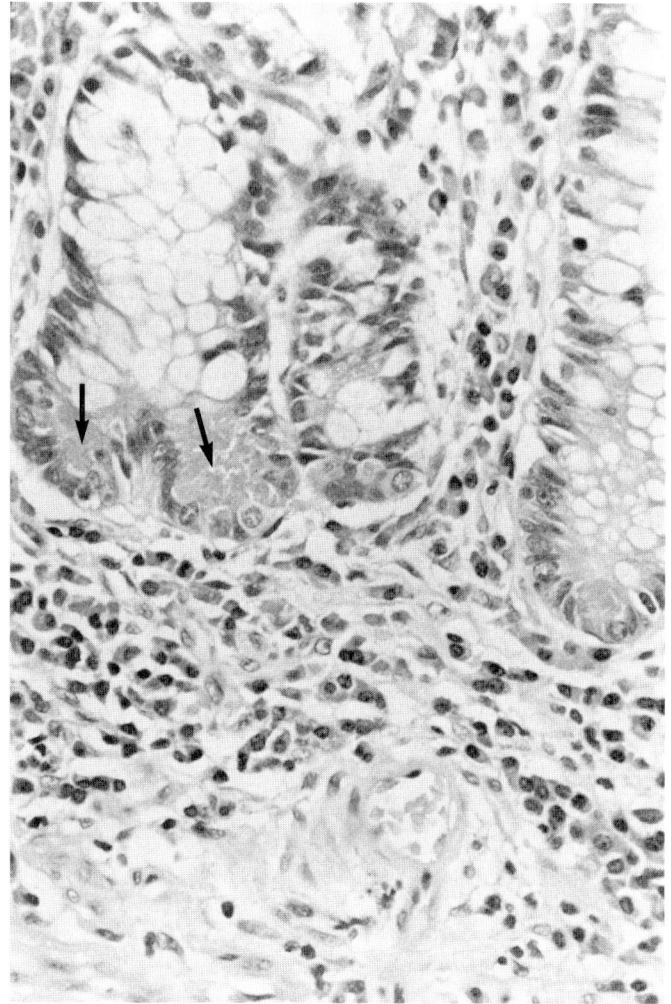

Fig. 38.1 Basal plasmacytosis and Paneth cell metaplasia in ulcerative colitis. Plasma cells are not normally present in the base of the colonic mucosa, but frequently expand this area in IBD. Paneth cells (arrowed) distal to the hepatic flexure indicate chronic irritation, as in IBD. Both of these features are useful in distinguishing IBD from AIC.

IBD patients had developed either focal or diffuse basal plasmacytosis. It had disappeared at the 1-year biopsy in half of those who had not yet relapsed. Absence of basal plasmacytosis does not rule out IBD, since only 69% of the IBD patients had this feature at their initial biopsy. Similarly, its presence does not in itself absolutely rule out AIC, being present in about 3% of those cases (Fig. 38.2).

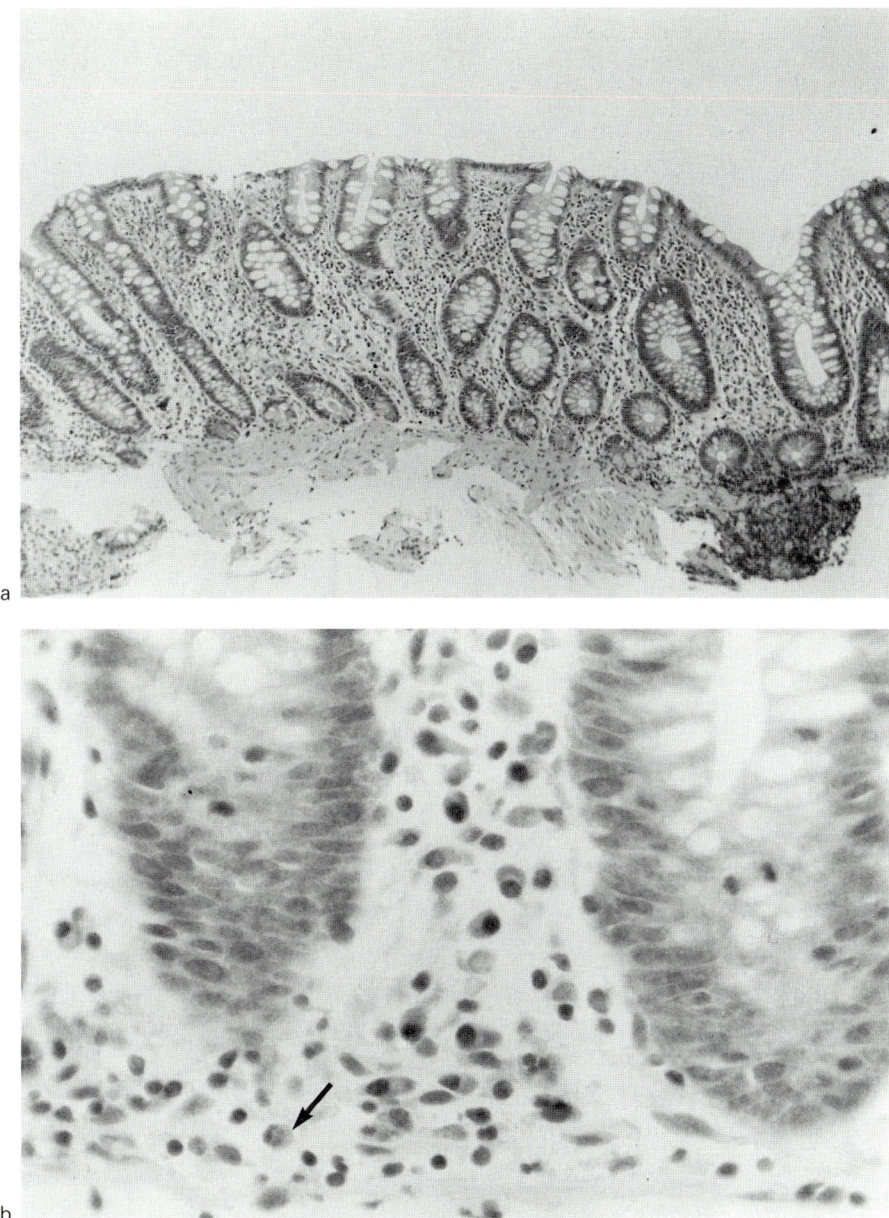

Fig. 38.2 Acute infectious colitis. Normal crypt architecture (**a**) accompanied by unusual finding of scattered deep plasma cells and rare neutrophil (arrowed) (**b**) in colonic biopsy from an elderly female with *E. Coli* 0157:H7 colitis.

Surawicz et al (1994) compared AIC and IBD patients who had had symptoms for less than 25 days. None of the AIC patients had basal plasmacytosis, compared to 71% of the acute-onset IBD patients. Basal lymphoid aggregates were also absent in the AIC patients, and found in almost half of the IBD group. An indirect indicator of chronic irritation is Paneth cell metaplasia, found occasionally in IBD but not in AIC (Schumacher et al 1994). Paneth cells can be normally found in the small bowel and right colon, as far as the region of the hepatic flexure. They are not normally present distal to this area (Fig. 38.1).

Architectural distortion is another important discriminant between AIC and IBD (Fig. 38.3) (Kumar et al 1982, Nostrant et al 1987, Janda et al 1991, Surawicz et al 1994, Schumacher et al 1994, Surawicz & Belic 1984). The specificity and sensitivity of this histologic change depends upon its definition. Rigorously defined, it is highly specific for IBD but at the expense of sensitivity. This is exemplified in Schumacher's study (Schumacher et al 1994), which defined crypt distortion as complete disorganization of crypts due to non-parallelism, more than two crypt branches in a medium-power field, at least twofold variation in crypt diameter, and usually an

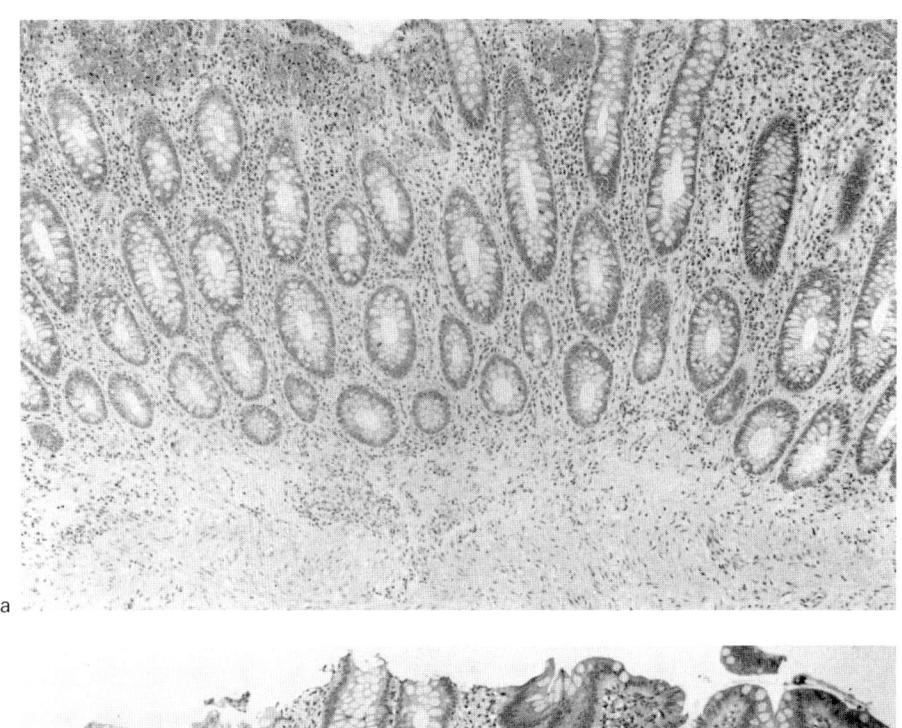
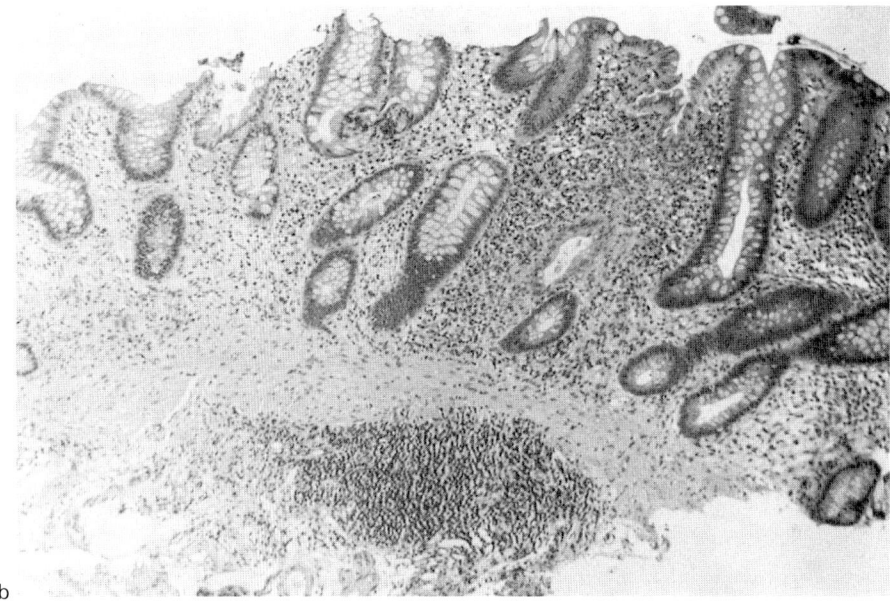

Fig. 38.3 (a) Normal crypt architecture in colonic biopsy from patient with acute infectious colitis due to *Shigella sonnei*. Compare with the distorted crypt architecture in (b), a colonic biopsy from a patient with active Crohn's disease. Crypt branching, non-parallelism of crypts, and irregular gland spacing are evident. A deep lymphoid aggregate is also present in the submucosa of (b).

increased distance between crypts and the muscularis mucosae. None of the IBD patients had crypt distortion within the first 2 weeks of symptoms. Not until after 4 months did most of them (78%) show this change on biopsy. Normal-appearing rectal mucosa can be found in established ulcerative colitis patients who have been treated with topical 5-ASA (Odze et al 1993). Others have also noted preservation of architecture in initial biopsies of up to one-third of IBD patients (Therkildsen et al 1989). In contrast, only one patient of Schumacher's AIC group had crypt distortion at the initial biopsy. This patient with *Salmonella typhi* also had basal plasmacytosis. The authors stressed that one or two vertical crypt branches, variation in the crypt diameter, and thinning out of crypts were fairly common in infectious colitis and should not be misinterpreted as crypt distortion. Surawicz also found that the presence of two or more branched glands was far more likely, although not specific, in IBD (8% vs 71%) (Surawicz et al 1994).

Another architectural derangement, villiform surface, identifies patients with IBD and is not seen in AIC (Fig. 38.4). However, it is not very sensitive, being found in

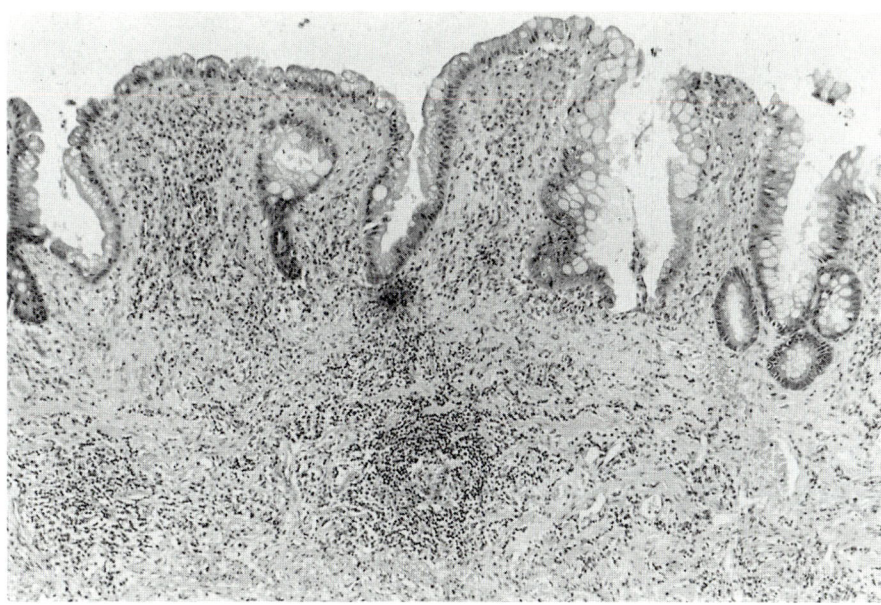

Fig. 38.4 Villiform surface of colonic biopsy from patient with ulcerative colitis. Architectural derangement of this severity is a feature of IBD, not AIC.

only about one-quarter of the biopsies (Surawicz et al 1994, Schumacher et al 1994). It is associated with marked inflammation. Crypt atrophy (crypts that are both widely spaced from each other and from the muscularis mucosa, as well as being shortened) is another helpful feature favoring IBD (Surawicz et al 1994, Schumacher et al 1994). It can be found in AIC, but only following known pathogens causing severe disease (e.g. *Shigella*, some *Salmonella*, *Cl. difficile*). Acute inflammation, without a concomitant increase in lymphocytes and plasma cells, seems to be mostly restricted to AIC (Fig. 38.5). IBD usually shows evidence of some chronic inflammation in the background, such as basal plasmacytosis or lymphoid aggregates (Surawicz et al 1994). Aphthoid ulcers are superficial erosions at the base of a crypt, and are often found over lymphoid aggregates. They are a classic feature of Crohn's disease but their presence is not pathognomonic. Many infections may also cause identical lesions. These include Campylobacter, Shigella, Salmonella, Yersinia, tuberculosis, and herpes virus (Mathan & Mathan 1991, Lewin et al 1992). Pseudomembranes may be a clue to an underlying infection. They may be seen both endoscopically and microscopically in *Clostridium difficile* infections, or severe cases of Shigella or Salmonella. Pseudomembranes that are seen only with the microscope and not recognized endoscopically are highly suggestive of verotoxic *E. coli* 0157 infection (Griffin et al 1990, Lewin et al 1992).

Epithelioid granulomas, a recognized feature of Crohn's disease, can be rarely found in infectious colitis, apparently in cases due to infection by Salmonella or Campylobacter (Surawicz et al 1994). They have also been found in rectal biopsies with Chlamydia proctitis (Surawicz et al 1986).

Our approach to the histological distinction between AIC and IBD concentrates on the assessment of architecture and chronic inflammation. When acute inflammation is present, but the architecture is not significantly distorted, and basal plasmacytosis is absent, we diagnose AIC. We remain comfortable with that diagnosis even when the architecture becomes deranged, as long as basal plasmacytosis or lymphoid aggregates are absent. Only when both features of architectural distortion and basal chronic inflammation are present do we diagnose IBD, in the context of the appropriate clinical setting.

We have repeatedly found that the greatest histological difficulty is in distinguishing AIC from early Crohn's disease. This reflects the marked focality of inflammation that is often present in both diseases. For instance, Crohn's disease and verotoxic *E. coli* may both affect the right colon preferentially, and both may be characterized by focal acute inflammation interspersed between patches of normal mucosa. In this setting, attention to the presence or absence of basal plasmacytosis or lymphoid aggregates is essential. Preliminary results published in a recent abstract found that focal cryptitis with either basal plasmacytosis or focal crypt distortion, but not both, was not predictive of IBD (Stern et al 1995). However, the combination of focal cryptitis with both crypt distortion and basal plasmacytosis was seen significantly more often in IBD patients. Numerous levels through the paraffin blocks may yield additional features that clarify the diagnosis (Fig. 38.6).

Histology of several colonic biopsies from the Henderson County outbreak of chronic diarrhea revealed a pattern of

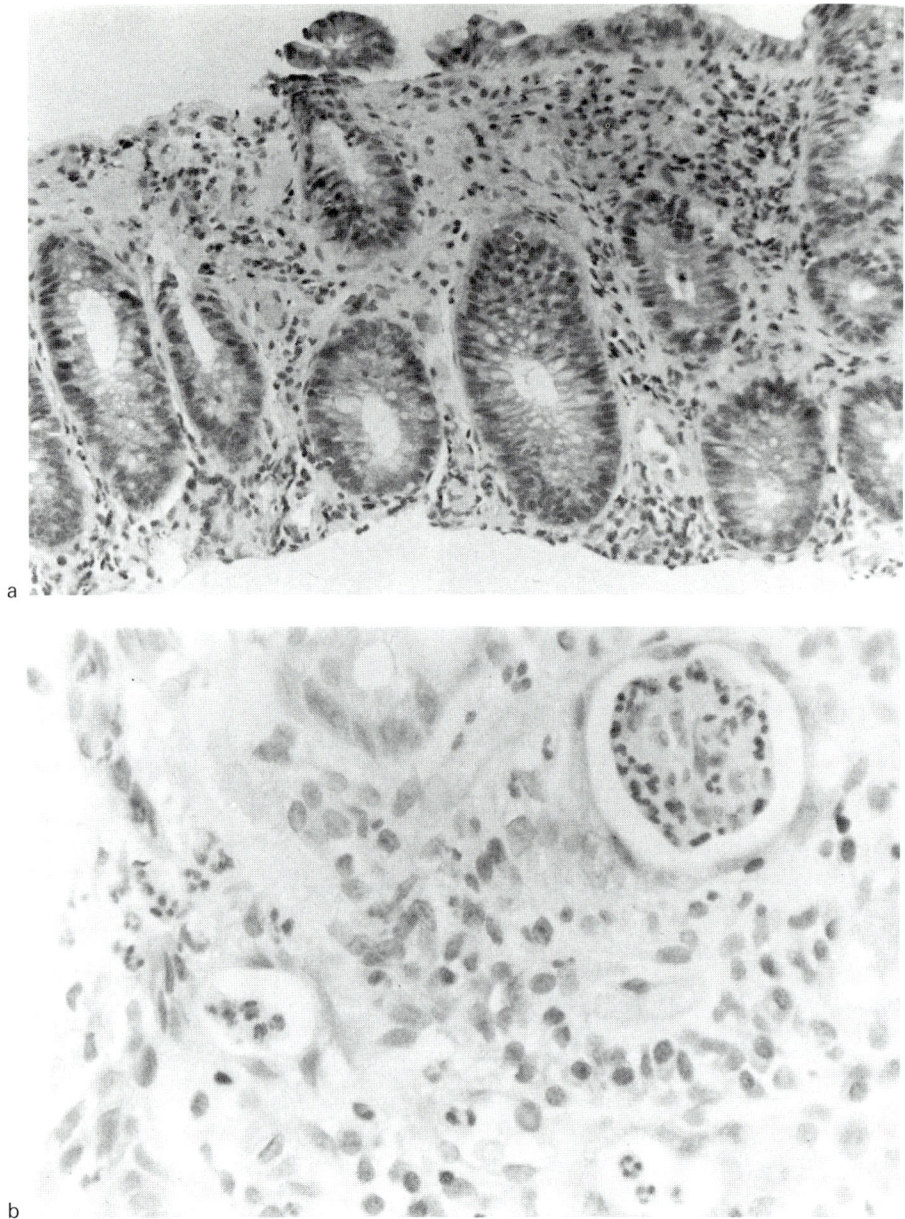

Fig. 38.5 Acute infectious-type colitis. Normal crypt architecture (**a**) with focal acute inflammation (**b**).

multifocal mild acute inflammation, with an excess of intraepithelial lymphocytes (Schumacher et al 1991). The biopsies lacked the architectural distortion of IBD. The features were reminiscent of lymphocytic colitis, but lacked the diffuse pattern more typical of that entity.

FAILURE TO IDENTIFY PATHOGEN

The diagnostic yield of organisms from routine stool cultures varies from 8 to 40% in patients with presumed infective diarrhea. Reference laboratories are usually set up to detect over 20 agents. Their recovery rate of infectious agents of gastroenteritis is frequently over 50%, and can be as high as 80% in certain risk groups, such as those with infantile diarrhea (Lewin et al 1992). If only three organisms are routinely cultured (Salmonella, Shigella and *Campylobacter jejuni*) the diagnostic yield can be as low as 8%. This rises to 15% in the presence of fever and/or bloody diarrhea, and to about 50% with the additional finding of numerous fecal neutrophils (Lewin et al 1992).

Approximately 30–50% of cases of AIC have positive stool cultures. *Campylobacter jejuni* is commonly isolated, being found in up to half of the cases. *Clostridium difficile* is also common, sometimes identified almost as frequently as *C. jejuni* in westernized countries. Also common are

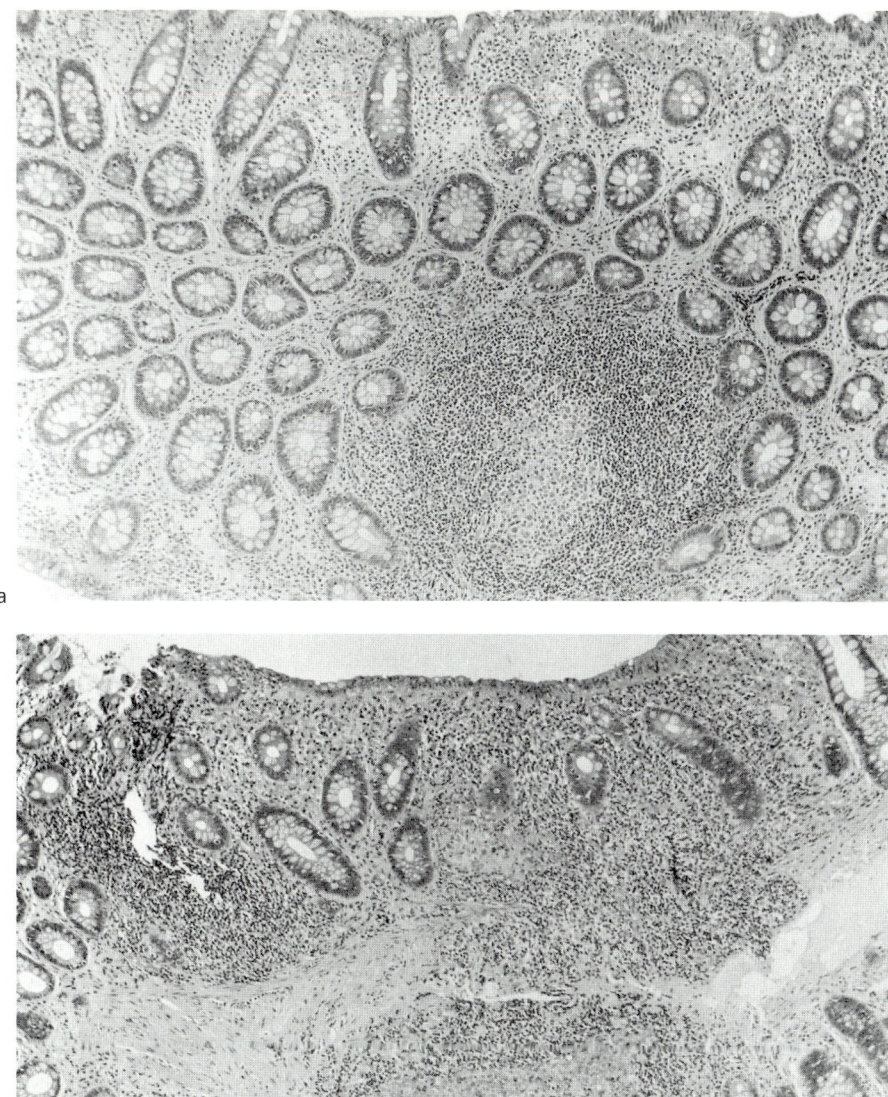

Fig. 38.6 AIC vs IBD. Additional tissue, such as that obtained from multiple biopsies or even just from deeper levels through a biopsy, may yield valuable information essential to the correct diagnosis. The initial level of this rectal biopsy (**a**) is suboptimally oriented, but the crypt architecture appears within normal limits. A single deep lymphoid follicle is present, and neutrophils were scattered throughout the lamina propria. Acute infectious-type colitis was initially diagnosed. Subsequent upper gastrointestinal biopsies showed features typical of Crohn's disease, prompting deeper levels through the colonic biopsy (**b**). This revealed mild architectural change with several deep lymphoid aggregates and follicles, as well as a small granuloma, features most in keeping with Crohn's disease.

Salmonella, *Shigella* and *Aeromonas* spp. Other organisms found less frequently include *E. coli*: 0157 H7, *Yersinia*, *Entamoeba histolytica* and *Staphylococcus aureus* (Kumar et al 1982, George et al 1985, Nostrant et al 1987, Therkildsen et al 1989, Surawicz et al 1994, Matsumoto et al 1994, Vinje et al 1995). Cultures of colonoscopically obtained biopsies are more than twice as often positive as stool cultures. Matsumoto et al (1994) prospectively evaluated 20 patients with cultures of stool and biopsy material. Enteric pathogens were found in only 20% when just the stool specimen was considered. The yield jumped to 50% for biopsy cultures. The combination resulted in an overall yield of 65% (Matsumoto et al 1994). In only one of the patients were both the biopsy and stool cultures positive (*Campylobacter jejuni*). Thus, the number of cases of so-called 'culture-negative' acute infectious colitis may be considerably reduced by culture of the tissue as well as stool. Schumacher et al (1993) identified positive microbial findings in 78% of AIC patients. This was achieved by culturing three stool samples, and a rectal swab or biopsy. In addition, toxin tests and serology were performed in samples from many of the subjects.

Both the culture-positive and culture-negative groups of AIC have the same clinical findings and biopsy features, and follow the same course (Kumar et al 1982).

Microbiology alone does not differentiate between AIC and inflammatory bowel disease. Bacterial contamination in ulcerative colitis may limit the usefulness of fecal cultures (Nostrant et al 1987) and about 13–20% of patients with active IBD may have concurrent infection (Schumacher et al 1993, Vinje et al 1995).

ISOLATION OF CANDIDATE PATHOGENS ONLY

Sometimes the clinical impression is of infection, but only organisms of uncertain pathogenicity are found, e.g. spirochetes, *Blastocystic hominis* and some bacteria. This can be a particular problem in patients with acquired immunodeficiency syndrome (AIDS).

EVOLUTION OF AIC INTO IBD

There is a small proportion of cases in which a previously healthy patient develops a documented infectious colitis, the symptoms of which do not resolve despite the disappearance or eradication of the inciting organism. The clinical picture eventually evolves into one resembling typical ulcerative colitis (Stewart 1950, Banks et al 1957, Acheson & Nefzger 1963, Lewin et al 1992). It is possible that the infection may either precipitate or unmask the disease in otherwise predisposed individuals (Bernhoft 1949, Banks et al 1957, Willoughby et al 1989, Jewell 1993, Vinje et al 1995). It is interesting that in some series over 60% of IBD patients with an acute or subacute onset fell ill in connection with travelling abroad, gastrointestinal infection, or treatment with antibiotics. They may have had altered intestinal flora that precipitated or aggravated the symptoms in latent IBD, resulting in a more acute, rather than insidious, onset (Vinje et al 1995). The organisms most frequently implicated include amebae, Shigella and Salmonella (Bernhoft 1949, Stewart 1950, Acheson & Nefzger 1963, Powell & Wilmot 1966, Lindeman et al 1967, Fung et al 1972, Dronfield et al 1974, Rampton et al 1983, Taylor-Robinson et al 1989, Sturgess et al 1992, Sung et al 1993). *Aeromonas* spp. and cytomegalovirus (CMV) have also recently been documented (Willoughby et al 1989, Dickinson et al 1989, Diepersloot et al 1990, Orvar et al 1993). The proportion of IBD cases preceded by infection is unknown. Brown et al (1992) recently sought microbial pathogens in feces of patients with initial presentation of active ulcerative colitis: no bacterial pathogens were identified using culture techniques (including staphylococci, *E. coli*, streptococci, *Bacillus cereus*, *Salmonella* spp, *Shigella* spp, *Aeromonas* sp, *Yersinia* sp, *Vibrio*, *Clostridium perfringens*, *Campylobacter* spp, and *Plesiomonas shigelloides*) (Brown et al 1992). Yet Schumacher et al (1993) found that 21% of IBD patients at initial presentation had positive microbial findings.

Other cases may evolve into a constellation of features resembling the irritable bowel syndrome. These have been referred to as 'functional post-dysenteric colitis' Stewart 1950, Powell & Wilmot 1966). Biopsies are normal or edematous. The temporal relationship may raise the question of a persistent toxin-related diarrhea.

The term 'ulcerative post-dysenteric colitis' has been used to describe patients with bloody diarrhea and colonic ulcerations that persist despite apparent eradication of the primary infection, usually *Entamoeba histolytica* (Stewart 1950, Powell & Wilmot 1966, Rampton et al 1983, Fung et al 1972). Symptoms may persist for many months. Some of these patients have probably had persistent infection, but laboratory methods may not have been sophisticated or sensitive enough to detect the organisms. Most cases somewhat resemble idiopathic ulcerative colitis, but differ in that they are not characterized by remissions and relapses; extraintestinal manifestations such as erythema nodosum and conjunctivitis are also absent (Powell & Wilmot 1966, Fung et al 1972). There remain occasional patients who appear to develop a postinfectious colitis indistinguishable from idiopathic ulcerative colitis (Rampton et al 1983). Rampton et al point out that although the infection may have unmasked a subclinical ulcerative colitis, it may also be possible that the subsequent chronic diarrhea was really the initial presentation of the disease (Rampton et al 1983). The prior infection may have been coincidental.

Aeromonas spp. are a recent addition to the list of possible precipitants of ulcerative colitis. (Willoughby et al 1989, Dickinson & Wright 1989) This organism usually causes an acute self-limiting enteritis which resolves in a couple of weeks, but frequently diarrhea may persist for longer than 30 days (Blaser 1986). Approximately 15% of patients with *Aeromonas*-related diarrhea have evidence of colonic involvement (George et al 1985). Three patients identified by Willoughby et al (1989) had acute *Aeromonas* colitis, then subsequently developed ulcerative colitis. However, one of those patients had previous episodes possibly representing mild ulcerative colitis. One patient reported by Dickinson (Dickinson & Wright 1989) developed diarrhea with fever while on holiday, and *Aeromonas hydrophila* was cultured. The histopathology was of an 'active non-specific proctitis'. Two weeks later, ulceration and mucosal thickening of the transverse and descending colon resembled Crohn's disease, although the pathology was equivocal. Six months later, colonoscopy showed pancolitis which histologically appeared to be Crohn's disease. The patient was asymptomatic for $3\frac{1}{2}$ years, then developed diarrhea. He had a pancolitis on colonoscopy and radiology. The pathologist favored a diagnosis of ulcerative colitis. Since the patient had no bowel symptoms before the infection, the authors postulated that the IBD was triggered by the infection. *Salmonella* spp. have also been the subject of reports linking them to the triggering of ulcerative colitis (Lindeman et al 1967, Dronfield et al 1974, Taylor-Robinson et al 1989). Some of the patients in these reports were diagnosed with ulcerative colitis within only weeks of documenting the infection; they remained free of symptoms after protracted treatment (Dronfield et al 1974, Taylor-Robinson et al 1989). Without a history of recurrent relapses, or details of the histological appearances of the biopsies, one must be reluctant to attach a diagnosis of ulcerative colitis to some of these patients. Many of the reports purporting an infectious cause or unmasking of ulcerative colitis fail to provide convincing evidence of IBD, and one must wonder if the patient's entire disease was solely due to an unusually long or fulminant infectious process (Dronfield et al 1974, Taylor-Robinson et al 1989).

DIAGNOSIS AND MANAGEMENT

The diagnosis of acute infectious-type colitis rests upon the constellation of history, clinical symptoms and their temporal relationships, cultures, and histopathology. (Surawicz et al 1994, Schumacher et al 1994, Vinje et al 1995).

Acute onset of symptoms within 24 hours, early fever within 1 week of onset of symptoms, and rapid improvement indicate AIC. Simultaneous stool and tissue cultures, as well as sigmoidoscopy with rectal biopsy, may help sort out those with a non-insidious onset of symptoms who are not rapidly improving. A positive culture, together with a biopsy lacking features of IBD, indicates infectious colitis. A 'positive' biopsy, regardless of the culture results, would strongly favor IBD if the patient did not have early fever or acute onset of symptoms.

It is the group with negative cultures and 'negative' biopsies that are the most difficult to diagnose and manage. Careful histologic examination, as outlined earlier, and maximizing culture yields by submitting biopsy tissue for microbiology, will ensure that the size of this group is minimized. If these patients do not improve rapidly, were afebrile or had fever later than 1 week after onset of symptoms, or had fewer than 4–6 bowel movements per 24 hours at onset, then IBD is probable. If they had early fever, or more than 10–12 bowel movements per 24 hours, then AIC is probable (Vinje et al 1995). There will always remain a small subset who will remain undiagnosed. Careful follow-up with repeat biopsies will eventually yield the diagnosis.

REFERENCES

Acheson E D, Nefzger D 1963 Ulcerative colitis in the United States army in 1944. Epidemiology: comparisons between patients and controls. Gastroenterology 44: 7–19

Banks B M, Korelitz B I, Zetzel L 1957 The course of nonspecific ulcerative colitis: review of twenty years' experience and late results. Gastroenterology 32: 983–1012

Bernhoft W H 1949 The relation of amebic dysentery to chronic ulcerative colitis. New York State Medical Journal 49: 1795–1796

Blaser M J 1986 Infectious diarrheas: acute, chronic, and iatrogenic. Annals of Internal Medicine 105: 785–787

Brown W J, Hudson M J, Patrick S et al 1992 Search for enteric microbial pathogens in patients with ulcerative colitis. Digestion 53: 121–128

Dickinson R J, Wright D G D 1989 Chronic colitis after Aeromonas infection. Gut 30: 1436

Dieperslloot R J A, Kroes A C M, Visser W, Jiwa N M, Rothbarth P H 1990 Acute ulcerative proctocolitis associated with primary cytomegalovirus infection. Archives of Internal Medicine 150: 1749–1751

Dronfield M W, Fletcher J, Langman M J S 1974 Coincident Salmonella infection and ulcerative colitis: problems of recognition and management. British Medical Journal 1: 99–100

Edwards F C, Truelove S C 1964 The course and prognosis of ulcerative colitis. Gut 5: 1–22

Evans J G, Acheson E D 1965 An epidemiological study of ulcerative colitis and regional enteritis in the Oxford area. Gut 6: 311–324

Farmer R G 1990 Infectious causes of diarrhea in the differential diagnosis of inflammatory bowel disease. Medical Clinics of North America 74: 29–38

Fung W P, Monteiro E H, Ang H B, Kho K M, Lee S K 1972 Ulcerative postdysenteric colitis. American Journal of Gastroenterology 57: 341–348

George W L, Nakata M M, Thompson J, White M L 1985 Aeromonas-related diarrhea in adults. Archives of Internal Medicine 145: 2207–2211

Griffin P M, Olmstead L C, Petras R E 1990 *Escherichia coli* 0157:H7-associated colitis. A clinical and histological study of 11 cases. Gastroenterology 99: 142–149

Janda R C, Conklin J L, Mitros F A, Parsonnet J 1991 Multifocal colitis associated with an epidemic of chronic diarrhea. Gastroenterology 100: 318–328

Jewell D P 1993 Ulcerative colitis. In: Sleisinger M H, Fordtran J S (eds) Gastrointestinal disease. W B Saunders, Philadelphia, pp 1305–1330

Kumar N B, Nostrant T T, Appelman H D 1982 The histopathologic spectrum of acute self-limited colitis. American Journal of Surgical Pathology 6: 523–529

Lewin K J, Riddell R H, Weinstein W M 1992 Gastrointestinal pathology and its clinical implications. Igaku-Shoin, New York

Lindeman R J, Weinstein L, Levitan R, Patterson J F 1967 Ulcerative colitis and intestinal salmonellosis. American Journal of Medical Science 254: 855–861

Mathan M M, Mathan V I 1991 Morphology of rectal mucosa of patients with shigellosis. Reviews of Infectious Diseases 13 (Suppl 4): S314–S318

Matsumoto T, Iida M, Kimura Y, Fujishima M 1994 Culture of colonoscopically obtained biopsy specimens in acute infectious colitis. Gastrointestinal Endoscopy 40: 184–187

Nostrant T T, Kumar N B, Appelman H D 1987 Histopathology differentiates acute self-limited colitis from ulcerative colitis. Gastroenterology 92: 318–328

Odze R, Antonioli D, Peppercorn M, Goldman H 1993 Effects of topical 5-aminosalicylic acid (5-ASA) therapy on rectal mucosal biopsy morphology in chronic ulcerative colitis. American Journal of

Surgical Pathology 17: 869–875
Orvar K, Murray J, Carmen G, Conklin J 1993 Cytomegalovirus infection associated with onset of inflammatory bowel disease. Digestive Diseases and Sciences 38: 2307–2310
Powell S J, Wilmot A J 1966 Ulcerative post-dysenteric colitis. Gut 7: 438–443
Rampton D S, Salmon P R, Clark C G 1983 Nonspecific ulcerative colitis as a sequel to amebic dysentery. Journal of Clinical Gastroenterology 5: 217–219
Schumacher G, Kollberg B, Sandstedt B 1994 A prospective study of first attacks of inflammatory bowel disease and infectious colitis. Histologic course during the 1st year after presentation. Scandinavian Journal of Gastroenterology 29: 318–332
Schumacher G, Kollberg B, Sandstedt B et al 1993 A prospective study of first attacks of inflammatory bowel disease and non-relapsing colitis. Microbiologic findings. Scandinavian Journal of Gastroenterology 28: 1077–1085
Schumacher G, Sandstedt B, Mollby R, Kollberg B 1991 Clinical and histologic features differentiating non-relapsing colitis from first attacks of inflammatory bowel disease. Scandinavian Journal of Gastroenterology 26: 151–161
Stern R A, Carpenter S L, Barnett J L, Greenson J K 1995 The clinical significance of focal active colitis. Gastroenterology 108: A922 (Abstract)
Stewart G T 1950 Post-dysenteric colitis. British Medical Journal i: 405–409
Sturgess I, Greenfield S M, Teare J, O'Doherty M J 1992 Ulcerative colitis developing after amoebic dysentery in a haemophiliac patient with AIDS. Gut 33: 408–410
Sung J Y, Chan K L, Hsu R, Liew C T, Lawton J W M 1993 Ulcerative colitis and antineutrophil cytoplasmic antibodies in Hong Kong Chinese. American Journal of Gastroenterology 88: 1993
Surawicz C M, Belic L 1984 Rectal biopsy helps to distinguish acute self-limited colitis from idiopathic inflammatory bowel disease. Gastroenterology 86: 104–113
Surawicz C M, Goodell S E, Quinn T C et al 1986 Spectrum of rectal biopsy abnormalities in homosexual men with intestinal symptoms. Gastroenterology 91: 645–649
Surawicz C M, Haggitt R C, Husseman M, McFarland L V 1994 Mucosal biopsy diagnosis of colitis: acute self-limited colitis and idiopathic inflammatory bowel disease. Gastroenterology 107: 755–763
Taylor-Robinson S, Miles R, Whitehead A, Dickinson R J 1989 Salmonella infection and ulcerative colitis. Lancet (i): 1145
Therkildsen M H, Jensen B N, Teglbjaerg P S, Rasmussen N 1989 The final outcome of patients presenting with their first episode of acute diarrhoea and an inflamed rectal mucosa with preserved crypt architecture. A clinicopathological study. Scandinavian Journal of Gastroenterology 24: 158–164
Vinje B, Gudmundsen T E, Halvorsen F A, Pedersen H K, Ostensen H 1995 Changes in diagnostic imaging routines of the stomach and the large bowel during the period between 1975 and 1992. Clinical Imaging 19: 57–59
Willoughby J M T, Rahman A F M S, Gregory M M 1989 Chronic colitis after Aeromonas infection. Gut 30: 686–690

39. Collagenous, microscopic and lymphocytic colitis

N. P. Mapstone   M. F. Dixon

INTRODUCTION

The past 20 years has seen increased accessibility of the large intestine to gastroenterologists using the colonoscope. Along with the increasing availability of multiple biopsies has come a recognition of 'new' diseases with subtle clinical features. Two such are collagenous colitis and lymphocytic colitis. These diseases characteristically cause watery diarrhea with a normal colonoscopic appearance but an abnormal colonic biopsy. Their features and relationship with a third potential diagnosis, microscopic colitis, are discussed below.

COLLAGENOUS COLITIS

This condition was first described by Lindstrom in 1976. Further case reports started appearing in 1980, but its acceptance as a discrete pathological entity has not been unopposed (Williams & Rhodes 1987). However, it is now well established and has a place in most modern textbooks.

Natural history

Collagenous colitis is rare, occurring in approximately 4/1000 patients undergoing biopsy for non-neoplastic disease at The Johns Hopkins Hospital in 1987 (Lazenby et al 1990). It is more common in women (male:female ratio 1:7.5) (Lazenby et al 1989). The mean age at presentation is 59, and most reports are of patients aged 40–70. However, the disease has been seen in an 89-year-old and pediatric cases have been reported: a 7-year-old (Busuttil 1989) and a 5-year-old (Perisic & Kokai 1989) have been diagnosed as having collagenous colitis. However, another case report in a child (Gremse et al 1993) was later claimed to be a misinterpretation of a normal colonic biopsy (Yardley et al 1993), illustrating the ease with which the condition can be overdiagnosed.

A familial form has been reported in two families, each with two members suffering from collagenous colitis (van Tilburg et al 1990), and one of these families had a history of autoimmune diseases.

Clinical features

Collagenous colitis presents with watery diarrhea and colicky abdominal pain of long duration and variable persistence. Clinical remissions may occur (Palmer et al 1986). The symptoms are very similar to those suffered in irritable bowel syndrome. Exceptional presentations have been documented: it has once been seen in a patient with a long history of constipation (Leigh et al 1993). In another patient, with no history of chronic diarrhea, it was an incidental finding in a resection for colonic carcinoma (Gardiner et al 1984). The diarrhea may have mucus, but blood is not seen in the stool and there is typically no history of weight loss or vomiting. Routine investigations for the cause of diarrhea, such as microbiology and radiology, are characteristically negative. Typically the colonoscopy will be macroscopically normal and although often suspected clinically, the diagnosis can only be confirmed by histological examination. There are occasional reports (Kingham et al 1986, Richieri et al 1993) of abnormal appearances at colonoscopy, with linear hemorrhagic lesions and loss of normal haustrations, but definite collagenous thickening on biopsy.

Many conditions present in a similar fashion to collagenous colitis, and some will have a macroscopically normal colonoscopy. The long list of diagnoses to be excluded includes laxative abuse, malabsorption, infection, ischemic colitis, irritable bowel syndrome, Crohn's disease and ulcerative colitis, hyperthyroidism, scleroderma, amyloidosis and diverticulosis.

There have been many case reports of collagenous colitis associated with other diseases. These include discoid lupus (Castanet et al 1994), rheumatoid arthritis (Farah et al 1985, Wengrower et al 1987, Widgren & MacGee 1990), monoarticular reactive arthritis (Roubenoff et al 1989), tropical sprue (Puri et al 1994), pulmonary fibrosis (Wiener 1986), multiple ileal carcinoids (Nussinson et al 1988), scleroderma (Esselinckx et al 1989), CRST syndrome (calcinosis, Raynaud's phenomenon, sclerodactyly, telangiectasia) (Kenesi et al 1991) and Hodgkin's lymphoma (van der Werf et al 1987). In one series, 10 of 15 patients with collagenous colitis had either thyroid disease or arthritis (Jessurun et al 1987).

Should biopsies be performed on patients with macroscopically normal colonoscopies? Having found no histological evidence of collagenous colitis in 89 of their patients with irritable bowel syndrome, MacIntosh et al (1992) concluded that biopsy was not helpful. However, negative diagnoses were made using rectal biopsies without colonoscopy in all but three of those patients. As will be noted below, sigmoidoscopy alone may miss a large proportion of patients with collagenous colitis. When biopsies of the hepatic flexure and the sigmoid were used in another study (Prior et al 1987) two cases of collagenous colitis were found in 180 patients with normal colonoscopies. It seems that, far from a rectal biopsy being superfluous at sigmoidoscopy, only full colonoscopic examination can definitively exclude the disease.

Radiology

Patients with collagenous colitis are usually reported as having normal barium enema examinations (Giardiello et al 1987). However, in one series of five patients with single and double contrast barium enemas three showed mucosal granularity and nodularity (Feczko & Mezwa 1991). Unfortunately these changes are non-specific, and similar appearances can be seen in other forms of colitis.

Other investigations

As with radiological examination, these patients may show a range of non-specific abnormalities that are unhelpful in diagnosing the condition. A proportion may have, for example, an elevated erythrocyte sedimentation rate (Kingham et al 1986) or eosinophilia. However, given the number of associated conditions these findings should be viewed with caution.

Microbiological examination for gut pathogens is negative in patients with collagenous colitis.

Histopathology

The defining feature of collagenous colitis seen on biopsy is a thickened subepithelial collagen layer (Fig. 39.1). Other, less constant, features include 'entrapment' of fibroblasts and capillaries in the collagen layer, an increased number of lymphocytes and plasma cells in the lamina propria, an increase in intraepithelial lymphocytes, and degeneration and separation of the epithelium from the basement membrane. The collagen band is easy to recognize and there is good concordance among pathologists in the diagnosis of the condition (Carpenter et al 1992).

The normal collagen layer is around 3 μm thick (Lee et al 1992), but it can be as much as 6.9 μm (Bogomoletz et al 1980). In collagenous colitis the layer is between 7 and 93 μm thick (Wang et al 1987). This thickening can be identified on standard hematoxylin and eosin stains, although some special techniques, such as Masson's trichrome (which stains the collagen green), or a reticulin stain will accentuate the abnormality. As a general rule the diagnosis should not be made if the collagen layer is less than 10 μm thick (Bogomoletz & Flejou 1991).

This thickening of this collagen 'table' is most prominent underlying the surface epithelium between the crypts, although some excess collagen can extend down the sides

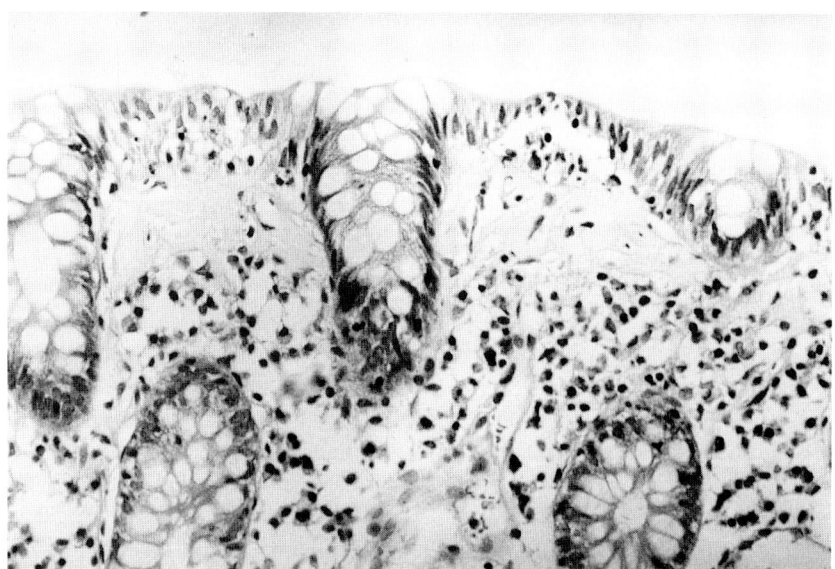

Fig. 39.1 Colonic biopsy from a patient with collagenous colitis. Note the thickened collagen band and entrapped capillaries. (Hematoxylin and eosin × 250)

of crypts. It may have a patchy distribution within the large bowel (Carpenter et al 1992) and only multiple biopsies can exclude the diagnosis. It may be that this patchy distribution accounts for some of the reports of spontaneous or post-therapeutic regression of the collagen band (Palmer et al 1986). It is now well recognized that the thickened band is more prominent in the colon than the rectum (Jessurun et al 1987, Carpenter et al 1992), and cannot be excluded on sigmoidoscopic examination alone. Some have found rectal and sigmoid biopsies to be diagnostic in 90% of patients with collagenous colitis (Armes et al 1992). However, another series of sequential biopsies from 33 patients (Tanaka et al 1992) indicated that rectal biopsy alone may only diagnose 27% of cases. If a sigmoid biopsy is included this figure rises to 71%, but there are still some patients who show the characteristic band only on more proximal colonic or cecal biopsies.

Excessive collagen deposition occasionally extends even more proximally, with the terminal ileum affected in one case (Lewis et al 1991), and the stomach and duodenum in another (Stolte et al 1990).

The collagen layer is not just thickened in collagenous colitis, it also shows qualitative differences (Lazenby et al 1990). It may have an indistinct, blurred lower border. Occasionally it is acellular. However, most cases show an accumulation of lymphocytes, capillaries and myofibroblasts embedded in the thickened collagen layer (Widgren et al 1988).

An inflammatory infiltrate is another constant feature of collagenous colitis (Lazenby et al 1990). A thickened collagen layer can be mimicked histologically by tangential sectioning, superficial alignment of epithelial nuclei, or slicing the edge of a normal crypt. If the thickened collagen layer is the only criterion used in the identification of this conditions, and no attention is paid to the inflammatory infiltrate, misdiagnoses will occur. The infiltrate includes lymphocytes, eosinophils, variable numbers of mast cells (Flejou et al 1984, Balazs et al 1988) and plasma cells. Neutrophils are not commonly seen. All cases show degeneration of the epithelium (Jessurun et al 1987), which may become detached from the underlying collagen layer. This epithelial damage appears to be independent of the thickness of the adjacent collagen band. Intraepithelial CD8-positive T lymphocytes (Armes et al 1992) are present in increased numbers (Jessurun et al 1987). In one study there was a mean of 21 lymphocytes per 100 epithelial cells (Lazenby et al 1989). The morphological similarities to celiac disease are therefore striking.

Electron microscopy (Balazs et al 1988) shows production of collagen fibres by pericryptal fibroblasts (Hwang et al 1986), which develop from proliferating myofibroblasts (Widgren et al 1988). Ultrastructural study demonstrates that the classic description of collagenous colitis as a thickening of the basement membrane is an oversimplification. It has been convincingly shown that the basal lamina is normal or even focally deficient (Hwang et al 1986), and that the thickening is adjacent to rather than incorporating, the basal lamina (Flejou et al 1984).

Immunohistochemistry shows the thickened collagen to be types 1 and 3, with no type 4 collagen, laminin or fibronectin (Flejou et al 1984). This has implications for the pathogenesis of the disease.

The histological differential diagnosis is from ischemic colitis, amyloidosis and progressive systemic sclerosis. In ischemic colitis there is a more diffuse fibrosis, with atrophy of crypts. In amyloidosis the hyaline appearance is seen around glands as well as beneath the surface, and may also affect vessels. Progressive systemic sclerosis also affects all basement membranes, and may involve the entire lamina propria.

Some thickening of the basement membrane zone has been suggested as a non-specific feature of many diseases, and as the cause of diarrhea in such diseases (Gledhill & Cole 1984). An extensive study of 1549 mucosal specimens (Wang et al 1988) found a thickened subepithelial collagen layer in 33, but only a quarter of these had a history of unexplained diarrhea. However, those patients who did have diarrhea tended to have much thicker collagen layers. The average basement membrane thickness for patients without a history of diarrhea was 11 µm, and some may not have been classified as collagenous colitis in routine diagnostic practice. This work suggests that the thicker the collagen layer the more accurate the diagnosis of collagenous colitis.

Pathology

The unanswered question regarding collagenous colitis is: what causes the thickened collagen band, the associated inflammation and the diarrhea?

A number of theories are propounded to explain the presence of the thickened collagen layer. Two older theories, that there is some innate disorder in collagen synthesis, and that the collagen is a product of seepage from the vessels (Kingham et al 1986), no longer fit the known features of the disease. Neither explains its purely intestinal distribution. The success of various drugs in individual patients, for example cholestyramine (Andersen et al 1993), has raised the possibility of a role for bacterial cytotoxins in the pathogenesis.

Currently it seems that most support is for the idea that the collagen is a byproduct of some component of the inflammatory infiltrate. Sequential biopsy examination in two patients (Teglbjaerg et al 1984) has shown an initial episode of chronic active inflammation followed by gradual deposition of collagen. It is reassuring that the collagen is mainly of type 3 (Flejou et al 1984), itself usually seen in the context of repair following some form of injury. However, many diseases cause inflammation of the gut, and few cause a thickened collagen band. Ulcerative colitis is the best example of a disease causing prolonged inflammation, yet it does not affect the colonic epithelial basement membrane. It has been suggested that the rapid cell turnover seen in ulcerative colitis does not allow the development of mature fibroblasts from the myofibroblasts in the pericryptal sheath (Kingham et al 1986). Thus the inflammation of collagenous colitis may stimulate the myofibroblasts to mature into fibroblasts and commence the production of collagen fibres.

If the collagen band is a consequence of the inflammation, what causes the inflammation itself? Apart from a few case reports (Chandratre et al 1987, Giardiello et al 1991), there appears to be no link with inflammatory bowel disease. It has been suggested that diarrhea itself can cause the inflammation. This seems unlikely, as many systemic diseases which cause diarrhea show no inflammation.

One suggested cause of the inflammation is the administration of non-steroidal anti-inflammatory drugs (NSAIDs). It has been reported following the long-term administration of NSAIDS in two patients (Giardiello et al 1990). A case controlled study (Riddell et al 1992) of 31 patients with collagenous colitis showed they were much more likely to have a history of NSAID use. Some even showed improvement of diarrhea following cessation of therapy.

NSAIDs increase the permeability of the gut to a number of compounds, and may facilitate the toxicity of some other agent, either immunological or chemical (Riddell et al 1992). There are, however many problems associated with proving that a rare disease is linked to the administration of a class of drug as common as NSAIDs. Not least is the association of collagenous colitis with autoimmune diseases, the very conditions for which many non-steroidals are taken. Indeed, the rarity of collagenous colitis would argue against the involvement of such a common form of medication. Alternatively, three cases have been reported following administration of a phlebotonic drug (cyclo 3 fort) (Beaugerie et al 1994), but this obviously does not explain the vast majority of instances of the disease.

Autoimmunity has been suggested by many as the cause of the inflammation. The fact that many sufferers from collagenous colitis also have autoimmune diseases affecting, for example, the thyroid gland and joints, is suggestive. The female preponderance and the response to steroids (Jessurun et al 1987) have also been adduced in support of the association. However, studies on HLA associations have been disappointing and have shown no association between collagenous colitis and HLA antigens (Giardiello et al 1992). Electron microscopic examination shows no evidence of antigen–antibody complexes in colonic biopsies showing the disease (Fausa et al 1985).

Finally, what causes the diarrhea? Is it the increased collagen, preventing the reabsorption of solutes (Flejou et al 1984)? One large study (Wang et al 1988) suggests some correlation between collagen thickness and degree of diarrhea. However, as noted above, the average collagen layer thickness of their patients without diarrhea was 11 μm, and some might not be classified as collagenous colitis. Other studies have shown no correlation between the thickness of the band and the severity of the diarrhea (Wang et al 1987). Indeed, an occasional observation is the persistence of the collagen layer in some patients whose diarrhea has subsided following treatment, although histological regression has also been seen in some treated patients The few studies of the diarrhea itself suggest that it is secretory. There may be some increase in 24-hour fecal fats (Giardiello et al 1987), and there is net fluid secretion in the colon (Giardiello et al 1987). However, in other studies all tests are normal.

One intriguing suggestion is that mast cells may have an important role in the disease. Mast cells have long been recognized in collagenous colitis (Flejou et al 1984, Balazs et al 1988) and a case report has highlighted their presence in a case of microscopic colitis (Baum et al 1989). In this patient the use of the antihistamine chlorpheniramine resulted in a marked improvement of symptoms. Studies on the effects of histamine on the neurons of the gut in experimental animals has confirmed that long-term exposure to histamine continues to stimulate these nerves (Tamura & Wood 1992), unlike other neurotransmitters such as serotonin. This provides a plausible 'effector' arm for the causation of long-term diarrhea. It is also documented that an excess of mast cells in other conditions, such as systemic mastocytosis (Brunning et al 1983), can result in prominent thickening of basement membranes by collagen. The similarities with asthma (in which there is often subepithelial thickening by type 3 collagen, an excess of mast cells, intraepithelial lymphocytes, a long-term history of excess mucus secretion by an epithelial surface, and a variable response to anti-inflammatory therapy) is also striking. A potential line of research would be to measure the number of mast cells in the colonic mucosa of patients with collagenous colitis whose diarrhea was either well established or, conversely, had subsided.

Treatment

Various treatments for collagenous colitis have been used, with varying degrees of success. Straightforward symptomatic treatment with antidiarrheal drugs such as loperamide has not been successful. Case reports have shown the efficacy in individual patients of drugs such as peptobismol (bismuth subsalicylate) (Girard & Keeffe 1987), omeprazole (Roblin et al 1991), metronidazole (Mogensen et al 1984) and cholestyramine (Andersen et al 1993).

As the inflammatory infiltrate is a characteristic feature of collagenous colitis, empirically it would seem logical to attempt treatment with anti-inflammatory drugs. Indeed, initial reports confirmed the efficacy in individual cases of drugs such as sulfasalazine (Weidner et al 1984, Farah et al 1985). There is no consensus on the utility of such medicines in collagenous colitis. Kingham et al (1986) reported that only one of six patients found any benefit from standard anti-inflammatory treatment. Indeed, natural remission may occur in some patients even without treatment (Debongnie et al 1984). However, most series (Carpenter et al 1992) suggest at least some benefit to a proportion of patients from prednisolone, sulfasalazine and 5-ASA. Thus Giardiello et al (1987) showed a reduction of symptoms in four of seven patients given anti-inflammatory treatment. Two of these patients also apparently lost their collagen band, and such reduction of histological appearances has been reported in other studies (Pieterse et al 1982, Carpenter et al 1992). Although prednisolone has reduced stool frequency in some patients (Sloth et al 1991), the diarrhea returns once the treatment is stopped and it should only be used for acute diarrheal episodes.

MICROSCOPIC/LYMPHOCYTIC COLITIS

Some doubts may exist about the pathogenesis of collagenous colitis. It is, however, a well defined condition with a good claim to be a distinct nosological entity. This status is not shared by microscopic colitis. The very name is a cause of contention. The term is readily confused with 'minimal change' colitis (Eliot et al 1982), i.e. histologically unambiguous ulcerative colitis in a patient with normal endoscopic and radiographic appearances. Some refer to it as microscopic colitis, some as microscopic/lymphocytic colitis, and some as lymphocytic colitis. There may even be separate diseases: lymphocytic colitis and microscopic colitis. For the purposes of the current discussion, the nomenclature used will be that of the original researchers being referred to. At the end of the chapter, the rights of the respective conditions to separate classification will be discussed.

Natural history

Microscopic colitis was initially described by Read (Read et al 1980) and Kingham (Kingham et al 1982), who documented a uniform increase in inflammatory cells in the lamina propria in patients with diarrhea. Many of the characteristics of microscopic colitis are similar to those of collagenous colitis. Thus the disease presents with a long history of watery diarrhea. Most investigations are normal and the colonoscopy is macroscopically normal, although there is one case report of microscopic colitis with a 'mucosal nodularity' in the colon (Glick et al 1989). The age profiles are similar, and microscopic colitis has been reported in children (Mashako et al 1990). Indeed, the similarities are such that some have suggested that microscopic colitis is an early stage of collagenous colitis. However, there are also major differences. The female preponderance of lymphocytic colitis is much lower (1.3:1) (Giardiello et al 1989), which fortifies its position as a discrete disease from collagenous colitis. This is further supported by studies of HLA associations (Giardiello et al 1992), which have found an increase in HLA A1 and a decrease in HLA A3 in lymphocytic colitis patients. There was, however, no significant excess of other HLAs commonly associated with autoimmune diseases. These HLA associations were not seen in patients with collagenous colitis.

Pathology

Although colonoscopy is normal, biopsy shows an increase in lymphocytes, plasma cells, mast cells (Baum et al 1989) and occasionally neutrophils (Bo-Linn et al 1985) in the lamina propria, with some degeneration of the overlying epithelium. There is, however, no evidence of thickening of the basement membrane zone, and no specific features of inflammatory bowel disease are present. There may or may not be an increase in lymphocytes within the overlying epithelium (Fig. 39.2). This feature has resulted in the use of the term 'lymphocytic colitis', which may or may not be a discrete disease entity. In lymphocytic colitis, intraepithelial T lymphocytes are increased to around 25 per 100 epithelial cells (Lazenby et al 1989). This compares with the five per 100 seen in the normal colon.

Biochemical investigation of patients with microscopic colitis shows a reduction in colonic absorption of fluids (Bo-Linn et al 1985), associated with a reduction in sodium and chloride absorption.

The histological similarity with collagenous colitis may result in diagnostic confusion. A diagnosis of microscopic colitis based on a rectal biopsy alone may be missing a collagen band in the more proximal colon, thus it would seem reasonable to require a more proximal biopsy before making the definitive diagnosis of microscopic colitis.

Treatment

As in collagenous colitis, publications concerning the treatment of microscopic colitis depend mainly upon individual case reports. Thus response to cholestyramine (Rampton & Baithun 1987) and chlorpheniramine (Baum et al 1989) has been documented in individual cases.

MICROSCOPIC VS. LYMPHOCYTIC VS. COLLAGENOUS COLITIS

Current feeling is divided as to the validity and nomenclature of these diseases. Two main bodies of opinion

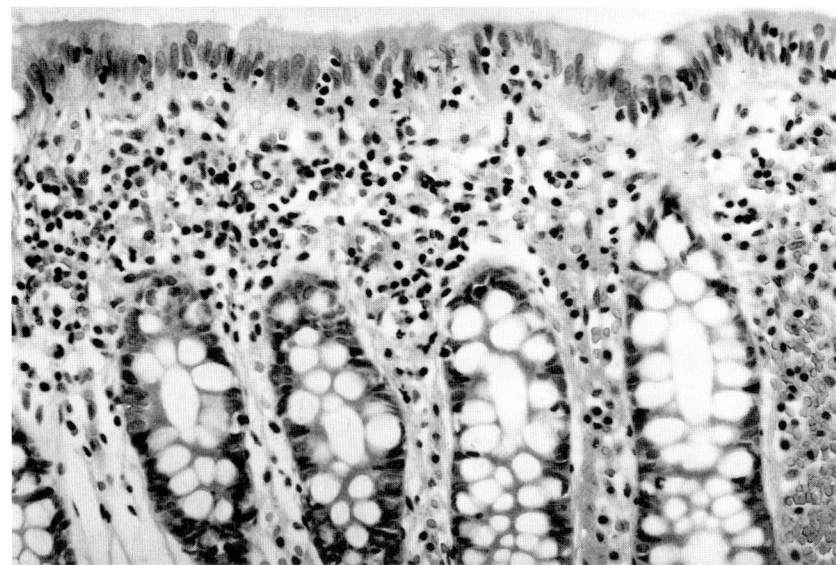

Fig. 39.2 Colonic biopsy showing increased intraepithelial lymphocytes in a case of lymphocytic colitis. (Hematoxylin and eosin × 250)

exist, with various subsets. They can be summarized as follows.

The one disease model. This suggests that most of these cases are collagenous colitis at varying stages of evolution. The similarities between the diseases are persuasive. Appearances identical to microscopic colitis can be seen following treatment and histological resolution of the thickened collagen band in collagenous colitis (Carpenter et al 1992). Review of five cases initially described as microscopic colitis by Kingham et al (1982) suggests that two were really collagenous colitis, one was inflammatory bowel disease and two were not further categorized (Levison et al 1993). Follow-up of nine cases of collagenous colitis for up to 5 years (Sylwestrowicz et al 1989) showed variations in collagen band thickness, with, sometimes, a microscopic colitis-like picture. Sylwestrowicz et al advocated grouping microscopic colitis and collagenous colitis together as 'watery diarrhea–colitis syndrome'. This group did, however, see one patient with a typical diarrhea history and 'microscopic colitis' picture on biopsy who, over 5 years, never showed any evidence of collagen thickening. When measurements of collagen table thickness are made in both groups no continuity is found, (Lee et al 1992), but rather two discrete groups of widths, suggesting the presence of two diseases. However, some cases of microscopic colitis may well be missed collagenous colitis. The missed cases may be a product of inadequate biopsies or non-recognition of the histology. Cases in one of the initial series of microscopic colitis (Bo-Linn et al 1985) were later considered to be mostly collagenous (Jessurun et al 1986). It has been suggested that lymphocytic colitis eventually develops into collagenous colitis, in a scenario analogous to that seen in celiac disease and collagenous sprue, but Giardiello et al (1989) found only one case of such progression in more than 18 studied.

The two disease model. This suggests that there are two diseases, i.e. collagenous colitis, and another characterized by the absence of a thickened collagen band and a normal colonoscopy. This model is confused by varying nomenclature. Some prefer to call it lymphocytic (Yardley et al 1990) and some prefer microscopic (Kingham 1991) colitis. Others call the disease microscopic (lymphocytic) colitis (Bogomoletz & Flejou 1991) or lymphocytic ('microscopic') colitis (Lazenby et al 1989). Lymphocytic colitis does differ in a number of ways from collagenous colitis, apart from the absence of a collagen layer. As noted above, there is a marked difference in sex ratio, and the HLA associations seen in lymphocytic colitis are absent in collagenous colitis.

There is much less support for the three-disease model, i.e. collagenous, lymphocytic (with intraepithelial lymphocytes) and microscopic (no intraepithelial lymphocytes) colitis. One study has found a distinct subset of microscopic colitis with a diffuse intraepithelial and intramucosal lymphocytic infiltrate (Mills et al 1993). The other cases of microscopic colitis, with a focal infiltrate and no intraepithelial lymphocytes, were often seen in patients with diverticulosis or polyps. Flejou and Bogomoletz (1993) suggested that lymphocytic and collagenous colitis were both forms of microscopic colitis, suggesting that there were some types of microscopic colitis which had neither an excess of intraepithelial lymphocytes nor subepithelial collagen, possibly related to NSAID use (Levison et al 1993).

It would seem to be most flexible for the purposes of research to acknowledge a difference between microscopic and lymphocytic colitis. Thus there may be a few patients with an appropriate clinical history, an excess of lymphocytes in the lamina propria, but no increase in intraepithelial lymphocytes (Bogomoletz & Flejou 1993). Calling these cases 'lymphocytic colitis' would confuse the picture. If future research shows that these cases are in fact inadequately sampled collagenous colitis, or an evolving stage of lymphocytic colitis, or indeed a mixture of conditions associated with many other diseases, no harm will be done. If, however, they are subsumed under the heading of lymphocytic colitis, the true identity of lymphocytic colitis may be obscured.

ASSOCIATIONS WITH OTHER DISEASE

Inflammatory bowel disease

Collagenous colitis has been seen in patients with ulcerative colitis (Giardiello et al 1991) and Crohn's disease (Chandratre et al 1987) in single case reports. Apart from these occasional instances there is no evidence of links between either collagenous or lymphocytic/microscopic colitis and inflammatory bowel disease.

Lymphocytic gastritis

The histological similarities between lymphocytic colitis and lymphocytic gastritis are evident, and an individual case report (Christ et al 1993) documents a patient with both diseases.

Celiac disease

The first reports of collagenous colitis associated with celiac disease (Eckstein et al 1988, Hamilton et al 1986) were of one or two cases respectively. The association was not surprising: the microscopic similarities between collagenous colitis and celiac disease/collagenous sprue were evident (intraepithelial lymphocytes, subepithelial collagen thickening, epithelial degeneration). In one series of nine patients with collagenous colitis or microscopic colitis (Sylwestrowicz et al 1989), one showed celiac disease and regression of colitis with gluten withdrawal, as was also seen in a case report (O'Mahony et al 1990). In another (Sylwestrowicz et al 1989) gluten withdrawal had no effect on the colitis. A stronger association was found in another study (Armes et al 1992), where review of 38 patients with collagenous colitis showed that four of 10 patients with small-bowel biopsies had celiac disease.

Two of the cases originally reported as having microscopic colitis and later reclassified as collagenous colitis (Levison et al 1993) showed subtotal villous atrophy on jejunal biopsy.

Lymphocytic colitis shows associations with celiac disease. When 39 patients with celiac disease had a colonoscopy (Wolber et al 1990), 12 had much-increased numbers of colonic intraepithelial T lymphocytes. Two also showed lymphocytic gastritis on gastric biopsy. However, only one of these 12 patients showed any reduction in colonic intraepithelial lymphocytes on a gluten-free diet. Review of the colonic biopsies of another 21 patients with celiac disease (DuBois et al 1989) showed five with lymphocytic colitis, of whom three showed no response to a gluten-free diet. There are, however, differences from celiac disease. Thus the antireticulin antibodies found in a third of patients with celiac disease are not found in patients with lymphocytic colitis (Greenson et al 1990).

The overlap between lymphocytic gastritis, celiac disease and collagenous/lymphocytic colitis could point to some common abnormality in the response to luminal antigen. The main site of involvement may be dictated by the nature of the antigen and its access to the mucosal immune system. Thus certain individuals only express an increase in intraepithelial lymphocytes or collagen deposition and perturbations of function at one site, whereas other individuals may show similar changes in the stomach and small and large intestines. It could be that lymphocytic/collagenous colitis is a reflection of a wider tendency to mount an atypical immune response in the gastrointestinal tract, and that the concept of a 'diffuse lymphocytic gastroenteritis' may eventually emerge.

REFERENCES

Andersen T, Andersen J R, Tvede M, Franzmann M B 1993 Collagenous colitis: are bacterial cytotoxins responsible? American Journal of Gastroenterology 88: 375–377

Armes J, Gee D C, Macrae F A, Schroeder W, Bhathal P S 1992 Collagenous colitis: jejunal and colorectal pathology. Journal of Clinical Pathology 45: 784–787

Balazs M, Egerszegi P, Vadasz G, Kovacs A 1988 Collagenous colitis: an electron microscopic study including comparison with the chronic fibrotic stage of ulcerative colitis. Histopathology 13: 319–328

Baum C A, Bhatia P, Miner P J 1989 Increased colonic mucosal mast cells associated with severe watery diarrhea and microscopic colitis. Digestive Diseases and Sciences 34: 1462–1465

Beaugerie L, Luboinski J, Brousse N et al 1994 Drug induced lymphocytic colitis. Gut 35: 426–428

Bogomoletz W V, Flejou J 1993 Microscopic colitis: A 'transatlantic' unifying concept. Gastroenterology 105: 1727

Bogomoletz W V, Flejou J F 1991 Newly recognized forms of colitis: collagenous colitis, microscopic (lymphocytic) colitis, and lymphoid follicular proctitis. Seminars in Diagnostic Pathology 8: 178–189

Bogomoletz W V, Adnet J J, Birembaut P, Feydy P, Dupont P 1980 Collagenous colitis: an unrecognised entity. Gut 21: 164–168

Bo-Linn G W, Vendrell D D, Lee E, Fordtran J S 1985 An evaluation of the significance of microscopic colitis in patients with chronic diarrhea. Journal of Clinical Investigation 75: 1559–1569

Brunning R D, McKenna R W, Rosai J 1983 Systemic mastocytosis: extracutaneous manifestations. American Journal of Surgical Pathology 7: 425–438

Busuttil A 1989 Collagenous colitis in a child. American Journal of Diseases of Children 143: 998–1000

Carpenter H A, Tremaine W J, Batts K P, Czaja A J 1992 Sequential histologic evaluations in collagenous colitis. Correlations with disease behaviour and sampling strategy. Digestive Diseases and Sciences 37: 1903–1909

Castanet J, Lacour J P, Ortonne J P 1994 Arthritis, collagenous colitis, and discoid lupus. Annals of Internal Medicine 120: 89–90

Chandratre S, Bramble M G, Cooke W M, Jones R A 1987 Simultaneous occurrence of collagenous colitis and Crohn's disease. Digestion 36: 55–60

Christ A D, Meier R, Bauerfeind P, Wegmann W, Gyr K 1993 Simultaneous occurrence of lymphocytic gastritis and lymphocytic colitis with transition to collagenous colitis. Schweizerische Medizinische Wochenschrift 123: 1487–1490

Debongnie J C, De G C, Caholessur M O, Haot J 1984 Collagenous colitis: a transient condition? Report of two cases. Diseases of the Colon and Rectum 27: 672–676

DuBois R N, Lazenby A J, Yardley J H, Hendrix T R, Bayless T M, Giardiello F M 1989 Lymphocytic enterocolitis in patients with 'refractory sprue'. Journal of the American Medical Association 262: 935–937

Eckstein R P, Dowsett J F, Riley J W 1988 Collagenous enterocolitis: a case of collagenous colitis with involvement of the small intestine. American Journal of Gastroenterology 83: 767–771

Eliot P R, Williams C B, Lennard-Jones J E et al 1982 Colonoscopic diagnosis of minimal change colitis in patients with a normal sigmoidoscopy and a normal air-contrast barium enema. Lancet i: 650–651

Esselinckx W, Brenard R, Colin J F, Melange M 1989 Juvenile scleroderma and collagenous colitis. The first case. Journal of Rheumatology 16: 834–836

Farah D A, Mills P R, Lee F D, McLay A, Russell R I 1985 Collagenous colitis: possible response to sulfasalazine and local steroid therapy. Gastroenterology 88: 792–797

Fausa O, Foerster A, Hovig T 1985 Collagenous colitis. A clinical, histological, and ultrastructural study. Scandinavian Journal of Gastroenterology 107 (Suppl): 8–23

Feczko P J, Mezwa D G 1991 Nonspecific radiographic abnormalities in collagenous colitis. Gastrointestinal Radiology 16: 128–132

Flejou J F, Bogomoletz W V 1993 Microscopic colitis: collagenous colitis and lymphocytic colitis. A single concept? Gastroenterologie Clinique et Biologique 17: 28–32

Flejou J F, Grimaud J A, Molas G, Baviera E, Potet F 1984 Collagenous colitis. Ultrastructural study and collagen immunotyping of four cases. Archives of Pathology and Laboratory Medicine 108: 977–982

Gardiner G W, Goldberg R, Currie D, Murray D 1984 Colonic carcinoma associated with an abnormal collagen table. Collagenous colitis. Cancer 54: 2973–2977

Giardiello F M, Bayless T M, Jessurun J, Hamilton S R, Yardley J H 1987 Collagenous colitis: physiologic and histopathologic studies in seven patients. Annals of Internal Medicine 106: 46–49

Giardiello F M, Hansen F C III, Lazenby A J et al 1990 Collagenous colitis in setting of nonsteroidal antiinflammatory drugs and antibiotics. Digestive Diseases and Sciences 35: 257–260

Giardiello F M, Jackson F W, Lazenby A J 1991 Metachronous occurrence of collagenous colitis and ulcerative colitis. Gut 32: 447–449

Giardiello F M, Lazenby A J, Bayless T M et al 1989 Lymphocytic (microscopic) colitis. Clinicopathologic study of 18 patients and comparison to collagenous colitis. Digestive Diseases and Sciences 34: 1730–1738

Giardiello F M, Lazenby A J, Yardley J H et al 1992 Increased HLA A1 and diminished HLA A3 in lymphocytic colitis compared to controls and patients with collagenous colitis. Digestive Diseases and Sciences 37: 496–499

Girard D E, Keeffe E B 1987 Therapy for collagenous colitis. Annals of Internal Medicine 106: 909

Gledhill A, Cole F M 1984 Significance of basement membrane thickening in the human colon. Gut 25: 1085–1088

Glick S N, Teplick S K, Amenta P S 1989 Microscopic (collagenous) colitis. American Journal of Roentgenology 153: 995–996

Greenson J K, Giardiello F M, Lazenby A J, Pena S A, Bayless T M, Yardley J H 1990 Antireticulin antibodies in collagenous and lymphocytic (microscopic) colitis. Modern Pathology 3: 259–260

Gremse D A, Boudreaux C W, Manci E A 1993 Collagenous colitis in children. Gastroenterology 104: 906–909

Hamilton I, Sanders S, Hopwood D, Bouchier I A 1986 Collagenous colitis associated with small intestinal villous atrophy. Gut 27: 1394–1398

Hwang W S, Kelly J K, Shaffer E A, Hershfield N B 1986 Collagenous colitis: a disease of pericryptal fibroblast sheath? Journal of Pathology 149: 33–40

Jessurun J, Yardley J H, Giardiello F M, Hamilton S R, Bayless T M 1987 Chronic colitis with thickening of the subepithelial collagen layer (collagenous colitis): histopathologic findings in 15 patients. Human Pathology 18: 839–848

Jessurun J, Yardley J H, Lee E L, Vendrell D D, Schiller L R, Fordtran J S 1986 Microscopic and collagenous colitis: different names for the same condition? Gastroenterology 91: 1583–1584

Kenesi L M, Chapelon A C, Fattah Z A, Naudin G, Godeau P 1991 The first case of CRST syndrome associated with collagenous colitis. Journal of Rheumatology 18: 1765–1767

Kingham J G 1991 Microscopic colitis. Gut 32: 234–235

Kingham J G, Levison D A, Ball J A, Dawson A M 1982 Microscopic colitis – a cause of chronic watery diarrhoea. British Medical Journal Clinical Research 285: 1601–1604

Kingham J G, Levison D A, Morson B C, Dawson A M 1986 Collagenous colitis. Gut 27: 570–577

Lazenby A J, Yardley J H, Giardiello F M, Bayless T M 1990 Pitfalls in the diagnosis of collagenous colitis: experience with 75 cases from a registry of collagenous colitis at the Johns Hopkins Hospital. Human Pathology 21: 905–910

Lazenby A J, Yardley J H, Giardiello F M, Jessurun J, Bayless T M 1989 Lymphocytic ('microscopic') colitis: a comparative histopathologic study with particular reference to collagenous colitis. Human Pathology 20: 18–28

Lee E, Schiller L R, Vendrell D, Santa A C, Fordtran J S 1992 Subepithelial collagen table thickness in colon specimens from patients with microscopic colitis and collagenous colitis. Gastroenterology 103: 1790–1796

Leigh C, Elahmady A, Mitros F A, Metcalf A, al-Jurf A 1993 Collagenous colitis associated with chronic constipation. American Journal of Surgical Pathology 17: 81–84

Levison D A, Lazenby A J, Yardley J H 1993 Microscopic colitis cases revisited. Gastroenterology 105: 1594–1596

Lewis F W, Warren G H, Goff J S 1991 Collagenous colitis with involvement of terminal ileum. Digestive Diseases and Sciences 36: 1161–1163

Lindstrom C G 1976 'Collagenous colitis' with watery diarrhoea – a new entity? Pathologia Europaea 11: 87–89

MacIntosh D G, Thompson W G, Patel D G, Barr R, Guindi M 1992 Is rectal biopsy necessary in irritable bowel syndrome? American Journal of Gastroenterology 87: 1407–1409

Mashako M N, Sonsino E, Navarro J et al 1990 Microscopic colitis: a new cause of chronic diarrhea in children? Journal of Pediatric Gastroenterology and Nutrition 10: 21–26

Mills L R, Schuman B M, Thompson W O 1993 Lymphocytic colitis. A definable clinical and histological diagnosis. Digestive Diseases and Sciences 38: 1147–1151

Mogensen A M, Olsen J H, Gudmand H E 1984 Collagenous colitis. Acta Medica Scandinavica 216: 535–540

Nussinson E, Samara M, Vigder L, Shafer I, Tzur N 1988 Concurrent collagenous colitis and multiple ileal carcinoids. Digestive Diseases and Sciences 33: 1040–1044

O'Mahony S, Nawroz I M, Ferguson A 1990 Coeliac disease and collagenous colitis. Postgraduate Medical Journal 66: 238–241

Palmer K R, Berry H, Wheeler P J et al 1986 Collagenous colitis – a relapsing and remitting disease. Gut 27: 578–580

Perisic V N, Kokai G 1989 Diarrhoea caused by collagenous colitis. Archives of Disease in Childhood 64: 867–869

Pieterse A S, Hecker R, Rowland R 1982 Collagenous colitis: a distinctive and potentially reversible disorder. Journal of Clinical Pathology 35: 338–340

Prior A, Lessells A M, Whorwell P J 1987 Is biopsy necessary if colonoscopy is normal? Digestive Diseases and Sciences 32: 673–676

Puri A S, Khan E M, Kumar M, Pandey R, Choudhuri G 1994 Association of lymphocytic (microscopic) colitis with tropical sprue. Journal of Gastroenterology and Hepatology 9: 105–107

Rampton D S, Baithun S I 1987 Is microscopic colitis due to bile-salt malabsorption? Diseases of the Colon and Rectum 30: 950–952

Read N, Krejs G J, Read M G 1980 Chronic diarrhea of unknown origin. Gastroenterology 78: 264–271

Richieri J P, Bonneau H P, Cano N, Di C J, Martin J 1993 Collagenous colitis: an unusual endoscopic appearance. Gastrointestinal endoscopy 39: 192–194

Riddell R H, Tanaka M, Mazzoleni G 1992 Non-steroidal anti-inflammatory drugs as a possible cause of collagenous colitis: a case-control study. Gut 33: 683–686

Roblin X, Becot F, Abinader J, Piquemal A, Monnet D, Carre J L 1991 Value of omeprazole in the treatment of collagenous colitis. Annales de Gastroenterologie et d'Hepatologie 27: 177–178

Roubenoff R, Ratain J, Giardiello F et al 1989 Collagenous colitis, enteropathic arthritis, and autoimmune diseases: results of a patient survey. Journal of Rheumatology 16: 1229–1232

Sloth H, Bisgaard C, Grove A 1991 Collagenous colitis: a prospective trial of prednisolone in six patients. Journal of Internal Medicine 229: 443–446

Stolte M, Ritter M, Borchard F, Koch S G 1990 Collagenous gastroduodenitis on collagenous colitis. Endoscopy 22: 186–187

Sylwestrowicz T, Kelly J K, Hwang W S, Shaffer E A 1989 Collagenous colitis and microscopic colitis: the watery diarrhea–colitis syndrome. American Journal of Gastroenterology 84: 763–768

Tamura K, Wood J D 1992 Effects of prolonged exposure to histamine on guinea pig intestinal neurons. Digestive Diseases and Sciences 37: 1084–1088

Tanaka M, Mazzoleni G, Riddell R H 1992 Distribution of collagenous colitis: utility of flexible sigmoidoscopy. Gut 33: 65–70

Teglbjaerg P S, Thaysen E H, Jensen H H 1984 Development of collagenous colitis in sequential biopsy specimens. Gastroenterology 87: 703–709

van der Werf S D, van Berge Henegouwen G P, Bronkhorst F B, Werre J M 1987 Chemotherapy responsive collagenous colitis in a patient with Hodgkin's disease: a possible paraneoplastic phenomenon. Netherlands Journal of Medicine 31: 228–233

van Tilburg A J, Lam H G, Seldenrijk C A et al 1990 Familial occurrence of collagenous colitis. A report of two families. Journal of Clinical Gastroenterology 12: 279–285

Wang H H, Owings D V, Antonioli D A, Goldman H 1988 Increased subepithelial collagen deposition is not specific for collagenous colitis. Modern Pathology 1: 329–335

Wang K K, Perrault J, Carpenter H A, Schroeder K W, Tremaine W J 1987 Collagenous colitis: a clinicopathologic correlation. Mayo Clinic Proceedings 62: 665–671

Weidner N, Smith J, Pattee B 1984 Sulfasalazine in treatment of collagenous colitis. Case report and review of the literature. American Journal of Medicine 77: 162–166

Wengrower D, Pollak A, Okon E, Stalnikowicz R 1987 Collagenous colitis and rheumatoid arthritis with response to sulfasalazine. A case report and review of the literature. Journal of Clinical Gastroenterology 9: 456–460

Widgren S, Jlidi R, Cox J N 1988 Collagenous colitis: histologic, morphometric, immunohistochemical and ultrastructural studies. Report of 21 cases. Virchows Archiv A, Pathological Anatomy and Histopathology 413: 287–296

Widgren S, MacGee W 1990 Collagenous colitis with protracted course and fatal evolution. Report of a case. Pathology, Research and Practice 186: 303–306

Wiener M D 1986 Collagenous colitis and pulmonary fibrosis. Manifestations of a single disease? Journal of Clinical Gastroenterology 8: 677–680

Williams G T, Rhodes J 1987 Collagenous colitis: disease or diversion? British Medical Journal Clinical Research 294: 855–856

Wolber R, Owen D, Freeman H 1990 Colonic lymphocytosis in patients with celiac sprue. Human Pathology 21: 1092–1096

Yardley J H, Lazenby A J, Giardiello F M, Bayless T M 1990 Collagenous, 'microscopic', lymphocytic, and other gentler and more subtle forms of colitis. Human Pathology 21: 1089–1091

Yardley J H, Lazenby A J, Kornacki S 1993 Collagenous colitis in children. Gastroenterology 105: 647–648

40. Other granulomatous diseases of the bowel

H. H. Tsai

INTRODUCTION

Granulomata are a pathological hallmark of Crohn's disease, and understanding the factors that lead to their formation should improve our understanding of Crohn's disease itself. There is a wide range of granulomatous diseases, some of completely unknown etiology, e.g. sarcoidosis, some with known antigens, e.g. tuberculosis, berylliosis, and some with well characterized underlying defects in phagocyte function, e.g. chronic granulomatous disease of childhood. The clinical manifestations of these conditions often overlap with each other and sometimes with Crohn's disease. They are therefore considered here, because of the need to recognize them as distinct from Crohn's disease, and also because they may help us to better understand the pathophysiology of Crohn's disease.

THE GRANULOMATOUS INFLAMMATORY RESPONSE

The granulomatous response is characterized by a localized collection of epithelioid cells, macrophages and lymphocytes. It is the host response to a persistent irritant or pathogen (Sheffield 1990) and is found in many infective, allergic, neoplastic and autoimmune disorders. Infective causes include schistosomiasis, tuberculosis, leprosy and fungal infections (Ridley 1974). Drugs and metals (barium, beryllium, copper) may also act as triggering agents (Boros 1980). Autoimmune diseases and diseases of uncertain etiology include sarcoidosis, primary biliary cirrhosis, Whipple's disease and Crohn's disease. The nature and evolution of the granuloma depends on the irritant involved and the immune competence of the host.

Cellular composition of a granuloma

The principal cells involved in granuloma formation are derived from circulating mononuclear phagocytes (macrophage/monocytes). These cells may change their morphology to form epithelioid cells. Aging macrophages may also fuse with newly arrived mononuclear cells to form multinuclear giant cells (Chambers 1978). The function of these differentiated macrophages remains unclear. Epithelioid cells may have a secretory role (Pertshuk et al 1981) but are poorly phagocytic, and giant cells are unable to phagocytose. This cohesive aggregation of cells is often surrounded by plasma cells and fibroblasts. It is usual to divide granulomatous responses into two classes, the foreign-body type granulomas induced by agents such as talc, silica and carageenan, and immune (hypersensitivity)-type epithelioid granulomas found in infective lesions. Epithelioid cell granulomas are differentiated from foreign body granulomas on light microscopy by the presence of lymphocytes which show close interactions with the epithelioid cells. These divisions are not absolute, as metals such as zirconium and beryllium induce immune-type granulomas, possibly via an autoimmune response.

The macrophages of the granuloma are derived from circulating monocytes, which originate from the bone marrow. The resident macrophage population may also participate and there is also some evidence of local macrophage multiplication (Dannenburg et al 1975). Macrophages contain peroxidase, esterase and lysozyme activity and express receptors for complement (C3) and immunoglobulin (Fc). As the stimulus is chronic, a granuloma contains macrophages at differing times of differentiation and maturation. These differently aged macrophages display varying phagocytic activity, HLA (Ia) antigen processing activity, Fc receptors and C3 receptors. Thus, in a typical granuloma both small and large macrophages, epithelioid and giant cells may all be present. Giant cells may represent the final fate of aging or dying macrophages.

Macrophages secrete a number of products in response to interferon-γ and other mediators. These secretory products include products that are preformed and released, such as lysozyme, lactoferrin, fibronectin, prostaglandins, C1Q, C2, C3, factor H and factor I (Nathan 1987). Others are induced by the antigen stimulus and include IL-1, angiotensins, angiogenesis factors, tumor necrosis factors (TNF), leukotriene C4 and hydrogen peroxide.

Macrophages play a vital role in microbial defense and the secretory products lactoferrin, pepsin G and lysozyme have an antimicrobial effect (Gordon et al 1974, Bennet & Kokocinsky 1978). Bactericidal oxygen radicals are also released. Macrophages possess a unique membrane-associated nicotinamide adenine dinucleotide phosphate (NADPH)-oxidase system, dormant in resting cells, which becomes activated upon exposure to the appropriate stimulus and catalyzes the one-electron reduction of molecular oxygen to superoxide, O_2^-. Oxidase activation involves the assembly in the plasma membrane, of membrane-bound and cytosolic constituents of the oxidase system, which are disassembled in the resting stage (Babior et al 1971). An inherited deficiency in the ability to mount this 'oxygen burst' as a result of a cytochrome defect is the basis of chronic granulomatous disease. Another product of macrophage activation is nitric oxide (Mathew & Wienstock 1994), which has the effect of locally improving blood supply.

Monocytes in culture are capable of differentiating into epithelioid cells (Sutton & Weiss 1966). Under electron microscopy epithelioid cells show a well developed rough endoplasmic reticulum and Golgi apparatus. There are also large numbers of secretory vacuoles. This suggests that these cells have a major secretory contribution. The products of their prolific secretory apparatus is uncertain. They do not contain acid phosphatase and are thus unlikely to be of lysosomal origin. However, mucopolysaccharides and angiotensin-converting enzymes have been found in their secretory vacuoles (Pertshuk et al 1981). Whether these cells participate in antigen processing is unclear. In sarcoid granulomas they appear to strongly express HLA-DR (Ia) antigens (Munro et al 1988), but this is not universally reported (Turk & Narayanan 1982). However, they do appear to interact closely with activated T lymphocytes (Unanue 1980).

In epithelioid cell (hypersensitivity) granulomas lymphocytes play a very important role. In mature granulomas there are two populations of lymphocytes, those that are scattered between epithelioid cells in the centre of the granuloma (mainly of the CD4 helper/inducer type) and a second population of mainly CD8 suppressor/ cytotoxic lymphocytes, forming a mantle around the inflammatory focus (Mishra et al 1983). This suggest that the granuloma forms a microenvironment that walls off the irritant.

The CD4 T cells are important as orchestrators of the granulomatous response and its resolution. Thymectomized mice and nude mice fail to mount a granulomatous response (Byram or von Lichtenberg 1977). Also, administration of anti-CD4 monoclonal antibody greatly diminishes the ability of the host to form granulomas (Mathew & Boros 1986). Interestingly, in acquired immune deficiency syndrome (AIDS), where there is a selective depletion of CD4 T cells, the patient is particularly vulnerable to organisms that normally invoke a granulomatous response, such as *Mycobacterium avium intracellulare*, *Toxoplasma gondii*, *Pneumocystis carinii* and cytomegalovirus. Furthermore, in granulomatous diseases such as Crohn's disease, resolution occurs in patients who develop AIDS (James 1988).

CD4 T cells orchestrate the granulomatous response by the secretion of various lymphokines. The type of lymphokine released depends on the disease process. In Crohn's disease, schistosomiasis and other helminthic infections, where eosinophils are commonly encountered, the CD4 cells secrete IL-5, an important eosinophil differentiation and growth factor (Yamamura et al 1991). There are varying cycles of inflammation and resolution (modulation), and this process is probably controlled by the T cells.

The function of B cells in Crohn's disease granulomas is not known. In some granulomas they appear to produce anti-idiotypic antibodies, which may be important in downregulation of the granuloma (Weinstock 1992). Eosinophils and mast cells are also commonly seen in association with granulomas in Crohn's disease. Eosinophils respond to CD4-produced IL-5, and this can be abolished by anti-IL-5 antibodies (Sher et al 1990). In schistosomiasis, eosinophils play an important role in the destruction of the parasite (James & Colley 1978). Their function in Crohn's disease is unknown. It is likely that mast cells control the local vascular flow through the granuloma (Varilek et al 1991).

Diagnostic value of granulomas in Crohn's disease

In Crohn's disease, granulomas may be found in any part of the intestine, from mouth to anus, but are particularly common in patients with rectal and anal disease (Chambers & Morson 1979). Although most extraintestinal manifestations of the disease are not granulomatous, rare cutaneous metastatic Crohn's disease may contain granulomas (Tweedie & McGann 1984).

Reported rates of granulomas detection vary from 50 to 70% (Morsan 1968, Schmitz-Moormann & Pittner 1984), depending on the tissue studied. Unless a large number of sections are taken at many levels, many may be missed. The lesions tend to occur in the submucosa, but may occur in all layers of the bowel. Hence the chance of picking up a granuloma on small focal colonoscopic biopsies is not likely to exceed 25% (Potzi et al 1989), but may be improved by biopsying adjacent to ulcerated areas. On resected surgical specimens, granulomas in mesenteric lymph nodes may be found in up to a quarter of cases (Geboes et al 1986). Mesenteric nodal granulomas are rare in the absence of intestinal disease, and an alternative diagnosis should then be sought (Cook 1972). The incidence of granulomas in Crohn's disease declines with the age of onset of disease (Schmitz-Moormann & Schag 1990; Kelly & Sutherland 1988).

Granulomas in Crohn's disease are associated with damage to intestinal vasculature. They occur close to or within vessels or lymphatics, and it has therefore been suggested that Crohn's disease represents a granulomatous vasculitis (Wakefield et al 1991) associated with thrombosis and possible microinfarction (Wakefield et al 1989).

Although the granuloma is the hallmark of Crohn's disease, their relative infrequency in biopsy specimens makes them less useful as a diagnostic tool. Other microscopic features are important, and the histological findings must be interpreted in the light of clinical context. However, the presence of non-caseating granulomas in the intestinal tract in western populations is highly suggestive of Crohn's disease. Other colonic diseases that produce granulomas include campylobacter, chlamydia, yersinia and tuberculosis (Surawicz 1968). Authorities disagree as to whether the presence of small numbers of granulomas in the presence of otherwise typical features of ulcerative colitis implies that the disease is not ulcerative colitis. It is probably wisest to accept that there is overlap, and some patients may switch from typical ulcerative colitis to typical Crohn's disease (Dwarakanath et al 1994) or remain indeterminate.

Prognostic value of granulomas in Crohn's disease

In children the presence of granulomas found in rectosigmoid biopsies has been reported to be associated with a poorer prognosis (Markowitz et al 1989). In adult Crohn's disease, two studies reported that patients with more granulomas in resected specimens have a better prognosis (Glass & Baker 1976, Chambers & Morson 1979), although a more recent study has failed to show such an association (Wolfsan et al 1982).

OTHER GRANULOMATOUS DISEASES OF THE BOWEL

Chronic granulomatous disease

Chronic granulomatous disease (CGD), first described in 1957 (Landing & Shrikey 1957, Berendes et al 1957), is a rare inherited disease characterized by recurrent life-threatening infections, hypergammaglobulinemia and widespread granulomatous lesions. It is characterized by the absence of respiratory burst activity in phagocytes of affected individuals. Although hereditary, it is also characterized by remarkable genetic and clinical heterogeneity. The molecular basis of this condition has been recently characterized (Thrasher et al 1994).

Clinical features

CGD is rare, affecting about 1 in 500 000 of the population. It is probably underdiagnosed, as milder forms of the disease exist. The presence of phenotypic heterogeneity suggests that several different genes may be involved. The original description of the disease was as an X-linked disorder but females with an identical syndrome were then reported (Azimi et al 1968, Quie et al 1968). Variable clinical manifestations may occur even in the same family. In general, those with the X-linked disease have a more severe clinical course.

Most patients are diagnosed in the first 2 years of life, although some are diagnosed in later childhood or even adulthood (Johnston & Newman 1977). The principal clinical feature is that of recurrent bacterial and fungal infections. Infections occur particularly on epithelial surfaces that are in contact with the external environment. Thus infections of the skin, mucous membranes, respiratory and alimentary tract are the most common. Affected individuals commonly present with lymphadenopathy, cutaneous infections, chest infections, diarrhea and pyrexia. Associated deep infections are also common, owing to hematological spread. These include osteomyelitis, hepatic abscesses, kidney infections and septicemia. Clinical examination may reveal hepatosplenomegaly, pallor and lymphadenopathy in a child that presents with failure to thrive.

The most common infective agents encountered are *Staphylococcus aureus* and *Aspergillus fumigatus*. Other important bacterial pathogens include *Pseudomonas cepacia*, which is potentially lethal (O'Neil et al 1986), *Candida albicans* and *Nocardia* spp. It is somewhat surprising that many other major pathogens are not more frequently encountered in CGD, given the fundamental defect of phagocyte function. This may be because of preservation of non-oxidant mechanisms of microbial killing, such as lysozyme (Odell & Segal 1991). It is notable that the principal CGD pathogens possess catalase (Mandell & Hook 1969) as a further handicap to oxidative killing.

With modern antibiotic therapy many affected children survive well into adulthood, and suffer the consequences of chronic inflammatory stimulation. These include the non-infective complications of glomerulonephritis, pulmonary fibrosis and granulomatous gastrointestinal obstructions.

Gastrointestinal lesions are particularly important. They may mimic Crohn's disease clinically, radiologically and histopathologically (Isaacs et al 1985). If the incorrect diagnosis is made the consequences may be disastrous, as corticosteroids would further immunocompromise the patient. Gastrointestinal involvement may include granulomatous narrowing of the gastric antrum (Griscom et al 1974), perianal fistulation, ileal disease and colitis. Children usually present in the first year of life, which should alert the physician as Crohn's disease in the first year of life is most unusual. A family history may be present. Patients with milder forms of CGD may present much later in life, and presentation of gastrointestinal manifestations well into the teens has been reported (Harris & Boles 1973).

Retrospective studies suggest a 10-year survival rate of between 50 and 70%, although those surviving beyond 20 years do very well (Mouy et al 1989, Finn et al 1990). The introduction of newer antibiotics and prophylactic antibiotic therapy is likely to improve the future prognosis of these patients.

Pathology and molecular pathology

The gastrointestinal lesions of CGD show granulomata with lipid-laden macrophages. Ileal lesions usually show infiltration of lipid-laden macrophages only, although rectal and gastric lesions tend to show granulomas (Ament & Ochs 1973). Occasionally, ileal lesions may display large non-caseating granulomas that infiltrate the muscular coat with prominent eosinophils. Fibrosis and transmural inflammation may be seen, and this may be indistinguishable from Crohn's disease histologically (Isaacs et al 1985).

The biochemical and molecular basis of CGD has been elucidated. The basic defect is a failure of phagocytic cells to mount an oxygen burst on opsonizing. Normal phagocytes increase their oxygen consumption 100-fold when stimulated (Behner & Nathan 1967). This has the effect of generating free radicals (O_2^-, H_2O_2 or HOCl) by which macrophages kill microbes (Weiss 1989). The generation of these oxygen nascents is catalyzed by the enzyme NADPH oxidase. This is a complex enzyme with four components, named after their protein type, (gp = glycoprotein, p = protein) followed by the molecular weight in kDa, and have the suffix *phox* to indicate that they are *p*hagocyte *ox*idases. Thus the four units are gp91-*phox*, p22-*phox*, p47-*phox* and p67-*phox*. All four subunits have now been sequenced. Defects in any of the subunits result in the phenotype.

In the inactive state the NADPH oxidase complex is disengaged, with the gp91-*phox* and p22-*phox* attached to the membrane and p47-*phox* and p67-*phox* in the cytosol (Leto et al 1991). Upon stimulation the cytosolic components translocate to the membrane portion, and with the participation of flavin (FAD) as electron donors catalyze the oxidative process. gp91-*phox* is located in chromosome X. Defects in this gene account for the X-linked cases of CGD and make up some 65% of patients (Dinnaer et al 1987). The rest of the autosomal cases have defects in any of the other three components of the enzyme. p22-*phox*, p47-*phox* and p67-*phox* are located in chromosomes 16, 7 and 1 respectively. Reported mutations include deletions, insertions, point mutations leading to premature stop codons, amino acid substitutions, and splice site defects (Curnutte 1993). Many mutations are unique to their families.

The molecular unveiling of CGD has opened up exciting prospects in the uncovering of other diseases in which granulomas play an important role, particularly its gastrointestinal mimic, Crohn's disease.

Diagnosis and clinical management

Anemia of chronic disease is frequent, but malabsorption of B_{12} owing to ileal disease may occur. Hypergammaglobulinemia is usual, with a high ESR. Leukocytosis suggests an infective episode.

Diagnosis is made by demonstrating a defect in respiratory burst activity in phagocytic cells. The most common screening test used is the dye nitroblue tetrazolium (NBT) microscope test (Ochs & Igo 1973). This assesses the ability of the cell to produce superoxide, which changes the colour of the dye from yellow to a blue precipitate. The test is only qualitative, and may also detect some female carriers of the X-linked disease. This is because some carriers have partial or even preferential inactivation of the normal gene. Carriers of the autosomal variety require genetic analysis for detection. Confirmation of diagnosis is made either by direct measurement of oxygen consumption, or measurement of superoxide production by chemiluminescence (Wyman et al 1987).

Clinical management takes the form of prevention and aggressive treatment of infection. General measures include immunization, avoidance of infection and adequate nutrition, especially of those with gastrointestinal manifestations, who may require enteral nutrition. The anemia responds to erythropoietin.

Prophylactic antibiotics (usually co-trimoxazole) are recommended and are effective in reducing bacterial infective episodes (Margolis et al 1990). Interferon-gamma (IFN-γ) appears to be effective in reducing the risk of serious infection, and may be considered in particularly at-risk patients (International Chronic Granulomatous Disease Study Group 1991).

Infective episodes are treated aggressively with the appropriate antibiotics, depending on pathogen and sensitivity. In many instances the pathogen is not isolated and empirical treatment with a combination of antipseudomonal antibiotics such as ceftazidime and ciprofloxacin is required, along with a broad-spectrum antibiotic active against Gram-positive organisms such as teicoplanin. Fungal infections require amphotericin intravenously, but the availability of itraconazole as an oral agent is now replacing the more toxic drug. Granulomatous intestinal disease may necessitate enteral feeding, but may respond to careful use of corticosteroids, provided prophylactic antibiotics are used as well (Thrasher et al 1994).

Although hemopoietic stem cell transplantation may be expected to work, the results are poor and associated with a high mortality (Kamani et al 1988). Gene therapy using a viral vector is an intriguing possibility for the future.

Malakoplakia

Malakoplakia was first noted by von Hansemann in 1900 in the bladder, but it was his assistant Michaelis, with Gutmann, who first published the findings of the characteristic inclusion bodies found in these lesions which now bear their names (Michaelis & Gutmann 1902). von Hasemann coined the word 'malakoplakia' (malakos = soft, plakos = plaques).

Malakoplakia usually affects the urinary tract, but it may also affect the gastrointestinal tract when it mimics Crohn's disease. It usually presents as solitary or multiple 'tumors' of the large bowel (Joyeuse et al 1971) but diffuse colonic involvement has also been reported (di Silvo & Bartlett 1971). Twenty-seven cases of gastrointestinal malakoplakia have so far been reported in the English literature (Joyeuse et al 1971, di Silvo & Bartlett 1971, Sanusi & Tio 1974, Ng & Ng 1993, Terner & Lattes 1965, Gonzales-Angulo et al 1965, Kuzma 1966, Yunis et al 1967, Finlay-Jones et al 1968, Rywlin et al 1969, Dockerty 1972, Ranchod & Kaln 1972, Wilkey & Rubel 1972, de la Garza et al 1973, Lewin et al 1974, Robert et al 1974, Lou & Teplitz 1974, Sinclair-Smith et al 1975, Chaudhry et al 1979, 1980, Satti et al 1985, El-Mouzan et al 1988, Moran et al 1989). All had colonic disease, although one had additional gastric involvement and three had ileal disease. The sites suggest that areas of bacterial colonization are important for the development of the condition. It occurs in association with malignancy or chronic debility, and in immunocompromised or immunosuppressed patients. Seven cases were associated with systemic diseases, including lymphoma, leukemia, tuberculosis, diabetes mellitus, cirrhosis, drug abuse and chronic chest disease. In 12 patients there was associated gastrointestinal disease, six with colorectal adenocarcinoma, two with adenomas, two with abdominal infections (tuberculosis and cytomegalovirus), and two with ulcerative colitis.

Renal tract malakoplakia is more common in women (female to male ratio 3:1), in whom the lesions develop in a younger age group (third to fifth decades) than in men (over 50 years) (Dobyan et al 1993).

The histology is characteristic, with infiltration by macrophages with ample cytoplasm containing abundant periodic acid–Schiff-positive granules, known as von Hansemann cells, and the presence of diagnostic extracytoplasmic or intracytoplasmic calcospherites, known as Michaelis–Gutmann bodies. These bodies are chemically identified as calcium hydroxyapatite in a glycolipid matrix (An et al 1974). The pathogenesis of these granules is unclear, but is likely to represent incomplete digestion of glycolipid by macrophage lysozymes. There is evidence that it represents an abnormal macrophage response to bacterial infection (Abdou et al 1977). It is common to find coliform bacteria in the macrophages, suggesting a macrophage defect in bacteria killing.

Control of bacterial infections is the mainstay of therapy. The recommended antibiotics are those that penetrate macrophages well, such as trimethoprim-sulphamathoxazole, rifampicin and ciprofloxacin (Dobyan et al 1993). Ascorbic acid and bethanecol may help restore macrophage function by increasing intracellular cGMP. Often very prolonged use of the antibiotics is required. If patients are receiving immunosuppressives then attempts should be made to withdraw them. Surgery may be required for bowel obstruction. Prognosis is dependent largely on the underlying pathology, as the majority of those with colonic malakoplakia succumb to the coexisting systemic or malignant disease. Patients with uncomplicated disease do well with antibiotic treatment, and some of those on immunosuppression have complete resolution of disease on withdrawal of the drugs. Extensive disease and multiorgan involvement carry a poor prognosis (Deridder et al 1977).

REFERENCES

Abdou N I, Napombejera C, Sagawa A 1977 Malakoplakia: evidence for a correctable monocyte lysosomal abnormality. New England Journal of Medicine 297: 1413

Ament M E, Ochs H D 1973 Gastrointestinal manifestations of chronic granulomatous disease. New England Journal of Medicine 288: 382–387

An T, Ferenczy A, Wilens S L, Melicow M M 1974 Observation of the formation of Michaelis–Gutmann bodies. Human Pathology 5: 753–758

Azimi P H, Bodenbender J G, Hintz R L, Kontras S B 1968 Chronic granulomatous disease in three female siblings. Journal of the American Medical Association 206: 2865–2870

Babior B M, Kipnes R S, Carnutte J T 1971 Biological defence mechanisms: the production of leukocytes of superoxide, a potential bacteriocidal agent. Journal of Clinical Investigation 52: 741–744

Behner R L, Nathan D G 1967 Leukocyte oxidase: defective activity in chronic granulomatous disease. Science 155: 835–836

Bennet R M, Kokocinsky T 1978 Lactoferrin content of peripheral blood cells. British Journal of Haematology 39: 509

Berendes H, Bridges R A, Good R A 1957 Fatal granulomatosis of childhood. Minnesota Medicine 40: 309–312

Boros D L 1980 The granulomatous inflammatory response. In: Boros D L, Yoshida T (eds) Basic and clinical aspects of granulomatous disorders. Elsevier, New York, pp 181–197

Byram J E, von Lichtenberg F 1977 Altered schistosome granuloma formation in nude mice. American Journal of Tropical Medicine and Hygiene 26: 944–956

Chambers T J 1978 Mutinucleated giant cells. Journal of Pathology 126: 125–148

Chambers T J, Morson B C 1979 The granuloma in Crohn's disease. Gut 20: 269

Chaudhry A P, Saigal K P, Intengan M, Nickerson P A 1979 Malakoplakia of the large intestine found incidentally at necropsy. Light and electron microscopic features. Diseases of the Colon and Rectum 22: 73–81

Chaudhry A P, Satchidanand S K, Anthone R, Baumler R A, Graeta J F 1980 An unusual case of supraclavicular and colonic malakoplakia – light and ultrastructural study. Journal of Pathology 131: 193–208

Cook M G 1972 The size and histological appearance of mesenteric lymph nodes in Crohn's disease. Gut 12: 970

Curnutte J T 1993 Chronic granulomatous disease: the solving of a clinical riddle at the molecular level. Clinical Immunology and

Immunopathology 67: S2–S15
Dannenburg A M, Ando M, Shima K, Tsuda T 1975 Macrophage turnover and activation in tuberculous granulomata. In: van Furth R (ed) Mononuclear phagocytes in immunity infection and pathology. Blackwell Scientific, Oxford, 959–980
de la Garza T, Nunez-Rasilla V, Alagra-Palafox R, Albores-Saavedra J 1973 Malakoplakia of the colon: report of the case with a review of eight previous reports. Diseases of the Colon and Rectum 16: 216–223
Deridder P A, Koff S A, Gikas P W, Heidelberger K P 1977 Renal malakoplakia. Journal of Urology 117: 428–432
Dinuaer M C, Orkin S H, Brown R, Jesiatis A J, Parkos C A 1987 The glycoprotein encoded by the X-linked chronic granulomatous disease locus is a component of the neutrophil cytochrome b complex. Nature 327: 717–720
Di Silvo T V, Bartlett E F 1971 Malakoplakia of the colon. Archives of Pathology 92: 167
Dobyan D C, Truong L D, Eknoyan G 1993a Renal malakoplakia reappraised. American Journal of Kidney Disease 22: 243–252
Dockerty M B 1972 Primary malakoplakia of the colon. Mayo Clinic Proceedings 47: 114–116
Dwarakanath A D, Nash J, Rhodes J M 1994 Conversion from ulcerative colitis to Crohn's disease associated with corticosteroid treatment. Gut 35: 1141–1144
El-Mouzan M I, Satti M B, Al-Quorain A A, El-Ageb A 1988 Colonic malakoplakia – occurrence in a family. Diseases of the Colon and Rectum 31: 390–393
Finlay-Jones L R, Blackwell J B, Papadimitrou J M 1968 Malakoplakia of the colon. American Journal of Clinical Pathology 50: 320–329
Finn A, Hadzic N, Morgan G, Strobel S, Levinsky R J 1990 Prognosis of chronic granulomatous disease. Archives of Diseases in Childhood 65: 942–945
Geboes K, van der Oord J, De Wolf-Peters C et al 1986 The cellular composition of granulomas in mesenteric lymph nodes from patients with Crohn's disease. Virchows Archiv 409: 679–692
Glass R E, Baker W N W 1976 Role of the granuloma in recurrent Crohn's disease. Gut 17: 75–77
Gonzales-Angulo A, Corral E, Garcia-Torres R 1965 Malakoplakia of the colon. Gastroenterology 48: 383–387
Gordon S, Todd J, Cohn Z A 1974 In vitro synthesis and secretion of lysozyme by mononuclear phagocytes. Journal of Experimental Medicine 139: 1228
Griscom N T, Kirkpatrick J A, Girdany B R, Berdon W E, Grand R J, Mackie G G 1974 Gastric antral narrowing in chronic granulomatous disease. Pediatrics 54: 456–460
Harris B H, Boles E T 1973 Intestinal lesions in chronic granulomatous disease of childhood. Journal of Pediatric Surgery 8: 955–961
International Chronic Granulomatous Disease Study Group 1991 A controlled trial of interferon gamma to prevent infection in chronic granulomatous disease. New England Journal of Medicine 324: 509–516
Isaacs D, Wright V M, Shaw D G, Raafat F, Walker-Smith J A 1985 Chronic granulomatous disease mimicking Crohn's disease. Journal of Pediatric Gastroenterology and Nutrition 4: 498–501
James S P 1988 Remission of Crohn's disease after human immunodeficiency virus infection. Gastroenterology 95: 1667–1669
James S L, Colley D G 1978 Eosinophil-mediated destruction of *Schistosoma mansoni* eggs. III. Lymphokine involvement in the induction of eosinophil function abnormalities. Cellular Immunology 38: 48–58
Johnston R B, Newman S L 1977 Chronic granulomatous disease. Pediatric Clinics of North America 24: 365–376
Joyeuse R, Lott J V, Michaelis M, Gumucio C C 1971 Malakoplakia of the colon and rectum: report of a case and review of the literature. Surgery 81: 189
Kamani N, August C S, Campbell D E, Nassan N F, Douglas S D 1988 Marrow transplantation in chronic granulomatous disease: an update with 6-year follow-up. Journal of Paediatrics 113: 697–700
Kely J, Sutherland L R 1988 The chronological sequence in the pathology of Crohn's disease. Journal of Clinical Gastroenterology 10; 28
Kuzma J P 1966 Polypoid lymphoid hyperplasia of the colon with malakoplakia. American Society of Clinical Pathology 9–13

Landing B H, Shrikey H S 1957 A syndrome of recurrent infection and infiltration of viscera by pigmented lipid histiocytes. Paediatrics 20: 431–438
Leto T L, Garrret M C, Fujii H, Nunoi H 1991 Characterization of neutrophil NADPH oxidase factors are p47-*phox* and p67-*phox* from recombinant baculoviruses. Journal of Biological Chemistry 266: 19812–19818
Lewin K J, Harell G, Lee A S, Crowley L 1974 Malakoplakia: an electronmicroscopy study: demonstration of bacilliform organisms in malakoplakic macrophages. Gastroenterology 66: 28–45
Lou T Y, Teplitz C 1974 Malakoplakia: pathogenesis and ultrastructural morphogenesis. A problem with altered macrophages (phagolysosomal) response. Human Pathology 5: 191–207
Mandell G L, Hook E W 1969 Leukocyte bacterial activity in chronic granulomatous disease: correlation of hydrogen peroxide production and susceptibility in intracellular killing. Journal of Bacteriology 100: 531–532
Margolis D M, Melnick D A, Alling D W, Gallin J I 1990 Trimethoprim-sulfamethoxazole prophylaxis in the management of chronic granulomatous disease. Journal of Infectious Diseases 162: 723–726
Markowitz J, Kahn E, Daum F 1989 Prognostic significance of epithelioid granulomas found in rectosigmoid biopsies at the initial presentation of pediatric Crohn's disease. Journal of Pediatric Gastroenterology and Nutrition 9: 182–186
Mathew R C, Boros D L 1986 Anti-LT3T4 antibody treatment suppresses hepatic granuloma formation and abrogates antigen-induced interleukin 2 production in murine schistosomiasis. Infection and Immunity 54: 820–826
Mathew R C, Wienstock J V 1994 Granuloma formation. In: Targan S R, Shanahan F (eds) Inflammatory bowel disease: from bench to bedside. Williams and Wilkins, Baltimore, pp 151–159
Michaelis L, Gutmann M 1902 Uber Einschlusse in Blasentumoren. Zeitschrift für Klinische Medizin 47: 208–215
Mishra B B, Poulter L W, Janossy G, James D G 1983 The distribution of lymphoid and macrophage like cell subsets of sarcoid and Kveim granulomata: possible mechanism of negative PPD reaction in sarcoidosis. Clinical and Experimental Immunology 54: 705–715
Moran C A, West B, Schartz I 1989 Malakoplakia of the colon associated with colonic adenocarcinoma. American Journal of Gastroenterology 84: 1580–1582
Morson B C 1968 Crohn's disease. Proceedings of the Royal Society of Medicine 61: 79–83
Mouy R, Fischer A, Vilmer E, Seger R, Griscelli C 1989 Incidence severity and prevention of infection in chronic granulomatous disease. Journal of Paediatrics 114: 555–560
Munro C S, Campbell D A, DuBois R M, Mitchell D N, Cole P J, Poulter L W 1988 Suppressor associated lymphocyte markers in lesions of sarcoidosis. Thorax 43: 471–474
Nathan C 1987 Macrophage secretory products. Journal of Clinical Investigation 79: 319–326
Ng I O, Ng M 1993 Colonic malacoplakia: unusual association with ulcerative colitis. Journal of Gastroenterology and Hepatology 8: 110
Ochs H D, Igo R P 1973 The NBT slide test: a simple screening method for detection of chronic granulomatous disease and female carriers. Journal of Paediatrics 83: 77–82
Odell E W, Segal A W 1991 Killing pathogens associated with chronic granulomatous disease by non-oxidative microbial mechanisms of human neutrophils. Journal of Medical Microbiology 34: 129–135
O'Neil K M, Herman J H, Modlin J F, Moxon E R, Chir B, Winkelstein J A 1986 *Pseudomonas cepacia*: an emerging pathogen in chronic granulomatous disease. Journal of Pediatrics 108: 940–942
Pertshuk L P, Silverstein E, Friedland J 1981 Immunohistologic diagnosis of sarcoidosis. Detection of angiotensin converting enzyme in sarcoid granulomas. American Journal of Clinical Pathology 75: 350–354
Potzi R, Walgram M, Klozner H, Gangl A 1989 Diagnostic significance of endoscopic biopsy in Crohn's disease. Endoscopy 21: 60–62
Quie P G, Kaplan E L, Page A R, Gruskay F L, Malawista S E 1968 Defective polynuclear-leukocyte function and chronic granulomatous disease in two female children. New England Journal of Medicine 278: 976–980
Ranchod M, Kaln L B 1972 Malakoplakia of the gastrointestinal tract. Archives of Pathology 94: 90–97

Ridley D S 1974 Histological classification and immunological spectrum of leprosy. Bulletin of the World Health Organization 51: 451

Robert J, Lagagce R, Delage C 1974 Malakoplakia of the colon associated with a villous adenoma: report of a case. Diseases of the Colon and Rectum 17: 668–671

Rywlin A M, Ravel R, Hurwitz A 1969 Malakoplakia of the colon. American Journal of Digestive Diseases 14: 491–499

Sanusi I D, Tio F O 1974 Gastrointestinal malakoplakia. Report of a case and review of the literature. American Journal of Gastroenterology 62: 356

Satti M B, Abu-Melha A, Taha O M A, Idrissi H Y 1985 Colonic malakoplakia and abdominal tuberculosis in a child – report of a case and review of the literature. Diseases of the Colon and Rectum 28: 353–357

Schmitz-Moormann P, Pittner P M 1984 The granuloma in Crohn's disease: a bioptical study. Pathology Research and Practice 178: 467–476

Schmitz-Moormann, Schag M 1990 Histology of the lower intestinal tract in Crohn's disease of children and adolescents. Multicentric paediatric Crohn's disease study. Pathology Research and Practice 186: 479–484

Sheffield E A 1990 The granulomatous inflammatory response. Journal of Pathology 160: 1–2

Sher A, Coffman R L, Hieny S, Scott P, Cheever A W 1990 Interleukin 5 is required for the blood and tissue eosinophilia but no granuloma formation induced by infection with *Schistosoma mansoni*. Proceedings of the National Academy of Sciences of the USA 87: 61–65

Sinclair-Smith C, Kahn L B, Cywes S 1975 Malakoplakia in childhood. Case report with ultrastructural studies and review of the literature. Archives of Pathology 99: 198–203

Surawicz C M 1968 The role of rectal biopsy in infectious colitis. American Journal of Pathology 12(Suppl 1): 81

Sutton J S, Weiss L 1966 Transformation of monocytes in tissue culture into macrophages, epithelioid cells and multinucleated giant cells: an electron microscopic study. Journal of Cell Biology 28: 303–332

Terner J Y, Lattes R 1965 Malakoplakia of colon and retroperitoneum. American Journal of Clinical Pathology 44: 20–31

Thrasher A J, Keep N H, Wientjes F, Segal A W 1994 Chronic granulomatous disease. Biochimica Biophysica Acta 1227: 1–24

Turk T L, Narayanan R B 1982 The origin, morphology and function of epithelioid cells. Immunobiology 161: 274–282

Tweedie J M, McGann B G 1984 Metastatic Crohn's disease of the thigh and forearm. Gut 25: 213

Unanue E R 1980 Cooperation between mononuclear phagocytes and lymphocytes in immunity. New England Journal of Medicine 303: 977–985

Varilek G, Weinstock J V, Pantazis N 1991 Isolated hepatic granulomas from mice infected with *Schistosoma mansoni* contain nerve growth factor. Infection and Immunity 59: 4443–4449

von Hasemann D 1903 Uber Malakoplakia der Harnblase. Virchows Archiv A Pathologie Anatomie Histopathologie 173: 302–308

Wakefield A J, Sankey E A, Dhillon A P et al 1991 Granulomatous vasculitis in Crohn's disease. Gastroenterology 100: 1279–1287

Wakefield A J, Sawyerr A M, Dhillon A P et al 1989 Pathogenesis of Crohn's disease: multifocial gastrointestinal infarction. Lancet 1: 1057–1062

Weinstock J V 1992 The granuloma and Crohn's disease. In: MacDermott R P, Stenson W F (eds) Inflammatory bowel diseases. Elsevier, New York pp 163–176

Weiss S J 1989 Mechanisms of disease: tissue destruction by neutrophils. New England Journal of Medicine 320: 365–376

Wilkey I S, Rubel L R 1972 Intestinal malakoplakia: report of a case. Pathology 4: 311–314

Wolfson D M, Sachar D B, Cohen A et al 1982 Granulomas do not affect post-operative recurrence rates in Crohn's disease. Gastroenterology 83: 405–409

Wyman M P, von Tscharner V, Deranleau D A, Bagiolini M 1987 Chemiluminescence detection of H_2O_2 production by human neutrophils during the respiratory burst. Annals of Biochemistry 165: 371–378

Yamamura M, Uyemura K, Deans R J et al 1991 Defining protective responses to pathogens: cytokine profiles in leprosy lesions. Science 254: 277–279

Yunis T J, Estevez J M, Pinzon G J, Moran T J 1967 Malakoplakia: discussion of pathogenesis and report of three cases including one of fatal gastric and colonic involvement. Archives of Pathology 83: 180–187

41. Gastrointestinal Behçet's disease

H. H. Tsai

This rare disease, characterized by oral and genital ulceration associated with uveitis, was probably first recognized by Hippocrates (Feigenbaum 1956). The first modern description was by Behçet, a Turkish dermatologist, in 1937, who suggested a viral etiology for the condition (Behçet 1937). Although recurrent oral aphthous ulceration is a universal feature of this disease, it is a vasculitic disorder that affects many organs, including the eyes, skin, muscle, joints, kidneys, pulmonary, cardiovascular, neurological and gastrointestinal systems.

INTERNATIONAL DIAGNOSTIC CRITERIA (1990)

To standardize the diagnosis for Behçet's disease, the International Study Group for Behçet's Disease published in 1990 the agreed criteria shown in (Table 41.1). There was initial concern that most of the patients (89%) evaluated for these criteria originated in Japan, Iran and Turkey. A recent study to assess the performance of these criteria in new patient groups determined their sensitivity in 300 patients with Behçet's disease from seven countries, and specificity in a group of 62 control patients from China, and found the criteria bearing up well (O'Neill et al 1994).

Table 41.1 International criteria for classification of Behçet's disease

Recurrence of minor, major aphthous, or herpetiform ulceration at least 3 times during a 12 month period*
Plus 2 of the following:
Recurrent genital aphthous ulceration or scarring
Eye lesions†
   Anterior or posterior uveitis
   Cells in vitreous humor on slit-lamp examination
   Retinal vasculitis
Skin lesions*
   Erythema nodosum
   Pseudofolliculosis or papulopustular lesions
   Acneform nodules
Positive pathergy test*
Development of an erythematous papule, >2 mm at site of injection 48 hours after oblique penetration of a 20–22 gauge sterile needle 5 mm into forearm skin

* Must be observed by a physician
† Must be observed by an ophthalmologist.

EPIDEMIOLOGY AND ETIOLOGY

Behçet's disease has been reported worldwide but is most common in Japan, with a prevalence of up to 1 in 1000. High prevalence has also been reported in the Mediterranean countries and Middle East. However, previously poor agreement of diagnostic criteria makes comparison difficult, although the new diagnostic criteria may help future epidemiological studies. It is generally regarded as a rare condition in Europe and North America, where a prevalence rate of 1 in 500 000 is usually quoted, but this is based on a Scottish report of only 15 patients (Jankowski et al 1992) and an estimate of 1–5 in 100 000 is probably more realistic. A recent study in Minnesota, USA, reported a prevalence of 1 in 15 000 (O'Duffy 1994).

The etiology of Behçet's disease remains unknown, but there is a significant association with HLA-B5 in Japanese and eastern Mediterranean patients. This is particularly true of the HLA-51 split (Mizuki et al 1992a) which was found in 57% of Japanese patients. This association, although significant, is not entirely convincing and is not found in northern European patients. The genes for tumor necrosis factors TNF-α and TNF-β lie close to the class I genes, and it has been suggested that the susceptibility gene may be TNF-β (Mizuki et al 1992b). The familial form of Behçet's disease was found to account for 8.7% of cases in a metanalysis and was associated with a lower incidence of vasculitis (Akpolat et al 1992).

Various environmental triggers have been suggested. There is an association with previous streptococcal infections (Niwa & Mizushima 1990), recent dental treatment (Mizushima et al 1988), and travel to high-incidence areas (Cooper et al 1989). Of particular interest is previous infection with *Streptococcus sanguis*, as there is evidence of antigenic cross-reactivity between the bacteria and oral mucosal antigens and the 65 kDa heat shock protein (Lehner et al 1991). Herpes simplex type I has also been implicated (Young et al 1988).

Many immunological abnormalities have been described. Autoantibodies directed against endothelial cells (Pivetti-

Pezzi et al 1992), mucosal epithelium and retina (Yamamoto et al 1993), and neutrophil cytoplasm (ANCA) (Yang et al 1993) have been reported. The role of these antibodies remain obscure. Tissue damage may be mediated by free radicals generated by mononuclear cells (Pronai et al 1990). The thrombotic tendency in Behçet's disease has been associated with alterations in Factor XII (Disdier et al 1992), protein S (Chafa et al 1992) and protein C (Shento et al 1992) levels and defective fibrinolysis (Atchison et al 1989). Patients with predominant vascular disease have increased circulating levels of von Willebrand's factor (Kagawa & Okubo 1993).

CLINICAL FEATURES OF INTESTINAL BEHÇET'S DISEASE

Typically, Behçet's disease runs a remittent course over a variable number of years, and eventually declines in activity. A small number of patients develop multiple organ vasculitis, which may result in multiple organ failure and death. In Japan and the Mediterranean countries, where the incidence is high, it predominantly affects young men and is a major cause of blindness, but in Europe and North America it is more common in women and tends to run a less aggressive course.

The oral lesions of Behçet's disease may be minor (<1 cm), major (>1 cm) or herpetiform, and it can be impossible to distinguish them from common oral aphthous ulcers (Main & Chamberlain 1992). Extraoral gastrointestinal involvement is present in 15–65% of patients with Behçet's disease, the pattern of which may often mimic Crohn's disease. Typically the mucosa is involved, with punched-out, fissuring or aphthoid ulcers, which may be solitary but are more often numerous. They are most often localized in the ileocecal region or diffusely spread throughout the colon (Kasahara et al 1981). The involvement is often segmental as in Crohn's disease, but stricturing and fibrotic reaction is unusual. The pattern of intestinal involvement has geographical variation, with ileocecal involvement common in Japan and colonic involvement the most commonly encountered gastrointestinal involvement in the West (Smith et al 1973, Shimizu et al 1979).

Vasculitis is a common feature, with lymphocytic infiltration of the small veins and venules (Baba et al 1976). However, histologically it may be difficult to differentiate from Crohn's disease, with non-specific inflammatory infiltrate being seen in the mucosa adjacent to ulcers and normal mucosa in between. Occasionally the inflammation may be transmural and granulomas may occasionally be present (O'Connell et al 1980).

Gastrointestinal lesions take two forms, mucosal inflammation or ischemia/infarction. Large vessel involvement of the mesenteric artery or its branches leads to ischemia and infarction, whereas small vessel disease is probably the mechanism for mucosal ulceration. Patients with inflammatory mucosal lesions present with features indistinguishable from those of inflammatory bowel disease (Armas et al 1992). In fact, the two conditions share many features as well as similar extraintestinal involvement, including pyoderma gangrenosum, uveitis, seronegative arthropathy and erythema nodosum. The stigmata of Behçet's disease may not become evident until well after the gastrointestinal features (Jong et al 1991). This has prompted some to suggest that inflammatory bowel disease and Behçet's disease may be variants of the same disease (Gedikolglu et al 1992). Anorectal fistulation and rectovaginal fistulation as well as enteroenteric fistulae are also seen in Behçet's disease, as in Crohn's (The et al 1989, Kyle et al 1991), and wound fistulation may also occur after laparotomy. Ileocecal involvement may present with a right iliac fossa mass with weight loss and anemia, mimicking cecal carcinoma. Intestinal Behçet's disease may also be complicated by amyloidosis in the gastrointestinal tract and kidney (Hamza et al 1988).

Useful diagnostic investigations may include contrast radiology, colonoscopy and CT examination of the abdomen. Barium enema or small-bowel enemas (enteroclysis) may show skip lesions and deep fissuring ulcers not dissimilar to Crohn's disease. Large-bowel lesions may also be confluent, as seen in ulcerative colitis (Iida et al 1993). Colonoscopic features also resemble Crohn's disease, with serpiginous, or aphthoid ulcers and pseudopolyposis (Toila et al 1989). Colonoscopic biopsies are often indistinguishable from inflammatory bowel disease histologically. Even with resected specimens the pathologist may not be able to distinguish between the two.

Patients who have intestinal ischemia or infarction usually present as an acute abdomen. There may be associated features of bowel obstruction, vomiting and constipation, or massive upper or lower gastrointestinal hemorrhage (Arora et al 1989).

Upper gastrointestinal involvement is less common. Ulceration of the esophagus and duodenum has been reported (Anti et al 1986), with the latter leading to pyloric stenosis (Satake et al 1986). These ulcers may bleed, perforate or fistulate (O'Duffy 1990a). Gastrointestinal involvement carries a poor prognosis: some 10% of cases will require surgical intervention, with consequent high morbidity and mortality (Bradbury et al 1994).

MANAGEMENT

The mainstay of therapy for Behçet's disease is medical. Treatment must be tailored to the individual patient, since the manifestations of the disease are so variable. The relative rarity of the disease and its wide spectrum makes it difficult to conduct double-blind controlled trials of treatment.

Non-steroidal anti-inflammatory drugs (NSAIDs) and corticosteroids are the mainstay of treatment for the rheumatological and inflammatory aspects of Behçet's disease. Skin and joint lesions respond to indomethacin (Simsek et al 1991). Systemic corticosteroids are required for more resistant arthritis, erythema nodosum or pyoderma gangrenosum. Vasculitis also responds to steroids, but antithrombotic therapy and anticoagulation is often indicated to prevent thrombotic episodes. Neurological complications require high-dose corticosteroids. Topically administered corticosteroids are also very helpful. Intra-articular and intraocular instillation of corticosteroids can be effective. However, uveitis, which can lead to blindness, does not always respond to corticosteroids. This has led to the use of powerful immunosuppressives, such as chlorambucil, cyclophosphamide and azathicoprine for patients with severe uveitis (O'Duffy 1990b, Tessler & Jennings 1990). More recently, cyclosporin (Saylan 1982) and FK506 (Jenkins et al 1989) have shown promise for the treatment of uveitis.

Treatment of gastrointestinal manifestations may need medical or surgical intervention. Oral lesions are an almost universal feature of the disease, and so oral hygiene is important. Topical corticosteroids and lignocaine are helpful for painful lesions. Large oral and genital ulcers often respond dramatically to thalidomide (200–400 mg/day) (Saylan 1982, Jenkins et al 1989). The tragic history of this drug, however, has made it unavailable in many countries. If used, it should be restricted to males only and the patient warned of the risk of drug-induced neuropathy. Safer, less teratogenic analogs of thalidomide may prove to be potent not only for Behçet's disease but perhaps for Crohn's disease and ulcerative colitis as well (Waters & Laing 1970, D'Arcy & Griffin 1994). Azathioprine may be used in patients with severe recurrent ulceration Yakzici et al 1990).

The colitis associated with Behçet's disease is usually treated with sulfasalazine at doses of 2–4 g/day. Although no controlled trials exist, it appears to be of benefit. During exacerbations or if the condition is not responsive to sulfasalazine, systemic corticosteroids may be added. Steroid enemas or foam preparations may also be useful. Cyclosporin is reported to be of no benefit in gastrointestinal Behçet's disease. Surgical intervention may be required in up to 10% of patients. Ileocecal disease may be successfully treated with resection (Abdullah & Keczkes 1989). Intestinal vasculitis and infarction leading to perforation is a surgical emergency and requires laparotomy. Patients in whom medical therapy has failed or who have extensive disease should be considered for surgery. Extensive gastrointestinal Behçet's disease has a high complication rate and surgery should be contemplated early in the course of the illness, as delay may prove fatal. Total colectomy and ileostomy is preferred for extensive colitis. Surgical excision margins should be wider than for inflammatory bowel disease, and a stoma preferred to primary anastomosis because of the high rate of anastomotic leak, perforation and fistulation (Matsumoto et al 1991).

REFERENCES

Abdullah A N, Keczkes K 1989 Behçet's syndrome with gastrointestinal tract involvement mimicking carcinoma of the caecum – a case report. Clinical and Experimental Dermatology 14: 459–461

Akpolat T, Koc Y, Yeniay I et al 1992 Familial Behçet's disease. European Journal of Medicine 1: 391–359

Anti M, Marra G, Rapaccini G L et al 1986 Esophageal involvement in Behçet's disease. Journal of Clinical Gastroenterology 8: 514–519

Armas J B, Davies J, Davies M, Lovell C, McHugh N 1992 Atypical Behçet's disease with peripheral erosive arthropathy and pyoderma gangrenosum. Clinical and Experimental Rheumatology 10: 177–180

Arora A, Tandon R K, Jain P et al 1989 Massive lower gastrointestinal bleeding as a presenting feature in Behçet's disease. Tropical Gastroenterology 10: 56–61

Atchison R, Chu P, Cater D R, Harris R J Powell R J 1989 Defective fibrinolysis in Behçet's syndrome: significance and possible mechanisms. Annals of Rheumatic Diseases 18: 410–414

Baba S, Maruta M, Ando K, Teramoto T, Endo I 1976 Intestinal Behçet disease: a report of five cases. Diseases of the Colon and Rectum 9: 428–440

Behçet H 1937 Uber rezidiviriende, aphtose, durch ein Virus verursachte Geschwire am Mund, am Auge und an den Genitalen. Dermatologiste Wochenschrift 105: 1152–1157

Bradbury A W, Milne A A, Murie J A 1994 Surgical aspects of Behçet's disease. British Journal of Surgery 81: 1712–1721

Chafa O, Fischer A M, Meriane F et al 1992 Behçet's syndrome associated with protein S deficiency. Thrombosis and Haemostasis 67: 1–3

Cooper C, Pippard E C, Sharp H, Wickham, Chamberlain M A, Barker D J 1989 Is Behçet's disease triggered by childhood infection? Annals of Rheumatic Diseases 48: 421–423

D'Arcy P F, Griffin J P 1994 Thalidomide revisited. Adverse Drug Reaction and Toxicology Review 13: 65–76

Diodier P, Harle J R, Monly A, Ailaud M F, Weiler P J 1992 Behçet's syndrome and factor XII deficiency. Clinical Rheumatology 11: 422–423

Feigenbaum A 1956 Description of Behçet's disease in the Hippocratic third book of endemic diseases. British Journal of Ophthalmology 40: 355–357

Gedikolglu G, Demiriz M, Gunhan O, Somuncu I, Finci R 1992 Enterocolitis in Behçet's syndrome. European Journal of Surgery 158: 515–517

Hamza M, Wechler B, Godeau P, Hamza H, Ayed K 1988 Intestinal amyloidosis: an unusual complication of Behçet's disease. American Journal of Gastroenterology 83: 793–794

Iida M, Kobayashi H, Matsumoto T et al 1993 Intestinal Behçet's disease: serial changes in radiography. Radiology 188: 65–69

International Study Group for Behçet's Disease 1990 Evaluation of diagnostic criteria in Behçet's disease: toward internationally agreed criteria. Lancet 335: 1078–1080

Jankowski J, Crombie I, Jankowski R 1992 Behçet's disease in Scotland. Postgraduate Medical Journal 68: 566–570

Jenkins J S, Allen R, Maurica P D L 1989 Thalidomide in giant orogenital ulceration. Lancet 2: 1424–1426

Jong H C, Rhee P L, Song I G, Choi K W, Kim C Y 1991 Temporal changes in the clinical type of diagnosis of Behçet's colitis in patients with aphthoid or punched out colonic ulcerations. Journal of Korean Medical Science 6: 313–318

Kagawa H, Okubo S 1993 Plasma coagulation and fibrinolysis parameters in patients with vascular Behçet's disease, and analysis of multimeric structure of von Willebrand factor (vWF). Ryumachi 33: 416–423

Kasahara Y, Tanaka S, Nishimo M, Umemura H, Shiraha S, Kuyama T 1981 Intestinal involvement in Behçet's disease: review of

136 surgical cases in the Japanese literature. Diseases of the Colon and Rectum 24: 103–106

Kyle S M, Yeong M L, Isbister W H, Clark S P 1991 Behçet's colitis: a differential diagnosis in inflammations of the large intestine. Australia and New Zealand Journal of Surgery 61: 547–550

Lehner T, Lavery E, Smith R, van Embden J, Mizushima Y 1991 Cross-rectivity between the 65 kDa heat shock protein, *Streptococcus sanguis* and the corresponding antibodies in Behçet's disease. Infection and Immunity 59: 1434–1441

Main D M G, Chamberlain M A 1992 Clinical differential of oral ulceration in Behçet's disease. British Journal of Rheumatology 31: 767–770

Matsumoto T, Uekusa T, Fukuda Y 1991 Vasculo-Behçet's disease: a pathologic study of eight cases. Human Pathology 22: 45–51

Mizuki N, Inoko H, Sugimura K et al 1992a Human leukocyte antigen serologic and DNA typing of Behçet's disease and its primary association with B51. Investigative Ophthalmology and Visual Science 33: 3332–3400

Mizuki N, Inoko H, Sugimura K et al 1992b Analysis of the TGFβ gene and the susceptibility to alloreactive NK cells in Behçet's disease. Investigative Ophthalmology and Visual Science 33: 3084–3090

Mizushima Y, Matsuda T, Hoshi K, Ohno S 1988 Induction of Behçet's disease symptoms after dental treatment and streptococcal skin test. Journal of Rheumatology 15: 1029–1030

Niwa Y, Mizushima Y 1990 Neutrophil-potentiating factors released from stimulated lymphocytes: special reference to the increase in neutrophil-potentiating factors from streptococcus-stimulated lymphocytes of the patients with Behçet's disease. Clinical and Experimental Immunology 79: 353–360

O'Connell D J, Courtney J V, Riddell R H 1980 Colitis of Behçet's syndrome – radiologic and pathologic features. Gastrointestinal Radiology 5: 173–179

O'Duffy J D 1990a Behçet's syndrome. New England Journal of Medicine 322: 326–328

O'Duffy J D 1990 Vasculitis in Behçet's disease. Rheumatic Diseases Clinics of North America 16: 423–431

O'Duffy J D 1994 Behçet's disease. Current Opinion in Rheumatology 6: 39–43

O'Neill T W, Rigby A S, Silman A J, Barnes C 1994 Validation of the International Study Group criteria for Behçet's disease. British Journal of Rheumatology 33: 115–117

Pivetti-Pezzi P, Priori R, Catarinelli G et al 1992 Markers of vascular injury in Behçet's disease associated with retinal vasculitis. Annals of Ophthalmology 24: 441–444

Pronai L, Ichikawa Y, Nakazawa H, Arimori S 1990 Superoxide scavenging activity of leukocytes in rheumatoid arthritis and Behçet's disease. Tokai Journal of Experimental and Clinical Medicine 15: 93–97

Satake K, Yada K, Ikehara T, Umeyama K, Inoue T 1986 Pyloric stenosis: an uncommon complication of Behçet's disease. American Journal of Gastroenterology 81: 816–818

Saylan 1982 Thalidomide in the treatment of Behçet's syndrome. Archives of Dermatology 118: 536

Shento N M, Ghosh K, Abdul Kader B, al Assad H S 1992 Extensive venous thrombosis in a case of Behçet's disease associated with heterozygous protein C deficiency. Thrombosis and Haemostasis 67: 283

Shizimu T, Ehrlich G E, Inaba K, Hyashi K 1979 Behçet's disease (Behçet's syndrome). Seminars in Arthritis and Rheumatism 8: 223–260

Simsek H, Dundar S, Telatar H 1991 Treatment of Behçet's disease. International Journal of Dermatology 30: 54–57

Smith G E, Kime L R, Pilcher J L 1973 The colitis of Behçet's disease: a separate entity? Colonoscopic findings and literature review. American Journal of Digestive Diseases 18: 987–1000

Tessler H H, Jennings T 1990 High-dose, short-term chlorambucil for intractable sympathetic ophthalmia and Behçet's disease. British Journal of Ophthalmology 74: 353–357

The L S, Green K A, O'Sullivan M M, Morris J S, Williams B D 1989 Behçet's syndrome: severe proctitis with rectovaginal fistula formation. Annals of Rheumatic Diseases 48: 779–780

Toila V, Abdullah A, Thiroomoorthi M C, Chang C H 1989 A case of Behçet's disease with intestinal involvement due to Crohn's disease. American Journal of Gastroenterology 84: 322–325

Waters M F, Laing A B, Ambikapathy A, Lennard-Jones J E 1970 Treatment of ulcerative colitis with thalidomide. British Medical Journal 1: 792

Yakzici H, Parzali H, Barnes C G et al 1990 A controlled trial of azothiaprine in Behçet's syndrome. New England Journal of Medicine 281–285

Yamamoto J H, Minami M, Inaba G, Masuda K, Mochizuki M 1993 Cellular immunity to retinal specific antigens in patients with Behçet's disease. British Journal of Ophthalmology 77: 584–589

Yang C W, Park I S, Kim S Y et al 1993 Antineutrophil cytoplasmic antibodies associated vasculitis and renal failure in Behçet's disease. Clinical and Experimental Immunology 8: 871–873

Young C, Lehner T, Barnes C G 1988 CD4 and CD8 cell responses to herpes simplex virus in Behçet's disease. Clinical and Experimental Immunology 73: 6–10

42. Tuberculosis of the gastrointestinal tract

P. Ghosh

INTRODUCTION

Gastrointestinal tuberculosis is said to be rare in the developed world, but over the last 10 years there has been a sharp increase in incidence in the west, reversing a downward trend observed for over 3 decades. This can be attributed partly to the HIV epidemic, but the increase in the non-HIV population may well be related to the increased number of homeless peoples and immigrants from endemic areas (Guth & Kim 1991, Probert et al 1992). The disease is endemic in the Indian subcontinent, the West Indies and South Africa. It is estimated that a third of the world's population is infected, with 10 million new cases of active disease occurring annually and accounting for 6% of deaths worldwide (Daniel 1994).

The success of pasteurization and tuberculin testing of dairy herds has virtually eliminated bovine tuberculosis. *Mycobacterium tuberculosis* is the common pathogen today. The past success of the campaign to eliminate *Mycobacterium tuberculosis* in developed countries has lulled many clinicians and radiologists into placing gastrointestinal tuberculosis too low on the list of differential diagnoses.

The HIV epidemic has dramatically changed the spectrum of tuberculosis. Fifty per cent of AIDS patients with tuberculosis have extrapulmonary manifestations; the disease progresses rapidly in this group, and multidrug-resistant organisms are common (Chaisson & Slutkin 1989, Braun et al 1990). *Mycobacterium avium intracellulare* (MAI) infection, rarely reported before the AIDS epidemic, has become a common concurrent infection in HIV-positive individuals with low CD4 counts. MAI (or *Mycobacterium avium* complex, MAC) is a ubiquitous organism and the gastrointestinal tract is the usual portal of entry. MAI predominantly affects the duodenum, and with increasing immunosuppression can proliferate and disseminate via the bloodstream.

PATHOLOGY

Gastrointestinal tuberculosis can be primary but it is most commonly secondary to a focus of infection elsewhere in the body. The usual mode of infection is by the ingestion of expectorated sputum. Hematogenous spread is rare. In women the infection may gain access via the genital tract. The mechanism of true primary infection of tuberculosis is unclear, but may be from ingestion of contaminated food.

The disease can present in three ways: peritoneal disease, macroscopic lesions of the GI tract and, rarely, a combination of both.

Peritoneal disease

Peritoneal disease usually occurs either by hematogenous spread from a primary focus or direct extension from caseous tuberculous nodes. It is rarely associated with either tuberculous salpingitis or intestinal tuberculosis. Cirrhotics and patients on continuous ambulatory peritoneal dialysis have an increased incidence of peritoneal tuberculosis (Cheng et al 1989). Evidence of active pulmonary tuberculosis is seen in around 14% of patients, with an abnormal chest X-ray in up to two-thirds (Marshall 1993). Other series, however, report coincidental pulmonary disease in less than 6% (Singh et al 1969).

There are two forms – the ascitic form, which may be acute, and the dry fibrinous variant, which is generally chronic. The ascitic fluid is thin, straw colored and may be bloodstained. The classic doughy abdomen is rare. The peritoneum is studded with tubercles varying from pinhead-sized lesions to lesions up to 1 cm in diameter. The omentum is thick and infiltrated, forming plaque-like masses. In chronic dry peritonitis, which occurs less commonly, there is matting of viscera, caseating necrosis and multiple adhesions, with very little free fluid.

Gastrointestinal tract

Gastrointestinal tract involvement includes focal ulcers, fibrotic change and hypertrophic lesions. Typical granulomas are seen histologically, characterized by epithelioid cells, Langhans'-type giant cells, fibrosis and caseation. Caseation is not always present, however, and was only found in a third of patients in one series (Hoon et al 1950). These granulomas may only be present in the regional lymph nodes, with non-specific changes in the bowel wall (Tandon & Prakash 1972). This can make the distinction from Crohn's disease difficult. In Anand's (1956) series only 10% of affected lymph nodes showed caseation.

The demonstration of acid-fast bacilli combined with suggestive histology establishes a definitive diagnosis. Auramine–rhodamine staining is helpful, as well as the more established Ziehl–Neelsen staining. Special stains for tuberculosis may fail to demonstrate acid-fast bacilli, although the lesion is otherwise typical of tuberculosis. In Findlay's series tubercle bacilli were demonstrated in 27% of patients.

Identification of tubercle bacilli

Blumberg (1928) emphasized that the demonstration of tubercle bacilli alone is not sufficient to establish the diagnosis of intestinal tuberculosis. In extensive pulmonary disease, swallowed sputum containing *Mycobacterium tuberculosis* may yield positive fecal cultures, but may not be associated with a lesion in the gastrointestinal tract. The converse is also true, namely that a tuberculous lesion can exist in the gastrointestinal tract although stool cultures are persistently negative. Every effort should be made to culture the organism from the sputum, ascitic fluid, gastric aspirate or endoscopic biopsy, as not only is this important for diagnosis but with increasing incidence of drug resistance, finding the appropriate drug sensitivity of the organism can be vital. Polymerase chain reaction (PCR) techniques have been used in the diagnosis of tuberculosis, but although it is a very sensitive test, at the present time PCR is unable to distinguish active disease from past infection, and culture remains the gold standard for assessing viability and thus infectivity (Kikuchi et al 1992, Andersen et al 1993).

PRESENTATION

In the UK the disease is predominantly seen in immigrants, mostly from the Indian subcontinent. It has also been reported in immigrants in North America, usually in Caucasians from Europe (Hill et al 1976, Schulze et al 1977). The disease most commonly occurs in the fourth decade and in Britain is more common in men than women, probably because there is a larger population of immigrant men, often living in overcrowded conditions. In third-world countries the disease is more common in women, possibly because they nurse infected family members.

Patients present with active gastrointestinal tuberculosis at varying intervals after immigration. In one series (Findlay et al 1979) the range was 6 months to 16 years, with the mean interval being 6 years. Phage typing of the tubercle bacilli usually reveals an organism characteristic of the immigrant's country of origin (Grange et al 1977).

Anorexia, weight loss, malaise and abdominal pain, typically in the right iliac fossa, are predominant symptoms. Diarrhea is less common and may be related to ulceration, lymphatic obstruction or bacterial overgrowth. The patient is generally malnourished. A tender mass may be felt in about 50% of cases, with the classic doughy abdomen being rather uncommon.

Investigation

A mild normocytic anemia and elevated ESR are common, but not universal. The serum albumin is usually low, partly owing to the effect of the acute-phase response and partly to increased protein loss from the gastrointestinal tract. Chest X-ray is normal in at least a third of patients. Radiological examination of the small intestine is often particularly helpful.

Heaf and Tine testing is positive in up to two-thirds of patients (Marshall 1993). Fecal fat collections, Schilling test and xylose tolerance tests may all be normal, even in the presence of extensive small-bowel disease.

Specific investigations

Crohn's disease can mimic tuberculosis and is often impossible to distinguish on X-rays. Hypersegmentation and flocculation of barium, accelerated transit and thickening of mucosal folds are often early signs. In more advanced cases ulceration and narrowing of the bowel are common, with a gaping ileocecal valve and shortening of the cecum and ascending colon. It is not unusual in such advanced cases to find a deformed cecum in a subhepatic location.

Ascitic fluid analysis reveals an exudate with an increased cell count consisting predominantly of lymphocytes. Bacteriologic study is not rewarding, with positive culture in less than 20% of cases (Marshall 1993). In one study, however, 83% of patients studied had positive cultures when 1 liter of ascitic fluid was centrifuged and used for culture (Singh et al 1969). Several studies have shown that ascitic fluid adenosine deaminase (ADA) activity is highly sensitive and fairly specific. High concentrations of ADA are present in T lymphocytes during a cellular immune response. ADA catalyzes the conversion of adenosine to inosine. Values above 33 U/l are said to be 100% sensitive and 95% specific for the diagnosis of tuberculosis (Voight et al 1989, Bhargava et al 1990). False positives have, however, been reported with lymphoproliferative disease, fungal peritonitis and mesotheliomas (Israel 1994). The value of ADA in AIDS patients remains unclear. The importance of PCR testing of ascitic fluid as a tool for clinical diagnosis remains to be determined.

Ultrasound and CT scans, although helpful in showing bowel thickening and lymph node enlargement, are rarely discriminatory (Balthazar et al 1990, Kedar et al 1994).

In endemic areas endoscopy and colonoscopy are often the procedures of choice, as they allow direct visualization of the involved bowel with cytologic and histologic confirmation (Bhargava et al 1985, Kochhar et al 1991).

Laparoscopy with directed biopsy is extremely useful for the diagnosis of tuberculous peritonitis. Laparoscopic findings of whitish 'miliary nodules' less than 5 mm in diameter scattered over the visceral and parietal peritoneum with adhesions allow a presumptive diagnosis in 85–95% of cases (Marshall 1993). Laparoscopy combined with targeted peritoneal biopsy helps to eliminate the need for diagnostic laparotomy (Wolfe et al 1979). Other authors have confirmed the value of peritoneal biopsy (Mehrotra et al 1966, Pimparker 1977). Laparoscopy is considerably easier in patients with ascites than those with fibrocaseous disease. It has much to offer when recurrent abdominal pain, abdominal mass, ascites, pyrexia or weight loss are presenting symptoms.

It is worth emphasizing that even at formal laparotomy the diagnosis of tuberculosis can be extremely difficult. The distinction between tuberculosis, Crohn's disease and carcinoma may be impossible without histological examination of biopsies from seedlings, strictures, glandular enlargement or cecal mass.

Serological tests have also been used. ELISA and a soluble antigen fluorescent antibody (SAFA) test have been shown to be 80% sensitive and over 90% specific (Bhargava et al 1986, 1992). If followed up by additional confirmative diagnostic tests, these relatively inexpensive tests could prove extremely useful as a preliminary test in suspected cases.

Lymphangiography is of limited value since abnormalities are often indistinguishable from those seen in metastatic disease, lymphomatous processes and non-specific reactive hyperplasia (Bettlestone et al 1977). Gallium-67 citrate scanning can occasionally be helpful, but a positive scan only suggests inflammation and is not pathognomonic of tuberculosis.

Oropharyngeal tuberculosis

Before the introduction of antituberculous therapy the tongue was affected in 1.2% of patients with pulmonary tuberculosis (Cawson 1960). The tonsils may also be involved (Cowan & Jones 1972). The larynx is now rarely affected, but formerly was frequently involved in extensive pulmonary tuberculosis.

Esophageal tuberculosis

Esophageal disease is exceedingly rare. Most instances are associated with direct spread from adjacent affected structures, such as mediastinal nodes, or a pulmonary focus (Dow 1981). It may be associated with a bronchoesophageal fistula, which will usually clear quickly after antituberculous therapy.

Gastric tuberculosis

Tuberculosis of the stomach is rare, accounting for less than 3% of gastrointestinal tuberculosis in one series (Findlay et al 1979); it was not seen in any of 102 patients reported by Vaidya and Sodhi (1978). Mukerjee and Singal (1979) reported an incidence of 2.8% of 500 patients operated on for abdominal tuberculosis. The low pH probably protects the stomach from swallowed tubercle bacilli. As in tuberculosis affecting any organ, gastric TB can occur in the absence of pulmonary disease. The antrum is commonly involved and the disease mimics peptic ulceration, gastric cancer, gastric lymphoma and gastric Crohn's disease.

Duodenal tuberculosis

Duodenal disease is rare (Findlay et al 1979, Marshall 1993). It occurs in three forms: the first is simple ulceration, and indeed tuberculous ulceration of the duodenum was described long before peptic ulceration; secondly, the duodenal mucosa may be infiltrated by a chronic inflammatory process without actual ulceration; thirdly, duodenal obstruction can result, with extrinsic pressure from an inflammatory mass of lymph nodes.

Clinical presentation is often similar to peptic ulcer disease. Although helpful, endoscopy and biopsy may not yield a definitive diagnosis, which is often made at surgery. In endemic areas early onset of gastric outlet obstruction in a patient with peptic ulcer disease should raise suspicion of tuberculosis (Ali et al 1993).

Jejunal, ileal and ileocecal tuberculosis

Jejunal and ileal disease are common forms of intestinal tuberculosis. Ileocecal disease is by far the most common lesion, affecting approximately two-thirds (Pimparker 1977, Findlay et al 1979), and is usually characterized by obstruction and a tender abdominal mass. The radiological appearances are a high-riding cecum with a string-like lesion of the terminal ileum (Fig. 42.1). Patients present with symptoms caused by the complications of small-intestinal disease: obstruction, pain, alteration in bowel habit and malabsorption. Nodular mucosa with ulcerations, which are often aphthous, can be seen on colonoscopy and ileoscopy (Fig. 42.2). PCR on the

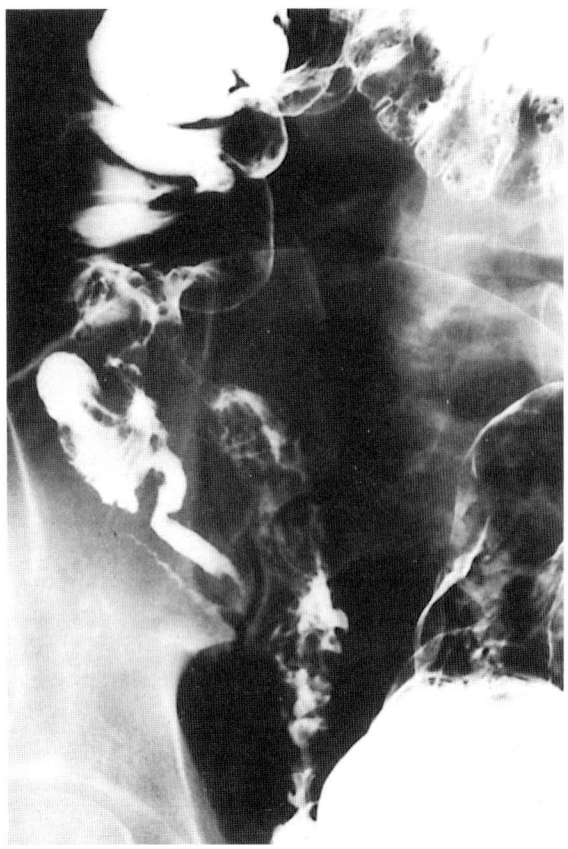

Fig. 42.1 Barium follow-through showing the typical contracted highly placed cecum with terminal ileal involvement by tuberculosis.

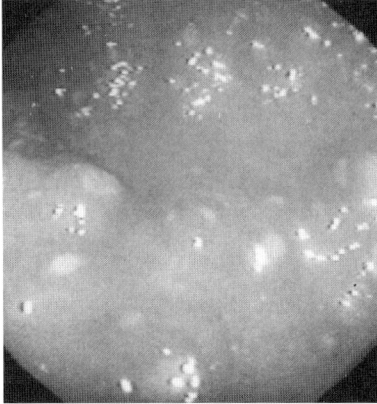

Fig. 42.2 Ileoscopy showing nodular mucosa with ulcerations in the terminal ileum. PCR on the biopsy specimen was positive for *Mycobacterium tuberculosis*. (Courtesy of Dr Anand, Houston, Texas) (See page xx.)

biopsy specimen can be helpful when biopsy and cultures are not diagnostic, as in this patient (Anand et al 1994).

Tuberculosis of the appendix

Tuberculous appendicitis is rare even in endemic areas. Shah et al (1967) studied 20 patients with ileocecal disease without finding any evidence of appendicular involvement. Anand (1956) found no evidence of tuberculosis of the appendix in a series of 50 patients. When the appendix is involved it is associated with low-grade intermittent pain, vomiting and diarrhea. These non-specific symptoms make it impossible to distinguish appendicular from ileocecal disease. A latent type of infection, where the appendix may look macroscopically normal, is a rarity (Patkin & Robinson 1964).

Tuberculous colitis

Tuberculous colitis, like Crohn's disease, can involve all layers of the bowel and frequently produces deep ulcers, which may progress to fistula or stricture formation. Colonic tuberculosis can present as hypertrophic lesions resembling malignancy, segmental ulcers, multiple focal strictures or long strictures (Figs 42.3, 42.4) (Hill et al 1976). There are isolated case reports in the literature of tuberculous pancolitis mimicking idiopathic ulcerative colitis (Ahuja et al 1976, Balikian et al 1977). Massive bleeding, obstruction, perforation and fistulae have all been described. Colonic involvement without ileal disease is uncommon (Abrams & Holden 1964). There are now several reports of tuberculous colitis and colon cancer occurring in the same individual (Fuyono 1972, Leong et

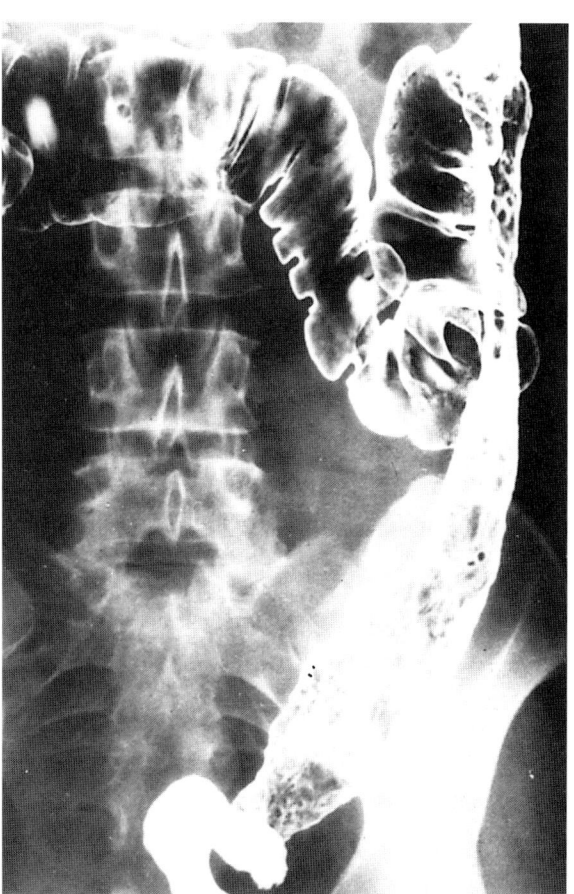

Fig. 42.3 Barium enema showing extensive distal colonic involvement.

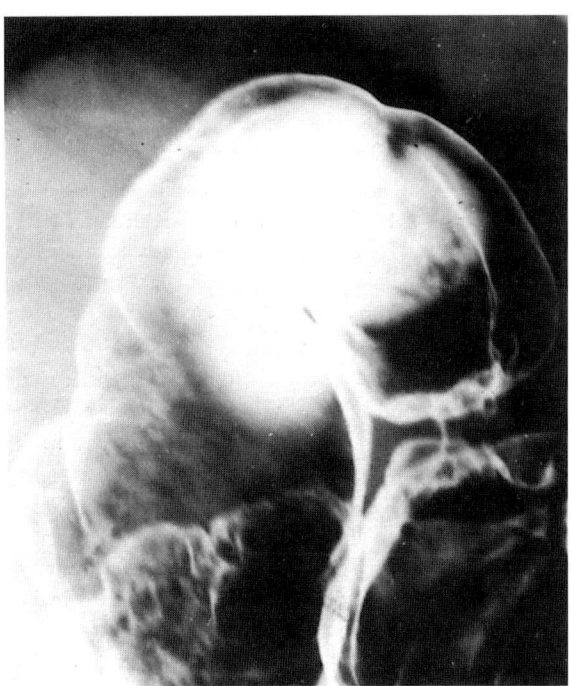

Fig. 42.4 Barium enema showing a stricture at the distal end of the transverse colon.

al 1993), although this occurrence may be coincidental. Colonoscopy is the diagnostic procedure of choice and allows for biopsy, cytology and culture (Bhargava et al 1983, Kochhar et al 1991).

Anorectal tuberculosis

Anorectal disease is uncommon and in the west is likely to be mistaken for Crohn's disease. It may present as ulcers resembling amebic ulcers with undermined edges or as hypertrophic lesions simulating rectal carcinoma (Gupta et al 1976). In the St Mark's hospital experience tuberculosis as a cause of fistula-in-ano declined from 16% in 1921 to 0.85% in 1969 (Logan 1969). However, in endemic areas tuberculosis continues to be a common cause of fistula-in-ano: it comprised 16% of such cases in a recent report from India (Shukla et al 1988).

Crohn's disease and gastrointestinal tuberculosis

The distinction between tuberculosis and Crohn's disease may be extremely difficult, even with endoscopy, surgery and histology. Some useful differentiating features are listed in Table 42.1. If an Asian patient presents with fever, anorexia, weight loss and abdominal pain a diagnosis of tuberculosis is more likely than Crohn's disease. The reverse is true for indigenous Caucasians. A patient with active pulmonary tuberculosis and gastrointestinal symptoms is unlikely to have coincidental Crohn's disease. The extraintestinal features of Crohn's disease, such as arthropathy and ankylosing spondylitis, sclerosing cholangitis and pyoderma gangrenosum, are not usually seen in tuberculosis. Both conditions are characterized by perianal fistulae and perianal disease. Lupus vulgaris is not found in Crohn's disease. Both conditions may involve the eyes. Mouth ulceration and oral involvement is not uncommon in Crohn's disease, but is much rarer in tuberculosis.

A precise diagnosis should be made whenever possible, as corticosteroids administered in the mistaken belief that a patient with tuberculosis has Crohn's disease could be hazardous.

Treatment

Diagnostic techniques have improved so that the need for surgical intervention is less common than formerly. The

Table 42.1 Differentiating features between tuberculosis and Crohn's disease

Characteristics	Tuberculosis	Crohn's
Etiology	*Mycobacterium tuberculosis*	Unknown
Internal fistulae	Rare	Common
Pulled-up cecum	Common	Rare
Anal lesions	Uncommon	Common
Anal ulcerations	Rare	Frequent
Extraintestinal features	Exceedingly rare	Arthropathy, sclerosing cholangitis, pyoderma gangrenosum
TB Tine	Positive (2/3)	Negative
Chest X-ray	Some abnormality in 1/3–2/3	Normal
Gross pathology	Miliary nodules in serosa. Circumferential strictures <3 cm	Eccentric long strictures in mesenteric border
Granulomas	Large, confluent with caseation. May be present in nodes when absent in bowel	Small. Absent in 25%. Not present in nodes when absent in bowel
Response to antitubercular drugs	Excellent	No/poor response
Risk of malignancy	? None	Yes

primary role of surgery is the management of complications, although it is still occasionally necessary for diagnosis (Anand 1956, Homan et al 1977).

Medical therapy

The recent emergence of drug-resistant strains of tuberculosis is of great concern. In New York City 33% of tuberculous isolates are resistant to one drug and 19% were resistant to both isoniazid (INH) and rifampicin (MMWR 1993). The current increase in drug resistance is felt to be largely due to poor compliance with medication. The spontaneous development of drug-resistant mutants to INH occurs in $1/10^6$ organisms. The probability of resistance to two drugs is assumed to be $1/10^{12}$. It has also been estimated that active tuberculous lesions have 10^9 organisms (MMWR 1993). Because administration of a single drug often leads to the development of bacterial populations resistant to that drug, effective regimens must include multiple drugs to which the organism is susceptible, preferably as directly observed therapy (DOT). However, since at the beginning of therapy the in vitro susceptibility is unknown, the Center for Disease Control now recommends a four-drug regimen with INH, rifampicin, pyrazinamide and ethambutol or streptomycin for 2 months (MMWR 1993). On this schedule at least 95% of patients will receive adequate therapy with at least two drugs to which the organism is susceptible. Following this treatment patients are continued on INH and rifampicin for a further 4 months as daily treatment, or two to three times a week as DOT (MMWR 1993). A longer course for 9 months or 6 months after being culture negative has been recommended for HIV-positive patients. For drug-resistant organisms two drugs to which the organism is sensitive must be continued throughout the duration of therapy. For the treatment of intestinal or peritoneal tuberculosis it is generally recommended that the duration of treatment should be extended to 9 months (MMWR 1993).

Antituberculous medications have side effects that may at times be life threatening. It is customary to give 10–20 mg of pyridoxine orally to prevent INH-induced peripheral neuropathy. Clinical hepatitis related to INH occurs in 1% of individuals, generally over 35 years of age and usually within 4–8 weeks of treatment (Harding & Bailey 1994). Rifampicin turns secretions orange, stains soft contact lenses, inhibits the effects of oral contraceptives and potentiates the hepatic side effects of INH. Ethambutol causes a usually reversible optic neuritis and is to be avoided in children, where precise visual testing may not be possible, and in patients with renal failure. Pyrazinamide increases uric acid levels and is hepatotoxic. Up to 10% of patients treated with streptomycin develop ototoxicity, with the vestibular component generally being affected first (Harding & Bailey 1994).

In multidrug-resistant cases second-line drugs should be considered. These include prothionamide, thiacetazone, cycloserine, capreomycin, kanamycin and ciprofloxacin. Many experimental drugs are currently under trial (Harding & Bailey 1994). Corticosteroids have been used on the premise that they may decrease fibrosis and hence stricturing, but their role is unclear. A single controlled trial showed corticosteroids to be useful in tuberculous peritonitis to avoid late intestinal obstruction (Singh et al 1969). A recent large series on gastrointestinal tuberculosis found that patients did well without steroids (Anand et al 1988), and most clinicians even in endemic areas do not use them.

The patient should be carefully monitored and, as an integral part of management, health visitors specially trained in the follow-up of tuberculous patients at home should supervise and ensure the regular consumption of antituberculous therapy and monitor for possible side effects. The major problem among the immigrant population is their frequent movement from one town to another, with return trips to Asia for prolonged spells. The direct family and cohabitees of affected patients should also be screened to exclude tuberculosis.

The patient's general condition should receive attention, with particular attention given to diet, and the correction of anemia and vitamin depletion. Hyperalimentation or parenteral nutrition may occasionally be necessary.

Surgical treatment

Surgical treatment has two major roles, first in the acute situation, where complications supervene, and secondly in the more chronic situation, where a diagnostic laparotomy is indicated.

Emergency surgical treatment is needed for free perforation of a tuberculous ulcer, perforation with abscess formation, intestinal obstruction due to cicatricial stenosis or shortening of the bowel mesentery resulting in kinking of the bowel, localized hypertrophic change and gastrointestinal hemorrhage (Kita et al 1977).

In the chronic situation the abdomen should be explored through a paramedian incision. If there is no mechanical obstruction or perforation an omental or lymph node biopsy should be carried out, and this tissue, together with any available peritoneal fluid, should be sent for culture. If tuberculosis is confirmed the patient should be started on a course of antituberculous drugs. The majority of patients with tuberculous strictures and chronic obstructive symptoms respond very well to antituberculous treatment and do not need surgery (Anand et al 1988).

When an acute obstruction occurs in the small intestine a localized resection should be undertaken, provided that the lesion is localized, or where there are multiple strictures confined to a short segment. However,

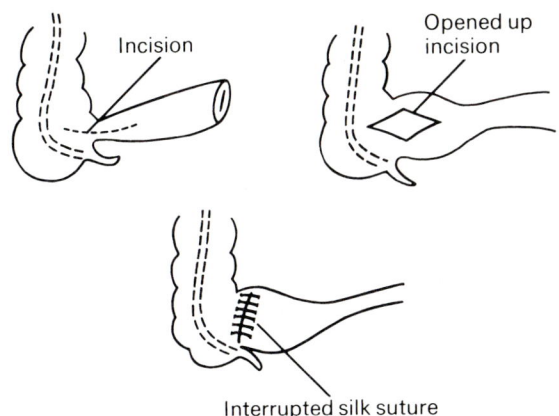

Fig. 42.5 Ileocecoplasty – the technique is the same as that for plastic correction of tuberculous strictures (Katariya et al 1977).

strictureplasty (Fig. 42.5) may be a very useful alternative if strictures are more widespread (Katariya et al 1977, Pujari 1979). The stenosed segment is incised longitudinally and sewn up along its antimesenteric border in a manner similar to a pyloroplasty. Katariya et al (1977) described successful results in 20 patients who had 36 strictures operated upon in this manner.

A right hemicolectomy is the treatment of choice for ileocecal disease with obstruction. Bypass ileotransverse colostomy should be avoided, and so should implantation of the proximal limb of the ileum into the transverse colon, since these procedures create a blind loop which is prone to sinus and abscess formation. Isolated colonic lesions (see Fig. 42.4) may be resected. The only real place for bypass surgery is in the patient with duodenal obstruction.

Perforation is rare, but can occur in any part of the gastrointestinal tract. Classic board-like rigidity is not always found. The presentation may be chronic, with pain, distension and tenderness. Although frequently extremely ill, patients are not always febrile. Simple double-layer closure with or without omental patching resection or, for ileocecal lesions, closure of the perforation with ileotransverse colostomy, is indicated. Sweetman and Wise (1959) suggest that the integrity of single closure is unpredictable, particularly where there is much granulation tissue and caseation. They also stress the surgical principle that when a perforation occurs secondary to a distal stricture the stenotic segment should be removed, provided the patient is fit enough. The mortality rate in perforation complicating abdominal tuberculosis was 30% in the series of Mukherjee and Mukherjee (1965), and can be as high as 50% (Sweetman & Wise 1959).

REFERENCES

Abrams J S, Holden W D 1964 Tuberculosis of the gastrointestinal tract. Archives of Surgery 89: 282–293

Ahuja S K, Gaiha M, Sachdev S et al 1976 Tubercular colitis stimulating ulcerative colitis. Journal of the Association of Physicians of India 24: 617–619

Ali W, Sikora S S, Banerjee D et al 1993 Gastroduodenal tuberculosis. Australia and New Zealand Journal of Surgery 63: 466–467

Anand S S 1956 Hypertrophic ileo-caecal tuberculosis in India with record of 50 hemicolectomies: Hunterian lecture. Annals of the Royal College of Surgeons of England 19: 205–222

Anand B S, Nanda R, Sachdev G K 1988 Response of tuberculous stricture to antituberculous treatment. Gut 29: 62–69

Anand B S, Schneider F E, El Zaatari F A K, Shawar R M, Clarridge J E, Graham D Y 1994 Diagnosis of intestinal tuberculosis by polymerase chain reaction on endoscopic biopsy specimens. American Journal of Gastroenterology 89: 2248–2249

Andersen A B, Thybo S, Godfrey-Faussett P, Stoker N G 1993 Polymerase chain reaction for detection of *Mycobacterium tuberculosis* in sputum. European Journal of Clinical Microbiology and Infectious Diseases 12: 922–927

Balikian J P, Uthman S M, Kabakian H A 1977 Tuberculous colitis. American Journal of Proctology 28: 75–79

Balthazar E J, Gordon R, Hulnick D 1990 Ileocaecal tuberculosis: CT and radiologic evaluation. American Journal of Roentgenology 154: 499–503

Bettlestone C A, Wieland W, Lewis E A, Itayemi S O 1977 Lymphogram in abdominal tuberculosis. Clinical Radiology 28: 653–658

Bhargava D K, Dasarathy S, Shrinivas et al 1992 Evaluation of enzyme-linked immunosorbent assay using mycobacterial saline extracted antigen for the serodiagnosis of abdominal tuberculosis. American Journal of Gastroenterology 87: 105–108

Bhargava D K, Gupta M, Nijhawan S et al 1990 Adenosine deaminase (ADA) in peritoneal tuberculosis: diagnostic value in ascitic fluid and serum. Tubercle 72: 193–197

Bhargava D K, Shriniwas, Tandon B N, Kiran U, Chawla T C, Kapur B M L 1986 Serodiagnosis of intestinal tuberculosis by the soluble antigen fluorescent antibody test (SAFA tests). Journal of Tropical Medicine and Hygiene 89: 61–65

Bhargava D K, Tandon H D Chawla T C, Shriniwas, Tandon B N, Kapur B 1985 Diagnosis of ileocaecal and colonic tuberculosis by colonoscopy. Gastrointestinal Endoscopy 31: 68–70

Blumberg A 1928 Pathology of intestinal tuberculosis. Journal of Laboratory and Clinical Medicine 13: 405–412

Braun M M, Byers R H, Heyward W L et al 1990 Acquired immunodeficiency syndrome and extrapulmonary tuberculosis in the United States. Archives of Internal Medicine 150: 1913–1916

Cawson R A 1960 Tuberculosis of the mouth and throat with special reference to the incidence and management since the introduction of chemotherapy. British Journal of Diseases of the Chest 56: 40–53

Chaisson R E, Slutkin G 1989 Tuberculosis and human immunodeficiency virus infection. Journal of Infectious Diseases 159: 96–100

Cheng I K P, Chan P C K, Chan M K 1989 Tuberculous peritonitis complicating long term peritoneal dialysis: report of 5 cases and review of the literature. American Journal of Nephrology 9: 155–161

Cowan D L, Jones G R 1972 Tuberculosis of the tonsil: case report and review. Tubercle 53: 255–258

Daniel T M 1994 Tuberculosis In: Isselbacher K J, Braunwald E, Wilson J D et al (eds) Harrison's principles of internal medicine, 13th edn. McGraw-Hill, New York, pp 710–718

Dow C J 1981 Oesophageal tuberculosis: four cases. Gut 22: 234–236

Findlay J M, Addison N V, Stevenson D K, Mirza Z A 1979 Tuberculosis of the gastrointestinal tract in Bradford, 1967–1977. Journal of the Royal Society of Medicine 72: 587–590

Fuyono S 1972 Colonic cancer complicating tuberculosis of the colon. Japanese Journal of Gastroenterology 8: 987–991

Gandhi B M, Bhargava D K, Irshad M, Chawla T C, Dube A, Tandon B N 1986 Enzyme linked protein-A: an ELISA for detection of IgG antibodies against *Mycobacterium tuberculosis* in intestinal tuberculosis. Tubercle 67: 21–224

Grange J M, Aber V R, Allen B W et al 1977 Comparison of strains of

Mycobacterium tuberculosis from British, Ugandan and Asian immigrant patients: a study in bacteriophage typing, susceptibility to hydrogen peroxide and sensitivity to the thiopen-2-carbonic acid hydrazide. Tubercle 58: 207–215

Gupta A S, Sharma V P, Rathi G L 1976 Ano-rectal tuberculosis simulating carcinoma. American Journal of Proctology 27: 22–28

Guth A A, Kim U 1991 The reappearance of abdominal tuberculosis. Surgery, Gynecology and Obstetrics 172: 432–436

Harding S M, Bailey W C 1994 Chemotherapy of tuberculosis In: Schlossberg D (ed) Tuberculosis, 3rd edn. Springer-Verlag, New York, pp 69–89

Hill G S Jr, Tabrisky J, Peter M E 1976 Tuberculous enteritis. Western Journal of Medicine 124: 440–445

Homan W P, Grafe W R, Dineen P 1977 A 44-year experience with tuberculous entercolitis. World Journal of Surgery 2: 245–250

Hoon J R, Dockerty M B, Pemberton J de J 1950 Collective review: ileocecal tuberculosis including a comparison of this disease with non-specific regional entercolitis and non-caseous tuberculated entercolitis. International Abstracts of Surgery in Surgery, Gynecology and Obstetrics 91: 417–440

Israel H L 1994 Tuberculous peritonitis. In: Schlossberg D (ed) Tuberculosis, 3rd edn. Springer-Verlag, New York, pp 193–199

Katariya R N, Sood S, Rao P G, Rao P L N G 1977 Strictureplasty for tubercular strictures of the gastrointestinal tract. British Journal of Surgery 64: 496–498

Kedar R P, Shah P P, Shivde R S, Malde H M 1994 Sonographic findings in gastrointestinal and peritoneal tuberculosis. Clinical Radiology 49: 24–29

Kikuchi Y, Oka S, Kimurra S, Mitamura K, Shimata K 1992 Clinical application of the polymerase chain reaction for the rapid diagnosis of mycobacterial tuberculosis infection Internal Medicine 31: 1016–1022

Kita R, Kim E, Yukawa K, Hayashi M, Yukawa E 1977 Treatment of intestinal tuberculosis. Gastroenterologia Japonica 12: 363–367

Kochhar R, Rajwanshi A, Goenka M K et al 1991 Colonoscopic fine needle aspiration cytology in the diagnosis of ileocaecal tuberculosis. American Journal of Gastroenterology 86: 102–104

Leong A F, Seow C F, Goh H S 1993 Colorectal cancer and intestinal tuberculosis. Annals of the Academy of Medicine of Singapore 22: 934–936

Logan V S D 1969 Anorectal tuberculosis. Proceedings of the Royal Society of Medicine 62: 27–30

Marshall J B 1993 Tuberculosis of the gastrointestinal tract and peritoneum. American Journal of Gastroenterology 88: 989–999

Mehrotra M P, Mathur K S, Agarwal A N 1966 Value of the peritoneal biopsy in clinically diagnosed cases of abdominal tuberculosis. Journal of the Association of Physicians of India 14: 625–628

MMWR 1993 Centers for Disease Control and Prevention. Initial therapy for tuberculosis in the era of multidrug resistance. Recommendations of the Advisory Council for the elimination of tuberculosis. 42: 1–8

Mukherjee P, Mukherjee S 1965 Tuberculous perforation of intestine. Surgical Journal of Delhi 1: 40–56

Mukerjee P, Singal 1979 Intestinal tuberculosis: 500 operated cases. Proceedings of the Association of Surgeons of East Africa 2: 70–75

Patkin M R, Robinson B L 1964 Tuberculosis of the appendix. British Journal of Clinical Practice 18: 741–742

Pimparker B D 1977 Abdominal tuberculosis. Journal of the Association of Physicians of India: 801–811

Probert C S J, Jayanthi V, Wicks A C, Carr-Locke D L, Garner P, Mayberry J F 1992 Epidemiological study of abdominal tuberculosis among Indian migrants and the indigenous population of Leicester, 1972–1989. Gut 33: 1085–1089

Pujari B D 1979 Modified surgical procedure in intestinal tuberculosis. British Journal of Surgery 66: 180–181

Schulze K, Warner H A, Murray D 1977 American Journal of Medicine 63: 735–745

Shah R C, Mehta K N, Jalundhawala J M 1967 Tuberculosis of the appendix. Journal of the Indian Medical Association 49: 138–140

Shukla H S, Gupta S C, Singh G et al 1988 Tubercular fistula in ano. British Journal of Surgery 75: 38–39

Singh M M, Bhargava A N, Jain K P 1969 Tuberculous peritonitis; an evaluation of pathogenic mechanisms, diagnostic procedures and therapeutic measures. New England Journal of Medicine 281: 1091–1094

Sweetman W R, Wise R A 1959 Acute perforated tuberculous enteritis; surgical treatment. Annals of Surgery 149: 143–148

Tandon H D, Prakash A 1972 Pathology of intestinal tuberculosis and its distinction from Crohn's disease. Gut 13: 260–269

Taylor A W 1945 Chronic hypertrophic ileocaecal tuberculosis and its relation to regional ileitis (Crohn's disease). British Journal of Surgery 33: 178–181

Vaidya M G, Sodhi J S 1978 Gastrointestinal tract tuberculosis: a study of 102 cases including 55 hemicolectomies. Clinical Radiology 29: 189–195

Voigt M D, Kalvaria I, Trey C, Berman P, Lombard C, Kirsch R E 1989 Diagnostic value of ascites adenosine deaminase in tuberculous peritonitis. Lancet 1: 751–754

Wolfe J H, Behn A R, Jackson B T 1979 Tuberculous peritonitis and role of diagnostic laparoscopy. Lancet 1: 852–853

43. Sexually transmitted diseases/HIV

M. S. Kapembwa   P. A. Batman   G. E. Griffin

GASTROINTESTINAL DISEASE IN AIDS

Gastrointestinal dysfunction is a major cause of morbidity and mortality in AIDS and may be attributed to several causes. Immunodeficiency characterized by severe CD4 lymphopenia predisposes to opportunistic infections and malignancies. However, gastrointestinal symptoms may also occur early in HIV infection and in patients lacking apparent evidence of immunodepression. This chapter focuses on some common gastrointestinal manifestations of HIV disease. A brief discussion on proctitis associated with the more traditional sexually transmitted infections, such as gonorrhea, syphilis, herpes simplex and cytomegalovirus (CMV), is also included.

Abdominal pain

Abdominal pain is an important non-specific symptom in HIV-infected patients and was found in 12.3% of a series of 235 North American patients with AIDS (Barone et al 1986). The major causes of abdominal pain are opportunistic enteropathogens and malignancy. The former, classically associated with diarrheal disease, include *Cryptosporidium* spp., *Isospora belli*, microsporidium, CMV, mycobacterium, salmonella, shigella and *Campylobacter* spp. Infections of the small bowel give rise to cramp-like pain localized to the periumbilical area, whereas colitic pain often localizes to the hypogastrium or lower quadrant, and is often described as gripping in character. However, localization of visceral pain is poor and cannot be used with any degree of certainty in diagnosing infection clinically, since many of these enteropathogens affect both the large and the small intestine.

HIV-related gastrointestinal malignancies such as Kaposi's sarcoma cause pain as a result of partial intestinal obstruction. Surgical exploration for diagnosis is, however, indicated only rarely in such cases because of the existence of cutaneous or other visceral manifestations of malignancy (Friedman et al 1985, Wilson et al 1989), but may be necessary in cases of complete obstruction (Potter et al 1984), severe bleeding or perforation (Frank & Raicht 1984) and intussusption (Hofstetter & Stollman 1988). Abdominal pain and guarding associated with the latter conditions carries the same significance in AIDS patients as in immunocompetent patients.

Odynophagia and dysphagia

Odynophagia (pain on swallowing) and dysphagia (difficulty in propelling food from the mouth to the stomach) are common and serious problems in HIV disease. Fortunately, most of the underlying causes are treatable. If left untreated, however, these symptoms will lead to an eating disorder characterized by weight loss and dehydration (Levine et al 1981).

Esophageal candidiasis is by far the most common cause of both symptoms and can be expected to occur in up to 75% of AIDS patients (Eras et al 1972), often coexisting with oral candidiasis. A double contrast barium swallow usually shows fine ulcerations and plaques, particularly in the distal esophagus. However, these findings are by no means specific and similar changes may be produced by herpes simplex esophagitis (Levine et al 1981). Definitive diagnosis is made by endoscopy, showing the characteristic white patches overlying shaggy, erythematous mucosa, with confirmation by the detection of spores and pseudohyphae within the epithelium and submucosa on histology. Other causes of odynophagia and dysphagia include esophageal ulceration or erosions due to CMV (Jacobson et al 1988) and HIV (Rabeneck et al 1986).

Dysphagia, which first involves solids and later liquids, usually suggests infiltrating masses such as Kaposi's sarcoma or lymphoma. These lesions produce symptoms on the basis of either simple mechanical obstruction or local nerve involvement. Occasionally diseases outside the esophagus, for example mediastinal lymphoma and various neurological conditions involving the brain stem, can cause difficulty in initiating the act of swallowing (personal observations) and a quick search should be made to exclude such conditions. For unknown reasons, Kaposi's sarcoma commonly affect the roof of the mouth and is a cause of serious morbidity in this position. Mediastinal tuberculosis may cause dysphagia by an extrinsic pressure effect and may result in tracheo oesophageal fistulation.

Nausea and vomiting

Nausea and vomiting may occur at any clinical stage of HIV disease, including the acute seroconversion illness associated with primary HIV infection (Cooper et al 1985). More often, these symptoms are encountered as side effects of the medication used to treat intercurrent infection or malignancy in patients with AIDS (Tuazon & Labriola 1987). Such symptoms may also be manifestations of opportunistic infection within the bowel or biliary tree. Finally, persistent vomiting is a feature of expanding CNS lesions and forms part of the multisymptom complex associated with terminal illness in patients with AIDS.

Diarrhea

Chronic diarrhea and severe weight loss with attendant CD4 lymphopenia are hallmarks of gastrointestinal disease in AIDS (Kotler et al 1984, Rolston et al 1989). Clinical observations seem to suggest distinct patterns of diarrhea in AIDS (Kotler 1987). Thus, patients with small-intestinal (enteropathic) diarrhea tend to produce voluminous, non-bloody stools of variable frequency (3–15 bowel movements per day) which are frothy, malodorous, and have a tendency to float suggestive of malabsorption. Diarrhea is usually intermittent at the onset and may be interspersed with long asymptomatic periods which become progressively shorter (personal observations). Stool volumes are classically decreased by fasting in this condition and tenesmus is not a feature. Though wasted, patients may look surprisingly well and have a normal appetite.

In contrast, bowel movements in patients with large-bowel diarrhea comprise small mucoid stools which occur frequently at regular intervals throughout the day and night. Fever and anorexia are common. Occasionally patients may present with features of both small-intestinal and colonic diarrhea. A severe secretory diarrhea is associated with specific opportunistic enteropathogens, for example cryptosporidia and microsporidia infections.

The pathogenesis of diarrhea in HIV infection is little understood, but suggested mechanisms include opportunistic enteric infection (Smith et al 1988), autonomic neuropathy (Batman et al 1991a), cytokine dysregulation in intestinal mucosa (Reka & Kotler 1993, Steffen et al 1993) small-intestinal bacterial overgrowth (Budhraja et al 1987) and HIV infection per se (Miller et al 1988). In African patients a syndrome of diarrhea and cachexia, often without evidence of opportunistic infection, has characteristically been associated with advanced HIV infection and has been descriptively referred to as 'Slim disease' (Serwadda et al 1985). The mechanism of wasting in such patients is the subject of intense debate, but it is likely to be multifactorial and not just representing malabsorption as was originally thought. Infection with *Mycobacterium tuberculosis*, for example, has been shown to be common among patients suffering from 'Slim disease' (Lucas et al 1994).

Jaundice

Although biochemical abnormalities of liver function are commonly seen in patients with AIDS or AIDS-related complex (ARC) (Schneiderman et al 1987), jaundice is encountered less often. Patients should be evaluated to exclude treatable parenchymatous and biliary tract disease, including hepatic abscess, calculous and acalculous gallbladder disease and postsurgical biliary strictures. Not all of these conditions are likely to be directly related to HIV infection.

Fever and right upper quadrant pain accompanying jaundice point to cholecystitis (Cello 1989). *Cryptosporidium* spp., CMV or *Mycobacterium avium-intracellulare* infections are frequently detected in patients with these features (Blumberg et al 1984, Horsburgh et al 1985). There is, however, no evidence for a cause and effect relationship between such infections and biliary tract disease. In a jaundiced patient the finding of markedly evelated alkaline phosphatase should prompt further investigation to exclude an intra- or extrahepatic cause of biliary tract obstruction, such as sclerosing cholangitis, papillary stenosis, bile duct lymphoma, Kaposi's sarcoma or portal lymphadenopathy. Although serological evidence of past hepatitis B viral infection among AIDS patients is high in most reported series (80–95%), the HBs Ag carrier state is seen in only 5–15% of patients (Lebovics et al 1985, Schneiderman et al 1987).

CMV gastrointestinal disease in AIDS

The disease spectrum associated with CMV infection within the gastrointestinal tract is wide and includes inflammation, bleeding, ulceration (Meiselman et al 1985) gangrene and perforation (DeRiso et al 1989). The liver and pancreas may be involved, but the most commonly affected sites are the esophagus, colon and anorectum.

Careful histological examination by an experienced pathologist is the most reliable and cost-effective means of making a diagnosis of CMV infection. Viral cultures are not helpful for diagnosis since false negative and false positive results are common (Zurlo et al 1993). The characteristic finding in intestinal mucosal biopsy is the CMV inclusion body present in swollen endothelial and smooth muscle cells of the muscularis mucosa (Culpepper-Morgan et al 1987, Rene et al 1988). However, it is the degree of inflammatory infiltrate and vasculitis present which appears to determine the severity of clinical illness, and consequently patient management.

Ganciclovir – 9(1-3-dihydroxy-2-propoxymethyl)guanine – a nucleoside analog which differs from acyclovir by a single hydroxyl side-chain, has established value in the treatment of CMV disease (Smee et al 1983, Chachoua et al 1987). The drug is given intravenously, starting with an induction course followed by maintenance therapy, and can cause severe bone marrow suppression. The latter makes concurrent treatment with zidovudine particularly problematic in AIDS patients. Foscarnet, a newer agent, is effective against CMV and has been shown to offer survival advantage over ganciclovir in one large study (Studies of Ocular Complications 1992). However, renal failure and hypocalcaemia are major side effects and tend to limit clinical use of this drug. Both ganciclovir and Foscarnet are virostatic agents and relapse of CMV disease following cessation of treatment is common owing to continuing immunosuppression. The value of long-term therapy in preventing the recurrence of CMV gastrointestinal disease, e.g. proctocolitis, has yet to be determined. Newer strategies for oral agents in treatment and prophylaxis of CMV infection are being evaluated.

Herpes simplex virus infection

The oropharynx and perianal areas are the most favored sites of primary infection or reactivation by herpes simplex virus (HSV). Early lesions are characterized by vesicles surrounded by an erythematous base which subsequently rupture to form small cropped ulcers which may coalesce. The major clinical problems in AIDS patients with HSV infection are ulcerative esophagitis (Agha et al 1986) and proctitis (Siegal et al 1981), both of which recur frequently and are extremely painful. Diagnostic confirmation by culture of swabs taken from the ulcer base or biopsy at endoscopy is highly desirable since the lesions may be indistinguishable clinically from those caused by CMV or HIV itself.

Acyclovir has been shown to significantly reduce symptoms and virus excretion in placebo-controlled, double-blind trials in patients with anogenital HSV infection (Mayers et al 1982, Mindel et al 1982), and is effective when used prophylactically to prevent recurrences (Douglas et al 1984).

Protozoal infections

Coccidial parasites

Coccidial parasites, in particular *Cryptosporidium* spp, *Isospora belli* and *Microsporidium* spp., are major opportunistic enteropathogens in AIDS (Soave & Johnson 1988, Orenstein et al 1990). Intestinal infection with any one of these microorganisms persisting for longer than 1 month in an HIV seropositive individual constitutes AIDS diagnosis (Centers for Disease Control 1986).

Cryptosporidiosis. *Cryptosporidium* spp. is widely recognized as a cause of self-limited acute gastroenteritis in immunocompetent individuals. In patients with AIDS, however, this parasite can infect both small- and large-intestinal mucosal surfaces. The illness is associated with severe and potentially life-threatening diseases, characterized by persistent diarrhea, malabsorption and weight loss (Current et al 1983). Biliary infection should be suspected when patients develop persistent vomiting and right upper quadrant abdominal pain in addition to diarrhea. The diagnosis of intestinal cryptosporidiosis rests with the detection of oocysts, in either stool or jejunal aspirate, using modified Ziehl–Neelsen stain. No effective chemotherapeutic agent is as yet available for cryptosporidiosis. However, a variety of antibiotics, including spiramycin, paromomycin and azithromycin, have been tried, with variable degrees of success. Lactose exclusion from the diet and oral cholestyramine may help reduce diarrhea.

Isospora belli. In contrast to chronic intestinal cryptosporidiosis, much less has been written about *Isospora belli* infections in humans. The parasite has been reported more frequently in AIDS patients from some areas of the developing world, such as east Africa or Haiti (DeHovitz et al 1986, Sewankambo et al 1987). The spectrum of infection in HIV seropositive individuals appears to be no different from that seen in cryptosporidiosis, although oocysts are less often detected in stool samples than cryptosporidial oocysts, which might result in some missed diagnosis. Intracellular stages of the parasite are, however, easily identified in small-intestinal biopsies. *Isospora belli* infection can be successfully treated with a combination of trimethoprim and sulfamethoxazole, (DeHovitz et al 1986), but prophylaxis is often indicated to prevent recurrences.

Microsporidiosis. Microsporidia are a complex group of unicellular parasites that have only recently been recognized as human pathogens (Desportes et al 1985). The organisms are being detected with increasing frequency in the small intestine of patients with AIDS and chronic diarrhea (Orenstein et al 1990, Rabeneck et al 1993). Infection with these parasites can result in nutrient malabsorption. Microsporidia were previously not easily detected in stools because of the minute size of the spores, and the hallmark of diagnosis rested with identification of the parasite within enterocytes in biopsy specimens using light or transmission electron microscopy (Peacock et al 1991). However, recent studies have demonstrated that, using stool concentration methods and chromotrope-based or fluorescent staining techniques (Weber et al 1992, Van Gool et al 1993), this enteroparasite can be detected in stool specimens with speed and accuracy; these methods might replace endoscopic biopsy as the diagnostic test of choice.

Mycobacteria avium intracellulare

Mycobacteria avium intracellulare (MAC) comprises two closely related slow-growing non-chromogenic mycobacteria (*Mycobacteria avium* and *Mycobacteria intracellulare*) that cannot be distinguished in most laboratories. In the developed world, MAC is by far the most common mycobacterium isolated from patients with AIDS, in contrast to the developing world where *Mycobacteria tuberculosis* predominates (Malebranche et al 1983, Roth et al 1985). MAC is probably acquired through ingestion of contaminated water (Goslee & Wolinsky 1976), but the organism is also found in soil and dust, raising the possibility of aerosol transmission.

In patients with AIDS, MAC is a systemic infection with widespread tissue involvement. The gastrointestinal tract, liver, spleen, bone marrow and lymph nodes are among the most commonly affected organs. Diarrhea, weight loss and malabsorption are major clinical manifestations and can produce an illness resembling Whipple's disease (Gillin et al 1983). MAC can present as mediastinal–esophageal fistulae with esophagitis (Goodman et al 1989), terminal ileitis mimicking Crohn's disease (Schneebaum et al 1987), or enlarged periportal lymph nodes causing extrahepatic biliary obstructive jaundice (Hawkins et al 1986). Disseminated MAC infection is often diagnosed on culture of the organism from blood during the course of a diagnostic screen for the source of fever.

The pathogenicity of MAC is the subject of intense debate. MAC infections tend to occur late in the course of HIV disease, when patients are severely lymphopenic (CD4 count less than 100 cells/cu. mm) (Modilevsky et al 1989). Failure of phagocytosis by macrophages due to diminished T-cell regulatory function is thought to be the main pathogenetic mechanism for MAC infection (Crowle et al 1992). MAC may be diagnosed by blood cultures or on jejunal biopsy, demonstrating typical acid-fast bacilli within the macrophages.

Therapy for MAC is problematic since, unlike *Mycobacterium tuberculosis*, the organisms are often resistant to standard first-line antituberculous drugs. Current therapy consists of combinations of drugs which have been shown to have variable bactericidal effects against the organism in vitro. Such drugs include rifabutin, clofazimine, ciprofloxacin, ethambutol, clarithromycin and azithyromycin.

HIV enteropathy

Clinical and laboratory evidence of nutrient malabsorption is seen in many HIV-infected patients in the absence of any identifiable enteropathogen or malignancy in the gastrointestinal tract. This observation has prompted several authors to raise the question of an enteropathy due to HIV (Kotler et al 1984, Gillin et al 1985, Miller et al 1988). Meticulous studies of jejunal mucosal architecture in such patients have almost universally documented partial villous atrophy at all clinical stages of HIV disease (Batman et al 1989, Greenson et al 1991, Kalil et al 1991). The overall effect of such enteropathy is malabsorption brought about by any of the following mechanisms:

1. Reduced surface area as a consequence of villous atrophy
2. Functional immaturity of enterocytes, evidenced by decreased or absent brush border disaccharidases (Kapembwa et al 1989, Ullrich et al 1989, Heise et al 1991)
3. Functional enterocyte damage, induced directly or indirectly by HIV (Nelson et al 1988, Fox et al 1989, Jarry et al 1990).

The etiology of villous atrophy in the jejunum of patients infected with HIV is not entirely clear, but most studies have shown that it is associated with hyperplasia of mucosal crypts (Batman et al 1989, Cummins et al 1990, Greenson et al 1991). Other work has shown villous atrophy with hyporegeneration of crypts and a consequent defect in maturation of enterocytes (Ullrich et al 1989). Jejunal villous atrophy, however, is a common morphological end-point of damage mediated by an immune response within the lamina propria (Elson et al 1977). In HIV-infected patients disturbance of crypt cell kinetics with villous atrophy may be attributed to such an immune response directed against lamina propria lymphocytes and macrophages expressing viral antigens (Jarry et al 1990).

The identification of microsporidia in jejunal biopsies and the stool of patients with AIDS-related diarrhea has raised doubts about the existence of HIV enteropathy (La Brooy 1993). However, recently it has been possible to infect lymphoid cells with HIV in the lamina propria of fetal intestinal explants maintained in tissue culture (Fleming et al 1992), and to demonstrate profound crypt cell hyperplasia in infected tissue (Batman et al 1994). This experimental model of HIV enteropathy suggests that jejunal crypt cell hyperplasia, induced indirectly by HIV-infected cells in the lamina propria, may force immature enterocytes on to the sides of villi, leading to a shift of the crypt–villus junction in a luminal direction, with a reduction in villus absorptive surface area. In addition, primary cultures of epithelial and mesenchymal cells derived from the bowel may replicate and establish HIV latency (Moyer et al 1990). Gastrointestinal physiology may be further compromised by autonomic neuropathy induced by HIV (Griffin et al 1988, Batman et al 1991b). These findings strongly suggest that HIV per se may influence intestinal mucosal structure and function.

Kaposi's sarcoma

Kaposi's sarcoma (KS) is a multicentric tumor arising spontaneously at several anatomical sites. The lesion is thought to be a vascular hyperplasia in its initial stages, rather than a true neoplasm (Roth et al 1992). The malignant proliferation that emerges is thought to be endothelial (Nadji et al 1981) in origin, but there is disagreement as to the type of endothelium from which KS arises, namely vascular (Modlin et al 1983, Rutgers et al 1986) or lymphatic (Beckstead et al 1985).

The detailed mechanism of oncogenesis is unclear. Epidemic KS is seen primarily in HIV-seropositive white homosexual males (Gottlieb et al 1981) and African patients (Bayley et al 1985). The tumour is rare in hemophiliacs and HIV-infected children, and experimental evidence indicates that it is stimulated by growth factors released from KS-primed cell cultures (Ensoli et al 1989), leading to speculation that a specific cofactor, possibly another sexually transmitted disease, is involved in pathogenesis (Beral et al 1990). Studies (Moore et al 1995) have now firmly implicated a Herpes virus in the aetiology of Kaposi's sarcoma in both HIV positive and negative individuals.

HIV-related KS presents a wide spectrum of disease severity, ranging from flat, brown macules or papules to large confluent skin lesions with multiple lymphadenopathy and visceral involvement. Approximately 40% of patients with cutaneous KS have gastrointestinal tract involvement (Friedman et al 1985). Rarely, gastrointestinal lesions can occur in the absence of KS in other locations (Lustbader & Sherman 1987). The diagnosis of intestinal KS is best made by visual inspection at endoscopy, although the radiographic features of KS have been well characterized (Wall et al 1984). Luminal lesions may appear as purple-red, diffuse or discrete nodules, with or without surrounding hemorrhage. Lymphadenopathy secondary to KS cannot be readily differentiated from either lymphoma or *Mycobacterium avium intracellulare* by CT appearance, and fine-needle aspiration biopsy may be necessary for a correct diagnosis. Endoscopic biopsies may give false negative results for KS due to inaccessible submucosal lesions (Friedman et al 1985).

KS is responsive to chemotherapy, but patients are often unable to tolerate aggressive therapy and succumb to opportunistic infection. The antimitotic agents commonly used include adriamycin, vincristine, bleomycin, and doxorubicin either alone or in combination. Patients with endoscopic evidence of KS tend to have decreased survival at 24 months (11%) compared to those without intestinal KS (88%) at time of presentation (Friedman et al 1985).

AIDS cholangiopathy

AIDS-related cholangiopathy is a well recognized complication of HIV infection. Radiologically and pathologically, AIDS cholangiopathy resembles primary sclerosing cholangitis (Schneiderman et al 1987). In addition, atypical HLA-DR expression on bile duct epithelial cells was demonstrated in patients with AIDS (Sieratzki et al 1986), prompting speculation that biliary tract injury in HIV disease is a consequence of immunological events directed against epithelial cells analogous, pathogenetically, to graft-versus-host disease and primary biliary cirrhosis (Takacs et al 1983, Ballardini et al 1984). Pain related to the biliary system is common in cryptosporidial infection.

EFFECT OF HIV ON ULCERATIVE COLITIS AND CROHN'S DISEASE: IMPLICATIONS FOR PATHOGENESIS OF IBD

AIDS has been described in patients with previously documented inflammatory bowel disease (IBD) (Dhar et al 1984, Liebowitz & McShane 1986, James 1988), and occasionally the gastrointestinal manifestations of HIV infection have been mistaken for IBD (Weber et al 1985, Caroline et al 1987, Schneebaum et al 1987, Biggs et al 1987). Progressive decline of CD4+ T cells as a result of AIDS was associated with clinical remission of Crohn's disease in one case (James 1988), suggesting that an intact cell-mediated immune response, and the CD4 lymphocyte in particular, may play a central role in the pathogenesis of IBD.

'Non-specific' inflammatory changes within the mucosa have been reported in the colon of AIDS patients with otherwise enteropathogen-negative chronic diarrhea (Hing et al 1992, Law et al 1992, Kotler et al 1993). However, the significance of this finding in terms of pathogenesis and progression of intestinal disease in HIV infection is unknown. Mucosal inflammation can alter permeability (Madara 1990), and Kapembwa et al (1991) have shown increased small-intestinal permeability in patients with advanced HIV infection. Such disruption of the mucosal barrier may have adverse physiological consequences, with increased uptake of luminal antigen, e.g. bacterial polysaccharide, leading to accelerated inflammatory activity, activation of immune cells and release of TNF (tumor necrosis factor) and other cytokines (Beutler et al 1986), which might in turn enhance HIV activation (Clouse et al 1989) and produce a self-perpetuating cycle.

Gonococcal proctitis

Anorectal gonococcal infection is thought to be transmitted almost entirely by receptive anal intercourse, and is an important cause of rectal inflammation in homosexual men. The term 'gay bowel syndrome' (Clouse et al 1989) was historically coined to describe this and other infectious diseases frequently affecting the gastrointestinal tract in the male homosexual population. However, it is important to recognize that proctitis can be associated with a variety of infections not exclusive to homosexual men, and the role of the bisexual in transmitting infection to the heterosexual partner must be appreciated.

A small amount of clear mucoid discharge at the anus is not uncommon in individuals practising receptive anorectal intercourse, and patients often have difficulty describing such symptoms, owing in part to embarrassment or worry about stigmatization. A sympathetic and non-judgmental approach by the physician is therefore most important in eliciting these symptoms. In addition, the use or an understanding of some of the 'street' vernacular, for example 'rimming' or 'fisting', helps clarify the history, particularly with regard to homosexual practice.

Anorectal gonorrhea is asymptomatic in approximately two-thirds of patients (Owen & Hill 1972, Kazal et al 1976, Klein et al 1977). When symptoms do occur they are often mild and non-specific. The most common complaints are mucoid rectal discharge, painful or difficult defecation, tenesmus, bleeding at defecation and pruritus ani. Disseminated gonococcal infections and local complications such as fistula formation and anorectal abscesses are rarely seen in 'gay bowel syndrome'.

Proctoscopic examination in patients with acute gonococcal proctitis is usually either normal or non-specific. The underlying mucosa may be erythematous, edematous and friable. Frank ulcerations are rarely seen. The rectal histological appearances of gonococcal proctitis are variable, and range from the less often seen destruction of crypts and infiltration by polymorphonuclear leukocytes in severe cases, to focal collections of acute inflammatory cells in the lamina propria with intercrypt edema in mild cases.

The diagnosis of rectal gonorrhea is made by isolation of *Neisseria gonorrhoeae* in rectal swab cultures plated on selective media. Gram-stain of rectal smears for intracellular diplococci has lower specifity and sensitivity than culture owing to the presence within the rectal microenvironment of non-pathogenic commensal neisseria, as well as other pathogenic *Neisseria* species such as *Neisseria meningitidis*. The latter gives rise to an illness not dissimilar to that of gonococcal proctitis (Judson et al 1978, Faur et al 1981, McKenna et al 1993).

In general, gonococcal infections of the rectum seem harder to treat adequately than gonococcal infections in other sites, except for the pharynx. Aqueous procaine penicillin, for decades the preferred therapeutic agent for gonococcal infection of all sites, is associated with a treatment failure rate of 2–5%. With the increasing emergence of penicillinase-producing *Neisseria gonorrhoeae*, the newer 4-quinolones (ciprofloxacin and ofloxacin) have become increasingly attractive as drugs of first choice in the treatment of gonorrhea. They may be used in penicillin-allergic patients and have the advantage over procaine penicillin of being given orally (Loo et al 1985). A test of cure and contact tracing, including the treatment of sexual partners, should be essential parts of any successful treatment program.

Syphilitic proctitis

Syphilitic infections of the rectum and anus may be primary or secondary. The primary chancre presents as a painless ulcer with raised edges on the perianal skin, and can mimic several conditions, namely anal fissure, fistula, idiopathic anorectal ulcer, colonic polyp or carcinoma (Quinn et al 1982). When present within the anal canal or rectum such lesions may be missed unless proctoscopic examination is performed. In contrast, lesions of secondary syphilis in the anorectal area appear as moist, hypertrophic papules (condylomata lata), and are often associated with the presence of a cutaneous skin rash on the palms and the soles of the feet, and patchy alopecia. Condylomata lata teem with spirochetes and are therefore highly infectious. The rash is a useful pointer to the diagnosis and serves to differentiate syphilitic condylomata from the edematous perianal skin tags of Crohn's disease and genital warts (condylomata acuminata).

The diagnosis of syphilitic proctitis can be extremely difficult. Dark-field microscopic examination of serum from the ulcer base for *Treponema pallidum* is confounded by the presence of non-pathogenic spirochetes in the rectum of up to 36% of homosexual men practising receptive intercourse (McMillan & Lee 1981). Laboratory confirmation is therefore the final arbiter, but serological tests may be negative in early syphilis. The fluorescent treponemal antibody (FTA) test provides a specific and sensitive means of detecting syphilis, and often gives the earliest positive result, followed by the Venereal Disease Research Laboratory (VDRL) and *Treponema pallidum* hemaglutination tests. Repeat serological testing should therefore be undertaken in suspicious cases where the first result is negative. In doubtful cases, silver staining of rectal biopsy specimens may reveal *Treponema pallidum* and thereby help to establish the diagnosis of syphilis, in addition to ruling out other causes of rectal ulceration. Histological changes in early syphilis comprise crypt distortion, granulomata (including giant cell formation) and infiltration of lymphocytes and plasma cells in the lamina propria (McMillan & Lee 1981). Vasculitic changes may also be seen (Nazemi et al 1975).

Early syphilis is treated by benzathine penicillin 2.4 m units intramuscularly (i.m.) given once weekly for up to a maximum of 3 weeks (i.e. total 7.2 m units), or aqueous procaine penicillin 1.2 m units i.m. for 10 days. An acute febrile reaction, often accompanied by headache, myalgia and hypotension, may occur after treatment (Jarisch–Herxheimer reaction) (Lancet 1977). There are no reliable methods for either predicting or preventing such reactions and patients should be warned of this complication. Oxytetracycline or erythromycin are useful alternatives in penicillin-allergic individuals.

Herpetic proctitis

Herpes simplex virus (HSV types I and II) are DNA viruses responsible for most cases of non-gonococcal proctitis in sexually active homosexual men (Quinn et al 1981, Laughon et al 1988). Type I virus classically produces lesions above the waist, and type II is associated with sexually transmitted infection below the waist.

The symptoms and signs of anogenital HSV infection are often related to the anatomical site of involvement. Anal lesions classically present with painful vesicular eruptions on an erythematous base, which subsequently rupture leaving shallow ulcers. Viral infection of the sacral ganglia can produce a radiculomyelopathy, with radiation of severe pain in the distribution of the sacral plexus (sacral syndrome) (Goldmeier 1985). Occasionally patients may develop urinary dysfunction, impotence and constipation. Following resolution of the primary attack of HSV infection individuals may remain well, with negative viral cultures, indefinitely; suffer recurrent episodes, often less severe and of shorter duration than the primary attack, with intermittent viral shedding, or become asymptomatic viral shedders for prolonged periods (Isselbacher et al 1980).

Material from anal ulcers and vesicles may be cultured for HSV and is diagnostic. Serological tests are of little help in the clinical management of anorectal HSV infection.

REFERENCES

Agha F P, Horchang H L, Nostrant T T 1986 Herpetic oesophagitis: a diagnostic challenge in immunocompromised patients. American Journal of Gastroenterology 81: 246–253

Ballardini G, Mirakian R, Bianchi F B et al 1984 Aberrant expression of HLA-DR antigens on bile duct epithelium in primary biliary cirrhosis: relevance to pathogenesis. Lancet 2: 1009–1013

Barone J E, Gingold S B, Nealon F T, Arvanitis L M 1986 Abdominal pain in patients with acquired immunodeficiency syndrome. Annals of Surgery 204: 619–623

Batman P A, Miller A R O, Forster S M, Harris J R W, Pinching A J, Griffin G E 1989 Jejunal enteropathy associated with human immunodeficiency virus infection: quantitative histology. Journal of Clinical Pathology 42: 275–281

Batman A P, Miller A R O, Sedgwick M P, Griffin G E G 1991a Autonomic denervation in jejunal mucosa of homosexual men infected with HIV. AIDS 5: 1247–1252

Batman A P, Miller A R O, Sedgwick M P, Griffin G E G 1991b Autonomic denervation in jejunal mucosa of homosexual men infected with HIV. AIDS 5: 1247–1252

Batman P A, Fleming S C, Sedgwick P M, MacDonald T T, Griffin G E 1994 HIV infection of human foetal intestinal explant cultures induces epithelial cell proliferation. AIDS 8: 161–167

Bayley A C, Downing R G, Cheingsong-Popov R et al 1985 HTLV-III serology distinguishes atypical and endemic Kaposi's sarcoma in Africa. Lancet i: 359–361

Beckstead J H, Wood G S, Fletcher V 1983 Evidence for the origin of Kaposi's sarcoma from lymphatic endothelium. American Journal of Pathology 119: 249–300

Beral V, Peterman T A, Berkelman R L, Jaffe H W 1990 Kaposi's sarcoma among persons with AIDS: a sexually transmitted infection? Lancet i: 123–128

Beutler B, Krochin N, Milsark I W, Luedke C, Cerami A 1986 Control of cachectin (tumor necrosis factor) synthesis: mechanisms for endotoxin resistance. Science 232: 977–980

Biggs B A, Crowe S M, Lucas C R, Ralston M, Thompson I L, Hardy K J 1987 AIDS-related Kaposi's sarcoma presenting as ulcerative colitis and complicated by toxic megacolon. Gut 28: 1302–1306

Blumberg R S, Kelsey P, Perrone T, Dickersin R, Laquaglia M, Ferruci J 1984 Cytomegalovirus – and cryptosporidium – associated acalculous cholecystitis. American Journal of Medicine 76: 1118–1123

Budhraja M, Levendoglu H, Kocka F, Mangkornkanok M, Sherer R 1987 Duodenal mucosal T-cell sub-population and bacterial cultures in acquired immune deficiency syndrome. American Journal of Gastroenterology 82: 427–431

Caroline D F, Hilpert P L, Russin V L 1987 CMV colitis mimicking Crohn's disease in patients with acquired immune deficiency syndrome (AIDS) Journal of the Canadian Association for Radiology 38: 227–228

Cello J P 1989 Acquired immunodeficiency syndrome cholangiopathy: spectrum of disease. American Journal of Medicine 86: 539–546

Centers for Disease Control 1986 Classification system for human T-lymphotropic virus type III/lymphadenopathy-associated virus infection. Morbidity and Mortality Weekly 35: 344

Chachoua A, Dieterich D, Krasinski K et al 1987 9-(1,3-dihydroxy-2-propoxymethyl) guanine in the treatment of cytomegalovirus gastrointestinal disease with the acquired immunodeficiency syndrome. Annals of Internal Medicine 107: 133–137

Clouse K A, Powell D, Washington I et al 1989 Monokine regulation of human immunodeficiency virus-1 expression in a chronically infected human T cell clone. Journal of Immunology 142: 431–438

Cooper D A, Gold J, Maclean P et al 1985 Acute AIDS retrovirus infection. Definition of a clinical illness associated with seroconversion. Lancet 1: 537–540

Crowle A J, Ross E R, Cohn D J L, Gilden J, May M H 1992 Comparison of the abilities of *Mycobacterium avium* and *Mycobacterium intracellulare* to infect and multiply in cultured human macrophages from normal and human immunodeficiency virus-infected subjects. Infection and Immunity 60: 3697–3703

Culpepper-Morgan J, Kotler D P, Tierney A R et al 1987 Evaluation of diagnostic criteria for disseminated cytomegalovirus infection in the acquired immune deficiency syndrome. American Journal of Gastroenterology 82: 1264–1270

Cummins A G, La Brooy T J, Stanley D P Rowland R, Shearman D J C 1990 Quantitative histological study of enteropathy associated with HIV infection. Gut 31: 317–321

Current L W, Reese N C, Ernst J V, Bailey W S, Heyman M B, Weinstein W M 1983 Human cryptosporidiosis in immunocompetent and immunodeficient persons: studies of an outbreak and experimental transmission. New England Journal of Medicine 308: 1252–1257

DeHovitz J A, Pape J W, Boncy M, Johnson W D 1986 Clinical manifestations and therapy of *Isospora belli* infection in patients with the acquired immunodeficiency syndrome. New England Journal of Medicine 315: 87–90

DeRiso A J, Kemeny M M, Torres R A, Oliver J M 1989 Multiple jejunal perforations secondary to cytomegalovirus in a patient with acquired immune deficiency syndrome. Case report and review. Digestive Diseases and Sciences 34: 623–629

Desportes I, Le Charpentier Y, Galian A et al 1985 Occurrence of a new microsporidian: *Enterocytozoon bieneusi* n.g., n.sp., in the enterocytes of a human patient with AIDS. Journal of Protozoology 32: 250–254

Dhar J M, Pidgeon N D, Burton A L 1984 AIDS in a patient with Crohn's disease. British Medical Journal 288: 1802–1803

Douglas J M, Crichlow C, Benedetti J 1984 A double-blind study of oral acyclovir for suppression of recurrences of genital herpes simplex virus infection. New England Journal of Medicine 310: 1551–1556

Elson C O, Reilly R W, Rosenberg I H 1977 Small intestinal injury in the graft versus host reaction: an innocent bystander phenomenon. Gastroenterology 72: 886–889

Ensoli M, Nakamura S, Salahuddin S Z et al 1989 AIDS – Kaposi's sarcoma-derived cells express cytokines with autocrine and paracrine growth effects. Science 243: 223–243

Eras P, Goldstein M J, Sherlock P 1972 Candida infection of the gastrointestinal tract. Medicine 51: 367–378

Faur Y C, Wilson M E, May P S 1981 Isolation of *Neisseria meningitidis* in patients in a gonorrhea screening program. A four year survey in New York city. American Journal of Public Health 71: 53–58

Fleming S C, Kapembwa M S, MacDonald T T, Griffin G E 1992 Direct *in vitro* infection of human intestine with HIV-1. AIDS 6: 1099–1104

Fox C H, Kotler D, Tierney A, Wilson C S, Fauci A S 1989 Detection of HIV-1 RNA in the lamina propria of patients with AIDS and gastrointestinal disease. Journal of Infectious Diseases 159: 467–471

Frank D, Raicht R F 1984 Intestinal perforation associated with cytomegalovirus infection in patients with AIDS. American Journal of Gastroenterology 79: 201–205

Friedman S L, Wright T L, Altman D F 1985 Gastrointestinal Kaposi's sarcoma in patients with acquired immunodeficiency syndrome: endoscopic and autopsy findings. Gastroenterology 89: 102–108

Gillin J S, Urmacher C, West R et al 1983 Disseminated *Mycobacterium avium intracellulare* infection in acquired immunodeficiency syndrome mimicking Whipple's disease. Gastroenterology 85: 1187–1191

Gillin J S, Shike M, Alcock N et al 1985 Malabsorption and mucosal abnormalities in the small intestine in the acquired immunodeficiency syndrome. Annals of Internal Medicine 102: 619–622

Goldmeier D 1985 Proctitis. In: Taylor-Robinson D (ed) Clinical problems in sexually transmitted diseases. New perspectives in clinical microbiology. Martinus Nijhoff, Dordrecht, pp 261–264

Goodman P, Pinero S S, Rance R M et al 1989 Mycobacterial esophagitis in AIDS. Gastrointestinal Radiology 14: 103–105

Goslee S, Wolinsky E 1976 Water as a source of potentially pathogenic mycobacteria. American Review of Respiratory Diseases 113: 287–292

Gottlieb G J, Ragaz A, Vogel J V et al 1981 A preliminary communication on extensively disseminated Kaposi's sarcoma in young homosexual men. American Journal of Dermatology 3: 111–114

Greenson J K, Belitsos P C, Yardley J H, Bartlett J G 1991 AIDS enteropathy: occult enteric infections and duodenal mucosal alterations in chronic diarrhoea. Annals of Internal Medicine 114: 366–372

Griffin G E, Miller A, Batman P et al 1988 Damage to jejunal intrinsic autonomic nerves in HIV infection. AIDS 2: 379–382

Hawkins C C, Gold J W, Whimbey E et al 1986 *Mycobacterium avium* complex infections in patients with acquired immunodeficiency syndrome. Annals of Internal Medicine 105: 184–188

Heise C, Dandekar S, Kumar P, Duplantier R, Donovan M R, Halsted H C 1991 Human immunodeficiency virus infection of enterocytes and mononuclear cells in human jejunal mucosa. Gastroenterology 100: 1521–1527

Hing M C, Goldschmidt C, Mathijs J M, Cunningham A L, Cooper D A 1992 Chronic colitis associated with human immunodeficiency virus infection. Medical Journal of Australia 156: 683–687

Hofstetter S R, Stollman N 1988 Adult intussusception in association with the acquired immune deficiency syndrome and intestinal Kaposi's sarcoma. American Journal of Gastroenterology 83: 1304–1305

Horsburgh C R, Mason U G, Farhi D C, Iseman M D 1985 Disseminated infection with *Mycobacterium avium-intracellulare*: a report of 13 cases and a review of the literature. Medicine 64: 36–48

Isselbacher K J, Adams R D, Braunwald E, Petersdorf R G, Wilson J D (eds) 1980 Harrison's principles of internal medicine, 9th edn. McGraw-Hill, New York, pp 849–851

Jacobson M A, O'Donnell J J, Porteous D et al 1988 Retinal and gastrointestinal disease due to cytomegalovirus in patients with the acquired immune deficiency syndrome: prevalence, natural history, and response to ganciclovir therapy. Quarterly Journal of Medicine 67: 473–486

James S P 1988 Remission of Crohn's disease after human immunodeficiency virus infection. Gastroenterology 95: 1667–1669

Jarry A, Cortez A, Rene' E, Muzeau F, Brousse N 1990 Infected cells and immune cells in the gastrointestinal tract of AIDS patients. An immunohistochemical study of 127 cases. Histopathology 16: 133–140

Judson F N, Ehret J M, Eickoff T C 1978 Anogenital infection with *Neisseria meningitidis* in homosexual men. Journal of Infectious Diseases 137: 458–463

Kalil M, Trajman A, Fonseca da Silva C et al 1991 Jejunal biopsy in HIV-infected patients. Journal of Acquired Immune Deficiency Syndromes 4: 930–937

Kapembwa M S, Batman P A, Fleming S C, Griffin G E 1989 HIV enteropathy. Lancet ii: 1521–1522

Kapembwa M S, Fleming S C, Sewankambo N et al 1991 Altered small intestinal permeability associated with diarrhoea in human immunodeficiency virus-infected Caucasian and African subjects. Clinical Science 81: 327–334

Kazal H L, Sohn N, Carrasco J I et al 1976 The gay bowel syndrome: clinico-pathologic correlations in 260 cases. Annals of Clinical and Laboratory Science 6: 184–192

Klein E I, Fisher L S, Chow A N et al 1977 Anorectal gonococcal infection. Annals of Internal Medicine 86: 340–346

Kotler P D, Gaetz P H, Lange M, Klein E B, Holt P R 1984 Enteropathy associated with the acquired immunodeficiency syndrome. Annals of Internal Medicine 101: 421–428

Kotler P D 1987 Diarrhoea in AIDS: diagnosis and management. Resident Staff Physician 33: 30–41

Kotler D P, Reka S, Clayton F 1993 Intestinal mucosal inflammation associated with human immunodeficiency virus infection. Digestive Diseases and Sciences 38: 1119–1127

La Brooy T J 1993 Enteropathy in HIV infection. Journal of Acquired Immune Deficiency Syndromes 6(Suppl 1): S16–S19

Lancet 1977. The Jarisch–Herxheimer reaction. Lancet i: 340–341

Laughon B E, Druckman D A, Vernon A et al 1988 Prevalence of enteric pathogens in homosexual men with and without acquired immunodeficiency syndrome. Gastroenterology 94: 984–993

Law L H C, Qassim M, Cunningham L A, Mulhall B, Grierson M J 1992 Non-specific proctitis: association with human immunodeficiency virus infection in homosexual men. Journal of Infectious Diseases 165: 150–154

Lebovics E, Thung S N, Schaffner F et al 1985 The liver in the acquired immunodeficiency syndrome: a clinical and histologic study. Hepatology 5: 293

Levine M S, Laufer I, Kressel H Y, Freidman H 1981 Herpes esophagitis. American Journal of Roentgenology 138: 863–866

Liebowitz D, McShane D 1986 Non-specific chronic inflammatory bowel disease in AIDS. Journal of Clinician Gastroenterology 8: 66–68

Loo P S, Ridgway G L, Oriel J D 1985 Single dose ciprofloxacin for treating gonococcal infections in men. Genitourinary Medicine 61: 302–305

Lucas S B, De Cock K M, Hounnou A et al 1994 Contribution of tuberculosis to Slim disease in Africa. British Medical Journal 308: 1531–1533

Lustbader I, Sherman A 1987 Primary gastrointestinal Kaposi's sarcoma in a patient with acquired immune deficiency syndrome. American Journal of Gastroenterology 82: 894–895

McKenna J G, Fallon R J, Moyes A, Young H 1993 Anogenital non-gonococcal neisseriae: prevalence and clinical significance. International Journal of Sexually Transmitted Diseases and AIDS 4: 8–12

McMillan A, Lee F D 1981 Sigmoidoscopic and microscopic appearance of the rectal mucosa in homosexual men. Gut 22: 1035–1041

Madara J L 1990 Pathobiology of the intestinal epithelial barrier. American Journal of Pathology 137: 1273–1281

Malebranche R, Guerin J M, Laroche C A et al 1983 Acquired immunodeficiency syndrome with severe gastrointestinal manifestations in Haiti. Lancet ii: 873–877

Meiselman M S, Cello J P, Margaretten W 1985 Cytomegalovirus colitis. Gastroenterology 88: 171–175

Meyers J D, Wade J C, Mitchell C D et al 1982 Multicenter collaborative trial of intravenous acyclovir for treatment of mucocutaneous herpes simplex virus infection in the immunocompromised host. American Journal of Medicine 73 (Suppl 1A): 229–235

Miller A R O, Griffin G E, Batman P et al 1988 Jejunal mucosal architecture and fat absorption in male homosexuals infected with human immunodeficiency virus. Quarterly Journal of Medicine 69: 1009–1019

Mindel A, Adler M W, Sutherland S, Fiddian A P 1982 Intravenous acyclovir treatment for primary genital herpes. Lancet i: 697–700

Modilevsky T, Sattler F R, Barnes P F 1989 Mycobacterial disease in patients with human immunodeficiency virus infection. Archives Internal Medicine 149: 2201–2205

Modlin R L, Hofman E M, Kempf R A et al 1983 Kaposi's sarcoma in homosexual men: an immunohistochemical study. Journal of the American Academy of Dermatology 8: 620

Moore P S, Chang Y 1995 Detection of Herpesvirus-like DNA sequences in Kaposi's sarcoma in patients with and those without HIV infection. New England Journal of Medicine 332: 1181–1191

Moyer P M, Huot I R, Ramirez A, Joe S, Meltzer S M, Gendelman E H 1990 Infection of human gastrointestinal cells by HIV-1. Aids Research and Human Retroviruses 6: 1409–1415

Nadji M, Morales A R, Ziegles-Weissman J, Penneys N S 1981 Kaposi's sarcoma: immunohistologic evidence for an endothelial origin. Archives of Pathology and Laboratory Medicine 105: 274–275

Nazemi M M, Musher D M, Schell R F, Milo S 1975 Syphilitic proctitis in a homosexual man. Journal of the American Medical Association 231: 389

Nelson A J, Reynolds-Kohler C, Margaretten W, Wiley A C, Reese E C, Levy A J 1988 Human immunodeficiency virus detected in bowel epithelium from patients with gastrointestinal symptoms. Lancet i: 259–262

Orenstein M J, Chiang J, Steinberg W, Smith D P, Rotterdam H, Kotler D P 1990 Intestinal microsporidiosis as a cause of diarrhoea in human immunodeficiency virus-infected patients: A report of 20 cases. Human Pathology 21: 475–481

Owen R L, Hill J L 1972 Rectal and pharyngeal gonorrhoea in homosexual men. Journal of the American Medical Association 220: 1315–1318

Peacock C S, Blanshard C, Tovey D G, Ellis D S, Gazzard B G 1991 Histological diagnosis of intestinal microsporidiosis in patients with AIDS. Journal of Clinical Pathology 44: 558–563

Potter D A, Danforth D N, Macher A M, Longo D L, Stweart L, Masur H 1984 Evaluation of abdominal pain in the AIDS patient. Annals of Surgery 199: 332–339

Quinn T C, Corey L, Chaffer R G et al 1981 The etiology of ano-rectal infections in homosexual men. American Journal of Medicine 71: 395–406

Quinn T C, Lukehart S A, Goodell S et al 1982 Rectal mass caused by *Treponema pallidum*: confirmation by immunofluorescent staining. Gastroenterology 82: 135–139

Rabeneck L, Bogko W J, McLean D M, McLeod W A, Wong K K 1986 Unusual oesophageal ulcers containing enveloped virus-like particles in homosexual men. Gastroenterology 90: 1882–1889

Rabeneck L, Gyorkey F, Genta R M, Gyorkey P, Foote L W, Risser J M H 1993 The role of *Microsporidia* in the pathogenesis of HIV related chronic diarrhoea. Annals of Internal Medicine 119: 895–899

Reka S, Kotler D P 1993 Detection and localisation of HIV RNA and TNF mRNA in rectal biopsies from patients with AIDS. Cytokine 5: 305–308

Rene E, Marche C, Chevalier T et al 1988 Cytomegalovirus colitis in patients with acquired immunodeficiency syndrome. Digestive Disease and Sciences 33: 741–750

Rolston K V, Rodriguez S, Hernandez M, Bodey G P 1989 Diarrhea in patients with the human immunodeficiency virus. American Journal of Medicine 86: 137–138

Roth R I, Owen R L, Keren D F 1985 Intestinal infection with *Mycobacterium avium* in acquired immunodeficiency syndrome (AIDS). Histological and clinical comparison with Whipple's disease. Digestive Diseases and Sciences 30: 497–504

Roth W K, Brandstetter H, Sturzl M 1992 Cellular and molecular features of HIV-associated Kaposi's sarcoma. AIDS 6: 895–913

Rutgers J L, Wieczorek R, Bonetti F et al 1986 The expression of endothelial cell surface antigens by AIDS-associated Kaposi's sarcoma: evidence for a vascular endothelial cell origin. American Journal of Pathology 122: 493–499

Schneebaum C W, Novick D M, Chabon A B, Strutynsky N, Yancovitz S R, Freund S 1987 Terminal ileitis asoscated with *Mycobacterium avium intracellulare* infection in a homosexual man with acquired immune deficiency syndrome. Gastroenterology 92: 1127–1132

Schneiderman D J, Cello J P, Laing F C 1987 Papillary stenosis and sclerosing cholangitis in the acquired immunodeficiency syndrome. Annals of Internal Medicine 106: 546–549

Schneiderman D J, Arenson D M, Cello J P et al 1987 Hepatic disease in patients with the acquired immune deficiency syndrome (AIDS). Hepatology 7: 925–930

Serwadda D, Sewankambo N K, Carswell J W et al 1985 Slim disease: a new disease in Uganda and its association with HTLV-III. Lancet ii: 849–852

Sewankambo N, Mugerwa R D, Goodgame R et al 1987 Enteropathic AIDS in Uganda. An endoscopic, histological and microbiological study. AIDS 1: 9–13

Siegal F P, Lopez C, Hammer G S et al 1981 Severe acquired immunodeficiency in male homosexuals manifested by chronic perianal ulcers of herpes simplex lesions. New England Journal of Medicine 305: 1439–1444

Sieratzki J, Thung S N, Gerber M A et al 1986 Aberrant HLA class II antigen expression on bile duct epithelium in patients with AIDS. Hepatology 6: 1155 A

Smee D F, Martin J C, Verheyden J P H et al 1983 Anti-herpes virus activity of the acyclic nucleoside 9-(1,3-dihydroxy-2-propoxymethyl) guanine. Antimicrobial Agents Chemotherapy 23: 676–682

Smith P D, Lane C H, Gill J V et al 1988 Intestinal infections in patients with the acquired immunodeficiency syndrome (AIDS): etiology and response to treatment. Annals of Internal Medicine 108: 328–333

Soave R, Johnson W D 1988 *Cryptosporidium* and *Isospora belli* infections. Journal of Infectious Diseases 157: 225–229

Steffen M, Reinecker H C, Petersen J et al 1993 Differences in cytokine secretion by intestinal mononuclear cells, peripheral blood monocytes and alveolar macrophages from HIV-infected patients. Clinical and Experimental Immunology 91: 30–36

Studies of Ocular Complications of AIDS Research Group, AIDS Clinical Trials Group 1992 Mortality in patients with the acquired immunodeficiency syndrome treated with either foscarnet or ganciclovir for cytomegalovirus retinitis. New England Journal of Medicine 326: 213–220

Takacs L, Szende B, Monostori E et al 1983 Expression of HLA-DR antigens on bile duct epithelial cells of rejected liver transplant. Lancet 1: 1500–1503

Tuazon C U, Labriola A M 1987 Management of infections and immunological complicatons of acquired immunodeficiency syndrome (AIDS). Current and future prospects. Drugs 33: 66–84

Ullrich R, Zeith M, Heise W, L'age M, Hoffken G, Reicken E O 1989 Small intestinal structure and function in patients infected with human immunodeficiency virus (HIV): evidence for HIV-induced enteropathy. Annals of Internal Medicine 111: 15–21

Van Gool T, Snijders F, Reiss P et al 1993 Diagnosis of intestinal and disseminated microsporidial infections in patients with HIV by a new rapid fluorescence technique. Journal of Clinical Pathology 6: 694–699

Wall W D, Friedman S L, Margulis A R 1984 Gastrointestinal Kaposi's sarcoma in AIDS: radiographic manifestations. Journal of Clinical Gastroenterology 6: 165–171

Weber J N, Carmichael D J, Boylston A, Munro A, Whitear W.P, Pinching A J 1985 Kaposi's sarcoma of the bowel presenting as apparent ulcerative colitis. Gut 26: 295–300

Weber R, Bryan R T, Owen R L et al 1992 Improved light microscopical detection of microsporidial spores and duodenal aspirates. New England Journal of Medicine 326: 161–166

Wilson S E, Robinson G, Williams R A et al 1989 Acquired immunodeficiency syndrome (AIDS): indicatons for abdominal surgery, pathology and outcome. Annals of Surgery 210: 428–434

Zurlo J J, O'Neill D, Polis A M et al 1993 Lack of clinical utility of cytomegalovirus blood and urine cultures in patients with HIV infection. Annals of Internal Medicine 118: 12–17

44. Amebic colitis

E. P. Variyam

Colitis caused by *Entamoeba histolytica* presents features that resemble ulcerative colitis, Crohn's colitis and colonic neoplasia. Specific therapy cures amebic colitis, therefore distinction of amebic colitis from idiopathic inflammatory bowel diseases is essential.

THE ORGANISM

A variety of amebae can colonize the human colon, but only *E. histolytica* is indisputably known to be pathogenic in humans (Walker & Sellards 1913). Based on biochemical, molecular and immunologic analysis of isolates and clinical manifestations in infected individuals, most researchers are 'dualists' who separate *E. histolytica* into two morphologically indistinguishable varieties (species), the more prevalent non-pathogenic variety (*E. dispar*), usually isolated from persons without invasive diseases, and the potentially pathogenic variety (true *E. histolytica*), which can cause invasive diseases such as colitis and liver abscess (Sargeaunt et al 1978, Gathiram & Jackson 1985, Blanc 1992, Diamond & Clark 1993, Petri et al 1994). However, others caution against separation into two species (Mirelman et al 1990) because of the presence in each variety of many markers of the other, albeit in smaller amounts, reports of convertibility of non-pathogenic to pathogenic (deemed to have resulted from laboratory contamination in the view of dualists), and the paucity of data on the status of the organisms in vivo. Dualists generally consider the two varieties to be mutually exclusive in a clinical infection. In a recent study mixed infection was detected in a majority by direct amplification from stool of DNA fragments of pathogenic and non-pathogenic varieties using polymerase chain reaction (PCR) (Acuna-Soto et al 1993). Careful longitudinal studies are needed to clarify the situation.

The life cycle of *E. histolytica* is simple (Dobell 1928). The vegetative forms – trophozoites – multiply in the colon lumen, most probably in the right colon. Under conditions not fully known (probably dependent on the transit time of luminal contents, fluid absorption and modification by various microbial and host hydrolases) the trophozoites develop into cysts that have a chitinous cell wall. Mature cysts have four nuclei. Cysts can survive for weeks to months in favorable environmental conditions of temperature and humidity (Walsh 1988). Infection is acquired by the ingestion of cysts from fecal contamination. The cyst wall is resistant to the action of gastric juice. The organism excysts in the distal ileum or colon and develops into trophozoites.

Worldwide, *E. histolytica* infection (including *E. dispar*) is estimated to exist in 10% of the population (Walsh 1988). High infection rates occur with crowding and inadequate sanitation, water supplies or hygiene. In developed nations infection rates are higher in immigrants from developing areas, the institutionalized (mentally retarded, demented elderly), frequent travellers to endemic areas and in male homosexuals (Walsh 1988).

PATHOGENESIS, PATHOLOGY

Even when infected with pathogenic *E. histolytica* most individuals are asymptomatic, with the trophozoites surviving in the colon lumen as a commensal (Gathiram & Jackson 1987, Variyam et al 1989). Factors that promote commensalism are not well known, but the colonic mucus gel layer (Chadee et al 1987) and microbial and host hydrolases (Variyam & Shah 1991) may be potential barriers to invasion. A variety of gastrointestinal symptoms have been ascribed to the presence of luminal amebic infection and termed 'chronic amebiasis' or 'non-dysenteric intestinal amebiasis'; careful analysis indicates that there is inadequate evidence to blame the ameba for causation of such symptoms, most of which are not distinguishable from those in irritable bowel syndrome (Variyam et al 1989). Approximately 10% of infected individuals develop invasive diseases, predominantly colitis (Gathiram & Jackson 1987) and to a lesser extent liver abscess. Little is known about the factors that transform the commensal ameba to one producing invasive diseases. The interval from acquiring infection to clinical presentation is highly variable, ranging from days to years (Walsh 1988). There is no information on the interval from the time of initial invasion to the development of symptoms. Colitis is the most frequent manifestation of invasive amebiasis. Liver abscess formation is believed to be caused by spread from the colon by way of the portal vein. Spread to the lungs, pleura, pericardial space, skin, urogenital tract and brain occurs infrequently.

Recent studies in animals and in vitro systems have contributed substantially to our understanding of the potential mechanisms of *E. histolytica*-induced tissue injury (Ravdin 1989). Adherence to the target cell is a required initial step (Ravdin & Guerrant 1981). Of the several adherence proteins identified, the one that is inhibitable by galactose or *N*-acetyl galactosamine ('ameba lectin') seems to play a key role (Horstman et al 1992, McCoy et al 1994). Mediators of target cell injury include amebapore (Lieppe & Muller-Eberhard 1994), a protein that is similar in its action to the pore-forming protein of cytotoxic lymphocytes, cysteine proteases, phospholipases and mediators that increase target cell intracellular calcium (Ravdin 1989). Amebic interactions with host immune cells may lead to additional tissue damage.

Any part of the colon may be affected in amebic colitis (Castro 1973). Diffuse involvement of the entire colon is seen in a third of cases, and segmental colitis is noted in the rest. The cecum and ascending colon are most frequently affected, followed by the sigmoid colon and rectum.

Classic descriptions of the pathology of amebic colitis are of ulcers that are flask-shaped and extend to the submucosal layer (Councilman & LaFleur 1891). However, ulcers may represent a late stage of colonic invasion (Prathap & Gilman 1970). The earliest abnormality in amebic colitis may be non-specific mucosal changes with glandular hyperplasia, neutrophil transmigration, stromal edema and hyperemia. Crypt abscesses are not seen and there is little exudate at the mucosal surface. The earliest specific lesion is a microscopic area of depression and ulceration in the interglandular epithelium, with loss of mucin from the surface epithelial cells, usually within an area of non-specific changes. Exuberant exudate is seen over the ulcer and amebae may be observed in the exudate. Later, more epithelial cell destruction is noted, with minimal inflammatory cell infiltration. Amebae are noted in the tissue with greater constancy at this stage. The late-stage lesion is the typical flask-shaped ulcer, with undermined mucosal edges and extending down to the level of the submucosa. Inflammatory cells are infrequent at this stage. A thick, layered exudate, consisting of acellular proteinaceous material, red cells and strands of fibrin, is present in the floor of the ulcer. A deeply eosinophilic zone of fibrinoid necrosis separates the exudate from the viable tissue. Amebae are seen at the edges of the necrosis and in the surface exudate. The mucosa between the ulcers may be normal or show changes of early invasion. In some chronic lesions a mass of granulation tissue – an ameboma – may form.

CLINICAL FEATURES OF AMEBIC COLITIS

There is considerable variation in the severity and mode of presentation of amebic colitis (Lewis & Antia 1969, Adams & MacLeod 1977). The onset is usually gradual, with most patients reporting symptoms for 1 month or less. Occasionally symptoms may last years, with intermittent bloody diarrhea. The daily bowel frequency is highly variable, from minimal increase to as many as >20, and dehydration may occur. Localized or diffuse abdominal pain is often present and tenesmus is frequent. Fever is inconstant. Severe colitis occurs in ~5% and toxic megacolon may be seen in ~0.5%. Peritonitis may complicate in ~3%. Amebomas may be seen in ~0.5%. Rarely, rectal bleeding without diarrhea may be the clinical presentation. Glucocorticoid therapy worsens clinical manifestations of amebic colitis (Eisert et al 1959). Whether ulcerative postdysenteric colitis really exists must await further study.

Endoscopic findings of early amebic colitis are diffuse mucosal edema, loss of vascular pattern and increased friability, and are not easily distinguishable from those of ulcerative colitis (Gilman & Prathap 1971, Pittman et al 1973). Typical late-stage lesions – ulcers separated by near-normal appearing mucosa in between – may be more readily distinguished. Asymmetrical involvement, with amebic granuloma formation and the existence of skip areas, may simulate the findings of Crohn's disease.

The radiological findings of amebic colitis are also variable (Cardoso et al 1977). Diffuse edema and superficial ulcerations may be noted in early lesions. The typical lesion of the late stages of the disease is the narrow-necked ulcer. Localized thickening of the bowel wall due to ameboma may be confused with Crohn's disease or carcinoma. Narrowing and shortening of the proximal colon in chronic amebic colitis may produce a characteristic conical cecum. Terminal ileum involvement is seen rarely as an extension of cecal disease.

DIAGNOSIS, DIFFERENTIATION FROM INFLAMMATORY BOWEL DISEASE

Amebic colitis must be considered in every patient being evaluated for inflammatory bowel disease (Pittman et al 1973, Tucker et al 1975, Giachinno et al 1978, Patel & DeRidder 1989, Larsson et al 1991). The degree of suspicion and the zeal of search must be based on the epidemiologic and clinical setting. Rare cases of coexistence of inflammatory bowel disease and *E. histolytica* infection have been described.

Careful microscopic examination of freshly passed stool remains the most available method for detecting amebic colitis. Stool examination must precede barium studies or the use of agents reported to interfere with microscopic detection (Bruckner 1992). The physician caring for the patient must be knowledgeable of laboratory testing protocol and its limitations. Preserved specimens are essential if a sample is not examined fresh (within 30 minutes of passage at room temperature, or 2 hours if refrigerated). The laboratory must be specifically alerted to the possibility of E. histolytica infection to perform appropriate additional steps.

The characteristic finding on examination of fresh stool in amebic colitis is the presence of motile trophozoites with directional movement and containing phagocytosed red cells (Gonzales-Ruiz et al 1994a). Methylene blue staining stops trophozoite motility, but allows recognition of nuclear morphology to enable distinction of amebae from host immune cells. Cysts can be identified by iodine stain. Their detection can be enhanced by concentration methods. Several monoclonal antibody-based systems (Stanley et al 1991, Gonzalez-Ruiz et al 1994b, Haque et al 1993, 1994) appear promising for the detection of fecal antigens or microscopy of the organisms, but are not yet widely available.

A variety of serological tests are available for the diagnosis of invasive amebiasis (Healy 1988). An indirect hemagglutination – (IHA) test and an enzyme immunoassay to detect antibodies to whole-cell amebic antigen are two of the most frequently used, but these tests are only 70–80% sensitive in amebic colitis. Furthermore, positive serology persists long after cure of the invasive disease. There is controversy regarding routine serological evaluation of all patients suspected to have idiopathic inflammatory bowel disease in areas where there is low prevalence of amebiasis. In one study of a cohort of inflammatory bowel disease patients routine testing of clinic patients using IHA did not reveal any new clinical cases of amebic colitis (Healy & Kraft 1972). However, it is likely that the study patients were probably carefully screened initially by stool microscopy. Although antibodies to several defined antigens can be detected in the serum (Stanley et al 1991) their clinical use is still limited.

Mucosal biopsy helps detect E. histolytica trophozoites (Prathap & Gilman 1970). Detection rates can be improved by biopsy of the edges of ulcers and by including the overlying exudate. Special stains (periodic acid–Schiff, iron hematoxylin) help identify the organisms with a greater degree of certainty.

TREATMENT

All patients with invasive amebiasis require treatment with tissue amebicides (Knight 1980). One of the nitroimidazoles (metronidazole, tinidazole, secnidazole) is the drug of choice for treatment of amebic colitis. The usual adult dose of metronidazole is 750 mg three times daily for 10 days. The drug may be administered parenterally if necessary. Alternative agents that require parenteral administration are emetine and dehydroemetine, which have cardiac toxicity. The above tissue amebicidal agents eliminate luminal infection in two-thirds of patients only. Agents that have ~90% efficacy in curing luminal infection (and their usual adult dosages) are diloxanide furoate (500 mg t.i.d. × 10 days), di-iodohydroxyquinoline (650 mg t.i.d. × 20 days) and paromomycin (500 mg t.i.d. × 7 days). One of these luminal agents is recommended as additional therapy in a patient with invasive amebiasis (McAuley et al 1992). Antiamebic therapy of all patients diagnosed to have inflammatory bowel disease is not recommended in developed countries.

REFERENCES

Acuna-Soto R, Samuelson J, DeGirolami et al 1993 Application of the polymerase chain reaction to the epidemiology of pathogenic and nonpathogenic Entamoeba histolytica. American Journal of Tropical Medicine and Hygiene 48: 58–70

Adams E B, MacLeod I N 1977 Invasive amebiasis. I. Amebic dysentery and its complications. Medicine 56: 315–323

Blanc D S 1992 Determination of taxonomic status of pathogenic and nonpathogenic Entamoeba histolytica zymodemes using isoenzyme analysis. Journal of Protozoology 39: 471–479

Bruckner D A 1992 Amebiasis. Clinical Microbiology Reviews 5: 356–369

Cardoso J M, Kimura K, Stoopen M et al 1977 Radiology of invasive amebiasis of the colon. American Journal of Roentgenology 128: 935–941

Castro H F 1973 Anatomic and pathological findings in amebiasis. Report of 320 cases. Amebiasis in man: epidemiology, therapeutics, clinical correlations and prophylaxis. Charles C Thomas, Springfield, IL, pp 44–68

Chadee K, Petri W A Jr, Ines D J, Ravdin J I 1987 Rat and human colonic mucins bind to and inhibit adherence lectin of Entamoeba histolytica. Journal of Clinical Investigation 80: 1245–1254

Councilman W T, LaFleur H A 1891 Amoebic dysentery. Johns Hopkins Hospital Reports 2: 395–548

Diamond L S, Clark G C 1993 A redescription of Entamoeba histolytica Schaudinn, 1903 (Emended Walker, 1911) separating it from Entamoeba dispar, Brumpt, 1925. Journal of Eukaryotic Microbiology 40: 340–344

Dobell C 1928 Researches on the intestinal protozoa of monkeys and man. Parasitology 20: 357–412

Eisert J, Hannibal J E Jr, Sanders S E 1959 Fatal amebiasis complicating corticosteroid management of pemphigus vulgaris. New England Journal of Medicine 261: 843–845

Gathiram V, Jackson T F H G 1985 Frequency distribution of Entamoeba histolytica zymodemes in a rural South African population. Lancet i: 719–721

Gathiram V, Jackson T F H G 1987 A longitudinal study of asymptomatic carriers of pathogenic zymodemes of Entamoeba histolytica. South African Medical Journal 72: 669–672

Giachinno J L, Pickleman, J, Bartizal J F, Banich F E 1978 The therapeutic dilemma of acute amebic and ulcerative colitis. Surgery, Gynaecology and Obstetrics 146: 599–603

Gilman R H, Prathap K 1971 Acute intestinal amoebiasis – proctoscopic appearances with histopathologic correlation. Annals of Tropical Medicine and Parasitology 65: 359–365

Gonzalez-Ruiz A, Haque R, Aguirre A et al 1994a Value of microscopy in the diagnosis of dysentery associated with Entamoeba histolytica.

Journal of Clinical Pathology 47: 236–239

Gonzalez-Ruiz A, Haque R, Rehman T et al 1994b Diagnosis of amebic dysentery by detection of *Entamoeba histolytica* fecal antigen by an invasive strain-specific, monoclonal antibody-based enzyme-linked immunosorbent assay. Journal of Clinical Microbiology 32: 964–970

Haque R, Kress K, Wood S et al 1993 Diagnosis of pathogenic *Entamoeba histolytica* infection using a stool ELISA based on monoclonal antibodies to the galactose-specific adhesin. Journal of Infectious Diseases 167: 247–249

Haque R, Neville L, Wood S, Petri W A Jr 1994 Detection of *Entamoeba histolytica* and *E. dispar* directly in stool. American Journal of Tropical Medicine and Hygiene 50: 595–596

Healy G R 1988 Serology. In: Ravdin J I (ed) Amebiasis. Human infection by *Entamoeba histolytica*. John Wiley, New York, pp 650–663

Healy G R, Kraft S C 1972 The indirect hemagglutination test for amoebiasis in patients with inflammatory bowel disease. American Journal of Digestive Diseases 17: 97–104

Horstmann R D, Leippe M, Tannich E 1992 Recent progress in the molecular biology of *Entamoeba histolytica*. Tropical Medicine and Parasitology 43: 213–218

Knight R 1980 The chemotherapy of amoebiasis. Journal of Antimicrobial Chemotherapy 6: 577–593

Larsson P, Olling S, Darle 1991 Amoebic colitis presenting as acute inflammatory bowel disease. European Journal of Surgery 157: 553–555

Lewis E A, Antia A U 1969 Amoebic colitis: review of 295 cases. Transactions of the Royal Society of Tropical Medicine and Hygiene 63: 633–638

Lieppe M, Muller-Eberhard H J 1994 The pore-forming peptide of *Entamoeba histolytica*, the protozoan parasite causing human amoebiasis. Toxicology 87: 5–18

McAuley J B, Herwaldt B L, Stokes S L et al 1992 Diloxanide furoate for treating asymptomatic *Entamoeba histolytica* cyst passers: 14 years' experience in the United States. Clinical Infectious Diseases 15: 464–468

McCoy J J, Mann B J, Petri W A Jr 1994 Adherence and cytotoxicity of *Entamoeba histolytica* or how lectins let parasites stick around. Infection and Immunity 62: 3045–3050

Mirelman D, Bracha R, Rozenblatt S, Garfinkel L I 1990 Repetitive DNA elements characteristic of pathogenic *Entamoeba histolytica* strains can also be detected after polymerase chain reaction in a cloned nonpathogenic strain. Infection and Immunity 58: 1660–1663

Patel A S, DeRidder 1989 Amebic colitis masquerading as acute inflammatory bowel disease: the role of serology in its diagnosis. Journal of Clinical Gastroenterology 11: 407–410

Petri W A Jr, Clark G C, Diamond L S 1994 Host–parasite relationships in amebiasis: conference report. Journal of Infectious Diseases 169: 483–484

Pittman F E, El-Hashimi, Pittman J C 1973 Studies of human amoebiasis. I. Clinical and laboratory findings in eight cases of acute amoebic colitis. Gastroenterology 65: 581–587

Prathap K, Gilman R 1970 The histopathology of acute intestinal amoebiasis. A rectal biopsy study. American Journal of Pathology 60: 229–245

Ravdin J I 1989 *Entamoeba histolytica*: from adherence to enteropathy. Journal of Infectious Diseases 159: 420–429

Ravdin J I, Guerrant R L 1981 Role of adherence in cytopathogenic mechanism of *Entamoeba histolytica*. Journal of Clinical Investigation 68: 1305–1313

Sanderson I R, Walker-Smith J A 1984 Indigenous amoebiasis: an important differential diagnosis of chronic inflammatory bowel disease. British Medical Journal iii: 823–824

Sargeaunt P G, Williams J E, Greene J D 1978 The differentiation of invasive and non-invasive. *Entamoeba histolytica* by isoenzyme electrophoresis. Transactions of the Royal Society of Tropical Medicine and Hygiene 72: 519–522

Stanley S L Jr, Jackson T F H G, Reed S et al 1991 Serodiagnosis of invasive amebiasis using a recombinant *Entamoeba histolytica* protein. Journal of the American Medical Association 266: 1984–1986

Tucker P C, Webster P D, Kilpatric Z M 1975 Amebic colitis mistaken for inflammatory bowel disease. Archives of Internal Medicine 135: 681–685

Variyam E P, Gogate P, Hassan M et al 1989 Nondysenteric intestinal amebiasis. Colonic morphology and search for *Entamoeba histolytica* adherence and invasion. Digestive Diseases and Sciences 34: 732–740

Variyam E P, Shah P S 1991 A novel host defense mechanism against enteric pathogens. Gastroenterology 100: A622

Walker E L, Sellards A W 1913 Experimental entamoebic dysentery. Philippine Journal of Science (Section B) 8: 253–330

Walsh J A 1988 Transmission of *Entamoeba histolytica* infection. In: Ravdin J I (ed) Amebiasis. Human infection by *Entamoeba histolytica*. John Wiley, Chichester, pp 106–119

45. Yersinia-related enteric disease
H. J. Freeman

Yersinia enterocolitica is a human pathogen that has been associated with a broad clinical and pathological spectrum of gastrointestinal diseases, from a self-limited gastroenteritis to a more invasive ileitis and/or colitis. Concomitant bacteremia or systemic extraintestinal features may be present. This organism is a non-lactose-fermenting, urease-positive, Gram-negative rod. A number of serotypes and biotypes of *Yersinia enterocolitica* have been described, as well as a number of newly recognized atypical or variant *Yersinia enterocolitica* species. For some *Yersinia* strains a variety of pathogenic mechanisms and virulence-defining factors have been detected, including the gene-directed ability to penetrate and invade intestinal epithelial cells and/or produce enterotoxin. This chapter will review the microbiological aspects of yersinia infection, including its characterization, isolation and serology. In addition, studies on pathogenesis and the role of specific virulence and host factors will be explored. Finally, clinical and pathological features of yersinia infection will be examined, including intestinal and extraintestinal changes as well as treatment.

HISTORICAL ASPECTS

In 1944 a new genus, *Yersinia*, was proposed to include the Gram-negative, anaerobic coccobacilli (van Loghem 1944); this followed its initial clinical isolation (Schleifstein & Coleman 1939). In 1964 *Yersiniae* were classified into three separate species: *Yersinia pestis*, *Yersinia pseudotuberculosis* and *Yersinia enterocolitica*. Subsequently, *Yersinia enterocolitica* was associated with clinical illness, first in a patient with acute terminal ileitis after its recovery from mesenteric lymph nodes (Carlsson et al 1964), and later with an appendicitis-like clinical illness and acute diarrheal disease; both culture-positive and seropositive *Yersinia enterocolitica* infections were defined (Winblad et al 1966). By 1966 a total of 23 cases had been reported (Wormser & Keusch 1981).

In 1967 the first North American isolate was described from a patient with gastroenteritis, but most cases continued to be detected in northern Europe (Toma & Lafleur 1981). Since then, the organism has been reported extensively on a global scale and the rate of detection has dramatically increased, especially in North America, often with small food-related epidemics (Martin et al 1982). Most patients present with acute abdominal pain and diarrhea. Others, however, may have chronic symptoms with extraintestinal features (i.e. polyarthritis), and occasionally invasive disease with bacteremia occurs.

MICROBIOLOGY

Organism characterization

The *Yersinia* genus is now known to include at least eight species, including three human pathogens, *Yersinia pestis*, *Yersinia pseudotuberculosis* and *Yersinia enterocolitica*, as well as three 'new' atypical species, *Yersinia frederiksenii*, *Yersinia intermedia* and *Yersinia kristensenii*. Two other species are solely aquatic isolates, *Yersinia ruckeri* and *Yersinia aldovae*. The 'new' atypical strains are variants of *Yersinia enterocolitica* and have been labeled *Yersinia enterocolitica*-like, based on biochemical reactions and DNA hybridization homology (Bercovier et al 1980, Brenner et al 1980, Ursing et al 1980).

Yersinia enterocolitica does not refer to a single species. Variants can be defined on the basis of seven biotypes, 33 'O' antigen (lipopolysaccharide) types and 19 'H' antigen (flagellar) types (Wauters 1981). Although this biotyping and serotyping system is valuable for epidemiologic studies of small outbreaks, a strong geographical distribution exists (i.e. 0:3 common in eastern Canada, 0:7.8 and 0:6.30 common in western Canada, 0:8 common in the United States, and 0:9 common in Europe) that may interfere with source identification. Other differentiating systems to define strains have been used, e.g. susceptibility to specific antibiotics and phage typing.

Selective isolation

There is a distinct possibility that increased detection rates are due to improved isolation methods. On conventional enteric media (i.e. SS, EMB, or MacConkey Agar), *Yersinia* growth may be suppressed or pinpoint in nature, allowing overgrowth by other enteric organisms (Feeley 1981). A medium (CIN medium) containing *c*efsulidin, *ir*gasan, and *n*ovobiocin was developed (Schiemann 1979) that appeared to be selective for *Yersinia*. On CIN medium *Yersinia* colonies are red, owing to mannitol fermentation, with a bullseye morphology (Simmonds et al 1987). It has also become appreciated that *Yersinia* will grow at temperatures lower than competing flora; as a result, cold enrichment at 4°C for 1–2 weeks has increased isolation (Pai et al 1979). However, a possible bias in the *Yersinia* isolated may result from cold enrichment, as some serotypes are more readily detected. Others have observed that *Yersinia enterocolitica* 0:3 was recovered more frequently from asymptomatic or convalescent patients with cold enrichment, but not in acutely ill patients with the same organism strains (Marks et al 1980).

Serologic detection

Serologic evaluation may be useful. A rise in serum titers of *Yersinia*-specific antibody occurs early in infection, mainly in IgA immunoglobulins. Commonly performed serological tests include a microagglutination assay and an ELISA method. Using the microagglutination assay, a titer of 1:128 in a previously healthy individual is considered suggestive of recent infection.

PATHOGENESIS

Mechanisms involved in the pathogenesis of *Yersinia*-related enteric disease have been extensively investigated. Currently, virulence may be defined with in vivo methods, such as animal models and cell culture methods, or with in vitro techniques (Noble et al 1989).

IN VIVO VIRULENCE CHARACTERISTICS

Animal models

Bacterial invasiveness has been assessed with an animal model where a loopful of bacterial suspension is inoculated under the eyelid of an adult guinea pig and invasion defined by the development of keratoconjunctivitis (Sereny 1955, Zink et al 1980). This method was originally used to identify virulent *Yersinia enterocolitica* strains, but some pathogenic strains failed to evoke a conjunctivitis response (Bakour et al 1985). The most commonly used animal for virulence testing is the mouse. Infected via numerous routes, i.e. cutaneous, intravenous, intragastric injection or peroral challenge, symptoms closely mimic those of humans and, after intravenous or intragastric inoculation, intestinal lesions develop that are histologically similar to those in humans (Carter 1975). After peroral challenge in mice, pathogenic effects may be defined on the basis of prolonged fecal excretion of viable organisms, diarrhea induction, and deep organ penetration after 48 hours (Bakour et al 1985). The latter permits semi-quantitative analysis, virulence grading (i.e. <10 organisms per spleen is considered avirulent, whereas 50–100 organisms per spleen is considered virulent), and correlates well with diarrhea in the mouse model.

Cell culture

Human cell culture lines have also been used to examine the virulence of various *Yersinia* strains. *Yersinia enterocolitica* attach and invade, but do not multiply inside HeLa cells, HEP-2 and Henle 407 epithelial cells (Devenish & Schiemann 1981). The ability to invade cells has been associated with a virulence plasmid (Vesikari et al 1981), whereas both invasion and attachment appear to be temperature dependent.

IN VITRO VIRULENCE CHARACTERISTICS

In vitro virulence-related phenomena have been recognized and assay methods developed to allow rapid screening for organisms present in food or water that induce clinical illness in animal models. No single in-vitro test of virulence, however, can reliably predict the onset or presence of symptoms in humans (Noble et al 1987).

Calcium dependence

This phenomenon was initially associated with virulent *Yersinia pestis* strains that required calcium for growth. Subsequently, a differential plating medium, magnesium oxalate agar (MOX) was developed that was deficient in calcium. With calcium starvation, virulent strains had reduced nucleotide triphosphate and adenylate energy metabolism; as a result cell division ceased and pinpoint colonies formed (Brubaker 1986). Later, calcium dependence was detected on a virulence-inducing plasmid in *Yersinia* species (Gemski et al 1980), and later mapped to a highly conversed 9 kb region in virulence plasmids (Portnoy & Falkow 1981).

Autoagglutination

Autoagglutination has been seen with mouse virulent strains of *Yersinia enterocolitica* at 37°C, but not at 25°C (Laird & Cavanaugh 1980) and associated with two outer membrane proteins, V and W (Carter 1981). Bacteria agglutinating at both temperatures are considered false positives. This virulence characteristic has been associated with temperature-dependent expression of plasmid-mediated proteins and reliably predicts virulence in the mouse.

Congo Red absorption

Congo Red absorption mimics ferric ion absorption. *Yersinia enterocolitica* do not produce exogenous siderophores, although a series of iron-regulated proteins are expressed under iron starvation conditions: the organisms depend on the uptake of siderophores or free ferric iron released into the environment. The absorption of the hemin-type dye Congo Red was associated with some virulent strains of *Yersinia enterocolitica* (Prpic et al 1983). A differential medium containing Congo Red may distinguish organisms that actively absorb dye and form red colonies from those that exclude dye and form white colonies. Dye uptake is associated with expression of an outer membrane protein and is not plasmid mediated.

Serum resistance

This characteristic was observed with mouse virulent strains of *Yersinia enterocolitica* that resisted the bactericidal activity of 10% normal human serum (Pai & DeStephano 1982). Because it was a stable characteristic, it could be examined in organisms stored for prolonged periods and was associated with plasmid carriage.

Plasmid carriage

Plasmid carriage was initially reported with a *Yersinia enterocolitica* 0:8 outbreak of enteric illness associated with chocolate milk ingestion (Zink et al 1980). The plasmid, 40–42 MDa, was associated with tissue invasiveness, animal virulence and calcium dependence (Gemski et al 1980, Portnoy et al 1981). In addition, plasmid carriage was associated with inhibition of normal phagocytosis, a chemiluminescence response of normal human neutrophils and human epithelial cell cytotoxicity (Gemski et al 1980, Portnoy et al 1981, Lian et al 1985).

Outer membrane proteins

Outer membrane proteins may be a mechanism of expression for plasmid-associated phenomena (Martinez 1983). There are seven temperature-inducible outer membrane proteins expressed, at least in part, on the cell surface (Bolin et al 1982). Some membrane proteins may have a role in serum resistance, autoagglutination and resistance to phagocytosis.

CHROMOSOMAL PROPERTIES

In addition to plasmid-mediated virulence factors, a number of chromosomally controlled properties may be important.

Surface characteristics

Lipopolysaccharide expression is important in enteric infections, but is not plasmid mediated in *Yersinia* species. Expression is temperature regulated, with organisms being 'smooth' at 25°C and 'rough' at 37°C. Rough morphology may unmask surface proteins, allowing increased intercellular interactions or resistance to some adverse environmental conditions. Fimbriae expression is also temperature but not plasmid controlled, with adherence via fimbriae greatest at 25°C. Iron-regulated proteins are also chromosomally encoded, and appear to be regulated by the environmental iron content.

Enterotoxin

Enterotoxin activity, as reflected in the suckling mouse assay, has been observed with *Yersinia enterocolitica* (Pai & Mors 1978) and atypical *Yersinia* species (Scholey & Freeman 1983). The toxin is chromosomally mediated but the significance is not clear since the toxin is produced at 25°C but not 37°C, for *Yersinia enterocolitica* (Pai & Mors 1978); interestingly, however, toxin activity is detectable for atypical *Yersinia* species at 37°C (Scholey & Freeman 1983).

HOST-RELATED FACTORS

Genetic determinants

Differences in resistance to yersinia infection are evident in different genetic mouse strains. This is specific for yersinia as genetic determinants conferring resistance to infection were unrelated to determinants conferring resistance to other enteric pathogens, i.e. *Salmonella* species (Hancock et al 1986).

Immunoprotection

Immunoprotection appears to play a role in resistance to yersinia infection. Intraperitoneal infection with plasmid-containing strains resulted in protection from infection on a subsequent intraperitoneal challenge with a plasmid-containing strain; however, infection with plasmid-free strains did not provide protection (Aulisio et al 1983).

Iron stores

Increased host iron stores have been associated with a greater risk of infection with *Yersinia enterocolitica*. Patients with iron overload (i.e. hemochromatosis), with or without desferrioxamine treatment, appear to be at increased risk for the development of bacteremia with enteric infection (Capron et al 1984, Robins-Browne & Prpic 1985). Iron overload and desferrioxamine appear to replace hydroxymate siderophores, which are absent in *Yersinia enterocolitica* strains (Noble & Freeman 1986).

CLINICAL AND PATHOLOGICAL FEATURES

Enteric disease

Yersinia enterocolitica infection predominantly leads to an enteric illness, commonly presenting in children as well as adults with acute-onset diarrhea, often with abdominal pain, nausea and vomiting, as well as fever (Black et al 1978, Leino & Kalliomaki 1974, Gutman et al 1973, Marks et al 1980, Tacket et al 1985). In some reports there is an apparent seasonal incidence, with a peak in late autumn and early winter, possibly related to the organism's ability to grow with enhanced virulence at cooler temperatures (Wormser & Keusch 1981). The acute enteric syndrome may last 1–2 weeks, often with watery, sometimes bloody, diarrhea. In most patients no endoscopic or histologic changes in the colonic mucosa are evident. In others a range of changes, including moderate to severe abnormalities, may be present. These may be focal or patchy, with so-called 'aphthoid' ulcers or deep linear, serpiginous and 'rake-like' ulcers; alternatively, diffuse mucosal inflammatory changes without significant ulceration may be evident. In some these focal or diffuse inflammatory changes may be indistinguishable from the features of Crohn's colitis or ulcerative colitis, respectively. Alternatively, yersinia infection may be 'superimposed' on pre-existing inflammatory bowel disease and may be responsible for a symptomatic exacerbation. Histological changes are usually not specific for an infectious colitis; features of both an acute and chronic process may be seen. Mucosal lymphoid aggregates or lymphoid nodules with focal and central necrosis may be seen (Bradford et al 1974). In occasional patients mucosal biopsies may also demonstrate granulomas with multinucleated giant cells. Less commonly, typical endoscopic and histologic features of pseudomembranous colitis are present (Simmonds et al 1987). In some a concomitant or copathogen may be detected; in patients with colitis recently treated with antibiotics, *Clostridium difficile* may be detected (Fishman et al 1989).

In the upper gastrointestinal tract inflammatory changes may be evident in the stomach and duodenum; in some patients single or multiple erosions and/or frank gastric and/or duodenal ulceration may be seen (Simmonds et al 1987). Barium imaging of the small intestine and/or endoscopic visualization of the ileal mucosa has also demonstrated ileal changes consistent with an ileitis (van Trappen et al 1980, Simmonds et al 1987). Persistent inflammatory changes in the distal ileum with ulceration resembling Crohn's disease of the ileum have been reported following treatment of yersinia infections (van Trappen et al 1980). In contrast to Crohn's disease, however, there were no skip lesions, fibrotic stenosis or fistulae. Earlier studies have suggested that patients with acute ileitis and either serologic or microbiologic evidence of *Yersinia enterocolitica* infection do not subsequently develop Crohn's disease; conversely, patients with Crohn's disease apparently do not have serologic or microbiologic evidence for previous yersinia infection (Persson et al 1976). Chronic gastrointestinal symptoms have also been recorded in some adults (Simmonds et al 1987). Abdominal pain, either intermittent or recurrent, nausea and/or vomiting, as well as chronic diarrhea, may occur. A multiplicity of different *Yersinia enterocolitica* serotypes may be present (Simmonds et al 1987).

Often, patients with *Yersinia enterocolitica* will present with an acute appendicitis-like syndrome (Gutman et al 1973, Marks et al 1980). Pathological findings at the time of surgery usually confirm the presence of appendiceal inflammation, although a normal appendix along with mesenteric lymphadenitis may be found (Leino & Kalliomaki 1974, Black et al 1978). In some patients with mesenteric adenitis an associated ileitis or colitis is present, often with nausea, vomiting and oral aphthous ulcers.

Invasive disease and bacteremia

Bacteremia is a rare occurrence, most frequently reported in patients with significant underlying diseases, including diabetes mellitus, renal failure, malignant disease and, in particular, cirrhosis with iron overload (Robins-Browne et al 1979, Noble & Freeman 1986). The high mortality (approximately 40%), reflects the severity of the underlying disease.

Bacteremia without diarrhea may occur with both hepatic and/or splenic abscesses (Reinicke & Korner 1977, Rabson et al 1975). Metastatic foci can occur in meninges (Sonnenwirth 1970), synovium (Spira & Kabins 1976, Taylor et al 1977), skin (Sonnenwirth 1970, Abramovitch & Butas 1973), lung (Sebes et al 1976, Taylor et al 1977), bone (Thirumoorthi & Dajani 1978), eye (Sonnenwirth, 1970, Chin & Noble 1977) and kidney (Sonnenwirth 1970).

Extraintestinal features

In addition to bacteremia and metastatic foci, other extraintestinal features have been observed. Very rarely, possibly 2–3 weeks after an episode of acute diarrhea, a reactive arthritis and a skin rash, occasionally resembling erythema nodosum or erythema multiforme, may develop reminiscent of a Reiter's-like syndrome. Carditis may occur (Agner et al 1978). Reactive synovitis or polyarthritis may also develop rarely, usually in association with the major histocompatibility antigen HLA-B27 (Toivanen et al 1985). Patients with reactive arthritis may also have high and persistent levels of IgA-anti-*Yersinia* antibodies, possibly owing to chronic stimulation of intestinal lymphoid tissues (Granfors & Toivanen 1986). Finally, an acute glomerulonephritis has been associated with yersinia infection (Forsstrom et al 1977, Friedberg et al 1978).

TREATMENT

Yersinia enterocolitica is susceptible to various agents, including tetracycline, aminoglycosides, trimethoprim-sulfamethoxazole and chloramphenicol (Gutman et al 1973, Raevuori et al 1978) and, more recently, its in-vitro susceptibility to the quinolones, including ciprofloxacin, was documented with multiple strains of the organism (Noble et al 1985). *Yersinia enterocolitica* strains have β-lactamase activities (Cornelis 1975) that may account for its very significant resistance to penicillin (Raevuori et al 1978). In addition, some strains have R-plasmids that code for resistance to specific antibiotics, including chloramphenicol, aminoglycosides and tetracycline (Kimura et al 1976).

Usually the acute enteric syndrome is self-limited and treatment is not required; in addition, antibiotics have no specific effect on the late complications of the disease, including arthritis (Ahvonen 1972). Patients with bacteremia or metastatic foci of infection require intravenous therapy, although the precise duration of intravenous treatment is unknown.

DIFFERENTIATION FROM INFLAMMATORY BOWEL DISEASE

Clinical features

There is generally little difficulty in distinguishing between yersinia enteritis and inflammatory bowel disease, especially Crohn's disease. The former tends to be a self-limited diarrheal illness, sometimes as part of a small outbreak, whereas the latter is usually associated with symptoms of intermittent intestinal obstruction, fistula formation and generalized wasting with malnutrition. In some adults, however, especially if the clinical course is chronic or prolonged, distinction may be more difficult. Diarrhea and abdominal pain may be present in both, and both may express common extraintestinal features, including peripheral arthritis, ankylosing spondylitis and erythema nodosum. Both may have similar associated laboratory changes, including anemia, an elevated white cell count, a reactive thrombocytosis and an elevated sedimentation rate. In both the peripheral arthritis has a similar distribution, but in Crohn's disease the peripheral arthritis is generally not associated with HLA-B27 and appears to parallel the activity of the underlying bowel disease; in contrast, yersinia arthritis is usually associated with HLA-B27 and follows a course independent of the course of the bowel disease. Some clinical features tend to occur more frequently in yersinia infection, e.g. exudative pharyngitis and lymphadenopathy, whereas other features typically occur only in patients with chronic inflammatory bowel disease, e.g. pyoderma gangrenosum and perianal fistulas.

The radiological and/or endoscopic changes of inflammatory bowel disease, particularly Crohn's disease, have some similarities to the changes observed in yersinia enterocolitis. In both, the distal ileum may be involved, with mucosal nodularity, coarse and irregular mucosal folds, ulceration and proximal luminal dilation. In most, but not all, patients with yersinia infection, these small-intestinal changes resolve after 3–4 months. Similarly, radiological and endoscopic changes in the colon may be seen that are common to both conditions, particularly aphthoid ulceration; again, these tend to resolve completely within weeks to months. In contrast, changes in Crohn's disease usually persist and may be complicated by fistula and stricture formation.

Pathological changes may be very similar in both conditions. In both, the gastric, small and large intestines may be involved, with an acute and/or chronic inflammatory process that is non-specific. Changes may be focal or diffuse. In yersinia infection, mucosal lymphoid aggregates may show central necrosis; rare granulomas or multinucleated giant cells, more typical of Crohn's disease, may be seen. In both yersinia enteritis and Crohn's disease, most severe changes may be seen in the distal ileum and/or colon. However, deep ulcerations with fissures, fistulization and perforation with abscess formation, and involvement of mesenteric fat are features usually associated with Crohn's disease.

REFERENCES

Abramovitch H, Butas C A 1973 Septicemia due to *Yersinia enterocolitica*. Canadian Medical Association Journal 109: 1112

Agner E, Larsen H J, Leth A 1978 *Yersinia enterocolitica* carditis as a differential diagnosis – and the prognosis of this disease. Scandinavian Journal of Rheumatism 7: 26

Ahvonen P 1972 Human yersiniosis in Finland. I. Bacteriology and serology. Annals of Clinical Research 4: 30

Aulisio C C G, Hill W E, Stanfield J T, Sellers R L 1983 Evaluation of virulence factor testing and characteristics of pathogenicity in *Yersinia enterocolitica*. Infection and Immunity 40: 330–335

Bakour R, Balligard G, Laroche G, Cornelis G, Wauters C 1985 A simple adult mouse test for tissue invasiveness in *Yersinia enterocolitica* strains of low experimental virulence. Journal of Medical Microbiology 19: 237–246

Bercovier D J, Ursing J, Brenner D J 1980 *Yersinia kristensenii*: a new species of enterobacteriaceae composed of sucrose negative strains (formerly called atypical *Yersinia enterocolitica* or *Yersinia enterocolitica*-like). Current Microbiology 4: 219–224

Black R E, Jackson R J, Tsai T et al 1978 Epidemic *Yersinia enterocolitica* infection due to contaminated chocolate milk. New England Journal of Medicine 298: 76–79

Bolin I, Norlander L, Wolf-Watz H 1982 Temperature inducible outer membrane protein of *Yersinia enterocolitica* is associated with the virulence plasmid. Infection and Immunity 37: 506

Bradford W D, Noce P S, Gutman L T 1974 Pathologic features of enteric infection with *Yersinia enterocolitica*. Archives of Pathology 98: 17

Brenner D J, Bercovier H, Ursing J, Alonso J M 1980 *Yersinia intermedia*: a new species of enterobacteriaceae composed of rhamnose positive, melibiose positive raffinose positive strains (formerly called *Yersinia enterocolitica* or *Yersinia enterocolitica*-like). Current Microbiology 4: 207–212

Brubaker R R 1986 Low-calcium response of virulent *Yersiniae*. Medicine Microbiology and Immunology 175: 43

Capron J P, Capron-Chivrac D, Tousson H 1984 Spontaneous *Yersinia enterocolitica* peritonitis in idiopathic hemochromatosis. Gastroenterology 87: 1372–1375

Carlsson M G, Ryd H, Sternby N H 1964 A case of human infection with *Pasteurella pseudotuberculosis* X. Acta Pathologica Microbiologica Scandinavica 62: 128

Carter P B 1975 Pathogenicity of *Yersinia enterocolitica* for mice. Infection and Immunity 11: 164

Carter P B 1981 Human *Yersinia enterocolitica* infection: laboratory models. In: Bottone E J (ed) *Yersinia enterocolitica* CRC Press, Boca Raton, Florida, pp 73–81

Chin G N, Noble R C 1977 Ocular involvement in *Yersinia enterocolitica* infection presenting as Parinaud's oculoglandular syndrome. American Journal of Ophthalmology 83: 19

Cornelis G 1975 Distribution of beta-lactamases A and B in some groups of *Yersinia enterocolitica* and their role in resistance. Journal of General Microbiology 91: 391

Devenish J A, Schiemann D A 1981 HeLa cell infection by *Yersinia enterocolitica*: evidence for lack of intracellular multiplication and development of a new procedure or quantitative expression of infectivity. Infection and Immunity 32: 48–55

Feeley J C 1981 Isolation techniques for *Yersinia enterocolitica*. In: Bottone E J (ed) *Yersinia enterocolitica* CRC Press, Boca Raton, Florida, pp 9–15

Fishman M J, Noble M A, Freeman H J 1989 Yersinia infection with *Clostridium difficile* colitis. Canadian Journal of Gastroenterology 3: 21–25

Forsstrom J, Viander M, Letonen A, Ekfors T 1977 *Yersinia enterocolitica* infection complicated by glomerulonephritis. Scandinavian Journal of Infectious Diseases 9: 253

Friedberg M, Larsen S, Denneberg T 1978 *Yersinia enterocolitica* and glomerulonephritis. Lancet 1: 498

Gemski P, Lazere J R, Casey T 1980 Plasmid associated with pathogenicity and calcium dependency of *Yersinia enterocolitica*. Infection and Immunity 27: 682–685

Granfors K, Toivanen A 1986 IgA-anti-*Yersinia* antibodies in *Yersinia* triggered arthritis. Annals of Rheumatic Diseases 45: 561

Gutman L T, Ottesen E A, Quan T J, Noce P S, Katz S L 1973 An interfamilial outbreak of *Yersinia enterocolitica* enteritis. New England Journal of Medicine 288: 1372–1377

Hancock G E, Schaedler R W, MacDonald T T 1986 *Yersinia enterocolitica* infection in resistant and susceptible strains of mice. Infections and Immunity 53: 26

Kimura S, Ikeda T, Eda T, Mitsui Y, Nakata K 1976 R plasmids from *Yersinia*. Journal of General Microbiology 97: 141

Laird W J, Cavanaugh D C 1980 Correlation of autoagglutination and virulence in *Yersiniae*. Journal of Clinical Microbiology 11: 430–432

Leino R, Kalliomaki J L 1974 Yersiniosis as an internal disease. Annals of Internal Medicine 81: 458–461

Lian C J, Pai C H 1985 Inhibition of human neutrophil chemiluminescence by plasmid-mediated outer membrane proteins of *Yersinia enterocolitica*. Infection and Immunity 49: 145–151

Marks M I, Pai C H, Lafleur L, Lackman L, Hammerberg O 1980 *Yersinia enterocolitica* gastroenteritis: a proposective study of clinical, bacteriologic, and epidemiologic features. Journal of Pediatrics 96: 26–31

Martin T, Kasian G F, Stead S 1982 Family outbreak of yersiniosis. Journal of Clinical Microbiology 16: 622–626

Martinez R J 1983 Plasmid-mediated and temperature-regulated surface properties of *Yersinia enterocolitica*. Infection and Immunity 41: 921

Noble M A, Freeman H J 1986 Which patients are at risk for *Yersinia* septicemia? Journal of Critical Illness 1: 8–9

Noble M A, Barteluk R, Freeman H J 1985 Antimicrobial sensitivity patterns for clinical isolates of *Yersinia enterocolitica*. Gastroenterology 88: 1519

Noble M A, Barteluk R, Freeman H J, Subramanian R, Hudson J B 1987 Clinical significance of virulence-related assays for *Yersinia* species. Journal of Clinical Microbiology 25: 802–807

Noble M A, Fletcher K M, Freeman H J 1989 *Yersinia enterocolitica* associated enteric disease. In: Freeman H J (ed) Inflammatory bowel disease, vol 2 CRC Press, Boca Raton, Florida, pp 85–97

Pai C H, Mors V 1978 Production of enterotoxin by *Yersinia enterocolitica*. Infection and Immunity 19: 908

Pai C H, DeStephano L 1982 Serum resistance associated with virulence in *Yersinia enterocolitica*. Infection and Immunity 35: 605–611

Pai C H, Sorger S, Lafleur L, Marks M 1979 Efficacy of cold enrichment techniques for recovery of *Yersinia enterocolitica* from human stools. Journal of Clinical Microbiology 9: 712–715

Persson S, Danielsson D, Kjellander J, Wallensten S 1976 Studies on Crohn's disease. I. The relationship between *Yersinia enterocolitica* infection and terminal ileitis. Acta Chirurgica Scandinavica 142: 84

Portnoy D A, Falkow S 1981 Virulence-associated plasmids from *Yersinia enterocolitica* and *Yersinia pestis*. Journal of Bacteriology 148: 877

Prpic J K, Robins-Browne R M, Davey R B 1983 Differentiation between virulent and avirulent *Yersinia enterocolitica* isolates using Congo Red agar. Journal of Clinical Microbiology 18: 486–490

Rabson A R, Hallett A F, Koornhof H J 1975 Generalized *Yersinia enterocolitica* infection. Journal of Infectious Diseases 131: 447

Raevuori M, Harvey S M, Pickett M J, Martin W J 1978 *Yersinia enterocolitica*: in vitro antimicrobial susceptibility. Antimicrobial Agents and Chemotherapy 13: 888

Reinicke V, Korner B 1977 Fulminant septicemia caused by *Yersinia enterocolitica*. Scandinavian Journal of Infectious Diseases 9: 249–251

Robins-Browne R M, Prpic J K 1985 Effects of iron and desferrioxamine on infection with *Yersinia enterocolitica*. Infection and Immunity 47: 774–779

Robins-Browne R M, Rabson A R, Koornhof H J 1979 Generalized infection with *Yersinia enterocolitica* and the role of iron. Contributions in Microbiology and Immunology 5: 277–282

Schiemann D A 1979 Synthesis of a selective medicine for *Yersinia enterocolitica*. Canadian Journal of Microbiology 25: 1298–1304

Schleifstein J I, Coleman M B 1939 An unidentified microorganism resembling *B. ligneiri* and *Past. pseudotuberculosis*, and pathogenic for man. New York State Journal of Medicine 39: 1749–1753

Scholey J, Freeman H J 1983 Diarrhea and *Yersinia fredriksenii*: demonstration of heat-stable enterotoxin activity in a human-derived strain. Clinical Investigative Medicine 6: 51

Sebes J I, Mabry E H, Rabinowitz J G 1976 Lung abscess and osteomyelitis of ribs due to *Yersinia enterocolitica*. Chest 69: 546

Sereny B 1955 Experimental *Shigella* keratoconjunctivitis. Acta Microbiologica Academy of Sciences (Hungary) 2: 293–296

Simmonds S D, Noble M A, Freeman H J 1987 Gastrointestinal features of culture-positive *Yersinia enterocolitica* infection. Gastroenterology 92: 112–117

Sonnenwirth A C 1970 Bacteremia with and without meningitis due to *Yersinia enterocolitica*, *Edwardsiella tarda*, *Comamonas terrigena*, and *Pseudomonas maltophila*. Annals of the New York Academy of Sciences 174: 488

Spira T J, Kabins S A 1976 *Yersinia enterocolitica* septicemia with septic arthritis. Archives of Internal Medicine 136: 1305

Tacket C O, Ballard J, Harris N et al 1985 An outbreak of *Yersinia enterocolitica* infections caused by contaminated tofu (soybean curd). American Journal of Epidemiology 121: 705–711

Taylor B G, Zafarzai M Z, Humphreys D W, Manfredi F 1977 Nodular pulmonary infiltrates and septic arthritis associated with *Yersinia enterocolitica* bacteremia. American Review of Respiratory Diseases 116: 525

Thirumoorthi M C, Dajani A S 1978 *Yersinia enterocolitica* osteomyelitis in a child. American Journal of Diseases of Children 132: 578

Toivanen A, Granfors K, Lahesman-Ramtala R, Leino R, Stahlberg T, Vuento R 1985 Pathogenesis of *Yersinia*-triggered reactive arthritis: immunological, microbiological and clinical aspects. Immunological Review 86: 47

Toma S, Lafleur L 1981 *Yersinia enterocolitica* infections in Canada 1966 to August 1978. In: Bottone E J (ed) *Yersinia enterocolitica* CRC Press, Boca Raton, Florida, pp 183–191

Ursing J, Brenner D J, Bercovier H 1980 *Yersinia fredriksenii*: a new species of enterobacteriaceae composed of rhamnose-positive strains (formerly called atypical *Yersinia enterocolitica* or *Yersinia enterocolitica*-like). Current Microbiology 4: 213–217

van Loghem J J 1944 The classification of the plague bacillus. Journal of Microbiology and Serology 10: 15

van Trappen G, Agg H O, Ponette E, Geboes K, Bertrand P H 1980 *Yersinia* enteritis and enterocolitis: gastroenterological aspects. Gastroenterology 72: 220–227

Vesikari T, Nurmi T, Maki M et al 1981 Plasmids in *Yersinia enterocolitica* serotypes 0:3 and 0:9, correlation with epithelial cell adherence in vitro. Infection and Immunity 33: 870

Wauters G 1981 Antigens of *Yersinia enterocolitica*. In: Bottone E J (ed) *Yersinia enterocolitica*. CRC Press, Boca Raton, Florida, pp 41–53

Winblad S, Nilehn B, Sternby N 1966 *Yersinia enterocolitica (Pasteurella X)* in human enteric infections. British Medical Journal December: 1363

Wormser G P, Keusch G T 1981 *Yersinia enterocolitica*: clinical observations. In: Bottone E J (ed) *Yersinia enterocolitica* CRC Press, Boca Raton, Florida, pp 83–93

Zink D L, Feeley J C, Wells J G, Vanderzant C, Vickery J C, O'Donovan G A 1980 Plasmid-mediated tissue invasiveness in *Yersinia enterocolitica*. Nature 283: 224–225

46. Ischemic colitis

M. G. Thomas

INTRODUCTION

The gut lives in equilibrium with its luminal environment, therefore any reduction in mucosal viability due to poor blood supply can result in bacterial invasion (Marston 1994). The colon has a relatively poor collateral blood supply compared to the small bowel. This, combined with the presence of pathogenic bacteria, makes focal ischemia more likely in the large bowel than in the small bowel (Marston 1994). Oxygen free radicals are produced in anaerobic conditions (by xanthine oxidase) and during tissue reperfusion: these radicals are highly destructive to cell membranes (Welch et al 1986, Magnusson et al 1990, Marston 1994). Once the intestinal mucosal barrier has been compromised the gut can deliver noxious substances into the systemic, portal and lymphatic circulations. Intestinal mucosa is very sensitive to ischemia and, as a consequence, mucosal changes develop within minutes of an ischemic injury (Thompson et al 1990). As yet, however, there is no reliable specific test for colonic ischemia.

The presenting symptoms and signs of ischemic colitis are often non-specific and numerous conditions can favor its development, hence it is frequently misdiagnosed (Roberts et al 1993). Often the correct diagnosis is only made with hindsight or with the aid of histopathology.

Clearly the primary event in the pathogenesis is a sudden decrease in colonic blood flow. Existing impaired segmental blood flow, such as that caused by atherosclerosis or vasculitis, can facilitate the development of colonic ischemia but is by no means a prerequisite, as illustrated by its development in athletes (Fogoros 1980, Roberts et al 1993). Uncommon causes of impaired colonic perfusion include cholesterol emboli (Moolenar et al 1989), hematological causes (Welch et al 1986, Magnusson et al 1990), therapeutic vasoconstriction (Schmitt & Wagner Thiessen 1987), anaphylactic shock (Travis et al 1991), sickle cell disease (Gage & Gagnter 1983) and *Schistosoma mansoni* infestation (Neves et al 1993). In general, however, most patients who develop ischemic colitis are elderly, and Morson (1988) suggests that in more than 50% of cases atherosclerotic disease of the mesenteric vessels is the primary cause. Indeed, the presence of pre-existing cardiovascular disease in elderly patients with abdominal pain and rectal bleeding should alert the clinician to the diagnosis.

In some cases of large-bowel ischemia there is no demonstrable blood vessel occlusion (Renton 1972). The development of mesenteric ischemia without vessel occlusion might be facilitated by a regional reduction in splanchnic blood flow, such as might occur following a hypotensive event (Renton 1972, Aldrete et al 1977). Ischemic colitis related to hypotension is rare in the young. An age-related increase in tortuosity of the colonic vessels might account for the increased incidence of non-occlusive colitis seen in the elderly (Binns & Isaacson 1978). Colonic 'long-vessel' tortuosity could cause mucosal ischemia by providing an increased resistance to flow, thus aggravating the effects of low blood flow (Binns & Isaacson 1978).

Broadly, there are two natural histories for large-bowel ischemia: first, gangrenous colitis, where the severity of ischemia is profound and rapidly progresses to focal or pan-colonic gangrene, or secondly, a more benign transient form which resolves without intervention.

ACUTE SEVERE ISCHEMIA

Spontaneous ischemic colitis can pursue a self-limiting, relatively benign course; sometimes, however, recovery is not complete and the disease progresses to dilatation, persistent colitis or gangrene.

Gangrenous ischemic colitis

Gangrene of the colon usually presents as an abdominal event in a severely ill patient, requiring prompt resuscitation and surgery. The diagnosis is rarely made before laparotomy. Acute gangrene frequently affects the splenic flexure or descending colon, and so resection with exteriorization and colonic lavage seems the safest course of action.

Colonic gangrene with obstruction

Extensive colonic gangrene can occur with obstructing colonic lesions and may represent a severe life-threatening complication. In a series of six cases of gangrene complicating colonic obstruction, the histology ranged from mucosal necrosis, to focal full-thickness necrosis with extensive mucosal erosions, to frank transmural gangrene (Teasdale & Mortensen 1983). The need for radical surgery is illustrated by Teasdale and Mortensen's series: the four patients treated by total abdominal colectomy survived, whereas two patients treated by defunctioning colostomy developed major complications and died (Teasdale & Mortensen 1983).

Colonic gangrene complicating obstruction appears to be a secondary phenomenon but its pathogenesis is unknown. A postulated sequence of events is that increased intraluminal pressure causes a reduction in mucosal blood flow with subsequent ischemia, and hence mucosal integrity deteriorates and allows bacterial proliferation within the colonic wall, which leads to frank gangrene (Boley et al 1969, Teasdale & Mortensen 1983).

Colonic dilatation of ischemic colitis

Dilatation complicating ischemic colitis may occur within a focal area of ischemia (Rosato et al 1969), proximal to an area of ischemia (Margolis et al 1979) or involve the whole length of the colon (Carr et al 1986). Clinically dilatation is usually associated with abdominal pain, and therefore might be confused with toxic megacolon in ulcerative colitis or Crohn's colitis. Indeed, in a series of nine patients where colonic dilatation complicated ischemia, abdominal pain and diarrhea were the main presenting features, with rectal bleeding occurring in only one patient (Carr et al 1986). At laparotomy the operative appearance of some forms of large-bowel ischemia is strikingly similar to fulminating inflammatory bowel disease (Eisenberg et al 1979, Margolis et al 1979). Although this relatively rare presentation of ischemia usually occurs in the elderly, it can occur in young patients, further adding to a potential diagnostic dilemma (Carr et al 1986). Dilatation of non-viable colon can result from transmural necrosis and, when encountered, there is usually little doubt that such obviously gangrenous tissue requires resection.

Colonic dilatation also complicates non-gangrenous ischemic colitis and occurs in the proximal non-diseased colon (Margolis et al 1979). Margolis reported three cases of functional obstruction of the transverse colon with dilatation secondary to segmental ischemia of the descending colon (Margolis et al 1979). In all three reported cases there were prodromal abdominal symptoms that lasted for at least 3 weeks prior to surgery, and all had large-bowel ischemia that spared the rectum. It has been suggested that the dilatation of apparently unaffected proximal bowel results from a functional obstruction to peristalsis by the focal ischemia (Margolis et al 1979, Carr et al 1986). In cases of toxic megacolon without gangrene, decompression by colostomy with or without ileostomy followed by interval resection has been advocated as a surgical strategy (Margolis et al 1979). However, difficulty in assessing viability may cause a management dilemma and thus favor resection.

Ischemic colitis following abdominal aortic surgery

Acute ischemic colitis is a well recognized complication of aortoiliac surgery, the reported incidence being approximately 2–9% in elective surgery rising to 17.6% after rupture of an aortic aneurysm (Bast et al 1990, Bjoerk & Hedberg 1994). Indeed, there is mounting evidence that intestinal ischemia may play a role in the postoperative irreversible shock and multiorgan failure associated with aortoiliac surgery (Antonsson & Fiddian-Green 1991). Non-invasive techniques such as mucosal pH monitoring or laser Doppler flowmetry have recently gained support in order to help predict the onset of ischemia and hence alert clinicians to possible major complications of aortic surgery (Krohg-Sorensen & Kvernebo 1989, Bjoerk & Hedberg 1994). A sigmoid tanometer that can detect colonic acidosis and the accumulation of CO_2 has been reported to be 100% sensitive and 86% specific for the development of ischemic colitis when intramucosal pH is less than 6.86 (Fiddian-Green et al 1986, Schiedler et al 1987). Bjoerk and Hedberg monitored intramucosal pH in the sigmoid colon of 34 patients undergoing abdominal aortic surgery, and claimed that all postoperative complications could be predicted using a sigmoid pH of 7.10 as the lower limit of normal (Bjoerk & Hedberg 1994). One of the fundamental issues that needs to be addressed in multiple organ failure is whether the primary insult is the onset of ischemic colitis or if the large bowel response is simply a regional manifestation of systemic events.

NON-GANGRENOUS COLITIS WITH RESOLUTION

Mild or transient ischemic colitis

Most patients with colonic ischemia (perhaps two-thirds) follow a clinical course leading to resolution, with or without colonic stricturing secondary to fibrosis (Roberts et al 1993, Marston 1994). Mild or moderate ischemia probably results from mucosal and submucosal underperfusion (Welch et al 1986); the muscularis propria is relatively avascular and thus may resist damage (Halligan et al 1994) or heal by fibrosis (Welch et al 1986). The clinical picture is of acute abdominal pain with regional peritoneal inflammation (often on the left side). The pain is accompanied by pyrexia, rectal bleeding, diarrhea and leukocytosis. Flexible sigmoidoscopy and gastrografin enema can aid the diagnosis. There is a well recognized left-sided predominance in large-bowel ischemia (Marston et al 1966, Boley & Schwartz 1971, Hagihara et al 1975); this might be due to the reduction in the diameter of the marginal artery seen from the right to the left side of the large intestine (Binns & Isaacson 1978). Ischemia occurs quite frequently at the splenic flexure (Marston et al 1966), but there is some dispute as to whether or not this site is at special risk (Williams & Wittenberg 1975, Binns & Isaacson 1978). The mild or transient forms of ischemic colitis carry an excellent prognosis. The favorable outcome is illustrated in a series of 33 in which a retrospective review concluded that surgical intervention should only have been necessary in two of the cases (Williams & Wittenberg 1975).

Rarer forms of ischemic colitis with resolution

Acute ischemic colitis can develop in athletes, and has been well documented in a female long-distance runner who showed colonoscopic and histological evidence of ischemia together with a reduction in the regional mesenteric flow measured by duplex scanning (Heer et al 1987). There was a resolution of symptoms and signs after the athlete tapered her running schedule. Small-bowel and colonic ischemia have also been reported in young women taking the oral contraceptive pill (Kilpatrick et al 1968, Cotton & Thomas 1971, Gelfand 1972).

HISTOPATHOLOGY

Histological features of colonic ischemia include extensive mucosal hemorrhage, dilated capillaries, patchy fibrosis and superficial erosions (Whitehead 1972). Regeneration has been reported to be associated with widespread fibrosis, submucosal hemosiderosis, crypt distortion, paneth cell metaplasia, goblet cell depletion and high mitotic counts (Carr et al 1986).

Ischemic enterocolitis can produce chronic strictures suggestive of Crohn's disease (Shepherd 1991). In the chronic phase histology may show chronic inflammation, microscopic fissures, crypt epithelial regeneration with distortion and chronic inflammation, all of which may be seen in chronic inflammatory bowel disease (Shepherd 1991). Some histological features are, however, more typical of ischemia rather than inflammatory bowel disease. These include the presence of hemosiderin-laden macrophages in the lamina propria, a relative paucity of chronic inflammatory cells, and selective damage to the more superficial epithelium of the crypt (Whitehead 1972, Morson et al 1990). In necrosis the early phase may involve the upper crypt and lamina propria, but transmural coagulative necrosis with intense polymorphonuclear infiltration is more common, and this infiltrate might be associated with a pseudomembrane (Carr et al 1986).

RADIOLOGY

Radiological evidence of large-bowel ischemia includes thumbprinting, saw-toothing, tubular narrowing and thickening of mucosal folds (Roberts et al 1993). Thumbprinting, which probably reflects submucosal edema with hemorrhage (Halligan et al 1994), is one of the earliest signs, being seen within 3 days of the onset of an attack on barium enema examination (Marston et al 1966). Radiological changes can, however, be transient in self-limiting forms of colitis (Roberts et al 1993).

Dilatation of the transverse colon without thumbprinting can complicate ischemic strictures of the descending colon (Margolis et al 1979). Robson emphasized the importance of considering ischemic colitis in elderly patients who had a dilated featureless colon on plain radiographs (Robson et al 1992). In addition, when a segment of ischemic colon is demonstrated on barium enema it is important to consider the association with a distal tumor (Halligan et al 1994).

COLONOSCOPIC APPEARANCE

Endoscopy in large-bowel ischemia often reveals lower rectal sparing, with edema and cyanosis occurring in the upper rectosigmoid. The endoscopic finding of submucosal hemorrhage or hematoma is very suggestive of an ischemic etiology. In addition, mucosal loss or fragility, edema, ulceration and pseudomembranes can occur in large-bowel ischemia and might aid the diagnosis (Roberts et al 1993). Ischemic colitis can, however, also be a complication of colonoscopy (Wheeldon & Grundman 1990).

CONCLUSION

Ischemic colitis usually occurs as a mild or transient regional ischemia affecting the left side of the colon, and most cases resolve without surgical intervention. In a small percentage of cases large-bowel ischemia pursues a fulminant course, requiring surgery for obstruction or gangrene.

The clinical, radiological and histological picture can resemble inflammatory bowel disease, and thus ischemic colitis should be considered as a differential diagnosis in patients with regional colonic pain associated with diarrhea or rectal bleeding.

REFERENCES

Aldrete J S, Han S Y, Laws H I, Kirklin J W 1977 Intestinal infarction complicating low cardiac output states. Surgery Gynecology and Obstetrics 144: 371–375

Antonsson J, Fiddian-Green R G 1991 The role of the gut in shock and multiple system organ failure. European Journal of Surgery 157: 3–12

Bast T J, van der Biezen J J, Scherpenisse J, Eikelboom B C 1990 Ischaemic disease of the colon and rectum after surgery for abdominal aortic aneurysm. A prospective study of the incidence and risk factors. European Journal of Vascular Surgery 4: 253–257

Binns J C, Isaacson P 1978 Age-related changes in the colonic blood supply: their relevance to ischaemic colitis. Gut 19: 384–390

Bjoerk M, Hedberg B 1994 Early detection of major complications after abdominal aortic surgery: predictive value of sigmoid colon and gastric intramucosal pH monitoring. British Journal of Surgery 81: 25–30

Boley S J, Schwartz S S 1971 Colonic ischaemia: reversible ischaemic lesion. In: Boley S J, Schwartz S S, Williams L F (eds) Vascular disorders of the intestine. Appleton Century Crofts, New York, pp 579–596

Boley S J, Agrawal G P, Warren A P et al 1969 Pathophysiological effects of bowel distension on intestinal blood flow. American Journal of Surgery 117: 228–234

Carr N D, Wells S, Haboubi N Y, Salem R J, Schofield P F 1986 Ischaemic dilatation of the colon. Annals of the Royal College of Surgeons of England 68: 264–266

Cotton P B, Thomas M L 1971 Ischaemic colitis and the contraceptive pill. British Medical Journal 3: 27–28

Eisenberg R L, Montgomery C K, Margolis A R 1979 Colitis in the elderly: ischaemic colitis mimicking ulcerative and grannulomatous colitis. American Journal of Radiology 133: 1113–1118

Fiddian-Green R G, Amelin P, Herrman J B et al 1986 Prediction of the development of sigmoid ischemia on the day of operation from indirect measurements of intramural pH in the colon. Archives of Surgery 85: 654–660

Fogoros R N 1980 'Runners trots'. Gastrointestinal disturbances. Journal of the American Medical Association 243: 1743–1744

Gage T P, Gagnter J M 1983 Ischaemic colitis complicating sickle cell crisis. Gastroenterology 84: 171–174

Gelfand M D 1972 Ischaemic colitis associated with a depot synthetic progesterone. American Journal of Digestive Diseases 17: 275–277

Hagihara P F, Parker J C, Griffin W O 1975 Spontaneous ischaemic colitis. Diseases of the Colon and Rectum 20: 236–251

Halligan M S, Saunders-B P, Thomas B M, Phillips R K 1994 Ischaemic colitis in association with sigmoid carcinoma: a report of two cases. Clinical Radiology 49: 183–184

Heer M, Repond F, Hany A, Sulser H, Kehl O, Jager K 1987 Acute ischaemic colitis in a female long distance runner. Gut 28: 896–899

Kilpatrick Z M, Silverman J F, Betancourt E, Farman J, Lawson J P 1968 Vascular occlusion of the colon and oral contraceptives. New England Journal of Medicine 278: 438–440

Krohg-Sorensen K, Kvernebo K 1989 Laser Doppler flowmetry in evaluation of colonic blood flow during aortic reconstruction. European Journal of Vascular Surgery 3: 37–41

Magnusson I, Rieger A, Nilsson R, Civalero L A 1990 Clinical appearances in severe ischaemic colitis. Case report. Acta Chirurgica Scandinavica 156: 241–245

Margolis I B, Faro R S, Howells E M, Organ C H 1979 Megacolon in the elderly: ischaemic or inflammatory? Annals of Surgery 190: 40–44

Marston A 1994 Ischaemia of the gut. In Misiewicz J J, Pounder R E, Venables C W (eds). Diseases of the gut and pancreas, 2nd edn. Blackwell Scientific, Oxford, pp 1007–1019

Marston A, Pheils M T, Thomas M L, Morson B C 1966 Ischaemic colitis. Gut 7: 1–15

Moolenar W, Kreuning J, Eulderink F, Lamers C B H W 1989 Ischemic colitis and acalculous necrotizing cholecystitis as rare manifestations of cholesterol emboli in the same patient. American Journal of Gastroenterology 84: 1421–1422

Morson B C 1988 A colour atlas of gastrointestinal pathology. Oxford University Press, Oxford, p 217

Morson B C, Dawson I M P, Day D W, Jass J R, Price A B, Williams G T 1990 Vascular disorders. In: Morson B C, Dawson I M P (eds) Gastrointestinal pathology. Blackwell Scientific, Oxford, pp 551–559

Neves J, Raso P, Pinto D de M, da Silva S P, Alvarenga R J 1993 Ischaemic colitis (necrotizing colitis, pseudomembranous colitis) in acute schistosomiasis mansoni: report of two cases. Transactions of the Royal Society of Tropical Medicine and Hygiene 87: 449–452

Renton C J C 1972 Non-occlusive intestinal infarction. Clinics in Gastroenterology 1: 655–673

Roberts J H, Mentha G, Rohner A 1993 Ischaemic colitis: two distinct patterns of severity. Gut 34: 4–6

Robson N K, Khan S M, Rawlinson J, Dewbury K C 1992 Ischaemic colitis: clinical, radiological and pathological correlation in three cases. Clinical Radiology 46: 337–339

Rosato E F, Rosata F E, Scott J et al 1969 Ischaemic dilatation of the colon. American Journal of Digestive Diseases 14: 922–928

Schiedler M G, Cutler B S, Fiddian-Green R G 1987 Sigmoid intramural pH for prediction of ischemic colitis during aortic surgery. A comparison with risk factors and inferior mesenteric artery stump pressures. Archives of Surgery 122: 881–886

Schmitt W, Wagner Thiessen E 1987 Ischaemic colitis in a patient treated with glypressin for bleeding oesophageal varices. Hepatogastroenterology 34: 134–136

Shepherd N A 1991 Pathological mimics of chronic inflammatory bowel disease. Journal of Clinical Pathology 44: 726–733

Teasdale C, Mortensen N J 1983 Acute necrotizing colitis and obstruction. British Journal of Surgery 70: 44–47

Thompson J S, Bragg L E, West W W 1990 Serum enzyme levels during intestinal ischaemia. Annals of Surgery 211: 369–373

Travis S, Davies D R, Creamer B 1991 Acute colorectal ischaemia after anaphylactic shock. Gut 32: 443–446

Welch G H, Shearer M A, Imrie C W, Andersson S R, Gilmour D G 1986 Total ischaemic colitis. Diseases of the Colon and Rectum 29: 410–412

Wheeldon N M, Grundman M J 1990 Ischaemic colitis as a complication of colonoscopy. British Medical Journal 301: 1080–1081

Whitehead R 1972 The pathology of intestinal ischaemia. Clinics in Gastroenterology 1: 613–637

Williams L F, Wittenberg J 1975 Ischaemic colitis: a useful clinical diagnosis, but is it ischaemia? Annals of Surgery 182: 439–446

47. Irradiation enterocolitis

G. S. W. Whiteley   P. F. Schofield

INTRODUCTION

When radiotherapy was first used, powdered radium contained in glass was applied to advanced tumors of the cervix, with later developments in the form of metal containers and needles to filter the rays once the physical characteristics of the radiation were established. Modern intracavitary and interstitial therapy are based on this principle, although in a much modified form (Papillon 1975, Schofield & James 1983, Cole & Hunter 1985), often using artificial radionuclides. The effective agent in both these treatment modalities is the gamma ray.

External beam irradiation, or teletherapy using X-rays, gained favor in the 1930s. Nowadays, X-rays generated from a megavoltage source, such as a linear accelerator or a telecobalt unit, can be precisely controlled as regards both dose and effective 'aiming' of the beam on to the tumor (James & Schofield 1985). Irrespective of the source of the ionizing radiation, whether X-rays or gamma rays, the effect on cells and tissues, both malignant and normal, is the same.

Shortly after the discovery of radium 100 years ago, and coincident with its use on malignant tumors, came the realization that normal tissues in the vicinity of the tumor could be affected by radiation. The early reports implicated vascular damage in the peritumor tissues. The study of the effects of ionizing radiation on tissues continues to develop, and consequently the safety of radiotherapy has been much improved. A major contribution was made by Tod, in Manchester, with the establishment of the now internationally recognized safe dosage regimens for X-ray therapy (Tod 1943).

The site of radiation injury is dependent on the region irradiated and the technique of the radiotherapy. The majority of radiation bowel disease (RBD) is due to pelvic irradiation, but it must be noted that esophageal disease may be caused by irradiation for bronchial carcinoma (Lepke & Libshitz 1982), and radiation disease affecting the stomach and duodenum is recognized following irradiation for lymphoma (Gallez-Marchal et al 1984). Owing to its widespread occupation of the peritoneal cavity the small intestine may be affected by any abdominal irradiation technique, although its mobility often mitigates the extent of the subsequent damage (Berthrong & Fajardo 1981).

The differential diagnosis of RBD includes coincident gastrointestinal disease, and indeed the diagnosis of RBD may be missed, partly because of the long period of time from radiotherapy to onset of symptoms.

PATHOLOGY (Table 47.1)

The pathological changes of radiation bowel disease may conveniently be considered in terms of early and late disease. Early disease is due to a direct effect on the intestinal mucosa, but late disease appears to have a vascular basis. While radiotherapy is in progress there is no structural change in the vasculature, but meganucleosis, eosinophilic abscesses and edema of the lamina propria occur (Haboubi et al 1988). In the later stages after radiotherapy, changes are seen which affect all types and sizes of vessels. The damage begins in the endothelium (Fajardo & Stewart 1973, Fonkalsrud et al 1977), although the whole vessel wall is subsequently affected. The formation of thrombus within these damaged vessels

Table 47.1 Histopathological changes in radiation bowel disease. After Haboubi and Hasleton (1989)

Early RBD	Late RBD
Epithelial changes	
Meganucleosis	Focal ulceration
Cell necrosis	Branching crypts
Eosinophilic abscesses	
Stromal changes	
Eosinophilic infiltrate	Vascular
Edema	ectasia
Fibroblastic reaction	microaneurysm
	thrombosis
	Xanthomatous reaction
	Fibrosis
	Hemosiderin

Table 47.2 Classification of radiation bowel disease

Early effects	Reaction during treatment or immediately after
Late effects	Several months later
Remote effects	Many years later

leads directly to occlusion, which may be compounded by a vasoconstrictive effect of thromboxane produced by the thrombus. The net effect is ischemia to the tissues supplied by these vessels, which is the basis of radiation damage.

CLINICAL FEATURES

The incidence of RBD after pelvic radiotherapy is reported to be 1–20% (Kjorstad et al 1983, Editorial 1984, Sherrah-Davies 1985). Schofield (Schofield et al 1983) has divided the gastrointestinal features into early, late and remote, according to the time period between radiotherapy and presentation (Table 47.2).

Early disease

This is the reaction to radiotherapy during and immediately after treatment. The most common feature is a rectal reaction which resolves spontaneously. A transient diarrhea usually occurs (Smith & DeCosse 1986) which requires, at the most, simple therapy. However, rarely the diarrhea is accompanied by septicemia or peritoneal irritation. Although many of these cases settle on conservative management, one must be aware of the possibility of a free perforation, which would require operative treatment. This possibility is increased if the patient is receiving coincident chemotherapy (Danjoux & Catton 1979). A further occasional problem is reactivation of quiescent inflammatory bowel disease, diverticular disease or gynecological inflammation.

Late disease

The timespan from radiotherapy to onset of symptoms may be months or years, and the differentiation between tumor recurrence and RBD is difficult. Although there may be a totally unrelated cause for bowel symptoms, it must be stressed that radiation-induced disease must be considered in the differential diagnosis. Concurrent chemotherapy, previous pelvic surgery and systemic conditions known to diminish vessel calibre, for example atherosclerosis, hypertension and diabetes mellitus, favor the development of RBD (DeCosse et al 1969).

Remote disease

The presentation of remote disease many years after radiotherapy is usually with either intestinal obstruction or malabsorption. Intestinal obstruction may be distal ileal or colorectal, the former presenting with colic and distension, usually with a history of vomiting and diarrhea. Plain abdominal X-ray will suggest the diagnosis of obstruction. At operation the lesion is found to be an ischaemic stricture. Colorectal strictures are usually in the sigmoid colon and typically present with features of an incomplete large-bowel obstruction.

The other remote problem due to ileal disease is malabsorption. Mechanisms include defective bile salt absorption by the damaged terminal ileum, or bacterial colonization of the ileum above a stricture. Megaloblastic anemia due to impaired vitamin B_{12} absorption may be a feature. Steatorrhea, as estimated by fecal fat excretion, is frequently found. Specifc tests such as a hydrogen breath test for small-bowel colonization (Rhodes et al 1979) or SeHCAT bile acid absorption test (Ludgate & Merrick 1985) may aid diagnosis.

There is some evidence of increased malignant risk inside the radiation field after many years (Black & Ackerman 1965, Sandler & Sandler 1983).

CLINICAL PRESENTATION (Table 47.3)

Most patients with RBD are in the 'late' group and fall into one of five categories of severity (Table 47.4). Grades I and II are relatively minor problems, and only the more severe grades require surgical management.

Rectal bleeding is common but generally not serious. Most patients will settle within the first 1–2 years. A small

Table 47.3 Presentation of RBD and its temporal relationship to therapy

Presentation	Time between XRT and onset
Early	
Acute proctitis	0–1 month
Acute enteritis	0–1 month
Late	
Rectal bleeding	4–12 months
Chronic abscess/intestinal obstruction	9–15 months
Anal/perineal pain	6–12 months
Fistula	1.5–2 years
Remote	
Stricture/malabsorption	2–20 years
Rectal malignancy	5–40 years

Table 47.4 The grading system for radiation disease. After Pilepich et al (1983)

Grade I	Minor symptoms which require no treatment
Grade II	The symptoms do not affect the performance status and can be managed by simple outpatient methods
Grade III	More severe symptoms altering the performance status. May have to be admitted for diagnostic procedures or minor surgery
Grade IV	Prolonged hospitalization and major surgical intervention
Grade V	Fatal complications

group present with more serious bleeding for which transfusion is necessary. If repeated transfusion is needed, or the bleeding is accompanied by abdominal pain, this frequently heralds the need for surgery (Gilinsky et al 1983).

Intestinal obstruction is a common presentation in patients with ileal disease. In the early stages physical signs cannot be elicited and radiological studies are unrewarding. These patients may progress with mild attacks before developing definite evidence of obstruction. In previously irradiated patients this picture is more likely to be due to RBD than recurrence or other causes of obstruction (Walsh & Schofield 1984).

Chronic perforation with abscess formation occurs as a consequence of slowly progressive ischemia, causing localized sepsis due to colonic necrosis which is walled off by local adhesions. The patient may experience colic and some distension, but symptoms of sepsis predominate over obstruction. Disturbances of bowel function and pain are usual. The signs of distension and an abdominal or rectal mass mislead the clinician into a diagnosis of recurrence rather than RBD. Further investigation is often unhelpful, and most cases come to operation. Operation is usually curative in RBD and can offer good palliation in the case of tumor recurrence.

Anal and perineal pain may occur owing to ulceration within the anal canal; may be intermittent or persistent (Schofield et al 1983). This problem usually occurs within a few months of treatment. All but the most minor ulcers usually require excisional surgery to relieve the pain. In the female patient there is a risk of fistula formation within a matter of months. Biopsy of these ulcers may merely speed the development of a fistula.

Fistulation of both the gastrointestinal and urinary tracts into the vagina may occur. Rectovaginal is the more common after radiotherapy (Smith & DeCosse 1986). The usual symptoms are of fecal leakage and perineal discomfort. Diagnosis is relatively simple, but an examination under anesthesia is often needed because of swelling or pain. In the presence of an established fistula a biopsy is necessary to differentiate between RBD or recurrence.

INVESTIGATIONS

Apart from the clinical assessment of the patient and the awareness of the possibility of RBD, investigations on a general level should include full hematological and biochemical profiles. Many such patients are anemic and have some degree of malnutrition. The specific aims of investigation are to differentiate between tumor recurrence and RBD, and to localize accurately the radiation changes.

Exclusion of distant metastases by chest radiography and liver ultrasonography is desirable. If possible, a tissue diagnosis by biopsy should be obtained as the possibility of coincident disease exists and the findings of coexisting recurrence and radiation bowel diseases should be remembered. However, it is often impractical to perform biopsy prior to early surgery. In this unit the presence of a raised platelet count is frequently noted with active RBD (Carr et al 1985).

The localization of the disease is usually clarified by sigmoidoscopy and occasionally colonoscopy together with radiological techniques (Mason et al 1970, Mendelson & Nolan 1985). For large-bowel lesions the radiological investigation of choice is the double contrast barium enema with multiple oblique views of the sigmoid colon. It is recommended that this procedure be augmented by the use of a muscle relaxant such as hyoscine butylbromide. For distal small-bowel lesions a plain X-ray combined with clinical suspicion may be all that is required. However, a small-bowel enema is the investigation of choice in obscure cases (Miller & Sellink 1979, Nolan 1985). Owing to the frequent involvement of the urinary tract in the disease process an assessment of the urinary tract is recommended when practicable.

Computerized tomography (CT) or nuclear magnetic resonance (NMR) scans have been used increasingly in recent years to investigate and evaluate the differences between radiation disease and recurrent disease. Whilst both these techniques are useful in the majority of cases there can be difficulties, and in some cases it has proved impossible to resolve the diagnosis before operation.

TREATMENT

Most patients with early symptoms are easily managed by symptomatic treatment and reassurance. In the few patients with early disease in whom a severe reaction occurs, intensive non operative management with intravenous fluids and nasogastric aspiration should be instituted. Surgery is rarely required, but exacerbation of preexisting bowel disease and the failure of conservative management leading to early perforation may herald the need for surgery.

In late disease there would appear to be no specific medical regimen which materially affects the outcome. Supportive measures in rectal bleeding include stool softeners, iron supplementation or blood transfusion. Laser treatment of rectal bleeding will benefit some patients (Ahlquist et al 1986). In late ileal disease with malabsorption, antibiotics to treat bacterial colonization, vitamin B_{12} replacement for deficiency states, and cholestyramine for bile salt diarrhea may be used.

However, surgery is usually indicated for severe symptoms. There are obvious indications for emergency surgery, for example total obstruction, free perforation or massive bleeding. In 40–50% of patients the presentation will be semiurgent, with sepsis, incomplete obstruction or fistula formation. In these patients management should be divided into three stages. Stabilization including resuscitative and nutritional measures is of paramount importance, with

Table 47.5 Operations for radiation bowel disease

Site	Operation	
	Defunction	Resection
Ileum	Exclusion bypass Exclusion and anastomosis	Ileocecal resection
Sigmoid colon	Colostomy	Sigmoid resection + colorectal anastomosis
Rectum	Colostomy	A-P excision of the rectum Proctectomy + coloanal

the correction of electrolyte abnormalities, fluid imbalance and anemia, followed by a period of total parenteral nutrition. The second stage is the definition of the extent of disease by diagnostic procedures, and the third stage is the operative management.

The operative management of RBD may be by bypass, but resection has become established as the treatment of choice (Gazet 1985, Schofield et al 1986, Galland & Spencer 1987), provided correct principles are followed (Table 47.5). We believe that RBD is progressive even after defunctioning (Anseline et al 1981). It is very unusual for a defunctioned rectum to heal sufficiently well for reanastomosis to be considered.

In early ileal disease operation is occasionally needed for acute enteritis with perforation. It is better to exteriorize both ends after resection and return after the acute illness. The resection in late ileal disease should be fairly wide owing to the diffuse nature of the disease. We usually resect 40–50 cm of small bowel in order to be above the damaged section (Carr et al 1984). Extensive right colonic resection is not necessary because the ascending colon is outside the irradiation field. There is no greater risk of leakage than in anastomosis for other disease, with figures of 0–6% being reported (Schofield 1986). If significant rectosigmoid disease is present at the time of surgery it should be corrected at that time.

In colonic disease the surgical procedure depends upon the presenting complaint. Severe persistent bleeding will require resection. Coloanal anastomosis is usually possible. In case of chronic perforation with abscess we feel that resection of the affected bowel is mandatory. When combined external beam and intracavitary radiation has been delivered it is unwise to leave any rectum, and a coloanal anastomosis should be employed with a covering colostomy which is closed at 3 months. If one modality has been delivered then low anterior resection is usually safe with a covering colostomy.

The management of fistula in our unit again relies on excision of the affected bowel. The procedure used depends upon the height of the fistula. For very high rectovaginal fistula a low anterior resection is carried out. Most fistulae are to the mid or low vagina. In these circumstances, although bowel continuity may be preserved by coloanal anastomosis, this is not always possible. If the sphincter mechanism is affected then there is little alternative but to perform abdominoperineal excision of the rectum with permanent colostomy.

Despite the significant morbidity of RBD it makes only a minor contribution to mortality. Survival figures after radiotherapy for carcinoma of the cervix indicate a 10-year survival of 52% in those patients suffering RBD, compared with 58% survival in those patients who did not suffer the disease (Harling & Balslev 1988).

REFERENCES

Ahlquist D A, Gastout C J, Viggiano T R, Pemberton J H 1986 Laser therapy for severe radiation induced rectal bleeding. Mayo Clinic Proceedings 61: 927–931

Anseline P F, Lavery I C, Fazio V W, Jagelman D G, Weakley F L 1981 Radiation injury of the rectum. Annals of Surgery 194: 716–724

Berthrong M, Fajardo L F 1981 Radiation in surgical pathology, part 2, alimentary tract. American Journal of Surgical Pathology 5: 153–178

Black W C, Ackerman L V 1965 Carcinoma of the large intestine as a late complication of pelvic radiotherapy. Clinical Radiology 16: 278–281

Carr N D, Hasleton P S, Schofield P F 1985 Platelet count in radiation bowel disease: An aid to diagnosis. British Journal of Surgery 72: 287–288

Carr N D, Pullen B R, Hasleton P S, Schofield P F 1984 Radiation bowel disease. Gut 25: 448–454

Cole M P, Hunter R D 1985 Female genital tract. In: Easson E C, Pointon R C S (eds) The radiotherapy of malignant disease. Springer-Verlag, Berlin, pp 280–309

Danjoux C E, Catton G E 1979 Delayed complications in colorectal carcinoma treated by combination radiotherapy and 5-fluorouracil – Eastern Cooperative (ECOG) pilot study. International Journal of Radiation Oncology Biology and Physics 5: 311–316

DeCosse J J, Rhodes R S, Wentz W B, Reagan J W, Dworken H J, Holden W D 1969 The natural history and management of radiation induced injury of the gastrointestinal tract. Annals of Surgery 170: 369–384

Editorial 1984 Radiation bowel disease. Lancet ii: 963–964

Fajardo L F, Stewart J R 1973 Pathogenesis of radiation-induced myocardial fibrosis. Laboratory Investigation 29: 244–257

Fonkalsrud E W, Sanchez M, Zerbuarel R, Mahoney A 1977 Serial changes in arterial structure following radiation therapy. Surgery, Gynecology and Obstetrics 145: 395–400

Galland R B, Spencer J 1987 Natural history and surgical management of radiation enteritis. British Journal of Surgery 74: 742–747

Gallez-Marchal D, Foyolle M, Henry-Amar M, Le Bourgeois J P, Rougier P, Cosset J M 1984 Radiation injuries of the gastrointestinal tract in Hodgkin's disease. Radiotherapy and Oncology 2: 93–99

Gazet J-C 1985 Parks colo-anal pull-through anastomosis for severe complicated radiation proctitis. Diseases of the Colon and Rectum 28: 110–114

Gilinsky N H, Burns D G, Barbezat G O, Levin W, Myers H S, Marks I N 1983 The natural history of radiation induced proctosigmoiditis: analysis of 88 patients. Quarterly Journal of Medicine 52: 40–53

Haboubi N Y, Hasleton P S 1989 Pathology of radiation injury. In: Schofield P F, Lupton E W (eds) The causation and management of pelvic radiation disease. Springer-Verlag, Berlin, pp 17–35

Haboubi N Y, Schofield P F, Rowland P 1988 The light and electron microscopic features of early and late phase radiation-induced proctitis. American Journal of Gastroenterology 3: 1140–1144

Harling H, Balslev I 1988 Long-term prognosis of patients with severe radiation enteritis. American Journal of Surgery 155: 517–519

James R D, Schofield P F 1985 Resection of 'inoperable' rectal cancer following radiotherapy. British Journal of Surgery 72: 279–281

Kjorstad K E, Martimbeau P W, Iversen T 1983 Stage 1B carcinoma of the cervix, the Norwegian Radium Hospital: results and complications. Gynecology and Oncology 15: 42–47

Lepke R A, Libshitz H I 1983 Radiation-induced injury of the oesophagus. Radiology 148: 375–378

Ludgate S M, Merrick M V 1985 The pathogenesis of post-irradiation chronic diarrhoea: measurement of SeHCAT and B_{12} absorption for differential diagnosis determines treatment. Clinical Radiology 36: 275–278

Mason G R, Dietrich P, Friedland G W, Hanks G E 1970 The radiological findings in radiation-induced enteritis and colitis. Clinical Radiology 21: 232–247

Mendelson R M, Nolan D J 1985 The radiological features of chronic radiation enteritis. Clinical Radiology 36: 141–148

Miller R E, Sellink J L 1979 Enteroclysis: the small bowel enema. How to succeed and how to fail. Gastrointestinal Radiology 4: 269–283

Nolan D J 1983 Radiological investigation of the small intestine. In: Whitehouse G H, Worthington B (eds) Techniques in diagnostic radiology. Blackwell Scientific, Oxford, pp 21–31

Papillon J 1975 Intracavitary irradiation of early rectal cancer for cure: a review of 186 cases. Cancer 36: 696

Pilepich M V, Pajak T, George F W et al 1983 Preliminary report on phase III RTOG studies of extended-field irradiation in carcinoma of the prostate. American Journal of Clinical Oncology (CCT) 6: 485–491

Rhodes J M, Middleton P, Jewell D P 1979 The lactulose hydrogen breath test as a diagnostic test for small-bowel bacterial overgrowth. Scandinavian Journal of Gastroenterology 14: 333–336

Sandler R S, Sandler D P 1983 Radiation induced cancers of the colon and rectum. Assessing the risk. Gastroenterology 84: 51–57

Schofield P F, Carr N D, Holden D 1986 The pathogenesis and treatment of radiation bowel disease. Journal of the Royal Society of Medicine 79: 30–32

Schofield P F, James R D 1983 Treatment of carcinoma rectum and anus. In: Irving M H, Beart R (eds) International medical reviews, Surgery 3, Gastroenterological surgery. Butterworths, London, pp 198–217

Schofield P F, Holden D, Carr N D 1983 Bowel disease after radiotherapy. Journal of the Royal Society of Medicine 76: 463–466

Sherrah-Davies E 1985 Morbidity after selectron therapy for cervical cancer. Clinical Radiology 36: 131–139

Smith D H, DeCosse J J 1986 Radiation damage to the small intestine. World Journal of Surgery 10: 189–194

Tod M C 1947 Optimum dosage in the treatment of cancer of the cervix by radiation. Acta Radiologica 28: 564–575

Walsh H P J, Schofield P F 1984 Is laparotomy for small bowel obstruction justified in patients with previously treated malignancy? British Journal of Surgery 71: 933–935

48. Ulcerative jejunoileitis

G. K. T. Holmes

INTRODUCTION

This uncommon and poorly understood condition is characterized by malabsorption and chronic ulcers, found mainly in the jejunum and ileum but rarely in the colon. It is referred to by a variety of different terms, including ulcerative jejunitis, chronic ulcerative non-granulomatous jejunitis, chronic non-specific ulcerative duodeno-jejunoileitis and chronic non-granulomatous ulcerative enterocolitis. Since ulcers are found in the small bowel and rarely elsewhere, ulcerative jejunoileitis is the preferred term. The etiology is unknown, but disturbances of factors which maintain the integrity of the intestinal mucosa (Wright 1993) or inappropriate immune responses to luminal antigens or components of the bowel wall may play a part. There is no evidence that infection has a primary role (Stuber et al 1971, Freeman & Cho 1984).

Patients divide into four groups: those with celiac disease or refractory sprue, those with normal small-bowel mucosa and those with lymphoma. In many cases it is impossible to decide whether patients have celiac disease or not, because there is no universally accepted definition, some stressing only the importance of a flat small-bowel mucosa but others requiring clear-cut responses to gluten withdrawal (Cooke & Holmes 1984). Even when clinical responses to a gluten-free diet and improvement in mucosal morphology are taken into account difficulties may remain, because in those with intestinal ulceration such responses are often temporary and incomplete.

CELIAC DISEASE

Almost all patients with jejunoileitis have flat small-intestinal biopsies, and in some series about half fulfil the requirements for diagnosing celiac disease with clinical and histological responses to gluten withdrawal (Bayless et al 1967, Modigliani et al 1979, Baer et al 1980). In a review of 47 cases, 17 were regarded as having celiac disease as judged by responses to gluten withdrawal, and another five because of strongly supporting evidence, such as a long history of malabsorption (Baer et al 1980). There are now many well documented cases (London et al 1961, Goulston et al 1965, Davidson 1969, Neale 1970, Moritz et al 1971, Stuber et al 1971, Dowling & Henry 1972, Jones & Gleeson 1973, Blau et al 1974, Connon et al 1975, Klaeveman et al 1975, Bateson et al 1979, Kavin 1981, Lamont et al 1982, Lance & Gazzard 1983, Robertson et al 1983, Venturatos et al 1984). The development of jejunoileitis may bring a patient with celiac disease to diagnosis but may also cause deterioration in patients with celiac disease previously well controlled on a gluten-free diet, as may happen with lymphoma (Holmes et al 1989).

REFRACTORY SPRUE

Patients with intestinal ulceration and flat small-bowel mucosa but in whom responses to gluten withdrawal have not been demonstrated or sustained, are regarded as having refractory or unclassified sprue (Collins & Isselbacher 1965, Jeffries et al 1968, Corlin & Pops 1972, Armstrong et al 1973, Mills et al 1980, Lamont et al 1982, Freeman & Cho 1984, Green et al 1993). This disorder is difficult to categorize, and whether or not it is related to celiac disease has generated much debate. Among the various case reports are patients with long histories of malabsorption, possible family histories of celiac disease and showing clinical reponse to a gluten-free diet, albeit only temporarily, who probably had celiac disease. Baer et al (1980) reported 11 cases of refractory sprue and speculated that most of these had celiac disease but the presence of intestinal ulceration had rendered them unresponsive to gluten withdrawal. In-vitro studies of jejunal tissue further support the concept that ulcerative jejunoileitis is a complication of celiac disease (Klaveman et al 1975).

NORMAL BIOPSIES

In the few patients with intestinal ulceration who have normal biopsies or only mild abnormalities away from the ulcers there appears to be no relationship to celiac disease (Jeffries et al 1968, Case Records 1969, Karz et al 1971, Modigliani et al 1979, Baer et al 1980, Costello et al 1991).

RELATIONSHIP TO LYMPHOMA

There may be an association between jejunoileitis and lymphoma. Both conditions may coexist in the same patient, and sometimes ulceration will be diagnosed before lymphoma becomes apparent (Freeman et al 1977, Bayless et al 1978, Baer et al 1980). It has been proposed that ulceration is a precursor of lymphoma due to neoplastic T cells (Isaacson & Wright 1978, Isaacson et al 1985).

CLINICAL FEATURES AND INVESTIGATIONS

Jejunoileitis affects older adults and presents with diarrhea, dehydration, weight loss, anorexia, anemia, edema, abdominal pain and fever. Steatorrhea, anemia and hypoalbuminemia are common. Osteomalacia and hemorrhagic manifestations due to malabsorption of vitamins D and K respectively, may be present. Symptoms may be of short duration. However, the disorder may be preceded by a long history of malabsorption indicative of celiac disease, or may cause the appearance of new symptoms in patients with established celiac disease previously well controlled on a gluten-free diet. At presentation patients are usually very unwell and it is wise to arrange admission for investigation and treatment because deterioration in health is relentless and valuable time is lost if attempts are made to manage cases as outpatients. Rarely symptoms may be mild (Kane & Parkins 1979). Presentation is often acute, with intestinal obstruction, perforation or hemorrhage from the gastrointestinal tract (Connon et al 1975).

Anemia is common and folate, ferritin and vitamin B_{12} concentrations should be assayed. A polymorphonuclear leukocytosis indicates infection or ulcer perforation. Prothrombin time should be measured. Hypoalbuminemia results from anorexia, malabsorption and protein-losing enteropathy, and is likely to be severe. Low serum calcium and elevated alkaline phosphatase concentrations indicate osteomalacia. Blood cultures are required in those with fever or leukocytosis.

Imaging

Both erect and supine plain X-ray of the abdomen may be normal or show appearances of small-bowel obstruction, with multiple fluid levels. The presence of air under the diaphragm indicates ulcer perforation. Barium studies of the small intestine in early cases may only show features of malabsorption, as seen in uncomplicated celiac disease, with bowel dilatation, flocculation, segmentation and effacement of the mucosal folds. Later, more diagnostic appearances become evident, with irregular luminal narrowing and dilatation of bowel proximal to strictures, which may be multiple (Fig. 48.1). Ulcers are not usually visualized (Armstrong et al 1973, Modigliani et al 1979, Lamont et al 1982). Abdominal ultrasound and CT scanning may reveal masses or enlarged lymph nodes, indicating malignancy or cavitating mesenteric lymph nodes, which may also complicate celiac disease (Holmes 1986).

Laparotomy

Laparotomy will be necessary in some cases to clarify the diagnosis, and in particular to differentiate jejunoileitis from lymphoma. The decision whether to perform a diagnostic laparotomy in a very ill patient can be difficult: laparotomy has probably been overused and has contributed to the high death rate. It is better to defer this and continue with intensive medical support, including prolonged parenteral nutrition. A marked clinical improvement with these measures may well render an operation unnecessary. Nevertheless, patients who are deteriorating on treatment will require exploration.

PATHOLOGY

A biopsy of the upper small intestine is required and is usually obtained by a fiber-optic endoscope. A flat mucosa indistinguishable from that found in celiac disease is seen in the majority of cases, although occasionally normal or near-normal villi are present. Small-bowel enteroscopy allows inspection and biopsy of the jejunum beyond the ligament of Treitz, and has the potential to diagnose ulcerative jejunoileitis (Green et al 1993). There is a small risk of intestinal perforation with this technique.

In ulcerative jejunoileitis a spectrum of change is evident in the small bowel at laparotomy. In early cases appearances may be normal, but later segments of varying length become reddened and indurated, with involvement of the mesentery and enlargement of the regional lymph nodes (Moritz et al 1971, Armstrong et al 1973). Peristalsis in the affected areas is defective (Lamont et al 1982). These changes can be reversible (Corlin & Pops 1972). As the disorder progresses the bowel becomes more diffusely narrowed or develops discrete, single or multiple strictures, with intervening dilated loops of bowel and the formation of diverticula (Mills et al 1980, Venturatos et al 1984). Strictures may rarely occur in the colon (Stuber et al 1971) and even in the esophagus (Connon et al 1975).

When the bowel is opened ulcers of varying sizes are seen, with intervening normal or atrophic mucosa, and strictures may be present. Ulcers may be superficial but can extent down to and through the serosa. The

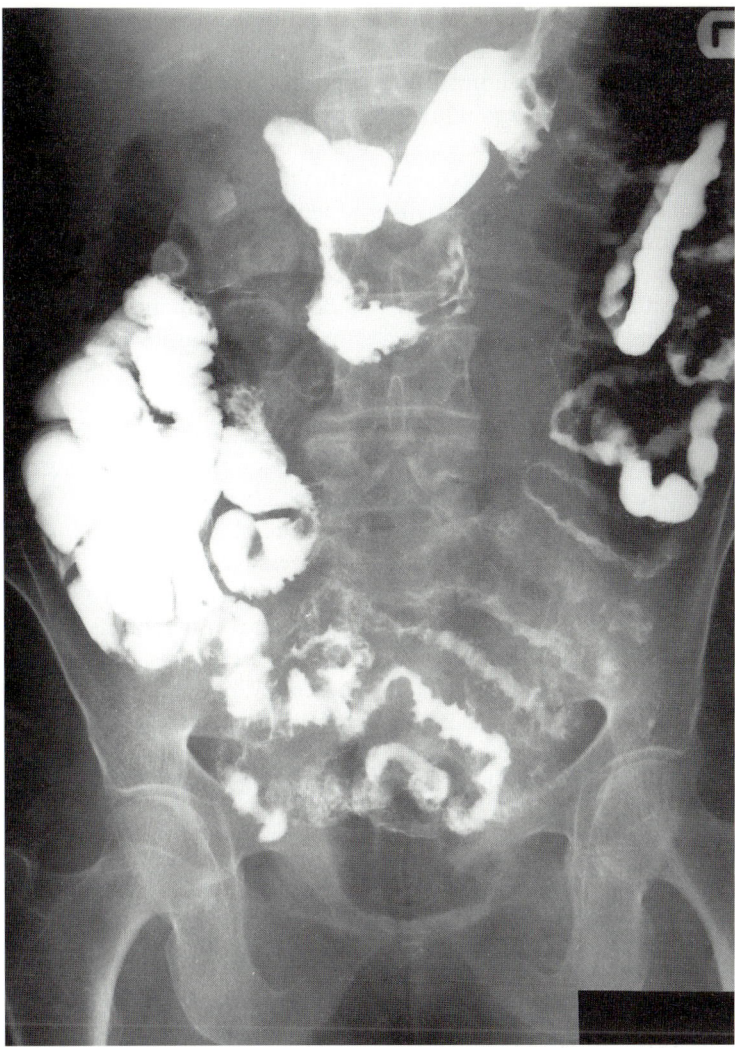

Fig. 48.1 Ulcerative jejunoileitis in a patient with celiac disease. On this radiograph the duodenum and entire small bowel show a very abnormal mucosal pattern with ulceration. Normal folds are absent and the wall of the small bowel is thickened, with narrowing of the lumen and separation of the loops. This patient was extremely ill and developed a serum albumin of 11 g/l. She received steroids and azathiaprine. Parenteral nutrition was continued for 3 months. A subsequent small-bowel follow-through showed virtually normal appearances. Six years after the diagnosis she is in good health and continues a strict gluten-free diet.

inflammatory infiltrate of the ulcers is made up of lymphocytes, plasma cells, polymorphonuclear leukocytes and histiocytes, and vasculitis may be present. Fibrosis and muscular hypertrophy are prominent features in some cases and are responsible for stricture formation. Giant cells and granulomas are not seen. Lymph nodes reveal only reactive hyperplasia. Bacteria may be recovered from the ulcers but their significance is uncertain.

DIFFERENTIAL DIAGNOSIS

Pointers to the diagnosis of ulcerative jejunoileitis are a history of malabsorption, a flat small-intestinal biopsy, widespread radiological and pathological abnormalities in the small bowel, particularly the jejunum, and no response to a gluten-free diet. There may be a prior diagnosis of celiac disease. If these features are considered the diagnosis if relatively easy, but there may be confusion with Crohn's disease and celiac disease complicated by malignancy. The differential diagnosis also includes bowel damage from the ingestion of non-steroidal anti-inflammatory drugs, intestinal tuberculosis, radiation enteritis, Whipple's disease, polyarteritis nodosa, and the Zollinger–Ellison syndrome.

Ulcerative jejunoileitis may be mistaken for Crohn's disease even at laparotomy (Case Records 1969, 1975).

Crohn's disease affecting the small bowel, however, tends to occur in a younger age group, is more likely to affect the distal ileum, jejunal biopsies are usually normal or show only mild, non-specific change, and granulomas, absent in jejunoileitis, are characteristic. Nevertheless, it is possible that some patients considered to have ulcerative jejunoileitis, particularly those with normal small-bowel biopsies, have a diffuse form of Crohn's disease (Cooke & Swan 1974). Patients with Crohn's disease who develop malignancy can be difficult to differentiate from those with ulcerative jejunoileitis without laparotomy.

Ulcerative jejunoileitis may be very difficult to differentiate from celiac disease complicated by small-intestinal lymphoma (Holmes et al 1989). Widespread abnormalities demonstrated radiologically would favor benign ulceration, but single or multiple shorter abnormal segments probably require a laparotomy for definitive diagnosis. Adenocarcinoma of the jejunum complicating celiac disease is less likely to cause diagnostic problems because an abdominal mass may be present, and only a single, short stricture with proximal dilatation of the bowel demonstrated by radiology (Holmes et al 1980).

There are many other causes and diseases associated with small-intestinal ulceration. Wayte and Helwig (1968) collected 59 patients with ulcers, 18 of whom had taken potassium chloride medication, but those with Crohn's disease were excluded. Boydstun et al (1981) reviewed a series of non-specific ulcers of the small bowel. The usual pathological features in all patients were simple punched-out ulcers or, more commonly, annular 'napkin ring' ulcers producing strictures 1–2 cm wide. Sometimes two or three similar constrictions were present, with dilated intervening bowel with normal mucosa. The ileum was the most common site of ulceration. These appearances are unlike those of ulcerative jejunoileitis. Patients were often considered incorrectly to have Crohn's disease. The length of bowel involved, however, is much shorter than would be the case for Crohn's disease, and patients tend to be older than those with newly diagnosed Crohn's disease. Pathological changes suggestive of Crohn's disease are absent.

TREATMENT

Of immediate concern, especially in those who present with severe diarrhea, are dehydration and electrolyte disturbances, particularly potassium deficiency. These abnormalities require urgent correction by intravenous replacement. Anemia as a result of bleeding or malabsorption will warrant transfusion. These simple measures make patients feel better and improve their general condition. Intravenous corticosteroids should be administered from the onset. This route avoids the uncertainties of gastrointestinal absorption. Debilitated patients are prone to infections, particularly pneumonia, which should be treated appropriately. Those who present acutely with ulcer perforation, intestinal obstruction or uncontrollable bleeding from the gastrointestinal tract will require early surgery. Subacute intestinal obstruction may settle on conservative management, but if this fails a stenosed, ulcerated segment of bowel will require resection, which may help to induce remission (Davidson 1969, Moritz et al 1971, Mills et al 1980).

Deficiencies of folic acid, vitamin B_{12}, ferritin and vitamins D and K should be corrected. An important aspect of treatment is the management of malnutrition. This is usually severe and should be corrected by parenteral feeding, which may be required for 2–3 months. Success is judged by weight gain and improvement in serum albumin. There should be no haste to discontinue parenteral nutrition as this approach rests the bowel and avoids symptoms of pain and bloating when patients try to eat. When enteral feeding is possible a gluten-free diet should be given to those who have a flat small-intestinal biopsy. Milk restriction may improve abdominal distension, wind and continuing diarrhea. Azathioprine is useful if corticosteroids are not controlling symptoms or large doses are necessary, or if the serum albumin remains stubbornly low. There are interesting reports of the value of omeprazole in Crohn's disease and ulcerative colitis (Valori & Cockel 1990, Heinzow & Schlegelberger 1994), and this has been used in jejunoileitis with apparent benefit (Kumar et al 1991).

The discovery of new peptide growth factors which appear to maintain the integrity of intestinal mucosa offers new means of treating ulcerative jejunoileitis. (Lemoine et al 1992). Small-bowel transplantation may extend hope to those with irreversible intestinal failure. These developments are still at a very early stage and their value in clinical practice remains to be determined.

PROGNOSIS

The prognosis of jejunoileitis is poor. In three series deaths were 13 of 16 cases (Bayless et al 1967), 20 of 32 (Mills et al 1980) and 23 of 33 patients (Baer et al 1980). Deaths are due to ulcer complications, malnutrition or postoperative problems. Many of these cases were managed at a time when the principles of intensive care and nutritional support were not as well understood as they are now, so that it should be possible to improve prognosis by using more modern approaches.

REFERENCES

Armstrong B K, Ammon R K, Finlay-Jones L R, Joske R A, Vivian A B 1973 A further case of chronic ulcerative enteritis. Gut 14: 649–652

Baer A N, Bayless T M, Yardley J H 1980 Intestinal ulceration and malabsorption syndromes. Gastroenterology 79: 754–765

Bateson M C, Clark J, Beck J S, Clark J, Baxby K, Bouchier I A D 1979 Extensive alimentary and genital ulceration, mesenteric cysts, malabsorption, T-lymphocyte depletion and subsequent anaplastic bladder carcinoma. Postgraduate Medical Journal 55: 836–839

Bayless T M, Kapelowitz R F, Shelley W M, Ballinger W F, Hendrix T R 1967 Intestinal ulceration – a complication of coeliac disease. New England Journal of Medicine 276: 996–1002

Bayless T M, Yardley J H, Baer A, Hendrix T R 1978 Intestinal ulceration, flat mucosa and malabsorption. Report of registry of 33 patients. In: McNichol B, McCarthy C F, Fottrell P F (eds) Perspectives in coeliac disease. MTP Press, Lancaster, pp 311–312

Blau J S, Stolzenberg J, Toffler R B 1974 Small bowel ulcerations – an unusual complication of coeliac disease. Journal of the Canadian Association of Radiologists 25: 77–78

Boydstun J S, Gaffey T A, Bartholomew L G 1981 Clinicopathologic studies of nonspecific ulcers of the small intestine. Digestive Diseases and Sciences 26: 911–916

Case Records of the Massachusetts General Hospital 1969 New England Journal of Medicine 280: 885–894

Case Records of the Massachusetts General Hospital 1975 New England Journal of Medicine 293: 712–717

Collins J R, Isselbacher K J 1965 The occurrence of severe intestinal mucosal damage in conditions other than coeliac disease (nontropical sprue). Gastroenterology 49: 425–432

Connon J J, McFarland J, Kelly A, Biggart J D, McLoughlin J 1975 Acute abdominal complications of coeliac disease. Scandinavian Journal of Medicine 10: 843–849

Cooke W T, Holmes G K T 1984 Definition and epidemiology In: Cooke W T, Holmes G K T (eds) Coeliac disease. Churchill Livingstone, Edinburgh, pp 11–22

Cooke W T, Swan C H J 1974 Diffuse jejuno-ileitis of Crohn's disease. Quarterly Journal of Medicine 43: 583–601

Corlin R F, Pops M A 1972 Nongranulomatous ulcerative jejunoileitis with hypogammaglobulinaemia. Gastroenterology 62: 473–478

Costello R W, Lyons D J, Fielding J F 1991 Ulcerative jejunitis: are we missing cases? Irish Journal of Medical Sciences 160: 342–343

Davidson A R 1969 Recurrent benign ileal ulcer occurring with the coeliac syndrome. British Medical Journal 3: 341

Dowling R H, Henry K 1972 Non-responsive coeliac disease. British Medical Journal 3: 624–631

Freeman H J, Weinstein W M, Shnitka T K, Piercey J R A, Wensel R H 1977 Primary abdominal lymphoma. Presenting manifestations of coeliac sprue or complicating dermatitis herpetiformis. American Journal of Medicine 63: 585–594

Freeman M, Cho S R 1984 Nongranulomatous ulcerative jejunoileitis. American Journal of Gastroenterology 79: 446–449

Goulston K J, Skyring A P, McGovern V J 1965 Ulcerative jejunitis associated with malabsorption. Australian Annals of Medicine 14: 57–64

Green J A, Barkin J S, Gregg P A, Kohen K 1993 Ulcerative jejunitis in refractory coeliac disease: enteroscopic visualisation. Gastrointestinal Endoscopy 39: 584–585

Heinzow U, Schlegelberger T 1994 Omeprazole in ulcerative colitis. Lancet 343: 477

Holmes G K T 1986 Mesenteric lymph node cavitation in coeliac disease. Gut 27: 728–733

Holmes G K T, Dunn G I, Cockel R, Brookes V S 1980 Adenocarcinoma of the small bowel complicating coeliac disease. Gut 21: 1010–1016

Holmes G K T, Prior P, Lane M R, Pope D, Allan R N 1989 Malignancy in coeliac disease – effect of a gluten free diet. Gut 30: 333–338

Isaacson P, Wright D H 1978 Malignant histiocytosis of the intestine. Its relationship to malabsorption and ulcerative jejunitis. Human Pathology 9: 661–667

Isaacson P G, O'Connor N T J, Spencer J et al 1985 Malignant histiocytosis of the intestine: a T-cell lymphoma. Lancet ii: 688–691

Jeffries G H, Steinberg H, Sleisenger M H 1968 Chronic ulcerative (nongranulomatous) jejunitis. American Journal of Medicine 44: 47–59

Jones P E, Gleeson M H 1973 Mucosal ulceration and mesenteric lymphadenopathy in coeliac disease. British Medical Journal 3: 212–213

Kane S P, Parkins R A 1979 Chronic ulcerative jejunitis without symptoms. Postgraduate Medical Journal 55: 215–217

Karz S, Guth P H, Polonsky L 1971 Chronic ulcerative jejunoileitis. American Journal of Gastroenterology 56: 61–67

Kavin H 1981 Coeliac disease complicated by chronic nongranulomatous ulcerative enterocolitis, nodular lymphoid hyperplasia and disseminated intravascular coagulation. Digestive Diseases and Sciences 26: 73–80

Klaeveman H L, Gebhard R, Sessoms C, Strober W 1975 In vitro studies of ulcerative ileojejunitis. Gastroenterology 68: 572–582

Kumar P J, Clark M L, Dawson A M 1991 Unresponsive subtotal villous atrophy, ulcerative jejunitis: treatment with omeprazole. In: Mearin ML, Mulder C J J (eds) Coeliac disease: 40 years gluten free. Kluwer Academic Publishers, Dordrecht, p 212

Lamont C M, Adams F G, Mills P R 1982 Radiology in idiopathic chronic ulcerative enteritis. Clinical Radiology 33: 283–287

Lance P, Gazzard B G 1983 Ulcerative enteritis and liver disease in a patient with coeliac disease. Gut 24: 433–437

Lemoine N R, Leung H Y, Gullick W J 1992 Growth factors in the gastrointestinal tract. Gut 33: 1297–1300

London D R, Bamforth J, Creamer B 1961 Steatorrhoea presenting with gastrointestinal protein loss. Lancet 2: 18–19

Mills P R, Brown I L, Watkinson G 1980 Idiopathic chronic ulcerative enteritis. Quarterly Journal of Medicine 49: 133–149

Modigliani R, Poitras P, Galian A et al 1979 Chronic non-specific ulcerative duodenojejuno-ileitis: report of four cases. Gut 20: 318–328

Moritz M, Moran J M, Patterson J F 1971 Chronic ulcerative jejunitis. Report of case and discussion of classification. Gastroenterology 60: 96–102

Neale G 1970 A case of malabsorption, intestinal mucosal atrophy and ulceration, cirrhosis and emphysema. British Medical Journal 3: 207–212

Robertson D A F, Dixon M F, Scott B B, Simpson F G, Losowsky M S 1983 Small intestinal ulceration: diagnostic difficulties in relation to coeliac disease. Gut 24: 565–574

Stuber J L, Wiegman H, Crosby I, Gonzalez G 1971 Ulcers of the colon and jejunum in coeliac disease. Radiology 99: 339–340

Valori R M, Cockel R 1990 Omeprazole for duodenal ulceration in Crohn's disease. British Medical Journal 300: 438–439

Venturatos S G, Hines C, Blalock J B 1984 Ulceration of the small intestine in a patient with coeliac disease. Southern Medical Journal 77: 520–522

Wayte D M, Helwig E B 1968 Small bowel ulceration – iatrogenic or multifactorial origin. American Journal of Clinical Pathology 49: 26–40

Wright N A 1993 Trefoil peptides and the gut. Gut 34: 577–579

49. Non-steroidal anti-inflammatory drug-induced enteritis

I. Bjarnason   A. Macpherson   A. B. Price

INTRODUCTION

Non-steroidal anti-inflammatory drugs (NSAIDs) cause a range of intestinal pathologies. The most severe side effects occur in the gastroduodenal region. Here NSAIDs are associated with characteristic (chemical gastritis) or incidental (chronic gastritis associated with Helicobacter) histological changes which are equally associated with ulcers, and which have the potential to perforate or bleed (Dixon et al 1986, Taha et al 1992, Quinn et al 1993). The most common site of damage is, however, the small intestine, where NSAIDs cause an enteritis in about 65% of patients (Bjarnason et al 1984, 1987a, 1993, Rooney et al 1986, Segal et al 1986). NSAID enteropathy is at times associated with substantial complications, namely small intestinal ulcers and strictures, in which case the clinician may be called upon to differentiate the disease from Crohn's disease.

CLINICAL FEATURES OF NSAID ENTEROPATHY

Most patients with NSAID enteropathy have no specific symptoms. Nevertheless, the enteropathy is clinically important as patients may bleed from the small intestine, contributing to the iron-deficiency anemia which is so common in rheumatic patients; they also have a protein-losing enteropathy which may cause hypoalbuminemia (Bjarnason et al 1987b). When sufficiently severe these complications may require treatment. The therapeutic options include metronidazole, sulfasalazine and misoprostol (Bjarnason & Macpherson 1994).

In the context of the present chapter it is important to note that uncomplicated NSAID enteropathy does not cause any radiological abnormalities. A problem arises, however, in relation to the differential diagnosis when iron deficiency is refractory, or when the more serious complications associated with the enteropathy appear, namely ulcers and strictures.

NSAID-INDUCED SMALL-INTESTINAL ULCERS

Small-intestinal ulcers caused by NSAIDs have been described in the clinical setting of severe, persistent or recurring iron-deficiency anemia (Shack 1966, Sturges & Krone 1973, Venturatos et al 1984, Madhok et al 1986). One such patient, which is a typical example, is worth describing. She was middle-aged and had had rheumatoid arthritis for almost 20 years, maintained solely on NSAIDs. In 1993 her hemoglobin had dropped below 8 g/dl and she required blood transfusion on a 4–6 weekly basis for the next 10 months. She improved temporarily following a course of metronidazole, which has been shown to be an effective treatment for straightforward NSAID enteropathy and blood loss (Bjarnason et al 1992), but the anemia recurred. Conventional studies did not identify the site of intestinal bleeding, but her small-bowel enema is shown in Figure 49.1. The small-intestinal resection specimen showed no fewer than eight ulcers, each flanked by early 'diaphragm' formation. The important clinical feature here is that although NSAID enteropathy is associated with small-intestinal bleeding, which contributes to iron-deficiency anemia, the search for ulcers need only be initiated if the anemia is severe, recurrent or refractory to conventional treatment for the enteropathy. In this case there was no suspicion of Crohn's disease, but in other cases it has not been so easy to distinguish the two conditions clinically.

The relatively few reports of NSAID-induced small-intestinal ulcers may only represent the tip of the iceberg, for enteroscopy studies show discrete mid small-intestinal ulcers in about 30% of patients taking NSAIDs (Morris et al 1992), and an impressive autopsy study showed that 28% of patients on long-term NSAIDs had small-intestinal ulcers (Allison et al 1992). The figure may be higher as some ulcers may easily have been missed because of autolysis.

NSAID-INDUCED STRICTURES

In the case of NSAID-induced small-intestinal strictures the symptoms have been more varied. Only rarely have patients presented with acute intestinal obstruction, in

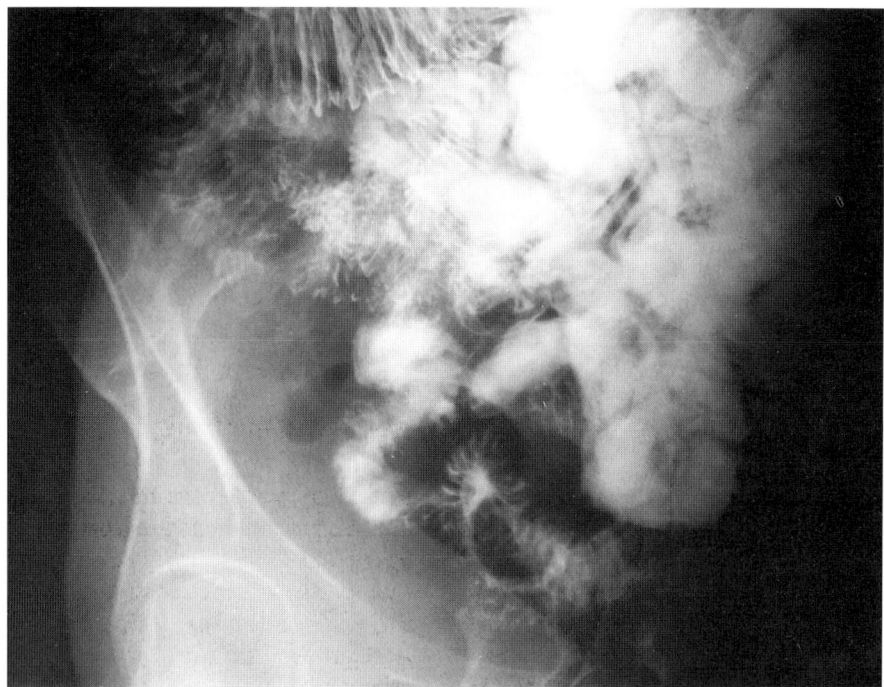

Fig. 49.1 Small-bowel enema in a patient with recurring iron deficiency anemia on NSAIDs. The main abnormality in this oblique view is a crescent or half-moon sign, which was interpreted as evidence of an ulcer.

which case there is no option but to proceed to surgery and the diagnosis is made (Johnson 1987, Sukumar 1987). More commonly, patients present with intermittent subacute small-intestinal obstruction (Sturges & Krone 1973, Neoptolemos & Locke 1983, Bjarnason et al 1988, Lang et al 1988). In these cases symptoms have often been vague. Not only is the abdominal pain intermittent and inconsistent in relation to food intake and severity, but there is also an overlap between the intestinal discomfort and pain that patients on NSAIDs commonly experience, which is not associated with strictures. In the dozen cases we have diagnosed there have usually been the additional findings of hypoalbuminemia or troublesome iron deficiency, perhaps indicating the severity of the enteropathy.

Patients on slow release diclofenac preparations are prone to develop colonic rather than small-intestinal strictures (Fellows et al 1992, Huber et al 1992, Monahan et al 1992, Halter et al 1993). These may present with symptoms identical to the small-intestinal strictures, but are easily diagnosed at colonoscopy.

RADIOLOGY

Uncomplicated NSAID enteropathy is not associated with any radiological abnormalities. Severe hypoalbuminemia may be associated with non-specific mucosal edema, which is seen as thickened folds. Figure 49.1 shows a typical case of a NSAID-induced small-intestinal ulcer. An angiographic examination showed a submucosal blush (Fig. 49.2), but still seven other ulcers were missed. Other authors describe similar findings or ulceration associated with significant spasm, in which case the picture may resemble an obstruction. Considering the frequency of enteroscopic ulcers in patients taking NSAIDs (Morris et al 1992), it would seem clear that most are missed on small-intestinal barium enemas.

In cases of NSAID-induced intestinal strictures the radiological findings have often mirrored the pathology findings (Levi et al 1990). There is a spectrum from single non-specific strictures that distort the bowel, which may or may not resemble Crohn's disease, to multiple ones pathognomic of what has been termed 'diaphragm' disease (Fig. 49.3). The latter are extremely difficult to diagnose, as the multiple thin septa look like exaggerated plicae circularis, which do not distort the bowel wall. In only the rarest cases does radiology resemble Crohn's disease (Fig. 49.4). In our experience half of the cases have had no detectable abnormal small-intestinal radiology, so it is to be hoped that enteroscopy may be an aid to the diagnosis in the future.

Depending on the clinical severity an exploratory laparotomy may be indicated. If pathology is demonstrated it may be easy to distinguish it from Crohn's disease, but there is currently no effective treatment for radiologically demonstrated NSAID-induced ulcers or strictures apart from surgery. One caveat, however, is the careful assessment of the patient who develops severe

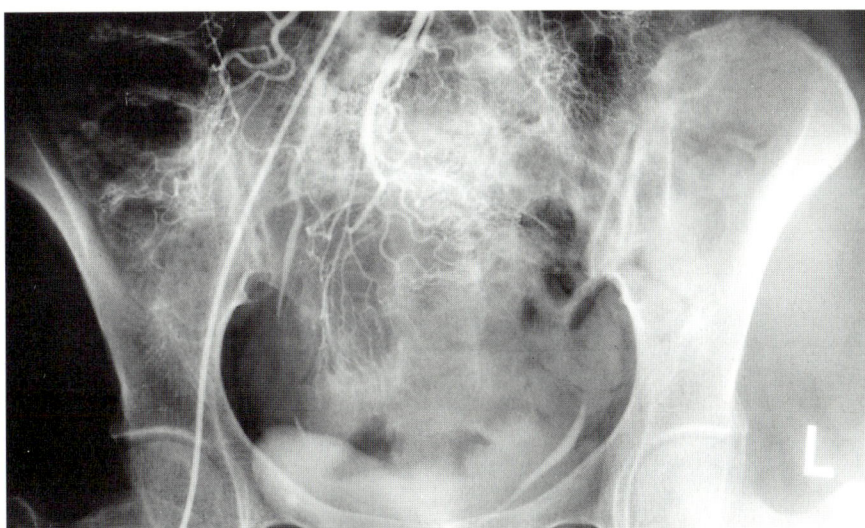

Fig. 49.2 Angiographic appearances of the ulcer shown in the patient in Figure 49.1, demonstrating a submucosal flush resembling a crescent, but no active bleeding.

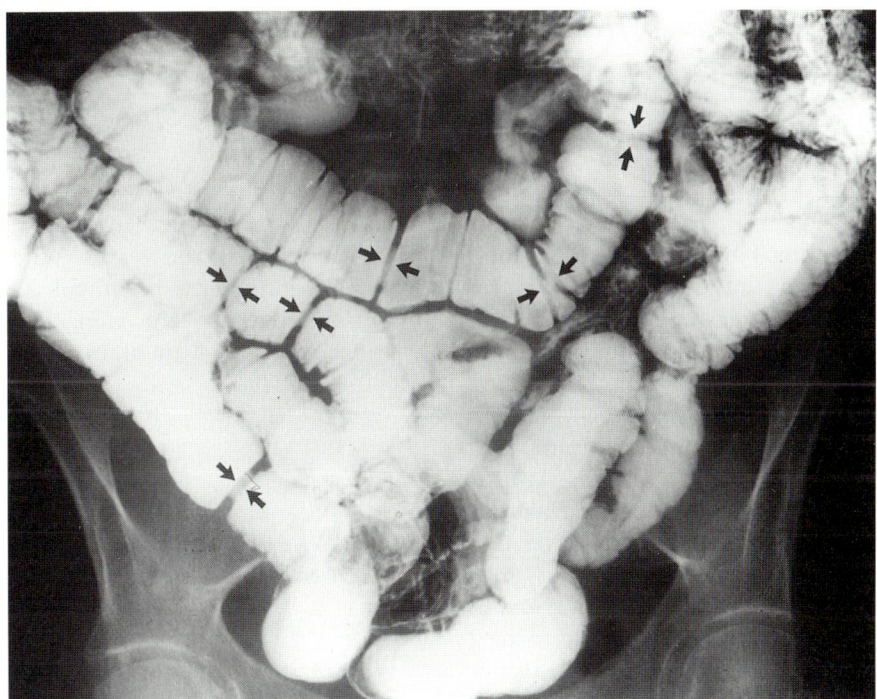

Fig. 49.3 Small-bowel enema from a patient with symptoms of subacute small-intestinal obstruction demonstrating multiple slit-like narrowings (between arrows), which at operation turned out to be 'diaphragm' strictures.

intestinal symptoms within weeks of commencing NSAID treatment, for this may be the emergence of pre-existing subclinical Crohn's disease which is known to be activated by such drugs.

PATHOLOGY

Histology of single ulcers has been unrewarding, the picture being non-specific, although a raised profile should prompt suspicion of a drug-induced lesion (Lang et al 1988). The raised profile is caused by fibromuscular expansion of the submucosa. The absence of any single diagnostic feature raises the differential diagnosis of other non-specific small-intestinal ulcerations, of which there are up to 50 causes, including Crohn's disease, tuberculosis, ischemia, celiac disease, lymphoma and idiopathic ulcerative jejunitis (Thomas & Williamson 1985).

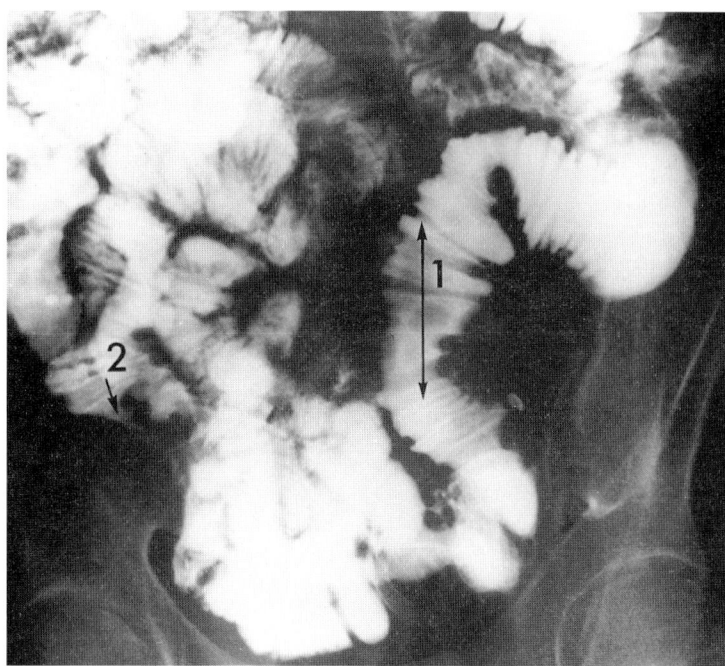

Fig. 49.4 Small-bowel follow-through from a patient on NSAIDs demonstrating (1) an irregular ileal segment with suspicion of mucosal ulceration, and (2) string sign close to the terminal ileum. Accordingly the patient was thought to have Crohn's disease, but multiple 'diaphragm' lesions were found at operation.

NSAID-associated strictures have been more common than ulcers, but this may be misleading as ulcers are commonly demonstrated at enteroscopy (Morris et al 1992). The strictures have a range of pathologies, from single non-specific broad hump-like strictures to the multiple thin concentric strictures of 'diaphragm' disease (Lang et al 1988). The former are presumably the end result of healing of the solitary ulcers, and indistinguishable from descriptions of potassium-induced strictures. Indeed, some of the documented cases of the latter had also been receiving NSAIDs. The 'diaphragms' may number up to 70, are typically concentric, thin, 2–4 mm septate-like projections, narrowing the lumen down to a few millimeters in most cases, as demonstrated in Figure 49.5, but at times causing complete obstruction. 'Diaphragm' disease is most often found in the mid small intestine, but in patients on slow-release diclofenac have tended to occur in the ascending colon.

Histopathologically the basic structure of the diaphragm resembles the normal plicae circularis. However, a zone of fibrosis immediately beneath, or merging with, the muscularis mucosa, as shown in Figure 49.6, is characteristic. The overlying mucosa shows varying degrees of inflammation and villus blunting, with or without shallow ulceration. Slips of muscularis may splay up into the lamina propria, but the mucosa along the side of the 'diaphragm' quickly returns to normal. The degree of submucosal fibromuscular obliteration seems to determine the profile of the lesions. When mild the distinction from plicae circularis is difficult. When florid the more hump-like outlines are seen. There is no associated vascular damage to medium or small vessels, although blood-flow studies and experimental work in animal

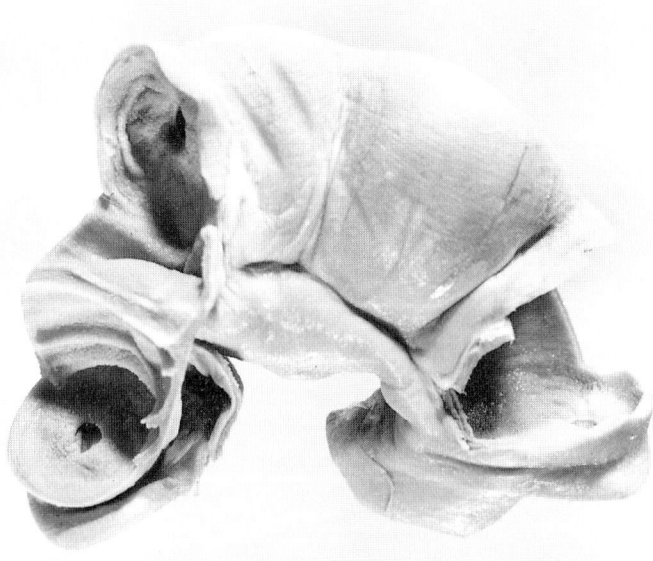

Fig. 49.5 A segment of small bowel with well formed 'diaphragms' dividing the lumen into compartments, but producing only slight serosal distortion.

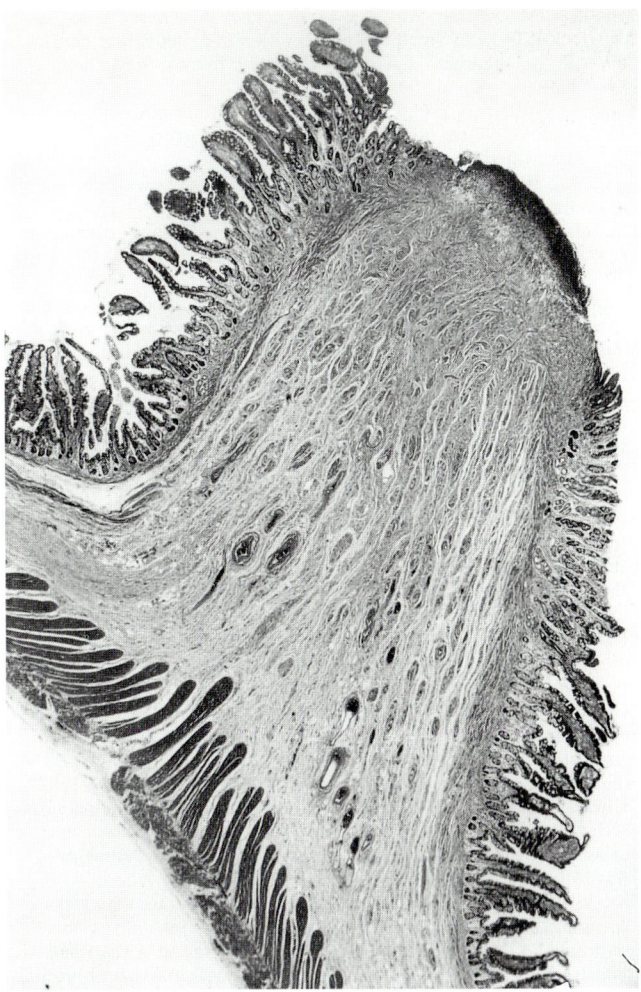

Fig. 49.6 The cross-section of a 'diaphragm' clearly shows it is predominantly an abnormality in the submucosa, where there is upwards tenting and fibrosis. Mucosal ulceration and inflammation is restricted to the apex. There is no widespread inflammatory infiltrate nor evidence of a vasculitis. The muscle coat is uninvolved and the illustration clearly shows why there is so little abnormality seen from the serosal aspects.

models implicate a role for vascular endothelium and neutrophil adhesion molecules (Wallace 1992, Wallace and Granger 1992, Whittle 1992). A full account of the pathogenesis of NSAID enteropathy is not appropriate here (Bjarnason et al 1993, Somasundaram et al 1994), but it has been suggested that there are two main stages to the damage. First there is predominantly biochemical damage, initiated by the common action of NSAIDs to uncouple oxidative phosphorylation (or inhibit electron transport along the respiratory chain). The immediate consequences are that calcium leaks from mitochondria, activating cellular proteases, endonucleases etc., and sets off a chain reaction of damage caused by oxygen-reactive species. In addition, reduced ATP production disrupts the integrity of paracellular junctions. The resulting increased intestinal permeability then translates the biochemical damage to the second-stage tissue reaction, which develops into an inflammatory reaction in response to luminal bacteria gaining access to the mucosa. Thus the participation of the vascular endothelium and neutrophils would appear to be a late pathogenic event in NSAID-induced damage to the intestine, and indeed an essential component of the inflammatory reaction rather than its immediate cause.

TREATMENT AND PROGNOSIS

Treatment of NSAID enteropathy and its common complications, namely blood and protein loss, is detailed elsewhere, but the choice is between metronidazole, sulfasalazine, 5-amino salicylates and misoprostol, depending on the clinical circumstances (Bjarnason & Macpherson 1994). In most patients a substantial improvement can be expected, and as with many other treatments the more severe the enteropathy the greater the apparent improvement.

There is no evidence, however, that the intestinal strictures regress or respond to medical treatment. So, in the case of radiologically demonstrated ulcers surgery should be contemplated because of the difficulties in distinguishing between the NSAID-induced lesion and a more sinister pathology. Resection is appropriate for the ulcers but strictureplasty may be adequate for most of the strictures.

DIFFERENTIAL DIAGNOSIS FROM CROHN'S DISEASE

NSAID enteropathy is not likely to be confused with Crohn's disease in the large majority of cases, because it is usually asymptomatic. Patients requiring NSAIDs may have activation of subclinical inflammatory bowel disease within days of ingestion (Kaufman & Taubin 1987), but NSAID enteropathy becomes evident only after a few months of treatment. Normal intestinal radiology and a mildly increased fecal excretion of ^{111}In leukocytes are characteristic of NSAID enteropathy.

In cases where small-intestinal radiology is abnormal, the single ulcer, lack of terminal ileal involvement and lack of bowel wall distortion are all in favor of NSAID damage, which again can be supported by a much lower ^{111}In leukocyte fecal excretion than in Crohn's disease.

REFERENCES

Allison M C, Howatson A G, Torrance C J, Lee F D, Russell R I 1992 Gastrointestinal damage associated with the use of nonsteroidal anti-inflammatory drugs. New England Journal of Medicine 327: 749–754

Bjarnason I, Macpherson A 1994 Treatment of nonsteroidal antiinflammatory drug induced damage to the small and large intestine. In: Bayless T M (ed) Current therapy in gastroenterology and liver disease, 4th edn. Mosby, St Louis, pp 295–298

Bjarnason I, Williams P, So A et al 1984 Intestinal permeability and inflammation in rheumatoid arthritis: effects of non-steroidal anti-inflammatory drugs. Lancet ii: 1171–1174

Bjarnason I, Zanelli G, Smith T et al 1987a Nonsteroidal anti-inflammatory drug induced intestinal inflammation in humans. Gastroenterology 93: 480–489

Bjarnason I, Zanelli G, Prouse P et al 1987b Blood and protein loss via small intestinal inflammation induced by nonsteroidal antiinflammatory drugs. Lancet 2: 711–714

Bjarnason I, Price A B, Zanelli G et al 1988 Clinico-pathological features of NSAID induced small intestinal strictures. Gastroenterology 94: 1070–1074

Bjarnason I, Hayllar J, Smethurst P, Price A B, Gumpel M J 1992 Metronidazole reduces inflammation and blood loss in NSAID enteropathy. Gut 33: 1204–1208

Bjarnason I, Hayllar J, Macpherson A J, Russell A S 1993 Side effects of nonsteroidal anti-inflammatory drugs on the small and large intestine. Gastroenterology 104: 1832–1847

Dixon M J, O'Connor H J, Axon A T R, King R F J G, Johnston D 1986 Reflux gastritis: a distinct histopathological entity? Journal of Clinical Pathology 39: 524–530

Fellows I W, Clarke J M, Roberts P F 1992 Non-steroidal anti-inflammatory drug-induced jejunal and colonic diaphragm disease: a report of two cases. Gut 33: 1424–1426

Halter F, Weber B, Huber T, Eigenmann F, Frey M, Rutchi C 1993 Diaphragm disease of the ascending colon associated with sustained release diclofenac. Journal of Clinical Gastroenterology 16: 74–80

Huber T, Ruchti C, Halter F 1992 Nonsteroidal antiinflammatory drug-induced colonic strictures: a case report. Gastroenterology 100: 1119–1122

Johnson F 1987 Recurrent small bowel obstruction with piroxicam. British Journal of Surgery 74: 654

Kaufman H J, Taubin H L 1987 NSAID activate quiescent inflammatory bowel disease. Annals of Internal Medicine 107: 513–516

Lang J, Price A B, Levi A J, Burk M, Gumpel J M, Bjarnason I 1988 Diaphragm disease: the pathology of non-steroidal anti-inflammatory drug induced small intestinal strictures. Journal of Clinical Pathology 41: 516–526

Levi S, DeLacey G, Price A B, Gumpel M J, Levi A J, Bjarnason I 1990 'Diaphragm like' strictures of the small bowel in patients treated with non-steroidal anti-inflammatory drugs. British Journal of Radiology 63: 186–189

Madhok R, Mackenzie J A, Lee F D, Bruckner F E, Terry T R, Sturrock R D 1986 Small bowel ulceration in patients receiving NSAIDs for rheumatoid arthritis. Quarterly Journal of Medicine 58: 53–58

Monahan W, Starnes E C, Parker A L 1992 Colonic strictures in a patient on long-term non-steroidal anti-inflammatory drugs. Gastrointestinal Endoscopy 38: 385–386

Morris A J, Wasson L A, Mackenzie J F 1992 Small bowel enteroscopy in undiagnosed gastrointestinal blood loss. Gut 33: 887–889

Neoptolemos J P, Locke T J 1983 Recurrent small bowel obstruction associated with phenylbutazone. British Journal of Surgery 70: 244–245

Quinn C M, Bjarnason I, Price A B 1993 Gastritis in patients on non-steroidal anti-inflammatory drugs. Histopathology 23: 341–348

Rooney P J, Jenkins R T, Smith K M, Coates G 1986 ^{111}Indium-labelled polymorphonuclear scans in rheumatoid arthritis – an important clinical cause of positive results. British Journal of Rheumatology 15: 167–170

Segal A W, Isenberg D A, Hajirousow V, Tolfree S, Clark J, Snaith M L 1986 Preliminary evidence for gut involvement in the pathogenesis of rheumatoid arthritis? British Journal of Rheumatology 25: 162–166

Shack M E 1966 Drug induced ulceration of and perforation of the small bowel. Arizona Medical Journal 23: 517–523

Somasundaram S, Hayllar J, Rafi S, Wrigglesworth J, Macpherson A, Bjarnason I 1995 The biochemical basis of NSAID-induced damage to the gastrointestinal tract: a review and a hypothesis. Scandinavian Journal of Gastroenterology 30: 289–299

Sturges H F, Krone C L 1973 Ulcers and strictures of the jejunum in a patient on long term indomethacin therapy. American Journal of Gastroenterology 59: 162–169

Sukumar L 1987 Recurrent small bowel obstruction with piroxicam. British Journal of Surgery 74: 186

Taha A S, Nakshabendi I, Lee F D, Sturrock R D, Russell R I 1992 Chemical gastritis and *Helicobacter pylori* related gastritis in patients receiving non-steroidal anti-inflammatory drugs: comparison and correlation with peptic ulceration. Journal of Clinical Pathology 45: 135–139

Thomas W E G, Williamson M D 1985 Enteric ulceration and its complications. World Journal of Surgery 9: 876–886

Venturatos S G, Hines C, Blalock J B 1984 Ulceration of the small intestine in a patient with coeliac disease. Southern Medical Journal 77: 520–522

Wallace J L 1992 Non-steroidal anti-inflammatory drug gastropathy and cytoprotection: pathogenesis and mechanisms re-examined. Scandinavian Journal of Gastroenterology 27 (Suppl. 192): 3–8

Wallace J L, Granger D N 1992 Pathogenesis of NSAID gastropathy: are neutrophils the culprits? Trends in Pharmacological Science 13: 129–130

Whittle B J R 1992 Protective mechanisms of the gastric mucosa. In: Gustsavsson S, Kumar D, Graham D Y (eds) The stomach. Churchill Livingstone, Edinburgh, pp 81–101

50. Diverticular disease

B. T. Jackson

Colonic diverticula were first described in the mid-19th century by Cruveilhier (1849). The pathological complications that may be associated with them, however, were not established until the early 20th century (Telling & Gruner 1916–17). It is uncertain whether symptomatic diverticular disease is truly a condition of the last 100 years or whether it existed, unrecognized, in earlier times.

CLINICAL FEATURES

A distinction must be drawn between asymptomatic colonic diverticula – a condition often referred to as diverticulosis – and the symptoms and complications that may result if the diverticula become inflamed. When symptoms occur the condition is usually known as diverticulitis. This may present either electively in the outpatient clinic or, acutely, as an emergency.

Elective presentation

Typically the patient complains of left-sided lower abdominal pain, often associated with abdominal bloating and a change in bowel habit. Small, hard, round pellets of stool are said to be characteristic, the so-called 'rabbit-pellet stool'. Abdominal examination is usually normal or, at most, exhibits tenderness in the left iliac fossa. There is considerable overlap with the presentation of irritable bowel syndrome, often the only difference being the presence or absence of diverticula demonstrated by contrast radiology. Some authors even go so far as to doubt whether the condition of symptomatic, but uncomplicated, diverticular disease exists (Thompson 1986).

Less often, a patient presents electively with a fistula. Colovesical fistula presenting with recurrent attacks of cystitis, pneumaturia or occasionally fecaluria is more common than colovaginal, colocutaneous or coloenteric fistulae, all of which can occur. Crohn's disease is a differential diagnosis in all patients who present with a fistula.

Emergency presentation

Acute diverticulitis presents with severe left lower abdominal pain, nausea and vomiting associated with a fever, tachycardia, abdominal tenderness and guarding, leukocytosis and a raised ESR. The colon may perforate locally, causing a palpable mass in the left iliac fossa. If free perforation into the peritoneal cavity occurs the patient will have the signs of generalized peritonitis, and air may be seen beneath the diaphragm on erect abdominal radiography. Stricture formation is not uncommon but this rarely progresses to cause intestinal obstruction. If obstruction does develop a coexisting carcinoma should be suspected. Hemorrhage may occur and can be severe. Although bleeding is a recognized complication of diverticular disease there is evidence that the vascular malformation angiodysplasia accounts for the majority of severe colonic bleeds (Boley et al 1977, 1984). Bleeding from diverticular disease occurs mainly in elderly patients, is often unassociated with other symptoms, and is more common in the right colon (Allison et al 1982).

IMAGING

Plain abdominal radiography is rarely of value except in patients with perforated acute diverticulitis, when air may be seen beneath the diaphragm.

The mainstay of radiological investigation is a double contrast barium enema. This may show uncomplicated diverticula, typically localized to the left colon or, less commonly, occurring throughout the entire colon (Fig. 50.1). More advanced disease will cause a saw-tooth appearance, which may on occasion mimic Crohn's disease (Fig. 50.2). Sigmoid stricturing caused by pericolic fibrosis may closely simulate a carcinoma (Fig. 50.3), and is sometimes radiologically indistinguishable from malignancy. Endoscopy and biopsy will usually distinguish between these conditions, but surgical resection and histological examination of the stricture may be required. A small coexisting carcinoma may be difficult to demonstrate in

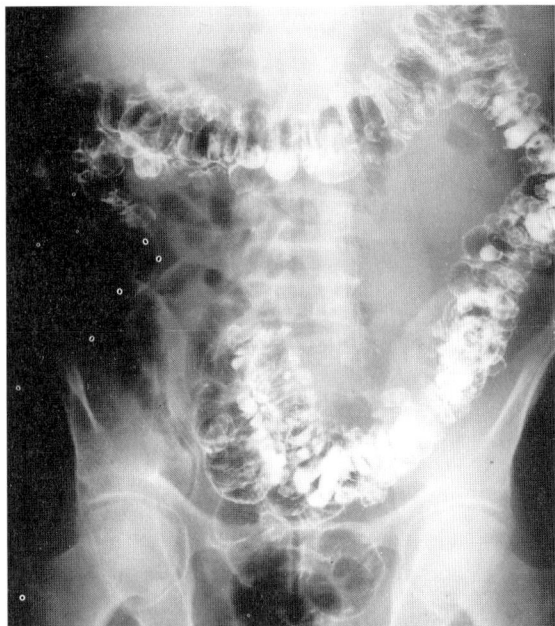

Fig. 50.1 Diverticular disease affecting the entire colon.

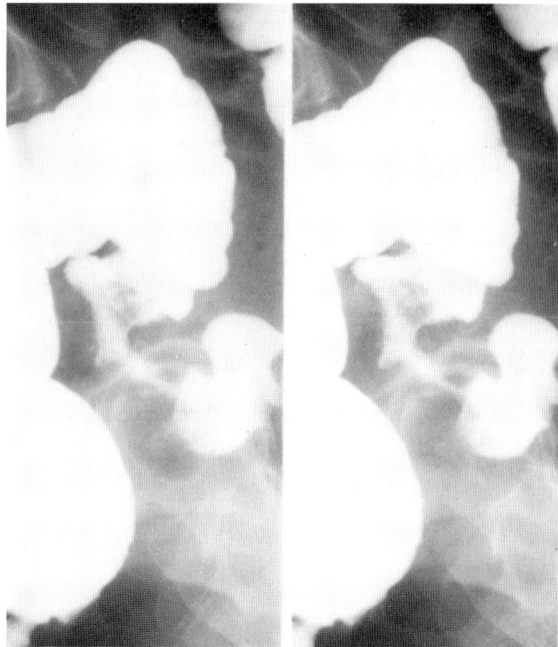

Fig. 50.3 A sigmoid stricture caused by diverticular disease but simulating carcinoma. Note the absence of obvious diverticula.

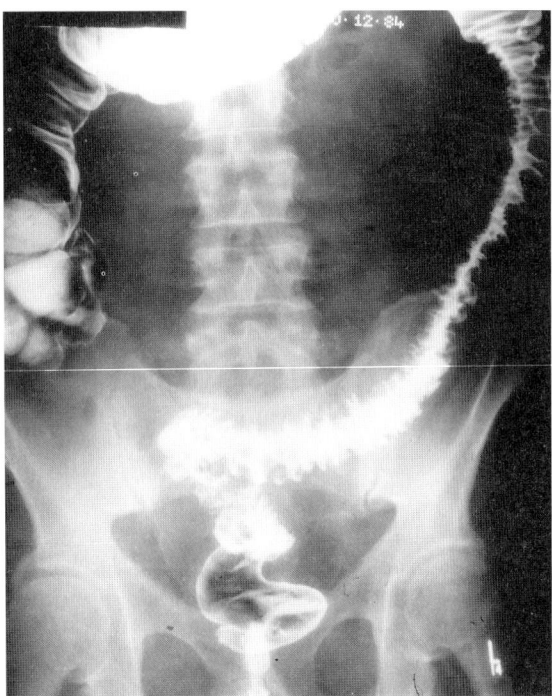

Fig. 50.2 Diverticular disease showing a saw-tooth appearance in the descending colon similar to the 'rosethorn' ulceration of Crohn's disease.

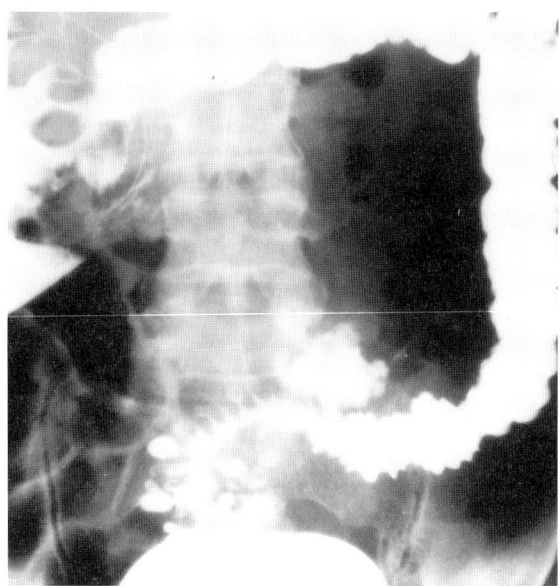

Fig. 50.4 A localized perforation in sigmoid diverticular disease.

sigmoid diverticular disease owing to distortion of the bowel and overlying loops of colon (Boulos et al 1985).

Extravasation of barium usually indicates a localized perforation (Fig. 50.4). Occasionally a fistula is outlined but cystoscopy is the investigation of choice in suspected cases of colovesical fistula. A long sinus is sometimes observed if infection tracks along tissue planes (Fig. 50.5).

Patients with continuing severe colonic bleeding may need visceral angiography to demonstrate the site of the bleeding before undergoing surgical operation (Baum et al 1973). If hemorrhage is less severe or intermittent, a radioactive ^{131}I-labeled red cell scan may localize the bleeding site (Berry et al 1988). Ultrasonography and CT scanning may be helpful in distinguishing between a pericolic abscess and a solid inflammatory mass in patients with acute diverticulitis (Schwerk et al 1992, McKee et al 1993).

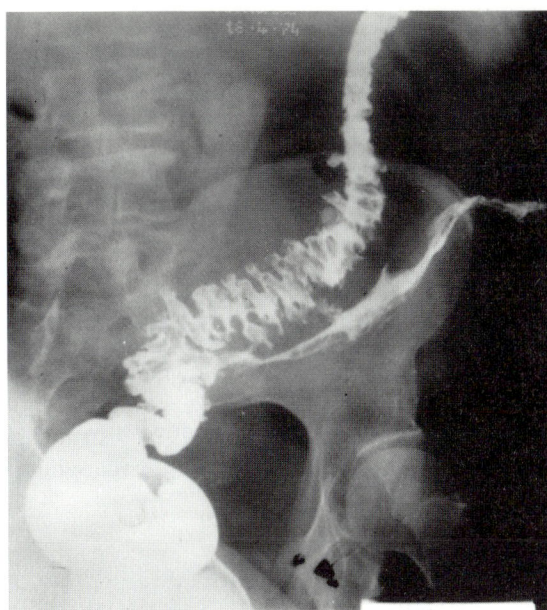

Fig. 50.5 Perforated sigmoid diverticular disease with a sinus extending into the lateral abdominal wall.

ENDOSCOPY

All patients should undergo sigmoidoscopy before a barium enema is performed in order to determine if rectal disease is present. Rigidity and fixity of the colon by symptomatic sigmoid diverticular disease may preclude the advancement of a rigid sigmoidoscope beyond the rectosigmoid junction, but a flexible instrument can usually be passed throughout the length of the sigmoid. Multiple diverticular openings may be seen within the lumen of the bowel.

Flexible endoscopy is essential if a stricture is shown on contrast radiology. Narrowing of the colonic lumen which fails to distend with introduced air suggests active diverticular disease. In contrast to malignancy, strictures caused by diverticular disease show no evidence of mucosal ulceration, but it may not be possible to observe more proximal pathology. Mucosal biopsy and brush cytology may be helpful in distinguishing between diverticular disease, Crohn's disease and carcinoma.

Total colonoscopy is normally indicated in patients with colonic hemorrhage to determine the source of the bleeding, but vision may be hampered by intraluminal blood (Boulos et al 1984).

PATHOLOGY

The prevalence of diverticula increases with age (Manousos et al 1967). However, there is a marked geographical variation, with a high prevalence in Europe and the USA and a virtual absence of the condition in many African and Asian countries. The prevalence in the UK is commonly said to be one-third of the population over the age of 60 (Parks 1968). There is no genetic or racial association, the differing prevalence being accounted for by different dietary habits. The site of the diverticula also has a geographical variation, with right-sided disease predominant in Japan and China, whereas sigmoid disease accounts for most symptomatic disease in the west (Sugihara et al 1984, Lee 1986). The rectum is never involved.

The etiology of colonic diverticula is generally accepted as being associated with a lifelong deficiency in dietary fiber (Heaton 1985). It is believed that such a diet results in a small stool, the propulsion of which requires a high intracolonic pressure over many years. The high pressure causes protrusion of the mucosa through weak areas of the sigmoid and descending colon. These weak areas occur at the site of blood vessels which penetrate the wall of the colon between the mesentery and the lateral taenia coli. However, structural changes in the colon that occur with increasing age may also play a part. It has been shown that aging is associated with a decreased tensile strength of the muscle fibers of the colon, this being most evident in the sigmoid and descending colon (Eastwood et al 1982). Furthermore, electron microscopy has shown that collagen fibers in the left colon are smaller than those in the right colon, and that this difference increases with age. The changes are more marked in patients with diverticular disease (Thompson et al 1987). There is also evidence that lack of exercise correlates with an increased risk for symptomatic diverticular disease (Aldoori et al 1995).

In addition to the mucosal protrusions through the wall of the colon, there is thickening of the circular muscle and the taenia. The elastin content of the taenia coli is increased by over 200%, which explains the concertina-like corrugations of the circular muscle (Whiteway & Morson 1985).

The cause of symptomatic diverticular disease is uncertain. Probably it is associated with feces becoming trapped in a diverticulum and causing mucosal ulceration and bacterial migration into the surrounding pericolic fat. An inflammatory process then results which, if long lasting, causes pericolic fibrosis. The penetrating artery of the colonic wall may be eroded and cause hemorrhage.

TREATMENT

It is possible that the regular intake of a high-fiber diet may prevent symptomatic diverticular disease (Heaton 1985) or even prevent the development of complications (Hyland & Taylor 1980). It is therefore sensible to suggest an increased intake of dietary fiber to patients with asymptomatic diverticular disease.

The treatment of painful diverticular disease consists principally of reassurance and explanation, together with a high-fiber diet (Painter 1975). This is most easily taken in the form of two tablespoons of natural unprocessed bran sprinkled on breakfast cereal. Coarse bran is a better fecal bulking agent than finely milled bran and is to be preferred, although it is less palatable (Kirwan et al 1974). Patients should be warned that an increase in colonic flatus may be a side effect. Antispasmodic agents such as mebeverine hydrochloride or propantheline bromide are also often prescribed. Surgical resection is rarely indicated.

Acute diverticulitis is treated with antimicrobials, including an agent that kills anerobic organisms such as metronidazole, analgesia and bed rest. Intravenous fluid and electrolyte replacement may be required. If complications develop more invasive treatment is indicated. A pericolic abscess requires drainage, which often can be carried out percutaneously using ultrasound or CT imaging to guide the drain (Hachigian et al 1992). Free perforation with peritonitis requires urgent laparotomy. A fistula requires elective surgical operation.

NATURAL HISTORY

Diverticular disease of the colon is common in the western world but only a minority of patients develop acute symptoms or complications. In most instances the disease runs a benign course, especially if a high dietary fiber intake is maintained (Parks 1969, 1975).

More than 80% of patients become symptom free after medical treatment of an episode of painful diverticular disease (Larson et al 1976), and despite the advanced age of many patients with complicated diverticular disease the immediate outcome of surgical operation is generally favorable (Tudor et al 1994). Not surprisingly, however, elderly patients who develop fecal peritonitis as a result of perforation have a poor prognosis unless operation is carried out within a very short time of the onset of symptoms.

Little is known about the long-term course of the disease after an episode of acute diverticulitis has been treated. Owing to the elderly age group concerned, many patients die of unrelated illness within a relatively short time of discharge from hospital. One study (Sarin & Boulos 1994) followed 164 patients admitted with acute diverticulitis or complications arising from it. Nine patients died (5%) and 11 were lost to follow-up. Of the remaining 144, the median follow-up period was 48 months (range 30–65 months). Thirty-nine patients (27%) died of unrelated causes and 13 (9%) were readmitted with further acute diverticular disease or its complications.

In another study (Farmakis et al 1994), 120 patients admitted with complicated diverticular disease were reviewed after a five-year follow-up. Twenty-nine (24%) had died from unrelated causes and 10 (8%) had died from recurrent complicated diverticular disease. Seventy patients were either asymptomatic at 5 years or had been so at their time of death from other causes. However, 40 (33%) patients remained sufficiently symptomatic to require medication. These authors argue in favor of elective surgical resection after the acute attack has settled with medical treatment. This opinion runs counter to the more traditional view that recurrent complicated diverticular disease is uncommon, and that the hazards of interval colectomy are not justified owing to the low risk of subsequent complications (Parks & Connell 1970, Sheppard & Keighley 1986, Jones 1992). Further population studies are needed before a consensus opinion can be given.

OVERLAP WITH CROHN'S DISEASE

The diagnosis of large-bowel Crohn's disease is usually straightforward but problems may arise if there is coexistent diverticular disease. It may be uncertain as to which of the conditions is causing symptoms, or occasionally the Crohn's disease may be unrecognized and the patient wrongly treated for diverticulitis. There is evidence that the complication rate is high in patients undergoing surgical operation for presumed diverticular disease when the diagnosis is actually Crohn's disease (Tchirkow et al 1983). Fortunately, the two conditions do not often coexist, Crohn's disease occurring in the elderly only infrequently.

The diagnosis of coexistent colonic Crohn's disease should be suspected if the symptoms are principally diarrhea and bleeding, as both of these are relatively uncommon in diverticular disease. Abdominal pain, a regular feature of diverticular disease, is unusual in Crohn's disease. The presence of anal disease such as fissures, fistulae or large edematous tags should always arouse suspicion of occult Crohn's disease (Lockhart-Mummery & Morson 1964). There is a marked female predominance in patients with combined Crohn's colitis and diverticular disease (Schmidt et al 1968).

The diagnosis of coexisting Crohn's colitis is usually made by rigid sigmoidoscopy and biopsy. However, although the rectum is often involved in large-bowel Crohn's disease this is by no means invariable. The disease can be segmental and confined to the colon. Rigid sigmoidoscopy is then inadequate to visualize the affected bowel and flexible sigmoidoscopy and biopsy are necessary. In patients with diverticular disease alone the colonic mucosa is seen to be intact, but ulceration will often be seen in patients with Crohn's disease.

REFERENCES

Aldoori W H, Giovannucci E L, Rimm E B et al 1995 Prospective study of physical activity and the risk of symptomatic diverticular disease in men. Gut 36: 276–282

Allison D J, Hemingway A P, Cunningham D A 1982 Angiography in gastrointestinal bleeding. Lancet ii: 30–33

Baum S, Rösch J, Dotter C T et al 1973 Selective mesenteric arterial infusions in the management of massive diverticular haemorrhage. New England Journal of Medicine 288: 1269–1272

Berry A R, Campbell W B, Kettlewell M G W 1988 Management of major colonic haemorrhage. British Journal of Surgery 75: 637–640

Boley S J, Brandt L J, Mitsudo S M 1984 Vascular lesions of the colon. Annals of Internal Medicine 29: 301–326

Boley S J, Sammartano R, Adams A, Dibiase A, Kleinhaus S, Sprayregen S 1977 On the nature and aetiology of vascular ectasias of the colon. Gastroenterology 72: 650–660

Boulos P B, Cowin A P, Karamanolis D G, Clark C G 1985 Diverticula, neoplasia or both? Early detection of carcinoma in sigmoid diverticular disease. Annals of Surgery 202: 607–609

Boulos P B, Karamanolis D G, Salmon P R, Clark C G 1984 Is colonoscopy necessary in diverticular disease? Lancet i: 95–113

Cruveilhier J 1849 Traité d'anatomie pathologique. Baillière, Paris

Eastwood M A, Watters D A K, Smith A N 1982 Diverticular disease – is it a motility disorder? Clinical Gastroenterology 11: 545–562

Farmakis N, Tudor R G, Keighley M R B 1994 The 5-year natural history of complicated diverticular disease. British Journal of Surgery 81: 733–735

Hachigian M P, Honickman S, Eisenstat T E, Rubin R J, Salvati E P 1992 Computed tomography in the initial management of acute left-sided diverticulitis. Diseases of the Colon and Rectum 35: 1123–1129

Heaton K W 1985 Diet and diverticulosis – new leads. Gut 26: 541–543

Hyland J M P, Taylor I 1980 Does a high fibre diet prevent the complications of diverticular disease? British Journal of Surgery 67: 77–79

Jones D J 1992 Diverticular disease. British Medical Journal 304: 1435–1436

Kirwan W O, Smith A N, McConnell A, Mitchell W D 1974 Action of different bran preparations on colonic function. British Medical Journal 4: 187–188

Larson D M, Master S S, Saro H M 1976 Medical and surgical therapy in diverticular disease. Gastroenterology 71: 734–736

Lee Y S 1986 Diverticular disease of the large bowel in Singapore. An autopsy survey. Diseases of the Colon and Rectum 29: 330–335

Lockhart-Mummery H E, Morson B C 1964 Crohn's disease of the large intestine. Gut 5: 493–509

McKee R F, Deignan R W, Krukowski Z H 1993 Radiological investigation in acute diverticulitis. British Journal of Surgery 80: 560–565

Manousos O N, Truelove S C, Lumsden K 1967 Prevalence of colonic diverticulosis in general population of the Oxford area. British Medical Journal 3: 762–763

Painter N S 1975 Diverticular disease of the colon. Heinemann, London

Parks T G 1968 Post-mortem studies on the colon with special reference to diverticular disease. Proceedings of the Royal Society of Medicine 61: 932–934

Parks T G 1969 Natural history of diverticular disease of the colon. A review of 521 cases. British Medical Journal 4: 639–642

Parks T G 1975 The natural history of diverticular disease of the colon. Clinical Gastroenterology 4: 53–69

Parks T G, Connell A M 1970 The outcome in 455 patients admitted for treatment of diverticular disease of the colon. British Journal of Surgery 57: 775–778

Sarin S, Boulos P B 1994 Long term outcome of patients presenting with acute complications of diverticular disease. Annals of the Royal College of Surgeons of England 76: 117–120

Schmidt G T, Lennard-Jones J E, Morson B C, Young A C 1968 Crohn's disease of the colon and its distinction from diverticulitis. Gut 9: 17–21

Schwerk W B, Schwarz S, Rothmund M D 1992 Sonography in acute colonic diverticulitis. A prospective study. Diseases of the Colon and Rectum 35: 1077–1084

Sheppard W A, Keighley M R B 1986 Audit of complicated diverticular disease. Annals of the Royal College of Surgeons of England 68: 8–10

Sugihara K, Muto T, Morioka Y, Asano A, Yamamoto T 1984 Diverticular disease of the colon in Japan – a review of 615 cases. Diseases of the Colon and Rectum 27: 521–537

Tchirkow G, Leveny I C, Fazio V W 1983 Crohn's disease in the elderly. Diseases of the Colon and Rectum 26: 177–181

Telling W G M, Gruner O C 1916–17 Acquired diverticula, diverticulitis and peri-diverticulitis of the large intestine. British Journal of Surgery 4: 468–530

Thompson H J, Busuttil A, Eastwood M A, Smith A N, Elton R A 1987 Submucosal collagen changes in normal colon and in diverticular disease. International Journal of Colorectal Disease 2: 208–213

Thompson W G 1986 Do colonic diverticula cause symptoms? American Journal of Gastroenterology 81: 613–614

Tudor R G, Farmakis N, Keighley M R B 1994 National audit of complicated diverticular disease: analysis of index cases. British Journal of Surgery 81: 730–732

Whiteway J, Morson B C 1985 Elastosis in diverticular disease of the sigmoid colon. Gut 26: 258–266

51. Diversion colitis
R. C. Evans

INTRODUCTION

An inflammatory process occurs in segments of colon which have been surgically excluded from the fecal stream, with rapid resolution on return to continuity. The presence of this inflammatory response was first recognized by Morson (Morson & Dawson 1972) and described by Glotzer, who introduced the term 'diversion-related colitis' (Glotzer et al 1981). The appearance of inflammation in an isolated segment of colon appears to be universal, but there is considerable variation in the time of onset after surgery, the extent of affected colon and its severity.

ETIOLOGY

The development of diversion colitis is independent of the pathology for which surgery was performed, and is seen following operations for conditions as diverse as inflammatory bowel disease, cancer, Hirchsprung's disease and the formation of a neovagina. Although the cause has been variously attributed to changes in bacterial flora or the development of pathogenic organisms, the strongest evidence is for a hypothesis linking the inflammatory response to deprivation of essential colonocyte nutrients. The colonic epithelium, unlike the small bowel, derives its respiratory fuel from the lumen in the form of short-chain fatty acids (SCFAs), of which the most important is believed to be butyrate (Scheppach 1994). SCFAs are derived from anerobic bacterial degradation of resistant starch and fiber (non-starch polysaccharide). It has been shown that not only is there a virtual absence of SCFAs in the diverted colon but remission of the disease can be obtained by instillation of physiological quantities of SCFAs into the affected segment (Harig et al 1989). In addition, analysis of changes in bacterial flora has revealed a reduction in strict anerobes and an increase in enterobacteria, which would lend support to this hypothesis (Neut et al 1989). It has been suggested that the variation in the severity of the disease could be explained on the basis of a difference in the ability of luminal bacteria to use other substrates, such as mucus, to form SCFAs. Pathogenic bacteria have not been isolated in this condition.

PRESENTATION

The majority of patients are asymptomatic, but may complain of bleeding, mucus discharge or pain, which can develop from a few months to over 10 years after surgery (Geraghty & Talbot 1991).

The condition is usually identified during endoscopic examination of the redundant colon and the features are variously reported as erythema, nodularity, friability, inflammatory polyps or aphthous ulceration. These features sometimes cause diagnostic difficulty, especially in patients with pre-existing ulcerative colitis or Crohn's disease. The inflammation may only affect the distal few centimeters of the rectum or extend throughout the isolated segment and stricture formation can occur. The appearances on barium examination range from mucosal nodularity/ulceration to inflammatory polyps (Glotzer et al 1981, Ma et al 1990, Haque et al 1993).

HISTOLOGY

There are no firm diagnostic criteria on histological examination in diversion colitis. In general the features are of a mild and non-specific inflammation which does not necessarily correlate to the clinical severity (Geraghty & Talbot 1991). The inflammation is confined to the mucosal layer, with crypt abscesses and mucin granulomas, although distortion of crypt architecture, if present, is mild and there is preservation of goblet cells. Follicular lymphoid hyperplasia is common and more florid than that seen in ulcerative colitis or Crohn's disease (Warren et al 1993). In severe cases, however, the findings are more likely to resemble those seen in ulcerative colitis.

MANAGEMENT

Although many cases go unnoticed, the finding of an inflamed redundant segment of colon may unnecessarily delay a restorative procedure. Where there has been no pre-existing inflammatory bowel disease and the endoscopic and/or pathological features are consistent with diversion colitis, the treatment of choice is restoration of continuity. If the clinical situation precludes surgery then butyrate enemas can be tried (Harig et al 1989). Steroids are unhelpful.

A difficult problem arises with the appearance of inflammation in a diverted segment when surgery has been undertaken for ulcerative colitis or Crohn's disease (Korelitz et al 1985). Histological features with mucosal inflammation alone and/or large lymphoid follicles would support a diagnosis of diversion colitis. A diagnostic trial of SCFA enemas can then be justified (Harig et al 1989).

In differentiating diversion colitis from ulcerative colitis the histological features of minimal crypt distortion, presence of goblet cells and large lymphoid follicles would again support a diagnosis of diversion colitis. Butyrate enemas have been shown to be effective in ulcerative colitis, which is associated with impaired SCFA metabolism, unlike Crohn's disease (Scheppach et al 1992). A comparison of the contrasting features between the three colitides is shown in Table 51.1.

Table 51.1 Differentiating features between diversion colitis, ulcerative colitis and Crohn's disease

	Diversion	Ulcerative	Crohn's
Follicular Lymphoid Hyperplasia	++	+	+
Crypt architecture distortion	–	++	+
Mucus depletion	–	++	+–
Steroid response	–	+	+
SCFA response	++	+	–

REFERENCES

Geraghty J M, Talbot I C 1991 Diversion colitis: histological features in the colon and rectum after defunctioning colostomy Gut 32: 1020–1023

Glotzer D J, Glick M E, Goldman H 1981 Proctitis and colitis following diversion of the faecal stream. Gastroenterology 80: 438–441

Haque S, Eisen R N, West A B 1993 The morphologic features of diversion colitis. Human Pathology 24: 211–218

Harig J M, Soergel K H, Komorowski R A et al 1989 Treatment of diversion colitis with short-chain-fatty acid irrigation. New England Journal of Medicine 320: 23–28

Korelitz B I, Cheskin L J, Soln N et al 1985 The fate of the rectal segment after diversion of the faecal stream in Crohn's disease. Journal of Clinical Gastroenterology 7: 37–43

Ma C K, Gotlieb C, Haas P A 1990 Diversion colitis: a clinicopathologic study of 21 cases. Human Pathology 21: 429–436

Morson B C, Dawson I M P 1972 Gastrointestinal pathology. Blackwell, London, p 485

Neut C, Colombel J F, Guillemot F et al 1989 Impaired bacterial flora in human excluded colon. Gut 30: 1094–1098

Scheppach W 1994 Effects of short chain fatty acids on gut morphology and function. Gut (Suppl 1): S35–S38

Scheppach W, Sommer H, Kirchner T et al 1992 Effect of butyrate enemas on the colonic mucosa in distal ulcerative colitis. Gastroenterology 103: 51–56

Warren B F, Shepherd N A, Bartolo D C C et al 1993 Pathology of the defunctioned rectum in ulcerative colitis. Gut 34: 514–516

52. Ileitis in the spondylarthropathies

M. De Vos H. Mielants C. Cuvelier

INTRODUCTION

A relationship between gut and joint pathology has long been recognized: as early as 1922 colectomy was proposed as treatment for rheumatoid arthritis (Smith 1922). It has become more and more evident that the gut plays a central role in the pathogenesis of many inflammatory arthritides (spondylarthropathies, blind loop syndrome, Whipple's disease, celiac disease). In other inflammatory joint diseases the gut is not primarily involved, but symptoms are due to inflammation of the mesenteric arteries with secondary vasculitic lesions (Henoch–Schönlein, rheumatoid arthritis, lupus erythematosus, periarteritis nodosa, scleroderma) or secondary to the intake of non-steroidal anti-inflammatory drugs (NSAIDs).

This chapter will concentrate on the evidence of intestinal inflammation in the spondylarthropathies.

SPONDYLARTHROPATHIES

Criteria

The concept of spondylarthropathy (SpA) was introduced by Wright and Moll in 1976 as 'seronegative polyarthritis'. Over the last two decades the concept has evolved into a distinct clinical entity, with specific classification criteria based on clinical observations, epidemiological, histological and genetic studies and radiographic evaluation (Dougados et al 1991) (Table 52.1). The absence of rheumatoid factor is a discriminating feature between SpA and rheumatoid arthritis (Wright & Moll 1976). However, overlap between the two entities has been reported. Rheumatoid nodules are characteristic for rheumatoid arthritis and are never found in SpA.

Locomotor manifestations

The locomotor manifestations are characterized by:

1. An axial involvement with the presence of inflammatory spinal pain (predominantly at night and at rest) in the dorsal or cervical region. The disease most commonly has an insidious onset before the age of 45, improves with exercise and is associated with morning stiffness. Limitation of movement in the lumbar and cervical region and reduced chest expansion are typical but not obligatory. Radiological evidence of sacroiliitis and spondylitis is frequent and includes squaring of the vertebrae, the presence of syndesmophytes and the development of arthritis of the lateral facet joints.
2. A peripheral inflammatory arthritis with a typical asymmetric pauciarticular pattern, with predominant involvement of the large and small joints of the lower limbs. Arthritis is mainly migratory and transient, resolving within 6–8 weeks. Recurrence is common. In rare cases arthritis becomes chronic and destructive
3. Enthesopathy, which is an inflammation of the insertion of the tendon, capsule or ligament to the bone. The insertions of the fascia plantaris and the Achilles tendon on the calcaneum, and/or the ligamentum patellae on the tibia are most frequently affected (Fig. 52.1).

Other features of the concept of spondylarthropathy are the clinical overlap between the different clinical entities that are encompassed (as will be described below) and its common association with other extraintestinal manifestations, such as uveitis, erythema nodosum and thrombophlebitis. Family studies have shown familial aggregation of the different clinical entities (Hochberg et al 1978, Mielants et al 1986b). The strong association of SpA with HLA B27 antigen supports the interrelationship between

Table 52.1 European Spondylarthropathy Study Group: criteria for classification of spondylarthropathy

Inflammatory spinal pain and/or asymmetric synovitis affecting lower limbs and one or more of following criteria:
Positive family history of SpA
Recent history of urethritis, cervicitis or acute diarrhea
Presence of alternating buttock pain, enthesopathy or sacroiliitis
Personal history of psoriasis or inflammatory bowel disease

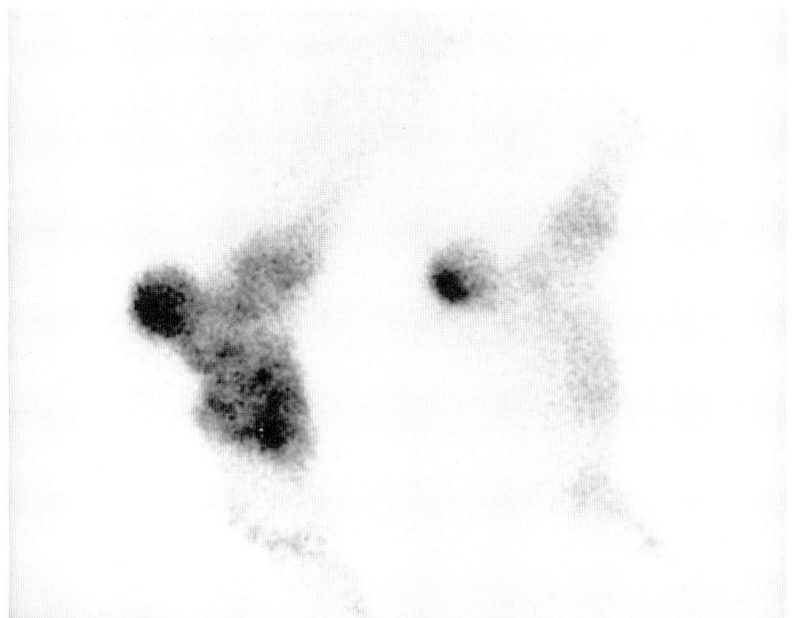

Fig. 52.1 A ^{99m}Tc dimethyl phosphonate scintigram of an enthesopathy with a bilateral inflammation of the fascia plantaris.

these different entities and suggests the participation of genetic factors in the etiopathogenesis of the disease. HLA B27 is particularly related to the presence of sacroiliitis and spondylitis.

Clinical entities

Several clinical entities are encompassed by the term spondylarthropathy: ankylosing spondylitis (AS), reactive arthritis (ReA), psoriatic arthritis, inflammatory bowel disease-related arthritis, some forms of juvenile chronic arthritis and a group of patients with undifferentiated SpA. The grouping of these clinical entities under one term is important because of a possible common etiopathogenetic role of the intestine and a similar treatment of the articular disease. For all these entities a relationship between gut and articular inflammation has been demonstrated.

Intestinal inflammation in spondylarthropathies

Enteropathic arthritis in inflammatory bowel disease (IBD)

The association between colitis and peripheral arthritis was first documented by Bargen in 1929 and the association with ankylosing spondylitis was recognized in 1958. Delineation of these two arthritic patterns was made by the Leeds group (Wright & Watkinson 1966).

Peripheral arthritis occurs in 15–20% of patients with Crohn's disease and 5–10% of patients with ulcerative colitis (Ansell & Wigley 1964, Haslock & Wright 1973, Münch et al 1986, Passo et al 1986). In both arthropathy seems to be related to the presence and the extent of colonic involvement (Greenstein et al 1976, Rankin et al 1979, Selby et al 1979, Moll 1985, Isdale & Wright 1989). The association between attacks of peripheral arthritis and relapses of bowel disease is most striking in ulcerative colitis (Gravallese & Kantrowitz 1988): colectomy can result in a complete articular remission (Wright & Watkinson 1965). In contrast, in Crohn's disease articular manifestations can precede intestinal symptoms by years (Haslock 1973). There is evidence that in some cases of SpA, Crohn's disease remains subclinical, joint and tendon inflammation being the only clinical manifestation of the disease (Mielants & Veys 1990). The simultaneous presence of other extraintestinal manifestations increases the susceptibility for arthritis (Greenstein et al 1976). The evolution of articular and intestinal disease are less clearly related in Crohn's disease than in ulcerative colitis. In Crohn's disease colectomy has no effect on arthritis (Isdale & Wright 1989).

The exact prevalence of sacroiliitis and spondylitis is difficult to estimate since the onset of this pathology is frequently insidious. Rates of 10–20% for sacroiliitis and 7–12% for spondylitis have been reported (Macrae & Wright 1973, Haslock & Wright 1973, Meuwissen et al 1978, Schorr-Resnick & Brandt 1988). Axial symptoms frequently precede overt bowel disease (Gravallese & Kantrowitz 1988). The clinical course is comparable with that of idiopathic AS and independent of the course of the bowel disease. Surgery has no effect on the axial disease (Dekker-Saeys et al 1978).

Pathology. Synovial fluid is sterile and consistent with an inflammatory arthritis, with a white cell count between 1500 and 50 000 cells/mm^3.

A limited number of histologic examinations of joint specimens have been performed, showing a non-specific synovitis (Bywaters & Ansell 1968, Soren 1966). Granulomatous non-erosive synovitis has also been described (Hermans et al 1984, Alh-Hadidi et al 1984, Toubert et al 1985).

HLA B27 association. In IBD-related arthritis association with HLA B27 antigen seems to be principally related to the presence of sacroiliitis and spondylitis: the prevalence of B27 in both populations is 5–38% and 30–75% respectively (Mallas et al 1976, Van den Berg-Loonen et al 1977, Huaux et al 1977). Although increased compared to a normal population (8%), these rates remain lower than in uncomplicated AS (90%). These data suggest that B27 increases the susceptibility to develop spondylitis and may operate in concert with an (as yet undefined) IBD gene to increase the likelihood of developing axial inflammation, but that the B27 gene is not a prerequisite (Khan et al 1980). An increased incidence of HLA B27–B44 association has been described in patients with Crohn's disease and AS (Purrmann et al 1988, Khan 1989). An increased prevalence of Bw62 has been reported in SpA with chronic gut inflammation as well as in patients with uncomplicated Crohn's disease (Mielants et al 1995b).

Enterogenic reactive arthritis

The term 'reactive arthritis' (ReA) has been proposed to describe aseptic arthritides developing soon after an infection elsewhere in the body (Ahvonen et al 1969, Aho & Leirisalo-Repo 1985). Reactive arthritis typically follows venereal (principally *Chlamydia trachomatis*) or enteric infections. The term 'Reiter's syndrome' implies the triad of arthritis, conjunctivitis or iritis and urethritis occurring either together or sequentially.

Dysenteric arthritis was already a well known disease in the 19th century. Poor hygienic conditions during World War I, with epidemic Shigella outbreaks, led to the classic observations of Reiter (1916). Arthritis was reported with a large epidemic of *Shigella flexneri* in 1948 (Paronen 1948). Later, Salmonella (Vairtiainen & Hurri 1964), *Yersinia enterocolitica* (Ahvonen et al 1969) and Campylobacter (Urmaen et al 1977) were also identified as arthritogenic agents. Arthritis associated with *Clostridium difficile* infection (Atkinson & McLeod 1988), *Giardia lamblia* (Woo & Panayi 1984) and Leptospira (Winter et al 1984) has also been reported, but their relationship with postenteric ReA remains to be determined. Septic arthritis cannot be excluded in some of these reports.

Postenteric arthritis is characterized by the abrupt onset of a peripheral arthritis 10–18 days after an infective episode with an arthritogenic microbe. These microorganisms have common features: they are invasive bacteria which penetrate into the epithelium, multiply intracellularly and produce inflammatory reactions.

Although arthritis usually develops 10–18 days after the intestinal infection, the interval may be as long as 3 months. The severity of the triggering infection has no influence on the presence or severity of joint symptoms: enteritis is often mild and sometimes asymptomatic. Diagnosis is made by recovering the microbe and/or by demonstrating antibody response. Joint symptoms usually take longer to subside than abdominal symptoms. Arthritis may become chronic in about 5% of cases. ReA is usually a non-destructive arthropathy, but erosive lesions have been described (Martel 1979, Mielants et al 1990). In these cases radiological differentiation from rheumatoid arthritis is only possible on the basis of the asymmetric and pauciarticular involvement of the joints.

Although back pain may occur in 30% of patients in the acute stage, sacroiliitis is only present in 6–9% most commonly in those with chronic or recurrent disease (Sairanen et al 1969, Maral et al 1981, Aho & Leirisalo-Repo 1985). Evolution to ankylosing spondylitis is rare but has been described in severe recurrent cases of ReA (Good 1979, Mielants et al 1995a).

Pathology. Synovial fluid is consistent with an inflammatory arthritis, with a white cell count between 4000 and 120 000 cells/ml. Although cultures are negative (Granfors et al 1989a, 1990, Merilahti-Palo et al 1991), the presence of microbial antigens has been demonstrated in the joints. In Yersinia-induced ReA, antigenic material was found in synovial fluid (Lahesmaa-Rantala et al 1987, Granfors et al 1989a) and in synovial membrane (Hammer et al 1990a). The presence of bacterial antigens in a synovial biopsy has been confirmed by immunohistology and immunoblotting for ReA secondary to *Yersinia enterocolitica* (Granfors et al 1989b, Merilahti-Palo et al 1991), *Salmonella enteritidis* and *typhimurium* (Granfors et al 1990), and *Chlamydia trachomatis* (Keat et al 1987, Schumacher et al 1988, Rahman et al 1992). Efforts to detect microbial DNA using polymerase chain reaction have been unsuccessful for enterogenic ReA (Toivanen et al 1990, Viitanen et al 1991) but successful for Chlamydia (Taylor-Robinson et al 1992). Persistance of virulent Yersinia in the intestinal mucosa and lymphatic tissue has been described in post-Yersinia ReA (De Koning et al 1989).

HLA B27 association. The prevalence of HLA B27 in ReA ranges between 60 and 80%. The presence of B27 increases 20–50 times the relative risk of developing ReA after an enteric bacterial infection (Aho 1989). Carriage of B27 influences not only the development of the disease but also its severity, extent and duration: B27-positive patients tend to have more severe disease and more axial symptoms (Leirisalo-Repo et al 1982).

Ankylosing spondylitis

Since the end of the 19th century AS has been recognized as a chronic inflammatory disorder affecting the axial skeleton and the large peripheral joints. Because of the insidious onset of the disease, clinical criteria have been proposed for its early diagnosis (Rome criteria: Kellgren et al 1963; New York criteria: Bennett & Burch 1968).

In addition to the well recognized association between AS and IBD, subclinical gut inflammation has been found in about 60% of AS patients (Mielants et al 1985, Cuvelier et al 1987, De Vos et al 1989, Simenon et al 1990, Leirisalo Repo et al 1994). In the largest study macroscopic lesions were rare (30%) and mostly confined to small erosions in the terminal ileum. In half the cases inflammation was only seen on microscopy, almost always in the ileum and ileocolon, and rarely in the colon alone (Cuvelier et al 1987, De Vos et al 1989). Lesions were not related to the intake of NSAIDs, since they were absent in patients with rheumatoid arthritis taking NSAIDs and present in AS patients not taking NSAIDs (De Vos et al 1989, Simenon et al 1990, Leirisalo-Repo et al 1994, Mielants et al 1995d). There was a strikingly high prevalence of gut lesions in patients were associated peripheral arthiritis. As long-term follow-up ileocolonoscopic studies demonstrated inflammation disappeared in all patients who went into clinical articular remission, but persisted in 68% of patients with persistent articular symptoms and associated peripheral arthritis. In patients with pure axial AS, gut histology returned to or remained normal (De Vos et al 1989, Mielants et al 1995c). In contrast, an evolution to full-blown IBD was observed in 10% of patients with AS associated with peripheral arthritis. These findings support a strong relationship between gut inflammation and the presence of peripheral arthritis, and illustrate the existence of overlaps between different entities of SpA.

Pathology. Histological study of intestinal biopsies in AS revealed two types of inflammation: in a minority of cases (12%) an acute inflammation was seen resembling an infectious enterocolitis, with a preserved normal mucosal architecture, infiltration of the epithelium with neutrophils and eosinophils, and infiltration of the lamina propria with polymorphonuclear cells (Fig. 52.2). More frequently (44% of patients) a chronic inflammation was found characterized by crypt distortion, villous blunting and fusion, increased mixed lamina propria cellularity and basal lymphoid aggregates in the lamina propria (Fig. 52.3). In some of these patients lesions were seen resembling early Crohn's disease, such as sarcoid granulomas, aphthoid ulcers and pyloric metaplasia (Cuvelier et al 1987, De Vos et al 1989). This chronic inflammation was more frequently associated with severe destructive joint lesions, principally of the hip (Mielants et al 1990) and with a higher risk of later evolution to full-blown IBD (De Vos et al 1994, Mielants et al 1995b).

HLA B27 association. The prevalence of HLA B27 antigen in AS patients is about 90%. Some clinical differences can be observed between B27-positive and B27-negative patients (Khan et al 1977, Linssen & Feltkamp 1988, Mielants et al 1993a). In HLA B27-negative patients, AS is later in onset; less frequently associated with acute anterior uveitis; more frequently associated with psoriasis and IBD; milder in course; without a tendency to familial aggregation. Moreover, subclinical chronic gut inflamma-

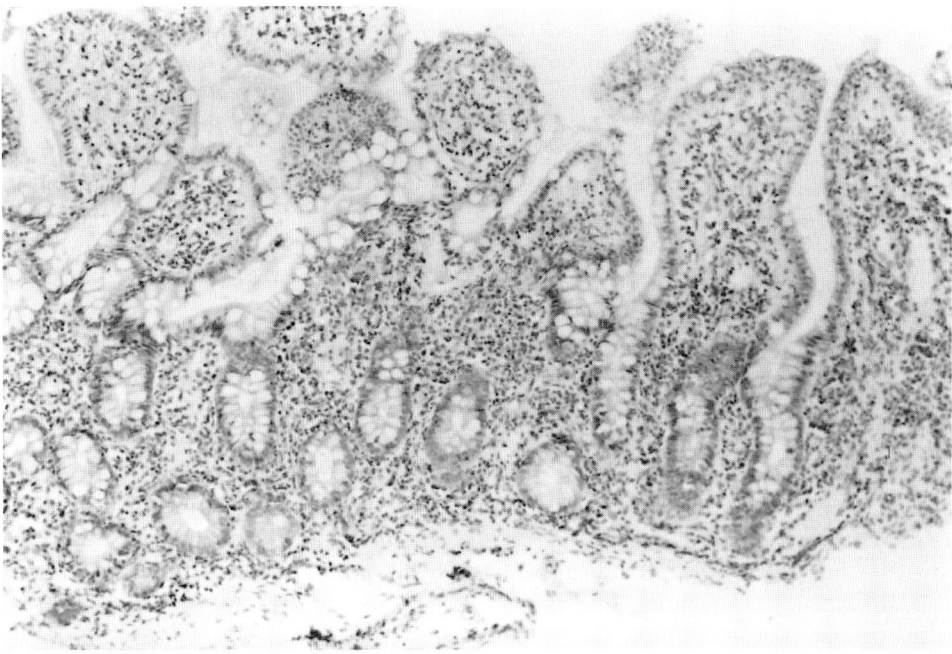

Fig. 52.2 Acute ileitis: the villus and crypt architectures are preserved. Villi are swollen by edema and increased mixed inflammatory cell infiltration featuring lymphocytes, plasma cells and polymorphonuclear cells. (Hematoxylin and eosin × 100)

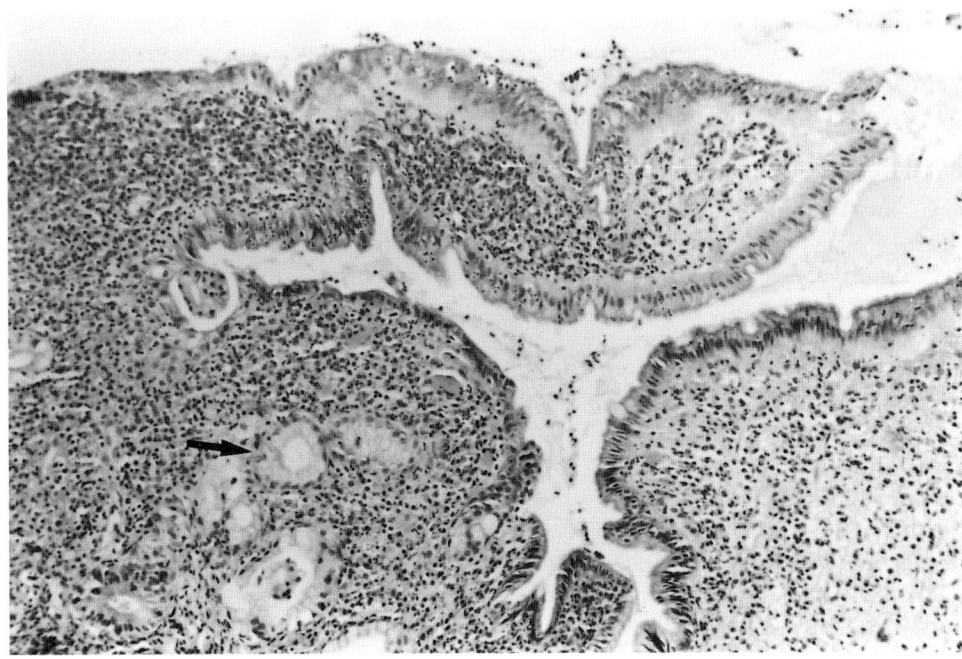

Fig. 52.3 Chronic ileitis: the villus and crypt architectures are altered. Villi are blunted, fused and irregular. Crypts are grouped and may show pseudopyloric metaplasia (arrow). The lamina propria shows a discontinuous inflammatory infiltrate consisting of mononuclear cells and granulocytes (Hematoxylin and eosin × 110)

tion is more frequently observed in B27-negative patients (De Vos et al 1989, Mielants et al 1993a).

Undifferentiated SpA

The term 'undifferentiated SpA' includes patients with the clinical, radiologic and genetic features of SpA who are not clearly classifiable into one of the known clinical entities (Hind 1982, Keat 1983, Burns & Calin 1984). This term includes patients who later develop a full clinical picture of associated disease, and also those with 'fruste' or overlap syndromes where the rheumatological diagnosis may be unclear.

Ileocolonoscopic studies in patients with undifferentiated SpA have demonstrated subclinical inflammation in 70% (Mielants et al 1985, Cuvelier et al 1987, De Vos et al 1989). Again, macroscopic lesions were rare (35%) and inflammation mostly confined to the terminal ileum. In a recent study of the long-term evolution of these patients 60% went into remission, 18% developed AS and 16% remained undifferentiated. Six percent developed rheumatoid arthritis and were probably initially misdiagnosed as SpA (Mielants et al 1995a).

Pathology. As in AS, histologic study of the subclinical gut inflammation revealed a similar distinction between acute and chronic inflammation (Cuvelier et al 1987). Both types were equally present and had no predictive value about the later evolution of the articular disease: clinical remission has been observed at a similar rate in the different histologic subgroups (De Vos et al 1994, Mielants et al 1995b). In contrast, evolution to full-blown IBD has only been observed in patients with initial chronic gut inflammation.

Repeat ileocolonoscopic studies demonstrated persistent active gut inflammation in 41% of patients with persistent active joint disease. All except one evolved to AS with peripheral arthritis. No gut inflammation appeared in patients with an initial normal histology, suggesting at least two different groups of undifferentiated SpA: one having a definite relation with gut pathology and another undefined group (De Vos et al 1994, Mielants et al 1995c).

HLA B27 association. In patients with undifferentiated SpA the prevalence of B27 is similar to that found in ReA (Mielants et al 1987). An increased prevalence of Bw62 has been observed in patients with associated chronic gut inflammation (Mielants et al 1987).

Psoriatic arthritis

Although psoriatic arthritis was described in 1818 (Alibert 1818), it was only recognized as a distinct articular disease in the middle of this century (Baker et al 1963). The classification criteria proposed by Moll and Wright in 1973 are widely accepted and distinguish five types of arthritis: distal interphalangeal arthritis, arthritis mutilans, symmetric polyarthritis, oligoarticular arthritis and axial involvement. Recognition of distal interphalangeal arthritis as a separate entity has been contested because this joint involvement is seen in all subgroups (Torre et al 1991).

As in other forms of SpA, evidence of subclinical gut inflammation has recently been reported (Schatteman et al 1995). However, the incidence was lower: macroscopic lesions were seen in only 11% of patients and microscopic inflammation in 15%. Inflammation was predominantly observed in patients with oligoarthritis (20%) and in patients with axial involvement (30%), and not in patients with polyarthritis.

Pathology. The inflammatory nature of psoriatic arthritis, the cellular infiltrates in skin and joint lesions and the deposits of immunoglobulins on epidermis support an immune mechanism (Gladman 1992). In the gut, acute and chronic inflammation as described in ReA and AS have been observed (Schatteman et al 1995).

HLA B27 association. The prevalence of B27 is increased only in patients with psoriatic arthritis and axial involvement (65%) and in patients with oligoarticular involvement (60%) (Gladman et al 1986). An increased incidence of HLA Bw62 in both subgroups of psoriatic arthritis has also been observed. These findings support the suggestion that both subgroups of psoriatic arthritis belong to the concept of spondylarthropathies, and that the gut plays a role in the etiopathogenesis, although less frequently than in other forms of SpA.

Juvenile chronic arthritis

The diagnosis of juvenile chronic arthritis (JCA) implies the presence of an arthritis in one or more joints for at least 3 months and before the age of 16 years. Several subtypes exist (EULAR classification) (Ansell 1978). One of these subtypes, with a late onset (after age of 9 years) and a strong asymmetric pauciarticular involvement of the joints, belongs to the concept of SpA. It predominantly affects males and is associated with HLA B27. Arthritis of the hip and sacroiliitis are frequent in the initial phase of the disease as well as during evolution. Diagnosis of AS is often impossible because of difficulties in the radiological interpretation of the sacroiliac joints in childhood. In this subgroup of late-onset JCA a high incidence (75%) of subclinical gut inflammation has been found (Mielants et al 1993b), confirming previous findings in adult SpA patients with a juvenile onset (Mielants et al 1987). A strong relationship has been observed between the persistence of joint or axial inflammation and the perpetuation of the gut inflammation.

Pathology. A similar incidence of acute and chronic inflammation has been observed in patients with late-onset JCA (Mielants et al 1993b). However, during further evolution in these patients only chronic lesions have been found, always associated with persistent inflammation of the locomotor system. Morever, this chronic inflammation has been related to axial complaints, the presence of sacroiliitis and evolution to AS. Evolution to full-blown IBD has been observed in some patients.

HLA B27 association. As with the other entities of SpA, HLA B27 antigen is frequently present in this subgroup of patients with JCA (Schaller et al 1976, Veys et al 1976).

Etiopathogenetic considerations

The close relationship observed between joint and gut inflammation in all forms of SpA and the high prevalence of the B27 phenotype are two important clues in the development of a common etiopathogenetic hypothesis. Two different, partially complementary, working hypotheses have been proposed.

Infective agents act as primary triggers. *Specific bacterial–host interactions between enterobacteria and HLA B27 as the initiating events.* Although no specific arthritogenic antigen has so far been found, several bacterial fragments may be responsible. Lipopolysaccharides (LPS), major surface components of all known arthritis causing microorganisms, are the prime candidates. Fractions of bacterial LPS have been found in the inflamed joints of patients with ReA (Granfors et al 1989b, 1990, Gronberg et al 1989, Merilahti-Palo 1991, Viitanen et al 1991). These fragments are always in a highly processed form but conserve their immunostimulating effects (Granfors 1992). A strong IgA response directed against LPS has been found in patients with Yersinia- and Shigella-triggered ReA (Granfors et al 1989a) and a strong IgM, IgG and IgA response in Salmonella-triggered ReA (Mäki-Ikola 1992).

Another intriguing bacterial candidate is *Klebsiella pneumoniae*. Although some authors have found an increased fecal Klebsiella carriage in patients with active AS (Ebringer et al 1977, 1978), other studies, using highly sensitive culture media, failed to confirm differences in isolation rates between AS and normal controls (Van Kregten et al 1991). Specific anti-Klebsiella antibodies have been reported during the acute phase of the disease (Trull et al 1983). Furthermore, an amino acid sequence has been identified in some *Klebsiella* species identical to a sequence of HLA B27.1 (now B*2705) (Schwimmbeck et al 1987). Antibodies to this shared sequence were found in the sera of AS patients (Schwimmbeck et al 1987). A reaction between rat antisera raised against Klebsiella amino acid sequence and synovial biopsies obtained from B27-positive patients has been demonstrated (Husby et al 1989). Other researchers have been unable to detect similar differences in cross-reactive antibodies in sera from AS and ReA patients and healthy blood donors (Tsuchiya et al 1989, De Vries et al 1990). The role of the B27 molecule in the pathogenesis of SpA has been investigated by introducing B27 and human $\beta 2$ microglobulin genes into rats (Hammer et al 1990b). Rats of two transgenic lines developed a multiorgan disease that included the gastrointestinal tract, peripheral and central joints, genital tract, skin, nails and heart. The most prevalent site of involvement appeared to be the gastrointestinal tract, with inflammation similar to that found in humans with SpA. Neither gastrointestinal nor joint lesions were observed in germ-free animals, supporting the strong relation between intestinal and joint disease (Breban et al 1994).

There have been general explanations proposed to account for the strong association between HLA B27 and SpA. The molecular mimicry hypothesis suggests that antimicrobial antibodies cross-react with B27 antigen because of antigenic homology (Ebringer et al 1976, Welsh et al 1980, van Bohemen et al 1984, Ebringer 1992) as discussed above for Klebsiella. The arthritogenic peptide model proposes that bacterial peptides prime a cytotoxic lymphocyte (CTL) response when presented by HLA B27. This CTL response cross-reacts with a structurally similar peptide derived from normal spinal tissue, which is also presented by the HLA B27 molecule (Khan 1992). However, bacterial infections usually do not generate cytotoxic lymphocytes but T-cell MHC class II-restricted responses. Therefore, this hypothesis requires an additional hypothesis that B27 molecules have an unusual antigen-presenting property. Recent studies of the binding of synthetic peptides to MHC class I molecules support this idea (Benjamin & Parham 1992).

Infective agents only perpetuate the disease. An excessive absorption of luminal factors induces an immunocascade responsible for gut inflammation and extraintestinal manifestations. This hypothesis is supported by the high incidence of subclinical gut inflammation and the evidence of an increased intestinal permeability (Smith et al 1985, Serrander et al 1986, Wendling et al 1990, Mielants et al 1991). This increase in permeability can be induced by drugs, by the disease itself or by genetic determinants. The inflammation can be an appropriate reaction to absorbed known and unknown antigens, or inappropriate and related to defective local immunoregulatory mechanisms. Indirect evidence for increased antigen handling is found in the terminal ileum of SpA patients: MHC class II antigen (HLA DR) expression is increased (Cuvelier et al 1990) the number of membranous (M) cells is elevated, and ruptures of these cells can be observed at the top of the lymphoid follicles (Cuvelier et al 1994). These interruptions in the gut epithelial lining can facilitate the access of the luminal content to the lymphoid tissue and stimulate T and B cell-mediated responses with activation of cytokine production and complement cascade. These phenomena could be sufficient to initiate joint inflammation in genetically predisposed patients.

Treatment

If bacterial antigens are part of the etiopathogenetic mechanism, antibiotic treatment against triggering infection can be considered. However, evidence of efficacy is lacking: antibiotic treatment is usually considered inefficient (Popert et al 1964, Stein et al 1980, Marsal et al 1981, Fryden et al 1990), although recent reports suggest a significant decrease in severity and duration of Chlamydia arthritis (Lauhio et al 1991, Leirisalo-Repo & Repo 1992). No beneficial effect has been reported in enteric ReA. So far the effects of long-term treatment have not been explored.

Symptomatic treatment of peripheral arthritis with NSAIDs and cautious use of local glucocorticoids is usually sufficient.

Sulfasalazine has been found effective in the treatment of the peripheral manifestations of AS (Nissila et al 1988) especially when gut inflammation is present (Mielants & Veys 1985, Zwillich et al 1988), in the treatment of ReA (Mielants et al 1986, Trnansky et al 1988) and in undifferentiated SpA (Mielants et al 1986a). Furthermore, sulfasalazine seems to have a beneficial effect on the clinical evolution of SpA, probably by healing the gut inflammation. However, it does not seem to prevent the evolution of undifferentiated Spa into full-blown IBD (De Vos et al 1994, Mielants et al 1995d).

Oral corticosteroids have minimal effect on the peripheral synovitis and no effect on the axial joint involvement. In IBD they should be used only as necessary to control the bowel disease.

Prognosis

The long-term prognosis of SpA is generally good. A number of prospective studies have confirmed the high remission rate in ReA (Sairanen et al 1969, Amor 1979, Good 1979, Leirisalo et al 1982, Leirisalo-Repo & Suoranta 1988, Herrlinger & Asmussen 1992): only about 20% of patients develop a chronic articular disease (Keat 1983). The prognosis seems better for the enterogenic forms (Sairanen et al 1969, Leirisalo-Repo et al 1987, Bremell et al 1991, Lindholm & Viskorpi 1991) than for urogenital ReA. Many authors also described a good prognosis for AS (Carette et al 1983, Mau et al 1988, Mielants et al 1995a). Others found a long-term remission in only 1% of patients (Kennedy et al 1993). This study concerned the evolution of non-treated patients; recent data on drug-treated patients give a remission rate of 20% (Mielants, unpublished data). A deterioration of radiological involvement has been observed in 17–23% of patients (Good 1979, Leirisalo et al 1982, Leirisalo-Repo & Suoranta 1988, Lindholm & Viskorpi 1991, Mielants et al 1995a). Most authors correlate the presence of HLA B27 with a poorer prognosis.

Transition between different forms of SpA has been observed: an evolution from ReA to AS has been found in 2–20% of patients, mostly in those who are B27-positive (Good 1979, Costello et al 1980, Leirisalo et al 1982, Leirisalo-Repo 1987, Lindholm & Viskorpi 1991, Bremell et al 1991, Herrlinger & Asmussen 1992, Mielants et al 1995a). Evolution from asymptomatic gut inflammation to full-blown IBD has been demonstrated in 6% of patients, always associated with an articular evolution to AS and unrelated to the presence of B27 (De Vos et al 1994, Mielants et al 1995a).

REFERENCES

Aho K 1989 Bowel infection predisposing to reactive arthritis. Baillière's Clinical Rheumatology 3: 303–319

Aho K, Leirisalo-Repo M 1985 Reactive arthritis. In Panayi G S (ed) Clinics in rheumatic diseases: the seronegative spondylarthropathies. W B Saunders Company, London, pp 25–40

Ahvonen P, Sievers K, Aho K 1969 Arthritis associated with *Yersinia enterocolitica* infection. Acta Rheumatologica Scandinavica 15: 323–332

Alh-Hadidi S, Khatib G, Chlatwal P, Khatib R 1984 Granulomatous arthritis in Crohn's disease. Arthritis and Rheumatism 27: 1061–1062

Alibert J L 1818 Précis théorique sur les maladies de la peau. Caille et Ravier, Paris

Amor B 1979 Reiter's syndrome: long-term follow-up data. Annals of Rheumatic Diseases 38 (Suppl): 32–33

Ansell B M 1978 Diagnostic criteria, nomenclature and classification. In: Munthe E (ed) The case of rheumatic children. Eular, Basel, pp 42

Ansell B M, Wigley R A D 1964 Arthritis manifestations in regional enteritis. Annals of Rheumatic Diseases 23: 64–72

Atkinson M H, McLeod B D 1988 Reactive arthritis associated with *Clostridium difficile* enteritis. Journal of Rheumatology 15: 520–522

Baker H, Golding D N, Thompson M 1963 Psoriasis and arthritis. Annals of Internal Medicine 58: 909–925

Bargen J A 1929 Complications and sequelae of chronic ulcerative colitis. Annals of Internal Medicine 3: 335–352

Benjamin B, Parham P 1992 HLA-B27 and disease: a consequence of inadvertent antigen presentation? Rheumatic Diseases Clinics of North American 18: 11–21

Bennett P H, Burch T A 1968 The epidemiological diagnosis of ankylosing spondylitis. In: Bennett P H, Wood P H N (eds) Population studies of the rheumatic diseases. Excerpta Medica New York, pp 305

Breban M, Hadavand R, Montanez S, Richardson J D, Hammer R E, Taurog J D 1994 HLA-B27 transgenic rats. Clinical and Experimental Rheumatology 12: 97–116

Bremell T, Bjelle A, Svedhem A 1991 Rheumatic symptoms following an outbreak of *Campylobacter* enteritis: a five year follow-up. Annals of the Rheumatic Diseases 30: 934–938

Burns T M, Calin A 1984 Undifferentiated spondylarthropathy. In: Calin A (ed) Spondylarthropathies. Grune & Stratton, Orlando, pp 253–264

Bywaters E G L, Ansell B M 1958 Arthritis associated with ulcerative colitis. Annals of Rheumatic Diseases 17: 169–183

Carette S, Graham D, Little H, Rubenstein J, Rosen P 1983 The natural disease course of ankylosing spondylitis. Arthritis and Rheumatism 26: 186–189

Costello P B, Alea J A, Kennedy A C, McCluskey R T, Green F A 1980 Prevalence of occult inflammatory bowel disease in ankylosing spondylitis. Annals of Rheumatic Diseases 39: 453–456

Cuvelier C, Barbatis C, Mielants H, De Vos M, Veys E, Roels H 1987 The histopathology of intestinal inflammation in relation to reactive arthritis. Gut 28: 394–402

Cuvelier C, Mielants H, De Vos M, Veys E M, Roels H 1990 Major histocompatibility class II antigen (HLA-DR) expression by ileal epithelial cells in patients with seronegative spondylarthropathies. Gut 31: 545–549

Cuvelier C A, Quatacker J, Mielants H, De Vos M, Veys E, Roels H J 1994 M-Cells are damaged and increased in number in inflamed human ileal mucosa. Histopathology 24: 417–426

Dekker-Saeys B J, Meuwissen S G M, van den Berg-Loonen E M, De Haas W H D, Agenant D, Tytgat G N J 1978 Prevalence of peripheral arthritis, sacroiliitis and ankylosing spondylitis in patients suffering from inflammatory bowel disease. Annals of Rheumatic Diseases 37: 33–35

De Koning J, Heesemann J, Hoogkamp-Korstanje J A A, Festen J J M, Houtman P M, Van Oijen P L M 1989 Yersinia in intestinal biopsy specimens from patients with seronegative spondylarthropathy: correlation with specific serum IgA antibodies. Journal of Infectious Diseases 159: 109–112

De Vos M, Cuvelier C, Mielants H, Veys E, Barbier F, Elewaut A 1989 Ileocolonoscopy in seronegative spondylarthropathy. Gastroenterology 96: 339–344

De vos M, Mielants H, Cuvelier C, Veys E, Elewaut A 1994 Long-term evolution of patients with spondylarthropathy and gut inflammation. Gastrotenterology 106: A671

De Vries D D, Dekker-Saeys A J, Gyodi E et al 1990 Failure to detect cross-reacting antibodies to HLA B27.5 and Klebsiella nitrogenase in sera from patients with ankylosing spondylitis and Reiter's syndrome. Scandinavian Journal of Rheumatology 87 (Suppl): 72–73

Dougados M, Van Der Linden S, Juhlin R et al 1991 The European Spondylarthropathy Study Group preliminary criteria for the classification of spondylarthropathy. Arthritis and Rheumatism 34: 1218–1227

Ebringer A 1992 Ankylosing spondylitis is caused by Klebsiella. Rheumatic Diseases Clinics of North America 18: 105–121

Ebringer R, Cooke D, Cawdell D R et al 1977 Ankylosing spondylitis: Klebsiella and HLA-B27. Rheumatology and Rehabilitation 16: 190–196

Ebringer A, Cowling P, Ngwa Suh N et al 1976 Cross-reactivity between *Klebsiella aerogenes* species and HLA-B27 lymphocyte antigens as an aetological factor in ankylosing spondylitis. In: Dausset Y, Svejgaard A (eds) HLA and diseases. Inserm, Paris, 58: 27

Ebringer R W, Cawdell D R, Cowling P, Ebringer A 1978 Sequential studies in ankylosing spondylitis. Association of *Klebsiella pneumoniae* with active disease. Annals of Rheumatic Diseases 37: 146–151

Frydén A, Bengtsson A, Foberg U et al 1990 Early antibiotic treatment of reactive arthritis associated with enteric infections: clinical and serological study. British Medical Journal 301: 1299–1302

Gladman D D 1992 Psoriatic arthritis: recent advances in pathogenesis and treatment. Rheumatic Diseases Clinics of North America 18: 247–256

Gladman D D, Anhorn K A B, Schachter R K, Mervart H 1986 HLA antigens in psoriatic arthritis. Journal of Rheumatology 13: 586–592

Good A E 1979 Reiter's syndrome: Long-term follow-up in relation to development of ankylosing spondylitis. Annals of Rheumatic Diseases 38(Suppl): 39–45

Granfors K 1992 Do bacterial antigens cause reactive arthritis? Rheumatic Diseases Clinics of North America 18: 37–48

Granfors K, Jalkanen S, von Essen R et al 1989a Yersinia antigens in synovial fluid cells from patients with reactive arthritis. New England Journal of Medicine 320: 216–221

Granfors K, Ogasawara M, Hill J L, Lahesmaa-Rantala R, Toivanen A, Yu D T 1989b Analysis of IgA anti-lipopolysaccharide antibodies in Yersinia-triggered reactive arthritis. Journal of Infectious Diseases 159: 1142–1147

Granfors K, Jalkanen S, Lindberg A A et al 1990 Salmonella lipopolysaccharide in synovial cells from patients with reactive arthritis. Lancet 335: 685–688

Gravallese E M, Kantrowitz F G 1988 Arthritic manifestations of inflammatory bowel disease. American Journal of Gastroenterology 83: 703–709

Greenstein A J, Janowitz H D, Sachar D B 1976 The extraintestinal complications of Crohn's disease and ulcerative colitis: a study of 700 patients. Medicine (Baltimore) 55: 401–412

Gronberg A, Fryden A, Kihlstrom E 1989 Humoral immune response to individual *Yersinia enterolitica* antigens in patients with and without reactive arthritis. Clinical and Experimental Immunology 76: 361–365

Hammer M, Zeidler H, Klisma S, Heeseman J 1990a *Yersinia enterocolitica* in the synovial membrane of patients with Yersinia-induced arthritis. Arthritis and Rheumatism 33: 1795–1800

Hammer R E, Maika S D, Richardson T A, Tang J P, Taurog J 1990b

Spontaneous inflammatory diseases in transgenic rats expressing HLA-B27 and human β2 microglobulin in animal model for B27 associated human disorders. Cell 63: 1099–1112

Haslock I 1973 Arthritis and Crohn's disease – a family study. Annals of Rheumatic Diseases 32: 479–486

Haslock I, Wright V 1973 The musculo-skeletal problems of Crohn's disease. Medicine (Baltimore) 52: 217–225

Hermans P J, Fievez M L, Descamps C L, Aupaiz M A 1984 Granulomatous synovitis and Crohn's disease. Journal of Rheumatology 11: 710–712

Herrlinger J D, Asmussen J U 1992 Long term prognosis in Yersinia arthritis: clinical and serological findings. Annals of Rheumatic Diseases 51: 1332–1334

Hind C R K 1982 Reactive arthritis. Postgraduate Medical Journal 58: 131–137

Hochberg M C, Bias W B, Arnett F C 1978 Family studies in HLA-B27 associated arthritis. Medicine 57: 463

Huaux J P, Fiasse R, De Bruyere M et al 1977 HLA-B27 in regional enteritis with and without ankylosing spondylitis or sacroiliitis. Journal of Rheumatology 4 (Suppl 3): 60–63

Husby G, Tsuchiya N, Schwimmbeck P L et al 1989 Cross-reactive epitope with *Klebsiella pneumoniae* nitrogenase in articular tissue of HLA-B27 positive patients with ankylosing spondylitis. Arthritis and Rheumatism 32: 437–445

Isdale A, Wright V 1989 Seronegative arthritis and the bowel. Baillière's Clinical Rheumatology 3: 285–301

Keat A, Dixey J, Sonnex C et al 1987 *Chlamydia trachomatis* and reactive arthritis: the missing link. Lancet 1: 72–74

Keat A E 1983 Reiter's syndrome and reactive arthritis in perspective. New England Journal of Medicine 309: 1606–1616

Kellgren J H, Jeffrey M R, Ball J 1963 The epidemiology of chronic rheumatism. Blackwell Scientific, Oxford, p 326

Kennedy L G, Edmond L, Calin A 1993 The natural history of ankylosing spondylitis. Does it burn? Journal of Rheumatology 20: 688–692

Khan M A 1989 HLA-B27 and B12 (B44) in Crohn's disease with ankylosing spondylitis. Journal of Rheumatology 16: 851–852

Khan M A 1992 An overview of clinical spectrum and heterogeniety of spondylarthropathies. Rheumatic Diseases Clinics of North America 18: 1–10

Khan M A, Kushner I, Braun W E 1977 Comparison of clinical features of HLA-B27 positive and negative patients with ankylosing spondylitis. Arthritis and Rheumatism 20: 909–912

Khan M A, Kushner I, Braun W 1980 Genetic heterogeneity in primary ankylosing spondylitis. Journal of Rheumatology 7: 383–386

Lahesmaa-Rantala R, Gransfors K, Isomaki H, Toivanen A 1987 Yersinia specific immune complexes in the synovial fluid of patients with Yersinia triggered reactive arthritis. Annals of Rheumatic Diseases 46: 510–514

Lauhio A, Leirisalo-Repo M, Lähdevirta J et al 1991 Double-blind, placebo-controlled study of three-month treatment with lymecycline in reactive arthritis, with special reference to Chlamydia arthritis. Arthritis and Rheumatism 34: 6–14

Leirisalo M, Skylv G, Kousa M et al 1982 Follow-up study on patients with Reiter's disease and reactive arthritis with special reference to HLA B27. Arthritis and Rheumatism 25: 249–259

Leirisalo-Repo M, Repo H 1992 Gut and spondyloarthropathies. Rheumatic Diseases Clinics of North America 18: 23–35

Leirisalo-Repo M, Suoranta H 1988 Ten-year follow-up study of patients with Yersinia arthritis. Arthritis and Rheumatism 31: 533–537

Leirisalo-Repo M, Skylv G, Kousa M 1987 Follow-up of Reiter's disease and reactive arthritis. Factors influencing the natural course and the prognosis. Clinical Rheumatology 6 (Suppl 2): 73–82

Leirisalo-Repo M, Turunen U, Stenman S, Helenius P, Seppälä K 1994 High frequency of silent inflammatory bowel disease in spondylarthropathy. Arthritis and Rheumatism 37: 23–31

Lindholm H, Viskorpi R 1991 Late complications after a *Yersinia enterolitica* epidemic: a follow-up study. Annals of Rheumatic Diseases 50: 694–696

Linssen A, Feltkamp T E W 1988 B27-positive diseases versus B27 negative disease. Annals of Rheumatic Diseases 47: 431–439

Macrae I, Wright V 1973 A family study of ulcerative colitis. Annals of Rheumatic Diseases 32: 16–20

Mäki-Ikola O, Yli-Kertulla U, Saario R, Toivanen P, Granfors K 1992 Salmonella specfic antibodies in serum and synovial fluid in patients with reactive arthritis. British Journal of Rheumatology 31: 25–29

Mallas E C, McIntosh P, Asquith P et al 1976 Histocompatibility antigens in inflammatory bowel disease: their clinical significance and their association with arthropathy with special reference to HLA B27. Gut 17: 906–910

Marsal L, Winblad S, Wollheim F A 1981 *Yersinia enterocolitica* arthritis in southern Sweden: a four-year follow-up study. British Medical Journal 283: 101

Martel W 1979 Radiological manifestations of Reiter's syndrome. Annals of Rheumatic Diseases 38 (Suppl 1): 12

Mau W, Zeidler H, Mau R et al 1988 Clinical features and prognosis of patients with possible ankylosing spondylitis. Results of a 10-year follow-up. Journal of Rheumatology 15: 1109–1114

Merilahti-Palo R, Söderström K O, Lahesmaa-Rantala R et al 1991 Bacterial antigens in synovial biopsy specimens in Yersinia triggered reactive arthritis. Annals of Rheumatic Diseases 50: 87–90

Meuwissen S G M, Dekker-Saeys B, Agenant D, Tytgat G N J 1978 Ankylosing spondylitis and inflammatory bowel disease. I. Prevalence of inflammatory bowel disease in patients suffering from ankylosing spondylitis. Annals of Rheumatic Diseases 37: 30–32

Mielants H, Veys E M 1985 HLA-B27 related arthritis and bowel inflammation. Part I: Sulphasalazine (Salazopyrin) in HLA-B27 related reactive arthritis. Journal of Rheumatology 12: 287–293

Mielants H, Veys E M, Cuvelier C, de Vos H, Botelberghe L 1985 HLA-B27 related arthritis and bowel inflammation. Journal of Rheumatology 12: 293–298

Mielants H, Veys E M 1990 The gut in the spondyloarthropathies. Journal of Rheumatology 17: 7–10

Miclants H, Veys E M, Joos R 1986a Sulphasalazine in the treatment of enterogenic reactive synovitis and ankylosing spondylitis with peripheral arthritis. Clinical Rheumatology 5: 80–83

Mielants H, Veys E M, Joos R et al 1986b Familial aggregation in seronegative spondylarthritis of enterogenic origin. A family study. Journal of Rheumatology 13: 126–128

Mielants H, Veys E M, Joos R, Cuvelier C, De Vos M, Proot F 1987 Late onset pauciarticular juvenile chronic arthritis: Relation to gut inflammation. Journal of Rheumatology 14: 459–465

Mielants H, Veys E M, Goethals K et al 1990 Destructive lesions of small joints in seronegative spondylarthropathies: relation to gut inflammation. Clinical and Experimental Rheumatology 8: 23–27

Mielants H, De Vos M, Goemaere S et al 1991 Intestinal mucosal permeability in inflammatory rheumatic diseases. Part II. Role of disease. Journal of Rheumatology 18: 394–400

Mielants H, Veys E M, Goemaere S, Cuvelier C, De Vos M 1993a A prospective study of patients with spondyloarthropathy with special reference to HLA-B27 and to gut histology. Journal of Rheumatology 20: 1353–1358

Mielants H, Veys E M, Cuvelier C et al 1993b Gut inflammation in children with late onset pauciarticular juvenile chronic arthritis and evolution to adult spondylarthropathy. A prospective study. Journal of Rheumatology 20: 1567–1572

Mielants H, Veys E M, De Vos M et al 1995a The evolution of spondylarthropathies in relation to gut histology. Part I: Clinical aspects. Journal of Rheumatology 22: 2266–2272

Mielants H, Veys E M, Cuvelier C et al 1995b The evolution of spondylarthropathies in relation to gut histology. Part II: Histological aspects. Journal of Rheumatology 22: 2273–2278

Mielants H, Veys E M, Cuvelier C 1995c The evolution of spondylarthropathies in relation to gut histology. Part III: Relation between gut and joint. Journal of Rheumatology 22: 2279–2289

Moll J M H 1985 Inflammatory bowel disease. Clinics in Rheumatic Diseases 11: 87–111

Moll J M H, Wright V 1973 Psoriatic arthritis. Seminars in Arthritis and Rheumatisim 3: 55–78

Münch H, Purrman J, Reis H E et al 1986 Clinical features of inflammatory joint and spine manifestations in Crohn's disease. Hepatogastroenterology 33: 123–127

Nissila M, Lethinen K, Leirisalo-Repo M et al 1988 Sulphasalazine in the treatment of ankylosing spondylitis. Arthritis and Rheumatism 31: 1111–1116

Paronen J 1948 Reiter's disease. A study of 344 cases observed in

Finland. Acta Medica Scandinavica 212 (Suppl): 1
Passo M H, Fitzgerald J F, Brandt K D 1986 Arthritis associated with inflammatory bowel disease in children. Relationship of joint disease to activity and severity of bowel lesion. Digestive Diseases and Sciences 31: 492–497
Popert A J, Gill A J, Laird S M 1964 A prospective study of Reiter's syndrome: an interim report on the first 82 cases. British Journal of Venereal Diseases 40: 160
Purrmann J, Zeidler H, Bertrams J et al 1988 HLA antigens in ankylosing spondylitis aasociated with Crohn's disease. Increased frequency of the HLA phenotype B27, B44. Journal of Rheumatology 15: 1658–1661
Rahman MU, Cheema M A, Schumacher H R, Hudson A P 1992 Molecular evidence for the presence of Chlamydia in the synovium of patients with Reiter's syndrome. Arthritis and Rheumatism 35: 521–529
Rankin G B, Watts H D, Melnyk C S, Kelley M L 1979 National cooperative Crohn's disease study: extraintestinal manifestations and perianal complications. Gastroenterology 77: 914–920
Reiter H 1916 Über eine bisher unerkannte Spirochäteninfektion (Spirochätosis Artritica). Deutsche Medizinische Wochenschrift 42: 1535
Sairanen E, Paronen I, Mähönen H 1969 Reiter's syndrome: a follow-up study. Acta Medica Scandinavica 185: 57–63
Schaller J G, Ochs H D, Thomas E D 1976 Characteristics of B27 positive patients with childhood onset of arthritis. Arthritis and Rheumatism 19: 820
Schatteman L, Mielants H, Veys E M et al 1995 Gut inflammation in psoriatic arthritis: a prospective ileocolonoscopic study. Journal of Rheumatology 22: 680–683
Schorr-Resnick B, Brandt L J 1988 Selected rheumatologic and dermatologic manifestations of inflammatory bowel disease. American Journal of Gastroenterology 83: 216–223
Schumacher H R Jr, Magge S, Cherian P V et al 1988 Light and electron microscopic studies on the synovial membrane in Reiter's syndrome. Immunocytochemical identification of chlamydial antigen in patients with early disease. Arthritis and Rheumatism 31: 937–946
Schwimmbeck P L, Yu D T Y, Oldstone M B A 1987 Autoantibodies to HLA B27 in the sera of HLA B27 patients with ankylosing spondylitis and Reiter's syndrome: molecular mimicry with *Klebsiella pneumoniae* as a potential mechanism of autoimmune disease. Journal of Experimental Medicine 166: 173–181
Selby W S, Kater R M, Heap T R, Gallagher N D 1979 Crohn's disease: a review of 122 cases. Australia and New Zealand Journal of Medicine 9: 145
Serrander R, Magnusson K E, Kihlström E 1986 Acute Yersinia infections in man increase permeability for low molecular polyethylene glycols. Scandinavian Journal of Infectious Diseases 18: 409–413
Simenon G, Van Gossum A, Adler M, Rickaert F, Appelboom T 1990 Macroscopic and microscopic gut lesions in seronegative spondylarthropathies. Journal of Rheumatology 17: 1491–1494
Smith M D, Gibson R A, Brooks P M 1985 Abnormal bowel permeability in ankylosing spondylitis and rheumatoid arthritis. Journal of Rheumatology 12: 299–305
Smith R 1922 Treatment of rheumatoid arthritis by colectomy. Annals of Surgery 76: 515–578
Soren A 1966 Joints affections in regional enteritis. Archives of Internal Medicine 117: 78
Stein H B, Abdullah A, Robinson H S, Ford D K 1980 Salmonella reactive arthritis in British Columbia. Arthritis and Rheumatism 23: 206
Taylor-Robinson D, Gilroy C B, Thomas B J, Keat A C S 1992 Detection of *Chlamydia trachomatis* DNA in joints of reactive arthritis patients by polymerase chain reaction. Lancet 340: 81–82
Toivanen P, Toivanen A 1990 Microbial antigens in the synovium in reactive arthritis. In: Reactive Arthritis workshop, Berlin 10–11 June. Deutsches RheumaForschungsZentrum, 48
Torre A J C, Rodriguez P A, Arribas C J M, Ballina G J, Riestra N J L, Lopez L 1991 Psoriatic arthritis (PA): clinical, immunological and radiological study of 180 patients. British Journal of Rheumatology 30: 245–250
Toubert A, Dougados M, Amor B 1985 Erosive granulomatous arthritis in Crohn's disease. (Letter) Arthritis and Rheumatism 28: 958
Trnansky K, Peliskova D, Vacha J 1988 Sulphasalazine in the treatment of reactive athritis. Scandinavian Journal of Rheumatology 67 (Suppl): 76–79
Trull A K, Ebringer R, Panayi G S, Colthorpe D, James DCO, Ebringer A 1983 IgA antibodies to *Klebsiella pneumoniae* in ankylosing spondylitis. Scandinavian Journal of Rheumatology 12: 249–253
Tsuchiya N, Husby G, Williams R C 1989 Studies of humoral and cell mediated immunity to peptides shared by HLA 27.1 and *Klebsiella pneumoniae* nitrogenase in ankylosing spondylitis. Clinical and Experimental Immunology 76: 354–360
Urmaen J D, Zurier R B, Rothfield N F 1977 Reiter's syndrome associated with *Campylobacter fetus* infection. Annals of Internal Medicine 86: 44
Vairtiainen J, Hurri L 1964 Arthritis due to *Salmonella typhimurium*. Report of 12 cases of migratory arthritis in association with *Salmonella typhimurium* infection. Acta Medica Scandinavica 175: 771
van Bohemen C G, Grumet F C, Zanen H C 1984 Identification of HLA-B27 M1 and M2 cross-reactive antigens in Klebsiella, Shigella, and Yersinia. Immunology 52: 607–610
Van Den Berg-Loonen E, Dekker-Saeys B J, Meuwissen S G D et al 1977 Histocompatibility antigens and other genetic markers in ankylosing spondylitis and inflammatory bowel disease. Journal of Immunogenetics 4: 167–175
van Kregten E, Huber-Bruning O, Vandebroucke J P et al 1991 No conclusive evidence of an epidemiological relation between Klebsiella and ankylosing spondylitis. Journal of Rheumatology 18: 384–388
Veys E M, Coigne E, Mielants H et al 1976 HLA and juvenile chronic polyarthritis. Tissue Antigens 8: 61
Viitanen A M, Arstila T, Lahesmaa R, Granfors K, Skurnik M, Tooivanen P 1991 Application of the polymerase chain reaction and immunofluorescence techniques on the detection of bacteria in Yersinia-triggered reactive arthritis. Arthritis and Rheumatism 34: 89–96
Welsh J, Avakian H, Cowling P et al 1980 Ankylosing spondylitis, HLA-B27 and Klebsiella. I: Crossreactivity studies with rabbit antisera. British Journal of Experimental Pathology 61: 85–91
Wendling G, Bidet A, Guidet M 1990 Intestinal permeability in ankylosing spondylitis. Journal of Rheumatology 17: 114–115
Winter R J, Richardson A, Lehner M J, Hoffbrand B I 1984 Lung abscess and reactive arthritis: rare complications of leptospirosis. British Medical Journal of Clinical Research 288: 448–449
Woo P, Panayi G S 1984 Reactive arthritis due to infestation with *Giardia lamblia*. Journal of Rheumatology 11: 719
Wright V, Moll J M H 1976 Seronegative polyarthritis. North-Holland, Amsterdam
Wright V, Watkinson G 1965 The arthritis of ulcerative colitis. British Medical Journal 2: 670–675
Wright V, Watkinson G 1966 Articular complications of ulcerative colitis. American Journal of Proctology 17: 107–115
Zwillich S G, Comer S S, Lee E et al 1988 Treatment of the seronegative spondylarthropathies with sulphasalazine. Journal of Rheumatology 15 (Suppl 16): 33–39

SECTION 4

Natural history and prognosis

53. Natural history of ulcerative colitis

H. Debinski   M. A. Kamm

INTRODUCTION

Ulcerative colitis is a disease with a broad clinical spectrum, affecting all age groups but with a predominance in the young and middle-aged. The majority of patients have a chronic intermittent course with recurrent attacks, or more rarely chronically active disease. A small group of patients have had only one attack with no recurrence of symptoms, and many of these may have had infective colitis which has not been identified by culture or biopsy. Some patients with distal colitis at the onset progress with time to more extensive disease.

The natural history of ulcerative colitis is most accurately studied by observing large and unselected groups of patients. Early epidemiological studies were limited by reliance on uncertain diagnostic criteria, poor definition of the population being studied, and lack of follow-up data. Many of the reports originated in tertiary referral centers, where the population was skewed by the inclusion of severe cases. A critical comparison of incidence and prevalence studies depends on complete ascertainment of cases, effective diagnostic verification and a clear statement of the source of the population.

In critically analyzing the natural history of this condition and using this information to decide on future management strategies, the timing of interventions and whether there have been structured management protocols needs to be carefully considered. In addition, progress in medical and surgical management has definitely influenced the course of ulcerative colitis and altered the natural history as we understand it. It is also possible that the disease manifestation, for example the proportion of patients with more extensive disease or the proportion of patients presenting with more severe disease, changes with time. Prior to the 1950s many patients died early in the course of their disease. The improvement in mortality since then is well illustrated in the Oxford series (Edwards & Truelove 1963a,b), in which there was a marked reduction in the mortality rate in patients presenting with their first attack, or relapse, over the course of only two decades. In the period 1938–1952 33% of patients with a severe episode (initial or relapse) died, compared to 27% in the period 1953–1962. More impressive was the reduction in mortality in those with an attack of moderate severity, the mortality rate falling from 20% to 4%. These changes occurred because of improvements in management, including general measures such as blood transfusion, parenteral therapy, electrolyte replacement and nutritional care, as well as specific measures such as drug treatment. An overall fall in mortality was also due to a greater proportion of patients presenting with mild attacks.

Several aspects of drug treatment have had a major impact on the course of the disease. The introduction of steroids greatly reduced the mortality in severe disease. Maintenance therapies with aminosalicylic or immunosuppressive drugs often effectively control disease over a long term. Such a reduction in disease activity may reduce the cancer risk, and will influence the approach to cancer surveillance. An aggressive surgical policy of early colectomy will select those patients with more extensive and severe disease, and reduce the cumulative cancer risk within a study cohort.

Over the last four decades an increasing proportion of patients have had appropriate treatment of acute exacerbations of their disease with corticosteroids, and then been compliant with maintenance therapy to prevent relapse. As a result we are now reviewing outcomes relating to the natural history of treated ulcerative colitis (Hodgson 1994), which may be altogether different from the time-honored views based on earlier studies.

FIRST ATTACK AND OUTCOME

From a large referral population Farmer et al (1993) have suggested that the major determinants of the natural history of ulcerative colitis are the extent and severity of the disease at the time of diagnosis. A large body of literature would support these simple principles.

Many studies have examined the prognosis for the first attack in both population and non-population based studies. Early non-population based studies have a certain uniformity in that they demonstrated that the majority of first attacks are mild and associated with a low mortality. Moderate to severe attacks only occur in 6–25% of patients (Edwards & Truelove 1963a,b, Sinclair et al 1983, Stonnington et al 1987b), affecting predominantly those with total colitis. Earlier studies reported a mortality rate of 23–33% in these more severe cases.

An early series from Oxford reported the outcome in 250 patients presenting for the first time. Of the 25 deaths (10%) 72% had severe disease (Edwards & Truelove 1963a,b). Mortality was directly related to severity; after 1952 no deaths were recorded in their series in patients with moderate or mild disease. Older age was also a poor prognostic indicator, with patients over 60 having a greater mortality rate (16% versus 9% in younger patients). In their series no deaths occurred in patients with distal disease, and 84% of patients presenting for the first time entered remission.

In a series from Leeds reported in the 1960s (Watts et al 1966a) 204 patients were treated for their first attack between 1952 and 1963. For these patients the overall mortality was 4% and the overall colectomy rate was 11%. Only 70% of patients entered complete remission. An end result during the first episode of either colectomy or death occurred in 36% with severe disease, 37% with total colitis, and 31% of those aged over 60. Severity, extent and age were the three main risk factors for either surgery or death.

The results from a population-based study are similar. In a study from Scotland covering the decade 1967–1976 (Sinclair et al 1983), in 537 patients with ulcerative colitis the outcome of the initial attack was clearly related to the severity and extent of disease. The initial episode was mild in 68%, moderate in 26% and severe in 6%. Based on barium studies only 11% had total colitis, 15% 'substantial' colitis (proximal to the sigmoid colon but not proximal to the hepatic flexure) and the majority (74%) had distal disease. Seventeen patients (3%) died during the acute initial attack, and more than half were over 70 years of age. Of the patients with severe disease only 40% entered remission, 4% had continuous symptoms, 31% underwent resection and 25% died of complications related to their disease.

Overall the outcome for the first attack in most older studies was similar, with 3–6% of all patients dying, 86–95% going into remission and 1–5% undergoing colectomy (Edwards & Truelove 1963a, b, Sinclair et al 1983). The adverse outcomes were usually in patients with pancolitis (total colitis) and severe disease, and more commonly in those presenting in advanced age.

More recently the routine use of steroids and other immunosuppressive drugs, together with closer observation and a lower threshold for surgery, has altered the outlook associated with the first episode. However, in a recent study Langholz et al (1992) found that even with optimal treatment the relative risk of death was 2.4 in the year of diagnosis compared to an age- and sex-matched population.

PROGNOSIS OF SUBSEQUENT ATTACKS

After the first episode most patients will have a recurrence of the disease, and the interest now lies in assessing the impact of 5-amino salicylic acid (5-ASA) compounds in reducing the risk of recurrence.

In one of the earlier English series (Edwards & Truelove 1963a, b) 64% of patients had a chronic course which was intermittent, 7% had a chronic continuous course and 8% died in the first attack of fulminant disease. Of the 18% that had only one attack most would probably have been infective in etiology. In a more recent American study (Stonnington et al 1987b) of 182 patients the overall course was assessed as transient (i.e. which did not relapse during a median follow-up of 14 years) in 28%, intermittent in 65% and unremitting in 5%. These data suggested that in community-based studies the course of the disease may be milder than that reported by specialist hospitals.

The best data relating to the prognosis of the subsequent course of ulcerative colitis come from a recent report from Copenhagen (Langholz et al 1994). Langholz et al described the course of an unselected cohort of patients comprising all patients drawn from a large local population diagnosed in a hospital setting as having ulcerative colitis. Patients were treated medically and surgically by well defined protocols (Langholz et al 1994). In particular these patients had fast access to their specialist as soon as a relapse occurred, and were managed on a continuous regimen of maintenance therapy with 5-ASA compounds.

Most patients with ulcerative colitis had subsequent flare-ups of their disease after the initial presentation. Twenty-three percent of patients had only one disease episode within the study period, but these particular patients had only been followed for a median observation period of 3 years (range 1–25 years). The majority (77%) of patients had a continuously active or acute relapsing course after the first attack. The median period of observation in the latter group was 10 years, with a range of 1–25 years.

Figure 53.1, derived from the Danish population study (Langholz et al 1994), demonstrates the clinical course after the first attack by looking at the cumulative probability with time of continuous activity from diagnosis, an intermittent course and a relapse-free course. By 7 years after the initial episode no patient was still experiencing a continuous chronically active course, suggesting that all patients had either achieved at least one period of remission or had undergone colectomy. In the Oxford series the cumulative probability of a continuously active course

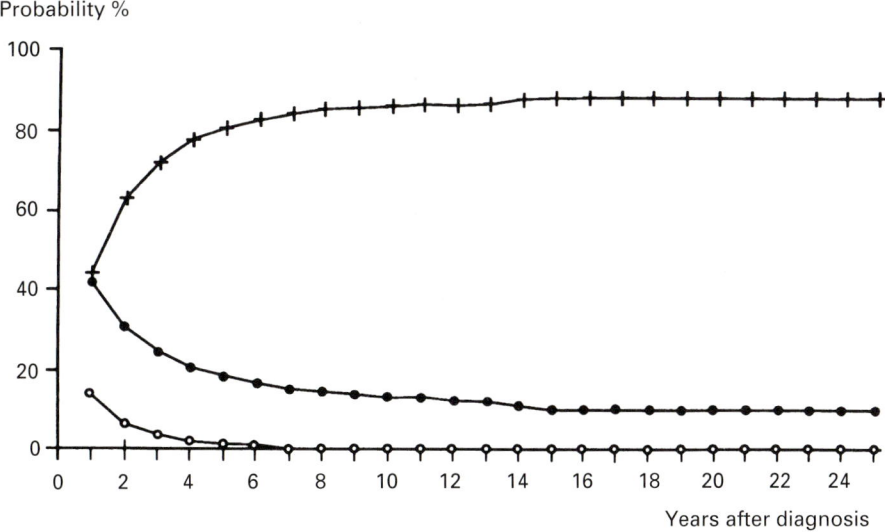

Fig. 53.1 The cumulative probabilities for having only one disease episode of ulcerative colitis (●), a course with continuous activity from diagnosis (○), and a course with intermittent activity from diagnosis (+). From Langholz et al (1994) with permission.

was also low, being 1% after 5 years and 0.1% after 25 years (Edwards & Truelove 1963a). In the Danish study the cumulative probability of a totally relapse-free course decreased with time, and was 18% after 5 years and 11% after 25 years (Langholz et al 1994). Similarly, in the Oxford study after 15 years only 4% of patients had not experienced a recurrence of their disease (Edwards & Truelove 1963a). The probability of having had an intermittent relapsing course was 90% after 25 years, a similar figure for the two studies.

Langholz et al (1994) highlighted that after 3 years from the first diagnosis 40–50% of patients were in clinical remission in any one year (Fig. 53.2). The proportion of patients with continuously active chronic disease gradually decreased with time from 50% 1 year after diagnosis to 25% 20 years after diagnosis. Seventy-five percent of the patients who had not undergone a colectomy were in remission late in the course of their disease. The proportion of patients in remission and relapse each year did not differ when analyzed according to the extent of disease

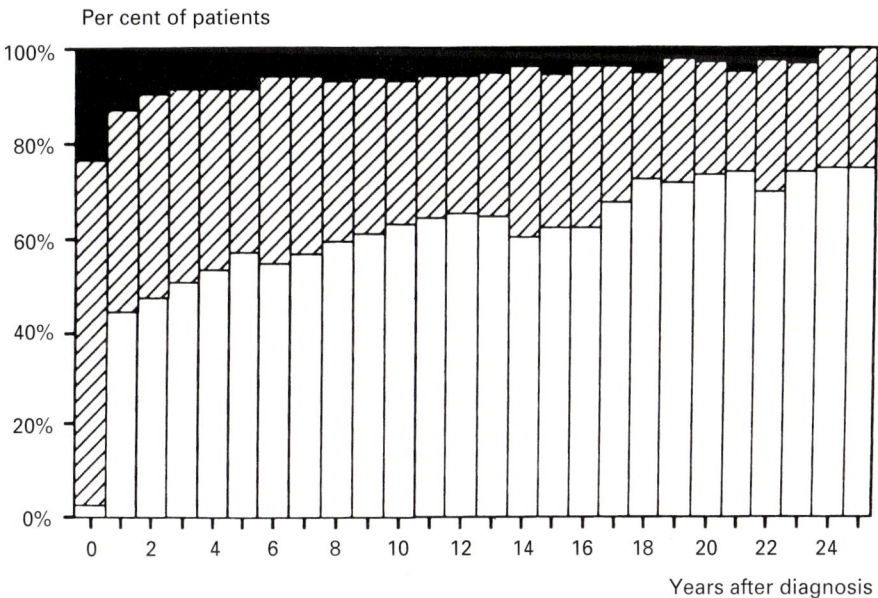

Fig. 53.2 The percentage of patients in remission (□), with continuous disease activity within the year (■), and with intermittent disease activity within the year (▨) in all years after diagnosis. The calculation is based on all study patients in the actual year of observation except for patients undergoing colectomy. From Langholz et al (1994) with permission.

(proctosigmoiditis, substantial colitis and total colitis). In summary, only a small proportion of patients have continuous activity in a year, and this proportion decreases with time.

Figure 53.3 demonstrates the probability of staying in remission from one year to the next, that is, short-term prognosis. For patients who are in remission for a year, the probability of maintaining that remission in the following year increases with time from approximately 75% to about 90% after 15 years.

Figure 53.4 demonstrates the cumulative probability for remaining in remission in each of the first 10 years of disease. The cumulative probability of a course without relapse is between 40 and 60% after 10 years of observation, once a patient has achieved remission, with a positive trend with increasing disease duration.

In order to view long-term outcome in a more meaningful way Langholz and colleagues also analyzed a subgroup of 600 of their patients who had not undergone colectomy but had been followed for at least 7 years. In this more representative group with chronic disease, over the 5-year period between years 3 and 7 after diagnosis 18% had active disease every year, 25% were in continuous remission, and 57% had intermittent activity. During that 5-year period relevant factors that independently predicted the subsequent course of illness were the previous disease course in the year of diagnosis plus the following 2 years (more earlier relapses predicted more relapses later in the disease); the calendar year (patients diagnosed in the 1960s had a more active course than those diagnosed in the 1980s); and the occurrence of systemic symptoms at diagnosis. The presence of initial fever and weight loss correlated inversely with the subsequent course: a higher proportion of patients with these symptoms had a subsequent quiescent course with remission throughout the 5-year period. Therefore, patients with initial high disease activity who responded to medical therapy and avoided colectomy were more likely to enter a prolonged period of remission.

The initial extent of disease did not affect the subsequent clinical course, apart from those with more extensive disease being more likely to undergo colectomy within the first few years (Langholz et al 1992).

EXTENT OF DISEASE

Prevalence of different disease extents

When examining the proportion of patients with different extents of disease at the time of diagnosis in population-based studies, the proportion of patients with proctitis, left-sided and extensive colitis varies considerably. Different centers have also varied in the proportion of patients with different disease severity at the time of diagnosis. Differences between centers may relate to selection bias of patients referred to hospital with distal disease, differences in evaluation or definition, or true geographical differences in disease manifestation.

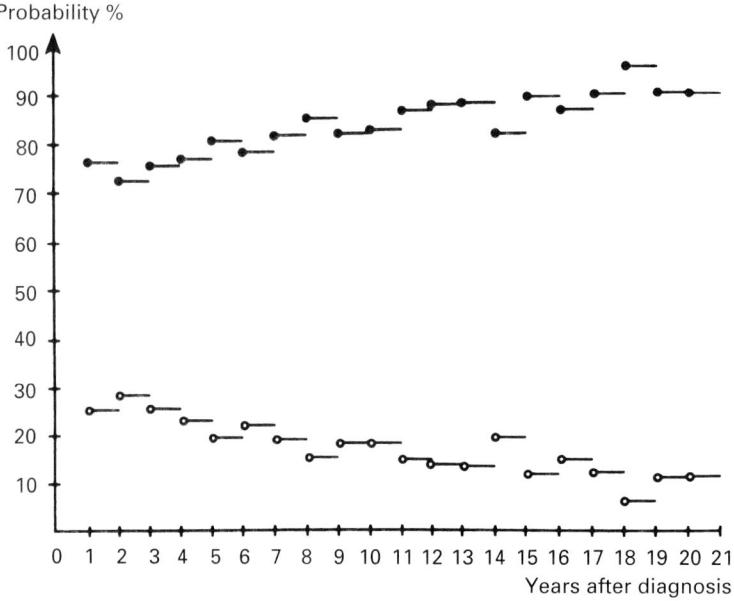

Fig. 53.3 One-year probabilities of staying in remission (●) and for having a relapse (○) for patients in remission the previous year. The point and the adherent line indicates the probability level within a year. The lines are not coherent, indicating that the analysis only deals with 2 consecutive years and does not allow comparison over a longer period than 2 years. From Langholz et al (1994) with permission.

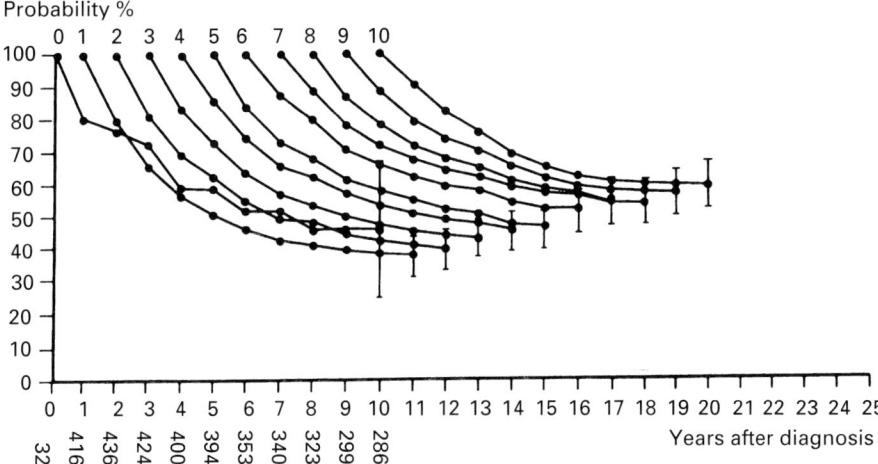

Fig. 53.4 Cumulative probability graphs for remaining in remission for each of the first 10 years of disease. The parallel graphs show the probabilities of staying in remission in a particular year and the following 10 years; 95% confidence intervals are indicated with bars at the end of each 10-year graph. From Langholz et al (1994) with permission.

In many early studies rigid proctoscopy was used to determine extent, making it likely that in some patients with more extensive disease this was underestimated. For example, in the early Cleveland Clinic series, consisting of patients with proctosigmoiditis, an upper limit of disease was visualized in only 127 of the 276 patients (Farmer & Brown 1972). The remainder had disease extending beyond 15 cm from the anus, with the examination being limited by factors such as bleeding and spasm (Farmer & Brown 1972). Understaging of disease extent may also occur if assessment is based solely on single contrast barium studies. It is also difficult to compare studies and assess the extent of disease when there have been variations in the frequency, quality and interpretation of radiological investigations. Colonoscopy is more likely to identify patients with extensive disease than radiological studies. Colonoscopy performed around the time of diagnosis, when the disease is at least partially active, will allow an upper limit of disease activity to be recorded and hence an accurate assessment of extent to be made. If colonoscopy is performed when the disease is in remission, understaging of extent is likely (Niv et al 1987). A possible further advantage of an initial staging colonoscopy is that biopsies can be taken throughout the entire colon, allowing definition of macroscopically normal but microscopically involved colon, although the significance of such microscopic changes is unknown.

In two population-based reports from Copenhagen (Langholz et al 1991) and Scotland (Sinclair et al 1983) only 11–18% of patients had total colitis, in contrast to rates of 28–36% reported from population-based studies in Uppsala, Sweden (Ekbom et al 1991), Rochester, USA (Stonnington et al 1987a), and Stockholm, Sweden (Brostrom et al 1987b).

Progression of disease extent

Patients with disease limited to the rectum or only part of the colon are often concerned that it will spread to involve the remainder of the large bowel. The same problems inherent in defining initial disease extent, as already described, apply to establishing the precise risk and extent of such disease progression.

A further difference between centers relates to the motivation for redefining the extent of disease in a patient population. In some centers patients are reinvestigated during periods of relapse for reasons of clinical management, whereas in other centers the extent of disease is more carefully followed as part of a cancer surveillance policy.

The published series vary enormously in the way that the anatomical extent of disease is defined. We have therefore included each series' definition to facilitate comparison.

The Leeds study of 204 patients included 50 with proctitis (Watts et al 1966b). It concluded that after a mean follow-up of 3.2 years 18 patients (36%) had disease extension, with seven developing total colitis (Watts et al 1966b). The Oxford (Edwards & Truelove 1963a,b) and Uppsala series (Samuelsson 1976) showed a spread of distal disease to left-sided in 8–19% of cases, and to total colitis in 2–15% of cases. In patients with initial left-sided disease, 14–18% progressed to total colitis. In Scotland an increase form distal to more extensive disease after 5 and 10 years of disease occurred in 12 and 30%, respectively (Sinclair et al 1983). All these studies of progression of disease extent are limited by differing periods of follow-up and lack of life-table analysis.

At St Mark's Hospital in London the progression of disease was assessed in 269 patients with ulcerative colitis treated between 1966 and 1975 (Ritchie et al 1978). The initial extent of disease was assessed within 6 months of the first onset of symptoms. Extent was determined by rigid proctosigmoidoscopy and the majority of patients underwent barium enema examination. Histological confirmation was available in 79% of cases. In 17% the precise extent of disease was not ascertained. At first presentation 28% of patients had proctitis, 29% had proctosigmoiditis, 12% had disease extending between the sigmoid colon and the hepatic flexure, and 14% had disease extending from proximal to the hepatic flexure (Fig. 53.5). The study included patients followed up for a maximum of 11 years. Of the 76 patients with proctitis five were noted to have had disease extension, three to the descending colon and two to the hepatic flexure. The cumulative probability after 5 years of extension to the descending colon was 5%, and to the right colon in 3%. Of the 79 patients with proctosigmoiditis progression was noted in 17. In these patients the cumulative probability after 5 years of extension to the descending colon was 18% and 7% who became extensive. Of the 33 patients with disease distal to the hepatic flexure but involving more than the rectosigmoid the cumulative probability at 5 years of progressing was 21% (Fig. 53.6). In summary, it would

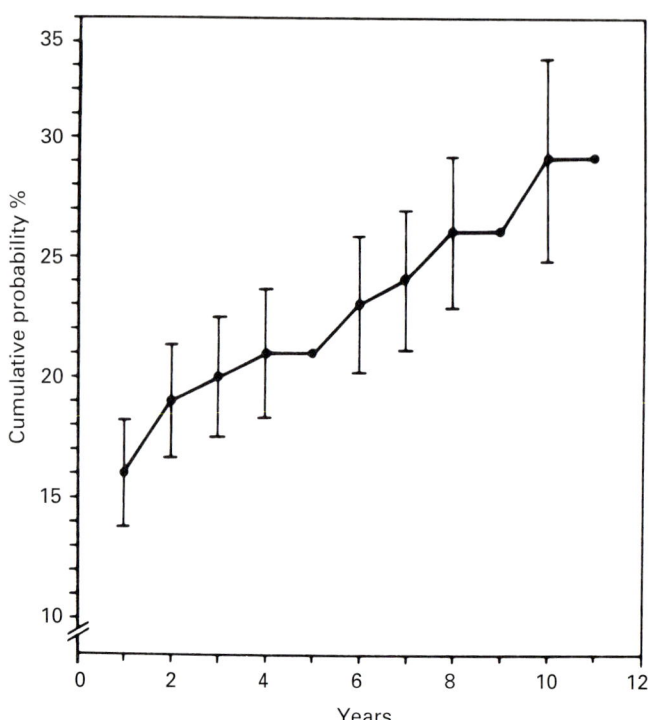

Fig. 53.6 Cumulative probability graphs for developing extensive colitis at follow-up. Within 3 months of presentation 16% have extensive colitis and this increases to 30% at 10 years. From Ritchie et al (1978) with permission.

appear from these data that over a 5-year period about 10% of patients with proctitis and about 20% of patients with more extensive disease will experience progression of their disease extent.

The data from the Cleveland Clinic would suggest a much higher rate of disease progression, partly related to a longer period of follow-up. From a large referral population Farmer et al (1993) studied the natural history of ulcerative colitis by following 1116 patients in whom ulcerative colitis had been diagnosed or confirmed at the Cleveland Clinic between 1960 and 1983. Of these 1116 46% had proctosigmoiditis, only 17% had left-sided colitis (to the splenic flexure), and 37% had pancolitis (colitis of the entire large intestine). After a mean follow-up of 13 years the disease had extended in 54% of the patients. This progression was determined even though two-thirds of the patients were asymptomatic, suggesting that subclinical progression may be common.

Overall, 70% of patients with left-sided disease and 34% of those with proctosigmoiditis extended their disease to develop pancolitis (Farmer et al 1993). Factors more likely to be associated with progression of extent were more severe initial disease, the extent of disease at diagnosis (left-sided disease was more likely to extend than proctitis alone), the presence of joint symptoms, younger age at diagnosis, and severe bleeding (which was probably a reflection of ongoing disease activity).

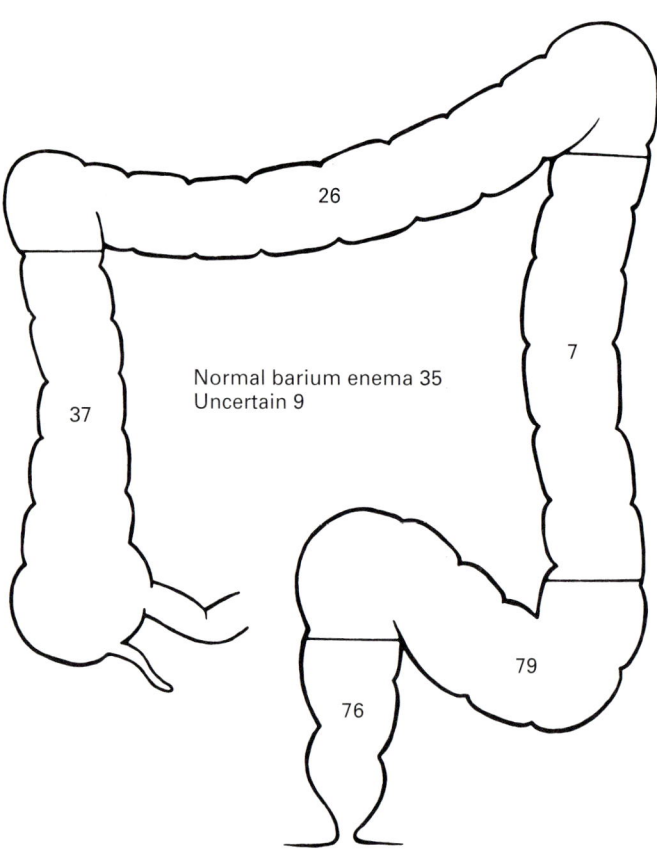

Fig. 53.5 The proximal limit of disease determined within 3 months of presentation in 269 patients. From Ritchie et al (1978) with permission.

The Scottish study (Sinclair et al 1983) has demonstrated that with continued follow-up an increasing proportion of patients will demonstrate disease progression. In their series 12% of patients had disease progression after 5 years, and 30% had progression after 10 years (Sinclair et al 1983).

All the previous series have relied predominantly on radiological assessment to define disease extent. A population-based colonoscopic surveillance study has suggested that macroscopic progression of disease extent occurs in as many as half of all patients with distal disease (Jones et al 1988).

Maintenance therapy and prevention of disease extension

It is unknown whether disease extension is related to the number or frequency of episodes of relapse, or to chronically active disease. It is therefore also not clear to what extent maintenance therapy prevents the extension of disease, although 5-ASA drugs and azathioprine are indisputably effective in substantially reducing the relapse rate. The widespread effective use of drugs to maintain remission may be changing the patter of disease extension.

CAPACITY TO WORK

The ability to work effectively is dependent on being physically well enough to cope with tasks, and not losing excessive time in treatment and convalescence. The need for hospitalization is maximal in the early years of the disease, although increasingly patients are being managed on an outpatient basis, with inpatient care reserved for those with acute severe or chronic refractory disease.

Even in the early Oxford study it was found that 90% of patients were living a near normal existence (Edwards & Truelove 1963a, b). A hospital-based study reported a cumulative admission rate of 11% in patients followed for 4.3 years (Watts et al 1966a,b)

Despite the fact that most patients relapse after the first year the outlook for a productive working life is good. The Copenhagen study involved an annual assessment of whether each patient had been fully capable of work – that is, in work for more than 11 months during the year (Langholz et al 1994). Of those patients of employable age (up to 67 years) 90% were fully capable of work. Of the 10% incapable of work, in only one-third was this related to colitis. The cumulative probability of staying fully capable of work for patients capable of work in the second year after diagnosis was 93% after 10 years, and 86% after 20 years.

Figure 53.7 demonstrates the working capacity in a population of patients with ulcerative colitis in relation to disease duration. For the small number of patients less than 65 years of age who were incapable of work in the second year of their illness, the cumulative probability of remaining so after the second year of diagnosis fell to 66% after 7 years (Langholz et al 1994).

Wyke et al (1988) looked at employment prospects and problems at work in a random sample of 170 patients with more extensive chronic inflammatory bowel disease, 75 of whom had ulcerative colitis. These patients were drawn from a hospital clinic with a special interest in inflammatory bowel disease. Patients were interviewed or

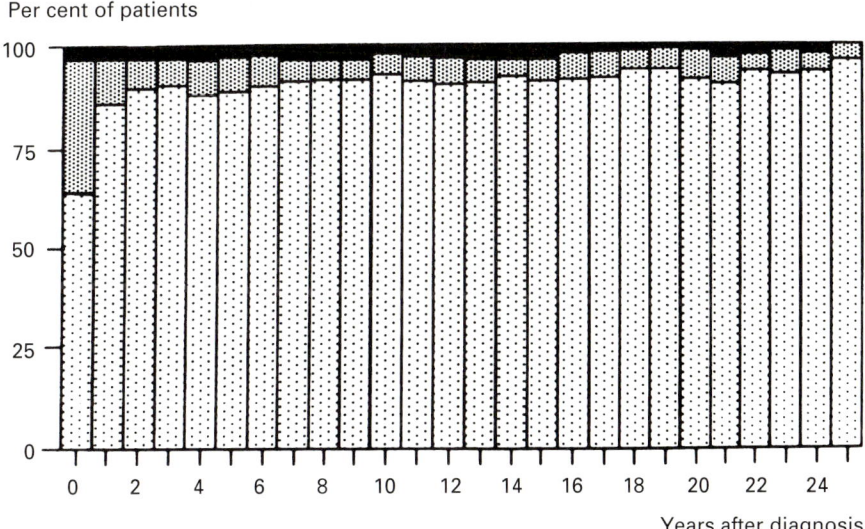

Fig. 53.7 Working capacity for all patients in relation to disease duration shown as percentage of prevalent patients. ■ = incapable because of ulcerative colitis, ▨ = partly incapable or incapable for other reason than ulcerative colitis, ▢ = fully capable. From Langholz et al (1994) with permission.

assessed by questionnaire on two occasions, in 1979 and 1985. Eighty-eight of them were men. This cohort is likely to have had a high proportion of patients with severe disease, as surgery had been carried out on 120 at the time of the initial interview for the study: fifty-three had had an ileostomy.

The outcome in terms of employment was similar for patients with Crohn's disease and those with ulcerative colitis (Wyke et al 1988). Even in this group of patients with apparently severe disease, at the beginning of the study 72% were working and only 1% were registered unemployed. After 6 years a similar proportion were working and 5% were unemployed. Continuity of employment was good, with 57% remaining in the same job, although changes in their work pattern (such as change of hours, retraining, and taking on lighter work) had been made by 72 patients, mainly because of their bowel disease.

After surgery 10% of patients completely changed and 22% modified their work; a few had to retrain or retire. Problems at work, in particular general malaise and arthritis, were experienced by 34 patients (28%). The authors concluded that in general the employment prospects and time off work were good, and employers should be encouraged to take an optimistic and supportive role.

COLORECTAL CANCER RISK AND ITS MODIFICATION BY DRUGS AND SURGERY

Accumulated evidence is conclusive that untreated ulcerative colitis predisposes to the development of colorectal cancer, and the risk is proportional to the duration and extent of disease (Greenstein et al 1979, Lashner 1992). However, the true magnitude of this risk is disputed. The reasons for variation in the estimated cancer risk between studies relate to differences in methodology, especially with respect to patient cohort, geographical factors, inclusion criteria, duration of follow-up and colectomy rates.

Population-based studies contain a greater proportion of patients with milder disease than studies reported from major centers (Stonnington et al 1987a). Early reports from tertiary referral centers described the development of cancer in up to 40% of all patients with ulcerative colitis. In these studies the patients at most risk were those with extensive colitis in whom disease duration was longer than 10 years. The disparity in reported cancer risk is highlighted in four population-based studies that have shown a cumulative cancer risk ranging from 1.3 to 24% at 20–25 years (Watts et al 1966b, Brostrom et al 1987a, Gilat et al 1988, Langholz et al 1992).

Work from St Mark's Hospital in London has suggested a cumulative 5–10% incidence of colorectal cancer in patients who have had ulcerative colitis for 20 years, and an incidence of 12–20% in those who have had their disease for 30 years (Lennard-Jones et al 1990). Along similar lines, a report which included a cohort of primary referrals to three major European institutions estimated a 12% cumulative cancer risk at 25 years (Gyde et al 1988).

This study estimated that the risk of colorectal cancer was increased twentyfold for patients with extensive colitis and fourfold for those with distal colitis, compared to the general population (Gyde et al 1988). The relative risk for cancer, compared to the general population, is highest in young patients with long-standing disease because of the relative rarity of spontaneous colorectal cancer in that age group.

Ekbom et al (1990) found that the absolute risk for developing colorectal cancer 35 years after a diagnosis of pancolitis was 30%, and 40% for those given this diagnosis at less than 15 years of age. Ekbom studied a population-based cohort of 3117 patients given a diagnosis of ulcerative colitis from 1922 through to 1983. Compared with the expected incidence in the general population, the incidence of colorectal cancer in the cohort was increased by an odds ratio of 5.7. Less extensive disease at diagnosis was associated with a lower risk; for patients with ulcerative proctitis the standardized odds ratio was 1.7; for those with left-sided colitis 2.8; and for those with pancolitis (extensive colitis, or inflammation of the entire colon) 14.8. Age and extent of disease at diagnosis were strong and independent risk factors for colorectal cancer. For each increase in age group at diagnosis (<15 years, 15–29 years, 30–39 years, 40–49 years, 50–59 years, and ≥ 60 years), the relative risk of colorectal cancer, adjusted for the extent of disease at diagnosis, decreased by about half.

Data about the cancer incidence in ulcerative colitis are also derived from surveillance programs. Lashner (1992) reviewed data from a single university-based surveillance program. The annual risk of developing cancer was found to rise exponentially with disease duration and to be approximately 2% after 20 years of disease and nearly 8% after 30 years of disease. More than 25% of patients who had disease for more than 25 years developed colorectal cancer (Lashner 1992). In practice, an accurate assessment of the cancer risk in patients whose disease exceeds 25 years is difficult, since patient numbers at risk are small and the confidence intervals correspondingly wide. For an individual patient a reasonable working estimate of the risk is 0.5–1.0% per year after the first decade of extensive ulcerative colitis.

The most important independent risk factors for developing colorectal cancer in ulcerative colitis appear to be duration of illness, younger age of onset and more extensive anatomical involvement (Ekbom et al 1990). Patients with proctitis or proctosigmoiditis have only a slightly increased cancer risk, whereas the cancer risk in left-sided disease is about four times that of the general population (Gyde et al 1988).

Whether tighter control of the disease prevents the development of cancer is not known, but some evidence is emerging that a high colectomy rate, combined with pharmacological prevention of relapse, contributes towards reducing the incidence of cancer. This is consistent with the suggestion of a protective effect of aspirin against sporadic colorectal cancer. In a population-based cohort of 3112 patients with ulcerative colitis, 102 cases of colorectal cancer and 196 matched controls without cancer were compared. Pharmacological therapy, particularly sulfasalazine, for at least 3 months at some stage during the illness, was associated with a significant protective effect (risk ratio 0.38; 95% confidence interval 0.20–0.69) independent of disease activity (Pinczowski et al 1994). In this study the risk of colorectal cancer was substantially lower among those patients who had completed at least one course of sulfasalazine, although most patients were in fact taking the drug as a long-term basis. The protective effect was unaffected by adjustment for age and disease activity.

As an extension of these findings it has been argued that with an active approach to medical and surgical treatment patients whose colons are left intact have no significantly increased risk of colorectal malignancy (Langholz et al 1992). In the hospital-based study of all patients with ulcerative colitis in the Copenhagen region, 1161 patients with ulcerative colitis diagnosed between 1962 and 1987 were followed up for a median of 12 years. Twenty-six deaths caused by ulcerative colitis or its complications occurred. Six patients developed colorectal cancer within the observation period, compared with the expected population number of 6.6; the relative risk for patients with ulcerative colitis was therefore 0.9. The calculated cumulative cancer incidence was 3.1% after 25 years (95% confidence limits 0.0–6.8). The calculated lifetime risk, between the ages of 0 and 74 years, for the development of colorectal cancer was 3.5% for ulcerative colitis patients compared with 3.7% for the Danish population. They concluded that the risk for developing cancer did not increase with disease duration, and is much lower than previously thought because of the lifelong use of sulfasalazine or mesalazine, combined with surgery when disease was poorly controlled. In this cohort the crude colectomy rate was 21%, and the cumulative colectomy rate 25 years after diagnosis was 32% for all patients with ulcerative colitis.

RISK OF COLECTOMY

Systemic and topical medical therapy must be appropriate to the patient's needs and lifestyle. The decision to proceed to surgery will be based on disease severity, the disability it produces, the perceived cancer risk, and the efficacy and tolerance of medications such as corticosteroids and immunosuppressives, including newer agents such as cyclosporin A. In the absence of a good index of disease severity which is universally accepted and adds uniformity to the interpretation of the results of clinical trials, the threshold for defining disease as intractable will be related to the philosophy of the medical and surgical team. This is reflected in the difference in colectomy rates between different centers.

Surgical colectomy rates are dependent on many variables. The extent and severity of disease at presentation are the most important factors for the risk of colectomy. Hence the finding that in both population- and non-population based studies the risk of colectomy is greatest in the first 2 years. The cumulative rate will be inversely related to the proportion of patients with distal colitis in a study cohort.

The factors affecting the colectomy rate were studied retrospectively in a population-based cohort of 1586 patients with ulcerative colitis treated in Stockholm County during the period 1955–1984. During a median period of observation of 13 years 514 patients were treated by colectomy. Ten percent of the 1586 patients had a colectomy during the first year after diagnosis, 4% during the second year and 1% during each subsequent year (Leijonmarck et al 1990). The 5-, 10- and 25-year cumulative colectomy rates were 20, 28 and 45% respectively. The main factor affecting the colectomy rate was the extent of disease at diagnosis. Patients with total colitis showed a 5-, 10- and 25-year cumulative colectomy rate of 32, 42 and 65% respectively.

The results were very similar in the Danish population-based series. Eighteen percent of the 1161 patients had pancolitis. The colectomy rate was 9% in the year of diagnosis, 3% per year in the following 4 years, and 1% per year from then on (Langholz et al 1994). The cumulative colectomy rate was 30% after 15 years. The initial extent of disease significantly influenced the colectomy probability, being 35% in total colitis, 19% in substantial colitis, and 9% in distal colitis within the first 5 years after diagnosis (Langholz et al 1992).

In Copenhagen and northeastern Scotland, an estimate of the cumulative colectomy rate highlights that it is highest during the first year of diagnosis, is still relatively common in the next 4 years, and thereafter is relatively low and constant. Surgery is most commonly required for severe and extensive disease, the two factors being related.

Surgery is indicated most commonly for fulminant disease or chronic active disease resistant to medical therapy. In the tertiary referral Cleveland Clinic series, within the first 2 years after diagnosis such fulminant disease also included colonic hemorrhage in 17% and toxic colitis in 13% of patients (Farmer et al 1993). These events occurred most commonly among patients with pancolitis, 61% of whom required a colectomy. Overall surgery was required for 38% of their patients. Primary indications for surgery in all their patients during the entire observation period included chronic or intractable disability (40%), fulminant medical failure (17%) and colonic dilatation (18%).

Surgery is undertaken initially for uncontrolled disease, but after 10 years is also undertaken for the added indications of cancer and precancerous changes. Over a 22-year period 401 patients with total ulcerative colitis for 10 years were entered into a surveillance program at St Mark's Hospital. Thirty-four of these required surgery for cancer or high-grade dysplasia (Lennard-Jones et al 1990).

A further factor which is likely to have influenced the colectomy rate over the last 15 years is the ability to have a proctocolectomy but retain continence through the creation of an ileoanal reservoir.

RISK OF DEATH

The prognosis of ulcerative colitis is very different from that of 50 years ago, when many patients died early in the course of their illness. In the Oxford series (Edwards and Truelove 1963a, b), which included patients from the pre-corticosteroid era, the survival probability for patients with total colitis was extremely poor, with only 45% surviving for 15 years after the onset of their disease. The mortality was especially high in the first years after diagnosis. In Stockholm County (Brostrom et al 1987b) there was a trend for improved survival in patients diagnosed in the period 1970–1979, compared to those diagnosed from 1955 to 1969. Similar findings have been reported in Uppsala (Ekbom et al 1992).

Recent studies present a more optimistic view of the outcome of ulcerative colitis (Stonnington et al 1987b, Langholz et al 1994), and this has implications in terms of relieving patient anxiety and the adoption of a more lenient approach in insurance assessment. If there are differences in survival between patients with ulcerative colitis and the general population in this the era of active treatment, then they are small and only apparent after subgroup analysis.

When comparing the mortality in patients with ulcerative colitis with the general population, neither the Scottish (Sinclair et al 1983) nor the Rochester (USA) (Stonnington et al 1987b) studies showed a difference when all patients were considered. Actuarial analysis by Sinclair and colleagues (1983) failed to demonstrate a difference between observed and expected mortality in 537 patients over 10 years. However, in the subgroup of 33 patients with extensive colitis presenting with an acute attack, the mortality of 30% in the first 2 years was excessive, but did not extend beyond 2 years. In the regional patient cohort from Rochester (Stonnington et al 1987b) 182 patients were followed up for a mean of 14 years. Life-table analysis showed that survival was similar to that expected for the general age- and sex-matched population (Stonnington et al 1987a, b).

In a well documented study from Uppsala, Sweden, relative survival was analysed for 2509 patients diagnosed with ulcerative colitis during the period 1965–1983 (Ekbom et al 1992). After 10 years survival was 96% of that expected. Patients with ulcerative proctitis, left-sided colitis and pancolitis at diagnosis had relative survival rates of 98%, 96% and 93% respectively. The standardized mortality ratio was significantly increased at 1.4. Inflammatory bowel disease was the main reason for this excess mortality. Colorectal cancer also increased mortality, although deaths from other cancers were no greater than expected. Unexpectedly, mortality from obstructive respiratory diseases, especially bronchitis, emphysema and asthma, was also significantly increased, with a standardized mortality ratio of 1.5. The incidence of other medical conditions was no greater than expected. In contrast, Gyde et al failed to demonstrate an increased respiratory or vascular mortality in a group of patients from Birmingham (Gyde et al 1982).

In the Danish study of 1161 ulcerative colitis patients (Langholz et al 1992), 149 deaths were observed of which 26 were caused by ulcerative colitis or its complications. In the year of diagnosis the relative risk of death was 2.4 ($P<0.001$). In this study the low mortality due to colitis of less than 0.8% tended to occur in a small number of patients with severe acute pancolitis. After the first year there was no significant difference in mortality between patients with colitis and a matched population derived from the Danish National Department of Statistics.

Earlier work had suggested that this early excess in ulcerative colitis mortality in Copenhagen occurred predominantly in men over 40 years of age who suffered cardiovascular complications related to surgery (Hendriksen et al 1985). Other work has suggested that in patients over 60 there is a marked increase in mortality during the first attack and subsequent relapse attacks (Edwards and Truelove 1963a, b, Sinclair et al 1983) but a more recent study has failed to confirm this (Langholz et al 1994).

Since steroids were introduced mortality rates have continued to fall with time (Brostrom et al 1987b). The overall mortality for men and women in the USA and in England has declined from the early 1960s (Sonnenberg 1986). This is true for all age groups, but especially younger patients. It is unknown whether the severity of initial presenting episodes has changed over the last 30 years.

In summary, it is only when patients with total colitis are assessed as a separate group that there are trends suggestive of excessive mortality, and this occurs mainly in relation to the first attack or early in the course of the illness. Survival of patients with ulcerative colitis is almost unaffected, provided that they are treated appropriately during acute attacks and remain compliant with 5-ASA maintenance therapy.

REFERENCES

Brostrom O, Lofberg R, Nordenvall B et al 1987a The risk of colorectal cancer in ulcerative colitis. An epidemiologic study. Scandinavian Journal of Gastroenterology 22: 1193–1199

Brostrom O, Monsen U, Nordenvall B et al 1987b Prognosis and mortality of ulcerative colitis in Stockholm County. Scandinavian Journal of Gastroenterology 22: 907–913

Edwards F C, Truelove S C 1963a The course and prognosis of ulcerative colitis. Part II. Long-term prognosis. Gut 4: 309–315

Edwards F C, Truelove S C 1963b The course and prognosis of ulcerative colitis. Part I. Short-term prognosis. Gut 4: 299–308

Ekbom A, Helmick C, Zack M et al 1990 Ulcerative colitis and colorectal cancer. A population-based study. New England Journal of Medicine 323: 1228–1233

Ekbom A, Helmick C, Zack M et al 1991 The epidemiology of inflammatory bowel disease: a large, population-based study in Sweden. Gastroenterology 100: 350–358

Ekbom A, Helmick C G, Zack M et al 1992 Survival and causes of death in patients with inflammatory bowel disease: a population-based study. Gastroenterology 103: 954–960

Farmer R, Brown C H 1972 Emerging concepts of proctosigmoiditis. Diseases of the Colon and Rectum 15: 142–146

Farmer R G, Easley K A, Rankin G B 1993 Clinical patterns, natural history, and progression of ulcerative colitis. A long-term follow-up of 1116 patients. Digestive Diseases and Sciences 38: 1137–1146

Gilat T, Fireman Z, Grossman A et al 1988 Colorectal cancer in patients with ulcerative colitis. A population study in central Israel. Gastroenterology 94: 870–877

Greenstein A J, Sachar D B, Smith H et al 1979 Cancer in universal and left-sided ulcerative colitis: factors determining risk. Gastroenterology 77: 290–294

Gyde S N, Prior P, Dew M J et al 1982 Mortality in ulcerative colitis. Gastroenterology 83: 36–43

Gyde S N, Prior P, Allan R N et al 1988 Colorectal cancer in ulcerative colitis: a cohort study of primary referrals from three centres. Gut 29: 206–217

Hendriksen C, Kreiner S, Binder V 1985 Long term prognosis in ulcerative colitis based on results form a regional patient group from the county of Copenhagen. Gut 26: 158–163

Hodgson H J F 1994 The natural history of treated ulcerative colitis. Gastroenterology 107: 300–302

Jones II W, Grogono J, Hoare A M 1988 Surveillance in ulcerative colitis: burdens and benefit. Gut 29: 325–331

Langholz E, Munkholm P, Nielsen O H et al 1991 Incidence and prevalence of ulcerative colitis in Copenhagen county from 1962 to 1987. Scandinavian Journal of Gastroenterology 26: 1247–1256

Langholz E, Munkholm P, Davidsen M et al 1992 Colorectal cancer risk and mortality in patients with ulcerative colitis [see comments]. Gastroenterology 103: 1444–1451

Langholz E, Munkholm P, Davidsen M et al 1994 Course of ulcerative colitis: analysis of changes in disease activity over years. Gastroenterology 107: 3–11

Lashner B A 1992 Recommendations for colorectal cancer screening in ulcerative colitis: a review of research from a single university-based surveillance program. American Journal of Gastroenterology 87: 168–175

Leijonmarck C E, Persson P G, Hellers G 1990 Factors affecting colectomy rate in ulcerative colitis: an epidemiologic study. Gut 31: 329–333

Lennard-Jones J E, Melville D M, Morson B C et al 1990 Precancer and cancer in extensive ulcerative colitis: findings among 401 patients over 22 years. Gut 31: 800–806

Niv Y, Bat L, Ron E 1987 Change in the extent of colonic-involvement in ulcerative colitis. A colonoscopic study. American Journal of Gastroenterology 82: 1046–1051

Pinczowski D, Ekbom A, Baron J et al 1994 Risk factors for colorectal cancer in patients with ulcerative colitis. Gastroenterology 107: 117–120

Ritchie J K, Powell-Tuck J, Lennard-Jones J E 1978 Clinical outcome of the first ten years of ulcerative colitis and proctitis. Lancet 1: 1140–1143

Samuelsson S M 1976 Ulcerative colitis in the County of Uppsala. Clinical, epidemiological, social and medical aspects (unpublished thesis). Acta Univ Uppsala

Sinclair T S, Brunt P W, Mowat N A G 1983 Nonspecific proctocolitis in northeastern Scotland: a community study. Gastroenterology 85: 1–11

Sonnenberg A 1986 Mortality from Crohn's disease and ulcerative colitis in England, Wales and the US from 1950 to 1983. Diseases of the Colon and Rectum 29: 624–629

Stonnington C M, Phillips S F, Melton L et al 1987a Chronic ulcerative colitis: incidence and prevalence in a community. Gut 28: 402–409

Stonnington C M, Phillips S F, Zinsmeister A R et al 1987b Prognosis of chronic ulcerative colitis in a community. Gut 28: 1261–1266

Watts J M, De Dombal F T, Watkinson G et al 1966a Early course of ulcerative colitis. Gut 7: 16–31

Watts J M, De Dombal F T, Watkinson G et al 1966b Long term prognosis of ulcerative colitis. British Medical Journal 1: 1447–1453

Wyke R J, Edwards F C, Allan R N 1988 Employment problems and prospects for patients with inflammatory bowel disease. Gut 29: 1229–1235

54. Natural history of Crohn's disease

A. Brzezinski   B. A. Lashner

Crohn's disease is an inflammatory bowel disease of unknown cause that can affect any segment of the gastrointestinal tract. It is a heterogeneous disease with many different clinical manifestations, which depend on disease location, anatomic extent, disease behavior, disease characteristics and operative history. Because the manifestations vary widely, discussing the natural history of Crohn's disease requires patients to be classified into more homogeneous groups, an exercise that is useful if it leads to prediction of the natural history so that intervention can be initiated to favorably alter the disease course.

IMPORTANCE OF STUDYING THE NATURAL HISTORY OF CROHN'S DISEASE

A chronic and recurrent illness, Crohn's disease is characterized by periods of activity and quiescence, the duration of which can vary dramatically among patient populations. The severity of the disease ranges from mild to fulminant. Morbidity can be substantial and includes sepsis, malnutrition, malabsorption, cancer and extraintestinal complications, such as pyoderma gangrenosum, erythema nodosum, arthritis, iritis and uveitis.

The mortality rate of patients with Crohn's disease is double that of the unaffected population and is highest during the first 5 years of disease (Truelove & Pena 1976, Prior et al 1981, Sonnenberg 1990). Approximately 6% of patients will die of complications directly related to Crohn's disease, a rate that is not related to the location or extent of disease (Weterman et al 1990, Ekbom et al 1992). Interestingly, patients with sedentary indoor occupations have the highest mortality (Sonnenberg 1990). In recent years survival has improved with the introduction of corticosteroids as a principal treatment. Undoubtedly mortality also has decreased because of improved surgical techniques, judicious use of antibiotics, and improved nutritional support. In earlier years the principal causes of mortality were amyloidosis, malnutrition and postoperative infections (Andrews et al 1989, Gitkind & Wright 1990, Weterman et al 1990). Currently, mortality occurs later in the course of the disease, and the principal causes of death are sepsis, perforation, pulmonary embolism and cancer. Perioperative deaths are related to emergency surgery only (Andrews et al 1989).

Treatment may have both a positive and negative impact on the patient's quality of life. Medical therapy includes 5-aminosalicylic acid (5-ASA), corticosteroids, antibiotics, nutritional modifications and immunosuppressive drugs – treatments that all have important benefits but also significant risks and side effects. Surgical treatment often is required for certain complications and for certain disease patterns, such as fibrostenotic disease. Treatment for Crohn's disease is currently based on patient symptoms and complications. Because management decisions depend on location, extent, types of complications, and disease course, a prognostic classification would be useful to identify patients most likely to benefit from a specific therapy at a specific time. Some progress has been made in identifying predictors of recurrence, and perhaps with early intervention the normal disease course might be favorably altered, with a concomitant decrease in morbidity and mortality. Therefore, studying the natural history of Crohn's disease is important.

The three main prognostically and therapeutically important groupings that have been proposed relate to location and extent of the disease, its principal characteristics (i.e. fibrostenotic, inflammatory or perforating), and the behavior of the disease (i.e. aggressive or indolent). Ideally, Crohn's disease patients would be classified according to one of these groups. In reality, a patient's symptoms and signs span several groups and confound even the best of intentions to classify.

PITFALLS IN STUDYING THE NATURAL HISTORY OF A HETEROGENEOUS DISEASE

Studies on the natural history of Crohn's disease are difficult to compare because of variability in study design, definitions of recurrence, relapse and remission, and multiple biases in studies. The effects of different criteria

Table 54.1 Definitions of recurrence in Crohn's disease

Definition method	Positive features	Negative features
Symptomatic recurrence	Highly sensitive, most patients included	Poor specificity, symptoms not always related to recurrence
Endoscopic, radiographic, or histologic recurrence	Good sensitivity, good specificity	Features may be due to postsurgical changes or tissue may be unobtainable
Reoperation rate	Excellent specificity, easy to quantify in a defined population	Poor sensitivity. Not all patients with recurrence require surgery and surgery may be necessary for other reasons

on the sensitivity and specificity of the diagnosis of recurrence are listed in Table 54.1. Furthermore, treatment may interfere with observations of the natural history. Since 1913, when Dalziel reported six patients with chronic interstitial enteritis who were successfully treated with resection, virtually no patient with Crohn's disease has been untreated. Those patients allocated to the placebo arms of large randomized clinical trials do not represent an untreated population (Meyers & Janowitz 1984): because placebo-treated patients are under close medical supervision, the placebo effect cannot be ignored.

Attempts to study the natural history of Crohn's disease by identifying homogeneous groups when the disease is heterogeneous are fraught with uncertainties. Studies of different populations are likely to vary widely because of differences in the referral filter, stability of the population, disease definition, and the quality of diagnostic testing (Sackett 1979). Studies from the United States are mostly from referral centers, where patients tend to have more complicated disease that requires surgery or innovative treatment measures. Patients in these populations may be more likely than others to have a specific type of disease (i.e. aggressive or fistulous) confined to a specific location. True rates of occurrence of Crohn's disease and disease complications in a more general population often cannot be estimated from referral centers. Alternatively, studies from Europe, especially Great Britain and Scandinavia, where large geographically defined populations of patients can be analyzed, incidence rates and classification of disease type are more likely to accurately reflect the true rates in a general population. Also, studies from Europe most often reflect a stable population free of migration, whereas in the US people migrate to warmer climates at older ages, which may influence rates of complications and surgery in those areas.

Disease definition and the sensitivity of diagnostic testing can profoundly bias study results (Sackett 1979). At tertiary care centers in the US strict diagnostic criteria often exist, and diagnostic testing is quite sensitive. Highly sensitive testing, at the expense of specificity, will include a high proportion of complicated or severe cases and exclude more subtle and less severe cases. Studies from tertiary centers in the US, therefore, often have a higher rate of complications and disease requiring surgery than populations representative of a geographic community. Concomitantly, European studies of Crohn's disease may report lower rates of complications and surgery as a result of the less sensitive and more specific diagnostic testing.

NATURAL HISTORY OF CROHN'S DISEASE ACCORDING TO PRINCIPAL LOCATION AND EXTENT OF DISEASE

Classifying Crohn's disease according to the principal location and extent of the disease is the time-honored approach and the one most useful to the surgeon. Unfortunately, even in a group of patients with similar anatomic location and extent, disease characteristics and behaviors differ widely. Although useful for surgery, grouping patients in this way is less useful for medical therapy.

At presentation approximately 40% of patients have ileocolonic disease, 28–30% have small-bowel disease only, 25–27% have colonic disease only, and 3% have isolated anorectal or perianal disease (Lock et al 1981). Only rarely do patients present with pure gastroduodenal disease.

Gastroduodenal disease

The stomach and duodenum are the principal locations of Crohn's disease in 0.5–4% of patients but almost all have evidence of Crohn's disease elsewhere in the gut. In such cases Crohn's disease may be difficult to distinguish from peptic ulcer disease and erosions caused by nonsteroidal anti-inflammatory drugs (Tootla et al 1976, Nugent et al 1977). Some recent series have reported a higher incidence (up to 15%), possibly related to the extreme sensitivity of diagnostic upper endoscopy testing rather than to a change in the spectrum of disease (Sachar et al 1992). Gastric involvement is usually confined to the antrum, and universal gastric involvement rarely occurs without evidence of Crohn's disease elsewhere in the gastrointestinal tract (Cary et al 1989). Symptoms and signs of upper gastrointestinal Crohn's disease include nausea, vomiting, epigastric pain that is moderately relieved with antacids, a small contracted stomach, or gastric outlet obstruction. Gastroduodenal Crohn's disease does not increase the risk for peptic ulcer disease, but omeprazole provides adequate symptomatic relief in some patients (Woolfson & Greenberg 1992).

Fistulous disease originating from the stomach or duodenum is very rare. More commonly, fistulae arise from more distal regions of the gastrointestinal tract (Farmer et al 1972, Jacobson et al 1985). Patients with gastrocolic fistulae can present with diarrhea and malabsorption because the gastric contents bypass the small intestine and empty into the colon; or with feculent vomitus or gastric outlet obstruction. The most common indication for surgical intervention in patients with gastric Crohn's disease is gastric outlet obstruction, a complication that occurs in approximately 30% of cases (Fielding et al 1970).

Duodenal Crohn's disease involves the second portion of the duodenum more often than the bulb. Fistulous disease is particularly common, and even a duodenobiliary fistula has been reported (Zarnow et al 1976). Patients with duodenal fistulae may have bacterial overgrowth and malabsorption. Patients with duodenal Crohn's disease are often treated with H_2-receptor antagonists or proton pump inhibitors with or without corticosteroids. Approximately 30% do not respond to medical treatment and require surgery (Murray et al 1984). Other indications for surgery in gastroduodenal Crohn's disease are intractable pain or upper gastrointestinal bleeding. Surgery for duodenal Crohn's disease carries substantial morbidity with important complications, such as duodenal fistulae, transection of the common bile duct, gastric outlet obstruction requiring reoperation, subphrenic abscess, or small-bowel obstruction – such complications occur in approximately one-third of patients with gastroduodenal disease.

Surgical mortality occurs in less than 5% of patients. In one study nine of 11 patients requiring a gastrojejunostomy to bypass an outlet obstruction had a good result, with immediate relief of symptoms (Ross et al 1983). However, reoperation is common. Seven of 10 patients followed for a mean of 13.9 years required further upper gastrointestinal tract surgery (Ross et al 1983). The average interval between the first and second operations was 7.7 years (range 11 months to 12.3 years). In all patients other areas of the gastrointestinal tract were also affected.

Ileocolonic disease

The ileocecal region is the most common site of inflammation when a patient initially presents with Crohn's disease. The most common symptoms of ileocecal disease are diarrhea, crampy abdominal pain and low-grade fever. Physical examination may reveal tenderness and a right lower quadrant abdominal mass. Occasionally patients are advised to undergo surgery for presumed appendicitis, but instead ileocecal Crohn's disease is found. In more than 90% of patients with ileocecal disease the diseased bowel must eventually be resected; the most common indications for surgery are internal fistulization with abscess and small-bowel obstruction (Farmer et al 1985).

The inflammatory mass in the ileocecal region is composed of bowel, mesentery and lymph nodes, some of which may contain granulomas. A localized abscess may obstruct the right ureter or extend locally to promote fistulization to the bladder, sigmoid colon, mesentery or skin. Patients with fibrostenotic disease of the ileocecal region often present with symptoms and signs of small-bowel obstruction, such as crampy abdominal pain, distension, vomiting and few bowel movements.

Small-bowel disease

In about 30% of patients with Crohn's disease only the small intestine is involved. In the majority of patients with small-bowel disease exclusively the terminal ileum is involved, and only a few have diffuse small-bowel involvement or jejunal disease. In the European Cooperative Crohn's Disease Study (ECCDS), patients with small-bowel disease tended to be older than patients with ileocolonic disease and had a worse outcome (Steinhardt et al 1985). At the Cleveland Clinic, after a mean follow-up of more than 13 years, 65.5% of patients in whom only the small bowel was affected required surgery, compared with 91.5% of patients with ileocolonic disease and 58% of patients with colonic disease (Farmer et al 1985). In over 60% of patients the indication for surgery was obstruction. Patients with jejunal disease had more frequent problems related to malabsorption and steatorrhea.

Regardless of whether patients receive surgical or medical treatment, 5- and 10-year survival rates for those with small-bowel disease only have been reported not to differ from survival rates in those with ileocolonic or colonic disease (Whelan et al 1985). The estimated median time to recurrence following a medically or surgically induced remission was 92 months. The rate of recurrence requiring a second surgery increased steeply during the first 3 years. Almost half the patients required a second operation within 10 years, and 38% of these required a third operation. A population-based study in Europe reported that the risk of recurrence requiring reoperation in patients with small-bowel Crohn's disease was as low as 25% at 10 years (Shivananda et al 1989).

In the pediatric population, after resection the median disease-free interval between flares of disease is 6 years for children in whom Crohn's disease is confined to the small bowel (Griffiths et al 1991). During disease-free intervals children who have not completed their growth gain height more rapidly and can enjoy a symptom- and medication-free period. The growth retardation in children with active Crohn's disease is believed to result from inflammatory disease of the small bowel, with malabsorption and malnutrition. Even though somatomedin-C deficiency has been implicated as an important factor in growth retardation, malabsorption almost certainly plays an important role (Kirschner & Sutton 1986).

Colonic disease

Crohn's disease is limited to the colon in approximately 25% of patients. The principal symptoms in inflammatory disease of the colon are diarrhea and hematochezia. Obstruction may occur in fibrostenotic disease, and fistulae to and from the colon are frequently found. For optimal medical and surgical management, distinguishing between the colitis seen with Crohn's disease and ulcerative colitis is important. The differentiation most often can be made colonoscopically, but fully 10% of patients with colitis cannot be classified and are described as having "indeterminate colitis." Endoscopic features typical of Crohn's disease include aphthous ulcers, discrete longitudinal ulcers, skip areas, strictures, fissures and fistulae. Interestingly, when followed over time so that indeterminate disease has an opportunity to declare itself, patients with indeterminate colitis most often emerge as having Crohn's colitis (Kirsner 1975). However, the long-term outcome and complication rate for patients undergoing ileal pouch–anal anastomosis who have indeterminate colitis at surgery do not differ from the outcome and complication rate of patients who have such surgery for ulcerative colitis (Pezim et al 1989). A confident diagnosis of Crohn's or ulcerative colitis is difficult to make in patients with indeterminate colitis who have emergency proctocolectomy, even after careful histopathologic review of the resected colon. Still, these patients have an excellent outcome after proctocolectomy and ileal pouch–anal anastomosis and should be strongly considered for such a procedure, if necessary (Wells et al 1991).

Approximately half the patients with Crohn's colitis will require surgery, with the most common indications being perianal disease and large-bowel obstruction (Farmer et al 1985). Postoperative mortality after elective colectomy for Crohn's disease is only 2%, but is higher if colectomy is accompanied by an ileorectal anastomosis (Ritchie 1990). Recurrence after colectomy is lower with ileostomy than with ileorectal anastomosis. As in ulcerative colitis, the risk of dysplasia and cancer occurring in Crohn's disease increases when colonic strictures are present. With transmural inflammation and subsequent wall thickening, patients with Crohn's colitis are not likely to develop toxic megacolon, although this complication has been noted in patients with disease of short duration, aggressive disease, or inflammatory as opposed to fibrostenotic disease.

Perianal fistulae are common findings in patients with Crohn's colitis. Interestingly, not all patients with perianal fistulae will have colonic Crohn's disease that is evident upon endoscopy. For perianal disease to occur, however, at least mild or purely microscopic rectal disease must be assumed to exist (Markowitz et al 1984). Approximately 10% of women with Crohn's colitis will develop a rectovaginal fistula.

Other disease sites

Symptoms and signs of Crohn's disease may develop before there is any evidence for intestinal disease. Nondeforming reactive polyarticular arthritis is the most common alternative presenting complaint (Michener et al 1990). Patients also often present with cholestatic liver disease, particularly pericholangitis or primary sclerosing cholangitis. Acute pancreatitis, even in the absence of fibrostenotic duodenal disease or choledocholithiasis, has been frequently reported and must now be considered an extraintestinal manifestation of Crohn's disease (Seyrig et al 1985, Lashner et al 1986, Spiess et al 1992, Tromm et al 1992, Eisner et al 1993). Similarly, oral ulcerations (usually with granulomas), ocular diseases such as episcleritis or uveitis, or cutaneous diseases such as psoriasis, erythema nodosum or pyoderma gangrenosum may be initial or early sites of Crohn's disease (Plauth et al 1991, Schuettenberg 1991). Patients with Crohn's disease who have a family medical history of psoriasis are more likely to develop psoriasis themselves (Lee et al 1990).

NATURAL HISTORY OF CROHN'S DISEASE ACCORDING TO DISEASE BEHAVIOR

Until 1971, studies on the natural history of Crohn's disease assumed that recurrence was homogeneous. DeDombal et al (1971) described two patterns of recurrence: type A had an aggressive course, with early surgery, a high risk of early recurrence and a poor prognosis, whereas type B had a more indolent course, later surgery, a lower risk of recurrence and a good prognosis. Recurrence was defined both symptomatically and with objective histopathologic or radiologic evidence of recurrent disease. Patients in whom disease was restricted to the colon most often had late recurrences, whereas patients with small-intestinal or ileocolonic disease most often had early recurrences. The cumulative risk of recurrence predicted by actuarial analysis was 15.5% at 1 year, 22.5% after 5 years, 35.3% after 10 years, and 52.3% after 20 years. Recurrence was significantly more frequent in patients who had surgery between ages 10 and 49 than those who were over age 50 at the time of the primary operation. Patients with early recurrence had a higher mortality and were more symptomatic than patients with late recurrence. Serum C-reactive protein and orosomucoid levels have also been found to increase in the 3 months before a documented recurrence, especially in inflammatory or aggressive disease (Wright et al 1987). However, the value of intervention to maintain remission in patients with abnormal laboratory values remains to be proven.

Age at symptom onset was believed to influence prognosis, with younger patients more often having aggressive disease. However, this theory was not supported by a large study of patients with Crohn's disease who had undergone surgery (Sachar et al 1983b). Despite the longer duration of disease before the first surgery, the rate of postoperative recurrence, as defined by radiological or surgical criteria, in older patients was similar to that in younger patients. At all ages the preoperative duration of disease had a direct effect on postoperative recurrence, so that patients with the longest duration of disease before surgery had the longest recurrence-free survival. The cumulative postoperative recurrence rate at 5 years in patients with indolent disease was 23%, compared to 65% for patients with more aggressive disease, as defined by preoperative duration of disease in Sachar's study. The relative risk of recurrence for patients with a 2-year remission duration compared to a 10-year remission duration was 1.5.

When the initial surgical indications were classified as perforating or non-perforating disease, the mean time to the first reoperation in patients with perforating disease was 4.7 years and was 8.8 years in patients with non-perforating disease (Farmer et al 1985). Perforating indications included acute free perforation, subacute perforation with abscess formation, and chronic perforation with internal fistula formation. Non-perforating indications included intestinal obstruction, disease that did not respond to medical therapy, hemorrhage, and toxic dilatation without perforation. More patients with perforating disease required a third operation than patients with non-perforating disease. The indications for surgery also varied according to the anatomical distribution of the disease. The principal indication for the first surgery in patients with ileitis or ileocolitis was perforating disease. Furthermore, recurrence in patients with ileitis or ileocolitis was usually perforating disease that occurred much earlier than in patients with colonic disease. Non-perforating disease was the most frequent indication for surgery in patients with colonic disease.

NATURAL HISTORY OF CROHN'S DISEASE ACCORDING TO DISEASE CHARACTERISTICS

Manifestations of Crohn's disease usually, but not always, follow the same pattern over time. The three principal disease patterns that have been described are fibrostenotic, inflammatory and perforating. A patient may have more than one pattern, but one pattern usually predominates (Sachar et al 1992). Furthermore, aggressive disease usually remains aggressive and indolent disease progresses slowly.

Exacerbations of disease activity

Crohn's disease is a naturally remitting and recurring disease. In the placebo arm of large randomized clinical trials, 8–44% of patients with active disease have spontaneous remission, with a mean time to remission of 4 months after entry (Meyers & Janowitz 1984). In the 20% of patients with indolent disease remission may be long-lasting, for more than 20 years after one or two flares. In patients with more aggressive disease 30% will relapse within 1 year, and 40% will relapse within 2 years. Patients with even more aggressive disease never achieve remission (Table 54.2).

Aggressive disease is usually inflammatory or perforating and is characterized by a short duration of disease before

Table 54.2 Comparison of aggressive and indolent disease in patients with Crohn's disease

Characteristic	Aggressive disease	Indolent disease
Disease type	Inflammatory Perforating	Fibrostenotic
Symptom duration before first surgery	Short	Long
Surgical indications	Inflammatory mass Fistula perforation	Obstruction Stricture Refractory to therapy
Recurrence rate after surgery	High	Low
Duration of remission	Short	Long
Need for second surgery	High	Low

the first surgery. Patients with aggressive disease often develop an inflammatory mass, with abscess and perforation (Basilisco et al 1989). Patients with an inflammatory mass, azotemia, elevated transaminase levels and elevated acute-phase reactants, including erythrocyte sedimentation rate, are likely to require early hospitalization and surgery (Brignola et al 1986, Visser et al 1990). The severity and bowel location of the relapse correspond closely with the initial attack (Wright 1992).

Indolent Crohn's disease is characterized by fibrostenotic disease and a long duration before the first surgery. The most important complications are fixed stenotic bowel segments, chronic active disease refractory to therapy, or fistulae (Table 54.2) (Basilisco et al 1989). Elevated acute-phase reactants do not accurately predict symptomatic recurrence in fibrostenotic or indolent disease (Wright et al 1987). Surgical treatment of indolent disease often produces prolonged remission.

Although the causes of recurrence and disease type are not known, recurrences are associated with a variety of factors, such as cigarette smoking, oral contraceptive use, non-steroidal anti-inflammatory drug use, and bacterial infection. Cigarette smokers and children exposed to passive smoking are more likely than controls to develop Crohn's disease initially (Silverstein et al 1989, Persson et al 1990, Lashner et al 1993). Half the patients with Crohn's disease are cigarette smokers: Such patients experience significantly more symptomatic days per month than non-smokers, and have a 60% higher relapse rate than non-smokers (Duffy et al 1990, Kurata et al 1992). Also, repeat surgery is more often required among smokers (Sutherland et al 1990). Smokers are also more likely to develop inflammatory and aggressive disease, whereas non-smokers and former smokers more often develop indolent and fibrostenotic disease (Duffy et al 1990). Smoking cessation should be a part of any therapeutic program for patients with Crohn's disease.

Although oral contraceptive users have no increased risk of developing Crohn's disease (Lashner et al 1989), women with Crohn's disease who smoke and use oral contraceptives have a higher risk of relapse than women who smoke and do not use oral contraceptives (Wakefield et al 1991). Relapses are most often inflammatory and located in the ileocolonic or colonic regions, regions that also are affected in multifocal thrombosis with local infarction (Wakefield et al 1991, Wright 1992). Enteric infections from *Clostridium difficile*, enteropathic *Escherichia coli* and *Campylobacter jejuni* that could account for a relapse are rarely found and so do not explain high relapse rates (Wever et al 1992).

Postoperative recurrence

In a large series the average annual frequency of Crohn's disease flares before surgery was 1.9 and after surgery was 1.7 (Pallone et al 1992). Postoperative complications are disturbingly similar to be complications that required the initial surgery – the natural history of a disease type is rarely altered by surgery (Greenstein et al 1988). Reoperation rates reach 50% for all disease sites and are even higher for fistulous or perianal disease (Whelan et al 1985). Over 75% of patients will have endoscopic evidence of recurrence at the anastomotic site at 1 year, and 20% will develop symptoms within 1 year of surgery (Rutgeerts et al 1990, Olaison et al 1992, Heimann et al 1993). Within 3 years 85% have endoscopic recurrence and 35% develop recurrent symptoms. Patients likely to have early recurrence are those with extensive resections, multiple anastomoses or both. When multiple sites are resected during a single surgery the risk of recurrence increases by 2.5 compared to patients with single-site disease (Michelassi et al 1991).

Before surgery inflammation most often extends distally from the initial site. After surgery disease usually recurs immediately proximal to the anastomosis. Factors that predict early recurrence are inflammatory and aggressive disease with high preoperative disease activity, multiple previous bowel resections, and a short duration of disease before surgery (Sachar et al 1983b, Lindor et al 1985, Rutgeerts et al 1990). Patients with aggressive disease are at greatest risk for reoperation in the first postoperative year, unlike patients with indolent disease (Agrez et al 1982). Microscopic disease at the resection margins, age at resection or oral contraceptive use alone are not reliable predictors of postsurgical recurrence (Sutherland et al 1992).

OTHER PROBLEMS OCCURRING IN THE NATURAL HISTORY OF CROHN'S DISEASE

Cancer

Patients with Crohn's disease have a 50% greater risk of developing cancer, either intestinal or extraintestinal (Ekbom et al 1991). Intestinal cancers are principally colorectal and small-bowel (usually ileal). Extraintestinal cancers are only modestly increased (10%) over those found in a control population, with the most common tumor type being squamous cell cancer of the skin (Ekbom et al 1991).

The relative risk of colorectal cancer in patients with Crohn's colitis is approximately 3 (Ekbom et al 1990a, 1992), and cancer occurs at a younger age than does sporadic small-bowel cancer (Hamilton 1985). Although patients with Crohn's colitis are at substantial risk for colorectal cancer, this risk is much lower than in patients with ulcerative colitis. Two typical patient profiles for colorectal cancer in Crohn's disease have been described (Ekbom et al 1990a, Kyle & Ewen 1992). One is that of a patient who develops cancer at a young age (less than 55 years old) and has had a long duration of inflammatory disease. Such patients have a poor prognosis. The other profile is that of an older patient with a short duration of fibrostenotic Crohn's disease; such patients have a more favorable prognosis.

Mucosal dysplasia has been found adjacent to colorectal cancer in Crohn's disease (Petras et al 1987). Distant dysplasia, an important feature of ulcerative colitis that allows for effective colorectal cancer surveillance, is usually absent in Crohn's colitis. Therefore, because patients with Crohn's disease are at less risk for cancer and because distant dysplasia is usually absent, surveillance is less likely to reduce cancer-related mortality than in patients with ulcerative colitis.

Small-bowel cancer is a rare complication of Crohn's disease. Compared to sporadic small-bowel cancer, cancer in Crohn's disease occurs at a younger age, is more common in the distal small bowel, occurs more often in men, and is rarely diagnosed before surgery (Lashner 1992). Because a surgical cure is rare, identifying preventable risk factors is important. Case series have suggested that unresected bowel loops with chronic inflammatory disease, fibrostenotic unresected disease, and chronic fistulous disease – all three types of behavior for Crohn's disease – are risk factors (Sachar 1983). A case-control study has suggested additional risk factors, including proximal (therefore extensive) small-bowel disease, hazardous industrial occupational exposures, and chronic immunosuppressive therapy (Lashner 1992). Confirmatory studies are needed before recommending limitations on exposures.

Fertility and pregnancy

Fertility, as determined by the number of children born to women, is diminished in patients with Crohn's disease: parity is inversely associated with the number of bowel resections (Nwokolo et al 1994). It is not clear, though, that abnormalities in reproductive physiology are widespread. Among women with Crohn's disease who are in a stable relationship 25% reported infrequent or no intercourse, principally because of disease symptoms such as abdominal pain and diarrhea, or fear of incontinence (Moody et al 1992). Dyspareunia is common, especially in women with perianal disease and fistulae. A right lower quadrant inflammatory mass may induce inflammation in the adjacent fallopian tube and cause infertility. Still, the reduced rate of deliveries is primarily the result of patient choice rather than sexual dysfunction or Crohn's disease activity (Baird et al 1990).

Pregnancy does not necessarily influence the course of Crohn's disease, nor is pregnancy associated with the development of new-onset Crohn's disease (Donaldson 1985, Ekbom et al 1990b). However, if an inflammatory flare should occur during pregnancy the relative risk of a premature birth is approximately 3 (Baird et al 1990). Inflammatory flares during pregnancy have been successfully treated using an elemental diet and no medication, resulting in the delivery of a full-term baby (Teahon et al 1991).

Quality of life

Issues regarding quality of life and psychology have a great impact on the course of Crohn's disease in both children and adults. Common and treatable psychologic illness can be overlooked by both clinicians and families (Engstron 1991). Over half of children with Crohn's disease exhibit signs of severe depression and anxiety, compared to only 15% of an unaffected population (Engstron & Lindquist 1991). Psychiatric symptoms in children correlate with the severity of disease. Anorexia nervosa is associated with Crohn's disease (Mailett & Murch 1990). Although children diagnosed with Crohn's disease by high school age lose more school days, they achieved similar academic success to peer-nominated or community controls, as measured by performance on standardized examinations and the proportion matriculating to college (Mayberry et al 1992).

Adults with Crohn's disease lose more time from work, although the proportion employed and career achievement levels are not diminished (Mayberry et al 1992). Compared to controls, high-school graduates with Crohn's disease are just as likely to be employed but have a higher rate of long-term unemployment, and one-third conceal their diagnosis from their employer (Mayberry et al 1992). Stressful events correlate with worsening signs and symptoms of Crohn's disease (Garrett et al 1991). In times of major stress the risk of exacerbation is more than twice the rate in patients with less stress (Duffy et al 1991). Furthermore, complications of Crohn's disease and reduced sexual intimacy correlate with poorer psychological function, poorer perception of health and well-being, and greater psychological stress (Drossman et al 1991).

CONCLUSIONS

Crohn's disease is so heterogeneous that the natural history cannot be predicted simply by determining the location of disease in the gastrointestinal tract. Disease behavior (aggressive versus indolent) and disease characteristics (inflammatory versus fibrostenotic versus perforating) also contribute greatly to the prognosis. Treatment success, too, may be predicted by a careful description of disease. Therefore, classifying a patient with Crohn's disease by anatomical extent is insufficient. Additional descriptions of disease characteristics and behavior are essential in predicting the natural history of Crohn's disease.

REFERENCES

Agrez M V, Valente R M, Pierce W et al 1982 Surgical history of Crohn's disease in a well-defined population. Mayo Clinic Proceedings 57: 747–752

Andrews H A, Lewis P, Allan R N 1989 Mortality in Crohn's disease – a clinical analysis. Quarterly Journal of Medicine 71: 399–405

Baird D D, Narendranathan M, Sandler R S 1990 Increased risk of preterm birth for women with inflammatory bowel disease. Gastroenterology 99: 987–994

Basilisco G, Campanini M, Cesana B, Ranzi T, Bianchi P 1989 Risk factors for first operation in Crohn's disease. American Journal of Gastroenterology 84: 749–752

Brignola C, Campieri M, Bazzocchi G et al 1986 A laboratory index for predicting relapse in asymptomatic patients with Crohn's disease. Gastroenterology 91: 1490–1494

Cary E R, Tremaine W J, Banks P M, Nagorney D M 1989 Isolated Crohn's disease of the stomach. Mayo Clinic Proceedings 14: 776–779

DeDombal F T, Burton I, Goligher J C 1971 Recurrence of Crohn's disease after primary excisional surgery. Gut 12: 519–527

Donaldson R M 1985 Management of medical problems in pregnancy – inflammatory bowel disease. New England Journal of Medicine 312: 1616–1619

Drossman D A, Leserman J, Li Z M, Mitchell C M, Zagami E A, Patrick D L 1991 The rating form of IBD patient concerns: a new measure of health status. Psychosomatic Medicine 53: 701–712

Duffy L C, Zielezny M A, Marshall J R et al 1990 Cigarette smoking and risk of clinical relapse in patients with Crohn's disease. American Journal of Preventive Medicine 6: 161–166

Duffy L C, Zielezny M A, Marshall J R et al 1991 Relevance of major stress events as an indicator of disease activity prevalence in inflammatory bowel disease. Behavioral Medicine 17: 101–110

Eisner T D, Goldman I S, McKinley M J 1993 Crohn's disease and pancreatitis. American Journal of Gastroenterology 88: 583–586

Ekbom A, Helmick C, Zack M, Adami H O 1990a Increased risk of large bowel cancer in Crohn's disease with colonic involvement. Lancet 336: 357–359

Ekbom A, Adami H O, Helmick C G, Jonzon A, Zack M M 1990b Perinatal risk factors for inflammatory bowel disease: a case-control study. American Journal of Epidemiology 132: 1111–1119

Ekbom A, Helmick C, Zack M, Adami H O 1991 Extracolonic malignancies in inflammatory bowel disease. Cancer 67: 2015–2019

Ekbom A, Helmick C G, Zack M, Holmberg L, Adami H O 1992 Survival and causes of death in patients with inflammatory bowel disease: a population-based study. Gastroenterology 103: 954–960

Engstron I 1991 Family interaction and locus of control in children and adolescents with inflammatory bowel disease. Journal of the American Acadamy of Child and Adolescent Psychology 30: 913–920

Engstron I, Lindquist B L 1991 Inflammatory bowel disease in children and adolescents: a somatic and psychiatric investigation. Acta Pediatrica Scandinavica 80: 640–647

Farmer R G, Hawk W A, Turnbull R B 1972 Crohn's disease of the duodenum (transmural duodenitis): clinical manifestations and report of 11 cases. American Journal of Digestive Diseases 17: 191–198

Farmer R G, Whelan G, Fazio V W 1985 Long-term follow-up of patients with Crohn's disease: relationship between clinical pattern and prognosis. Gastroenterology 88: 1818–1825

Fielding J F, Toye D K M, Beton D C, Cooke W T 1970 Crohn's disease of the stomach and duodenum. Gut 11: 1001–1006

Garrett V D, Brantley P J, Jones G N, McKnight G T 1991 The relation between daily stress and Crohn's disease. Journal of Behavioral Medicine 14: 87–96

Gitkind M J, Wright S C 1990 Amyloidosis complicating inflammatory bowel disease: a case report and review of the literature. Digestive Diseases and Sciences 35: 906–908

Greenstein A J, Lachman P, Sachar D B et al 1988 Perforating and non-perforating indications for repeated operations in Crohn's disease: evidence for two clinical forms. Gut 29: 588–592

Griffiths A M, Wesson D E, Shandling B, Corey M, Sherman P M 1991 Factors influencing postoperative recurrence of Crohn's disease in childhood. Gut 32: 491–495

Hamilton S R 1985 Colorectal carcinoma in patients with Crohn's disease. Gastroenterology 89: 398–407

Heimann T M, Greenstein A J, Lewis B, Kaufman D, Heimann D M, Aufses A H 1993 Prediction of early symptomatic recurrence after intestinal resection in Crohn's disease. Annals of Surgery 218: 294–298

Jacobson I M, Schapiro R H, Warshaw A L 1985 Gastric and duodenal fistulas in Crohn's disease. Gastroenterology 89: 1347–1352

Kirschner B S, Sutton M M 1986 Somatomedin-C levels in growth-impaired children and adolescents with inflammatory bowel disease. Gastroenterology 91: 830–836

Kirsner J B 1975 Problems in the differentiation of ulcerative colitis and Crohn's disease of the colon: the need for repeated diagnostic evaluation. Gastroenterology 68: 187–191

Kurata J H, Kantor-Fish S, Frankl H, Godby P, Vadheim C M 1992 Crohn's disease among ethnic groups in a large health maintenance organization. Gastroenterology 102: 1940–1948

Kyle J, Ewen S W 1992 Two types of colorectal carcinoma in Crohn's disease. Annals of the Royal College of Surgeons of England 74: 387–390

Lashner B A 1992 Risk factors for small bowel cancer in Crohn's disease. Digestive Diseases and Sciences 37: 1179–1184

Lashner B A, Kane S V, Hanauer S B 1989 Lack of association between oral contraceptives and Crohn's disease: a community-based matched case-control study. Gastroenterology 97: 1442–1447

Lashner B A, Kirsner J B, Hanauer S B 1986 Acute pancreatitis associated with high concentration lipid emulsion during total parenteral nutrition for Crohn's disease. Gastroenterology 90: 1039–1041

Lashner B A, Shaheen N J, Hanauer S B, Kirschner B S 1993 Passive smoking is associated with an increased risk of developing inflammatory bowel disease in children. American Journal of Gastroenterology 88: 356–359

Lee F I, Bellary S V, Francis C 1990 Increased occurrence of psoriasis in patients with Crohn's disease and their relatives. American Journal of Gastroenterology 85: 962–963

Lindor K D, Fleming C R, Ilstrup D M 1985 Preoperative nutritional status and other factors that influence surgical outcome in patients with Crohn's disease. Mayo Clinic Proceedings 60: 393–396

Lock M R, Farmer R G, Fazio V M, Jagelman D G, Lavery I C, Weakley F L 1981 Recurrence and reoperation for Crohn's disease: the role of disease location in prognosis. New England Journal of Medicine 304: 1586–1588

Mailett P, Murch S 1990 Anorexia nervosa complicating inflammatory bowel disease. Archives of Diseases of Childhood 65: 298–300

Markowitz J, Daum F, Aiges H et al 1984 Perianal disease in children and adolescents with Crohn's disease. Gastroenterology 86: 829–833

Mayberry M K, Probert C, Srivastava E, Rhodes J, Mayberry J F 1992 Perceived discrimination in education and employment by people with Crohn's disease: a case-control study of educational achievement and employment. Gut 33: 312–314

Meyers S, Janowitz H D 1984 'Natural history' of Crohn's disease: an analytic review of the placebo lesson. Gastroenterology 87: 1189–1192

Michelassi F, Balestracci T, Chappell R, Block G E 1991 Primary and recurrent Crohn's disease: experience with 1379 patients. Annals of Surgery 214: 230–238

Michener W M, Caulfield M, Wyllie R, Farmer R G 1990 Management of inflammatory bowel disease: 30 years of observation. Cleveland Clinic Journal of Medicine 37: 685–691

Moody G, Probert C S, Srivastava E M, Rhodes J, Mayberry J F 1992 Sexual dysfunction amongst women with Crohn's disease: a hidden problem. Digestion 52: 179–183

Murray J J, Schoetz D J, Nugent F W, Coller J A, Veidenheimer M C 1984 Surgical management of Crohn's disease involving the duodenum. American Journal of Surgery 147: 58–65

Nugent F W, Richmond M, Park S K 1977 Crohn's disease of the duodenum. Gut 18: 115–120

Nwokolo C U, Tan W C, Andrews H A, Allan R N 1994 Surgical resections in parous patients with distal ileal and colonic Crohn's disease. Gut 35: 220–223

Olaison G, Smedh K, Sjodahl R 1992 Natural course of Crohn's disease after ileocolic resection: endoscopically visualized ileal ulcers preceding symptoms. Gut 33: 331–335

Pallone F, Boirivant M, Stazi M A, Cosintino R, Prantera C, Torsoli A 1992 Analysis of clinical course of postoperative recurrence in Crohn's disease of the distal ileum. Digestive Diseases and Sciences 37: 215–219

Persson P G, Ahlbom A, Hellers G 1990 Inflammatory bowel disease and tobacco smoke: a case-control study. Gut 31: 1377–1381

Petras R E, Mir-Madjlessi S H, Farmer R G 1987 Crohn's disease and intestinal carcinoma: a report of 11 cases with emphasis on associated epithelial dysplasia. Gastroenterology 93: 1307–1314

Pezim M E, Pemberton J H, Beart R W, et al 1989 Outcome of 'indeterminate' colitis following ileal pouch–anal anastomosis. Diseases of the Colon and Rectum 32: 653–658

Plauth M, Jenss H, Meyle J 1991 Oral manifestations of Crohn's disease: an analysis of 79 cases. Journal of Clinical Gastroenterology 13: 29–37

Prior P, Gyde S N, Cooke W T, Waterhouse J A H, Allan R N 1981 Mortality in Crohn's disease. Gastroenterology 80: 307–312

Ritchie J K 1990 The results of surgery for large bowel Crohn's disease. Annals of the Royal College of Surgeons of England 72: 155–157

Ross T M, Fazio V M, Farmer R G 1983 Long-term results of surgical treatment for Crohn's disease of the duodenum. Annals of Surgery 197: 399–406

Rutgeerts P, Goboes K, Vantrappen G, Beyls J, Kerremans R, Hiele M 1990 Predictability of the postoperative course of Crohn's disease. Gastroenterology 99: 956–963

Sachar D B 1983 New concepts of cancer. Mount Sinai Journal of Medicine 50: 133–137

Sachar D B, Andrews H, Farmer R G, et al 1992 Proposed classification of patient subgroups in Crohn's disease. Working team report 4. Gastroenterology International 3: 141–154

Sachar D B, Wolfson D M, Greenstein A J, Goldberg J, Styczynski R, Janowitz H D 1983 Risk factors for postoperative recurrence of Crohn's disease. Gastroenterology 85: 917–921

Sackett D L 1979 Bias in analytic research. Journal of Chronic Diseases 32: 51–63

Schuettenberg S P 1991 Nodular scleritis, episcleritis, and anterior uveitis as ocular complications of Crohn's disease. Journal of the American Optometric Association 62: 377–381

Seyrig J A, Jian R, Modigliani R et al 1985 Idiopathic pancreatitis associated with inflammatory bowel disease. Digestive Diseases and Sciences 30: 1121–1126

Shivananda S, Hordjik M L, Pena A S, Mayberry J F 1989 Crohn's disease: risk of recurrence and reoperation in a defined population. Gut 30: 990–995

Silverstein M D, Lashner B A, Hanauer S B, Evans A A, Kirsner J B 1989 Cigarette smoking in Crohn's disease. American Journal of Gastroenterology 84: 31–33

Sonnenberg A 1990 Occupational mortality of inflammatory bowel disease. Digestion 46: 10–18

Spiess S E, Braun M, Vogelzang R L, Craig R M 1992 Crohn's disease of the duodenum complicated by pancreatitis and common bile duct obstruction. American Journal of Gastroenterology 87: 1033–1036

Steinhardt H J, Loeschke K, Kasper H, Holtermuller K H, Schafer H 1985 European Cooperative Crohn's Disease Study (ECCDS): clinical features and natural history. Digestion 31: 97–108

Sutherland L R, Ramcharan S, Bryant H, Fick G 1990 Effect of cigarette smoking on recurrence of Crohn's disease. Gastroenterology 98: 1123–1128

Sutherland L R, Ramcharan S, Bryant H, Fick G 1992 Effect of oral contraceptive use on reoperation following surgery for Crohn's disease. Digestive Diseases and Sciences 37: 1377–1382

Teahon K, Pearson M, Levi A J, Bjarnason I 1991 Elemental diet in the management of Crohn's disease during pregnancy. Gut 32: 1079–1081

Tootla F, Lucas R J, Bernacki E G, Tabor H 1976 Gastroduodenal Crohn's disease. Archives of Surgery 111: 855–857

Tromm A, Huppe D, Micklemield G H, Schwegler U, May B 1992 Acute pancreatitis complicating Crohn's disease: a mere coincidence or causality? Gut 33: 1289–1291

Truelove S C, Pena A S 1976 Course and prognosis of Crohn's disease. But 17: 192–201

Visser N D, Bryant H E, Hershfield N B 1990 Predictors of hospitalization early in the course of Crohn's disease: a pilot study. Gastroenterology 39: 380–385

Wakefield A J, Sawyer A M, Hudson M, Dhillon A P, Pounder R E 1991 Smoking, the oral contraceptive pill, and Crohn's disease. Digestive Diseases and Sciences 36: 1147–1150

Wells A D, McMillan I, Price A B, Ritchie J K, Nicholls R J 1991 Natural history of indeterminate colitis. British Journal of Surgery 78: 179–181

Weterman I T, Beimond I, Pena A S 1990 Mortality and causes of death in Crohn's disease: review of 50 years' experience in Leiden University Hospital. Gut 31: 1387–1390

Wever P, Koch M, Heizmann W R, Scheurlen M, Jenss H, Hartmann F 1992 Microbic superinfection in relapse of inflammatory bowel disease. Journal of Clinical Gastroenterology 14: 302–308

Whelan G, Farmer R G, Fazio V W, Goormastic M 1985 Recurrence after surgery in Crohn's disease: relationship to location of disease (clinical pattern) and surgical indication. Gastroenterology 88: 1826–1833

Woolfson K, Greenberg G R 1992 Symptomatic improvement of gastroduodenal Crohn's disease with omeprazole. Canadian Journal of Gastroenterology 6: 21–24

Wright J P 1992 Factors influencing first relapse in patients with Crohn's disease. Journal of Clinical Gastroenterology 15: 12–16

Wright J P, Young G O, Tigler-Wybrandi N 1987 Predictors of acute relapse of Crohn's disease: a laboratory and clinical study. Digestive Diseases and Sciences 32: 164–170

Zarnow H, Grant T H, Spellberg M, Levin B 1976 Unusual complications of regional enteritis: duodenobiliary fistula and hepatic abscess. Journal of the American Medical Association 235: 1880–1881

SECTION 5

Therapeutic options

55. Sulfasalazine and the new salicylates

L. R. Sutherland

INTRODUCTION

Discovery of sulfasalazine

The discovery of the value of sulfasalazine in the treatment of ulcerative colitis is yet another example of medical serendipity. Nana Svartz, a Swedish physician, thought that the inflammatory response in ulcerative colitis and rheumatoid arthritis was most pronounced in the 'connective tissues', and that either might have a bacterial etiology. Since the ability of the salicylates to be effective in connective tissue diseases such as arthritis was well known, her concept was to link a salicylate with a sulfa, the only available antimicrobial known to have an effect against streptococci. The result was the new compound sulfasalazine, an antibiotic (sulfapyridine) linked with an anti-inflammatory (5-aminosalicylic acid, 5-ASA) by a diazo bond (Svartz 1988). These observations provided the first therapeutic agent for the treatment of ulcerative colitis, but it was not until the 1950s that her work became widely known. The first randomized placebo-controlled trials of sulfasalazine for ulcerative colitis were performed in the early 1960s.

For many years the basic pharmacology of sulfasalazine was unknown. The first important observations emphasized the role of gut bacteria (Schroder et al 1973) in sulfasalazine metabolism, and that taking 5-ASA by mouth was not associated with significant fecal 5-ASA levels (Peppercorn & Goldman 1973).

The next issue was to determine the active agent, sulfapyridine or 5-ASA. Azad Khan and colleagues (1977) in a randomized, 2-week trial of enemas containing either sulfasalazine (2 g), sulfapyridine (1.3 g) or 5-ASA (0.7 g), demonstrated that 5-ASA was the active moiety of sulfasalazine. These observations were confirmed by van Hees and associates (1980) using 5-ASA (200 mg), sulfapyridine (300 mg) or placebo suppositories. A third study by German investigators compared 3 g of either sulfasalazine or sulfapyridine tablets and 5-ASA suppositories in patients with Crohn's disease or ulcerative colitis, and confirmed the efficacy of 5-ASA (Klotz et al 1980).

Another early question in the evolution of 5-ASA therapy was the determination as to whether all salicylates had similar therapeutic properties for patients with inflammatory bowel disease. A placebo-controlled trial of sodium salicylate enemas in 19 patients with ulcerative colitis demonstrated that not all salicylates were effective (Campieri et al 1978).

The new aminosalicylates

Since 5-ASA taken by mouth is rapidly absorbed in the upper gastrointestinal tract, a variety of delivery systems to release the drug at different locations within the gut have been developed (Table 55.1). Broadly speaking they can be divided into three groups: pH dependent, microspheres, and azo-prodrugs (which require bacterial action for release). As the various formulations differ in where they release 5-ASA, it is not possible to write a generic prescription. Trade names are required for the following discussion.

pH dependent

These formulations consist of a core of 5-ASA covered by a thin coat of a pH-dependent resin. At the specified

Table 55.1 Classification of the aminosalicylates

pH dependent
Asacol
Claversal/Mesasal/Salofalk/Rowasa

Microspheres
Pentasa

Prodrugs
Sulfasalazine
Olsalazine (Dipentum)
Balsalazide (Colazide)
Ipsalazine

Others
N-acetyl-5-aminosalicylic acid
4-aminosalicylic acid

luminal pH the resin dissolves and the drug is released. For Asacol the pH-dependent resin is Eudragit-S, which should dissolve at pH of >7. It is used primarily for the treatment of colonic disease, specifically ulcerative colitis. Recent clinical trials have also suggested that it may be effective in maintaining remission in Crohn's disease, including patients with terminal ileal disease.

For Claversal (Mesasal, Salofalk) the pH resin is Eudragit-L, which should dissolve at pH >6. Release of 5-ASA is expected within the terminal ileum. This preparation is used for the management of patients with either Crohn's disease or ulcerative colitis. Rowasa is similar to Claversal except that the resin is Eudragit-L100, which dissolves at pH >5.

The pH pattern of release in either the terminal ileum or the colon is based in part on a study of two normal volunteers and seven patients with a variety of gastrointestinal disorders. The report suggested that the gut luminal pH rose to 7 or higher as the ileocecal region was reached (Meldrum et al 1972). This concept has been challenged recently by Raimundo and colleagues (1992). A pH-sensitive radiotelemetry capsule was used to measure gastrointestinal pH in patients with active ulcerative colitis, colitis in remission, and a control population. Similar pH profiles could be obtained in both the proximal and distal small intestine for controls and colitics. However, the pH in the right colon of pancolitics, regardless of disease activity, was significantly decreased compared to controls (4.6 versus 6.7, $P<0.02$). In approximately 25% of patients the pH of >7 was sustained for less than 30 minutes. Such alterations in colonic pH might explain why patients may from time to time report passing undissolved capsules.

Microspheres

Pentasa consists of microgranules of 5-ASA coated with a semipermeable ethylcellulose membrane, which begins to dissolve in the stomach and duodenum shortly after ingestion. This preparation should deliver the drug to all areas of the gut. Although approximately 60% of Pentasa is released in the small intestine, sufficient medication is still available to be effective in the treatment of colonic disease.

Azo-bond prodrugs

Sulfasalazine was the first azo-bond prodrug. Since many of the side effects related to sulfasalazine were thought to be related to the sulfapyridine carrier, it is not surprising that consideration would be given to attaching 5-ASA to other carriers via an azo bond, which would then be split by colonic bacteria. The most novel compound in this category is olsalazine (Dipentum), which consists of two 5-ASA molecules linked by a diazo bond.

Other compounds, particularly using benzoic acid derivatives as carriers, have been developed (Chan et al 1983). Balsalazide (Colazide) links 5-ASA to 4-aminobenzoyl-β-alanine; ipsalazide is 5-ASA joined with 4-aminobenzoylglycine. Benzalazine combines 5-ASA with *p*-aminobenzoic acid, an essential substrate for folic acid synthesis (Fleig et al 1988).

PHARMACOKINETICS

Only 25–33% of sulfasalazine taken by mouth is absorbed from the gastrointestinal tract: 10% of the dose given can be retrieved from urine and the remainder, including its metabolites, may be recovered from the feces. *N*-acetyl-5-aminosalicylic acid is the major metabolite of 5-ASA but does not appear to have clinical activity (see below).

Controversial pharmacokinetic issues regarding salicylates include lack of consensus as to which metabolite or body compartment (fecal, mucosal, circulatory) is important, and difficulty in extrapolating from in-vitro or in-vivo studies involving normal volunteers to studies in patients with varying inclusion criteria.

Examples of the problems include a study of 5-ASA and *N*-acetyl-5-aminosalicylic acid levels measured in colonic biopsies. Although differences in mucosal concentrations were found for the various formulations (De Vos et al 1992), all are effective clinically. Similarly, although diarrhea alters the release of 5-ASA (Rijk et al 1992b), clinically significant differences between the newer compounds are not apparent.

An important issue in the pharmacokinetics of the topical preparations is the effect of the enema medium on absorption. Plasma concentrations of 5-ASA were significantly higher in patients given 5-ASA in a neutral buffer, whereas patients receiving 5-ASA in a mildly acidic solution (pH 4.8) had levels approximating those expected with oral sulfasalazine (Bondesen et al 1984).

MECHANISMS OF ACTION

The potential mechanisms of action for either sulfasalazine or 5-ASA have recently been reviewed (Greenfield et al 1993). They include alterations in eicosanoid metabolism, scavenging of free radicals, and immunologic and metabolic effects.

Many of the in-vitro effects occur at drug concentrations that may not be achieved in vivo. Alterations in various inflammatory markers could reflect the healing, anti-inflammatory properties of the drug rather than the specific therapeutic mode of action. Another possible confounder is that various studies used normal human colonic tissues, whereas others worked with biopsies taken from patients with ulcerative colitis. Extrapolating the effects seen in normals to mechanisms of action for patients might be inappropriate.

Alterations in eicosanoid metabolism

Arachidonic acid is a 20-carbon polyunsaturated fatty acid ubiquitous in cell membranes. The eicosanoids derived from the metabolism of arachidonic acid may be broadly divided into those which are generated through the cyclo-oxygenase pathway (prostaglandins, prostacyclin and thromboxane A_2) and those which are derived from the 5-lipoxygenase pathway (5-HPETE and leukotrienes (LT)).

The effects of the aminosalicylates on prostaglandin production appear to be dose dependent. Higher concentrations of 5-ASA result in the inhibition of prostaglandin (PGE_2) production (Sharon et al 1978), whereas at lower concentrations production of prostaglandins may be stimulated (Hawkey et al 1985). The effect of modification of prostaglandin levels on disease activity is controversial. NSAIDs (non-steroidal anti-inflammatory drugs), which are potent inhibitors of prostaglandins, have been implicated as a potential cause of flares of ulcerative colitis (Rampton et al 1983).

The products of lipoxygenation of arachidonic acid include the leukotrienes (LT), potent chemotactic agents having effects on vascular permeability and neutrophil function. Inhibition of LTB_4 production by either sulfasalazine or 5-ASA can be demonstrated, but possibly at concentrations higher than that which might be expected physiologically. The role of the inhibition of lipoxygenase has also been assessed using more specific inhibitors such as zileuton, which did not demonstrate convincing evidence of clinical activity (Hawkey et al 1994, Peppercorn et al 1994).

Free radical scavengers

Free radicals or reactive oxygen metabolites oxidize proteins, nucleic acids and cell membranes, and have been implicated in ulcerative colitis. They may be produced during the synthesis of prostaglandins or released by monocytes and neutrophils. Tamai and associates (1991) demonstrated that 5-ASA has free radical scavenging properties in vitro. It appears to complex with free radicals, preventing them from oxidizing cysteine. In-vivo studies suggest that the aminosalicylates are effective in attenuating the damage caused by reactive oxygen metabolites (Keshavarzian et al 1990). Metabolites produced by interactions between aminosalicylates and free radicals have been demonstrated in the stools of patients with ulcerative colitis treated with sulfasalazine (Ahnfelt-Ronne et al 1990).

Immunologic effects

It is possible that the mechanism of action by which the aminosalicylates exert their effect is not related to the inflammatory cascade, but rather through alterations in the immunologic repertoire. Potential mechanisms of action have been reviewed (Greenfield et al 1993) and include effects on antibody and cytokine secretion, alterations in interleukin-1 (IL-1) release, HLA-DR expression and lymphocyte function.

IL-1 is an important cytokine in the acute inflammatory response, having effects on neutrophils, protein synthesis, adhesion molecules and the synthesis of other interleukins. 5-ASA inhibits the release of IL-1 and appears to decrease the mucosal concentrations of IL-1 (Rachmilewitz et al 1992).

Metabolic effects

Roediger and associates (1989) suggest that 5-ASA could exert its effect via colonocyte metabolism. Specifically, they report that 5-ASA suppressed in-vitro colonocyte fatty acid oxidation. Although this effect was apparent for 5- and 3-ASA, 4-ASA had little effect. Since 4-ASA has a therapeutic efficacy similar to 5-ASA, this putative mechanism of action may not be important.

Summary of mechanism of action

The mechanism of action of the aminosalicylates will probably not be known for some time, but it is safe to suggest that the final explanation will be multifactorial. Studies should evaluate sulfasalazine, as well as 5- and 4-ASA. Effects which are limited to one compound and not others, particularly when comparing 5- and 4-ASA, are unlikely to be clinically important. Studies which suggest that intact sulfasalazine has effects give credence to physicians who feel that the parent drug has intrinsic therapeutic properties.

ADVERSE EFFECTS OF THE AMINOSALICYLATES

Sulfasalazine

As might be expected from a compound that contains a sulfa group, side effects are common (Table 55.2): approximately 20% of patients taking sulfasalazine complain of adverse events. Common side effects include nausea, vomiting, headache and anorexia, which may be alleviated by taking the coated form.

Adverse effects involving almost every organ system have been reported (Peppercorn 1984). Many of these reactions are related to serum levels of sulfapyridine and can be expected to occur more commonly in patients who are slow acetylators or who are taking a higher dose of medication. Various skin rashes have been described, including toxic epidermal necrolysis. Pulmonary complications include fibrosing alveolitis, bronchospasm and

Table 55.2 Side effects of the aminosalicylates

Unique to sulfasalazine
Gastrointestinal
    Nausea, vomiting
    Anorexia
    Dyspepsia
Hematological
    Hemolysis
    Neutropenia
    Agranulocytosis
    Folate malabsorption
Male infertility
Neuropathy

Common to all aminosalicylates
General
    Headache
    Fever, rash
Gastrointestinal
    Exacerbation of colitis
    Pancreatitis
    Inflammatory liver disease
    Watery diarrhea (olsalazine)
Other
    Pericarditis
    Pneumonitis
    Nephritis

allergic pneumonitis. A variety of hepatic lesions have been documented, including granulomatous hepatitis, acute hepatitis, cholestasis and a mixed hepatitic/cholestatic picture. Episodes of acute pancreatitis have been reported.

Hematological complications associated with sulfasalazine therapy vary, and include red cell aplasia and megaloblastic anemia related to folate malabsorption. Hemolytic anemia associated with either glucose-6-phosphate dehydrogenase deficiency or Heinz bodies, methemoglobinemia and sulfhemoglobinemia have been reported. Neutropenia, agranulocytosis and thrombocytopenia have also been documented.

Sulfasalazine has effects on male fertility. In one study most men had significantly lower sperm density, abnormal motility and morphology within 2 months of initiation of sulfasalazine therapy. Two months after withdrawal sperm function approached pretreatment values (Levi et al 1981). Substitution of sulfasalazine by 5-ASA is associated with a return towards normal sperm characteristics (Kjaergaard et al 1989).

The newer aminosalicylates

Assuming that most sulfasalazine side effects were related to sulfapyridine, it was anticipated that there would be fewer side effects associated with the newer delivery systems. This assumption has been generally correct: 80–90% of patients considered to be sulfasalazine sensitive will tolerate 5-ASA (Campieri et al 1984b, Turunen et al 1987).

The newer compounds are not totally free of adverse events, however. If the adverse event related to sulfasalazine was severe, caution should be exercised before switching the patient to a new preparation. On rare occasions pancreatitis or skin rashes and hepatotoxicity due to sulfasalazine have recurred with non-sulfa aminosalicylates (Poldermans & van Blankenstein 1988, Hautekeete et al 1992). In addition, isolated case reports document a variety of 5-ASA toxicities, including myocarditis, neuropathy and pancreatitis.

5-ASA is somewhat similar to phenacetin in chemical structure. Concerns have been expressed about alterations in renal function, particularly in patients receiving high doses of aminosalicylates. The peak serum 5-ASA level may be an important determinant of potential toxicity, but this has not been confirmed.

Despite few reports of significant renal toxicity, it is not clear which tests of renal function are relevant to determine the risk. Riley and colleagues (1992) were unable to demonstrate evidence of nephrotoxicity in patients taking either maintenance 5-ASA (0.8–2.4 g/day) or sulfasalazine (2–3 g/day). German investigators measuring urine proteins, α_2-microglobulin, IgG and tubular enzymes suggest that subtle evidence of renal tubular dysfunction can be demonstrated in patients taking 3 g or more of 5-ASA daily (Schreiber et al 1994b).

Exacerbation of diarrhea and abdominal symptoms within a few days after the initiation of 5-ASA therapy has been reported (Austin et al 1984). Patients often give a history of similar complaints when treated with sulfasalazine.

Diarrhea, however, has been a particular problem with olsalazine. In one trial (Wright et al 1993) 16% of osalazine-treated patients were withdrawn because of increased diarrhea. Subsequently it has been shown that olsalazine stimulates sodium, chloride and water secretion in the distal ileum (Goerg et al 1987). Fluid excretion is dose dependent (Sandberg-Gertzen et al 1986). Patients with ulcerative colitis may be particularly limited in their ability to reabsorb water across an inflamed colon, thereby lowering the threshold for diarrhea. Gradual titration of the dose and taking olsalazine with meals may reduce the incidence of diarrhea.

THERAPEUTIC TRIALS

Before reviewing the essential trials evaluating sulfasalazine and 5-ASA, it is important to consider the issue of possible type II or β errors. Many of the trials, particularly those comparing two forms of active therapy, have insufficient sample size to detect clinically significant differences. In this case an assumption that two treatments are equivalent may not be correct. In addition, it is important to consider the variable end points used, making comparisons between trials quite difficult.

This section will first consider the randomized controlled trials of the aminosalicylates in ulcerative colitis (active disease or maintenance of remission), followed by the trials in Crohn's disease (active disease or maintenance of remission). The trials using topical therapy either actively or for maintenance of remission in ulcerative colitis will be reviewed. Trials involving other aminosalicylates will also be covered.

ULCERATIVE COLITIS

Active disease

Sulfasalazine versus placebo

The first placebo-controlled randomized trial of sulfasalazine for active ulcerative colitis was performed by Baron and colleagues (1962). Patients were randomly allocated to 3 weeks of either sulfasalazine (1 g for 1 week followed by 0.5 g for 2 weeks), salicylazosulfadimidine (another sulfa-aminosalicylate combination thought to be better tolerated) or placebo. After the initial 30 patients were enrolled it became apparent that the majority of participants were not entering remission. An interim analysis demonstrated that the placebo and salicylazosulfadimidine were both ineffective. A further 20 patients were randomized to either placebo or sulfasalazine. The results of the trial have been confirmed several times. Approximately 80% of patients responded to sulfasalazine compared to 35% of placebo-treated patients. Side effects resulted in the withdrawal from the trial by 20% of those randomized to sulfasalazine.

5-ASA versus placebo

The major placebo-controlled studies involving at least 4 weeks of therapy for active ulcerative colitis include studies of olsalazine (Dipentum) (Hetzel et al 1986, Robinson et al 1988, Feurle et al 1989, Zinberg et al 1990), Asacol (Schroeder et al 1987, Sninsky et al 1991) Pentasa (Hanauer et al 1993a) and Rowasa (Sutherland et al 1990). As would be expected, the majority of trials show a statistically significant benefit compared to placebo (Fig. 55.1). The Zinberg (1990) and Hetzel (1986) trials were probably prone to type II errors, as they included small numbers of patients. The study by Feurle and colleagues (1989) had a sufficient sample size but utilized different endpoints from other studies.

When the results of the placebo-controlled studies are grouped according to the dose of 5-ASA given, a dose–response curve can be demonstrated: higher doses are associated with a better clinical response (Sutherland et al 1993). Whether or not greater benefit could be realized from even higher doses is not clear.

5-ASA versus sulfasalazine

Other trials compared the newer compounds with sulfasalazine. They include comparisons with olsalazine

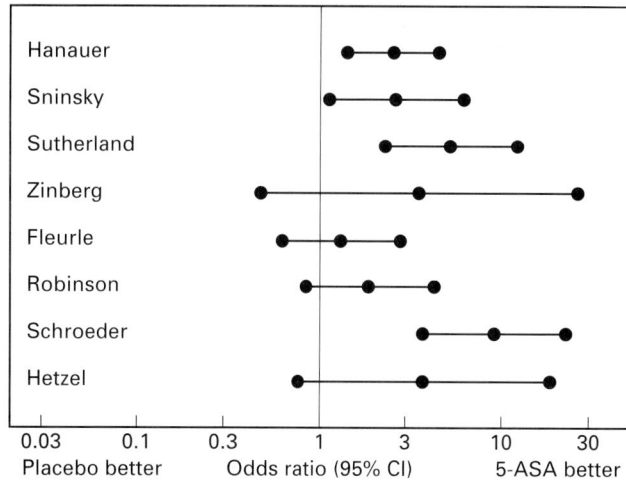

Fig. 55.1 Odds ratios for the major studies comparing 5-ASA and placebo in patients with active ulcerative colitis.

(Dipentum) (Willoughby et al 1988, Rao et al 1989, Rijk & Tongerson 1991), Asacol (Bresci et al 1990, Riley et al 1988b), Claversal (Andreoli et al 1987, Rachmilewitz 1989) and benzalazine (Fleig et al 1988). As can be seen in Figure 55.2, the results do not provide statistically significant evidence for superiority of the newer preparations over sulfasalazine.

However, as regards side effects, more trials demonstrate a benefit for 5-ASA over sulfasalazine than the reverse, although the exclusion criteria for many of these trials included intolerance to sulfasalazine, which would minimize differences in the adverse event profile. In the only study of newly diagnosed patients with ulcerative colitis (Rao et al 1989), intolerance to sulfasalazine was twice that of 5-ASA.

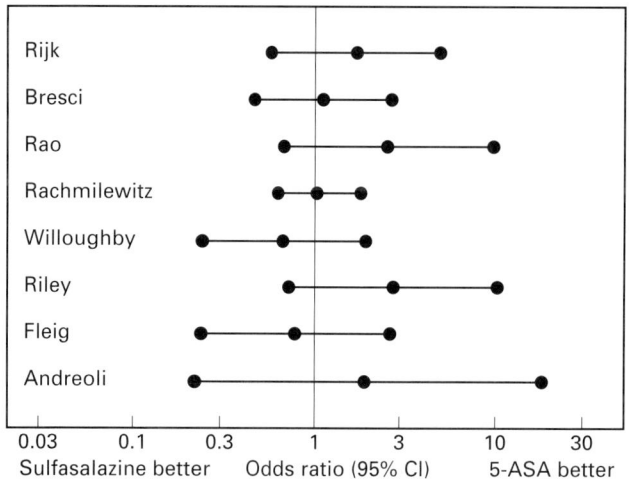

Fig. 55.2 Odds ratios for the major studies comparing sulfasalazine and 5-ASA for treatment of active ulcerative colitis.

Maintenance therapy

Sulfasalazine versus placebo

Ulcerative colitis is characterized by its propensity to relapse. After reviewing their experience in Oxford, Edwards & Truelove (1963) concluded that 80% of patients who enter remission will relapse within the next year. Misiewicz and associates (1965) were the first to assess the remission-sustaining properties of sulfasalazine. In their trial of 67 patients randomly allocated to 2 g of sulfasalazine or placebo, 24 of 34 (71%) sulfasalazine-treated patients remained in remission for a year, compared to 8 of 33 (24%) placebo-treated patients ($P<0.001$).

The next issues relating to the use of sulfasalazine for maintenance concerned the optimum dose and duration of therapy. The Oxford group (Azad Khan et al 1980) conducted a randomized trial of ulcerative colitis patients, already in remission, who received a 6-month course of either 1, 2 or 4 g of sulfasalazine. Significant differences in relapse rates were demonstrated for 1 g compared to either 2 or 4 g-treated patients. There was a trivial reduction (14% to 9%) in the relapse rates for the patients assigned to 4 g sulfasalazine compared to 2 g daily, but nearly 40% of patients allocated to the 4 g treatment arm complained of side effects. It was not possible to compare side effects across treatment groups, as participants had already proved that they tolerated 2 g of sulfasalazine daily. The authors concluded that 2 g of sulfasalazine was the optimum dose for maintenance. However, the 4 g regimen might be considered for treatment failures.

Dissanayake & Truelove (1973) examined the effect of duration of sulfasalazine therapy on the risk of relapse in a trial of 64 patients in remission currently taking 2 g of sulfasalazine. Patients were randomized either to continue sulfasalazine or to placebo. After 6 months relapse was common in the placebo-treated patients (over 50%), but the relapse rate did not differ when patients were stratified by the duration of their remission on sulfasalazine (< or >3 years in remission). The message would appear to be that lifelong therapy with an aminosalicylate is required to maintain remission.

The concept of continuous therapy with sulfasalazine or other 5-ASAs has been challenged. In a small trial patients in remission were randomized either to continue their daily 2 g sulfasalazine or were told to take a higher dose, 3 g/day, at the commencement of typical colitis symptoms. After 1 year 30% of those taking continuous sulfasalazine relapsed, compared to 39% of the 'on-demand' group (Dickinson et al 1985). The possibility of a type II error should be considered in evaluating this study.

5-ASA versus placebo

There are three placebo-controlled studies of 5-ASA for maintenance of remission in ulcerative colitis. A South African study of olsalazine (Dipentum) 2 g/day demonstrated a significant increase in time to relapse (Wright et al 1993). Pentasa 4 g/day was effective in maintaining remission (Miner et al 1992). Asacol at 0.8 and 1.6 g/day has also been shown to be effective compared to placebo for the maintenance of remission (Hanauer et al 1994).

5-ASA versus sulfasalazine

The relapse prevention properties of sulfasalazine and the newer 5-ASAs have also been compared in a variety of clinical trials, including comparisons with Asacol (Dew et al 1982, Riley et al 1988a), balsalazide (McIntyre et al 1988), Claversal, Mesasal, Salofalk (Andreoli et al 1987, Porro et al 1989, Rutgeerts & International Study Group, 1989), Dipentum (Ireland et al 1988, Rijk et al 1992a, Kiilerich et al 1992) and Pentasa (Mulder et al 1988a, Gionchetti et al 1990). The odds ratios for treatment effect are shown in Figure 55.3. In contrast to studies comparing sulfasalazine with 5-ASA for active disease, the treatment effect trend, although not quite reaching statistical significance, is towards a slight benefit for sulfasalazine compared to 5-ASA. Again there may be a selection bias, in that most patients would have been prevalent cases already known to be tolerant to sulfasalazine.

5-ASA, other issues

Other studies have examined the effects of various doses of 5-ASA. For example, a recent trial comparing daily Pentasa 1.5 g and 3 g showed a trend towards superiority for the higher dose (Fockens et al 1993). Studies with balsalazide (Colazide) did not reveal any differences between 3 and 6 g/day (Green et al 1992).

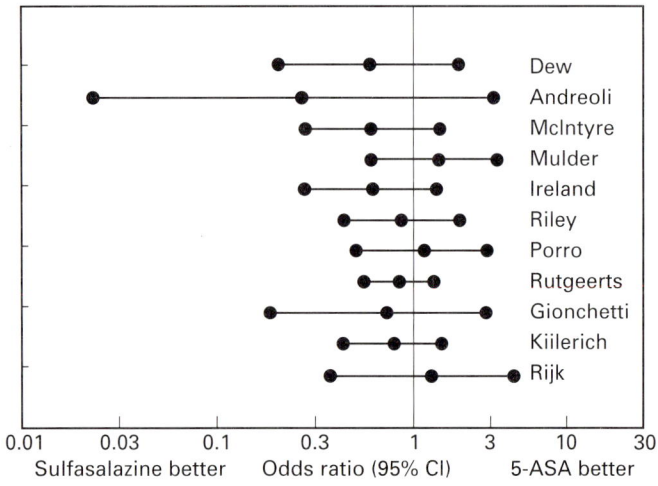

Fig. 55.3 Odds ratios for the major studies comparing sulfasalazine and 5-ASA for maintenance of remission in patients with ulcerative colitis.

An Irish trial compared two 5-ASA preparations, olsalazine (Dipentum, 1 g/day) and Asacol (1.2 g/day) for maintenance of remission. Dipentum was superior but the trial can be faulted for not employing a double-dummy technique (i.e. patients knew which medication they were taking). Moreover, it is also not clear whether there was a selection bias in favour of olsalazine in that many of the patients might have already demonstrated their tolerance of olsalazine (Courtney et al 1992).

The benefit of topical therapy for refractory patients has been challenged. The early trials consisted of patients refractory to oral sulfasalazine. The introduction of the oral aminosalicylates and the use of higher doses might produce different results. In a small randomized double-dummy trial comparing Asacol 3.2 g/day (equivalent to 8 g of sulfasalazine) and prednisolone (20 mg) enemas, no differences in clinical response could be detected (Cobden et al 1991).

Summary

The aminosalicylates should be considered to be first-line drugs for the treatment of mild to moderately active ulcerative colitis. Relatively high doses are required (3.0–4.8 g/day, depending on the preparation). As these regimens are equivalent to 8–12 g of sulfasalazine per day, it is surprising that a definite therapeutic benefit over sulfasalazine has not been clearly demonstrated.

The aminosalicylates are the only medications shown to be effective in maintaining remission in ulcerative colitis. The newer 5-ASAs offer an alternative for patients who are intolerant of sulfasalazine.

Two meta analyses report similar results: 5-ASA is superior to placebo and equivalent to sulfasalazine for the treatment of active disease; and 5-ASA is equivalent to sulfasalazine for maintenance of remission (Sutherland et al 1993, Ricca Rosellini et al 1993).

A broader issue is whether or not patients currently tolerant to sulfasalazine or newly diagnosed patients should be offered one of the newer preparations. The practice of excluding sulfasalazine-intolerant patients from most studies minimizes the superior adverse event profile of the 5-ASAs. The decision depends in part on physician patient concerns related to the risk of a serious adverse event – admittedly low – with sulfasalazine compared to the increased cost of the newer medications. In the sulfasalazine-tolerant there is little evidence that the new preparations are more effective than sulfasalazine.

CROHN'S DISEASE

Although sulfasalazine has been available for over four decades, there are surprisingly few trials of its utility either in the treatment of active Crohn's disease or for maintenance of remission. The early trials are also compromised by the inclusion of patients with only terminal ileal disease. Although it is possible that bacterial overgrowth occurs in patients with small-bowel Crohn's disease, thus providing a mechanism for the splitting of the diazo bond, it is unlikely that sufficient 5-ASA could be released from sulfasalazine to be effective in the small bowel. However, a therapeutic effect for the parent compound prior to the splitting of the azo bond remains a possibility.

Active disease

Sulfasalazine versus placebo

The largest placebo-controlled trials of sulfasalazine were the National Cooperative Crohn's Disease Study (NCCDS) (Summers et al 1979) and the European Cooperative Crohn's Disease Study (ECCDS) (Malchow et al 1984). The NCCDS is one of the best-known multi-center trials of the therapy of Crohn's disease. Patients with active disease were randomly assigned to one of four 17-week treatment regimens, including prednisone (up to 0.75 mg/kg/day), sulfasalazine (1 g/15 kg/day), azathioprine (2.5 mg/kg/day) or placebo. Sulfasalazine demonstrated clinical efficacy in patients with colonic or ileocecal disease, but not in those with isolated small-bowel disease.

Similar results were seen in the ECCDS, a 6–18-week trial during which patients were randomized to either high-dose methylprednisolone (48 mg/kg/day, tapering), sulfasalazine (3 g/day), a combination of both, or placebo. Life-table analysis demonstrated efficacy in patients with colonic or ileocecal disease, but not those with isolated small-bowel disease.

5-ASA versus placebo

Pentasa has been assessed in three placebo-controlled trials which suggest that dose of 4 g per day will be required for the treatment of active disease. Pentasa (1.5 g/day) was ineffective in placebo-controlled trials of either 6 (Mahida & Jewell 1990) or 16 weeks' duration (Rasmussen et al 1987). However, in a large multicenter North American trial involving 310 patients 4 g Pentasa was superior to placebo, with 43% of patients entering remission compared to 18% of those on placebo (Singleton et al 1993). Patients with disease confined to the small intestine had the best response.

A preliminary report suggests that Asacol may be effective in the treatment of active disease. Although it is not clear what proportion of patients were taking corticosteroids concurrently, 45% of patients randomized to Asacol 3.2 g/day entered remission compared to 22% on placebo (Tremaine et al 1993).

There are few studies of 5-ASA in the pediatric population. A small crossover trial of 8-week treatment courses of either up to 3 g/day of Pentasa or placebo in 14 children with disease confined to the terminal ileum has recently been reported. Although the final results did not reach statistical significance, there was a trend towards improvement in CDAI (Crohn's Disease Activity Index), with fewer dropouts during the 5-ASA treatment courses than in the placebo courses (Griffiths et al 1993).

5-ASA versus corticosteroids

A variety of recent studies have compared the usefulness of 5-ASA with corticosteroids for patients with active Crohn's disease. Unfortunately most of the trials are relatively small, and their statistical power is insufficient to allow firm conclusions to be reached.

In one 12-week trial Salofalk (3 g/day) was compared to the combination of sulfasalazine (3 g/day) and methylprednisolone (40 mg/day, tapering by weekly increments of 4 mg). Outcome was excellent, with remission rates of greater than 80% in both groups. Examination of the life tables suggests that the response to Salofalk was slightly slower in the early weeks of the trial (Maier et al 1990). Similar findings were reported by Canadian investigators, who compared prednisone (50 mg/day, tapering by 5 mg increments each week) with Salofalk 3 g daily (Martin et al 1990). Although there was a more rapid decline in CDAI in the prednisone-treated patients, by 8 weeks the responses were similar. The effect of Salofalk was most apparent in patients with disease confined to the small intestine. Salofalk 4.5 g/day was as effective as 6-methylprednisolone in an 8-week trial involving 34 patients with active disease (Gross et al 1994). If these findings could be confirmed in larger studies, it is possible that many patients, concerned about side effects related to steroid use, might opt for 5-ASA treatment and would accept a slower onset of action.

Sulfasalazine versus metronidazole

The Cooperative Crohn's Disease Study in Sweden compared the efficacy of sulfasalazine (3 g/day) with metronidazole (400 mg daily) for mild to moderately active Crohn's disease in a 16-week trial which utilized a crossover design for treatment failures (Ursing et al 1982). As a group, sulfasalazine-treated patients did as well as those receiving metronidazole. However, in the small subgroup of treatment failures (15 patients) all seven sulfasalazine failures responded to metronidazole, compared to only two of eight metronidazole failures who received sulfasalazine.

5-ASA in combination with corticosteroids

The various trials executed by the ECCDS have utilized the combination of methylprednisolone (48 mg/day, with a tapering dose) as their reference standard medical therapy. Remission rates after 6 weeks have ranged from 73 to 80% (Malchow et al 1984, 1990, Lochs et al 1991).

Dutch investigators performed a 16-week trial to examine the effect of the addition of a relatively low dose of corticosteroids (30 mg/day, tapering to 10 mg after 8 weeks) to sulfasalazine (4–6 g/day, depending on tolerance). As in the 5-ASA studies cited above, the addition of steroids induced a prompter reduction in disease activity at the 8-week assessment. The benefit, however, was not apparent by the conclusion of the trial. Patients who had more active disease appeared to do better on the combination (Rijk et al 1991).

The utility of routinely adding sulfasalazine (1 g/15 kg/day) to prednisone therapy (adjusted by disease activity) in patients with active Crohn's disease has also been assessed in an 8-week trial. Surprisingly, the prednisone-treated patients entered remission more frequently and more rapidly than those randomized to the combination. In the maintenance or remission phase of the study a steroid-sparing effect for sulfasalazine could not be demonstrated (Singleton et al 1979).

The potential steroid-sparing effects of the aminosalicylates have also been studied for Pentasa. In a compassionate use program, a mean reduction in prednisone use of 5 mg/day for patients with active disease and 11 mg/day for patients who entered into remission was documented (Hanauer et al 1993b).

Maintenance therapy

The failure of patients to remain in remission following either medical or surgical therapy remains an important issue in the therapy of Crohn's disease. A variety of trials, initially using sulfasalazine and more recently incorporating the newer preparations, have been carried out.

Sulfasalazine versus placebo

The first trials of sulfasalazine as maintenance therapy failed to demonstrate a significant benefit. This may have been due to the relatively small numbers of patients. Participants varied in terms of disease location, previous surgeries and length of time already in remission (Sutherland 1991).

The largest studies of sulfasalazine for maintaining remission are the NCCDS (Phase II), which compared 1.5 g/day sulfasalazine with placebo (Summers et al 1979), the ECCDS (Malchow et al 1984) and a large German study which both used 3 g/day sulfasalazine (Ewe et al 1989). Neither the NCCDS nor the ECCDS could demonstrate any benefit for sulfasalazine use. The German study, however, demonstrated that sulfasalazine provided a reduction in recurrence for at least the first 24 months following surgery. By the third year of the study there was insufficient statistical power to detect subtle differences (Ewe et al 1989). How did this study differ from the others? First, it was the largest – almost double that of the ECCDS and one-third larger than the NCCDS. This enhanced the statistical power to detect modest effects. Secondly, and probably more important, all the patients in the study had undergone a recent resection for Crohn's disease and therapy was initiated within 3 months of surgery.

5-ASA versus placebo

A variety of trials have assessed the efficacy of the newer 5-ASA preparations for the maintenance of remission of Crohn's disease. Trials are ongoing and some investigators have succumbed to the temptation to report interim analyses or incomplete results. A few trials have not used a placebo but rather simply randomized to either treatment or no therapy at all. From a methodological point of view this presents potential problems for biasing the trial results.

Results are conflicting. Definitions of outcome vary and include symptomatic recurrence, endoscopic recurrence or the requirement for repeat surgery. Although endoscopic recurrence has only rarely been used as an endpoint, it has much to recommend it (Rutgeerts et al 1990). Outstanding issues include the correct dosage, disease location and the appropriate time to initiate therapy. Results are displayed in Figure 55.4.

Claversal–Mesasal–Salofalk. The International Mesalazine Study Group (1990) reported the first large trial of Claversal 1.5 g/day for maintaining remission in 222 patients with Crohn's disease. After 12 months of follow-up, an approximately 33% reduction in recurrence rate, defined as a CDAI>200, was apparent for the 5-ASA-treated patients compared to those on placebo. The effect was particularly evident in the subgroups of patients with only ileal disease and a history of prior resection.

A second trial of Claversal studied a higher dose (3 g/day) and focused on endoscopic recurrence at 12 weeks following 'curative resection' for Crohn's disease. Therapy commenced within 15 days following surgery. At colonoscopy, 12 weeks later, only a modest decrease in endoscopic recurrence rates (50% versus 63%, P NS) could be demonstrated for Claversal-treated patients compared to those receiving placebo (Florent et al 1992).

Israeli investigators have also reported, in abstract form, that a 5-ASA preparation similar to Claversal, in a dose of 1 g/day, significantly reduced the clinical relapse rate after a 12-month follow-up in patients with ileal disease (Arber et al 1994).

McLeod and colleagues (1994) randomly assigned 177 patients to either 3 g/day of Salofalk or placebo within 2 months of resection with no obvious residual disease. Patients were followed for up to 7 years, with annual colonoscopies or barium enemas as well as clinical assessment. Life-table analysis revealed significant differences in clinical recurrence at 3 years (27% 5-ASA versus 47% placebo).

Pentasa. The Groupe d'Etudes Thérapeutiques des Affections Inflammatoires Digestives (GETAID) evaluated Pentasa 2 g/day in 161 patients with Crohn's disease. Patients were stratified by the duration of the current remission into two groups: less than or greater than 3 months. After 24 months of therapy significant differences in recurrence, defined as CDAI>200, were noted only in the patients who had recently entered remission. Seventy-one percent of placebo-treated patients relapsed compared to 55% on Pentasa (Gendre et al 1993).

Other studies involving Pentasa have not been as encouraging. Brignola and associates (1992) reported that Pentasa 2 g/day was no better than placebo in patients at high risk of relapse according to their laboratory index. Bondesen and the Danish 5-ASA Group (1991) found no benefit for 3 g of Pentasa per day in 202 patients with Crohn's disease in remission. This study, reported only in abstract form however, had a low recurrence rate (29%) for both active and control groups, suggesting that the patient population might not have been at high risk for recurrence.

Asacol. Prantera and others (1992) report a 12-month placebo-controlled study of Asacol 2.4 g/day in 125 patients, all of whom had had a previous flare of Crohn's disease within the past 24 months. The majority had disease localized to the terminal ileum. A reduction in clinical recurrence after 12 months of follow-up (CDAI>150 and 100 points above baseline) was evident, with 35 of 64 (55%) Asacol-treated patients remaining in remission compared to 39% on placebo. In agreement

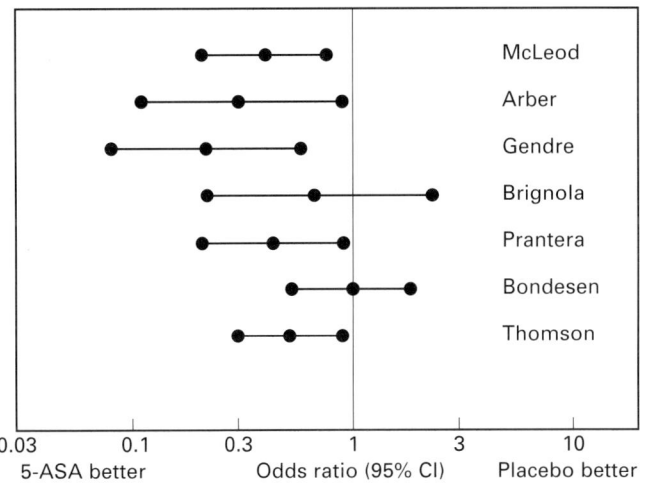

Fig. 55.4 Odds ratios for the major placebo-controlled studies evaluating 5-ASA for the prevention of clinical recurrence in patients with Crohn's disease.

with other studies, patients with either ileal disease or a history of bowel resection were more likely to respond. In contrast to other studies, which suggested that 5-ASA was most effective in patients who had recently entered remission, patients who were in remission for more than 9 months also benefited.

Summary

In contrast to the situation with ulcerative colitis, the newer 5-ASA preparations could represent an exciting advance in the therapy of Crohn's disease. For the treatment of moderately active disease the 5-aminosalicylates are not clinically as rapid in their onset of action as the corticosteroids. However, there is growing evidence that after 8 weeks of therapy many patients do as well on 5-ASA as on corticosteroids. As in ulcerative colitis, the higher dose ranges (3.0–4.8 g/day) need to be used.

The potential efficacy of 5-ASA for maintaining remission in Crohn's disease is intriguing. Two meta-analyses of the utility of maintenance therapy have reported similar results. 5-ASA will reduce the risk of a recurrence in the first year of therapy by approximately 30–40% (Messori et al 1994, Steinhart et al 1994). Patients with a recent resection might represent a group which would particularly benefit from 5-ASA therapy.

TOPICAL THERAPY

As the initial studies to determine the active moiety of sulfasalazine used either suppositories or enemas, it is not surprising that there are additional trials evaluating topical therapy with either 4- or 5-ASA for ulcerative colitis. Topical therapy provides a high concentration of drug to the area that needs it the most (i.e. the rectum or sigmoid colon). Studies with ^{99m}Tc demonstrate that instillation of a 100 ml enema results in consistent delivery to the splenic flexure (Campieri et al 1986, Tiel-van Buul et al 1991). Another potential benefit of topical therapy has been the claim that there is only minimal absorption of drug across the inflamed mucosa.

Active disease

Sulfasalazine versus placebo

Fruhmorgen and Demling (1980) were among the first to demonstrate that sulfasalazine enemas were effective in the treatment of ulcerative colitis. They also noted that the addition of oral sulfasalazine to the treatment regimen did not result in an enhanced therapeutic benefit. Other investigators confirmed the efficacy of sulfasalazine enemas and noted that they were tolerated by patients who were intolerant to oral sulfasalazine (Lennard-Jones 1984, Campieri et al 1984b).

5-ASA versus placebo

The first placebo-controlled studies of 5-ASA enemas assessed their efficacy in patients already resistant to topical corticosteroids. Friedman and associates (1986) demonstrated that 4 g 5-ASA enemas were effective in this situation. Other trials soon followed. In the largest multi-center trial significant improvement was demonstrated in 63% of 5-ASA-treated patients compared to 29% of those randomized to placebo (Sutherland et al 1987).

A study of a 2-week course of olsalazine 1 g enemas failed to demonstrate superiority over placebo in 60 patients with mildly active distal ulcerative colitis (Selby et al 1985). The authors speculated that perhaps there was insufficient time for bacteria to split the diazo bond linking the two 5-ASA molecules. Moreover, the placebo response rate in this study was high (43%).

Other investigators have focused on the utility of enemas containing less 5-ASA. Powell-Tuck and associates (1986) compared 1 and 2 g 5-ASA enemas in 25 patients and found equivalent efficacy. They suggested that a trial of 275 patients would be required to detect a statistically significant difference of 20% between the two groups. Such a trial will probably not be done.

Therapy with 5-ASA suppositories (Williams et al 1987) is effective for patients with disease confined to the distal colon. Perhaps not too surprisingly, patients preferred suppositories to enemas in terms of practicality and ease of compliance (Campieri et al 1988). Recently foams have also been shown to be effective, and are preferred to enemas by patients with active ulcerative colitis (Campieri et al 1993).

5-ASA versus corticosteroids

The first large-scale comparative trials of 5-ASA demonstrated that enemas containing 4 g of 5-ASA were superior to 100 g hydrocortisone enemas. Responses were prompt, with most patients (93%), demonstrating clinical improvement within 2 weeks of initiation of therapy (Campieri et al 1981). A second study from the same group reported similar results a few years later (Campieri et al 1987). Danish investigators indicated that enemas of either 1 g 5-ASA or 25 mg prednisolone were similarly effective (Danish 5-ASA Group 1987). A Dutch study compared 3 g 5-ASA enemas with 30 mg prednisolone enemas and could not detect a significant difference between the two (Mulder et al 1988b).

Maintenance therapy

5-ASA versus placebo

5-ASA enemas are effective in maintaining remission. Biddle and associates (1988) reported that 1 g 5-ASA enemas maintained remission for a year in 75% of patients, compared to 15.4% of placebo-treated patients. Enemas containing either 2 or 4 g of 5-ASA were equally effective in maintaining remission in patients who had already achieved remission of 4 g enemas (Sutherland & Martin 1987).

Compliance with long-term enema use for maintenance of remission may not be optimal. Alternative dosing schedules have been assessed. A comparison of 4 g 5-ASA enemas taken the first week of each month to sulfasalazine (2 g daily) failed to detect significant differences in relapse rates over the next 24 months (D'Albasio et al 1990). Others have suggested that 4 g 5-ASA enemas taken every third night provide better relapse prevention than 5-ASA tablets 1.5 g daily (Mantzaris et al 1994). Miner and colleagues (1994) found that 5-ASA enemas taken either nightly, every other night or every third night, were more effective than placebo in a 24-week trial involving 157 patients. There was also a suggestion that widening the interval between enemas increased the risk of relapse.

5-ASA suppositories have been used for maintenance of remission. In one placebo-controlled study of 65 patients with ulcerative proctitis in remission, 45% of those receiving a nightly 500 mg suppository remained in remission, compared to 9% of placebo-treated patients (Hanauer et al 1992).

Summary

The introduction of topical therapy has been an important advance in the management of patients with distal ulcerative proctosigmoiditis. In a meta-analysis of topical therapy, 5-ASA was effective compared to placebo for active disease as assessed by clinical, endoscopic and histologic criteria. Similar results were found for maintenance of remission. An insufficient number of patients has been studied to draw definitive conclusions about the comparative benefits of topical 5-ASA and corticosteroids (Marshall & Irvine 1994).

OTHER AMINOSALICYLATES

N-acetyl-5-aminosalicylic acid

N-acetyl-5-aminosalicylic acid is the major metabolite of 5-ASA. Three studies have evaluated its potential in the treatment of active ulcerative colitis. Willoughby and associates (1980) compared N-acetyl-5-ASA (equivalent to 2 g sulfasalazine) enemas to placebo in a group of patients only half of whom were in clinical relapse at the time of study entry. The remainder had only sigmoidoscopic or histologic evidence of disease activity. Patients were allowed to continue oral sulfasalazine. Although the N-acetyl-5-ASA-treated patients improved, the sample size was not sufficient to demonstrate clinical superiority.

A second study of a 2-week course of enemas containing similar amounts of N-acetyl-5-ASA failed to show any advantage over placebo (Binder et al 1981). A third trial of suppositories compared to 5-ASA suppositories failed to demonstrate any significant benefit (Van Hogezand et al 1988). It has been suggested that N-acetyl-5-ASA does not cross the colonic epithelium, explaining its superior in-vitro versus in-vivo properties.

4-aminosalicylic acid

4-ASA or PAS differs from 5-ASA only in the location of the amino group. It has been used for decades in the treatment of tuberculosis and is reportedly more stable in solution and less expensive than 5-ASA. Although PAS intolerance is reported in the tuberculosis literature, it has been suggested this is not a major problem as the doses used in antimycobacterial therapy are much higher (12 g/day) than those used in inflammatory bowel disease (4 g/day) (Brown 1987).

Ulcerative colitis

4-ASA enemas versus placebo The use of 4-ASA enemas for distal proctosigmoiditis has been assessed by three placebo-controlled studies. Selby and associates (1984) reported a 2-week trial in patients with active distal ulcerative colitis, comparing initially 1 g and subsequently 2 g 4-ASA enemas with placebo. When both treatment groups were combined and compared to placebo, statistically significant differences were demonstrated and a dose response was apparent (41%, 73%, 90%, χ^2 for trend, $P\ 0.003$).

These encouraging results could not be confirmed by Gandolfo and associates (1987), who randomized 47 patients with distal disease to a 2-week treatment course of either placebo or 1 or 2 g enemas twice daily. The results were surprising, in that whereas the 1 g enema patients demonstrated improvement, the 2 g-treated patients did not. Possible explanations included the chance of a type II error related to the small sample size or that the higher concentration of 4-ASA irritated the rectal mucosa and caused the symptoms to worsen.

Ginsberg and colleagues (1988) performed a randomized placebo-controlled study of 25 patients with active left-sided colitis. Patients were assigned to either 2 g 4-ASA or placebo. These results were more encouraging: after 8 weeks of treatment 83% of 4-ASA-treated patients demonstrated improvement compared to 15% of those receiving placebo.

4-ASA versus 5-ASA or corticosteroid enemas
4-ASA enemas have been compared to enemas of either 5-ASA or prednisolone. Campieri and associates (1984a) evaluated the efficacy of 2 weeks of enemas containing either 4 g of 5-ASA or 2 g of 4-ASA. Similar clinical

efficacy (81% versus 77%) could be demonstrated for either treatment assignment. It is possible that the sample size did not have sufficient statistical power to detect a subtle difference in response.

O'Donnell and associates (1992) compared the efficacy of a 6-week course of 2 g 4-ASA or 20 mg prednisolone enemas in 45 patients with active distal ulcerative colitis. Twenty percent dropped out because of deterioration. Clinical response was modest, with complete remission occurring in only 37.5% of 4-ASA patients and 23.8% of steroid-treated patients. The relatively small enema size (50 ml) may have influenced the results.

4-ASA tablets Ginsberg and associates (1992) gave 4 g of 4-ASA coated with Eudragit S and L designed to dissolve at pH 6.8, to 40 patients with active ulcerative colitis. After 12 weeks of therapy 11 of 20 (55%) treated patients were better, compared to 1 of 20 (5%) on placebo. The authors noted that in a subgroup of patients with distal disease who had previously responded to topical 4-ASA, the response tended to be slower and not as complete.

Crohn's disease

4-ASA tablets Schreiber (1994a) used a similar oral preparation and compared its relapse-maintaining properties with the 5-ASA preparation (Claversal) in Crohn's disease. Both groups received 1.5 g/day of medication. After 12 months of follow-up the relapse rates were essentially identical for both groups, 36% and 38%. They concluded that 1.5 g of 4-ASA was as effective as 1.5 g 5-ASA for maintenance of remission in Crohn's disease. However, given the relatively high relapse rate, an alternative interpretation might be that both treatments were equally ineffective.

SUMMARY

4-ASA has clinical efficacy in patients with inflammatory bowel disease, but with the large number of 5-ASA preparations currently available, it is difficult to imagine where it might fit into the therapeutic armamentarium unless significant cost savings could be anticipated.

REFERENCES

Ahnfelt-Ronne I, Nielsen O H, Christensen A, Langholz E, Binder V, Riis P 1990 Clinical evidence supporting the radical scavenger mechanism of 5-aminosalicylic acid. Gastroenterology 98: 1162–1169

Andreoli A, Cosintino R, Trotti R, Berri F, Prantera C 1987 5-aminosalicylic-acid (5-ASA) vs salazopyrin (SASP) in the oral treatment of active ulcerative colitis (UC) and in remission. Clinical Controversies in Inflammatory Bowel Disease, Abstract 170

Arber N, Odes S H, Fireman Z et al 1994 A controlled double blind multicentre study of the effectiveness of 5-aminosalicylic acid in patients with Crohn's disease in remission. Gastroenterology 106: A646 Abstract

Austin C A, Cann P A, Jones T H, Holdsworth C D 1984 Exacerbation of diarrhoea and pain in patients treated with 5-aminosalicylic acid for ulcerative colitis. Lancet 1: 917–918

Azad Khan A K, Piris J, Truelove S C 1977 An experiment to determine the active therapeutic moiety of sulphasalazine. Lancet ii: 892–895

Azad Khan A K, Piris J, Truelove S C, Howes D T 1980 An optimum dose of sulphasalazine for maintenance treatment in ulcerative colitis. Gut 21: 232–240

Baron J H, Connell A M, Lennard-Jones J E, Jones F A 1962 Sulphasalazine and salicylazosulphadimidine in ulcerative colitis. Lancet i: 1094–1096

Biddle W L, Greenberger N J, Swan J T, McPhee M S, Miner P B Jr 1988 5-aminosalicylic acid enemas: effective agent in maintaining remission in left-sided ulcerative colitis. Gastroenterology 94: 1075–1079

Binder V, Halskov S, Hvidberg E et al 1981 A controlled study of 5-acet-aminosalicylic (5-Ac-ASA) as enema in ulcerative colitis. Scandinavian Journal of Gastroenterology 16: 1122 Abstract

Bondesen S, Danish 5-ASA Group 1991 Mesalazine (Pentasa) as prophylaxis in Crohn's disease. A multicenter, controlled trial. Scandinavian Journal of Gastroenterology 26 (Suppl 183): 68 Abstract

Bondesen S, Nielsen O H, Jacobsen O et al 1984 5-aminosalicylic acid enemas in patients with active ulcerative colitis. Influence of acidity on the kinetic pattern. Scandinavian Journal of Gastroenterology 19: 677–682

Bresci G, Carrai M, Venturini G, Gambardella L 1990 Therapeutic effectiveness and tolerance of 5-aminosalicylic acid in short term treatment of patients with ulcerative colitis at a low or medium phase of activity. International Journal of Tissue Reactions 12: 243–246

Brignola C, Iannone P, Pasquali S et al 1992 Placebo-controlled trial of oral 5-ASA in relapse prevention of Crohn's disease. Digestive Diseases and Sciences 37: 29–32

Brown R 1987 Safety and efficacy of para-aminosalicylic acid (PAS; 4-ASA) in the treatment of ulcerative colitis: new clinical findings. Advances in Therapy 4: 279–297

Campieri M, Gionchetti P, Belluzzi A et al 1987 Efficacy of 5-aminosalicylic acid enemas versus hydrocortisone enemas in ulcerative colitis. Digestive Diseases and Sciences 32: 675–705

Campieri M, Gionchetti P, Belluzzi A et al 1988 5-aminosalicylic acid as enemas or suppositories in distal ulcerative colitis. Journal of Clinical Gastroenterology 10: 406–409

Campieri M, Lanfranchi G A, Bazzocchi G et al 1978 Salicylate other than 5-aminosalicylic acid ineffective in ulcerative colitis [letter]. Lancet ii: 993

Campieri M, Lanfranchi G A, Bazzocchi G et al 1981 Treatment of ulcerative colitis with high-dose 5-aminosalicylic acid enemas. Lancet ii: 270–271

Campieri M, Lanfranchi G A, Bertoni F et al 1984a A double-blind clinical trial to compare the effects of 4-aminosalicylic acid to 5-aminosalicylic acid in topical treatment of ulcerative colitis. Digestion 29: 204–208

Campieri M, Lanfranchi G A, Brignola C, Bazzocchi G, Minguzzi M R, Calari M T 1984b 5-aminosalicylic acid as rectal enema in ulcerative colitis patients unable to take sulphasalazine. Lancet i: 403

Campieri M, Lanfranchi G A, Brignola C et al 1986 Retrograde spread of 5-aminosalicylic acid enemas in patients with acute ulcerative colitis. Diseases of the Colon and Rectum 29: 108–110

Campieri M, Paoluzi P, D'Albasio G, Brunetti G, Pera A, Barbara L 1993 Better quality of therapy with 5-ASA colonic foam in active ulcerative colitis: a multicenter comparative trial with 5-ASA enema. Digestive Diseases and Sciences 38: 1843–1850

Chan R P, Pope D J, Gilbert A P, Sacra P J, Baron J H, Lennard-Jones J E 1983 Studies of two novel sulfasalazine analogs, ipsalazide and balsalazide. Digestive Diseases and Sciences 28: 609–615

Cobden I, Al-mardini H, Zaitoun A, Record C O 1991 Is topical therapy necessary in acute distal colitis? Double-blind comparison of high-dose oral mesalazine versus steroid enemas in the treatment of active distal ulcerative colitis. Alimentary Pharmacology and Therapeutics 5: 513–522

Courtney M G, Nunes D P, Bergin C F et al 1992 Randomised comparison of olsalazine and mesalazine in prevention of relapses in ulcerative colitis. Lancet 339: 1279–1281

D'Albasio G, Trallori G, Ghetti A et al 1990 Intermittent therapy with high-dose 5-aminosalicylic acid enemas for maintaining remission in ulcerative proctosigmoiditis. Diseases of the Colon and Rectum 33: 394–397

Danish 5-ASA Group 1987 Topical 5-aminosalicylic acid versus prednisolone in ulcerative proctosigmoiditis. Digestive Diseases and Sciences 32: 598–602

De Vos M, Verdievel H, Schoonjans R, Praet M, Bogaert M, Barbier F 1992 Concentrations of 5-ASA and Ac-5-ASA in human ileocolonic biopsy homogenates after oral 5-ASA preparations. Gut 33: 1338–1342

Dew M J, Hughes P, Harries A D, Williams G, Evans B K, Rhodes J 1982 Maintenance of remission in ulcerative colitis with oral preparation of 5-aminosalicylic acid. British Medical Journal 285: 1012

Dickinson R J, King A, Wight D G D, Hunter J O, Neale G 1985 Is continuous sulfasalazine necessary in the management of patients with ulcerative colitis? Results of a preliminary study. Diseases of the Colon and Rectum 28: 929–930

Dissanayake A S, Truelove S C 1973 A controlled therapeutic trial of long-term maintenance treatment of ulcerative colitis with sulphasalazine (salazopyrin). Gut 14: 923–926

Edwards F, Truelove S C 1963 The course and prognosis of ulcerative colitis II. Long-term prognosis. Gut 4: 309–315

Ewe K, Herfarth C, Malchow H, Jesdinsky H J 1989 Postoperative recurrence of Crohn's disease in relation to radicality of operation and sulfasalazine prophylaxis: a multicentre trial. Digestion 42: 224–232

Fedorak R N, Empey L R, MacArthur C, Jewell L D 1990 Misoprostol provides a colonic mucosal protective effect during acetic acid-induced colitis in rats. Gastroenterology 98: 615–625

Feurle G E, Theuer D, Velasco S et al 1989 Olsalazine versus placebo in the treatment of mild to moderate ulcerative colitis: a randomized double blind trial. Gut 30: 1354–1361

Fleig W E, Laudage G, Sommer H, Wellmann W, Stange E F, Riemann J 1988 Prospective, randomized, double-blind comparison of benzalazine and sulfasalazine in the treatment of ulcerative colitis. Digestion 40: 173–180

Florent C, Cortot A, Quandale P et al 1992 Placebo-controlled trial of Calversal (C) in the prevention of early endoscopic relapse after 'curative' resection for Crohn's disease (CD). Gastroenterology 102: A623 Abstract

Fockens P, Mulder C J J, Ferwerda J, Tytgat G N J, Dutch Pentasa Study Group 1993 Relapse prevention of ulcerative colitis: double-blind comparison of 1.5 g vs 3 g oral mesalazine (Pentasa). Gastroenterology 104: A701 Abstract

Friedman L S, Richter J M, Kirkham S E, DeMonaco H J, May R J 1986 5-aminosalicylic acid enemas in refractory distal ulcerative colitis: a randomized, controlled trial. American Journal of Gastroenterology 81: 412–417

Fruhmorgen P, Demling L 1980 On the efficacy of ready made-up commercially available salicylazosulphapyridine enemas in the treatment of proctitis, proctosigmoiditis and ulcerative colitis involving rectum, sigmoid and descending colon. Hepatogastroenterology 27: 473–476

Gandolfo J, Farthing M J, Powers G et al 1987 4-aminosalicylic acid retention enemas in treatment of distal colitis. Digestive Diseases and Sciences 32: 700–704

Gendre J P, Mary J Y, Florent C et al 1993 Oral mesalazine (Pentasa) as maintenance treatment in Crohn's disease: a multicentre placebo-controlled study. Gastroenterology 104: 435–439

Ginsberg A L, Beck L S, McIntosh T M, Nochomovitz L E 1988 Treatment of left-sided ulcerative colitis with 4-aminosalicylic acid enemas. Annals of Internal Medicine 108: 195–199

Ginsberg A L, Davis N D, Nochomovitz L E 1992 Placebo-controlled trial of ulcerative colitis with oral 4-aminosalicylic acid. Gastroenterology 102: 448–452

Gionchetti P, Campieri M, Belluzzi A et al 1990 Pentasa in maintenance treatment of ulcerative colitis [letter; comment]. Gastroenterology 98: 251

Goerg K J, Wanitschke R, Gabbert H, Breiling J, Franke M, Meyer zum Buschenfelde K H 1987 Azodisalicylate (azodisal sodium) causes intestinal secretion. Digestion 37: 79–87

Green J R B, Swan C H J, Rowlinson A E et al 1992 A three-year prospective study of the maintenance of remission of ulcerative colitis by a new 5-ASA releasing agent, Balsalazide. Gastroenterology 102: A631 Abstract

Greenfield S M, Punchard N A, Teare J P, Thompson R P H 1993 Review article: The mode of action of the aminosalicylates in inflammatory bowel disease. Alimentary Pharmacology and Therapeutics 7: 369–383

Griffiths A, Koletzko S, Sylvester F, Marcon M, Sherman P 1993 Slow-release 5-aminosalicylic acid therapy in children with small intestinal Crohn's disease. Journal of Pediatric Gastroenterology and Nutrition 17: 186–192

Gross V, Roth M, Fischbach W et al 1994 Comparison between high-dose 5-aminosalicylic acid (5-ASA) and 6-methylprednisolone in active Crohn's disease. Gastroenterology 106: A694 Abstract

Hanauer S, Borgen L, Reiss L 1992 Maintenance treatment of ulcerative proctitis with mesalazine suppositories: results of a multicenter two year controlled trial. Gastroenterology 102: A634 Abstract

Hanauer S, Powers B, Robinson M et al 1994 Maintenance of remission of ulcerative colitis by mesalazine (Asacol) vs placebo. Gastroenterology 106: A696 Abstract

Hanauer S B, Schwartz J, Robinson M et al 1993a Mesalazine capsules for treatment of active ulcerative colitis: results of a controlled trial. American Journal of Gastroenterology 88: 1188–1197

Hanauer S B, Krawitt E L, Robinson M, Rick G G, Safdi M A, Pentasa Crohn's Disease Compassionate Use Study Group 1993b Long-term management of Crohn's disease with mesalazine capsules (Pentasa). American Journal of Gastroenterology 88: 1343–1351

Hautekeete M L, Bourgeois N, Potvin P et al 1992 Hypersensitivity with hepatotoxicity to mesalazine after hypersensitivity to sulfasalazine. Gastroenterology 103: 1925–1927

Hawkey C J, Boughton-Smith N K, Whittle B J 1985 Modulation of human colonic arachidonic acid metabolism by sulfasalazine. Digestive Diseases and Sciences 30: 1161–1165

Hawkey C J, Gassull M A, Lauritsen K et al 1994 Efficacy of zileuton, a 5-lipoxygenase inhibitor, in the maintenance of remission in patients with ulcerative colitis. Gastroenterology 106: A697 Abstract

Hetzel D J, Shearman D J C, Bochner F et al 1986 Azodisalicylate (olsalazine) in the treatment of active ulcerative colitis. A placebo controlled clinical trial and assessment of drug disposition. Journal of Gastroenterology and Hepatology 1: 257–266

International Mesalazine Study Group 1990 Coated oral 5-aminosalicylic acid versus placebo in maintaining remission of inactive Crohn's disease. Alimentary Pharmacology and Therapeutics 4: 55–64

Ireland A, Mason C H, Jewell D P 1988 Controlled trial comparing olsalazine and sulphasalazine for the maintenance treatment of ulcerative colitis. Gut 29: 835–837

Keshavarzian A, Morgan G, Sedghi S, Gordon J H 1990 Role of reactive oxygen metabolites in experimental colitis. Gut 31: 786–790

Kiilerich S, Ladefoged K, Rannem T, Ranlov P J, Danish Olsalazine Study Group 1992 Prophylactic effects of olsalazine v sulphasalazine during 12 months' maintenance treatment of ulcerative colitis. Gut 33: 252–255

Kjaergaard N, Ambrosius Christensen L, Lauritsen J G, Norby Rasmussen S, Honoré Hansen S 1989 Effects of mesalazine substitution on salicylazosulfapyridine-induced seminal abnormalities in men with ulcerative colitis. Scandinavian Journal of Gastroenterology 24: 891–896

Klotz U, Maier K, Fischer C Heinkel K 1980 Therapeutic efficacy of sulphasalazine and its metabolites in patients with ulcerative colitis and Crohn's disease. New England Journal of Medicine 303: 1499–1502

Lennard-Jones J E 1984 Medical treatment of ulcerative colitis. Postgraduate Medical Journal 60: 797–802

Levi A J, Toovey S, Hudson E 1981 Male infertility due to sulphasalazine. Gastroenterology 80: 1208 Abstract

Lochs H, Steinhardt H J, Klaus-Wentz B et al 1991 Comparison of enteral nutrition and drug treatment in active Crohn's disease. Results of the European Cooperative Crohn's Disease Study IV. Gastroenterology 101: 881–888

McIntyre P B, Rodrigues C A, Lennard-Jones J E et al 1988 Balsalazide in the maintenance treatment of patients with ulcerative colitis, a double-blind comparison with sulphasalazine. Alimentary Pharmacology and Therapeutics 2: 237–243

McLeod R S, Wolff B G, Steinhart H J et al 1994 Delayed recurrence following surgery for Crohn's disease (CD). Gastroenterology 106: A733 Abstract

Mahida Y R, Jewell D P 1990 Slow-release 5-amino-salicylic acid (Pentasa) for the treatment of active Crohn's disease. Digestion 45: 88–92

Maier K, Frick H-J, von Gaisberg U, Tuefel T, Klotz U 1990 Clinical efficacy of oral mesalazine in Crohn's disease. Canadian Journal of Gastroenterology 4: 13–18

Malchow H, Ewe K, Brandes J W et al 1984 European Cooperative Crohn's Disease Study (ECCDS): results of drug treatment. Gastroenterology 86: 249–266

Malchow H, Steinhardt H J, Lorenz-Meyer H et al 1990 Feasibility and effectiveness of a defined formula diet regimen in treating active Crohn's disease. Scandinavian Journal of Gastroenterology 25: 235–244

Mantzaris G J, Hatzis A, Petraki K, Spiliadi C, Triantaphyllou G 1994 Intermittent therapy with high-dose 5-aminosalicylic acid enemas maintains remission in ulcerative proctitis and proctosigmoiditis. Diseases of the Colon and Rectum 37: 58–62

Marshall J K, Irvine E J 1994 Topical aminosalicylate (ASA) therapy for distal ulcerative colitis: a meta-analysis. Gastroenterology 106: A1037 Abstract

Martin F, Sutherland L R, Beck I T et al 1990 Oral 5-ASA versus prednisone in short term treatment of Crohn's disease: a multicentre controlled trial. Canadian Journal of Gastroenterology 4: 452–457

Meldrum S J, Watson B W, Riddle H C, Bown R L, Sladen G E 1972 pH-profile of gut as measured by radiotelemetry capsules. British Medical Journal 1: 104–106

Messori A, Brignola C, Trallori G et al 1994 Effectiveness of 5-aminosalicylic acid for maintaining remission in patients with Crohn's disease: a meta-analysis. American Journal of Gastroenterology 89: 692–698

Miner P B Jr, Daly R, Nester T, Rowasa Study Group 1994 The effect of varying dose intervals of mesalamine enemas on the prevention of relapse in distal ulcerative colitis. Gastroenterology 106: A736 Abstract

Miner P B Jr, Schwartz J, Aora S et al 1992 Maintenance of remission in ulcerative colitis (UC) patients with controlled-release mesalamine capsules (Pentasa). Gastroenterology 102: A666 Abstract

Misiewicz J J, Lennard-Jones J E, Connell A M, Baron J H, Jones F A 1965 Controlled trial of sulphasalazine in maintenance therapy for ulcerative colitis. Lancet 1: 185–188

Mulder C J J, Tytgat G N J, Weterman I T et al 1988a Double-blind comparison of slow-release 5-aminosalicylate and sulfasalazine in remission maintenance in ulcerative colitis. Gastroenterology 95: 1449–1453

Mulder C J J, Tytgat G N J, Wiltink E H H, Houthoff H J 1988b Comparison of 5-aminosalicylic acid (3 g) and prednisolone phosphate sodium enemas (30 mg) in the treatment of distal ulcerative colitis. Scandinavian Journal of Gastroenterology 23: 1005–1008

O'Donnell L J D, Arvind A S, Hoang P et al 1992 Double blind, controlled trial of 4-aminosalicylic acid and prednisolone enemas in distal ulcerative colitis. Gut 33: 947–949

Peppercorn M, Das K, Elson C O et al 1994 Zileuton, a 5-lipoxygenase inhibitor, in the treatment of active ulcerative colitis, a double-blind, placebo controlled trial. Gastroenterology 106: A751

Peppercorn M A 1984 Sulfasalazine. Pharmacology, clinical use, toxicity, and related new drug development. Annals of Internal Medicine 101: 377–386

Peppercorn M A, Goldman P 1973 Distribution studies of salicylazosulfapyridine and its metabolites. Gastroenterology 64: 240–245

Poldermans D, van Blankenstein M 1988 Pancreatitis induced by disodium azodisalicylate. American Journal of Gastroenterology 83: 578–580

Porro G B, Ardizzone S, Fasoli R, Petrillo M, Desideri S 1989 Comparison of mesalazine with sulphasalazine in prophylactic treatment of ulcerative colitis. Gut 30: A1467 Abstract

Powell-Tuck J, MacRae K D, Healy M J R, Lennard-Jones J E, Parkins R A 1986 A defence of the small clinical trial: evaluation of three gastroenterological studies. British Medical Journal 292: 599–602

Prantera C, Pallone F, Brunetti G, Cottone M, Miglioli M, Italian IBD Study Group 1992 Oral 5-aminosalicylic acid (Asacol) in the maintenance treatment of Crohn's disease. Gastroenterology 103: 363–368

Rachmilewitz D 1989 Coated mesalazine (5-aminosalicylic acid) versus sulphasalazine in the treatment of active ulcerative colitis: a randomised trial. British Medical Journal 298: 82–86

Rachmilewitz D, Karmeli F, Schwartz L W, Simon P L 1992 Effect of aminophenols (5-ASA and 4-ASA) on colonic interleukin-1 generation. Gut 33: 929–932

Raimundo A H, Evans D F, Rogers J, Silk D B 1992 Gastrointestinal pH profiles in ulcerative colitis. Gastroenterology 102: A681 Abstract

Rampton D S, McNeil N I, Sarner M 1983 Analgesic ingestion and other factors preceding relapse in ulcerative colitis. Gut 24: 187–189

Rao S S C, Dundas S A C, Holdsworth C D, Cann P A, Palmer K R, Corbett C L 1989 Olsalazine or sulphasalazine in first attacks of ulcerative colitis? A double blind study. Gut 30: 675–679

Rasmussen S N, Lauritsen K, Tage-Jensen U et al 1987 5-aminosalicylic acid in the treatment of Crohn's disease. A 16 week double-blind, placebo-controlled, multicenter study with Pentasa. Scandinavian Journal of Gastroenterology 22: 877–883

Ricca Rosellini S, Valpiani D, Spada M et al 1993 5-aminosalicylic acid and sulphasalazine in acute and maintenance treatment of ulcerative colitis. An updated meta-analysis of randomized trials. Gastroenterology 104: A769 Abstract

Rijk M C M, Tongerson J H M 1991 The efficacy and safety of sulfasalazine and olsalazine in patients with active ulcerative colitis. Gastroenterology 100: A243 Abstract

Rijk M C, Van Hogezand R A, Van Lier H J J, Van Tongeren J H M 1991 Sulphasalazine and prednisone compared with sulphasalazine for treating active Crohn's disease. Annals of Internal Medicine 114: 445–450

Rijk M C, van Lier H J, van Tongeren J H 1992a Relapse-preventing effect and safety of sulfasalazine and olsalazine in patients with ulcerative colitis in remission: a prospective double-blind, randomized multicentre study. American Journal of Gastroenterology 87: 438–442

Rijk M C M, Van Schaik A, Van Tongeren J H M 1992b Disposition of mesalazine from mesalazine-delivering drugs in patients with inflammatory bowel disease, with and without diarrhoea. Scandinavian Journal of Gastroenterology 27: 863–868

Riley S A, Lloyd D R, Mani V 1992 Tests of renal function in patients with quiescent colitis: effects of drug treatment. Gut 33: 1348–1352

Riley S A, Mani V, Goodman M J, Herd M E, Dutt S, Turnberg L A 1988a Comparison of delayed-release 5-aminosalicylic acid (mesalazine) and sulfasalazine as maintenance treatment for patients with ulcerative colitis. Gastroenterology 94: 1383–1389

Riley S A, Mani V, Goodman M J, Herd M E, Dutt S, Turnberg L A 1988b Comparison of delayed release 5 aminosalicylic acid (mesalazine) and sulphasalazine in the treatment of mild to moderate ulcerative colitis relapse. Gut 29: 669–674

Robinson M, Gitnick G, Balant L, Das K, Turkin D 1988 Olsalazine in the treatment of mild to moderate ulcerative colitis. Gastroenterology 84: A381 Abstract

Roediger W E W, Deakin E J, Walker G, Nance S H 1989 Assessment of salicylate derivatives for potential use in ulcerative colitis: proposal for a new action of 5-aminosalicylic acid? Pharmacology 39: 39–45

Rutgeerts P, International Study Group 1989 Comparative efficacy of coated, oral 5-aminosalicylic acid (Claversal) and sulphasalazine for maintaining remission of ulcerative colitis. Alimentary Pharmacology and Therapeutics 3: 183–191

Rutgeerts P, Geboes K, Vantrappen G, Beyls J, Kerremans R, Hiele M 1990 Predictability of the postoperative course of Crohn's disease. Gastroenterology 99: 956–963

Sandberg-Gertzen H, Jarnerot G, Kraaz W 1986 Effect of azodisal sodium and sulphasalazine on ileostomy output of fluid and PGE_2 and $PGF_{2\alpha}$ in subjects with a permanent ileostomy. Gut 27: 1306–1311

Schreiber S, Howaldt S, Raedier A 1994a Oral 4-aminosalicylate acid versus 5-aminosalicylic acid slow release tablets. Double blind, controlled pilot study in the maintenance treatment of Crohn's ileocolitis. Gut 35: 1081–1085

Schreiber S, Raedler A, Howaldt S, Zehnter W, Daerr W H, Kruis W

1994b 5-aminosalicylate related renal dysfunction in IBD. Gastroenterology 106: A770 Abstract

Schroder H, Lewkonia R M, Price Evans D A 1973 Metabolism of salicylazosulfapyridine in healthy subjects and in patients with ulcerative colitis. Effects of colectomy and of phenobarbital. Clinical Pharmacology and Therapeutics 14: 802–809

Schroeder K W, Tremaine W J, Ilstrup D M 1987 Coated oral 5-aminosalicylic acid therapy for mildly to moderately active ulcerative colitis. New England Journal of Medicine 317: 1625–1629

Selby W S, Bennett M K, Jewell D P 1984 Topical treatment of distal ulcerative colitis with 4-amino-salicylic acid enemas. Digestion 29: 231–234

Selby W S, Barr G D, Ireland A, Mason C H, Jewell D P 1985 Olsalazine in active ulcerative colitis. British Medical Journal 291: 1373–1375

Sharon P, Ligumsky M, Rachmilewitz D, Zor U 1978 Role of prostaglandins in ulcerative colitis. Enhanced production during active disease and inhibition by sulfasalazine. Gastroenterology 75: 638–640

Singleton J W, Hanauer S B, Gitnick G L et al 1993 Mesalazine capsules for the treatment of active Crohn's disease: results of a 16-week trial. Gastroenterology 104: 1293–1301

Singleton J W, Summers R W, Kern F et al 1979 A trial of sulfasalazine as adjunctive therapy in Crohn's disease. Gastroenterology 77: 887–897

Sninsky C A, Cort D H, Shanahan F et al 1991 Oral mesalazine (Asacol) for mildly to moderately active ulcerative colitis. Annals of Internal Medicine 115: 350–355

Steinhart A H, Hemphill D J, Greenberg G R 1994 Sulfasalazine and mesalazine for the maintenance therapy of Crohn's disease: a meta-analysis. Gastroenterology 106: A778 Abstract

Summers R W, Switz D M, Sessions J T Jr et al 1979 National Co-operative Crohn's Disease Study: results of drug treatment. Gastroenterology 77: 847–869

Sutherland L R 1991 Editorial: 5-aminosalicylates for prevention of recurrence in patients with Crohn's disease: Time for a reappraisal? Journal of Clinical Gastroenterology 13: 5–7

Sutherland L R, Martin F 1987 5-aminosalicylic acid enemas in the maintenance of remission in distal ulcerative colitis and proctitis. Canadian Journal of Gastroenterology 1: 3–6

Sutherland L R, Martin F, Greer S et al 1987 5-aminosalicylic acid enema in the treatment of distal ulcerative colitis, proctosigmoiditis, and proctitis. Gastroenterology 92: 1894–1898

Sutherland L R, Robinson M, Onstad G et al 1990 A double-blind, placebo controlled, multicentre study of the efficacy and safety of 5-aminosalicylic acid tablets in the treatment of ulcerative colitis. Canadian Journal of Gastroenterology 4: 463–467

Sutherland L R, May G R, Shaffer E A 1993 Sulfasalazine revisited: a meta-analysis of 5-aminosalicylic acid in the treatment of ulcerative colitis. Annals of Internal Medicine 118: 540–549

Svartz N 1988 Sulfasalazine: II. some notes on the discovery and development of salazopyrin. American Journal of Gastroenterology 83: 497–503

Tamai H, Kachur J F, Grisham M B, Gaginella T S 1991 Scavenging effect of 5-aminosalicylic acid on neutrophil-derived oxidants. Possible contribution to the mechanism of action in inflammatory bowel disease. Biochemical Pharmacology 41: 1001–1006

Tiel-van Buul M M C, Mulder C J J, Van Royen E A, Wiltink E H H, Tytgat G N J 1991 Retrograde spread of mesalazine (5-aminosalicylic acid)-containing enema in patients with ulcerative colitis. Clinical Pharmacokinetics 20: 247–251

Tremaine W J, Schroeder K W, Harrison J W, Harrison A R, Zinsmeister A R 1993 A randomized, double-blind, placebo-controlled trial of oral 5-ASA (Asacol) in the treatment of symptomatic Crohn's colitis and ileocolitis. Gastroenterology 104: A792 Abstract

Turunen U, Elomaa I, Anttila V J, Seppala K 1987 Mesalazine tolerance in patients with inflammatory bowel disease and previous intolerance or allergy to sulphasalazine or sulphonamides. Scandinavian Journal of Gastroenterology 22: 798–802

Ursing B, Alm T, Barany F et al 1982 A comparative study of metronidazole and sulfasalazine for active Crohn's disease: the Cooperative Crohn's Disease Study in Sweden. II. Result. Gastroenterology 83: 550–562

Van Hees P A M, Bakker J H, Van Tongeren J H M 1980 Effect of sulphapyridine, 5-aminosalicylic acid, and placebo in patients with idiopathic proctitis: a study to determine the active therapeutic moiety of sulphasalazine. Gut 21: 632–635

Van Hogezand R A, Van Hees P A M, Van Gorp J P W M et al 1988 Double-blind comparison of 5-aminosalicylic acid and acetyl-5-aminosalicylic acid suppositories in patients with idiopathic proctitis. Alimentary Pharmacology and Therapeutics 2: 33–40

Williams C N, Haber G, Aquino J A 1987 Double-blind, placebo-controlled evaluation of 5-ASA suppositories in active distal proctitis and measurement of extent of spread using ^{99m}Tc-labeled 5-ASA suppositories. Digestive Diseases and Sciences 32 (Suppl): 71S–75S

Willoughby C P, Piris J, Truelove S C 1980 The effect of topical N-acetyl-5-aminosalicylic acid in ulcerative colitis. Scandinavian Journal of Gastroenterology 15: 715–719

Willoughby C P, Cowan R E, Gould S R, Machell R J, Stewart J B 1988 Double-blind comparison of olsalazine and sulphasalazine in active ulcerative colitis. Scandinavian Journal of Gastroenterology (Suppl 148): 40–44

Wright J P, O'Keefe E A, Cuming L, Jaskiewicz K 1993 Olsalazine in maintenance of clinical remission in patients with ulcerative colitis. Digestive Diseases and Sciences 38: 1837–1842

Zinberg J, Molinas S, Das K M 1990 Double-blind placebo-controlled study of olsalazine in the treatment of ulcerative colitis. American Journal of Gastroenterology 85: 562–566

56. Corticosteroids

V. Binder   J. Brynskov

INTRODUCTION

The adrenal cortex secretes corticosteroids which traditionally are divided into those with a predominant effect on sodium retention (mineralocorticoids) and those with a predominant effect on immune functions and hepatic glycogen disposition (glucocorticoids). The potent anti-inflammatory properties of glucocorticoids were first described in rheumatoid arthritis patients in 1949, which led to clinical trials in numerous other chronic inflammatory disorders, including inflammatory bowel disease (Truelove & Witts 1955). Although many advances have been made in the management of patients with inflammatory bowel disease, glucocorticoids are still the mainstay of the medical treatment of both moderate to severe ulcerative colitis and Crohn's disease. This chapter deals with general aspects of glucocorticoid pharmacology and the optimal use of these drugs in patients with inflammatory bowel disease.

GLUCOCORTICOIDS

Mode of action

Glucocorticoids have a profound influence on intermediate metabolic processes, which accounts for their widespread physiological and pharmacological actions.

Protein metabolism: glucocorticoids decrease protein synthesis in extrahepatic tissues and promote protein catabolism, which may contribute to impaired wound healing as well as growth retardation in children treated with these drugs.
Carbohydrate metabolism: glucocorticoids increase gluconeogenesis and inhibit transportation of glucose into cells, as well as intracellular phosphorylation, which result in hyperglycemia and secondarily increased insulin secretion.
Fat metabolism: glucocorticoids induce hypercholesterolemia and increase the amounts of free fatty acids in the blood. Furthermore, they cause redistribution of body fat, with an increase in fat deposits in the face (moon face) and the back of the neck (buffalo hump) and with a loss of fat from the extremities.
Calcium metabolism: glucocorticoids inhibit both calcium absorption from the gastrointestinal tract and renal calcium reabsorption. This results in secondary hyperparathyroidism, with increased osteoclast activity and bone reabsorption. The concomitant decrease in osteoblast activity and the formation of osteoid tissue are presumedly the cause of osteoporosis which complicates long-lasting glucocorticoid treatment. The effects on osteoid tissue contribute further to growth retardation in children.
Mineralocorticoid effects: sodium and water retention and hypokalemic alkalosis may occur to some degree during treatment with hydrocortisone, but much less frequently than with mineralocorticoids. Synthetic glucocorticoids are practically free of mineralocorticoid effect.
Immunosuppressive effect: this overwhelming clinical and pharmacological importance of glucocorticoids is the clinically well known capacity to suppress both typical humoral (e.g. allergic reactions) and typical cell-mediated immune responses (e.g. transplant rejection). The doses necessary for an immunosuppressive or anti-inflammatory effect are far greater than the daily physiological production of these hormones. Since therapeutic efficacy and side effects are closely correlated, this implies that side effects are unavoidable, even at low pharmacological doses, which limits the usefulness of glucocorticoids in the treatment of chronic diseases.

Glucocorticoids diffuse passively into the cell cytoplasm, where each molecule forms a complex with a specific intracellular glucocorticoid receptor, present in almost all cells in the organism. The glucocorticoid-receptor complex becomes activated after the release of heat shock proteins, compounds with yet unknown functions. The complex then regulates genomic transcription by binding to certain glucocorticoid-responsive elements on DNA. By controlling cellular synthesis of mRNA, the production of certain signal proteins is decreased and that of others increased. There is considerable evidence to suggest that several of the anti-inflammatory/immunosuppressive effects of glucocorticoids may be ascribed to regulation of the transcription and production of cytokines (Brattsand 1993). Cytokines are soluble antigen-non-specific, non-antibody proteins generated by leukocytes (and other cells) which play an important role as intercellular mediators in immunoinflammatory reactions, including those involved in inflammatory bowel disease (Brynskov et al 1992, 1994). Glucocorticoids inhibit the production in vitro of key proinflammatory cytokines such as interleukin (IL)-1 (Goode et al 1991, Ligumski et al 1990, Pullman et al 1992), IL-6 (Andus et al 1991), and tumor necrosis factor (Braegger et al 1992). IL-1 itself influences the pituitary–adrenal axis by raising ACTH (adrenocorticotrophic hormone) and glucocorticoid levels, suggesting a natural, built-in anti-inflammatory feedback mechanism between the hormone and the immune system (Besedovski et al 1986). Furthermore, glucocorticoids block the production of IL-8, a potent neutrophil chemoattractant (Tobler et al 1992), the synthesis of proinflammatory/immunoregulatory cytokines such as interferon-gamma (Arya et al 1984) and IL-2 (Goodwin et al 1986), and that of 'allergic' cytokines, i.e. IL-4 and IL-5 (Schmidt et al 1994).

Glucocorticoids have additional pharmacological effects which also may be pertinent to inflammatory bowel disease, even though the precise mechanisms involved are not well understood. These effects include suppression of the formation of proinflammatory arachidonic acid metabolites, i.e. prostaglandin E_2 and leukotriene B4 (Lauritsen et al 1986) and platelet-activating factor (Eliakim et al 1988). These effects may in part be ascribed to inhibition of IL-1 synthesis, but other pathways may also be present. Glucocorticoids stimulate the production of lipocortin, which reduces phospholipase A_2 activity, and thereby the formation of prostaglandins (Goodwin et al 1986). Selective inhibition of prostaglandin E_2 production, by blocking the cyclo-oxygenase pathway with NSAIDs, may, however, worsen inflammatory bowel disease. Furthermore, inhibition of leukotriene B4 production by a specific inhibitor of the lipoxygenase pathway (e.g. zileuton) provides only a modest therapeutic gain, which seems somewhat disproportionate to the well documented role of this metabolite as a marker of ulcerative colitis disease activity in vivo (Lauersen et al 1994).

Structure–activity relationship

The biological potency of a glucocorticoid compound depends on its absorption, protein binding, rate of metabolic transformation, rate of excretion, ability to traverse membranes, and the intrinsic effectiveness of the molecule at its site of action. Adrenocortical cells take up cholesterol, which is an essential element in the formation of the classic sterol skeleton shared by all steroids (Fig. 56.1). Modifications of this structure have resulted in the development of a wide range of synthetic glucocorticoids, which differ from the basic cortisol molecule in terms of relative anti-inflammatory as opposed to sodium retaining potency, relative binding affinity for the intracellular glucocorticoid receptor, and pharmacokinetics. Particular effort has been made to construct a glucocorticoid with a topical effect and without systemic effects. This can be achieved either by high local adherence and low absorption, or by rapid hepatic degradation to metabolites without glucocorticoid effects, or a combination thereof.

Cortisone was the first-introduced glucocorticoid for the treatment of inflammatory bowel disease (Truelove & Witts 1955), even though it is now recognized as a prodrug, which, however, is rapidly reduced in the liver to hydrocortisone.

Hydrocortisone, i.e. *cortisol*, is the major physiologically secreted glucocorticoid, which is also available as a drug for medical treatment, primarily as substitution therapy in adrenal insufficiency. Hydrocortisone is also used in pharmacological doses, especially intravenously.

Prednisone, one of the first synthetic glucocorticoids, also requires hepatic hydroxylation to prednisolone before it exerts its effect.

Prednisolone is probably still the most widely used synthetic glucocorticoid and was designed specifically for oral use. It has a relative anti-inflammatory potency about four times that of cortisol and a slightly less relative sodium retaining potency. Prednisolone has a higher bioavailability (80%) than cortisol (50%) and a lower hepatic clearance, which make this drug most useful for systemic oral treatment of inflammatory bowel disease. Prednisolone differs only from cortisol by having a double bond at the C 1–2 position (Fig. 56.1). Prednisolone-21-phosphate is suitable for intravenous administration. In patients with active ulcerative colitis the mean plasma peak prednisolone levels are initially higher after an intravenous bolus injection, but decrease rapidly below the relatively constant plasma levels recorded after continuous infusion, and even approach the concentrations observed following single-dose oral administration. Constant intravenous infusion of 60 mg prednisolone per 24 hours produced plasma levels twice as high compared to oral administration of 40 mg per day (Fig. 56.2). Although gastrointestinal absorption of oral prednisolone in ulcerative colitis patients can be delayed, total absorption is complete and does not differ from healthy controls (Elliot et al 1980, Berghouse et al 1982, Milsap et al 1983).

In patients with active Crohn's disease, oral absorption of prednisolone has variously been reported to be normal, even in the presence of mucosal damage (Tanner et al 1981), or moderately decreased (Shaffer et al 1983). The possible absorption defect is, however, of a magnitude which should not give clinical consequences for oral use.

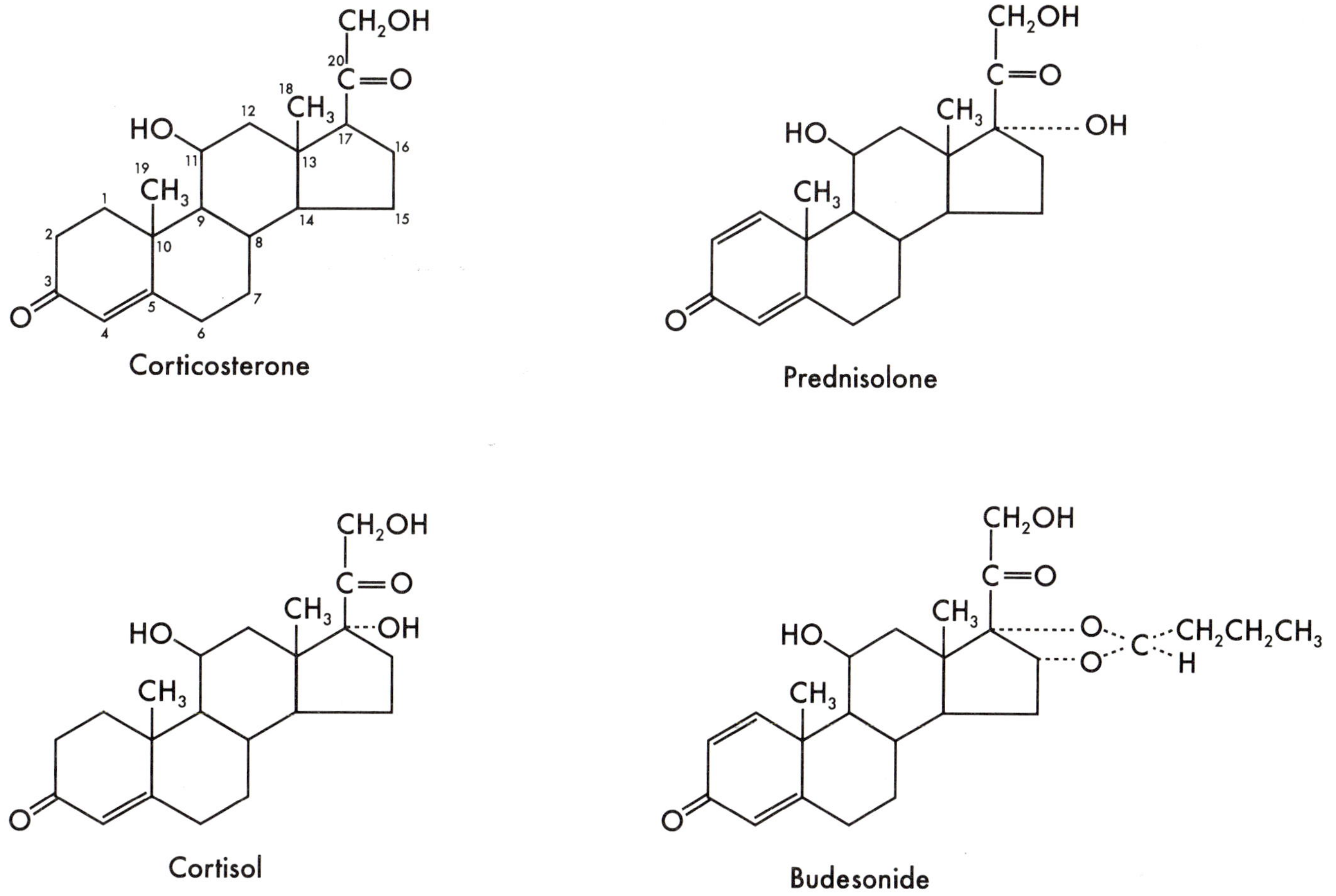

Fig. 56.1 Chemical structure of natural glucocorticoids, corticosterone and cortisol (left) and selected synthetic derivatives, prednisolone and budesonide (right).

Methylprednisolone has an effect profile like that of prednisolone, but is slightly more potent; 20 mg methylprednisolone is thus equivalent to 25 mg prednisolone. The anti-inflammatory effect is five times that of cortisol. Methylprednisolone can be used intravenously as well as orally.

Triamcinolone, betamethasone and dexamethasone are much more potent glucocorticoids owing to a high binding affinity for the glucocorticoid receptor, but the side effects are proportionally severe. From these drugs, however, the highly potent 'dermatologic formulations' betamethasone valerate and beclomethasone dipropionate were developed. More pertinent for the treatment of inflammatory bowel disease is the observation that topical selectivity for mucus membranes could be further improved by lipophilic C-17 α substitution as exemplified by budesonide (Fig. 56.1), which originally proved efficacious, as inhalation, in bronchial asthma (Clissold & Heel 1984).

Budesonide has a relative affinity for the glucocorticoid receptor which is nearly 200 times that of cortisol and a clearance 4–5 times greater than cortisol and prednisolone. This high first-pass liver metabolism explains the low oral bioavailability of budesonide (11%) compared with cortisol (55%) and prednisolone (80%) (Clissold & Heel 1984, Brattsand 1993). The effect of budesonide is thus predominantly topical, and the drug can be administered as an aerosol for bronchial asthma and allergic rhinitis, as an enema for distal inflammatory bowel disease, and as a sustained-release tablet for ileal release (controlled ileal release, CIR).

Fluticasone propionate, a fluorinated corticosteroid, with low bioavailability due to poor absorption from the gastrointestinal tract and a high first-pass metabolism, has pharmacological properties which seemed promising. However, a controlled study comparing fluticasone with prednisolone in oral treatment of mild to moderate Crohn's disease found prednisolone to be superior in colonic and ileocolonic Crohn's disease. An equal effect of the two drugs was observed only in ileitis cases (Wright et al 1993). Similarly, a placebo-controlled trial in active left-sided ulcerative colitis showed no effect; further development of fluticasone in this area seems to have been abandoned (Angus et al 1992).

Tixocortol pivalate is a thiol-derivative of cortisol which is also cleared by first-pass degradation in the liver, suggesting fewer systemic glucocorticoid effects, and it has

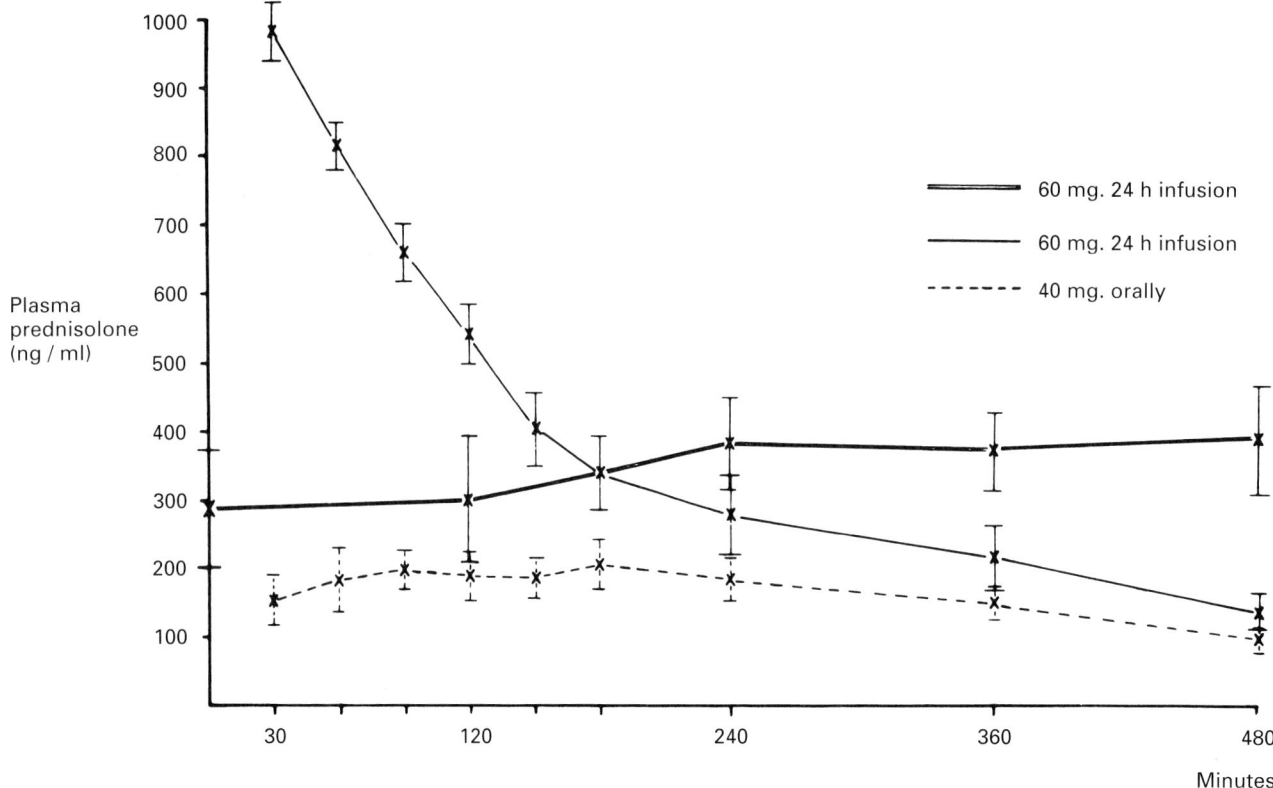

Fig. 56.2 Comparison of plasma prednisolone after prednisolone 40 mg orally and prednisolone (as prednisolone-21-phosphate) 20 mg intravenous bolus or 60 mg per 24 hour infusion (data reproduced from Berghouse et al 1982).

been tested as a rectal enema in patients with ulcerative colitis. The results, which have been presented in abstracts only, suggest that tixocortol pivalate is as effective as hydrocortisone enemas (Hanauer et al 1986).

Adrenocorticotrophic hormone (ACTH)

Endogenous adrenocortical steroid synthesis is stimulated by ACTH, a 39-amino acid peptide produced by the adenohypophysis. Physiological ACTH-induced release of natural glucocorticoids (cortisol, corticosterone; Fig. 56.1) leads in turn to a downregulation of ACTH production via a built-in negative feedback system. Clinical trials have shown that parenteral ACTH is at least as effective as oral cortisone (Truelove & Witts 1959) or intravenous cortisol in the treatment of active ulcerative colitis (Kaplan et al 1975, Powell-Tuck et al 1977, Meyers et al 1983). However, ACTH treatment is little used today, if ever, owing to the inconvenience of intramuscular injection, the unpredictable adrenal response in previously steroid-treated patients (Meyers et al 1983), and because it also stimulates the release of mineralocorticoids and androgens.

CURRENT CLINICAL PRACTICE

Ulcerative colitis

Since the introduction of glucocorticoids for active ulcerative colitis combined with a more active surgical approach in case of treatment failure, there has been a marked reduction in the mortality of patients with severe ulcerative colitis (Jewell 1989).

From the early studies of Baron et al (1962) it appears that there is a dose–response correlation. The improvement rate was twice as high after 40 and 60 mg of prednisolone per day as after 20 mg orally in outpatients with ulcerative colitis. Any dose of 40 mg (or above) per day of prednisolone thus seems to be fully effective (Fig. 56.3).

It remains difficult to identify the glucocorticoid-resistant patient rapidly, since 'if glucocorticoids do not help, they harm'. Although more recent clinical studies are not identical in terms of patient selection and endpoints, a relatively uniform pattern has nevertheless emerged.

In severe ulcerative colitis, i.e. patients with both severe bowel symptoms and systemic symptoms such as fever, weight loss etc., the overall clinical remission rates after a short course of high-dose glucocorticoids range from 41 to 60% (Kristensen et al 1974, Truelove et al 1978, Meyers et al 1983, Järnerot et al 1985, Kjeldsen 1993). Pulse therapy with high-dose methylprednisolone (1 g once daily) has been tried in a small open study in patients with severe ulcerative colitis, without beneficial effect (Rosenberg et al 1990), and this treatment regimen has thus not been adapted. The appropriate length of the initial high-dose treatment period is uncertain. Truelove

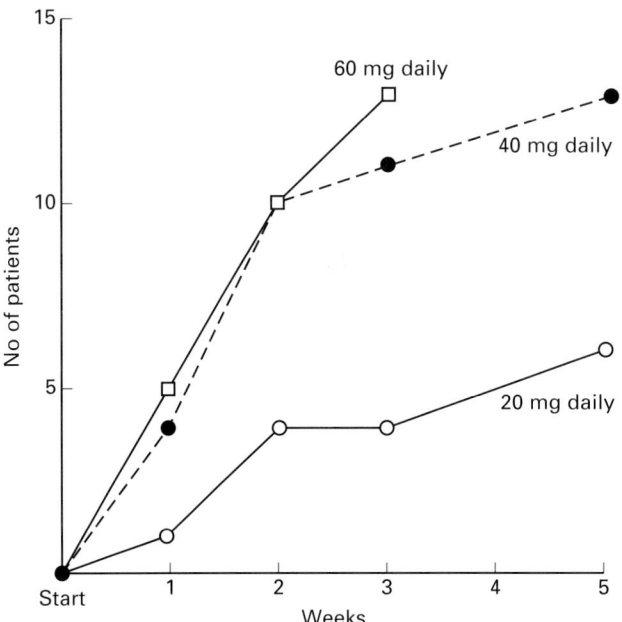

Fig. 56.3 Number of patients whose disease was in remission at different times after starting treatment with prednisolone 60, 40 and 20 mg daily. Data reproduced from Baron et al (1962).

et al (1978) found that 60% of the patients treated were in already clinical remission after 5 days of combined treatment with intravenous prednisolone-21-phosphate and total parenteral nutrition; 15% were improved and 25% unchanged or worse. Järnerot et al (1985), using a similar treatment regimen, found that 59% of their own patients (i.e. not referred from other hospitals) went into remission, as judged by both clinical and endoscopic criteria. Using this definition, two-thirds of the responders achieved remission within 5 days and the remaining one-third were already substantially improved, and subsequently achieved full remission.

In our own population-based study of course and prognosis in ulcerative colitis (Langholz et al 1994) we had a colectomy rate of 28% in the initial attack of the disease in patients with total colitis, treated with prednisolone orally in a starting dose of 1–2 mg/kg (60–80 mg/day). This indicates indirectly a success rate of about 70% for medical treatment, since our treatment policy in severe cases of ulcerative colitis is to advise colectomy in case of medical treatment failure.

Moderate or mild ulcerative colitis responds much better to high-dose glucocorticoid treatment. A remission rate of 89% was reported by Järnerot et al (1985) and of 83% by Kjeldsen (1993). All responding patients were substantially improved within 5 days of treatment, and two-thirds were already in clinical remission within these few days; one-third subsequently remitted.

In conclusion, from these data it appears that systemic treatment with glucocorticoids is highly effective in ulcerative colitis. The effect is rapid and patients who have not responded with substantial improvement within 5 days are unlikely to respond at all. The more active the disease, the lower response rate.

Practical recommendation for treatment

Based on the published clinical trials and series, a general recommendation for treatment of severe ulcerative colitis is prednisolone in a dose of 1–2 mg/kg per day, normally 60–80 mg, given orally if gastric emptying is normal; otherwise intravenously. The treatment should be started immediately after hospitalization, and the patient should be under close observation for life-threatening complications such as toxic megacolon or perforation. If no improvement is observed within 5–7 days, colectomy is advised. Acute severe ulcerative colitis is still a potentially dangerous condition. Previous studies (Edwards & Truelove 1963, Devroede et al 1971) reported a mortality of 30% in the first attack of severe ulcerative colitis. Recent studies, where the patients were treated according to these principles, have reported mortality rates of only 1–2% in the first year and a normal survival thereafter (Ritchie et al 1978, Langholz et al 1992). If improvement occurs the prednisolone dose can be tapered gradually over 6–10 weeks to the lowest dose where the patient remains in remission. We normally reduce the dose from 80 mg to 60 mg after 5–7 days, from 60 mg to 40 mg after a further 3–5 days, and then to 30 mg; from then on the dose is reduced by 5 mg/day per week to 15 mg. From then on further tapering is carried out at 2.5 mg reduction every week. If the patient suffers troublesome side effects the dose can be reduced more rapidly to a level of 10–15 mg and then maintained for at least 4–5 weeks before further reduction.

Among patients who respond to intensive steroid treatment for an acute attack of the disease and go into remission, 42% can expect to have a relapse within the following year and 70% within 3 years (Järnerot et al 1985).

From our own study of disease course and predictive factors in ulcerative colitis we found that patients with severe disease at diagnosis who responded to medical treatment had a no more serious course as regards the frequency of relapse than patients who presented with less severe or less extensive disease (Langholz et al 1994).

Patients with a chronic continuous disease course – about 20% of cases – are less suited to glucocorticoid treatment because tapering of the drug will be followed immediately by a return of symptoms, and long-term treatment with even small doses of glucocorticoid almost inevitably has severe side effects. In children growth retardation is a major consideration, and in adults the well known glucocorticoid effects on osteoid tissue, as well as the other serious adverse effects, are important. Osteonecrosis is a rare but serious consequence of steroid treatment.

If ulcerative colitis patients cannot be kept in clinical remission using maintenance treatment with 5-ASA preparations, they will often be advised within the first few years to undergo colectomy. In our own series, less than 5% of the unoperated patients suffered continuous active disease during the first 5 years (Langholz et al 1994). Long-term treatment with azathioprine is another option for these patients.

As relapse prevention, maintenance treatment with systemic glucocorticoids has no effect in inactive ulcerative colitis (Truelove & Witts 1959).

Topical treatment in distal ulcerative colitis

Topical instillation of glucocorticoids is clinically attractive because it increases the drug concentration at the site of local inflammation and reduces the risk of systemic effects. The benefit of local treatment with a hydroxycortisone or prednisolone water-based enema is well documented in placebo-controlled trials in patients with distal ulcerative colitis (Truelove 1958, Watkinson 1958). A clinical remission rate of about 75% after 3 weeks of treatment has been reported, but later studies using budesonide suggest that treatment should be continued for up to 8 weeks if immediate remission is not obtained (Bianchi Porro et al 1994). There is, however, no convincing evidence from comparative trials that more potent glucocorticoids, such as betamethasone 17-valerate (A Multicentre Trial 1971), beclomethasone dipropionate (van der Heide et al 1988, Mulder et al 1989), or even budesonide (Danish Budesonide Study Group 1991, Bianchi Porro et al 1994) are more efficacious.

The proximal spread of an enema is variable and depends on the volume of the enema and particularly on the presence of rectal discomfort and tenesmus. Although the splenic flexure, or even the ascending colon, may be reached occasionally (Matts & Gaskel 1961), topical treatment is generally unreliable in patients with extensive disease. However, for the large group of patients with proctosigmoiditis it is safe to assume that this area is tracked by a rectal enema provided that the patient is able to retain it. If not, a glucocorticoid foam preparation is convenient for patients and has been shown to be as efficacious as enema for equivalent glucocorticoid doses (Ruddel et al 1980). Foam preparations which do not distend the rectal ampulla minimize rectal discomfort and thus pave the way for subsequent enema administration. A further advantage of foam administration is that it can be retained during use in the day time. The ease of foam administration is offset by the limited proximal penetration which usually only extends to the mid-sigmoid colon (Farthing et al 1979).

For pure proctitis cases, a controlled trial has shown that prednisolone suppositories are superior to placebo (Lennard-Jones et al 1962).

Mode of action of topically applied glucocorticoids

Methods to measure systemic absorption, such as circulating glucocorticoid levels or the amount of radioactivity in the urine following administration of a labeled drug (Lee et al 1980) provide inconsistent results as to whether glucocorticoids applied topically have a predominantly local effect or whether they exert their action systemically after absorption. However, prednisolone metasulfobenzoate enemas, from which prednisolone is poorly absorbed, have proved as effective as conventional prednisolone but with lower blood prednisolone levels (Lee et al 1980, McIntyre et al 1985). These data, which suggest that the effect is primarily topical, are substantiated by the observation that enemas containing steroids with a rapid first-pass hepatic degradation, such as tixocortol (Hanauer et al 1986), beclomethasone dipropionate (van der Heide et al 1988) and budesonide (Danielsson et al 1992, Thomsen et al 1994), are effective despite no or minimal suppression of the hypothalamic–pituitary–adrenal axis, which is considered to be a marker of systemic glucocorticoid bioactivity.

These 'new-generation' topical steroid preparations have a clinical role in cases of distal ulcerative colitis which is refractory to 5-ASA preparations, where long and repeated steroid treatment courses are needed. There is no evidence for a superior effect on the disease but the fewer steroid side effects are an advantage for the occasional patient who requires long-lasting topical glucocorticoid treatment. The higher cost is justified in such cases.

Crohn's disease

Early reports of a favourable effect of glucocorticoids in regional enteritis (Sparberg & Kirsner 1966) were followed by two large placebo-controlled studies: the National Cooperative Crohn's Disease Study from the USA (Summers et al 1979) and the European Cooperative Crohn's Disease Study (Malchow et al 1984), which both confirmed the significant effect of glucocorticoids compared to placebo in patients with active disease. The prednisone dose in the American study was 0.5–0.75 mg/kg/day for 4 months. Remission was achieved within 1 week in 13% of patients, within 2 weeks in 21%, and within 4 weeks in 32%. The cumulative remission rate during the 4-month treatment course continued to rise, and 61% of the patients were in remission after 16 weeks. By comparison 28% of patients on placebo were in remission after 16 weeks. Although not reaching remission 30% of the patients improved clinically within 1 week and almost 60% within 4 weeks.

In the European study a dose of 6-methylprednisolone, equivalent to 60 mg prednisolone per day, was used initially, tapered over 6 weeks to 10 mg; 83% of the patients obtained remission within 6 weeks, compared to 38% on placebo. The rate of remission and improvement week by week was not reported. In a second part of the study patients in remission were given maintenance therapy with equivalent to 10 mg prednisolone for up to 2 years. No relapse-preventing effect of steroid treatment could be demonstrated. In Crohn's disease, therefore, the effect of glucocorticoid treatment is delayed compared to ulcerative colitis.

Since the inflammatory process in Crohn's disease is more chronic and less ulcerative than the inflammation in severe ulcerative colitis, the risk of acute perforation is low. This implies that it is acceptable to await improvement for longer than 1–2 weeks, which is the maximum for patients with severe ulcerative colitis. In a recent study from our group, we assessed the number of steroid responders, steroid failures and steroid-dependent patients. The outcome of the first steroid treatment course, in a regional unselected group of newly diagnosed patients with Crohn's disease, showed that complete clinical remission was achieved within 30 days in 48%, partial remission in 32% and no response was found in 20% (Munkholm et al 1993). Of primary responders 55% remained improved after cessation of treatment, whereas 45% relapsed within 1 month after cessation or during tapering of the treatment. No correlation was found between localization of disease, age, sex or clinical symptoms, and the outcome of the treatment, which in summary resulted in a prolonged steroid response in 44%, steroid dependency in 36% and steroid resistance in 20% of the patients. These results indicate that about one-third of patients with Crohn's disease, i.e. those who respond to steroids but cannot be withdrawn, are in need of an alternative to conventional glucocorticoid treatment. This could be either a 'new steroid' – topically delivered and therefore with fewer side effects – such as budesonide, or an immunosuppressive drug as azathioprine. For the patient who does not respond at all to glucocorticoid treatment (20% in our study) surgical resection of the diseased bowel segment(s) should be considered, and for those with widespread disease, azathioprine or rarely cyclosporin may be considered. With current conservative surgical practice, even in patients who are operated on several times, with resection of stenotic inflamed segments, short bowel syndromes seldom occur. The risk of this complication occurs more commonly when a necessary operation is postponed and intersegmental fistulae develop. In such cases, extensive small-bowel resection may result.

Topical treatment of Crohn's disease

The rectosigmoid colon

Although the role of glucocorticoid enemas in distal Crohn's disease apparently has not been subjected to clinical trials, this treatment modality is currently used in those patients along the same lines as in distal ulcerative colitis.

Ileocecal Crohn's disease

The recent development of an oral delayed-release budesonide capsule, which transports and releases the drug in the ileocecal region, has provided a new therapeutic option for patients with Crohn's disease, and corroborated the potential of topical treatment in this condition. In a controlled study budesonide (CIR) capsules 9 mg daily were found to be superior to placebo at 8 weeks: remission occurred in 51% of the patients compared to 20% on placebo. Except for moon face, which was reported in 7% of the patients, compared to 2% of patients on placebo, no significant differences between possible glucocorticoid side effects were found in patients treated with budesonide and patients treated with placebo. However, both basal and corticotrophin-induced plasma cortisol levels were found to be somewhat suppressed (Greenberg et al 1994). Another recent controlled trial comparing budesonide CIR to prednisolone in patients with Crohn's disease confirmed that budesonide CIR 9 mg/day did affect the pituitary–adrenal axis by suppressing morning cortisol levels, but significantly less than prednisolone in a dose of 10 mg/day or higher (Rutgeerts et al 1994). The clinical efficacy of budesonide CIR was slightly lower than that of prednisolone. One budesonide 45% of patients were brought into clinical remission after 2 weeks of treatment, and 52% after 8 weeks. The corresponding figures for prednisolone were 56% and 66%. The Crohn's Disease Activity Index score (CDAI) decreased in both treatment groups. After 10 weeks of treatment the budesonide group had decreased from a mean score of 275 to 175, compared to the prednisolone group, which decreased from 279 to 136.

A combination of these data suggests that clinically relevant improvement may be achieved with mainly topically acting glucocorticoid preparations such as budesonide, administered orally. However, the effect is less than can be achieved with standard systemic glucocorticoid treatment, but so are the side effects. As a continuation of the controlled study of budesonide CIR versus prednisolone in active Crohn's disease, the relapse-preventing effect of budesonide has been investigated against placebo (Löfberg et al 1994). The treatment period was 12 months, and the trial comprised patients who had been brought into clinical remission in the first study. The relapse rates after 12 months of treatment were not significantly different in patients on budesonide CIR 6 mg per day (59%), budesonide 3 mg per day (74%) or placebo (63%). The median time to relapse was, however, significantly longer (271 days) in the group on budesonide CIR 6 mg per day than in the placebo-treated patients (146 days). These results indicate that a treatment modality such as budesonide

CIR, with fewer steroid adverse effects than conventional glucocorticoid treatment, can profitably be sustained for some months further than what is acceptable for treatment with prednisolone. As with the observations regarding systemically active glucocorticoids, it is unlikely that relapse-preventing effects will be expected.

REFERENCES

A Multicentre Trial 1971 Betamethasone 17-valerate and prednisolone 21-phosphate retention enemata in proctitis. British Medical Journal 3: 84–86

Andus T, Gross V, Cäsar I et al 1991 Activation of monocytes during inflammatory bowel disease. Pathobiology 59: 166–170

Angus P, Snook J A, Reid M, Jewell D P 1992 Oral fluticasone propionate in active ulcerative colitis. Gut 33: 711–714

Arya S K, Wong-Staal F, Gallo R C 1984 Dexamethasone-mediated inhibition of human T cell growth factor and gamma interferon messenger RNA. Journal of Immunology 133: 273–276

Baron J H, Connell A M, Kanaghinis T G, Lennard-Jones J E, Avery Jones F A 1962 Out-patient treatment of ulcerative colitis. Comparison between three doses of oral prednisolone. British Medical Journal 2: 441–443

Berghouse L M, Elliot P R, Lennard-Jones J E, English J, Marks V 1982 Plasma prednisolone levels during intravenous therapy in acute colitis. Gut 23: 980–984

Besedovski H, del Rey A, Sorkin E, Dinarello C A 1986 Immunoregulatory feedback between interleukin-1 and glucocorticoid hormones. Science 223: 652–654

Bianchi-Porro G, Prantera C, Campieri M et al 1994 Comparative trial of methylprednisolone and budesonide enemas in active distal ulcerative colitis. European Journal of Gastroenterology and Hepatology 6: 125–130

Braegger C P, Nicholls S, Murch S H, Stephens S, MacDonald T T 1992 Tumor necrosis factor alpha in stools as a marker of intestinal inflammation. Lancet 339: 89–91

Brattsand R L 1993 Steroid development: a case of enhanced selectivity for the bowel wall. Research and Clinical Forums 15: 17–31

Brynskov J, Nielsen O H, Ahnfelt-Rønne I, Bendtzen K 1992 Review: Cytokines in inflammatory bowel disease. Scandinavian Journal of Gastroenterology 27: 897–906

Brynskov J, Nielsen O H, Ahnfelt-Rønne I, Bendtzen K 1994 Cytokines (immunoinflammatory hormones) and their natural regulation in inflammatory bowel disease (Crohn's disease and ulcerative colitis): a review. Digestive Diseases 12: 290–304

Clissold S P, Heel R C 1984 Budesonide. A preliminary review of its pharmacodynamic properties and therapeutic efficacy in asthma and rhinitis. Drugs 28: 485–518

Danish Budesonide Study Group 1991 Budesonide enema in distal ulcerative colitis. A randomized dose-response trial with prednisolone enema as positive control. Scandinavian Journal of Gastroenterology 26: 1225–1230

Danielsson Å, Löfberg R, Persson T, et al 1992 A steroid enema, budesonide, lacking systemic effects for the treatment of distal ulcerative colitis or proctitis. Scandinavian Journal of Gastroenterology 27: 9–12

Devroede G J, Taylor W F, Jackman R J, Stickler G B 1971 Cancer risk and life expectancy of children with ulcerative colitis. New England Journal of Medicine 285: 17–21

Edwards F C, Truelove T C 1963 The course and prognosis of ulcerative colitis. Gut 4: 299–315

Eliakim R, Karmeli F, Rasin E, Rachmilewitz D 1988 Role of platelet-activating factor in ulcerative colitis: enhanced production during active disease and inhibition by sulphasalazine and prednisolone. Gastroenterology 95: 1167–1172

Elliot P R, Powell-Tuck J, Gillespie P E et al 1980 Prednisolone absorption in acute colitis. Gut 21: 49–51

Farthing M J G, Rutland M D, Clark M L 1979 Retrograde spread of hydrocortisone containing foam given intrarectally in ulcerative colitis. British Medical Journal 2: 822–824

Goode H F, Rathbone B J, Kelleher J, Walker B E 1991 Monocyte zinc and in vitro prostaglandin E_2 and interleukin-1β production by cultured peripheral blood monocytes in patients with Crohn's disease. Digestive Diseases and Sciences 36: 627–633

Goodwin J S, Atluru D, Sierakowski S, Lianos E A 1986 Mechanism of action of glucocorticoids: inhibition of T cell proliferation and interleukin 2 production is reversed by leukotriene B4. Journal of Clinical Investigation 77: 1244–1250

Greenberg G R, Feagan B G, Martin F 1994 Oral budesonide for active Crohn's disease. New England Journal of Medicine 331: 836–841

Hanauer S B, Kirsner J B, Barrett W E 1986 The treatment of left-sided ulcerative colitis with tixocortol pivalate. Gastroenterology 90 (Suppl): 1449A

Järnerot G, Rolny P, Sandberg-Gertzen H 1985 Intensive intravenous treatment of ulcerative colitis. Gastroenterology 89: 1005–1013

Jewell D P 1989 Corticosteroids for the management of ulcerative colitis and Crohn's disease. Gastroenterology Clinics of North America 18: 21–34

Kaplan H P, Portnoy B, Binder H J, Amatruda T, Spiro H 1975 A controlled evaluation of intravenous adrenocorticotrophic hormone and hydrocortisone in the treatment of acute colitis. Gastroenterology 69: 91–95

Kjeldsen J 1993 Treatment of ulcerative colitis with high doses of oral prednisolone. The rate of remission, the need for surgery, and the effect of prolonging the treatment. Scandinavian Journal of Gastroenterology 1993: 28: 821–826

Kristensen M, Koudal G, Fischerman K, Jarnum S 1974 High dose prednisolone treatment in severe ulcerative colitis. Scandinavian Journal of Gastroenterology 9: 177–183

Lauersen L S, Lauritsen K, Bukhave K, Rask-Madsen J et al 1994 Selective 5-lipoxygenase inhibition by zileuton in the treatment of relapsing ulcerative colitis: a randomized double-blind, placebo-controlled multicentre trial. European Journal of Gastroenterology and Hepatology 6: 209–215

Lauritsen K, Lauersen L S, Bukhave K, Rask-Madsen J 1986 Effects of topical 5-aminosalicylic acid and prednisolone on prostaglandin E_2 and leukotriene B4 levels determined by equilibrium in vivo dialysis of rectum in relapsing ulcerative colitis. Gastroenterology 91: 837–844

Langholz E, Munkholm P, Davidsen M, Binder V 1992 Colorectal cancer risk and mortality in patients with ulcerative colitis. Gastroenterology 103: 1444–1451

Langholz E, Munkholm P, Davidsen M, Binder V 1994 Course of ulcerative colitis: analysis of changes in disease activity over years. Gastroenterology 107: 3–11

Lee D A H, Taylor M, James W H T, Walker G 1980 Rectally administered prednisolone – evidence for a predominantly local action. Gut 21: 215–218

Lennard-Jones, Baron J H, Connell A M, Avery Jones F 1962 A double blind controlled trial of prednisolone-21-phosphate suppositories in the treatment of idiopathic proctitis. Gut 3: 207–210

Ligumski M, Simon P L, Karmeli F, Rachmilewitz D 1990 Role of interleukin 1 in inflammatory bowel disease – enhanced production during active disease. Gut 31: 686–689

Löfberg R, Rutgeerts P, Malchow et al 1994 Budesonide CIR for maintenance of remission in ileocecal Crohn's disease. A European multicenter placebo controlled trial. Gastroenterology 106 (Suppl): A722

McIntyre P B, Macrae F A, Berghouse L, English J, Lennard-Jones J E 1985 Therapeutic benefits from a poorly absorbed prednisolone enema in distal colitis. Gut 26: 822–824

Malchow H, Ewe K, Brandes J W et al 1984 European cooperative Crohn's disease study: results of drug treatment. Gastroenterology 86: 249–266

Matts S G F, Gaskell K H 1961 Retrograde colonic spread of enemata in ulcerative colitis. British Medical Journal 2: 614–617

Meyers S, Sachar D B, Goldberg J D, Janowitz H D 1983 Corticotropin versus hydrocortisone in the intravenous treatment of ulcerative colitis. A prospective, randomized, double-blind clinical trial. Gastroenterology 85: 351–357

Milsap R L, George D E, Szefler S J, Murray K A, Lebenthal E, Jusko W J 1983 Effect of inflammatory bowel disease on absorption and disposition of prednisolone. Digestive Diseases and Sciences 28: 161–168

Mulder C J J, Endert E, van der Hiede H et al 1989 Comparison of beclomethasone dipropionate (2 and 3 mg) and prednisolone sodium phosphate enemas (30 mg) in the treatment of ulcerative proctitis. An adrenocortical approach. Netherlands Journal of Medicine 35: 18–24

Munkholm P, Langholz E, Davidsen M, Binder V 1993 Frequency of glucocorticoid resistance and dependency in Crohn's disease. Gut 35: 360–362

Powell-Tuck J, Buckell N A, Lennard-Jones J E 1977 A controlled comparison of corticotrophin and hydrocortisone in the treatment of severe proctocolitis. Scandinavian Journal of Gastroenterology 12: 971–975

Pullman W E, Elsbury S, Kobayashi M, Hapel A J, Doe W F 1992 Enhanced mucosal cytokine production in inflammatory bowel disease. Gastroenterology 102: 529–537

Ritchie J K, Powell-Tuck J, Lennard-Jones J E 1978 Clinical outcome of the first ten years of ulcerative colitis and proctitis. Lancet 1: 1140–1143

Rosenberg W, Ireland A, Jewell D P 1990. High-dose methylprednisolone in the treatment of active ulcerative colitis. Journal of Clinical Gastroenterology 12: 40–41

Ruddel W S J, Dickinson R J, Dixon M F, Axon A T R 1980 Treatment of distal ulcerative colitis (proctosigmoiditis) in relapse: comparison of hydrocortisone enemas and rectal hydrocortisone foam. Gut 21: 885–889

Rutgeerts P, Löfberg R, Malchow H et al 1994 A comparison of budesonide with prednisolone for active Crohn's disease. New England Journal of Medicine 331: 842–845

Schmidt J, Fleissner S, Heimann-Weitschat I, Lindstaedt R, Szelenyi I 1994 The effect of different corticosteroids and cyclosporin A on interleukin-4 and interleukin-5 release from murine Th2-type T cells. European Journal of Pharmacology 260: 247–250

Shaffer J A, Williams S E, Turnberg L A, Houston J B, Rowland M 1983 Absorption of prednisolone in patients with Crohn's disease. Gut 24: 182–186

Sparberg M, Kirsner J B 1966 Long-term corticosteroid therapy for regional enteritis: an analysis of 58 courses in 54 patients. American Journal of Digestive Diseases 11: 865–880

Summers R W, Switz D M, Sessions J T et al 1979 National Cooperative Crohn's Disease Study: results of drug treatment. Gastroenterology 77: 847–869

Tanner A R, Halliday J, Powell L W 1981 Serum prednisolone levels in Crohn's disease and coeliac disease following oral prednisolone administration. Digestion 21: 310–315

Thomsen O Ø, Andersen T, Langholz E et al 1994 Lack of adrenal gland suppression with budesonide enema in active distal ulcerative colitis: a prednisolone-controlled 8-week study. European Journal of Gastroenterology and Hepatology 6: 507–511

Tobler A, Meier R, Seitz M, Dewald B, Baggiolini M, Fey F 1992 Glucocorticoids downregulate gene expression of GM-CSF, NAP-1/IL-8, and IL-6, but not M-CSF in human fibroblasts. Blood 79: 45–51

Truelove S C 1958 Treatment of ulcerative colitis with local hydrocortisone hemisuccinate sodium. A report on a controlled therapeutic trial. British Medical Journal 2: 1072–1076

Truelove S C, Willoughby C P, Lee E G, Kettlewell M G W 1978 Further experience in the treatment of severe attacks of ulcerative colitis. Lancet 2: 1086–1088

Truelove S C, Witts L J, Cortisone in ulcerative colitis 1955 Final report on a therapeutic trial. British Medical Journal 2: 1041–1048

Truelove S C, Witts L J 1959 Cortisone and corticotrophin in ulcerative colitis. British Medical Journal 1959: 1: 387–394

van der Heide H, van den Brandt-Gradel V, Tytgat G N J et al 1988 Comparison of beclomethasone dipropionate and prednisolone 21-phosphate enemas in the treatment of ulcerative proctitis. Journal of Clinical Gastroenterology 10: 169–172

Watkinson 1958 Treatment of ulcerative colitis with topical hydrocortisone hemisuccinate sodium. British Medical Journal 2: 1077–1082

Wright J P, Jarnum S, Schaffalitzky de Muckadell O, Keech M L, Lennard-Jones J E 1993 Oral fluticasone propionate compared with prednisolone in treatment of active Crohn's disease: a randomized double-blind multicentre study. European Journal of Gastroenterology and Hepatology 5: 499–503

57. Immunosuppressive drugs in inflammatory bowel disease

A. B. Hawthorne

INTRODUCTION

Inflammatory bowel disease is characterized by an upregulated intestinal immune system with uncontrolled inflammatory activity. Corticosteroid drugs are still the most potent therapy for active intestinal inflammation, but for patients who fail to respond, and for those who develop side effects or who require long-term corticosteroid treatment, immunosuppressive drugs are important alternatives. The possible benefits always need to be balanced against the risks of side effects, and in ulcerative colitis (where colectomy offers a 'cure') there has been greater reluctance to use these agents than in Crohn's disease. Because of the unpredictable course of inflammatory bowel disease valid conclusions can only be drawn from well designed double-blind controlled trials. It is important to define clearly the type of patient that has been shown to respond, and not to assume that the conclusions can be extrapolated to other states of disease activity. This chapter considers the role of azathioprine, 6-mercaptopurine, cyclosporin and methotrexate in the treatment of inflammatory bowel disease using evidence from controlled trials, and will detail the toxicity of these drugs.

AZATHIOPRINE AND 6-MERCAPTOPURINE

These imidazole purine analogs are the most widely used immunosuppressive agents in inflammatory bowel disease. Their clinical effects are probably identical (Present 1989), but their exact mode of action is unknown (Hawthorne & Hawkey 1989). They alter lymphocyte function and reduce lamina propria plasma cells, as well as affecting natural killer cell function, but there is also an anti-inflammatory action. Azathioprine and 6-mercaptopurine have been in use since the 1960s. The use of 6-mercaptopurine in ulcerative colitis was first reported in 1962 (Bean 1962) and in Crohn's disease in 1969 (Brooke et al 1969). There have been a number of controlled trials in both Crohn's disease and ulcerative colitis (Tables 57.1 and 57.2). Results have been conflicting and trials can only be properly interpreted when it is realized that these drugs are extremely slow in onset of action, with a mean response time of 3 months (Present et al 1980).

Active Crohn's disease

Two early studies failed to show any benefit in patients with severe or unresponsive disease (Rhodes et al 1971, Klein et al 1974). The trials were probably too short to demonstrate benefit (Table 57.1), and crossover design, at a time when the drug might have had an effect, may also have obscured any benefit. A 6-month study in 20 patients used prednisolone dose as the endpoint and showed a clear corticosteroid-sparing effect of azathioprine (Rosenberg et al 1975a). The National Cooperative Crohn's Disease Study was a double-blind comparison of sulfasalazine versus azathioprine versus prednisolone versus placebo (Summers et al 1979). Fifty-nine patients with active Crohn's disease received azathioprine 2.5 mg/kg for 17 weeks; no significant difference from placebo was found. However, in 37% of patients corticosteroid treatment had been stopped in the 2 weeks before trial entry, which biased the trial against azathioprine, particularly given its slow onset of action. Only 43 of the 59 patients completed the 17-week trial. The study by Present et al (1980) in New York showed a dramatic benefit in the treatment of chronic active disease using 6-mercaptopurine in patients who were deemed unresponsive to corticosteroids or sulfasalazine. Sixty of the 83 patients were also receiving prednisolone (mean dose 20 mg daily). The trial was for 2 years, with crossover at 12 months in some patients. Overall 71% of courses of 6-mercaptopurine led to improvement, compared to 13% of placebo courses. There was a significant benefit in closure of fistulae, and reduction or cessation of corticosteroids. This trial clearly showed the slow onset of action, with a mean response time of 3.1 months. A more recent placebo-controlled study in 42 patients with active Crohn's disease showed benefit when azathioprine (2.5 mg/kg/day) was added to high-dose

Table 57.1 Controlled trials of azathioprine/6-mercaptopurine in Crohn's disease

Trial	Design	Duration	Number	Comments	Outcome
Active disease					
Rhodes et al 1971	P-C crossover	2 + 2 months	16	Duration too short to show benefit	O
Klein et al 1974	P-C crossover	4 + 4 months	26	Duration too short to show benefit	O
Rosenberg et al 1975	P-C	6 months	20	All patients on prednisolone	+(steroid sparing)
Summers et al 1979	Pl. vs aza. vs SASP. vs prednisolone	4 months	59 (aza.) 77 (Pl.)	Many stopped prednisolone prior to entry. Short duration	O
Present et al 1980	P-C crossover in some	2 years	83	Delayed response (3 months) Treatment improved symptoms, and closed fistulae	+(steroid sparing)
Ewe et al 1993	P-C	4 months	42	All received prednisolone 60 mg at entry, reducing to 10 mg over 8 weeks	+
Maintenance therapy					
Willoughby et al 1971	P-C	24 weeks	22	Some entered in relapse and received high-dose prednisolone initially	+
O'Donoghue et al 1978	P-C withdrawal trial	1 year	51	Patients in remission on aza. for 6 months + prior to entry	+
Summers et al 1979	Pl. vs aza. vs SASP. vs prednisolone	1 or 2 years	54 (aza.) 101 (Pl.)	Low dose of azathioprine (1 mg/kg/day)	O
Candy et al 1994	P-C	15 months	63	Active disease at entry: all received prednisolone for 3 months, and if in remission entered healing phase	+

P-C, placebo-controlled; Pl., placebo; aza., azathioprine; SASP., sulfasalazine

Table 57.2 Controlled trials of azathioprine in ulcerative colitis

Trial	Design	Duration	Number	Comments	Outcome
Acute relapse					
Jewell & Truelove 1974	P-C	1 month	80	Too short to show benefit. All received prednisolone with high response rate	O
Caprilli et al 1975	Aza. vs SASP	3 months	20	Comparison with SASP, no placebo group	Aza = SASP
Chronic active disease					
Rosenberg et al 1975	P-C	6 months	30	All patients on prednisolone	+ (steroid-sparing)
Kirk & Lennard-Jones 1982	P-C	6 months	44	All patients on prednisolone	+ (steroid-sparing)
Maintenance therapy					
Jewell & Truelove 1974	P-C	1 year	80	Continuation of acute study. All on steroids initially	Borderline benefit
Hawthorne et al 1992	P-C withdrawal trial	1 year	79	Majority in remission on aza. at entry	+

P-C, placebo-controlled; Aza., azathioprine; SASP., sulfasalazine

prednisolone (Ewe et al 1993). Both groups received prednisolone 60 mg at entry, tapering to a maintenance dose of 10 mg at 8 weeks. If symptoms became worse the prednisolone dose could be increased. At 4 months 76% of patients on azathioprine were in remission, compared to 38% on placebo. Overall, prednisolone consumption was lower in the azathioprine group.

In summary, purine analogs have no place as monotherapy in acute relapse of Crohn's disease because of their slow onset of action. They are, however, very useful in chronic active disease, where azathioprine 2 mg/kg/day, or 6-mercaptopurine 1.5 mg/kg/day, have been shown to reduce disease activity, increase the rate of remission, and have a corticosteroid-sparing effect. Concurrent prednisolone should not be withdrawn for the first 2–3 months of therapy.

Maintenance therapy in Crohn's disease

Several trials have addressed the question of maintenance therapy with azathioprine. The first (Willoughby et al 1971), studied ten patients who had already achieved remission with prednisolone, and a further 12 patients in relapse who initially received high-dose prednisolone to achieve remission at the start of the trial. The relapse rate was dramatically lower in those taking azathioprine. Very similar results were reported in a recent abstract from South Africa (Candy et al 1994), where 63 patients with active disease received a healing course of prednisolone for 3 months, but were also randomized to receive 2.5 mg/kg azathioprine or placebo. Those in remission (45 in all) at 3 months continued for a 1-year maintenance phase, and the overall remission rate at 1 year was 42.4% with azathioprine, compared to 6.6% with placebo. In a different trial design (O'Donoghue et al 1978) patients in remission on azathioprine were randomized to continue the drug or switch to placebo for 1 year (or until relapse). Five percent on azathioprine relapsed compared to 41% on placebo. In the National Cooperative Crohn's Disease Study (Summers et al 1979) a smaller dose of 1 mg/kg daily was used over a 2-year period, and no significant benefit was seen in comparison to placebo.

It is not known how long azathioprine should be continued in quiescent disease, but a survey of long-term treatment from Paris (Lemann et al 1994) showed that two-thirds of patients remained in remission at 5 years, and suggested that relapse was more likely in females and younger patients, whereas disease site did not influence relapse rate.

In summary, azathioprine does maintain long-term remission in Crohn's disease at a dose of 2 mg/kg daily, both in patients who have achieved remission on azathioprine and also in those with a corticosteroid-induced remission. The benefit has to be weighed against the risk of significant long-term side effects, discussed below.

Azathioprine in active ulcerative colitis

In ulcerative colitis there has always been a greater reluctance to use azathioprine or 6-mercaptopurine, because of potential toxicity. The optimum treatment for severe or chronic active disease has been felt to be colectomy, with elimination of diseased mucosa and removal of the long-term risk of carcinoma. There have been a number of case reports and uncontrolled studies but only four controlled studies in active disease. The first and largest, performed in Oxford (Jewell & Truelove 1974), was a double-blind trial in 80 patients with active ulcerative colitis. All patients were treated with prednisolone 20 mg daily plus prednisolone enemas for outpatients and 40 mg intravenously plus hydrocortisone enemas for inpatients. Patients received either azathioprine 2.5 mg/kg daily or identical placebo. The effect of treatment for active disease was assessed at 1 month, and there was no benefit from the addition of azathioprine. Once again, 1 month was insufficient time to show any benefit from azathioprine treatment, and in view of the high response rate in patients not receiving the drug this trial was too small to detect whether it had occurred. In a smaller study from Rome, Caprilli et al compared 20 patients with acute ulcerative colitis treated with either azathioprine or sulfasalazine and found no difference between the two drugs (Caprilli et al 1975).

Two further trials have explored the treatment of chronic active colitis (Table 57.2). Kirk and Lennard-Jones (1982) studied 44 patients who were taking an average of 22 mg prednisolone daily. There was no improvement in disease activity, but there was a significant reduction in prednisolone dose in the azathioprine group. However, there were large numbers of side effects (nausea in particular), and only 15 in the active group were analyzed. Rosenberg et al (1975b), from Chicago, reported a study similar to his Crohn's disease trial with 30 patients who were taking 10 mg or more of prednisolone. Significantly more patients were able to stop corticosteroids in the azathioprine group. The clinical courses were identical.

Azathioprine therefore has an important role in chronic active disease, where it enables the reduction or cessation of corticosteroids, but it is too slow-acting to be helpful in acute relapse. Patients with frequent relapses, or who are unable to achieve complete remission with prednisolone, particularly those with left-sided or distal disease, often have considerable disruption of their lifestyle and yet do not wish to consider colectomy, with the prospect of ileostomy or a pouch procedure. Many of these patients can achieve prolonged remission on azathioprine, with improved quality of life. Until recently, however, evidence that azathioprine is effective in maintaining established remission has been lacking.

Maintenance treatment in ulcerative colitis

Jewell and Truelove, in their Oxford trial, continued treatment with azathioprine after remission was achieved. There was a trend towards benefit, which did not achieve significance at the 5% level. A recent trial has, however, shown evidence of benefit in maintaining remission in ulcerative colitis (Hawthorne et al 1992). The design was similar to the Crohn's disease study by O'Donoghue et al (1978). Seventy-nine patients taking azathioprine for at least 6 months were randomized to continue the drug or switch to an identical placebo. Sixty-seven patients were in remission, and the remainder had chronic stable or corticosteroid-dependent disease. In the remission group the relapse rate was 36% for those continuing azathioprine, significantly better than the 59% relapse rate for the placebo group. For the 12 patients with chronic stable disease there was no benefit in continuing azathioprine. This trial confirms encouraging uncontrolled reports of remission maintenance, using 6-mercaptopurine (Present et al 1988, Adler & Korelitz 1990). The withdrawal design of course selected patients who had already responded to azathioprine by achieving remission on the drug. Whether the benefit of maintenance therapy can be generalized to all patients with ulcerative colitis is unknown. Once again, risks of toxicity have been a deterrent to their widespread use.

Side effects of azathioprine/6-mercaptopurine

The adverse effects of azathioprine/6-mercaptopurine can be divided into three areas: bone marrow suppression, short-term, and long-term effects.

Azathioprine causes a variable degree of macrocytosis, which is not deemed a side effect. The fall in total white cell count is dose dependent and usually improves with dose reduction. Bone marrow toxicity develops in approximately 5% of patients (Connell et al 1993). Severe reactions are rare if the azathioprine dose does not exceed 2 mg/kg/day, or 1.5 mg/kg/day for 6-mercaptopurine. Bone marrow toxicity can occur at any stage during therapy, as illustrated by the patient who developed severe pancytopenia and died after 10 years on azathioprine (O'Donoghue et al 1978). The drug should be introduced at a low dose, e.g. 50 mg daily, and increased gradually, with weekly or fortnightly blood count monitoring until the dose is stabilized, then monthly or 2-monthly for the duration of therapy. If the total white cell count falls below $3 \times 10^9/l$, or platelet count below $120 \times 10^9/l$, the drug should be discontinued or the dose reduced until the blood count normalizes, and then reintroduced cautiously. Monitoring cannot totally prevent marrow suppression, which can be sudden in onset (Connell et al 1993), and patients should be aware that unusual symptoms or signs of infection necessitate an early blood count.

Five to ten percent of patients stop treatment because of side effects, and the majority of these occur in the first month (Table 57.3). Nausea or vomiting is the most common problem, especially if the dose is increased too rapidly. The nausea can be minimized by taking the drug after food. Pancreatitis is not dose related and generally recurs on rechallenge (Present et al 1989). Arthralgia can be related to azathioprine, and diarrhea is a rare side effect that can be confused with a flare-up of disease (Cox et al 1988). Hypersensitivity reactions can occasionally be severe, with rash, fever, hypotension and abnormal liver function tests (Major & Moore 1985). Allopurinol blocks the metabolism of 6-mercaptopurine, and the azathioprine or 6-mercaptopurine dose should be halved.

A theoretical risk of long-term treatment is that of infection. Present et al (1989) studied 396 inflammatory bowel disease patients taking 6-mercaptopurine. Infections

Table 57.3 Short-term side effects of azathioprine/6-mercaptopurine in inflammatory bowel disease

	Frequency	Comments
Bone marrow suppression	2–5%	Dose dependent, responding to dose reduction. Commonest on starting treatment, but can occur at any time
Nausea/vomiting	3%	Dose related, occurs early
Pancreatitis	2–3%	In first month of treatment; often recurs on rechallenge
Allergic/hypersensitivity	2%	Fever/rash/joint pain/abdominal pain. In first month
Hepatic damage	rare	Cholestasis or hepatitis
Diarrhea	rare	

were recorded in 7.4%. These included viral infections with cytomegalovirus, herpes zoster (mild encephalitis in one case), hepatitis A and B; and bacterial infections such as liver abscess, pneumonia and septic phlebitis. There were no deaths. All such events have been reported in inflammatory bowel disease without immunosuppressive treatment, and the risk is probably no greater than for patients on high-dose prednisolone.

The development of neoplasia is the other long-term concern. In transplant recipients there is an increased incidence of lymphoma in patients taking azathioprine. Cerebral lymphomas occur more frequently than would be expected by chance. It has been suggested that the risk of neoplasia is a particular feature of transplant patients; however, a prospective survey of 1349 non-transplant patients on azathioprine (Kinlen et al 1979), including 280 patients with inflammatory bowel disease, also showed a significant increase in non-Hodgkin's lymphoma, squamous skin carcinoma and other tumors (overall risk increased 1.6-fold). It is possible that the increased risk is due to the underlying disease process rather than the drug therapy. This is borne out by a preliminary report from St Mark's Hospital (Connell et al 1994) of 755 patients with inflammatory bowel disease taking azathioprine. This showed that the overall risk of neoplasia was not increased compared to the general population, but the incidence of colorectal, anal and cervical cancers was increased. The incidence of colorectal cancer in ulcerative colitis patients taking azathioprine was no greater than in other ulcerative colitis patients who had not used the drug, and therefore likely to be due to the disease process rather than the treatment. The development of a cerebral lymphoma in an inflammatory bowel disease patient on 6-mercaptopurine was directly attributed to the drug (Present et al 1989). The increased risk of neoplasia, although likely to be very small, must be borne in mind when considering long-term use of these drugs.

Azathioprine and 6-mercaptopurine may be taken by women of childbearing potential. Although they cross the placenta, there are many reports of successful outcome of pregnancy in women taking these drugs (Present 1989, Alstead et al 1990). There are, however, reports of fetal bone marrow suppression (Dewitte et al 1984). Women who wish to conceive should be counselled fully about the risks and benefits. If it is possible to stop the drug then this is preferable, but where the drug is important in controlling disease activity women should be reassured that continuing treatment is compatible with the delivery of a healthy baby. There is no indication for termination of pregnancy as the risk of teratogenicity is very small.

Conclusions

The purine analogs will never be a first-line therapy in inflammatory bowel disease because of their long delay in onset of action. Their use will always involve a balance of risks, and the patient should be fully informed about toxicity and given clear information about the importance of regular monitoring.

In Crohn's disease they are indicated in chronic active disease that fails to respond to corticosteroids, or where prednisolone dose cannot be reduced below 15 mg, particularly if side effects are a problem. They may have a role in healing fistulae, and when used prior to surgery may reduce the extent of bowel resection needed. They should be used to maintain remission, but only in patients with previous extensive or troublesome chronic active disease.

In ulcerative colitis chronic unresponsive corticosteroid-dependent disease and frequent relapses (more than three over 2 years) are an indication for azathioprine/6-mercaptopurine. In an older patient with long-standing total colitis, because of the risk of neoplasia the balance of risks might favour colectomy, whereas azathioprine/6-mercaptopurine have a major role in younger patients with more recent onset of disease, who wish to avoid surgery at all costs. Left-sided disease more commonly fails to respond fully to corticosteroids or 5-aminosalicylic acid preparations, and purine analogs are particularly useful here. There is no evidence that disease site influences the response to these drugs. At present maintenance therapy should be restricted to patients who have achieved remission using the drugs. They should be continued for a minimum of 2–3 years, but the overall duration of benefit may be much longer.

CYCLOSPORIN

Cyclosporin is a cyclic undecapeptide extracted from the soil fungus *Tolypocladium inflatum gams*. The drug inhibits cellular immunity by blocking interleukin-2, and interleukin-2 receptor production by helper T cells (Hess et al 1982). It also inhibits production of B-cell activating factors and interferon-gamma by helper T cells (Reed et al 1988).

Pharmacology

Cyclosporin is strongly hydrophobic, with maximum absorption 3–4 hours after oral administration (Brynskov et al 1992). Absorption from the small bowel follows zero-order kinetics and is a function of contact time. Absorption also requires bile, and is reduced in biliary diversion (Venkataramanan et al 1985). Brynskov's paper shows that disposition kinetics are normal in Crohn's disease, but reduced bioavailability necessitates close monitoring of blood levels, and intravenous treatment should be considered in patients with rapid gut transit. There is negligible absorption from the colon when cyclosporin is given as an enema (Sandborn & Tremaine 1992), and this is not increased in proctosigmoiditis (Ranzi et al 1989). Trough concentrations of cyclosporin are used to adjust dosage. Whole blood levels are more reproducible than serum or plasma because there is a variable (e.g. temperature-dependent) uptake of cyclosporin by erythrocytes or lipoproteins. High-performance liquid chromatography or monoclonal radioimmunoassay, which are specific for native cyclosporin, give a narrow therapeutic

Table 57.4 Controlled studies of cyclosporin in inflammatory bowel disease

Trial	Design	Number	Dose (mg/kg/day)	Comments	Outcome
Crohn's disease: active					
Brynskov et al 1989	Placebo-controlled 3 months	71	5–7.5	Improvement by two weeks	+
Crohn's disease: maintenance of remission					
Archambault et al 1992	Placebo-controlled 18 months	305	4.8	14% withdrawn due to toxicity	O
Ulcerative colitis: i.v. treatment of active disease					
Lichtiger et al 1994	Placebo-controlled	20	4	Patients who had failed 7 days of i.v. corticosteroid	+
Ulcerative colitis: enema treatment for left-sided disease					
Sandborn et al 1994	Placebo-controlled 4 weeks	40	350 mg enema	Mild to moderate disease activity	+

window (150–300 ng/ml), whereas polyclonal radio-immunoassay gives a much wider range (200–800 ng/ml) (Sandborn & Tremaine 1992).

Cyclosporin is metabolized by cytochrome P450 enzymes in liver and small-bowel mucosa. Cyclosporin levels are therefore increased by ketoconazole, erythromycin, doxycycline, oral contraceptives, propafenone and some calcium-channel blockers, including diltiazem, nicardipine and verapamil. Levels are reduced by enzyme-inducing drugs such as phenytoin, carbamazepine, barbiturates and rifampicin.

Cyclosporin in active Crohn's disease

In the first placebo-controlled trial in active disease (Table 57.4), Brynskov et al (1989) enrolled patients with corticosteroid-resistant disease in six hospitals. A third were taking prednisolone (5–20 mg daily) and the dose was left unchanged during the trial. Improvement was defined by a grading score derived from wellbeing, symptoms and signs, and intestinal and extraintestinal complications. At the end of this period, 22 of the 37 on cyclosporin had improved (59%) versus 11 of 34 on placebo (32%). Responders started to improve at about 2 weeks.

There are no controlled studies of the use of cyclosporin in fistulous Crohn's disease, but there is some anecdotal evidence of healing of fistulae resistant to corticosteroids, azathioprine or metronidazole (Sandborn & Tremaine 1992, Hanauer & Smith 1993). In the latter study, using intravenous treatment, response occurred at a mean of 3.6 days. Two patients subsequently developed obstruction, which may be because of rapid healing and stricture formation (as has been postulated in 6-mercaptopurine therapy).

Maintenance therapy in Crohn's disease

In a continuation of Brynskov's trial in active Crohn's disease, cyclosporin (or placebo) was gradually withdrawn from responders in the following 3 months, and at 6 months 14 from the cyclosporin group (38%) and five (15%) from the placebo remained improved (a significant difference). Patients on corticosteroids were more likely to remain improved at the end of the tapering period. At 1 year (i.e. 6 months after stopping cyclosporin) there was no difference between the groups (Brynskov et al 1991). This raises the question of long-term maintenance therapy after achieving remission. Low-dose long-term therapy (2 mg/kg/day) was not effective in maintaining remission in the study by Lobo et al (1991). In a preliminary report of a large multicenter Canadian trial (305 patients), a mean dose of 4.8 mg/kg was no better than placebo in preventing worsening or relapse (Archambault et al 1992). There was a 14% withdrawal due to toxicity of cyclosporin. There is little evidence of benefit in maintaining remission.

Cyclosporin in ulcerative colitis

The first controlled trial (Lichtiger et al 1994) planned to recruit 42 patients who had failed at least 7 days of parenteral corticosteroids, using 4 mg/kg daily or placebo by continuous intravenous infusion. The study was terminated early because nine of 11 patients (82%) on cyclosporin improved compared to none of nine on placebo. Mean response time was 7 days. This dramatic benefit was confirmed in five of the nine on placebo who crossed over to open-label intravenous cyclosporin, with all responding. The same group showed in an open label continuation study that nine of 13 responders to intravenous therapy (69%) were in remission off corticosteroids after a further 6 months of oral cyclosporin (Kornbluth et al 1994), and many subsequently remained in remission off treatment (Lichtiger & Present 1992). It is not clear whether oral treatment in acute disease would be as effective as intravenous. Follow-on studies of 'responder' patients will always show up a drug in a favorable light. Further well designed controlled trials are needed to evaluate the role of cyclosporin in achieving complete remission, the optimum length of treatment, and the relapse rate on stopping treatment.

Cyclosporin enemas in ulcerative colitis

There is very little systemic absorption of cyclosporin when administered as an enema, hence fewer side effects. After considerable enthusiasm based on uncontrolled studies, Sandborn et al (1994) enrolled 40 patients with mild to moderately active left-sided colitis to receive cyclosporin enemas 350 mg daily (made up in a vehicle of carboxymethylcellulose and sorbitol), or placebo. At 4 weeks there was no difference between groups. This well designed study showed up the dangers of reporting uncontrolled studies in inflammatory bowel disease. The lack of effect of topical cyclosporin may be because local immunosuppression is not enough to prevent the inflammatory process, or because the vehicle (also used in the other studies) did not deliver a sufficient dose of cyclosporin to the colonic mucosa.

Side-effects of cyclosporin

Side effects are shown in Table 57.5. The major problem is nephrotoxicity. There is an invariable 20% reduction in glomerular filtration rate owing to vasoconstriction of afferent arterioles, but this is reversible. Tubular dysfunction can occur, with consequent hypomagnesemia or hyperkalemia. A few patients have histological changes in the kidney, with irreversible loss of renal function. This depends on cyclosporin dose and maximal creatinine concentration. The risk appears to be low if the dose is kept below 5 mg/kg and serum creatinine does not rise

Table 57.5 Side effects of cyclosporin

	Frequency (%)	Comment
Renal impairment	Majority	20% reduction in GFR in most patients. GFR returns to normal 2 weeks after stopping drug. Irreversible in some
Hypertrichosis	50	Maximal along spine, upper arms and face. Depilatory creams effective. Rarely a severe cosmetic problem. Resolves within weeks or months of stopping drug
Paresthesia	20	Burning in hands or feet. Associated tremor. Resolves on dose reduction
Hypertension	8	
Nausea and vomiting	8	
Headache	4	
Hepatotoxicity	2	Cholestasis
Gingival hyperplasia	2	
Lymphoma		5 lymphomas in 5700 patients with autoimmune disease receiving cyclosporin up to 1993

GFR, glomerular filtration rate

more than 30% above baseline. The dose should be halved if this occurs or creatinine rises above 140 mmol/l, regardless of trough cyclosporin levels. More uncommon side effects include confusion, seizures, hyperuricemia and hyperlipidemia.

Summary

In contrast to the purine analogs, cyclosporin is potent and fast-acting in both acute Crohn's disease and ulcerative colitis. Because of nephrotoxicity the drug should only be used in patients who do not respond to high-dose corticosteroids, and close monitoring of renal function and drug levels is mandatory. In extensive small-bowel Crohn's disease intravenous administration may be necessary. In ulcerative colitis further studies are required to assess whether oral therapy is as effective as intravenous. Early relapse may occur after stopping cyclosporin, and some authors recommend tapering the dose (Brynskov et al 1992), but there is no evidence that this is helpful. Neither is there evidence as yet of a role in maintaining remission, either in ulcerative colitis or in Crohn's disease, and the ongoing risk of irreversible renal damage would be a major deterrent. The use of purine analogs to maintain a cyclosporin-induced remission seems attractive. There are no studies of combined use, and as the mechanisms of action differ completely, side effects would not necessarily rule out starting both drugs together.

METHOTREXATE

Methotrexate is a folic acid antagonist that has molecular homology to interleukin-1 (IL-1) and interferes with its inflammatory actions. The only controlled trial using methotrexate in Crohn's disease has been reported in abstract form (Arora et al 1992). Thirty-two patients who had been on prednisolone 10 mg or more for at least 6 months were randomized to receive low-dose oral pulse methotrexate (5 mg three times a week) for a year. Attempts were made to taper the prednisolone. More patients on placebo had flare-up of disease (12 of 15, 80%) than on methotrexate (six of 13, 46%). Three patients on methotrexate had side effects (one with pneumonitis, two with severe gastrointestinal effects), and there was a rise in liver enzymes in the methotrexate group. This confirms the results of an open study which had suggested a benefit in Crohn's disease and ulcerative colitis (Kozarek et al 1989). A larger controlled trial from the North American Crohn's Study Group has demonstrated the ability of 25 mg administered parenterally to allow steroid withdrawal in 40% of steroid-dependent Crohn's patients compared to 19% of placebo-treated patients. The efficacy in comparison to purine analogs or cyclosporin is unknown.

Side effects may be a major limiting factor for this drug. Methotrexate impairs liver function and can cause irreversible hepatic fibrosis, although this is rare until the total dose exceeds 1.5 g. It also causes bone marrow suppression (dose related and prevented by folinic acid), pneumonitis, megaloblastic anemia, nausea, vomiting and anorexia. Folic acid supplementation is advisable.

OTHER IMMUNOSUPPRESSIVE TREATMENTS

No other immunosuppressive or immunomodulatory therapy has been shown to be effective in controlled trials. The future does, however, hold the prospect of more selective assaults on the immune response. Monoclonal antibody therapy can be specifically targeted at T-cell subpopulations to modulate immune response. An example is anti-CD4 therapy, reported to improve active Crohn's disease and ulcerative colitis when infused repeatedly over 7 days (Emmrich et al 1991). It is hoped that a range of monoclonal agents will shortly be developed. In the meantime, purine analogs and occasionally cyclosporin have a useful place in the therapeutic armamentarium in inflammatory bowel disease.

REFERENCES

Adler D J, Korelitz B I 1990 The therapeutic efficacy of 6-mercaptopurine in refractory ulcerative colitis. American Journal of Gastroenterology 85: 717–722

Alstead E M, Ritchie J K, Lennard-Jones J E, Farthing M J G, Clark M L 1990 Safety of azathioprine in pregnancy in inflammatory bowel disease. Gastroenterology 99: 443–446

Archambault A, Feagan B, Fedorak R et al 1992 The Canadian Crohn's relapse prevention trial (CCRPT). Gastroenterology 102: A591

Arora S, Katkov W N, Cooley J et al 1992 A double-blind, randomized, placebo-controlled trial of methotrexate in Crohn's disease. Gastroenterology 102: A591

Bean R H D 1962 The treatment of chronic ulcerative colitis with 6-mercaptopurine. Medical Journal of Australia 2: 592–593

Brooke B N, Hoffmann D C, Swarbrick E T 1969 Azathioprine for Crohn's disease. Lancet 2: 612–614

Brynskov J, Freund L, Norby Rasmussen S et al 1989 A placebo-controlled, double-blind, randomized trial of cyclosporine therapy in active chronic Crohn's disease. New England Journal of Medicine 321: 845–850

Brynskov J, Freund L, Norby Rasmussen S et al 1991 Final report on a placebo-controlled, double-blind, randomized multicentre trial of cyclosporine treatment in active chronic Crohn's disease. Scandinavian Journal of Gastroenterology 26: 689–695

Brynskov J, Freund L, Campanini M C, Kampmann J P 1992 Cyclosporin pharmacokinetics after intravenous and oral administration in patients with Crohn's disease. Scandinavian Journal of Gastroenterology 27: 961–967

Candy S, Wright J P, Gerber M, Adams G, Gerig M, Goodman R 1994 A double blind controlled study of azathioprine in the treatment and maintenance of remission in Crohn's disease. Gastroenterology 106: A659

Caprilli R, Carratu R, Babbini M 1975 A double-blind comparison of the effectiveness of azathioprine and sulfasalazine in idiopathic proctocolitis. Digestive Diseases 20: 115–120

Connell W R, Kamm M A, Ritchie J K, Lennard-Jones J E 1993 Bone marrow toxicity caused by azathioprine in inflammatory bowel disease: 27 years of experience. Gut 34: 1081–1085

Connell W R, Kinlen L J, Ritchie J K, Balkwill A, Lennard-Jones J E, Kamm M A 1994 Cancer risk from azathioprine in inflammatory bowel disease. Gastroenterology 106: A667

Cox J A, Daneshemend T K, Hawkey C J, Logan R F A, Walt R P 1988 Devastating diarrhoea due to azathioprine: management difficulty in inflammatory bowel disease. Gut 29: 686–688

Dewitte D B, Buick M K, Cyran S E, Maisells M J 1984 Neonatal pancytopaenia and severe combined immunodeficiency associated with antenatal administration of azathioprine and prednisolone. Pediatrics 105: 625–628

Emmrich J, Seyfarth M, Fleig W E, Emmrich F 1991 Treatment of inflammatory bowel disease with anti-CD4 monoclonal antibody. Lancet 338: 570–571

Ewe K, Press A G, Singe C C et al 1993 Azathioprine combined with prednisolone or monotherapy with prednisolone in active Crohn's disease. Gastroenterology 105: 367–372

Hanauer S B, Smith M B 1993 Rapid closure of Crohn's disease fistulas with continuous intravenous cyclosporin A. American Journal of Gastroenterology 88: 646–649

Hawthorne A B, Hawkey C J 1989 Immunosuppressive drugs in inflammatory bowel disease. Drugs 38: 267–288

Hawthorne A B, Logan R F A, Hawkey C J et al 1992 Randomised controlled trial of azathioprine withdrawal in ulcerative colitis. British Medical Journal 305: 20–22

Hess A D, Tutshka P J, Santos G W 1982 Effect of cyclosporin A on human lymphocyte responses in vitro. III. CsA inhibits the production of T lymphocyte growth factors in secondary mixed lymphocyte responses but does not inhibit the response of primed lymphocytes to TCGF. Journal of Immunology 128: 355–359

Jewell D P, Truelove S C 1974 Azathioprine in ulcerative colitis: final report on controlled therapeutic trial. British Medical Journal 4: 627–630

Kinlen L J, Sheil A G R, Peto J, Doll R 1979 Collaborative United Kingdom–Australasia study of cancer in patients treated with immunosuppressive drugs. British Medical Journal 2: 1461–1466

Kirk A P, Lennard-Jones J E 1982 Controlled trial of azathioprine in chronic ulcerative colitis. British Medical Journal 284: 1291–1292

Klein M, Binder H J, Mitchell M, Aaronson R, Spiro H 1974 Treatment of Crohn's disease with azathioprine: a controlled evaluation. Gastroenterology 66: 916–922

Kornbluth A, Lichtiger S, Present D, Hanauer S 1994 Long-term results of oral cyclosporin in patients with severe ulcerative colitis. Gastroenterology 106: A714

Kozarek R A, Patterson D J, Gelfand M D, Botoman V, Ball T J, Wilske K R 1989 Methotrexate induces clinical and histologic remission in patients with refractory inflammatory bowel disease. Annals of Internal Medicine 110: 353–356

Lemann M, Tai R, Bouhnik Y et al 1994 Long-term outcome of patients with Crohn's disease successfully treated with azathioprine or 6-mercaptopurine. Gastroenterology 106: A719

Lichtiger S, Present D H 1992 Cyclosporin A in the treatment of severe ulcerative colitis. Gastroenterology 102: A653

Lichtiger S, Present D H, Kornbluth A, Hanauer S 1994 Cyclosporin in severe ulcerative colitis refractory to steroid therapy. New England Journal of Medicine 330: 1841–1845

Lobo A J, Juby L D, Rothwell J et al 1991 Long-term treatment of Crohn's disease with cyclosporine: the effect of a very low dose on maintenance of remission. Journal of Clinical Gastroenterology 13: 42–45

Major G A C, Moore P G 1985 Profound circulatory collapse due to azathioprine. Journal of the Royal Society of Medicine 78: 1052

O'Donoghue D P, Dawson A M, Powell-Tuck J, Bown R L, Lennard-Jones J E 1978 Double-blind withdrawal trial of azathioprine as maintenance treatment for Crohn's disease. Lancet 2: 955–957

Present D H 1989 6-mercaptopurine and other immunosuppressive agents in the treatment of Crohn's disease and ulcerative colitis. Gastroenterology Clinics of North America 18: 57–71

Present D H, Chapman M L, Rubin P H 1988 Efficacy of 6-mercaptopurine in refractory ulcerative colitis. Gastroenterology 94: A359

Present D H, Korelitz B I, Wisch J L, Glass J L, Sachar D B, Pasternack B S 1980 Treatment of Crohn's disease with 6-mercaptopurine. New England Journal of Medicine 302: 981–987

Present D H, Meltzer S J, Krumholz M P, Wolke A, Korelitz B I 1989 6-mercaptopurine in the management of inflammatory bowel disease: short- and long-term toxicity. Annals of Internal Medicine 111: 641–649

Ranzi T, Campanini M C, Velio P, Quarto di Palo F, Bainchi P 1989 Treatment of chronic proctosigmoiditis with cyclosporin enemas. Lancet 2: 97

Reed J C, Prystowsky M B, Nowell P C 1988 Regulation of gene expression in lectin-stimulated or lymphokine-stimulated T lymphocytes. Transplantation 46(Suppl): 85S–89S

Rhodes J, Beck P, Bainton D, Campbell H 1971 Controlled trial of azathioprine in Crohn's disease. Lancet 2: 1273–1276

Rosenberg J L, Levin B, Wall A J, Kirsner J B 1975a A controlled trial of azathioprine in Crohn's disease. Digestive Diseases 20: 721–726

Rosenberg J L, Wall A J, Levin B, Binder H J, Kirsner J B 1975b A controlled trial of azathioprine in the management of chronic ulcerative colitis. Gastroenterology 69: 96–99

Sandborn W J, Tremaine W J 1992 Cyclosporin treatment of inflammatory bowel disease. Mayo Clinic Proceedings 67: 981–990

Sandborn W J, Tremaine W J, Schroeder K W et al 1994 A placebo-controlled trial of cyclosporine enemas for mildly to moderately active left-sided ulcerative colitis. Gastroenterology 106: 1429–1435

Summers R W, Switz D M, Sessions J T et al 1979 National cooperative Crohn's disease study: results of drug treatment. Gastroenterology 77: 847–869

Venkataramanan R, Burckhart G J, Ptachcinski R J 1985 Pharmacokinetics and monitoring of cyclosporine following orthotopic liver transplantation. Seminars in Liver Disease 5: 357–368

Willoughby J M T, Beckett J, Kumar P, Dawson A M 1971 Controlled trial of azathioprine in Crohn's disease. Lancet 2: 944–946

58. Inflammatory mediators

C. J. Hawkey

INTRODUCTION

Rational treatment in inflammatory bowel disease is hampered by our ignorance of the causes of ulcerative colitis and Crohn's disease. Although there is some evidence in support of adhesive *Escherichia coli* in ulcerative colitis (Burke & Axon 1988), measles virus in Crohn's disease (Wakefield et al 1989) and atypical mycobacteria in Crohn's disease (McFadden et al 1987), all of these proposals are controversial and/or antimicrobial treatments have not been effective. Several host abnormalities have been claimed as central to pathogenesis. Mucus synthesis is reduced in patients with ulcerative colitis (Cope et al 1988) and mucus glycoproteins are abnormal (Rhodes 1989). Metabolism of butyrate by colonocytes is abnormal (Roediger 1980) and the epithelial barrier is leaky (Katz et al 1989). However, with the possible exception of butyrate metabolism (Steinhart et al 1994) none of these abnormalities have led to new therapies. Treatments, both existing and prospective, are therefore often targeted at mediators or mechanisms of inflammation that are important in the pathophysiology of inflammatory bowel disease.

Regardless of the initiating event, the mucosa during a relapse of inflammatory bowel disease (whether ulcerative colitis or Crohn's disease) is characterized by a state of intense immune and inflammatory activation (Hawkey et al 1992). Intestinal macrophages are activated (Mahida et al 1989a, Wardle et al 1993) (Fig. 58.1) and antigen pre-

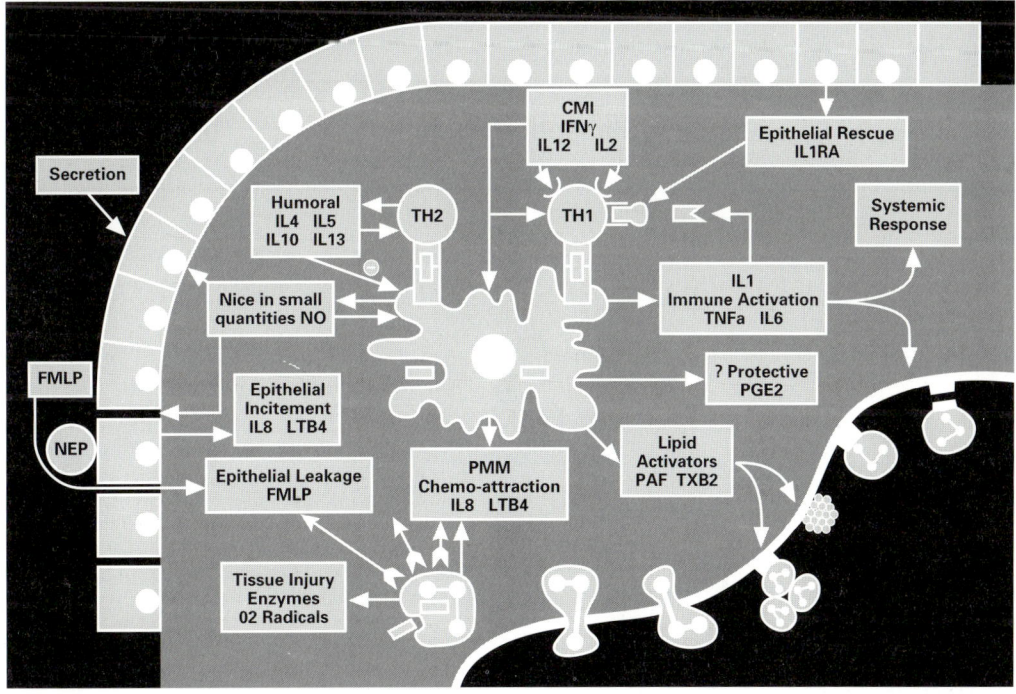

Fig. 58.1 Components of the immune and inflammatory response which represent targets for therapeutic intervention. There is some evidence that most of the events shown occur in active IBD, but in some cases this is uncertain or contentious (see text).

sentation is increased (Mahida et al 1988). Activated macrophages have increased antigen-presenting activity and produce increased amounts of interleukin (IL)-1 (Mahida et al 1989b), IL-6 (Mahida et al 1991, Reinecker et al 1993) and tumor necrosis factor (TNF)α (Nicholls et al 1993, Murch et al 1993), which can stimulate further cytokine production and synthesis of eicosanoids. Other functions of these cytokines include induction of local adhesion molecules and systemic changes such as decreased synthesis of albumin, increased synthesis of acute-phase proteins, release of platelets from the bone marrow, expression of endothelial procoagulant activity and suppression of erythropoietin production (Beagley & Elson 1992, Gasche et al 1994). IL-1 also acts as an accessory signal when antigen is presented to T-cell receptors in the presence of CD4 molecules, leading to clonal expansion with enhanced local expression and systemic release of IL-2 receptors (Mahida et al 1990). Clonal expansion is also normally associated with increased production of IL-2 by T cells, but this has not been unequivocally shown in inflammatory bowel disease, and many studies show an apparent paradoxical lowering of mucosal IL-2 levels and production (Beagley & Elson 1992, Breese et al 1993, McCabe et al 1993, Matsurra et al 1993).

There is some evidence that epithelial cells downregulate mucosal inflammation and that this may be lost in active inflammatory bowel disease. Downregulating mechanisms include a natural antagonist to IL-1, the IL-1 receptor antagonist (Dinarello 1991, Cominelli et al 1990, 1994). Ulcerative colitis is associated with a polymorphism of this gene (Mansfield et al 1994) and there is a relative deficiency during active disease (Nishiyama et al 1994). Another manifestation of this loss of immune downregulation by epithelial cells is shown by their increased expression of HLA antigens, with increased antigen-presenting activity (Mayer & Shilen 1987) and increased antibody-dependent cellular cytotoxicity (Hibi et al 1993). Although these phenomena imply synthesis of γ interferon this, like IL-2, is not always increased and may paradoxically be lowered (Beagley & Elson 1992, Breese et al 1993, McCabe et al 1993, Matsurra et al 1993).

Relapse of inflammatory bowel disease is characterized by neutrophil invasion. Increased adhesion molecule expression is likely to play a part in facilitating this process (Podolsky et al 1993, Balsitis et al 1994), but a chemoattractant stimulus is needed to achieve migration into the lamina propria (Cole et al 1993). During active disease there is increased release of platelet-activating factor (Eliakim et al 1988, Denizot et al 1992, Ferraris et al 1993, Travis & Jewell 1994a, Gross et al 1995) (Fig. 58.2) and of arachidonic acid, with metabolism to the chemoattractant leukotriene (LT) B4 as well as to

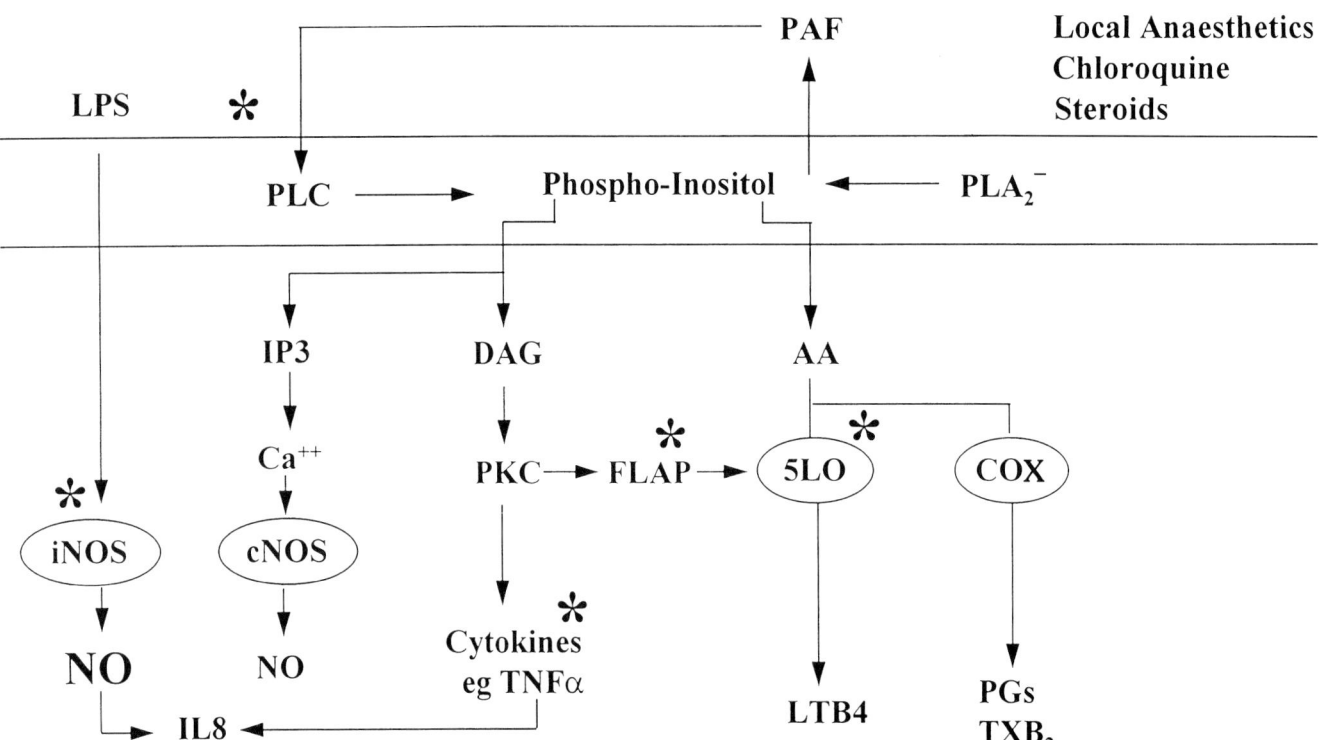

Fig. 58.2 A simplified schema in which cell surface and intracellular events which represent targets for therapeutic intervention are indicated. PAF–Platelet activating factor; PL–Phospholipase; LPS–Lipopolysaccharide; NOS–Nitric oxide synthase; I–Inducible; C–Constitutive; DAG–Diacyl glycerol; FLAP–5 lipoxygenase activating protein; 5LO–5 lipoxygenase; COX–Cyclooxygenase; PKC–Protein kinase.

prostaglandins and thromboxane (Rampton & Hawkey 1984, Sharon & Stenson 1984). Other chemoattractants found in increased amounts in active inflammatory bowel disease include activated complement (Ahrenstedt et al 1992), chemotactic bacterial peptides (Von Ritten et al 1989) and IL-8 and related chemokines (Mahida et al 1992, Raab et al 1993, Harada et al 1994, Mitsuyama et al 1994, Mazzucchelli et al 1994, McLaughlan et al 1995). Although these may derive from activated macrophages and neutrophils, probably providing a secondary amplification stimulus, epithelial cells are increasingly recognized as a source of both IL-8 and LTB-4 (Jung et al 1995, Dias et al 1992), with the possibility that, from this source, they may act as primary initiators of inflammation.

MEDIATOR-TARGETED TREATMENT – GENERAL ISSUES

In theory, treatment targeted at mediators or immunoinflammatory mechanisms might attempt to enhance or suppress them. Immunoenhancement strategies have not been conspicuously successful. Levamisole (Hermanowicz et al 1987, Sachar et al 1987) has had little effect in ulcerative colitis or Crohn's disease, and BCG is equally without benefit. Two patients treated with IL-2 for renal tumors who also had Crohn's disease deteriorated (Sparano et al 1993). Interferons have yet to show clear benefit (Vantrappen et al 1980, Yoshida et al 1988, Hadziselimovic et al 1992, Sumer et al 1992, Wirth et al 1993, Hanauer et al 1994, Davidsen et al 1995).

If the correct strategy is to suppress inflammatory mediators, the next question is whether treatment should attempt to suppress the many mechanisms that lead to inflammation, or to selectively target a relevant mechanism. The latter approach motivates much new drug development, but whether this strategy is correct will only become clear when a number of designer molecules have been assessed. Those who favor a blanket approach point to corticosteroids, which have multiple anti-inflammatory mechanisms including reduction in synthesis and release of eicosanoids, platelet-activating factor and many cytokines. Salicylates have also been shown to affect numerous potentially inflammatory mechanisms, albeit at high concentrations (Travis & Jewell 1994b). However, showing that high concentrations of salicylates can affect these processes does not, as is often asserted, prove that they act at multiple sites in vivo. It is just as likely that much is known about therapeutically irrelevant activities because the pivotal one has not yet been identified. Corticosteroids are particularly effective during established relapse when blanket suppression of inflammation seems conceptually apt. By contrast, first principles might suggest that inhibiting a discrete event that was pivotal in the initiation of relapse would be a sound strategy for maintenance of remission.

A final issue which remains unsettled is whether ulcerative colitis and Crohn's disease are best viewed as discrete entities or two ends of an inflammatory spectrum. Certainly most drugs which work in ulcerative colitis do so in Crohn's disease, although there are suggestions (see below) that some (e.g. methotrexate: Choi & Targan 1994, Debinski & Kamm 1995, Feagan et al 1995) may prove to be more valuable in Crohn's disease whereas others (e.g. cyclosporin) may be more valuable in ulcerative colitis (Davidsen et al 1995, Debinski & Kamm 1995, Lichtiger et al 1994).

Existing treatments

The mode of action of existing treatments may help to guide the selection of future designer molecules. The multiple actions of corticosteroids and salicylates have already been discussed. Azathioprine, active in both ulcerative colitis (Hawthorne et al 1992c) and Crohn's disease (Present et al 1980), probably acts by depletion of subgroups of lymphocytes (Hawthorne & Hawkey 1989). The mode of action of cyclosporin is more precisely understood. This drug interferes with the process by which activated T cells synthesize both IL-2 and IL-2 receptors and stimulate their own clonal expansion (Kahan 1989, Hodgson 1991). Its therapeutic value in inflammatory bowel disease is thus a prototypical example of the success of targeting IL-2-mediated lymphocyte stimulation. Clinically, current evidence for the activity of cyclosporin is better for ulcerative colitis than for Crohn's disease (Fig. 58.3) (Debinski & Kamm 1995, Choi & Targan 1994, Lichtiger et al 1994, Lobo et al 1994). Conversely, limited experience with methotrexate suggests that it is better in active Crohn's disease than ulcerative colitis (Debinski & Kamm 1995, Choi & Targan 1994, Feagan et al 1995). Methotrexate is a folic acid antimetabolite but, interestingly, is also structurally related to IL-1 and can interfere with its role as an accessory signal to T-cell clonal expansion (Wardle & Turnberg 1994).

Developing treatments

The major advances that have occurred in the understanding of inflammation in recent decades are now yielding a plethora of drugs targeted at immune stimulation or inflammation. Unfortunately, all too often, encouraging small open studies of new treatment in inflammatory bowel disease have been followed by controlled studies showing no benefit. In the next section potential new treatments are characterized by the mediators at which they are targeted: cytokines, lipid mediators, nitric oxide, radical scavengers and miscellaneous mediators of uncertain significance. Some of these new therapies, particularly those aimed at cytokines, are complex peptides which are more expensive to produce and more difficult to administer

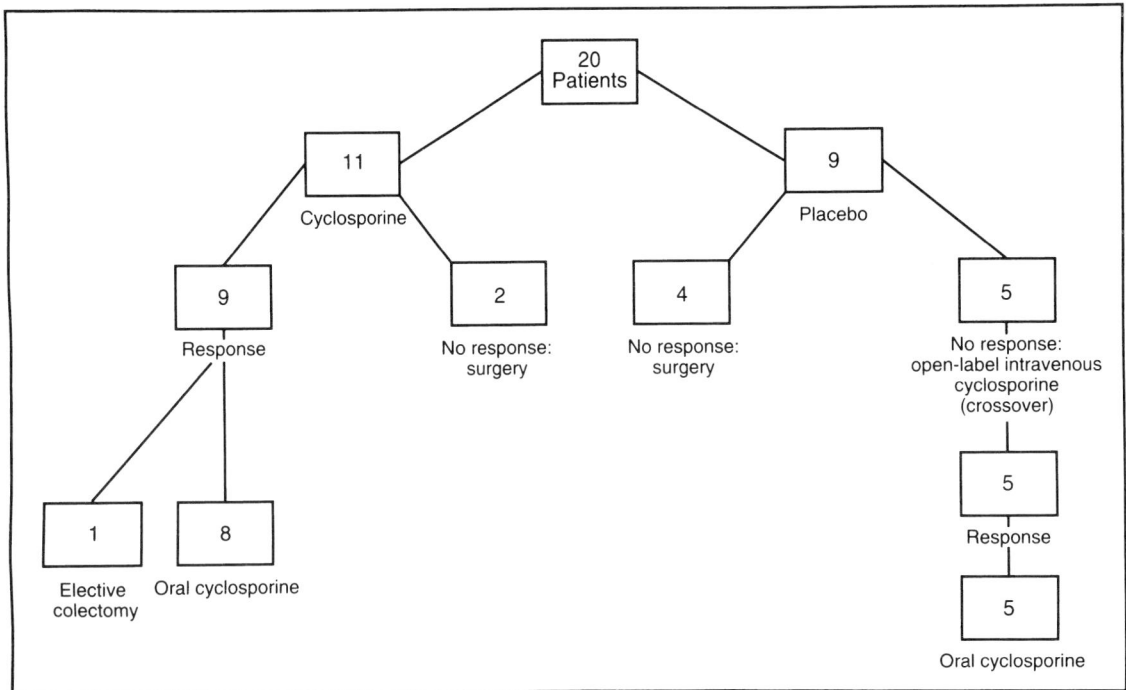

Fig. 58.3 Effectiveness of cyclosporine in ulcerative colitis. Reproduced from N Eng J Med 1994; 330: 841 with permission.

than traditional organic molecules. Many of them are available for treatment in inflammatory bowel disease only because they have been developed either for other inflammatory conditions or for use in septic shock.

TREATMENTS TARGETED AT CYTOKINES AND THE IMMUNE RESPONSE

Interleukin-1

Interleukin-1 is synthesized by many cells, including monocytes, tissue macrophages, lymphocytes, fibroblasts, vascular endothelium and smooth muscle, and has a wide range of biological activities on many different target cells, including B cells, T cells and monocytes (Dinarello 1991, 1993). There are two distinct molecular forms, IL-1α and IL-1β which, despite low sequence homology, bind to the same transmembrane glycoprotein receptor and have similar biological properties. IL-1β is released as an inactive precursor and activated by a cysteine protease IL-1-converting enzyme (ICE) (Ceretti et al 1992, Thornberry et al 1992). The immunostimulatory and proinflammatory actions of IL-1 are antagonized by the natural related peptide IL-1 receptor antagonist, levels of which are increased in inflammatory bowel disease, though to a much lesser extent than IL-1, resulting in an imbalance (Cominelli et al 1992, 1994, Hyams et al 1994).

Therapeutic possibilities

The pivotal role of IL-1 in the mucosal immune response and its increased production and the relative deficiency of IL-1 receptor antagonist in active inflammatory bowel disease makes IL-1 an obvious target for anti-inflammatory development. Four strategies are possible. The natural IL-1 receptor antagonist has been cloned, sequenced and synthesized. It had anti-inflammatory activity in a rabbit model of colitis (Cominelli et al 1990, 1992, Ferretti et al 1994) (Fig. 58.4), and is currently undergoing trials in inflammatory conditions, including inflammatory bowel disease in humans (Henderson & Blake 1992). One disadvantage of this compound is that it has to be given parenterally and, (because of relatively weak binding to the IL-1 receptor, compared to IL-1 itself) in high doses. An alternative would be to synthesize a non-peptide receptor antagonist, but as yet none is available for clinical trials. A third, potentially easier, approach would be to develop inhibitors of ICE which release mature IL-1β from its inactive proenzyme. A cowpox virus inhibitor of ICE has been shown to inhibit host inflammatory responses (Ray et al 1992), and ICE inhibitors are under development but have not yet been investigated in inflammatory bowel disease. A final approach would be to use soluble IL-1 receptors to mop up excess IL-1.

Interleukin-6

Interleukin-6 is a 26 kDa protein which shares many of the properties of IL-1. Synthesis of IL-6 is increased in active inflammatory bowel disease (Mahida et al 1991, Ross 1993a, Mazlam et al 1994, Raab et al 1994, Hyams et al 1993) and is an attractive target for therapy, although no drugs are yet available.

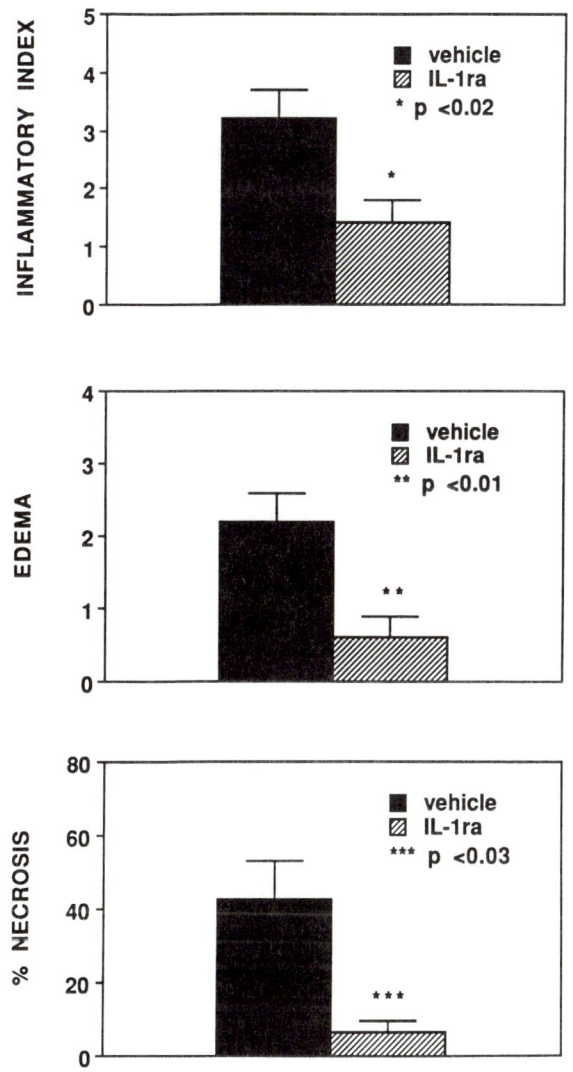

Fig. 58.4 Anti-inflammatory activity of IL-1 receptor antagonist in a rabbit model of colitis. Reproduced from Cominelli et al, J Clin Invest 1990; 86: 972 with permission.

Tumor necrosis factorα

Tumor necrosis factorα is secreted by activated monocytes, macrophages and other cells including, T and B lymphocytes and fibroblasts. Acting via two receptors, it is selectively cytotoxic and promotes immune and inflammatory responses and mediates a number of the systemic manifestations of inflammation. Circulating stool and mucosal levels of TNFα are probably increased in active inflammatory bowel disease, and may form a useful index of inflammation (Nicholls et al 1993, Murch et al 1993).

Therapeutic possibilities

Because TNFα is pivotal in inflammatory responses it is a natural target for treatment. As yet TNF receptor antagonists have not been developed. However, several monoclonal antibodies have been produced and used in the context of septic shock.

Evidence for efficacy in inflammatory bowel disease

Two open studies have suggested that single doses of the chimeric CA2 TNFα antibody can reduce Crohn's disease activity for up to 2 months or longer (Derkx et al 1993, van Dullemen et al 1994). (Fig. 58.5). However many of these patients were taking relatively high doses of steroids. A recent controlled study using a bio-engineered human TNFα monoclonal antibody (CDP 571) has also shown benefit in a blinded controlled study (Stack et al 1996).

Interleukin-2

Interleukin-2, or T-cell growth factor, is synthesized by T cells which have been activated under the stimulus of

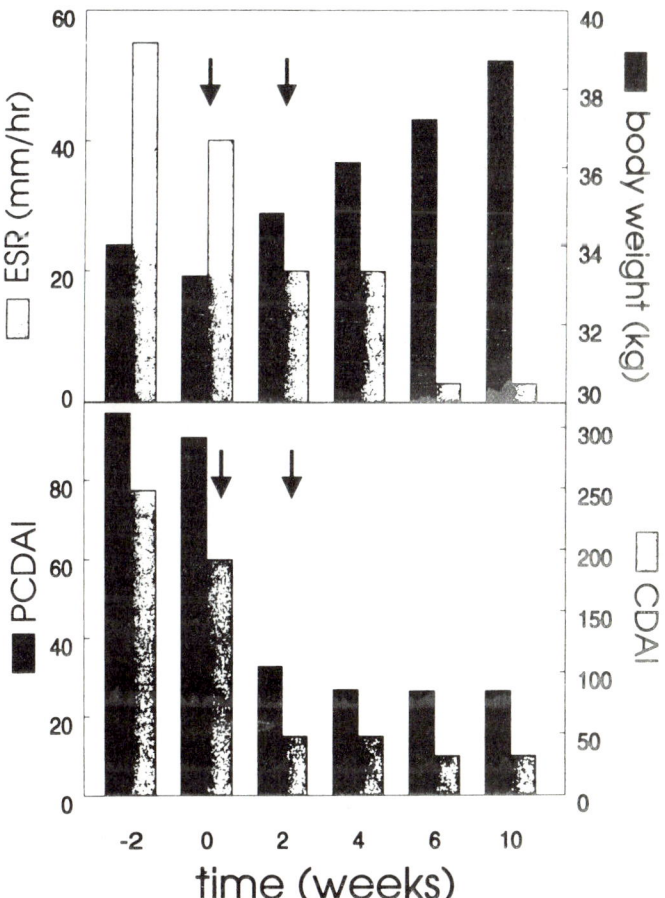

Fig. 58.5 Response to anti TNFα antibody in Crohn's disease. Reproduced from Lancet; 1993 342: 174 with permission.

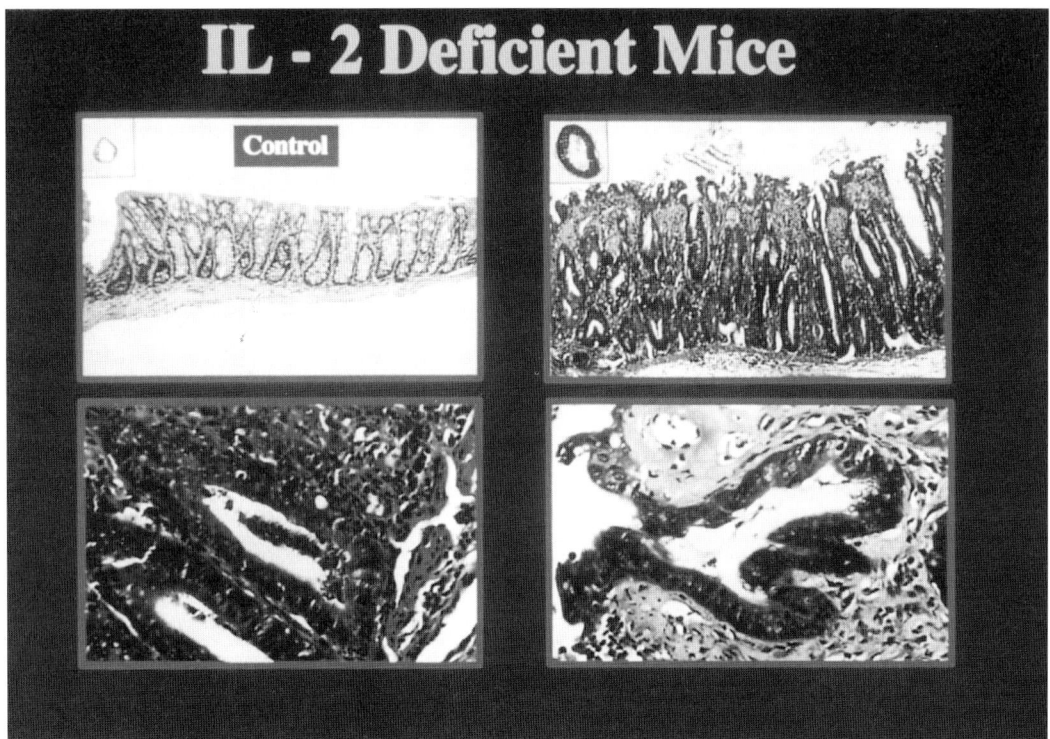

Fig. 58.6 Colitis in IL-2 knockout mice. Adapted from Cell 1993; 75: 253 with permission.

antigen presentation with IL-1 as an accessory signal. The autocrine clonal expansion it stimulates, acting via IL-2 receptors which are transiently expressed at the same time, is an immune amplifying step which offers a number of potentially immunosuppressive targets. However, the role of IL-2 remains somewhat cryptic in inflammatory bowel disease. Many studies have found reduced rather than increased levels (though this may be secondary) with, if anything, higher levels in ulcerative colitis than Crohn's disease. Paradoxically, IL-2 knockout mice develop colonic inflammation similar to ulcerative colitis (Fig. 58.6) (Sadlack et al 1993, Kuhn et al 1993, Strober & Ehrhardt 1993, Shanahian 1994), and two patients treated with IL-2 for renal tumors experienced exacerbation of their concurrent Crohn's disease (Sparano et al 1993). Taken at face value these data are confusing, suggesting that increased IL-2-dependent processes might be beneficial in ulcerative colitis and harmful in Crohn's disease.

Therapeutic possibilities

Despite these conceptual problems, the therapeutic value of cyclosporin in both ulcerative colitis and Crohn's disease is a prototypical illustration of the value of suppressing IL-2-mediated processes. A potential target is the CD4 antigen on T-helper cells, which acts as the receptor for class 1 HLA antigens during activation of these T cells on exposure to foreign antigens. In addition, the expression of IL-2 receptors offers a means by which toxins can be selectively targeted at lymphocytes undergoing clonal expansion.

Evidence for efficacy in inflammatory bowel disease

Three small open studies with two different monoclonal antibodies directed against CD4 (Fig. 58.7) antigens over periods between 7 and 16 months have been impressive, with remission or steroid dose reduction in about three-quarters of patients (Emmrich et al 1991, Deusch et al 1993, Stronkhorst et al 1993). CD4-positive cells declined, although the occurrence of chills and fever in some patients raised the specter of immunodeficiency leading to infection.

A number of intriguing molecules targeted at the IL-2 receptor have been developed. These include a monoclonal antibody and chimeric IL-2 toxins (Strom et al 1993), which bind to the IL-2 receptor, are internalized, and thereby selectively kill the cells which express IL-2 receptors. These molecules have been given to humans. They are well tolerated and there is some evidence of value in other inflammatory conditions (Strom et al 1993). Evidence of efficacy in inflammatory bowel disease is as yet no more than rumoured.

Interferons

α and β interferons are related inducible secreted proteins which confer resistance to viruses, inhibit cell proliferation

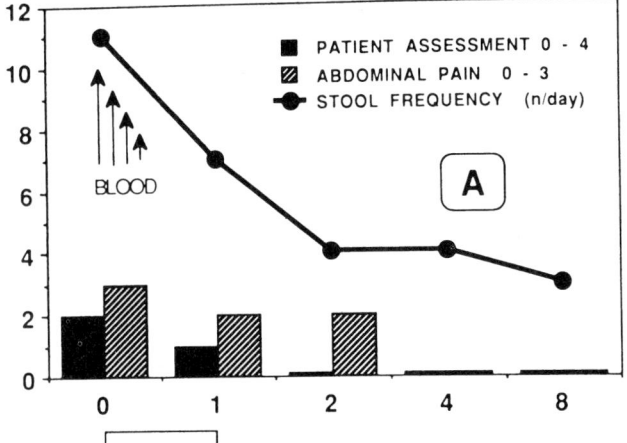

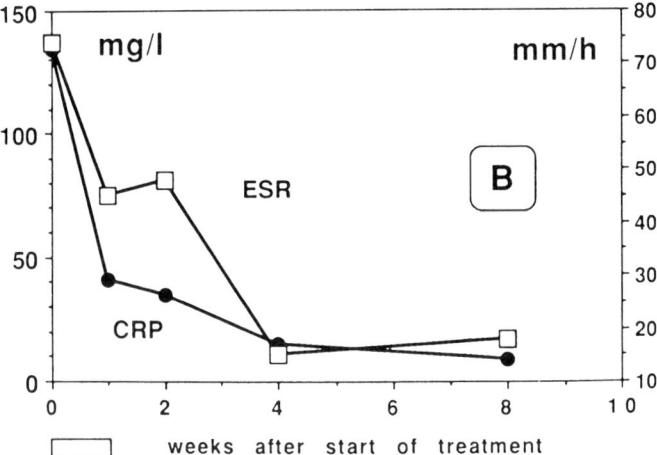

Fig. 58.7 Response of a patient with ulcerative colitis to seven infusions of a humanized anti-CD4 monoclonal antibody. Reproduced from Lancet 1991; 338: 570 with permission.

and regulate expression of cell MHC class 1 antigens. Gamma interferon possesses similar activity and has many other actions in the regulation of immune and inflammatory responses.

Therapeutic possibilities

Although these multiple properties, along with uncertainties about the levels of interferons in inflammatory bowel disease, make their therapeutic potential hard to predict, a number of small studies have been conducted (Vantrappen et al 1980, Yoshida et al 1988, Hadziselimovic et al 1992, Sumer et al 1992, Wirth et al 1993, Hanauer et al 1994, Davidsen et al 1995). Eleven out of 19 patients with Crohn's disease treated with α or β interferon, and 13 out of 15 with colitis, reported in five small open studies, appeared to benefit. Despite an increase in 2' 5' oligoadenylate synthetase no changes were seen in inflammatory markers. Controlled studies will be required before α or β interferon can be seen to have any role in inflammatory bowel disease. In one study of gamma interferon no patients out of five with Crohn's disease benefited.

Colony-stimulating factors

These include granulocyte and macrophage colony-stimulating factor and granulocyte colony-stimulating factor, activity of which is increased in inflammatory bowel disease. These are potential targets, since corticosteroids inhibit production whereas neutralizing antibodies have been effective in model systems of inflammation (Henderson & Blake 1992).

Interleukin-8

Interleukin-8 is a small inflammatory cytokine synthesized by a number of cells, including monocytes, macrophages, lymphocytes and PMNs, but also colonic epithelial cells. Acting through a high and a low infinity receptor it functions as a potent neutrophil chemoattractant and activator. Levels of IL-8 are elevated in active ulcerative colitis, though possibly less so in Crohn's disease (Mahida et al 1992, Raab et al 1993, Harada et al 1994, Mitsuyama et al 1994, Mazzucchelli et al 1994, McLaughlan et al 1995). Synthesis is suppressed by corticosteroids and IL-8 is an attractive target for therapeutic manipulation, as its epithelial source (Jung et al 1995) makes it potentially an early chemoattractant trigger. However, although natural antibodies exist and may regulate systemic inflammatory responses in inflammatory bowel disease (Mahida et al 1992), no therapies are yet available.

THERAPIES TARGETED AT LIPID MEDIATORS

Active inflammatory bowel disease is characterized by greatly enhanced release of arachidonic acid, with metabolism to increased levels of prostaglandins and leukotrienes, particularly LTB-4 and thromboxane (TX) A_2 and B_2 (Rampton & Hawkey 1984). This is accompanied by increased release of platelet-activating factor (PAF) (Gross et al 1995, Travis & Jewell 1994a, Eliakim et al 1988, Denizot et al 1992, Ferraris et al 1993) which in turn, by activating phospholipase, induces further release of arachidonic acid and enhancement of the inflammatory cascade. Eicosanoids have become a major focus for drug development, since they have been recognized for a long time, are known to play a role in the action of existing drugs such as non-steroidal anti-inflammatory drugs, and can be relatively easily targeted by enzyme inhibitors.

Leukotriene B4

In particular a number of inhibitors of the synthesis or action of the highly chemoattractant molecule LTB4 have been developed. Although enhanced local elaboration of

LTB4 may not be primary but largely derived from invading neutrophils, it is nevertheless both synthesized by epithelial cells and quantitatively the most important stimulus in the inflamed mucosa to continuing neutrophil chemoattraction (Cole et al 1993, Boughton-Smith et al 1983, Sharon et al 1978). Since up to half the body's daily production of neutrophils emigrates through the gut in active ulcerative colitis and Crohn's disease, this makes LTB4 a logical target for drug development.

Therapeutic possibilities

Eicosanoids in general and LTB4 in particular can in theory be inhibited at several sites. Release of substrate arachidonic acid can be blocked by corticosteroids, chloroquine and lignocaine (Mayer et al 1992, Mayer & Sachar 1992, Bjorck et al 1989, Anasetti et al 1992). Fish oil can be used to supplement the membrane content of eicosapentaenoic acid (EPA), which is metabolized to less inflammatory 5-lipoxygenase compounds such as LTB5 (Ross 1993b, Hawthorne et al 1992b). Finally, a new generation of selective 5-lipoxygenase inhibitors is available. These include drugs affecting the redox potential, direct inhibitors of the enzyme (Hawthorne et al 1992a) and inhibitors of a natural 5-lipoxygenase-activating protein (FLAP) (Dixon et al 1990).

Evidence for activity

Arachidonic acid release. Steroids inhibit the release of arachidonic acid, acting through a natural inhibitor (lipocortin) of phospholipase activity (see Fig. 58.2). The success of corticosteroids in treating inflammatory bowel disease could be taken as evidence for the success of this approach, although steroids have numerous other actions, making this difficult to assess. Other inhibitors of arachidonic acid release include chloroquine and lignocaine. In one open study topical chloroquine improved one out of ten patients with ulcerative colitis (Mayer & Sachar 1992); in another lignocaine was associated with a high response (Bjorck et al 1989). However, these drugs also have other actions, with chloroquine inhibiting T-helper cell activity and lignocaine affecting the neural component of inflammation (Anasetti et al 1992). Moreover, a double-blind study of hydroxychloroquine 400 mg q.d.s. showed no benefit compared to placebo in active ulcerative colitis (Mayer et al 1992). Controlled studies of local anesthetics are also under way.

Substrate availability. Fish oil has been used in four studies (Ross 1993). In the largest study, 87 patients received fish oil, providing 4.5 g of EPA daily for 1 year, or olive oil as placebo (Hawthorne et al 1992b). EPA was selectively incorporated into the rectal mucosa and this was maintained for a year and was associated with an approximate halving of ex-vivo LTB4 production by neutrophils (Fig. 58.8). However, trends to clinical benefit were very weak, although patients taking fish oil who had active disease were able to reduce steroids to a greater extent than controlled patients receiving olive oil. Several smaller studies have produced more optimistic data (Salomon et al 1990, Stenson et al 1992, Grimminger et al 1993), but overall a role for fish oil seems limited.

5-lipoxygenase inhibitors. A number of 5-lipoxygenase inhibitors have been produced for use in

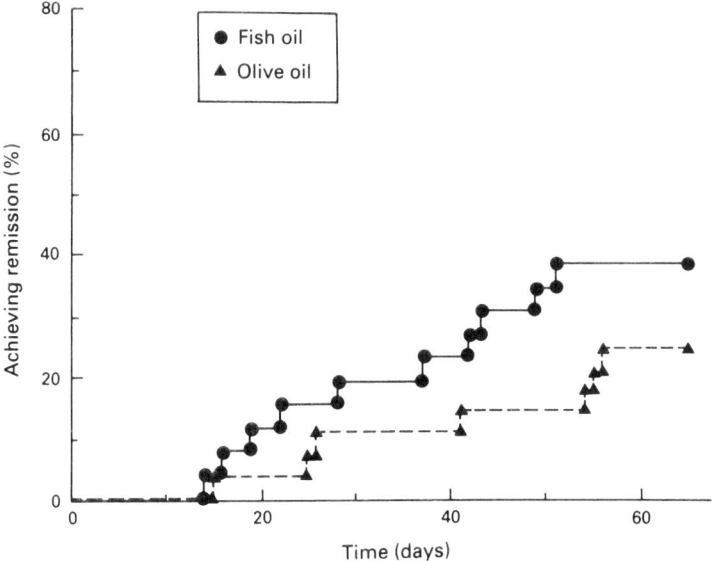

Fig. 58.8 Response to fish oil in patients with ulcerative colitis. Differences in achieving and maintaining remission compared to placebo did not reach statistical significance, but there was a small but significant steroid-sparing effect. Reproduced from Gut 1992; 33: 922 with permission.

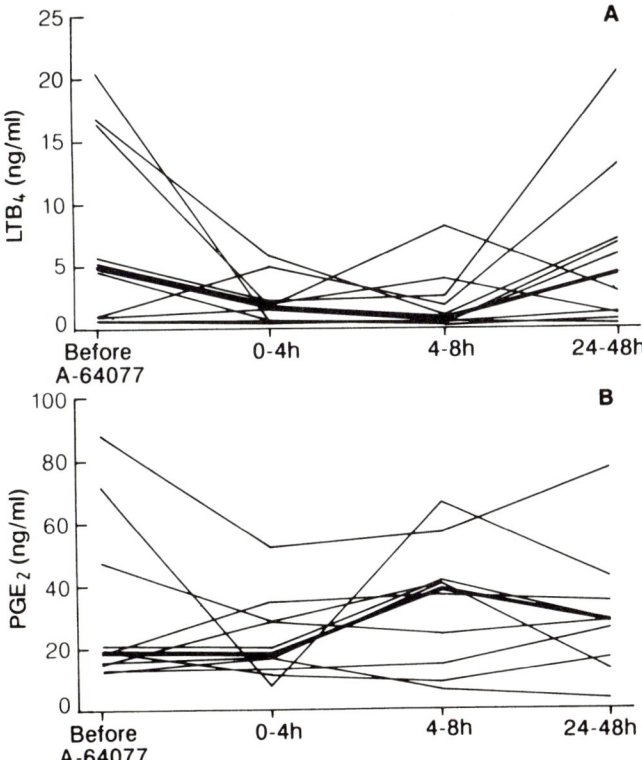

Fig. 58.9 Selective reduction of leukotriene B4 release into rectal dialysates with zileuton. Reproduced from Lancet 1990; 335: 683 with permission.

ulcerative colitis, asthma, psoriasis and other conditions. The first to be evaluated in ulcerative colitis was zileuton, which produced a selective fall in the release of LTB4 into rectal dialysates when single doses were given orally to patients with active proctitis (Laursen et al 1990) (Fig. 58.9). Zileuton has therefore undergone extensive phase 2 and 3 clinical trials in inflammatory bowel disease. An initial phase 2 study using 800 mg twice daily over 4 weeks found that a clinical response occurred significantly more often in patients receiving zileuton compared to placebo, but only if they were not receiving salicylates (Collawn et al 1992). Since salicylates have been shown to be moderately potent inhibitors of the 5-lipoxygenase enzyme, it was possible that this masked benefit in these patients. Four phase 3 studies, two in relapse and two in remission, using higher doses and more frequent administration, were conducted. In one study zileuton 600 mg q.d.s. was compared to mesalazine 400 mg q.d.s. and placebo for their ability to maintain remission over 6 months in ulcerative colitis (Hawkey et al 1994). In this study 6-month relapse rates were 57% for placebo recipients, 46% for those receiving zileuton and 37% for those receiving mesalazine. Benefit with mesalazine was clearly significant, but that with zileuton only marginal ($P=0.09$). Another maintenance study showed less effect. Likewise, of two large phase 3 studies in active disease, one was marginally positive and one showed no difference compared to placebo. In the most positive study zileuton 600 mg q.d.s. induced remission in 30% versus 23% of patients receiving placebo in the management of active ulcerative colitis (Peppercorn et al 1994). Zileuton therefore probably has marginal therapeutic effects in ulcerative colitis, but at the doses used these were insufficient to be of clinical interest. These disappointing results may have arisen because zileuton is a relatively ineffective inhibitor of the 5-lipoxygenase enzyme.

FLAP inhibitor. The 5-lipoxygenase enzyme is interesting in that it is activated by transport to the cell membrane by an activating protein. A highly potent 5-lipoxygenase-activating protein (FLAP) inhibitor has been developed (Hillings et al 1992) and is under evaluation in inflammatory bowel disease.

Thromboxane

Thromboxane A_2 is a potent but short-lived activator of platelets and, to a lesser extent, PMNs (Rampton & Collins 1993). It is derived from platelets, but also from macrophages and neutrophils. Increased levels of its stable degradation product TX B_2 can be detected in active inflammatory bowel disease (Mayer & Sachar 1992).

Therapeutic possibilities

Drugs are available which both inhibit synthesis of thromboxane selectively and act as receptor antagonists. In animal models such thromboxane synthesis inhibitors and receptor antagonists have been effective in reducing inflammation (Vilaseca et al 1990).

Evidence for efficacy

Low doses of aspirin inhibit the release of thromboxane into rectal dialysates by about 25% (Cole et al 1994) (Casellas 1992), suggesting that some mucosal thromboxane is platelet derived. Ridogral and picotamide, thromboxane receptor antagonists, have also been evaluated pharmacodynamically and, rather surprisingly, been shown to reduce colonic levels of thromboxane B_2 (Casellas 1992, Collins et al 1994). Two recent studies in abstract only have suggested that inhibition of thromboxane can reduce activity during relapse of ulcerative colitis (Collins et al 1994).

Platelet-activating factor antagonists

Platelet-activating factor (PAF) is synthesized by neutrophils and macrophages and released with arachidonic acid under the influence of phospholipase A_2; it also causes further release of substrate for eicosanoid synthesis by activating phospholipase C. Platelet-activating factor production is stimulated by IL-1 and TNFα, and mediates neutrophil chemoattraction and degranulation, platelet aggregation and increased vascular permeability. There is increased production of PAF in inflammatory bowel disease (Gross et al 1995, Travis & Jewell 1994a, Eliakim et al 1988, Denizot et al 1992, Ferraris et al 1993), and its pivotal role in eicosanoid metabolism makes it a logical target.

Evidence for efficacy

Several PAF antagonists have been developed. They are generally well tolerated, but one small study (Malchow et al 1994) showed no benefit in active ulcerative colitis. Other PAF antagonists are under controlled evaluation (Tubaro et al 1993, Sandberg-Gertzen 1993, Deshpande et al 1994).

Prostaglandins

Enhanced prostaglandin synthesis has long been recognized in inflammatory bowel disease. Since prostaglandins are vasodilators and enhance endothelial permeability, with fluid transudation and enhancement of leukocyte diapedesis, it was postulated that inhibiting prostaglandin synthesis could be of benefit in inflammatory bowel disease. In fact, the reverse appears to be the case. Systematic studies of flurbiprofen and other non-steroidal anti-inflammatory drugs (NSAIDs) in active ulcerative colitis showed no therapeutic benefit, with evidence of deterioration in some patients and a fall in the mucosal potential difference (Casellas et al 1993, Rampton & Sladen 1981). A number of epidemiological studies have associated NSAID usage and paracetamol with relapse of inflammatory bowel disease (Rampton et al 1983). Such studies suggest that prostaglandins could therefore be beneficial in active inflammatory bowel disease, either as a result of (ill defined) cytoprotection, by stimulation of mucosal restitution, or by suppression of lymphocyte activation. These considerations led to evaluation of prostaglandins themselves as potential therapeutic agents. Rioprostil, mistropostol and dimethyl PGE_2 have been shown in animal models of colitis to have cytoprotective properties (Wallace et al 1985, Allgayer et al 1989, Fedorak et al 1990), but dimethyl PGE_2 was of no value in humans with ulcerative colitis, probably because its stimulation of fluid secretion outweighed any benefits.

Complement

Complement activation results in the production of chemotactic fragments such as C5A. One study has suggested therapeutic benefit from K76 inhibitor of complement activity in ulcerative colitis (Ketano et al 1992).

Nitric oxide

Nitric oxide produced in small amounts by its constitutive enzyme has been shown in animal models to be protective to the intestinal epithelium (Stark & Szurszewski 1992). However, when the inducible enzyme is induced by lipopolysaccharide and cytokines, much larger quantities of nitric oxide are produced which enhance mucosal permeability and promote inflammation. Substrate antagonists such as L NAME or LNMMA can prevent or reverse inflammation in animal models of inflammatory bowel disease (Collins et al 1994).

Nitric oxide biosynthesis is increased in the mucosa in active ulcerative colitis (Middleton et al 1993, Boughton-Smith et al 1993) and the disease was the setting for the first identification of the inducible enzyme in humans (Middleton et al 1993) (Fig. 58.10). The increased production of nitric oxide can be detected in the colonic lumen (Lundberg et al 1994) and in mesenteric blood (Rees et al 1995). Nitric oxide impairs peristaltic activity and has

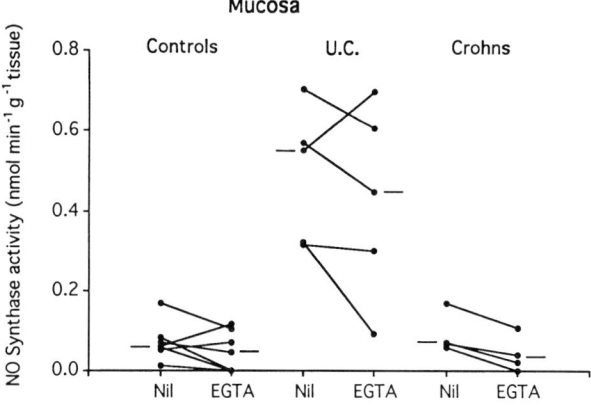

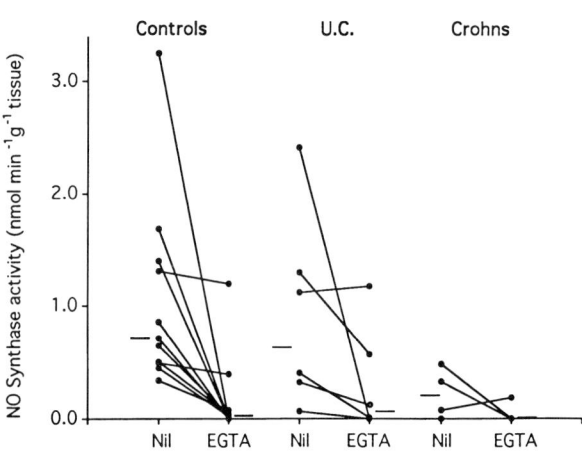

Fig. 58.10 Increased inducible nitric oxide synthase in ulcerative colitis. There is little reduction in the activity in the presence of the calcium chelator EGTA, characteristic of the inducible form of nitric oxide synthase. Reproduced from Lancet 1993; 342: 338 with permission.

been implicated in the pathogenesis of toxic megacolon (Casellas et al 1993). There is intense activity to develop selective inhibitors of iNOS, but none has yet been evaluated in humans with inflammatory disease.

Radical scavengers

Degranulation and release of enzymes such as elastase, and the synthesis of reactive oxygen molecules (ROM) are believed to be the main mechanism by which neutrophils produce mucosal damage in active ulcerative colitis. Increased production of ROM (Simmonds & Rampton 1993, Simmonds et al 1992, Williams et al 1990) has been demonstrated in active ulcerative colitis. In open studies superoxide dismutase improved ten of 12 patients with ulcerative colitis (Petkau 1986) and Crohn's disease (Szegli et al 1986). More recently a small open study of multiple antioxygen vitamin treatment has reported encouraging results in ulcerative colitis (Millar et al 1994a), and iron chelation has been suggested as a way of reducing radical levels (Millar et al 1994b).

Another approach has been to use allopurinol, which inhibits the xanthine oxidase pathway of ROM synthesis, together with the scavenger DMSO. An open study claimed impressive results (Salim 1992) but was later withdrawn. Benefit in pouchitis has also been reported (Levin et al 1992).

Growth factors

Increased expression of epidermal growth factor with associated expression of other growth factors, including trefoils, is a feature of the novel cell lineage which develops at the site of gastrointestinal ulcers, including those caused by Crohn's disease (Wright et al 1990). Epidermal growth factor has enhanced healing of inflamed colonic mucosa in an animal model (Procaccino et al 1994, Luck & Bass 1993), and the evaluation of epidermal growth factor and other bioengineered growth factor molecules in inflammatory bowel disease can be expected in the future.

Mediators of uncertain significance

One of the main epidemiological findings in inflammatory bowel disease has been the association of Crohn's disease with smoking, and of ulcerative colitis with non-smoking. The mediators of these effects of smoking are not known, but nicotine has been used on a pragmatic basis in ulcerative colitis. In a controlled study of 72 patients (Pullan et al 1994), nicotine patches delivering 15–25 mg of nicotine per day were more effective in inducing clinical remission than placebo. However, in another study nicotine patches did not maintain remission (Thomas et al 1995).

Clonidine, the centrally acting α_2 agonist, has been used in ulcerative colitis (Lechin et al 1985) where it appeared to be as effective as prednisolone. Whether any therapeutic activity was mediated via central control of inflammatory or by effects on gut motility is uncertain.

SUMMARY

There is intense activity in the investigation of designer molecules aimed at particular inflammatory targets in active inflammatory bowel disease, but as yet there have been too many small uncontrolled studies and too few large controlled ones for much progress to have been made. As yet, results with lipoxygenase inhibition have been disappointing, raising the possibility that a 'fire blanket' affecting multiple sites of inflammation may be more appropriate than a magic bullet. If, however, the promising early results targeting the early stages of immune activation are confirmed, they will represent a new approach to the treatment of inflammatory bowel disease and, coincidentally, help to identify which pathological processes are important.

REFERENCES

Ahrenstedt O, Knutson L, Nilsson B, Nilsson-Ekdahl K, Odlind B, Hallgren R 1992 Enhanced local production of complement components in the small intestines of patients with Crohn's disease. New England Journal of Medicine 322: 1345–1349

Allgayer H, Deschryver K, Stenson W F 1989 Treatment with 16,16'-dimethyl prostaglandin E_2 before and after induction of colitis with trinitrobenzenesulfonic acid in rats decreases inflammation. Gastroenterology 96: 1290–1300

Anasetti C, Hansen J A, Waldmann T et al 1992 Treatment of acute graft versus host disease with a humanized monoclonal antibody specific for the IL-2 receptor. Blood 80: 373A

Balsitis M, Morrell K, Mahida Y R, Hawkey C J 1994 Cell adhesion molecule expression by colonic mucosa in ulcerative colitis. European Journal of Gastroenterology and Hepatology 6: 351–358

Beagley K W, Elson C O 1992 Cells and cytokines in mucosal immunity and inflammation. Gastroenterology 21: 347–366

Bjorck S, Dahlstrom A, Ahlman H 1989 Topical treatment of ulcerative proctitis with lidocaine. Scandinavian Journal of Gastroenterology 24: 1061–1072

Boughton-Smith N K, Evans S M, Hawkey C J et al 1993 Differential changes in nitric oxide synthase activity in ulcerative colitis and Crohn's disease. Lancet 342: 338–340

Boughton-Smith N K, Hawkey C J, Whittle B J R 1983 The biosynthesis of lipoxygenase and cyclo-oxygenase products from arachidonic acid in human colonic mucosa. Gut 24: 1176–1182

Breese E, Braegger C P, Corrigan C J, Walker-Smith J A, MacDonaly T T 1993 Interleukin-2 and interferon gamma secreting T cells in normal and diseased human intestinal mucosa. Immunology 78: 127–131

Burke D A, Axon A T R 1988 Adhesive *Escherichia coli* in inflammatory bowel disease and infective diarrhoea. British Medical Journal 297: 102–104

Casellas F 1992 In vivo quantitation of intracolonic eicosanoic acid release in active ulcerative colitis after inhibition of thromboxane synthetase by ridogrel. Gastroenterology 102: A2437

Casellas F, Papo M, Guarner F 1993 A selective thromboxane synthetase inhibitor improves chronic ulcerative colitis. Gastroenterology 104: A677

Casellas F, Mourelle M, Guarmer F, Papo M, Mlagelda J R 1993 Toxic megacolon in chronic ulcerative colitis is associated with the induction of nitric oxide synthase. Gut 34: 525–530

Ceretti D P, Koz C J, Mosley B et al 1992 Molecular cloning of the interleukin-1β converting enzyme. Science 256: 97–100

Choi P M, Targan S R 1994 Immunomodulator therapy in inflammatory bowel disease. Digestive Diseases and Sciences 39: 1885–1892

Cole A T, Hyman-Taylor P, Hawkey C J 1994 Low dose aspirin: selective inhibition of rectal dialysis thromboxane B_2 in healthy volunteers. Alimentary Pharmacology and Therapeutics 8: 521–526

Cole A T, Pilkington B J, McLaughlan J, Hawkey C J 1993 Interleukin-8 bioactivity in mucosal homogenates from active colitis. Gastroenterology 104: A683

Collawn C, Rubin P, Perez N et al 1992 Phase II study of the safety and efficacy of a 5-lipoxygenase inhibitor in patients with ulcerative colitis. American Journal of Gastroenterology 87: 342–346

Collins C E, Forbes A, Rampton D S 1994 An open trial of anti platelet therapy in active Crohn's disease using picotamide, a thromboxane antagonist. Gut 35: S28

Cominelli F, Bortolami M, Pizarro T T et al 1994 Rabbit interleukin-1 receptor antagonist. Cloning, expression, functional characterization and regulation during intestinal inflammation. Journal of Biological Chemistry 269: 6962–6971

Cominelli F, Fiocchi C, Eisenberg S P, Bortolami M 1992 Imbalance of IL-1 and IL-2 receptor antagonists in the intestinal mucosa of Crohn's disease and ulcerative colitis patients. Gastroenterology 102: A609

Cominelli F, Nast C C, Clark B D et al 1990 Interleukin gene expression, synthesis and effect of specific IL-1 receptor blockade in rabbit immune complex colitis. Journal of Clinical Investigation 86: 972–980

Cope G F, Heatley R V, Kelleher J, Axon A T R 1988 In vitro mucus glycoprotein production by colonic tissue from patients with ulcerative colitis decreased when inactive. Gut 29: 229–234

Davidsen B, Munkholm P, Schlichting P, Nielsen O H, Krarup H, Bonnevie-Nielsen V 1995 Tolerability of interferon alpha-2b, a new possible treatment of active Crohn's disease. Alimentary Pharmacology and Therapeutics 9: 75–79

Debinski H S, Kamm M A 1995 Novel drug therapies in inflammatory bowel disease. European Journal of Gastroenterology and Hepatology 7: 169–182

Denizot Y, Chaaussade S, Nathan N, Colombel J F, Bossant M J, Cherouki N 1992 PAF acether and acetylhydrolase in stool of patients with Crohn's disease. Digestive Diseases and Sciences 37: 432–437

Derkx B, Taminiau J, Radema S et al 1993 Tumour necrosis factor antibody treatment in Crohn's disease. Lancet 342: 173–174

Deshpande Y, Longo W E, Chandel B et al 1994 Effect of platelet activating factor and its antagonists on colonic dysmotility and tissue levels of colonic neuropeptides. European Journal of Pharmacology 256: 113–115

Deusch K, Mauthe B, Reiter C, Reithmuller G, Classe M 1993 CD4-antibody treatment of inflammatory bowel disease: one year follow-up. Gastroenterology 104: A691

Dias V C, Wallace J L, Parsons H G 1992 Modulation of cellular phospholipid fatty acid and leukotriene B-4 synthesis in the human intestinal cell (CaCo-2). Gut 33: 622–627

Dinarello C A 1991 Interleukin-1 and interleukin-1 antagonism. Blood 77: 1627–1652

Dinarello C A 1993 Modalities for reducing interleukin 1 activity in disease. Immunology Today 14: 260–264

Dixon R A F, Diehl R E, Opas E et al 1990 Requirement of a 5-lipoxygenase activating protein for leukotriene synthesis. Nature 343: 282–284

Eliakim R, Karmeli F, Razin E, Rachmilewitz D 1988 Role of platelet activating factor in ulcerative colitis. Gastroenterology 95: 1167–1172

Emmrich J S, Eyfarth M, Fleig W E, Emmerich F 1991 Treatment of inflammatory bowel disease with anti-CD4 monoclonal antibody. Lancet 338: 570–571

Feagan B G, Rochon J, Fedorak R N et al 1995 Methotrexate for the treatment of Crohn's disease. New England Journal of Medicine 332: 292–297

Fedorak R N, Empey L R, MacArthur C, Jewell L D 1990 Misoprostol provides a colonic mucosal protective effect during acetic acid induced colitis in rats. Gastroenterology 98: 615–625

Ferraris L, Karmeli F, Eliakim R, Klein J, Fiocchi C, Rachmilewitz D 1993 Intestinal epithelial cells contribute to the enhanced generation of platelet activating factor in ulcerative colitis. Gut 34: 665–668

Ferretti M, Casini-Raggi V, Pizarro T T, Eisenberg S P 1994 Neutralization of endogenous IL-1 receptor antagonist exacerbates and prolongs inflammation in rabbit immune colitis. Journal of Clinical Investigation 94: 449–453

Gasche C, Reinisch W, Lochs H et al 1994 Anaemia in Crohn's disease. Importance of inadequate erythropoietin production and iron deficiency. Digestive Diseases and Sciences 39: 1930–1934

Grimminger F, Fuhrer D, Papavassilis C et al 1993 Influence of intravenous n-3 lipid supplementation on fatty acid profiles and lipid mediator generation in a patient with severe ulcerative colitis. European Journal of Clinical Investigation 23: 706–715

Gross V, Andus T, Daig R, Aschenbrenner E, Scholmerich J, Falk W 1995 Regualtion of interleukin-8 production in a human colon epithelial cell line (HT-29). Gastroenterology 108: 653–661

Hadziselimovic F, Emmons L R, Schaub U 1992 Interferon alfa-2a (Roferon) treatment of inflammatory bowel disease in children and adolescents. Falk Symposium, Basel 65: 10

Hanauer S B, Baert F J, Robinson M 1994 Interferon treatment in mild to moderate active Crohn's disease: preliminary results of an open label pilot study. Gastroenterology 106: A696

Harada K, Toyonaga A, Mitsuyama K, Sasaki E, Tanikawa K 1994 Role of cytokine induced neutrophil chemoattractant, a member of the interleukin-8 family, in rat experimental colitis. Digestion 55: 179–184

Hawkey C J, Gassul M, Lauritsen K et al 1994 Efficacy of zileuton, a 5-lipoxygenase inhibitor, in the maintenance of remission in patients with ulcerative colitis. Gastroenterology 106: A697

Hawkey C J, Mahida Y R, Hawthorne A B 1992 Therapeutic interventions in gastrointestinal disease based on an understanding of inflammatory mediators. Agents and Actions Special Conference Issue: C23–26

Hawthorne A B, Hawkey C J 1989 Immunosuppressive drugs in inflammatory bowel disease. Drugs 38: 267–288

Hawthorne A B, Boughton-Smith N K, Whittle B J H, Hawkey C J 1992a Colorectal leukotriene B4 synthesis in vitro in inflammatory bowel disease. Inhibition by the selective 5-lipoxygenase inhibitor BWA4C. Gut 33: 513–517

Hawthorne A B, Deneshmend T K, Hawkey C J et al 1992b Treatment of ulcerative colitis with fish oil supplementation: a prospective 12-month randomised trial. Gut 33: 922–928

Hawthorne A B, Logan R F A, Hawkey C J et al 1992c Randomized controlled trial of azathioprine withdrawal in ulcerative colitis. British Medical Journal 305: 20–22

Henderson B, Blake S 1992 Therapeutic potential of cytokine manipulation. Trends in Pharmacological Sciences 13: 145–152

Hermanowicz A, Sliwinski Z, Nowak A, Gajos L 1987 The effect of levamisole on the maintenance of remission of ulcerative colitis. Scandinavian Journal of Gastroenterology 22: 367–371

Hibi T, Ohara M, Watanabe M et al 1993 Interleukin 2 and interferon gamma augment anticolon antibody dependent cellular cytotoxicity in ulcerative colitis. Gut 34: 788–793

Hillings J, Kjeldsen J, Laursen L S et al 1992 Selective blockade of rectal leukotriene B_4 and systemic leukotriene production by a single, oral dose of MK-591 in patients with active ulcerative colitis. A double blind placebo controlled study. Gastroenterology 106: A698

Hodgson H J F 1991 Cyclosporin in inflammatory bowel disease. Alimentary Pharmacology and Therapeutics 5: 343–350

Hyams J S, Fitzgerald J E, Treem W R, Wyzga N, Kreutzer D L 1993 Relationship of functional and antigenic interleukin 6 to disease activity in inflammatory bowel disease. Gastroenterology 104: 1285–1292

Hyams J S, Fitzgerald J E, Wyzga N, Treem W R, Justinich C J, Kreutzer D L 1994 Characterization of circulating interleukin-1 receptor antagonist expression in children with inflammatory bowel disease. Digestive Diseases and Sciences 39: 1893–1899

Jung H C, Eckmann L, Yang S K et al 1995 A distinct array of pro inflammatory cytokines in expressed in human colon epithelial cells in response to bacterial invasion. Journal of Clinical Investigation 95: 55–65

Kahan B D 1989 Cyclosporine. New England Journal of Medicine 321: 1725–1738

Katz K D, Hollander D, Vadheim C M et al 1989 Intestinal permeability in patients with Crohn's disease and their healthy relatives. Gastroenterology 97: 927–931

Ketano A, Matsumoto T, Nakamura S et al 1992 New treatment of ulcerative colitis with K-76. Diseases of the Colon and Rectum 35: 560–567

Kuhn R, Lohler J, Rennick D, Rajewsky K, Muller W 1993 Interleukin-10 deficient mice develop chronic enterocolitis. Cell 75: 263–274

Laursen L S, Naesdal J, Bukhave K, Lauritsen K, Rask-Madsen J 1990 Selective 5-lipoxygenase inhibition in ulcerative colitis. Lancet 335: 683–685

Lechin F, Van der Dijs B, Insausti C L et al 1985 Treatment of ulcerative colitis with clonidine. Journal of Clinical Pharmacology 25: 219–226

Levin K E, Pemberton J H, Phillips S F, Zinmeister A R, Pezim M E 1992 Role of oxygen free radicals in the aetiology of pouchitis. Diseases of the Colon and Rectum 35: 452–456

Lichtiger S, Present D H, Kornbluth A et al 1994 Cyclosporine in severe ulcerative colitis refractory to steroid therapy. New England Journal of Medicine 330: 1841–1845

Lobo A J, Juby L D, Rothwell J, Poole T W, Axon A T R 1994 Long term treatment of Crohn's disease with cyclosporin – the effect of very low dose on maintenance of remission. Journal of Clinical Gastroenterology 13: 42–46

Luck M S, Bass P 1993 Effect of epidermal growth factor on experimental colitis in the rat. Journal of Pharmacology and Experimental Therapeutics 264: 984–990

Lundberg J O N, Hellstrom P M, Lundberg J M, Alving K 1994 Greatly increased luminal nitric oxide in ulcerative colitis. Lancet 344: 1673–1674

McCabe R P, Secrist H, Botney M, Egan M, Peters M G 1993 Cytokine mRNA expression in intestine from normal and inflammatory bowel disease patients. Clinical Immunology and Immunopathology 66: 52–58

McFadden J, Butcher P, Thompson J et al 1987 Crohn's disease: isolated mycobacteria are identical to *Mycobacterium paratuberculosis* and determined by DNA probes that distinguish between mycobacterial species. Journal of Clinical Microbiology 25: 796–801

McLaughlan J, Seth R, Robins A et al 1995 Use of a new enzyme linked PCR assay to show increased inducible nitric oxide synthase and interleukin 8 mRNA in ulcerative colitis. Gut 36: A56

Mahida Y R, Gallagher A, Kurlak L, Hawkey C J 1990 Plasma and tissue interleukin-2 receptor levels in inflammatory bowel disease. Clinical and Experimental Immunology 82: 75–80

Mahida Y R, Gallagher A, Kurlak L, Hawkey C J 1991 High circulating levels of interleukin-6 in Crohn's disease. Gut 32: 1531–1534

Mahida Y R, Lindley I, Ceska M, Effenberger F, Kurlak L, Hawkey C J 1992 Enhanced synthesis of NAP/IL-8 in active ulcerative colitis. Clinical Science 82: 273–275

Mahida Y R, Wu K C, Jewell D P 1988 Characterization of antigen presenting activity of intestinal mononuclear cells isolated from normal and inflammatory bowel disease colon and ileum. Immunology 65: 543–549

Mahida Y R, Wu K C, Jewell D P 1989a Respiratory burst activity of intestinal macrophages in normal and inflammatory bowel disease. Gut 30: 1362–1370

Mahida Y R, Wu K, Jewell D P 1989b Enhanced production of interleukin-1β by mononuclear cells isolated from mucosa with active ulcerative colitis of Crohn's disease. Gut 30: 835–838

Malchow H, Ewe K, Goebell H, Wellmann W, Leimer H G, Kempe R 1994 Failure of the specific PAF antagonist apafant in the treatment of ulcerative colitis. Gastroenterology 106: A728

Mansfield J C, Holden H, Tarlow J K et al 1994 Novel genetic association between ulcerative colitis and the anti inflammatory cytokine interleukin-1 receptor antagonist. Gastroenterology 106: 637–642

Matsurra T, West G A, Youngman K R, Klein J S, Fiocchi C 1993 Immune activation genes in inflammatory bowel disease. Gastroenterology 104: 448–458

Mayer L, Sachar D B 1992 Efficacy of chloroquine in the treatment of inflammatory bowel disease. Gastroenterology 102: A661

Mayer L L, Shilen R 1987 Evidence for function of Ia molecules on gut epithelial cells in man. Journal of Experimental Medicine 166: 1471–1483

Mayer L, Sachar D B, Present D H et al 1992 Randomized double blind placebo controlled trial of hydroxychloroquine in the treatment of ulcerative colitis. Gastroenterology 102: A661

Mazlam M Z, Hodgson H J 1994 Interrelations between interleukin-6, interleukin-1 beta, plasma C-reactive protein values, and in vitro C-reactive protein generation in patients with inflammatory bowel disease. Gut 35: 77–83

Mazzucchelli L, Hauser C, Zgraggen K et al 1994 Expression of interleukin-8 gene in inflammatory bowel disease is related to the histological grade of active inflammation. American Journal of Pathology 144: 997–1007

Middleton S J, Shorthouse M, Hunter J O 1993 Increased nitric oxide synthesis in ulcerative colitis. Lancet 341: 465–466

Millar A D, Blake D R, Rampton D S 1994a An open trial of antioxidant nutrient therapy in active ulcerative colitis. Gut S29: T113

Millar A D, Blake D R, Rampton D S 1994b Iron chelation in ulcerative colitis: a new antioxidant approach. Gut S50: F198

Mitsuyama K, Toyonaga A, Sasaki E et al 1994 IL-8 as an important chemoattractant for neutrophils in ulcerative colitis and Crohn's disease. Clinical and Experimental Immunology 96: 432–436

Murch S H, Braegger C P, Walker-Smith J A, MacDonald T T 1993 Location of tumour necrosis factor alpha by immunohistochemistry in chronic inflammatory bowel disease. Gut 34: 1705–1709

Nicholls S, Stephens S, Braegger C P, Walker-Smith J A, MacDonald T T 1993 Cytokines in stools of children with inflammatory bowel disease of infective diarrhoea. Journal of Clinical Pathology 46: 757

Nishiyama T, Mitsuyama K, Toyonaga A, Sasaki E, Tanikawa K 1994 Colonic mucosal interleukin 1 receptor antagonist in inflammatory bowel disease. Digestion 55: 368–373

Podolsky D K, Lobb R, King N et al 1993 Attenuation of colitis in the cotton-top tamarin by anti alpha 4 integrin monoclonal antibody. Journal of Clinical Investigation 92: 372–380

Peppercorn M, Das K, Elson C et al 1994 Zileuton, a 5-lipoxygenase inhibitor in the treatment of active ulcerative colitis: a double blind placebo controlled trial. Gastroenterology 106: A751

Petkau A 1986 Scientific basis for the clinical use of superoxide dismutase. Cancer Treatment Review 13: 17–44

Present D H, Korelitz B I, Wisch J L et al 1980 Treatment of Crohn's disease with 6-mercaptopurine. New England Journal of Medicine 302: 981–987

Procaccino F, Reinshagen M, Hoffmann P et al 1994 Protective effect of epidermal growth factor in an experimental model of colitis in rats. Gastroenterology 107: 12–17

Pullan R, Rhodes J, Ganesh S et al 1994 Transdermal nicotine for active ulcerative colitis. New England Journal of Medicine 330: 811–815

Raab Y, Gerdin B, Ahlstedt S, Hallgren R 1993 Neutrophil mucosal involvement is accompanied by enhanced local production of interleukin-8 in ulcerative colitis. Gut 34: 1203–1206

Raab Y, Hallgren R, Gerdin B 1994 Enhanced intestinal synthesis of interleukin-6 is related to the disease severity and activity in ulcerative colitis. Digestion 55: 44–49

Rampton D S, Collins C E 1993 Review article: thromboxane in inflammatory bowel disease – pathogenic and therapeutic implications. Alimentary Pharmacology and Therapeutics 7: 357–367

Rampton D A, Hawkey C J 1984 Prostaglandins in ulcerative colitis (progress report). Gut 25: 1399–1413

Rampton D S, Sladen G E 1981 Prostaglandin synthesis inhibitors in ulcerative colitis: flurbiprofen compared with conventional treatment. Prostaglandins 21: 417–425

Rampton D S, McNeil N I, Sarner M 1983 Analgesic ingestion and other factors preceding relapse in ulcerative colitis. Gut 24: 187–189

Ray C A, Black R A, Kronheim S R et al 1992 Viral inhibition of inflammation – cowpox virus encodes an inhibitor of the interleukin-1β converting enzyme. Cole 69: 597–604

Rees D C, Satsangi J, Travis S P L, Cornelissen P L, White J, Jewell D P 1995 Serum concentrations of nitric oxide metabolites in severe acute ulcerative colitis. European Journal of Gastroenterology and Hepatology 7: 227–230

Reinecker H C, Steffen M, Witthoeft T et al 1993 Enhanced secretion of tumour necrosis factor-alpha, IL-6, and IL-1 beta by isolated lamina propria mononuclear cells from patients with ulcerative colitis and Crohn's disease. Clinical and Experimental Immunology 94: 174–181

Rhodes J M 1989 Colonic mucus and mucosal glycoproteins: the key to colitis and cancer. Gut 30: 1660–1666

Roediger W E W 1980 The colonic epithelium in ulcerative colitis: an energy deficient disease? Lancet ii: 712–715

Ross E 1993a The role of marine fish oils in the treatment of ulcerative colitis. Nutrition Reviews 51: 47–49

Ross E 1993b The role of marine fish oils in the treatment of ulcerative colitis. Nutrition Reviews 51: 47

Sachar D B, Rubin K P, Gumaste V 1987 Levamisole in Crohn's disease: a randomized double-blind, placebo controlled clinical trial. American Journal of Medicine 82: 536–539

Sadlack B, Merz H, Schorle H, Schimpl A, Feller A C, Horak I 1993 Ulcerative colitis like disease in mice with a disrupted interleukin-2 gene. Cell 75: 253–261

Salim A S 1992 Role of oxygen delivered free radical scavengers in the management of recurrent attack of ulcerative colitis a new approach. Journal of Laboratory and Clinical Medicine 119: 710–717

Salomon P, Kornbluth A A, Janowitz H D 1990 Treatment of ulcerative colitis with fish oil n-2-w-fatty acid: an open trial. Journal of Clinical Gastroenterology 12: 157–161

Sandberg-Gertzen H 1993 An open trial of cedemin, a Gingko biloba extract with PAF antagonistic effects for ulcerative colitis. American Journal of Gastroenterology 88: 615–616

Shanahian F 1994 Gene-targeted immunologic knockouts: new models of inflammatory bowel disease. Gastroenterology 107: 312–314

Sharon P, Stenson W F 1984 Enhanced synthesis of leukotriene B-4 by colonic mucosa in inflammatory bowel disease. Gastroenterology 86: 453–460

Sharon P, Ligumsky M, Rachmilewitz D, Zor U 1978 Role of prostaglandins in ulcerative colitis. Enhanced production during active disease and inhibition by sulfasalazine. Gastroenterology 75: 638–648

Simmonds N J, Rampton D S 1993 Inflammatory bowel disease: a radical view. Gut 34: 865–868

Simmonds N J, Allen R E, Stevens T J, van Someren R N M, Blake D R, Rampton D S 1992 Chemiluminescence assay of reactive oxygen metabolites in inflammatory bowel disease. Gastroenterology 103: 186–196

Sparano J A, Brandt L J, Dutcher J P, DuBois J S, Atkins M B 1993 Symptomatic exacerbation of Crohn's disease after treatment with high dose interleukin-2. Annals of Internal Medicine 118: 617–618

Stack W, Mann S, Roy A, Heath P, Sopwith M, Freeman J, Holmes G, Long R, Forbes A, Kamm M, Hawkey C J 1996 The effects of CDP571, an engineered human IgG4 anti-TNFα antibody in Crohn's disease. Gut (Suppl 1) 38: T107

Stark M E, Szurszewski 1992 Role of nitric oxide in gastrointestinal and hepatic function and disease. Gastroenterology 103: 1928–1949

Steinhart A H, Brezinski A, Baker J P 1994 Treatment of refractory ulcerative proctosigmoiditis with butyrate enemas. American Journal of Gastroenterology 89: 179–183

Stenson W F, Cort D, Rodger S J et al 1992 Dietary supplementation with fish oil in ulcerative colitis. Annals of Internal Medicine 116: 609–614

Strober W, Ehrdhardt R O 1993 Chronic intestinal inflammation: an unexpected outcome in cytokine or T cell receptor mutant mice. Cell 75: 203–205

Strom T B, Kelley V R, Murphy J R, Nichols J, Woodworth T G 1993 Interleukin-2 receptor directed therapies: antibody or cytokine based targeting molecules. Annual Review of Medicine 44: 343–353

Stronkhorst A, Rodema S, ten Berge I 1993 Phase I multiple-dose study of chimeric monoclonal MT412 (anti CD-4) antibodies in Crohn's disease. Gastroenterology 104: A784

Sumer N, Beyler A R, Palabiyikoglu M et al 1992 The effect of interferon-alpha-2a on clinical endoscopic findings in chronic active ulcerative colitis. Hellenic Journal of Gastroenterology 341: 1362–1366

Szegli G, Herold A, Negut E et al 1986 Clinical efficacy of a new anti inflammatory drug with free radicals scavenging properties. Archives Roumaines de Pathologie Experimentale et de Microbiologie 45: 75–89

Thomas G A O, Rhodes J, Mani V et al 1995 Transdermal nicotine as maintenance therapy for ulcerative colitis. New England Journal of Medicine 332: 992–998

Thornberry N A, Bull H G, Calaycay J R et al 1992 A novel heterodimeric cysteine protease is required for interleukin-1β processing in monocytes. Nature 356: 768–774

Travis S P, Jewell D P 1994a The role of platelet activating factor in the pathogenesis of gastrointestinal disease. Prostaglandins, Leukotrienes and Essential Fatty Acids 50: 103–113

Travis S P L, Jewell D P 1994b Salicylates for inflammatory bowel disease. Baillière's Clinical Gastroenterology 8: 203–231

Tubaro E, Santiangeli C, Cavallo G et al 1993 Effect of a new de-N-acetyl-lysoglycosphingolipid on chemically induced inflammatory bowel disease: possible mechanism of action. Naunyn-Schmiedebergs Archives of Pharmacology 348: 670–678

van Dullemen H M, Hommes D W, Meenan J et al 1994 Complete remissions of steroid refractory Crohn's disease after administration of monoclonal TNF antibody cA2. Gastroenterology 106: A1054

Vantrappen G, Coremans G, Billiau A 1980 Treatment of Crohn's disease with interferon. A preliminary clinical trial. Acta Clinica Belgica 35: 238–242

Vilaseca J, Salas A, Guarner F, Rodriguez R, Malagelada J R 1990 Participation of thromboxane and other eicosanoid synthesis in the course of experimental inflammatory colitis. Gastroenterology 98: 269–277

Von Ritten C, Gisham M B, Granger D N 1989 Sulphasalazine metabolites and dapsone attenuate formyl methionyl phenylalanine induced mucosal injury in rat ileum. Gastroenterology 96: 811–816

Wakefield A J, Dhillon A P, Rowles P M, Sawyeer A M, Pittilo R M, Lewis A A M 1989 Pathogenesis of Crohn's disease multifocal gastrointestinal infarction. Lancet 2: 1057–1062

Wallace J L, Whittle B J R, Boughton-Smith N K 1985 Prostaglandin protection of rat colonic mucosa from damage induced by ethanol. Digestive Diseases and Sciences 30: 866–876

Wardle T D, Turnberg L A 1994 Potential role for interleukin-1 in the pathophysiology of ulcerative colitis. Clinical Science 86: 619–626

Wardle T D, Hall L, Turnberg L A 1993 Interrelationships between inflammatory mediators released from colonic mucosa in ulcerative colitis and their effects on colonic secretion. Gut 34: 503–508

Williams J G, Hughes L E, Hallett M B 1990 Toxic oxygen metabolite production by circulating phagocytic cells in inflammatory bowel disease. Gut 31: 187–193

Wirth H P, Zala Meyenberger C, Jost R, Amman R, Munch R 1993 Alpha-interferon therapy in Crohn's disease initial clinical results. Schweitzer Medizinische Wochenschrift 123: 1384–1388

Wright N A, Pike C, Elia G 1990 Induction of a novel epidermal growth factor – secreting cell lineage by mucosal ulceration in human gastrointestinal stem cells. Nature 343: 82–85

Yoshida T, Higa A, Sakamoto H et al 1988 Immunological and clinical effects of interferon gamma on Crohn's disease. Clinical and Laboratory Immunology 25: 105–108

59. Dietary manipulations – elemental and enteral

C. O'Morain   M. O'Sullivan

ENTERAL NUTRITION AND INFLAMMATORY BOWEL DISEASE

Enteral nutritional support is frequently required in patients with inflammatory bowel disease (IBD) because of malnutrition. This is caused by several factors, including poor nutritional intake, protein losses into the gut, malabsorption (due to active disease or previous resection), increased energy requirements and drug–nutrient interactions. Chronic weight loss and malnutrition is more common in Crohn's disease than ulcerative colitis and can be reversed by the provision of appropriate nutritional support. Several studies have shown that enteral nutrition has a role in inducing remission in Crohn's disease. In contrast, no such therapeutic effect has been demonstrated in patients with ulcerative colitis, in whom the role of enteral nutrition is to maintain or improve nutritional status where appropriate.

ENTERAL NUTRITION IN CROHN'S DISEASE

Total parenteral nutrition (TPN) has been used as primary therapy in Crohn's disease (see Chapter 60). A randomized controlled trial (Greenberg et al 1988) of 51 patients with active Crohn's disease found no significant difference in the number of remissions achieved after 21 days treatment with TPN, polymeric enteral feed or peripheral parenteral nutrition with oral diet. At 1 year there was no significant difference between the three groups in the number of patients in remission. Remission can be achieved more economically and with fewer complications with enteral diets. It is widely accepted that the enteral route is preferable for feeding most groups of patients. For more than a decade, research has set out to evaluate the therapeutic role of enteral formulae (elemental, peptide based and polymeric) in the management of Crohn's disease.

Role of elemental diets in Crohn's disease

Elemental diets were originally designed for use in the US manned space program and gastroenterologists began using such diets when preparing patients for surgery. Some of these patients who had Crohn's disease inadvertently found their symptoms improving, suggesting that the elemental diet might play a primary role in the treatment of this disease.

An elemental diet provides nutrients in their simplest form: protein as amino acids, carbohydrate as glucose or maltodextrins and fat as short-chain triglycerides.

Elemental diets have been evaluated as primary therapy in Crohn's disease. Four prospective randomized controlled trials show elemental diets to be as effective as steroids in achieving short-term remission (Table 59.1). These and other studies are often confounded by relatively small numbers of patients who are not homogeneous in nature. Patients with small-bowel Crohn's disease appear to do best with an elemental diet, whereas those with disease complicated by fistula or perianal involvement tend to require further treatment to maintain diet-induced remission (Teahon et al 1990).

Table 59.1 Elemental diets versus steroids in the treatment of Crohn's disease

Reference	Patients (n)	Duration (weeks)	Remission rates (%)	
			Diet group	Steroid group
O'Morain 1984	21	4	81	80
Saverymuttu et al 1985	32	1.5	94	100
Seidman et al 1986	18	3	78	68
Hunt et al 1989	29	4	100	100

Practical use of an elemental diet

An elemental diet regimen requires a team approach, involving patient, dietitian, nurse and physician. Patients with Crohn's disease often require hospitalization during acute exacerbation of the disease, which allows supervision and support in the initial stages of the diet. Compliance may be difficult for many patients in the early stages of the diet, but once symptomatic improvement begins they usually find the diet more acceptable. Unpalatability is the most important practical disadvantage. The elemental diet can be administered orally as a drink, or via a nasogastric tube. The concentration of the feed is increased gradually over a number of days to minimize diarrhea induced by the high osmolarity of the feed.

The patient is allowed no other food, but in our unit water, black tea and coffee, minerals, boiled sweets and glucose polymers are allowed in addition. The regimen is designed to meet the individual patient's nutritional requirements. Patients who fail to show clinical improvement within 7–10 days may be assigned alternative treatment. If some clinical improvement is seen we generally encourage patients to continue on the diet for 3–4 weeks (O'Morain & McGuinness 1994).

Peptide-based diets

The nitrogen source of peptide-based (or oligopeptide) enteral formulae consists of a mixture of peptides of varying lengths with or without amino acids. Di- and tri-peptides are believed to be better absorbed than free amino acids. These diets have a lower osmolarity than elemental formulae and tend to be more palatable and less expensive. The possibility of reduced osmotic load and better nitrogen absorption would suggest a superior therapeutic response to elemental formulae.

Controlled trials show conflicting results. A large controlled trial by Lochs and colleagues (1991) showed peptide-based diets to be less effective than steroids in inducing remission in active Crohn's disease. Overall, 47% of the diet group did not achieve remission. Smaller studies have shown peptide diets to be similar to elemental diets (Table 59.2).

In a recent meta-analysis of trials to date (Fernandez-Banares et al 1994a, Griffiths et al 1995) peptide-based diets were shown to be significantly inferior to steroids in inducing remission in patients with Crohn's disease.

Polymeric diets in Crohn's disease

Several controlled trials have evaluated the effect of polymeric diets in Crohn's disease. Some, but not all, have shown these to be as effective as elemental diets (Table 59.3). A recent study found polymeric diets as effective as steroids in inducing remission in Crohn's disease (Gonzalez-Huix et al 1993). The interpretation and comparison of individual trials remains difficult

Table 59.2 Peptide-based diets in Crohn's disease

Reference	Diet	No	Remission (%)
Lochs et al 1991	PP v S	107	53 v 79
Sanderson et al 1987	PP v S	17	88 v 86
Middleton et al 1991	PP v EL	29	87 v 92
Royall et al 1994	PP v EL	40	75 v 84

EL, elemental formula; S, steroids; PP, peptide-based enteral formula

Table 59.3 Polymeric diets in Crohn's disease

Reference	Diet	No	Remission (%)	Relapse (%)
Giaffer et al 1990	PM v EL	30	36 v 75	—
Raouf et al 1991	PM v EL	24	82 v 78	—
Rigaud et al 1991	PM v EL	30	73 v 66	77 v 66 (12 mo)
Park et al 1991	PM v EL	14	71 v 29	66 v 100 (12 mo)
Gonzalez-Huix et al 1993	PM v S	32	80 v 88	42 v 67 (12 mo)

PM, polymeric enteral formula; EL, elemental formula; S, steroids

because of a large number of variable factors, including sample size, composition of enteral formulae, disease site and extent, outcome measure and length of follow-up.

According to two meta-analyses of randomized controlled trials (Fernandez-Banares et al 1994a, Griffiths et al 1995) data available to date show that steroids are better than enteral nutrition to induce remission in active Crohn's disease. These results are more evident when peptide-based diets are administered, but they are not conclusive when either elemental or whole protein-based diets are employed (Fernandez-Banares et al 1994a). However, Griffiths and colleagues found that there was no difference between efficacy of elemental versus non-elemental formulae.

MODE OF ACTION OF AN ELEMENTAL DIET

The mechanism by which elemental diets induce remission is not yet clear. A number of theories have been suggested.

Medical bypass. The elemental diet is almost completely absorbed in the proximal intestine, leaving only endogenous matter to enter the remainder of the intestine. This mechanism may allow the diseased section of the gut to rest and the inflammation to subside.

Flora alterations. An elemental diet may benefit patients by inducing a positive change in bowel flora. We have found no difference in amount or type of fecal flora before and after treatment with elemental diet, although this is a very inaccurate mode of assessment. In a controlled study two groups of patients received TPN and steroids, with sulfasalazine and metronidazole where appropriate (Wellmann et al 1986). One group also randomly received whole-gut lavage with 18L saline over 2 hours followed by 4g of 5-aminosalicylic acid on two occasions in the first week. The lavage group were found to have a significantly more rapid fall in Crohn's disease activity and circulating endotoxin, with a shorter duration of hospital stay. It is thus possible that an elemental diet may induce an improvement by reducing circulating endotoxin.

Mucosal permeability. It may be that an abnormality of mucosal permeability in Crohn's disease allows microbial or dietary antigens access to the mucosa, resulting in the observed alteration in immune function and possibly causing the chronic inflammation seen. In a study of intestinal permeability as assessed by polyethylene glycol 400 (PEG 400), chromium-labeled ethylenediaminetetraacetic acid (^{51}Cr EDTA) and lactulose/rhamnose, a significant increase in the urinary excretion of these probes occurred in Crohn's patients, indicating increased permeation (O'Morain et al 1986). Another study involving the use of an elemental diet as treatment showed that a significant decrease in urinary excretion of EDTA and lactulose/rhamnose occurred, and thus the authors concluded that the elemental diet decreased intestinal permeability. Conflicting results of altered intestinal permeability in relatives of Crohn's patients have been reported, depending on the probe used, reflecting the different permeation pathways used by each probe.

A reduction in protein exudation into the gut has also been reported after treatment with elemental diet (Logan et al 1981).

Amino acids. Elemental diets were initially introduced as primary treatment of active Crohn's disease because of their hypoallergenicity. It was considered that whole proteins may act as dietary antigens, increasing immune stimuli in the gut (O'Morain et al 1984). A number of studies show that polymeric diets induce similar remission rates to elemental diets. This suggests that the therapeutic effect of the elemental diet cannot be due solely to the presence of amino acids.

There is increasing interest in the amino acids glutamine and arginine in enteral feeds. Glutamine has multiple functions, including acting as a principal fuel for the enterocyte (Windmueller 1982). Although classed as a non-essential amino acid, glutamine may become essential in certain disease-stressed states. Steroids have been shown to increase intestinal utilization and stimulate muscle release of glutamine (Souba et al 1985). In patients with Crohn's disease glutamine requirements may be higher than normal.

Arginine has been shown to have an effect on immune function. It is suggested that it stimulates T-cell response and improves and preserves immune function (Barbul et al 1981, Daly et al 1988). Both glutamine and arginine are present in elemental feeds but have only recently been added to specific commercially available polymeric formulae.

Nutritional effect

Undernutrition, even when uncomplicated by disease, leads to a number of disturbances, including depression, irritability, anxiety and reduced concentration levels, all of which are reversed by refeeding (Keys et al 1950). Malnutrition can also impair physiological function. It may be that the provision of adequate nutrition improves nutritional status and wellbeing, and therefore effects clinical improvement (Harries et al 1983). Improvement in disease parameters usually occurs before improvements

Table 59.4 Fat composition of enteral diets in Crohn's disease

Reference	Formula type	Fat (%)	Fat type	Outcome
O'Morain et al 1984	EL	1.3	Linoleic	EL = S
Lochs et al 1991	PP	12	65% Linoleic	PP < S
Giaffer et al 1990	EL	1.3	Linoleic	EL > PM
	PM	36	80% Linoleic	
Park et al 1991	EL	15	60% MUFA	PM > EL
	PM	19	60% MUFA	
Royall et al 1994	EL	1.3	Linoleic	PP = EL
Gonzalez-Huix et al 1993	PM	32	50% MUFA	PM = S

EL, elemental enteral diet; PP, peptide-based enteral diet; PM, polymeric enteral diet; S, steroids; MUFA, monounsaturated fatty acids
Fat (%) = fat expressed as % of total energy (calories)
Modified from Fernandez-Banares et al (1994b), with permission.

in nutritional parameters, questioning a more fundamental role for elemental diets. It is likely that elemental diets result in clinical improvements in some patients via a combination of primary and nutritional effects.

ROLE OF FAT COMPOSITION OF ENTERAL DIETS IN CROHN'S DISEASE

The fat composition of enteral diets may influence therapeutic response (Table 59.4). Elemental diets are low in fat. In contrast, polymeric diets contain more fat and generally more linoleic acids. Linoleic acid is the parent compound of ω-6 polyunsaturated fatty acids and is a precursor for the synthesis of eicosanoids of the highest proinflammatory activity. When this is put in the context of enteral trials in Crohn's disease, three main points emerge (Fernandez-Banares et al 1994b):

1. Low-fat diets were associated with good outcome
2. Diets with higher quantities of fat were associated with less favorable results
3. Diets with high or intermediate fat content, but containing large proportions of monounsaturated fatty acids, were more favorable.

The fat composition of enteral feeds used in studies is often not clearly indicated. Further controlled trials are required to determine the exact role of fat composition of enteral diets in Crohn's disease, but reduced amounts of linoleic acid may be beneficial.

EXCLUSION DIETS IN CROHN'S DISEASE

Patients with Crohn's disease may have an inappropriate reaction to food. This might explain why patients on elemental diets frequently relapse soon after recommencing a normal diet, and prompted researchers in Cambridge to investigate the use of staged reintroduction of food in maintaining the remission achieved by an elemental diet. A small prospective controlled trial of 20 patients with active Crohn's disease treated with an unrefined carbohydrate or an exclusion diet, following induction of remission with TPN or elemental diet, showed encouraging results (Alun Jones et al 1985). This study led to a larger multicenter trial in which 136 patients with active Crohn's disease were treated with an elemental diet (Riordan et al 1993): 43 (31%) refused to continue the elemental diet for 14 days, but of the 93 who did 78 (84%) went into remission. These were stratified for disease site and randomized to receive either steroids or an exclusion diet. Steroids were gradually withdrawn if appropriate. Disease relapse at 2 years was significantly greater in the group of patients receiving steroids (79%) than those following the exclusion diet (62%). It may well be that certain foods act as secondary aggravating factors in Crohn's disease, rather than having any primary role in the disease process.

This approach requires immense dedication on the part of patient, family, dietitian and physician, and it may take years for the patient to return to a normal diet. Whether other centres can show equally promising results remains to be seen. In practice the difficulty lies in the complexity of this regimen and the time and staff required to effectively and exhaustively manage and follow up patients.

CROHN'S DISEASE IN CHILDREN

Growth retardation is a common manifestation of Crohn's disease in children, caused by insufficient calorie intake, malabsorption and steroid therapy. In a randomized trial of 18 pediatric patients, Seidman et al (1986) showed treatment with an elemental diet alone for 3 weeks to be as effective as steroids in inducing remission. However, such diets did not sustain remission. A controlled trial by Sanderson et al (1987) showed semi-elemental diets ($n = 8$) to be as effective as steroid treatment ($n = 9$) in children with Crohn's disease. Linear growth was significantly greater in children treated with the elemental diet.

Studies also show that peptide-based diets may be as effective as steroids in inducing remission in children with Crohn's disease (Polk et al 1992, Seidman et al 1993). The latter study employed intermittent semi-elemental diets as the sole nutrient source for 1 of 4 months during a 1-year period. There were significant improvements in disease activity and height and weight velocity, with a significant decrease in prednisone intake. In our center we tend to use elemental diets.

Enteral nutrition as primary treatment, particularly in children with Crohn's disease, offers therapy free from side effects and with the potential to improve growth and nutritional status.

OPTIMAL COMPOSITION OF ENTERAL FORMULAE IN CROHN'S DISEASE

Elemental, peptide and whole protein-based formulae differ with regard to nitrogen component. However, this is seldom the only difference: for example differences in fat composition, as shown in Table 59.4. The question remains as to which component(s) of the enteral diet influence therapeutic response. Factors such as nitrogen and lipid source, amino acid and fatty acid composition, other constituents and ingredients may be important. Better understanding of these and other factors may help to determine the optimal composition of enteral diets specific to the management of patients with Crohn's disease.

CONCLUSION

Enteral nutrition, does not have a primary therapeutic role in the management of patients with ulcerative colitis. To date, its role remains one of improving or maintaining nutritional status.

Elemental, peptide-based and polymeric enteral formulae have all been shown to have the ability to induce remission in patients with Crohn's disease with varying degrees of success. Deducing which formula is most effective is not easy. Results still tend to favor the elemental diet, which we continue to use in our unit.

Steroids remain the mainstay of medical management of Crohn's disease. Enteral nutrition, however, offers a therapy free from side effects and with an ability to induce remission rates often comparable to those achieved with steroids. Patients frequently require no specific treatment when remission is achieved with enteral nutrition.

Preventing relapse in patients with Crohn's disease remains a challenge in patients treated with enteral diets, and indeed with drug therapy. Challenges for the future of enteral nutrition in Crohn's disease include prolonging disease remission and establishing the optimal composition of formulae specific to the management of this disease.

REFERENCES

Alun Jones V, Dickinson R J, Workman E, Wilson A J, Freeman A H, Hunter J O 1985 Crohn's disease: maintenance of remission by diet. Lancet ii: 177–180

Barbul A, Sisto D A, Wasserkrug H L et al 1981 Arginine stimulates lymphocyte immune response in healthy human beings. Surgery 90: 244–251

Daly J M, Reynolds J V, Thom A et al 1988 Immune and metabolic effects of arginine in the surgical patient. Annals of Surgery 208: 512–523

Fernandez-Banares F, Cabre E, Esteve M, Gassull M A 1994a How effective is enteral nutrition in inducing clinical remission in active Crohn's disease? A meta-analysis of the randomised controlled trials. Clinical Nutrition 13 (Suppl 1): 15 [Abstract]

Fernandez-Banares F, Cabre E, Gonzalez-Huix F, Gassull M A 1994b Enteral nutrition as primary therapy in Crohn's disease. Gut (Suppl 1): S55–S59

Giaffer M H, North G, Holdsworth C D 1990 Controlled trial of polymeric versus elemental diet in treatment of active Crohn's disease. Lancet 335: 816–819

Gonzalez-Huix F, de Leon R, Fernandez-Banares F et al 1993 Polymeric enteral diets as primary treatment of active Crohn's disease. A prospective steroid-controlled trial. Gut 34: 778–782

Greenberg G R, Fleming C R, Jeejeebhoy K N, Rosenberg I H, Sales D, Tremaine W J 1988 Controlled trial of bowel rest and nutritional support in the management of Crohn's disease. Gut 29: 1309–1315

Griffiths A M, Ohlsson A, Sherman P M, Sutherland L R 1995 Meta-analysis of enteral nutrition as a primary treatment of active Crohn's disease. Gastroenterology 108(4): 1056–1067

Harries A D, Jones L A, Denis V, Fifield R, Heatley R V, Newcombe R G 1983 Controlled trial of supplemented oral nutrition in Crohn's disease. Lancet 1: 887–890

Hunt J B, Payne-James J J, Palmer K R et al 1989 A randomized controlled trial of elemental diet and prednisolone as primary therapy in acute exacerbations of Crohn's disease. Gastroenterology 96: 224 [Abstract]

Keys A, Brozek J, Henschel A, Mickelson O, Taylor H L 1950 The biology of human starvation. University of Minnesota Press, Minneapolis

Lochs H, Steinhardt H J, Klaus-Wentz B et al 1991 Comparison of enteral nutrition and drug treatment in active Crohn's disease: results of the European Cooperative Crohn's Disease Study IV. Gastroenterology 101: 881–888

Logan R F A, Gillon J, Ferrington C, Ferguson A 1981 Reduction of gastrointestinal protein loss by elemental diet in Crohn's disease of the small bowel. Gut 22: 381–387

Middleton S I, Riordan A M, Hunter J O 1991 Peptide based diet: an alternative to elemental diet in active Crohn's disease. Gut 32: A578

O'Morain C, McGuinness A 1994 Current therapy in gastroenterology and liver disease, 4th edn. Mosby, St Louis, pp 278–281

O'Morain C, Segal A W, Levi A J 1984 Elemental diet as primary treatment of acute Crohn's disease. British Medical Journal 288: 1859–1862

O'Morain C, Abelow A C, Lakshman C R, Fleischner G M 1986 Chromium 51-ethylenediaminetetraacetate test. A useful test in the assessment of inflammatory bowel disease. Journal of Laboratory Clinical Medicine 108: 430–435

Park R H R, Galloway A, Danesh B J Z, Russell R I 1991 Double-blind controlled trial of elemental and polymeric diets as primary therapy in active Crohn's disease. European Journal of Hepatology and Gastroenterology 3: 483–490

Polk B, Hattner A T, Kerner J A 1992 Improved growth and disease activity after intermittent administration of a defined formula diet in children with Crohn's disease. Journal of Parenteral and Enteral Nutrition 16: 499–504

Raouf A H, Hildrey V, Daniel J et al 1991 Enteral feeding as sole treatment for Crohn's disease: controlled trial of whole protein v amino acid based feed and a case study of dietary challenge. Gut 32: 702–707

Rigaud D, Cosnes J, Le Quintrec Y, Rene E, Gendre J P, Mignon M 1991 Controlled trial comparing two types of enteral nutrition in treatment of active Crohn's disease: elemental v polymeric diet. Gut 32: 1492–1497

Riordan A M, Hunter J O, Cowan R E et al 1993 Treatment of active Crohn's disease by exclusion diet: East Anglian Multicentre Controlled Trial. Lancet 342: 1131–1134

Royall D, Jeejeebhoy K N, Baker J et al 1994 Comparison of amino acid v peptide based enteral diets in active Crohn's disease: clinical and nutritional outcome. Gut 35: 783–787

Sanderson I R, Udeen S, Davies P S W, Savage M O, Walker-Smith J A 1987 Remission induced by an elemental diet in small bowel Crohn's disease. Archives of Disease in Childhood 61: 123–127

Saverymuttu S, Hodgson H J F, Chadwick V S 1985 Controlled trial comparing prednisolone with an elemental diet plus non-absorbable antibiotics in active Crohn's disease. Gut 26: 994–998

Seidman E G, Bouthillier L, Weber A M, Roy C C, Morin C L 1986 Elemental diet versus prednisone as primary treatment of Crohn's disease. Gastroenterology 90: 1625 [Abstract]

Seidman E, Griffiths A, Jones A, Issenman R 1993 Canadian Collaborative Paediatric Crohn's disease study group. Gastroenterology 104: 778 [Abstract]

Souba W W, Smith R J, Wilmore D W 1985 Effects of glucocorticoids on glutamine metabolism in organs. Metabolism 34: 450–456

Teahon K, Bjarnason J, Pearson M, Levi A J 1990 Ten years' experience with an elemental diet in the management of Crohn's disease. Gut 31: 1133–1137

Wellmann W, Fink P C, Benner F et al 1986 Endotoxinaemia in active Crohn's disease: treatment with whole gut irrigation and 5-aminosalicylic acid. Gut 27: 814–820

Windmueller H G 1982 Glutamine utilization by the small intestine. Advanced Enzymology 53: 201–237

60. Dietary manipulation – parenteral

I. D. A. D'Agata   E. G. Seidman

INTRODUCTION

The concept of providing nutrients intravenously to ill patients who cannot eat normally dates back to the 17th century, when Sir Christopher Wren and Robert Boyle injected animals with various substances, including oil and wine. The first successful intravenous administration of a substance in humans occurred in 1831, when a Scottish physician administered a salt solution to a man dying of cholera (Wilkinson 1963). Other attempts remained plagued by technical difficulties until the 1960's, when it was finally shown that total parenteral nutrition (TPN) could be used safely in humans (Lawson 1965). Shortly thereafter, Dudrick and colleagues (1968) demonstrated, first in beagle puppies and then in an infant, that the continuous infusion of hypertonic dextrose and amino acids via deep venous catheters could provide sufficient daily calories, ensuring adequate nutrition and growth. TPN thus became established as an effective and relatively safe means by which to prevent and reverse the metabolic consequences of malnutrition. Since then, TPN has greatly improved the quality of life of humans with a non-functional gut, allowing them to lead fairly independent and fulfilling lives.

TPN IN MALNUTRITION

Malnutrition is common in inflammatory bowel disease (IBD), particularly in Crohn's disease involving the small bowel (Seidman 1989). It has been estimated that most adult patients with Crohn's disease weigh about 10% less than ideal body weight when first examined. Over two-thirds of hospitalized pediatric patients with Crohn's disease have weight loss, hypoalbuminemia and anemia, and are in negative nitrogen balance prior to beginning therapy. The mechanisms contributing to inadequate caloric intake and micronutrient deficiencies are numerous, and include anorexia, extensive bowel disease impairing digestion and absorption, short gut due to surgical resections, and bacterial overgrowth. Nutrient losses occur by way of protein exudation from the inflamed gut, through bleeding, as well as mineral and vitamin losses through malabsorption. Not uncommonly patients with IBD limit their own diet, and iatrogenic dietary restrictions further reduce their intake. Parenteral nutrition support has thus been widely utilized for IBD patients over the last 20 years. Dudrick noted that of the first six patients successfully treated with TPN, two had severe IBD and would not have survived without using this novel technique. In view of the higher costs and the much greater risk of serious complications, it is now generally agreed that TPN use should be restricted to those situations where the enteral route cannot be employed, or has failed. Current indications for TPN in patients with IBD are summarized in Table 60.1.

TPN AND BOWEL REST IN IBD

Bowel rest with concomitant administration of TPN has traditionally been considered beneficial in the management of patients with severe IBD. The goals of this regimen are to induce clinical remission, avoid surgical resection, and correct or maintain nutritional status. Bowel rest allows for decreased gastrointestinal secretion and motility, and eliminates any antigenic stimulation by food, theoretically leading to diminished inflammation of the bowel. It may also help by avoiding unpleasant gastrointestinal symptoms associated with food intake at a time when the bowel is severely inflamed. The use of TPN as an adjunctive treatment to correct malnutrition is well established. However, the role of bowel rest using TPN to reverse disease activity in IBD remains controversial. TPN and bowel rest have not proved of benefit in reducing disease activity in patients with ulcerative colitis. The results are generally more encouraging in patients with Crohn's disease. However, data supporting a statistically significant effect are generally lacking. Most studies evaluating the effects of TPN and bowel rest in patients with ulcerative colitis have been either retrospective or non-controlled. Reilly and colleagues (1978) noted that on long-term follow-up 91% of patients eventually required

Table 60.1 Guidelines for TPN use in inflammatory bowel disease

Adults	Children
Crohn's disease	
Category A: Bowel rest for acute exacerbations of disease 　　　　　High-output fistulae 　　　　　High-grade obstruction 　　　　　Enteral treatment failure resulting in: 　　　　　　　inability to normalize nutritional status 　　　　　　　unacceptable GI symptoms Category B: Adjunctive therapy for malnutrition due to anorexia, 　　　　　diarrhea, abdominal pain, bloating, distension or side 　　　　　effects of medications	Category A: Nutrition support for patients with growth failure 　　　　　Near-complete bowel obstruction 　　　　　High-output fistula 　　　　　Gastrointestinal bleed 　　　　　Short bowel syndrome 　　　　　Malnutrition resulting from enteral treatment failure
Ulcerative colitis	
Category B: Adjunctive therapy in acute exacerbations 　　　　　of disease for: 　　　　　　malnutrition 　　　　　　perioperative support	Category C: Malnutrition resulting from enteral treatment failure

Category A:　Signifies that there is good research-based evidence to support the recommendation.
Category B:　Signifies that there is fair research-based evidence to support the recommendation.
Category C:　The recommendation is based on expert opinion and panel consensus.
Adapted from　ASPEN Board of Directors 1993

colectomy. Mullen and co-workers (1978) reported that 62% eventually needed surgery. In another retrospective study, Jarnerot and colleagues (1985) found that only 32% of patients with ulcerative colitis went into remission after 6 days of TPN, but that with prolongation of therapy for up to 18 days this proportion rose to 63%. The few prospective studies reported to date have failed to show a benefit of TPN and bowel rest in patients with ulcerative colitis. Elson and colleagues (1980) observed that 60% of patients did not improve on TPN and eventually required colectomy. A prospective randomized controlled trial by Dickinson and colleagues (1980) also reported this regimen to be ineffective. A similar conclusion was reached in 1986 by McIntyre et al. TPN is, however, an important adjunctive treatment in malnourished hospitalized ulcerative colitis patients unable to meet their nutrient requirements otherwise.

Patients with Crohn's disease seem to respond better to TPN and bowel rest. Most of the reported data are retrospective or prospective but uncontrolled studies (Muller et al 1983, Ostro et al 1985). Remission rates reported are considerably higher than those described in patients with ulcerative colitis. Patients with Crohn's colitis appear to respond less well to TPN and bowel rest than those with small-bowel involvement or ileocolitis, but specific data are lacking. Certain series have indicated that symptomatic response is independent of disease location (Ostro et al 1985, Lerebours et al 1986). Controversy also exists regarding the long-term outcome of TPN and bowel rest in patients with Crohn's disease. Although Shiloni and colleagues (1989) found that half of the patients who had initially gone into remission required surgery 6–72 months later, Sitzmann and co-workers (1990) reported that 75% of their patients remained in sustained remission for 15–100 months. Lerebours and colleagues (1986) also observed high recurrence rates in both steroid-resistant and steroid-dependent patients with Crohn's disease. However, the recurrences after TPN were mild and responded well to standard medical therapy. Furthermore, a small number of patients did experience a prolonged remission, thereby avoiding surgery. One randomized prospective study compared the ability of TPN and an enteral elemental diet to induce remission in 36 patients with active Crohn's disease (Alun Jones 1987). The rate of remission was similar in the two groups (84% and 89%). The two nutritional therapies were equally effective in improving laboratory parameters and the disease activity index. In 1988, Greenberg and colleagues conducted a prospective controlled trial in which patients with Crohn's disease who had failed conventional medical therapy (including steroids) were randomly assigned to receive 3 weeks of TPN, enteral nutrition or an oral diet. Although clinical improvement occurred in the patients on TPN, comparable remission rates were observed in the three groups (42%, 52% and 56% respectively). The authors concluded that bowel rest may not be essential to achieving remission in patients with steroid-resistant Crohn's disease.

PREOPERATIVE TPN

TPN may be of benefit for Crohn's disease patients who require bowel resection. Rombeau and colleagues (1982) found that patients who received TPN preoperatively had significantly fewer complications than those who did not. Lashmer and colleagues (1989) reported that patients receiving preoperative TPN required shorter segments of bowel to be resected. Nutritional support of patients with Crohn's disease improves their muscle performance (Christie & Hill 1990) and this finding is associated with a decrease in postoperative complications (Zeiderman & MacMahon 1989).

GROWTH FAILURE

Nearly 25% of patients with IBD present in the pediatric age group and growth failure affects one-third of such patients (Seidman et al 1987). Growth retardation is the most common extraintestinal manifestation of pediatric Crohn's disease. Delays in sexual maturation typically accompany the abnormal growth pattern, affecting the child's self-esteem. These children thus often have difficulties dealing with peer perceptions, and school performance may decline. In the prepubertal adolescent the potential for growth is limited because of progressive bone maturation and epiphyseal fusion. It is therefore important to intervene aggressively and early in IBD complicated by growth failure. The aim of nutritional therapy in the pediatric patient is thus both to provide adequate nutrition to permit growth, as well as to decrease disease activity, so as to avoid chronic therapy with steroids.

The main cause of growth retardation in pediatric IBD is malnutrition, and dietary intake inadequate to meet the overall nutrient requirements of the growing child or adolescent is the most important factor (Seidman 1989). Corticosteroid therapy has also been implicated in the growth failure that causes a high incidence of permanent short stature in adults whose Crohn's disease began in childhood (Markowitz et al 1993). Nevertheless, steroid use probably has a less important role than inadequate nutrient intake (Motil et al 1993). Increased energy requirements due to inflammation also have a secondary role in the genesis of malnutrition in pediatric IBD. In fact, energy balance studies have failed to demonstrate that the IBD inflammatory process per se significantly alters metabolic needs in the absence of fever (Chan et al 1986, Motil et al 1982). Although the enteral route of feeding is to be preferred whenever possible in this patient population as well, children who are profoundly malnourished may benefit from a short course of TPN prior to switching over to enteral alimentation. In order to achieve catch-up growth a sustained use of nutritional supplementation is needed (Seidman 1989). An added difficulty of enteral feeds in both children and adults is that long-term compliance with oral supplements is poor. Children are rarely willing to drink elemental or even polymeric formulae due to their inherent unpleasant taste, and hence almost always require nocturnal continuous nasogastric feeds (Seidman 1989). However, the use of flavor packets has recently been shown to enhance the oral intake of peptide-based diets in children with Crohn's disease (Bouthillier et al 1995). Nevertheless, the barometer of success must always be measured in terms of growth velocity. If enteral supplements fail to reverse growth failure, home TPN should be considered (De Potter et al 1992).

FISTULAE AND SHORT GUT

Enterocutaneous fistulae are among the most troublesome complications of Crohn's disease. TPN may aid in closing fistulae by providing nutritional support while reducing the necessity for enteral feeding, thereby allowing wound healing to occur. Unfortunately, no prospective randomized trials comparing TPN to medical therapy have yet been performed, and the current literature reports a wide variability in closure rates. These discrepancies may be ascribed to the fact that fistulae of various types are included in the studies. Nevertheless, it appears that post-operative fistulae caused by anastomotic leaks or occurring at the site of drainage heal reasonably well, whereas those consequent to active bowel wall inflammation generally do not respond favorably. Long-term closure of fistulae in Crohn's disease was reported in only 30% of patients, and most eventually required surgery (Hawker et al 1983, Gouma et al 1988). One clear advantage to patients with high-output fistulae is that home TPN has become quite accessible thereby shortening hospital stay. Patients with Crohn's disease who have undergone multiple resections and consequently suffer from short bowel syndrome may clearly benefit from TPN in the home (Stokes et al 1988, Vanderhoof et al 1992). Recently, Galandiuck and co-workers (1990) reviewed their experience with patients suffering from Crohn's disease who were on home TPN for high stoma output or short bowel syndrome and found that nutritional status was improved and steroid dosages were reduced.

COMPLICATIONS

Significant morbidity is associated with prolonged TPN use (Galandiuck et al 1990). This is in contrast with earlier reported findings by Strobel and co-workers (1979), who had observed few complications associated with home TPN use. The yearly reported frequency of catheter occlusion was low in one large series (Matuchansky et al 1992). Septic complications are minimized when proper antiseptic techniques are employed. Nevertheless, the risk of developing catheter-related sepsis is higher for patients receiving long-term TPN therapy and in younger patients (Herfindal et al 1992). In a review of 102 pediatric patients on home TPN, Vargas and colleagues (1987) noted that the two most common indications were short gut (33%) and IBD (23%). Thirty-one patients died while on TPN; 13 of these deaths were TPN related, with sepsis and liver failure being the most common causes.

TPN is commonly associated with abnormal liver function. A recent prospective study found that 61% of patients had abnormal liver function parameters, although these were generally mild and mainly consisted of elevated gamma-glutamyl transpeptidase (Abad-Lacruz et al 1990). Hepatic dysfunction as a result of nutritional support in IBD is far more common in patients receiving treatment via the parenteral than the enteral route. The complete loss of enteric stimulation in patients on TPN is the main determinant in the development of cholestasis (Quigley et al 1993). In a prospective study by Messing and co-workers (1983), ultrasonography was used to monitor the development of biliary sludge and gallstones in patients on TPN. Within 12 days of starting therapy, 61% of previously normal studies revealed the presence of sludge. After 6 weeks of TPN sludge was present in all patients. Gallstones developed in six of 14 early sludge formers, and three patients required surgery. Roslyn and colleagues (1983) found that cholelithiasis developed in 35% of patients who had been on TPN for 3 months or more, and that this was more common in patients with ileal disease (39%) than in those without (25%). Long-term TPN may thus precipitate cholelithiasis in patients with Crohn's disease who are predisposed to hepatobiliary complications. The only truly effective treatment for TPN-related liver disease is discontinuation of therapy, and even then cases of chronic liver disease, including cirrhosis, have been reported. Recently, ursodeoxycholic acid has been employed to prevent or resolve sludge gallstones, with some success, but controlled studies are lacking.

The ability to provide patients with hyperalimentation parenterally may, in certain situations, be deleterious. Excessive calorie provision in the face of severe malnutrition has been strongly linked to the pathogenesis of the 'refeeding' syndrome (Seidman & Pineault 1994). Electrolyte imbalances (potassium, phosphorus etc.) may result in cardiac arrhythmias and death may ensue. The dictum 'more is not necessarily better' certainly applies to TPN use, as hepatic steatosis may occur in normally nourished individuals provided with an imbalanced calorie/nitrogen intake. Therefore, in using TPN the clinician must always balance the risks and benefits, tailoring the decision to use TPN, as well as its composition, to each patient's individual needs. Indeed, IBD patients frequently have micronutrient as well as macronutrient deficiencies (Seidman 1989). These must be screened for and supplemented as needed. Serial evaluation of vitamin and micronutrient status is important in those patients undergoing long-term TPN (Seidman & Pineault 1994). Zinc, selenium and iron concentrations are often low in such patients (Main et al 1982, Rannem et al 1992).

MECHANISMS OF ACTION

Although TPN can be helpful in the management of patients with IBD, the mechanisms by which it achieves clinical improvement remain unclear. It may be due to the enhanced provision of calories and specific micronutrients, or to the removal of putative intraluminal antigenic stimuli that perpetuate the chronic inflammatory process characteristic of IBD (Seidman 1989). There are some theoretical concerns regarding the lack of enterocyte stimulation during prolonged bowel rest and TPN therapy (Seidman 1994). Reversible alterations in the intestinal microflora and villous atrophy occur during prolonged TPN therapy. There is currently a great deal of interest in modifying the composition of standard TPN formulations so as to provide certain specific gut nutrients. For example, the absence of glutamine and short-chain fatty acids from present-day TPN formulations appears to contribute to mucosal atrophy and favor bacterial translocation, enhancing the risk of Gram-negative sepsis. Adding these critical gut nutrients to TPN preparations has been associated with attenuation of gut atrophy and decreased bacterial translocation (Souba et al 1990, Seidman 1994). There is also evidence of decreased secretory IgA production after prolonged periods of TPN, further impairing gut barrier function. Gut non-utilization may lead to mucosal colonization with pathogenic bacteria, an increased local inflammatory response and the enhanced release of cytokines and bacterial translocation (Alverdy & Burke 1992). Glutamine, which is absent from standard TPN solutions, has been shown to enhance gut secretory IgA production.

CONCLUSION

Given the present state of knowledge, TPN use in patients with IBD should generally be limited to a few indications. Although there are some potential adverse consequences associated with its use, it is unquestionable that TPN can be of paramount aid in the management of carefully selected cases. TPN should only be utilized if attempts to employ enteral hyperalimentation (i.e. elemental diets) have failed or are contraindicated. Even then its use should be restricted to medical teams with the experience and knowledge to apply this therapy safely, in view of its potential life-threatening complications. The hope is that further research will improve our ability to safely employ TPN and limit complications, improving the quality of life for patients who require its use.

REFERENCES

Abad-Lacruz A, Gonzalez-Huix F, Esteve M et al 1990 Liver function test abnormalities in patients with inflammatory bowel disease receiving artificial nutrition: a prospective, randomized study of total enteral nutrition vs total parenteral nutrition. Journal of Parenteral and Enteral Nutrition 14:618–621

Alun Jones V 1987 Complications of total parenteral nutrition and elemental diet in the induction of remission of Crohn's disease. Digestive Diseases and Sciences 32:100S–107S

Alverdy J C, Burke D 1992 Total parenteral nutrition: iatrogenic immunosuppression. Nutrition 8: 359–365

ASPEN Board of Directors 1993 Guidelines for the use of parenteral and enteral nutrition in adult and pediatric patients. Journal of Parenteral and Enteral Nutrition 17:15A

Bouthillier L, Herzog D, Parent P, Seidman E 1995 Evolving use of elemental formulas in the treatment of pediatric Crohn's disease.

Journal of Parenteral and Enteral Nutrition (Abstract in press)
Chan A T H, Fleming C R, O'Fallon W M, Huizenga K H 1986 Estimated vs measured basal energy requirements in patients with Crohn's disease. Gastroenterology 91: 75–78
Christie P M, Hill G L 1990 Effect of intravenous nutrition on nutrition and function in acute attacks of inflammatory bowel disease. Gastroenterology 99: 730–736
De Potter S, Goulet O, Lamor M et al 1992 263 patient-years of home parenteral nutrition in children. Transplantation Proceedings 24: 1056–1057
Dickinson R J, Aston M J, Axon A T R, Smith R C, Yeung C K, Hill G L 1980 Controlled trial of intravenous hyperalimentation and bowel rest as an adjunctive to the routine therapy of acute colitis. Gastroenterology 79: 199–204
Dudrick S J, Wilmore D W, Vars H M et al 1968 Long term total parenteral nutrition with growth development and positive nitrogen balance. Surgery 64: 134–142
Elson C O, Layden T J, Nemchansky B A, Rosenberg J L, Rosenberg I H 1980 Evaluation of total parenteral nutrition in inflammatory bowel disease. Digestive Diseases and Sciences 25: 42–48
Galandiuk S, O'Neill M, MacDonald P et al 1990 A century of hyperalimentation for Crohn's disease. American Journal of Surgery 159: 540–545
Gouma D J, Van Meyenfelt M F, Ruflart M, Soeters P B 1988 Preoperative parenteral nutrition in severe Crohn's disease. Surgery 103: 648–652
Greenberg G R, Fleming C R, Jeejeebhoy K N et al 1988 Controlled trial of bowel rest and nutritional support in the management of Crohn's disease. Gut 29: 1309–1315
Hawker P C, Gevel J C, Keighley M R B et al 1983 Management of enterocutaneous fistulas in Crohn's disease. Gut 4: 284–287
Herfindal E T, Bernstein L R, Wong A F, Hogue I W, Parbenian J A 1992 Complications of hyperalimentation. Clinical Pharmacokinetics 11: 543–548
Jarnerot G, Rovny P, Sandberg–Gerton H 1985 Intravenous therapy of ulcerative colitis. Gastroenterology 85: 1005–1013
Lashmer B A, Evan A A, Hanyer S B 1989 Preoperative total parenteral nutrition for bowel resection in Crohn's disease. Digestive Diseases and Sciences 34: 741–748
Lawson L J 1965 Parenteral nutrition in surgery. British Journal of Surgery 52: 795–800
Lerebours E, Messing B, Chevalier B et al 1986 An evaluation of total parenteral nutrition in the management of steroid dependent and steroid resistant patients with Crohn's disease. Journal of Parenteral and Enteral Nutrition 10: 274–278
MacIntyre P B, Powell-Tuck J, Wood S R et al 1986 Controlled trial of bowel rest in the therapy of severe acute colitis. Gut 27: 481–484
Main A N H, Hall M J, Russell R I, Fell G S, Mills P R, Sherkin A 1982 Clinical experience of zinc supplementation during intravenous nutrition in Crohn's disease: value of serum and urine zinc measurements. Gut 23: 984–991
Markowitz J, Grancher K, Rosa J, Aiges H, Daum F 1993 Growth failure in pediatric inflammatory bowel disease. Journal of Pediatric Gastroenterology and Nutrition 16: 373–380
Matuchansky C, Messing B, Jeejeebhoy K N, Beau P, Beliah M, Allard J P 1992 Cyclical parenteral nutrition. Lancet 340: 588–592
Messing B, Bories C, Kustlinger F, Bernier J J 1983 Does TPN induce gallbladder sludge formation and lithiasis? Gastroenterology 84: 1012–1019
Motil K J, Grand R J, Davis-Kraft L, Ferlic L L, O' Brian-Smith E 1993 Growth failure in children with inflammatory bowel disease: a prospective study. Gastroenterology 105: 681–691
Motil K J, Grand R J, Muletskos C J, Young R 1982 The effect of disease, drug, and diet on whole body protein metabolism in adolescents with Crohn's disease and growth failure. Journal of Pediatrics 101: 345–351
Mullen J L, Hargrove W C, Dudrick S J et al 1978 Ten years' experience with intravenous hyperalimentation and inflammatory bowel disease. Annals of Surgery 187: 523–528
Muller J M, Keller H W, Erasmi H, Pichlmaier H 1983 Total parenteral nutrition as the sole therapy in Crohn's disease: a prospective study. British Journal of Surgery 70: 40-43
Ostro M J, Greenberg G R, Jeejeebhoy K N 1985 Total parenteral nutrition and complete bowel rest in management of Crohn's disease. Journal of Parenteral and Enteral Nutrition 9: 282–287
Quigley E M M, Marsh M N, Shaffer J L, Martin R S 1993 Hepatobiliary complications of total parenteral nutrition. Gastroenterology 104: 286–301
Rannem T, Ladefoged K, Hylander E, Hegnoj J, Jarnum S 1992 Selenium status in patients with Crohn's disease. American Journal of Clinical Nutrition 56: 933–937
Reilly J, Ryan J A, Strole W, Fisher J E 1978 Hyperalimentation in inflammatory bowel disease. American Journal of Surgery 131: 192–200
Rombeau L R, Williamson C E, Mullen J L 1982 Preoperative intravenous parenteral nutrition and surgical outcome in patients with inflammatory bowel disease. American Journal of Surgery 143: 139–143
Roslyn J J, Pitt H A, Mann L L, Ament M E, Den Besten L 1983 Gallbladder disease in patients on long term parenteral nutrition. Gastroenterology 84: 148–154
Seidman E 1994 Gastrointestinal benefits of enteral feeds. In: Baker S, Baker R, Davis A (eds) Pediatric enteral nutrition. Chapman & Hall, New York, pp 46–66
Seidman E, Pineault M 1994 Nutritional considerations in pediatric enteric neuromuscular disease. In: Hyman P E, DiLorenzo C (eds) Pediatric gastrointestinal motility. Academy Professional Information Services (in press)
Seidman E G 1989 Nutritional management of inflammatory bowel disease. Gastroenterology Clinics of North America 17: 129–155
Seidman E G, Roy C C, Weber A M, Morin C L 1987 Nutritional therapy of Crohn's disease in childhood. Digestive Diseases and Sciences 32: 82S–88S
Shiloni G, Cevonado E, Fraund H R 1989 Role of total parenteral nutrition in therapy of Crohn's disease. American Journal of Surgery 137: 180–185
Sitzmann J V, Lenverge R L, Bayless T M 1990 Favourable response to parenteral nutrition and medical therapy in Crohn's disease. Gastroenterology 99: 1647–1652
Souba N W, Klimberg S V, Plumley D A et al 1990 The role of glutamine in maintaining a healthy gut and supporting the metabolic response to injury and infection. Journal of Surgical Research 48: 383
Stokes M A, Almond D J, Pettit S H et al 1988 Home parenteral nutrition: a review of 100 patient years of therapy in 76 consecutive cases. British Journal of Surgery 75: 481–483
Strobel C T, Byrne W J, Ament M E 1979 Home parenteral nutrition in children with Crohn's disease: an effective management alternative. Gastroenterology 77: 272–279
Vanderhoof J A, Lagnas A N, Pinch L W, Thompson J S, Kaufmann S S 1992 Short bowel syndrome. Journal of Pediatric Gastroenterology and Nutrition 14: 359–370
Vargas J H, Ament M E, Berquist W E 1987 Long term home parenteral nutrition in pediatrics: ten years' experience in 102 patients. Journal of Pediatric Gastroenterology and Nutrition 6: 24–32
Wilkinson A W 1963 Historical background of intravenous feeding. Nutrition and Diet 5: 295–297
Zeiderman M R, MacMahon M J 1989 The role of objective measurement of skeletal muscle function in the preoperative patient. Clinical Nutrition 8: 161 – 166

SECTION 6

Ulcerative colitis

61. Medical management of mild and moderately active ulcerative colitis

J. E. Smithson   D. P. Jewell

This chapter considers current medical management of mild to moderately active ulcerative colitis in an outpatient setting. The approach to disease in remission and the treatment of severe attacks are covered in other chapters in this section. Idiopathic proctitis is regarded here as the most limited form of ulcerative colitis rather than as a distinctive disease entity. For this reason the principles of treatment outlined apply equally, irrespective of disease extent, although distal disease is clearly most amenable to topical therapy. The chapter is summarized in the form of algorithms (Figs 61.1 and 61.2) for managing initial and recurrent attacks of ulcerative colitis.

DIAGNOSIS

Optimal management of active ulcerative colitis depends first upon making an accurate diagnosis. Important differential diagnoses for the patient who presents with an initial attack characterized by rectal bleeding, altered bowel habit and mucosal inflammation include Crohn's disease, infectious colitis, pseudomembranous colitis and sexually transmitted disease. Nevertheless, the clinical features and sigmoidoscopic appearance, together with stool culture and microscopy, will be sufficient in most cases to allow a confident diagnosis of ulcerative colitis and the prompt initiation of treatment. At the initial consultation a variety of features may provide important clues to the underlying diagnosis; these are summarized in Table 61.1.

Although the correct diagnosis will be made in most cases, infective causes of colitis may be overlooked or may cause diagnostic confusion. For amebiasis to be excluded a freshly voided 'hot stool' must be examined by the microbiologist. Any delay in transporting the specimen will lead to loss of motility of the amebae and the diagnosis may be missed. For this reason it has been argued that stool samples or mucosal scrapes should be examined in the clinic immediately after transfer to prewarmed glass slides. The coincidence of salmonella infection and ulcerative colitis may also cause problems in

Table 61.1 Discriminating clinical features in the differential diagnosis of ulcerative colitis

Clinical features at presentation	Consider diagnosis
History of weeks or more Previous undiagnosed episodes Positive family history of IBD Extraintestinal manifestations Onset after stopping smoking Diffuse mucosal inflammation	Ulcerative colitis
Abdominal pain and mass Perianal disease Symptoms disproportionate to degree of rectal inflammation	Crohn's disease
Rapid onset Dietary history Travel history	Bacillary and amebic colitis
History of antibiotic use Mucosal pseudomembrane	Pseudomembranous colitis
History of excessive straining Discrete mucosal ulceration	Solitary rectal ulcer syndrome
Sexual history	Gonococcal and chlamydial infection, other venereal causes of proctitis
Previous radiotherapy to sacrum, prostate or cervix	Radiation colitis
Iatrogenic immunosuppression or AIDS	CMV colitis

diagnosis and management, particularly if a patient is presenting for the first time. Dronfield et al (1974) described five cases in whom there was delay in recognizing this combination. One of the patients died from salmonella septicemia following treatment with corticosteroids. Another source of diagnostic problems is patients returning from tropical countries with a first attack of bloody diarrhea. A quarter of such patients who were seen at the Hospital for Tropical Diseases, London, between 1978 and 1984 were found to have ulcerative colitis rather than amebic or bacillary dysentery (Harries et al 1985). The importance of close liaison between infectious disease clinicians and gastroenterologists in caring for these patients is clear. Diagnostic pitfalls may also be encountered with sexually transmitted causes of proctitis: gonococcal infection in particular may resemble idiopathic ulcerative proctitis (McMillan et al 1983a,b). Therefore, a sexual history may be relevant and, if venereal proctitis is suspected, swabs should be taken and inoculated on to appropriate selective media. Finally, cytomegalovirus colitis in patients with AIDS may give rise to endoscopic appearances easily confused with those of ulcerative colitis (Rene et al 1988). Histological examination reveals characteristic giant cells with intranuclear inclusion bodies. The correct diagnosis may not be recognized, however, if the underlying condition of AIDS is unsuspected. Treatment with corticosteroids in these circumstances may have severe consequences.

ASSESSMENT OF DISEASE SEVERITY

The importance of assessing disease severity is twofold. First, it allows identification of patients with severe attacks who require hospital admission for intensive treatment. Secondly, it provides a useful starting point for deciding on an individual's therapy. Indices for measuring disease activity must therefore be accurate, simple and robust. The index outlined by Truelove and Witts (1955), illustrated in Table 61.2, remains the standard for most clinicians. The systems described by Powell-Tuck et al (1978) and Rachmilewitz (1989) incorporate extra features, including sigmoidoscopic appearance and abdominal pain, and allow a numerical score to be assigned which may be especially useful in the context of clinical trials. Irrespective of the index employed, it is important to question patients about the total number of bowel actions in a full 24-hour period, since nocturnal symptoms may be underestimated. Fecal incontinence should also be directly ascertained, since this symptom may not be volunteered by patients, but if present should influence the physician to treat the attack more aggressively. Useful laboratory markers indicating a severe rather than a mild attack include leukocytosis, hypoalbuminemia and raised serum C-reactive protein and orosomucoids.

Table 61.2 Truelove and Witts' (1955) criteria for disease severity

Clinical features	Severity
Up to four bowel actions daily No systemic disturbance	Mild
Intermediate between mild and severe	Moderate
Six or more bloody bowel motions daily Pulse rate greater than 90 bpm Fever greater than 37.5°C Haemoglobin less than 10.5 g/dl ESR greater than 30 mm/h	Severe

ASSESSMENT OF DISEASE EXTENT

Disease severity is the primary determinant of therapy for active ulcerative colitis, but knowledge of the colonic extent of disease is useful for tailoring treatment to the needs of the individual patient. Since there is a positive correlation between severity and extent of disease (Watts et al 1966a,b), patients with mild to moderate grades of activity are more likely to have involvement of the distal colon only. Other clinical findings outlined below are helpful in determining disease extent without recourse to formal imaging.

The initial attack

During the initial presenting attack, unless the upper limit of inflammation can be clearly identified at rigid sigmoidoscopy the extent of colonic involvement will be unknown. However, at least half of those patients presenting with ulcerative colitis for the first time will have distal disease, that is, inflammation limited to the rectum or rectum and sigmoid colon (Both et al 1983, Sinclair et al 1983, Nordenvall et al 1985). A history of formed or semiformed stools together with mild to moderate activity also suggests distal disease. Plain radiography of the abdomen provides further help since fecal residue tends not to accumulate in segments of inflamed mucosa (Bartram 1976). In some clinics unprepared flexible sigmoidoscopy is performed routinely at presentation, allowing more confident estimation of colonic involvement. In general, full colonoscopy and double contrast barium enema are not indicated during an acute attack in view of the potential risks of bowel perforation. The role of isotope-labeled white cell scanning has been advocated as a non-invasive method of assessing the extent of active disease (Saverymuttu et al 1986), but others have found a poor correlation with endoscopic findings (Leddin et al 1987).

Recurrent attacks

For the patient presenting with a relapse of ulcerative colitis, disease extent will usually have been determined at an earlier date, either by barium enema or by colonoscopy. The latter is the method of choice, since not only does it avoid ionizing radiation but it provides histological confirmation of involvement, which may be more extensive than appreciated radiologically. It will also allow the early detection of epithelial dysplasia. Although previous imaging is useful in guiding medical therapy, disease extent may be underestimated as a result of the progressive colonic involvement typical of ulcerative colitis. Distal disease may extend to involve more proximal parts of the colon in up to 30% of patients within 20 years of initial diagnosis (Powell-Tuck et al 1977, Sinclair et al 1983).

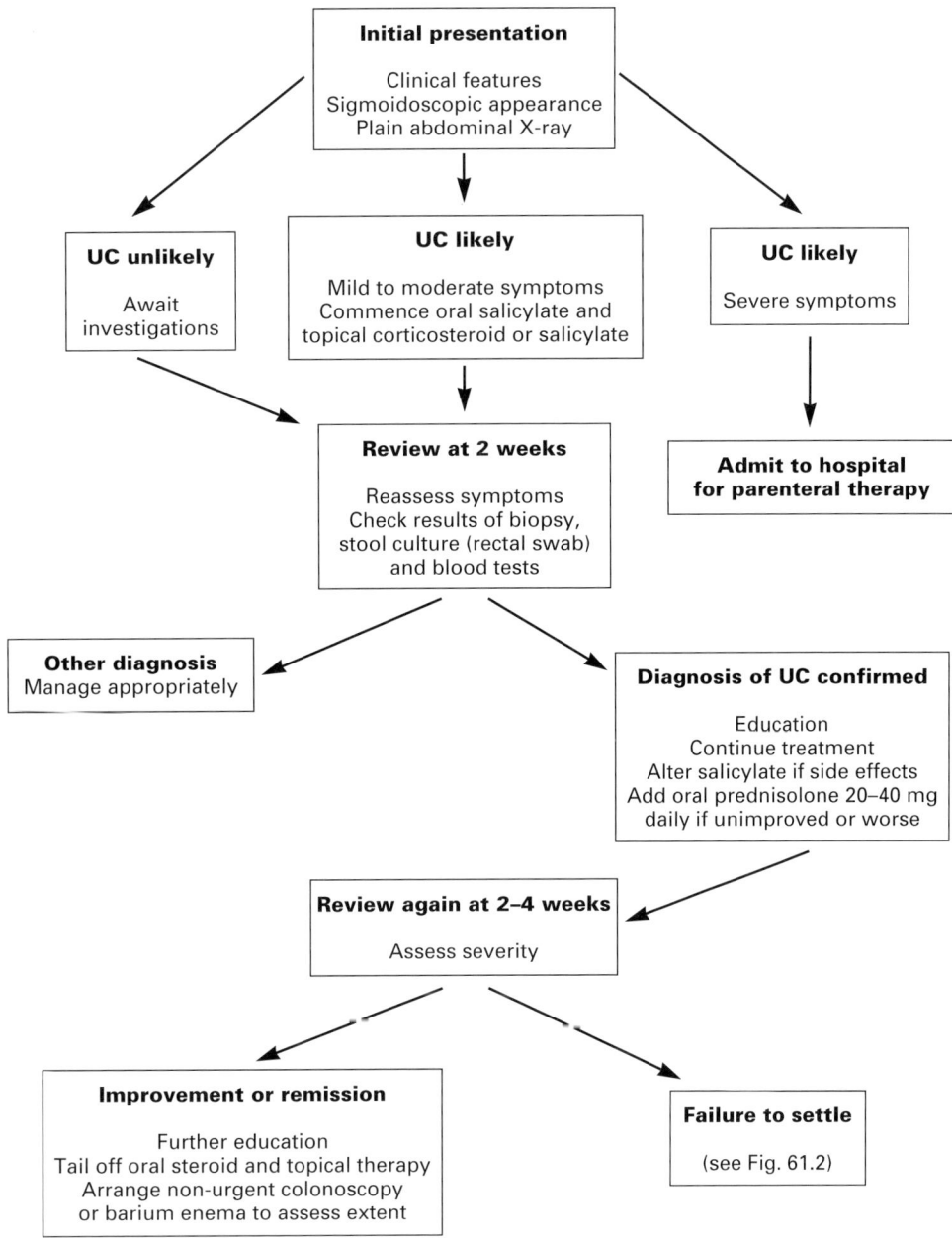

Fig. 61.1 Algorithm for managing initial attack of ulcerative colitis.

APPROACHES TO TREATMENT

General considerations and supportive measures

There is evidence that prompt initiation of therapy improves the clinical outcome (Meyers et al 1988). Many clinicians encourage patients to commence treatment on their own initiative and to attend the next available outpatient clinic. It is helpful if patients have a telephone number allowing them to contact a member of the team for advice.

An important aspect of the specialist clinic is that it provides a forum for education. Information leaflets and contact addresses for local and national self-help groups can be provided, together with counselling by doctors and gastrointestinal nurses. In view of the lack of serious psychological morbidity reported in the majority of patients (Gruner et al 1978), formal psychiatric support is rarely needed. Regular outpatient review may help to foster a sense of trust between the patient and the medical team, and allows continuing education as well as an opportunity for consolidating the diagnosis in uncertain cases and detecting complications of the disease.

Malnutrition in patients with mild and moderately active ulcerative colitis is extremely unusual, and if

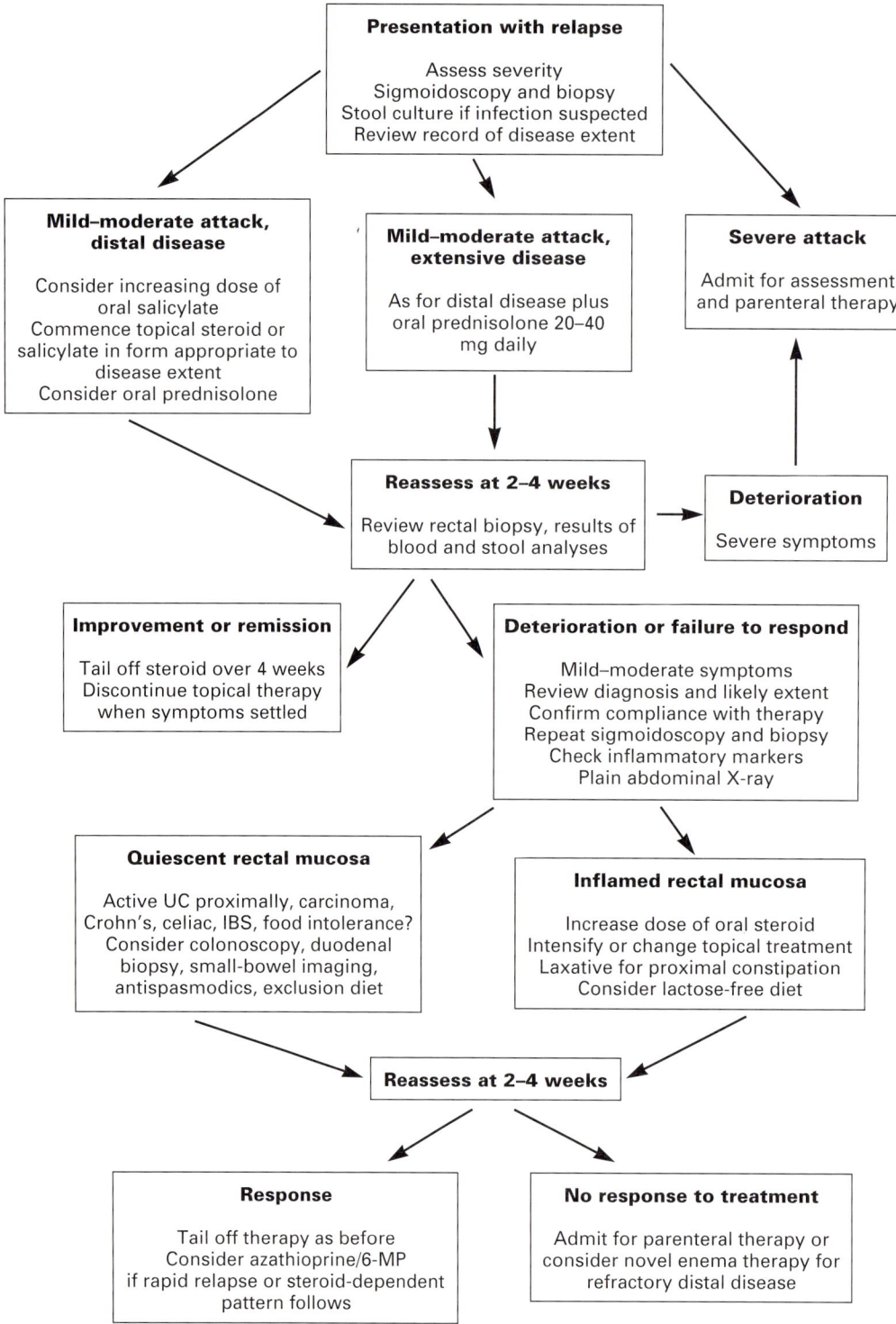

Fig. 61.2 Algorithm for managing relapse of ulcerative colitis.

present should alert the clinician to the possibility of alternative diagnoses (Crohn's disease, cancer, celiac disease). Iron deficiency anemia may occur as a consequence of long-standing colonic bleeding and should be treated. Since many patients with ulcerative colitis are intolerant of oral iron, a total dose infusion intravenously is often the best way of replacing iron stores. Antidiarrheal drugs are discouraged for several reasons. First, by delaying intestinal transit they may interfere with the delivery of oral salicylates to the colon. Secondly, they may disguise the severity of an attack and theoretically may predispose to colonic dilatation, although this rarely appears to happen in practice. Finally, diarrhea in ulcerative colitis usually reflects active disease, and persistent symptoms indicate a need for an intensification or change in therapy rather than simple symptomatic control.

Dietary measures

Understandably, many patients with ulcerative colitis may feel that their diet is in some way to blame for their disease. However, this has not been borne out in general by clinical trials. Complete dietary exclusion ('bowel rest') in patients with severe colitis did not improve the outcome in two separate studies (Dickinson et al 1980a, McIntyre et al 1986). The description of several patients in whom ulcerative colitis appeared to be provoked by cow's milk (Truelove 1961) led to a clinical trial of a milk-free diet in active disease (Wright & Truelove 1965). Approximately one in five patients benefited from milk exclusion, although lactose malabsorption rather than milk allergy is the likely explanation in this group (Pena & Truelove 1973, Busk et al 1975). Most clinicians would reserve a milk-free or lactose-free diet for those patients with ongoing abdominal discomfort and diarrhea despite apparent improvement in colonic inflammation. Careful dietary assessment is necessary before starting a diet to ensure that an adequate intake of calcium and protein will be maintained. Alternatively, if hypolactasia has been formally demonstrated by lactose hydrogen breath testing, lactase supplements can be added to milk at meal times (Rosado et al 1984). No studies have shown that the intake of dietary fiber influences the outcome of active ulcerative colitis. However, it would seem wise to encourage patients to follow a high fiber diet in order to avoid constipation.

DRUG TREATMENT

Standard therapy with corticosteroids and salicylates

For more than 30 years corticosteroids and salicylates have formed the cornerstone of the medical therapy of active disease. Both groups of drugs appear to act via several different mechanisms involved in the immune/inflammatory cascade, which accounts for their potent effects (Parillo & Fauci 1979, Greenfield et al 1993). In view of the variety of different preparations now available for both oral and topical use, there is a large number of possible permutations for combination therapy. Oral salicylates will be employed in most attacks, either at the standard maintenance dose or at higher doses, which are probably more effective during an acute attack (see below). Treatment with oral steroids is usual in moderate attacks, and should be introduced early on in mild attacks if other therapy is ineffective. Topical treatment with either corticosteroids or salicylates is usually employed in all attacks, irrespective of disease extent. Even in extensive ulcerative colitis they may produce symptomatic benefit by reducing distal inflammation, thus improving rectal compliance and the sense of urgency to defecate.

Salicylates

Most controlled clinical trials have included patients with both mild and moderately active disease, and in practice the approach to treatment in both is similar. The aim is to induce remission as quickly as possible with a minimum of side effects. Early studies demonstrated the efficacy of sulfasalazine as monotherapy in active disease (Baron et al 1962b), although it is less effective than corticosteroids (Lennard-Jones et al 1960, Truelove et al 1962). Since then, numerous trials have indicated that the newer salicylates are at least as effective as sulfasalazine in acute ulcerative colitis. Examples include comparisons with olsalazine (Willoughby et al 1988) and delayed-release preparations of mesalazine (Riley et al 1988, Rachmilewitz 1989). Meta-analysis of the published trials in active disease supports the concept of increased efficacy at higher doses (Sutherland et al 1993), but the benefits gained may be outweighed by side effects. Since the efficacy of sulfasalazine and the newer 5-ASA preparations is broadly similar, irrespective of their formulation and delivery system, the choice of oral salicylate tends to be determined by the side-effect profile and local prescribing practices.

The emergence during the 1980s of topical salicylate preparations represented an important advance in the therapy of distal disease. In comparative trials daily 5-ASA enemas containing doses of up to 3 g were as effective as topical corticosteroids (Danish 5-ASA Group 1987, Mulder et al 1988), and superior efficacy was claimed for higher doses (Campieri et al 1981, 1987). There were also reports of good response rates in patients refractory to corticosteroid enemas (Friedman et al 1986, Guarino et al 1987). The choice of formulation has increased more recently to include 5-ASA suppositories and foam preparations, which are effective and well tolerated by patients (Campieri et al 1988, 1993, Williams et al 1987). Whether to use a 5-ASA or corticosteroid preparation as first-line topical therapy remains open to debate. The choice of agent will usually be determined by availability, cost and acceptability to the patient. Some experimentation is often necessary to establish the most effective treatment for a given individual.

Corticosteroids

It was shown in early trials that the efficacy of corticosteroids was greater than sulfasalazine in acute ulcerative colitis (Lennard-Jones et al 1960, Truelove et al 1962). For this reason steroids should be employed in all but the mildest of attacks. The route and mode of administration of corticosteroids will depend on the extent of disease and patient tolerance. It has long been known that disease limited to the rectum or distal colon may be effectively treated by topical steroids without recourse to oral therapy (Truelove 1958, Watkinson 1958). When inflammation is clearly limited to the rectum prednisolone in the form of suppositories is appropriate, but involvement extending to and beyond the sigmoid colon should be treated with retention enemas. Foam suspensions of hydrocortisone have been shown to be as effective as liquid enemas in distal disease, and are better tolerated by patients (Ruddell et al 1980, Somerville et al 1985). However, retrograde colonic spread of liquid enemas (Swarbrick et al 1974, Wood et al 1985) is greater than that of foam enemas, which cannot be expected to penetrate effectively beyond the sigmoid colon (Farthing et al 1979, Hay et al 1979). Nevertheless, patients with active disease may find it difficult to retain liquid enemas, of which the typical volume is 100 ml. This reflects the increase in rectal sensitivity and marked decrease in compliance which has been demonstrated in the presence of active colitis (Rao et al 1987a). Hence a reasonable approach in disease involving the sigmoid colon and beyond is to use a foam enema initially and then to progress to a liquid preparation of increasing volume.

An important development has been the introduction of corticosteroids with low systemic bioavailability for topical use. As a consequence of either poor absorption or extensive local or first-pass hepatic metabolism, these new agents do not give rise to appreciable circulating levels of exogenous steroid, and thus avoid possible adrenal suppression and other unwanted steroid side effects. Enemas of budesonide and prednisolone metasulfobenzoate have been shown to be at least as effective as standard prednisolone phosphate in patients with active distal disease (McIntyre et al 1985, Danielsson et al 1987, Danish Budesonide Study Group 1991) and are now commercially available in several countries. Similar encouraging results have been obtained with tixocortol pivalate (Hanauer et al 1986) and beclomethasone dipropionate (van der Heide et al 1988), although neither preparation has entered widespread use.

Left-sided and more extensive colitis responds better to oral than to topical corticosteroid therapy (Lennard-Jones et al 1960, Misiewicz et al 1964), so that a combination of oral and local treatment is most appropriate in this setting. Oral steroids should also be used in those patients with distal disease who fail to settle promptly with topical therapy. An early dose-ranging trial demonstrated that 40 mg daily was more effective than 20 mg daily and gave rise to fewer side effects than 60 mg daily (Baron et al 1962a). The dose of oral prednisolone employed varies between clinicians but typical current practice is to use a dose of between 20 mg and 40 mg daily for 4–6 weeks and then taper off. The best response to oral corticosteroid is seen in patients with mild disease in their first attack, the majority of whom will be in symptomatic remission after 6 weeks (Truelove & Witts 1955). The efficacy of standard and enteric-coated oral prednisolone is similar, although the latter is preferred to reduce the incidence of upper gastrointestinal side effects.

Combined topical therapy

A recent randomized controlled trial of a combined enema of beclomethasone (3 mg) and 5-ASA (1 g) showed that combination therapy was superior to either treatment alone (Mulder et al 1994), with no side effects reported. Further trials of combined corticosteroid and salicylates administered topically would appear to be warranted. This approach to treatment may prove to be of particular value in patients with previously refractory distal disease (see below).

Suggested regimens of corticosteroids and salicylates for the treatment of mild and moderately active ulcerative colitis are shown in Table 61.3.

Chronic active disease

The approach outlined above for the management of acute attacks will result in remission being achieved in the majority of patients. Nevertheless, in formal clinical trials up to half of patients treated with corticosteroid equivalent to prednisolone 40 mg daily failed to achieve remission after 4–8 weeks (Truelove & Witts 1955, Baron et al 1962a, Powell-Tuck et al 1978). Among those patients not entering remission, different patterns of disease may emerge. For those with refractory extensive colitis which displays little or no response to therapy, the preferred option is hospital admission for parenteral treatment and consideration of surgery. Other patients may exhibit a steroid-dependent pattern, which is characterized by an initial response followed by relapse on tapering the dose of oral prednisolone. This group, together with those who tend to relapse as soon as steroids are discontinued, may benefit from the addition of immunosuppressive therapy. The value of both azathioprine and its active metabolite 6-mercaptopurine (6-MP) as steroid-sparing agents in chronic active disease has been demonstrated in a number of clinical trials (Rosenberg et al 1975, Kirk & Lennard-Jones 1982, Adler & Korelitz 1990). The doses employed varied between 1.5 and 2.5 mg/kg daily. The typical time to onset of action was approximately 2 months, and up to half of the patients treated overall were able to achieve steroid-free remission. A subsequent study has highlighted the benefit of continuing treatment

Table 61.3 Suggested regimens for treatment with salicylate and corticosteroid preparations in mild to moderately active ulcerative colitis

	Mild	Moderate
Proctitis	Oral salicylate Corticosteroid and/or salicylate suppository or foam/liquid enema	Oral salicylate Oral prednisolone 20–40 mg daily Corticosteroid and/or salicylate suppository or foam/liquid enema
Proctosigmoiditis	Oral salicylate Corticosteroid and/or salicylate foam/liquid enema	Oral salicylate Oral prednisolone 20–40 mg daily Corticosteroid and/or salicylate foam/liquid enema
Left-sided and extensive colitis	Oral salicylate Oral prednisolone 20–40 mg daily Corticosteroid and/or salicylate foam/liquid enema	Oral salicylate Oral prednisolone 20–40 mg daily Corticosteroid and/or salicylate foam/liquid enema

Combined oral and topical therapy is suggested for all grades of disease, although treatment by either route alone may also be effective. Salicylate doses may be increased from maintenance to therapeutic levels, side effects allowing. Oral prednisolone should be tapered off after 4 weeks and discontinued after approximately 8 weeks. Continued maintenance on low-dose prednisolone is not recommended.

once remission has been reached, since withdrawal of azathioprine leads to a significant relapse rate (Hawthorne et al 1992). Common clinical practice is to commence azathioprine or 6-MP at doses of up to 2 and 1.5 mg/kg daily respectively (usual maximum 150 mg), and to maintain concurrent oral corticosteroid treatment for at least 1 month before tapering it off. There are no clear guidelines as to how long to continue azathioprine or 6-MP thereafter. Concern about bone-marrow suppression and possible carcinogenicity (see below) influences many clinicians to withdraw immunosuppression after a period of 2–3 years if treatment has been successful. Alternatively, if no useful steroid-sparing effect has become evident by 6 months, it seems reasonable to assume lack of efficacy and withdraw the drug.

The principles outlined above apply to chronic active or steroid-dependent ulcerative colitis of any extent. However, for patients with distal disease a variety of novel topical treatments have increased the therapeutic options available to the clinician. These are discussed in greater detail in the following section.

Proctitis and proctosigmoiditis: special considerations

Refractory distal disease

For ulcerative colitis limited to the distal colon which is refractory to standard or immunosuppressive therapy, there is a natural reluctance on the part of clinicians and patients to resort to colectomy. This has stimulated investigators to develop new topical treatments, although none have been shown convincingly to benefit the subgroup of patients who are refractory to conventional therapy. Many of the agents described below have been associated with a positive response in open label studies. However, when subjected to randomized trials against placebo or other drugs the results have often been less impressive. Thus clinicians should be aware that a high placebo response rate is not unusual for trials of topical therapy, and this needs to be borne in mind when evaluating uncontrolled data.

The recognition of the efficacy of cyclosporin A in preventing rejection of transplanted organs led to its use in various diseases thought to have an immunological basis. Encouraging results were reported from open trials in refractory disease with cyclosporin A enemas using doses up to 350 mg daily, although a tendency to relapse following discontinuation of therapy was a common finding (Brynskov et al 1989, Sandborn et al 1993a, Winter et al 1993). However, when subjected to a randomized placebo-controlled trial in mild to moderately active left-sided ulcerative colitis, cyclosporin A enemas showed no convincing benefit (Sandborn et al 1994). Eight out of 20 patients in the treatment group improved, compared to nine of 20 given placebo. The value of cyclosporin enemas in refractory distal disease therefore remains unproven, and a multicenter controlled trial will be necessary to address this issue. In the meantime, it would seem reasonable to use cyclosporin enemas in patients with rectosigmoid disease unresponsive to other measures, since systemic absorption of the drug is minimal and side effects were not prominent in the studies described above. Patients are provided with powdered cyclosporin and shown how to add this to the enema vehicle (carboxymethylcellulose sodium 630 mg, sorbitol 5.5 g in 100 ml sterile water), allowing them to make up the enemas at home prior to use.

Observations suggesting abnormal butyrate metabolism of the colonic epithelium in ulcerative colitis have supported the concept of an 'energy-deficiency disease' (Roediger 1980, Chapman et al 1994). Trials of butyrate enemas (80–100 mmol) in refractory left-sided colitis have yielded promising results (Scheppach et al 1992, Steinhardt et al 1994). Ten out of ten and three of seven patients respectively with distal colitis unresponsive to other therapy improved according to a variety of different parameters. In the first of these studies, randomized crossover treatment with placebo was ineffective. However, true blinding of butyrate treatment is very difficult because of its characteristic strong odor, and thus trials may become biased towards the treatment arm. No adverse effects have been noted to date with topical butyrate, and hence this mode of treatment may be worth trying.

Two studies have indicated the efficacy of the arsenical compound acetarsol in suppository form for treating proctitis. An early randomized trial demonstrated that 500 mg acetarsol daily was at least as effective as prednisolone suppositories: 18 out of 20 patients with idiopathic proctitis showed improvement during the 3-week course of treatment (Connell et al 1965). More recently, an open study of ten patients with 'intractable' proctitis was described (Forbes et al 1989). The same dose of acetarsol was employed and nine patients achieved clinical remission within 2 weeks. The only side effect noted during the treatment course of 4 weeks was a single episode of thrombocytosis, although potentially hazardous levels of blood and urinary arsenic were noted in several patients. Acetarsol suppositories are not commercially available but may be prepared by the hospital pharmacy (Lennard-Jones 1984).

The well known therapeutic effects of sucralfate in the upper gastrointestinal tract prompted studies of its use in distal colitis. Riley et al (1989) compared a daily enema of 4 g with 20 mg enemas of prednisolone metasulfobenzoate (PMSB). Although sucralfate-treated patients responded, the effect was less than in those given PMSB. Kochar et al (1990) tried sucralfate enemas (2 g daily) in a group of patients with ulcerative diseases of the distal colon of various etiologies which were refractory to topical therapy with corticosteroids. All five patients with ulcerative proctitis improved, but measures of clinical and histological disease activity were not described.

The proven efficacy of bismuth salts in the treatment of peptic ulcer disease has led to trials of topical therapy in distal ulcerative colitis. Bismuth subsalicylate enemas 700–800 mg twice daily produced clinical and sigmoidoscopic remission in six out of 15 patients with distal disease, previously refractory to conventional therapy, who were treated for 8 weeks in an open trial (Ryder et al 1990). A subsequent controlled trial showed that bismuth citrate-carbomer enemas were as effective as 5-ASA enemas in a group of unselected patients with distal ulcerative colitis (Pullan et al 1993). Approximately half of those treated with bismuth achieved remission and no problems with toxicity were reported.

It has been suggested that some cases of proctitis may have an allergic basis and that they can be distinguished by the finding of increased numbers of IgE-positive plasma cells in the rectal mucosa (Rosekrans et al 1980). Although treatment with oral disodium cromoglycate (DSCG) was associated with clinical improvement in these patients, other trials of oral DSCG in unselected patients with active ulcerative colitis have been disappointing (Buckell et al 1978, Binder et al 1981). Topical treatment with DSCG enemas in active distal disease was associated with a positive clinical response in two trials (Heatley et al 1975, Grace et al 1987), although in the former study the effect was no greater than that of standard prednisolone enemas.

An impressive response rate to topical treatment with lidocaine gel (800 mg daily) has been reported in a large but uncontrolled series (Bjorck et al 1992). Of 77 patients with distal disease – many of whom had been refractory to previous treatment – nearly all responded to lidocaine, although subsequent relapse rates were high. The mechanism of action is unclear, but may reflect the importance of neural and immune interactions in the generation of inflammation. As yet little is known of this area in the context of inflammatory bowel disease. Ropivacaine, a local anesthetic of the same class as lidocaine, is currently under clinical trial.

In conclusion, clinicians now have a wide choice of alternative topical therapies in ulcerative colitis. From the available data, it would appear that bismuth, butyrate, cyclosporin A and possibly sucralfate enemas can be used safely and with a good chance of improvement in patients with refractory distal disease. Nevertheless, further controlled studies and toxicity data are clearly required. For disease limited to the rectum, acetarsol suppositories have demonstrable efficacy in short courses but their use is likely to be curtailed by fears of toxicity.

Motility disturbance and proximal constipation

Several observers have noted disturbances of colonic motility in active ulcerative colitis. Using radio-opaque markers Rao et al (1987b) showed that transit in the proximal colon was delayed in patients with active colitis, irrespective of disease extent. Clinically this may be a more significant problem in patients with distal disease. Plain radiography suggests that approximately 30% of patients with active distal ulcerative colitis will have proximal colonic stasis as judged by fecal residue in the right colon (Lennard-Jones et al 1962, Jalan et al 1970).

The physiological basis for this phenomenon of 'proximal constipation' in patients with active distal disease remains unexplained. Patients may complain of abdominal bloating and discomfort, and although frequently opening their bowels to pass blood and mucus, may not pass recognizable stools. Palpation may elicit tenderness or an ill-defined mass on the right side of the abdomen, and fecal loading of the proximal colon can readily be confirmed by plain radiography. Empirical treatment with bulking agents or mild laxatives will provide relief in many instances. It should be remembered that lactulose may cause a fall in intraluminal pH and therefore interfere with the release of pH-dependent salicylate formulations. For more stubborn constipation an alternative approach is to use sodium picosulphate or similar osmotic laxative in single or repeated doses. Clearly this treatment is inappropriate in the presence of mechanical obstruction caused by a distal colonic stricture. Whether relief of proximal constipation actually promotes healing of active distal ulcerative colitis as well as providing symptomatic improvement is open to question. In theory it will enhance the colonic transit of orally administered salicylates, and thus enable higher levels to be achieved distally.

Failure to respond to medical therapy

There are a number of reasons, other than refractory disease, which may account for a failure of response to standard treatment.

First, it is important to establish that the patient is compliant. There is understandable reluctance in some cases to take oral corticosteroids, and patients with newly diagnosed ulcerative colitis may find it difficult or distasteful to use topical preparations. Care needs to be taken in explaining the rationale and technique for using rectally administered drugs. Prewarming of liquid enemas by placing the container in a basin of water may be useful for patients who experience difficulty or discomfort on administering large volumes of 100 ml or more. Alternatively, a switch to foam or suppositories may be better tolerated in the initial stages of treating active distal disease. Liquid enemas are best administered while lying on the left side at bedtime. Subsequent alterations in posture will promote retrograde spread of the enema (Matts & Gaskell 1961).

Secondly, it should be considered whether there are additional causes of persistent symptoms other than active colitis. In this context repeat sigmoidoscopy is useful to confirm ongoing macroscopic inflammation. Even if the appearances of the rectal mucosa are unremarkable, histology may reveal persisting active disease and thus biopsies should always be taken. Continuing diarrhea in the absence of active rectal inflammation should raise the possibility of proximal extension of previously limited disease, or suggest alternative diagnoses. Colonic carcinoma, Crohn's colitis and celiac disease may all be responsible for ongoing symptoms; hence colonoscopy or barium enema and distal duodenal biopsy have a role in managing this group of patients. Persisting diarrhea is a recognized dose-dependent side effect of treatment with salicylates, and in some cases sulfasalazine and 5-ASA drugs may exacerbate or precipitate active disease (Adler 1982, Schwartz et al 1982, Austin et al 1984). For similar reasons non-steroidal anti-inflammatory drugs and broad-spectrum antibiotics should be used with care in patients with ulcerative colitis (Isgar et al 1983, Kaufmann & Taubin 1987). Thus it is important to review the drug history of patients with ongoing symptoms and consider selectively withdrawing those agents considered as potential causes. Hypolactasia or specific food intolerances are other possibilities to consider, and lactose-free or formal exclusion diets may be worthwhile in these circumstances. Irritable bowel syndrome may also cause confusion and should be managed in the conventional manner. Finally, exclusion of venereal causes of proctitis (especially gonococcal and chlamydial infection) should also be considered.

Treatment of extraintestinal manifestations in active disease

The extraintestinal manifestations of ulcerative colitis are dealt with in detail elsewhere in this volume. Those which reflect the activity of colonic disease include arthritis (not ankylosing spondylitis or sacroiliitis), episcleritis, uveitis, erythema nodosum and oral aphthous ulceration. Clustering of ocular and skin manifestations together with arthritis is a well known phenomenon (Kelley 1962, Palumbo et al 1973) and presumably reflects a common underlying genetic predisposition, although none has as yet been described. In general these extraintestinal manifestations respond to treatment of the underlying colitis. An important exception to this rule is uveitis which, unlike episcleritis, may threaten visual acuity as a result of the development of posterior synechiae. Evidence of past or present uveitis was reported in nearly 12% of one large series (Wright et al 1965). The onset of uveitis tends to be acute and painful, with blurring of vision and headaches. Suspected cases should be referred for urgent ophthalmic assessment for slit lamp examination to allow appropriate treatment with topical steroids and mydriatics. When arthralgia is slow to settle, simple analgesics, judiciously used non-steroidal inflammatory drugs or oral corticosteroids may be necessary for symptomatic relief. Troublesome mouth ulcers can be treated with analgesic mouthwashes or corticosteroid lozenges.

Adverse effects of standard medical therapy

It is important to counsel patients at the outset of treatment regarding the potential side effects of their medication. Recognition of a serious adverse event in association with the treatment of ulcerative colitis should be notified to the appropriate body (the Committee on Safety of Medicines in the UK, Food and Drug Administration in the USA). This principle applies equally to widely described as well as rare reactions. The most clinically prominent and serious reactions ascribed to drugs used in ulcerative colitis are discussed here, together with data relating to screening and prevention.

Salicylates

A full description of adverse events which can be ascribed to the oral aminosalicylates is found elsewhere in this volume. Common to this group are problems with headache, nausea and exacerbation of diarrhea, all of which appear to be dose dependent and thus are more prevalent at the higher doses which may be used in active disease. If these side effects are encountered with sulfasalazine they may be ameliorated by changing to the enteric-coated preparation. Diarrhea may be especially troublesome with olsalazine, which has been shown to stimulate sodium and water secretion in the terminal ileum (Goerg et al 1987). Patients experiencing this problem should be advised to take their medication with food or to reduce the dose.

Adverse reactions to sulfasalazine are common, occurring in up to half of those taking therapeutic doses (Taffet & Das 1983). The majority of reactions unique to sulfasalazine are dose related and so tend to occur in patients of slow-acetylator status in whom hepatic metabolism of the sulfapyridine moiety is relatively impaired. It is not usual clinical practice to test for acetylator phenotype but to reduce or withdraw sulfasalazine when suspected side effects occur. Periodic full blood counts are advisable to screen for megaloblastic anemia due to folate deficiency and Heinz body hemolytic anemia, both of which are more common at higher doses of sulfasalazine (Das et al 1973, van Hess et al 1979, Grieco et al 1986, Logan et al 1986). It is also advisable to check the blood count in the first 3 months after initiating therapy, when the rare but potentially fatal complication of agranulocytosis has been reported to occur (Jamshidi et al 1972). Oligospermia with sulfasalazine is well recognized but appears to be reversible on withdrawing the drug (Levi et al 1979) and does not recur when mesalazine is substituted (Kjaergaard et al 1989). In general, side effects other than those ascribed to the salicylate moiety tend not to recur when changing from sulfasalazine to a 5-ASA preparation, although there have been occasional case reports of recurrent severe hypersensitivity reactions (Poldermans & van Blankenstein 1988, Hautekeete et al 1992).

Nephrotoxicity is emerging as a serious potential complication of treatment with the delayed-release preparations of mesalazine, which tend to give rise to high peak serum levels of 5-ASA. An early indication of this problem was the finding of a reversible rise in serum creatinine in two patients taking 2.4 g daily of Asacol in a study of active disease (Riley et al 1988). The effect appears to be unpredictable, and it is not clear whether simple tests of renal function or measurements of urinary protein excretion will be useful in detecting patients at risk. A study of creatinine clearance and urinary protein and tubular enzyme excretion failed to show any differences between a group of patients maintained on doses of mesalazine up to 2.4 g daily compared to others taking sulfasalazine (Riley et al 1992). Until more is known of the mechanism of renal damage, it is advisable to avoid delayed-release 5-ASA preparations in patients with pre-existing renal disease or diabetes, and in the elderly.

Systemic absorption of rectally administered salicylates is low. In one study 10% of the administered dose of 5-ASA was recovered in the urine of patients with active disease compared to 19% in those in remission (Campieri et al 1985). Accordingly, side effects with topical treatment are uncommon, and most patients intolerant of or allergic to oral sulfasalazine are able to use 5-ASA enemas without ill effect (Campieri et al 1984). The main problems encountered with topical preparations relate to pain or discomfort on insertion of plastic tubing, or the delivery of large-volume enemas.

Corticosteroids

The adverse effects of steroids are well known and reflect unwanted systemic effects of this group of agents in a variety of different organ systems. Most problems are encountered with oral treatment, but significant systemic absorption of topical corticosteroids is also recognized (Powell-Tuck et al 1976, Sampson & Brooke 1963, Cann & Holdsworth 1987) and could thus potentially contribute to side effects if continued over a prolonged period. There seems little justification for continuing treatment with corticosteroids for more than 3 months at a time, and long-term steroid therapy for chronic active disease should be discouraged, even at doses below 10 mg prednisolone equivalent daily by mouth.

With increasing numbers of middle-aged and elderly patients who have been treated with corticosteroids there is some concern regarding the effects of prolonged or repeated courses of therapy on bone mass. The first study of hormone replacement therapy (HRT) in post-menopausal women with inflammatory bowel disease demonstrated improvements in both radial and spinal bone density over a 2-year period (Clements et al 1993). The small number of patients treated with prednisolone as well as HRT during this period had lower rates of change of spinal bone density. Clearly, controlled studies will be required to assess the efficacy of HRT in preventing corticosteroid-induced osteoporosis. For patients other than postmenopausal women, recommended measures for preventing osteoporosis include adequate dietary intake of calcium and vitamin D, moderate exercise and cessation of smoking. The potential role of vitamin D supplementation, sodium fluoride and biphosphonates in treating established osteoporosis in ulcerative colitis remains uncertain, although studies in other chronic steroid-sensitive diseases may provide useful indicators. Greater understanding of the causes and prevention of osteoporosis may lead to measurements of bone density becoming routine for identifying those patients at high risk of developing osteoporosis or bone fractures.

Azathioprine and 6-mercaptopurine

As a result of side effects, approximately 10% of patients in two large studies were unable to take these drugs when administered for Crohn's disease at doses of up to 2.5 mg/kg (Singleton et al 1979, Present et al 1980). Nausea, fever, leukopenia, myalgia and pancreatitis are well recognized reactions, but others, including hepatotoxicity and polyneuropathy, have also been described. Toxicity is more likely if allopurinol is also being taken, since this inhibitor of xanthine oxidase delays the metabolism of azathioprine and 6-MP. When introducing these drugs for the first time it may be advisable to commence at a low dose (0.5–1 mg/kg) and increase to the full maintenance dose over a period of weeks, side effects allowing.

Perhaps the major concern regarding azathioprine and 6-MP is their potential for bone marrow suppression. In the largest series reported to date, the St Mark's group found that 3.8% of 739 patients treated with azathioprine 2 mg/kg/day for up to 11 years developed leukopenia, of whom two died from septicemia (Connell et al 1993). An important observation was that bone marrow toxicity could occur at any time during treatment, even after many years without previous adverse effects. It is thought that the susceptibility of a small group of patients to myelotoxicity is due to a genetically determined low level of activity of the enzyme thiopurine-methyltransferase (TPMT), which partly inactivates 6-MP by methylation (Lennard et al 1989). It is not common practice to assay the levels of TPMT before commencing azathioprine or 6-MP, but rather to check the full blood count at weekly intervals for the first month after commencing the drugs, and monthly thereafter for the duration of treatment.

Another concern regarding long-term therapy with azathioprine is whether it predisposes to neoplasia, especially non-Hodgkin's lymphoma, which is a recognized problem in patients following organ transplantation. Among the cohort of 755 patients reviewed by Connell et al (1994) who had been treated with azathioprine for up to 15 years and were followed up for a median of 9 years, no excess cancer risk was detected and there were no lymphomas. These data are reassuring, but longer-term follow-up will be necessary for confirmation.

Whether azathioprine has teratogenic potential in patients with inflammatory bowel disease remains unknown. However, several normal pregnancies have occurred during treatment with this drug (Alstead et al 1989) and there are no reports of teratogenicity from other groups of patients treated with azathioprine and 6-MP. Whether to advise withdrawal of these drugs before conception is planned is at present uncertain, and will depend on the wishes of the patient as well as the consequences of disease relapse. Stopping azathioprine or 6-MP during gestation is likely to be more hazardous, since relapse may threaten the outcome of the pregnancy (Willoughby & Truelove 1980, Jarnerot 1982).

Novel agents for the treatment of active ulcerative colitis

Several different classes of drugs are currently under investigation. Of these perhaps the most promising are the new corticosteroids, which have much lower bioavailability than their conventional counterparts. Increased understanding of the pathophysiology of ulcerative colitis has also led to the development of new agents which are designed to influence specific pathways in the immune–inflammatory cascade. The following description of new compounds highlights those which may have particular clinical potential.

Immunosuppressants

The role of cyclosporin enemas is discussed above in the context of refractory distal disease. Intravenous cyclosporin for severe disease is considered in detail elsewhere in this volume. There is little other than anecdotal data concerning the use of oral cyclosporin in active ulcerative colitis. However, in a recently published placebo-controlled trial investigating the effect of oral cyclosporin on primary sclerosing cholangitis, it was found that there was a significant clinical improvement in coexisting ulcerative colitis (Sandborn et al 1993b). Disease activity was measured by the Truelove–Witts criteria during the treatment period, which was at least 1 year. The initial dose used was 5 mg/kg/day which was reduced to a mean of 4.1 mg/kg/day because of dose adjustments to maintain trough blood levels between 80 and 120 ng/ml. Side effects were common with cyclosporin: at least a quarter of patients reported headache and paresthesiae, and tremor, gingival hyperplasia, severe nausea, hypertension and renal impairment were also recorded. Despite this discouraging side-effect profile no controlled trial has yet been undertaken in patients with chronic active or refractory disease who might perhaps be expected to gain most benefit from treatment. Use of this agent should be limited to the context of clinical trials until further data are available.

The role of methotrexate has also been investigated recently in patients with inflammatory bowel disease. Experience to date in ulcerative colitis has been limited to two uncontrolled studies which suggested some response in patients with refractory disease during intramuscular treatment. A dose of 25 mg was given weekly for 12 weeks, followed by conversion to oral therapy (Kozarek et al 1989, 1992). Placebo-controlled trials are clearly required.

A pilot study of humanized antitumor necrosis factor monoclonal antibodies has been reported recently in a small number of patients with Crohn's disease (van Dullemen et al 1994). The results were extremely encouraging and side effects were minimal. Similar results were found in another small pilot study of anti-CD4 monoclonal antibodies in patients with refractory inflammatory bowel disease (Emmrich et al 1991). It is anticipated that controlled trials of these agents will follow soon in both Crohn's disease and ulcerative colitis.

Corticosteroids with low bioavailability

The potential advantages of the new corticosteroids with low bioavailability are clear, and rectal preparations with demonstrable efficacy and minimal side effects have become established in some countries for the treatment of distal ulcerative colitis. Development of the same agents in oral form is under progress and early trial data are now available. A preliminary open label study of enteric-coated prednisolone metasulfobenzoate in active ulcerative colitis suggested very low systemic absorption and a favorable clinical response (Ford et al 1992). A placebo-controlled trial of oral fluticasone proprionate 20 mg daily showed it to be ineffective in active ulcerative colitis (Angus et al 1992), and a subsequent study using the same dose demonstrated less efficacy than a standard tapering dose of oral prednisolone (Hawthorne et al 1993). Since fluticasone is poorly absorbed and is subject to high first-pass hepatic metabolism it would seem reasonable to carry out further dose-ranging studies, but further development of this drug has been halted. A stable oral formulation of budesonide is now available and trial data are awaited with interest.

Anti-inflammatory drugs

The recognition that a variety of potent lipid-derived inflammatory mediators are found at high levels in active ulcerative colitis has stimulated interest in drugs which interfere with specific steps in lipid metabolism. These include inhibitors of the arachidonic acid pathway, which gives rise to prostaglandins and leukotrienes, and antagonists of platelet-activating factor. There are no data as yet to suggest that the new anti-inflammatories have greater efficacy than corticosteroids or the salicylates in the treatment of ulcerative colitis. One of the new compounds is zileuton, a selective inhibitor of 5-lipoxygenase, which has recently been subjected to clinical trial. In a double-blind study 25% of patients with moderately active ulcerative colitis treated with a dose of 2.4 g daily achieved clinical remission, compared to 13% of those on a lower dose and 7% treated with placebo (Peppercorn et al 1994). Further trials at higher doses and comparisons with standard therapy will be required before the therapeutic role of zileuton is established. However, trials with a more potent 5-lipoxygenase-activating protein (FLAP) inhibitor produced nearly 100% LTB_4 inhibition without significant impact on symptoms or mucosal inflammation.

Nicotine

Epidemiological observations which demonstrated an inverse relationship between smoking habits and the incidence of ulcerative colitis raised the possibility that agents in cigarette smoke were exerting a therapeutic effect in the disease. Transdermal nicotine has subsequently been shown to improve active disease in a placebo-controlled trial (Pullan et al 1994): 17 out of 35 treated patients entered remission during a 6-week period compared to nine of 37 given placebo. Unfortunately, the same group failed to demonstrate a maintenance benefit from continuing on the same nicotine patch. Problematic side effects included nausea, headache and sleep disturbance, but these results are of considerable interest and may lead to the development of new approaches to treatment. Nicotine patches and chewing gum which are currently available on prescription for helping patients to stop smoking are not licensed for use in ulcerative colitis.

Antibiotics

Several investigators have explored the role of broad-spectrum antibiotics on the assumption that the colonic flora may play a role in perpetuating inflammation. A number of studies have demonstrated the presence of increased numbers of enteroadherent coliforms in ulcerative colitis (Dickinson et al 1980b, Burke & Axon 1988, Giaffer et al 1992). It is postulated that the quality of adhesiveness to epithelial cells may confer pathogenicity. Intravenous regimens have been ineffective in controlled trials in patients with severe disease (Chapman et al 1986, Mantzaris et al 1994), but oral tobramycin was reported to improve the outcome in a double-blind study when added for 1 week to standard steroid therapy (Burke et al 1990). At present the role of antibiotic treatment in ulcerative colitis remains uncertain, but better understanding of the relationship between enteric bacteria and the colonic epithelium may lead to powerful new therapeutic approaches.

REFERENCES

Adler D J, Korelitz B I 1990 The therapeutic efficacy of 6-mercaptopurine in refractory ulcerative colitis. American Journal of Gastroenterology 85: 717–722

Adler R B 1982 Sulphasalazine-induced exacerbation of ulcerative colitis. New England Journal of Medicine 307: 315

Alstead E M, Ritchie J K, Lennard-Jones J E, Farthing M J F, Clark M L 1989 Pregnancy in inflammatory bowel disease patients on azathioprine. Gut 30: 718

Angus P, Snook J A, Reid M, Jewell D P 1992 Oral fluticasone propionate in active distal ulcerative colitis. Gut 33: 711–714

Austin C A, Cann P A, Jones T H, Holdsworth C D 1984 Exacerbation of diarrhoea and pain in patients treated with 5-aminosalicylic acid for ulcerative colitis. Lancet i: 917–918

Baron J H, Connell A M, Kanaghinis T G, Lennard-Jones J E, Jones F A 1962a Out-patient treatment of ulcerative colitis: comparison between three doses of oral prednisolone. British Medical Journal ii: 441–443

Baron J H, Connell A M, Lennard-Jones J E, Jones F A 1962b Sulphasalazine and salicylazosulphadimidine in ulcerative colitis. Lancet i: 1094–1096

Bartram C I 1976 Plain abdominal X-ray in acute colitis. Proceedings of the Royal Society of Medicine 69: 617–618

Binder V, Elsborg L, Greibe J et al 1981 Disodium cromoglycate in the treatment of ulcerative colitis and Crohn's disease. Gut 22: 55–60

Bjorck S, Dahlstrom A, Johansson L, Ahlman H 1992 Treatment of the mucosa with local anaesthetics in ulcerative colitis. Agents and Actions (Special Conference Issue): C60–75

Both H, Torp-Pedersen K, Kreiner S, Hendriksen C, Binder V 1983 Clinical appearances at diagnosis of ulcerative colitis and Crohn's disease in a regional patient group. Scandinavian Journal of Gastroenterology 18: 987–991

Brynskov J, Freund L, Thomsen O O, Andersen C B, Rasmussen S N, Binder V 1989 Treatment of refractory ulcerative colitis with cyclosporin enemas. Lancet i: 721–722

Buckell N A, Gould S R, Day D W, Lennard-Jones J E, Edwards A M 1978 Controlled trial of disodium cromoglycate in chronic persistent ulcerative colitis. Gut 19: 1140–1143

Burke D A, Axon A T R 1988 Adhesive *Escherischia coli* in inflammatory bowel disease and infective diarrhoea. British Medical Journal 297: 102–104

Burke D A, Axon A T R, Clayden S A, Dixon M F, Johnston D, Lacey R W 1990 The efficacy of tobramycin in the treatment of ulcerative colitis. Alimentary Pharmacology and Therapeutics 4: 123–129

Busk H E, Dahlerup B, Lytzen T, Binder V, Gudmandhoyer E 1975 The incidence of lactose malabsorption in ulcerative colitis. Scandinavian Journal of Gastroenterology 10: 263–265

Campieri M, Gionchetti P, Belluzzi A et al 1987 Efficacy of 5-aminosalicylic acid enemas versus hydrocortisone enemas in ulcerative colitis. Digestive Diseases and Sciences 32: 675–705

Campieri M, Gionchetti P, Belluzzi et al 1988 5-aminosalicylic acid as enemas or suppositories in distal ulcerative colitis. Journal of Clinical Gastroenterology 10: 406–409

Campieri M, Lanfranchi G A, Bazzocchi G et al 1981 Treatment of ulcerative colitis with high-dose 5-aminosalicylic acid enemas. Lancet ii: 270–271

Campieri M, Lanfranchi G A, Boschi S et al 1985 Topical administration of 5-aminosalicylic acid enemas in patients with ulcerative colitis. Studies on rectal absorption and excretion. Gut 26: 400–405

Campieri M, Lanfranchi G A, Brignola C, Bazzocchi G, Minguzzi M R, Calari M T 1984 5-aminosalicylic acid as rectal enema in ulcerative colitis patients unable to take sulphasalazine. Lancet i: 403

Campieri M, Paoluzi P, D'Albasio G, Brunetti G, Pera A, Barbara L 1993 Better quality of therapy with 5-ASA colonic foam in active ulcerative colitis. A multicenter comparative trial with 5-ASA enema. Digestive Diseases and Sciences 38: 1843–1850

Cann P A, Holdsworth C D 1987 Systemic absorption from hydrocortisone foam enema in ulcerative colitis. Lancet i: 922–923

Chapman M A S, Grahn M F, Boyle M A, Hutton M, Rogers J, Williams N S 1994 Butyrate oxidation is impaired in the colonic mucosa of sufferers of quiescent ulcerative colitis. Gut 35: 73–76

Chapman R W, Selby W S, Jewell D P 1986 Controlled trial of intravenous metronidazole as an adjunct to corticosteroids in severe ulcerative colitis. Gut 27: 1210–1212

Clements D, Compston J E, Evans W D, Rhodes J 1993 Hormone replacement therapy prevents bone loss in patients with inflammatory bowel disease. Gut 34: 1543–1546

Connell L M, Lennard-Jones J E, Misiewicz J J, Baron J H, Avery Jones F 1965 Comparison of acetarsol and prednisolone-21-phosphate suppositories in the treatment of idiopathic proctitis. Lancet i: 238–239

Connell W R, Kamm M A, Dickson M, Balkwill A M, Ritchie J K, Lennard-Jones J E 1994 Long-term neoplasia risk after azathioprine treatment in inflammatory bowel disease. Lancet 343: 1249–1252

Connell W R, Kamm M A, Ritchie J K, Lennard-Jones J E 1993 Bone marrow toxicity caused by azathioprine in inflammatory bowel disease: 27 years of experience. Gut 34: 1081–1085

Danielsson A, Hellers G, Lyrenas E et al 1987 A controlled randomized trial of budesonide versus prednisolone retention enemas in active distal ulcerative colitis. Scandinavian Journal of Gastroenterology 22: 987–992

Danish Budesonide Study Group 1991 Budesonide enema in distal ulcerative colitis. A randomized dose–response trial with prednisolone enema as a positive control. Scandinavian Journal of Gastroenterology 26: 1225–1230

Danish 5-ASA Group 1987 Topical 5-aminosalicylic acid versus prednisolone in ulcerative proctosigmoiditis. Digestive Diseases and Sciences 32: 598–602

Das K M, Eastwood M A, McManus J P A, Sircus W 1973 Adverse reactions during salicylazosulfapyridine therapy and the relation with drug metabolism and acetylator phenotype. New England Journal of Medicine 289: 491–495

Dickinson R J, Ashton M G, Axon A, Smith R C, Yeung C K, Hill G L 1980a Controlled trial of intravenous hyperalimentation and total bowel rest as an adjunct to the routine therapy of acute colitis. Gastroenterology 79: 1199–1204

Dickinson R J, Varian S A, Axon A T R, Cooke E M 1980b Increased incidence of faecal coliforms with in vitro adhesive and invasive properties in patients with ulcerative colitis. Gut 21: 787–792

Dronfield M W, Fletcher J, Langman M J S 1974 Coincident salmonella infections and ulcerative colitis: problems of recognition and management. British Medical Journal i: 99–100

Emmrich J, Seyfarth M, Fleig W E, Emmrich F 1991 Treatment of inflammatory bowel disease with anti-CD4 monoclonal antibody. Lancet 338: 570–571

Farthing M J G, Rutland M D, Clark M L 1979 Retrograde spread of hydrocortisone containing foam given intrarectally in ulcerative colitis. British Medical Journal 2: 822–824

Forbes A, Britton T C, House I M, Gazzard B G 1989 Safety and efficacy of acetarsol suppositories in unresponsive proctitis. Alimentary Pharmacology and Therapeutics 3: 553–556

Ford G A, Oliver P S, Shepherd N A, Wilkinson S P 1992 A Eudragit-coated prednisolone preparation for ulcerative colitis: pharmacokinetics and preliminary therapeutic usage. Alimentary Pharmacology and Therapeutics 6: 31–40

Friedman L S, Richter J M, Kirkham S E, DeMonaco H J, May R J 1986 5-Aminosalicylic acid enemas in refractory distal ulcerative colitis: a randomized, controlled trial. American Journal of Gastroenterology 81: 412–417

Giaffer M H, Holdsworth C D, Duerden B I 1992 Virulence properties of *Escherichia coli* strains isolated from patients with inflammatory bowel disease. Gut 33: 646–650

Goerg K J, Wanitschke R, Gabbert H, Breiling J, Franke M, Meyer zum

Buschenfelde K H 1987 Azodisalicylate (azodisal sodium) causes intestinal secretion. Digestion 37: 79–87
Grace R H, Gent A E, Hellier M D 1987 Comparative trial of sodium cromoglycate enemas with prednisolone enemas in the treatment of ulcerative colitis. Gut 28: 88–92
Greenfield S M, Punchard N A, Teare J P, Thompson R P H 1993 Review article: The mode of action of the aminosalicylates in inflammatory bowel disease. Alimentary Pharmacology and Therapeutics 7: 369–383
Grieco A, Caputo S, Bertoli A, Caradonna P, Greco A V 1986 Megaloblastic anaemia due to sulphasalazine responding to drug withdrawal alone. Postgraduate Medical Journal 62: 307–308
Gruner O P, Naas R, Glone E, Flatmark A, Fretheim B 1978 Mental disorders in ulcerative colitis. Diseases of the Colon and Rectum 21: 37–39
Guarino J, Chatzinoff M, Berk T, Friedman L S 1987 5-aminosalicylic acid enemas in refractory distal ulcerative colitis: long-term results. American Journal of Gastroenterology 82: 732–737
Hanauer S, Kirsner J B, Barrett W E 1986 The treatment of left-sided ulcerative colitis with tixocortol pivalate. Gastroenterology 90: 1449
Harries A D, Myers B, Cook G C 1985 Inflammatory bowel disease: a common cause of bloody diarrhoea in visitors to the tropics. British Medical Journal 291: 1686–1687
Hautekeete M L, Bourgeois N, Potvin P et al 1992 Hypersensitivity with hepatotoxicity to mesalazine after hypersensitivity to sulfasalazine. Gastroenterology 103: 1925–1927
Hawthorne A B, Logan R F, Hawkey C J et al 1992 Randomised controlled trial of azathioprine withdrawal in ulcerative colitis. British Medical Journal 305: 20–22
Hawthorne A B, Record C O, Holdsworth C D et al 1993 Double blind trial of oral fluticasone propionate v prednisolone in the treatment of active ulcerative colitis. Gut 34: 125–128
Hay D J, Sharma H, Irving M H 1979 Spread of steroid-containing foam after intrarectal administration. British Medical Journal i: 1751–1753
Heatley R V, Calcraft B J, Rhodes J, Owen E, Evans B K 1975 Disodium cromoglycate in the treatment of chronic proctitis. Gut 16: 559–563
Isgar B, Harman N, Whorwell P J 1983 Factors preceding relapse of ulcerative colitis. Digestion 26: 236–238
Jalan K N, Walker R J, Prescott R J, Butterworth S T G, Smith A N, Sircus W 1970 Faecal stasis and diverticular disease in ulcerative colitis. Gut 11: 688–696
Jamshidi K, Arlander T, Garcia M C, Windschitl H W, Swain W R 1972 Azulfidine agranulocytosis with bone marrow megakaryocytosis, histiocytosis and plasmacytosis. Minnesota Medicine 55: 545–548
Jarnerot G 1982 Fertility, sterility and pregnancy in chronic inflammatory bowel disease. Scandinavian Journal of Gastroenterology 17: 1–4
Kaufmann H J, Taubin H L 1987 Nonsteroidal anti-inflammatory drugs activate quiescent inflammatory bowel disease. Annals of Internal Medicine 107: 513–516
Kelley M L 1962 Skin lesions associated with chronic ulcerative colitis. American Journal of Digestive Diseases 7: 255–272
Kirk A P, Lennard-Jones J E 1982 Controlled trial of azathioprine in chronic ulcerative colitis. British Medical Journal 284: 1291–1292
Kjaergaard N, Christensen L A, Lauritsen J G, Rasmussen S N, Hansen S H 1989 Effects of mesalazine substitution on salicylazosulfapyridine-induced seminal abnormalities in men with ulcerative colitis. Scandinavian Journal of Gastroenterology 24: 891–896
Kochar R, Mehta S K, Aggarwal R, Dhar A, Patel F 1990 Sucralfate enema in ulcerative rectosigmoid lesions. Diseases of the Colon and Rectum 33: 49–51
Kozarek R A, Patterson D J, Gelfand M D, Ball T J, Botoman V A 1992 Long-term use of methotrexate in inflammatory bowel disease. Gastroenterology 102: A648
Kozarek R A, Patterson D J, Gelfand M D, Botoman V A, Ball T J, Wilske K R 1989 Methotrexate induces clinical and histologic remission in patients with refractory inflammatory bowel disease. Annals of Internal Medicine 110: 353–356
Leddin D J, Paterson W G, DaCosta L R et al 1987 Indium-111-labeled autologous leukocyte imaging and fecal excretion. Digestive Diseases and Sciences 32: 377–387
Lennard L, van Loon J A, Weinshilboum R M 1989 Pharmacogenetics of acute azathioprine toxicity: relationship to thiopurine methyltransferase genetic polymorphism. Clinical Pharmacology and Therapeutics 46: 149–154
Lennard-Jones J E 1984 Medical treatment of ulcerative colitis. Postgraduate Medical Journal 60: 797–802
Lennard-Jones J E, Langman M J S, Avery Jones F 1962 Faecal stasis in proctocolitis. Gut 3: 301–305
Lennard-Jones J E, Longmore A J, Newell A C, Wilson C W E, Jones F A 1960 An assessment of prednisolone, salazopyrine and topical hydrocortisone hemisuccinate used as out-patient treatment for ulcerative colitis. Gut 1: 217–222
Levi A J, Fisher A M, Hughes L, Hendry W F 1979 Male infertility due to sulphasalazine. Lancet ii: 276–278
Logan E C M, Williamson L M, Ryrie D R 1986 Sulphasalazine associated pancytopaenia may be caused by acute folate deficiency. Gut 27: 868–872
McIntyre P B, Macrae F A, Berghouse L, English J, Lennard-Jones J E 1985 Therapeutic benefits from a poorly absorbed prednisolone enema in distal ulcerative colitis. Gut 26: 822–824
McIntyre P B, Powell-Tuck J, Wood S R et al 1986 Controlled trial of bowel rest in the treatment of severe acute colitis. Gut 27: 481–485
McMillan A, Gilmour H M, Slatford K, McNeillage G J C 1983a Proctitis in homosexual men. A diagnostic problem. British Journal of Venereal Diseases 59: 260–264
McMillan A, McNeillage G, Gilmour H M, Lee F D 1983b Histology of rectal gonorrhoea in men, with a note on anorectal infection with *Neisseria meningitidis*. Journal of Clinical Pathology 36: 511–514
Mantzaris G J, Hatzis A, Kontogiannis P, Triadaphyllou G 1994 Intravenous tobramycin and metronidazole as an adjunct to corticosteroids in acute, severe ulcerative colitis. American Journal of Gastroenterology 89: 43–46
Matts S G F, Gaskell K H 1961 Retrograde colonic spread of enemata in ulcerative colitis. British Medical Journal ii: 614–616
Meyers S, Sachar D B, Present D H, Janowitz H D 1987 Olsalazine in the treatment of ulcerative colitis among patients intolerant of sulfasalazine: a prospective, randomized, placebo-controlled, double-blind, dose-ranging clinical trial. Gastroenterology 93: 1255–1262
Misiewicz J J, Connell A M, Lennard-Jones J E, Jones F A 1964 Comparison of oral and rectal steroids in the treatment of proctocolitis. Proceedings of the Royal Society of Medicine 57: 561–562
Mulder C, Tytgat G, Wiltink E, Houthoff H J 1988 Comparison of 5-aminosalicylic acid (3 g) and prednisolone phosphate sodium enemas (30 mg) in the treatment of distal ulcerative colitis. Scandinavian Journal of Gastroenterology 23: 1005–1008
Mulder C J J, Fockens P, van der Heide H, Tytgat G N J 1994 A controlled randomized trial of beclomethasondiproprionate (3 mg) versus 5-aminosalicylic acid (1 g) versus the combination of both (3 mg/1 g) as retention enemas in active distal ulcerative colitis. Gastroenterology 106: A739
Nordenvall B, Brostrom O, Berglund M et al 1985 Incidence of ulcerative colitis in Stockholm County 1955–1979. Scandinavian Journal of Gastroenterology 20: 783–790
Palumbo P J, Ward L E, Sauer W G, Scudamore H H 1973 Musculoskeletal manifestations of inflammatory bowel disease – ulcerative and granulomatous colitis and ulcerative proctitis. Mayo Clinic Proceedings 48: 411–416
Parillo J E, Fauci A S 1979 Mechanisms of glucocorticoid action on immune processes. Annual Reviews of Pharmacology and Toxicology 19: 179–201
Pena A S, Truelove S C 1973 Hypolactasia and ulcerative colitis. Gastroenterology 64: 400–404
Peppercorn M, Das K, Elson C et al 1994 Zileuton, a 5-lipoxygenase inhibitor, in the treatment of active ulcerative colitis: a double-blind, placebo controlled trial. Gastroenterology 106: A751
Poldermans D, van Blankenstein M 1988 Pancreatitis induced by disodium azodisalicylate. American Journal of Gastroenterology 83: 578–580
Powell-Tuck J, Brown R L, Lennard-Jones J E 1978 A comparison of oral prednisolone given as single or multiple daily doses for active proctocolitis. Scandinavian Journal of Gastroenterology 13: 833–837

Powell-Tuck J, Lennard-Jones J E, May C S, Wilson C G, Paterson J W 1976 Plasma prednisolone levels after administration of prednisolone-21-phosphate as a retention enema in colitis. British Medical Journal i: 193–195

Powell-Tuck J, Ritchie J K, Lennard-Jones J E 1977 The prognosis of idiopathic proctitis. Scandinavian Journal of Gastroenterology 12: 727–732

Present D H, Korelitz B I, Wisch N, Glass J L, Sachar D B, Pasternack B S 1980 Treatment of Crohn's disease with 6-mercaptopurine: a long-term randomized double-blind study. New England Journal of Medicine 302: 981–987

Pullan R D, Ganesh S, Mani V et al 1993 Comparison of bismuth citrate and 5-aminosalicylic acid enemas in distal ulcerative colitis: a controlled trial. Gut 34: 676–679

Pullan R D, Rhodes J, Ganesh S et al 1994 Transdermal nicotine for active ulcerative colitis. New England Journal of Medicine 330: 811–815

Rachmilewitz D 1989 Coated mesalazine (5-aminosalicylic acid) versus sulphasalazine in the treatment of active ulcerative colitis: a randomised trial. British Medical Journal 298: 82–86

Rao S S C, Read N W, Davidson P A, Bannister J J, Holdsworth C D 1987a Anorectal sensitivity and responses to rectal distension in patients with ulcerative colitis. Gastroenterology 93: 1270–1275

Rao S S C, Read N W, Holdsworth C D 1987b Studies on the mechanism of bowel disturbance in ulcerative colitis. Gastroenterology 93: 934–940

Rene E, Marche C, Chevalier T et al 1988 Cytomegalus virus colitis in patients with acquired immunodeficiency syndrome. Digestive Diseases and Sciences 33: 741–750

Riley S A, Gupta I, Mani V 1989 A comparison of sucralfate and prednisolone enemas in the treatment of active distal ulcerative colitis. Scandinavian Journal of Gastroenterology 24: 1014–1018

Riley S A, Lloyd D R, Mani V 1992 Tests of renal function in patients with quiescent colitis: effects of drug treatment. Gut 33: 1348–1352

Riley S A, Mani V, Goodman M J, Herd M E, Dutt S, Turnberg L A 1988 Comparison of delayed-release 5 aminosalicylic acid and sulphasalazine in the treatment of mild to moderate ulcerative colitis. Gut 29: 669–674

Roediger W E W 1980 The colonic epithelium in ulcerative colitis: an energy deficiency disease? Lancet 2: 712–715

Rosado J L, Solomons N W, Lisker R, Bourges H 1984 Enzyme replacement therapy for primary adult lactase deficiency. Gastroenterology 87: 1072–1082

Rosekrans P C M, Meijer C J L M, Van der Wal A M, Lindeman J 1980 Allergic proctitis, a clinical and immunopathological entity. Gut 21: 1017–1023

Rosenberg J L, Wall A J, Levin B, Binder H J, Kirsner J B 1975 A controlled trial of azathioprine in the management of chronic ulcerative colitis. Gastroenterology 69: 96–99

Ruddell W, Dickinson R J, Dixon M F, Axon A 1980 Treatment of distal ulcerative colitis (proctosigmoiditis) in relapse: comparison of hydrocortisone enemas and rectal hydrocortisone foam. Gut 21: 885–889

Ryder S D, Walker R J, Jones H, Rhodes J M 1990 Rectal bismuth subsalicylate as therapy for ulcerative colitis. Alimentary Pharmacology and Therapeutics 4: 333–338

Sampson P A, Brooke B N 1963 Absorption of hydrocortisone from the large bowel. Lancet i: 701–702

Sandborn W J, Tremaine W J, Schroeder K W et al 1994 A placebo-controlled trial of cyclosporine enemas for mildly to moderately active left-sided ulcerative colitis. Gastroenterology 106: 1429–1435

Sandborn W J, Tremaine W J, Schroeder K W, Steiner B L, Batts K P, Lawson G M 1993a Cyclosporine enemas for treatment-resistant, mildly to moderately active, left-sided ulcerative colitis. American Journal of Gastroenterology 88: 640–645

Sandborn W J, Wiesner R H, Tremaine W J, Larusso N F 1993b Ulcerative colitis disease activity following treatment of associated primary sclerosing cholangitis with cyclosporin. Gut 34: 242–246

Saverymuttu S H, Camilleri M, Rees H, Lavender J P, Hodgson H J, Chadwick V S 1986 Indium-111 granulocyte scanning in the assessment of disease extent and disease activity in inflammatory bowel disease. A comparison with colonoscopy, histology and fecal indium-111 granulocyte excretion. Gastroenterology 90: 1121–1128

Scheppach W, Sommer H, Kirchner T et al 1992 Effect of butyrate enemas on the colonic mucosa in distal ulcerative colitis. Gastroenterology 103: 51–56

Schwartz A G, Targan S R, Saxon A, Weinstein W M 1982 Sulphasalazine induced exacerbation of ulcerative colitis. New England Journal of Medicine 306: 409–412

Sinclair T S, Brunt P W, Mowat N A G 1983 Nonspecific proctocolitis in Northeastern Scotland: a community study. Gastroenterology 85: 1–11

Singleton J W, Law D H, Kelley M L, Mekhijian H S, Sturdevant R A L 1979 National Co-operative Crohn's Disease Study: adverse reactions to study drugs. Gastroenterology 77: 870–882

Somerville K W, Langman M J S, Kane S P, MacGilchrist A J, Watkinson G, Salmon P 1985 Effect of treatment on symptoms and quality of life in patients with ulcerative colitis: comparative trial of hydrocortisone acetate foam and prednisolone 21-phosphate enemas. British Medical Journal 291: 866

Steinhardt A H, Brezinski A, Baker J P 1994 Treatment of refractory ulcerative proctosigmoiditis with butyrate enemas. American Journal of Gastroenterology 89: 179–183

Sutherland L R, May G R, Shaffer E A 1993 Sulfasalazine revisited: a meta-analysis of 5-aminosalicylic acid in the treatment of ulcerative colitis. Annals of Internal Medicine 118: 540–549

Swarbrick E T, Loose H, Lennard-Jones J E 1974 Enema volume as an important factor in successful topical corticosteroid treatment of colitis. Journal of the Royal Society of Medicine 67: 23–24

Taffet S L, Das K M 1983 Sulfasalazine – adverse effects and desensitisation. Digestive Diseases and Sciences 28: 833–842

Truelove S C 1958 Treatment of ulcerative colitis with local hydrocortisone hemisuccinate sodium: a report on a controlled therapeutic trial. British Medical Journal ii: 1072–1077

Truelove S C 1961 Ulcerative colitis provoked by milk. British Medical Journal i: 154–160

Truelove S C, Watkinson G, Draper G 1962 Comparison of corticosteroid and sulphasalazine therapy in ulcerative colitis. British Medical Journal ii: 1708–1711

Truelove S C, Witts L J 1955 Cortisone in ulcerative colitis. Final report on a therapeutic trial. British Medical Journal ii: 1041–1048

van der Heide H, van den Brandt-Gradel V, Tytgat G N J et al 1988 Comparison of beclomethasone dipropionate and prednisolone 21-phosphate enemas in the treatment of ulcerative proctitis. Journal of Clinical Gastroenterology 10: 169–172

van Dullemen H M, Hommes D W, Meenan J et al 1994 Complete remissions of steroid-refractory Crohn's disease after administration of monoclonal anti- TNF antibody cA2. Gastroenterology 106: A1054

van Hess P A, van Elferen L W, van Rossum J M, van Tongeren J H 1979 Hemolysis during salicylazosulfapyridine therapy. American Journal of Gastroenterology 70: 501–505

Watkinson G 1958 Treatment of ulcerative colitis with topical hydrocortisone hemisuccinate sodium: a controlled trial employing restricted sequential analysis. British Medical Journal ii: 1077–1082

Watts M J, de Dombal F T, Watkinson G, Goligher J C 1966a Early course of ulcerative colitis. Gut 7: 16–31

Watts M J, de Dombal F T, Watkinson G, Goligher J C 1966b Long term prognosis of ulcerative colitis. British Medical Journal i: 1447–1453

Williams C N, Haber G, Aquino J A 1987 Double-blind, placebo-controlled evaluation of 5-ASA suppositories in active distal proctitis and measurement of extent of spread using ^{99m}Tc-labeled 5-ASA suppositories. Digestive Diseases and Sciences 32 (Suppl): 71S–75S

Willoughby C P, Truelove S C 1980 Ulcerative colitis and pregnancy. Gut 21: 469–474

Willoughby C P, Cowan R E, Gould S R, Machell R J, Stewart J B 1988 Double-blind comparison of olsalazine and sulphasalazine in active ulcerative colitis. Scandinavian Journal of Gastroenterology 23 (Suppl 148): 40–44

Winter T A, Dalton H R, Merrett M N, Campbell A, Jewell D P 1993 Cyclosporin retention enemas in refractory distal ulcerative colitis and 'pouchitis'. Scandinavian Journal of Gastroenterology 28: 701–704

Wood E, Wilson C G, Hardy J G 1985 The spreading of foam and solution enemas. International Journal of Pharmaceutics 25: 191–197

Wright R, Truelove S C 1965 A controlled therapeutic trial of various diets in ulcerative colitis. British Medical Journal ii: 138–141

Wright R, Lumsden K, Luntz M H, Sevel D, Truelove S C 1965 Abnormalities of the sacroiliac joints and uveitis in ulcerative colitis. Quarterly Journal of Medicine 34: 229–236

62. Management of acute severe colitis

D. Present

INTRODUCTION

Although there is still some debate regarding the optimal technique for managing severe acute colitis, a thorough review and application of the lessons learned from the literature will lead the clinician to successful treatment in the majority of patients. Severe colitis complicates both Crohn's disease and ulcerative colitis, and in early series the mortality ranged from 25 to 35%. More recent data have shown that in specialist centers with teams of experienced gastroenterologists and surgeons working together, the mortality rate has fallen to approximately 1% (Jewell et al 1991). Between 5 and 15% of patients will develop fulminant colitis (with or without toxic megacolon), and it is important to stress that one-third will develop this complication with their first attack (Jalan et al 1969). In a large representative series colectomy was required in 37% of patients during their attack of fulminant disease. (Jarnerot et al 1985)

The incidence of severe acute colitis is probably decreasing, perhaps due to the changing epidemiology in which 50% of all new patients present with only distal ulcerative colitis. Another factor might be better management of active disease, with earlier institution of appropriate medical therapy. Despite the decreasing incidence, this potentially life-threatening complication requires a comprehensive medical regimen, with knowledge of all available therapeutic modalities and the appropriate timing for surgical intervention.

CLINICAL FEATURES

These have been well defined by Truelove and Witts (1955) and include six or more grossly bloody stools daily, with a mean evening temperature of more than 99.5°F (37.5°C) or temperature of 100°F (37.8°C) on at least 2 of 4 days, tachycardia with a pulse rate of 90 or greater, hemoglobin of 9 g/dl or less, and an elevated sedimentation rate of 30 mm/h or greater. Other investigators have added other valuable criteria, such as an increased serum orosomucoid, a lowered serum albumin and abdominal pain or tenderness.

Many of these criteria and clinical findings can be altered by corticosteroids and/or antibiotics. Fever may be totally suppressed by high-dose oral steroids and fever patterns may take the form of night sweats. If topical steroids and/or topical 5-ASA (5-aminosalicylic acid) have been administered a patient may have a fulminant course without significant bleeding. This may also occur in patients with severe acute Crohn's colitis. Diarrhea may be diminished with the ingestion of potent anti-diarrheals or narcotic pain medications, and when patients develop toxic megacolon bowel movements may be reduced to fewer than six daily, although the colitis may be very severe.

Other abnormalities with fulminant colitis include metabolic alkalosis, as measured by arterial pH and a decrease in stool pH and bicarbonate, with a fall in potassium/sodium ratio and an increase in lactate and the weight of a 24-hour stool collection (Caprilli et al 1987).

Physical findings also may be greatly modified in the presence of medication. For example, a patient being treated with high-dose corticosteroids may have a free perforation of the bowel with minimal findings. A more common physical finding with severe colitis is localized tenderness over the colon. If rebound tenderness is present this may be a sign of an impending perforation. Fulminant severe colitis is often associated with accumulations of air in the large and small bowel, and this can be suspected by the tympanitic sound when the upper abdomen is percussed.

RADIOGRAPHIC FEATURES

An abdominal X-ray series is essential in the diagnosis and management of severe ulcerative colitis. The examination should include prone and supine films to exclude free air (perforation). Classic findings in severe ulcerative colitis include mucosal irregularity and thickening of the bowel wall, with the presence of mucosal islands. A report examining specific radiological criteria noted that irregularity of the mucosal edge and increased thickness of the colon wall were the most useful in predicting the extent of the process (Prantera et al 1991). A tubular appearance may not reflect the extent of activity since this is an expression of burnt-out disease. The authors noted that the extent of disease could be defined accurately in over 80% of patients based on a plain abdominal film. Recent studies have also shown that a significant increase in small-intestinal gas can predict those patients who will develop toxic megacolon. When multiple loops of small intestine remain distended there may be a need for surgical intervention (Chew et al 1991).

The abdominal X-ray at presentation or in the course of an acute flare-up can demonstrate dilatation of the colon. When the transverse colon distends to 6 cm or greater, toxic megacolon can be diagnosed. It is not the degree of dilatation that is the major factor, but rather the degree of toxicity. The greatest dilatation is usually seen in the transverse colon, which may extend to 9–15 cm (Norland & Kirsner 1969). The colon wall appears irregular and scalloped, once again with mucosal islands and occasional radiolucent linear ulcerations. The latter may represent ulcerations with undermining and may be a forerunner of perforation. Air may become free or may track and present itself in a subcutaneous manner or, when the perforation occurs in the retroperitoneal area, may present as pneumomediastinum (Halpert 1987).

ENDOSCOPIC FEATURES

Colonoscopy has been used in clinical decision making (Alemyehu & Jarnerot 1991) as well as for decompression in the management of severe ulcerative colitis and toxic megacolon (Banez et al 1987). In the author's experience colonoscopy has no role in the management of these patients, since the decision regarding the need for surgery can be made on the basis of clinical examination, laboratory findings and plain radiographs. The mucosa will appear inflamed in all cases, and even the authors of the larger series (Alemyehu & Jarnerot 1991) note a disparity between the symptoms and the mucosal inflammation at colonoscopy. We therefore recommend endoscopy only when the differential diagnosis is uncertain. We do not use endoscopic techniques for monitoring progress or for decision making. The author has seen megacolon precipitated on several occasions following passage of an endoscope.

DIFFERENTIAL DIAGNOSIS

Although the majority of patients who present with severe colitis have either Crohn's disease or non-specific ulcerative colitis, other disorders must be excluded, especially if the patient has not been seen before the development of this complication (Present 1993).

PRECIPITATING FACTORS AND PATHOGENESIS

In Crohn's disease the inflammatory process is transmural, whereas in uncomplicated ulcerative colitis the inflammation is limited to the mucosa. In ulcerative colitis, as the disease progresses in severity the inflammation extends to involve the submucosa and may be associated with necrosis. In fulminant disease or toxic megacolon the process become transmural and may result in microperforations. Sealed-off perforations have been noted at surgery. This extensive process may impair motility, with destruction of the myenteric plexus. Factors which appear to predispose patients to the development of fulminant colitis and toxic megacolon have been reviewed in several papers (Hanan & Hanauer 1988). In the author's experience the most common trigger in developing this complication is stopping medication, including sulfasalazine or other 5-ASA agents, or a too-rapid tapering of steroids after an episode of severe colitis. It is important for clinicians (as well as patients) not to decrease or prematurely discontinue medications until there is a clinical, laboratory and endoscopic remission. Stopping smoking recently has been recognized as a trigger of activity in patients with ulcerative colitis (Bub et al 1993). In this report almost 90% of patients exacerbated their colitis within 1 year of stopping smoking. Other triggering factors include barium enema or colonoscopy. Whether the procedure itself or the required preparation is the trigger is uncertain. Double contrast barium enema should not be carried out in patients with active inflammatory bowel disease, as air insufflation may open up sealed-off perforations or even produce a toxic megacolon. Superimposed bacterial infections such as salmonellosis, shigellosis and campylobacter may all precipitate fulminant colitis. Recently, human immunodeficiency virus has been reported as triggering toxic megacolon (Beaugerie et al 1994) and both amebiasis and superimposed *Clostridium difficile* colitis may also precipitate an acute attack.

Several medications may predispose to toxic megacolon once an acute attack of severe colitis has occurred. These include anticholinergics, antidiarrheals (loperamide, diphenoxylate) and narcotics (codeine, deodorized tincture of opium, demerol). Antidepressant agents with strong anticholinergic effects have also been implicated. Several studies have reported that severe electrolyte disturbances, potassium depletion, magnesium depletion and fluid and electrolyte loss may also result in abnormal motility in the large bowel, and lead to a toxic megacolon.

GENERAL MEDICAL MANAGEMENT

Hospital admission is mandatory when there is a diagnosis of severe acute colitis. Management should be through a team approach and a surgeon should be consulted at the time of diagnosis. Patients should be seen by the team at least three or four times daily in case there is deterioration and surgery is required. Diagnostic procedures should include a complete blood count with differential, biochemical profile and sedimentation rate. If the diarrhea has been of prolonged duration then serum magnesium should be estimated. If cyclosporin is to be considered in the future, serum cholesterol should be drawn before this medication is instituted. Stools should be sent for culture, ova and parasites and *Cl. difficile*. If antibiotics are administered during the hospital stay and the patient is not responding to therapy then a repeat stool for *Cl. difficile* should be performed somewhere between 4 and 7 days. An obstructive series should be ordered on admission and performed daily, or at a minimum of every other day, until the patient shows significant clinical response.

Physical examination should be carried out by both medical and surgical teams to evaluate for abdominal tenderness, rebound tenderness, percussion for distension and possible loss of hepatic dullness. A recording should be kept of the number and character of the stools, including the presence or absence of blood. Optional studies include the measurement of stool weight and electrolytes, arterial pH or ^{111}In-labeled granulocyte scan. I do not believe these studies are necessary for the majority of patients. Vital signs should be recorded at least four times daily, and more frequently if the patient appears to be deteriorating.

Intravenous fluids should be administered and electrolyte abnormalities should be corrected. Patients should be transfused if anemia is significant (hemoglobin ≥9 g/dl). If bleeding is persistent, but especially if the patient has been taking antibiotics, blood studies should be performed to exclude a clotting defect. Anticholinergics should not be administered initially and parenteral narcotics should be avoided. These medications may tend to confuse the clinical picture since severe pain is not a common symptom in patients with severe colitis. Patients should not be given oral fluids and food for the first 24–48 hours after admission to the hospital. After they are stabilized, patients with ulcerative colitis can be fed unless there is significant small or large-bowel distension. There is no evidence to suggest that bowel rest and total parenteral nutrition is effective and there are two controlled trials in the literature which fail to demonstrate any benefit (Dickinson et al 1980, McIntyre et al 1986). In the McIntyre trial a higher percentage of patients with ulcerative colitis who were fed had a better result and avoided surgery. In contrast, Crohn's disease has been reported as showing a good response to total parenteral nutrition, which appears to play an independent therapeutic role in quieting the inflammatory process (Muller et al 1983). Parenteral nutrition should only be used in severe colitis when there is evidence of long-standing nutritional depletion.

In these days of high technology we often forget that the patient must have emotional support during this frightening, severe, acute illness. There is great fear of surgery and an ostomy, especially in patients who are experiencing their first attack. A compassionate, caring physician–nurse–social work team is required.

MEDICATIONS FOR ACUTE SEVERE COLITIS

Corticosteroids have been shown to be effective in both acute ulcerative colitis (Truelove & Witts 1955) and Crohn's disease (Shephard et al 1986). The question in the early literature as to whether steroids should be introduced initially in the acute phase (Meyers & Janowitz 1978), is no longer disputed. Most patients are already taking oral steroids prior to admission and accumulated evidence fails to confirm the contention that colonic perforation may be greater when the patient is receiving steroids. For those patients who have been receiving oral steroids hydrocortisone is administered in a dose of 100 mg intravenously every 6–8 hours, or methylprednisolone may be administered intravenously in a dose of 6–15 mg every 6 hours. There is no evidence to support the contention that higher doses are more effective (Rosenberg et al 1990). It is the author's experience that continuous administration of intravenous steroids is more effective than pulse therapy, but there are no double-blind controlled data to support this theory. There is a single well designed controlled trial demonstrating that adrenocorticotrophic (ACTH) hormone administered in a dose of 40 units every 8 hours by continuous intravenous infusion was more effective than intravenous hydrocortisone administration (100 mg every 8 hours) if the patient had not been receiving prior steroid therapy (Meyers et al 1983). For those patients who were already on steroid therapy the intravenous hydrocortisone was more effective than the ACTH.

As part of the therapeutic regimen rectal administration of a 100 mg hydrocortisone enema twice daily is recommended. Enemas are helpful in reducing tenesmus and urgency, but many patients cannot retain the medication. In this situation hydrocortisone foam can be administered twice daily until the enema can be retained. Steroids will produce significant fluid retention, especially in those patients with hypoalbuminemia, and so excessive sodium should be avoided. Diuretics are contraindicated because of the significant potassium loss associated with high-dose steroid administration. Another potential steroid complication is psychosis, which requires early diagnosis, a reduction of the steroid dosage and psychiatric consultation, with the administration of potent antipsychotic medication.

Antibiotics

In their initial studies Truelove and Jewell (1974) administered intravenous antibiotics in the treatment of fulminant colitis. However, two controlled trials, using metronidazole (Chapman et al 1986) and vancomycin (Dickinson et al 1985) showed no benefit. Conversely, a recent uncontrolled trial in seven patients with severe ulcerative colitis suggested benefits (Peppercorn 1993). In view of the fact that there are significant ulcerations in the bowel wall allowing invasion by luminal bacteria, with release of cytokines and the potential for sepsis, the author advocates the use of antibiotics in fulminant colitis, using a broad-spectrum regimen such as metronidazole 500 mg every 8 hours and an aminoglycoside (dosage based on weight) and ampicillin in a dose of 1–2 g every 6 hours. A third-generation cephalosporin is an alternative option. There may be an extra advantage in the use of metronidazole if the patient has Crohn's disease. As noted above, if the patient has not responded clinically within 1 week, repeat stool studies for *Cl. difficile* should be obtained.

Sulfasalazine, 5-aminosalicylic acid

There is no indication for initiating sulfasalazine or the newer 5-ASA agents in the midst of an episode of severe ulcerative colitis: these agents should be introduced only after the patient has responded and is leaving the hospital. Allergy to these agents may confuse the clinical picture, and there are no trials demonstrating the efficacy of topical 5-ASA agents during the acute phase. Steroid enemas are therefore preferred.

Immunosuppressives

Both 6-mercaptopurine and azathioprine have shown efficacy in controlled and uncontrolled trials in the treatment of ulcerative colitis and Crohn's disease (Present 1989). However, they have no role in the treatment of severe acute colitis, since the mean response time is slightly over 3 months. These drugs should not be initiated since an allergic reaction or leukopenia may confuse the clinical picture. When the patient has responded and has left the hospital, the use of either 6-MP or azathioprine may avert the high risk of recurrence of active disease within the next year (Kornbluth et al 1991).

Methotrexate, which has also shown efficacy in uncontrolled trials in ulcerative colitis (Kozarek 1993) and in a controlled trial in Crohn's disease (Feagan et al 1995), also takes several weeks to show any response and is therefore not indicated in the management of acute severe colitis.

Intravenous cyclosporin may be effective in severe active ulcerative colitis patients who have failed 10 days of intravenous steroids (Lichtiger & Present 1990). A recent double-blind controlled trial (Lichtiger et al 1994) has confirmed the uncontrolled data, with an initial acute response rate of over 80%. Both the uncontrolled and controlled data have demonstrated that cyclosporin has a low toxicity rate when used for a short time. When patients have shown no response to intensive steroid therapy within 7–10 days we advise instituting intravenous cyclosporin while maintaining the intensive steroid regimen. Response to intravenous cyclosporin is usually noted within 1 week in responding patients. Cyclosporin levels should be maintained in a high therapeutic range (100–400 ng/ml as measured by monoclonal antibody). The long-term role of cyclosporin is uncertain, and relapse is seen in approximately 30% (*Editor's note: up to 60%*) of patients over the next 6 months. The role of 6-MP or azathioprine in maintaining the response induced by cyclosporin is at present uncertain.

A recent uncontrolled trial using intravenous cyclosporin in the treatment of acute steroid-refractory Crohn's disease has shown initial success in 75% of patients (Santos et al 1995). The mean time to response was 9 days, and although some patients relapsed in the chronic phase the authors concluded that the cyclosporin was effective, with a rapid onset of action.

COMPLICATIONS OF SEVERE ACUTE COLITIS

As noted above, steroids may produce severe electrolyte complications, psychoses and fluid retention. There have also been reports of adrenal hemorrhage associated with intravenous ACTH (Kornbluth et al 1990). Cyclosporin is associated with electrolyte abnormalities (low magnesium) and seizures if the patient has a low serum cholesterol. Decreased renal function requires careful monitoring.

Massive hemorrhage is uncommon in severe acute colitis, and more often occurs when the rectal segment is left intact after a subtotal colectomy.

Free perforation may occur at any time and is an indication for immediate colectomy. The diagnosis must be suspected in patients who have persistent fever despite receiving high-dose corticosteroids. On clinical examination a loss of hepatic dullness should prompt emergency abdominal radiography, with an upright view to look closely for free air under the diaphragm.

Toxic megacolon may complicate 1.6–22% of cases of severe ulcerative colitis (Edwards & Truelove 1964). The worldwide incidence of toxic megacolon appears to be decreasing, perhaps because of improved medical therapy. Mortality rates range from 0 (Neschis et al 1968) to 45% (Jalan et al 1969). Some studies (Katzka et al 1979) have reported no mortality, again probably owing to intensive medical management by experienced teams. The medical management is similar to that outlined above, with the addition of two therapeutic modalities designed to decompress the dilated colon (Present 1991) which have been advocated by some groups.

Because of the increased accumulation of intestinal air (Caprilli et al 1987, Chew et al 1991) we recommend the passage of a long intestinal tube rather than nasogastric tube decompression (Huizenga 1975, Present et al 1988). If the X-rays demonstrate early megacolon and increased small-intestinal gas we position the tube in the duodenum under fluoroscopic guidance. Air tends to accumulate in the transverse colon in supine patients because it is the most anterior portion of the large intestine. We therefore roll the patient into a prone position on a flattened bed for 15 minutes every 2–3 hours to redistribute colonic air (Kramer & Wittenberg 1981). The patient is then advised to pass gas and fluid in this position. Only a rare patient will require the passage of a thin soft rubber catheter to facilitate this evacuation. With this rolling technique patients will usually experience significant relief from colonic distension within 24–48 hours. A study of 19 consecutive patients showed decompression in all (Present et al 1988). Our clinical experience suggests that with the passage of a long tube, the rolling technique and intensive medication, toxic megacolon rarely requires acute surgery. The colon will usually decompress and allow the physician a longer period of time to treat with steroids or cyclosporin in an attempt to bring the colitis into remission.

OUTCOME – MEDICAL AND SURGICAL

Predicting the outcome of acute severe colitis and toxic megacolon (Greenstein et al 1985) has been difficult. The remission rate in a large series of severe colitis was 56% for severe attacks, 87% for moderate attacks and 92% for mild attacks (Jarnerot et al 1985). Variables in addition to severity include the presence of excessive amounts of intestinal gas, distension of the colon or toxic megacolon, degrees of alkalosis and the rapidity of response to steroids. It was initially advised that if the patients did not respond to 5 days of intravenous steroids they should undergo surgery (Truelove & Jewell 1974). However, more recent studies have noted that it may take as many as 10 days to show a response (Meyers et al 1987, Jewell et al 1991). More recently cyclosporin data have demonstrated an 80% response in patients who had failed 10 days of intravenous steroids. On the other hand, the surgical options have increased dramatically in the last several years (Pemberton et al 1987), with a significant fall in mortality. Patients now have the option of undergoing an ileoanal anastomosis. This procedure is rarely performed in a single stage when the disease is severely active, but can be completed as a two or three-stage procedure. The concept that this alternative procedure is a 'cure' for ulcerative colitis is also not accurate. The technical failure rate is approximately 5–6% in all major centers performing this procedure (Pemberton et al 1987). In addition, pouchitis occurs with increased frequency as large series provide long-term follow-up. The incidence is now in the 50–60% range for a single episode of pouchitis (Lohmuller et al 1990). Finally, chronic pouchitis requiring continuous therapy is now being seen in somewhere between 2 and 5% of patients with ileoanal anastomosis with a proximal pouch (Sandborn 1994).

The author's conclusion is that since over 80% of patients can be spared a colectomy during an acute attack of severe colitis, intensive medical therapy is warranted in all patients. However, the appropriate timing for surgery is crucial and if a patient does not show a response after 7–10 days of intravenous steroid therapy, either cyclosporin should be initiated immediately or colectomy should be performed. Likewise, if there is no response to intravenous cyclosporin within 7 days an urgent colectomy is indicated. Significant deterioration at any time during medical therapy is an indication for surgery. A combined experienced surgical–medical team will be required to make these difficult decisions. The intensive medical management is outlined in Tables 62.1 and 62.2.

Table 62.1 Monitoring the patient with severe acute colitis

1. Hospitalize immediately. Obtain surgical consultation
2. Physical examination by the medical and surgical team two or more times daily, including evaluation for abdominal tenderness, rebound tenderness and percussion for loss of hepatic dullness and upper abdominal tympany
3. Recording of vital signs four times daily
4. Recording of the frequency and character of bowel movements daily
5. Blood studies to include complete blood count, sedimentation rate, serum electrolytes, serum albumin and other chemistries every 24–48 hours. If cyclosporin is used additional magnesium, cholesterol and cyclosporin levels
6. Daily or every other day obstructive series
7. Adequate fluid, blood and electrolyte replacement
8. Avoidance of narcotics, antidiarrheals and anticholinergics
9. Food restriction for the first 24–48 hours
10. Total parenteral nutrition 'only for Crohn's disease' and patients with long-term nutritional depletion
11. Passage of a long intestinal tube for accumulation of air in the colon, toxic megacolon and/or excessive small-intestinal gas
12. Rolling technique for severe colitis with any increased colonic air and/or toxic megacolon
13. Emotional support for the patient and family by a compassionate medical team

Table 62.2 Specific medical therapy for severe acute colitis

1. Intravenous administration of hydrocortisone 300 mg or ACTH 120 units if the patient has not already been receiving steroids. The infusion should be continuous
2. Hydrocortisone enemas twice daily unless the patient cannot retain them; in this case use hydrocortisone foam twice daily
3. Broad-spectrum intravenous antibiotics (metronidazole, ampicillin and an aminoglycoside) or third-generation cephalosporin
4. Avoidance of the institution of sulfasalazine, 5-ASA agents, 6-mercaptopurine/azathioprine and methotrexate
5. Intravenous cyclosporin 4 mg/kg/day by continuous infusion if the patient has shown no improvement in 7–10 days
6. Surgical intervention in 7–10 days if cyclosporin is not initiated
7. Surgery for free perforation, massive bleeding or significant deterioration at any time during intensive steroid or cyclosporin therapy

REFERENCES

Alemyehu G, Jarnerot G 1991 Colonoscopy during an attack of severe ulcerative colitis is a safe procedure and of great value in clinical decision-making. American Journal of Gastroenterology 86: 187–190

Banez A V, Yamanish I F, Crans C A 1987 Endoscopic colonic decompression of toxic megacolon. Placement of colonic tube and steroid colon clysis. American Journal of Gastroenterology 82: 692–694

Beaugerie L, Ngo Y, Goujard F et al 1994 Etiology and management of toxic megacolon in patients with human immunodeficiency virus. Gastroenterology 107: 858–863

Bub C, Friedman A, Rubin P H, Bodian C, Present D H 1993 Cessation of smoking is more likely to activate ulcerative colitis than Crohn's colitis. Gastroenterology 104: Abstract 103; 1

Caprilli R, Vernia P, Latella G, Torsoli A 1987 Early recognition of toxic megacolon. Journal of Clinical Gastroenterology 9: 160–164

Chapman R W, Selby W S, Jewell D P 1986 Controlled trial of intravenous metronidazole as an adjunct to corticosteroids in severe ulcerative colitis. Gut 27: 1210–1212

Chew C N, Nolan D J, Jewell D P 1991 Small bowel gas in ulcerative colitis. Gut 32: 1535–1537

Dickinson R J, Ashton M G, Axon A T R, Smith R C, Yeung C K, Hill G L 1980 Controlled trial of intravenous hyperalimentation and total bowel rest as an adjunct to the routine therapy of acute colitis. Gastroenterology 79: 1199–1204

Dickinson R J, O'Connor H J, Tinder I et al 1985 Double blind controlled trial of oral vancomycin as adjunctive therapy in acute exacerbations of ulcerative colitis. Gut 26: 1380–1384

Edwards F C, Truelove S C 1964 The course and prognosis of ulcerative colitis. Part 3 – Complications. Gut 5: 1–22

Feagan B G, Rochon J, Fedorak R et al 1995 Methotrexate for the treatment of Crohn's disease. New England Journal of Medicine 332: 292–297

Greenstein A J, Sachar D B, Gibas A et al 1985 Outcome of toxic dilatation in ulcerative colitis and Crohn's colitis. Journal of Clinical Gastroenterology 7: 137–144

Halpert R D 1987 Toxic dilatation of the colon. Radiologic Clinics of North America 25: 147–154

Hanan I M, Hanauer S B 1988 Fulminant colitis in toxic megacolon. Journal of Intensive Care Medicine 3: 164–170

Huizenga K A 1975 Medical treatment and prognosis of some local complications of chronic ulcerative colitis and Crohn's disease. In: Kirsner J B, Shorter R G (eds) Inflammatory Bowel Disease, Lea and Febiger, Philadelphia, pp 301–305

Jalan K N, Circus W, Cord W I et al 1969 An experience with ulcerative colitis: toxic dilation in 55 cases. Gastroenterology 57: 68–82

Jarnerot G, Rolny P, Sandberg-Gertzen H 1985 Intensive intravenous treatment of ulcerative colitis. Gastroenterology 89: 1005–1013

Jewell D P, Caprilli R, Mortensen N, Nicholls R J, Wright J P 1991 Indications and timing of surgery for severe ulcerative colitis. Gastroenterology International 4: 161–164

Katzka I, Katz S, Morris E 1979 Management of toxic megacolon: the significance of early recognition and medical management. Journal of Clinical Gastroenterology 1: 307–311

Kornbluth A A, Salomon P, Bharuch A S, Janowitz H D 1991 The efficacy of current medical therapy for severe ulcerative colitis: an analytic review of the defined trials. American Journal of Gastroenterology 86: 1356 Abstract

Kornbluth A A, Salomon P, Sachar D B et al 1990 ACTH induced adrenal hemorrhage: a complication of therapy masquerading as an acute abdomen. Journal of Clinical Gastroenterology 12: 371–377

Kozarek R A 1993 Review article: Immunosuppressive therapy for inflammatory bowel disease. Alimentary Pharmacology and Therapy 7: 117–123

Kramer P, Wittenberg J 1981 Colonic gas distribution in toxic megacolon. Gastroenterology 80: 433–437

Lichtiger S, Present D H 1990 Preliminary report: Cyclosporine in treatment of severe active ulcerative colitis. Lancet 2: 16–19

Lichtiger S, Present D H, Kornbluth A A et al 1994 Cyclosporin in severe ulcerative colitis refractory to steroid therapy. New England Journal of Medicine 330: 1841–1845

Lohmuller J C, Pemberton J H, Dozois R R, Ilstrup D M, Van Heerden J 1990 Pouchitis and extraintestinal manifestations of inflammatory bowel disease after ileal pouch–anal anastomosis. Annals of Surgery 211: 622–629

McIntyre P B, Powell-Tuck J, Wood S R et al 1986 Controlled trial of bowel rest in the treatment of severe acute colitis. Gut 27: 481–485

Meyers S, Janowitz H D 1978 The place of steroids in the therapy of toxic megacolon. Gastroenterology 75: 729–731

Meyers S, Lerer P, Feuer E J et al 1987 Predicting the outcome of corticoid therapy for acute ulcerative colitis. Journal of Clinical Gastroenterology 9: 50–54

Meyers S, Sachar D B, Goldberg J D et al 1983 Corticotropin versus hydrocortisone in the intravenous treatment of ulcerative colitis. Gastroenterology 85: 251–357

Muller J M, Keller H W, Erasin H 1983 Total parenteral nutrition as the sole therapy in Crohn's disease–a prospective study. British Journal of Surgery 70: 40–43

Neschis M, Siegelman S S, Parker J G 1968 Diagnosis and management of the megacolon of ulcerative colitis. Gastroenterology 55: 251–259

Norland C C, Kirsner J B 1969 Toxic dilatation of colon (toxic megacolon). Etiology, treatment and prognosis in 42 patients. Medicine 48: 229–250

Pemberton J H, Kelly K A, Beart R W, Dozois R R, Wolff B G, Ilstrup D M 1987 Ileal pouch–anal anastomosis for chronic ulcerative colitis: long term results. Annals of Surgery 206: 504–513

Peppercorn M A 1993 Are antibiotics useful in the management of nontoxic severe ulcerative colitis? Journal of Clinical Gastroenterology 17: 14–17

Prantera C, Lorenzetti R, Cerro P, Davoli M, Brancato G, Fanucci A 1991 The plain abdominal film accurately estimates extent of active ulcerative colitis. Journal of Clinical Gastroenterology 13: 231–234

Present D H 1989 6-mercaptopurine and other immunosuppressive agents in the treatment of Crohn's disease and ulcerative colitis. Clinics in Gastroenterology of North America 18: 57–72

Present D H 1991 Fulminant colitis. Seminars in Gastrointestinal Disease 2: 107–114

Present D H 1993 Toxic megacolon. Medical Clinics of North America 77: 1129–1148

Present D H, Wolfson D, Gelernt I M, Rubin P H, Bauer J, Chapman M L 1988 Medical decompression of toxic megacolon by 'rolling'. A new technique of decompression with favorable long term follow up. Journal of Clinical Gastroenterology 10: 485–490

Rosenberg W, Ireland A, Jewell D P 1990 High dose methylprednisolone in the treatment of active ulcerative colitis. Journal of Clinical Gastroenterology 12: 40–41

Sandborn W J 1994 Pouchitis following ileal pouch–anal anastomosis: definition, pathogenesis and treatment. Gastroenterology 107: 1856–1860

Santos J V, Baudet J A, Casellas F J, Guarna L A, Vilaseca J M, Malagelada J R B 1995 Intravenous cyclosporin for steroid refractory attacks of Crohn's disease: short and long term results. Journal of Clinical Gastroenterology 20: 207–210

Shephard A J, Barr G D, Jewell D P 1986 Use of an intravenous steroid regimen in the treatment of acute Crohn's disease. Journal of Clinical Gastroenterology 8: 154–159

Truelove S C, Jewell D P 1974 Intensive intravenous regimen for severe attacks of ulcerative colitis. Lancet 1: 1067–1070

Truelove S C, Witts L J 1955 Cortisone in ulcerative colitis. Final report on a therapeutic trial. British Medical Journal 2: 1041–1048

63. Treatment of ulcerative colitis in remission

G. Järnerot   H. Sandberg-Gertzén   C. Tysk

Once a patient has developed ulcerative colitis, recurrent attacks are likely. To reduce the risk of recurrence many different therapeutic agents have been tried, only a few of them yielding benefit. The most important of these are described below.

SULFASALAZINE–5-ASA

Pharmacokinetics

Sulfasalazine, although originally developed by Nanna Svartz for the treatment of rheumatoid arthritis (Svartz 1942), has for years also been used for inflammatory bowel disease. Sulfasalazine consists of a salicylate radical linked to sulfapyridine by an azo bond. The azo bond is split by the colonic bacteria, with the liberation of 5-aminosalicylic acid (5-ASA) and sulfapyridine. The sulfapyridine is almost completely absorbed from the colon, metabolized, and excreted in the urine (Peppercorn & Goldman 1973). Most of the side effects of sulfasalazine have been ascribed to the sulfapyridine moiety and correlate with its serum concentration, whereas 5-ASA is poorly absorbed from the colon.

For many years it was not known whether the pharmacological effects of sulfasalazine resided in the complete molecule or in one of its two metabolites, but in 1977 it was demonstrated that in ulcerative colitis 5-ASA was the active moiety (Azad Khan et al 1977). The acetylated form of 5-ASA has been proved ineffective in ulcerative colitis (Binder et al 1981).

The knowledge that 5-ASA is the pharmacologically active moiety in sulfasalazine has led to the development of new 5-ASA-based sulfa-free drugs. Oral 5-ASA is rapidly absorbed from the small intestine, acetylated and excreted in the urine, and does not reach the colon in appreciable quantities (Nielsen & Bondesen 1983). To overcome the rapid absorption of 5-ASA from the small intestine, various release preparations have been manufactured. Other azo compounds have also been synthesized, using a carrier other than sulfapyridine. 5-ASA has been given the generic name of mesalazine. The mesalazine preparations on the market have been formulated in different ways, resulting in different pharmacokinetic properties; thus it is necessary to evaluate each product. Table 63.1 shows the characteristics of the most commonly used compounds.

Clinical studies

The main therapeutic role of sulfasalazine has always been maintaining remission of the disease. In the first placebo-

Table 63.1 Formulations and sites of 5-ASA release with various new 5-ASA-based drugs

Generic name	Trade name	Formulation	Thickness of coating	Solubility	Sites of release
Mesalazine	Pentasa	Individually coated microgranules compressed into tablets. Ethylcellulose coating	Probably not relevant	Little influenced by pH	Duodenum, jejunum, ileum, colon
Mesalazine	Claversal Mesasal Salofalk	Eudragit L 100 coated	?	pH ≥6	Jejunum, ileum, colon
Mesalazine	Asacol	Eudragit-S coating	80–130 µm	pH ≥7	Terminal ileum, colon
Olsalazine	Dipentum	Gelatine capsules	Not relevant	Not influenced by pH	Colon
Balsalazine	Colazide	Tablets	Not relevant	Not influenced by pH	Colon

controlled maintenance trial the placebo relapse rate was 73% over 1 year, compared with 21% in the sulfasalazine group (Misiewicz et al 1965). Relapse rates on treatment are unrelated to the time previously spent on sulfasalazine, which led to the recommendation that, if tolerated, the drug should be continued for life (Dissanayake & Truelove 1973).

A dose–response study of sulfasalazine in the doses 1, 2 or 4 g daily showed the two higher doses to be more effective (Azad Khan et al 1980). The results indicated that 4 g might be better than 2 g daily, but the side effects increased considerably and the differences found did not reach statistical significance. An optimal dose of 2 g has been chosen, although individual patients may require higher maintenance doses to prevent relapse.

There are three factors to consider when choosing which drug to use: effectiveness; which formulation delivers 5-ASA to the colon with the fewest systemic effects; and safety. These aspects have been reviewed (Järnerot 1994).

1. A meta-analysis was unable to show that any of the new sulfa-free 5-ASA-based formulations was more efficient than sulfasalazine (Sutherland et al 1993).
2. It appears from a critical evaluation of published results that for maintenance treatment a minimum of 0.8 g 5-ASA should be delivered to the colon daily. For olsalazine this is achieved with a daily dose of 1 g/day and for balsalazide 2.5–3 g/day. Both these drugs are azo compounds, where 5-ASA is delivered only to the colon. For Asacol a daily dose of 1.2 g and for Pentasa and Claversal (Salofalk) 1.5–1.75 g appears adequate.
3. All new salicylates are better tolerated than sulfasalazine, but there are very few direct comparisons of the tolerance of the various new salicylates. One showed that the withdrawal rates in clinical trials because of side effects were similar in olsalazine and Asacol studies (Järnerot 1988). One study compared olsalazine, balsalazide and Asacol in sulfasalazine-intolerant patients: 91% tolerated at least one of the preparations, 42% all three and 70% two of three (Giaffer et al 1992). Nine percent of the patients experienced an adverse reaction to all preparations, indicating that 5-ASA and not the sulfa moiety in sulfasalazine can be the cause of intolerance.

Adverse effects

An appreciable minority of patients cannot tolerate sulfasalazine in therapeutic doses (Das et al 1973). Many of the common side effects are dose related, such as headache, nausea and general malaise. Rashes, adenitis and fever are also common. Some male patients suffer from reversible infertility (Toth 1979). A few side effects, although infrequent, are dangerous, such as exfoliative dermatitis and agranulocytosis.

5-ASA can induce diarrhea with or without blood, as well as idiosyncratic reactions such as pericarditis and pancreatitis (Järnerot 1989). However, the main concern with the mesalazine preparations has been nephrotoxicity, which mainly becomes manifest as interstitial nephritis (Ruf-Ballauf et al 1989). Animal studies have shown that 5-ASA is nephrotoxic (Calder et al 1972). This problem seems to be restricted to the formulations that depend on pH for release. Only two cases have been reported during the 50 years that sulfasalazine has been in use (Dwarakanath et al 1992). We are not aware of any published report with Pentasa, so far. It is assumed that this is an idiosyncratic reaction. If so, one would have expected that many more cases would be reported over the years that sulfasalazine has been in use. This also makes it unlikely that the nephritis is caused by a high renal load over the years. It therefore seems plausible that the reaction is caused by high serum peaks of 5-ASA. Such peaks can be reached with the pH-dependent drugs provided that the patient has an unsuitable small-gut pH environment that allows early release of the 5-ASA.

This risk is probably also influenced by gastric emptying, which may be delayed if the patient takes snacks between meals. These gastric juice-resistant tablets may then leave the stomach at night (Ewe et al 1992). If this happens, and the total daily dose is emptied at night in a patient whose intestinal environment allows early release of the tablets, nephrotoxic serum peaks may be reached. If this hypothesis is correct, this side effect, although rare, is avoidable.

Olsalazine can induce diarrhea, which is a definite concern. In the initial study 12.5% of patients treated with 1 g/day olsalazine were withdrawn because of diarrhea (Sandberg-Gertzén et al 1986) and in another placebo-controlled study using 2 g/day olsalazine 15.6% had to quit (Wright et al 1993). In neither study was olsalazine given directly after meals or introduced gradually, which seems to reduce the risk of diarrhea. There also seems to be a dose-related risk. In a dose-ranging study, 9% of patients taking 0.5 g or 1.0 g/day olsalazine withdrew because of diarrhea compared with 19% of those taking a 2 g dose (Travis et al 1994). Furthermore, the risk might be greater in patients with extensive disease (Sandberg-Gertzén et al 1986), although this could not be confirmed in two other studies (Ireland et al 1988, Travis et al 1994). In practice, and considering all kinds of patients, the withdrawal rate because of diarrhea was 6.3% (Järnerot 1988).

4-AMINOSALICYLIC ACID

4-ASA is a stable compound and differs from 5-ASA only in the position of the amino group, which is in the 4 or para position instead of the 5 or meta position as in 5-ASA (Fig. 63.1). 4-ASA has been used extensively in

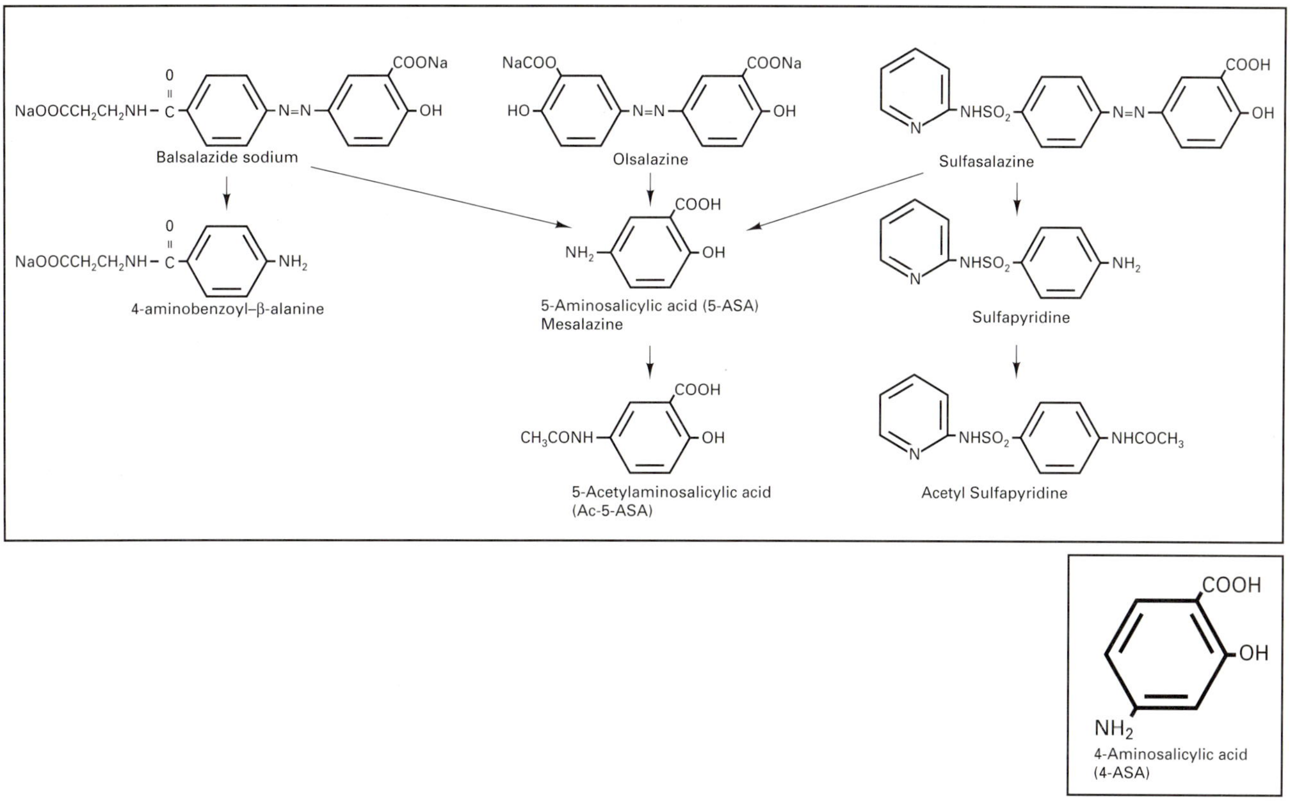

Fig. 63.1

the management of tuberculosis for over 40 years. As an enema 4-ASA is better than placebo (Selby et al 1984) and equivalent to 5-ASA (Campieri et al 1984) in the treatment of active distal ulcerative colitis. A small placebo-controlled trial of enteric-coated 4-ASA tablets in active ulcerative colitis proved it to be useful (Ginsberg et al 1992). We are not aware of any trial of 4-ASA as maintenance treatment. However, there is reason to believe that it is comparable to 5-ASA.

TOPICAL 5-ASA TREATMENT

The anti-inflammatory effect of 5-ASA is exerted from the luminal side of the gut. Various new formulations aim at delivering 5-ASA to the site of inflammation. Theoretically, the concentration of 5-ASA in the distal colon might be low when the drug is given orally. Studies have shown that a 100 ml enema spreads retrogradely to the splenic flexure, whereas foam preparations and suppositories stay within the rectosigmoid region. Thus topical treatment should ensure a sufficient luminal concentration in the distal part of the colon.

Pharmacokinetics

Bondesen et al (1984) found that enemas containing 1 g 5-ASA were rapidly absorbed from a neutral solution, sometimes resulting in plasma concentrations exceeding those found on oral sulfasalazine treatment. The uptake from a slightly acidic enema was reduced, with plasma levels similar to those seen during sulfasalazine medication. Campieri et al (1985) used 4 g enemas with a pH 5.5–5.8 and 2 g enemas with pH 6.1–6.3, and found 5-ASA to be absorbed to a variable extent with mean peak plasma concentrations higher than during oral sulfasalazine medication. The absorption seemed to be lower during relapse. Jacobsen et al (1991) studied the commercially available 5-ASA Pentasa: 1 g enemas or suppositories were given twice daily to healthy volunteers, and only 15 and 10% respectively was recovered in the urine in steady state, with very low plasma concentrations. Thus, after rectal instillation the absorption seems to be dependent on disease activity, 5-ASA concentration, the pH of the enema and the total volume given. Consequently, lower doses, small volumes and an acidic pH should minimize absorption and the risk of systemic side effects.

Clinical studies

Three uncontrolled studies (Guarino et al 1987, Sutherland & Martin 1987, Campieri et al 1989) report on the prophylactic use of 5-ASA rectally, but the results are difficult to interpret. Biddle and co-workers (1988) randomized 25 patients in remission to either placebo or 1 g 5-ASA enema daily. The following year three out of 12 patients on 5-ASA and 11 out of 13 on placebo relapsed. The results are impressive, considering that the patients were initially treated for refractory disease. These findings were substantiated by D'Arienzo et al (1990), who double-blindly randomized 30 patients in complete remission to either 5-ASA suppositories 400 mg twice daily or placebo. During the following 12 months 92% in the 5-ASA group and 21% in the placebo group remained in remission. D'Albasio et al (1990) studied intermittent treatment for relapse prevention: 29 patients were allotted to 4 g 5-ASA enema for the first 7 days of each month and were compared to 31 patients given sulfasalazine 2 g orally per day. During the first year, nine relapsed in the 5-ASA group and 12 in the sulfasalazine group. After 2 years the cumulative relapse rate was 45% on 5-ASA and 43% on sulfasalazine. The study lacks a placebo group and is to small to detect a type II error, but the frequency of relapses remained within the expected range seen on different oral 5-ASA preparations. Mantzaris et al (1994) have compared oral mesalazine 0.5 g three times daily or 4 g of 5-ASA enema every third night in 40 patients suffering distal ulcerative colitis or ulcerative proctitis. After 2 years 68% on oral medication had relapsed, compared to 26% on topical treatment.

Adverse effects

In one of the studies half of the patients complained of anal irritation due to the enema (Biddle et al 1988). None of the other studies referred to reported any intolerance or side effect. Idiosyncratic reactions are independent of the dose given and cannot be avoided by using the rectal route, and there has been a report on pancreatitis during sulfasalazine medication later challenged by 5-ASA enema (Isaacs & Murphy 1990).

IMMUNOSUPPRESSANTS

Immunological mechanisms are central in the pathogenesis of ulcerative colitis, but it is not clear whether the observed mucosal or systemic immunological abnormalities are of primary importance or secondary to disease activity. Although a large number of patients with ulcerative colitis have been treated with immunosuppressive therapy since 1962 (Bean 1962), still the place of this therapy in ulcerative colitis is debated. It has been used more frequently in patients with severe Crohn's disease, whereas in most unresponsive cases with a severe attack of ulcerative colitis or with a chronic continuous course surgical therapy remains the preferred option. However, in older patients who are poor surgical risks or in patients with recent onset of the disease who psychologically find surgery unacceptable, a trial with immunosuppressive therapy may be justified.

AZATHIOPRINE/6-MERCAPTOPURINE

Azathioprine and 6-mercaptopurine are purine analogs which inhibit nucleic acid synthesis. Azathioprine is converted to 6-mercaptopurine and they can therefore be expected to have similar clinical effects and side effects. 6-mercaptopurine is converted intracellularly to its biologically active nucleotide thioinosinic acid, by the enzyme hypoxanthine guanine phosphoribosyltransferase. Further breakdown of the drugs to their urinary metabolite, 6-thiouric acid, requires xanthine oxidase. The concomitant use of allopurinol inhibits this enzyme and the breakdown of azathioprine and 6-mercaptopurine is reduced, so toxic levels may occur unless the dose is reduced. Severe myelotoxicity may be associated with low thiopurine methyltransferase activity. The activity of this enzyme is genetically determined and the incidence of homozygotic deficiency is 1:300 in the general population, which corresponds to the frequency of severe myelotoxicity in azathioprine therapy (Connell et al 1993).

Pharmacologic effects

The major effect of azathioprine is probably related to its effect on plasma cells and lymphocytes. A 50% reduction of plasma cells in rectal lamina propria, a reduction in peripheral blood lymphocytes and a reduction of NK cell cytotoxic activity has been reported during therapy with azathioprine. No major changes in the proportion of T and B cells have been seen (Hawthorne & Hawkey 1989).

Clinical studies

Five controlled studies of azathioprine in ulcerative colitis have been published, yielding conflicting results (Table 63.2). In a double-blind placebo-controlled study of 80 patients with a recent attack of ulcerative colitis, Jewell and Truelove (1974) found that the addition of azathioprine in a daily dose of 2.5 mg/kg to a standard course of corticosteroids was of no value in the acute attack. The remission frequency after 1 month's treatment was equal in both groups. During maintenance therapy for 12 months, patients on azathioprine had a non-significant tendency to a lower relapse rate. In the study by Rosenberg et al (1975) 30 patients with chronic active steroid-dependent disease were randomized to azathioprine 1.5 mg/kg or placebo. After 6 months a significant reduction of the steroid dose was seen in the azathioprine group, without clinical or endoscopic benefit. A steroid-sparing effect of azathioprine was also reported by Kirk and Lennard-Jones (1982). Comparing a daily dose of azathioprine 2.5 mg/kg with sulfasalazine 65 mg/kg for 3 months in an acute attack of ulcerative colitis, no significant difference was seen (Caprilli et al 1975). In this study no corticosteroids were given, in contrast to other trials. Valuable data emerge

Table 63.2 Controlled studies of azathioprine (aza) in ulcerative colitis

Reference	Design	Dose of aza (mg/kg/day)	Duration (months)	No of patients	Results
Jewell & Truelove 1974	DB-Plac	2.5	12	Aza 40, Plac 40	Aza has no effect in acute attack; after 1 year a reduced relapse rate which did not reach statistical significance
Rosenberg et al 1975	DB-Plac	1.5	6	Aza 16, Plac 14	In aza a significant reduction of steroids but no symptomatic or endoscopic improvement
Caprilli et al 1975	DB-SASP	2.5	3	Aza 10, SASP 10	No difference in clinical efficacy
Kirk & Lennard-Jones 1982	DB-Plac	2–2.5	6	Aza 24, Plac 20	In aza a significant reduction of steroids
Hawthorne et al 1992b	DB-Plac withdrawal	100 mg/day	12	Aza 38, Plac 41	Relapse rate 35% (aza) 59% (plac)

DB, double-blind; Plac, placebo; SASP, sulfasalazine

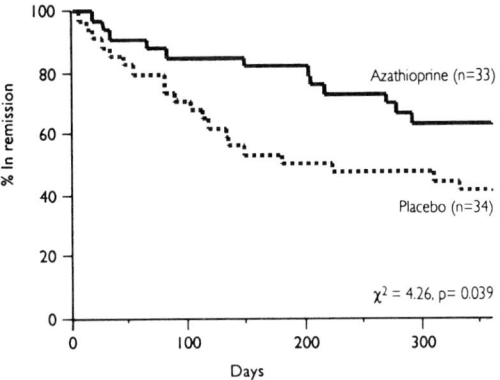

Fig. 63.2

from a double-blind placebo-controlled withdrawal study in which 67 patients, who had been treated with azathioprine for a minimum of 6 months, and who had been in remission for at least 2 months, were randomized to continued azathioprine or placebo (Hawthorne et al 1992b). A significant higher relapse rate in placebo-treated patients (59%) was found compared to patients who continued azathioprine therapy (36%) (Fig. 63.2). For the subgroup of patients with a long remission (more than 6 months) the benefit was still evident.

In addition, data from uncontrolled reports support the value of azathioprine in chronic resistant disease, and 50–80% of these selected patients responded to immunosuppressant therapy (Table 63.3). Similar results have been reported in an open pediatric study (Verhave et al 1990), but the role of immunosuppressants in children is still uncertain.

Adverse reactions

There is a great concern regarding toxicity and neoplastic complications during azathioprine or 6-mercaptopurine therapy in inflammatory bowel disease. Nausea is a common reason for early drug intolerance. Short- and long-term toxicity of 6-mercaptopurine was reviewed in 396 patients with inflammatory bowel disease of whom 120 had ulcerative colitis (Present et al 1989). Pancreatitis was seen in 3.3% of the cases, and occurred in most patients within the first month of therapy. It is not dose dependent and always recurs after reintroduction of therapy. Allergic reactions, including fever, rash and arthralgia, occurred in 2% of the patients, generally within the first weeks of therapy. There is a cross-reaction between azathioprine and 6-mercaptopurine in these respects. Infectious complications were seen in 7.4% of the patients, whereas serious hepatotoxic reactions were fairly uncom-

Table 63.3 Uncontrolled studies of azathioprine (aza) or 6-mercaptopurine (6-MP) in ulcerative colitis

Reference	Design	Drug dose (mg/kg/day)	Duration (months)	No of cases	Results
Theodor et al 1981	Retrosp	Aza–3		35	Remission in 33 out of 53 (62%) given courses
Present et al 1988	Open	6-MP		60	Remission in 24 patients, moderate improvement in 17, no effect in 15, side effects in 4; in 34 steroids were reduced
Lobo et al 1990	Retrosp	Aza–1.9	0.25–66	47	Remission in 13/28 with severe resistant UC Reduced steroids in 12/19 with steroid-dependent UC
Steinhart et al 1990	Retrosp	Aza–1.48	2–40	16	12/16 (75%) patients responded
Adler & Korelitz 1990	Retrosp	6-MP	4–67	81	Clinical response in 67/81 (83%) patients
Verhave et al 1990	Open	Aza–2.0	–24	9 children	Complete response in 6, partial in 1 and none in 2 children
Bianchi-Porro et al 1991	Open	Aza–2.0	4–24	14	After 1 year 7/14 patients in remission

Retrosp, retrospective

mon. Diarrhea induced by azathioprine occurs infrequently but is important to recognize as it may be confused with a recurrence of the disease (Cox et al 1988).

The risk of neoplastic complications after long-term therapy has been subject of several studies. In their extensive review, Present et al (1989) found neoplastic complications in 3.1% of the patients. In a population-controlled study of 755 patients with inflammatory bowel disease, of whom 282 had ulcerative colitis, no overall excess of cancer was seen in patients treated with azathioprine for a median period of 12.5 months and followed for a median period of 9 years (Connell et al 1994). An increased frequency of colorectal cancer was observed but other malignancies, including lymphoma, were not increased compared to the general population. The frequency of colorectal cancer was similar in patients treated with azathioprine as in patients without immuno-suppressant therapy. Leukopenia was the most common sign of myelotoxicity, and in milder asymptomatic forms therapy was withheld until the leukocyte count returned to normal; therapy was then reintroduced in a lower dose. Profound bone marrow suppression requiring hospitalization occurred in 2% of the patients (Present et al 1989). Myelotoxicity may occur at any time during treatment, as was shown in 739 patients treated with azathioprine for a median period of 12 months (Connell et al 1993). Asymptomatic leukopenia was found in 37 patients (5%), which caused a reduction of the dose. In nine patients (1%) severe leukopenia (white blood count $<2.0\times10^9/l$) was found, and five of them developed sepsis, pneumonia or mild upper respiratory infections. Two of the patients with sepsis died. Myelotoxicity occurred at any time from 2 weeks to 11 years of therapy, and either occurred suddenly or progressed over several months.

METHOTREXATE

Methotrexate is a folic acid antagonist used in psoriasis and rheumatoid arthritis. In an open study of 21 patients with refractory inflammatory bowel disease, methotrexate was given as a 25 mg intramuscular injection weekly for 12 weeks, followed by a tapering oral dose. Sixteen (76%) of the patients achieved remission after 12 weeks (Kozarek et al 1989). Extended data including 67 patients show a response rate in 70% of all treated patients with ulcerative colitis (Kozarek et al 1992). Previous failure to respond to azathioprine or 6-mercaptopurine did not preclude a response to methotrexate, although colectomy was required in three out of six patients with ulcerative colitis (Kozarek et al 1991). Prolonged follow-up for 59 weeks showed, however, that only 40% of the patients who responded to parenteral therapy maintained remission on oral therapy, and half of the patients required colectomy (Kozarek et al 1992, Kozarek 1993). Possibly, the long-term efficacy of methotrexate therapy is better in Crohn's disease (Kozarek 1993). So far, no controlled data are available in ulcerative colitis and concerns about toxicity limit its use. Hypersensitivity pneumonitis and liver toxicity are specific adverse reactions of methotrexate which must be considered in addition to gastrointestinal intolerance, myelotoxicity and teratogenesis.

In another study methotrexate was given orally in a weekly dose of 15 mg for 18 weeks, which seemed less effective as five out of eight patients with ulcerative colitis did not respond and four patients had a subsequent colectomy (Baron et al 1993).

CYCLOSPORIN A

Cyclosporin A is widely used to prevent transplant rejection. It inhibits the immune response by blocking the synthesis of interleukin-2 and the helper T-cell function is impaired. Intravenous infusion of cyclosporin has induced rapid remission and obviated the need for acute colectomy in a high proportion of patients with corticosteroid-resistant severe attacks of ulcerative colitis (Lichtiger et al 1994). The series are small and the long-term effect, however, remains uncertain (Baert & Hanauer 1994, Kornbluth et al 1994, Actis et al 1994). The effect of cyclosporin enemas in mildly to moderately active distal colitis has been a disappointment (Sandborn et al 1994). Still, many questions remain on the efficacy and safety of cyclosporin in the treatment of ulcerative colitis. More data on long-term therapy are required and the use of cyclosporin as maintenance therapy is still limited to controlled studies.

FISH-OIL SUPPLEMENTATION

Prostaglandin E_2 and leukotriene B4 are metabolites of arachidonic acid via the cyclo-oxygenase pathway and the lipoxygenase pathway respectively. Increased levels of prostaglandin E_2 and leukotriene B4 are found in active ulcerative colitis. Diets containing high levels of ω-3 fatty acids such as eicosapentaenoic acid and docosahexaenoic acid are known to modify leukotriene production, resulting in a reduced production of leukotriene B4 and an increased production of leukotriene B5, which has reduced chemotactic properties compared to leukotriene B4. Dietary fish-oil supplementation has improved patients with other inflammatory diseases such as rheumatoid arthritis. Five placebo-controlled double-blind studies have addressed this question in ulcerative colitis (Lorenz et al 1989, Stenson et al 1992, Hawthorne et al 1992a, Aslan & Triadafilopoulos 1992, Greenfield et al 1993). Despite reduced levels of leukotriene B4 and, in some studies, histopathologic improvement, no clinical benefit of dietary fish-oil supplementation for 4–12 months was seen in patients with ulcerative colitis.

CORTICOSTEROIDS

The relapse-preventing properties of systemic corticosteroids were studied in two early controlled studies. Truelove and Witts (1959) found no effect of 25 mg cortisone twice daily for 1 year compared to placebo, and a later study on prednisone 5 mg three times daily also showed disappointing results (Lennard-Jones et al 1965). Thus, there is no rationale for continued corticosteroid treatment once remission is achieved. Whether higher doses of the newer steroids with a high degree of first-pass metabolism diminishing the risks of side effects may alter this practice remains to be proven.

DISODIUM CROMOGLYCATE

This drug has been used extensively in the treatment of allergic conditions. At first it appeared as though it was beneficial in ulcerative colitis (Heatley et al 1975), but later large-scale controlled therapeutic trials showed it to be without value (Willoughby et al 1979).

ANTIDIARRHEALS

Agents aimed at reducing diarrhea should be avoided in an acute stage of colitis as they may contribute to the development of toxic megacolon. The situation may be different in the maintenance treatment. Some patients with ulcerative colitis in remission also suffer from irritable bowel syndrome. In such patients symptomatic treatment with a bulking agent may be helpful (Hallert et al 1991). In patients with inactive disease, where tenesmus is common, loperamide or diphenoxylate may decrease this socially disturbing symptom.

CLINICAL ADVICE

In a patient with ulcerative colitis who has been brought into remission the aim is to reduce the occurrence of future relapse. Maintenance treatment of ulcerative colitis is long lasting, often lifelong. So far, the mainstay of treatment is 5-ASA-based drugs. A drug should be prescribed which most reliably delivers 5-ASA to the colon.

If a patient is being treated with sulfasalazine and suffers no adverse effects, there is no need to switch to another compound, except in cases of male infertility.

In new cases a sulfa-free compound should be chosen to avoid the rare, but very serious, sulfa-related side effects of agranulocytosis, exfoliative dermatitis and sulfonamide-induced hepatotoxicity. The pH-release dependent formulations should not be used routinely in order to minimize the risk of renal lesions. Among the new drugs the most reliable deliverers of 5-ASA to the colon are olsalazine and balsalazide. In a patient who does not tolerate either of these two compounds a mesalazine formulation can be tried. Of these, Pentasa seems the most appropriate as it does not cause high serum peak concentrations of 5-ASA.

Sulfasalazine has been shown to be of great value as a second-line treatment in rheumatoid arthritis and pelvo-spondylitis (McConkey et al 1980). This effect is mediated by its sulfapyridine moiety. Thus, in a patient suffering from ulcerative colitis in combination with any of these joint diseases sulfasalazine may still be considered as the first option, even in a new case.

In a patient with an ileorectal anastomosis treatment with an azo bond-containing compound must be considered unsatisfactory. It is far from certain that the azo bond is split by gut bacteria in such a patient. Therefore maintenance treatment with 5-ASA as enema, foam or suppository appears more appropriate. Similarly, patients with high relapse rate of proctitis or proctosigmoiditis, in spite of oral therapy, may benefit from topical therapy. In patients who prefer oral treatment Pentasa is probably the drug of choice.

Corticosteroids are of no value as maintenance treatment.

In patients with unresponsive disease or a high relapse rate in spite of 5-ASA, or who cannot tolerate 5-ASA, azathioprine or 6-mercaptopurine are worth trying. From clinical experience it seems definite that there exists at least a subgroup of patients who benefits from such therapy. It also appears logical to combine azathioprine or 6-mercaptopurine with 5-ASA, if possible. Azathioprine may be used in a daily dose of 2 mg/kg. 6-mercaptopurine used to be given in a daily dose of 1–1.5 mg/kg, but in recent reports an initial dose of 50 mg/day has been given and adjusted depending on the clinical response (Present et al 1989). Concomitant use of corticosteroids in tapering doses is necessary initially, as the effects of both drugs develop slowly and it may take months until the full effect is achieved. Regular checks of full blood count and liver tests are required. At present the optimal duration of treatment is unknown. The relapse rate in patients who discontinue therapy, however, is probably high, as was illustrated by the withdrawal study by Hawthorne et al (1992b). In another study ten out of 13 patients had a relapse when 6-mercaptopurine was stopped after 1 year of clinical remission (Present et al 1988).

PREGNANCY AND LACTATION

In a pregnant woman with ulcerative colitis the various treatments can be broadly divided into those that are safe, those that should only be used if there is a strong indication, and those that should be avoided (Table 63.4). There is a general consensus that corticosteroids can be used during pregnancy exactly as in a non-pregnant woman.

Similarly, sulfasalazine can be used safely and does not cause congenital abnormalities (Järnerot 1982). However, sulfasalazine is known to reduce the serum folate con-

Table 63.4 Treatment for inflammatory bowel disease during pregnancy and lactation

Pregnancy

Can be used safely	Can possibly be used when indication strong	Should be avoided due to insufficient data
Corticosteroids Sulfasalazine Mesalazine	Azathioprine	Cyclosporin Olsalazine Metronidazole Diphenoxylate Loperamide

Lactation

Can be used safely	Sufficient data lacking but possibly safe
Corticosteroids Sulfasalazine Mesalazine Olsalazine Metronidazole Diphenoxylate Loperamide	Azathioprine Cyclosporin

centration (Franklin & Rosenberg 1973). Folate deficiency has been connected with congenital neural crest lesions, so an extra supply of folic acid should be considered in a fertile woman. The main concern with sulfasalazine has been the theoretical risk of inducing kernicterus due to the sulfa moiety, which competes with bilirubin for binding sites on albumin. However, this risk is negligible as bilirubin and sulfapyridine do not generally have the same binding sites on albumin. Very high serum sulfapyridine concentrations are needed to displace bilirubin from its albumin-binding site. Such high concentrations are not achieved with therapeutic doses of sulfasalazine (Järnerot et al 1981). Mesalazine preparations can probably be used safely during pregnancy, including those dependent on pH for release (Habal et al 1993). About 2% of unsplit olsalazine is normally absorbed, giving rise to very low serum concentrations of olsalazine. Whether this carries a risk for the fetus is unknown at present. Only a handful of pregnancies in olsalazine-treated women are known. So far, no untoward events have been reported.

No studies exist addressing this question for topical 5-ASA. From a theoretical point of view a low-dose low-volume enema with a slightly acidic pH should be without risk, as the plasma concentration of 5-ASA should not exceed that seen during oral sulfasalazine medication.

When there is a strong indication, azathioprine and 6-mercaptopurine can probably be used to treat pregnant women. To date, no complications have been noted. Successful pregnancies have been reported for transplant patients treated with azathioprine or 6-mercaptopurine, and 14 women with inflammatory bowel disease receiving azathioprine (2 mg/kg) had 16 uncomplicated pregnancies and normal children (Alstead et al 1990). However, caution is advised with the use of azathioprine in pregnancy.

During breastfeeding, corticosteroids, sulfasalazine, mesalazine, olsalazine, diphenoxylate and loperamide can all be used safely. However, incomplete data are available for azathioprine and cyclosporin, so their use for the treatment of ulcerative colitis in lactating women should be avoided if possible.

REFERENCES

Actis G C, Ottobrelli A, Lagget M, Pera A, Pinna-Pintor M, Verme G 1994 Intravenous cyclosporin for refractory ulcerative colitis. A phase II study to reduce dose and toxicity. Gastroenterology 106: A642

Adler D J, Korelitz B I 1990 The therapeutic efficacy of 6-mercaptopurine in refractory ulcerative colitis. American Journal of Gastroenterology 85: 717–722

Alstead E M, Ritchie J K, Lennard-Jones J E, Farthing M J G, Clark M L 1990. Safety of azathioprine in pregnancy in inflammatory bowel disease. Gastroenterology 99: 443–446

Aslan A, Triadafilopoulos G 1992 Fish oil fatty acid supplementation in active ulcerative colitis: a double-blind, placebo-controlled, cross-over study. American Journal of Gastroenterology 87: 432–437

Azad Khan A K, Piris J, Truelove S C 1977 An experiment to determine the active therapeutic moiety of sulphasalazine. Lancet 1: 892–895

Azad Khan A K, Howes D T, Piris J, Truelove S C 1980 Optimum dose of sulphasalazine for maintenance treatment of ulcerative colitis. Gut 21: 232–240

Baert F, Hanauer S 1994 CyA in severe steroid-resistant UC: long-term results of therapy. Gastroenterology 106: A648

Baron T H, Truss C D, Elson C O 1993. Low-dose oral methotrexate in refractory inflammatory bowel disease. Digestive Diseases and Sciences 38: 1851–1856

Bean R H D 1962 The treatment of chronic ulcerative colitis with 6-mercaptopurine. Medical Journal of Australia 2: 592–593

Bianchi-Porro G, Petrillo M, Ardizzone S, Dersideri S 1991 Azathioprine in the treatment of ulcerative colitis. Journal of Clinical Gastroenterology 13: 113–114

Biddle W L, Greenberger N J, Swan J T, McPhee M S, Miner P B 1988 5-Aminosalicylic acid enemas: effective agent in maintaining remission in left-sided ulcerative colitis. Gastroenterology 94: 1075–1079

Binder V, Halskov S, Hvidberg E et al 1981 A controlled study of 5-acet-aminosalicylic acid as enema in ulcerative colitis. Scandinavian Journal of Gastroenterology 16: 1122 Abstract

Bondesen S, Haagen Nielsen O, Jacobsen O et al 1984 5-Aminosalicylic acid enemas in patients with active ulcerative colitis. Influence of acidity on the kinetic pattern. Scandinavian Journal of Gastroenterology 19: 677–682

Calder J C, Funder C C, Green C R, Ham K N, Tauge J D 1972 Nephrotoxic lesions from 5-aminosalicylic acid. British Medical Journal 1: 152–154

Campieri M, Gionchetti P, Beluzzi A et al 1989 5-Aminosalicylic acid suppositories in the management of ulcerative colitis. Diseases of the Colon and Rectum 32: 398–399

Campieri M, Lanfranchi G A, Bertoni F et al 1984 A double-blind clinical trial to compare the effects of 4-aminosalicylic acid to 5-aminosalicylic acid in topical treatment of ulcerative colitis. Digestion 29: 204–208

Campieri M, Lanfranchi G A, Boschi S et al 1985 Topical administration of 5-aminosalicylic acid enemas in patients with ulcerative colitis. Studies on rectal absorption and excretion. Gut 26: 400–405

Caprilli R, Carratu R, Babbini M 1975 A double-blind comparison of the effectiveness of azathioprine and sulfasalazine in idiopathic proctocolitis. Preliminary report. Digestive Diseases 20: 115–120

Connell W R, Kamm M A, Lennard-Jones J E, Ritchie J K 1993 Bone marrow toxicity from azathioprine: twenty-seven year experience in inflammatory bowel disease. Gut 34: 1081–1085

Connell W R, Kamm M A, Dickson M, Balkwill A M, Ritchie J K,

Lennard-Jones J E 1994 Long-term neoplasia risk after azathioprine treatment in inflammatory bowel disease. Lancet 343: 1249–1252

Cox J A, Daneshmend T K, Hawkey C J, Logan R F A, Walt R P 1988 Devastating diarrhoea due to azathioprine: management difficulty in inflammatory bowel disease. Gut 29: 686–688

D'Albasio G, Trallori G, Ghetti A et al 1990 Intermittent therapy with high-dose 5-aminosalicylic acid enemas for maintaining remission in ulcerative proctosigmoiditis. Diseases of the Colon and Rectum 33: 394–397

D'Arienzo A, Panarese A, D'Armiento F P et al 1990 5-Aminosalicylic acid suppositories in the maintenance of remission in idiopathic proctitis or proctosigmoiditis: a double-blind placebo-controlled clinical trial. American Journal of Gastroenterology 85: 1079–1082

Das K M, Eastwood M A, McManus J P A, Sircus W 1973 Adverse reactions during salicylazo-sulphapyridine therapy and the relation with drug metabolism and acetylator phenotype. New England Journal of Medicine 289: 491–495

Dissanayake A S, Truelove S C 1973 A controlled therapeutic trial of long-term maintenance treatment in ulcerative colitis with sulphasalazine (Salazopyrine) Gut 14: 923–926

Dwarakanath A D, Michael J, Allan R N 1992 Sulphasalazine induced renal failure. Gut 33: 1006–1007

Ewe K, Press A G, Bollen S, Schuku I 1992 Gastric emptying of indigestible tablets in relation to compositions and time of ingestion of meals studied by metal detector. Digestive Diseases and Sciences 36: 146–152

Franklin J L, Rosenberg I H 1973 Impaired folic acid absorption in inflammatory bowel disease: effects of salicylazosulphapyridine (Azulfidine). Gastroenterology 64: 517–525

Giaffer M H, O'Brien C J, Holdsworth C D 1992 Clinical tolerance to three 5-aminosalicylic acid releasing preparations in patients with inflammatory bowel disease intolerant or allergic to sulphasalazine. Alimentary Pharmacology and Therapeutics 6: 51–59

Ginsberg A L, Davis W D, Nochomovitz L E 1992 Placebo-controlled trial of ulcerative colitis with oral 4-aminosalicylic acid. Gastroenterology 102: 448–452

Greenfield S M, Green A T, Teare J P et al 1993 A randomized controlled study of evening primrose oil and fish oil in ulcerative colitis. Alimentary Pharmacology and Therapeutics 7: 159–166

Guarino J, Chatzinoff M, Berk T, Friedman L S 1987 5-Aminosalicylic acid enemas in refractory distal ulcerative colitis: long term results. American Journal of Gastroenterology 82: 732–737

Habal F M, Hui G, Greenberg G R 1993 Oral 5-aminosalicylic acid for inflammatory bowel disease in pregnancy: safety and clinical course. Gastroenterology 105: 1057–1060

Hallert C, Kaldma M, Petersson B G 1991 Ispaghula husk may relieve gastrointestinal symptoms in ulcerative colitis in remission. Scandinavian Journal of Gastroenterology 26: 747–750

Hawthorne A B, Hawkey C J 1989 Immunosuppressive drugs in inflammatory bowel disease. A review of their mechanisms of efficacy and place in therapy. Drugs 38: 267–288

Hawthorne A B, Daneshmend T K, Hawkey C J et al 1992a Treatment of ulcerative colitis with fish oil supplementation: a prospective 12 month randomised controlled trial. Gut 33: 922–928

Hawthorne A B, Logan R F A, Hawkey C J et al 1992b Randomised controlled trial of azathioprine withdrawal in ulcerative colitis. British Medical Journal 305: 20–22

Heatley R V, Calcraft B J, Rhodes J, Owen E, Evans B K 1975 Disodium cromoglycate in the treatment of chronic proctitis. Gut 16: 559–563

Ireland A, Mason C H, Jewell D P 1988 A controlled trial comparing olsalazine and sulphasalazine for the maintenance treatment of ulcerative colitis. Gut 29: 835–837

Isaacs K L, Murphy D 1990 Pancreatitis after rectal administration of 5-aminosalicylic acid. Journal of Clinical Gastroenterology 12: 198–199

Jacobsen B A, Abildgaard K, Rasmussen H H 1991 Availability of mesalazine (5-aminosalicylic acid) from enemas and suppositories during steady-state conditions. Scandinavian Journal of Gastroenterology 26: 378–384

Järnerot G 1982 Fertility, sterility and pregnancy in chronic inflammatory bowel disease. Scandinavian Journal of Gastroenterology 17: 1–4

Järnerot G 1988 Clinical tolerance of olsalazine. Scandinavian Journal of Gastroenterology 23(Suppl 148): 21–23

Järnerot G 1989 Newer 5-aminosalicylic acid based drugs in chronic inflammatory bowel disease. Drugs 37: 73–86

Järnerot G 1994 New salicylates as maintenance treatment in ulcerative colitis. Gut 35: 1155–1158

Järnerot G, Andersen S, Esbjörner E, Sandström B, Brodersen R 1981 Albumin reserve for binding of bilirubin in maternal and cord serum under treatment with sulphasalazine. Scandinavian Journal of Gastroenterology 16: 1049–1055

Jewell D P, Truelove S 1974 Azathioprine in ulcerative colitis: final report on controlled therapeutic trial. British Medical Journal 4: 627–630

Kirk A P, Lennard-Jones J E 1982 Controlled trial of azathioprine in chronic ulcerative colitis. British Medical Journal 284: 1291–1292

Kornbluth A, Lichtiger S, Present D, Hanauer S 1994 Long-term results of oral cyclosporin in patients with severe ulcerative colitis: a double-blind, randomized, multicenter trial. Gastroenterology 106: A714

Kozarek R A 1993 Review article: immunosuppressive therapy for inflammatory bowel disease. Alimentary Pharmacology and Therapeutics 7: 117–123

Kozarek R A, Patterson D J, Gelfand M D, Botoman V A, Ball T J, Wilske K R 1989 Methotrexate induces clinical and histologic remission in patients with refractory inflammatory bowel disease. Annals of Internal Medicine 110: 353–356

Kozarek R A, Patterson D J, Botoman V A, Ball T J, Gelfand M D 1991 Methotrexate use in inflammatory bowel disease patients who have failed azathioprine or 6-mercaptopurine. Gastroenterology 100: A222

Kozarek R A, Patterson D J, Gelfand M D, Ball T J, Botoman V A 1992 Long-term use of methotrexate in inflammatory bowel disease: severe disease 3, drug therapy 2, seventh inning stretch. Gastroenterology 102: A648

Lennard-Jones J E, Misiewicz J J, Connell A M, Baron J H, Avery Jones F 1965 Prednisone as maintenance treatment for ulcerative colitis in remission. Lancet 1: 188–189

Lichtiger S, Present D H, Kornbluth A et al 1994 Cyclosporin in severe ulcerative colitis refractory to steroid therapy. New England Journal of Medicine 330: 1841–1845

Lobo A J, Foster P N, Burke D A, Johnston D, Axon A T R 1990 The role of azathioprine in the management of ulcerative colitis. Diseases of the Colon and Rectum 33: 374–377

Lorenz R, Weber P C, Szimnau P, Heldwein W, Strasser T, Loeschke K 1989 Supplementation with n-3 fatty acids from fish oil in chronic inflammatory bowel disease; a randomised, placebo-controlled, double-blind cross-over trial. Journal of Internal Medicine 225(Suppl 1): 225–232

McConkey B, Amos R S, Durham S, Forster P J G, Huball S 1980 Sulphasalazine in rheumatoid arthritis. British Medical Journal 1: 442–444

Mantzaris G J, Hatzis A, Petraki K, Spiliadi C, Triantaphyllou G 1994 Intermittent therapy with high-dose 5-aminosalicylic acid enemas maintains remission in ulcerative proctitis and proctosigmoiditis. Diseases of the Colon and Rectum 37: 58–62

Misiewicz J J, Lennard-Jones J E, Connell A M, Baron J H, Avery-Jones F 1965 Controlled trial of sulphasalazine in maintenance therapy for ulcerative colitis. Lancet 1: 185–188

Nielsen O H, Bondesen S 1983 Kinetics of 5-aminosalicylic acid after jejunal instillation in man. British Journal of Clinical Pharmacology 16: 738–740

Peppercorn M A, Goldman P 1973 Distribution of salicylazosulphapyridine and its metabolites. Gastroenterology 64: 240–245

Present D H, Chapman M L, Rubin P H 1988 Efficacy of 6-mercaptopurine (6MP) in refractory ulcerative colitis. Gastroenterology 94: A359

Present D H, Melyzer S J, Krumholz M P, Wolke A, Korelitz B I 1989 6-mercaptopurine in the management of inflammatory bowel disease: short- and long-term toxicity. Annals of Internal Medicine 111: 641–649

Rosenberg J I, Wall A J, Levin B, Binder H J, Kirsner J B 1975 A controlled trial of azathioprine in the management of chronic ulcerative colitis. Gastroenterology 69: 96–99

Ruf-Ballauf W, Hofstädter F, Kreutz K 1989 Akute interstitielle Nephritis durch 5-Aminosalicylsäure? Internist 30: 262–264

Sandberg-Gertzén H, Järnerot G, Kraaz W 1986 Azodisal sodium in the treatment of ulcerative colitis: a study of tolerance and relapse-prevention properties. Gastroenterology 90: 1024–1030

Sandborn W J, Tremaine W J, Schroeder K W et al 1994 A placebo-controlled trial of cyclosporine enemas for mildly to moderately active left-sided ulcerative colitis. Gastroenterology 106: 1429–1435

Selby W S, Bennett M K, Jewell D P 1984 Topical treatment of distal ulcerative colitis with 4-aminosalicylic acid. Digestion 29: 231–234

Steinhart A H, Baker J P, Brzezinski A, Prokipchuk E J 1990 Azathioprine therapy in chronic ulcerative colitis. Journal of Clinical Gastroenterology 12: 271–275

Stenson W F, Cort D, Rodgers J et al 1992 Dietary supplementation with fish oil in ulcerative colitis. Annals of Internal Medicine 116: 609–614

Sutherland L R, Martin F 1987 5-aminosalicylic acid enemas in the maintenance of remission in distal ulcerative colitis and proctitis. Canadian Journal of Gastroenterology 1: 3–6

Sutheraland L R, May G R, Shaffer E A 1993 Sulphasalazine revisited: a metaanalysis of 5-aminosalicylic acid in the treatment of ulcerative colitis. Annals of Internal Medicine 118: 540–549

Svartz N 1942 Salazopyrin, a new sulfanilamide preparation. Acta Medica Scandinavica 110: 557–598

Theodor E, Niv Y, Bat L 1981 Imuran in the treatment of ulcerative colitis. American Journal of Gastroenterology 76: 262–266

Toth A 1979. Reversible toxic effect of salicylazosulphapyridine on semen quality. Fertility and Sterility 31: 538–540

Travis S P L, Tysk C, De Silva H J, Sandberg-Gertzén H, Jewell D P, Järnerot G 1994 The optimum dose of olsalazine for maintaining remission in ulcerative colitis. Gut 35: 1282–1286

Truelove S C, Witts L J 1959 Cortisone and corticotropin in ulcerative colitis. British Medical Journal 1: 387–394

Verhave M, Winter H S, Grand R J 1990 Azathioprine in the treatment of children with inflammatory bowel disease. Journal of Pediatrics 117: 809–814

Willoughby C P, Heyworth M F, Piris J, Truelove S C 1979 Comparison of disodium cromoglycate and sulphasalazine as maintenance therapy for ulcerative colitis. Lancet 1: 119–122

Wright J P, O'Keefe E A, Cuming L, Jaskiewicz K 1993 Olsalazine in maintenance of clinical remission in patients with ulcerative colitis. Digestive Diseases and Sciences 38: 1837–1842

SECTION 7

Crohn's disease

64. Crohn's disease of the upper gastrointestinal tract

C. Lamers

This section provides guidance in the medical management of Crohn's disease. The avid reader will have digested the various theories of pathogenesis (Section 1) and concluded that at present medical treatment has to be prescribed for a disease of unknown cause. Medical management includes an understanding of the diagnostic aspects of Crohn's disease (radiology, endoscopy, histopathology and laboratory markers) and disorders which can be confused with Crohn's disease (Sections 2 and 3), together with an overview of the natural history (Section 4) and drug treatment, including the role of enteral and parenteral nutrition (Section 5). This section draws these threads together and provides guidelines for the management of Crohn's disease at different sites in the gastrointestinal tract.

DEFINITION

Although Crohn's disease usually affects the distal small bowel and colon, upper gastrointestinal involvement has received considerable attention recently. The prevalence depends on the definition used for the diagnosis. In most studies upper gastrointestinal Crohn's disease has been defined using criteria proposed by Nugent and Roy (1989). The diagnosis is established by one of two criteria: the histological presence of non-caseating granuloma or granulomatous inflammation with or without obvious Crohn's disease elsewhere in the intestinal tract, and without evidence of systemic granulomatous disorder, or documented Crohn's disease elsewhere in the intestinal tract and radiological and/or endoscopic findings of diffuse inflammatory change in the upper gastrointestinal tract consistent with Crohn's disease. However, the clinical significance of this diagnostic definition should not be overestimated. Many Crohn's disease patients will have one of these two criteria, provided that a thorough and careful upper gastrointestinal diagnostic work-up is carried out, including multiple deep endoscopic biopsies each with multiple sections for histological evaluation. These relatively common features contrast with the clinical symptoms of the upper gastrointestinal tract in Crohn's disease, which are uncommon. Recent studies have suggested that small gastroduodenal lesions can be found in more than 70% of patients with Crohn's disease when precise endoscopic evaluation of the upper gastrointestinal tract is included. In a Japanese study endoscopic findings consistent with Crohn's disease were discovered in the stomach in 75% and in the duodenum in 42% (Tanaka et al 1986). In that study granulomas were detected in 83% in the stomach and 76% in the duodenum by making 62 serial sections on average from each biopsy specimen. Crohn's disease of the stomach and duodenum appears also to occur frequently in children. Mashako et al (1989) showed that 42% of children with Crohn's disease had endoscopic lesions suggestive of Crohn's disease involvement, histologically confirmed by the presence of specific granuloma in over 90% of the cases. Only a minority of these patients had clinical symptoms due to the involvement of the upper gastrointestinal tract. The relatively high prevalence of upper gastroduodenal lesions in asymptomatic patients and the frequent occurrence of symptoms unrelated to Crohn's disease makes it hard to determine whether upper gastrointestinal symptoms in an individual patient with Crohn's disease are due to Crohn's disease of the upper gastrointestinal tract or not.

When applying the diagnostic criteria of Nugent and Roy (1989) the prevalence of Crohn's disease of the upper gastrointestinal tract in the IBD registry of the Department of Gastroenterology of Leiden University Hospital, The Netherlands, comprising 940 documented cases of Crohn's disease, was 49/940 (5.2%). This figure is in line with the prevalence reported in other studies (0.5–13%), in which only symptomatic patients with Crohn's disease have undergone upper gastrointestinal endoscopy and/or double contrast radiography (Dancygier & Frick 1992). A particularly high prevalence of upper gastrointestinal Crohn's disease has been reported in children and adolescents (Lenaerts et al 1989, Mashako et al 1989).

CROHN'S DISEASE OF THE ESOPHAGUS

Symptoms, diagnosis, complications

Crohn's disease of the esophagus is rare. The first reports of isolated non-specific granulomatous lesions in the esophagus were published by Franklin & Taylor (1950) and Heffernon & Kepkay (1954). The total number of reported cases is now close to 100. In our registry of 940 patients with Crohn's disease seven (7%) had esophageal involvement, while Geboes et al (1986) reported nine cases of lesions in the esophagus among 500 Crohn's disease patients (1.8%). Usually Crohn's disease of the esophagus is associated with active Crohn's disease elsewhere, in some cases only detected some time after the esophageal lesion. Patients usually present with dysphagia, odynophagia, pyrosis and substernal chest pain. Progressive painful dysphagia, the most common symptom, can become very severe within a few weeks to several months, and severe weight loss may occur. In the mouth aphthous ulcers may accompany aphthoid lesions in the esophagus (Geboes et al 1986). Extraintestinal manifestations and critical illness have been reported in patients with esophageal Crohn's disease lesions and involvement of multiple segments of the gastrointestinal tract (Geboes et al 1986).

The diagnosis is based on symptoms, double contrast radiography and endoscopy with serial sections of deep endoscopic biopsies. Two stages of Crohn's disease of the esophagus have been distinguished (Huchzermeyer et al 1976, Geboes et al 1986). In stage I inflammatory changes predominate and the esophagitis is mild or, more often, erosive ulcerative, whereas stage II is characterized by stenoses similar to those resulting from reflux esophagitis or a malignant tumor.

Radiological investigation of the esophagus may reveal thickened mucosal folds or cobblestones, segmental asymmetric irregularity of the wall, and aphthous or intramural ulcers, predominantly in the distal part. In advanced cases tubular stenosis develops in the middle or distal third. Occasional cases show intramural fistulous tracts and esophagobronchial fistulae (Cynn et al 1975). Filiform polyps may occur after severe esophagitis (Cockey et al 1985).

Endoscopic features are in general non-specific and include hyperemia, granularity, slight friability of the mucosa, and nodular thickening of the folds or cobblestones in the middle or distal part of the esophagus. Erosions and ulcers, aphthoid or deep, surrounded by normal or slightly diseased mucosa may also be found (Geboes et al 1986). Echoendoscopy may reveal a disrupted wall and transmural infiltration (Leurs et al 1987). However, the ultrasonographic findings are non-specific and may resemble those of a carcinoma (Dancygier & Frick 1992). Biopsy specimens are often too small to confirm the diagnosis of Crohn's disease of the esophagus. Routine histology usually reveals focal inflammation in the epithelium and lamina propria, and additional serial sections are needed to demonstrate granulomas (Geboes et al 1986). The differential diagnosis comprises reflux esophagitis, mycotic infection, herpes virus esophagitis and malignant disease. The main complication is severe obstruction due to fibrosis; rarely, esophagobronchial fistulae may occur (Cynn et al 1975).

Management of esophageal Crohn's disease

Little is known about the medical management of esophageal Crohn's disease. Furthermore, very little is known about the natural history of Crohn's disease lesions in the esophagus, since the majority of patients are treated with anti-inflammatory or immunosuppressive drugs for disease elsewhere. In fact, in most patients with Crohn's disease of the esophagus the clinical picture is determined by symptoms of the accompanying distal Crohn's disease. Gastroesophageal reflux disease (GORD) is also common, making it difficult to relate gastroesophageal symptoms such as heartburn, retrosternal pain and dysphagia to Crohn's disease involvement of the esophagus. Treatment of Crohn's disease with immunosuppressive drugs renders the esophagus susceptible to mycotic or virus infections.

In stage I esophageal Crohn's disease, where inflammatory and erosive ulcerative lesions are present, drug therapy is beneficial in alleviating symptoms, healing the mucosa and retarding the progression of the disease. However, in stage II Crohn's disease of the esophagus, where stenosis leads to obstructive complaints, endoscopic dilatation or resection of the stenotic esophagus may be needed. When stenosing esophageal Crohn's disease hampers adequate food intake, a liquid or semiliquid diet may be helpful. In rare cases with severe obstruction parenteral nutrition is required. Drug therapy for stage I esophageal Crohn's disease may be divided into those drugs directly modulating the inflammatory process, such as anti-inflammatory and immunosuppressive agents, and adjunctive therapy indirectly influencing the esophageal lesion and the symptoms, such as gastric antisecretory drugs and mucosa protective agents. Most patients with stage I Crohn's disease of the esophagus are successfully treated by corticosteroids. Geboes et al (1986) reported the treatment of seven patients with aphthoid lesions with prednisone in a dose of 30–50 mg/day. All esophageal symptoms readily disappeared after a few days. Endoscopy performed after 2 weeks in three patients and at a later stage in four patients showed complete disappearance of the lesions. D'Heans et al (1994) observed three patterns of evolution of esophageal Crohn's disease. About half of the patients had no relapse, a quarter had persistent lesions despite corticosteroid therapy, and a quarter had recurrent lesions after initial resolution. In contrast to other reports (Gelfand & Krone 1968, Niv 1988), Geboes et al (1986) also reported good results with sulfasalazine in two patients. Such an effect is surprising, since sulfasalazine requires conversion to active metabolites by bacterial enzymes to exert its local activity. It is unlikely that enteric-coated 5-aminosalicylic acid preparations or olsalazine would exert a local effect in the esophagus. Experience with immunosuppressive drugs such as cyclosporin or 6-mercaptopurine is anecdotal. Beck et al (1995) reported a case of Crohn's disease-associated esophageal disease who failed to respond to oral or intravenous corticosteroids but responded rapidly to cyclosporin A.

The indirect approach using powerful gastric antisecretory drugs as adjunctive therapy has attracted considerable interest. Two patients with Crohn's disease and ulcerative lesions in the esophagus were treated with the proton pump inhibitor omeprazole, which induced rapid symptomatic relief but no macroscopic evidence of healing (Przemioslo & Mee 1994). Reduction of gastroesophageal acid reflux by omeprazole may have diminished irritation of the esophageal lesions by luminal acid. However, Beck et al (1995) reported two patients with esophageal Crohn's disease who failed to respond to either the H_2-receptor antagonist ranitidine or the proton pump inhibitor omeprazole. It is likely that gastric antisecretory therapy is only effective in those patients with esophageal Crohn's disease who have appreciable gastroesophageal reflux. Little is known about the effect of the mucosal protective drug sucralfate. When given in a suspension form this might protect the esophageal mucosa from luminal irritants. Dasnoy et al (1993) reported a rapid response following combined treatment with corticosteroids and sucralfate in a Crohn's disease patient with esophageal lesions. In stage II esophageal Crohn's disease, where stenoses and occasionally fistulae predominate, surgical resection is often needed. However, in selected cases endoscopic bouginage may relieve symptoms. Recently, Mathis et al (1994) reported a case of Crohn's disease of the esophagus in whom gradual dilation of the stricture and sealing of fistulae appeared to be successful. About 40–50% with grade II esophageal Crohn's disease involvement will eventually require surgical therapy (Dancygier & Frick 1992).

CROHN'S DISEASE OF THE STOMACH AND DUODENUM

Symptoms, diagnosis, complications

The first report of duodenal involvement in a patient with regional jejunitis was published by Gottlieb and Alpert in 1937. Since then at least 300 cases have been reported (Nugent & Roy 1989). In our department 46 cases of gastric and/or duodenal involvement have been identified among 940 registered patients with Crohn's disease, a prevalence of 4.9%. In earlier reports from our department covering 226 and 760 patients, the prevalence was 1.8 and 4.5%, respectively (Weterman 1976, 1990).

The duodenum is usually involved more often than the stomach. In our series gastric lesions were found in 1.9% and duodenal lesions in 4.1%, while changes in both were found in 1.7%. In most cases gastroduodenal lesions are associated with more distal disease. The gastroduodenal region is rarely the first site to be involved. In some the stomach or duodenum is involved because of contiguity with adjacent ileal or colonic disease (Rutgeerts et al 1980).

In nearly all cases epigastric pain or dyspepsia is the predominant symptom, which mimics peptic ulcer or non-ulcer dyspepsia. In more advanced disease, most have symptoms due to obstructive lesions, (epigastric distress, early satiety, nausea, vomiting and weight loss). Only a few cases of hematemesis or melena have been described (Wise et al 1971, Johnson & Delaney 1972, Tootla et al 1976, Nugent et al 1977). In a series of 89 patients with duodenal Crohn's disease Nugent and Roy (1989) reported abdominal pain in 79%, weight loss in 64%, nausea/vomiting in 61% and hemorrhage in 17%.

The antrum is usually involved and the lesion frequently extends to the proximal duodenum. Early lesions, erosions and aphthous ulcers are best detected by double contrast radiography or endoscopy (Laufer et al 1976, Ariyama et al 1980, Levine 1987). Thickened antral folds, nodularity, deep irregular ulcers or cobblestones may also be demonstrated. Hypomotility and delay in emptying of the stomach, with some degree of pyloric obstruction, is seen in more advanced cases. Tubular narrowing and a 'ram's horn' appearance (Farman et al 1975) or, when stomach and duodenum are both involved, a pseudo-Billroth 1 configuration has been described (Thompson et al 1975). Every part of the duodenum can be involved (Frandsen et al 1980) but the second part is most commonly affected. Abnormal folds, stenosis and ulceration are the main radiographic features (Miller et al 1979). Different types of ulcer, such as aphthous, longitudinal, transverse and deep, can be found. Fissures and pseudodiverticula are occasionally seen, but fistula formation is rare (Rutgeerts et al 1980).

At endoscopy, early minute gastroduodenal lesions are described as patchy erythema, aphthoid erosion and verrucous change (Tanaka et al 1986). More advanced lesions include thickened antral folds, diffuse granularity, diffuse or mucosal erosions, stellate, serpiginous, linear or deep ulcers, and cobblestones (Alcantara et al 1993, Moonka et al 1993). When narrowing occurs the site may be prepyloric, in the duodenal bulb, or in the second part of the duodenum. Several authors have compared endoscopy and radiography in the diagnosis of Crohn's disease of the stomach or duodenum. Rutgeerts et al (1980) concluded that radiology and endoscopy of the gastroduodenal region are complementary. Endoscopy allowed better visualization of the mucosal defects, whereas other features such as diminished expansion and contiguity of lesions were demonstrated better by barium meal examination. In contrast, Mashako et al (1989) reported that endoscopic and histological evidence of Crohn's disease of the upper gastrointestinal tract is often present despite an absence of radiological changes. Non-caseating granuloma or granulomatous inflammation is frequently found in serial sections of biopsies from endoscopically involved mucosa (Tanaka et al 1986). However, granulomas may also be present in endoscopically normal tissue, although they may be absent in endoscopically characteristic lesions (Nugent & Roy 1989). The significance of active inflammatory changes reported in gastric biopsies of asymptomatic Crohn's disease patients has to be reconsidered in the light of the present knowledge of *Helicobacter pylori*-associated gastritis (Korelitz et al 1981, El-Omar et al 1994). Furthermore, the diagnostic value of an increased number of IgM-containing cells in the lamina propria in gastric and duodenal biopsies of Crohn's disease patients without gastric complaints awaits further study (Van Spreeuwel et al 1982). ^{99m}Tc HMPAO-labeled leukocyte scintigraphy may identify gastric involvement in a patient with intestinal Crohn's disease (Prats et al 1994).

Crohn's disease of the stomach has to be distinguished from *Helicobacter pylori*-associated and NSAID-induced gastric or duodenal ulcers, erosive or varioliforme gastritis, distal gastric cancer, lymphoma and various granulomatous diseases.

Obstruction is the most common complication of gastric or duodenal Crohn's disease. Fistulae arising from the stomach or duodenum are, however, extremely rare. Almost all gastric or duodenal fistulae originate from diseased small or large bowel (Murray et al 1984, Jacobson et al 1985, Klein et al 1987). Rutgeerts et al (1980) described two cases of fistula between a narrow duodenal bulb and the common bile duct. Massive upper gastrointestinal tract hemorrhage is rare in Crohn's disease (Paget et al 1972, Tootla et al 1976, Nugent et al 1977, Bruyns et al 1979).

A case of malignancy complicating duodenal Crohn's disease has been reported (Meiselman et al 1987).

Management of gastroduodenal Crohn's disease

Since the etiology of Crohn's disease is unknown, no specific therapy is available. As for Crohn's disease in other parts of the gastrointestinal tract, medical treatment for mucosal inflammatory changes should be tried first. However, most patients with gastroduodenal Crohn's disease are treated with anti-inflammatory or immunosuppressive drugs because of associated distal disease. Since upper gastrointestinal Crohn's disease is usually accompanied or preceded by distal Crohn's disease requiring medical therapy, no data are available regarding the natural history of untreated gastroduodenal Crohn's disease.

The medical therapy for gastroduodenal therapy comprises anti-inflammatory or immunosuppressive drugs on the one hand and adjunct gastric antisecretory or mucosa-protecting agents on the other. Most patients achieve good results with corticosteroids, which may be given in intermittent courses (Nugent & Roy 1989). A combination of corticosteroids with sulfasalazine or 5-aminosalicylic acid (5-ASA) has been advocated (Kuntz et al 1988), but the pharmacokinetic profile makes the latter unlikely to be efficacious in gastroduodenal Crohn's disease lesions. Theoretically, non-enteric coated mono-5-ASA or non-enteric coated budesonide may be of considerable therapeutic interest in such patients. Budesonide is a potent glucocorticosteroid which, after absorption, is converted to inactive metabolites by liver enzymes, thereby reducing the risk of corticosteroid-associated side effects (Brattsand 1990). Recently, the efficacy of an enteric-coated form of budesonide has been demonstrated in ileocecal Crohn's disease, with little suppression of plasma cortisol levels and few side effects (Greenberg et al 1994, Rutgeerts et al 1994). Reports on azathioprine (Nugent & Roy 1989, Kuntz et al 1988, Bianchi Porro et al 1991), 6-mercaptopurine (Griffiths et al 1989) and metronidazole (Nugent & Roy 1989), which are mainly used for simultaneous distal disease, are scanty and do not allow specific conclusions to be drawn. Similarly, no conclusion can be drawn regarding the immunosuppressant cyclosporin.

Gastric antisecretory therapy is usually used in combination with corticosteroids. Antacids or H_2-receptor antagonists have been used with variable success (Murray et al 1984, Nugent & Roy 1989, Griffiths et al 1989). Recently, Valori and Cockel (1990) reported two cases of duodenal ulceration in Crohn's disease that were unresponsive to high-dose H_2-receptor antagonists but healed when treated with the proton pump inhibitor omeprazole. Omeprazole is capable of maintaining high intragastric pH for long periods and is effective in H_2-receptor antagonist-resistant peptic ulceration. The authors recommended the long-term use of this drug in duodenal Crohn's disease in order to prevent pyloric or duodenal stenosis. In addition, they felt that acid inhibition therapy is more likely to heal duodenal ulceration associated with Crohn's disease than corticosteroid therapy, which may lead to complications such as perforation or hemorrhage (Valori & Cockel 1990). Similar positive results using omeprazole were reported by Woolfson and Greenberg (1992). These authors treated four patients with ileal Crohn's disease, weight loss and ulceration of the antrum or duodenum with 40 mg/day omeprazole, resulting in rapid pain relief and weight gain. Follow-up endoscopy showed ulcer healing in one, partial healing in two and no change in the fourth patient. Withdrawal of the drug resulted in relapse of ulceration in three of the four patients, but all responded to long-term omeprazole for up to 3 years (Woolfson & Greenberg 1992). Bianchi Porro et al (1991) treated four Crohn's disease patients with gastric or duodenal ulcerations. Based on the variable results obtained, the authors suggested that omeprazole may be efficacious only in those cases in which the ulcer is of a peptic nature and not in those cases in which the ulcer is Crohn's disease related. The distinction between peptic ulcer and ulcer lesions secondary to Crohn's disease is notoriously difficult (Bianchi Porro et al 1991) but attracts little attention. However, it is of clinical importance as peptic ulceration can be permanently healed by the eradication of *Helicobacter pylori* with antibiotics (Marshall et al 1988). Interestingly, the prevalence of positive *H. pylori* serology was low (10%) in patients who were currently receiving or had received sulfasalazine, but the patients on 5-ASA or olsalazine (45%) had a prevalence of seropositivity similar to the control subjects (52%; El-Omar et al 1994). It was suggested that sulfasalazine treatment leads to eradication of *H. pylori* infection. Since *H. pylori* infection is a prerequisite for peptic ulcer, patients on sulfasalazine are probably less susceptible to peptic ulceration. Eradication therapy with an appropriate antibiotic regimen may be indicated in those Crohn's disease patients who have gastroduodenal ulceration of possible peptic origin. However, triple-therapy regimens with combinations of amoxicillin, metronidazole, clarithromycine, tetracyclin or bismuth compounds are probably more effective in eradicating *H. pylori* than monotherapy with sulfasalazine (Dixon 1995). Omeprazole may be added to this antibiotic regimen to induce rapid symptomatic relief and possibly to increase the efficacy of antibiotics (Dixon 1995). Data on the mucosa protective agent sucralfate in gastroduodenal Crohn's disease are scanty and do not allow specific conclusions (Griffiths et al 1989, Valori & Cockel 1990). Eventually between 10 and 40% of patients with gastroduodenal Crohn's disease require surgical intervention (Dancygier & Frick 1992, Kuntz et al 1988, Nugent & Roy 1989). The most frequent indication for surgery is gastroduodenal obstruction, whereas major hemorrhage, extensive fistula formation or suspicion of malignancy may warrant resection. If bypass surgery is performed no additional vagotomy should be done because of the risk of severe side effects (Nugent & Roy 1989). In case of anastomotic ulceration after bypass surgery treatment with gastric antisecretory drugs such as omeprazole is likely to be effective. Dilatation of strictures and strictureplasty may be viable treatment options in selected patients with stenosing gastroduodenal Crohn's disease (Nugent & Roy 1989, Shepherd et al 1985).

REFERENCES

Alcántara M, Rodriguez R, Potenciano J L M, Carrobles J L, Muñoz C, Gomez R 1993 Endoscopic and bioptic findings in the upper gastrointestinal tract in patients with Crohn's disease. Endoscopy 25: 282–286

Ariyama J, Wehlin L, Lindstrom C G, Wenkert A, Roberts G M 1980 Gastro-duodenal erosions in Crohn's disease. Gastrointestinal Radiology 5: 121–125

Beck P L, Lay T E, Blustein P K 1995 Esophageal Crohn's disease: treat the inflammation, not just the symptoms. Digestive Diseases and Sciences 40: 837–838

Bianchi Porro G, Ardizzone S, Petrillo M, Desideri S 1991 Omeprazole for peptic ulcer in Crohn's disease. American Journal of Gastroenterology 86: 245–246

Brattsand R 1990 Overview of newer glucocorticosteroid preparations for inflammatory bowel disease. Canadian Journal of Gastroenterology 4: 407–414

Bruyns F, Lubbers E J C, van Tongeren J H M 1979 Major haemorrhage in Crohn's disease. Netherlands Journal of Medicine 22: 67–71

Cockey B M, Jones B, Bayless Th M, Shauer A B 1985 Filiform polyps of the esophagus with inflammatory bowel disease. American Journal of Radiology 144: 1207–1208

Cynn W S, Chon H, Gureghian P A, Levin B L 1975 Crohn's disease of the esophagus. American Journal of Roentgenology, Radium Therapy and Nuclear Medicine 125: 359–364

Dancygier H, Frick B 1992 Crohn's disease of the upper gastrointestinal tract. Endoscopy 24: 555–558

Dasnoy Ph, Mathieu J L, De Plean A, Rajan A, Fiasse R 1993 Maladie de Crohn de l'oesophage. A propos d'un cas. Acta Gastro-Enterologica Belgica LVI: 347–351

D'Heans G, Rutgeerts P, Geboes K, Vantrappen G 1994 The natural history of esophageal Crohn's disease: three patterns of evolution. Gastrointestinal Endoscopy 40: 296–300

Dixon J S 1995 *Helicobacter* eradication: unravelling the facts. Scandinavian Journal of Gastroenterology 30(Suppl 212): 48–62

El-Omar E, Penman I, Cruikshank G et al 1994 Low prevalence of *Helicobacter pylori* in inflammatory bowel disease: association with sulphasalazine. Gut 35: 1385–1388

Farman J, Faegenburg D, Dallelmand S, Kuo Chen C 1975 Crohn's disease of the stomach: the 'ram's horn' sign. American Journal of Roentgenology, Radium Therapy and Nuclear Medicine 123: 242–251

Frandsen P J, Jarnum S, Malmstrom J 1980 Crohn's disease of the duodenum. Scandinavian Journal of Gastroenterology 15: 683–688

Franklin R H, Taylor S 1950 Non-specific granulomatous (regional) esophagitis. Journal of Thoracic and Cardiovascular Surgery 19: 292–297

Geboes K, Janssens J, Rutgeerts P, Vantrappen G 1986 Crohn's disease of the esophagus. Journal of Clinical Gastroenterology 8: 31–37

Gelfand M D, Krone C H L 1968 Dysphagia and esophageal ulceration in Crohn's disease. Gastroenterology 55: 510–514

Gottlieb C H, Alpert S 1937 Regional jejunitis. American Journal of Roentgenology 38: 881–883

Greenberg G R, Feagan B G, Martin F et al 1994 Oral budesonide for active Crohn's disease. New England Journal of Medicine 331: 836–841

Griffiths A M, Alemayehu E, Sherman P 1989 Clinical features of gastroduodenal Crohn's disease in adolescents. Journal of Pediatric Gastroenterology and Nutrition 8: 166–171

Heffernon E W, Kepkay P H 1954 Segmental esophagitis, gastritis and enteritis. Gastroenterology 26: 83–88

Huchzermeyer G, Paul F, Seifert E, Frolich H, Rasmussen C H W 1976 Endoscopic results in five patients with Crohn's disease of the esophagus. Endoscopy 8: 75–81

Jacobson I M, Schapiro R H, Warshaw A L 1985 Gastric and duodenal fistulas in Crohn's disease. Gastroenterology 89: 1347–1352

Johnson F W, Delaney J P 1972 Regional enteritis involvement of the stomach. Archives of Surgery 105: 434–437

Klein S, Greenstein A J, Sachar D B 1987 Duodenal fistulas in Crohn's disease. Journal of Clinical Gastroenterology 9: 46–49

Korelitz B I, Waye J D, Kreuning J et al 1981 Crohn's disease in endoscopic biopsies of the gastric antrum and duodenum. American

Journal of Gastroenterology 76: 103–109
Kuntz H D, Schwegler U, May M, May B 1988 Der morbus Crohn des oberen gastrointestinaltrakts. Medizinische Klinik 22: 760–762
Laufer I, Trueman T, de Sa D 1976 Multiple superficial gastric erosions due to Crohn's disease of the stomach. Radiologic and endoscopic diagnosis. British Journal of Radiology 49: 726–728
Lenaerts C, Roy C C, Vaillancourt M, Weber A M, Morin C L, Seidman E 1989 High incidence of upper gastrointestinal tract involvement in children with Crohn's disease. Pediatrics 83: 777–781
Leurs P B, Mulder A W, Bartelsman J W F M 1987 Een jonge vrouw met de ziekte van Crohn in de slokdarm. Nederlands Tijdschrift voor Geneeskunde 131: 955–958
Levine M S 1987 Crohn's disease of the upper gastrointestinal tract. Radiologic Clinics of North America 25: 79–91
Marshall B J, Goodwin C S, Warren J R et al 1988 Prospective double-blind trial of duodenal ulcer relapse after eradication of *Campylobacter pylori*. Lancet ii: 1437–1441
Mashako M N L, Cezard J P, Navarro J et al 1989 Crohn's disease lesions in the upper gastrointestinal tract: correlation between clinical, radiological, endoscopic, and histological features in adolescents and children. Journal of Pediatric Gastroenterology and Nutrition 8: 442–446
Mathis G, Sutterlütti K, Dirschmid K, Feuerstein M, Zimmerman G 1994 Crohn's disease of the osophagus: dilatation of stricture and fibrin sealing of fistulas. Endoscopy 26: 508
Meiselman M S, Ghahremani G G, Kaufman M W 1987 Crohn's disease of the duodenum complicated by adenocarcinoma. Gastrointestinal Radiology 12: 333–336
Miller E M, Moss A A, Kresel H Y 1979 Duodenal involvement with Crohn's disease. A spectrum of radiologic abnormality. American Journal of Gastroenterology 17: 107–116
Moonka D, Lichtenstein G R, Levine M S, Rombeau J L, Furth E E, MacDermott R P 1993 Giant gastric ulcers: an unusual manifestation of Crohn's disease. American Journal of Gastroenterology 88: 297–299
Murray J J, Schoetz D J Jr, Nugent F W, Coller J A, Veidenheimer M C 1984 Surgical management of Crohn's disease involving the duodenum. American Journal of Surgery 147: 58–65
Niv Y 1988 Esophageal involvement in Crohn's disease. American Journal of Gastroenterology 83: 205
Nugent F W, Roy M A 1989 Duodenal Crohn's disease: an analysis of 89 cases. American Journal of Gastroenterology 84: 249–254
Nugent F W, Richmond M, Park S K 1977 Crohn's disease of the duodenum. Gut 18: 115–120
Paget E T, Owens P, Peniston W O, Mathewson C 1972 Massive upper gastrointestinal tract hemorrhage. A manifestation of regional enteritis of the duodenum. Archives of Surgery 104: 397–400
Prats E, Banzo J, Abós Olivares M D, Freile E 1994 Gastric Crohn's disease detected by Tc-99m HMPAO mixed leukocyte scan. Clinical Nuclear Medicine 19: 243–244
Przemioslo R T, Mee A S 1994 Omeprazole in possible esophageal Crohn's disease. Digestive Diseases and Sciences 39: 1594–1595
Rutgeerts P, Löfberg R, Malchow H et al 1994 A comparison of budesonide with prednisolone for active Crohn's disease. New England Journal of Medicine 331: 842–845
Rutgeerts P, Onette E, Vantrappen G, Geboes K, Broeckhaert L, Talloen L 1980 Crohn's disease of the stomach and duodenum: a clinical study with emphasis on the value of endoscopic biopsies. Endoscopy 12: 288–294
Shepherd A F I, Allan R N, Dykes P W et al 1985 The surgical treatment of gastroduodenal Crohn's disease. Annals of the Royal College of Surgeons of England 67: 381–384
Tanaka M, Kimura K, Sakai H, Yoshida Y, Saito K 1986 Long-term follow-up for minute gastroduodenal lesions in Crohn's disease. Gastrointestinal Endoscopy 32: 206–209
Thompson W M, Cockrill H, Price R P 1975 Regional enteritis of the duodenum. American Journal of Roentgenology, Radium Therapy and Nuclear Medicine 123: 252–261
Tootla F, Lucas R J, Bernacki E G, Tabor H 1976 Gastroduodenal Crohn's disease. Archives of Surgery 111: 855–857
Valori R M, Cockel R 1990 Omeprazole for duodenal ulceration in Crohn's disease. British Medical Journal 300: 438–439
Van Spreeuwel J P, Lindeman J, Van der Wal A M, Weterman I T, Kreuning J, Meyer C J L M 1982 Morphological and immunohistochemical findings in upper gastrointestinal biopsies of patients with Crohn's disease of the ileum and colon. Journal of Clinical Pathology 35: 934–940
Weterman I T 1976 Course and long-term prognosis of Crohn's disease. MD Thesis, Leiden, W D Weinema B V, Delft
Weterman I T 1990 Oral, oesophageal and gastro-duodenal Crohn's disease In: Allan R N, Keighley M R B, Alexander-Williams J, Hawkins C (eds) Inflammatory bowel diseases. Churchill Livingstone, London, pp 319–327
Wise L, Kyriakos M, McCown A, Ballinger W F 1971 Crohn's disease of the duodenum. A report and analysis of eleven new cases. American Journal of Surgery 121: 184–194
Woolfson K, Greenberg G R 1992 Symptomatic improvement of gastroduodenal Crohn's disease with omeprazole. Canadian Journal of Gastroenterology 6: 21–24

65. Crohn's disease of the small intestine – ileum and right colon

R. N. Allan

Medical management of Crohn's disease is much more than the manipulation of a number of specific drugs. Indeed, drug treatment plays a relatively small part in the management of many patients. The analysis and re-analysis of symptoms to determine their underlying cause provides a secure base to determine whether medical or surgical treatment is appropriate and then, in discussion, to help both the patient and their family to come to terms and accept what at times is unpalatable and difficult treatment. The diagnosis of Crohn's disease may come initially as a relief to the patient and their family, since symptoms have often been present for some time before the diagnosis is established. That relief is rapidly replaced by anxiety concerning the long-term prognosis and the impact on the patient and the family, particularly because it is a disorder of unknown cause with frequent relapses in young adults, anticipating an era in life of vigorous good health.

PRESENTATION

The majority of patients with Crohn's disease (60–70%) present with disease involving the distal ileum which often extends into the cecal pole or the proximal ascending colon. The nature of the disease at this site requires careful evaluation before a decision can be made about appropriate medical or surgical treatment.

The presentation ranges widely, from an acute onset in the severely ill patient to intermittent recurrent problems over many years. A careful history, physical examination and investigation enables the nature of the disease to be defined to provide a basis for subsequent management.

Obstructive symptoms

Most patients with distal ileal disease present with intermittent obstructive symptoms, with colicky abdominal pain, nausea and vomiting, but are otherwise in good health. The involved segment may only involve a few centimeters of the distal ileum and cecal pole with stricture formation and probably represents a late stage in the natural history of the disease. The initially inflamed mucosal disease has, over a period of months or years, largely healed, except for a residual short fibrous stricture. In these patients the number, frequency and severity of the obstructive episodes will determine management. The shorter and narrower the stricture formation and the more frequent and severe the attacks of pain, the more likely that surgical treatment is appropriate. A history of food bolus obstruction (after ingestion of vegetable stalks, orange pith or nuts) should be sought, since removing these items from the diet may be sufficient to minimize recurrent symptoms. Physical examination is usually normal and the patient looks fit and well, except during episodes of pain when there may be tenderness in the right iliac fossa. Perianal disease, aphthous ulcers or finger clubbing help to confirm the diagnosis. Laboratory indices, including hemoglobin, acute-phase proteins and serum albumin, are usually normal. A few patients even with radiological evidence of tight stricture formation have few symptoms and no active treatment is indicated for them.

Inflammatory mucosal disease

Some patients present with right iliac fossa discomfort, change in bowel habit, malaise, anorexia and weight loss; on radiological examination they have inflammatory mucosal disease of a variable length of the distal ileum and right colon, but no stricture formation. The severity and frequency of symptoms should be assessed, particularly how much the symptoms affect normal activity. There is some evidence that initially extensive ileal disease may heal with time, often with stricture formation, which may eventually be amenable in the symptomatic patient to either a short resection or strictureplasty. On examination the patient may be thin, sometimes with fever and tachycardia, with tenderness in the right iliac fossa.

Laboratory indices, including hemoglobin, acute-phase proteins and serum albumin, are usually abnormal and the severity of these changes is a useful guide to the severity and extent of the inflammatory mucosal response.

The key feature in this group is to avoid early resection of long segments of the small intestine. Initial medical treatment enables eventual surgical treatment to be restricted to strictureplasty or resection of short segments of small intestine.

Combined obstructive symptoms and inflammatory mucosal disease

Some patients have symptoms and radiological changes of inflammatory mucosal disease and evidence of single or multiple short strictures. A careful history in this group will determine whether the predominant symptoms arise from recurrent obstructive episodes or inflammatory mucosal disease. Anti-inflammatory medical treatment combined with the relief of short strictures by strictureplasty may be needed to maximize the benefit of medical and surgical treatment.

Presentation with right iliac fossa mass

The symptomatic patient with a right iliac fossa mass presents a challenge in both diagnosis and management. Radiological evidence usually suggests the diagnosis of Crohn's disease, although lingering diagnostic doubt, and particularly the difficulty of excluding tuberculosis, will influence management. The right iliac fossa mass is usually tender and in the presence of sepsis the acute-phase proteins are strikingly elevated. The distinction between inflammatory change in the gut and mesentery or a local abscess is important, and can be made by an indium-labeled leukocyte scan. In both disorders there is inflammatory activity at the site of the mass 4 hours after giving the labeled leukocytes, but persistent abnormality at 24 hours only occurs in the presence of an abscess. If the evidence for Crohn's disease is clear cut, with typical radiological appearances and no evidence of abscess formation, then medical treatment is appropriate. Any diagnostic doubt or evidence of abscess formation suggests that surgical treatment is necessary.

Fistula formation

Patients may first present with fistula formation, but this is more commonly a feature of recurrent ileal disease after an initial surgical resection. Fistulae originate in the gut immediately proximal to a stricture of the distal ileum and are often associated with secondary sepsis in the fistulous track. The track may present superficially as an enterocutaneous fistula, or erode into the bladder as an enterovesical fistula; rarely in females, usually after hysterectomy, it may present as an enterovaginal fistula. Although medical treatment of this group may include antimicrobial therapy to treat the secondary infection, surgery is the treatment of choice. Enteroenteric fistulae, usually between adjacent loops of small bowel, may be identified radiologically. Their presence does not alter management, except that they usually occur proximal to short strictures in the gut and the underlying strictures themselves give rise to recurrent obstructive symptoms, which commonly require surgical treatment.

Mimicking acute appendicitis

Some patients present acutely with symptoms consistent with acute appendicitis, although in many a careful history reveals antecedent abdominal symptoms. If distal ileal Crohn's disease is found at appendectomy then the appendix is usually removed and the stump oversewn. This presentation may be associated with a right iliac fossa mass, where the approach has already been outlined.

Metabolic problems

It is uncommon for patients with distal ileal disease to have metabolic problems at presentation. Diarrhea is not a major feature, so that fluid and electrolyte imbalance is rare. Iron deficiency anemia may need treatment. The sequelae of ileal resection, including bile salt malabsorption and B_{12} deficiency, will be considered later.

Disease at other sites

Although most patients with distal ileal disease have discrete disease at this site, disease may also be present at other sites, particularly in the perineum, the large intestine or even in the mouth or duodenum. The nature of the disease at each site will similarly need a careful analysis.

Presentation with other problems

Presentation with other problems is uncommon. The associated disorder of renal stones usually occurs in patients with persistent diarrhea, gallstones in those who have had extensive ileal resection, and duodenal ulcer in patients who in the past had been treated by extensive small-bowel resection.

DIAGNOSIS AND DIFFERENTIAL DIAGNOSIS

The initial diagnosis may be based on radiological features alone, and alternative possibilities such as tuberculosis must be considered and re-evaluated in the symptomatic patient. Symptoms may be due not to the underlying Crohn's disease, but to superimposed secondary infection with organisms such as *Campylobacter* or *Clostridium difficile*, which can be eradicated with specific antimicrobial treatment.

MEDICAL VERSUS SURGICAL TREATMENT

Both medical and surgical treatment have potential benefits and disadvantages. The benefits of both can be maximized by the experienced physician and surgeon working as a team in the best interests of the patient.

In the symptomatic patient with distal ileal disease, the nature of the underlying disease can be characterized by the history, physical examination, laboratory indices and radiological and endoscopic assessment.

Free perforation, massive hemorrhage, abscess and fistula formation are the province of the surgeon. The medical management is determined by the nature of the underlying disease.

APPROACHES TO MEDICAL MANAGEMENT

Symptomatic relief

Diarrhea is a common problem, and in addition to treatment of the underlying problems symptomatic relief is often helpful. Double-blind controlled studies have demonstrated that loperamide decreases both stool frequency and weight (Pelemans & Vantrappen 1976, Mainguet & Fiasse 1977). Loperamide (Tytgat & Huibregste 1975) and codeine phosphate (Newton 1978) both reduce ileostomy output and, by inference, are likely to be helpful in controlling diarrhea. Diphenoxylate is helpful, but less effective than the other two drugs.

Obstructive symptoms

Most patients with distal ileal Crohn's disease have radiological evidence of a short stricture and present with subacute obstructive episodes lasting 12–24 hours. Most of these episodes settle spontaneously without treatment. If they are severe enough to warrant admission, then nil by mouth, intravenous fluids for 24–48 hours and analgesia usually results in complete resolution of symptoms. Avoiding large food boluses should minimize some of these episodes. The authors rarely prescribe drug treatment for these patients. Three or four episodes of severe obstructive symptoms are a reasonable basis for recommending local resection or strictureplasty for short strictures (< 5 cm). No treatment is required in patients with a short stricture and few or minimal symptoms. The patient and their family should be reminded to inform their medical advisers, should their symptoms recur, that they have distal ileal Crohn's disease.

Inflammatory mucosal disease and combined obstructive and inflammatory features

Most patients with ileal disease have already developed stricture formation by the time of their initial presentation, but some are symptomatic with inflammatory mucosal disease only. Others have combined obstructive and inflammatory features and are usually treated, at least initially, with drugs. If the obstructive features become predominant then laparotomy and strictureplasty or local resection of the fibrous strictures can be carried out and drug treatment continued for the residual disease.

Sulfasalazine

Both the National Cooperative Crohn's Disease Study and the European Cooperative Crohn's Disease Study showed that for ileocecal disease, sulfasalazine 1 g per 15 kg per day was just superior to placebo over a treatment period of 4 months. The benefit, however, is not sustained and the significant benefit is lost some time between 4 months and 2 years. It has a useful role in the mildly symptomatic patient, particularly where the patient expects the doctor to make a positive contribution. In addition it enables the physician to observe the progress of the disease over several months.

5-Aminosalicylic acid (5-ASA)

It seemed likely that the new 5-ASA derivatives might be delivered to the principal site of inflammatory mucosal activity and that the higher doses (following the elimination of the carrier, sulfapyridine) might enhance the benefits of the parent compound sulfasalazine. The initial studies of Pentasa in a small dose of 1.5 g per day proved ineffective (Rasmussen et al 1987, Mahida & Jewell 1990). However, the large multicenter North American trial involving a large number of patients receiving 4 g of Pentasa per day proved this to be superior to placebo, with more than twice as many patients entering remission (Singleton et al 1993).

Corticosteroids

Both the National Cooperative Crohn's Disease Study from the USA (Summers et al 1979) and the European Cooperative Crohn's Disease Study (Malchow et al 1984) confirmed the significant short-term benefit of glucocorticoids in ileocecal Crohn's disease when compared with placebo. In a recent study of corticosteroids in newly diagnosed Crohn's disease, complete clinical remission was achieved in 30 days in 48% of patients, partial remission in 32% and no response in 20% (Munkholm et al 1993). Nearly half the patients relapsed within a month after reducing or withdrawing corticosteroid treatment.

The recent development of an oral delayed-release budesonide capsule which releases the drug predominantly in the ileocecal region has considerable potential for ileocecal Crohn's disease. Recent studies suggest that budesonide is associated with fewer side effects, but this is in part explained by its reduced potency compared with standard corticosteroid therapy (Greenberg et al 1994, Rutgeerts et al 1994).

Immunosuppressive therapy

Immunosuppressive therapy is rarely appropriate for acute disease and will be considered later for maintenance therapy.

Enteral/elemental feeding

Controlled studies have shown that elemental or enteral feeding has a benefit similar to that of oral corticosteroids, although the response is rather slower, somewhat less marked and the remission period shorter. The benefits are greater for patients with small-bowel disease than those with large-intestinal involvement. They are particularly useful in symptomatic children, where it is important to avoid corticosteroids and the associated growth failure.

MAINTENANCE THERAPY

Sulfasalazine

The NCCDS (Summers et al 1979) and the ECCDS (Malchow et al 1984) could find no benefit for sulfasalazine compared to placebo as maintenance treatment.

5-Aminosalicylic acid

There is some evidence that 5-ASA is helpful for maintaining remission in patients with Crohn's disease. The International Mesalazine Study Group in 1990, reported a 33% reduction in recurrence rates after 12 months' treatment. In patients treated with Pentasa immediately after going into remission there was some significant benefit for maintenance therapy over a period of 24 months (Gendre et al 1993). Prantera and colleagues (1992) also reported benefit over a 12-month period using Asacol 2.5 g per day.

The benefit of 5-ASA as maintenance therapy is not as clear-cut as the benefits in ulcerative colitis, but two meta-analyses of the value of maintenance therapy have reported similar results. 5-ASA will reduce the risk of a recurrence in the first year of therapy by approximately 30–40% (Messori et al 1994, Steinhart et al 1994).

Corticosteroids

The primary role of corticosteroids is for acute exacerbations of disease, and there is little evidence that maintenance therapy is effective except for a small subset of patients who were identified in the ECCDS. In those patients who relapse on reducing or withdrawing corticosteroid therapy immunosuppressive therapy should be considered.

Immunosuppressive therapy as maintenance treatment

O'Donoghue et al (1978) studied patients with Crohn's disease in remission on azathioprine who were randomized either to continue the drug or were switched to placebo: 5% of the azathioprine group relapsed, compared to 41% on placebo after 12 months. In patients initially treated with oral prednisolone with the addition of azathioprine or placebo, the remission rate after 1 year was much higher in those patients continuing with azathioprine compared to those taking placebo (Candy et al 1994). The duration of benefit is uncertain, but a long-term analysis suggested that two-thirds of patients remained in remission at 5 years (Lemann et al 1994). The benefit has to be weighed against the risk of significant long-term side effects.

Enteral/elemental feeding

Maintenance therapy with enteral or elemental feeding is probably impractical for most adults with symptomatic Crohn's disease.

Right iliac fossa mass

Presentation is usually acute and, provided local abscess formation can be confidently excluded, short-term treatment with oral prednisolone is appropriate. If there is doubt about the diagnosis, then oral prednisolone should be combined with antimicrobial therapy. Evidence of abscess formation is an indication for surgical drainage and resection of the underlying ileal Crohn's disease.

Fistula formation

Persistent enterocutaneous, enterovesical or enterovaginal fistulae are an indication for surgical treatment. Initially, however, patients may require antimicrobial treatment for secondary sepsis, intravenous fluid and electrolyte repletion if they have lost large volumes of intestinal fluid via the fistula, and the correction of anemia with hematinics or blood transfusion.

Outcome of short-term appraisal and treatment

Most patients come to surgical treatment (either resection or strictureplasty) within the first year after diagnosis because they develop recurrent severe obstructive symptoms due to short fibrous strictures associated with distal ileal Crohn's disease. Other patients are treated surgically because of abscess or fistula formation complicating fibrous stricture formation due to either resection or strictureplasty.

About 10–15% of patients remain well with little or no medical treatment, despite radiological evidence of inflammatory mucosal disease or stricture formation. A small number of patients with extensive ileal disease (perhaps 5% of the total group) have persistent symptoms and need to be considered for medium-term low-dose oral corticosteroids combined with immunosuppressive therapy, or even medium-term enteral therapy, particularly in childhood. What is the value of medical management in the postsurgical group?

Management after initial ileal resection

Most patients who undergo initial ileal resection are rapidly restored to good health, with complete resolution of their symptoms and no sequelae. They should be encouraged to resume normal activities as soon as possible, and alerted to the fact that they may develop recurrent disease, usually confined to a small segment of bowel at or around the anastomosis. The timing of the recurrence is unpredictable, although the mean interval is of the order of 10–15 years. They should be alerted to the fact that they may develop obstructive symptoms, in which case they should seek expert medical advice.

The expectation that an individual undergoing initial resection at the age of 30 will need two to three further local resections in their lifetime, and will otherwise be fit and well in the intervening years, is both factually correct and reassuring.

Prophylactic treatment after resection

Neither the NCCDS (Summers et al 1979) nor the ECCDS (Malchow et al 1984) could find any evidence of benefit for sulfasalazine in reducing recurrent disease after an initial ileal resection.

A modest reduction in recurrence rates for at least 2 years after resection was suggested by a large German study (Ewe et al 1989). The patients that did respond had been started on sulfasalazine within 3 months of resection.

5-Aminosalicylic acid

A study of Claversal in a dose of 3 g per day, started within 2 weeks of resection, showed no difference between the active treatment and placebo in an evaluation based on endoscopic recurrence at 12 weeks. A preliminary study suggested that the improvement might be maintained for a period of 12 months (Arber et al 1994). McLeod and colleagues (1994) randomly assigned 177 patients to either 3 g per day of Salofalk or placebo within 2 months of resection. The patients were followed up for up to 7 years, and at 3 years there were significant differences in clinical recurrence: 27% for 5-ASA versus 47% for placebo. These data are encouraging, but perhaps not yet strong enough to warrant the routine use of 5-ASA treatment after ileal resection outside clinical trials.

Corticosteroid and immunosuppressive therapy

The NCCDS (Summers et al 1979) found no evidence that continuous low-dose oral prednisolone or azathioprine was effective in reducing recurrence rates after resection. Budesonide has so far only been evaluated for the treatment of active disease.

Strictureplasty or local resection in the presence of residual disease

In some patients stricture formation can be relieved by strictureplasty or local resection, but with clear evidence at surgery that there is residual mucosal disease. There is little evidence that mucosal disease per se should be treated in the absence of symptoms, but if the residual disease is symptomatic then these symptoms, together with evidence of laboratory indices of activity, will provide a reasonable basis for treatment along the lines outlined for treatment of inflammatory mucosal disease.

Medical management of recurrent disease

Recurrent disease is disappointing for both the patient, their family and the physician. However, the impact of recurrent disease has often been overemphasized and its occurrence is usually surrounded with undue pessimism. For most patients recurrent disease is readily treated and is much less of a clinical and management problem than at the initial presentation.

Since the underlying diagnosis has already been established, the patient and their family are well informed about the disease, are aware that it might recur, and recognize the likely symptoms. There is rarely any significant delay in defining the problem and thus deciding on an appropriate course of action. Recurrent disease is variable, and patients should be investigated and the nature of the recurrence defined. They usually present as one of several well defined problems.

Short fibrous stricture at or around the anastomosis. Most patients with recurrent Crohn's disease after an initial ileal resection present with short-lived attacks of colicky abdominal pain, and are otherwise well between these recurrent episodes. Radiologically there is usually clear evidence of a short fibrous stricture at or around the anastomosis. The episodes of pain can be precipitated by food bolus, so that vegetable stalks, nuts and mushrooms should be avoided.

Although there is often endoscopic evidence of early recurrence in the form of aphthous ulcers at or around the anastomosis, there is usually a long interval from the initial resection to presentation with symptomatic recurrence (median 15 years). The shorter this interval the greater the disappointment and anxiety among the patient and the family. However, irrespective of the interval, if the patient develops recurrent symptoms a further local resection or strictureplasty usually resolves the problem. Early recurrence with short fibrous stricture has as good a long-term outlook following the second resection as the group of patients in whom the interval is much longer.

A few patients with recurrent disease will have only one or two episodes of colicky abdominal pain and no further symptoms for many years. No medical treatment is necessary in this group.

Inflammatory mucosal recurrence. In a few patients the recurrence involves a long segment of the ileum but no evidence of stricture formation. Presenting symptoms include malaise, abdominal discomfort, diarrhea and weight loss. The approach to medical treatment is along the lines outlined for inflammatory mucosal disease.

Fistula formation. A few patients with recurrent ileal disease present with enterocutaneous, enterovaginal or enterovesical fistulae. The most common form of presentation is as an enterocutaneous fistula arising at the site of the initial surgery. The fistulous track arises immediately proximal to stricture formation, and if the fistula persists then local resection of the stricture along with the fistulous track is the only effective way to resolve the problem.

Recurrent disease at other sites. Patients with ileal disease occasionally develop recurrent disease, either diffusely in the small bowel or extensively in the large intestine. In those who develop extensive disease in the large intestine, a careful review of earlier radiological evidence often identifies minor changes such as aphthous ulcers which had been previously overlooked. These patients with diffuse small-bowel disease or extensive Crohn's colitis should be treated as those with primary disease at these sites.

Major problems associated with recurrent disease

A handful of patients in any center provide a major challenge in the management of recurrent disease. The problems include diffuse recurrent disease, recurrent fistula formation, often associated with sepsis, and incomplete response to medical treatment. This group of patients needs constant re-evaluation, some of their problems can occasionally be resolved. In particular, it is easy to overlook local stricture formation and focal intra-abdominal sepsis. The evidence from controlled studies is not clear cut, but a small subset of such patients seem to respond to long-term treatment with small doses of corticosteroids, with or without the addition of immunosuppressive therapy such as azathioprine or 6-mercaptopurine.

METABOLIC SEQUELAE OF ILEAL DISEASE OR RECURRENT ILEAL DISEASE

Anemia. Blood loss from ileal or recurrent ileal disease may lead to iron deficiency anemia. An above-average proportion of patients with Crohn's disease seem to be intolerant of oral iron preparations, either because of indigestion or because iron therapy frequently exacerbates the diarrhea.

B_{12} deficiency. Extensive ileal disease or extensive ileal resection (the latter should now be uncommon) may lead to a macrocytic anemia secondary to B_{12} deficiency. B_{12} supplements are needed in a minority of such patients, so 1000 µg of vitamin B_{12} intramuscularly every 3–4 months is more than adequate.

Bile salt-induced diarrhea. Patients with extensive ileal disease or after extensive ileal resection have impaired bile acid absorption, so that the bile acids previously absorbed in the ileum pass into the colon, where they induce colonic mucosal secretion of sodium and water, with secondary watery diarrhea with urgency and frequency. Cholestyramine (Questran) one to two sachets per day can sometimes dramatically improve these troublesome symptoms.

Bile acid depletion and malabsorption. In patients with extensive ileal disease, bile salt loss with excessive fecal excretion may lead to a malabsorption pattern which can be ameliorated in part by reducing the fat intake in the diet.

Fluid and electrolyte depletion. Persistent diarrhea associated with ileal disease or following ileal resection may be associated with potassium depletion, and a few patients require regular potassium supplements. It is well recognized that serum potassium measurements are a poor guide to total body potassium. The simplest guide to potassium depletion is to measure its excretion in the urine. In practice the simple addition of potassium supplements to the medical regimen is sensible.

Magnesium depletion. Severe diarrhea can result in hypomagnesemia, with symptoms that resemble hypocalcemia. Supplements of magnesium can be given orally.

Other metabolic problems

Bile salt depletion and biliary sludge, which may occur in the postoperative period, are both associated with an increased incidence of gallstones and this diagnosis should be considered in patients with Crohn's disease presenting with atypical abdominal pain.

Patients with persistent diarrhea are more prone to renal stones, and this diagnosis should not be overlooked and simply labeled as abdominal pain associated with recurrent Crohn's disease.

In patients who have had extensive small-bowel resection there is an increased incidence of peptic ulcer, presumably because gastrin is poorly metabolized following extensive resection.

Chronic pancreatic disease

A few patients develop chronic pancreatitis in association with small-bowel Crohn's disease, giving rise to abdominal pain and steatorrhea.

OVERVIEW OF ILEAL DISEASE

Most patients present in young adult life with a short fibrous stricture in the distal ileum, and undergo resection within the first year of diagnosis. They then require two to three further resections in their lifetime and are well between these recurrent episodes.

A minority of patients have early recurrent disease, but after a second resection the long-term prognosis is as good as the primary group. A few patients have either extensive disease or extensive recurrent disease, and it is these few patients who give the disease a bad name, whereas the majority who are fit and well tend to be forgotten.

REFERENCES

Arber N, Odes S H, Fireman Z 1994 A controlled double blind multicentre study of the effectiveness of 5-aminosalicylic acid in patients with Crohn's disease in remission. Gastroenterology 106: A646

Candy S, Wright J P, Gerber M, Adams G, Gerig M, Goodman R 1994 A double blind controlled study of azathioprine in the treatment and maintenance of remission in Crohn's disease. Gastroenterology 106: A659

Ewe K, Herfarth C, Malchow H, Jesdinsky H J 1989 Postoperative recurrence of Crohn's disease in relation to radicality of operation and sulphasalazine prophylaxis: a multicentre trial. Digestion 42: 224–232

Gendre J P, Mavy J Y, Florent C 1993 Oral melsamine (Pentasa) as maintenance treatment in Crohn's disease: a multicentre placebo controlled study. Gastroenterology 104: 435–439

Greenberg G R, Feagan B G, Martin F 1994 Oral budesonide for active Crohn's disease. New England Journal of Medicine 331: 836–841

Lemann M, Tai R, Bouhnik Y 1994 Long term outcome of patients with Crohn's disease successfully treated with azathioprine or 6-mercaptopurine. Gastroenterology 106: A719

McLeod R S, Wolff B G, Steinhart H J 1994 Delayed recurrence following surgery for Crohn's disease. Gastroenterology 106: A733

Mahida Y R, Jewell D P 1990 Slow release 5-amino-salicylic acid (Pentasa) for the treatment of active Crohn's disease. Digestion 45: 88–92

Mainguet P, Fiasse R 1977 Double-blind placebo-controlled study of loperamide (Imodium) in chronic diarrhoea caused by ileocolic disease or resection. Gut 18: 575–579

Malchow H, Ewe K, Brandes J W 1984 European Co-operation Crohn's disease study: results of drug treatment. Gastroenterology 86: 249–266

Messori A, Brignola C, Trallori G 1994 Effectiveness of 5-amino-salicylic acid for maintaining remission in patients with Crohn's disease: A meta-analysis. American Journal of Gastroenterology 89: 692–698

Munkholm P, Langholz E, Davidson M, Binder V 1993 Frequency of glucocorticoid resistance and dependency in Crohn's disease. Gut 35: 360–362

Newton C R 1978 Effect of codeine phosphate, lomotil and isogel on ileostomy function. Gut 19: 377–383

O'Donoghue D P, Dawson A M, Powell-Tuck J, Bown R C, Lennard-Jones J E 1978 Double blind withdrawal trial of azathioprine as maintenance treatment for Crohn's disease. Lancet 2: 955–957

Pelemans W, Vantrappen G 1976 A double blind crossover comparison of loperamide with diphenoxylate in the symptomatic treatment of chronic diarrhoea. Gastroenterology 70: 1030–1034

Prantera C, Pallone F, Brunetti G, Coltone M, Miglioli M 1992 Oral 5-amino-salicylic acid (Asacol) in the maintenance treatment of Crohn's disease. Gastroenterology 103: 363–368

Rasmussen S N, Lauritsen K, Tage-Jensen U 1987 5-amino-salicylic acid in the treatment of Crohn's disease. Scandinavian Journal of Gastroenterology 22: 877–883

Rutgeerts P, Lofberg R, Malchow H 1994 A comparison of budesonide with prednisolone for active Crohn's disease. New England Journal of Medicine 331: 842–845

Singleton J W, Hanauer S B, Gitnick G L 1993 Mesalazine capsules for the treatment of active Crohn's disease: results of a 16 week trial. Gastroenterology 104: 1293–1301

Steinhart A H, Hemphill O J, Greenberg G R 1994 Sulphasalazine and mesalazine for the maintenance therapy of Crohn's disease: A meta-analysis. Gastroenterology 106: A778

Summers R W, Switz D M, Session J T 1979 National Cooperative Crohn's disease study: results of drug treatment. Gastroenterology 77: 847–869

Tytgat G N, Huibregtse K 1975 Loperamide and ileostomy output: placebo-controlled double-blind crossover study. British Medical Journal ii: 667

66. Crohn's disease of the small intestine diffuse jejunal ileitis

R. N. Allan

In many patients with apparently focal disease there is evidence of microscopic and pathophysiological involvement, suggesting that Crohn's disease is a diffuse lesion of the gastrointestinal tract in which the sites of macroscopic disease, demonstrated either radiologically, at endoscopy or at laparotomy, are merely the most severely affected sites.

In a few patients there is macroscopic evidence of diffuse small-bowel disease, where much or all of the jejunum and ileum is abnormal; patients with extensive jejunal disease should probably also be included in this category. The occasional patient with a short segment of jejunal disease should be managed along the lines outlined for patients with distal ileal Crohn's disease.

Crohn's disease was originally thought to be a disorder confined to the distal ileum, but diffuse jejunoileitis was first recognized and reported by Crohn and Yunich in 1941. There have since been few published studies of such patients, but they suggest that the incidence varies between 3 and 10% (van Patter et al 1954, Crohn & Yarnis 1958, Jones & Lennard-Jones 1966).

Cooke and Swan (1974) reported a series of 18 patients with Crohn's disease presenting with diffuse jejunoileitis between 1944 and 1970, of whom six died, five of these being related to the underlying Crohn's disease. They noted that conservative surgical management was an important development, since extensive small-bowel resection was associated with increased mortality.

The major recent improvement in management has been the suppression of inflammatory activity with medical treatment, and the use of strictureplasty or limited resection to relieve recurrent obstructive symptoms due to fibrous stricture. This approach has improved the long-term outlook for such patients, although the morbidity is usually high in the first few years after diagnosis.

We have recently analyzed the long-term outcome among 34 patients with diffuse jejunoileitis, and this study provides the basis for this chapter (Tan & Allan 1993).

SITE OF DISEASE AT PRESENTATION

Most patients with diffuse jejunoileitis present with extensive disease, though 10–15% of patients develop diffuse jejunoileitis several years after presenting initially with apparently focal macroscopic disease elsewhere, either in the distal ileum or large intestine.

In nearly a quarter of patients the disease extends to include the duodenum, and a third also have large-intestinal involvement.

INCIDENCE OF DIFFUSE JEJUNOILEITIS

The proportion of patients with diffuse jejunoileitis in our adult series was 5.7%.

The incidence of diffuse jejunoileitis in childhood is higher (21% in one published series), although there may be some selection bias in this figure (Puntis et al 1984).

Thus the majority of patients present in childhood or adolescence, although not exclusively so. The oldest patient in our series with diffuse jejunoileitis was 57 years of age at diagnosis.

PRESENTATION

Most patients present with severe persistent abdominal symptoms that warrant early investigation, and the diagnosis can usually be readily established since simple blood results are usually abnormal, with anemia, low serum albumin and elevated acute-phase proteins, together with typical radiological changes in the jejunum and ileum. In a few patients the initial symptoms are mild and further investigation is only appropriate once the symptoms become more severe. This initially mild presentation probably accounts for the mean interval between the onset of symptoms and diagnosis of some 2.5 years.

Most children and adolescents also present with abdominal symptoms, but these are often associated with weight loss and growth retardation. Presentation with weight loss of growth retardation alone is rare, although in patients presenting with abdominal symptoms it is often possible to identify growth failure occurring 2–3 years before the onset of abdominal symptoms.

Patients can usually be grouped according to their symptoms and radiological appearances into those with systemic disturbance associated with diffuse inflammatory change without focal stricture formation, and those with intermittent recurrent obstructive episodes due to either single or multiple short fibrous strictures. Both symptoms may coexist, but it is usually clear which is the predominant problem.

Some of the symptoms may arise because of fluid and electrolyte depletion or various forms of anemia, which need to be identified and corrected.

The typical patient with diffuse jejunoileitis is thin, with evidence of recent weight loss, sometimes with systemic disturbance including fever and tachycardia. Some patients have finger clubbing and koilonychia, and there may be perianal disease or aphthous ulcers in the mouth.

DIAGNOSIS AND DIFFERENTIAL DIAGNOSIS

The diagnosis is often based initially on radiological features. Multiple duodenal biopsies may be helpful in identifying typical features of Crohn's disease, including non-caseating granulomas, and also to exclude celiac disease. The possibility of infection such as giardiasis and tuberculosis needs to be considered and excluded. Multiple strictures in the small bowel may be complicated by enteroenteric fistulae or local abscess formation. This is particularly likely in patients with systemic disturbance and an abdominal mass, when a CT or indium-labeled leukocyte scan is important. Occasionally alternative explanations of abdominal pain should be considered, including peptic ulcer, renal stones and gallstones, all of which occur more commonly in patients with Crohn's disease than among the general population. Radiological and endoscopic investigations are helpful in defining the extent of disease, and the degree of anemia, fall in serum albumin and degree of elevation of acute-phase proteins in defining severity.

Anemia is usually a combination of iron and folate deficiency, and the possibility of bacterial overgrowth, particularly in patients with multiple strictures, should be considered.

MEDICAL MANAGEMENT

The nature of the disease, the short- and long-term morbidity and the likely impact on the individual need to be discussed with both the patient and their family, as it often involves reappraisal of training and education and work plans. Most patients have high morbidity in the first few years, but the long-term prognosis is good.

Drug treatment of inflammatory mucosal disease

At presentation the predominant symptoms are usually those of mucosal inflammatory disease. Because the prevalence of this type of disease is low no controlled drug trials have been carried out in these patients. It is assumed, although as yet unproven, that the results of drug trials carried out in patients with active Crohn's disease can be applied to patients with diffuse jejunoileitis.

The role of sulfasalazine and the new salicylates in the treatment of active Crohn's disease has been summarized by Sutherland (Chapter 55). In practice, most adult patients presenting with diffuse jejunal ileitis have severe symptoms and are treated with oral corticosteroids, usually prednisolone, in doses of 20–40 mg daily depending on body weight, tapered over the course of a few months depending on their symptomatic response and laboratory indices.

Some patients with diffuse jejunal ileitis need long-term low-dose oral corticosteroids, and there is some evidence of long-term benefit in this subgroup, as defined in the ECCDS (Malchow et al 1984). For those patients with chronic persistent symptoms, when the dose of oral prednisolone is either reduced or withdrawn azathioprine 2 mg/kg can be used both as a steroid-sparing agent and as an anti-inflammatory in its own right.

The duration of azathioprine therapy in quiescent disease is uncertain, but a survey of long-term treatment from Paris (Lemann et al 1994) showed that two-thirds of patients remained in remission at 5 years, and suggests that relapse is more likely in females and younger patients. The benefit has to be weighed against the risks of significant long-term side effects, such as bone marrow toxicity, nausea, vomiting, pancreatitis and arthralgia. In patients with diffuse jejunoileitis the benefits of medium-term azathioprine probably outweighs the hazards.

In childhood or adolescent-onset diffuse jejunoileitis enteral feeding is commonly the primary treatment of choice, and there is good evidence that the best response to enteral feeding is obtained in young people with small-bowel disease (see Chapter 59). Occasionally the severity of the disease is such that prolonged nutritional support is required, and of our adult patients six have received total parenteral nutrition, although usually as a supportive measure for postoperative complications, rather than as sustained medical treatment for severe disease.

Obstructive symptoms

Some patients at their initial presentation, and most patients during the course of follow-up, develop recurrent subacute obstructive episodes caused by stricture formation. In our series more than a third of patients had had their first laparotomy within 12 months from diagnosis, and half had been treated surgically within 3 years.

At laparotomy the object is to relieve the tightest strictures by strictureplasty, leaving residual narrowed areas, some of which will heal whereas others will progress to stricture formation and eventually require further surgical treatment. The annual operative rate in years 2–5 from diagnosis was 15% per year, but with time there is evidence that the disease may 'burn itself out'.

After 10 years from diagnosis the annual operative rate fell to 5.2%, and after 15 years it fell further to 2.6%. Only three patients had had more than four operations after a mean follow-up of 16 years.

Mortality

Two of the 34 patients died, one of a spontaneous perforation of the jejunum and the other of bronchogenic carcinoma.

At the close of the study, 24 of the 32 patients were well and symptom free, and not receiving any specific medical treatment; eight had abdominal symptoms including pain, diarrhea or high ileostomy output, of whom three were taking corticosteroid treatment and one azathioprine. None of the 32 patients were receiving nutritional support.

Long-term outcome

It is encouraging for both patients and their doctors that the disease becomes less aggressive with time and that the surgical intervention rates fall with increasing length of follow-up. Even so, the operative rates are high in the first 10 years after diagnosis. Most patients have recurrent problems, with high morbidity, particularly in the early years, which is reflected in the fact that nearly a third require psychiatric help for severe anxiety or depression. The excess mortality has largely been eliminated and there was only one disease-related death in our series.

SUMMARY

Diffuse jejunoileitis is a disorder of high morbidity, particularly in the early years, commonly requiring surgical intervention, but medium- to long-term optimism is justified as most patients can now be restored to good health with minimal symptoms, despite the high morbidity of the early years after diagnosis.

REFERENCES

Cooke W T, Swan C H J 1974 Diffuse jejuno-ileitis of Crohn's disease. Quarterly Journal of Medicine 179: 583–601

Crohn B B, Yarnis H 1958 Regional ileitis, 2nd edn. Grune & Stratton New York

Crohn B B, Yunich A M 1941 Ileojejunitis. Annals of Surgery 113: 371–380

Jones J H, Lennard-Jones J E 1966 Corticosteroids and corticotrophin in the treatment of Crohn's disease. Gut 7: 181–187

Lemann T, Tai R, Bouhnik Y et al 1994 Long term outcome of patients with Crohn's disease successfully treated with azathioprine or 6-mercaptopurine. Gastroenterology 106: A719

Malchow H, Ewe K, Brandes J W 1984 European Cooperative Crohn's disease study: results of drug treatment. Gastroenterology 86: 249–266

Puntis J, McNeish A S, Allan R N 1984 Long term prognosis of Crohn's disease with onset in childhood and adolescence. Gut 25: 329–336

Tan W C, Allan R N 1993 Diffuse jejunoileitis of Crohn's disease. Gut 34: 1374–1378

van Patter W N, Bargen J A, Dockerty M B et al 1954 Regional enteritis. Gastroenterology 26: 347–450

67. Crohn's disease of the large intestine

J. R. Lowes

INTRODUCTION

It is more than 60 years since Burrill Crohn and colleagues described the clinical and pathological features of the condition that we now recognize as Crohn's disease of the terminal ileum (Crohn et al 1932). It was nearly 30 years later that Brooke (1959) postulated the coexistence of ileal and colonic disease, and Lockhart-Mummery and Morson (1960) described the features of colonic disease without overt ileal disease. These workers highlighted the difference between Crohn's colitis and idiopathic ulcerative colitis, and this distinction still needs to be made clinically in patients with inflammatory bowel disease.

DISTINCTION BETWEEN CROHN'S AND ULCERATIVE COLITIS

The distinction between isolated colonic Crohn's disease and ulcerative colitis is important for several reasons. Appropriate epidemiological data can only be generated if patients are accurately categorized into the appropriate disease group. The potential benefit of new therapeutic agents needs to be assessed in patient subgroups that are defined as accurately as possible. Finally, in considering surgical therapy it is important to make the distinction between Crohn's disease of the colon and ulcerative colitis, particularly if ileoanal pouch construction is to be performed.

The clinical symptoms and signs of Crohn's disease of the colon and ulcerative colitis can be very similar. Arthralgia, anorexia and weight loss are more common in Crohn's disease than in ulcerative colitis, but are of little value in distinguishing between the two in individual cases. Morphological distinction between the two conditions has been addressed in a number of studies.

Macroscopic appearances

The distribution of the diseased mucosa throughout the colon provides clues to the underlying pathological process, but these are unreliable. Rectal sparing, which in the past has been thought a feature of colonic Crohn's disease, can also occur in ulcerative colitis, particularly but not exclusively after treatment with topical steroids (Bernstein et al 1993). Using microscopic features as the gold standard, macroscopic features are unreliable in distinguishing between the two diseases (Palnaes Hansen et al 1990). This study showed that cobblestone mucosa is more common in Crohn's disease, and pseudopolyposis is more common in ulcerative colitis, but there is considerable overlap with both of these features. Discontinuous involvement of the colonic mucosa and stricture formation were observed with equal frequency in both diseases.

Microscopic appearances

The early descriptive histologic work of Morson and others emphasized the distinguishing histological features of the disease (Lindner et al 1963, Lockhart-Mummery & Morson 1964, Janowitz & Present 1966, Howel-Jones et al 1966, Hawk et al 1967, Lennard-Jones et al 1968 Farmer et al 1968, Glotzer et al 1970). These important features are:

Transmural inflammation
Serositis
Microscopic fissuring
Submucosal lymphedema.

Granulomas are to be found in only about half the patients with Crohn's disease (Hawk et al 1967, Farmer et al 1968)

The importance of colonic biopsy in the diagnosis of colonic Crohn's disease cannot be overstated (Chambers & Morson 1980), and the increasing frequency with which granulomas are found in the more distal colon remains one of the histopathological enigmas in this condition (Chambers & Morson 1979).

EPIDEMIOLOGY

Epidemiological studies of the incidence and prevalence of Crohn's disease have not been site specific. There have been few studies looking at factors that affect the site of disease within the gastrointestinal tract. An interesting study from Sweden examined the effect of smoking on disease localization in Crohn's disease (Lindberg et al 1992). Smoking did not offer the same protection that has been observed in ulcerative colitis, and in fact appeared to have an adverse effect on the course of the disease. Smokers required more operations and developed more fistulae and abscesses than never-smokers.

Studies from both Europe and the United States are in broad agreement about the proportion of patients with each form of Crohn's disease. Approximately 40% of patients present with ileocecal disease, 30% with disease confined to the small bowel, and 25% with purely colonic involvement (Farmer et al 1975, Hellers 1979, Mekhijian et al 1979a).

DISTRIBUTION OF DISEASE AND MODES OF PRESENTATION

There are broadly three main subgroups of anatomical localization of colonic Crohn's disease: ileocolitis, distal left-sided colitis, and extensive and total colitis.

Although the term 'Crohn's disease' implies a tight clinical definition, in practice a wide variety of clinical and pathological features exist, of which any one patient will manifest a small number. As the disease may affect any part of the gut from mouth to anus, it is not surprising that differing clinical presentations are produced, depending upon the region of the gastrointestinal tract involved. It should be emphasized that although macroscopic evidence of Crohn's disease is limited to a relatively restricted part of the gastrointestinal tract, if investigation is pursued relentlessly other areas of involvement can be found that are clinically 'silent' (Goodman et al 1976, Dunne et al 1977). This phenomenon has recently been extended to include the oral cavity, as patients with active disease elsewhere in the gastrointestinal tract have increased oral inflammation, as demonstrated by oral pan-tomography (Halme et al 1993). Anal disease is often present in patients with Crohn's colitis, and the presence of anal and perianal disease may provide a useful clue to the underlying diagnosis. However, despite the evidence of the diffuse nature of the disease, clinically there are three main patterns of disease involvement in the colon.

Ileocolitis. This is dealt with in Chapter 65.

Distal left-sided colitis. The disease presents usually as diarrhea, weight loss and/or rectal bleeding. Pyrexia and an inflammatory abdominal mass may be present. Although population studies have not shown a preponderance of colonic Crohn's disease in the elderly (Rose et al 1988), other series have tended to suggest that there *is* an increased incidence of distal colonic disease in the elderly (Fabricius et al 1985, Carr & Schofield 1982). The sigmoid and distal descending colon appear to be predominantly affected. The association of the affected segment with the territory supplied by the inferior mesenteric artery has lent support to the hypothesis that an ischemic component is important in the etiology of the mucosal lesion. Ischemic colitis must be considered in the differential diagnosis of left-sided colitis. This can usually be recognized by its characteristic radiological appearances, and like Crohn's disease, can lead to stricture formation, particularly at the splenic flexure (Marston 1994).

Acute complications, including colonic perforation, have been described in patients with left-sided disease (Carr & Schofield 1982, Fabricius et al 1985). It is possible that these complications are due to delay in presentation, as patients often have symptoms prior to their acute presentation.

Isolated Crohn's proctitis tends to behave in a less dramatic fashion and in general appears to have a benign prognosis (Carr & Schofield 1982).

Total and/or extensive colitis. In these cases the macroscopic involvement may range from total colitis, which is difficult to distinguish from ulcerative colitis on macroscopic features alone, to patchy focal or segmental colitis, which strongly suggests Crohn's disease because of its discontinuous distribution.

Disease at this site presents predominantly as diarrhea, the severity of which tends to be correlated with the severity of colonic disease. Systemic features are usually present and often include weight loss, lethargy and malaise.

The severity of symptoms at presentation is extremely variable and can range from a mild increase in stool frequency through to a fulminant colitis, with all the attendant risks of toxic megacolon and perforation that are seen in other forms of fulminant colitis (Greenstein et al 1975, 1985, Fazio 1980). Bloody diarrhea can be a feature, depending upon the severity of mucosal inflammation. A pre-existing or concomitant diagnosis of small-bowel Crohn's disease makes the diagnosis easier. Perianal Crohn's disease, which is present in over 30% of cases (Farmer et al 1975), also helps distinguish between the two conditions.

Although abdominal pain is more of a feature of Crohn's disease than ulcerative colitis, symptoms of intestinal obstruction are uncommon in isolated colonic disease compared to ileocolonic involvement.

Typical symptoms of patients presenting with colonic Crohn's disease are demonstrated in the series from the Cleveland Clinic, outlined in Table 67.1.

CONDITIONS SEEN IN ASSOCIATION WITH CROHN'S COLITIS

As with Crohn's disease at other sites, extraintestinal manifestations of the disease may be present. Patients with colitis and ileocolitis have an increased chance of developing arthritis and erythema nodosum (Farmer et al 1979, Rankin et al 1979). One extraintestinal manifestation is frequently associated with another, and patients with arthritis

Table 67.1 Symptoms at presentation of 615 cases of Crohn's disease at the Cleveland Clinic (Farmer et al 1975)

	Ileocolic	Small bowel	Large bowel
Diarrhea	4+	4+	4+
Abdominal pain	3+	3+	3+
Bleeding	1+	1+	2+
Weight loss (≥ 20% body weight)	1+	1+	1+
Perianal disease	2+	+	2+
Arthritis	+	+	1+

Proportion of patients with each symptom:
4+, > 75%; 3+, 50–75%; 2+, 25–50%; 1+, 0–25%; +, ≤ 5%

frequently may have uveitis and erythema nodosum as well (Rankin et al 1979).

About half the elderly patients with Crohn's disease also have diverticular disease (Ritchie & Lennard-Jones 1976, Fabricius et al 1985). This is probably similar to the general population, but can mean the diagnosis is difficult to make on radiological grounds.

ASSESSMENT OF DISEASE ACTIVITY

Numerous methods have been developed to assess disease activity. The National Cooperative Crohn's Disease Study (NCCDS) produced one of the first indices, the Crohn's Disease Activity Index (CDAI) (Mekhijian et al 1979b), and others have followed (Harvey & Bradshaw 1980, Van Hees et al 1980). The large number perhaps indicates that there is no one satisfactory method of clinically categorizing disease activity. Such indices have largely been used in the context of clinical trials, and have not been widely taken up in clinical practice.

Assessment of patients remains rather empirical and must take into account a range of factors:

The severity of the acute attack
The possibility of complications: sepsis, perforation, fistula
The chronicity of the problem
The risks of surgery.

Severity of the acute attack. Crohn's colitis can be categorized into inactive or mild, moderate or severe attacks in a similar fashion to the initial descriptions of severity described for ulcerative colitis by Truelove and Witts (1960):

Mild: four or fewer motions per day. Little rectal bleeding. No systemic upset or anemia (hemoglobin >10.5 g/dl)
Moderate: more than four motions per day, no anemia or systemic upset
Severe: more than four bowel actions per day, with systemic upset such as fever, tachycardia colonic tenderness, low serum albumin (<30 g/l) or weight loss (>3 kg).

Failure to control a severe acute attack with intensive medical therapy is an indication for emergency surgery.

Possibility of complications: stricture, sepsis, perforation, fistula. Some complications of Crohn's disease of the colon, such as strictures or fistulae, can be asymptomatic but are identified during radiological or endoscopic assessment. Fistulae and strictures require therapy only if they are causing symptoms. A high index of suspicion is required to detect sepsis, as this may be difficult to distinguish from active disease. The presence of pyrexia and/or an inflammatory mass should prompt investigation into the possibility of an associated abscess. Sepsis makes medical therapy with immunosuppressive therapy hazardous.

Chronicity of the problem. The natural history of Crohn's colitis is for the disease to relapse and remit. The chronicity of the disease results in a heavy psychological toll on the patient, and significant associations between psychosocial stress and disease activity have been recorded (Greene et al 1994).

The requirement for repeated courses of immunosuppression therapy and the side effects of drug therapy constitute important clinical information in evaluating an acute exacerbation of the disease, and in particular assessing the necessity and timing of surgical intervention.

Risks of surgery. The risks of surgery for Crohn's colitis have fallen in parallel with advances in patient management in successive decades (Andrews et al 1989b). It is difficult to be precise about the reasons for this improvement, but possibilities include earlier operations on less ill patients, advances in the recognition and control of sepsis, better nutritional support, and recognition and prophylaxis against thromboembolic complications. Nevertheless, a small but significant morbidity and mortality is associated with surgical resection. Elective proctocolectomy is associated with a surgical mortality of between 2 and 4%. Previous surgery, and in particular the value of retaining the colon in patients who have undergone extensive small-bowel resection, should be considered when considering colonic surgery in patients with Crohn's colitis.

INVESTIGATIONS

Attempts to correlate clinical, endoscopic and biochemical estimations of disease activity are still difficult. Only weak correlation exists between clinical and endoscopic indices, and between these indices and biochemical markers (Cellier et al 1994).

Laboratory assessment

The main laboratory indicators are listed in Table 67.2. Platelet count in particular is a useful marker of inflammation (Harries et al 1983). Serum albumin concentration can be decreased in severe attacks of colitis, and acute-

Table 67.2 Laboratory markers of disease activity

Hemoglobin
White blood count
   Polymorphonuclear
     Lymphocyte
Platelet count
Plasma viscosity
Erythrocyte sedimentation rate

Albumin
C-reactive protein
α_1-acid glycoprotein
α_1-antitrypsin (fecal and serum)

phase proteins elevated. An interesting and as yet unexplained difference between colonic and ileal Crohn's disease is the behavior of the erythrocyte sedimentation rate in acute relapses. Sachar and colleagues (1990) have shown a correlation with disease activity in the colon, less good with ileocolonic disease, and an inverse correlation with ileal disease.

Endoscopic assessment

The endoscopic examination of the colonic mucosa is useful in a variety of situations, as outlined in Table 67.3.

Diagnosis

Endoscopy can give useful clues as to the diagnosis. Aphthous ulcers in the colon are an early macroscopic lesion pathognomonic of Crohn's disease, but their significance is uncertain (Ni & Goldberg 1986). Discontinuity and asymmetry of mucosal involvement are features of colonic Crohn's disease as opposed to ulcerative colitis, and this can be assessed endoscopically. It can be difficult to distinguish between Crohn's disease and other colitides macroscopically, but endoscopy allows a series of biopsies to be taken throughout the colon. Such colonic series can reveal discontinuity in microscopic inflammation throughout the colon, in addition to other features that make the diagnosis of Crohn's disease more likely. Pathognomonic features can be present in macroscopically normal bowel (Schmitz-Moorman et al 1985).

Endoscopy is generally considered inferior to contrast radiology in the demonstration of fistulae, but is of value in the evaluation of fistulae into the colon. In these circumstances colonoscopy can determine if there is active disease in the colon, and in the case of colocolic fistulae whether there is activity at one or both ends of the fistula, therefore determining the required resection.

Therapy

Primary strictures of the colon are rarely symptomatic. More recently, dilatation of anastomotic strictures in the colon has been performed with some success following ileocecal resection (Blomberg 1992).

Radiological assessment

Contrast radiology. The double contrast barium enema examination is the standard by which other imaging techniques need to be measured. The characteristic features of Crohn's colitis are described in Chapter 54. The earliest lesion recognized by the examination is the aphthoid ulcer, but more typically the radiological features are asymmetric deep ulceration and discontinuous disease. Barium contrast radiology is the optimum method for demonstrating fistulae involving the colon.

Computerized tomography (CT). CT scanning can be of value in assessing extraluminal masses, which can represent abscesses. Oral water-soluble contrast is used to outline the lumen of the bowel, thus allowing assessment of other intra-abdominal masses. Both CT and ultrasound scanning techniques can miss intra-abdominal masses (Cybulaky & Tam 1990).

Ultrasound. The use of ultrasound to assess patients with colonic disease is increasing but is likely to remain dependent upon enthusiastic exponents for some time. Like CT, it is useful in identifying extramural sepsis related to active inflammatory disease, but can also give useful information about inflammatory activity within the mucosa (Wijers et al 1992, Brignola et al 1993). Retrograde instillation of water into the colon allows ultrasonographic examination of distinct layers of the colon wall. High levels of sensitivity and specificity in differentiating ulcerative colitis from Crohn's disease by this method have been claimed (Limberg & Oswald 1994). Endoluminal ultrasound can also be used to distinguish between ulcerative colitis and Crohn's colitis by examining the depth of mucosal involvement (Hildebrandt et al 1992).

Radioisotope scanning. Isotope-labeled leukocyte scans cannot make the diagnosis of Crohn's disease. However, isotope-labeled leukocytes, and in particular neutrophils, have been used to demonstrate active inflammatory activity, and the use of delayed scanning after 24 hours can be helpful in distinguishing active disease from abscess formation. Furthermore, the scintigraphic measurement of stool samples is an objective method of evaluating inflammatory activity. ^{111}In and ^{99m}Tc isotopes have been employed (Saverymuttu et al 1986, Pullman et al 1988, Sciarretta et al 1993).

Table 67.3 Indications for endoscopic examination of the colon in Crohn's disease

Establishing a diagnosis
Assessing disease activity
Obtaining tissue for histological analysis
Examining areas of equivocal mucosa identified on barium contrast examinations especially strictures
Cancer surveillance
Dilatation of strictures
Assessing area of bowel involved in fistula

COMPLICATIONS

Toxic dilatation

It was initially thought that toxic dilatation was rare in Crohn's disease, but this was probably due to misdiagnosis of some fulminant cases as being due to ulcerative colitis, and only more chronic cases being recognized as Crohn's colitis. Toxic dilatation may occur in Crohn's colitis as in ulcerative colitis, particularly in those cases with a short preceding history (Buzzard et al 1974). The incidence of toxic megacolon in colonic disease is in the range 5–10%.

Hemorrhage

Frank and sometimes massive hemorrhage requiring emergency transfusion may complicate Crohn's colitis (Rubin et al 1980).

Anemia

Iron deficiency anemia is common (Hoffbrand et al 1968). Not all microcytic anemias are iron deficient and iron supplementation is often prescribed on the strength of a microcytic blood film. Microcytic anemia secondary to a chronic inflammatory response is often encountered (Dyer et al 1972, Sahay et al 1993). Horina et al (1993) reported three out of three cases of anemia secondary to chronic inflammation that responded to recombinant erythropoietin therapy, but the majority of such cases respond to adequate medical or surgical control of the disease. It is important to make a full hematological assessment, including an examination of the bone marrow in difficult cases, as the reasons for anemia may be quite varied. In addition to iron deficiency, folate deficiency, hemolysis secondary to drug therapy and B_{12} malabsorption secondary to coincident ileal disease or resection may also be important.

Sepsis

Intra-abdominal abscesses develop within the mesentery in association with active disease. These present with fever, leukocytosis, and in some cases a palpable mass. Antibiotics may help resolve some in the short term, but they frequently relapse on cessation of therapy and require surgery, usually with resection of the appropriate portion of diseased bowel. Abscesses frequently adhere to adjacent intra-abdominal structures and may drain via fistulae.

Fistula

Abnormal communications between Crohn's-affected tissue and other intra-abdominal or pelvic organs is relatively common. Fistulae have been observed in up to 20% of cases of pure colitis and 40% of cases of ileocolitis (Farmer et al 1976). Perianal fistulae are common in colonic disease, occurring in approximately 35% of cases of colonic or ileocolonic disease (Farmer et al 1975). Enteroenteric and enterocutaneous fistulae are more common in ileocolic disease (34%) than in either isolated colonic (16%) or small-bowel disease (17%).

Enteroenteric fistulae can be difficult to diagnose. In cases involving ileocolonic or colocolic communication, the macroscopic involvement of the gut with Crohn's disease can be confined to only one of the participating viscera, and when resectional surgery is required simple closure of a hole in macroscopically normal bowel with resection of the diseased segment may be all that is required. Where other segments of bowel are involved in active Crohn's disease more extensive resectional surgery may be required. Colonoscopic assessment of the bowel provides useful information about the involvement of the colon and helps to answer the question whether the colon is primarily involved with Crohn's disease or an 'innocent victim' of a fistula arising from active Crohn's disease elsewhere in the gastrointestinal tract.

Fistulae into the ileum can present with features of bacterial overgrowth, but more commonly are found incidentally, either radiologically or at surgery, when investigating patients at initial presentation or with subsequent relapse. Reviewing the presentation of colonic fistulae into the upper gastrointestinal tract, only 83 gastrocolic and duodenocolic fistulae have been described in the literature (27 gastric, 52 duodenal, and four both) (Pichney et al 1992). Fecal vomiting can occur in up to one-third of gastrocolic fistulae, but it is a rare presentation of a duodenocolic fistula. Barium enema is more sensitive in making the diagnosis than barium meal (McDaniel et al 1982).

Fistulae between the small bowel and distal large bowel usually present as intractable diarrhea because the large quantity of dihydroxy bile acids delivered into the colon results in a secretory state in the sigmoid colon.

Metabolic problems

Sodium, potassium and water loss. Salt and water depletion is a common problem in patients with intractable diarrhea. If a secretory state develops because of ileocolonic fistulae, or cholorrhetic diarrhea secondary to previous ileal resection, particularly severe sodium, potassium and water losses may occur in patients with Crohn's colitis. Oral (or in severe cases parenteral) supplementation is required. Potassium depletion may be insidious and may result in muscle weakness, fatiguability and malaise.

Magnesium. Magnesium deficiency is common in severe Crohn's disease. Symptoms develop insidiously and include ataxia, vertigo, muscle weakness and depression (Hanna et al 1960). Low serum magnesium concentration is always associated with deficiency, but many patients with total body magnesium deficiency will have normal serum levels (Dunn & Walser 1966, Heaton 1969, Barnes 1969, Main et al 1981).

Supplementation can be given orally, but care is required as many magnesium salts may exacerbate diarrhea. Magnesium glycerophosphate orally is usually well tolerated.

Zinc. The clinical syndrome of frank zinc deficiency, with acrodermatitis and diminished taste acuity, is rarely seen in Crohn's colitis. Plasma zinc levels may be low (McClain et al 1980), but this may not represent true zinc deficiency as serum levels are related to plasma albumin levels and tissue levels of zinc may be in the normal range (Ainley et al 1988). Zinc deficiency is probably best assessed by measuring tissue levels, such as in hair (Solomons et al 1977). Supplementation with 200 mg zinc sulphate daily may return zinc levels and the level of zinc-dependent hormones to the normal range (Brignola et al 1993).

Trace elements. Deficiencies of trace elements such as selenium, molybdenum, manganese and copper, although important in patients receiving parenteral nutrition, are rarely of clinical significance in patients with uncomplicated colonic Crohn's disease.

Osteoporosis and osteomalacia. Osteomalacia is closely associated with other features of malnutrition in Crohn's disease (Harries et al 1985), but osteoporosis is seen in up to 30% of patients and is correlated with mean lifetime corticosteroid dose. The risk factors for developing osteomalacia and osteoporosis in colonic Crohn's disease are listed in Table 67.4.

Renal complications

Renal stones, both urate and oxalate, are increased in frequency in patients with Crohn's colitis compared to the general population (Gelzayd et al 1968). Urate stones may be present in increased frequency secondary to dehydration from chronic diarrhea. Oxalate stones are more frequently associated with steatorrhea and Crohn's disease of the small intestine, but increased oxalate absorption may occur secondary to the mucosal lesion, which leads to an increased incidence of oxalate stones in colitis also.

Enterovesical fistulae may present as recurrent urinary tract infections, or more floridly with pneumaturia or the passage of feces per urethram. They are more common in men than in women, who have the uterus interposed between the colon and the bladder. They may be difficult to demonstrate and a variety of imaging techniques may need to be employed, such as CT scanning, cystoscopy, barium studies and colonoscopy.

Renal amyloid is a rare complication of long-standing Crohn's colitis which may be asymptomatic or lead to the nephrotic syndrome or renal failure (Werther et al 1960).

MEDICAL THERAPY

Medical therapy is used to treat acute attacks of the disease and also to maintain remission.

The spontaneously relapsing and remitting nature of Crohn's disease is one of the many reasons why drug therapy needs to be evaluated in the context of a controlled clinical trial. The National Cooperative Crohn's Disease Study (NCCDS) in 1979 remains the major study, in which the majority of current therapeutic regimens have their roots (Summers et al 1979). This double-blind placebo-controlled randomized trial studied the effects of sulfasalazine, prednisone and azathioprine compared to placebo.

Corticosteroids – acute disease

In the NCCDS prednisone was found to induce remission more effectively than placebo. However, if the subgroup of patients with purely colonic disease was studied no significant results were obtained, probably owing to the small number of patients available for study. The European Cooperative Crohn's Disease Study (ECCDS), the second large multicenter study of randomized treatments in Crohn's disease, showed a significant therapeutic effect in colonic Crohn's disease with 6-methylprednisolone (Malchow et al 1984). This study highlighted the dangers of corticosteroid therapy in the treatment of patients with inflammatory masses, which should be regarded as clinical signs indicating the need for further investigation to exclude active sepsis within the abdomen. The treatment of severe acute attacks of Crohn's disease has been studied by the Oxford group with a regimen similar to that advocated for severe acute ulcerative colitis, employing intravenous prednisolone and a rectal infusion of hydrocortisone hemisuccinate (Truelove & Jewell 1974, Shepherd et al 1986). The majority of patients can be brought into remission with this regimen.

Corticosteroids – maintenance therapy

The NCCDS failed to show any benefit for the use of maintenance therapy with prednisone at a dose of 0.25 mg/kg/day (Summers et al 1979). However, the ECCDS differed, and showed a beneficial effect of 8 mg daily of 6-methylprednisolone (Malchow et al 1984).

Table 67.4 Risk factors for developing osteoporosis and osteomalacia

Osteomalacia
Inadequate intake of calcium and vitamin D
Loss of protein-bound metabolites of vitamin D
Depleted bile salt pool leading to occult steatorrhea

Osteoporosis
Corticosteroid therapy
Inactivity
Secondary amenorrhea
Renal stones
Renal failure
Thrombosis

Studies of prednisolone absorption in Crohn's disease have been performed on a small number of subjects; although there appears to be decreased amount of urinary recovery of steroids in patients with predominantly ileal disease (Shaffer et al 1983), serum levels of prednisolone in patients with predominantly colonic disease were not significantly different from controls (Tanner et al 1981).

5-aminosalicylates – acute disease

The NCCDS showed that in patients with colonic disease sulfasalazine was significantly better than placebo in inducing remission, provided they had a short duration of symptoms (<6 months) and no previous medical or surgical therapy (Summers et al 1979). The benefit of sulfasalazine in acute Crohn's colitis was further supported by other controlled trials (Van Hees et al 1981, Ursing et al 1982). Two important studies were the starting point for further developments in the clinical pharmacology of inflammatory bowel disease. The splitting of the sulfasalazine diazo bond by bacterial azoreductase to release 5-aminosalicylic acid (5-ASA) and sulfapyridine was demonstrated by Peppercorn and Goldman (1972). It was subsequently demonstrated that colonic 5-aminosalicylic acid was the active therapeutic moiety of the parent compound (Azad-Khan et al 1977). The development of alternative delivery systems for 5-ASA into the colon that avoided some of the unwanted side effects of the sulfonamide moiety was a natural progression. Mesalazine, 5-ASA in a variety of pH-dependent delivery capsules; olsalazine, two molecules of 5-ASA linked by a diazo bond; and balsalazide, 5-ASA linked by a diazo bond to alanine, are available. Mesalazine (as Pentasa or Salofalk), particularly at the relatively high dose of 4 g daily, has been shown to be effective as a single agent in the treatment of acute Crohn's disease of the ileum and colon (Martin et al 1990, Singleton et al 1993). Large controlled trials of the treatment of acute Crohn's colitis with olsalazine and basalazide have not been published.

5-aminosalicylates – maintenance therapy

The prevention of disease relapse with oral 5-ASA preparations is more contentious (Greenberger & Miner 1994, Messori et al 1994). The NCCDS and the ECCDS did not show any benefit in using sulfasalazine for the maintenance of remission (Summers et al 1979, Malchow et al 1984). It is possible that the lack of benefit from sulfasalazine was due to the dose administered: using sulfasalazine, dosage is limited by the side effects of the sulfapyridine moiety at higher doses.

The use of mesalazine to prevent relapse has been attempted in a number of studies (Hanauer et al 1993, Gendre et al 1993), but no clear message about maintenance therapy has yet emerged. Patients entering such studies are heterogeneous: a number will have recently undergone a variety of medical or surgical interventions which will affect their response to treatment.

Metronidazole

There is a paucity of adequate controlled clinical trial data on the use of metronidazole in the treatment of specific subgroups of patients with Crohn's disease. A recent placebo-controlled trial of metronidazole, 10 or 20 mg/kg/day (Sutherland et al 1991) has recently confirmed earlier studies suggesting that the drug was of value in acute Crohn's colitis (Ursing & Kamme 1975, Blichfeldt et al 1978, Ursing et al 1982). It is particularly of value in the presence of perianal disease. It is not clear whether its mode of action is related to its antibacterial properties or to some other property. Many patients and physicians find it a difficult drug to employ in the medium and long term because of untoward side effects, particularly nausea and neurotoxicity. Enthusiasts claim that by careful adjustment of dosage many patients can be treated (Ursing 1991).

Immunosuppression

The relapsing and remitting nature of the disease and the unacceptable long-term effects of corticosteroid therapy has prompted the search for agents which might control disease activity over a longer period, with a more acceptable side-effect profile. The evidence for activation of immunological mechanisms led to the study of immunosuppressive agents in Crohn's disease.

Azathioprine and 6-mercaptopurine

Initial uncontrolled studies were enthusiastic about the value of azathioprine in Crohn's disease (Brooke et al 1969, 1973). Controlled studies which came later were not so encouraging (Willoughby et al 1971, Rhodes et al 1971, Klein et al 1974, Summers et al 1979). However, these studies may be criticized for the dose of azathioprine used and the relatively short duration of therapy before assessment. Encouragement to persist with the use of azathioprine, or its active metabolite 6-mercaptopurine, came from controlled studies of 6-mercaptopurine by Present and colleagues (1980) and a controlled withdrawal study by O'Donoghue and colleagues (1978). This latter study showed that azathioprine was of value in maintaining remission of the disease, as there was a significantly higher relapse rate in those randomized to receive placebo compared to azathioprine. Azathioprine is now widely used in the treatment of chronically active Crohn's disease, and the most widely employed dose is 2 mg/kg/day. Agranulocytosis is the side effect that causes the greatest concern, and regular estimations of the white blood cell count are essential. Other side effects include nausea, pancreatitis and photosensitive skin rashes.

Cyclosporin – acute disease

The impact of cyclosporin in preventing graft rejection in transplantation medicine led to experimentation in other clinical areas where immunosuppression was beneficial. Experience with azathioprine in Crohn's disease suggested that cyclosporin was worthy of study in the same situation. Anecdotal evidence that it was of benefit was first reported by Allison and Pounder (1984), and a subsequent controlled clinical trial by Brynskov and colleagues (1989, 1991) suggested that it was of some benefit to a group of patients that were resistant to or intolerant of corticosteroids. Another trial which also looked at patients with chronically active Crohn's disease (the majority with colonic or ileocolic involvement) could not show any anti-inflammatory or steroid-sparing effect (Jewell et al 1994). However, these trials were carried out on a particularly difficult group of patients and it was difficult to separate the beneficial effects of co-prescribed corticosteroids from any potential benefit due to the cyclosporin.

Cyclosporin – maintenance therapy

The use of long-term low-dose cyclosporin as a prophylactic agent has been studied in a randomized controlled trial. No benefit in terms of symptom control or reduced need for concomitant therapy was demonstrated (Feagan et al 1994).

Cyclosporin is a difficult drug to handle. It requires careful monitoring of drug levels and has several dangerous and unpleasant side effects. It is nephrotoxic and may cause hypertension, paresthesia and hirsutism. The therapeutic benefit from its use in the treatment of Crohn's disease seems small and the costs, as measured by side effects and therapeutic monitoring, are high. It is unlikely to gain widespread use in the treatment of chronic active Crohn's colitis. Anecdotal reports of its effectiveness in the treatment of fistulae are of interest (Present & Lichtiger 1994), but should be supported by controlled data of its effectiveness before being widely used.

Methotrexate

A limited number of uncontrolled studies employing oral or parenteral methotrexate have shown some evidence of effectiveness in controlling active Crohn's colitis (Kozarek et al 1989, Baron et al 1993). The doses that have been used have been below what is normally considered an immunosuppressive dose, and more controlled studies are required to support these claims. In the small number of cases studied the side effects have been mild.

NUTRITIONAL THERAPY

Nutritional therapy in Crohn's colitis can be considered either as supportive or as having a primary therapeutic role.

Supportive therapy

An acute attack of colitis is frequently associated with a marked catabolic state, often with considerable weight loss. Patients with Crohn's colitis may also suffer from chronic protein-calorie malnutrition. Multiple factors are involved, not least the inflammatory process, but also poor intake and associated malabsorption secondary to associated ileal disease or small-bowel surgery (Powell-Tuck et al 1984, Reilly et al 1976, Harries et al 1982, Jones et al 1984). This should be routinely assessed, and as a minimum patients should have their body mass index recorded at sequential clinic attendance. In children growth retardation is a predominant feature of Crohn's disease (Kelts et al 1979), and rate of growth should be regularly monitored. Although malnutrition is a significant problem in Crohn's disease and there is evidence that nutritional support can correct some of the deficiencies (Harries & Heatley 1983, Gassull et al 1986), there is no evidence that correcting the nutritional problems modifies the disease process. However, there have been attempts to modify the disease process by addressing therapeutic regimens to nutritional issues.

Parenteral nutrition

Total parenteral nutrition (TPN) is attractive as a form of therapy for Crohn's disease. It offers the potential to maintain an adequate nutritional intake while allowing the gastrointestinal tract to rest. Furthermore, it excludes any putative dietary component that may be important in the etiology or pathogenesis of the disease. However, a prospective randomized controlled trial comparing TPN with enteral or part enteral, part parenteral nutrition has shown that parenteral nutrition *per se* has no therapeutic benefit over other forms of nutritional support, and that bowel rest is not important in establishing remission (Greenberg et al 1988).

TPN is not without hazard, and its use in the treatment of isolated Crohn's colitis is rarely required. It is sometimes required in the treatment of patients who have short bowel syndrome following extensive ileal resection, or when acute or subacute intestinal obstruction precludes adequate nutritional support via the enteral route.

Elemental diet

A number of studies have examined the role of elemental or chemically defined diets in the treatment of Crohn's disease (O'Morain et al 1984, Saverymuttu et al 1985, Sanderson et al 1987, Lochs et al 1991, Gorard et al 1993). The evidence suggests that such diets are as effective as corticosteroids in inducing remission, irrespective of initial nutritional state, but that they are unpalatable. Administering the nitrogen source as partial digests of whole protein (i.e. mixtures containing free amino acids and oligopeptides) is no better. Treatment with polymeric diets containing whole proteins remains controversial, and owing to the variety of regimens employed and the endpoints measured, no consistent results have been obtained (Park et al 1991, Raouf et al 1991, Rigaud et al 1991, González-Huix et al 1993) They have not been shown to be effective in inducing remission compared to an elemental diet (Giaffer et al 1990). There is some evidence that distal Crohn's proctocolitis treated with an elemental diet has a particularly high relapse rate on cessation of therapy (Teahon et al 1990).

The suggestion that elemental diets allow repair of damaged epithelium, by altering factors in favor of intestinal repair as opposed to damage by luminal aggressive factors, is interesting (Teahon et al 1991). It suggests that given the differing nutritional requirements of the enterocyte through the gut (Roediger 1982), differing forms of elemental diet may be beneficial in different sites of disease. Short-chain fatty acids produced by bacterial fermentation in the colon are the main energy source for colonocytes (Roediger 1980), and although butyrate enemas are effective in the treatment of patients with distal ulcerative colitis, controlled data for the use of this form of treatment in colonic Crohn's disease are awaited.

Refined or unrefined carbohydrate?

Following on from the observation that patients with Crohn's disease have a significantly increased consumption of refined carbohydrate prior to diagnosis (Thornton et al 1979), a multicenter study of a diet containing unrefined carbohydrate, high in fiber, was undertaken (Ritchie et al 1987). Such a diet would appear to put unnecessary restrictions on a patient's intake without any benefit in outcome.

MEDICAL VERSUS SURGICAL THERAPY

There are a few definite indications for surgical intervention in the management of Crohn's colitis. These include fulminant colitis failing to respond to medical therapy, toxic dilatation, perforation, and symptomatic fistulae. The indications for surgery in the more common chronic undulating form of the disease are more difficult to define. The disadvantages of continuous medical therapy – side effects, recurrent attacks, failure to control disease – have to be weighed against the risks of surgical intervention, the disadvantages of a permanent ileostomy, or ileorectal anastomosis. The balance between these two options varies a great deal between different centers, and is heavily influenced by patient, physicians and surgeons involved. A study from Cardiff examined the timing of ileocolonic resection and anastomosis from the patient's perspective. Patients' views on the timing of their own surgical intervention in ileocolonic disease would suggest that a majority would have preferred earlier intervention, although those who had undergone previous resections were more likely to indicate that the timing of their surgery was correct. This study has many potential flaws, not least that some patients may be reluctant to express a difference of opinion to their medical attendants about their care, but no patient expressed the view that their surgical intervention was too early (Scott & Hughes 1994). It is important that surgery is not viewed as a failure of medical treatment but rather as one of various therapeutic options available. Whenever possible surgery should be elective, and patients medically as fit as possible, with sepsis under control and metabolic complications corrected to minimize the risks involved.

The decision between medical and surgical therapy is also dependent upon the operation proposed. More conservative surgical techniques may be less physically or psychologically demanding than older, more radical procedures.

One of the least radical operations for colonic Crohn's disease is some form of defunctioning ileostomy, either a split or a loop. This diversion of the fecal stream can induce remission of colonic disease and may be used for a variety of reasons (Harper et al 1983). It gives the patient the opportunity to experience life with an ileostomy; it may give them a chance to have a 'drug holiday': to experience life for a period of months without the need for repeated courses of corticosteroids or immunosuppressants; it allows an acute exacerbation of Crohn's colitis to resolve, allowing a safer interval colectomy, although nowadays this is seldom required. The major disadvantage of this therapy is the high recurrence rate on restoring intestinal continuity, and the risk of cancer developing in the defunctioned colon, particularly in young patients who refuse any further surgical treatment after a defunctioning procedure.

Resection of an involved segment of colon – usually left-sided, including proctectomy for isolated rectal disease – is controversial, being associated with a high recurrence rate of approximately 60% at 10 years (Allan et al 1989). Panproctocolectomy for colorectal disease is associated with a 23% chance of reoperation for recurrent small-bowel disease after 10 years in the series from the General Hospital, Birmingham (Scammell et al 1987).

PROGNOSIS

The short-term natural history of Crohn's colitis can be measured by the outcome of placebo-treated groups. The NCCDS and ECCDS give some of the best data in this respect. From these studies it would appear that about 20% of patients will go into spontaneous remission, which will be maintained in around 60% of subjects at 2 years (Summers et al 1979).

Consideration of the overall prognosis in Crohn's colitis has to take in several measures that contribute to quality of life.

Mortality

Hospital-based studies, often from centers with a large tertiary referral component to their case load, have in the past tended to suggest that Crohn's disease carried an excess mortality (Truelove & Peña 1976, Storgaard et al 1979, Prior et al 1981). Several epidemiological studies have more recently drawn attention to the slight effects that inflammatory bowel disease has on mortality (Binder et al 1985, Ekbom et al 1992, Probert et al 1992), and that improvements presumably related to antibiotics and surgical techniques have reduced mortality in recent years (Andrews et al 1989b). A Swedish study showed that survival was 96% of that expected for patients with Crohn's disease, with a standardized mortality ratio of 1.6 (Ekbom et al 1992). Colonic disease has a slightly worse prognosis than ileal or ileocolonic disease, and an ileoanal anastomosis or more than one resection had an adverse effect on survival (Probert et al 1992).

Operation rate

Failure to respond to medical measures, chronic ill health, anorectal disease or acute complications are the main indications for surgical intervention in Crohn's colitis. Patients with colonic disease do not require surgical intervention as commonly as patients with ileocolic disease (Farmer et al 1975), and intractable disease is a much more common indication for surgery than Crohn's disease at other sites. In the Cleveland Clinic series approximately 40% of patients with colonic disease had required operation at 10 years (Farmer et al 1985). In the Birmingham series (Andrews et al 1989a) 49 out of 130 patients with distal Crohn's colitis had been treated without surgical intervention after a mean follow-up of 8 years. At 10 years after onset of symptoms 55% of patients had undergone surgery. The operations performed are shown in Table 67.5. Age at diagnosis did not affect operation rate.

Eleven of the patients undergoing segmental colectomy did not require any further surgery, three required a completion panproctocolectomy, and one a right hemicolectomy. Patients with extensive colitis have a slightly higher expectation of an operation, with 63% having undergone surgery within 10 years of the onset of symptoms in

Table 67.5 Initial operations for 130 patients with distal Crohn's colitis at the General Hospital, Birmingham, 1944–1986. Data from Andrews et al (1989a)

No operation	49
Panproctocolectomy	17
Colectomy and ileorectal anastomosis	9
Colectomy and end ileostomy	10
Segmental colectomy	15
Right hemicolectomy or terminal ileal resection	15
Ileostomy alone	12
Other	3

Table 67.6 Initial operations for 145 patients with extensive Crohn's colitis at the General Hospital, Birmingham, 1944–1986. Data from Andrews et al (1989a)

No operation	30
Panproctocolectomy	27
Colectomy and ileorectal anastomosis	47
Colectomy and end ileostomy	13
Right hemicolectomy or terminal ileal resection	12
Ileostomy alone	10
Other	6

the same series. The operations performed are shown in Table 67.6.

There is clearly a significant morbidity and mortality linked with surgical intervention, and the more radical the procedure the greater the risk. As in small-bowel Crohn's disease the panenteric nature of the disease has led to the evolution of less aggressive surgical procedures being employed where appropriate.

Quality of life

Although the morbidity and mortality associated with Crohn's colitis are falling, there remains evidence of significant impairment of the quality of life. Patients with Crohn's disease have more evidence of psychological stress than patients with ulcerative colitis, and this relates to the severity of their symptoms (Drossman et al 1991, 1992). As the disease tends to affect a relatively young population the socioeconomic implications are significant, and although the majority of patients are well there remain a small number who are chronically disabled by the disease. There is evidence of increased unemployment, missed schooling, and the need to call upon disability pensions in a small proportion of patients (Mayberry et al 1992, Sonnenberg 1992).

Disease recurrence

The recurrence of disease after surgery remains a significant problem. In left-sided or distal disease, defunctioning operations are associated with the need for further surgery. In the Birmingham series, reoperation rates for recurrent disease were 1, 10 and 21% at 2, 5 and 10 years respectively after panproctocolectomy. The reoperation rates after the less radical colectomy and ileorectal anastomosis are understandably much higher, at 27, 46 and 60% at the same 2-, 5- and 10-year intervals (Andrews et al 1989a).

CONCLUSIONS

Crohn's colitis is now a well recognized clinical entity. Acute disease and its complications of malnutrition, sepsis and metabolic upset are amenable to medical therapy in the majority of cases, although colonic perforation remains one of the few life-threatening manifestations of the disease. The more difficult problems now lie in maintaining remission with well tolerated and efficacious therapies. Surgery at present offers the best prospect of a prolonged remission, but unfortunately the best results are obtained with the most radical forms of surgery. Although better management of the acute disease has led to significant reductions in mortality, there remains a significant physical, social and psychological morbidity, which must be addressed in the future.

REFERENCES

Ainley C C, Cason J, Carlsson L K, Slavin B M, Thompson R P H 1988 Zinc status in inflammatory bowel disease. Clinical Science 75: 227–283

Allan A, Andrews H, Hilton C et al 1989 Segmental colonic resection is an appropriate operation for short skip lesions due to Crohn's disease in the colon. World Journal of Surgery 13: 611–616

Allison M C, Pounder R E 1984 Cyclosporin for Crohn's disease. Lancet i: 902–903

Andrews H A, Lewis P, Allan R N 1989a Prognosis after surgery for colonic Crohn's disease. British Journal of Surgery 76: 1184–1190

Andrews H A, Lewis P, Allan R N 1989b Mortality in Crohn's disease – a clinical analysis. Quarterly Journal of Medicine 71: 399–405

Azad-Khan A K, Piris J, Truelove S C 1977 An experiment to determine the active therapeutic moiety of sulphasalazine. Lancet ii: 892–895

Barnes B A 1969 Magnesium conservation: a study of surgical patients. Annals of the New York Academy of Science 162: 786–801

Baron T H, Truss C D, Elson C O 1993 Low dose oral methotrexate in refractory inflammatory bowel disease. Digestive Diseases and Sciences 3810: 1851–1856

Bernstein C N, Shanahan F, Anton P A, Weinstein W M 1993 Patchy involvement, including rectal sparing occurs in ulcerative colitis. Gastroenterology 104: A668

Binder V, Hendriksen C, Kreiner S 1985 Prognosis in Crohn's disease, based on results from a regional patient group from the county of Copenhagen. Gut 26: 146–150

Blichfeldt P, Blomhoff J P, Myhre E, Gjone E 1978 Metronidazole in Crohn's disease: a double blind cross-over clinical trial. Scandinavian Journal of Gastroenterology 13: 123–127

Blomberg B 1992 Endoscopic treatment modalities in inflammatory bowel disease. Endoscopy 24: 578–581

Brignola C, Belloli C, Iannone P, De Simone G, Corbelli C, Levorato M 1993 Comparison of scintigraphy with indium-111 leukocyte scan and ultrasonography in assessment of X-ray demonstrated lesions of Crohn's disease. Digestive Diseases and Sciences 383: 433–437

Brooke B N 1959 Granulomatous disease of the intestine. Lancet ii: 745–749

Brooke B N, Hoffman D C, Swarbrick E T 1969 Azathioprine for Crohn's disease. Lancet ii: 612–614

Brooke B N, Javet S L, Davidson O W 1973 Further experience with azathioprine for Crohn's disease. Lancet ii: 1050–1053

Brynskov J, Freund L, Rasmussen S N et al 1989 A placebo controlled, double blind, randomized trial of cyclosporine A in patients with severe active Crohn's disease refractory to conventional therapy. New England Journal of Medicine 321: 845–850

Brynskov J, Freund L, Rasmussen S N et al 1991 Final report on a placebo controlled, double blind, randomized trial of cyclosporin A in active chronic Crohn's disease. Scandinavian Journal of Gastroenterology 26: 689–695

Buzzard A J, Baker W N W, Neeham P R G, Warren R E 1974 Acute toxic dilatation of the colon in Crohn's disease. Gut 15: 416–419

Carr N, Schofield P F 1982 Inflammatory bowel disease in the older patient. British Journal of Surgery 69: 223–225

Cellier C, Sahmoud T, Froguel E, Adenis A, Belaiche J, Bretagne J-F 1994 Correlations between clinical activity, endoscopic severity, and biologic parameters in colonic or ileocolonic Crohn's disease. A prospective multicentre study of 121 cases. Gut 35: 231–235

Chambers T J, Morson B C 1979 The granuloma in Crohn's disease. Gut 20: 269–274

Chambers T J, Morson B C 1980 Large bowel biopsy in the differential diagnosis of inflammatory bowel disease. Investigational Cell Pathology 3: 159–173

Crohn B B, Ginzberg L, Oppenheimer G D 1932 Regional ileitis, a pathological and clinical entity. Journal of the American Medical Association 99: 1323–1329

Cybulaky I J, Tam P 1990 Intra-abdominal abscesses in Crohn's disease. American Surgeon 56: 678–682

Drossman D A, Leserman J, Mitchell C M, Li Z M, Zagami E A, Patrick D L 1991 Health status and health care use in persons with inflammatory bowel disease: a national sample. Digestive Diseases and Sciences 36: 1746–1755

Drossman D A, Li Z M, Leserman J, Patrick D L 1992 Ulcerative colitis and Crohn's disease. Health status scales for research and clinical practice. Journal of Clinical Gastroenterology 15: 104–112

Dunn M J, Walser M 1966 Magnesium depletion in normal man. Metabolism 15: 884–895

Dunne W T, Cooke W T, Allan R N 1977 Enzymatic and morphometric evidence of Crohn's disease as a diffuse lesion of the gastrointestinal tract. Gut 18: 290–291

Dyer N H, Child J A, Mollin D L, Dawson A M 1972 Anaemia in Crohn's disease. Quarterly Journal of Medicine 41: 419–436

Ekbom A, Helmick C J, Zack M, Holmberg L, Adami H-O 1992 Survival and causes of death in patients with inflammatory bowel disease: a population based study. Gastroenterology 103: 954–960

Fabricius P J, Gyde S N, Shouler P, Keighley M R B, Alexander-Williams J, Allan R N 1985 Crohn's disease in the elderly. Gut 26: 461–465

Farmer R G, Hawk W A, Turnbull R B 1968 Regional enteritis of the colon: a clinical and pathological comparison with ulcerative colitis. American Journal of Digestive Diseases 13: 501–514

Farmer R G, Hawk W A, Turnbull C D 1975 Clinical patterns in Crohn's disease: a statistical study of 615 cases. Gastroenterology 68: 627–635

Farmer R G, Hawk W A, Turnbull R B Jr 1976 Indications for surgery in Crohn's disease. Analysis of 500 cases. Gastroenterology 71: 245–250

Farmer R G, Whelan G, Fazio V W 1985 Long term follow up of patients with Crohn's disease. Gastroenterology 88: 1818–1825

Fazio V W 1980 Toxic megacolon in ulcerative colitis and Crohn's colitis. Clinical Gastroenterology 9: 389–407

Feagan B G, McDonald J W, Rochon J et al 1994 Low-dose cyclosporine for the treatment of Crohn's disease. The Canadian Crohn's disease relapse prevention trial. New England Journal of Medicine 330: 1846–1851

Gassull M A, Abad A, Cabre E, Gonzalez-Huiz F, Gine J J, Dolz C 1986 Enteral nutrition in inflammatory bowel disease. Gut 27: 76–80

Gelzayd E A, Breuer R I, Kirsner J B 1968 Nephrolithiasis in inflammatory bowel disease. American Journal of Digestive Diseases 13: 1927–1934

Giaffer M H, North G, Holdsworth C D 1990 Controlled trial of polymeric versus elemental in treatment of active Crohn's disease. Lancet 335: 816–819

Glotzer D J, Gardner R C, Goldman H, Hinrichs H R, Rosen H, Zetzel L 1970 Comparative features and course of ulcerative colitis and granulomatous colitis. New England Journal of Medicine 282: 582–587

González-Huix F, De Leon R, Fernández-Bañares F et al 1993 Polymeric enteral diets as primary treatment of active Crohn's disease. A prospective steroid-controlled trial. Gut 34: 778–782

Goodman M J, Skinner J A, Truelove S C 1976 Abnormalities of the apparently normal bowel mucosa in Crohn's disease. Lancet i: 275–278

Gorard D A, Hunt J B, Payne-James J J et al 1993 Initial response and subsequent course of Crohn's disease treated with elemental diet or prednisolone. Gut 34: 1198–1202

Greenberg G R, Fleming C R, Jeejeebhoy K N, Rubernberg I N, Sales D, Tremaine W J 1988 Controlled trial of bowel rest and nutritional support in the management of Crohn's disease. Gut 29: 1309–1315

Greenberger N J, Miner P B 1994 Is maintenance therapy effective in Crohn's disease? Lancet 344: 900–901

Greene B R, Blanchard E B, Wan C K 1994 Long term monitoring of psychosocial stress and symptomatology in inflammatory bowel disease. Behaviour Research and Therapy 322: 217–226

Greenstein A J, Kark A E, Dreiling D A 1975 Crohn's disease of the colon III: Toxic dilatation of the colon in Crohn's disease. American Journal of Gastroenterology 63: 117–128

Greenstein A J, Sachar B D, Gibas A et al 1985 Outcome of toxic dilatation in ulcerative colitis and Crohn's disease. Journal of Clinical Gastroenterology 7: 137–143

Halme L, Meurman J H, Laine P, von Smitten K, Syrjanen S, Lindqvist C 1993 Oral findings in patients with active or inactive Crohn's disease. Oral Surgery, Oral Medicine, Oral Pathology 762: 175–181

Hanna S, Harrison M, MacIntyre I, Fraser R 1960 The syndrome of magnesium deficiency in man. Lancet ii: 172–176

Harper P H, Truelove S C, Lee E C G, Kettlewell M G W, Jewell D P 1983 Split ileostomy and ileo-colostomy for Crohn's disease of the colon and ulcerative colitis: a 20 year survey. Gut 24: 106–110

Harries A D, Heatley R V 1983 Nutritional disturbances in Crohn's disease. Postgraduate Medical Journal 59: 690–697

Harries A D, Brown R, Heatley R V et al 1985 Vitamin D status in Crohn's disease: association with nutrition and disease activity. Gut 26: 1197–1203

Harries A D, Fitzsimons E, Fifield R, Dew M J, Rhodes J 1983 A simple measure of activity in Crohn's disease. British Medical Journal 286: 1476

Harries A D, Jones L, Heatley R V, Rhodes J, Fitzsimmons E 1982 Mid-arm circumference as a simple means of identifying malnutrition in Crohn's disease. British Medical Journal 285: 1317–1318

Harvey R F, Bradshaw J M 1980 A simple index of Crohn's disease activity. Lancet i: 514

Hawk W A, Turnbull R B, Farmer R G 1967 Regional enteritis of the colon. Distinctive features of the entity. Journal of the American Medical Association 201: 738–746

Heaton F W 1969 The kidney and magnesium homeostasis. Annals of the New York Academy of Science 162: 775–785

Hellers G 1979 Crohn's disease in Stockholm County, 1955–1974. A study of epidemiology, results of surgical treatment and long term prognosis. Acta Chirurgica Scandinavica 490: 1–84

Hildebrandt U, Kraus J, Ecker K W, Schmid T, Schuder G, Feifel G 1992 Endosonographic differentiation of mucosal and transmural non-specific inflammatory bowel disease. Endoscopy 24: 359–363

Hoffbrand A V, Stowart J S, Booth C C, Mollin D L 1968 Folate deficiency in Crohn's disease: incidence, pathogenesis, and treatment. Lancet ii: 71–75

Horina J H, Petritsch W, Schmid C R, Reicht G, Wenzl H, Silly H 1993 Treatment of anaemia in inflammatory bowel disease with recombinant human erythropoietin: results in three patients. Gastroenterology 1046: 1828–1831

Howel-Jones J, Lennard-Jones J E, Lockhart-Mummery H E 1966 Experience in the treatment of Crohn's disease of the large intestine. Gut 7: 448–452

Janowitz H D, Present D H 1966 Granulomatous colitis – pathogenic concepts. Gastroenterology 51: 778–784

Jewell D P, Lennard-Jones J E, Cyclosporin Study Group of Great Britain and Ireland 1994 Oral cyclosporin for chronic active Crohn's disease: a multicentre controlled trial. European Journal of Gastroenterology and Hepatology 6: 499–505

Jones L A, Harries A D, Rhodes J 1984 Normal energy intake in undernourished patients with Crohn's disease. British Medical Journal 288: 193

Kelts D G, Grand R, Shen G, Watkins J B, Werlin S L, Boehme C 1979 Nutritional basis of growth failure in children and adolescents with Crohn's disease. Gastroenterology 76: 720–727

Klein M, Binder J H, Mitchell M, Aaronson R, Spiro H 1974 Treatment of Crohn's disease with azathioprine: a controlled evaluation. Gastroenterology 66: 916–922

Kozarek R A, Patterson D J, Gelfand M D et al 1989 Methotrexate induces clinical and histological remission in patients with refractory inflammatory bowel disease. Annals of Internal Medicine 110: 353–356

Lennard-Jones J E, Lockhart-Mummery H E, Morson B C 1968 Clinical and pathological differentiation of Crohn's disease and proctocolitis. Gastroenterology 54: 1162–1170

Limberg B, Oswald B 1994 Diagnosis and differential diagnosis of ulcerative colitis and Crohn's disease by hydrocolonic sonography. American Journal of Gastroenterology 897: 1051–1057

Lindberg E, Järnerot G, Huitfeldt B 1992 Smoking in Crohn's disease: effect on localisation and clinical course. Gut 33: 779–782

Lindner A E, Marshak R H, Wolf B S, Janowitz H D 1963 Granulomatous colitis. A clinical study. New England Journal of Medicine 269: 379–385

Lochs H, Steinhardt H J, Klaus-Wentz B et al 1991 Comparison of enteral nutrition and drug treatment in active Crohn's disease. Results of the European Cooperative Crohn's Disease Study IV. Gastroenterology 101: 881–888

Lockhart-Mummery H E, Morson B C 1960 Crohn's disease (regional enteritis) of the large intestine and its distinction from ulcerative colitis. Gut 1: 87–105

Lockhart-Mummery H E, Morson B C 1964 Crohn's disease of the large intestine. Gut 5: 493–509

McClain C, Soutor C, Zieve I 1980 Zinc deficiency: a complication of Crohn's disease. Gastroenterology 78: 272–279

McDaniel N T Jr, Bluth E L, Ray J E 1982 Gastrocolic fistula in Crohn's disease. American Journal of Gastroenterology 77: 588–589

Main A N H, Morgan R J, Russell R I et al 1981 Magnesium deficiency in chronic inflammatory bowel disease and requirements during intravenous nutrition. Journal of Parenteral and Enteral Nutrition 5: 15–19

Malchow H, Ewe K, Brandes J W et al 1984 European Co-operative Crohn's Disease Study (ECCDS): results of drug treatment. Gastroenterology 86: 249–266

Marston A 1994 Ischaemia of the gut. In: Misiewicz J J, Pounder R E, Venables C W (eds) Diseases of the gut and pancreas, 2nd edn. Blackwell Scientific, Oxford, pp 1007–1019

Martin F, Sutherland L, Beck I T et al 1990 Oral 5-ASA versus prednisone in short term treatment of Crohn's disease: a multicentre controlled trial. Canadian Journal of Gastroenterology 4: 452–457

Mayberry M K, Probert C, Srivastava E, Rhodes J, Mayberry J F 1992 Perceived discrimination in education and employment by people with Crohn's disease: a case control study of educational achievement and employment. Gut 33: 312–314

Mekhijian H S, Switz D M, Watts H D, Deren J J, Katon R N, Beman F M 1979a National Cooperative Crohn's disease study: factors determining recurrence of Crohn's disease after surgery. Gastroenterology 77: 907–913

Mekhijian H S, Switz D M, Melnyk C S, Rankin G B, Brooks R K 1979b Clinical features and natural history of Crohn's disease. Gastroenterology 77: 898–906

Messori A, Brignola C, Trallori G et al 1994 Effectiveness of 5-aminosalicylic acid for maintaining remission in patients with Crohn's disease: a meta-analysis. American Journal of Gastroenterology 89: 811–818

Ni X Y, Goldberg H I 1986 Aphthoid ulcers in Crohn's disease: radiographic course and relationship to bowel appearance. Radiology 158: 589–596

O'Donoghue D P, Dawson A M, Powell-Tuck J, Brown R J, Lennard-Jones J E 1978 Double blind withdrawal trial of azathioprine as maintenance treatment for Crohn's disease. Lancet ii: 955–977

O'Morain C A, Segal A W, Levi A J 1984 Elemental diet as primary treatment of acute Crohn's disease: a controlled trial. British Medical Journal 281: 1859–1862

Palnaes Hansen C, Hegnhoj J, Moller A, Brauer C, Hage E, Jarnum S 1990 Ulcerative colitis and Crohn's disease of the colon. Is there a macroscopic difference? Annales Chirurgiae et Gynaecologiae 792: 78–81

Park R H R, Galloway A, Danesh B J Z, Russell R I 1991 Double blind controlled trial of elemental diet and polymeric diets as primary treatment in active Crohn's disease. European Journal of Gastroenterology and Hepatology 3: 483–490

Peppercorn M A, Goldman P 1972 The role of intestinal bacteria in the metabolism of salicylazosulphapyridine. Journal of Pharmacology and Experimental Therapeutics 181: 555–562

Pichney L S, Fantry G T, Graham S M 1992 Gastrocolic and duodenocolic fistulas in Crohn's disease. Journal of Clinical Gastroenterology 153: 205–211

Powell-Tuck J, Garlick P J, Lennard-Jones J E, Waterlow J C 1984 Rates of whole body protein synthesis and breakdown increase with the severity of inflammatory bowel disease. Gut 25: 460–464

Present D H, Lichtiger S 1994 Efficacy of cyclosporine in the treatment of the fistula of Crohn's disease. Digestive Diseases and Sciences 392: 374–380

Present D H, Korelitz B I, Wisch N et al 1980 Treatment of Crohn's disease with 6-mercaptopurine: a long term randomized double blind study. New England Journal of Medicine 302: 981–987

Prior P, Gyde S, Cooke W T, Waterhouse J A H, Allan R N 1981 Mortality in Crohn's disease. Gastroenterology 80: 307–312

Probert C S J, Jayanthi V, Wicks A C B, Mayberry J F 1992 Mortality from Crohn's disease in Leicestershire 1972–1989: an epidemiological community based study. Gut 33: 1226–1228

Pullman W E, Sullivan P J, Barratt P J, Lising J, Booth J A, Doe W F 1988 Assessment of inflammatory bowel disease activity by technetium 99m phagocyte scanning. Gastroenterology 95: 989–996

Rankin G B, Watts H D, Melnyck C S, Kelly M L 1979 National Cooperative Crohn's Disease Study: extraintestinal manifestations and perianal complications. Gastroenterology 77: 914–920

Raouf A H, Hildrey V, Daniel J et al 1991 Enteral feeding as sole treatment for Crohn's disease: controlled trial of whole protein versus aminoacid based feed and a case study of dietary challenge. Gut 32: 702–707

Reilly J, Ryan J A, Strole W E, Fischer J E 1976 Hyperalimentation in inflammatory bowel disease. American Journal of Surgery 131: 192–200

Rhodes J, Bainton D, Beck P, Campbell H 1971 Controlled trial of azathioprine in Crohn's disease. Lancet ii: 1273–1276

Rigaud D, Cosnes J, Le Quintrec Y, René E, Gendre J P, Mignon M 1991 Controlled trial comparing two types of enteral nutrition in the treatment of active Crohn's disease: elemental versus polymeric trial. Gut 32: 1492–1497

Ritchie J K, Lennard-Jones J E 1976 Crohn's disease of the distal large bowel. Gastroenterology 11: 433–436

Ritchie J K, Wadsworth J, Lennard-Jones J E, Rogers E 1987 Controlled multicentre therapeutic trial of an unrefined carbohydrate, fibre rich diet in Crohn's disease. British Medical Journal 295: 517–520

Roediger W E W 1980 Role of anaerobic bacteria in the metabolic welfare of the colonic mucosa in man. Gut 21: 793–798

Roediger W E W 1982 Utilization of nutrients by isolated epithelial cells of the rat colon. Gastroenterology 83: 424–429

Rose J R, Roberts G M, Williams G T, Mayberry J F, Rhodes J 1988 Cardiff Crohn's disease jubilee: the incidence over 50 years. Gut 29: 346–351

Rubin M, Herrington J I, Schneider R 1980 Regional enteritis with major gastrointestinal haemorrhage as the initial manifestation. Archives of Internal Medicine 140: 217–219

Sachar D B, Luppescu N E, Bodian C, Shlien R D, Fabry T L, Gumaste V V 1990 Erythrocyte sedimentation as a measure of Crohn's disease activity: opposite trends in ileitis versus colitis. Journal of Clinical Gastroenterology 126: 643–646

Sahay R, Prangnell D R, Scott B B 1993 Inflammatory bowel disease and refractory anaemia (myelodysplasia). Gut 34: 1630–1631

Sanderson I R, Udeen S, Davies P S W, Savage M O, Walker-Smith J A 1987 Remission induced by an elemental diet in small bowel Crohn's disease. Archives of Diseases of Childhood 61: 123–127

Saverymuttu S, Hodgson H J F, Chadwick V S 1985 Controlled trial comparing prednisolone with an elemental diet plus non-absorbable antibiotics in active Crohn's disease. Gut 26: 994–998

Saverymuttu S H, Camillieri M, Rees H, Lowender J P, Hodgson H J F, Chadwick V S 1986 Indium 111-granulocyte scanning in the assessment of disease extent and disease activity in inflammatory bowel disease. Gastroenterology 90: 1121–1128

Scammell B, Andrews H, Allan R N et al 1987 Results of proctocolectomy for Crohn's disease. British Journal of Surgery 74: 671–674

Schmitz-Moormann P, Himmelmann G W, Brandes J W 1985 Relationships between clinical data and histology of the large bowel in Crohn's disease and ulcerative colitis. Pathology Annual 20: 281–301

Sciarretta G, Furno A, Mazzoni M, Basile C, Malaguti P 1993 Technetium-99m hexamethyl propylene amine oxime granulocyte scintigraphy in Crohn's disease: diagnostic and clinical relevance. Gut 34: 1364–1369

Scott N A, Hughes L E 1994 Timing of ileocolonic resection for Crohn's disease – the patient's view. Gut 35: 656–657

Shaffer J A, Williams S E, Turnberg L A, Houston J B, Rowland M 1983 Absorption of prednisolone in patients with Crohn's disease. Gut 24: 182–186

Shepherd H, Barr G, Jewell D 1986 Use of an intravenous steroid regimen in the treatment of acute Crohn's disease. Journal of Clinical Gastroenterology 8: 154–159

Singleton J W, Hanauer S B, Gitnick G L et al 1993 Mesalazine capsules for the treatment of active Crohn's disease: results of a sixteen week trial. Pentasa Crohn's Disease Study Group. Gastroenterology 104: 1293–1301

Solomons N W, Rosenberg I H, Sandstead H H, Vo-Khactu K P 1977 Zinc deficiency in Crohn's disease. Digestion 16: 87–95

Sonnenberg A 1992 Disability and need for rehabilitation among patients with inflammatory bowel disease. Digestion 51: 168–178

Storgaard L, Bischoff N, Henriksen F W, Fischerman K, Jarnum S 1979 Survival rate in Crohn's disease and ulcerative colitis. Scandinavian Journal of Gastroenterology 14: 225–230

Summers R W, Switz D M, Sessions J T Jr et al 1979 National Cooperative Crohn's Disease Study: results of drug treatment. Gastroenterology 77: 847–869

Sutherland L, Singleton J W, Sessions J T et al 1991 Double blind, placebo controlled trial of metronidazole in Crohn's disease. Gut 32: 1071–1075

Tanner A, Halliday J, Powell L 1981 Serum prednisolone levels in Crohn's disease and coeliac disease following oral prednisolone administration. Digestion 21: 310–315

Teahon K, Bjarnason I, Pearson M, Levi A J 1990 Ten years experience with an elemental diet in the management of Crohn's disease. Gut 31: 1133–1137

Teahon K, Smethurst P, Pearson M, Levi A J, Bjarnason I 1991 The effect of elemental diet on intestinal permeability and inflammation in Crohn's disease. Gastroenterology 101: 84–89

Thornton J R, Emmett P M, Heaton K W 1979 Diet and Crohn's disease: characteristics of the pre-illness diet. British Medical Journal 2: 762–764

Truelove S C, Jewell D P 1974 Intensive intravenous regimen for severe attacks of ulcerative colitis. Lancet i: 1067–1070

Truelove S C, Peña A S 1976 Course and prognosis of Crohn's disease. Gut 17: 192–201

Truelove S C, Witts L J 1960 Cortisone and corticotrophin in ulcerative colitis. British Medical Journal 1: 464–467

Ursing B 1991 Metronidazole in Crohn's disease. In: Inflammatory bowel disease, diagnosis and treatment. Gitnick G (ed) Igaku-Shoin, New York, pp 347–358

Ursing B, Kamme C 1975 Metronidazole for Crohn's disease. Lancet i: 775–777

Ursing B, Alm T, Bárány F et al 1982 A comparative study of metronidazole and sulfasalazine for active Crohn's disease: The Cooperative Crohn's Disease Study in Sweden II: Result. Gastroenterology 83: 550–562

Van Hees P A M, Val Elteren P H, Van Lier H J J, Van Tongeren J H M 1980 An index of inflammatory activity in patients with Crohn's disease. Gut 21: 279–286

Van Hees P A M, Van Lier H J J, Van Elteren P H et al 1981 Effect of sulphasalazine in patients with active Crohn's disease: a controlled double blind study. Gut 22: 404–409

Werther J L, Schapira A, Rubinstein O et al 1960 Amyloidosis in regional enteritis: a report of five cases. American Journal of Medicine 29: 416–423

Wijers O B, Tio T L, Tygat G N 1992 Ultrasonography and endosonography in the diagnosis and management of inflammatory bowel disease. Endoscopy 246: 559–564

Willoughby J M T, Kumar P J, Beckett J, Dawson A M 1971 Controlled trial of azathioprine in Crohn's disease. Lancet ii: 944–947

68. Perianal Crohn's disease

R. S. McLeod   Z. Cohen

Gabriel described multinucleated giant cells in the tissues of patients with rectal fistulae approximately 10 years prior to the classic description of Crohn's disease by Crohn, Ginsburg and Oppenheimer (Gabriel 1921, Crohn et al 1932). However, the association of perianal disease with Crohn's disease was not recognized initially (Bissell 1934). Subsequently, it was recognized that perianal lesions may precede the intestinal manifestations by many years (Gray et al 1965).

Although the significance of perianal lesions was not appreciated initially, their significance is now well recognized, partly because of their frequency and partly because of their morbidity. Thus, management of perianal disease is often an important component of the overall management of the Crohn's patient.

FREQUENCY OF PERIANAL DISEASE

There is great variation in the reported frequency of perianal lesions, probably owing to differences in the intensity of the search made for anal lesions and in the definitions of what constitutes perianal Crohn's disease. In addition, most reviews have been performed retrospectively.

Rates ranging from 43 to 92% have been reported (Fielding 1972, Rankin et al 1979). In a retrospective study, Fielding reviewed 167 patients and found that 80% had perianal complications (Fielding 1972). However, broad criteria, which included the presence of skin maceration and skin tags, were used to define perianal disease. The National Crohn's Cooperative Disease Study (NCCDS) was a prospective study which reported on the prevalence of perianal disease (Rankin et al 1979). Only fissures, fistulae and abscesses were considered. Overall, of the 569 patients entered into the study, 36% gave a history of perianal disease before randomization, including 14% who had perianal complications at the time of randomization. During the study an additional 70 (12%) developed perianal complications.

The site of the intestinal disease appears to influence the rate of perianal disease. The literature consistently documents an increased frequency of perianal lesions in large-bowel disease. In the NCCDS, 46.7% of patients with colonic disease had perianal lesions, compared with 25.5% of those with disease confined to the small bowel (Rankin et al 1979). In the Fielding series, again using his broader criteria, 92% of patients with colonic disease had perianal lesions and 74% with small-bowel disease had perianal lesions (Fielding 1972). In both series, patients with ileocolic disease had intermediate rates of perianal disease.

CLINICAL FEATURES

Buchmann and Alexander-Williams classified perianal disease into the following categories: skin lesions, anal canal lesions and fistulae (Buchmann & Alexander-Williams 1980). Skin lesions include maceration, erosion, ulceration, superficial abscess formation and skin tags. Such lesions are usually due to diarrhea and local irritation, resulting in maceration and subsequent ulceration and subcutaneous abscess formation. Skin tags are edematous corrugated perianal skin. They tend to be larger, thicker and harder than those seen in the non-Crohn's patient, and often have a bluish hue.

The anal canal lesions include fissures, ulcers and stenosis. Fissures tend to be broad based and deep, with undermining of the edges. There may be associated large skin tags and a cyanotic hue to the surrounding skin. They tend to be multiple and placed eccentrically around the anal canal, in contrast to idiopathic fissures which lie in the midline. Despite their appearance they tend to be relatively asymptomatic, unless there is associated sepsis.

A minor degree of anal stenosis due to contracture of the anal canal from long-standing diarrhea may be observed in many patients. More severe stenosis is usually due to scarring following long-standing anal ulceration or surgery. Whereas mild stenosis is usually not clinically significant, advanced cases may cause outflow obstruction.

Fistulae and abscesses may be cryptogenic in origin. These tend to be low-lying fistulae which are simple to treat. Others, resulting from penetration of ulcers or fissures in the rectum and anal canal, tend to be more complex, with high internal openings or multiple indirect tracts. External openings may extend to the scrotum, labia, buttocks and thighs. The fistulae tend to be indurated and cyanotic and, despite their appearance, tend to be asymptomatic unless there is associated sepsis. In a review of the St Mark's Hospital experience with 125 perianal Crohn's fistulae, approximately one-third were low (superficial, intersphincteric or low transsphincteric), one-quarter were rectovaginal, and the remainder were extrasphincteric, had inter- or transsphincteric extensions, or were unclassified (Marks et al 1981). Hobbiss and Schofield reported on a series of 26 patients, 22 of whom had low fistulae (Hobbiss & Schofield 1982).

Rectovaginal fistulae may result from direct penetration by anal canal or rectal wall fissures or ulcers into the vagina. They are a relatively frequent complication of severe perianal Crohn's disease, with reported rates of 3.5–23% (Lockhart-Mummery 1975, Ritchie & Lennard-Jones 1976). Once again, these wide ranges reflect differences in patient populations. Rectovaginal fistulae tend to be low lying but may have multiple side tracts, including anovaginal or anoperineal fistulae. Some may be asymptomatic, whereas others result in varying amounts of gas or fecal discharge being passed through the vagina, or tenderness in the posterior vaginal wall.

DIAGNOSIS

The diagnosis is usually obvious from inspection of the perianal region of patients with Crohn's disease. However, because perianal disease may precede intestinal manifestations, a high degree of suspicion is required in patients who present for treatment of their perianal lesions and have atypical lesions or symptoms related to the gastrointestinal tract. Other diseases which must be considered in the differential diagnosis are sexually transmitted diseases, perianal leukemia, perianal tuberculosis and anal cancer, and appropriate investigations must be undertaken to rule these out.

Perianal disease is unusual in patients with ulcerative colitis. Even in those with perianal lesions who have endoscopic and histologic pictures consistent with ulcerative colitis, one should suspect the diagnosis of Crohn's disease.

Various investigations are available for studying the perianal disease. Generally fistulograms are of limited value. Transanal ultrasound may be valuable in detecting abscesses or delineating fistula tracts. Unfortunately, some patients may not tolerate this procedure, but in such cases intraoperative ultrasound can be performed if available. In a small series of patients with perianal Crohn's disease who underwent transanal ultrasound at our institution, physicians felt that their clinical decision making was altered in four of ten patients and strengthened in 24 of 29 by the results of the examination (Solomon et al 1994).

Magnetic resonance imaging (MRI) has also been shown to be of use in accurately identifying complex fistula tracts and localizing abscesses. The advantage of MRI is that it is non-invasive and painless. However, it may not be readily available in all centers. Jenss et al compared the MRI results to the operative findings in 34 patients with Crohn's disease and suspected perianal complications (Jenss et al 1992). All abscesses were documented by MRI, including eight that had been unsuspected clinically. Although MRI was not more accurate in documenting simple fistula tracts, it did prove to be more accurate in determining the relation of complex fistulae to the sphincter and pelvic floor musculature.

Evaluation of the gastrointestinal tract radiologically and endoscopically is indicated in patients in whom the diagnosis of Crohn's disease is suspected because of gastrointestinal symptoms or unusual perianal findings. Barium small-bowel enema (enteroclysis) is preferable to upper gastrointestinal follow-through examination in assessing the mucosal pattern. Colonoscopy is the preferred examination for the colon and rectum. In those patients where the gastrointestinal disease does not appear to be active, full examination of the gastrointestinal tract is unnecessary. However, as a minimum all patients require a proctosigmoidoscopic examination to assess the rectal mucosa, since decisions may differ depending on whether or not there is rectal disease.

MANAGEMENT

In view of the wide spectrum of perianal lesions, treatment is often variable and must be individualized. Often surgical and medical measures must be combined, especially in those patients with complex disease. Treatment may vary depending on the severity of the symptoms. Other considerations include the nutritional status, and the extent and severity of the disease in the remainder of the gastrointestinal tract. The concerns and expectations of the patient must also be considered in the decision making. In patients who have relatively few symptoms, despite what appears to be very severe perianal disease, the goal should be alleviation of their symptoms rather than eradication of the disease.

General measures

Although treatment may vary according to the specific lesions in the individual patient, certain general measures may be of benefit to most patients. These may include improvement of the nutritional status, treatment of the proximal gastrointestinal disease, and local skin measures including sitz baths, anesthetic ointments and frequent dressing changes.

Patients who are nutritionally depleted may require supplementation with parenteral or enteral nutrition. Parenteral nutrition may be preferable since diarrhea can be exacerbated by enteric feeding. By decreasing the stool frequency there may be improvement in the anal lesions. There are some reports of long-term improvement following treatment with elemental or parenteral feeding (Calam et al 1980, Teahon et al 1990). However, more often there is an exacerbation of the perianal disease as food is reintroduced and patients begin passing stool. Thus, the main indication for parenteral nutrition and elemental diets should be to improve the nutritional status and decrease local perianal sepsis prior to more definitive surgery.

There are also reports suggesting that surgical treatment of proximal gastrointestinal disease may result in improvement of the perianal disease (Hellers et al 1980, Heuman et al 1981, Orkin & Telander 1985). Heuman et al reviewed 20 patients who had perianal disease and underwent a proximal bowel resection (Heuman et al 1981). Complete healing of the perianal disease occurred within 3 months of the resection in 12 patients (60%). Healing occurred in 80% of those patients who did not develop a recurrence of their disease, but in none of those patients who subsequently developed a recurrence. In 43 patients reviewed by Hellers, 20 (47%) had spontaneous healing of anal fistulae after resection of their intestinal disease (Hellers et al 1980). However, in 7 (35%) the fistulae reopened within 2–5 years. In reviewing the Mayo Clinic experience in children, Orkin and Telander noted that only five of 19 (29%) of patients with intestinal and perianal disease had improvement in their perianal disease following intestinal resection and primary anastomosis (Orkin & Telander 1985). The above series are all retrospective and uncontrolled, with small numbers of patients, and it is the authors' view that an intestinal resection should not be performed unless warranted because of intestinal symptomatology.

Management of specific lesions

Hemorrhoids and skin tags

True internal hemorrhoids occur infrequently in patients with Crohn's disease. On the other hand, external skin tags occur frequently. Should patients develop symptomatic internal hemorrhoids a conservative approach should be adopted, including the prescription of sitz baths and local preparations such as cortisone suppositories. If patients are also suffering from diarrhea, this should be treated either medically or with symptomatic treatments, such as antidiarrheal agents.

Surgical management of hemorrhoids is contraindicated in patients with Crohn's disease. Wounds tend to heal poorly and there is a risk of damaging the sphincters or causing anal stenosis. A review of the experience at St Mark's Hospital revealed that of 20 patients treated for hemorrhoids, there were complications in 11 (Jeffrey et al 1977). Six patients required proctectomy because of complications related to the hemorrhoidectomy.

Skin tags are usually asymptomatic, but may cause some discomfort and difficulty with hygiene. Treatment should be limited to local therapy. Excision should be avoided because of the same risks associated with hemorrhoidectomy.

Anal stenosis

A mild degree of anal stenosis is usually well tolerated by patients because of the loose or soft stool they pass as a result of more proximal disease. Only rarely is anal dilatation indicated. Stool softeners may also be beneficial.

Anal fissures

Fissures with characteristics typical of the idiopathic fissure-in-ano occur infrequently. The etiology is probably similar to that of an idiopathic fissure. Such fissures usually respond to sitz baths, regulation of bowel movements with bulking agents, cortisone suppositories or treatments directed to the disease. Surgical intervention should be avoided. In the rare instance where the fissure persists and there is no associated anal or rectal disease, a limited internal sphincterotomy may be performed but it should be done with extreme caution.

The more typical wide-based fissures seen in Crohn's disease are often associated with rectal disease or severe perianal disease, including fistulae. If they are painful there may be associated sepsis, and they may respond to antibiotic therapy. If, on the other hand, the fissure is asymptomatic, no treatment is warranted.

Abscesses and fistulae

Although a conservative approach to the treatment of perianal Crohn's disease is usually advocated, abscesses require drainage, similar to abscesses seen in the non-Crohn's patient. Abscesses should be suspected in patients with perianal disease who complain of pain in fissures and fistulae which were previously asymptomatic. In these patients one should not hesitate to perform an examination under anesthesia. This may be helpful in assessing the extent of disease and determining whether there is an abscess. There is no case for treating abscesses with antibiotics alone. Occasionally in patients where there is considerable cellulitis, broad-spectrum antibiotics may be necessary.

Fistulae tend to be the most difficult perianal lesions to treat, and often both medical and surgical modalities must be employed. Initial treatment will depend on the symptomatology, the complexity of the fistula and whether there is associated rectal disease. Although many gastroenterologists treat simple fistulae with repeated courses of antibiotics when the patient becomes symptomatic, these fistulae are often amenable to surgery and can be eradicated without risk of incontinence or delayed wound healing. Several series have reported excellent results (Bergstrand et al 1980, Bernard et al 1986, Hobbiss & Schofield 1982, Marks et al 1981, Sohn et al 1980).

Complex fistulae or those occurring in the presence of severe rectal disease must be approached differently. It is unusual that they can be eradicated surgically without leading to significant morbidity. Thus, the aim of treatment should be palliative, to eliminate sepsis and hence symptoms. A combined surgical/medical approach is often required. Thus, abscesses may be drained and long-term drains and setons inserted prior to initiating medical management. Surgical management will be discussed in a later chapter; discussion here will be limited to the results of medical management.

Antibiotics may be used in the short or long term. Metronidazole has been widely used for acute exacerbations of perianal Crohn's disease since Ursing and Kamme's first report on patients with active Crohn's disease (Ursing & Kamme 1975). It is unknown whether its effect is entirely due to its antimicrobial action, or whether it has some more specific effect on the Crohn's disease process.

Encouraging results have been reported from two other uncontrolled trials, but there have been no randomized controlled trials in patients with perianal disease. Bernstein et al reported their experience in 21 consecutive patients with chronic unremitting perianal Crohn's disease who had symptoms present for more than 5 years (Bernstein et al 1980). Patients received metronidazole 20 mg/kg/day. Symptomatic improvement occurred within 2 weeks in 90%, with the remaining 10% noting improvement by 6–8 weeks. Using photography to document healing, there was complete or partial healing of 83% of lesions at 8 and 12 weeks. Brandt et al followed this group of patients plus nine others and noted a recurrence of symptoms in 78% within 4 months of cessation of metronidazole (Brandt et al 1982).

Jakobovits and Schuster reported on a group of eight consecutive patients with intractable chronic perianal fistula treated with metronidazole, and reported that 50% of the fistulae closed (Jakobovits & Schuster 1984).

The role of metronidazole is controversial. Because these trials are uncontrolled it is difficult to know whether the improvement was due to the metronidazole or simply to the natural history of the disease. It does appear that metronidazole must be used continuously. There are side effects, including paresthesias, which are almost always reversible. Patients often complain of gastrointestinal symptoms, a metallic taste and an antabuse effect, so they may not be able to take alcohol.

Ciprofloxacin is a fluoroquinolone antibiotic with a broad spectrum of bacterial coverage, including Gram-negative aerobic organisms. Ciprofloxacin has been used to treat gastrointestinal infections since the mid 1980s, although its use in Crohn's disease has been reported only more recently. Ciprofloxacin is appealing for the treatment of Crohn's disease because high intestinal luminal concentrations can be achieved and there is a low incidence of adverse reactions.

Two small uncontrolled trials have shown some benefit with ciprofloxacin in severe perianal Crohn's disease. Turunen et al reported the results of eight patients with continuously active perianal Crohn's disease previously treated with metronidazole and various surgical procedures (Turunen et al 1989). All patients who were treated with ciprofloxacin (in doses of 1000–1500 mg for 3–12 months) showed improvement in physician and patient goal assessments. Wolf reported the disappearance of perianal pain in four of five patients with acute perianal Crohn's disease after 4 days to 5 weeks of ciprofloxacin treatment (Wolf 1990). There was healing of fissures in three patients, one patient with a perianal fistula became asymptomatic, and another with a rectovaginal fistula had partial closure.

Combination therapy with metronidazole and ciprofloxacin has been advocated based on the rationale that metronidazole is effective against anerobic organisms, whereas ciprofloxacin is effective against Gram-negative organisms. Solomon et al (1993) retrospectively reviewed the results of 14 patients who had complex fistula (9), anal canal ulceration (6), rectovaginal fistula (1) or abscesses (5). After 12 weeks of treatment with ciprofloxacin 1000–1500 mg/day and metronidazole 500–1500 mg/day, there was improvement in nine and healing in three; one patient was unchanged and one worsened, necessitating defunctioning with an ileostomy. Unfortunately, however, symptoms recurred in most patients once treatment was stopped, so nine of 14 required continuous or repeat treatment.

Imuran and 6-mercaptopurine have also been used in the treatment of perianal fistulous disease. Korelitz reported that 56% of perirectal fistulae were improved or closed following treatment with 6-mercaptopurine, a metabolite of Imuran (Korelitz & Present 1985). The long-term use of Imuran must be considered carefully. It is an immunosuppressive agent with potentially serious side effects. A response is usually not observed before 3 months of therapy. Markowitz et al reported on 44 adolescents who received 6-mercaptopurine, for their gastrointestinal disease (Markowitz et al 1990): 40% of these patients had perianal fistulae at the start of treatment, but only 14% while on therapy. In addition, no new fistulae developed. These authors, however, fail to report whether the fistula was eradicated or whether symptoms were simply alleviated.

Cyclosporin is another immunosuppressive agent which has been used extensively in patients undergoing transplantation. There is limited experience with cyclosporin A in the treatment of Crohn's disease fistulae. One of the potential difficulties in using this drug is the variable absorption when it is given orally, particularly in patients with Crohn's disease, who may have gastrointestinal involvement or have had prior intestinal resections. Present and Lichtiger reported on 16 patients, ten of whom had perirectal fistulae and two had rectovaginal fistulae (Present & Lichtiger 1994). All were given a 2-week course of intravenous cyclosporin followed by orally administered medication. Four of the patients with perirectal disease and one with a rectovaginal fistula were said to have closed their fistulae after 2 weeks. After a mean follow-up of 12 months, seven of the ten patients with perirectal fistulae remained on cyclosporin, with approximately half improved and half having fistulae closure. Both of the patients with rectovaginal fistulae relapsed, with one requiring surgery. Hanauer and colleagues reported on three patients with perianal fistulae who were treated with oral cyclosporin (Hanauer & Smith 1993). Relapses were seen in two of the three after 3 weeks and 7 months. They also reported that one of the five patients in the series developed a mycotic aneurysm. Thus, these data suggest that cyclosporin may be beneficial in minimizing the symptoms of perianal disease but, like metronidazole, it is unlikely that it will lead to eradication of the fistula.

Most surgeons would argue that simple fistulae, even in Crohn's disease, can usually be eliminated with surgery without the risk of incontinence and without the possible side effects of immunosuppressive agents. Thus, while data about their efficacy are limited, it would seem that if they are to be employed it should only be in patients with complex fistulous disease where local surgical treatment is not an option.

SUMMARY

Discussion in this chapter has been limited to the medical therapy of perianal Crohn's disease. However, treatment usually needs to be individualized depending on the perianal manifestations and symptoms, the site and severity of the underlying gastrointestinal disease, and the general status of the patient. In patients with complex disease multimodality therapy, including both surgical and medical treatments, is usually required. Thus, as is true of most aspects of the treatment of Crohn's disease, a cooperative team approach between surgeon and gastroenterologist is necessary for optimal results.

REFERENCES

Bergstrand O, Ewerth S, Hellers G, Holmstrom B, Willman J, Wallberg P 1980 Outcome following treatment of anal fistulae in Crohn's disease. Acta Chirurgia Scandinavica 500 (Suppl): 43–44

Bernard D, Morgan S, Tasse D 1986 Selective surgical management of Crohn's disease of the anus. Canadian Journal of Surgery 29: 318–322

Bernstein L H, Frank M S, Brandt L J et al 1980 Healing of perineal Crohn's disease with metronidazole. Gastroenterology 79: 357–365

Bissell A D 1934 Localized chronic ulcerative colitis. Annals of Surgery 99: 957–966

Brandt L J, Bernstein L H, Boley S J et al 1982 Metronidazole therapy for perineal Crohn's disease. A followup study. Gastroenterology 83: 383–387

Buchmann P, Alexander-Williams J 1980 Classification of perianal Crohn's disease. Clinical Gastroenterology 9: 323–329

Calam J, Cacoks P E, Walker R J 1980 Elemental diets in the management of Crohn's perianal fistulae. Journal of Parenteral and Enteral Nutrition 4: 4–8

Crohn B B, Ginzburg L, Oppenheimer G D 1932 Regional enteritis: a pathological and clinical entity. Journal of the American Medical Association 95: 1323–1329

Fielding J F 1972 Perianal lesions in Crohn's disease. Journal of the Royal College of Surgeons (Edinburgh) 1717: 32–37

Gabriel W B 1921 Results of an experimental and histological investigation into seventy-five cases of rectal fistulae. Proceedings of the Royal Society of Medicine (London) 14: 156–161

Gray B K, Lockhart-Mummery H E, Morson B C 1965 Crohn's disease of the anal region. Gut 6: 515–524

Hanauer S B, Smith M B 1993 Rapid closure of Crohn's disease fistulas with continuous intravenous cyclosporin A. American Journal of Gastroenterology 88: 646–649

Hellers G, Bergstrand O, Ewerth S, Helmstrom B 1980 Occurrence and outcome after primary treatment of anal fistulae in Crohn's disease. Gut 21: 525–527

Heuman R, Bolin T, Sjodahl R et al 1981 The incidence and course of perianal complications and arthralgia after intestinal resection with restoration of continuity for Crohn's disease. British Journal of Surgery 68: 528–530

Hobbiss J H, Schofield P F 1982 Management of perianal Crohn's disease. Journal of the Royal Society of Medicine (London) 75: 414–417

Jakobovits J, Schuster M 1984 Metronidazole therapy for Crohn's disease and associated fistulae. American Journal of Gastroenterology 79: 533–540

Jeffrey P J, Ritchie J L, Parks A G 1977 Treatment of hemorrhoids in patients with inflammatory bowel disease. Lancet 1: 1084–1085

Jenss H, Starlinger M, Skaleij 1992 Magnetic resonance imaging in perianal Crohn's disease [Letter]. Lancet 340: 1286

Korelitz B I, Present D H 1985 Favorable effect of 6-mercaptopurine on fistulae of Crohn's disease. Digestive Diseases and Sciences 30: 58–64

Lockhart-Mummery H E 1975 Crohn's disease: anal lesions. Diseases of the Colon and Rectum 18: 200–202

Markowitz J, Rosa J, Grancher K, Aiges H, Daum 1990 Long-term 6-mercaptopurine treatment in adolescents with Crohn's disease. Gastroenterology 99: 1347–1351

Marks C G, Ritchie J K, Lockhart-Mummery H E 1981 Anal fistulas in Crohn's disease. British Journal of Surgery 68: 525–527

Orkin B A, Telander R L 1985 The effect of intraabdominal resection and fecal diversion on perianal disease in pediatric Crohn's disease. Journal of Pediatric Surgery 20: 343–347

Present D H, Lichtiger S 1994 Efficacy of cyclosporine in treatment of fistula of Crohn's disease. Digestive Diseases and Sciences 39: 374–380

Rankin G B, Watts D, Melnyk C S et al 1979 National Cooperative Crohn's Disease Study: extraintestinal manifestations and perianal complications. Gastroenterology 77: 914–920

Ritchie J K, Lennard-Jones J E 1976 Crohn's disease of the distal large bowel. Scandinavian Journal of Gastroenterology 11: 433

Sohn N, Korelitz B I, Weinstein M A 1980 Anorectal Crohn's disease: definitive surgery for fistulas and recurrent abscesses. American Journal of Surgery 139: 394–397

Solomon M J, McLeod R S, O'Connor B I, Steinhart A H, Greenberg G R, Cohen Z 1993 Combination ciprofloxacin and metronidazole in severe perianal Crohn's disease. Canadian Journal of Gastroenterology 7: 571–573

Solomon M J, McLeod R S, Cohen E K, Simons M F, Wilson S 1994 Reliability and validity studies of endoluminal ultrasonography for anorectal disorders. Diseases of the Colon and Rectum 37: 546–551

Teahon K, Bjarnason I, Pearson M, Levi A J 1990 Ten years' experience with an elemental diet in the management of Crohn's disease. Gut 31: 1133–1137

Turunen U, Farkkila M, Seppala K 1989 Long-term treatment of perianal or fistulous Crohn's disease with ciprofloxacin. Scandinavian Journal of Gastroenterology 24 (Suppl 148): 144

Ursing B, Kamme C 1975 Metronidazole for Crohn's disease. Lancet i: 775–777

Wolf J 1990 Ciprofloxacin may be useful in Crohn's disease. Gastroenterology 92: 2 (Abstract)

SECTION 8

Inflammatory bowel disease – special problems

69. Extraintestinal manifestations of inflammatory bowel disease

A. Weiss   L. Mayer

INTRODUCTION

Inflammatory bowel disease is a systemic disorder. Although patients most commonly present with abdominal symptoms, management of the extraintestinal manifestations often plays an important role in their care. These conditions may precede recognition of the underlying bowel disorder, and at times are the dominant complaint. The relationship of these extraintestinal manifestations to both ulcerative colitis and Crohn's disease has long been recognized (Crohn 1925, Bargen 1929) and may involve every organ system. Hepatobiliary disorders are discussed elsewhere.

Reviews of large series of patients (Greenstein et al 1976) have helped to categorize and define which patients may be at risk. For example, patients with small-bowel disease are more likely to develop malabsorption (predisposing to osteopenia and cholelithiasis) and enterovesical fistulae. There is still no clear understanding of the mechanism which initiates these manifestations and their relationship to the underlying bowel disease.

Several large studies report an overall incidence of extraintestinal manifestations ranging from 25 to 36% (Greenstein et al 1976, Rankin 1990).

A wide variety of rare extraintestinal manifestations have been reported. The premise of their association with inflammatory bowel disease rests either on the relative rarity of the condition itself, such as amyloid, a clear pathological correlation such as non-caseating granulomas in an extraintestinal site, or a pattern clearly associating it with active bowel disease.

The presence of extraintestinal symptoms in association with inflammatory colitis does not in itself establish a diagnosis of either Crohn's disease or ulcerative colitis. Behçet's disease may present with ulcerative lesions of the colon in association with oral and genital lesions, ocular, dermatological and arthritic lesions (Kyle et al 1991). A reactive arthritis may be seen in association with Campylobacter, Yersinia and other enteric infections (Danzi 1988). Arthritis and pyoderma gangrenosum have been reported in patients in association with diverticular disease (Klein et al 1988). Steroids, salicylates, 5-ASA derivatives and immunosuppressants may all be associated with extraintestinal side effects. This possibility must be excluded before ascribing a systemic complaint to the underlying inflammatory bowel disease.

Extraintestinal manifestations have been categorized in several ways usually as related to or independent of underlying disease activity. Certain symptoms are recognized as direct sequelae of the bowel disease, such as anemia from gastrointestinal blood loss or renal oxalate stones secondary to fat malabsorption. Malabsorption, nephrolithiasis and gallstones are more frequently associated with small-bowel disease, but also occur with large-bowel disease.

Certain extraintestinal manifestations occur together. The triad of joint–eye–skin involvement is the most common array of symptoms (Table 69.1). Approximately one-quarter of those affected present with multiple manifestations (Greenstein et al 1976, Rankin 1990). Extraintestinal manifestations are more common in Crohn's disease than ulcerative colitis (Danzi 1988). In

Table 69.1   Incidence of major extraintestinal manifestations

	Ulcerative colitis					Crohn's disease			
	Greenstein et al 1976 (202 pts)	Kildebo et al 1990 (179 pts)	Greenstein et al 1976 (498 pts)			Farmer et al 1975 (615 pts)			Rankin et al 1979 (569 pts)
			Colitis	Ileocolitis	Enteritis	Colitis	Ileocolitis	Enteritis	Combined
Joint	26%	23%	39%	26%	14%	21%	5%	4.5%	19%
Skin	19%	2%	11%	3%	3%	0%	1.6%	0%	4.6%
Eye	4%	6%	13%	4%	1%	0%	0%	0%	3.5%

Crohn's disease this group of manifestations is more strongly associated with colonic involvement. Around 20% of these patients will also have perianal disease (Rankin 1990). Most reports suggest that the incidence of extraintestinal manifestations is higher in patients with total colitis. One recent study reported that the incidence of extraintestinal manifestations was greater in patients with left-sided colitis (Kildebo et al 1990).

MUSCULOSKELETAL

Arthritis is the most common extraintestinal manifestation of inflammatory bowel disease, occurring in about 20% of all patients (Gravallese & Kantrowitz 1988). There are two common forms, colitic or enteropathic peripheral arthritis, and a form of ankylosing spondylitis which resembles Reiter's syndrome or psoriatic arthritis. This may be associated with bilateral symmetrical sacroiliitis, which can also occur independently.

Colitic arthritis

Colitic arthritis is more common in colonic disease than in small-bowel Crohn's disease. The characteristic peripheral arthropathy affects large joints in a migratory asymmetrical pattern (Ansell 1976). As many as six joints may be involved at any one time (McEwen et al 1962). Polyarticular attacks occur most of the time and a migratory pattern is seen in about half the patients (Gravallese & Kantrowitz 1988). The knees are more commonly affected than the hips, ankles, wrists and elbows (Palumbo et al 1973, Ansell 1976). There is no clear association with gender (Gravallese & Kantrowitz 1988), age or onset of disease (Wright et al 1965), although most cases of arthritis associated with bowel disease occur in young adults.

The arthritis runs a self-limited course lasting 6–12 weeks, although recurrences are common in association with relapses of the bowel disease. Frequently a flare may be heralded by the onset of arthritis and many patients develop a pattern of joint pain antedating diarrhea, bleeding or abdominal pain. Symptomatically the patient may note only arthralgias, although swelling and inflammation may also occur. Residual or progressive joint damage has been reported (Ford & Vallis 1959, McEwen et al 1962, Clark et al 1971) but is rare. Several cases have been reported of a persistent erosive granulomatous monoarthritis in patients with Crohn's disease (Tomlinson & Jayson 1981, Lindström et al 1972, Frayha et al 1975, Hermans et al 1984). The erythrocyte sedimentation rate is always elevated, but rheumatoid factor is negative. The synovial fluid is turbid, with an elevated white blood count (10 000–50 000/cm), protein, sugar and viscosity are normal, although there is a poor mucin clot. The histological changes of the synovium are non-specific (Bywaters & Ansell 1958).

Concurrent skin and ocular manifestations are common. The triad of peripheral arthritis, erythema nodosum and iritis is well recognized (Goldgraber & Kirsner 1969, Palumbo et al 1973). This is more common in pediatric patients and may be the first sign of IBD.

Treatment is conservative. Therapy directed towards the underlying disease will usually also control the arthritis. Mild analgesia or anti-inflammatory medication is used to control the pain. Corticosteroids are only needed occasionally. The arthritic complaints wax and wane with the activity of the bowel disease. Any agent used to treat the bowel disease should therefore ameliorate the joint symptoms. We have observed several patients with IBD with an acute arthropathy attributable to high-dose steroid therapy. These patients present with sudden onset of severe, usually monoarticular, pain, most commonly in the knee, but no objective evidence of inflammation of the joint except for mild swelling. Analgesia is usually required until the steroid dose can be tapered.

Axial arthropathy

Two syndromes of axial arthropathy have been described. The first is a spondylitis which is indistinguishable from idiopathic ankylosing spondylitis and the second is an isolated sacroiliitis.

Ankylosing spondylitis occurs in 2–6% of patients with either Crohn's disease or ulcerative colitis. The prevalence is 20–30-fold greater than the risk in the general population (Brewerton et al 1974, Russell 1977). Conversely, 10–20% of cases of ankylosing spondylitis occur in patients with ulcerative colitis (Acheson 1960, Lukash & Johnson 1975). The spondylitis seen in IBD is common in females (up to 40%) (Russell 1977), unlike primary ankylosing spondylitis, which has a male/female ratio of 8–9:1 (Palumbo et al 1973).

Components of this syndrome include sacroiliitis, which tends to be slowly progressive and unrelated to disease activity. Although the initial symptoms of spondylitis usually occur after the onset of bowel symptoms, they can antedate the diagnosis of IBD by many years (Palumbo et al 1973). Presenting features include low back pain, at times confused with sciatica, early morning stiffness and a typical stooped posture. Once the spine becomes involved the typical findings of stiffness and limited movement develop. These may be accompanied by an arthritis involving the hips, shoulders and knees. Unlike with colitic arthritis, however, there can be permanent damage to these joints (Gravallese & Kantrowitz 1988). IBD patients with spondylitis may develop aortic incompetence or atrioventricular conduction abnormalities (Lukash & Johnson 1975). In a recent study, ileocolonoscopy was performed in a group of patients with spondylitis but no symptoms of IBD. Inflammatory changes in the colon and ileum were observed in 44% and changes consistent with Crohn's disease in 26% (Leirisalo-Repo et al 1994).

The spondylitis of inflammatory bowel disease is HLA-B27 antigen related. The incidence of the antigen itself is not increased in patients with IBD, but 50–70% of those with spondylitis are positive (Gravallese & Kantrowitz 1988). This is lower than the positive rate of 90% seen in patients with primary ankylosing spondylitis, suggesting that the increased risk in IBD patients is not solely due to genetic factors. Indeed, only 5–10% of patients who are HLA B27 antigen-positive develop spondylitis (Brewerton et al 1974, Russell 1977). The families of inflammatory bowel disease patients have an increased risk of spondylitis or sacroiliitis.

Asymptomatic sacroiliitis is common, with radiologic changes in 15% of patients and 68% of patients with abnormalities which may be documented by bone scan (McEwen et al 1962). Recent studies of unselected patients with IBD have found an incidence of only 3.7% (Dekker-Saeys et al 1978). Sacroiliitis alone is not associated with an increased incidence of HLA B27, and may not progress to spondylitis (Hyla et al 1976, Gravallese & Kantrowitz 1988).

Salicylates and other anti-inflammatory drugs are helpful to relieve pain and stiffness. Physical therapy and exercise programs are useful. Resection of the underlying bowel disease does not alter the outcome: there are numerous reports of ankylosing spondylitis starting or progressing after colectomy.

Clubbing and hypertrophic osteoarthropathy

Hypertrophic osteoarthropathy includes clubbing, periostosis with pain and new bone formation, synovitis, and autonomic dysfunction (sweating of palms and soles) (Farman et al 1976). Clubbing is a painless phenomenon that occurs more commonly with Crohn's disease than ulcerative colitis (Fielding & Cooke 1971, Perry et al 1972, Kirshner et al 1978). Clubbing usually correlates well with disease activity (Kitis et al 1979). Periostosis is seen more commonly with Crohn's disease and correlates with disease activity (Janowitz 1989). It presents as a dull aching of the hands, feet, arms, legs and spine. X-rays reveal periosteal new bone formation (Gravallese & Kantrowitz 1988). Non-steroidal anti-inflammatory agents and treatment of the underlying bowel disease are helpful.

Osteoporosis and osteomalacia

Patients receiving prolonged treatment with steroids, those with small-bowel disease or following extensive small-intestinal resection are all at increased risk of impaired bone mineralization. The exact prevalence is unclear. Late complications of osteoporosis and osteomalacia include vertebral crush fractures and kyphosis. The best approach is prevention, with close attention to the patient's nutritional status and serum levels of calcium, phosphorus and vitamin D. It is best to diagnose these deficiencies early, since no form of replacement therapy effectively replaces losses in bone volume (Jackson & Rosenberg 1989). Calcium and vitamin D regimens should also be instituted in premenopausal patients who are on chronic corticosteroid therapy. Estrogen replacement therapy is helpful in the postmenopausal patient.

SKIN AND MUCOUS MEMBRANES

Oral lesions

Aphthous stomatitis is the most commonly reported lesion, usually involving the soft palate, buccal mucosa and tongue (Greenstein et al 1976, Plauth et al 1991). These lesions tend to parallel disease activity, especially in Crohn's disease. Granulomatous involvement of the oral mucosa in Crohn's disease, although rare, is well documented (Plauth et al 1991).

DERMATOLOGIC MANIFESTATIONS

More than 40 different cutaneous disorders have been reported in patients with IBD (Apgar 1991), including erythema multiforme, eczema and urticaria. Erythema nodosum and pyoderma gangrenosum are common and are seen in approximately 5% of cases.

Erythema nodosum

Erythema nodosum is a common manifestation of systemic diseases and may be drug related. It occurs in up to 4% of patients with ulcerative colitis and 15% of patients with Crohn's disease (Basler 1980, Apgar 1981). It is the most common extraintestinal manifestation in children (Basler 1980). There is a definite relationship with activity of the underlying bowel disease, although there is no correlation with severity. The lesions may precede bowel activity. They often coexist with peripheral arthritis and respond to therapy of the underlying bowel disease. The lesions are characteristically located on the anterior tibial surface, although they may be found on the lateral and posterior surfaces and upper extremities as well. They consist of raised red tender nodules, ranging in size from 1 to several centimeters, usually subsiding in a few days, leaving a temporary brownish discoloration of the skin.

Histologically the lesions are a panniculitis or vasculitis and are indistinguishable from erythema nodosum associated with other disorders. Therapy once again should be directed at the underlying bowel disease, although non-steroidal anti-inflammatory agents are helpful for the pain. Colectomy is never considered a therapeutic option.

Pyoderma gangrenosum

Nearly half the cases of pyoderma gangrenosum occur in patients with ulcerative colitis (Perry 1969, Thornton et al 1980), although it may also occur in Crohn's disease (Levitt et al 1991). It is an uncommon complication, with an incidence of 2% in one large series (Mir-Madjlessi et al 1985). Although bowel disease is usually active, there is no clear correlation with activity and pyoderma gangrenosum may occur after colectomy (Cook & Lorincz 1962, Mir-Madjlessi et al 1985).

Pyoderma presents as a cutaneous ulceration of the lower extremity, face or oral cavity. The fully developed lesion is a large, deep ulcer with an advancing border which is rolled or undermined. The center is necrotic and infected. Multiple lesions are common, with the lower limbs most commonly affected. Their appearance at sites of trauma (pathergy) is well documented (Finkel & Janowitz 1981). Pyoderma usually occurs in long-standing bowel disease.

Numerous therapies have been employed with varying degrees of success, including systemic, topical and intralesional steroids, topical antibiotics and the immunosuppressants cyclosporin and FK-506 (Abu-Elmgad et al 1991, Elgart et al 1991, O'Donnell & Powell 1991).

Colectomy has a variable effect on pyoderma. One retrospective review noted that pyoderma tended to resolve if colonic disease was moderate to severe, but not in mild cases (Talansky et al 1983).

Metastatic Crohn's disease

Non-caseating granuloma of the skin is rare (Lebwohl 1984). Lesions can occur in the form of erythematous nodules, plaques or ulcers (Shum & Guenther 1990), and may affect the face, arms, lower extremities and vulva, as well as muscle and bone (Kremer et al 1984, Lebwohl 1984, Tweedie & McCann 1984, Shum & Guenther 1990). The diagnosis is usually straightforward in the setting of established Crohn's disease, but occasionally a mistaken diagnosis of cutaneous sarcoid has been made (McGillis & Huntley 1989). Treatment is directed at the underlying bowel disease and may include systemic steroids. Great care should be taken to distinguish this entity from extensive perianal disease, where steroids are contraindicated.

OCULAR

The most common ocular complications include uveitis, which is limited to the anterior chamber of the eye, episcleritis, denoting inflammation of the collagenous shell of the eye, and occasionally a deeper inflammation or scleritis.

The incidence of ocular findings depends on patient selection and whether common conditions which may be incidental are included (Ellis & Gentry 1964, Billson et al 1967). In one series of 332 patients with Crohn's disease (Hopkins et al 1974) ocular complaints occurred in 6.2%.

In a pediatric population without ocular symptoms (Hofley et al 1993) inflammation of the anterior chamber was found in 6.2% of patients with Crohn's disease. There was a strong association with colonic involvement, but no clear association with disease activity. None of the 50 children with ulcerative colitis had any abnormalities.

Episcleritis, presenting as a localized tender elevated area of dilated vessels, occurs in 3–4% of IBD patients and is more common in Crohn's disease than in ulcerative colitis (Greenstein et al 1976, Knox et al 1984). Symptoms are generally mild, with burning and itching being the main symptoms. Both episcleritis and scleritis are related to disease activity, and therapy is directed at the underlying bowel disease. Topical steroids are also effective. Ulceration of the cornea can occur and usually requires combined topical and systemic steroids to achieve resolution (Knox et al 1984).

Uveitis is a more serious complication. Its incidence is similar to that of episcleritis (0.5–3.0%) (Hopkins et al 1974, Daum et al 1979). Uveitis may precede development of colonic disease and is correlated with exacerbation of disease (Wright et al 1965, Billson et al 1967). Association with arthritis, stomatitis and erythema nodosum is well documented (Wright et al 1965, Billson et al 1967, Goldgraber & Kirsner 1969; Palumbo et al 1973). Recurrent episodes are common (Korelitz & Coles 1967).

Although some patients may be asymptomatic, the classic presentation is of sudden onset of headache and blurred vision. Slit-lamp examination reveals inflammatory changes in the anterior chamber. Treatment includes therapy of the underlying bowel disease, topical steroids and cycloplegics.

A specific keratopathy of Crohn's disease has been described (Knox et al 1980). Inflammation of the posterior segment of the eye is rare, occurring in less than 0.1% of cases (Ernst et al 1991) of patients with either Crohn's disease or ulcerative colitis.

Secondary ocular complications include night blindness and reduced tear formation, which occurs secondary to malnutrition owing to an inability to absorb fat-soluble vitamin A. Cataracts and glaucoma may occur as a result of chronic steroid use (Knox et al 1984).

BRONCHOPULMONARY

Pulmonary disease is rare, with fewer than 200 cases reported in the literature. Kraft et al (1976) described six patients with inflammatory bowel disease (five with ulcerative colitis) who had chronic bronchitis and bronchiectasis, apparently unrelated to smoking, environmental factors or medication. Fibrosing alveolitis was first described by

Turner-Warwick (1968). This complication has been well described with sulfasalazine therapy (Jones & Malone 1972, Davies & MacFarlane 1974). Pulmonary vasculitis has also been reported, with and without eosinophilia (Isenberg et al 1968, Forrest & Sherman 1975).

Eade et al (1977, 1980) reported reduced CO_2 diffusing capacity in patients with IBD; however, Johnson et al (1978) found no abnormalities after correcting for hemoglobin levels. More recently, Douglas et al (1989) reported abnormalities in diffusing capacity, residual volume and functional residual capacity in one-third of patients with IBD. In this study, however, half of patients had pulmonary symptoms and many were smokers. Indium labeling of neutrophils has demonstrated that granulocyte migration to the lung occurs in patients with active IBD, although the clinical implications of this finding are unclear (Jonker et al 1992).

Camus et al (1993) reviewed 33 patients with pulmonary pathology which they felt could be attributed to IBD in the absence of a childhood history of pulmonary disease, environmental or occupational risk factors. Common pulmonary diseases such as asthma, chronic bronchitis and emphysema which might have represented a chance association of disease were excluded. The mean age of diagnosis of the pulmonary disease postdated that of the inflammatory bowel disease by 7 years; however, as a group there were no features that distinguished these patients from IBD patients without pulmonary involvement. Seventy percent had evidence of other extraintestinal manifestations, most commonly arthritis, but seven patients also had pyoderma. Sixty percent had inactive gastrointestinal disease at time of diagnosis, 10% had active disease and 28% were postcolectomy.

Three patterns of disease were seen. Half had large airway disease, including subglottic stenosis, chronic bronchitis and bronchiectasis. Histologically these lesions were characterized by neutrophilic infiltrates and mucosal ulcerations, and were more commonly associated with ulcerative colitis than with Crohn's disease. Patients presented with a chronic productive cough, with periodic exacerbations unresponsive to antibiotics. Inhaled or systemic steroids tended to be effective in controlling symptoms. There were occasional examples of small airway disease, chronic bronchiolitis – bronchiolitis obliterans – tending to present with dyspnea, a dry cough and pleuritic chest pain. Primary interstitial lung disease is described but could not be clearly separated from reactions to the use of ASA or sulfa drugs. Two patients with ulcerative colitis developed multiple cavitary nodules whose histology resembled pyoderma gangrenosum.

PLEUROPERICARDITIS

Pericarditis in association with inflammatory bowel disease was first described by Young in 1967. Only 20 cases have been described in the literature (Patwardhan et al 1983). Therapy includes aspirin and NSAIDS, steroids and, if necessary, drainage of effusions.

Hematological features

Anemia

Iron deficiency anemia can occur from chronic blood loss or following surgery. In patients with significant ileal disease or resection B_{12} deficiency may occur, and folate deficiency can occur in proximal small-bowel disease or with sulfasalazine treatment (Ormerod 1967). Autoimmune hemolytic anemia has been reported (Lorber et al 1955, Balint et al 1963, Shasahty et al 1977, Altman et al 1979). Treatment of autoimmune disease is usually with high-dose steroids, although splenectomy and even total proctocolectomy has been used.

Coagulation

Increased activity of coagulation factors V and VII and VIII (Lam et al 1975, Lake et al 1978) has been reported, which may return to normal with control of the underlying disease. Reduced levels of antithrombin III have been reported (Lam et al 1975). Increased levels of fibrinopeptide A (Edwards et al 1987) and impaired fibrinolytic activity have also been described (Kwaan et al 1969). Thrombocytosis is commonly seen; however, a review by Talbot et al (1986) found no association between increased platelet count and thromboembolic events. Webberly et al (1993) reported abnormal spontaneous platelet aggregation in 18 out of 40 patients with Crohn's disease and 17 out of 64 patients with ulcerative colitis, which did not change with disease activity. In this series this abnormality was found in 7 of 8 patients with thromboembolic events. Increased levels of β-thromboglobulin and thromboxane B2 were also reported.

Blood samples from patients with Crohn's disease (or ulcerative colitis) may form clots in response to endotoxin, a phenomenon not seen in healthy subjects (Juhlin et al 1980). Patients with Crohn's disease have decreased levels of protein S (Aadland et al 1994). The presence of anticardiolipin antibody and thrombosis in a patient with Crohn's disease has also been reported (Vianna et al 1992).

VASCULAR COMPLICATIONS

An increased risk of arterial and venous thrombosis was originally reported by Bargen and Barker in 1936. The reported incidence has been as high as 39% in autopsy series, although clinically it is seen in only 1–3% of patients admitted to the hospital for IBD. The Mayo clinic (Talbot et al 1986) reviewed the prevalence of arterial and venous thrombotic events in more than 7000 patients admitted to their hospital over a 10-year period. Excluding patients with underlying diabetes, obesity or known atherosclerotic disease, they reported an incidence of 1.3% in patients with IBD. An additional 17 patients had thromboembolic events complicating vasculitis. The majority of these events were deep venous thrombosis, pulmonary emboli or both. Half occurred after surgery, an incidence similar to that of postoperative patients in general. A subset of patients had a history of recurrent deep vein thrombosis or pulmonary embolus in association with active disease.

Other associated features include cerebrovascular, myocardial infarct, mesenteric, peripheral arterial and venous occlusions. Most infarct patients had significant cardiac risk factors. Interestingly, all peripheral arterial events occurred in patients with active Crohn's disease. Overall mortality was high (25%), although over half of these occurred in the setting of postoperative sepsis.

Johns (1991) reviewed the literature of 42 reported cases of cerebrovascular thrombotic events in association with IBD. He concluded that these events represented a true association with the primary disease because of the average young age of the patients (30.7 years), predisposition to unusual events, such as dural sinus thrombosis, and the absence of other clinical risk factors.

Several mechanisms have been described which might explain an increased tendency for thromboembolic events in patients with inflammatory bowel disease. Some, such as dehydration and prolonged immobilization, are obviously not specific to IBD. Large-vessel cerebral vasculitis has been described, in which neurological symptoms are prominent (Soloway et al 1970, Yassinger 1976, Chapman et al 1978).

RENAL AND GENITOURINARY

Genitourinary complications include metabolic problems, usually urinary tract calculi, and inflammatory complications, including retroperitoneal abscess and fibrosis, ureteral obstruction and fistula formation.

Nephrolithiasis

The incidence of renal stones is higher in Crohn's disease (6–18%), particularly in patients with ileal disease or following resection (Gelazyd et al 1968, Banner 1987) than in patients with ulcerative colitis (2–3%) (Deren et al 1962, Grossman & Nugent 1967). This compares with an incidence of 0.09% in patients hospitalized without IBD (Banner 1987). Most stones are calcium oxalate (Banner 1987), although urate stones are also found more frequently than in the general population. Small-intestinal malabsorption increases the risk of oxalate stones by allowing free oxalate to enter the colon, where it is absorbed (the actively inflamed colonic mucosa in ulcerative colitis is still capable of absorbing oxalate). Colectomy also increases the risk of renal stones (Deren et al 1962, Maratka & Nedbal 1964), presumably owing to decreased urinary volume and dehydration. Large losses of alkaline fluid from the gastrointestinal tract leads to acidification of the urine, which promotes the formation of uric acid stones. In one series from Japan, the incidence of uric acid stones in ulcerative colitis patients who underwent colectomy was 20% (Fukushima et al 1982). Contributing factors include diarrhea or high ileostomy output with a metabolic acidosis and reduced intestinal absorption of sodium with reduced urinary sodium, all of which promote stone formation. Prolonged bed rest may increase calcium mobilization and excretion. Steroids and fever also increase urate excretion.

Preventative measures include adequate intake of oral fluids and reduction of ileostomy water losses with antidiarrheal medications. If urine pH is low, alkalinization with sodium bicarbonate is useful. Urinary tract infections should be treated promptly.

Obstructive inflammatory or suppurative processes related to the bowel may involve the retroperitoneal space and lead to hydroureter or hydronephrosis. This complication is seen exclusively in Crohn's disease. The tendency of Crohn's disease to involve the terminal ileum accounts for a predilection of this complication for the right kidney and ureter (Banner 1987). Ureteral obstruction may be transient, resolving with control of the intraperitoneal process.

Bladder and genital complications have long been recognized in patients with Crohn's disease, owing to direct fistulization from the bowel into the bladder or vagina. Symptoms include urinary frequency, dysuria, pneumaturia, dyspareunia or the passage of fecal material in the urine or through the vagina. Males may be at greater risk for bladder fistula than females, as the uterus tends to protect the bladder from the inflammatory process (Banner 1987).

AMYLOID

Amyloid is a well recognized cause of death in patients with Crohn's disease (Verbanck 1979). One early series reported a 25% incidence of amyloid in patients with Crohn's disease (Werther et al 1960). However reviews of larger series of patients combining pre- and postmortem diagnosis put the true incidence at less than 1% (Greenstein et al 1992). Amyloid has been reported in ulcerative colitis (Rand et al 1980) but the incidence is significantly less than in Crohn's disease, approximately 0.07% (Greenstein et al 1992). There is a clear predilection for renal involvement which presents as the nephrotic syndrome (Shorvon 1977), and death is usually due to renal disease (Greenstein et al 1992). Other presentations include enteropathy, hepatosplenomegaly, cardiomyopathy and amyloidosis. Remissions after colectomy have been reported (Fitchen 1975), but surgical mortality in these patients is excessively high (Greenstein et al 1992). Colchicine has no proven benefit but should be tried in all IBD patients presenting with amyloid as it has been effective in a small number of cases.

Pancreatitis

Pancreatitis is rare in association with IBD. In most cases it is attributable to medications such as sulfasalazine, 6-mercaptopurine or azathioprine, parenteral nutrition or sclerosing cholangitis. In Crohn's disease acute pancreatitis has been reported in association with gastroduodenal and ampullary involvement (Legge et al 1971, Altman et al 1983, Newman et al 1987, Speiss et al 1992), implying that the underlying cause is obstruction secondary to acute inflammation. Meyers et al (1987) reported a case of severe pancreatitis in a patient with ileocolonic disease that resolved after resection. Recently, a case of granulomatous pancreatitis has been reported in a patient with gastroduodenal Crohn's disease (Geschwantler et al 1995).

Although pancreatic disease is uncommon in patients with Crohn's disease, it is intriguing to note that studies of pancreatic function in such patients have demonstrated exocrine deficiency in a third of cases (Angelini et al 1988, Piontek et al 1990), and autopsy series noted acinar dilatation and periductular fibrosis in one-third of patients (Chapin et al 1956). In addition, several authors have noted the presence of autoantibodies to pancreatic acinar cells in patients with Crohn's disease (Stöcker et al 1987, Piontek et al 1990). The clinical implications of these findings are unclear. The role of pancreatic inflammation and insufficiency in the symptoms of Crohn's disease merits further study (Piontek et al 1990).

PATHOGENESIS OF EXTRAINTESTINAL MANIFESTATIONS

Several different mechanisms have been examined to explain the occurrence of extraintestinal manifestations in IBD, including malabsorption/malnutrition, bacterial antigens, cryoproteins and immune complexes.

Bacterial antigens have been thought to be relevant since arthritis–dermatitis syndromes are seen in other intestinal inflammatory diseases where there is an increased antigen load, as in bacterial colitis, diverticular disease, jejunoileal bypass and patients who have undergone ileal pouch–anal anastomosis for familial polyposis. Increased bowel permeability to luminal antigens is seen in patients with inflammatory bowel disease (Danzi 1988). However, studies have found no evidence of bacteremia or endotoxin in inflammatory bowel disease (Aoki 1978).

Cryoproteins have been implicated as the cause of necrotic skin lesions in both Crohn's disease and ulcerative colitis (Mayer et al 1981), but cannot explain the other manifestations.

Immune complexes are a logical cause, since many of the extraintestinal symptoms are consistent with a serum sickness-type reaction. The recent identification of a tissue-bound immune complex consisting of IgG immunoglobulin and a colonic epithelial protein occurring in patients with ulcerative colitis is of interest (Takahashi & Das 1985). A monoclonal antibody has been developed against the epithelial cell antigen that cross-reacts with an antigen on chondrocytes, biliary epithelium and the ciliary process of the eye (Bhagat & Das 1994, Mandal et al 1994). Recent reports by Halstenen and Brandzaeg have reported that activated complement components colocalize with the anti-40 kDa antibody on colonic epithelium in vivo. Activated complement components, despite not causing direct tissue destruction, can recruit and activate neutrophils and mast cells, resulting in nonspecific tissue injury. This is a plausible explanation for inflammation at remote sites. No similar antibody has been reported in Crohn's disease, although this may reflect the fact that ulcerative colitis is a more B-cell or antibody-driven disorder, whereas Crohn's disease appears to represent a T cell-driven type of response. It is certainly plausible that T cell-mediated tissue injury occurs at extraintestinal sites, but no clear evidence for this exists at the present time.

REFERENCES

Aadland E, Odegaard O R, Roseth A, Try K 1994 Free protein S deficiency in patients with Crohn's disease. Scandinavian Journal of Gastroenterology 29: 333–335

Abu-Elmagd K, Jegasothy B V, Ackerman C D et al 1991 Efficacy of FK 506 in the treatment of recalcitrant pyoderma gangrenosum. Transplantation Proceedings 23: 3328–3329

Acheson E D 1960 An association between ulcerative colitis, regional enteritis and ankylosing spondylitis. Quarterly Journal of Medicine 29: 48–489

Altman A R, Maltz C R, Janowitz H D 1979 Auto immune hemolytic anemia in ulcerative colitis. Digestive Diseases and Sciences 24: 282–285

Altman A, Meyers S, Sachar D B, Janowitz H D 1979 Crohn's ileocolitis, cutaneous gangrene and cryoglobulinemia. Mount Sinai Journal of Medicine 46: 293–296

Altmann H S, Phillips F, Bank S et al 1983 Pancreatitis associated with duodenal Crohn's disease. American Journal of Gastroenterology 78: 174–177

Angelini G, Cavalini G, Bovo P et al 1988 Pancreatic function in chronic inflammatory bowel disease. International Journal of Pancreatology 3: 185–193

Ansell B M 1976 In: Dumonde D C (ed) Infection and immunology of rheumatic diseases. Blackwell, Oxford, pp 129–132

Aoki K 1978 Endotoxins in inflammatory bowel disease. Acta Medicina Okayama 32: 147

Apgar J T 1991 Newer aspects of inflammatory bowel disease and its cutaneous manifestations: a selective review. Seminars in Dermatology 10: 138–147

Balint J A, Hammock W J, Paton T B 1963 Association of ulcerative colitis and red blood cells coated with auto-immune antibody. American Journal of Digestive Diseases 8: 537–544

Banner M P 1987 Genitourinary complications of inflammatory bowel disease. Radiologic Clinics of North America 25: 199–209

Bargen J A 1929 Complications and sequelae of chronic ulcerative colitis. Annals of Internal Medicine 3: 335–352

Bargen J A, Barker N W 1936 Extensive arterial and venous thrombosis complicating chronic ulcerative colitis. Archives of Internal Medicine 58: 17–31

Basler R S W 1980 Ulcerative colitis and the skin. Medical Clinics of North America 64: 941–954

Bhagat S, Das K 1994 A shared and unique peptide in the human colon, eye and joint detected by a monoclonal antibody. Gastroenterology 107: 103–108

Billson F A, deDombal F T, Watkinson G, Goligher J C 1967 Ocular complications of ulcerative colitis. Gut 8: 102–106

Bowen G E, Kirsner J B 1965 The arthritis of ulcerative colitis and regional enteritis ('intestinal arthritis'). Medical Clinics of North America 49: 17–32

Brewerton D A, Carffrey M, Nichols A, Walters D, James D C O 1974 HL-A 27 and arthropathies associated with ulcerative colitis and psoriasis. Lancet 1: 956–957

Brewerton D A, James D C O 1975 Histocompatibility antigen (HLA27) and disease. Seminars in Arthritis and Rheumatism 4: 191–203

Bywaters E G L, Ansell B M 1958 Arthritis associated with ulcerative colitis – a clinical and pathological study. Annals of Rheumatic Disease 17: 169–183

Camus P, Piard F, Ashcroft T, Gal-Anthony A, Colby T V 1993 The lung in inflammatory bowel disease. Medicine 72: 151–183

Chapin L E, Scudamore H H, Baggenstoss A H et al 1956 Regional enteritis: associated visceral changes. Gastroenterology 30: 404–415

Chapman R, Dawe C, Whorewell P J, Wright R 1978 Ulcerative colitis in association with Takayasu's disease. American Journal of Digestive Disease 23: 660

Clark R L, Muhletaler C A, Margulies S I 1971 Colitic arthritis, clinical and radiographic manifestations. Diagnostic Radiology 101: 585–594

Collins C E, Cahill M R, Newland A C, Rampton D S 1994 Platelets circulate in an activated state in inflammatory bowel disease. Gastroenterology 106: 840–845

Cook T J, Lorincz A L 1962 Pyoderma gangrenosum appearing ten years after colectomy and apparent cure of chronic ulcerative colitis.

Crohn B B 1925 Ocular lesions complicating ulcerative colitis. American Journal of Medical Sciences 169: 260–267

Danzi T 1988 Extraintestinal manifestations of idiopathic inflammatory bowel disease. Archives of Internal Medicine 148: 297–302

Daum F, Gould H B, Gold D et al 1979 Asymptomatic transient uveitis in children with inflammatory bowel disease. American Journal of Diseases of Children 133: 170–171

Davies D, MacFarlane A 1974 Fibrosing alveolitis and therapy with sulphasalazine. Gut 15: 185–188

Dekker-Saeys B J, Meuwissen S G M, Van Der Berg-Loonen E M et al 1978 Prevalence of peripheral arthritis, sacroileitis and ankylosing spondylitis in patients suffering from inflammatory bowel disease. Annals of Rheumatic Disease 37: 33–35

Deren J J, Porush J G, Levitt M F, Khilnani M T 1962 Nephrolithiasis as a complication of ulcerative colitis and regional enteritis. Annals of Internal Medicine 56: 843–853

Douglas J G, McDonald C F, Leslie M J, Gillon J, Crompton G K, McHardy G J 1989 Respiratory impairment in inflammatory bowel disease: does it vary with disease activity? Respiratory Medicine 83: 389–394

Eade O E, Smith C L, Alexander J R, Whorwell D J 1980 Pulmonary function in patients with inflammatory bowel disease. American Journal of Gastroenterology 73: 154–156

Eade O E, Smith C L, Whorwell P J 1977 Pulmonary function in inflammatory bowel disease. Gut 18: A423

Edwards R L, Levine J B, Green R, Duffy M, Matthews E, Brande W 1987 Activation of blood coagulation in Crohn's disease. Increased fibrinopeptide A levels and enhanced generation of monocyte tissue factor activity. Gastroenterology 92: 329–337

Elgart G, Stover P, Larson K et al 1991 Treatment of pyoderma gangrenosum with cyclosporine: results in seven patients. Journal of the American Academy of Dermatology 24: 83–86

Ellis P P, Gentry J H 1964 Ocular complications of ulcerative colitis. American Journal of Ophthalmology 58: 779–785

Ernst B B, Lowder C Y, Meisler D M, Gutman F A 1991 Posterior segment manifestations of inflammatory bowel disease. Ophthalmology 98: 1272–1280

Farman J, Twersky J, Fierst S 1976 Ulcerative colitis associated with hypertrophic osteoarthropathy. American Journal of Digestive Disease 21: 130–135

Farmer R G, Hawk W A, Turnbull R B 1975 Clinical patterns in Crohn's disease: a statistical study of 615 cases. Gastroenterology 68: 627–635

Fielding J F, Cooke W T 1971 Finger clubbing and regional enteritis. Gut 12: 442–444

Finkel S I, Janowitz H D 1981 Trauma and the pyoderma gangrenosum of inflammatory bowel disease. Gut 22: 410–412

Fitchen J H 1975 Amyloidosis and granulomatous ileocolitis. New England Journal of Medicine 292: 352–353

Ford D K, Vallis D G 1959 The clinical course of arthritis associated with ulcerative colitis and regional enteritis. Arthritis and Rheumatism 2: 526–536

Forrest J A H, Sherman D J C 1975 Pulmonary vasculitis and ulcerative colitis. American Journal of Digestive Disease 20: 482–486

Frayha R, Stevens M B, Bayless T M 1975 Destructive monoarthritis and granulomatous synovitis as the presenting manifestations of Crohn's disease. Johns Hopkins Medical Journal 137: 151–155

Fukushima T, Ishiguro N, Matsuda Y et al 1982 Clinical and urinary characteristics of urolithiasis in ulcerative colitis. American Journal of Gastroenterology 77: 238–240

Gelazyd E A, Breuer R I, Kirsner J B 1968 Nephrolithiasis in inflammatory bowel disease. American Journal of Digestive Disease 13: 1027–1034

Geschwantler M, Kegelbauer G, Klose W, Bibus B, Tscholakoff D, Weiss W 1995 The pancreas as a site of granulomatous inflammations in Crohn's disease. Gastroenterology 108: 1246–1249

Goldgraber M B, Kirsner J B 1969 Gangrenous skin lesions associated with chronic ulcerative colitis. A case study. Gastroenterology 39: 94–103

Gravallese E M, Kantrowitz F G 1988 Arthritic manifestations of inflammatory bowel disease. American Journal of Gastroenterology 83: 703–709

Greenstein A J, Janowitz H D, Sachar D B 1976 The extraintestinal complications of Crohn's disease and ulcerative colitis: a study of 700 patients. Medicine 55: 401–411

Greenstein A J, Sachar D B, Panday A K N et al 1992 Amyloidosis and inflammatory bowel disease. A fifty year experience with 25 patients. Medicine 71: 261–270

Grossman M S, Nugent F W 1967 Urolithiasis as a complication of chronic diarrheal disease. American Journal of Digestive Disease 12: 491–498

Hermans P J, Fievez M L, Descamps L 1984 Granulomatous arthritis in Crohn's disease. Journal of Rheumatology 11: 710–712

Hofley P, Roarty J, McGinnity G et al 1993 Asymptomatic uveitis in children with chronic inflammatory bowel diseases. Journal of Pediatric Gastroenterology and Nutrition 17: 397–400

Hopkins D J, Horan E, Burton I L et al 1974 Ocular disorders in a series of 332 patients with Crohn's disease. British Journal of Ophthalmology 58: 732–740

Hyla J F, Franck W A, Davis J S 1976 Lack of association of HLA B27 with radiographic sacroiliitis in inflammatory bowel disease. Journal of Rheumatology 3: 196–200

Isenberg J J, Goldstein H, Korn A R, Ozeran R S, Rosen V 1968 Pulmonary vasculitis an uncommon complications of ulcerative colitis. New England Journal of Medicine 279: 1376–1377

Jackson W D, Rosenberg I H 1989 Osteoporosis and osteomalacia. In: Bayless T (ed) Current management of inflammatory bowel disease. BD Decker, Toronto, pp 179–183

Janowitz H 1989 Extraintestinal manifestations. In: Bayless T (ed) Current management of inflammatory bowel disease. B D Decker, Toronto, pp 157–159

Johns D R 1991 Cerbrovascular complications of inflammatory bowel disease. American Journal of Gastroenterology 86: 367–370

Johnson N M I, Mee A S, Jewell D P, Clarke S W 1978 Pulmonary function in inflammatory bowel disease. Digestion 18: 416–418
Jones G R, Malone D N S 1972 Sulphasalazine induced lung disease. Thorax 27: 713–717
Jonker N D, Peters A M, Carpani de Kaski M, Hodgson H J, Lavender J P 1992 Pulmonary granulocyte margination is increased in patients with inflammatory bowel disease. Nuclear Medicine Communications 12: 806–810
Juhlin L, Krause U, Shelley W B 1980 Endotoxin induced microclots in ulcerative colitis and Crohn's disease. Scandinavian Journal of Gastroenterology 15: 311–314
Kildebo S, Norgaard K, Aronsen O, Breckan R, Burghol P G, Jorde E
Kirschner B, Volnchet O, Rosenberg I H 1978 Growth retardation in inflammatory bowel disease. Gastroenterology 75: 504–511
Kitis G, Thompson H, Allan R N 1979 Finger clubbing in inflammatory bowel disease: its prevalence and pathogenesis. British Medical Journal 2: 825–828
Klein S, Mayer L, Present D H, Youner K D, Cerulli M A, Sachar D B 1988 Extraintestinal manifestations in patients with diverticulitis. Annals of Internal Medicine 108: 700–702
Knox D L, Schachat A P, Mustonen E 1984 Primary secondary and coincidental complications of Crohn's disease. Ophthalmology 91: 163–173
Knox D L, Snip R C, Stark W J 1980 The keratopathy of Crohn's disease. American Journal of Ophthalmology 90: 862–865
Korelitz B I, Coles R S 1967 Uveitis (iritis) associated with ulcerative colitis and granulomatous colitis. Gastroenterology 52: 78–82
Kraft S C, Earle F H, Roesler M, Eaterly J R 1976 Unexplained broncho-pulmonary disease with inflammatory bowel disease. Archives of Internal Medicine 136: 454–459
Kremer M, Nussenson E, Steinfeld M, Zuckerman P 1984 Crohn's disease of the vulva. American Journal of Gastroenterology 79: 376
Kwaan H C, Cocco A, Mendeloff A I, Astrupp T 1969 Fibrinolytic activity in the normal and inflamed rectal mucosa. Scandinavian Journal of Gastroenterology 4: 441–445
Kyle S M, Yeoung M L, Ibister W H, Clark S P 1991 Beçet's colitis: a differential diagnosis in inflammations of the large intestine. Australia and New Zealand Journal of Surgery 61: 47–55
Lake A M, Stauffer J Q, Stuart M J 1978 Hemostatic alterations in IBD: response to therapy. American Journal of Digestive Disease 23: 897–902
Lam A T, Borde I T, Inwood M J, Thomson S 1975 Coagulation studies in ulcerative colitis and Crohn's disease. Gastroenterology 68: 345–251
Lebwohl M, Fleischmajer R, Janowitz H, Present D, Prioleau P G 1984 Metastatic Crohn's disease. Journal of the American Academy of Dermatology 10: 33–38
Legge D A, Hoffman H N, Carlson H C 1971 Pancreatitis as a complication of regional enteritis of the duodenum. Gastroenterology 61: 834–837
Leirisalo-Repo M, Turunen U, Stenman S, Helenius P, Seppala K 1994 High frequency of silent inflammatory bowel disease in spondylarthropathy. Arthritis and Rheumatism 37: 23–31
Levitt M D, Ritchie J K, Lennard-Jones J E, Phillips R K S 1991 Pyoderma gangrenosum in inflammatory bowel disease. British Journal of Surgery 78: 676–678
Lindström C, Wramsby I, Östberg G, 1972 Granulomatous arthritis in Crohn's disease. Gut 13: 257–259
Lohmuller J L, Pemberton J H, Dozois R R, Ilstrup D, van Heerden J 1990 Pouchitis and extraintestinal manifestations of inflammatory bowel disease after ileal pouch–anal anastomosis. Annals of Surgery 211: 622–627
Lorber M, Schwarts L I, Wasserman L R 1955 Association of antibody-coated red blood cells with ulcerative colitis. American Journal of Medicine 19: 887–894
Lukash W M, Johnson R B (eds) 1975 The systemic manifestations of inflammatory bowel disease. C C Thomas, Illinois
McEwen C, Ling C, Kirsner J B 1962 Arthritis accompanying ulcerative colitis. American Journal of Medicine 33: 923–941
McGillis S T, Huntley A C 1989 Metastatic Crohn's disease. Western Journal of Medicine 151: 203–205
Mandal A, Dasgupta A, Jeffers L et al 1994 Autoantibodies in sclerosing cholangitis against a shared peptide in biliary and colon epithelium. Gastroenterology 106: 185–192
Maratka Z, Nedbal J 1964 Urolithiasis as a complication of the surgical treatment of ulcerative colitis. Gut 5: 214–217
Mayer L, Meyers S, Janowitz H D 1981 Cryoproteinemia in the cutaneous gangrene of Crohn's disease: a report of two cases. Journal of Clinical Gastroenterology 3: 17–21
Meyers S, Greenspan J, Greenstein A J et al 1987 Pancreatitis coincident with Crohn's ileocolitis. Diseases of the Colon and Rectum 30: 119–122
Mir-Madjlessi S H, Taylor J S, Farmer R G 1985 Clinical course and evolution of erythema nodosum and pyoderma gangrenosum in chronic ulcerative colitis: a study of 42 patients. American Journal of Gastroenterology 80: 615–620
Newman L H, Wellinger J R, Present D H, Aufses A H 1987 Crohn's disease of the duodenum associated with pancreatitis: a case report and review of the literature. Mount Sinai Journal of Medicine 54: 429–432
O'Donnell B, Powell F C 1991 Cyclosporine treatment of pyoderma gangrenosum. Journal of the American Academy of Dermatology 24: 141–143
Ormerod T P 1967 Observations on the incidence and cause of anemia in ulcerative colitis. Gut 8: 107
Palumbo P J, Ward L E, Sauer W G, Scudamore H H 1973 Musculoskeletal manifestations of inflammatory bowel disease – ulcerative and granulomatous colitis and ulcerative proctitis. Mayo Clinic Proceedings 48: 411–416
Patwardhan R V, Heilpern R J, Brewster A C, Darrah J J 1983 Pleuropericarditis: an extraintestinal complication of inflammatory bowel disease. Report of three cases and review of literature. Archives of Internal Medicine 143: 94–96
Perry H O 1969 Pyoderma gangrenosum. Southern Medical Journal 62: 899–908
Perry P M, Evans G A, Davies J D 1972 Regional ileitis, ulcerative colitis and clubbed fingers. Diseases of the Colon and Rectum 15: 278–279
Piontek M, Hengels K J, Strohmeyer G 1990 Editorial: Crohn's disease: what about the pancreas? Journal of Clinical Gastroenterology 12: 491–493
Plauth M, Jenss H, Meyle J 1991 Oral manifestations of Crohn's disease. Journal of Clinical Gastroenterology 13: 29–37
Rand J A, Brandt L J, Baker N H, Lynch J 1980 Ulcerative colitis complicated by amyloid. American Journal of Gastroenterology 74: 185–188
Rankin G B 1990 Extraintestinal and systemic manifestations of inflammatory bowel disease. Medical Clinics of North America 74: 39–50
Russell A S 1977 Arthritis, inflammatory bowel disease and histocompatibility antigens. Annals of Internal Medicine 86: 820–821
Shasahty G G, Rath C E, Britt E J 1977 Autoimmune hemolytic anemia associated with ulcerative colitis. American Journal of Hematology 3: 199–208
Shorvon P J 1977 Amyloidosis and inflammatory bowel disease. American Journal of Digestive Disease 22: 209–213
Shum D T, Guenther L 1990 Metastatic Crohn's disease. Archives of Dermatology 126: 645–648
Soloway M, Moir T W, Linton D W 1970 Takayasu's arteritis: report of a case with unusual findings. American Journal of Cardiology 25: 258
Speiss S E, Braun M, Vogelzgang R L, Craig R M 1992 Crohn's disease of the duodenum complicated by pancreatitis and common bile duct obstruction. American Journal of Gastroenterology 87: 1033–1036
Stöcker W, Otte M, Ulrich S et al 1987 Autoimmunity to pancreatic juice in Crohn's disease. Scandinavian Journal of Gastroenterology 22: 41–52
Takahashi F, Das K M 1985 Isolation and characterisation of a colonic autoantigen specifically recognised by colon tissue bound immunoglobulin G from idiopathic ulcerative colitis. Journal of Clinical Investigation 76: 311–318
Talansky A, Meyers S, Greenstein A J, Janowitz H D 1983 Does intestinal resection heal the pyoderma gangrenosum of inflammatory bowel disease? Journal of Clinical Gastroenterology 5: 207–210
Talbot R W, Heppell J, Dozois R R, Beart R W Jr 1986 Vascular complications of inflammatory bowel disease. Mayo Clinic Proceedings 61: 40–145

Thorton J R, Teague R H M, Low-Beer T S, Read A E 1980 Pyoderma gangrenosum and ulcerative colitis. Gut 21: 347–248

Tomlinson I W, Jayson M I V 1981 Erosive Crohn's arthritis. Journal of the Royal Society of Medicine 74: 540–542

Turner-Warwick M 1968 Fibrosing alveolitis and chronic liver disease. Quarterly Journal of Medicine 145: 133–149

Tweedie J H, McCann B G 1984 Metastatic Crohn's disease of the thigh and forearm. Gut 25: 213

Verbanck J, Lamiere N, Praet M, Ringoin A, Elewart A, Barbier F 1979 Renal amyloidosis as complication of Crohn's disease. Acta Clinica Belgica 34: 6–13

Vianna J L, D'Cruz D P, Khamashta M A, Asherson R A, Hughes G R V 1992 Anticardiolipin antibodies in a patient with Crohn's disease and thrombosis. Clinical and Experimental Rheumatology 10: 165–178

Webberly M J, Hart M T Melikian V 1993 Thromboembolism in IBD: role of platelets. Gut 34: 247–251

Werther J L, Shapira A, Rubinstein O, Janowitz H D 1960 Amyloidosis in regional enteritis. A report of 5 cases. American Journal of Medicine 29: 416–423

Wright R, Lumsden K, Luntz M H, Sevel D, Truelove S 1965 Abnormalities of the sacroiliac joints and uveitis in ulcerative colitis. Quarterly Journal of Medicine 34: 229–236

Yassinger S 1976 Association of inflammatory bowel disease and large vascular lesions. Gastroenterology 71: 844

Young P C 1967 Colonic and systemic manifestations of chronic ulcerative colitis. Medical Clinics of North America 51: 1011–1013

70. Oral manifestations of Crohn's disease

J. Hamburger

INTRODUCTION

Oral Crohn's disease was first described in 1969 by Dudeney and Todd, but Varley (1973) first reported the occurrence of oral lesions in the absence of intestinal disease. Although a relatively unusual manifestation of Crohn's disease, a number of cases have since been reported. Basu and Asquith (1980) estimated the prevalence of oral manifestations of Crohn's disease at between 4 and 14%.

NOMENCLATURE

The term 'oral Crohn's disease' has frequently been used to describe a constellation of clinical features that includes diffuse facial and labial swelling, oral ulceration, oral mucosal hyperplasia and, in some cases, VIIth nerve palsy. However, such features are common to a number of different disorders. In an attempt to rationalize terminology, Wiesenfeld et al (1985) proposed the term 'orofacial granulomatosis' to describe these clinical features that may present without identifiable coexisting disease. Tyldesley (1979) also preferred the use of the term 'orofacial granulomatosis' to 'oral Crohn's disease' in the absence of intestinal involvement, although a number of these patients will subsequently develop intestinal Crohn's disease.

DIFFERENTIAL DIAGNOSIS

Oral Crohn's disease must be differentiated from the other known causes of orofacial granulomatosis, such as hypersensitivity reactions, Melkersson–Rosenthal syndrome, cheilitis granulomatosa (Miescher 1945), sarcoidosis and mycobacterial infections (tuberculosis and leprosy).

Other possibilities include angioedema and focal infection of the orofacial tissues (Worsae et al 1982). Scully et al (1993), reported a case of a T-cell lymphoma masquerading as oral Crohn's disease, and James and Ferguson (1986) described a case of orofacial granulomatosis, presenting initially as cervical lymphadenopathy, which was originally diagnosed and treated as tuberculosis.

The reported frequency of Crohn's disease as a cause of orofacial granulomatosis varies considerably between authors. Wiesenfeld et al (1985) quoted a frequency of 10%, whereas Williams et al (1991) reported an incidence of 48%. Such wide variation may in part be explained by the observation that oral Crohn's disease often predates intestinal disease. Ghandour and Issa (1991) described an example of oral Crohn's disease that predated the onset of intestinal disease by 9 years. Plauth et al (1991) stated that oral lesions preceded intestinal disease in 60% of patients, and Williams et al (1991) reported that 9 out of 14 patients with orofacial granulomatosis subsequently developed intestinal Crohn's.

CLINICAL FEATURES

In a review by Plauth et al (1991) of 79 patients with oral Crohn's disease, the median age at presentation was 22 years, with a range 6–57 years and a male preponderance of 1.85:1, this ratio increasing to 3:1 in the 16–30 year age group. This male predilection is not seen in Crohn's disease patients in general (Mendeloff & Calkins 1988), nor is it apparent in childhood-onset Crohn's disease (Barton et al 1989). The series of 29 patients described by Williams et al (1991) had a median age and age range similar to those described by Plauth, with 10 patients under 20 years of age at diagnosis; 8 of these were children in the first decade of life.

The clinical features are variable but the main characteristics are:

Oedematous diffuse swelling of the face and lips
Angular cheilitis
Cobblestone appearance to the mucosa
Linear ulceration
Mucosal tagging/localized swellings
Hyperplastic gingivitis
Aphthous ulceration.

Initially there may be unilateral or bilateral swelling of the lips (Fig. 70.1) or orofacial tissues, often intermittent but rarely regressing completely. As the condition progresses the swelling becomes more persistent as a result of fibrosis, which also accounts for the furrowing that contributes to the typical cobblestone appearance (Fig. 70.2).

The lips may be dry, crusted and sore, and are frequently associated with angular cheilitis which is analogous to anal fissuring (Field & Tyldesley 1989). The painful deep linear ulcers that often occur in the buccal sulci (Fig. 70.3) are similar to those seen in intestinal disease. Tissue tags and folds of hyperplastic tissue resembling denture granulomata are also a feature (Fig. 70.4). The hyperplastic gingivitis is quite unlike that seen in other conditions, involving the free and attached gingivae and extending on to the alveolar mucosa (Fig. 70.5).

Orofacial disease activity is generally independent of disease activity elsewhere in the gut, and ESR and C-reactive protein are poor markers of active orofacial

Figs 70.1–70.5 – see page xxi.

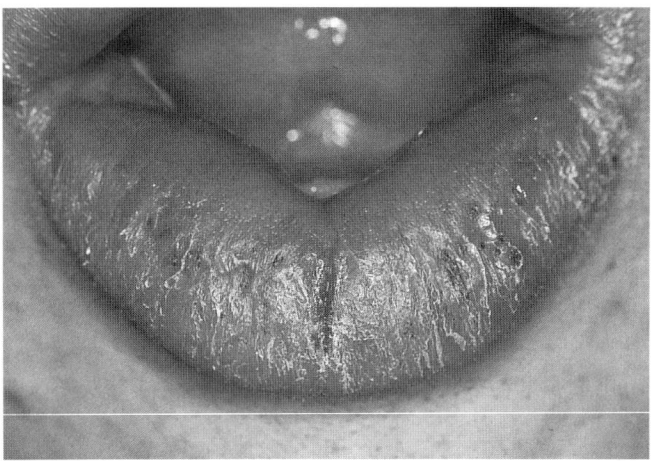

Fig. 70.1 Diffuse bilateral labial swelling, dryness and crusting in an adolescent with oral Crohn's disease.

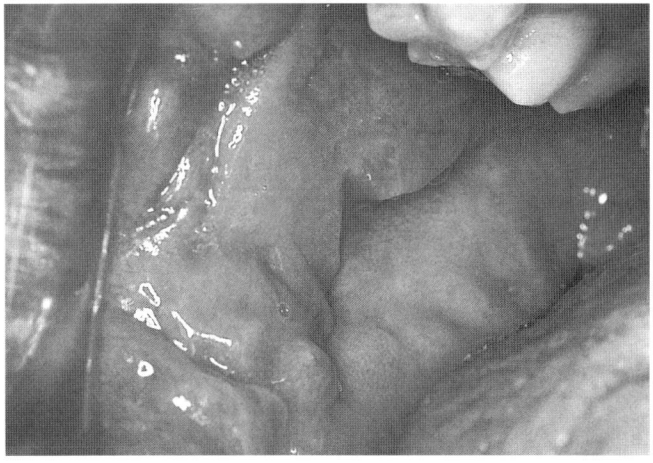

Fig. 70.2 Typical cobblestone appearance of the buccal mucosa in a 36-year-old male with previously undiagnosed intestinal Crohn's disease.

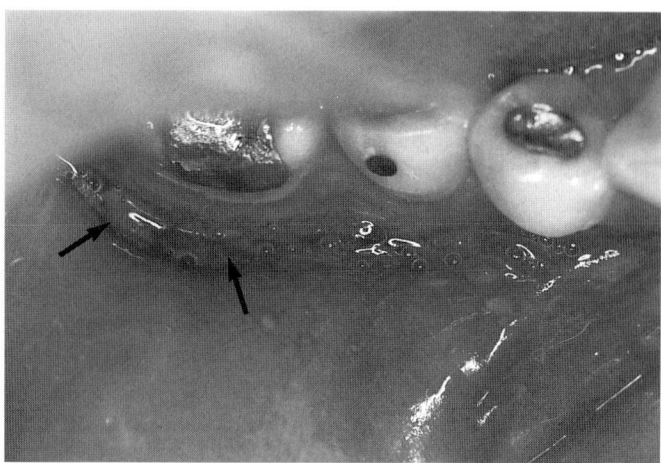

Fig. 70.3 Deep linear ulcer in the buccal sulcus of a 24-year-old male with intestinal Crohn's disease.

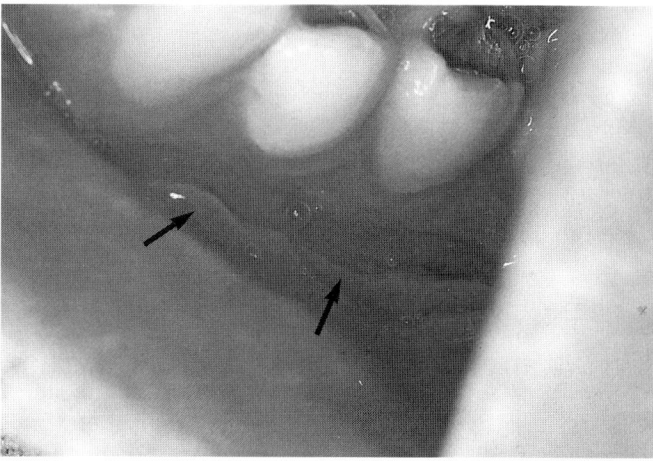

Fig. 70.4 Hyperplastic tissue folds seen in the labial sulcus of the same patient as shown in Fig 70.3.

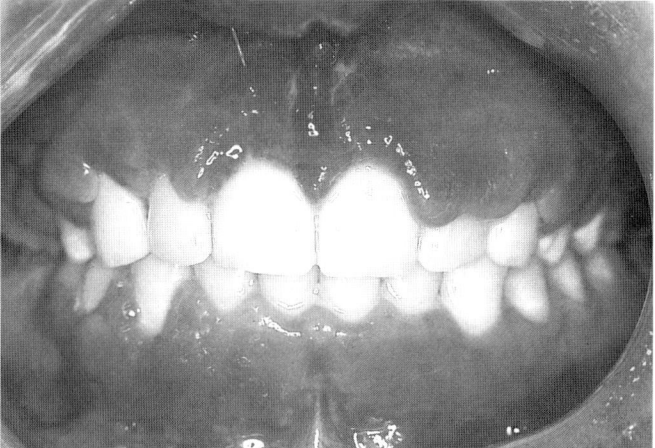

Fig. 70.5 Hyperplastic gingivitis in a patient with orofacial granulomatosis.

disease (Williams et al 1991). In contrast, aphthous ulceration, which occurs in 10–20% of cases, tends to be associated with active intestinal disease (Basu et al 1975).

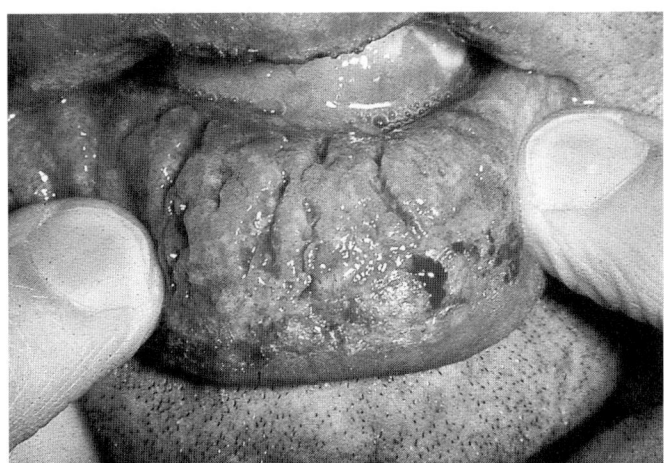

Fig. 70.6 Pyostomatitis vegetans of the lower labial mucosa. (Reproduced with permission from Basu & Chesner 1990). (See page xxi.)

Pyostomatitis vegetans (Fig. 70.6), characterized by mucosal erythema and edema, together with multiple small yellow pustules, is a rare oral manifestation of inflammatory bowel disease. Although particularly linked with ulcerative colitis, several cases have also been reported in association with Crohn's disease (Cataldo et al 1981, Ballo et al 1989 Ficarra et al 1993).

INVESTIGATIONS

Although the clinical features of orofacial granulomatosis are characteristic, confirmation of the diagnosis should be made by biopsy of involved tissue. The biopsy specimen should extend down to muscle, as the non-caseating epithelioid granulomata are often deeply located. They may be found in a perivascular distribution, bulging into vessels and lymphatics, producing obstruction. Intercellular edema, lymphangiectasia and perivascular cuffing of lymphocytes are also features. The histological features of oral Crohn's disease do not differ from those seen in other causes of orofacial granulomatosis, nor do they distinguish between those patients with intestinal Crohn's disease and those without such lesions (Tyldesley 1979). Patients therefore need to be further investigated to exclude the other known causes of orofacial granulomatosis.

Ivanyi et al (1993) suggested that the presence of serum antibody to the mycobacterial 65 kDa stress protein may be of diagnostic value for oral Crohn's disease, but this awaits confirmation.

TREATMENT

Treatment is often unrewarding and no overall consensus has emerged. Many of the reported treatment data apply to orofacial granulomatosis in general rather than oral Crohn's disease in particular, and are often based on uncontrolled open trials involving small groups of patients. Plauth et al (1991) reported that topical steroid therapy was just as effective as systemic steroid therapy, producing complete remission in 50% patients, although a tendency to over report successful cases was acknowledged. Williams et al (1991), however, found no benefit from topical steroids. Systemic steroids are of value in managing the oral ulceration and accompanying pain, but do not provide permanent reduction in the mucosal edema.

Although exclusion diets may be of some benefit in the management of intestinal Crohn's (Alun-Jones et al 1985), few data exist on their use in the management of oral Crohn's disease. James et al (1986) reported a 60% incidence of atopy in patients with orofacial granulomatosis, whereas Patton et al (1985) found 18% of patients with orofacial granulomatosis to be intolerant of certain food substances, including cinnamonaldehyde, cocoa and coloring agents. Exclusion diets were shown to be of value in some of these patients (Patton et al 1985, Ferguson & McFadyen 1986), but Williams et al (1991) found them to be of no value in patients with oral Crohn's disease. Intralesional triamcinolone was first advocated as a treatment for cheilitis granulomatosa (Cerimele & Serri 1965). Tyldesley (1979) found the technique unhelpful, suggesting that since the swelling was probably a result of blocked lymphatic drainage, local infiltrations were unlikely to be successful. High-volume intralesional triamcinolone (administered under local anesthesia) was found to be of value in five patients with orofacial granulomatosis not related to allergic causes, but the authors did not indicate whether any of these patients had oral Crohn's disease (Sakuntabhai et al 1993). Williams and Greenberg (1991) also reported successful use of intralesional triamcinolone in cheilitis granulomatosa, and stressed the importance of eliminating foci of dental infection while maintaining a high level of oral hygiene. However, the use of intralesional steroids is not without hazard, including degenerative changes in skeletal muscle (Williams 1959), necrosis and fibrosis (Krutchkoff & James 1978). Krutchkoff & James (1978) reported success with surgical reduction of the lip swelling when combined with intralesional triamcinolone. Cessation of the triamcinolone resulted in recurrence of labial swelling, however, thus suggesting the need for continued postoperative intralesional steroids. In general, surgical reduction of the swollen tissues is of dubious value, being unreliable and of limited duration (Worsae et al 1982).

A variety of other drugs have been used in the management of orofacial granulomatosis in general, including danazol (Madanes & Farber 1982), metronidazole (Wiesenfeld et al 1985), clofazimine (Podmore & Burrows 1986, Schlegel-Gomez et al 1989), minocycline (Veller Fornasa et al 1992) and hydroxychloroquine (Allen et al 1990). They have produced no significant therapeutic benefit in oral Crohn's disease. Similarly, Williams et al (1991) found that cyclosporin, azathioprine and sulfasalazine were also of no value.

PROGNOSIS

The long-term behavior of oral Crohn's disease is variable. Typically the clinical features are persistent, with episodes of acute exacerbation. However, the condition remits spontaneously in approximately 25% of patients, particularly in younger individuals (Williams et al 1991). Field and Tyldesley (1989) suggested that the labial and buccal swelling gradually resolved over a 10-year period, the prognosis being little influenced by attempts at treatment.

REFERENCES

Allen C M, Camisa C, Hamzeh S, Stephens L 1990 Cheilitis granulomatosa: report of six cases and review of the literature. Journal of the American Academy of Dermatology 23: 444–450

Alun-Jones V, Dickinson R J, Workman E, Wilson A J, Freeman A H, Hunter J O 1985 Crohn's disease: maintenance of remission by diet. Lancet ii: 177–180

Ballo F S, Camisa C, Allen C M 1989 Pyostomatitis vegetans. Report of a case and review of the literature. Journal of the American Academy of Dermatology 21: 381–387

Barton J R, Gillon S, Ferguson A 1989 Incidence of inflammatory bowel disease in Scottish children between 1968 and 1983: marginal fall in ulcerative colitis, three-fold rise in Crohn's disease. Gut 30: 618–622

Basu M K Asquith P 1980 Oral manifestations of inflammatory bowel disease. Clinics in Gastroenterology 9: 307–321

Basu M K, Asquith P, Thompson R A, Cooke W T 1975 Oral manifestations of Crohn's disease. Gut 16: 249–254

Basu M K, Chesner I M 1990 Diseases of the gastrointestinal tract. In: Jones J H, Mason D K (eds) Oral manifestations of systemic disease. Baillière Tindall, London, pp 783–799

Cataldo F, Covino M C, Tesone P E 1981 Pyostomatitis vegetans. Oral Surgery, Oral Medicine, Oral Pathology 52: 172–177

Cerimele D, Serri F 1965 Intra-lesional injection of triamcinolone for the treatment of cheilitis granulomatosa. Archives of Dermatology 92: 695

Dudeney T P, Todd I P 1969 Crohn's disease of the mouth. Proceedings of the Royal Society of Medicine 62: 1237–1238

Ferguson M M, McFadyen E E 1986 Orofacial granulomatosis: a 10 year review. Annals of the Academy of Medicine of Singapore 15: 370–377

Ficarra G, Cicchi P, Amorosi A, Piluso S 1993 Oral Crohn's disease and pyostomatitis vegetans. An unusual association. Oral Surgery, Oral Medicine, Oral Pathology 75: 220–224

Field E A, Tyldesley W R 1989 Oral Crohn's disease revisited-a 10-year review. British Journal of Oral and Maxillofacial Surgery 27: 114–123

Ghandour K, Issa M 1991 Oral Crohn's disease with late intestinal manifestations. Oral Surgery, Oral Medicine, Oral Pathology 72: 565–567

Ivanyi L, Kirby A, Zakrzewska, J M 1993 Antibodies to mycobacterial stress protein in patients with orofacial granulomatosis. Journal of Oral Pathology and Medicine 22: 320–322

James J, Ferguson M M 1986 Orofacial granulomatosis presenting clinically as tuberculosis of cervical lymph nodes. British Dental Journal 161: 17–19

James J, Patton D W, Lewis L J, Kirkwood E M, Ferguson M M 1986 Orofacial granulomatosis and clinical atopy. Journal of Oral Medicine 41: 29–30

Krutchkoff D, James R 1978 Cheilitis granulomatosa. Successful treatment with combined local triamcinolone injections and surgery. Archives of Dermatology 114: 1203–1206

Madanes A Z, Farber M 1982 Danazol. Annals of Internal Medicine 96: 625–630

Mendeloff A I, Calkins B M 1988 The epidemiology of idiopathic inflammatory bowel disease. In: Kirsner J B, Shorter R G (eds) Inflammatory bowel disease. Lea and Febiger, Philadelphia, pp 3–34

Miescher G 1945 Uber essentielle granulomatöse Makrocheille (cheilitis Granulomatosa). Dermatologica 91: 57–85

Patton D W, Ferguson M M, Forsyth A, James J 1985 Orofacial granulomatosis: a possible allergic basis. British Journal of Oral and Maxillofacial Surgery 23: 235–242

Plauth M, Jenss H, Meyle J 1991 Oral manifestations of Crohn's disease. An analysis of 79 cases. Journal of Clinical Gastroenterology 13: 29–37

Podmore P, Burrows D 1986 Clofazimine – an effective treatment for Melkersson-Rosenthal syndrome or Miescher's cheilitis. Clinical and Experimental Dermatology 11: 173-178

Sakuntabhai A, MacLeod R I, Lawrence C M 1993 Intralesional steroid injection after nerve block anaesthesia in the treatment of orofacial granulomatosis. Archives of Dermatology 129: 477–480

Schlegel-Gomez R, Ozen I Y, Peters K-P, Simon M Jr, Hornstein O-P 1989 Morbus Crohn – Erstmanifestation im oralen und anogenitalen Bereich. Hautarzt 40: 451–455

Scully C, Eveson J W, Witherow H, Young A H, Tan R S, Gilby E D 1993 Oral presentation of lymphoma: Case report of T-cell lymphoma masquerading as oral Crohn's disease and review of the literature. Oral Oncology, European Journal of Cancer 29B 3: 225–229

Tyldesley W R 1979 Oral Crohn's disease and related conditions. British Journal of Oral Surgery 17: 1–9

Varley E W B 1973 Crohn's disease of the mouth: report of three cases. Oral Surgery, Oral Medicine, Oral Pathology 33: 570

Veller Fornasa C, Catalano P, Peserico A 1992 Minocycline in granulomatous cheilitis: experience with 6 cases. Dermatology 185: 220

Wiesenfeld D, Ferguson M M, Mitchell D N et al 1985 Oro-Facial Granulomatosis – A Clinical and Pathological Analysis. Quarterly Journal of Medicine 54(213): 101–113

Williams A J, Wray D, Ferguson A 1991 The clinical entity of orofacial Crohn's disease. Quarterly Journal of Medicine 79: 451–458

Williams P M, Greenberg M S 1991 Management of cheilitis granulomatosa. Oral Surgery, Oral Medicine, Oral Pathology 72: 436–439

Williams R S 1959 Triamcinolone myopathy. Lancet i: 698–701

Worsae N, Christensen K C, Schiodt M, Reibel J 1982 Melkersson-Rosenthal syndrome and cheilitis granulomatosa. A clinicopathologic study of 33 patients with special reference to their oral lesions. Oral Surgery, Oral Medicine, Oral Pathology 54: 404–413

71. Hepatobiliary disease

R. Chapman

INTRODUCTION

The association between colonic ulceration and liver disease was first described in 1874 by Thomas, who reported the case of a young man who died of a 'much enlarged, fatty liver in the presence of ulceration of the colon'. The association was confirmed by Lister (1889), who reported a patient with ulcerative colitis and secondary diffuse hepatitis. It has since emerged that there is a close relationship between inflammatory bowel disease and various hepatobiliary disorders. The major hepatobiliary diseases seen in association with inflammatory bowel disease, namely primary sclerosing cholangitis, cirrhosis, cholangiocarcinoma and most cases of chronic active hepatitis, probably represent different aspects of the same spectrum of hepatobiliary disease (Table 71.1).

PREVALENCE OF LIVER DISEASE

The prevalence of liver disease in patients with ulcerative colitis and Crohn's disease has varied widely in different series, probably influenced by the number of patients included who have severe, active or extensive inflammatory bowel disease, and the methods used for assessment of liver dysfunction.

Abnormal liver function tests are found in more than half of patients with inflammatory bowel disease requiring surgery, and are due to a number of factors, including malnutrition, sepsis and blood transfusions, with the attendant risk of subsequent viral infection. However, significant liver disease is much less common. The true prevalence of hepatobiliary abnormality is difficult to determine, as it would involve obtaining liver histology and cholangiography on an unselected group of patients with inflammatory bowel disease. Studies in most series have therefore relied upon detecting persistent abnormalities on serum biochemical testing before proceeding to hepatic biopsy or endoscopic retrograde cholangiography (ERCP). In an early study from Oxford (Perrett et al 1971a) 5–6% of patients with ulcerative colitis had significant histological abnormalities on hepatic histology, compared to 10% of patients with Crohn's disease. Schrumpf et al (1982a) studied a group of 336 unselected Norwegian patients with ulcerative colitis. All those with persistently abnormal liver function tests were investigated by means of cholangiography. More than 14% of patients were found to have some form of hepatobiliary disease, and 5% (later updated to 7.5%) of all patients had primary sclerosing cholangitis, although most were asymptomatic.

More recently, a large study has been carried out by Olsson et al (1991), who identified all patients over the age of 16 years old with a diagnosis of ulcerative colitis in five well defined catchment areas of Sweden, representing 12.7% of the Swedish population and exactly 1500 patients. Recent liver function tests were obtained in 94% of the patients and 65 of the 72 with abnormal serum alkaline phosphatase values had endoscopic retrograde cholangiograms performed. Primary sclerosing cholangitis was diagnosed in 55 (3.7%). The prevalence of the disease was 5.5% in patients with substantial colitis (proximal to the splenic flexure) and only 0.5% in patients with distal colitis. A further large study has been performed in Stockholm, Sweden, of 1274 patients with ulcerative colitis

Table 71.1 Hepatobiliary diseases associated with inflammatory bowel disease

	Ulcerative colitis	Crohn's disease
Primary sclerosing cholangitis (PSC)	+	+
Small-duct PSC (pericholangitis)	+	+
Chronic active hepatitis	(+)	–
Cirrhosis	+	+
Cholangiocarcinoma	+	(+)
Hepatocellular carcinoma	(+)	–
Fatty liver	+	+
Granulomas	(+)	+
Amyloidosis	(+)	+
Gallstones	–	+*
Hepatic abscess	–	+
Primary biliary cirrhosis	(+)	–

+, definite association; (+), possible association;
–, no association;
*, Crohn's disease involving the terminal ileum

who had been diagnosed between 1955 and 1979 (Broome et al 1994). Eleven percent showed signs of hepatobiliary disease on serum biochemistry. Follow-up study was performed on all 142 patients with abnormal liver function and ulcerative colitis between 1989 and 1991. Sixty had developed normal liver function as judged from test results, whereas the remaining 74 still had evidence of hepatobiliary disease. In 21 patients the cause of the liver function abnormality was due to hepatitis B or C virus transmitted by blood transfusions. Twenty-nine (2.3%) of the patients developed primary sclerosing cholangitis and 12 of this group died during the study period.

In summary, approximately 3–7.5% of all patients with inflammatory bowel disease will have significant hepatobiliary disease. Although the number of patients with hepatobiliary abnormality is approximately the same for both ulcerative colitis and Crohn's disease, severe significant liver disease is much more commonly seen with patients with ulcerative colitis, and when it occurs in Crohn's disease it is usually associated with extensive colonic involvement.

PRIMARY SCLEROSING CHOLANGITIS

Primary sclerosing cholangitis is a chronic cholestatic liver disease characterized by an obliterative inflammatory fibrosis which usually involves the whole biliary tree (Fig. 71.1). The changes are sometimes localized to either the extra- or the intrahepatic bile ducts and the degree of involvement in different segments of the biliary tract varies considerably from patient to patient. Once considered a rare disease, the advent of improved cholangiographic techniques such as ERCP has enabled the diagnosis to be made without resort to laparotomy. A much larger number of cases of sclerosing cholangitis have now been diagnosed, and a much wider clinical and pathological spectrum has emerged than was previously appreciated (Chapman et al 1980, Wiesner & LaRusso 1980, Helzberg et al 1987).

Relationship with ulcerative colitis

There is a close relationship between primary sclerosing cholangitis and inflammatory bowel disease, particularly ulcerative colitis. Approximately 70% of all patients with primary sclerosing cholangitis have coexisting ulcerative colitis (Table 71.2) and primary sclerosing cholangitis is the most common form of chronic liver disease associated with ulcerative colitis. A number of studies from different parts of the world have reviewed the clinical features of patients with ulcerative colitis and primary sclerosing cholangitis (Chapman et al 1980, Schrumpf et al 1982a, Olsson et al 1991, Broome et al 1994). The findings from these studies have been remarkably consistent. Paradoxically, the colitis is usually total in over 90% of patients, but is symptomatically mild (often without rectal bleeding) and characterized by prolonged remissions. Patients with ulcerative colitis and primary sclerosing cholangitis have a male predominance, with a male:female ratio of 2:1, which contrasts with the slight female predominance found overall in ulcerative colitis (Edwards & Truelove 1963). Although the symptoms of ulcerative colitis usually develop before those of sclerosing cholangitis, in some patients, the primary sclerosing cholangitis may precede the symptoms of colitis by up to 4 years. The outcome of the hepatobiliary disease is completely unrelated to the activity, severity or clinical course of the colitis. In particular, colectomy does not affect the clinical progression or the mortality of patients with primary sclerosing cholangitis, and liver disease may even develop some years after total colectomy (Chapman et al 1980, Cangemi et al 1989).

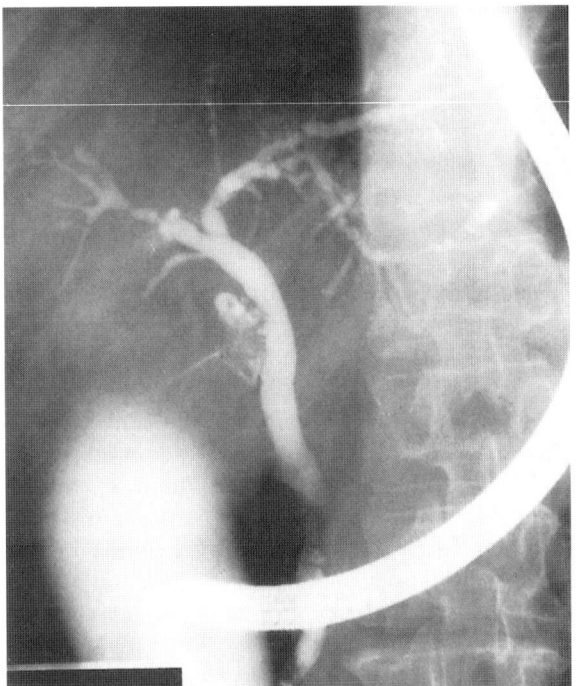

Fig. 71.1 Endoscopic cholangiogram showing generalized beading and stricturing of the intra- and extrahepatic bile ducts; the diagnostic changes of primary sclerosing cholangitis.

Table 71.2 Prevalence of inflammatory bowel disease in patients with primary sclerosing cholangitis

Institution (year published)		Number of patients	% with inflammatory bowel disease
Royal Free Hospital	(1980)	29	72
Mayo Clinic	(1980)	50	70
Yale	(1987)	53	62
King's College Hospital (children)	(1987)	13	77
King's College Hospital (adults)	(1991)	81	72
Pittsburgh	(1990)	66	71

The increased frequency of bile duct cancer, including carcinoma of the gallbladder, in patients with ulcerative colitis is well established (Ritchie et al 1974). Carcinoma of the bile duct may also develop in patients with long-standing primary sclerosing cholangitis and ulcerative colitis. It seems likely that all patients with ulcerative colitis developing biliary cancer have underlying sclerosing cholangitis and this will be discussed later.

There are fewer reports of primary sclerosing cholangitis associated with Crohn's disease, and the prevalence of primary sclerosing cholangitis in patients with Crohn's colitis is less than 1% (Olsson et al 1991). The prevalence of bile duct carcinoma is not increased in Crohn's disease. The explanation for these differences is unclear but may be related to the lower prevalence of total colonic involvement in patients with Crohn's disease.

It has recently been proposed that primary sclerosing cholangitis may be a risk factor for the development of dysplasia of the colon and DNA aneuploidy (Broome et al 1992). It is unclear whether this simply reflects the association of primary sclerosing cholangitis and total long-standing colitis or whether it is related to the underlying hepatobiliary disease.

Epidemiology

The prevalence of primary sclerosing cholangitis is unknown, although in patients with ulcerative colitis it is of the order of 2.4–7.5%. Prevalence in the United States has been estimated at 2–7 cases per 100 000 population, based on a prevalence of ulcerative colitis of 40–225 cases per 100 000 population. This estimate has been confirmed by the results from Olsson et al (1991), who calculated the prevalence of ulcerative colitis and primary sclerosing cholangitis as 171 and 6.3 cases per 100 000 population respectively. These results probably underestimate the real prevalence of primary sclerosing cholangitis, as the disease can occur in patients with normal serum levels of alkaline phosphatase and 20–30% of patients have no associated inflammatory bowel disease. Primary sclerosing cholangitis is more common than previously suspected, and the prevalence is of the same order as that for primary biliary cirrhosis.

Etiology

The cause of primary sclerosing cholangitis is unknown, but any proposed etiological mechanism must incorporate its close association with ulcerative colitis. A number of hypotheses have been proposed to explain the association between colonic disease and biliary tract inflammation and fibrosis (Table 71.3). Warren et al (1965) suggested that the primary event is a chronic low-grade portal venous infection which may occur in some patients with ulcerative colitis (Eade & Brooke 1969). This, could lead

Table 71.3 Possible causes of primary sclerosing cholangitis

Portal bacteremia
Abnormal bile acids
Absorbed colonic toxins
Viral infections
Copper toxicity
Immunological mechanisms
Genetic predisposition
Ischemic arteriolar injury

in turn to chronic biliary tract inflammation. However, Palmer et al (1980) were unable to show any significant bacteremia in the portal blood of patients undergoing surgery for severe ulcerative colitis. Furthermore, Ludwig et al (1981) have shown that portal phlebitis is mild or absent in liver biopsies from patients with primary sclerosing cholangitis, and cultures of liver biopsies have not revealed any organisms. This hypothesis cannot explain why sclerosing cholangitis may occur several years before the onset of ulcerative colitis, and does not improve after either remission of the colitis or following colectomy.

A second hypothesis is that primary sclerosing cholangitis associated with ulcerative colitis is caused by reaction to toxic bile acids, such as lithocolic acid, arising from bacterial action in the diseased colon (Carey 1964). Abnormal bile acids could be absorbed directly into the portal blood and produce a portal tract inflammation, but three studies have shown no major abnormality in bile acid metabolism in patients with primary sclerosing cholangitis and/or ulcerative colitis (Siegel et al 1977, Dew et al 1980, Holzbach et al 1980).

Ludwig et al (1981) suggested that primary sclerosing cholangitis may be caused by a virus, since cholangitis and biliary atresia may be induced in weaning mice, primates, and possibly in human infants, after infection with reovirus type III. Recent studies have failed to find any evidence of past or current infection with this virus. The same group proposed that the excess liver copper found in patients with primary sclerosing cholangitis may have a role in either initiating or perpetuating the disease process (Gross et al 1985), although excess liver copper is found in chronic cholestasis from any cause. In conclusion, none of these hypotheses satisfactorily explains the development of biliary disease in patients with ulcerative colitis.

Recent studies have suggested that genetic and immunological factors are important in the pathogenesis of primary sclerosing cholangitis. Three sets of siblings from three families have been described with primary sclerosing cholangitis and ulcerative colitis (Quigley et al 1983). Furthermore, the frequency of HLA B8, DR3 and DR52A is much higher in primary sclerosing cholangitis patients than in controls (Schrumpf et al 1982b, Chapman et al 1983). More recently, HLA-DR52a, which is closely associated with the HLA B8 DR3 haplotype by linkage disequilibrium, has been shown to be the most closely associated HLA allele in primary sclerosing cholangitis and is present in nearly 60% of patients (Farrant et al 1992). Other studies have found that the prevalence of HLA-DR2 is increased in those patients who are HLA B8, DR3 negative (Donaldson et al 1991). However, the HLA gene confirming the primary HLA-associated susceptibility to primary sclerosing cholangitis remains to be established. This finding not only confirms the role of genetic factors but also suggests that the disease may be immunologically mediated, as the HLA B8 and DR3 haplotype is associated with a number of autoimmune diseases such as autoimmune chronic active hepatitis, myasthenia gravis and thyrotoxicosis. Although the prevalence of HLA B8 and DR3 is not increased in patients with ulcerative colitis, such a patient who is unfortunate enough to possess the HLA B8 and DR3 haplotype, has a tenfold increase in the relative risk of developing primary sclerosing cholangitis.

The potential importance of immunological factors has been emphasized by the number of recent reports which have shown humoral and cellular abnormalities in primary sclerosing cholangitis. The cellular immune abnormalities include depressed levels of circulating or suppressor T cells in serum and large increases in the numbers of both suppressor and helper T cells in the portal tracts of patients with primary sclerosing cholangitis (Whiteside et al 1985), an inhibition of leukocyte migration in response to biliary antigens (McFarlane et al 1979), and aberrant expression of HLA DR antigens on biliary epithelium in the early stages of the disease (Chapman et al 1988). Humoral immune defects include increased levels of circulating immune complexes in the blood (Bodenheimer et al 1983), defective clearance of immune complexes (Minuk et al 1986) and the demonstration of circulating autoantibodies against colonic epithelium (Chapman et al 1986), neutrophil nuclei (Snook et al 1989) and antineutrophil cytoplasmic antibodies 9ANCA0 (Duerr et al 1991, Lo et al 1992).

Perinuclear antineutrophil cytoplasmic antibodies (ANCA) have been detected in the sera of 26–85% of patients with primary sclerosing cholangitis with or without ulcerative colitis, and in up to 68% with ulcerative colitis alone (Duerr et al 1991, Lo et al 1992). Current data suggest that the ANCA-reactive antigens are similar and may be indicative of a common immunopathological mechanism. As for ulcerative colitis, no correlation exists between disease activity and ANCA in primary sclerosing cholangitis (Lo et al 1994). Unfortunately, the antigen(s) specific to mature neutrophils have not been isolated and it is not yet clear whether ANCA have pathogenic, diagnostic or prognostic significance or are merely an epiphenomenon.

The present evidence suggests that primary sclerosing cholangitis is an immunologically mediated disease, probably triggered in genetically susceptible subjects by acquired toxic or infectious agents which could gain access through the colonic mucosa.

Clinical features

Primary sclerosing cholangitis is mainly a disease of young males, with a male:female ratio of 2:1. The majority of patients present between the ages of 25 and 40 years, although the disease has been diagnosed at all ages between 1 and 90 years! The clinical presentation commonly includes fatigue, intermittent jaundice, weight loss, right upper quadrant abdominal pain and pruritus (Chapman et al 1980, Helzberg et al 1987). Despite the name of the disease, only a few patients suffer attacks of acute cholangitis, which usually follow reconstructive biliary surgery or some form of endoscopic interventional therapy.

Some patients with primary sclerosing cholangitis may present with an established cirrhosis and portal hypertension without any previous symptoms of cholangitis or cholestasis. These patients may be diagnosed and treated as cryptogenic cirrhosis for many years before the diagnosis is established.

Physical examination is abnormal in about half the symptomatic patients at presentation. Common abnormalities include hepatosplenomegaly and jaundice, although jaundice often only appears late in the course of the disease. The stigmata of liver disease, including spider naevi, palmar erythema and finger clubbing, are uncommon. An increasing number of asymptomatic patients with primary sclerosing cholangitis are being diagnosed in whom physical examination is normal. The diagnosis is usually made incidentally when a persistently raised serum alkaline phosphatase is found in a patient with ulcerative colitis.

Laboratory investigations

Serum biochemical tests usually indicate cholestasis. However, the levels of alkaline phosphatase and bilirubin may vary widely in an individual patient during the course of the disease, increasing, for example, during periods of acute cholangitis and falling after appropriate therapy. Sometimes the levels may fluctuate for no apparent reason. Modest elevations in serum transaminase are usually found. Hypoalbuminemia and clotting abnormalities are only found at a late stage.

The diagnostic role of ANCA in primary sclerosing cholangitis have already been discussed. Low titers of serum antinuclear and smooth muscle antibodies have been found in patients with primary sclerosing cholangitis, but they have no diagnostic significance; serum mitochondrial antibody is invariably absent (Chapman et al 1980). Increased serum IgM concentrations are seen in about half of symptomatic patients, and the levels of IgM are similar to those observed in patients with primary biliary cirrhosis. Elevation of IgG is found in about a third of adult patients tested. High levels of serum IgG are frequently observed in children with primary sclerosing cholangitis (El-Shabrawi et al 1987).

Radiographic features

Endoscopic cholangiography is the best method of demonstrating the biliary system in patients with sclerosing cholangitis. Although in skilled hands the bile ducts can be visualized by percutaneous transhepatic angiography, this technique is difficult in sclerosing cholangitis and carries a significant morbidity. The cholangiographic appearances are diagnostic and consist of multiple stricturing and dilatation (beading) of the intrahepatic and extrahepatic bile ducts (MacCarty et al 1983) (Fig. 71.1).

Occasionally involvement may be limited to the intrahepatic ducts alone or, more rarely, in patients with concurrent ulcerative colitis only the extrahepatic bile ducts may be abnormal (Rabinovitz et al 1990). Small diverticuli along the common bile duct are diagnostic and found in about 25% of patients (Wells et al 1980) (Fig. 71.2).

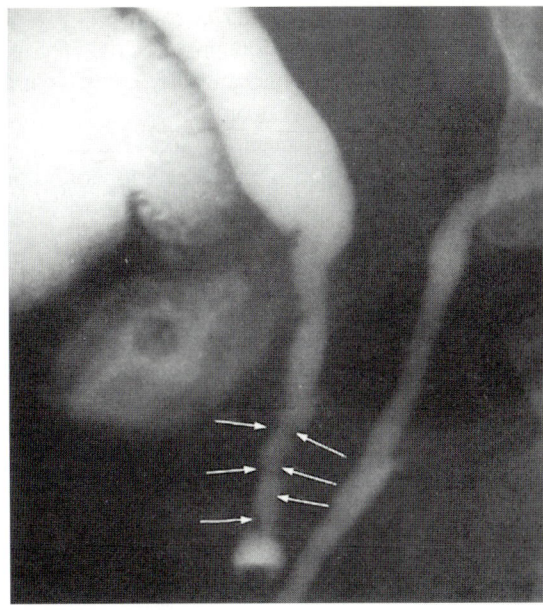

Fig. 71.2 Endoscopic cholangiogram from a patient with primary sclerosing cholangitis showing a strictured lower common bile duct with small diverticulae present (arrows).

Pathological features

Extrahepatic bile ducts appear macroscopically as thickened cords, although the overall diameter is not usually increased. In cross-section the lumen is narrow and the wall may be up to eight times the usual thickness. The inflammation and dense concentric fibrosis usually affect the submucosa and outer layers of the bile ducts, leaving the mucosa largely unaffected.

The histological appearances of the liver biopsy are not usually diagnostic, although some form of biliary disease can usually be identified, indicating the need for cholangiography (Chapman et al 1980). Ludwig et al (1981) proposed a histological staging system for hepatic involvement, where stage I is characterized by enlargement of the portal tracts with periductal fibrosis, inflammation and bile ductular proliferation (Fig. 71.3). In the second stage tongues of connective tissue grow into the periportal liver parenchyma. This process leads to the formation of the fibrous septa linking portal tracts (stage III), and finally in stage IV a fully developed biliary

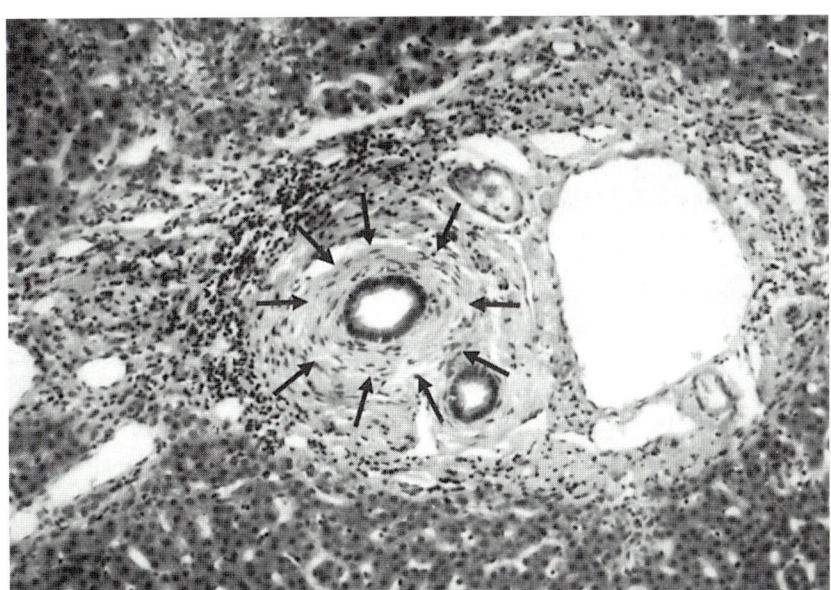

Fig. 71.3 An expanded portal tract with chronic inflammatory cells and marked periductular concentric fibrosis (arrows).

cirrhosis. As with primary biliary cirrhosis, as the disease progresses an obliterative cholangitis leads to complete replacement of intralobular bile ducts by connective tissue, i.e. vanishing bile duct syndrome, similar to PBC and chronic graft-versus-host disease (Chapman et al 1980, Ludwig et al 1981). Piecemeal necrosis, copper and protein accumulation in the liver are similar to those found in other chronic cholestatic liver diseases. Copper levels may increase without morphological evidence of cholestasis (Gross et al 1985). There is a poor correlation between the histological and cholangiographic findings, as the hepatic changes can be focal and variable in different parts of the liver. Bile duct dysplasia may precede the development of cholangiocarcinoma, analogous to chronic dysplasia in primary sclerosing cholangitis (Martins et al 1994).

Treatment

There is no curative treatment for primary sclerosing cholangitis but a plethora of medical, endoscopic and surgical approaches have been advocated. Treatment can be divided into the management of cholestasis, the management of the complications, and specific treatments of the disease process.

Management of cholestasis

Symptomatic patients are frequently troubled by pruritus. This is best managed initially by cholestyramine and the dose should be increased until the pruritus is relieved. In addition, fat-soluble vitamin replacement is necessary for the jaundiced patient and this should be given by monthly intramuscular injections. Metabolic bone disease (usually osteoporosis) is a frequent complication of advanced primary sclerosing cholangitis. No effective treatment is available for the prevention or management of osteopenia.

Management of complications

Broad-spectrum antibiotics such as ciprofloxacin should be given for acute attacks of cholangitis but they have no proven prophylactic value and should not be used long term except in patients with recurrent cholangitis. If cholangiography shows a well defined obstruction to the main extrahepatic bile ducts mechanical relief must be considered. In many patients the best therapeutic approach is the placing of a prosthesis (stent) through the obstruction. This may be placed non-operatively by the percutaneous transhepatic route or at ERCP (Johnson et al 1987). Balloon dilatation of the strictures before stenting may prove useful in those few patients with well defined localized strictures, and can lead to a striking improvement in both symptoms and serum biochemistry (May et al 1985). The development of small biliary stones and sludge can lead to sudden clinical or biochemical deterioration. In these patients endoscopic sphincterotomy with extraction of the biliary debris is beneficial. Some authors have advocated endoscopic biliary drainage, but no long-term controlled results have been reported.

Patients with primary sclerosing cholangitis and chronic ulcerative colitis treated by colectomy may develop peristomal varices, which can bleed profusely (Wiesner et al 1986). No effective measures are available once they have developed, although local measures such as injection of sclerosants have been tried.

Specific treatments

Medical treatment of primary sclerosing cholangitis has included uncontrolled trials of corticosteroids, immunosuppressive drugs, cholecystogogs and antibiotics, either alone or in combination. The results have been universally disappointing, although assessment of treatment in this uncommon disease is difficult because the clinical course fluctuates, survival is variable and some patients may remain asymptomatic for many years.

The role of corticosteroid therapy in primary sclerosing cholangitis is unclear. There have been no controlled trials of steroid therapy, but many patients with sclerosing cholangitis, particularly those who also have ulcerative colitis, will have received corticosteroids. Corticosteroids have been used both topically and systemically in small and generally uncontrolled trials in sclerosing cholangitis. A controlled trial of nasobiliary lavage with corticosteroids or placebo produced no significant benefit (Allison et al 1986). However, a small uncontrolled study showed benefit in seven of 10 patients with sclerosing cholangitis who received biliary lavage with prednisolone (Grijm et al 1986).

Good results with prednisolone have been reported in some pilot studies (Burgert et al 1984), but no benefit was seen in patients treated with prednisolone and colchicine for 2 years at the Mayo Clinic (Lindor et al 1991). Controlled trials with bone-sparing agents are needed before this treatment can be widely recommended in view of the risk of bone disease being accentuated by steroid therapy.

A number of immunosuppressive agents have been tried, either alone or in combination, including penicillamine, methotrexate and cyclosporin. No benefit has been demonstrated. In addition, treatment with ursodeoxycholic acid is being assessed in clinical trials. Early results have shown an improvement in biochemistry but no effect on symptoms or histology (Wiesner 1994).

Orthotropic liver transplantation is the only option available in young patients with primary sclerosing cholangitis and advanced liver disease. Although the initial reports were unfavorable, the 4-year survival rate is 70% in 75 patients who were transplanted at the University of Pittsburgh (Esquivel et al 1988). These results compare favorably with the survival rates for other forms of chronic liver disease. So far there have been fewer than ten cases of primary sclerosing cholangitis recurring in the transplanted liver. However, patients with primary sclerosing cholangitis and ulcerative colitis are at increased risk for the development of colon cancer after transplantation. Annual colonoscopic surveillance has been recommended in this group (Wiesner 1994).

Natural history

In the majority of patients primary sclerosing cholangitis is a progressive disease. The median survival time from diagnosis is approximately 12–17 years (Broome et al 1992), and both symptomatic and asymptomatic patients have a shorter survival period than a matched controlled population. Patients usually die in hepatic failure with progressive cholestatic jaundice. However, approximately 10–20% of patients with long-standing primary sclerosing cholangitis develop bile duct carcinoma, which often follows an aggressive course (Adlund et al 1987, Farrant et al 1991, Broome et al 1994). Prognostic models have been developed in order to predict the clinical course of the hepatobiliary disease, but no model has been of value in the individual patient, although most studies have shown that an elevated serum bilirubin level at presentation is associated with a poor prognosis (Dickson et al 1992). Further models are being developed to facilitate the timing of liver transplantation and to evaluate the usefulness of monitoring the effect of experimental therapy on disease progression.

SMALL-DUCT PRIMARY SCLEROSING CHOLANGITIS

A few patients with ulcerative colitis will have persistently abnormal cholestatic liver function tests, together with typical histological appearances such as concentric fibrosis, but with normal bile ducts at cholangiography. The term 'small-duct primary sclerosing cholangitis' has been proposed to replace the term 'pericholangitis' in this group of patients, as the evidence suggests that these conditions are part of the same disease spectrum. Out of a group of 64 ulcerative colitis patients with abnormal liver function tests, five fulfilled the above criteria (Boberg et al 1994). Wee and Ludwig (1985) described two patients who progressed from small-duct primary sclerosing cholangitis to develop extrahepatic biliary involvement typical of sclerosing cholangitis. In addition, patients with either large or small-duct sclerosing cholangitis have an increased risk of developing cholangiocarcinoma.

For many years the term 'pericholangitis' has been synonymous with involvement of the liver in inflammatory bowel disease (Mistilis 1965, Mistilis et al 1965). Some patients with pericholangitis progressed to cirrhosis of the liver and cholangiocarcinoma (Bowden et al 1959).

Pericholangitis has been used as a histological diagnosis to describe inflammatory reactions in the portal zones of the liver together with periductular inflammation and fibrosis. However, most patients with histological pericholangitis will have cholangiographic appearances diagnostic of large-duct primary sclerosing cholangitis at ERCP (Blackstone & Nemchausky 1978), thus the term pericholangitis has become redundant and most authorities feel that it should be abandoned in the context of liver abnormality in primary sclerosing cholangitis.

CHRONIC ACTIVE HEPATITIS

Chronic active hepatitis has been reported in association with ulcerative colitis (Olsson & Hulten 1975). However, histological evidence of piecemeal necrosis can accompany the classic bile duct changes of primary sclerosing cholangitis on cholangiography (Chapman et al 1980), and the majority of patients with chronic active hepatitis and inflammatory bowel disease probably have either large- or small-duct primary sclerosing cholangitis.

CIRRHOSIS

The incidence of cirrhosis associated with inflammatory bowel disease varies in different series from 1 to 5% (Edwards & Truelove 1963, Perrett et al 1971a, Dew et al 1979, Schrumpf et al 1980). Most patients are reported to have biliary cirrhosis, but since patients with sclerosing cholangitis can present with portal hypertension and established cirrhosis without preceding symptoms, many of these patients probably have end-stage primary sclerosing cholangitis. Not all patients with cirrhosis and inflammatory bowel disease will have primary sclerosing cholangitis, however, and it is possible that some cases may be due to chronic hepatitis C associated with previous blood transfusions (Broome et al 1994).

CHOLANGIOCARCINOMA

The first case of a biliary tract cancer and ulcerative colitis was reported by Parker and Kendall in 1954. Since that time the association between cholangiocarcinoma and ulcerative colitis has been well established (Rosen et al 1991). A large study from the Cleveland Clinic has reported a prevalence rate of 0.5% (Mir-Madjlessi et al 1987). The relative risk of developing bile duct cancer in ulcerative colitis is approximately 20–30 times that of the general population.

Bile duct cancer develops in patients with long-standing total colitis. Colectomy does not protect against the development of the tumor, which can occur as long as 20 years after colectomy. Early studies did not always report evidence of associated hepatobiliary diseases (Ritchie et al 1974), but more recent studies have shown that most patients have either large- or small-duct primary sclerosing cholangitis, which may precede the development of carcinoma by many years (Mir-Madjlessi et al 1987). Five of 12 patients at the Mayo Clinic who died from primary sclerosing cholangitis, and who came to postmortem, had cholangiocarcinoma which was multifocal in some (Wee et al 1985). It is not known why some patients with primary sclerosing cholangitis develop biliary cancer. Bile duct carcinoma has been reported in association with Crohn's disease, but is rare (Berman et al 1980).

The clinical presentation of bile duct cancer is of progressive cholestatic jaundice. Cholangiography usually reveals bile duct stricture, although the distinction from focal primary sclerosing cholangitis can be difficult or impossible before surgery. Less than 10% survive for more than 2 years. The tumor usually pursues a progressive course and the prognosis is poor. Patients with primary sclerosing cholangitis who develop a cholangiocarcinoma should not be considered for liver transplant, as the survival figures are very poor. Patients with biliary dysplasia should be offered a transplant to pre-empt the development of cancer (Martins et al 1994).

FATTY CHANGE

Fatty liver is often reported as the most common type of hepatobiliary lesions in patients with inflammatory bowel disease. It has been recorded in 45% of patients with ulcerative colitis and in 40% of patients with Crohn's disease undergoing colectomy (Eade 1970, Eade et al 1971a, b), but the presence of fatty liver reflects the general state of health of the patient and the severity of the underlying colitis rather than any other specific factors. In an unselected series fatty liver was found in only 6.3% and 4% of patients with ulcerative colitis and Crohn's disease respectively (Perrett et al 1971a, b). Moreover, the incidence of fatty change in patients with ulcerative colitis at postmortem is similar to that of other debilitated patients (Palmer et al 1964).

There are no symptoms associated with fatty liver, although hepatomegaly may be present. Treatment of the underlying bowel disorder and improvement in the general health of the patient leads to resolution of the fatty change. There is no evidence that the lesion progresses to chronic liver disease such as cirrhosis. In view of improvements in the management of inflammatory bowel disease, the incidence of fatty change is probably much lower now than previously recorded.

GALLSTONES

Patients with Crohn's disease of the small bowel have an increased incidence of gallstones. The reported incidence in patients with Crohn's ileitis, ileal resection or intestinal bypass ranges from 13 to 34% (Heaton & Read 1969, Cohen et al 1971). However, the incidence of gallstones in ulcerative colitis and in patients with Crohn's disease confined to the colon is about 5%, and does not differ from that in the general population. The increased rate of gallstone formation in patients with inflammation or following resection of the terminal ileum is due to reduced bile salt absorption, decreased biliary bile salt concentration and relative increases in biliary cholesterol. This increases cholesterol precipitation in the gallbladder and results in gallstone formation.

AMYLOIDOSIS

Hepatic amyloidosis is a rare complication and is found in less than 1% of patients with inflammatory bowel disease. It is much more commonly associated with Crohn's disease than ulcerative colitis. Although regression of amyloidosis has been reported after colectomy (Fausa et al 1977), the prognosis is poor in most patients.

GRANULOMAS

Granulomas are occasionally seen in the liver biopsy specimens of patients with Crohn's disease, sometimes associated with a moderate elevation of serum alkaline phosphatase (Mauer et al 1967, Eade 1970). There have been a few isolated reports of hepatic granulomas occurring in association with ulcerative colitis, but the relationship remains unproven.

LIVER ABSCESS

Intra-abdominal abscess is a frequent complication of Crohn's disease. The development of hepatic abscess in association with inflammatory bowel disease is well documented but rare. The abscesses are often multiple and carry a high mortality (Greenstein et al 1985). Streptococci, especially *Streptococcus milleri*, are the most frequent organisms isolated from the abscesses (Mir-Madjlessi et al 1986).

PRIMARY BILIARY CIRRHOSIS

Five patients have been described with concomitant ulcerative colitis and primary biliary cirrhosis. This may represent a true association but is more likely to have occurred by chance (Kato et al 1985, Bush et al 1987).

REFERENCES

Aadland E, Schrumpf E, Fausa O, Elgjo K, Heilo A, Aakhus T 1987 Primary sclerosing cholangitis: a longterm follow-up study. Scandinavian Journal of Gastroenterology 2: 655–664

Allison M C, Buroughs A K, Noone P, Summerfield J A 1986 Biliary lavage with corticosteroids in primary sclerosing cholangitis. Journal of Hepatology 3: 118–122

Berman M D, Falchuk K'R, Trey C 1980 Carcinoma of the biliary tree complicating Crohn's disease. Digestive Diseases and Sciences 25: 795–797

Blackstone M O, Nemchausky B A 1978 Cholangiographic abnormalities in ulcerative colitis associated pericholangitis which resemble sclerosing cholangitis. Digestive Diseases and Sciences 23: 5769–5785

Boberg K M, Schrumpf E, Fause O et al 1994 Hepatobiliary disease in ulcerative colitis. An analysis of 18 patients with hepatobiliary lesions classified as small duct primary sclerosing cholangitis. Scandinavian Journal of Gastroenterology 29: 744–752

Boden R W, Rantin J G, Goulston S J, Morrow W 1959 The liver in ulcerative colitis: the significance of raised serum alkaline phosphatase levels. Lancet 2: 245–248

Bodenheimer H C, La Russo N F, Thayer W R et al 1985 Elevated circulating immune complexes in primary sclerosing cholangitis. Gastroenterology 88: 166–170

Broome U, Lindberg G, Lofberg R 1982 Primary sclerosing cholangitis in ulcerative colitis – a risk factor for the development of dysplasia and DNA anuploidy. Gastroenterology 1087–1080

Broome U, Glaumann H, Hellers G, Nilsson B, Sorstat J, Hultcrantz R 1994 Liver disease in ulcerative colitis: an epidemiological and follow-up study in the county of Stockholm. 35: 84–89

Burgert S L, Brown B P, Kirkpatrick R B, La Brecque D R 1984 Positive corticosteroid response in early primary sclerosing cholangitis. Gastroenterology 86: 1037 (Abstract)

Bush A, Mitchison H, Walt R et al 1987 Primary biliary cirrhosis and ulcerative colitis. Gastroenterology 92: 2009–2013

Cangemi J R, Wiesner R H, Beaver S J et al 1989 The effect of proctocolectomy for chronic ulcerative colitis on the natural history of primary sclerosing cholangitis. Gastroenterology 96: 790–794

Carey J B 1964 Bile acids, cirrhosis and human evolution. Gastroenterology 46: 490–492

Chapman R W, Arborgh B A, Rhodes J M et al 1980 Primary sclerosing cholangitis – a review of its clinical features, cholangiography and hepatic histology. Gut 21: 870–877

Chapman R W, Kelly P M A, Heryet A, Jewell D P, Fleming K A 1988 Expression of HLA-DR antigens on bile-duct epithelium in primary sclerosing cholangitis. Gut 29: 422–427

Chapman R W, Cottone M, Selby W S, Jewell D P 1986 Serum autoantibodies, ulcerative colitis and primary sclerosing cholangitis. Gut 27: 86–91

Chapman R W, Varghese Z, Gaul R, Patel G, Kokinon N, Sherlock S 1983 Association of primary sclerosing cholangitis with HLA-B8. Gut 24: 38–41

Cohen S, Kaplan M, Glottlieb L, Patterson J 1971 Liver disease and gallstones in regional enteritis. Gastroenterology 60: 243–245

Dew M J, Henegouwen G P, van B Huybregts A W M, Allan R N 1980 Hepatotoxic effect of bile acids in inflammatory bowel disease. Gastroenterology 78: 1398–1401

Dew M J, Thompson H, Allan R N 1979 The spectrum of hepatic dysfunction in inflammatory bowel disease. Quarterly Journal of Medicine 48: 113–135

Dickson E R, Murtaugh P A, Wiesner R H, Grambsch P M, Fleming T R, Ludwig J 1992 Primary sclerosing cholangitis: refinement and validation of survival models. Gastroenterology 103: 1893–1901

Donaldson P T, Farrant J M, Wilkinson M L, Hayllar K, Portmann B C, Williams R 1991 Dual association of HLA DR2 and DR3 with primary sclerosing cholangitis. Hepatology 13: 129–133

Duerr R H, Targan S R, Landers C J, LaRusso N F, Lindsey K L, Wiesner R H 1991 Neutrophil cytoplasmic antibodies: a link between primary sclerosing cholangitis and ulcerative colitis. Gastroenterology 100: 1381–1385

Eade M N 1970 Liver disease in ulcerative colitis. I. Analysis of operative liver biopsy in 138 consecutive patients having colectomy. Annals of Internal Medicine 72: 457–487

Eade M N, Brooke B N 1969 Portal bacteraemia in cases of ulcerative colitis submitted to colectomy. Lancet 1: 1008–1009

Eade M N, Cooke W T, Williams J A 1971a Liver disease in Crohn's disease. A study of 100 consecutive patients. Scandinavian Journal of Gastroenterology 6: 199–204

Eade M N, Cooke W T, Brooke B N, Thompson H 1971b Liver disease in Crohn's colitis. A study of 21 consecutive patients having colectomy. Annals of Internal Medicine 74: 518–528

Edwards F C, Truelove S C 1963 The course and prognosis of ulcerative colitis. Gut 4: 209–308

El-Shabrawi M, Wilkinson M L, Portmann B, Mieli-Vergani G, Chong S K F, Williams R, Mowat A P 1987 Primary sclerosing cholangitis in childhood. Gastroenterology 92: 1226–1235

Esquivel C O, Marsh J W, Fan Thiel D H 1988 Liver transplantation for chronic cholestatic liver disease in adults and children. Gastroenterology Clinics of North America 17: 145–155

Farrant J M, Doherty D G, Donaldson P T et al 1992 Amino acid substitutions at position 38 of the DRB polypeptide susceptibility to and protection from primary sclerosing cholangitis. Hepatology 16: 390–395

Fausa O, Nygaard K, Elgio K 1977 Amyloidosis and Crohn's disease. Scandinavian Journal of Gastroenterology 12: 657–662

Greenstein A J, Sachar D B, Lowenthal D, Goldofsky E, Aufses A H 1985 Pyogenic liver abscess in Crohn's disease. Quarterly Journal of Medicine 56: 505–518

Grijm R, Huibregtse K, Bartelsman J et al 1986 Therapeutic investigations in primary sclerosing cholangitis. Digestive Diseases and Sciences 31: 792–798

Gross J B Jr, Ludwig J, Wiesner R H et al 1985 Abnormalities in tests of copper metabolism in primary sclerosing cholangitis. Gastroenterology 89: 272–278

Heaton K W, Read A E 1969 Gallstones in patients with disorders of terminal ileum and disturbed bile salt metabolism. British Medical Journal 3: 494–496

Helzberg J H, Petersen J M, Boyer J L 1987 Improved survival with primary sclerosing cholangitis. Gastroenterology 92: 1869–1875

Holzbach R T, Marsh M E, Freedman M R, Fazio V W, Lavery I C, Jagelman D A 1980 Portal vein bile acids in patients with severe inflammatory bowel disease. Gut 21: 428–435

Johnson G K, Grenen J E, Venu R P, Hogan W J 1987 Endoscopic treatment of biliary duct strictures in sclerosing cholangitis: follow-up assessment of a new therapeutic approach. Gastrointestinal Endoscopy 33: 9–12

Kato Y, Morimoto H, Unousa M et al 1985 Primary biliary cirrhosis and chronic pancreatitis in patients with ulcerative colitis. Journal of Clinical Gastroenterology 7: 425–427

LaRusso N, Wiesner R, Ludwig J et al 1988 Prospective trial of penicillamine in primary sclerosing cholangitis. Gastroenterology 95: 1036–1042

Lindor K D, Wiesner R H, Colwell L J, Steiner B L, Beaver S, LaRusso N F 1991 The combination of prednisolone and colchicine in patients with primary sclerosing cholangitis. American Journal of Gastroenterology 85: 57–61

Lister J D 1889 A specimen of diffuse ulcerative colitis with secondary diffuse hepatitis. Transactions of the Pathology Society of London 50: 130–135

Lo S K, Fleming K A, Chapman R W 1992 Prevalence of antineutrophil antibody in primary sclerosing cholangitis and ulcerative colitis using an alkaline phosphatase technique. Gut 33: 1370–1375

Lo S K, Fleming K A, Chapman R W 1994 A 2 year follow-up study of antineutrophil antibody in primary sclerosing cholangitis. Journal of Hepatology 21: 974–978

Ludwig J, Barham S S, LaRusso N F, Elveback L R, Wiesner R H, McCall J T 1981 Morphologic features of chronic hepatitis associated with primary sclerosing cholangitis and chronic ulcerative colitis. Hepatology 1: 632–640

MacCarty R L, LaRusso N F, Wiesner R H, Ludwig J 1983 Cholangiographic and pancreatographic features of primary sclerosing cholangitis. Radiology 149: 39–44

McFarlane I G, Wojcicka B M, Tsantoulas D C, Portmann B C, Eddleston A L W F, Williams R 1979 Leucocyte migration inhibition in response to biliary antigens in primary biliary cirrhosis, sclerosing cholangitis and other chronic liver diseases. Gastroenterology 76: 1333–1340

Martins E R, Fleming K W, Garrido M C, Hine K R, Chapman R W 1994 Superficial thrombophlebitis, dysplasia and cholangiocarcinoma in primary sclerosing cholangitis. Gastroenterology 107: 537–542

Mauer H L, Hughes R W, Jarrett H F, Mosenthal 1967 Granulomatous hepatitis associated with regional enteritis. Gastroenterology 53: 301–305

May G R, Bender C E, LaRusso N F, Wiesner R H 1985 Non operative dilatation of dominant strictures in primary sclerosing cholangitis. American Journal of Radiology 145: 1061–1064

Minuk G Y, Hershfield N B, Lee W Y et al 1986 Reticuloendothelial system FC receptor-mediated clearance of IgG-tagged erythrocytes from the circulation of patients with idiopathic ulcerative colitis and chronic liver disease. Hepatology 6: 1–5

Mir-Madjlessi S H, Farmer R G, Sivak M V 1987 Bile duct carcinoma in patients with ulcerative colitis. Digestive Diseases and Sciences 32: 145–154

Mir-Madjlessi S H, McHenry M C, Farmer R G 1986 Liver abscess in Crohn's disease. Gastroenterology 91: 987–993

Mistilis S P 1965 Pericholangitis and ulcerative colitis: I pathology, aetiology and pathogenesis. Annals of Internal Medicine 63: 1–16

Mistilis S P, Dkyring A P, Goulston S J M 1965 Pericholangitis and ulcerative colitis: II Clinical aspects. Annals of Internal Medicine 63: 17–26

Olsson R, Hulten L 1975 Concurrence of ulcerative colitis and chronic active hepatitis. Clinical courses and results of colectomy. Scandinavian Journal of Gastroenterology 10: 331–335

Olsson R, Danielsson A, Jarnerot G, Lindstrom E, Loof L, Rolny P, Ryden B-O, Tysk C, Wallerstedt S 1991 Prevalence of primary sclerosing cholangitis in patients with ulcerative colitis. Gastroenterology 100: 1319–1323

Palmer K R, Duerden B I, Holdsworth C D 1980 Bacteriological and endotoxin studies in cases of ulcerative colitis submitted to surgery. Gut 21: 851–854

Palmer W L, Kirsner J B, Goldgraber M B, Fuenter S S 1964 Disease of the liver in chronic ulcerative colitis. American Journal of Medicine 36: 856–866

Parker R G F, Kendall E J C 1954 The liver in ulcerative colitis. British Medical Journal 2: 1030–1033

Perrett A D, Higgins G, Johnston H H, Massarella G, Truelove S C, Wright R 1971a The liver in ulcerative colitis. Quarterly Journal of Medicine 40: 211–238

Perrett A D, Higgins G, Johnston H H, Massarella G, Truelove S C, Wright R 1971b The liver in Crohn's disease. Quarterly Journal of Medicine 40: 187–209

Quigley E M M, LaRusso N F, Ludwig J, MacSween R N M, Birnie G G, Watkinson G 1983 Familial occurrence of primary sclerosing cholangitis and ulcerative colitis. Gastroenterology 85: 1160–1165

Rabinovitz M, Gavalier J S, Schade R R, Dindzans V J, Chien M-C, Van Thiel D H 1990 Does primary sclerosing cholangitis occurring in association with inflammatory bowel disease differ from that occurring in the absence of inflammatory bowel disease? A study of 66 subjects. Hepatology 11: 7–11

Ritchie J K, Allan R N, Macartney J et al 1974 Biliary tract carcinoma associated with ulcerative colitis. Quarterly Journal of Medicine 43: 263–279

Rosen C B, Nagorney D M, Wiesner R H, Coffey R J Jr, La Russo N F 1991 Cholangiocarcinoma complicating primary sclerosing cholangitis. Annals of Surgery 213: 21–25

Schrumpf E, Elgio K, Fuasa Q, Gjone F, Kolmannskog F, Ritland S 1980 Sclerosing cholangitis in ulcerative colitis. Scandinavian Journal of Gastroenterology 15: 689–697

Schrumpf E, Fausa O, Kolmannskog F, Elgjo K, Ritland S, Gjone E 1982a Sclerosing cholangitis in ulcerative colitis. A follow-up study. Scandinavian Journal of Gastroenterology 17: 33–39

Schrumpf E, Fausa O, Forre O, Doblong J H, Ritland S, Thorsby E 1982b HLA antigens and immunoregulatory T cells in ulcerative colitis associated with hepatobiliary disease. Scandinavian Journal of Gastroenterology 17: 187–191

Siegel J H, Barnes S, Morris J S 1977 Bile acids in liver disease associated with inflammatory bowel disease. Digestion 15: 469–481

Snook J A, Chapman R W, Fleming K, Jewell D P 1989 Antineutrophil nuclear antibody in ulcerative colitis, Crohn's disease and primary sclerosing cholangitis. Journal of Immunology (in press)

Thomas C H 1873 Ulceration of the colon with a much enlarged fatty liver. Transactions of the Pathology Society of Philadelphia 4: 87–88

Warren K W, Athanassiales S, Monge J I 1966 Primary sclerosing cholangitis. American Journal of Surgery 111: 23–38

Wee A, Ludwig J 1985 Pericholangitis in chronic ulcerative colitis: Primary sclerosing cholangitis of the small ducts? Annals of Internal Medicine 102: 581–587

Wee A, Ludwig J, Coffey R J et al 1985 Hepatobiliary carcinoma associated with primary sclerosing cholangitis and chronic ulcerative colitis. Human Pathology 16: 719–726

Wells I P, Wheeler P G, Laws J W, Williams R 1980 A new appearance of the common bile duct in sclerosing cholangitis. British Journal of Radiology 53: 502–504

Whiteside T L, Lasky S, Si L, VanThiel D H 1985 Immunologic analysis of mononuclear cells in liver tissues and blood of patients with primary sclerosing cholangitis. Hepatology 5: 468–474

Wiesner R H 1994 Current concepts in primary sclerosing cholangitis. Mayo Clinic Proceedings 69: 969–982

Wiesner R H, LaRusso N F 1980 Clinicopathologic features of the syndrome of primary sclerosing cholangitis. Gastroenterology 79: 200–206

Wiesner R H, LaRusso N F, Dozois R R, Beaver S J 1986 Peristomal varices after proctocolectomy in patients with primary sclerosing cholangitis. Gastroenterology 90: 316–322

72. Inflammatory bowel disease in childhood

C. M. Evans   R. M. Beattie   J. A. Walker-Smith

INTRODUCTION

Chronic inflammatory bowel disease in childhood includes Crohn's disease and ulcerative colitis and other, less well defined, entities such as indeterminate colitis, microscopic colitis and Behçet's enterocolitis.

The advent of safe endoscopy in pediatric practice over the past decade, even for very small infants, has transformed the pediatrician's ability to make an accurate diagnosis. Total colonoscopy, with inspection of the distal 5–10 cm of terminal ileum, can now be achieved in most children. Multiple biopsy of the colon and terminal ileum permits accurate histological diagnosis and has led to the recognition of other disorders, such as food-sensitive colitis (Jenkins et al 1984).

CROHN'S DISEASE

First reports of Crohn's disease in children

Dr Burrill Crohn made his very first observation of ileitis over 60 years ago in a child, a 14-year-old-boy (Crohn 1934). In his 1949 monograph, Crohn mentions a girl of 13 years described by Abercrombie in 1828 as a likely case, and reports six children under the age of 10 years at onset of disease in his personal series of 222 cases. However, Schiff (1945) first described a series of children with Crohn's disease (48 cases), culled from the world literature. He took particular care to exclude other disorders of the gastrointestinal tract resembling Crohn's disease, and established the condition as a childhood illness for the first time. Schiff also documented all the clinical features in children previously described in adults, including the classic triad of abdominal pain, weight loss and diarrhea.

In 1954, a report of 600 patients with Crohn's disease from the Mayo Clinic included 85 who had developed the disorder before 16 years of age. Moseley et al (1960) reviewed 28 pediatric cases and pointed out that lack of awareness of the disease in children frequently led to diagnostic delay: over half of their series had remained undiagnosed for a year or more after onset of symptoms.

Silverman (1966) stressed the effect of Crohn's disease upon growth and emphasized that children with the disorder may first present with short stature. O'Donoghue and Dawson (1977), in the first detailed study of children with Crohn's disease in the United Kingdom, also emphasized the frequent delay in making a diagnosis. Several further studies from St Bartholomew's Hospital have since described the features of Crohn's disease in childhood (Chong et al 1982, Sanderson & Walker-Smith 1985, Sanderson 1986).

Epidemiology and genetics

There have been few epidemiological studies directed at the pediatric age group. Ferguson et al (1986) conducted a postal survey on behalf of the British Paediatric Gastroenterology Group and recorded 447 children with Crohn's disease in the United Kingdom out of an estimated childhood population of 15 314 300, a prevalence of 4.91 per 100 000. However, this must have been an underestimate, since only 29% of the cases in Scotland recorded in the Scottish Hospital In-patient Statistics databank appeared in the survey. The true prevalence in the United Kingdom, therefore, may be nearer to ten per 100 000 children.

In Malmo, Brahme et al (1975) reported an incidence in children of 2.5 cases per 100 000 per year between 1958 and 1973, a figure similar to that found in adults (Ferguson et al 1986). The rise in incidence of Crohn's disease in adults has also been reported in children, even after allowing for improvements in diagnosis. Hellers (1979) noted that the incidence in Stockholm in children under 19 years of age increased from 2.5 per 100 000 between 1955 and 1959 to ten per 100 000 between 1970 and 1974. There is also evidence that the disease has increased threefold in Britain over the past two decades (Barton et al 1989). Figure 72.1 shows the rise in new cases of Crohn's disease per annum referred to the pediatric inflammatory bowel disease clinic at St Bartholomew's Hospital during the past 20 years.

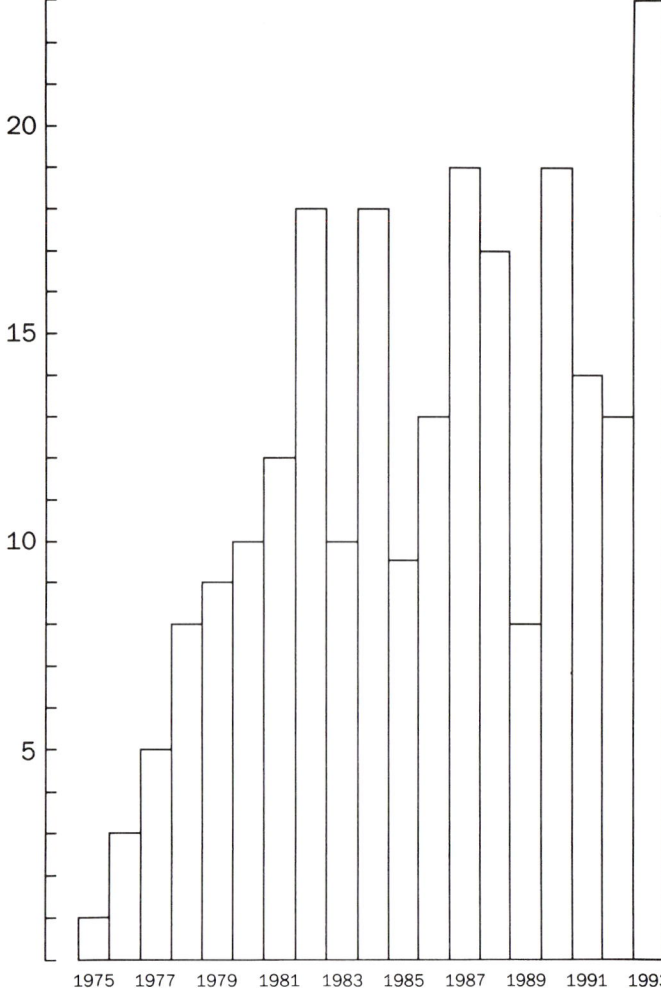

Fig. 72.1 Children with Crohn's disease. New referrals seen at St Bartholomew's Hospital, London

The geographical distribution of Crohn's disease is of great interest, being most prevalent in northwest Europe and North America. Among ethnic groups the condition is found in American caucasians and negroes, but not in African blacks. Exposure to a western environment, therefore, seems to be an important etiological factor. In the United Kingdom, black children of West Indian origin now account for 13% of the pediatric cases attending St Bartholomew's Hospital (Walker-Smith et al 1986). It was once considered so unusual to diagnose Crohn's disease in this ethnic group that individual case reports were published (Wallis & Walker-Smith 1976). In addition, increasing numbers of British children of Indian subcontinent origin are also presenting with the disease (Salim & Evans, unpublished observations), whereas the disorder is almost unknown in indigenous Asian children.

There is considerable variation in the prevalence of Crohn's disease among different caucasian groups. For example, 30% of the children attending the pediatric inflammatory bowel disease clinic at St Bartholomew's Hospital are of Jewish origin, far in excess of the number expected on demographic grounds.

With regard to environmental factors which may be of importance in the etiology of inflammatory bowel disease, cigarette smoking is known to increase the risk of developing Crohn's disease in adults (Calkins 1989). One recent study has also suggested a link between exposure to environmental cigarette smoke ('passive smoking') and an increased risk of developing the disease in childhood (Lashner et al 1993).

Children with Crohn's disease are more likely to have a family member with chronic inflammatory bowel disease than would be expected by chance. In a survey of 91 children attending St Bartholomew's Hospital (Sanderson et al 1986), 9% of first-degree and 6% of second-degree relatives were affected. This may be an underestimate, as some of the normal siblings of the children interviewed may yet develop the disease. There was an intermingling of Crohn's disease, ulcerative colitis and indeterminate colitis in these families, suggesting that the disorders may have a related genetic basis.

Further evidence that genetic factors are of importance in the etiology of Crohn's disease is that the great majority of identical twins are concordant for the disorder, whereas most non-identical twins are discordant.

Pathology in children

Crohn's disease may affect any part of the alimentary tract from mouth to anus. However, proximal small-bowel involvement appears to be more common in children than in adults. Table 72.1 indicates the major site of disease in 100 children diagnosed at St Bartholomew's Hospital, of whom 19 had pathology confined to the small bowel.

The gross pathology of the intestine in Crohn's disease is characteristic. The wall of the affected bowel becomes thickened, which may produce narrowing of the lumen and stricture formation leading to complete obstruction. In addition there is often longitudinal and transverse ulceration of the intestinal mucosa, which produces the characteristic 'cobblestoning' of the bowel surface.

Table 72.1 Major site of involvement in 100 children with biopsy-proven Crohn's disease seen at St Bartholomew's Hospital

Mouth alone	3
Extensive small bowel disease	5
Terminal ileum alone	14
Ileocecal disease	21
Ileocolonic disease	24
Colon alone	21
Extensive small bowel and colonic involvement	10
Perineum alone	2

Microscopic sinuses may pass from the ulcerated mucosal surface deep into the intestinal wall.

Histologically the lesions of Crohn's disease are typically transmural, with submucosal thickening being particularly characteristic. There is usually a diffuse inflammation of the submucosa consisting of acute and chronic inflammatory cells and often, but not always, epithelioid granulomata containing giant cells. In many cases the lymphoid follicles of the bowel also contain granulomas, and a granulomatous reaction has been described in the regional lymph nodes.

Morson (1968) has suggested that the frequency with which the terminal ileum and anal region are involved in Crohn's disease is explained by the fact that both of these areas are rich in lymphoid aggregates.

Clinical features of Crohn's disease in children

Most children with Crohn's disease present in early adolescence, with a mean age at diagnosis of 12 years. The condition is very uncommon before 7 years of age, and affects both sexes equally (Bender 1977). Isolated cases have been described in infancy; however, the accuracy of these early diagnoses and their relationship to Crohn's disease in older children is uncertain.

The early clinical manifestations of disease may be subtle and non-specific. Systemic features such as growth failure, pyrexia of unknown origin and weight loss may predominate, whereas gastrointestinal symptoms may be minimal or non-existent (Silverman 1966, Chrispin & Tempany 1967). This may account for the frequent delay in diagnosing Crohn's disease in childhood (Moseley et al 1960, Burbige et al 1975).

The first detailed clinical study of Crohn's disease in children reported from Britain was by O'Donoghue and Dawson (1977). Thirty-two patients were studied, all of whom presented with symptoms before their 16th birthday. In this series gastrointestinal complaints were the dominant feature, but unexplained fever and growth failure were frequent problems. The classic triad of abdominal pain, diarrhea and weight loss occurred commonly, and fever was reported more often than is usually seen in adult patients. As in previous studies there was a significant mean delay in diagnosis (2.9 years).

In a multicenter European study (Bender 1977) analysis of the symptoms of 155 children presenting with Crohn's disease revealed a similar picture, with abdominal pain in 90%, anorexia in 84% and diarrhea in 73%. Table 72.2 shows the incidence of clinical features at diagnosis of disease in 54 children referred to St Bartholomew's Hospital (Chong et al 1982).

Gastrointestinal manifestations

Gastrointestinal symptoms include abdominal pain, anorexia and diarrhea. Pain may be periumbilical in location or centered in one or other iliac fossa, depending on the site of disease. Periumbilical pain suggests small-bowel involvement, and is typically colicky in nature and exacerbated by eating. Pain located in the right iliac fossa is usually secondary to disease of the terminal ileum, and may be severe enough to present as an acute abdomen (pseudoappendicitis). Left-sided and infraumbilical pain of a crampy nature points to colonic disease, particularly if relieved by defecation.

Perianal disease is usually painless, but may cause steady, persistent localized pain in some patients. A tender abdominal mass may be palpable in up to 20% of children at presentation, usually located in the right lower quadrant and composed of loops of inflamed bowel. Occasionally the mass may indicate abscess formation.

Anorexia associated with Crohn's disease can be severe, prompting an erroneous diagnosis of anorexia nervosa, particularly when there is marked weight loss (Gryboski et al 1968). The diagnostic confusion is further compounded by the fact that the two disorders may coexist (Mallett & Murch 1990).

Most patients have chronic diarrhea of varying severity. However, diarrhea of acute onset may also occur, suggesting an infective enteritis, particularly if associated with nausea and vomiting. Nocturnal diarrhea is common, but urgency, soiling and tenesmus are unusual. Bloody diarrhea also occurs in Crohn's disease, particularly when the colon is involved, but is much less common than in ulcerative colitis. Fresh blood on the surface of the stool may be secondary to the presence of an anal fissure. Rarely, hemorrhage from a segment of ulcerated bowel may be severe and require urgent resuscitation, with a blood transfusion and emergency surgery to arrest bleeding.

Chronic constipation may cause diagnostic confusion, particularly when regarded as the cause of the child's abdominal pain. Nausea, dyspepsia and epigastric

Table 72.2 Incidence of clinical features at diagnosis of Crohn's disease in 54 children attending St Bartholomew's Hospital (data from Chong et al 1982)

Symptoms		Signs	
Abdominal pain	85%	Weight loss	52%
Weight loss	78%	Growth retardation	46%
Anorexia	75%	Perianal abnormality	46%
Lethargy	75%	Tender abdomen	34%
Diarrhea	72%	Pallor	32%
Poor growth	43%	Abdominal distension	32%
Rectal bleeding	28%	No significant	
Perianal symptoms	25%	abnormality	10%
Urgency of		Mouth lesions	8%
defecation	25%	Finger clubbing	8%
Tenesmus	25%	Abdominal mass	6%
Fever	22%	Erythema nodosum	6%
Nausea/vomiting	22%	Peripheral edema	6%
Constipation	20%	Uveitis	4%
Skin rashes	15%	Toxic megacolon	0%
Joint pains	10%	Rectal prolapse	0%
Mouth ulcers	8%	Jaundice	0%

tenderness may be present when there is involvement of the duodenum, which may be attributed to peptic ulceration. In addition, a child with diffuse small-bowel Crohn's disease may present with a chronic malabsorption syndrome or features of a protein-losing enteropathy.

About 10% of children will have lesions in the mouth at presentation. These can vary from mild, recurrent aphthous ulcers on the tongue, fauces, palate or buccal mucosa to marked swelling and ulceration of the lips, gums and buccal mucosa. Linear ulceration at the reflection of the buccal mucosa on to the gum is often seen. Another common finding is cracking and fissuring at the corners of the mouth (angular cheilitis).

Perianal Crohn's disease is common in children (Palder et al 1991): over 50% of cases have some perianal abnormality, which can take a variety of forms. There may be one or more anal fissures, which are usually painless. Perianal excoriation and skin tags are common and perianal abscesses may also occur. More severe involvement may lead to fistula-in-ano or an ischiorectal abscess requiring surgical drainage. When perianal disease occurs as the sole manifestation of Crohn's disease in children, diagnosis is often significantly delayed (Wallis & Walker-Smith 1976). Diagnostic confusion can also arise between perianal Crohn's disease and the lesions seen in child sexual abuse, where the presenting abnormalities may be very similar (Evans & Walker-Smith 1988).

Systemic manifestations

The systemic impact of Crohn's disease in the pediatric age group is significant (Rankin et al 1979). At diagnosis, approximately two-thirds of patients will both look and feel systemically unwell. Anorexia, lethargy, change in personality, fever, pallor and weight loss may dominate the clinical picture, with few gastrointestinal symptoms, particularly in those with small-bowel disease. The most significant systemic complication of the disease in children, however, is its effect on growth and maturity (Kirschner et al 1978). At diagnosis, up to a quarter of patients are below the third centile for height and nearly half are significantly underweight (Evans & Walker-Smith 1989). In children of appropriate age, significant delay of pubertal development will be found in at least one-third.

Growth failure and poor nutritional status are probably secondary to a combination of an inadequate calorie intake (Kelts et al 1979, Kirschner et al 1981) and active bowel inflammation (Motil et al 1993). Severe nutritional insufficiency may also result from bacterial overgrowth in the bowel (blind-loop syndrome) and losses from enteric fistulae. Some studies have suggested that malabsorption alone does not contribute significantly to growth failure (Kelts et al 1979, Kirschner et al 1981), although protein, mineral and trace element losses are all increased in the presence of active bowel inflammation (Motil et al 1985, Murch et al 1993a). Long-term corticosteroid therapy is a potent suppressor of linear growth (Friedmann & Strang 1966), and this may play a role in some children. The etiology of growth failure is discussed in greater detail later (see complications), and has been well reviewed by Brain and Savage (1994).

Growth failure accompanied by unexplained fever, anemia and other constitutional disturbances in a child with elevated acute-phase proteins or erythrocyte sedimentation rate should always raise the possibility of Crohn's disease. A similar clinical picture in an adolescent with delayed puberty should also arise suspicion of the disease. Crohn's disease is much more likely to suppress growth and puberty than is ulcerative colitis (Kirschner et al 1978).

Fever occurs in up to one-quarter of children, and may well occur more frequently but remain undiagnosed. It is usually low grade and intermittent, often recurring at a particular time of the day. Occasionally, a child will present with a high, swinging pyrexia associated with a striking tachycardia, a general appearance often described as 'toxic'.

Finger clubbing is found in about 10% of children with Crohn's disease at presentation, and erythema nodosum in approximately 6% (Table 72.1). Other dermatological manifestations include pyoderma gangrenosum and papulonecrotic lesions, both of which are rare (Greenstein et al 1976). Skin lesions are usually, though not always, most active during relapses of intestinal disease. Pyoderma gangrenosum may prove refractory to treatment and require intensive long-term local and systemic therapy.

Arthralgia and arthritis are common findings, occurring in up to 15% of children (Lindsey & Schaller 1974), and may precede bowel symptoms by months or even years. Larger joints tend to be most commonly affected, such as the knee, hip, ankle and wrist, usually in a monoarticular fashion. Joint destruction and deformity are very rare, however. Ankylosing spondylitis has been reported in children with Crohn's disease, particularly in association with HLA B27 (Passo et al 1986).

Anterior uveitis (iritis) is an uncommon but important finding in association with Crohn's disease in children, and requires careful follow-up. There is no apparent relationship between the activity of bowel disease and ocular inflammation (Hofley et al 1993). Other ophthalmological problems include conjunctivitis and episcleritis.

Liver disease is a rare complication of Crohn's disease in children, but chronic active hepatitis, pericholangitis and liver abscesses have all been reported. Hepatic complications may precede bowel symptoms (Kane et al 1980), with the child presenting with pruritis secondary to hyperbilirubinemia. Renal calculi are found in up to 6% of children with Crohn's disease (Greenstein et al 1976): they are usually composed of calcium oxalate, owing to enhanced absorption of oxalate through inflamed bowel mucosa. Secondary amyloidosis has also been reported in the pediatric literature (Kirschner & Samanowitz 1986).

Psychiatric problems are common in children with Crohn's disease (Szajnberg et al 1993), particularly in adolescence. The emotional sequelae of chronic inflammatory bowel disease in childhood have been well documented by Bruce (1986). Most children are remarkably stoical, but occasionally some will become anxious and depressed. Contributory factors include missing school because of illness or hospital admissions, feeling embarrassed about the nature of their symptoms, difficulty in forming relationships within their peer group, undesirable side effects related to treatment, and the prospect of having to accept a long-term stoma.

Bruce has also described the 'infantilizing' effect of chronic inflammatory bowel disease in some families: parental preoccupation with their child's bowel habits may become positively unhealthy, leading them to treat their adolescent offspring as if they were still at the toilet training stage. As a result, a minority of children come to regard themselves as chronic invalids and play up their symptoms accordingly.

Many of the systemic manifestations described above also occur in ulcerative colitis (see later). Overall, however, extraintestinal complications of inflammatory bowel disease are significantly more common among children with Crohn's disease than those with ulcerative colitis.

Diagnosis

Confirming a diagnosis of Crohn's disease in childhood is based on a combination of clinical, radiological, endoscopic and histopathological parameters (Chong et al 1982). A practical approach to diagnosis is illustrated in Figure 72.2. A detailed clinical assessment includes a complete history and physical examination, with particular attention to weight, growth and pubertal development, and a number of blood tests.

A presumptive diagnosis is usually made when radiological investigations demonstrate the typical abnormalities of Crohn's disease in a child with compatible clinical features. A definite diagnosis can subsequently, be

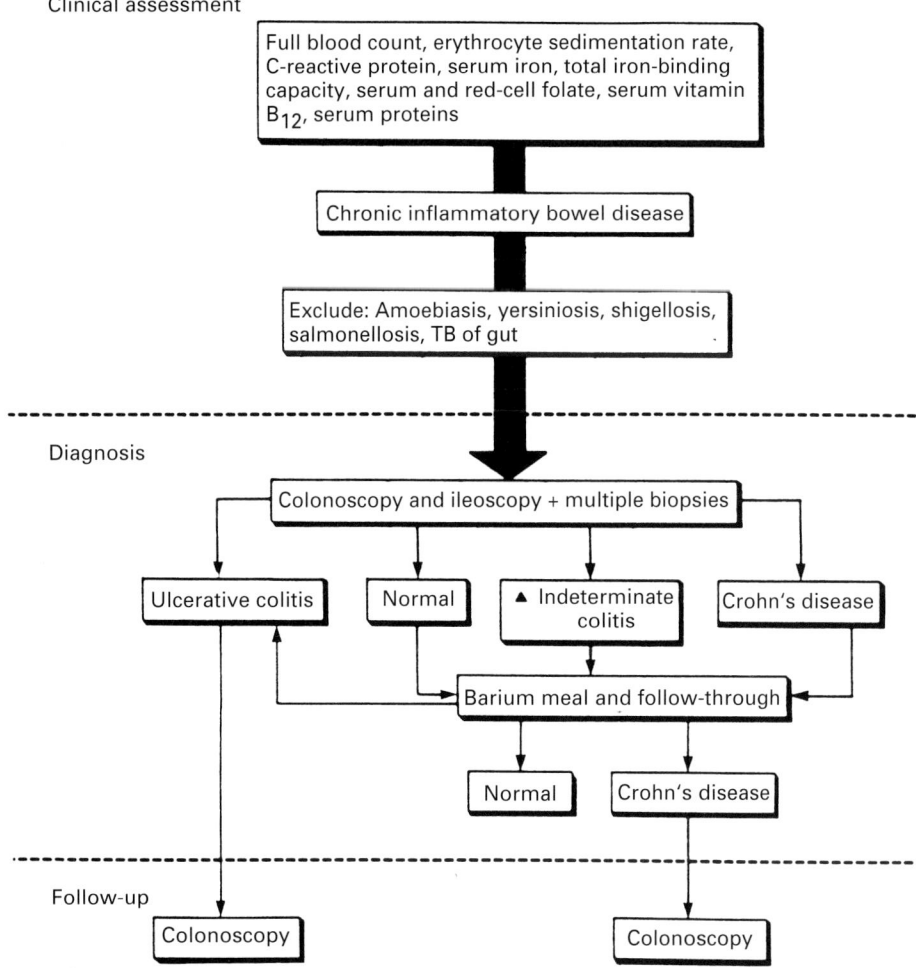

Fig. 72.2 A practical approach to the diagnosis of Crohn's disease.

Table 72.3 Histological diagnosis of chronic inflammatory bowel disease in children (Chong et al 1985)

Definite ulcerative colitis
Acute inflammation with severe crypt cell distortion and diffuse goblet cell (mucus) depletion. Inflammation is diffuse and solely mucosal. Vascularity is increased

Probable ulcerative colitis
(a) Diffuse mucosal inflammation with only mild or moderate crypt distortion, mucosal atrophy or mucus depletion. (b) Diffuse acute and chronic inflammation with increased vascularity but little mucus depletion, suggesting resolving phase

Indeterminate colitis
Some features suggestive of both ulcerative colitis and Crohn's disease

Probable Crohn's disease
One or more of the following features present: (a) focal inflammation; (b) submucosal or transmural inflammation; (c) lymphocyte aggregates (without germinal centers); (d) mucus retention in the presence of more than minimal inflammation

Definite Crohn's disease
Any or all of the above, together with either (a) non-caseating granulomata or (b) fissuring ulceration.

established when the characteristic histological abnormalities are found in endoscopic biopsies (Williams et al 1982) or in bowel removed at surgery. Biopsy of oral or anal lesions may also be of value for diagnostic purposes.

We recommend total colonoscopy with ileal biopsy in all children with suspected inflammatory bowel disease. This enables direct visualization of the colonic and ileal mucosa, from which multiple biopsies can be obtained. Following endoscopy we perform a barium meal and follow-through, using acceleration and compression techniques to visualize the terminal ileum adequately (McLean & Bartram 1990). Barium or 'instant' enemas are no longer performed as a first-line investigation in children referred to St Bartholomew's Hospital, but are useful for specific indications, such as the assessment of fulminant colitis and colonic strictures (Thomas 1979). A firm diagnosis should be possible in most patients following the above investigations, with histology remaining the final arbiter.

Some authorities demand the demonstration of non-caseating granulomas in biopsies of the bowel mucosa or submucosa before accepting a diagnosis of Crohn's disease. However, in a large retrospective histopathological study of 385 children with clinically proven Crohn's disease (Schmitz-Moormann & Schag 1990) granulomas were only present in the colonic biopsies of 42%. Others consider patchy inflammatory changes, with granulation tissue containing epithelioid cells and giant cells, as sufficient evidence, even in the absence of definite granulomas. Table 72.3 outlines the histological findings commonly found in colitis and relates them to the likely diagnosis (Chong et al 1985).

Differential diagnosis

The presenting clinical picture in Crohn's disease and ulcerative colitis is often similar, and biopsy histology may be the only means of differentiating between the two conditions. Bacterial and parasitic infections must be excluded, particularly *Yersinia enterocolitica* (O'Morain 1981), campylobacter, salmonella, shigella, enteropathogenic *Escherichia coli* (Pai 1984) and amebic colitis (Sanderson & Walker-Smith 1984). Ileocecal tuberculosis should also be considered, particularly in certain predisposed ethnic groups. Behçet's syndrome (see later) may cause a colitis resembling Crohn's disease (Chong et al 1986).

In some children hyperplasia of lymphoid follicles within the terminal ileum can simulate the radiological abnormalities seen in early Crohn's disease. This condition, known as lymphoid nodular hyperplasia (LNH), is a relatively common finding in children and is of unknown etiology. The child may present with a clinical syndrome resembling inflammatory bowel disease, with abdominal pain, diarrhea and rectal bleeding. The disorder can be distinguished from Crohn's disease with certainty by direct visualization and biopsy of the terminal ileum at colonoscopy. LNH usually runs a benign course, with a high rate of spontaneous remission.

Chronic granulomatous disease (CGD) is an important differential diagnosis of Crohn's disease in younger children. This rare disorder of childhood is characterized by recurrent infections with catalase-positive bacteria, which the patient's neutrophils can phagocytose but not kill. The mucosa of both small and large bowel is often chronically inflamed and contains granulomas (Harris & Boles 1973). The condition may present with chronic diarrhea, perianal suppuration and growth retardation. It is distinguished from Crohn's disease by demonstrating a flat response to the nitroblue tetrazolium (NBT) test. CGD should be considered in any child presenting with clinical features of Crohn's disease at a very early age (Isaacs et al 1985).

In the past, general practitioners and pediatricians alike have often been slow to consider the possibility of Crohn's disease in a child, leading to long delays in confirming the diagnosis. Fortunately, increasing awareness that the condition exists in childhood, coupled with better diagnostic techniques, has resulted in a significant reduction in the interval between presentation and diagnosis.

Investigations

A full blood count may reveal anemia due to either blood loss or poor nutritional intake. The serum iron and ferritin levels are often low. Folate deficiency is usually due to poor dietary intake, but may occur secondary to malabsorption from extensive small-bowel disease. Thus a low serum folate may be a pointer to disease of the small intestine (Chong et al 1982). Frank megaloblastic anemia due to vitamin B_{12} deficiency is rare in children with Crohn's disease, despite the frequency of terminal ileal pathology. However, a Schilling test for B_{12} absorption may be abnormal. Thrombocytosis is common and a useful marker of active disease.

The erythrocyte sedimentation rate (ESR) is usually elevated, but may be normal despite clinically active disease. Acute-phase proteins, such as C-reactive protein (CRP), α-acid glycoprotein and $α_1$-antitrypsin, correlate well with disease activity (Campbell et al 1982). In particular, the CRP is of value in predicting early relapse in asymptomatic or mildly symptomatic patients. We routinely monitor both the ESR and CRP as indicators of disease activity in all our pediatric patients.

Hypoalbuminemia may be present due to enteric protein losses, and is occasionally severe enough to cause edema. Malabsorption is rare, despite the frequency of small-bowel involvement in childhood Crohn's disease, but serum electrolytes, minerals and trace elements, such as zinc and magnesium, may be low in long-standing disease.

Serology should be checked to exclude antibodies to *Yersinia enterocolitica* (ELISA technique) and *Entamoeba histolytica* (fluorescent antibody test). Stools should be examined for ova, cysts and parasites and cultured for enteric pathogens. A Mantoux and chest X-ray should be performed to look for tuberculosis.

A plain abdominal X-ray may reveal abnormal segments of bowel in Crohn's disease, but barium contrast studies are required to delineate the extent and nature of bowel involvement. However, barium radiographs may not be helpful in the early stages of the disease (Silverman 1966). The earliest change seen radiologically is aphthoid ulceration, which may deform the normal fold pattern of the mucosa. In more severe disease there is deep linear ulceration and edema of the bowel wall, leading to the typical 'rosethorn' ulceration and 'cobblestoning' of the mucosa seen on barium studies. The affected bowel becomes narrowed and subsequent fibrosis may produce stenotic lesions of the bowel ('string sign of Kantor'). In addition, gross thickening of the bowel wall produces wide separation of adjacent loops of gut radiologically. Asymmetrical involvement of the bowel is characteristic of Crohn's disease, producing the classic 'skip lesions' seen in contrast studies. An X-ray of the wrist should be performed in all children with suspected Crohn's disease to determine the bone age. This is generally delayed by a mean of 2 years at time of diagnosis.

Fiberoptic colonoscopy with multiple biopsies is now the investigation of choice in children with suspected Crohn's disease of the large bowel and/or terminal ileum. The main advantage of colonoscopy over barium enema is the ability to take biopsy material to provide a definitive histological diagnosis. The procedure can be performed quite safely in children under intravenous sedation following standard bowel preparation. A recent audit of 191 new pediatric referrals to St Bartholomew's Hospital with suspected inflammatory bowel disease or unexplained rectal bleeding confirmed the high diagnostic yield of endoscopy: 104 examinations were abnormal and provided histological confirmation of the disease involved in each case (Evans, unpublished observations).

Colonoscopy readily demonstrates the extent and severity of Crohn's disease of the colon and terminal ileum in children. The earliest lesion visible macroscopically is the aphthoid ulcer, a 1–2 mm lesion which occurs directly over mucosal lymphoid follicles. More advanced disease causes diffuse or segmental hyperemia and friability of the mucosa, with loss of the normal vascular pattern. Severe inflammation leads to the formation of deep linear ulcers, with sloughing and cobblestoning of the mucosa. Characteristically the lesions are patchy in distribution, with intervening areas of normal-looking mucosa; however, in fulminating disease the whole colon may become friable and ulcerated. Endoscopy may also reveal the presence of inflammatory strictures.

Complications of Crohn's disease in childhood

Delay of growth and pubertal development

The association of Crohn's disease with growth retardation and delayed sexual maturation is extremely important. The cause of growth impairment is not clear, but is likely to be multifactorial: poor nutrition, malabsorption, 'toxic bowel', circulating inflammatory mediators, endocrine abnormalities and corticosteroid therapy may all play a part. It is of concern that two recent studies (Markowitz et al 1993a, Hildebrand et al 1994) have shown that permanent impairment of linear growth leading to a reduction in ultimate adult height is a common finding in childhood Crohn's disease. In contrast, however, Ferguson and Sedgwick (1994) have recently reported normal adult height achievement in most young people with inflammatory bowel disease who were growth retarded in their teenage years.

Earlier studies demonstrated a suboptimal growth hormone response to hypoglycemic stress in a minority of children with Crohn's disease (McCaffery et al 1974a, b, Chong et al 1984) and an impaired plasma gonadotrophin response to stimulation (Green et al 1977), both suggestive of hypopituitarism. Farthing et al (1981) investigated nocturnal growth hormone and gonadotrophin secretion in five growth-retarded children with Crohn's disease; in three, mean growth hormone levels were reduced, but the normal pulsatile pattern of growth hormone secretion was preserved. Nocturnal growth hormone secretion correlated significantly with disease activity, severity and gonadotrophin secretion, but not with growth velocity.

More recently, Braegger et al (1993) have shown no significant difference in urinary growth hormone excretion between growth-impaired children with chronic inflammatory bowel disease and normal controls. Thus, it seems that, although hypothalamic–pituitary function may be depressed in growth-retarded children with Crohn's disease, growth hormone secretion is normal. In addition, administration of human growth hormone to growth-retarded children with chronic inflammatory bowel disease is usually ineffective (McCaffery et al 1974a, b).

However, other studies have shown that insulin-like growth factor-1 (IGF-1), which mediates the effects of growth hormone in the periphery, is reduced in active inflammatory bowel disease and returns to normal levels following treatment (Thomas et al 1993b). IGF-1 is bound in the circulation to various carrier proteins, including IGF-binding proteins 1 and 3. IGF-BP3 is also reduced in active Crohn's disease, and also improves to normal levels following therapy (Camacho-Hubner et al 1993). Thus, growth impairment in active inflammatory bowel disease may be related to reduction of growth hormone effectiveness at the peripheral level, rather than through impaired secretion.

Recently, much interest has centered on the role of circulating inflammatory cytokines, such as tumor necrosis factor-α (TNFα), as potential mediators of growth suppression in children with chronic inflammatory bowel disease (Murch et al 1991). Some studies have shown TNF and other proinflammatory cytokines to be raised in the serum, gut and stools of children with active bowel disease (Braegger et al 1992, Murch et al 1993b), returning to normal following treatment. This may be one explanation for the rapid improvement in growth velocity usually observed in growth-retarded children with Crohn's disease following surgical resection of diseased bowel (Lipson et al 1990, McLain et al 1990).

Other complications

Intestinal obstruction is a common complication of small-bowel Crohn's disease in children, as are fistulae and abscess formation. All may require surgical intervention.

Toxic megacolon and colonic perforation may occasionally complicate Crohn's colitis in children, and we have also seen one child with spontaneous perforation of the ileum.

Studies in adults with long-standing Crohn's disease suggest a higher than expected incidence of intestinal carcinoma, but this is much lower than in chronic ulcerative colitis. One large study in adults (Binder et al 1985) has estimated a cancer risk of only 0.56% by 10 years after diagnosis. The relative risk of developing malignancy in Crohn's disease beginning in childhood has not been accurately determined, but individual cases have been reported (Michelassi et al 1993).

Management of Crohn's disease

The approach to the treatment of Crohn's disease in childhood will depend upon the severity of the presenting illness and the frequency and nature of subsequent relapses. Most newly diagnosed cases will require hospital admission to initiate treatment, and admission with bed rest is advisable in children with severe disease. Patients with mild to moderate relapses can often be managed on an outpatient basis. A careful explanation of the nature of the disorder, its possible implications and the need for continuing treatment and medical supervision should be given to the child and parents. It should be emphasized that the child's illness should interfere as little as possible with normal family life. Continuing psychological counselling and support are important.

All patients should have a full auxological and dietary assessment. A nutritious, balanced diet should be advised to optimize growth, and formal dietetic counseling is therefore advisable. Calorie supplementation may be necessary in children with anorexia, and vitamin, mineral and trace element supplements are required in some cases. Highly specialized forms of dietary therapy may have a significant impact in children with Crohn's disease and are discussed below.

The aim of therapy is to induce and maintain a remission of the patient's symptoms and disease activity. There are three basic forms of treatment: drugs, enteral nutrition and surgery. In addition, total parenteral nutrition may be required as an adjunct in malnourished children with severe disease.

Drug treatment

Medications used in the management of Crohn's disease in childhood are basically the same as those used to treat adult patients.

The first-line drugs are sulfasalazine (Salazopyrin) and mesalazine (Asacol, Pentasa), which are generally used to induce remission in patients with mild disease (Malchow et al 1984). Used alone, sulfasalazine is most useful for inducing and maintaining remission in patients with mild colonic disease. It is less effective in the treatment of small-bowel involvement (Summers et al 1979, Malchow et al 1984). More recently, mesalazine has been introduced and is a form of 5-aminosalicylic acid which lacks the sulfur component found in sulfasalazine. This drug is as effective as sulfasalazine in inducing and maintaining remission in children with mild chronic inflammatory bowel disease of the colon, but with fewer adverse effects (Barden et al 1989). It also appears to have a beneficial effect in diffuse small-bowel Crohn's disease (Griffiths et al 1993).

The dose of sulfasalazine recommended for use in children is 50 mg/kg/day in two to four divided doses, and that for mesalazine is 20 mg/kg/day in two divided doses. Nausea, vomiting and headaches are relatively common side effects, and patients should be warned that sulfasalazine discolors the urine. Serious side effects are uncommon, and more frequent with sulfasalazine. They include allergic reactions, exfoliative dermatitis, hemolytic anemia, transient oligospermia and bone marrow suppression.

Children with more severe disease usually require therapy with corticosteroids, which have been shown to be more effective than sulfasalazine in inducing remission in adult patients (Summers et al 1979). Systemically administered prednisolone is effective for treating acute exacerbations of Crohn's disease and will induce a good remission in the majority of children. Prednisolone is given orally at a dosage of 1–2 mg/kg per day (maximum dose 40 mg daily) until remission is achieved, which usually takes 3–4 weeks. The dosage is then gradually reduced over a period of 6–8 weeks, daily at first, then on alternate days (Table 72.4). In the most severe cases, where a rapid therapeutic response is desired, intravenous therapy with hydrocortisone may be given, 5–10 mg/kg per day in four divided doses. Treatment is then continued with oral prednisolone at the dosage described above. Once remission of disease has been achieved with prednisolone, the aim should be to discontinue steroid therapy completely and maintain remission with sulfasalazine/mesalazine alone.

Rectal steroids are useful in children with proctitis and distal colonic disease; their use is discussed under the management of ulcerative colitis. Topical steroid creams (e.g. Scheriproct) may be helpful in the management of mild perianal disease.

Unfortunately, a minority of children will remain steroid dependent, with the consequent risk of adverse effects from long-term therapy. The most worrying complication associated with chronic steroid use in children is growth suppression (Friedmann & Strang 1966). The risk of this occurring can be minimized, but not always prevented, by using an alternate-day steroid regimen at the lowest possible dosage to maintain adequate remission. Untreated, chronically active bowel inflammation is more likely to cause growth suppression than steroid therapy. Indeed, some children actually experience an increase in growth velocity while taking corticosteroids, as their disease becomes less active. However, severe osteoporosis can occur in a minority of children requiring long-term high-dose therapy. Accordingly, a balance between symptomatic relief and the side effects of chronic steroid usage must be reached in these children.

The role of immunosuppressive therapy for Crohn's disease in childhood is unproven. Both azathioprine (Verhave et al 1990) and 6-mercaptopurine (Perrault et al 1991) have been advocated for use as steroid-sparing agents in children with signs of steroid toxicity and for severe, extensive disease unresponsive to conventional therapy and not amenable to surgery. Studies in adults have suggested that azathioprine is ineffective at a dose of 1 mg/kg per day (Summers et al 1979), but may produce an improvement in disease activity at dosages approaching 2 mg/kg per day (Lennard-Jones 1981). If used, the drug should be continued for at least 3 months to assess the therapeutic response adequately.

Azathioprine therapy should not be undertaken lightly. There are a number of potentially serious complications, although these are rare in practice. An influenza-like illness may occur shortly after commencing treatment, but this is usually self-limiting and not an indication for drug withdrawal. Bone marrow suppression, particularly leukopenia, may occur and therefore regular blood counts should be performed while treatment continues. Pancreatitis is another rare complication. Fortunately, long-term use of azathioprine in childhood does not seem to be associated with toxic effects on the reproductive system, as have been described for cyclofosfamide. The development of lymphoma remains a potential, albeit unknown, risk.

Table 72.4 Drugs used in the treatment of chronic inflammatory bowel disease

5-aminosalicylic acid derivatives	
Sulfasalazine	May be given orally or per rectum. 500 mg plain or enteric-coated tabs available
	Elixer (250 mg per 5 ml) may also be prepared
	Enemas contain 3 g in 100 ml of vehicle
	500 mg suppositories also available
	Acute relapse: 40–60 mg/kg/day in 3–4 doses
	Maintenance: 20–30 mg/kg/day in 2–3 doses
	Treatment continued until 2 years of remission
Mesalazine	400 mg enteric-coated capsules available
	Dosage: 20 mg/kg/day
	Maintenance treatment as for sulfasalazine
Corticosteroids	
ACTH	Intramuscular injection used during acute relapse 2 iu/kg/day for 5 days, followed by prednisolone
Prednisolone	May be given orally or per rectum
	Orally: 1–2 mg/kg/day in 2–3 doses for 4 weeks, then gradually reduced to alternate days
	Enema: Prednisolone-2, 1-phosphate, 5–10 mg tabs in 25–50 ml water × 1–2 daily via a Jacques catheter
Hydrocortisone acetate 10% (Colifoam)	Aerosol foam enema administered via the supplied applicator × 1–2 daily. Each dose contains 125 mg hydrocortisone acetate
Predsol	Available as enema or 5mg suppositories. Enema contains 20 mg prednisolone in 100 ml vehicle
	Administer enema × 1 daily, suppositories × 2 daily
Azathioprine	Immunosuppressive, used as a steroid-sparing agent
	Administered orally. 50 mg tablets available
	Dosage: 2 mg/kg/day as a single dose
	Monitor blood count closely
Metronidazole	Used for treatment of perianal disease
	Administered orally. 200 and 400 mg tabs available
	Dosage: 15 mg/kg/day in × 3 divided dose.

Recently, interest has been aroused in the use of cyclosporin A in the management of adult patients with Crohn's disease which has proved refractory to conventional therapy (Brynskov et al 1989, Hodgson 1991, Sandborn & Tremaine 1992). This powerful immunosuppressive drug is commonly used to combat rejection following organ transplantation. A recent randomized controlled trial in children at St Bartholomew's Hospital (Nicholls et al, in press) showed oral cyclosporin to be as effective as conventional therapy in the management of acute relapses of Crohn's disease, but not superior. In addition, there were problems with drug absorption and renal toxicity.

Metronidazole has been used to good effect in adult patients with perianal Crohn's disease (Bernstein et al 1980). It is sometimes beneficial in children with severe anal complications which have not responded to other medications. One study has also reported an improvement in both small-bowel and colonic disease in adult patients given a 4-month course of the drug (Ursing et al 1982). The dose is usually 15 mg/kg/day. Peripheral neuropathy has been reported in adults on long-term therapy, for which the clinician should remain vigilant.

Crohn's disease of the mouth in childhood may prove very resistant to treatment. Angular cheilitis may respond to the application of a topical steroid cream, such as triamcinolone acetonide (Adcortyl cream, Squibb). Aphthous stomatitis may be helped by the use of triamcinolone in a carboxymethylcellulose gelatin paste (Adcortyl in Orabase, Squibb) or hydrocortisone sodium succinate lozenges (Corlan, Glaxo) applied topically to the ulcers. More severe oral disease can be treated by direct injection of corticosteroids into the lesions or with oral prednisolone.

Symptomatic medications have a limited role in the treatment of inflammatory bowel disease in children. Antidiarrheal drugs, such as loperamide and codeine phosphate, may provide symptomatic relief in mild relapses, and abdominal pain is sometimes helped by an antispasmodic such as mebeverine. However, in general therapy should be aimed at controlling symptoms by reducing disease activity rather than by masking its effects.

New therapeutic strategies currently under investigation in Crohn's disease include anti-CD4 monoclonal antibody therapy (Emmrich et al 1991), interferon α2a therapy (Hadziselomovic & Emmons 1990) and antitumor necrosis factor (TNF) monoclonal antibody therapy (Derkx et al 1993).

Enteral nutrition

Elemental diets were first developed at the National Institute of Health in the United States as part of the space exploration program. Studies showed that animals fed a simple diet composed of sugars, amino acids and medium-chain fatty acids only, continued to grow and reproduce normally (Greenstein et al 1957). Later work in healthy human volunteers, given an elemental diet as their sole source of nutrition for 19 weeks, revealed no ill effects (Winitz et al 1965). Stephens and Randall (1969) noted reversal of weight loss in an adult patient with Crohn's disease treated with an elemental diet. Elemental diets then found favor among surgeons, who used them in adult patients with Crohn's disease to improve their nutritional status prior to surgery (Voitk et al 1973, Rocchio et al 1973).

Subsequently, the complete cessation of normal dietary intake and its replacement with an elemental diet, either given orally or via a nasogastric tube, has been used as first-line management in Crohn's disease. Giorgini et al (1973) demonstrated resolution of terminal ileal inflammation in a child with Crohn's disease, using barium follow-through radiography before and after treatment with an elemental diet. Studies in adults have also revealed definite evidence of disease remission following elemental diets (Axelsson & Jarnum 1977, O'Morain 1979, O'Morain et al 1980, Logan et al 1981).

A number of studies have now shown elemental diets to be very effective in the management of children with Crohn's disease. Navarro et al (1982) reported their successful use in children with severe malnutrition and persistent symptoms despite conventional medical therapy, particularly as a transitional feeding regimen following total parenteral nutrition. Morin et al (1980) reported clinical improvement and an acceleration in growth in four growth-retarded children with Crohn's disease treated with an elemental diet. Two other studies (Morin et al 1982, O'Morain et al 1983) have also reported a significant clinical response to this therapy in children.

Sanderson et al (1987), at St Bartholomew's Hospital, have demonstrated that an elemental diet (Flexical, Mead Johnson) is as effective as high-dose steroid therapy in inducing remission of symptoms in children with Crohn's disease of the small bowel. In addition, growth acceleration was superior in the elemental diet group, a finding confirmed by Thomas et al (1993a) in a more recent report which included patients with colonic disease. Two other studies (Belli et al 1988, Polk et al 1992) have also demonstrated an improvement in growth, weight gain and disease activity by the use of long-term intermittent therapy with an elemental diet over a 12-month period.

The method of administering the elemental diet is not crucial for its efficacy (Sanderson 1986). However, as the majority of children are anorexic prior to starting therapy and as most of the preparations used are highly unpalatable, administration via a nasogastric tube is usually required. In the past we have used Flexical at St Bartholomew's Hospital as the elemental diet of choice. This is a semi-elemental preparation available in powder form for reconstitution with water, and contains corn syrup, hydrolyzed casein, soya oil, modified tapioca starch, medium-chain triglycerides, vitamins and minerals. It contains 9.9% protein, 66.9% carbohydrate and 15% fat by volume, and is gluten-and lactose-free.

The reconstituted solution is usually drip-fed via the nasogastric route and given overnight, where possible, to enable the child to attend school during the day if well enough. Treatment should be started in hospital under the close supervision of a dietitian and then continued at home. No food other than Flexical is allowed for a total of 6 weeks, following which food is slowly reintroduced in a controlled manner over a further 6 weeks (Sanderson et al 1987). The volume of Flexical is gradually reduced as the calorie intake from food increases. Ideally, the child is back on a normal diet after 3 months and remains in remission.

Elemental diets are most suitable for treating children with predominantly small-bowel disease. In our experience this regimen is less effective in the management of disease confined to the large bowel. The majority of children tolerate elemental diets remarkably well; nevertheless, considerable willpower is required to refrain from eating during the initial 6 weeks of treatment.

More recently, polymeric diets have been used to induce remission in both small- and large-bowel Crohn's disease. Published work in adult patients suggests a similar efficacy and relapse rate to elemental formulae and steroid therapy (Rigaud et al 1991, Gonzalez-Huix 1993). The main advantage of a polymeric formula compared to an elemental or semielemental one is that it contains whole protein and, as a consequence, is more palatable. Our own experience at St Bartholomew's Hospital using a casein-based polymeric feed suggests that this diet is as effective and better tolerated than the semielemental formula (Flexical) used previously (Beattie et al 1994, in press).

Surgery

Surgery is usually reserved for the management of complications of Crohn's disease, such as intestinal obstruction, fistulae and anorectal problems. It is not a curative therapy, as disease tends to recur elsewhere in the bowel. Early surgery should be considered for localized disease when medical therapy yields suboptimal results. Surgery may also be indicated for the relief of symptoms where medical treatment has failed, and for extraintestinal complications, such as growth failure. Farmer and Michener (1979) found that 69% of 522 patients with Crohn's disease starting in childhood required surgery within a mean of 7.7 years of diagnosis. Puntis et al (1984) reported an even higher figure of 87% when children were followed for 15 years.

Resection of a 'toxic mass' of inflamed bowel in Crohn's disease frequently leads to a marked improvement in the child's overall condition, at least in the short term. In addition there may be a rapid acceleration in growth velocity postoperatively (Wesson & Schandling 1981, Lipson et al 1990). The timing of surgery with respect to reversing growth failure is important, however: an adolescent in advanced puberty at the time of surgery is unlikely to show a significant response, whereas results can be dramatic in the pre- or early pubertal child (Evans et al 1991).

Until recently there have been few reports of the outcome of surgery for Crohn's disease in childhood. A retrospective study of 167 children with histologically proven Crohn's disease attending St Bartholomew's Hospital between 1979 and 1988 (Davies et al 1990) showed that 67 (40%) had required surgery. The main indications were failure of medical treatment, intestinal obstruction, growth failure and localized sepsis. There were 44 males and 23 females; mean age at first operation was 13.6 years and average follow-up after surgery was 3.5 years. Patients were divided into four groups on the basis of main disease location: panenteric disease involving both small and large bowel ($n=3$); small-bowel disease only ($n=7$); localized ileocecal disease ($n=30$); large-bowel and perianal disease ($n=27$). The three patients with panenteric disease had lesions involving the mouth, small bowel, colon and perineum. These unfortunate children required 14 surgical procedures between them, mainly for failure of medical treatment and perianal disease. Postoperative morbidity was high and the results of surgery disappointing.

The seven children with disease localized to the jejunum and proximal ileum required surgery for chronic abdominal pain and/or subacute intestinal obstruction. All had jejunal resections, and a right hemicolectomy was also required in three children. Results of surgery were good, with a low morbidity and lengthy remission in six of the seven cases. One child required a second operation for small-bowel relapse.

The 30 children with localized disease of the terminal ileum or ileocecal region were treated by extended right hemicolectomy. The results were impressive: 24 children (80%) were well and asymptomatic at a mean of 3.4 years after surgery, and most had experienced a significant acceleration of growth and puberty. The remaining six cases developed radiological evidence of small-bowel recurrence, one of whom required further small-bowel resection 5 years after the primary operation.

In the 27 children with Crohn's colitis the results of surgery were mixed. Patients could be subdivided into three groups according to the type of surgery performed:

1. Four children with severe rectal and perianal disease were given a defunctioning loop ileostomy to divert the fecal flow, in an attempt to heal their perianal lesions. Only one child benefited from this approach, whereas

the other three subsequently required further, more radical surgery.

2. Seven children had segmental resections of the colon, four of whom required further colonic surgery. The total number of surgical procedures for the group as a whole was 13. Postoperative morbidity was high and six patients relapsed with recurrence of disease at the site of the primary anastamosis.

3. Best results were obtained in the 16 children who had a subtotal colectomy, ileostomy and mucus fistula as the primary procedure: 15 (94%) were well at follow-up ranging from 18 months to 9 years, although persistence of disease in the rectal stump had caused minor problems in some. Only one child required further surgery, for a small-bowel relapse.

In the above series mortality from surgery was zero. However, the postoperative morbidity varied considerably. The overall relapse rate following surgery was 30% at a mean of 3.5 years after the primary operation. Surgery was very successful in children with disease confined to the ileocecal region, in whom relief of symptoms was usually followed by sustained remission and an acceleration of growth (Fig. 72.3). Surgery also proved successful in patients with diffuse jejunal disease for the relief of obstruction.

In Crohn's colitis subtotal colectomy with ileostomy and mucus fistula was the clear operation of choice, as limited segmental resections of the colon were almost invariably followed by rapid recurrence of disease at the site of anastamosis. Diversion of the fecal flow for severe perianal disease proved disappointing; this approach is therefore not recommended. In children with widespread panenteric disease surgery appears to have little to offer over medical therapy, apart from dealing with localized complications.

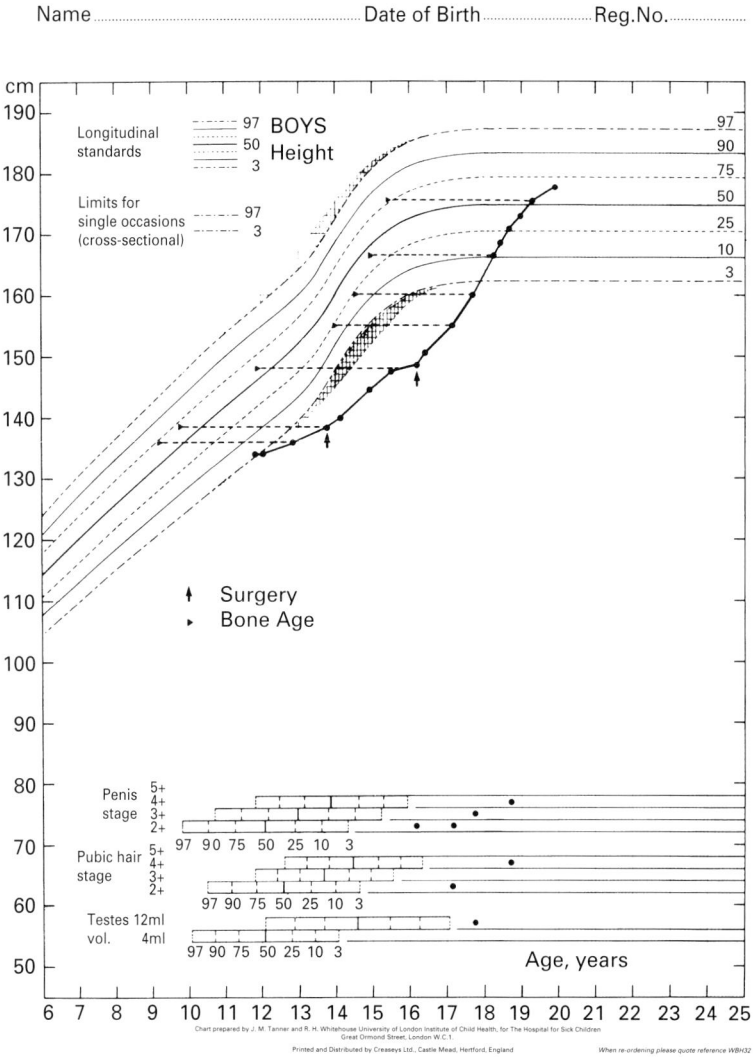

Fig. 72.3 Acceleration in growth and pubertal advancement following surgery in a child with Crohn's disease.

Total parenteral nutrition (TPN)

Parenteral nutrition has been largely superseded by enteral therapy with elemental diets in the management of children with chronic inflammatory bowel disease. However, TPN may be required in severely ill and malnourished children, particularly prior to bowel resection. In such patients total (or partial) parenteral feeding can be administered preoperatively via a central venous catheter to restore adequate nutritional status (Rombeau et al 1982). This will improve outcome following surgery, particularly in relation to growth (Lake et al 1985). TPN may also be required in patients with profusely discharging bowel fistulae, to rest the bowel and allow the lesions to heal (Greenberg et al 1976). Intestinal inflammation often subsides rapidly after commencing therapy with TPN, but tends to relapse just as quickly on restarting oral feeds.

In chronically ill malnourished children who are deemed unfit for surgery, long-term TPN at home is a feasible therapeutic option (Strobel et al 1979). Home TPN may also be indicated for children with malabsorption secondary to 'short gut syndrome', a consequence of widespread small-bowel Crohn's disease and/or extensive bowel resection. Such treatment requires intensive supervision, however, and should only be attempted by a specialist center with the necessary experience and expertise.

Indications for different treatment regimens

The decision regarding which of the above treatment modalities should be used in an individual child with Crohn's disease can be difficult. At present we manage children with extensive small-bowel disease with a polymeric diet, provided this can be tolerated and the child is compliant. Subsequent small-bowel relapses may also respond to dietary therapy, which will often induce repeated remissions in the same child. However, in some patients the therapeutic response may become less impressive with each attempt. If symptoms persist, or the interval between dietary therapy and subsequent relapse is short, an alternative form of management should be tried. This usually involves corticosteroids, with or without azathioprine.

Crohn's colitis and disease involving both large and small bowel is best managed in the first instance with drug therapy – usually a combination of steroids, a 5-aminosalicylate derivative and, in a minority, azathioprine. In a severely ill child intravenous hydrocortisone can be given prior to starting oral steroid therapy to achieve a more rapid remission. The management of toxic dilatation of the colon is discussed under ulcerative colitis.

Children with localized disease of the terminal ileum or ileocecal region may be suitable for early surgery, with the aim of removing all diseased bowel. However, medical therapy will induce a satisfactory remission in many of these children and surgery can then be reserved for the management of complications, such as drug-resistant disease, growth delay and bowel obstruction.

Follow-up of patients

Careful long-term follow-up is a vital part of the management of all children with Crohn's disease. The most effective way of monitoring progress is by regular review in a specialist pediatric inflammatory bowel disease clinic, with a full assessment of disease activity at each attendance. A detailed history of the patient's symptoms since their previous visit should be obtained and a full clinical examination performed. Blood should be obtained at each visit for a full blood count, erythrocyte sedimentation rate, C-reactive protein, total serum proteins and albumin. In children with clinical evidence of poor growth or malabsorption the serum iron, ferritin, folate and B_{12} should be carefully monitored. Bone age estimations should be performed at least 6-monthly in children with significant delay of growth and puberty.

Serial fiberoptic colonoscopy is of value in patients with known Crohn's disease who relapse frequently. The extent and severity of colonic disease can be reassessed and compared with previous findings to plan the most appropriate therapy. A repeat barium follow-through examination may yield useful information during relapses, but consideration should be given to the high dose of radiation involved with repeated studies.

Combined clinics between the pediatric gastroenterologist and other specialists, such as an endocrinologist, surgeon or psychiatrist, are helpful in tackling the variety of problems encountered in childhood Crohn's disease in a coordinated fashion. In addition, a shared care program with the patient's local general pediatrician may be desirable for children living remote from the referral center or who find travelling difficult.

Prognosis

The current management of Crohn's disease in childhood is not always satisfactory. However, with modern treatment regimens many children can be maintained in remission and are able to lead a normal, active life.

The long-term prognosis for Crohn's disease is often better than might seem possible during childhood, when the patient can become resigned to a life of chronic ill-health. Puntis et al (1984) have shown that 38 of 67 patients (56%) who developed Crohn's disease in childhood were well, with no significant recurrence of disease, at a mean follow-up interval of 15 years after diagnosis. Fourteen (21%) had no evidence of active disease at all and only six (9%) were still symptomatic. Outcome was best in children with disease confined to the ileocecal region (38 cases), of whom 36 (95%) were managed by early surgery. In addition, although 21 patients had shown evidence of poor growth at some point in childhood, only ten of these developed permanent growth retardation. Four patients (6%) died during the 15-year follow-up period.

Farmer and Michener (1979) looked at outcome in over 500 cases of Crohn's disease diagnosed before 20 years of age. The mean duration of follow-up for the whole series was 7.7 years; 67% of those studied had required bowel resection and 2% had died, usually of sepsis following surgery. In a large group of adult patients from the same center, however, the mortality rate was higher (12%), but over a longer duration of follow-up (Farmer et al 1985); most deaths occurred within 5 years of diagnosis and were related to bowel fistulae, intraperitoneal sepsis, bowel perforation and toxic megacolon. However, this high mortality rate has not been observed in recent pediatric reports. Kirschner (1988) has reported a zero mortality rate among almost 200 children with Crohn's disease who attended the Wyler Children's Hospital in Chicago between 1975 and 1988. In our own experience there have been no deaths among the 212 children with biopsy-proven Crohn's disease attending the pediatric inflammatory bowel disease clinic at St Bartholomew's Hospital since 1975 (Evans & Beattie, unpublished observation).

Up to half of young adult patients with Crohn's disease beginning in childhood have said that their quality of life is not as good as that of their peer group (Farmer et al 1985). In another study (Sorenson et al 1987), however, there were no obvious differences between the two groups in terms of factors directly influencing quality of life, such as marriage, parenthood, education, employment and leisure activity.

ULCERATIVE COLITIS

First reports of ulcerative colitis in children

Helmholtz, in 1923, reported the first case of ulcerative colitis in a child. The first report from Britain (Bourne 1926) surveyed the world literature and only nine other 'well authenticated' pediatric cases had been published. Bourne was familiar with ulcerative colitis in adult patients, so failure to recognize the disease is unlikely to account for the rarity of childhood cases reported at this time (Walker-Smith 1986). Since then, many reports have described ulcerative colitis in children from developed countries, including the United Kingdom (Kirsner et al 1955, Broberger & Lagercrantz 1966, Chong & Walker-Smith 1984).

Epidemiology and genetics

Although ulcerative colitis appears to be more common in children today than it was 70 years ago, the prevalence is not increasing as fast as Crohn's disease (Barton et al 1989). Ferguson et al (1986) have estimated the prevalence of ulcerative colitis in British children to be 6.86 per 100 000.

The geographical distribution of ulcerative colitis is similar to Crohn's disease. The disorder is relatively common in northwest Europe and North America, but much less so in the developing world. However, there have been a number of reports suggesting that ulcerative colitis occurs more commonly in adults in the Indian subcontinent than previously thought (Tandon et al 1965). In addition, increasing numbers of British children of Indian subcontinent origin have presented to the inflammatory bowel disease clinic at St Bartholomew's Hospital in the past decade (Salim and Evans, unpublished observations), as well as children from Afro-Caribbean families (Walker-Smith 1986). This suggests that environmental factors present in industrialized societies may be of etiological significance.

Hereditary factors also appear to be important in ulcerative colitis, as in Crohn's disease, and the two disorders may share a common genetic basis. It has been speculated that ulcerative colitis develops in patients with a partial predisposing genotype, and Crohn's disease in those with the full genotype (McConnell et al 1986). However, it is likely that environmental factors also play a key role in the development of the disease. Tysk et al (1988) have found that the prevalence of ulcerative colitis amongst twins in Stockholm is similar to that in the general population.

Pathology in children

In adults the inflammatory process in ulcerative colitis typically begins in the rectum and then spreads more proximally along the colon to a variable degree. In children the rectum may be relatively spared (Markowitz et al 1993b), with more severe disease occurring in the transverse, descending and sigmoid colon.

Initially the inflammatory process is confined to the colonic mucosa, which becomes hyperemic, friable and granular in appearance at endoscopy. As the disease progresses multiple ragged ulcers develop, together with a mucopurulent exudate and spontaneous bleeding from the increasingly friable mucosa. Eventually the mucosa becomes hyperplastic and 'pseudopolyp' formation may occur.

Histologically, in early disease the mucosal lamina propria is heavily infiltrated with plasma cells and there is a depletion of goblet cells in the colonic crypts and surface epithelium. As the disease becomes more active, the mucosa becomes populated with polymorphonuclear leukocytes, which infiltrate individual crypts to form crypt abscesses. Distortion of the crypt architecture occurs and the surface epithelium becomes flattened and ulcerated.

Table 72.5 Incidence of clinical features at time of diagnosis of ulcerative colitis in 28 children attending St Bartholomew's Hospital (data from Chong & Walker-Smith 1984)

Symptoms		Signs	
Diarrhea	100%	No significant	
Rectal bleeding	95%	abnormality	54%
Abdominal pain	72%	Weight loss	46%
Urgency	60%	Pallor	46%
Anorexia	56%	Tender abdomen	32%
Weight loss	52%	Growth retardation	14%
Lethargy	43%	Abdominal distension	14%
Tenesmus	43%	Mouth lesions	11%
Nausea and vomiting	16%	Perianal abnormality	7%
Psychological		Jaundice	4%
symptoms	12%	Toxic dilatation	4%
Poor growth	5%	Rectal prolapse	4%

In severe disease the inflammatory process penetrates the muscularis mucosae into the submucosa, forming deeper abscesses and, by this stage, obvious mascroscopic ulceration is visible at endoscopy. In fulminating disease inflammation involves the whole of the bowel wall and may result in perforation of the colon.

Clinical features of ulcerative colitis in children

Ulcerative colitis may begin in infancy, but the mean age of onset in childhood is around 10 years. The sex incidence is equal. The major clinical features are summarized in Table 72.5. The illness typically presents with bloody diarrhea and crampy, lower abdominal pain. These symptoms tend to prompt urgent medical attention, thus leading to an early diagnosis. Gastrointestinal symptoms are more common than systemic manifestations in the early stages of disease.

Acute relapses of ulcerative colitis can be classified as mild, moderate or severe, depending on such factors as stool frequency, the presence of abdominal tenderness and the degree of systemic disturbance. This classification helps in deciding on the most appropriate form of management for individual patients.

The inflammatory process involves the rectum in most children, with a varying degree of proximal colonic extension. Pancolitis is the most common form, accounting for 57% of a series of 62 children attending St Bartholomew's Hospital (Evans, unpublished observations). In the same series, disease localized to the left colon (distal to the splenic flexure) was seen in 22% of children and disease limited to the rectum only was present in 21%. The extent and severity of inflammation may influence the course of the disease and the features at presentation. Children with pancolitis tend to run a more severe course than those with more limited disease.

Gastrointestinal manifestations

Diarrhea is present in almost all children from an early stage. Loose, frequent, watery stools containing a large amount of mucus and varying quantities of fresh blood are characteristic. Diarrhea tends to be most troublesome in the early morning, but in severe cases may also be nocturnal. The passage of fresh blood per rectum may precede the onset of diarrhea, particularly if disease is confined to the distal colon. Urgency of defecation is a common complaint, occasionally resulting in fecal incontinence. Paradoxically, a small number of children with ulcerative colitis present with constipation.

Crampy, lower abdominal pain is common, sometimes localized to the left iliac fossa. Pain is often exacerbated by eating (due to the gastrocolic reflex), may be maximal prior to and during defecation, and is usually relieved by the passage of stool and flatus. Tenesmus is a common associated complaint.

Anorexia is a presenting feature in half of affected children at diagnosis, and is often directly related to disease severity. Weight loss does occur, but is less common and less severe than in Crohn's disease (Kirschner 1988). Vomiting is uncommon in ulcerative colitis and indicates severe disease when present.

Perianal disease occurs less frequently in ulcerative colitis than Crohn's disease (10% cf. 43%). A chronic fissure-in-ano or perianal suppuration are occasional findings, but perianal fistulae are very rare. Perianal excoriation due to diarrhea is a common problem.

Systemic manifestations

Extraintestinal manifestations of ulcerative colitis occur less frequently in children than in adult patients. The systemic features of the illness are similar to those found in Crohn's disease, but occur less often.

Although many children are obviously unwell at presentation, in some the complaints may be subtle, such as an increased desire for sleep or lack of endurance during exercise. Chronic, active ulcerative colitis in childhood may arrest growth and maturation, but less so than with Crohn's disease. Between 5 and 10% of cases will have evidence of growth retardation at presentation (height below the third centile), compared with nearly one-third of those with Crohn's disease (Kirschner et al 1978).

Arthritis, with joint swelling and tenderness, occurs in just under 10% of children with ulcerative colitis, usually affecting large joints such as the knees, hips, ankles, shoulders and wrists. Joint deformity and destruction are rare. Arthritis may precede gastrointestinal symptoms, as in Crohn's disease, but joint problems are usually most troublesome during an acute flare-up of the colitis.

Other extraintestinal manifestations of ulcerative colitis seen in childhood include finger clubbing, skin lesions, stomatitis, ophthalmic problems and hepatobiliary disease (Greenstein et al 1976). Erythema nodosum is the most common skin lesion, but is seen in less than 5% of cases.

Pyoderma gangrenosum is an extremely rare dermatological feature of the disease in children. Aphthous stomatitis affects less than 2% of children and is much less common than in Crohn's disease. Conjunctivitis and iritis are found in approximately 4% of children with ulcerative colitis, and tend to be seen more commonly in patients with skin and joint problems.

Sclerosing cholangitis, the characteristic hepatobiliary lesion of adult ulcerative colitis, rarely occurs in childhood. Chronic active hepatitis is occasionally seen and may progress despite colectomy (Kane et al 1980). One study of 34 children with ulcerative colitis (Nemeth et al 1990) reported a surprisingly high incidence of abnormal liver function tests (60%) and abnormal liver biopsies (24%), but no correlation was found with the extent, duration or treatment of colonic disease.

Diagnosis

The rapid onset of gastrointestinal symptoms in most children with ulcerative colitis, particularly bloody diarrhea, tends to result in early referral from the general practitioner and prompt investigation. Most children are diagnosed within 6 months of their first symptoms.

A provisional diagnosis of ulcerative colitis in children is usually made on the basis of the typical clinical features, although distinction from Crohn's disease may be difficult on clinical grounds alone. The diagnostic approach discussed previously for Crohn's disease should be followed (see Fig. 72.1).

A detailed clinical assessment should be performed, followed by the appropriate blood tests and stool cultures, before proceeding on to a barium follow-through examination and a colonoscopy. A definite diagnosis, however, can only be made by observing the characteristic histological changes of ulcerative colitis in colonic biopsies obtained at endoscopy (see Table 72.2).

Investigations

Stool cultures are important, as bloody diarrhea of acute onset may indicate an infective colitis. Several stool specimens should be cultured to exclude colitis due to shigella, salmonella, campylobacter and enteropathogenic *Escherichia coli* (Pai 1984). Stools should also be examined for ova, cysts and parasites, and serological testing performed to exclude amebic dysentery due to *Entamoeba histolytica* (Sanderson & Walker-Smith 1984).

A full blood count will reveal mild to moderate anemia in most patients, usually of the hypochromic, microcytic variety due to iron deficiency from chronic blood loss. Occasionally a Coombs-positive hemolytic anemia may occur in association with ulcerative colitis. A leukocytosis and thrombocytosis are often present in active disease, and the erythrocyte sedimentation rate is elevated in about 50% of children at presentation. Acute-phase proteins, such as the serum C-reactive protein, are also useful markers of disease activity (Campbell et al 1982), but are usually less highly elevated than in Crohn's disease and may be normal despite extensive inflammation. Serum iron and ferritin levels should also be measured, together with the total protein and albumin levels. Liver function tests may be abnormal in the occasional child with hepatobiliary complications. Tests of small-bowel function are normal.

Diagnostic colonoscopy with multiple biopsies has generally replaced the barium enema for investigating suspected colonic disease in children. However, double contrast barium studies may provide adequate visualization of the colonic mucosa where endoscopy is unavailable (Stringer et al 1986a). The appearances may be normal initially (Ament 1975), but later there is loss of the normal colonic haustral pattern, with mucosal irregularity. In long-standing disease the colon becomes shortened and featureless, and occasionally a colonic stricture may develop. In approximately 10% of cases the terminal ileum will appear abnormal radiologically due to backwash ileitis. A barium follow-through examination should be performed to exclude small-bowel Crohn's disease, particularly if the colonic biopsy histology is equivocal.

Endoscopy with multiple biopsies will confirm the diagnosis of ulcerative colitis in most cases and indicate the severity and extent of disease. Inflamed bowel will appear hyperemic and friable, with loss of the normal vascular pattern, but macroscopic ulceration is rarely seen (Chong et al 1984). However, in severe disease areas of denuded mucosa may be visible. Inflammatory polyps (pseudopolyps) are seen in chronic disease, when the whole colon may be shortened and poorly distensible. Colonoscopy is also of value in the surveillance of patients with long-standing disease for the development of colonic carcinoma. The characteristic histological features of ulcerative colitis are outlined in Table 72.3.

Complications of ulcerative colitis in childhood

Children with severe pancolitis are most at risk of developing acute toxic dilatation of the colon (toxic megacolon). This is a serious condition that can evolve quickly over a matter of hours. Between 2 and 4% of children with total colitis will develop this complication at some stage (Kirschner 1988). Rapid onset of fever, pallor and tachycardia, together with abdominal pain, distension and tenderness, may indicate that toxic dilatation is occurring. Dilatation may affect the whole colon or a single segment, and will usually exceed 6 cm in diameter on a plain abdominal radiograph (Norland & Kirsner 1969).

The main complication of toxic megacolon is perforation of the bowel leading to peritonitis, which is associated with a high mortality rate. High-dose corticosteroid therapy may obscure the typical signs of bowel perforation and peritonitis, so extreme vigilance is required. The diagnosis can be confirmed by demonstrating massive colonic dilatation on plain abdominal X-ray; barium enema and colonoscopy should be avoided if possible, because of the risk of perforation. Treatment includes intravenous fluids, parenteral corticosteroids and broad-spectrum antibiotics. Emergency surgery with colectomy and ileostomy may be required as a life-saving procedure.

Severe diarrhea in ulcerative colitis can lead to rapid disturbances in fluid and electrolyte balance and acid–base status. Major acute hemorrhage from ulcerated colonic mucosa is uncommon, but may occasionally require emergency blood transfusion and surgery.

Colonic carcinoma is a well recognized complication of long-standing ulcerative colitis, with an incidence of between 8.7 and 20% at 20 years after diagnosis (Devroede et al 1971, Michener et al 1979). Detailed analysis of a series of 30 patients with ulcerative colitis who subsequently developed colonic carcinoma was reported by Greenstein et al (1979). Two-thirds of the patients had pancolitis, in whom the cancer risk was 11 times that of the general population. The remaining patients with left-sided colonic disease had a cancer risk three times that expected. However, the incidence of malignancy was not greater among those patients who had presented in childhood. A few cases have been reported in whom colectomy has been required in early adult life for colonic cancer complicating long-standing ulcerative colitis beginning in childhood (Michener et al 1979, Greenstein et al 1979).

Management of ulcerative colitis

The general principles involved in the management of ulcerative colitis in children are similar to those in Crohn's disease. Care should be taken to explain the nature of the illness to the child and parents, and to discuss the likely disease course, treatment options and prognosis.

As in Crohn's disease, the aim of therapy is to induce and maintain a long-lasting remission of symptoms to allow the child to live a normal, active life. Treatment is with drugs and/or surgery. The choice of therapy will depend on the severity of the presenting illness and the frequency of subsequent relapses. When considering the most appropriate treatment to use in the individual child, it is helpful to divide ulcerative colitis into three grades of disease severity – mild, moderate and severe – as the severity of disease has a direct influence on management and outcome.

Mild ulcerative colitis

Mild disease is characterized by mild to moderate diarrhea, often containing blood and mucus. First-line treatment consists of oral sulfasalazine (50 mg/kg/day) or mesalazine (20 mg/kg/day), which may be sufficient to induce and maintain remission in many children with mild colitis. Treatment is usually continued for a period of 1–2 years after presentation or last relapse, but may be discontinued sooner in mild cases. The side effects of the 5-aminosalicylate derivatives have been discussed earlier (management of Crohn's disease).

Children with a mild proctitis or distal colitis which does not extend beyond the splenic flexure at colonoscopy can often be managed successfully with steroid enemas, in addition to sulfasalazine or mesalazine. Rectal steroids can be given once or twice daily, either as hydrocortisone acetate 10% in a foam aerosol (Colifoam) or as prednisolone-21-phosphate tablets dissolved in 25–50 ml of water and given via a fine-bore Jacques catheter. This approach may obviate the need for oral steroid therapy. Some centers also advocate the use of 5-aminosalicylate enemas in children, particularly for those who find the oral preparation difficult to tolerate.

Moderate ulcerative colitis

Moderately severe disease is characterized by more troublesome diarrhea, blood and mucus per rectum, cramping lower abdominal pain, fever, anemia, anorexia and, occasionally, weight loss. These children almost always require high-dose steroid therapy to induce a remission. Oral prednisolone 1–2 mg/kg per day (maximum dose 40 mg daily) should be prescribed for an initial period of 3–4 weeks, following which the dose is gradually tapered off over 6–8 weeks if successful remission is achieved. Sulfasalazine or mesalazine alone may then be sufficient to maintain remission once disease activity has subsided. If the child is too ill to tolerate oral prednisolone, initial therapy can be started with intravenous hydrocortisone (5–10 mg/kg per day in four divided doses).

As with mild colitis, treatment with one of the steroid enema preparations described above may help symptoms associated with distal disease, such as tenesmus or urgency.

Severe ulcerative colitis and toxic megacolon

Children presenting with severe ulcerative colitis should be regarded as a medical emergency, because of the risk of developing toxic dilatation of the colon. Most patients show signs of marked systemic toxicity in addition to severe gastrointestinal symptoms.

Werlin and Grand (1977) proposed the following criteria for establishing a diagnosis of severe colitis in children:

1. Gross bloody diarrhea (> 5 motions per day)
2. Fever (>38°C)
3. Tachycardia (>90 beats/min)

4. Anemia (Hct<30%)
5. Hypoalbuminemia (<30 g/dl)
6. Toxic dilatation of the colon.

Children should be considered to have severe colitis if they satisfy four of the first five criteria, or criterion 6 alone.

Children with severe colitis require immediate hospitalization. A careful clinical examination should be performed on admission and repeated regularly. Ominous signs include increasing abdominal distension; worsening abdominal pain with guarding, rebound tenderness and rigidity; a rising pulse rate and fever; and a general deterioration in the child's condition. A plain abdominal radiograph on admission is essential to determine the diameter of the colon, and this may need to be repeated regularly. Samples should be taken for a full blood count, ESR, C-reactive protein, electrolytes, calcium and albumin. Compatible blood should be cross-matched in case transfusion is required for anemia, severe rectal bleeding or emergency surgery.

The medical management of severe colitis and toxic megacolon in children is similar to that in adults. Patients should be kept nil by mouth and given intravenous fluids to correct water and electrolyte losses. Broad-spectrum antibiotics are usually prescribed parenterally (Booth & Harries 1984) and transfusions of blood, plasma or albumin solutions may all be required. Intravenous hydrocortisone should be started at a dose of 10 mg/kg per day in four divided doses, and continued until the child is well enough to restart oral fluids. Oral prednisolone (1–2 mg/kg/day) can then be substituted for the parenteral hydrocortisone.

Most children responding to medical therapy do so within a few days, but some may take over a week. Up to 50% of children will require urgent surgery (Werlin & Grand 1977), but it is difficult to predict at presentation which patients will respond to medical therapy and thus avoid colectomy.

The role of immunosuppressive therapy in the management of children with ulcerative colitis has not been well established. However, the potential risk of long-term immunosuppressive therapy resulting in malignancy needs careful consideration in a condition which is curable by surgery. Azathioprine has been used in children, mainly as a steroid-sparing agent, and does seem to benefit some patients. Kirschner et al (1987) have reported dramatic success with cyclosporin A in two adolescents with severe, acute colitis unresponsive to parenteral steroids and total parenteral nutrition. Both patents achieved a marked clinical and histological remission of their disease within 2 weeks of starting cyclosporin A at a dosage of 6 mg/kg per day. However, Treem et al (1991) administered cyclosporin to six children with ulcerative colitis and, although all showed a transient improvement, four had required colectomy within 8 months. In addition, reports of the use of cyclosporin in adult patients with colitis are not encouraging (Lichtiger & Present 1990).

Nutritional therapy

The same general recommendations regarding an adequate diet apply in ulcerative colitis as in Crohn's disease. However, elemental diets are not as effective in inducing remission in ulcerative colitis (Sanderson 1986), although there have been no controlled trials in children to confirm this. Nutritional support by mouth or by the parenteral route may be indicated in malnourished children during or after a relapse.

Parenteral nutrition has been used in the management of adults with ulcerative colitis, but experience in children is not so well documented. TPN seems less effective in inducing remission in children with ulcerative colitis than in Crohn's disease. The main role of TPN in both conditions is to restore nutritional status, particularly prior to surgery, rather than to directly alter the long-term course of the disease. Seashore et al (1982) evaluated the role of TPN in 22 children with severe active inflammatory bowel disease (eight with ulcerative colitis) who were given 2–4 weeks' intravenous nutrition with complete bowel rest. Four of the patients with ulcerative colitis improved sufficiently to avoid colectomy, three within a week, but two of these subsequently relapsed. Similar results were reported by Werlin and Grand (1977) in 19 adolescents with severe inflammatory bowel disease, 14 of whom had ulcerative colitis; 32% improved on TPN, but only 5% (one patient) achieved a sustained remission of more than 2 years.

Surgery

Indications for acute surgical intervention in children with ulcerative colitis include life-threatening conditions such as toxic megacolon, colonic perforation, intestinal obstruction and massive hemorrhage. Failure of medical treatment with persistence of symptoms, particularly in children under 3 years of age, is another indication for colectomy. In addition, surgery is occasionally required primarily for growth failure, but this is much less common than in Crohn's disease.

Total colectomy is curative in ulcerative colitis but leaves the child with an ileostomy. Most centers now perform subtotal colectomy in children, raising an ileostomy and mucus fistula but leaving the rectum in situ. This procedure preserves the rectum for an ileorectal anastomosis later (Telander & Perrault 1980). The continent ileostomy pioneered by Kock (1969) has now been superceded by the ileal pouch procedure. The pouch is constructed from the ileum prior to anastomosing it to the anus, and acts as a fecal reservoir, thus helping to reduce stool frequency (Telander & Perrault 1980, Odigwe et al 1987, Morgan et al 1987, Perrault et al 1988). It is currently felt to be the surgical procedure of choice in children (Telander et al 1990).

Follow-up

The long-term management of children with ulcerative colitis should, ideally, be carried out in a specialist pediatric inflammatory bowel disease clinic. The general principles involved in monitoring the child's progress apply as in Crohn's disease (see earlier). Regular clinic reviews are required to assess disease activity and growth, during which routine blood sampling should be performed to look for evidence of early subclinical relapse. In addition, serial endoscopy is of value in assessing disease activity/extent and in surveillance for the development of colonic malignancy in long-standing colitis.

Prognosis

As in adults, the course of ulcerative colitis in children is unpredictable. Typically, the condition is characterized by recurrent episodes of acute relapse followed by remission, but it may also present as a chronic low-grade smouldering colonic inflammation. Many children remain well and asymptomatic for months, or even years, after the initial attack, but their disease may flare up again at any time. Between 60 and 70% of children report chronic symptoms (Michener et al 1979), but most of these can be kept well with medical therapy and correctly timed surgical intervention.

The prognosis for patients developing ulcerative colitis in childhood appears to be no different from that of cases diagnosed in adult life (Keventer et al 1978). Outcome is dependent on disease extent, severity and duration. Early studies of long-term outcome for childhood ulcerative colitis were pessimistic: Devroede et al (1971) reported a 2% mortality rate and a 20% risk of colonic malignancy within 10 years of diagnosis in a large retrospective study of children presenting with the disease over a 50-year period. However, Michener et al (1979), in a study of long-term outcome in 336 children with ulcerative colitis diagnosed before 20 years of age, found the incidence of colonic cancer to be much lower (8.7%) 20 years after diagnosis. More recently, Hendriksen et al (1985) calculated a cumulative cancer risk in Danish patients with ulcerative colitis of only 1.4% at 18 years after diagnosis.

The number of children requiring colectomy for ulcerative colitis has fallen over the past 30 years. In Michener's (1979) study 49% of cases required surgery between 1955 and 1965, but the figure had fallen to 26% by 1965–1974. At St Bartholomew's Hospital, 17 of the 70 children (24%) with biopsy-proven ulcerative colitis seen between 1975 and 1988 have required colectomy before their 17th birthday (Evans, unpublished observations).

BEHÇET'S ENTEROCOLITIS

Behçet's syndrome is a chronic multisystem disease of unknown etiology characterized by four distinct clinical features: oral ulceration, skin lesions (e.g. erythema nodosum, thrombophlebitis), ulceration of the genitalia and inflammatory ocular disease (conjunctivitis, iritis). The condition is rare in childhood and occurs most frequently in Japan and the Middle East. In adult patients an incomplete form of the syndrome has been described in association with arthropathy (Mason & Barnes 1969) and/or inflammatory bowel disease (Smith et al 1973, Kasahara et al 1981). In addition, intestinal involvement in the form of a chronic enterocolitis has been reported in children with the condition (Lebowohl et al 1977, Okabe et al 1980, Stringer et al 1986a, b, Chong et al 1988).

In children, Behçet's colitis characteristically presents at an early age (under 2 years) and at least three neonatal cases have been reported (Lewis & Priestley 1986). Interestingly, the neonatal form only occurs in infants born to affected mothers and usually resolves within 2 months of birth. A familial form of the disease is well recognized (Dundar et al 1985), particularly in siblings of consanguinous parentage, which suggests a genetic predisposition. In addition, distinct clinical variants of the syndrome seem to be related to geographical location (Chong et al 1988).

The clinical features of Behçet's colitis may resemble those of Crohn's disease, with chronic diarrhea, rectal bleeding and poor growth being prominent. In addition, aphthous stomatitis and perianal ulceration occur. Examination of the colon by radiography and endoscopy frequently reveals the presence of multiple deep discrete 'flask-shaped' ulcers, together with non-specific chronic inflammation of a patchy nature. It may be difficult to distinguish Behçet's colitis from both Crohn's disease and amebiasis at endoscopy.

Histological confirmation may also prove difficult because the microscopic features overlap with Crohn's colitis. However, the characteristic flask-shaped ulcers, the normal intervening mucosa, evidence of a vasculitis and the lack of epithelioid granulomas are all suggestive of Behçet's colitis (Watanabe et al 1979, Chong et al 1988).

Treatment of Behçet's colitis in children may prove difficult. A trial of steroid therapy is usually attempted, but review of the literature suggests that subtotal colectomy with ileostomy is often required to control symptoms. However, oral ulceration and perianal disease may persist despite colectomy, and growth may remain suboptimal. There are case reports suggesting that cyclosporin A may induce remission in adults with Behçet's disease (French-Constant et al 1983), but this has yet to be confirmed in children.

INTRACTABLE ENTEROCOLITIS OF INFANCY

Sanderson et al (1991) have described a series of five children with a disorder similar to, but distinct from, Behçet's disease named 'intractable ulcerating enterocolitis of infancy'. All five children presented in the first year of life with intractable diarrhea and ulcerating stomatitis; four had severe perianal ulceration in addition. Diffuse inflammatory changes were present in both small- and large-bowel biopsies, which was not typical of either Behçet's disease or Crohn's disease. Medical treatment was unsuccessful and all five children required colectomy. As four of the five children were born to consanguinous parents (and two were siblings), the disorder may represent a distinct form of hereditary enterocolitis.

INDETERMINATE COLITIS

The distinction between Crohn's disease and ulcerative colitis may prove particularly difficult in children presenting with inflammatory bowel disease confined to the colon. The term 'indeterminate colitis' has been proposed (Chong et al 1985) to describe a colitis in which the characteristic histopathological features of Crohn's disease or ulcerative colitis are not evident (see Table 72.2). Further investigation at a later date may lead to a definite histological diagnosis, but in some cases of indeterminate colitis a firm diagnosis is never made (Price 1978).

Of the 282 children with biopsy-proven chronic inflammatory bowel disease diagnosed at St Bartholomew's Hospital between 1975 and 1988, 39 (14%) had indeterminate colitis at presentation. Of these, 18 were followed up for at least 5 years, of whom six developed Crohn's disease or ulcerative colitis, six remained 'indeterminate' and six had a spontaneous remission of disease (Evans & Keck, unpublished observations).

The management of indeterminate colitis is similar to that previously described for ulcerative colitis.

MICROSCOPIC COLITIS

Occasionally, patients with symptoms suggestive of chronic inflammatory bowel disease have no evidence of macroscopic disease at colonoscopy or on a barium radiograph of the bowel. However, histological examination of biopsy specimens obtained at endoscopy reveals an active inflammatory process, i.e. a microscopic colitis. This phenomenon has been reported in both adults (Kingham et al 1982) and children (Sanderson et al 1985). Seven (4.5%) of the 191 new referrals endoscoped at St Bartholomew's Hospital between 1985 and 1988 had histological abnormalities in the absence of macroscopic disease (Evans, unpublished observation). This demonstrates the importance of obtaining biopsy material for histology purposes at endoscopy, even when the colon appears normal macroscopically.

Microscopic colitis in childhood may be due to Crohn's disease, ulcerative colitis, indeterminate colitis or Behçet's disease. The condition has also been reported in association with celiac disease, cow's milk protein intolerance (Jenkins et al 1984) and chronic granulomatous disease (Harris & Boles 1973 – see earlier). The management is that of the underlying cause.

CONCLUSION

The present limitations in the management of chronic inflammatory bowel disease in childhood can only be overcome by further fundamental research. Organizations such as the Crohn's in Childhood Research Association (CICRA) and the National Association for Crohn's and Colitis (NACC) in the United Kingdom, and the Ileitis Foundation in the United States, currently provide much of the momentum for further research in this field. In addition, they provide a focus for information and mutual support for patients with chronic inflammatory bowel disease and their families.

Acknowledgement

We wish to thank the Crohn's in Childhood Research Association (CICRA) for their generous funding of a research fellowship in pediatric gastroenterology based at St Bartholomew's Hospital, London.

REFERENCES

Axelsson C, Jarnum S 1977 Assessment of the therapeutic value of an elemental diet in chronic inflammatory bowel disease. Scandinavian Journal of Gastroenterology 77: 272–279

Barton J R, Gillon S, Ferguson A 1989 Incidence of inflammatory bowel disease in Scottish children between 1968 and 1982: threefold rise in Crohn's disease. Gut 30: 618–622

Bartram C I, Kumar P 1981 Clinical radiology in gastro-enterology. Blackwell Scientific Publications, Oxford

Beattie R M, Schiffrin E J, Donnet-Hughes A et al 1994 Polymeric nutrition as the primary therapy in children with small bowel Crohn's disease. Alimentary Pharmacology and Therapeutics (in press)

Belli D C, Seidman E, Bouthillier L 1988 Chronic intermittent elemental diet improves growth failure in children with Crohn's disease. Gastroenterology 94: 603–610

Bender S W 1977 Crohn's disease in children: initial symptomatology. Acta Paediatrica Belgica 30: 193

Bernstein L H, Frank M S, Brandt L J et al 1980 Healing of perianal Crohn's disease with metronidazole. Gastroenterology 79: 357–365

Binder V, Hendrikson C, Kreiner S 1985 Prognosis in Crohn's disease – based on results from a regional patient group from the county of Copenhagen. Gut 26: 146–150

Booth I W, Harries J T 1984 Inflammatory bowel disease in childhood. Gut 25: 188–202

Bourne G 1926 Chronic ulcerative colitis in children. Archives of Disease in Childhood 1: 175–181

Braegger C P, Nicholls S W, Murch S H et al 1992 Tumour necrosis factor alpha in stool as a marker of intestinal inflammation. Lancet 339: 89–91

Braegger C P, Torresani T, Murch S H et al 1993 Urinary growth hormone in growth-impaired children with chronic inflammatory bowel disease. Journal of Pediatric Gastroenterology and Nutrition 16: 49–52

Brahme F, Lindstrom C, Wenckert A 1975 Crohn's disease in a defined population. An epidemiological study of incidence, prevalence, mortality and secular trends in the city of Malmo, Sweden. Gastroenterology 69: 342–351

Brain C E, Savage M O 1994 Growth and puberty in chronic inflammatory bowel disease. In: Chronic inflammatory bowel disease in childhood. Baillière's Clinical Gastroenterology 8: 83–100

Broberger O, Lagercrantz L 1966 Ulcerative colitis in childhood and adolescence. Advances in Paediatrics 14: 9

Bruce T 1986 Emotional sequelae of chronic inflammatory bowel disease in children and adolescents. Clinics in Gastroenterology 15: 71–89

Brynskov J, Freund L, Rasmussen S N et al 1989 A placebo-controlled, double-blind, randomized trial of cyclosporine therapy in active chronic Crohn's disease. New England Journal of Medicine 321: 845–850

Burbige E J, Huang S S, Bayless T M 1975 Clinical manifestations of Crohn's disease in children and adolescents. Pediatrics 55: 866–871

Calkins B M 1989 A meta-analysis of the role of smoking in inflammatory bowel disease. Digestive Diseases and Sciences 34: 1841–1854

Camacho-Hubner C, Beattie R M, Brain C R et al 1993 The effect of enteral diet or steroid therapy on insulin-like growth factor-1 (IGF-1) and IGF-binding proteins in inflammatory bowel disease. Journal of Endocrinology 139: S97

Campbell C A, Walker-Smith J A, Hindocha P et al 1982 Acute phase proteins in chronic inflammatory bowel disease in childhood. Journal of Pediatric Gastroenterology and Nutrition 1: 193–201

Chong S K F, Walker-Smith J A 1984 Ulcerative colitis in childhood. Journal of the Royal Society of Medicine 77 (Suppl 3): 21–25

Chong S K F, Bartram C I, Campbell C A et al 1982 Chronic inflammatory bowel disease in childhood. British Medical Journal 284: 101–103

Chong S K F, Blackshaw A J, Boyle S A et al 1985 Histological diagnosis of chronic inflammatory bowel disease in childhood. Gut 26: 69–74

Chong S K F, Blackshaw A J, Morson B C et al 1986 A prospective study of colitis in infancy and childhood. Journal of Pediatric Gastroenterology and Nutrition 5: 352–358

Chong S K F, Grossman A, Walker-Smith J A et al 1984 Endocrine dysfunction in children with Crohn's disease. Journal of Pediatric Gastroenterology and Nutrition 3: 529–535

Chong S K F, Walker-Smith J A, Blackshaw A J et al 1983 Colitis in early infancy and childhood: a prospective study. Gut 24: A462–A463

Chong S K F, Wright V M, Nishigame T et al 1988 Infantile colitis: a manifestation of intestinal Behçet's Syndrome. Journal of Pediatric Gastroenterology and Nutrition 7: 622–627

Chrispin A R, Tempany E 1967 Crohn's disease of the jejunum in children. Archives of Disease in Childhood 42: 631

Crohn B B 1934 The broadening concept of regional ileitis. American Journal of Digestive Diseases 1: 97–99

Crohn B B 1949 Regional ileitis. Staples Press, London

Davies G, Evans C M, Shand W S et al 1990 Surgery for Crohn's disease in childhood: influence of site of disease and operative procedure on outcome. British Journal of Surgery 77: 891–894

Derkx B, Taminau J, Radema S et al 1993 Tumour necrosis factor antibody treatment in Crohn's disease. Lancet 342: 173

Devroede G J, Taylor W F, Sauer W G et al 1971 Cancer risk and life expectancy of children with ulcerative colitis. New England Journal of Medicine 285: 17–21

Driscoll R H, Rosenberg I H 1978 Total parenteral nutrition in inflammatory bowel disease. Medical Clinics of North America 62: 185–201

Dundar S V, Genccalp U, Simcsek H 1985 Familial cases of Behçet's disease. British Journal of Dermatology 113: 319–321

Emmrich J, Seyfarth M, Fleig W E et al 1991 Treatment of inflammatory bowel disease with anti-CD4 monoclonal antibody. Lancet 338: 570–571

Evans C M, Walker-Smith J A 1988 Management of sexual abuse (correspondence). Archives of Disease in Childhood 63: 678–679

Evans C M, Walker-Smith J A 1989 Recording growth and development in children with inflammatory bowel disease. British Medical Journal 298: 1312–1313

Evans C M, Kirk J W M, Savage M O, Walker-Smith J A 1991 Growth after gut resection for Crohn's disease. Archives of Disease in Childhood 66: 370

Farmer R G, Michener W M 1979 Prognosis of Crohn's disease with onset in childhood or adolescence. Digestive Diseases and Sciences 24: 752

Farmer R G, Whelan G, Fazio V W 1985 Long-term follow-up of patients with Crohn's disease. Relationship between the clinical pattern and prognosis. Gastroenterology 88: 1818

Farthing M J G, Campbell C A, Walker-Smith J A et al 1981 Nocturnal growth hormone and gonadotrophin secretion in growth retarded children with Crohn's disease. Gut 22: 933–938

Ferguson A, Sedgwick D M 1994 Juvenile onset inflammatory bowel disease: height and body mass index in adult life. British Medical Journal 308: 1259–1263

Ferguson A, Rifkind E A, Doig C M 1986 Prevalence of chronic inflammatory bowel disease in British children. In: McConnell R, Rozen P, Langman M, Gilat T (eds) Frontiers of Gastrointestinal Research Vol. 11: 68–73

French-Constant C, Wolman R, James G D 1983 Cyclosporin in Behçet's disease. Lancet ii: 454–455

Friedmann M, Strang L B 1966 Effect of long term cortico-steroids and corticotrophin on the growth of children. Lancet ii: 568–569

Giorgini G L, Stephens R V, Thayer W R 1973 The use of 'medical bypass' in the therapy of Crohn's disease: report of a case. American Journal of Digestive Diseases 18: 153–157

Gonzales-Huix F, de Leon R, Fernandez-Banares F et al 1993 Polymeric enteral diets as primary treatment of active Crohn's disease: a prospective steroid controlled trial. Gut 34: 778–782

Green J R B, O'Donoghue D P, Edwards C R W et al 1977 A case of apparent hypopituitarism complicating chronic inflammatory bowel disease in childhood adolescence. Acta Paediatrica Scandinavica 66: 643

Greenberg G R, Haber G B, Jeejeebhoy K N 1976 Total parenteral nutrition (TPN) and bowel rest in the management of Crohn's disease. Gut 17: 828

Greenstein A J, Janowitz H D, Sachar D B 1976 The extra-intestinal complications of Crohn's disease and ulcerative colitis: a study of 700 patients. Medicine 55: 401

Greenstein A J, Sachar D B, Pucillo A 1979 Cancer in universal and left-sided ulcerative colitis: clinical and pathological features. Mount Sinai Journal of Medicine 46: 25

Greenstein J P, Birnbaum S M, Winitz M et al 1957 Quantitative nutritional studies with water-soluble chemically defined diets. I. Growth, reproduction and lactation in rats. Archives of Biochemistry and Biophysics 72: 396–456

Griffiths A, Koletzko S, Sylvester F et al 1993 Slow-release 5-aminosalicylic acid therapy in children with small intestinal Crohn's disease. Journal of Pediatric Gastroenterology and Nutrition 17: 186–192

Gryboski J D, Katz J, Sangree M H et al 1968 Eleven adolescent girls with severe anorexia. Clinical Pediatrics 7: 684

Hadziselomovic F, Emmons L R 1990 Letters to the editor. Journal of the American Medical Association 264: 2741

Harries J T, Lloyd J 1971 Azathioprine in the treatment of Crohn's disease. Acta Paediatrica Scandinavica 60: 376

Harris B H, Boles E T 1973 Intestinal lesions in chronic granulomatous disease of childhood. Journal of Pediatric Surgery 8: 955

Hellers G 1979 Crohn's disease in Stockholm County 1955–1974. A study of epidemiology, results of surgical treatment and long-term prognosis. Acta Chirurgica Scandinavica Supplement 490

Helmholz H F 1923 Chronic ulcerative colitis in childhood. American Journal of Diseases in Childhood 26: 418–430

Hendriksen C, Kreiner S, Binder V 1985 Long-term prognosis in ulcerative colitis – based on results from a regional patient group from

the county of Copenhagen. Gut 26: 158–163
Hildebrand H, Karlberg J, Kristiansson B 1994 Longitudinal growth in children and adolescents with inflammatory bowel disease. Journal of Pediatric Gastroenterology and Nutrition 18: 165–173
Hodgson H J F 1991 Cyclosporine in inflammatory bowel disease. Alimentary Pharmacology and Therapeutics 5: 343–350
Hofley P, Roarty J, McGinnity G et al 1993 Asymptomatic uveitis in children with chronic inflammatory bowel disease. Journal of Pediatric Gastroenterology and Nutrition 17: 397
Hollander D, Vadheim C M, Brettholz E et al 1986 Increased intestinal permeability in patients with Crohn's disease and their relatives. Annals of Internal Medicine 105: 883
Isaacs D, Wright V M, Shaw D G et al 1985 Chronic granulomatous disease mimicking Crohn's disease. Journal of Pediatric Gastroenterology and Nutrition 4: 498–502
Jenkins H R, Pincott J R, Soothill J F et al 1984 Food allergy: the major cause of infantile colitis. Archives of Disease in Childhood 59: 326–329
Kane W, Miller K, Sharp H L 1980 Inflammatory bowel disease presenting as liver disease in childhood. Journal of Pediatrics 97: 775–778
Kasahara Y, Tanaka S, Nishino M et al 1981 Intestinal involvement in Behçet's disease. Review of 136 surgical cases. Diseases of the Colon and Rectum 24: 103–106
Kelts D J, Grand R J, Shen G et al 1979 Nutritional basis of growth failure in children and adolescents with Crohn's disease. Gastroenterology 76: 720–727
Keventer J, Ahlman H, Hulton L 1978 Cancer risk in extensive ulcerative colitis. Annals of Surgery 188: 824–828
Kingham J G C, Levinson D A, Ball J A et al 1982 Microscopic colitis – a cause of chronic watery diarrhoea. British Medical Journal 285: 1601–1604
Kirschner B S 1988 Inflammatory bowel disease in children. Pediatric Clinics of North America 34: 189–208
Kirschner B S, Samanowitz W 1986 Secondary amyloidosis in Crohn's disease of childhood. Journal of Pediatric Gastroenterology and Nutrition 5: 816–821
Kirschner B S, Klich J R, Kalman S S et al 1981 Reversal of growth retardation in Crohn's disease with therapy emphasising oral nutritional restitution. Gastroenterology 80: 10–15
Kirschner B S, Voinchet O, Rosenberg I H 1978 Growth retardation in children with inflammatory bowel disease. Gastroenterology 75: 504
Kirschner B S, Whitington P F, Black D B 1987 Cyclosporin-induced remission in severe colitis unresponsive to corticosteroid therapy (abstract). Pediatric Research 21: 271A
Kirsner J B, Rakin H F, Palmer W L 1955 Ulcerative colitis in children: observations in selected patients. American Journal of Diseases in Childhood 90: 141–152
Kock N G 1969 Intra-abdominal 'reservoir' in patients with permanent ileostomy. Archives of Surgery 99: 223–231
Lake A M, Kim S, Mathis R K et al 1985 Influence of preoperative parenteral alimentation of post-operative growth in adolescent Crohn's disease. Journal of Pediatric Gastroenterology and Nutrition 4: 182
Lashner B A, Shaheen N J, Hanauer et al 1993 Passive smoking is associated with an increased risk of developing inflammatory bowel disease in children. American Journal of Gastroenterology 88: 356–359
Lebowohl O, Forde K, Berdon W et al 1977 Ulcerative oesophagitis and colitis in a pediatric patient with Behçet's syndrome. American Journal of Gastroenterology 68: 550–555
Lennard-Jones J E 1981 Azathioprine and 6-mercaptopurine have a role in the treatment of Crohn's disease. Digestive Diseases and Sciences 26: 364
Lewis M A, Priestley B L 1986 Transient neonatal Behçet's disease. Archives of Disease in Childhood 61: 805–806
Lichtiger S, Present D H 1990 Preliminary report: cyclosporin in the treatment of severe active ulcerative colitis. Lancet 336: 16–19
Lindsey C B, Schaller J G 1974 Arthritis associated with inflammatory bowel disease in childhood. Journal of Pediatrics 84: 16
Lipson A B, Savage M O, Davies P S W 1990 Acceleration of linear growth following intestinal resection for Crohn's disease. European Journal of Paediatrics 149: 687–690
Lloyd-Still J D, Green C 1979 A clinical scoring system for chronic inflammatory bowel disease in children. Digestive Diseases and Sciences 24: 620–624
Logan R F A, Gillon J, Ferrington C et al 1981 Reduction of intestinal protein loss by elemental diet in Crohn's disease of the small bowel. Gut 22: 383–387
McCaffery T D, Nast R, Lawrence A M et al 1974a Severe growth retardation in children with inflammatory bowel disease. Pediatrics 45: 386
McCaffery T D, Nasr K, Laurence A M et al 1974b Effect of administered human growth hormone on growth retardation in inflammatory bowel disease. Journal of Digestive Diseases 9: 411–416
McConnell R B 1980 Inflammatory bowel disease: newer views of genetic influences. In: Berk (ed) Developments in digestive diseases. Lea and Febiger, Philadelphia, pp 129–138
McConnell R B, Shaw J M, Whibley E J et al 1986 Inflammatory bowel disease. Frontiers of gastrointestinal research, vol II. Karger, Basel, 1–11
McLain B I, Davidson P M, Stokes K B et al 1990 Growth after gut resection for Crohn's disease. Archives of Disease in Childhood 65: 760–762
McLean A, Bartram C I 1990 Prone compression with the pneumatic paddle during barium studies. Clinical Radiology 41: 5–8
Malchow H, Ewe K, Brandes J W et al 1984 European Cooperative Crohn's Disease Study (ECCDS): results of drug treatment. Gastroenterology 86: 249–273
Mallett P, Murch S H 1990 Anorexia nervosa complicating inflammatory bowel disease. Archives of Disease in Childhood 65: 298–300
Markowitz J, Grancher K, Rosa J et al 1993a Growth failure in pediatric inflammatory bowel disease. Journal of Pediatric Gastroenterology and Nutrition 16: 373–380
Markowitz J, Kahn E, Grancher K et al 1993b Atypical recto-sigmoid histology in children with newly diagnosed ulcerative colitis. American Journal of Gastroenterology 88: 2034–2037
Mason R M, Barnes C G 1969 Behçet's syndrome with arthritis. Annals of Rheumatic Diseases 28: 95–103
Michelassi F, Testa G, Pomidor W J et al 1993 Adenocarcinoma complicating Crohn's disease. Diseases of the Colon and Rectum 36: 654–661
Michener W M, Farmer R G, Mortimer E A 1979 Long-term prognosis of ulcerative colitis with onset in childhood or adolescence. Journal of Clinical Gastroenterology 1: 301
Morgan R A, Manning P B, Coran A G 1987 Experience with the straight endorectal pull-through for the management of ulcerative colitis and familial polyposis in children and adults. Annals of Surgery 206: 595–599
Morin C L, Roulet M, Roy C C et al 1980 Continuous elemental enteral alimentation in children with Crohn's disease and growth failure. Gastroenterology 79: 1205–1210
Morin C L, Roulet M, Weber A et al 1982 Continuous elemental alimentation in the treatment of children and adolescents with Crohn's disease. Journal of Parenteral and Enteral Nutrition 6: 194–199
Morson B C 1968 Histopathology of Crohn's disease. Proceedings of the Royal Society of Medicine 61: 79
Moseley J E, Marshak R H, Wolf B S 1960 Regional enteritis in children. American Journal of Roentgenology 84: 532–539
Motil K J, Altschuler S I, Grand R J 1985 Mineral balance during nutritional supplementation in adolescents with Crohn's disease and growth failure. Journal of Pediatrics 107: 473
Motil K J, Grand R J, Davis-Kraft L et al 1993 Growth failure in children with inflammatory bowel disease: a prospective study. Gastroenterology 105: 681–691
Murch S H, Braegger C P, Walker-Smith J A et al 1993b Location of tumour necrosis factor alpha by immunohistochemistry in chronic inflammatory bowel disease. Gut 34: 1705–1709
Murch S H, Lamkin V A, Savage M O et al 1991 Serum concentrations of tumour necrosis factor alpha in childhood chronic inflammatory bowel disease. Gut 32: 913–917
Murch S H, MacDonald T T, Walker-Smith J A 1993a Disruption of sulphated glycosaminoglycans in intestinal inflammation. Lancet 341: 711–714

Navarro J, Vargas J, Cezard J P et al 1982 Prolonged constant rate elemental nutrition in Crohn's disease. Journal of Pediatric Gastroenterology and Nutrition 1: 541–546

Nemeth A, Ejderhamn J, Glaumann et al 1990 Liver damage in juvenile inflammatory bowel disease. Liver 10: 239–248

Nicholls S W, Domizio P, Williams C B et al 1995 Cyclosporin A as initial therapy for Crohn's disease. Archives of Disease in Childhood (in press)

Norland C C, Kirsner J B 1969 Toxic dilatation of the colon (toxic megacolon): etiology, treatment and prognosis in 42 patients. Medicine 48: 229–250

Odigwe L, Sherman P M, Filler R et al 1987 Straight ileo-anal anastamosis and ileal pouch–anal anastamosis in the surgical management of idiopathic ulcerative colitis and familial polyposis coli in children: follow-up and comparative analysis. Journal of Pediatric Gastroenterology and Nutrition 6: 426–429

O'Donoghue D P, Dawson A M 1977 Crohn's disease in childhood. Archives of Disease in Childhood 52: 627

O'Donoghue D P, Powel-Tuck J, Brown R C et al 1978 Double blind withdrawal trial of azathioprine as maintainence treatment for Crohn's disease. Lancet ii: 955–957

Okabe M, Hiraki M, Chiba Y 1980 Behçet's disease in a one year-old child. Japanese Journal of Pediatrics 33: 549–552

O'Morain C 1979 Elemental diet in the treatment of Crohn's disease. Proceedings of the Nutritional Society 38: 403–408

O'Morain C 1981 Acute ileitis. British Medical Journal 283: 1075

O'Morain C, Segal A W, Levi A J 1980 Elemantal diets in the treatment of acute Crohn's disease. British Medical Journal 281: 1173–1175

O'Morain C, Segal A W, Levi A J et al 1983 Elemental diet in acute Crohn's disease. Archives of Disease in Childhood 53: 44

O'Morain C, Segal A W, Levi A J 1984 Elemental diet as primary treatment of acute Crohn's disease: a controlled trial. British Medical Journal 288: 1859–1862

Pai C H 1984 Sporadic cases of haemorrhagic colitis associated with *Escherichia coli*: H7. Annals of Internal Medicine 101: 738

Palder S B, Shandling B, Bilik R et al 1991 Perianal complications of pediatric Crohn's disease. Journal of Pediatric Surgery 26: 513–515

Passo M H, Fitzgerald J F, Brandt K D 1986 Arthritis associated with inflammatory bowel disease in children: relationship of joint disease to activity and severity of bowel lesion. Digestive Diseases and Sciences 31: 492

Perrault J, Greseth J L, Tremaine W J 1991 6-mercaptopurine therapy in selected cases of corticosteroid-dependent Crohn's disease. Mayo Clinic Proceedings 66: 480–484

Perrault J, Telander R L, Zinsmeister A R et al 1988 The endorectal pull-through procedure in children and young adults: a follow-up study. Journal of Pediatric Gastroenterology and Nutrition 7: 89–94

Polk D B, Hattner J A, Kerner J A Jr 1992 Improved growth and disease activity after intermittent administration of a defined formula diet in children with Crohn's disease. Journal of Parenteral and Enteral Nutrition 16: 499–504

Price A B 1978 Overlap in the spectrum of non-specific inflammatory bowel disease – 'colitis intermediate'. Journal of Clinical Pathology 56: 74–77

Puntis J, McNeish A S, Allan R N 1984 Long-term prognosis of Crohn's disease with onset in childhood and adolescence. Gut 25: 329–336

Rankin G B, Watts H D, Melnyk C J et al 1979 National Cooperative Crohn's Disease Study – extraintestinal manifestations and perianal complications. Gastroenterology 77: 914–920

Rigaud D, Cosnes J, le Quintrec Y et al 1991 Controlled trial comparing two types of enteral nutrition in treatment of active Crohn's disease: elemental v polymeric diet. Gut 32: 1492–1497

Rocchio M A, Mo Cha C J, Haas K F 1973 Use of chemically defined diets in the management of patients with acute inflammatory bowel disease. American Journal of Surgery 127: 469–475

Rombeau J C, Barot L R, Williamson C E et al 1982 Preoperative total parenteral nutrition and surgical outcome in patients with inflammatory bowel disease. American Journal of Surgery 143: 139

Sandborn W J, Tremaine W J 1992 Cyclosporine treatment of inflammatory bowel disease. Mayo Clinic Proceedings 67: 981–990

Sanderson I R 1986 Chronic inflammatory bowel disease. Clinics in Gastroenterology 15: 71–89

Sanderson I R, Walker-Smith J A 1984 Indigenous amoebiasis: an important differential diagnosis of chronic inflammatory bowel disease. British Medical Journal 289: 823

Sanderson I R, Walker-Smith J A 1985 Crohn's disease in childhood. British Journal of Surgery 72 (Suppl): S87–90

Sanderson I R, Boyle S, Walford N et al 1985 Abnormal histology in children with macroscopically normal appearance at colonoscopy (Abstract). 57th Meeting of the British Paediatric Association, York

Sanderson I R, Chong S F K, Walker-Smith J A 1986 Family occurrence of chronic inflammatory bowel disease. In: Rozen P, McConnell R (eds) Epidemiology and genetics of inflammatory bowel disease

Sanderson I R, Risdon R A, Walker-Smith J A 1991 Intractable enterocolitis of infancy. Archives of Disease in Childhood 66: 295–299

Sanderson I R, Udeen S, Davies P S W et al 1987 Remission induced by an elemental diet in small bowel Crohn's disease. Archives of Disease in Childhood 61: 123–127

Schaffer J A, Williams S E, Turnberg C A et al 1983 Absorption of prednisolone in patients with Crohn's disease. Gut 24: 182–186

Schiff E 1945 Die regionale Enteritis. Annales Paediatrici 165: 281–311

Schmitz-Moormann P, Schag M 1990 Histology of the lower intestinal tract in Crohn's disease of children and adolescents. Multicentre Paediatric Crohn's Disease Study. Pathology, Research and Practice 186: 479–484

Seashore H J, Hillemeier A C, Gryboski J D 1982 Total parenteral nutrition in the management of inflammatory bowel disease in children: a limited role. American Journal of Surgery 143: 504

Silverman F N 1966 Regional enteritis in children. Australian Paediatric Journal ii: 20

Smith G E, Kime L R, Loren Pitcher J 1973 The colitis of Behçet's disease. A separate entity. Digestive Diseases 18: 987–1000

Sorenson V Z, Olsen B G, Binder V 1987 Life prospects and quality of life in patients with Crohn's disease. Gut 28: 382

Stephens R V, Randall H T 1969 Use of a concentrated balanced liquid elemental diet for nutritional management of catabolic states. Annals of Surgery 170: 642–667

Stringer D A, Sherman P M, Jakowenko N 1986a Correlation of double-contrast high-density barium enema, colonoscopy and histology in children with special attention to disparities. Pediatric Radiology 16: 298–301

Stringer D A, Cleghorn G J, Durie P R et al 1986b Behçet's syndrome involving the gastrointestinal tract – a diagnostic dilemma in childhood. Pediatric Radiology 16: 131–134

Strobel C T, Byrne W J, Ament M E 1979 Home parenteral nutrition in children with Crohn's disease: an effective management alternative. Gastroenterology 77: 272–279

Summers R W, Switz D M, Sessions J T Jr et al 1979 National Cooperative Crohn's Disease Study: results of drug treatment. Gastroenterology 77: 827–828

Szajnberg N, Krall V, Davis P et al 1993 Psychopathology and relationship measures in children with inflammatory bowel disease and their parents. Child Psychiatry and Human Development 23: 215–232

Tandon B N, Mathur A K, Mohapatra L N 1965 A study of the prevalence and clinical pattern of non-specific ulcerative colitis in Northern India. Gut 6: 448–453

Telander R L, Perrault J 1980 Total colectomy with rectal mucosectomy and ileo-anal anastomosis for chronic ulcerative colitis in children and young adults. Mayo Clinic Proceedings 55: 420

Telander R L, Spencer M, Perrault J et al 1990 Long-term follow-up of the ileoanal anastamosis in children and young adults. Surgery 108: 717–723

Thomas A G, Taylor F, Miller V 1993a Dietary intake and nutritional treatment in childhood Crohn's disease. Journal of Pediatric Gastroenterology and Nutrition 17: 75–81

Thomas A G, Holly J M, Taylor F et al 1993b Insulin-like growth factor-1, insulin-like growth factor binding protein-1 and insulin in childhood Crohn's disease. Gut 34: 944–947

Thomas B M 1979 The instant enema in inflammatory bowel disease of the colon. Clinical Radiology 30: 165–173

Treem W R, Davis P M, Hyams J S 1991 Cyclosporine treatment of severe ulcerative colitis in children. Journal of Pediatrics 119: 994–997

Ursing B, Alm T, Barany F et al 1982 A cooperative study of metronidazole and sulfasalazine for active Crohn's disease: the Cooperative Crohn's Disease Study in Sweden. II. Result. Gastroenterology 83: 550

Verhave M, Winter H S, Grand R J (1990) Azathioprine in the treatment of children with inflammatory bowel disease. Journal of Pediatrics 117: 809–814

Voitk A J, Echave B, Feller J H 1973 Experience of elemental diets in the treatment of inflammatory bowel disease. Is this primary therapy? Archives of Surgery 107: 329–333

Walker-Smith J A 1986 Commentary. Archives of Disease in Childhood 61: 958–959

Walker-Smith J A, Benfield G F A, Montgomery R D et al 1986 Chronic inflammatory bowel disease in immigrants in the United Kingdom. In: McConnell R, Rozen P, Langman M, Gilat T (eds) Frontiers of gastrointestinal research: the genetics and epidemiology of inflammatory bowel disease Vol 11: 18–25

Wallis S M, Walker-Smith J A 1976 An unusual case of Crohn's disease in a West Indian child. Acta Paediatrica Scandinavica 65: 749

Watanabe I, Kuwabara N, Fukada Y 1979 Histopathological studies in intestinal Behçet's disease. Stomach and Intestine 7: 903–913

Werlin S C, Grand R J 1977 Severe colitis in children and adolescents: diagnostic course and treatment. Gastroenterology 73: 828–837

Wesson D E, Schandling B 1981 Results of bowel resection for Crohn's disease in the young. Journal of Pediatric Surgery 16: 449

Williams C B, Laage N J, Campbell C A et al 1982 Total colonoscopy in children. Archives of Disease in Childhood 57: 49–53

Winitz M, Graff J, Gallagher N et al 1965 Evaluation of chemicals as nutrition for man-in-space. Nature 205: 741–743

73. Inflammatory bowel disease, the oral contraceptive pill and pregnancy

R. N. Allan

This chapter opens with a review of the role of the oral contraceptive pill in the pathogenesis of inflammatory bowel disease and fertility in inflammatory bowel disease patients. The next section is concerned with inflammatory bowel disease and pregnancy, including the impact of ulcerative colitis and Crohn's disease on both the fetus and the mother, and the safety of drug treatment during pregnancy. The outcome of surgical treatment during pregnancy and the problems that may be encountered in patients with an ileostomy or ileoanal pouch is then considered. The chapter closes with a review of the short- and long-term prognosis of ulcerative colitis and Crohn's disease after parturition.

ORAL CONTRACEPTIVE PILL AND PATHOGENESIS

Several large studies have shown a small but consistent increase in the prevalence of ulcerative colitis and Crohn's disease among users of the oral contraceptive pill compared to non-users, but despite the large number of patients studied, the differences between the groups did not reach statistical significance. For example, in the study by Logan and colleagues (1989) the relative risk of developing Crohn's disease when users were compared with non-users was 1.7, and a 1.3-fold risk for patients with ulcerative colitis. Neither reached statistical significance.

Lesko et al (1985) found a 1.9-fold relative risk among patients with Crohn's disease who used the oral contraceptive pill compared with non-users. The excess risk was greatly increased in recent users (relative risk 4.3) compared to ex-users (relative risk 1.2). Most studies have consistently shown that this small excess relative risk returns to normal when the oral contraceptives are stopped.

These data suggest that the oral contraceptive pill is safe and only rarely associated with the development of ulcerative colitis or Crohn's disease. The data are probably best interpreted as suggesting that a small subset of individuals develop a pill-related colitis indistinguishable from ulcerative colitis and Crohn's colitis, which resolves on withdrawing the oral contraceptive pill. It seems sensible to advise withdrawal of the oral contraceptive pill in patients with ulcerative colitis or Crohn's disease who have not responded to standard therapy, provided of course that alternative contraceptive measures are offered at the same time.

FERTILITY IN WOMEN

Ulcerative colitis

Several excellent clinical studies have shown that fertility in women with ulcerative colitis is normal and no different from that in the general population. Thus in a large series of married women with ulcerative colitis, 81% conceived normally, 12% voluntarily avoided pregnancy, 2% of husbands had oligospermia and 5% were unable to have children. These figures are equivalent to the general population, for example 10% of UK marriages are childless (Willoughby & Truelove 1980).

Crohn's disease

There is good evidence that fertility in women with Crohn's disease is impaired. Mayberry and Weterman (1986) undertook an extensive European study and showed that patients with Crohn's disease had only half the number of children produced by healthy control couples. There are several good reasons which might explain this finding, but the exact explanation has not yet been defined. The possibilities include the severity of disease, avoiding pregnancy on medical advice, dyspareunia, particularly in the presence of severe perianal disease, and impaired ovulation or fallopian tube blockage following pelvic sepsis complicating Crohn's disease.

FERTILITY IN MEN

It is well recognized that fertility may be affected in men taking sulfasalazine, by reducing both the total sperm count and sperm motility, but that this effect is reversible after withdrawing the drug (Cann & Holdsworth 1984). The sulfapyridine moiety is probably responsible, since this problem is not found with other 5-ASA preparations. There is evidence that active Crohn's disease may cause oligospermia in some men, and thus directly account for infertility.

IMPACT OF INFLAMMATORY BOWEL DISEASE ON PREGNANCY

Ulcerative colitis – impact on the fetus

Many studies have shown that pregnancy in ulcerative colitis usually results in a normal full-term baby. The incidence of low birth weight or fetal abnormality is no greater than that expected in the general population.

Willoughby (1990) summarized the 14 major studies on the outcome of pregnancy in women with ulcerative colitis, and showed that of 1466 pregnancies a normal live birth resulted in 1238 (84%). The incidence of spontaneous abortion (8%), therapeutic abortion (5%), congenital abnormalities (1%) and stillbirth (1%) is similar to that observed in the healthy population.

Impact on the mother

In patients with established ulcerative colitis in remission at the time of conception, the disease is likely to remain quiescent throughout pregnancy and the puerperium. Active disease at the time of conception is more likely to be associated with recurrence of symptoms during pregnancy, particularly during the first trimester. In the past relapse of disease in the puerperium was thought to be common, but this has not been substantiated in practice. Ulcerative colitis occasionally arises for the first time during pregnancy.

Crohn's disease – impact on the fetus

Excellent data on Crohn's disease and pregnancy are available from a recent study by Woolfson and colleagues (1990). They studied 78 pregnancies in 50 patients with Crohn's disease. The incidence of spontaneous abortion, babies small for dates, premature birth, respiratory distress and fetal abnormality was similar to that expected in the general population.

At the time of conception 79% had inactive Crohn's disease and in general a poorer fetal outcome was found in patients with active disease at the time of conception. There was no evidence that appropriate medical or surgical treatment adversely affected the outcome for the fetus.

Crohn's disease – impact on the mother

The outlook for the mother is particularly favorable if their Crohn's disease is quiescent at the time of conception, when most (70%) remain symptom-free during pregnancy and the puerperium. Individual case reports have been described of Crohn's disease presenting either during pregnancy or shortly after delivery, but both these events are rare.

The overall prospects for pregnancy in Crohn's disease are good, but patients should avoid becoming pregnant when their disease is active, since it impairs the outcome of both the pregnancy and the underlying Crohn's disease.

SURGICAL TREATMENT DURING PREGNANCY

Several individual case reports and small series report a satisfactory outcome in pregnant patients undergoing surgery for their inflammatory bowel disease, but the reported numbers are too small to draw reliable conclusions.

PREGNANCY IN ILEOSTOMY PATIENTS

Willoughby (1990) summarized nine studies of patients with ulcerative colitis who became pregnant after surgical treatment which included an ileostomy. Among 119 pregnancies the outcome for the fetus was similar to that expected in the general population. Among the 119 pregnancies there were 18 stoma problems, including intestinal obstruction (9), stoma prolapse (5), leakage around the stoma (2), intussusception (1) and one further undefined problem.

Individual case reports and small series of patients with ileoanal pouches who have undergone successful and uneventful pregnancy have been reported, and are summarized by Metcalf et al (1985).

DRUG TREATMENT DURING PREGNANCY

Sulfasalazine

Although high-dose sulfonamides can cause congenital abnormalities in the offspring of pregnant rats, there are no published reports of sulfasalazine-associated congenital abnormalities in humans. Indeed, extensive studies of sulfasalazine in pregnancy have shown no adverse effect on the chances of producing a normal child (Nielson et al 1984). Recent studies of oral 5-amino salicylic acid (5-ASA) for inflammatory bowel disease in pregnancy have shown that its use is safe for both the fetus and the mother (Habal et al 1993).

Metronidazole

There are no large reports of the use of metronidazole during pregnancy in patients with inflammatory bowel disease. However, there are several large studies of pregnant patients taking metronidazole during pregnancy for trichomonas vaginalis. No adverse effect on the fetus was found. In particular, birth weight, the incidence of stillbirths and congenital abnormalities were exactly as would be expected in the general population (Piper et al 1993).

Immunosuppressive therapy

There are no large studies of the use of azathioprine during pregnancy in patients with inflammatory bowel disease. The nearest equivalent are the data analyzed from those women receiving azathioprine during pregnancy following renal transplantation. The data collected from 49 papers describe the outcome of 434 pregnancies in 375 women, of which 356 (82%) resulted in overtly normal infants, a figure close to that expected in the general population (P M Davies 1994, personal communication).

BREASTFEEDING IN IBD PATIENTS TAKING SULFASALAZINE

Sulfasalazine and sulfapyridine are secreted into breast milk, and theoretically sulfasalazine could bind to circulating albumin and displace unconjugated bilirubin. However, it is now clear that sulfasalazine binds to albumin at sites other than high-affinity sites for bilirubin, and is not therefore a risk factor for the development of kernicterus in the breastfed infant (Jarnerot et al 1981).

LONG-TERM OUTCOME AFTER PREGNANCY

Ulcerative colitis

The symptomatic pattern of ulcerative colitis in the first pregnancy cannot be used to predict the symptomatic pattern in subsequent pregnancies.

Crohn's disease

Interesting evidence is emerging that parity in women with Crohn's disease improves the long-term outcome, in that women in the postpartum period have fewer exacerbations and undergo fewer resections than non-parous controls with Crohn's disease. This beneficial effect was evident in patients with both distal ileal and colonic Crohn's disease. In non-parous patients with ileal disease after a mean follow-up of 15 years, the mean number of resections per patient was 1.5 compared with a mean resection rate of 1.2 in those who had been pregnant before diagnosis.

The interval from first to second resection was 10 years in non-parous patients and 13 years in parous patients. Similar data were evident in patients with colonic Crohn's disease, where the number of resections per patient was fewer in those who had been pregnant before diagnosis and the interval from first to subsequent resection was much longer (Nwokolo et al 1994). The mechanism for this protective effect of pregnancy on the outcome of Crohn's disease is uncertain, but pregnancy could influence the natural history of the disease either by decreasing immune responsiveness or by retarding fibrous stricture formation, which is the most common indication for surgical intervention, particularly in patients with distal ileal disease.

REFERENCES

Cann P A, Holdsworth C D 1984 Reversal of male infertility on changing treatment from sulphasalazine to 5 amino salicylate. Lancet 1: 1119

Habal F M, Hui G, Greenberg G R 1993 Oral 5-aminosalicylic acid for inflammatory bowel disease in pregnancy: safety and clinical course. Gastroenterology 105: 1057–1060

Jarnerot G, Anderson S, Esbjorner E, Sandstrom B, Brodersen R 1981 Albumin reserve for binding of bilirubin in maternal and cord serum under treatment with sulphasalazine. Scandinavian Journal of Gastroenterology 16: 1049–1055

Lesko S M, Kaufman D W, Rosenberg L et al 1985 Evidence for an increased risk of Crohn's disease in oral contraceptive users. Gastroenterology 89: 1046–1049

Logan R F A, Kay C R, Scott L 1989 The pill, smoking and inflammatory bowel disease: results from the RCGP oral contraceptive study. International Journal of Epidemiology 18: 105–107

Mayberry J F, Weterman I T 1986 European survey of fertility and pregnancy in women with Crohn's disease: a case-control study by European collaborative group. Gut 27: 821–825

Metcalf A, Dozois R R, Beart R W, Wolff B G 1985 Pregnancy following ileal pouch–anal anastomosis. Diseases of the Colon and Rectum 28: 859–861

Nielson O H, Andreasson B, Bondesen S, Jacobson O, Jarnum S 1984 Pregnancy in Crohn's disease. Scandinavian Journal of Gastroenterology 19: 724–732

Nwokolo C U, Tan W C, Andrews H A, Allan R N 1994 Surgical resections in parous patients with distal ileal and colonic Crohn's disease. Gut 35: 220–223

Piper J M, Mitchell E F, Ray W A 1993 Prenatal use of metronidazole and birth defects: no association. Obstetrics and Gynaecology 82: 348–352

Willoughby C P 1990 Fertility, pregnancy and inflammatory bowel disease. In: Allan R N, Keighley M R B, Hawkins C F, Alexander-Williams J (eds) Inflammatory bowel diseases, 2nd edn Churchill Livingstone, Edinburgh, pp 547–558

Willoughby C P, Truelove S C 1980 Ulcerative colitis and pregnancy. Gut 21: 469–474

Woolfson K, Cohen Z, McLeod R S 1990 Crohn's disease and pregnancy. Diseases of the Colon and Rectum 33: 869–873

74. Cancer risk in ulcerative colitis and Crohn's disease – strategies to avoid cancer deaths

J. E. Lennard-Jones

INTRODUCTION

A complete Swedish follow-up study of 4776 patients with inflammatory bowel disease (IBD) seen between 1965 and 1983 showed that there were 684 deaths compared to 481 expected (Ekbom et al 1992). The causes of death related to the gastrointestinal tract were 159 from IBD, mainly during the first 2 years after diagnosis, 50 from colorectal cancer, 20 from non-alcohol related hepatobiliary disease, and 42 from other conditions. These figures confirm those of other studies, which show that the mortality from IBD relative to the general population is low (SMR 1.4, 95% CI 1.3–1.5) and that the most common cause of death is acute disease soon after diagnosis. The number of deaths from colorectal cancer complicating IBD is numerically small, but it is one of the two most common causes of late death from related disorders. The purpose of this chapter is to discuss how the number of deaths from colorectal cancer can be reduced.

POSSIBLE STRATEGIES TO REDUCE CANCER DEATHS

Prophylactic surgery

Removal of the colon and rectum before the development of cancer is an effective preventive measure. However, most patients who are well, or who experience only minimal symptoms, do not accept surgical treatment purely to avoid the development of cancer because the risk does not seem great enough. Similarly, most clinicians would not advise surgical treatment, with its uncertainties of outcome, for a symptomless patient unless they were convinced that the risk of that person already having a cancer, or of developing one within a short period, was very high. All clinicians, however, are prepared to advise surgical treatment for severe or disabling colitis, when the symptomatic outcome is likely to be better than before operation; the cancer risk may be an additional factor in this recommendation.

Clinical supervision

Supervision means repeated clinical assessment of a patient's symptoms, disability and treatment, with reinvestigation if new symptoms develop or there is a change in clinical state. Patients are encouraged to seek early advice for any new symptoms that develop between regular visits.

Screening investigations

Screening implies an occasional investigation among a population of patients to detect precancer or cancer. In the context of colitis it means endoscopy with biopsy, with or without barium enema, for a patient who has not been fully investigated for many years.

Cancer surveillance

Surveillance can be defined as a regular program of investigation in patients without symptoms due to cancer. The first investigation is of necessity a screening procedure.

The rationale of surveillance is based on observations that dysplastic epithelial change often occurs at a distance from carcinoma in ulcerative colitis, and less commonly in Crohn's disease, suggesting that it is a precancerous phase of disease. The hypothesis on which pilot studies have been based is that the recognition of dysplasia might enable colectomy to be performed in particularly high-risk subjects before carcinoma develops or, as a second-best option, that a finding of dysplasia might act as a marker for symptomless carcinoma elsewhere in the colon and thus increase the likelihood of curative surgery. The success of a surveillance program can be judged only by the demonstration that it reduces cancer mortality. This proof has not so far been possible.

ULCERATIVE COLITIS

Recognition of high-risk patients

Any cancer screening or surveillance program in ulcerative colitis is most likely to find precancer or cancer in patients with a greater risk of cancer than other patients with the disease.

Extent of disease

Many studies have shown that the risk of cancer is little, if at all, greater than normal among patients with proctitis. When disease is limited to the left side of the colon the risk overall is about four times, and when it also affects the transverse or right colon it is about 20 times that in the general population (Gyde et al 1988).

Definitions of the extent of colitis vary in the literature, but if the term 'extensive' colitis is taken as macroscopic inflammation of part or all of the colon proximal to the splenic flexure, this accords with many published series.

Histological abnormalities often extend proximal to the apparent upper limit of inflammation as judged by barium enema or endoscopy. At present, in the absence of data to the contrary, it seems best to judge the upper limit of inflammation by visual changes on endoscopy or air contrast barium enema. The upper limit is most easily assessed when the colitis is active; when quiescent, evidence of previous proximal inflammation may be shown by mucosal atrophy, scarring or inflammatory polyp formation.

Duration of disease

Although cancer occasionally develops during the first few years after the onset of colitis, there is an extensive literature which shows that the risk rises to become clinically significant in patients with extensive colitis 8–10 years or more after the first symptoms (Gyde et al 1988).

Age of onset

There is controversy as to whether onset of ulcerative colitis during childhood or adolescence increases the cancer risk. The extent of colitis tends to be greater among children than adults, thus increasing the proportion of children at higher risk. It is not certain whether the risk per patient year for children or young people with extensive colitis is greater than in adults. However, since life expectancy is long the lifetime risk is likely to be greater than in older people. Lastly, the relative risk compared with the general population of the same age is greatly raised because colorectal carcinoma is so rare among healthy young people. For all these reasons, the cancer risk among young people with colitis needs special attention.

Presence of stricture(s)

A stricture may not only indicate long-standing chronic disease but also be a manifestation of carcinoma. In one series of 70 strictures in 59 patients, 17 (24%) proved to be malignant. Factors suggesting malignancy were appearance late in the disease course, location proximal to the splenic flexure, and association with symptoms of obstruction (Gumaste et al 1992).

Retained rectum and/or distal colon after surgical treatment

Several series have shown that the retained rectum after colectomy and ileorectal anastomosis is at risk of developing carcinoma. Clinical experience suggests that a similar risk applies to the defunctioned rectum and/or distal colon after colectomy.

Association with primary sclerosing cholangitis (PSC)

A case control study has shown that patients with primary sclerosing cholangitis and ulcerative colitis have a greater risk of developing colorectal carcinoma or dysplasia than matched patients with ulcerative colitis alone (Broomé et al 1995). The patients with primary sclerosing cholangitis also have an increased risk of cholangiocarcinoma.

Limitations of dysplasia

Experience of dysplasia as a clinical marker of precancer or cancer has now shown that it is a useful prognostic test but that it has limitations, which must be clearly appreciated if histological findings are to be interpreted correctly.

Is dysplasia present or absent?

The 'threshold' for diagnosis of dysplasia can vary with time and from one pathologist to another. Blinded review by two experienced pathologists of biopsies regarded as showing dysplasia in earlier years showed that changes regarded previously as mild or low-grade dysplasia are now often considered a reaction to inflammation (Connell et al 1994a). Agreement between these pathologists as to whether dysplasia was present or absent was good, but not totally concordant. The raised threshold for diagnosis of low-grade dysplasia in recent years has increased its specificity with little loss of sensitivity.

If present, is dysplasia low or high grade?

A consensus classification introduced in 1983 (Riddell et al 1983) has not removed all uncertainty and several blinded reviews have shown that agreement is only fair. For example, in a recent study, although one experienced pathologist identified 22 biopsies as showing high-grade dysplasia, another recorded only ten as high grade, nine as low grade and three as being indefinite or negative for dysplasia (Connell et al 1994a).

Dysplasia is patchy

The current concept of spreading areas of clonal pre-cancerous change explains the patchy distribution of dysplasia. Since endoscopic biopsies sample only a small proportion of the total colonic mucosal area, dysplasia can be missed. Targeted biopsies of any elevated lesion, plaque, stricture or unusual ulcer increase the diagnostic rate. One study has suggested that 33 biopsies from the whole colon are needed to give a 90% certainty of detecting dysplasia if it is present (Rubin et al 1992).

Dysplasia is not always present at a distance from a carcinoma

Three studies have shown that about one-quarter of carcinomas are not associated with dysplasia detectable by biopsy in mucosa away from the tumor (Ransohoff et al 1985, Taylor et al 1992, Connel et al 1994c). Thus if no dysplasia is found it does not exclude the presence of carcinoma now or in the future.

Dysplasia as a marker of carcinoma

In flat mucosa all are agreed that high-grade dysplasia is associated with a carcinoma, often unrecognized before operation, in about 40% of cases. Low-grade dysplasia can also be associated with a carcinoma, but its predictive value is at present uncertain and may be as high as 20% (Bernstein et al 1994).

On the surface of an elevated lesion

When dysplasia is found on the surface of an elevated lesion, a decision has to be made as to whether the lesion is a manifestation of widespread dysplasia or is an isolated adenoma. If dysplasia is found elsewhere in the colon, or the lesion is part of an extensive broad-based elevation, the former is the case; the likelihood of carcinoma is about 40% and colectomy is indicated (Bernstein et al 1994, Connell et al 1994a). If there is no evidence of dysplasia elsewhere and the lesion is localized, particularly if it is pedunculated, or is situated above the upper limit of colitis in a person of middle age or older, it is probably an isolated adenoma and can safely be removed endoscopically (Nugent et al 1991, Connell et al 1994a).

Dysplasia as a precursor of carcinoma

Cases are reported of patients with high-grade dysplasia who remain free of carcinoma over many years (Jonsson et al 1994). In general, the likelihood of synchronous carcinoma precludes follow-up unless a patient declines operation or there is some other reason against it. These rare cases illustrate the fact that advice has to be given on grounds of probability rather than certainty. After a finding of low-grade dysplasia, our own data suggest that the cumulative probability of carcinoma or high-grade dysplasia during the next 5 years is about 50% (Connell et al 1994a).

Factors affecting the mortality of carcinoma complicating colitis

Pathological stage

Several series have shown that the mortality of carcinoma complicating colitis is very similar to that of carcinoma occurring in the general population, and 5-year crude survival rates of 30–55% have been reported. Thus a diagnosis of carcinoma complicating colitis does not necessarily mean that the patient will die from it.

As in sporadic carcinoma, the prognosis depends on the pathological stage of the lesion. In a series of 120 patients, among those with carcinomas confined to the bowel wall (Dukes A), the crude survival rate at 5 and 10 years was 91% and 82% respectively; when the carcinoma had extended outside the wall but had not involved lymph nodes (Dukes B) the figures were 88% and 88%; and when the tumor had invaded the draining lymph nodes (Dukes C) the survival was 28% and 23% (Connell et al 1994c). These figures suggest that early diagnosis should improve prognosis.

Symptomless or symptomatic

Dukes A and B tumors are found most commonly before symptoms develop, and presentation with symptoms from the tumor tends to be associated with Dukes C or disseminated tumors and a correspondingly poor prognosis. Thus, in our own surveillance program among 332 patients, 11 were discovered to have a symptomless cancer (8 Dukes A, 1B, 2C), all of whom survive. In contrast, six presented with symptomatic cancer (four Dukes C, two disseminated tumors), four of whom died.

Results of clinical supervision with a vigorous medical and surgical policy

In a community-based study characterized by early medical treatment of active colitis, prolonged aminosalicylate treatment of quiescent disease, operation when oral corticosteroid treatment failed, and a surgical bias towards the treatment of extensive colitis, the occurrence of carcinoma did not exceed that expected in the general population (Langholz et al 1992). These results in a center which treats all known cases of colitis in its area, with open access to a hospital clinic allowing rapid treatment of relapse and a research-based follow-up program, demonstrate the results of vigorous medical and surgical management. One aim of a clinical follow-up program is to gain the confidence of patients so that they are prepared to accept surgical treatment for severe acute or chronic extensive colitis; this measure alone is likely to reduce the cancer risk.

Results of episodic screening investigations

Investigation or reinvestigation of patients with a long history of colitis newly referred back to hospital is a valuable procedure. Among 213 patients whose symptoms began 8–39 years previously, examined for the first time at the Lahey Clinic by colonoscopy (Nugent et al 1991), 18 were found to have definite dysplasia, 20 to have indefinite dysplasia and 175 were found to have no dysplasia. A carcinoma was subsequently diagnosed during follow-up in seven of those with dysplasia, compared with two of those without dysplasia. Our own findings at the first surveillance colonoscopy in patients with extensive colitis and a mean disease duration of 15.5 years have been similar: three of 332 patients had high-grade dysplasia or a dysplastic mass (two with Dukes A carcinoma at operation), 41 had dysplasia but no detected tumor, and 288 had no dysplasia. Among those who remained in the surveillance program, 18% of those with dysplasia developed carcinoma, compared to 3% of the patients without dysplasia ($P < 0.01$) (Connell et al 1994a).

Results of pilot surveillance programs

Colonoscopy was introduced in the early 1970s and sufficient time has now elapsed for pilot studies to be assessed. Details of series published between 1990 and 1994 are shown in Table 74.1. The results divide into two groups, depending on whether the program was conducted at a hospital with a regional catchment area or at a tertiary referral center. In the former, the diagnosis of high-grade dysplasia or carcinoma has been uncommon and the effectiveness of the program can be questioned on the basis 'much effort, little result'. At the two tertiary centers the results have been disappointing because fatal carcinomas have occurred, and the effectiveness of the program can be questioned for this reason.

Hospitals serving one region

At three centers, one in Finland and two in Sweden (Löfberg et al 1990, Jonsson et al 1994, Leidenius et al 1991) it is stated that all or the majority of patients came from the hospital's catchment area; at an English center (Lynch et al 1993) this is also likely to have been the case. At these four centers 429 patients were studied over 12–14 years and 1844 colonoscopies were performed. As a result, 11 patients were advised to undergo operation for dysplasia and seven carcinomas were diagnosed, only two of which were successfully removed at a symptomless stage. One fatal carcinoma developed in a patient who defaulted from follow-up (Lynch et al 1993). The other four occurred, despite great efforts to detect and follow up every patient with long-standing ulcerative colitis by colonoscopy and biopsy, in a defined Swedish catchment area of 65 000 inhabitants. One symptomatic cecal carcinoma was diagnosed 9 years after onset of the disease before the first surveillance colonoscopy, two others in symptomatic elderly patients with long histories of disease not previously included in the program, and one in a patient with high-grade dysplasia who declined advice to accept operation until it became essential owing to the severity of inflammation.

In one series only two patients were operated upon for high-grade dysplasia; two others with high-grade dysplasia declined operation and had not developed overt cancer

Table 74.1 Surveillance programs published between 1990 and 1994

Country (Reference)	No. of patients	Years (19–)	Disease extent	Duration (> = yrs)	No. of colonoscopies	Operation for dysplasia	Carcinoma (Dukes Grade*)	Cancer deaths	Cancer Outside series
Sweden (Löfberg et al 1990)	72	73–88	Total	8	291	9	1 A	0	NK
Sweden (Jonsson et al 1994)	131	77–91	LS + EXT	6–10	632	2	4 2B 1C1?	1	0
Finland (Leidenius et al 1991)	66	76–89	LS + EXT	7	182	0	0	0	NK
England (Lynch et al 1993)	160	78–90	EXT	8	739	0	2[†] 1A 1?	1[†]	7
England (Connell et al 1994a)	332	71–91	EXT	10	1316	12	20[§] 8A 3B 6C 3 Dis	5[§]	33
USA (Nugent et al 1991)	213	74–86	LS + EXT	8	NK	12	10 1A 3B 4C 2?	6	22[††]

* Duke's grade is stated for the most advanced tumor if more than one was present
[†] 1 fatal carcinoma occurred in a patient who defaulted from surveillance
[§] 3 carcinomas (1 death) occurred in patients who defaulted from surveillance
[††] This figure is taken from Choi et al (1993), who describe 22 patients with symptomatic carcinoma diagnosed at the same hospital during the period 1974–1991. By the time of this report 19 carcinomas had been detected in the surveillance program, excluding 3 from the 1991 report
LS, left-sided colitis; EXT, extensive colitis; DIS, disseminated carcinoma; NK, not known

4 and 13 years after this diagnosis (Jonsson et al 1994). Therefore, high-grade dysplasia is not an infallible indication of incipient carcinoma. Another report questions the validity of low-grade dysplasia as a marker of premalignant change (Lynch et al 1993). A third series illustrates the problem of defining the presence or absence of dysplasia (Leidenius et al 1991).

Tertiary referral centers

The two series from tertiary referral centers are characterized by a relatively large number of cancers diagnosed and of patients treated surgically for dysplastic change. In one series only four of ten carcinomas (Nugent et al 1991) and in the other 11 of 20 carcinomas were Dukes A or B stage (Connell et al 1994a); cancer deaths occurred in both series. One center considered that 21 of 332 patients had benefited from the program, 12 operated upon for dysplasia confirmed in the operation specimen and nine treated surgically for symptomless cancer at a stage of Dukes A or B (Connell et al 1994a).

Mortality compared with symptomatic carcinoma outside surveillance programs

Some encouragement is provided by three studies which have shown that patients with cancers detected during endoscopic surveillance had a lower mortality than those with carcinomas presenting outside such a program, many of which tumors were symptomatic (Choi et al 1993, Giardiello et al 1993, Connell et al 1994c). However, these findings are not conclusive evidence that surveillance is beneficial because cancers developing outside a program occur in a population of unknown size and characteristics.

Outcome using chromosomal and genetic markers

All results described are based on programs using dysplasia as the only marker of neoplastic change. Preliminary follow-up studies suggest that the addition of flow cytometry to detect aneuploidy may improve results by recognition of chromosomal abnormalities before histological dysplasia is recognizable, and by strengthening the diagnosis of dysplasia when both occur in the same patient (Löfberg et al 1992, Rubin et al 1992). It is too early to conclude how much improvement in outcome may be found when aneuploidy or other markers of genetic instability (Burmer et al 1992) are combined with dysplasia in surveillance programs.

Patients with carcinoma outside surveillance programs

Despite considerable effort to recruit all eligible patients, carcinoma has occurred in patients not included in the program at three centers. These have been patients not recruited (Connell et al 1994a), elderly patients with long-standing quiescent colitis (Jonsson et al 1994), patients whose carcinoma developed early in the disease course before the start of surveillance (Lynch et al 1993), patients whose colitis was diagnosed before the start of the program and who were lost to follow-up (Lynch et al 1993), patients though to have distal colitis or proctitis but whose disease had extended without recognition of the fact (Lynch et al 1993, Connell et al 1994a), and patients with a retained rectum or distal colon after colectomy (Connell et al 1994a). In two series the number of these patients with carcinoma exceeded the number who developed carcinoma during surveillance. Such patients had already been treated at, or were under the care of, the hospitals concerned. In addition, patients are referred from elsewhere with unrecognized or unsupervised colitis and present with symptomatic cancers (Choi et al 1993, Connell et al 1994a). These facts suggest that it is impracticable to attempt cancer surveillance for every patient with long-standing extensive colitis.

CROHN'S DISEASE

Small-bowel disease

There is an increased incidence of cancer in small-bowel disease, especially in a bypassed segment, but the total number of cases reported is less than 100. Surveillance is not feasible but the possibility of carcinoma should be considered when symptoms recur in long-standing quiescent disease.

Crohn's colitis

Evidence is increasing that the cancer risk in extensive Crohn's colitis is similar to that in extensive ulcerative colitis, especially in young people (Gillen et al 1994). Dysplasia appears less common in Crohn's disease than ulcerative colitis, although it does occur. The limited success of surveillance programs in ulcerative colitis discourages clinicians from initiating similar studies in Crohn's colitis, where the incidence of dysplasia is less. Current opinion suggests that patients with chronic Crohn's colitis should be encouraged to report new symptoms, and these should be investigated by endoscopy and/or radiology. Strictures are common in Crohn's colitis, and can be due to carcinoma. There should be particular vigilance if the stricture is known to have developed recently. All strictures should be investigated by multiple biopsies and cytological brushing. The known cancer risk in chronic Crohn's colitis is an added indication, especially in young people, for surgical treatment if this is also indicated on grounds of ill-health or symptomatic disability.

Anorectal disease

Squamous carcinoma of the anus or adenocarcinoma of the anorectal junction can develop in association with chronic anal or perianal lesions of Crohn's disease. The development of an unusual anal ulcer, anorectal stricture or area of induration in a chronic fistula should raise the possibility of a complicating carcinoma (Connell et al 1994b).

RECOMMENDATIONS FOR CLINICAL PRACTICE IN ULCERATIVE COLITIS

Contribution of careful treatment and clinical follow-up to minimizing cancer risk

To minimize the cancer risk in ulcerative colitis is only one aspect of overall management. Regular clinical assessment should lead to prolonged quiescence of disease and maintenance of general health. An important aspect of medical follow-up is to advise surgical treatment for severe acute attacks, chronic symptomatic disability or ill-health unresponsive to medical measures. An appreciation of the potential benefit of modern surgical treatment minimizes not only disability from the disease but also the cancer risk.

Detection of high-risk group

About one in 120 patients develops carcinoma annually after the 10th year of disease if inflammation, detectable by macroscopic endoscopic or radiological appearance (Gyde et al 1988, Lennard-Jones et al 1990) has at some time involved the colon proximal to the splenic flexure.

To detect this high-risk group every colitic should undergo flexible sigmoidoscopy 8–10 years after onset of symptoms. Those in whom an upper limit of disease is apparent do not need colonoscopy. When an upper limit of disease is not apparent, colonoscopy should be advised.

If a patient is seen with a history of colitis exceeding 10 years, who has not been investigated for at least 2 years, reinvestigation is indicated as above.

Advice to patients with proctitis or left-sided colitis

Patients with proctitis can be reassured that their risk of carcinoma is no greater than in the general population, and those with left-sided colitis that the risk is not greatly increased. They should be encouraged to seek medical advice if their symptoms change. Flexible sigmoidoscopy is indicated for new symptoms or a relapse which is severe enough to suggest that the inflammation has extended to involve a greater proportion of the colon than previously. If annual clinical follow-up is instituted this should include flexible sigmoidoscopy and biopsy.

Advice to patients with retained rectum or distal colon after surgical treatment

Any patient with the rectum and/or distal colon retained after previous surgery should be advised to accept annual follow-up to include digital, sigmoidoscopic and biopsy examination of the retained segment.

Advice to patients with extensive colitis

Patients shown to have present or past (judged by scarring or inflammatory polyps) 'extensive' colitis by colonoscopy with a history exceeding 10 years should be assessed clinically. If the disease is chronic and clinically disabling, surgical treatment should be advised. If symptoms are slight or absent, or if advice to accept operation is declined, the available options to minimize the cancer risk should be discussed. All patients should be advised to seek advice if new symptoms develop.

Cancer surveillance by regular endoscopic examination with biopsies is not mandatory. In terms of medical resources it is of unproven value and is impracticable for every patient. If medical resources allow, regular endoscopic surveillance can be offered. Such a program entails acceptance by the patient of regular clinical assessment and endoscopy, even if symptoms are slight or absent, and includes an understanding that surgical treatment will be advised if definite dysplasia or carcinoma is detected. It must also be made clear that surveillance has not been proven to reduce the cancer risk and cannot be guaranteed to do so. However, surveillance does offer a reasonable chance of reducing cancer mortality by surgical treatment at a stage of either precancer or symptomless cancer. If surveillance is an available option, the patient's wishes should decide whether or not it is undertaken.

Conduct of surveillance program

Flexible sigmoidoscopy or colonoscopy

At least two-thirds of tumors or dysplastic changes occur in the rectosigmoid (Connell et al 1994c). Regular flexible sigmoidoscopy is thus a potentially useful measure. Adequate bowel preparation can be obtained by a single dose of laxative (Picolax) on the previous evening or a phosphate enema in the clinic. A search should be made for any broad-based elevated lesion, plaque, stricture or unusual ulcer with a raised edge. Targeted biopsies of suspicious lesions and biopsies of flat mucosa at 10 cm intervals (preferably four-quadrant) on withdrawal of the instrument, including rectal biopsies, should be taken.

Colonoscopy, if available and accepted, should be performed similarly. Clearly colonoscopy has the advantage over flexible sigmoidoscopy that the whole colon can be examined. It is the preferable option if availability and patient acceptance permit.

Optimal interval between examinations

The best frequency of examination is undecided, but interval cancers do occur if colonoscopy is performed once every 2 years (Connell et al 1994a). Annual examination therefore appears desirable. If this is difficult to arrange or is unacceptable to the patient, then a compromise in which annual flexible sigmoidoscopy is complemented by colonoscopy every second or third year appears a reasonable plan. Such a program has not been tested in practice.

Indications for surgical treatment

Indications for surgical treatment are carcinoma, high-grade dysplasia or dysplasia on the surface of a broad-based elevated lesion unsuitable for endoscopic removal or associated with dysplasia elsewhere in the colon. Both these types of dysplasia are associated with carcinoma in about 40% of cases. Low-grade dysplasia in flat mucosa is an indication for surgery provided that the pathological diagnosis is unequivocal, and preferably made on more than one occasion or in different parts of the large bowel. Such patients may have an associated undetected carcinoma and have about a 50% chance of developing carcinoma or high-grade dysplasia during the next 5 years. In practice, a finding of low-grade dysplasia in flat mucosa is usually an indication for repeat examination within about 6 months, before a decision is made about the need for colectomy.

Policy on finding an adenomatous polyp

A localized dysplastic polyp can be removed endoscopically provided that there is no evidence of dysplasia affecting the surrounding mucosa or elsewhere in the colon, and particularly if it is pedunculated or situated proximal to the colitis in normal mucosa.

RECOMMENDATIONS FOR CLINICAL PRACTICE IN CROHN'S DISEASE

The possibility of carcinoma should be considered in any patient with long-standing Crohn's disease, particularly anorectal and/or colonic disease, who develops new symptoms. There should be a bias towards surgical treatment in younger patients with extensive colonic disease who have recurrent or persistent symptoms.

FUTURE RESEARCH

Assessment of new methods

Future research at specialized centers should assess new methods of detecting precancerous change in the epithelium, including brushings (Melville et al 1988) or washings to increase the sampling area, cytometry to detect chromosomal changes, and immunohistological or molecular biological techniques to detect gene abnormalities. Such techniques should not be introduced into routine practice until they have been thoroughly evaluated in prospective research studies.

Difficulty of controlled trials

Once the current limitations of histological assessment of dysplasia have been improved by sampling larger areas of mucosa than is possible with routine biopsy forceps and by the detection of chromosomal and gene abnormalities, a case control study of cancer surveillance should be designed to assess whether or not such a program can reduce colorectal cancer mortality in ulcerative colitis. The difficulties of obtaining a statistically significant result from a controlled study should not be underestimated. Present estimates suggest that the cumulative incidence of carcinoma is about 12% during the period 10–25 years after onset of disease. At least one-third of such patients who develop cancer outside a surveillance program are cured by surgical treatment. A controlled trial of surveillance would thus have to demonstrate a fall in mortality from about 8% to say 4% in a group of patients with extensive colitis who are not treated surgically early in the disease course, and who do not die from causes other than colorectal cancer over the 25-year period from onset of disease. Follow-up would need to be prolonged to avoid lead-time bias. To achieve sufficient statistical power such a study would need to involve about 500 patients in each study group, all studied regularly over a period of 10 or more years at many centers.

The composition of the control group would be difficult to determine. Should such patients be under regular clinical supervision and, if so, what should be the indication for endoscopy and biopsy? Ideally, a group of patients not under regular supervision should be used as a control, and compared with two other groups, one under clinical supervision and the other under regular endoscopic surveillance.

Ethical problems of informed patient consent are likely to make it difficult to randomize patients into different groups at each center. It is more likely that the outcome of different policies adopted by each collaborating center will have to be compared.

CONCLUSION

Since a controlled evaluation of cancer surveillance in colitis will be difficult to organize and take many years to produce a result, it is likely that a decision whether or not to advise a cancer surveillance program for individual patients will depend, as at present, on the assessment of pilot studies of new methods introduced to supplement the techniques currently in use.

REFERENCES

Bernstein C N, Shanahan F, Weinstein W M 1994 Are we telling patients the truth about surveillance colonoscopy in ulcerative colitis? Lancet 343: 71–74

Broomé U, Löfberg R, Veress B, Eriksson L S 1995 Primary sclerosing cholangitis and ulcerative colitis – evidence for increased neoplastic potential. Hepatology 22: 1404–1408

Burmer G C, Rabinovitch P S, Haggitt R C et al 1992 Neoplastic progression in ulcerative colitis: histology, DNA content, and loss of a p53 allele. Gastroenterology 103: 1602–1610

Choi P M, Nugent F W, Schoetz D J Jr, Silverman M L, Haggitt R C 1993 Colonoscopic surveillance reduces mortality from colorectal cancer in ulcerative colitis. Gastroenterology 105: 418–424

Connell W R, Lennard-Jones J E, Williams C B, Talbot I C, Price A B, Wilkinson K H 1994a Factors affecting the outcome of endoscopic surveillance for cancer in ulcerative colitis. Gastroenterology 107: 934–944

Connell W R, Sheffield J P, Kamm M A, Ritchie J K, Hawley P R, Lennard-Jones J E 1994b Lower gastrointestinal malignancy in Crohn's disease. Gut 35: 347–352

Connell W R, Talbot I C, Harpaz N et al 1994c Clinicopathological characteristics of colorectal carcinoma complicating ulcerative colitis. Gut 35: 1419–1423

Ekbom A, Helmick C G, Zack M, Holmberg L, Adami H-O 1992 Survival and causes of death in patients with inflammatory bowel disease: a population-based study. Gastroenterology 103: 954–960

Giardiello F M, Gurbuz A K, Bayless T M, Yardley J H 1993 Colorectal cancer (CRC) in ulcerative colitis (UC): effect of a cancer prevention strategy on survival. Gastroenterology 104: A705

Gillen C D, Andrews H A, Prior P, Allan R N 1994 Crohn's disease and colorectal cancer. Gut 35: 651–655

Gumaste V, Sachar D B, Greenstein A J 1992 Benign and malignant colorectal strictures in ulcerative colitis. Gut 33: 938–941

Gyde S N, Prior P, Allan R N et al 1988 Colorectal cancer in ulcerative colitis: a cohort study of primary referrals from three centres. Gut 29: 206–217

Jonsson B, Åhsgren L, Andersson L O, Stenling R, Rutegard J 1994 Colorectal cancer surveillance in patients with ulcerative colitis. British Journal of Surgery 81: 689–691

Langholz E, Munkholm P, Davidsen M, Binder V 1992 Colorectal cancer risk and mortality in patients with ulcerative colitis. Gastroenterology 103: 1444–1451

Leidenius M, Kellokumpu I, Husa A, Riihela M, Sipponen P 1991 Dysplasia and carcinoma in longstanding ulcerative colitis: an endoscopic and histological surveillance programme. Gut 32: 1521–1525

Lennard-Jones J E, Melville D M, Morson B C, Ritchie J K, Williams C B 1990 Precancer and cancer in extensive ulcerative colitis; findings among 401 patients over 22 years. Gut 31: 800–806

Löfberg R, Broström O, Karlén P, Tribukait B, Öst A 1990 Colonoscopic surveillance in long-standing total ulcerative colitis: a 15-year follow-up study. Gastroenterology 99: 1021–1031

Löfberg R, Broström O, Karlén P, Öst Å, Tribukait B 1992 DNA aneuploidy in ulcerative colitis: reproducibility, topographic distribution and relation to dysplasia. Gastroenterology 102: 1149–1154

Lynch D A F, Lobo A J, Sobala G M, Dixon M F, Axon A T R 1993 Failure of colonoscopic surveillance in ulcerative colitis. Gut 34: 1075–1080

Melville D M, Richman P I, Shepherd N A, Williams C B, Lennard-Jones J E 1988 Brush cytology of the colon and rectum in ulcerative colitis: an aid to cancer diagnosis. Journal of Clinical Pathology 41: 1180–1186

Nugent F W, Haggitt R C, Gilpin P A 1991 Cancer surveillance in ulcerative colitis. Gastroenterology 100: 1241–1248

Ransohoff D F, Riddell R H, Levin B 1985 Ulcerative colitis and colonic cancer: problems in assessing the diagnostic usefulness of mucosal dysplasia. Diseases of the Colon and Rectum 28: 383–388

Riddell R H, Goldman R H, Ransohoff D F et al 1983 Dysplasia in inflammatory bowel disease: standardized classification with provisional clinical applications. Human Pathology 14: 931–966

Rubin C E, Haggitt R C, Burmer G C et al 1992 DNA aneuploidy in colonic biopsies predicts future development of dysplasia in ulcerative colitis. Gastroenterology 103: 1611–1620

Taylor B A, Pemberton J H, Carpenter H A et al 1992 Dysplasia in chronic ulcerative colitis: implications for colonoscopic surveillance. Diseases of the Colon and Rectum 35: 950–956

75. Surgical management of cancer occurring in inflammatory bowel disease

A. J. Greenstein   S. Balasubramanian

INTRODUCTION

The increased risk of colorectal cancer with ulcerative colitis is well established (Edwards & Truelove 1964, Kewenter et al 1978, Greenstein et al 1979, Prior et al 1982), especially for those with pancolitis and early age at onset (Ekbom et al 1990a). The association of cancer with Crohn's disease remains more controversial. Both small (Frank & Shorey 1973, Hoffman et al 1977) and large bowel (Ekbom et al 1990b, Weedon et al 1973, Greenstein et al 1981, Gyde et al 1980, Korelitz 1983) adenocarcinoma have been found to occur in a greater than expected incidence in Crohn's disease, especially in Crohn's colitis and with early age at onset (Weedon et al 1973, Ekbom et al 1990b). Several population-based studies have, however, failed to find such an increase (Binder et al 1985, Kvist et al 1986). Although earlier reports found no excess of extraintestinal cancers in inflammatory bowel disease (IBD) (Gyde et al 1980), a later study (Greenstein et al 1985) noted an increased frequency for perianal squamous cell cancers (Slater et al 1984, Connell et al 1994) in Crohn's disease, leukemia in ulcerative colitis, and lymphoma in both.

The main emphasis in this chapter will be on the intestinal cancers. New unpublished data will be presented based upon a study of 151 intestinal cancers derived from 3326 IBD patients, 1406 with ulcerative colitis and 1920 with Crohn's disease, with a few additional cases obtained from our pathology department.

INDICATIONS FOR SURGERY

The extraordinary difficulty of diagnosing cancer in IBD may affect our ability to evaluate patients for surgical intervention, and hence lead to delayed diagnosis. The problems include:

1. 'Invisibility', with difficulty in appreciating cancers macroscopically (Fleming & Pollak 1975) or endoscopically. A significant number of cancers are only recognized microscopically on histopathological examination of the resected specimen
2. Failure to appreciate that symptoms of IBD may be identical to those of cancer
3. Inability to diagnose underlying cancer within, or proximal to, a stricture
4. Excluded segments in Crohn's disease which may mask a cancer.

Ulcerative colitis

Surgical indications for colorectal cancer in ulcerative colitis include:

1. Dysplasia in patients in surveillance programs, including high-grade dysplasia, low-grade dysplasia in the absence of acute inflammation, and a dysplasia-associated lesion or mass (DALM)
2. A stricture that cannot be passed
3. A poorly compliant patient for whom surveillance is unreliable
4. Carcinoma proven by endoscopic biopsy
5. Patients may be operated upon for other indications: fulminating colitis, toxic megacolon etc.

Crohn's disease

Surveillance is now advised by many gastroenterologists for Crohn's disease as well as for ulcerative colitis. Surgical indications include:

1. Dysplasia or DALM. Surveillance may be confounded by the presence of pseudopolyps and the difficulty of differentiating the dysplasia of the adenomatous polyps
2. Inability to pass a stricture at colonoscopy
3. Cancer diagnosed by histopathology
4. An excluded loop, especially with recrudescence of symptoms in long-standing disease (Greenstein et al 1978).

GENERAL PRINCIPLES OF SURGERY FOR IBD

The procedure of choice for ulcerative colitis without complicating cancer is total proctocolectomy, preferably carried out in one stage. This may be with or without the construction of a pelvic pouch with rectal mucosal stripping or stapling, and with ileoanal pull-through with or without a proximal defunctioning loop ileostomy. For seriously ill patients with toxic megacolon, fulminating colitis, perforation, hypoalbuminemia, and on high-dose steroids, primary subtotal colectomy with Brooke ileostomy and Hartmann closure of the rectum is preferred. Proctectomy with construction of a pelvic pouch can then be carried out electively, at a later date. In cases in which there is doubt regarding pathology subtotal colectomy allows a definitive diagnosis to be made by histological examination of the operative specimen.

In Crohn's colitis, on the other hand, except when the disease is universal and severe perianal disease present, segmental resection with reanastomosis is the preferred method of treatment. Although there is a high recurrence rate for colocolostomy, or ileosigmoidostomy, the more limited resections allow the patient to preserve the rectum, maintain intestinal continuity, and avoid a permanent ileostomy. Ileoanal pouch construction for Crohn's disease is contraindicated. In indeterminate colitis pelvic pouch construction appears to be successful, with results as good as those for ulcerative colitis (Pezim et al 1989).

Colorectal cancer

The surgery for cancer in IBD is based on the principles which have evolved for cancer surgery in general: wide excision with lymphadenectomy.

Between 1960 and 1989 a total of 147 patients with cancer occurring in IBD were seen at the Mount Sinai Medical Center in New York City. There were 100 patients with colorectal cancer in ulcerative colitis (Sugita et al 1993), and 30 with large-bowel adenocarcinoma in Crohn's disease. An additional 19 patients were seen with small-bowel cancer (Ribeiro et al 1992). The four groups of surgical procedures required for these patients included total proctocolectomy with end ileostomy or pelvic pouch, subtotal colectomy with or without reanastomosis, segmental resection, and palliative procedures, including diversionary colostomy or ileostomy. The surgical procedures in our 130 patients with ulcerative colitis and Crohn's disease complicated by colorectal cancer are listed in Table 75.1.

Total proctocolectomy

This was the procedure of choice in 51% of our patients with ulcerative colitis with colorectal cancer. In only eight of these patients was a pelvic pouch constructed simultaneously. In earlier years it was believed that the presence of complicating colorectal cancer was a contraindication to restorative proctocolectomy with pelvic pouch construction. As survival in ulcerative colitis colorectal cancer is as good as in de novo colorectal cancer, with an overall 5-year survival rate of approximately 52%, and survival for early cancers (stages A and B, which constitute 55% of our ulcerative colitis colorectal cancers) is 85–100% (Sugita et al 1993), one may carry out restorative

Table 75.1 Surgical procedures for colorectal cancer in inflammatory bowel disease

	Ulcerative colitis		Crohn's disease
Total proctocolectomy		51 (51%)	5 (17%)
with ileostomy	43 (43%)		5 (17%)
with pelvic pouch	8 (8%)		0 (0%)
Subtotal colectomy		25 (25%)	5 (17%)
with ileostomy	11 (11%)		4 (14%)
with reanastomosis	14 (14%)		1 (3%)
Segmental resection		14 (14%)	14 (46%)
ileocolic	0 (0%)		2 (6%)
right colectomy	7 (24%)		1 (3%)
left colectomy	1 (0%)		4 (14%)
sigmoid / ant. res.	1 (1%)		1 (3%)
proctect/Hartmann	0 (0%)		1 (3%)
abdominoperineal	5 (5%)		5 (16%)
Palliative procedure		5 (5%)	5 (17%)
ileostomy	1 (1%)		3 (10%)*
colostomy/Hartmann	4 (4%)†		2 (7%)
Unresectable		5 (5%)	1 (3%)
inoperable/biopsy	4 (4%)		1 (3%)
laparotomy	1 (1%)		0 (0%)
Total		100 (100%)	30 (100%)

* One with proximal jejunojejunostomy and ileoileostomy
† One following recurrence of a rectovesical fistula after a decade-long quiescent interval

proctocolectomy for early colorectal cancer complicating ulcerative colitis, with the exception of distal colorectal and anorectal cancer (Connell et al 1994). If there is doubt regarding the stage, a subtotal colectomy can be done as the primary procedure, and final pathology awaited.

In Crohn's disease total proctocolectomy is generally reserved for those with extensive or universal colitis, especially those with perianal disease in whom reconstruction of intestinal continuity is inadvisable.

Subtotal colectomy

Subtotal colectomy was carried out in 25% of our ulcerative colitis patients for colonic cancer above the rectosigmoid. This is the preferred surgical procedure for patients who are ill, have severe active disease in addition to the cancer, are on steroids, hypoalbuminemic and severely anemic. It is of interest that 14 of our ulcerative colitis patients who had a subtotal colectomy could be safely reanastomosed by ileosigmoidostomy or ileoproctostomy, as the rectal disease was relatively quiescent. An anastomotic disruption occurred in only one patient. Total colectomy would be advised today.

In Crohn's disease complicated by carcinoma subtotal colectomy was carried out in 17%, a proportion somewhat less than that in our ulcerative colitis patients.

Segmental resection

Right, left or distal abdominoperineal resection was the preferred surgical therapy for Crohn's colitis a segmental disease. In fact, in this series seven cases of colorectal cancer occurred in patients with regional enteritis localized to the small bowel (Greenstein et al 1987). These cases were clearly ideal for segmental resection, which was carried out in 14 patients, 46% of the series. It is of interest that 21% of the ulcerative colitis cases, including seven having right colectomy and 14 subtotal colectomy, had sufficiently quiescent colitis to have colonic resection with reanastomosis. Most of these were carried out in earlier years, and some of these patients may have been candidates for restorative proctocolectomy today. When proctectomy is carried out for rectal cancer with or without restorative proctocolectomy radical excision of the mesorectum is mandatory.

Palliative procedures

In less than 5% of cases in each series the cancers were so advanced that the patients were inoperable. Palliative diversionary ostomy without resection was also necessary in an additional 5% of ulcerative colitis patients, and in 17% of the patients with Crohn's disease. The large number of unresectable cancers in Crohn's colitis was contributed to by the five patients with cancers in excluded loops. This operation was carried out frequently at the Mount Sinai Hospital in the past, but is no longer done today. In most other series cancers in excluded loops are less common.

Table 75.2 Surgical procedures for small-bowel cancer in Crohn's disease

Resection	15 (79%)
small-bowel resection	2 (11%)
with ileostomy	1 (5%)
with strictureplasty	1 (5%)
ileocolic resection and reanastomosis	11 (58%)
Palliative procedures	4 (21%)
bypass/diversion	
ileotransverse colostomy	1 (5%)
jejunostomy	2 (11%)
inoperable	1 (5%)
Total	19 (100%)

SMALL-BOWEL CANCER IN CROHN'S ENTERITIS (Table 75.2)

Segmental resection was the preferred surgical therapy for Crohn's enteritis in 79% of patients. Unlike the patients with colorectal cancer, only one patient developed cancer in non-diseased bowel. The four patients requiring palliative diversion, or being inoperable, constituted 21% of the total series, a similar proportion to the six of 30 patients (20%) with Crohn's disease colorectal cancer. Again, this was contributed to by the five cancers that occurred in excluded loops (Greenstein et al 1978, Ribeiro et al 1992).

RETICULOENDOTHELIAL TUMORS

Lymphomas

Lymphomas, either colonic or extraintestinal (Greenstein et al 1992), occur occasionally in both Crohn's disease and ulcerative colitis. It has been suggested that the incidence is above that expected (Greenstein et al 1985). For intestinal lymphomas local excision is required. This should be followed by radiotherapy when indicated, and chemotherapy, which is the definitive therapy for extraintestinal lymphoma (Greenstein et al 1992).

Leukemias

Leukemias occur in ulcerative colitis (Greenstein et al 1985) and occasionally may exacerbate the hemorrhage due to ulceration. In cases of this type total proctocolectomy is mandatory for massive hemorrhage, and this should be followed by appropriate chemotherapy, (Fabry et al 1980, Greenstein et al 1985).

CANCERS OF THE ANORECTUM

Low rectal adenocarcinomas in both forms of IBD, and squamous cell cancers of the anus in Crohn's disease, usually with perianal disease, are treated by radical abdominoperineal resection of the rectum, including the sphincter muscles when resectable (Slater et al 1984, Connell et al 1994). Early or advanced squamous cell cancers may be treated by local excision, or radical excision with or without radical lymphadenectomy prior to radiotherapy and chemotherapy.

PERI-ILEOSTOMY CANCERS

Cancers occurring at the site of an ileostomy are rare, but a number have been reported. Radical excision with transposition of the ileostomy is required (Suarez et al 1988).

STRICTURE CANCERS

Cancers occurring in association with strictures constitute a particularly difficult diagnostic problem in both Crohn's (Yamazaki et al 1991) and ulcerative colitis (Gumaste et al 1992), in which the incidence of malignancy in strictures is approximately 30% and 5% respectively. When the diagnosis of cancer cannot be ruled out, surgical resection is indicated.

Small-bowel cancer should be ruled out in all patients with multiple strictures in jejunoileitis, in whom strictureplasty is performed (Ribeiro et al 1992).

CANCER OCCURRING WITH FISTULAE

This association has long been recognized (Lightdale et al 1975, Greenstein et al 1978, Church et al 1985). Unfortunately, such cancers are often unresectable. However, it is possible on occasion to carry out radical cancer 'en bloc' resections, including the bowel on either side. This principle should be applied whenever the possibility of fistula cancer exists, even if unproven. Even if a complete cure is not possible a longer period of palliation may be attained.

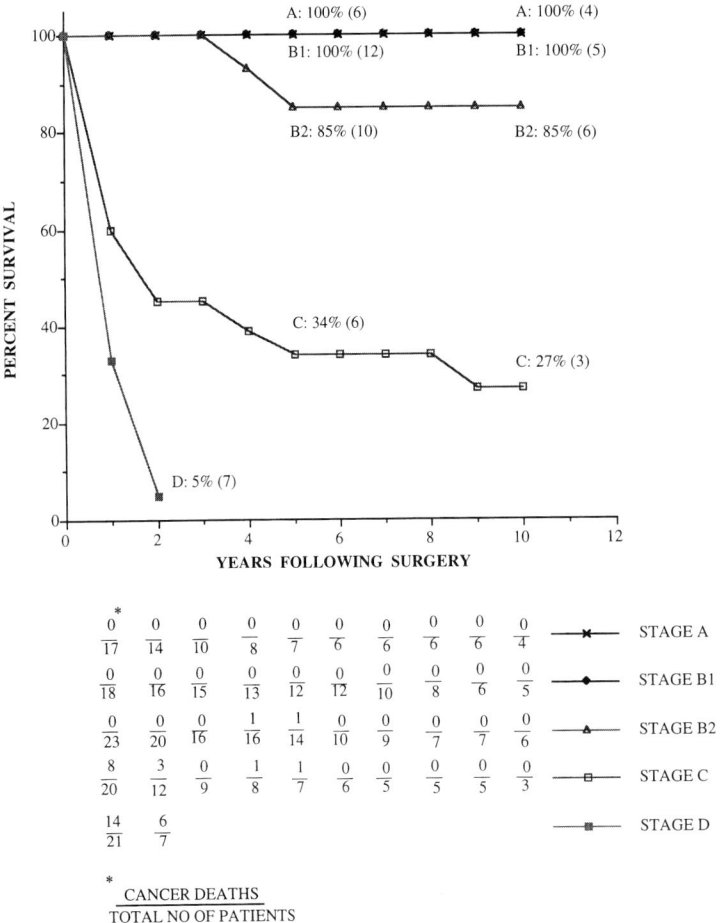

Fig. 75.1 Postoperative actuarial survival in 99 patients with ulcerative colitis-associated colorectal cancer according to cancer stage by Astler-Coller's criteria. There is a statistically significant difference between all five groups ($P<0.0001$); and between stage B2 and stage C ($P<0.0001$); and between stage C and stage D ($P<0.04$) Overall 5-year actuarial survival was 52%. (Reprinted with permission from Sugita et al 1993)

LONG-TERM OUTCOME FOLLOWING SURGERY

Survival following surgical resection is best in colorectal cancer. Although early series suggested a poor long-term outcome for ulcerative colitis colorectal cancer, recent studies have shown that survival is similar to that for de novo colorectal cancer. We have found a 45% 5-year survival for colorectal cancer in Crohn's disease, which increases to 56% if cancers in excluded loops are excluded (Ribeiro et al 1996). This is comparable to the 52% survival for our 100 ulcerative colitis patients (Fig. 75.1) (Sugita et al 1993). For small-bowel cancer survival is much poorer, at best 23% at 3 years and 0% for cancers in excluded bowel (Figs 75.2, 75.3) (Ribeiro et al 1992).

CONCLUSION

Surgery for cancer in inflammatory bowel disease is based on a combination of the general principles for the surgery

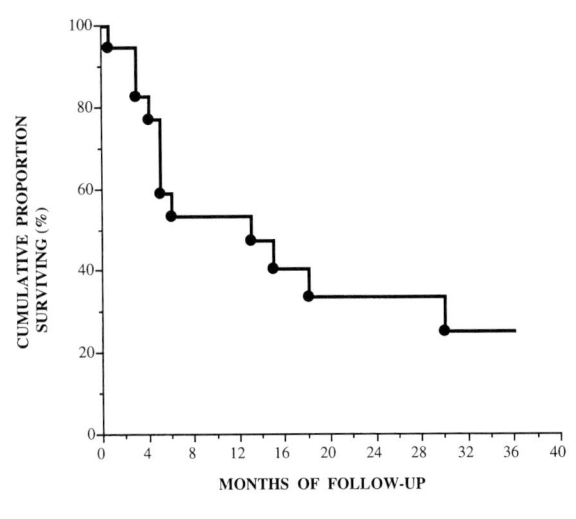
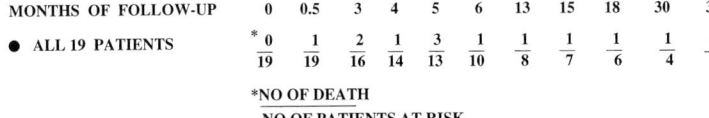

Fig. 75.2 Survival curve calculated by the Kaplan–Meier method for 19 patients with small-bowel carcinoma complicating Crohn's disease. (Reprinted with permission from Ribeiro et al 1991)

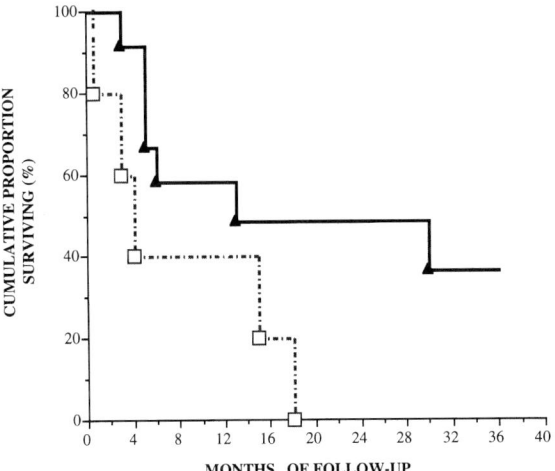
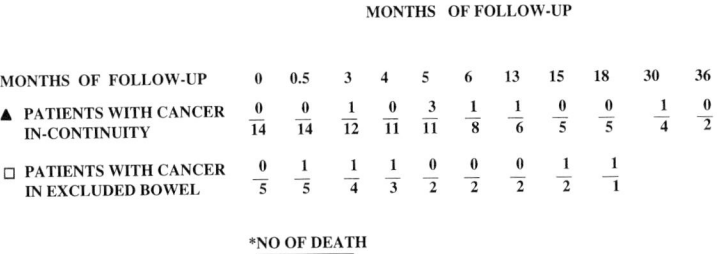

Fig. 75.3 Survival curves for five patients with cancer in excluded bowel, and the 14 patients with cancer in non-excluded bowel. The difference did not reach statistical significance. (Reprinted with permission from Ribeiro et al 1991)

of IBD without cancer, and radical excisional cancer surgery. Resection of the mesentery and lymphadenectomy should be carried out according to general cancer principles. Postoperative survival for colorectal cancer is good, (approximately 50%), compared with the poor (less than 23%) survival for small-bowel cancer.

REFERENCES

Binder V, Hendriksen C, Kreiner S 1985 Prognosis in Crohn's disease, based on results from a regional patient group from the county of Copenhagen. Gut 26: 146–150

Church J M, Weakley F L, Fazio V W, Sebek B A, Achkar E, Carwell M 1985 The relationship between fistulas in Crohn's disease and associated carcinoma. Report of four cases and a review of the literature. Diseases of the Colon and Rectum 28: 361–366

Connell W R, Sheffield M A, Kamm M A, Ritchie J K, Hawley P R, Lennard-Jones J E 1994 Lower gastrointestinal malignancy in Crohn's disease. Gut 35: 347–352

Edwards F C, Truelove S C 1964 The course and prognosis of ulcerative colitis IV. Carcinoma of the colon. Gut 5: 15–22

Ekbom A, Helmick C, Zack M, Adami H-O 1990a Ulcerative colitis and colorectal cancer. New England Journal of Medicine 323: 1228–1233

Ekbom A, Helmick C, Zack M, Adami H-O 1990b Increased risk of large bowel cancer in Crohn's disease with colonic involvement. Lancet 336: 357–359

Fabry T L, Sachar D B, Janowitz H D 1980 Acute myelogenous leukemia in patients with ulcerative colitis. Journal of Clinical Gastroenterology 2: 225–227

Fleming K, Pollak A 1975 A case of 'Crohn's carcinoma'. Gut 16: 533–537

Frank J D, Shorey B A 1973 Adenocarcinoma of the small bowel as a complication of Crohn's disease. Gut 14: 120–124

Greenstein A J, Gennuso R, Sachar D B et al 1985 Extraintestinal cancers in inflammatory bowel disease. Cancer 56: 2914–2921

Greenstein A J, Meyers S, Szporn A, Slater G, Janowitz H D, Aufses A H Jr 1987 Colorectal cancer in regional ileitis. Quarterly Journal of Medicine 62: 33–40

Greenstein A J, Mullin G E, Strauchen J A et al 1992 Lymphoma in inflammatory bowel disease: a study of 9 cases. Cancer 69: 1119–1123

Greenstein A J, Sachar D B, Pucillo A et al 1978 Cancer in Crohn's disease after diversionary surgery: a report of seven carcinomas occurring in excluded bowel. American Journal of Surgery 135: 86–90

Greenstein A J, Sachar D B, Smith H, Janowitz H D, Aufses A H Jr 1981 A comparison of cancer risk in Crohn's disease and ulcerative colitis. Cancer 48: 2742–2745

Greenstein A J, Sachar D B, Smith H et al 1979 Cancer in universal and left-sided ulcerative colitis: factors determining risk. Gastroenterology 77: 290–294

Gumaste V, Sachar D B, Greenstein A J 1992 Benign and malignant colorectal strictures in ulcerative colitis. Gut 33: 938–941

Gyde S N, Prior P, Macartney J C, Thompson H, Waterhouse J A H, Allan R N 1980 Malignancy in Crohn's disease. Gut 21: 1024–1029

Hoffman J P, Taft D A, Wheelis R F, Walker J H 1977 Adenocarcinoma in regional enteritis of the small intestine. Archives of Surgery 112: 605–611

Kewenter J, Ahlman H, Hulten L 1978 Cancer risk in extensive ulcerative colitis. Annals of Surgery 188: 824–828

Korelitz B 1983 Carcinoma of the intestinal tract in Crohn's disease: results of a survey carried out by the National Foundation for ileitis and colitis. American Journal of Gastroenterology 78: 44–46

Kvist N, Jacobsen O, Norgaard P et al 1986 Malignancy in Crohn's disease. Scandinavian Journal of Gastroenterology 21: 82–86

Lightdale C J, Stern S S, Posner G, Sherlock P 1975 Carcinoma complicating Crohn's disease: report of seven cases and review of the literature. American Journal of Medicine 59: 262–268

Pezim M E, Pemberton J H, Beart R W 1989 Outcome of indeterminate colitis following pouch–anal anastomosis. Diseases of the Colon and Rectum 32: 653–658

Prior P, Gyde S N, Macartney J C, Thompson H, Waterhouse J A H, Allan R N 1982 Cancer morbidity in ulcerative colitis. Gut 23: 490–497

Ribeiro M B, Greenstein A J, Heimann T M, Yamazaki Y, Aufses A H Jr 1992 Adenocarcinoma of the small intestine in Crohn's disease. Surgery, Gynecology and Obstetrics 173: 343–350

Ribeiro M B, Greenstein A J, Sachar D B et al 1996 Colorectal adenocarcinoma in Crohn's disease. Annals of Surgery 223: 186–193

Slater G, Greenstein A J, Aufses A H 1984 Anal carcinoma in patients with Crohn's disease. Annals of Surgery 199: 348–350

Suarez V, Alexander-Williams J, O'Connor H J et al 1988 Carcinoma developing in ileostomies after 25 or more years. Gastroenterology 95: 205–208

Sugita A, Greenstein A J, Ribeiro M B et al 1993 Survival with colorectal cancer in ulcerative colitis: a study of 102 cases. Annals of Surgery 218: 189–195

Weedon D D, Shorter R G, Ilstrup D M, Huizenga K A, Taylor W F 1973 Crohn's disease and cancer. New England Journal of Medicine 289: 1099–1102

Yamazaki Y, Ribeiro M B, Sachar D B, Aufses A H Jr, Greenstein A J 1991 Malignant colorectal strictures in Crohn's disease. American Journal of Gastroenterology 86: 882–885

SECTION 9

Surgical principles

76. Incisions and surgical approaches in surgery for inflammatory bowel disease

M. R. B. Keighley

INCISIONS

There are three principles with the surgeon should bear in mind when making an incision for the treatment of inflammatory bowel disease: accessibility, extensibility and security (Maingot 1969). Vertical incisions are used most frequently for both elective and emergency surgery. These are usually either midline or paramedian. Muscle-splitting vertical incisions are no longer popular. Also, pararectal incisions are virtually never used today as they sever the nerves supplying the rectus muscle, causing paralysis and weakness.

An overriding consideration in planning an incision is its effect on a potential stoma site. Transverse or oblique incisions may be used for local resections of the right and left colon in conditions such as malignant disease, but they are ill advised in patients with Crohn's disease because of the risk of recurrence requiring reoperation and the eventual need for a stoma. Interestingly, transverse incisions are not associated with less pain, wound dehiscence or respiratory complications than midline incisions (Greenall et al 1980a,b).

The choice between the two most commonly used vertical incisions, paramedian and midline, is largely a matter of personal preference, but midline incisions have become more popular: they allow easier repeated access, do not infringe on a stoma site on either side of the abdomen, and in terms of strength probably do not differ from paramedian incisions. It is the view of this author that a midline incision is preferable for all operations in Crohn's disease. It may seem unsightly and may be more likely to cause a keloid scar, but it does not transgress potential stoma sites, can be reopened with ease, heals well and does not paralyse muscle (Poticha 1978). Furthermore, a midline incision can be easily extended if it is too small.

PATIENT POSITION

The Lloyd Davies position is very useful for almost all operations for inflammatory bowel disease. Admittedly it takes a little longer to set up than the supine position, but it has many valuable advantages. The Lloyd Davies position with the legs in Allen stirrups provides much better access to the pelvis and the pelvic floor; it is the only way to perform synchronous combined excision of the rectum and, most importantly, it allows access to the colon and rectum at operation. Access to the anus is necessary for the treatment of coexisting perianal disease, particularly abscess drainage, the exploration of complex fistulae and the use of setons in high fistulae. Access to the anus also allows peroperative endoscopy, which may be very useful in assessing the extent of the disease or in the localization of bleeding from inflammatory disease. Access to the anus is necessary if intraluminal circular stapling devices are needed for low anastomoses. Anal mucosectomy or intra-anal polypectomy combined with rectal excision is only feasible with the patient in the Lloyd Davies position. Access to the anus also allows peroperative anal ultrasonography, which may prove very useful for complex sepsis and fistulae. One very useful advantage of the position is to confirm the proximal or distal end of a loop of bowel, particularly in the presence of multiple adhesions in the pelvis. If a proximal stoma is to be raised it is very embarrassing if the wrong end is delivered to the abdominal wall! By clamping the bowel and insufflating air from the rectum, the distal segment can be varified without having to mobilize all the bowel from the pelvis, a procedure that might be hazardous and could result in iatrogenic injury (Keighley & Williams 1993).

FURTHER PRINCIPLES IN THE SURGERY OF INFLAMMATORY BOWEL DISEASE

Surgery of inflammatory bowel disease may involve a high reoperation rate. Therefore, ease of access for repeated operations must be considered.

All patients with inflammatory bowel disease may eventually require an intestinal stoma and its site should not be compromised, particularly if there have been previous operations with scars.

Surgery in Crohn's disease is panenteric in nature and therefore resections can never cure. Consequently, in Crohn's disease the aim of surgery is to resect obstruction, fistulae and abscess in the small bowel, while preserving as much of the small intestine as possible, hence the principle of miniresection and strictureplasty for small-bowel disease. By contrast, in large-bowel disease miniresections tend to be associated with a high recurrence rate.

Where possible anal sphincter function should be preserved: certainly surgical treatment should avoid rendering a patient incontinent (see Chapter 81). Therefore, surgical treatment for anal lesions should be used sparingly and highly selectively, but early and complete drainage is mandatory for anorectal sepsis to preserve function.

Surgical treatment must be safe and there should be appropriate measures to prevent bleeding, infection, anastomotic breakdown, fistula and thromboembolism. Any preoperative bleeding diathesis should be corrected and preoperative or peroperative and antiembolism prophylaxis instituted (see Chapter 78). Antibiotic prophylaxis is advised in all patients, but the duration of antibiotic cover may have to be prolonged if there is established sepsis at operation (see Chapter 77). Established sepsis should be treated by resection of the causative pathology, which is usually due to panmural Crohn's disease; there should be adequate drainage of pus and bowel defunction is usually necessary as well.

USEFUL 'RULES'

1. **Minimize the risk of sepsis**. Apart from antibiotic cover and peritoneal lavage, avoid using open drains and avoid non-absorbable suture materials in the peritoneal cavity.
2. **Avoid leaks and fistulae**. Do not be tempted to perform an anastomosis in the presence of sepsis or if there is any doubt about the viability of the bowel. If in doubt, protect an anastomosis by raising a proximal stoma. Staples are probably best avoided in Crohn's disease: all anastomoses must be constructed with care and we prefer the extramucosal technique, since it inverts and causes the least compromise to luminal diameter.
3. **Do not compromise stoma sites**. Midline incisions are best: avoid placing drains through potential stoma sites. Avoid scarring of incisions by minimizing sepsis and using inert suture material for closure of the abdominal wall.
4. **Preserve small bowel**. Use miniresections and strictureplasties where indicated in Crohn's disease. The technique 'pinching' allows the safe separation of loops of bowel in an inflammatory mass or round an abscess. Do not try to resect mesenteric lymph nodes and divide the mesenteric blood supply close to the bowel in order to avoid having to resect an ischemic segment of uninvolved Crohn's disease. Whenever possible, use end-to-end anastomoses.
5. **Minimize sexual dysfunction**. Look for and preserve the presacral nerves in the pelvis. Keep close to the anterior rectum and behind Denonvillier's fascia. Do not allow the perineal operator to enter the presacral fascia, since stripping this from below will damage the nervi erigentes. Keep close to the anorectum during perineal dissection, as this will prevent perineal scarring.
6. **Preserve anal function**. Avoid stretching the anorectum and do not divide striated muscle. Establish early drainage of sepsis and never operate on the anus unless there is a good indication. Avoid creating anal wounds in Crohn's disease.
7. **Avoid urological injury**. Identify the ureters before entering the pelvis and in patients with retroperitoneal disease; stents may help in identification and ureters should be taped in difficult cases. To avoid renal damage keep close to the bowel, especially in the upper descending colon. Preserve the bladder and avoid segmental bladder resection in enterovesical fistula. Keep close to the anorectum during proctectomy in order to minimize urethral damage. Suprapubic catheter drainage is probably superior to prolonged urethral catheterization.

REFERENCES

Greenall M J, Evans M, Pollock A V 1980a Midline or transverse laparotomy? A random controlled clinical trial. Part 1: Influence on healing. British Journal of Surgery 67: 188–190

Greenall M J, Evans M, Pollock A V 1980b Midline or transverse laparotomy. A random controlled trial. Part 2: Influence on postoperative pulmonary complications. British Journal of Surgery 67: 191–194

Keighley M R B, Williams N S 1993 Surgery of the anus, rectum and colon. WB Saunders London

Maingot R 1969 Abdominal operations, 5th edn. Appleton-Century-Crofts, New York

Poticha S M 1978 The midline incision in patients with Crohn's disease. Surgery, Gynecology and Obstetrics 146: 435–436

77. Antimicrobials and their use in surgery for inflammatory bowel disease

M. R. B. Keighley

Sepsis still remains the most common cause of hospital death in inflammatory bowel disease (Allsop & Lee 1978, Stephen & Loewenthal 1979, Fry et al 1980, Andrews et al 1991). The principal infective complications are septicemia, peritonitis, abdominal or pelvic abscess, wound sepsis and synergistic gangrene.

Risk factors for postoperative infection include age, malnutrition, obesity, renal disease, anergy, diabetes and certain drugs, blood transfusion, long operations, open drains and established sepsis at the time of operation. Elderly patients have an increased risk of infection (Claesson & Holmlund 1988). Malnutrition is thought to be associated with an increased risk of infection, but this has not been absolutely established either in our own practice or from other centers. However, malnourished patients tend to be immunocompromised and septic (Holter et al 1976, Goodgame 1980, Higgens et al 1980a). Obesity is associated with a greater risk of infection, particularly for patients undergoing rectal excision (DeGennaro et al 1978, Stone 1983). Renal disease is thought to increase the risk of infection, particularly from organisms such as *Pseudomonas aeruginosa* (Dobkin et al 1978) as well as from viral and fungal infections, but many of these people are immunocompromised, being immunosuppressed after transplantation, or at risk of sepsis if they are on chronic ambulatory peritoneal dialysis or on a hemodialysis program. Patients with coexisting malignant disease also have an increased susceptibility to infection. In these patients host defense mechanisms are also impaired (Pietsch et al 1977, Brown et al 1982). Diabetes mellitus is also a risk factor for sepsis (Goodson & Hunt 1979). Anergy and impaired reticuloendothelial function (Saba & Joffe 1980) increase the risk of infection (Christou et al 1985) since both are compromised in advanced malignancy, diabetes, established sepsis and malnutrition.

There are certain drugs which increase the risk of infection: antimicrobials may cause superinfection with staphylococci, resistant Gram-negative organisms and yeasts. Steroids probably increase the risk of infection (Knudsen et al 1976, Allsop & Lee 1978) but proof that steroid administration is an independent variable for sepsis has been difficult to establish conclusively (Keighley & Williams 1993). Blood transfusion has been shown to increase the risk of infection, but it may on the other hand protect against recurrence in Crohn's disease (Tartter 1988, Peters et al 1989). Cancer chemotherapy may increase the risk of sepsis, and previous radiotherapy impairs wound healing (Sparso et al 1986).

There are certain surgical factors which increase the risk of infection: contamination unquestionably increases the risk of localized infection in the peritoneal cavity and in the surgical incision (Pollock & Evans 1986, Claesson et al 1986, Tornqvist et al 1987). Long operations are associated with an increased risk of infection, and if a single-dose prophylaxis is used the concentration of antibiotic in serum may have fallen well below its therapeutic level by the end of the surgical procedure. There is no evidence that wound protection reduces the risk of infection, and the data on shaving with respect to sepsis are unclear. Open drains certainly increase the risk of infection but closed suction drains probably do not (Higson & Kettlewell 1978, Simchen et al 1984).

BACTERIA RESPONSIBLE FOR INFECTIONS IN INFLAMMATORY BOWEL DISEASE

Normally surgery on the small intestine is only complicated by aerobic bacterial species, since the small bowel is rarely colonized with high counts of anaerobes; hence the organisms most commonly isolated from wounds are *Escherichia coli*, *Klebsiella* species, *Proteus* species, non-hemolytic streptococci and enterococci. However, Crohn's disease causes obstruction and fistulae; under these circumstances there is colonization from anaerobic bacteria, which is responsible for colonic organisms causing postoperative sepsis as well (Arabi et al 1978, Ambrose et al 1984). Operations involving the colon immediately incur a risk of anaerobic infections since they are the principal bacteria within the large bowel. The dominant organisms causing postoperative infections after resections on the large bowel or in the obstructed small bowel are *Bacteroides fragilis*, *Clostridium* species, peptococcus and peptostreptococci (Keighley & Burdon 1979).

CHOICE OF ANTIMICROBIALS

To provide appropriate cover against the dominant enteric organisms that may cause postoperative infection it is important to provide broad-spectrum cover against the aerobic Gram-negative organisms as well as the anerobic Gram-positive and Gram-negative bacteria. Metronidazole remains the most appropriate agent for almost all anaerobic bacteria (Willis et al 1977), and therefore should be combined with an agent which is non-toxic and which is effective against the aerobic Gram-positive and Gram-negative bacteria which may be encountered.

Agents effective against aerobic bacteria within the bowel

Aminoglycosides. The aminoglycosides have traditionally been used for both prophylaxis and therapy. They are effective against Gram-positive cocci and against most Gram-negative organisms. They are potentially toxic and may need to be monitored by repeated serum assay. They still have a role in therapy but are rarely used for prophylaxis.

Cephalosporins. The cephalosporins are used extensively for prophylaxis and therapy. Their range of activity depends on each agent's own spectrum of cover. Agents such as cefuroxime are effective against most Gram-negative organisms but have little activity against Gram-positive bacteria, but the product is cheap and is used widely for prophylaxis. By contrast, agents such as cefotaxime, with a wider spectrum of activity, tend to be reserved for life-threatening infections requiring therapy.

Quinolones. The quinolones, particularly agents such as ciprofloxacin, are extremely effective against Gram-negative organisms, although resistance is beginning to emerge. They probably have an important place in prophylaxis and therapy.

Tetracyclines. Tetracyclines used to be used particularly for antibiotic lavage (Krukowski & Matheson 1983), but the increasing emergence of resistant organisms has reduced their effectiveness. Tetracycline lavage has never been adequately tested by randomized controlled studies (Silverman et al 1986).

Monobactams. Monobactams include agents such as aztreonam. They may have a role for therapy in the future.

Imipenems. This group of antimicrobials have a very broad spectrum of activity and are very active. They should be reserved for life-threatening infections.

PROPHYLAXIS OR THERAPY

The term prophylaxis should be confined to operations undertaken in the absence of any established sepsis. Hence, antibiotic cover for Crohn's disease complicated by an abscess or a fistula is not prophylaxis but therapy. For the same reason, the term antimicrobial prophylaxis can hardly be applied to emergency colectomy for fulminating colitis where there is already infection in the tissues of the bowel and the possibility of perforation before the operation commences.

Prophylaxis

The term prophylaxis is appropriate for elective resections in uncomplicated disease. There are certain principles which should be adhered to, as follows:

1. Bowel preparation should be meticulous and complete. We have investigated a wide variety of different regimens. Catharsis with magnesium sulfate is effective but poorly tolerated; whole bowel irrigation, although effective, is an assault that most patients will not accept and there are potential biochemical complications; oral electrolyte preparations with an osmotic agent require patients to drink large volumes of fluid, which many find difficult and the preparation is generally inferior to our standard regimen, which is two sachets of sodium picosulphate (Picolax) 36 hours before operation, followed by fluids only by mouth. If fluids cannot be tolerated an intravenous infusion should be commenced (Keighley & Williams 1993).
2. Surgical technique should also be meticulous; there should be avoidance of dead space, ischemic tissues, trauma and excessive blood loss, and anastomoses must be constructed with great care and preferably tested to ensure that they are airtight.
3. Theatre discipline. A disciplined operating theatre team is almost invariably associated with lower rates of infections than a team that is not committed to colorectal surgery or not used to performing colorectal operations routinely.
4. Audit. The process of audit reduces the risk of infection simply by a process of surveillance.
5. Antimicrobial prophylaxis should be by the intravenous route and should be given just before the operation commences. The dose of antibiotic must be one that achieves high therapeutic serum concentrations throughout the operation (Keighley & Burdon 1979). Antibiotic administration must therefore be repeated if the operation is very prolonged. The aim of prophylaxis is to achieve high serum concentrations and high tissue concentrations at the time of potential bacterial inoculation. There is no evidence that prolonged antimicrobial exposure beyond the duration of the operation further reduces

the risk of infection unless there is established sepsis at the time of surgery. The following issues have now been proved from randomized controlled clinical trials:

(a) Intravenous antimicrobial prophylaxis aimed to provide high serum and tissue levels at the time of operation is superior to oral antimicrobial therapy aimed at reducing the flora of the colon (Keighley et al 1979, Kaiser et al 1983, Weawer et al 1986, Lau et al 1988, Beggs et al 1982, Playforth et al 1988)
(b) Single-dose or 24-hour cover only for prophylaxis in colorectal surgery is just as effective as prolonged antimicrobial exposure (Higgens et al 1980b, Giercksky et al 1982, Goransson et al 1984, Juul et al 1987)
(c) In contaminated surgical procedures, or where there is established sepsis at the time of operation, prolonged antibiotic cover gives lower rates of sepsis than short-term antimicrobial exposure (Hares et al 1982)
(d) Use of an antianerobe (usually metronidazole) with a broad-spectrum agent effective against aerobic Gram-negative bacteria, is more effective than either type of antimicrobial used alone (Morris et al 1983, Hares et al 1981, Tudor et al 1988, Weaver et al 1986).

Therapeutic antibiotic

In certain circumstances operations are undertaken in the presence of coexisting sepsis, as in patients with enterocutaneous fistulae, enteroenteric fistulae complicated by abscess, in patients with emergency fulminating colitis, reoperations in the presence of coexisting sepsis and emergency operations for hemorrhage. Under these circumstances the overwhelming evidence is that antimicrobial exposure should be prolonged for at least 3 days, and often longer depending upon severity of contamination, host defense factors, and the virulence of the organisms encountered at the initial operation. In most patients with complex inflammatory bowel disease antimicrobial cover probably should be extended for at least 3 if not 5 days (Allsop & Lee 1978, Higgens et al 1980a, Hares et al 1982).

Other important principles of therapy for emergency surgery or surgery associated with established infection are:

1. Adequate debridement of devitalized tissues
2. Avoidance of intestinal anastomoses
3. Adequate drainage of localized collections of pus, preferably using closed suction drain systems, with or without irrigation
4. Irrigation of the peritoneal cavity with saline during the procedure. However, somewhat surprisingly, there is no evidence that peritoneal lavage with antimicrobial agents reduces the risk of infection. Indeed, the use of intraperitoneal antibiotics in the presence of peritonitis may cause rapid absorption and dangerously high serum concentrations (Stephen & Loewenthal 1978, Ericsson et al 1978)
5. Grossly contaminated wounds should be left open
6. Laparostomy (leaving the peritoneal cavity open) may be employed in life-threatening situations but it creates problems of its own and should not be undertaken lightly. Most patients require a prolonged period of ventilation, total parenteral nutrition, repeated abdominal debridement and large 'wound manager' bags to cover exposed bowel. Furthermore, there is a risk of fistula formation, bleeding, bowel obstruction and prolonged colonization by resistant bacteria
7. Patients with enterocutaneous fistula or prolonged ileus require nutritional support, usually by total parenteral nutrition delivered through a dedicated subclavian catheter
8. Close surveillance is required to detect persistent intra-abdominal sepsis, which should be drained either percutaneously (or, in the case of pelvic sepsis, per rectum or per vaginam) or, if multifocal and inaccessible, by repeat laparotomy.

REFERENCES

Allsop JR, Lee ECG 1978 Factors which influenced post-operative complications in patients with UC or Crohn's disease of the colon on corticosteroids. Gut 19: 729–734

Ambrose N S, Johnson M, Burdon D W, Keighley M R B 1984 Incidence of pathogenic bacteria from mesenteric lymph nodes and ileal serosa during Crohn's disease surgery. British Journal of Surgery 71: 623–625

Andrews H A, Keighley M R B, Alexander-Williams J, Allan RN 1991 Strategy for management of distal ileal Crohn's disease. British Journal of Surgery 78: 679–682

Arabi Y, Dimock F, Burdon D W, Alexander-Williams J, Keighley M R B 1978 Influence of bowel preparation and antimicrobials on colonic microflora. British Journal of Surgery 65: 555–559

Beggs F D, Jobanputra R S, Holmes J T 1982 A comparison of intravenous and oral metronidazole as prophylactic in colorectal surgery. British Journal of Surgery 69: 226–227

Brown R, Bancewicz J, Hamid J et al 1982 Failure of delayed hypersensitivity skin testing to predict post-operative sepsis and mortality. British Medical Journal 284: 851–853

Christou N V, Boisvert G, Broadhead M, Meakins J L 1985 The techniques of measurement of the delayed hypersensitivity skin test response for the assessment of bacterial host resistance. World Journal of Surgery 9: 798–806

Claesson B E B, Holmlund D E W 1988 Predictors of intra-operative bacterial contamination and post-operative infection in elective colorectal surgery. Journal of Hospital Infection 11: 127–135

Claesson B E B, Filipsson S, Holmlund D E W, Matzsch T W, Wahlby L 1986 Selective cefuroxime prophylaxis following colorectal surgery based on intra-operative dipslide culture. British Journal of Surgery 73: 953–957

DeGennaro V A, Corman M L, Coller J A, Pribek M C, Veidenheimer M C 1978 Wound infections after colectomy. Diseases of the Colon and Rectum 21: 567–572

Dobkin J F, Miller M H, Steigbiegel N H 1978 Septicaemia in patients on chronic haemodialysis. Annals of Internal Medicine 88: 28–33

Ericsson C D, Duke J H Jr, Pickering L K 1978 Clinical pharmacology of intravenous and intraperitoneal aminoglycoside antibiotics in the prevention of wound infections. Annals of Surgery 188: 66–70

Fry D E, Pearlstein L, Folton R L, Polk H C Jr 1980 Multiple system organ failure: the role of uncontrolled infection. Archives of Surgery 115: 16–140

Giercksky K E, Danielson S, Garberg O et al 1982 A single dose tinidozole and doxycycline prophylaxis in elective surgery of colon and rectum. Annals of Surgery 195: 227–231

Goodgame J T 1980 A critical assessment of the indication for total parenteral nutrition. Surgery, Gynecology and Obstetrics 151: 433–441

Goodson W H III, Hunt T K 1979 Wound healing and the diabetic patient. Surgery, Gynecology and Obstetrics 149: 600–608

Goransson G, Nilsson-Ehle I, Olsson S A et al 1984 Single versus multiple dose doxycycline prophylaxis in elective colorectal surgery. Acta Chirurgica Scandinavica 150: 245–249

Hares M M, Bentley S, Burdon D W, Allan R N, Keighley M R B 1982 Clinical trials of the efficacy and duration of antibacterial cover for elective resection in IBD. British Journal of Surgery 69: 215–217

Hares M M, Green F, Youngs D, Bentley S, Burdon D W, Keighley M R B 1981 Failure of antimicrobial prophylaxis with cefoxitin or metronidazole and gentamicin in colorectal surgery: is mannitol to blame? Journal of Hospital Infection 2: 127–133

Higgens C S, Allan R N, Keighley M R B, Arabi Y, Alexander-Williams J 1980a Sepsis following operation for inflammatory intestinal disease. Diseases of the Colon and Rectum 23: 102–105

Higgens A F, Lewis A, Moore P, Hole M 1980b Single and multiple dose cotrimoxazole and metronidazole in colorectal surgery. British Journal of Surgery 67: 90–92

Higson R H, Kettlewell M G W 1978 Parietal wound drainage in abdominal surgery. British Journal of Surgery 65: 326–329

Holter A R, Rosen H M, Fischer J E 1976 The effects of hyperalimentation on major surgery in patients with malignant diseases: a prospective study. Acta Chirurgica Scandinavica 446 (Suppl): 86–87

Juul P, Klaaborg K E, Kronborg O 1987 Single or multiple doses of metronidazole and ampicillin in elective colorectal surgery. A randomized trial. Diseases of the Colon and Rectum 30: 526–528

Kaiser A B, Herrington J L, Jacobs J K, Mulherin J L Jr, Roach A C, Sawyers J L 1983 Cefoxitin versus erythromycin, neomycin and cefazolin in colorectal operations. Annals of Surgery 198: 525–530

Keighley M R B, Burdon D W 1979 Antimicrobial prophylaxis in surgery. Pitman Press, London

Keighley M R B, Williams N S 1993 Surgery of the anus, rectum and Colon. W B Saunders, London

Keighley M R B, Alexander-Williams J, Arabi Y, Youngs D 1979 Comparison between systemic and oral antimicrobial prophylaxis in colorectal surgery. Lancet i: 894–897

Knudsen L, Christiansen L, Jarnum S 1976 Early complications in patients previously treated with corticosteroids. Scandinavian Journal of Gastroenterology 11 (Suppl 27): 123–128

Krukowski Z H, Matheson M A 1983 The management of peritoneal and parietal contamination in abdominal surgery. British Journal of Surgery 70: 440–441

Lau W Y, Chu K W, Poon G P, Ho K K 1988 Prophylactic antibiotics in elective colorectal surgery. British Journal of Surgery 75: 782–785

Morris D L, Hares M M, Voogt R J, Burdon D W, Keighley M R B 1983 Metronidazole need not be combined with an aminoglycoside when used for prophylaxis in elective colorectal surgery. Journal of Hospital Infection 4: 65–69

Peters W R, Fry R D, Fleshman J W, Kodner I J 1989 Multiple blood transfusions reduce the recurrence rate of Crohn's disease. Diseases of the Colon and Rectum 32: 749–753

Pietsch J B, Meakins J L, McLean L D 1977 The delayed hypersensitivity response: application in clinical surgery. Surgery 82: 349–355

Playforth M J, Smith G M R, Evans M, Pollock A V 1988 Antimicrobial bowel preparation: oral, parenteral or both? Diseases of the Colon and Rectum 31: 90–93

Pollock A V, Evans M 1986 Addition of oral neomycin and metronidazole lowers sepsis when used with systemic metronidazole and augmentin in colorectal surgery. Proceedings of the World Congress of Gastroenterology, San Paulo

Saba T M, Joffe E 1980 Plasma fibronectin (opsonic glycoprotein): its synthesis by vascular endothelial cells and role in cardiopulmonary integrity after trauma as related to reticuloendothelial function. American Journal of Medicine 68: 577–594

Silverman S H, Ambrose N S, Youngs D J, Shepherd A F I, Roberts A P, Keighley M R B 1986 The effect of peritoneal lavage with tetracycline solution in post-operative infection. Diseases of the Colon and Rectum 29: 165–169

Simchen E, Shapiro M, Sacks T G, Michel J, Durst A, Eyal Z 1984 Determinants of wound infection after colon surgery. Annals of Surgery 199: 260–265

Sparso B H, Van der Masse H, Kristensen D et al 1984 Complications following post-operative combined radiation and chemotherapy in adenocarcinoma of the rectum and rectosigmoid. Cancer 54: 2363–2366

Stephen M, Loewenthal J 1979 Generalised infective peritonitis. Surgery, Gynecology and Obstetrics 147: 231–234

Stone H H 1983 Antibiotics in colon surgery. Surgical Clinics of North America 63: 3–9

Tartter P I 1988 Blood transfusion and infection complications following colorectal cancer surgery. British Journal of Surgery 75: 789–792

Tornqvist A, Forsgren A, Leandoer L, Ursing J 1987 Identification and antibiotic prophylaxis of high risk patients in elective colorectal surgery. World Journal of Surgery 65: 77–79

Tudor R G, Haynes I, Youngs D J, Burdon D W, Keighley M R B 1988 Comparison of short-term antibiotic cover with a third-generation cephalosporin against conventional five-day therapy using metronidazole with an aminoglycoside in emergency and complicated colorectal surgery. Diseases of the Colon and Rectum 31: 28–32

Weaver M, Burdon D W, Youngs D J, Keighley M R B 1986 Oral neomycin and erythromycin compared with single dose systemic metronidazole and ceftriaxone prophylaxis in elective colorectal surgery. American Journal of Surgery 151: 437–442

Willis A T, Ferguson I R, Jones P H et al 1977 Metronidazole in prevention and treatment of bacteroids infections in elective colonic surgery. British Medical Journal 1: 607–610

78. Thromboembolism in inflammatory bowel disease – etiology, prophylaxis and treatment

W. R. Fleming   W. A. Kmiot

ETIOLOGY

General features

Venous thromboembolic disease was first recognized in 1936 to be a significant contributor to the morbidity and mortality of inflammatory bowel disease (IBD) (Bargen & Barker 1936). Increasingly frequent reports have since emerged detailing thrombotic complications in IBD, with a reported incidence in clinical studies from 1.3% (Talbot et al 1986) to 6.4% (Edwards & Truelove 1964), and 39% of patients in a postmortem study (Graef et al 1966). Thromboembolic complications of IBD have been reported in both arterial and venous systems, but arterial thromboses account for less than one-third of reported events. Thromboses in IBD tend to occur spontaneously in young patients, often at unusual sites, and occur more frequently during exacerbations of the underlying disease. Thromboembolic events affecting mesenteric and peripheral vessels (Talbot et al 1986, Novotny et al 1992), portal (Brinberg et al 1991, Crowe et al 1992) and hepatic veins (Maccini et al 1989, Chesner et al 1991), cardiac vessels (Talbot et al 1986), cerebral arteries and sinuses (Kiff & Denton 1989, Johns 1991, Garcia-Monco & Gomez-Beldarrain 1991, Musio et al 1993), gonadal veins (Jain & Jeffrey 1991) and retinal vessels (Knox et al 1984, Ruby and Jampol 1990) have been reported. Not only may IBD be associated with thrombotic phenomena but a causal relationship of thrombosis, vasculitis and multifocal microinfarction has been proposed as an important factor in the etiology of Crohn's disease (Wakefield et al 1989).

Role of thrombosis in pathogenesis of IBD

In a study of resected specimens from 15 patients with Crohn's disease (Wakefield et al 1989), a focal vascular injury confined to intramural vessels supplying Crohn's-affected bowel was found, suggesting a possible pathogenic mechanism. The authors suggested that the vascular damage in the muscularis propria resulted in the activation of the monocyte and vascular endothelial cellular procoagulant pathway, producing localized thrombosis and microinfarction. In another study of rectal biopsies the same group noted the presence of mucosal capillary thromboses, particularly in patients with ulcerative colitis (Dhillon et al 1992), although their significance was uncertain. Abnormal platelet function, owing to activation and hyperaggregability, may support the hypothesis of a microvascular thrombotic cause in the pathogenesis of IBD (Webberley et al 1993, Collins et al 1994). Activated hyperaggregable platelets may be important in a number of ways: they may promote neutrophil recruitment and chemotaxis, amplifying the inflammatory cascade; platelet aggregates may add to microinfarction by occluding the bowel microcirculation; and activated platelets release platelet-derived growth factor, a potent chemotactic mediator for fibroblasts, which may contribute to stricture formation (Collins et al 1994).

Etiology of thromboembolism in IBD

Patients with inflammatory bowel disease appear to have a thrombotic tendency, although the cause for this hypercoagulability is unclear, with some authors disputing its existence at all (Knot et al 1983). Virtually every aspect of the coagulation system has been studied for abnormalities, but even though a number have been found their significance in the etiology of clinical thrombotic complications remains elusive. Abnormalities in the coagulation system found in patients with active disease include elevated levels of coagulation factors V and VIII and fibrinogen (Lee et al 1968, Lake et al 1978, Leardi et al 1983, Talbot et al 1986), thrombocytosis (Morowitz et al 1966, Talstead et al 1970) and decreased levels of antithrombin III (Ghosh et al 1983). A deficiency in the vitamin K-dependent natural anticoagulant protein S has also been noted (Aadland et al 1992), but this appears to be an acute-phase response only.

A major problem in assessing etiology is deciding whether hemostatic system changes are a response to acute inflammation or genuinely reflect a hypercoagulable state. The increased clotting factors and platelets tend to return to normal during disease remission (Lake et al 1978, Knot et al 1983). However, Conlan and co-workers did find abnormalities in fibrinolysis and elevated levels of circulating immune complexes in patients in remission, concluding that these changes may increase the risk of thrombosis, especially if compounded by the acute inflammatory response of active disease (Conlan et al 1989).

More recently, attention has returned to the role of platelets not only in mediating mucosal inflammation, but also in promoting thrombosis. Past studies have shown that activation of platelets results in the release of chemotactic agents for inflammatory cells, such as platelet factor IV (Simi et al 1987), platelet-activating factor (Eliakim et al 1988) and arachidonic acid metabolites such as prostaglandin E_2 and thromboxane (Lauritsen et al 1988, Webberley et al 1993). In a Birmingham study of 104 patients with IBD, platelet aggregation, and in particular spontaneous aggregation, was found to be markedly active in a high proportion of patients with IBD, and spontaneous aggregation was observed in seven of eight patients with previous thromboembolism (Webberley et al 1993). This was recently supported in a study of 88 patients with IBD, which noted increased numbers of circulating platelet aggregates and found that platelets circulated in an activated state, regardless of the level of disease activity, thereby increasing the risk of thrombosis (Collins et al 1994). This has led to the suggestion that platelet-activation inhibitors may be useful in the treatment of IBD.

THROMBOEMBOLISM PROPHYLAXIS

General features

Because of the higher reported incidence of thromboembolic disease in patients with IBD and the possibility of microthrombosis playing a role in its etiology, prophylaxis against deep venous thrombosis (DVT) is important as clinical diagnosis of early DVT may be difficult (Davidson et al 1992, Kilpatrick et al 1993), treatment may be prolonged and hazardous, and the mortality of embolic complications may be high.

In order to design preventive measures, high-risk groups within the population of patients with IBD should be identified. The risk of thrombosis is increased with age, female gender, duration of immobility, especially if combined with surgery (Simi et al 1990), oral contraceptives (Quinn et al 1992), pregnancy, malignancy and surgery in the region of the pelvis or lower limbs (Treasure & Griffin 1990). Prophylactic measures taken to diminish the risk of venous thrombosis can be conveniently divided into non-pharmacological and pharmacological modalities, although in very high-risk groups a combination will be needed.

Non-pharmacological modalities

Graduated compression stockings. By using elastic graduated compression stockings the risk of DVT in the postoperative patient can be reduced by more than half (Jeffery & Nicolaides 1990, Wells et al 1994). In a meta-analysis of 1752 patients undergoing moderate-risk surgery, definitive conclusions could not be drawn about the value of combining stockings with other prophylactic measures, such as heparin, nor whether the current trend towards the use of knee-high stockings changed the risk. However, the use of graduated compression stockings is very variable, ranging from under 3% to over 79% of patients (Wells et al 1994). Stocking usage should be combined with active leg exercises, early ambulation and avoidance of prolonged periods of bed-rest in order to increase venous blood flow.

Intraoperative measures. In patients undergoing surgery active measures should be undertaken to prevent the formation of thrombi in the legs while the patient is anesthetized. Electrically stimulated contraction of the calf muscles, intermittent calf compression with pneumatic boots and the use of motorized foot maneuvers will all decrease the risk of thrombosis. Pneumatic compression boots not only increase venous blood flow but may stimulate endogenous fibrinolytic activity as well (Knight & Dawson 1976).

Interruption of the inferior vena cava. Inferior vena caval interruption, using a filter device such as a bird's nest or Greenfield filter, can trap potentially fatal emboli before they reach the lungs. The three main indications for the use of such a device are: contraindications to anticoagulant therapy; recurrent pulmonary embolism despite anticoagulation; in unusual circumstances as prophylaxis for extremely high-risk patients with established DVT (Goldhaber & Morpurgo 1992). They can be inserted percutaneously under local anesthesia and are 97% effective in preventing recurrent pulmonary emboli while maintaining high patency rates (Goldstone 1991).

Pharmacological modalities

Low-dose subcutaneous heparin. In the International Multicentre Trial, a controlled randomized study involving over 4000 patients, low-dose subcutaneous heparin in a dose of 5000 U 2 hours preoperatively and every 8 hours thereafter for 7 days was found to be significantly effective in reducing the incidence of fatal pulmonary embolism. Non-fatal emboli and DVT were also less common in the heparin group, although there was a slight increase in the number of wound hematomas (International

Multicentre Trial 1975). This finding was confirmed using meta-analysis of 78 controlled trials involving over 15 000 patients, with a 40% reduction in non-fatal and 64% reduction in fatal pulmonary embolisms (Collins et al 1988).

Low molecular weight heparins. Low molecular weight heparins (LMWH) are fragments of standard heparin produced by enzymatic or chemical depolymerization. They have a higher bioavailability at low doses and an extended plasma half-life, meaning that they can possibly be used in once-daily injections. Their main advantage is the reported lower frequency of bleeding for an equivalent antithrombotic effect (Hirsh 1992). In clinical studies LMWHs are safe and effective, with a significant reduction in thromboembolic deaths and non-fatal scan-detected thrombi (Mohr et al 1992). In addition, LMWHs appear to be at least as effective as standard heparin in the treatment of established thrombosis, with the added advantage of subcutaneous administration instead of continuous infusion.

Low-dose warfarin. Very low-dose warfarin (1 mg daily) has been shown to be effective in reducing the incidence of venous thrombosis in patients undergoing major surgery, but the potential for bleeding problems requires further study (Poller et al 1987).

Antiplatelet therapy. Drugs that suppress platelet function, such as aspirin or dypyridamole, prevent platelet aggregation, which is largely unaffected by conventional anticoagulants. Meta-analysis of controlled trials shows that 2 weeks of antiplatelet therapy in surgical patients produces a highly significant reduction in the incidence of DVT and pulmonary embolism. By acting on another part of the coagulation system, antiplatelet agents may be more effective in combination with standard anticoagulant prophylaxis than when used alone (Antiplatelet Trialists' Collaboration 1994).

Dextran 40 or 70 may be given as an infusion during or after surgery, its mechanism of action being a combination of plasma volume expansion and antiplatelet activity. It appears to have a limited role in thrombosis prophylaxis because of the incidence of side effects, including volume overload and anaphylaxis. It is probably best used in patients unable to receive heparin because of bleeding or allergic reactions, such as heparin-induced thrombocytopenia (Goldhaber & Morpurgo 1992).

TREATMENT OF DVT

General features

Once a clinical diagnosis of clear-cut deep venous thrombosis has been made, treatment should be commenced with anticoagulants and confirmation of the diagnosis undertaken by phlebography. The objectives of treatment are to prevent the formation of further thromboses, to prevent the extension and embolization of existing thrombus, and to minimize valvular damage. More commonly the diagnosis is unclear after clinical assessment, and investigation must be undertaken before treatment is begun. The choice of investigation includes radionuclide venography, scanning with labeled fibrinogen, Doppler and duplex ultrasound, and contrast venography.

Contrast venography has been regarded as the 'gold standard' in the past but has a risk of contrast allergy and may actually induce DVT (Bettmann et al 1987). Using fibrinogen labeled with ^{125}I, which is taken up preferentially by forming thrombus, early thrombi can be detected by external scanning over the veins. It appears to be sensitive enough to detect small thrombi in the venous sinuses of the calf, but is less useful in detecting pre-existing thrombi that are not actively incorporating fibrinogen, and in detecting pelvic and common femoral DVT. Ultrasound assessment, preferably with color Doppler, has become a widely preferred initial investigation in the diagnosis of acute DVT (Robertson & Kelly 1993). Ultrasound has the advantage of being relatively cheap, quick and readily available, but is more difficult to perform in the calf veins and in veins affected by previous DVT. Contrast venography with ^{99m}Tc-RBC may be performed when ultrasound is unavailable or inadequate.

Treatment modalities

When DVT has been diagnosed general measures should be instituted to reduce pain and swelling and also the risk of embolization. The patient should be confined to bed with leg elevation until the acute symptoms have resolved, followed by ambulation in graduated compression stockings. The specific treatment of choice is anticoagulation, unless there are specific contraindications. The aims of treatment are to prevent extension of the thrombus, prevent the formation of new thrombi and diminish the risk of pulmonary embolization. By allowing the natural fibrinolytic process to act unopposed, anticoagulation may also help speed the dissolution of the thrombus.

Heparin. Heparin acts quickly to prevent thrombus extension by preventing the action of thrombin and the formation of thromboplastin. It is given intravenously in a dose sufficient to maintain the activated partial thromboplastin time (APTT) at 1.5–2.5 times the control. A loading dose of 10 000 units with a continuous infusion of 1000–2000 units per hour is usually sufficient, and the dosage should be monitored by daily APTT estimation (Goldstone 1991). Bleeding is an uncommon complication, being most likely to occur in fresh surgical wounds or in the gut or urinary tract, and generally reflects an excessive dose of heparin.

Warfarin. Coumarin derivatives such as warfarin act by inhibiting the synthesis of vitamin K-dependent clotting factors in the liver. Warfarin has a slow onset of action and a long half-life, making it more suited to long-term therapy after heparin has been stopped. A course of 3 months' therapy allows collaterals to develop and covers the period when recurrence is most likely to occur (Goldstone 1991). Because of the wide range of drug interactions that can complicate treatment, careful monitoring by the measurement of prothrombin time (INR) should be undertaken to maintain a level two to three times greater than control.

Fibrinolytic drugs. Urokinase, streptokinase and recombinant tissue plasminogen activator act directly on the thrombus by converting plasminogen to plasmin, which has a specific proteolytic effect on fibrin and fibrinogen. Their use is extremely limited in venous thrombosis of the extremities, but is more common in arterial thrombosis and embolism. Bleeding complications are more troublesome than with heparin, particularly in patients who have had surgery within the previous fortnight (Treasure & Griffin 1990).

REFERENCES

Aadland E, Odegaard O R, Roseth A, Try K 1992 Free protein S deficiency in patients with chronic inflammatory bowel disease. Scandinavian Journal of Gastroenterology 27: 957–960

Antiplatelet Triallists' Collaboration 1994 Collaborative overview of randomised trials of antiplatelet therapy-III: reduction in venous thrombosis and pulmonary embolism by antiplatelet prophylaxis among surgical and medical patients. British Medical Journal 308: 235–246

Bargen J A, Barker N W 1936 Extensive arterial and venous thrombosis complicating chronic ulcerative colitis. Archives of Internal Medicine 58: 17–31

Bettmann M A, Robbins A, Braun S D, Wetzner S, Dunnick N R, Finkelstein J 1987 Contrast venography of the leg: diagnostic efficacy, tolerance, and complication rates with ionic and nonionic contrast media. Radiology 165: 113–116

Brinberg D E, Stefansson T B, Greicius F A, Kahlam S S, Molin C 1991 Portal vein thrombosis in Crohn's disease. Gastrointestinal Radiology 16: 245–247

Chesner I M, Muller S, Newman J 1991 Ulcerative colitis complicated by Budd–Chiari syndrome. Gut 27: 1096–1100

Collins C E, Cahill M R, Newland A C, Rampton D S 1994 Platelets circulate in an activated state in inflammatory bowel disease. Gastroenterology 106: 840–845

Collins R, Scrimgeour A, Yusuf S, Peto R 1988 Reduction in fatal pulmonary embolism and venous thrombosis by perioperative administration of subcutaneous heparin: overview of results of randomized trials in general, orthopedic and urologic surgery. New England Journal of Medicine 318: 1162–1173

Conlan M G, Haire W D, Burnett D A 1989 Prothrombotic abnormalities in inflammatory bowel disease. Digestive Diseases and Sciences 34: 1089–1093

Crowe A, Taffinder N, Layer G T, Irvine A, Nicholls R J 1992 Portal vein thrombosis in a complicated case of Crohn's disease. Postgraduate Medical Journal 68: 291–293

Davidson B L, Elliott C G, Lensing A W A 1992 Low accuracy of color Doppler ultrasound in the detection of proximal leg vein thrombosis in asymptomatic high-risk patients. Annals of Internal Medicine 117: 735–738

Dhillon A P, Anthony A, Sim R et al 1992 Mucosal capillary thrombi in rectal biopsies. Histopathology 21: 127–133

Edwards F C, Truelove S C 1964 The course and prognosis of ulcerative colitis. III. Complications. Gut 5: 1–22

Eliakim R, Karmeli F, Razin E, Rachmilewitz D 1988 Role of platelet-activating factor for ulcerative colitis. Enhanced production during active disease and inhibition by sulfasalazine and prednisolone. Gastroenterology 95: 1167–1172

Garcia-Monco J C, Gomez-Beldarrain M 1991 Superior sagittal sinus thrombosis complicating Crohn's disease. Neurology 41: 1324–1325

Ghosh S, Mackie M J, McVerry B A, Galloway M, Ellis A, McKay J 1983 Chronic inflammatory bowel disease, deep venous thrombosis and antithrombin activity. Acta Haematologica 70: 50–53

Goldhaber S Z, Morpurgo M 1992 Diagnosis, treatment and prevention of pulmonary embolism. Report of the WHO/International Society and Federation of Cardiology Task Force. Journal of the American Medical Association 268: 1727–1733

Goldstone J 1991 Veins and lymphatics. In: Way L W (ed) Current surgical diagnosis and treatment. Appleton & Lange, Norwalk, USA, pp 768–792

Graef V, Bagenstoss A H, Sauer W G, Spittell J A Jr 1966 Venous thrombosis occurring in nonspecific ulcerative colitis: a necropsy study. Archives of Internal Medicine 117: 377–382

Hirsh J 1992 Overview of low molecular weight heparins and heparinoids: basic and clinical aspects. Australia and New Zealand Journal of Medicine 22: 487–495

International Multicentre Trial 1975 Prevention of fatal postoperative pulmonary embolism by low doses of heparin. Lancet 2: 45–51

Jain K A, Jeffrey R B Jr 1991 Gonadal vein thrombosis in patients with acute gastrointestinal inflammation: diagnosis with CT. Radiology 180: 111–113

Jeffery P C, Nicolaides A N 1990 Graduated compression stockings in the prevention of postoperative deep vein thrombosis. British Journal of Surgery 77: 380–383

Johns D R 1991 Cerebrovascular complications of inflammatory bowel disease. American Journal of Gastroenterology 86: 367–370

Kiff R S, Denton G W 1989 Fatal cerebral venous thrombosis complicating acute ulcerative colitis. American Journal of Gastroenterology 84: 577–578

Kilpatrick T K, Lichtenstein M, Andrews J, Gibson R N, Neerhut P, Hopper J 1993 A comparative study of radionuclide venography and contrast venography in the diagnosis of deep venous thrombosis. Australia and New Zealand Journal of Medicine 23: 641–645

Knight M T N, Dawson R 1976 Effect of intermittent compression of the arms on deep venous thrombosis in the legs. Lancet 2: 1265–1268

Knot E A R, Ten Cate J W, Leeksma O C H, Tytgat G N, Vreeken J 1983 No evidence for a prethrombotic state in stable chronic inflammatory bowel disease. Journal of Clinical Pathology 36: 1387–1390

Knox R L, Schachat A P, Mustonsen E 1984 Primary, secondary and coincidental ocular complications of Crohn's disease. Ophthalmology 91: 163–173

Lake A M, Stauffer J Q, Stuart M J 1978 Hemostatic alterations in inflammatory bowel disease. Response to therapy. Digestive Diseases and Sciences 23: 897–902

Lauritsen K, Laursen L S, Bukhave K, Rask-Madsen J 1988 In vivo profiles of eicosanoids in ulcerative colitis, Crohn's colitis, and *Clostridium difficile* colitis. Gastroenterology 95: 11–17

Leardi S, Amoroso A, Afeltra A, Ferri G M, Tebano M T, Simi M, Speranza V 1983 Blood coagulation alterations and thromboembolism in Crohn's disease. Italian Journal of Surgical Science 13: 197–201

Lee J C L, Spittell J A Jr, Sauer W G, Owen C A, Thompson J H 1968 Hypercoagulability associated with chronic ulcerative colitis. Changes in blood coagulation factors. Gastroenterology 54: 76–84

Maccini D M, Berg J C, Bell G A 1989 Budd–Chiari syndrome and Crohn's disease. An unreported association. Digestive Diseases and Sciences 34: 1933–1936

Mohr D N, Silverstein M D, Murtaugh P A, Harrison J M 1992 Prophylactic agents for venous thrombosis in elective hip surgery. Meta-analysis of studies using venographic assessment. Archives of Internal Medicine 153: 2221–2228

Morowitz D A, Allen L W, Kirnsner J B 1966 Thrombocytosis in chronic inflammatory bowel disease. Annals of Internal Medicine 68: 1013–1021

Musio F, Older S A, Jenkins T, Gregorie E M 1993 Case report: cerebral venous thrombosis as a manifestation of acute ulcerative colitis. American Journal of Medical Science 305: 28–35

Novotny D A, Rubin R J, Slezak F A, Porter J A 1992 Arterial thromboembolic complications of inflammatory bowel disease. Report of three cases. Diseases of the Colon and Rectum 35: 193–196

Poller L, McKernan A, Thomson J M, Elstein M, Hirsch P J, Jones J B 1987 Fixed minidose warfarin: a new approach to prophylaxis against venous thrombosis after major surgery. British Medical Journal 295: 1309–1312

Quinn D A, Thompson T, Terrin M L et al 1992 A prospective investigation of pulmonary embolism in women and men. Journal of the American Medical Association 268: 1689–1696

Robertson P L, Kelly M J 1993 Diagnosis of deep venous thrombosis: the role of selected investigational modalities. Australia and New Zealand Journal of Medicine 23: 635–637

Ruby A J, Jampol L M 1990 Crohn's disease and retinal vascular disease. American Journal of Ophthalmology 110: 349–353

Simi M, Leardi S, Tebano M T, Castelli M, Costantini F M, Speranza V 1987 Raised plasma concentrations of platelet factor 4 (PF4) in Crohn's disease. Gut 28: 336–338

Simi M, Leardi S, Minervini S, Pietroletti R, Schietroma M, Speranza V 1990 Early complications after surgery for Crohn's disease. Netherlands Journal of Surgery 42: 105–109

Talbot R W, Heppell J, Dozois R R, Beart R W Jr 1986 Vascular complications of inflammatory bowel disease. Mayo Clinical Proceedings 61: 140–145

Talstead I, Rootweit K, Gijone E 1970 Thrombocytosis in ulcerative colitis and Crohn's disease. Scandinavian Journal of Gastroenterology 8: 135–138

Treasure T, Griffin S 1990 Postoperative thromboembolic disease: a tantalizing enigma. In: Hadfield J, Hobsley M, Treasure T (eds) Current surgical practice, Vol 5. Edward Arnold, London, pp 39–51

Wakefield A J, Sawyerr A M, Dhillon A P et al 1989 Pathogenesis of Crohn's disease: multifocal gastrointestinal infarction. Lancet 2: 1057–1062

Webberley M J, Hart M T, Melikian V 1993 Thromboembolism in inflammatory bowel disease: role of platelets. Gut 34: 247–251

Wells P S, Lensing A W A, Hirsh J 1994 Graduated compression stockings in the prevention of postoperative venous thromboembolism. A meta-analysis. Archives of Internal Medicine 154: 67–72

79. A team approach

M. H. Irving   N. A. Scott

The contents of this book demonstrate the breadth of the manifestations, investigations and treatments of inflammatory bowel disease (IBD). Long gone are the days when Crohn's disease and ulcerative colitis were footnotes in textbooks of medicine and surgery, and when the treatment was primarily excisional surgery. Today's medical and surgical gastroenterologists are faced with patients whose symptoms may include skin disorders, arthritides and ocular problems as well as the more usual gastrointestinal manifestations. Today, the medical gastroenterologist has a wide range of pharmacological products which can be used for treatment of IBD, either simultaneously or sequentially. Similarly, the surgeon, as well as having to be an expert in the nutritional support of patients under his care, has an increasing variety of surgical techniques to offer the patient. Although the necessity for collaboration between medical and surgical gastroenterologists has been accepted for many years as being in the best interests of the patient, it is now apparent that a number of other medical specialties and members of the paramedical professions should be incorporated into the therapeutic team if an optimal service is to be provided. For the past 20 years the surgical and medical gastroenterological units at Hope Hospital have developed a system, which continues to evolve, for the management of patients with IBD. This has involved an increasing role for radiologists and specialized nurses in particular and, a central place for the patient's view in the overall management of their disease. We believe that our experience has produced a harmonious atmosphere in which to deliver care, especially to the patient afflicted with a complicated pattern of disease. The essential events and components of this team approach are as follows.

THE OUTPATIENT CONSULTATION

The first point of contact with specialist care for most patients with IBD will be an outpatient consultation with a medical or surgical gastroenterologist. The medical gastroenterologist will tend to be consulted by patients with diarrhea associated with abdominal pain, weight loss and anemia, whereas the surgeon will tend to see those patients referred with abdominal or perianal sepsis, abdominal masses and rectal bleeding.

The team approach should begin at this stage, with the medical and surgical gastroenterologists holding simultaneous clinics in adjacent consulting suites, thus allowing easy cross-consultation and referral. It is not our practice to have combined clinics with patients being seen by both specialists at the same time, as we believe this builds in unnecessary delays and can be confusing to patients, who almost invariably need an individual explanation of their problem and the treatment options available. However, for both medical and surgical gastroenterologist this process can be enhanced by additional consultation with a nurse specialist in gastroenterology or, where appropriate, a stoma care nurse who can elaborate at leisure on what has been said. In appropriate cases the nurse specialist can assume the task of ensuring a seamless run-through of a patient's care, from initial consultation through hospital admission to discharge back into the community.

HOSPITAL ADMISSION: ELECTIVE AND EMERGENCY

Patients are admitted electively for the management of problematic disease or for operation. Emergency admissions tend to be for abdominal pain, attacks of intestinal obstruction, often associated with intra-abdominal abscess formation, gastrointestinal bleeding, rapid weight loss, uncontrollable diarrhea or exacerbations of perineal sepsis. Wherever possible elective and emergency admissions should be to a specialist gastrointestinal ward. Many hospitals choose to make this a combined medical and surgical ward. This has not been our practice, for we believe that surgical and medical management require different knowledge, skills and attitudes, and are best undertaken separately but preferably in adjacent wards, which facilitates easy interchange of staff and patients.

The management of patients with IBD should be based on locally agreed medical and nursing protocols, which should themselves be founded on research-based optimum practice guidelines. An example of the effect of such a protocol on the good management of acute colitis is the insistence that all patients admitted with this condition under the medical gastroenterologists are seen in joint consultation with a surgical gastroenterologist within 24 hours, to agree a management regimen in the event of the patient's continued deterioration into a state of disintegrative colitis (toxic megacolon). Soon after admission the medical team will write up the admission history and examination and will describe a plan of investigation and treatment to be approved by the senior medical staff. The patient should receive an explanation of the situation that has been found, and the proposed investigations and treatment. Once this has been agreed the plan should be discussed with the nursing staff, who will construct their own plans for instigating it.

THE WEEKLY MEETING

The key to our team working is the weekly meeting, where the medical and surgical staff meet with other specialties to agree the management of problematic patients and to discuss instances where treatment has not gone as planned or adverse events have occurred.

The meeting is of particular value in discussing with radiologists the nature and order of radiological investigations. Patients needing medical or surgical treatment can be referred from one team to another, and where one team is at an impasse detailed debate can bring forward new ideas. The nursing and paramedical perspectives on management can also be brought into the debate. Where appropriate, and when the patient is able to collaborate and understand, they can be invited to the meeting to hear their case discussed and to contribute to the debate. The weekly meeting is of educational as well as practical value, enabling knowledge to be shared and concepts to be developed.

The technique can be used even by those with a limited practice in gastroenterology, the minimum requirement being a physician and surgeon with an interest in gastroenterology sharing their discussions with a radiologist and the relevant nursing staff.

THE WARD ROUND

Day-to-day team work is expressed through the ward rounds. It is at this point that the medical, pharmacy and nursing staff collaborate to carry forward the patient's treatment plan. The practice, sometimes observed, of doctors and nurses undertaking separate rounds and communicating only by means of written notes is the antithesis of team work, and exists only to be condemned.

At ward rounds complex investigations can be planned so they can be carried out with maximum effectiveness. This applies particularly to investigations such as fistulography, which for maximum effect will need preparation of the patient by the nursing staff and joint discussion between senior clinical staff and the radiologist.

THE INTESTINAL FAILURE UNIT

The pinnacle of team collaboration at Hope Hospital is the Intestinal Failure Unit, which concentrates on the treatment of patients who cannot support their nutritional state because of extensive bowel disease, fistulation, short bowel syndrome, motility disorder or sepsis. The principal reason for admission to the unit is intestinal failure due to Crohn's disease. Such patients usually have a healthy cardiorespiratory and renal system but require high-risk treatments such as proximal intestinal diversion (jejunostomy) or intravenous feeding. In the absence of a facility for managing such situations patients are likely to be admitted to an intensive care unit, which is an inappropriate and high-risk area for such treatments. The simplest form of intestinal failure unit is a high-dependency area which allows the specialist nursing staff to give the highest-quality nursing care, particularly to stomas and intravenous lines, according to locally agreed protocols. The quality of care that can be obtained with such specialist nursing care is demonstrated in Figure 79.1, which shows an intestinal fistula and intravenous line in close proximity yet where line infection is prevented using regimens which will prevent exit site infections as well as intraluminal contamination.

In a unit such as ours, with a high tertiary referral load, such a facility will need to be large, with its own dedicated nursing and ancillary staff. Patients referred to such a

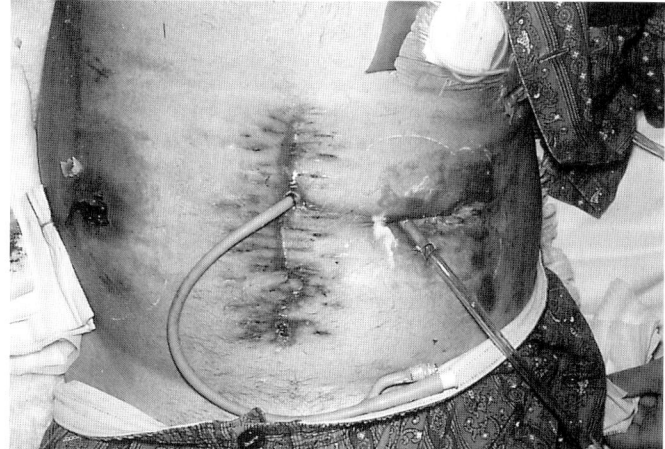

Fig. 79.1 High-output fistula adjacent to tunneled subclavian intravenous feeding line. The latter remained uninfected throughout the patient's course of treatment as a consequence of the maintenance of strict catheter care protocols.

unit, often from a long distance, will of necessity be unwell and traumatized by their experiences. They may well have lost confidence in the medical profession and, more importantly, in themselves.

Such patients need special management, perhaps the most important part of which is what we call 'the hour-long explanation'. Once the patient has been assessed in detail, the most senior clinician in charge of the patient sits down alone with the patient and explains in detail the problem as it is seen from the medical point of view. Every effort is made to outline a plan of action that the patient can follow, and it is emphasized to the patient that they can accept, reject or delay all or part of the plan as they see fit. In this way some control is restored to the patient. The hour-long discussion also affords the patient the opportunity to see the problems faced by those looking after him, and to realize the need for some investigations to be repeated. 'We must understand your problems but you must also understand ours' is a sentence that will inevitably emerge during such discussion.

Patients are then introduced to the other members of the team who will be involved with their care, and the confidence-building process resumes.

Patients with the severity of illness that warrants tertiary referral to an intestinal failure unit are likely to need prolonged treatment, often for 3–4 months and occasionally up to a year. During this time the maintenance of morale is a key feature if success is to be achieved. Factors that aid this process include the limitation of intravenous feeding to a proportion of the day, e.g. night-time only, access to exercise, and the opportunity to have showers and excursions out of the hospital with relatives or friends, the latter sometimes being hospital visitors.

MEMBERS OF THE TEAM

Medical practitioner

The roles of the medical staff are obvious but will be diminished unless they can work harmoniously one with another and with the non-medical members of the team. All members of the team should remember that respect is something to be earned and not expected as a right. This applies particularly to the medical practitioners. Respect is freely afforded to those who are patently good at their job, who listen to and are considerate of the views of others, particularly their patients, and who are willing to respond to calls for assistance without delay. Perhaps the greatest respect is accorded to those who, however experienced and senior, are willing to admit ignorance and error and to consider advice from wherever it is proffered. Perhaps the most effective phrase that can be used by doctors building a team is 'What is your opinion?' when addressing those with whom they have to work.

The importance of the patient's family practitioner must never be forgotten. At the very least high-quality and timely information should be sent to the family practitioner whenever a patient is discharged from hospital. In complex cases the direct involvement of the family practitioner at the weekly meeting can be invaluable.

Nursing staff

High-calibre nursing staff of all grades are the key to successful team working. They are the people who have the closest and continual contact with the patient, and without their collaboration the often taxing treatments that have to be delivered will not be successful. To this end it is important that the senior members of the nursing staff involved with the patient's care are involved in discussions about therapeutic regimens. Where possible, a nurse specialist in gastroenterology should be involved in the team. Such nurses, who often have long experience of nursing patients with inflammatory bowel disease, will have the time to discuss in detail the proposed treatments and to ensure that they are delivered. They are also capable of undertaking certain specialized tasks, such as dilatation of rectal strictures etc.

Stoma care nurses

Stoma care nurses are an essential part of the team. Their training means that they can deal with both the mechanical and the psychological problems associated with the presence of a stoma. They can also help by introducing patients to someone who has undergone the procedure and lived with a stoma, and to the relevant patient organization such as the Ileostomy Association and the National Association for Colitis and Crohn's Disease.

Nutritional support nurses

It is important that nutritional therapy, particularly parenteral nutrition, is delivered by nurses specially trained to avoid the complications associated with intravenous feeding. Maximum effectiveness is achieved by concentrating patients who need intravenous feeding on one ward. However, if this is not possible then the hospital should establish a focal point from where intravenous feeding is coordinated, and whence nurses can supervise intravenous feeding in the hospital. The nutritional support nurses work in close collaboration with the dietitian to ensure the efficacy of enteral feeding.

Pharmacist

The pharmacist is a key member of the team, responsible for ensuring the compatibility of the components of intravenous regimens and advising on how specific deficits in trace metal and vitamin provision can be addressed.

Dietitian

The dietitian has a crucial role in monitoring the overall nutritional state of the patient, and is probably the best person to record and maintain nutritional measurements such as anthropometric data. The dietitian also advises on and supervises the introduction of specialized enteric feeding regimens.

Additional key medical support staff

In addition to those already listed, together with the medical gastroenterologist and the dedicated colorectal surgeon, are a further group of key medical personnel. Such staff include a dedicated radiologist or team of radiologists, a committed pathologist, a psychologist and, if possible, a microbiologist who will regularly advise on hospital-acquired and nosocomial infections.

CONCLUSION

The best results for patients are obtained by collaboration between the key members of the team. It should never be forgotten that the patient is at the center of that team.

80. Surgical maneuvers in Crohn's disease – a personal guide

J. Alexander-Williams

BACKGROUND

The particular pathological features of Crohn's disease that affect the technique of operation are its slowly progressive nature which resembles, yet differs from, tuberculosis and diverticulitis. In Crohn's disease there are often edematous tissue planes that usually make gentle finger-guided separation feasible. In addition there are major technical problems due to complex tracking of abscesses in tissue planes and the tendency to form satellite abscesses.

Some parts of the dissection are pure pleasure, as the tissue planes separate, but there are other areas of excitement and technical challenge. Having operated on many hundreds of patients with Crohn's disease over the last 30 years, no other surgical technical exercise has given me greater pleasure or satisfaction.

I have also observed that Crohn's disease is less likely to form impenetrable intraperitoneal adhesions than, say, diverticulitis or starch peritonitis. In Crohn's disease, separating adherent loops of gut is relatively simple. It is also of interest that although patients may require multiple operations, often through the same scar, it is relatively uncommon for them to develop wound herniae.

LAPAROTOMY AND ACCESS

The first operation for Crohn's disease on any individual patient is usually straightforward. I do not shave the abdomen except when performing a proctectomy. I operate with the patient in the supine position. I tend to site the incision over the point of maximum tenderness or palpable mass. I generally prefer low transverse incisions, particularly in young people, who wish to avoid unsightly abdominal scars. However, the most important consideration is to avoid any potential stoma sites: paramedian or oblique wounds are inappropriate. For reoperations I generally use the old wound.

During reoperation the immediate danger is that the gut may be adherent behind the previous scar. This is particularly so if there has been previous wound sepsis or a fistula. For this reason it is safest to make the initial laparotomy approach through the old wound, as far away as possible from the site of any dense or thickened scar, which may indicate such problems. I always use cutting diathermy because it avoids bleeding and allows the muscle wall of any adherent gut to be identified easily, and so avoid making an incision through it.

I usually start at the least scarred end of the wound and, having cut with diathermy through the fibrous scar, I elevate the edges of the scar with tissue forceps. I then incise gently, a millimeter at a time, until either the peritoneal cavity is entered or the gut muscle is seen. If the gut seems to be adherent, I turn my attention to another part of the wound, usually at the opposite end. Gentle finger pressure will often move adherent gut away and facilitate entry into the peritoneal cavity. As soon as a cavity is entered the index finger gently enlarges the hole and pushes the gut further away. As the gut is pushed from behind the scar, the incision can slowly be enlarged.

The surgeon's finger gradually enlarges the peritoneal access by sweeping round and gently teasing gut away from the parietal peritoneum. Sweeping movements are made in all directions. Provided the gut separates easily and readily, progress will be fast. However, once resistance to gentle finger dissection stops, I turn my attention elsewhere and approach from some other direction in which dissection is easier. With a gentle slow technique it is extremely rare to make a hole in the gut, even when it is firmly adherent to some part of the wound.

It is always best to work around any point of difficulty and gently push the gut away, where there is the least resistance. It is interesting to note that gut which initially seems to be firmly stuck, often ceases to be a problem when tackled from another direction.

MANAGING TOUGH ADHESIONS

Sometimes there is an area of dense adhesion that cannot be dissected by gentle finger pressure or incision. Often this can be separated by a pinching maneuver (Fig. 80.1). When the adhesion is too dense to be separated by a pinch, particularly when the tissue planes are edematous, I often use closed curved scissors in what I describe as a 'tyre lever' maneuver (Fig 80.2).

With even tougher adhesions, particularly where there has been a satellite abscess or a fistula track, gut cannot be prised away from the parietes even with the tyre lever maneuver. Under these circumstances I remove a small patch of the patient's abdominal wall attached to the bowel. This I call the 'postage stamp' maneuver (Fig 80.3).

AIDS TO DISSECTION

When there are multiple loops of bowel stuck to each other or to the peritoneum, I aid dissection by exaggerating the tissue planes, either by the injection of saline or, in recent years, by the injection of carbon dioxide gas. Carbon

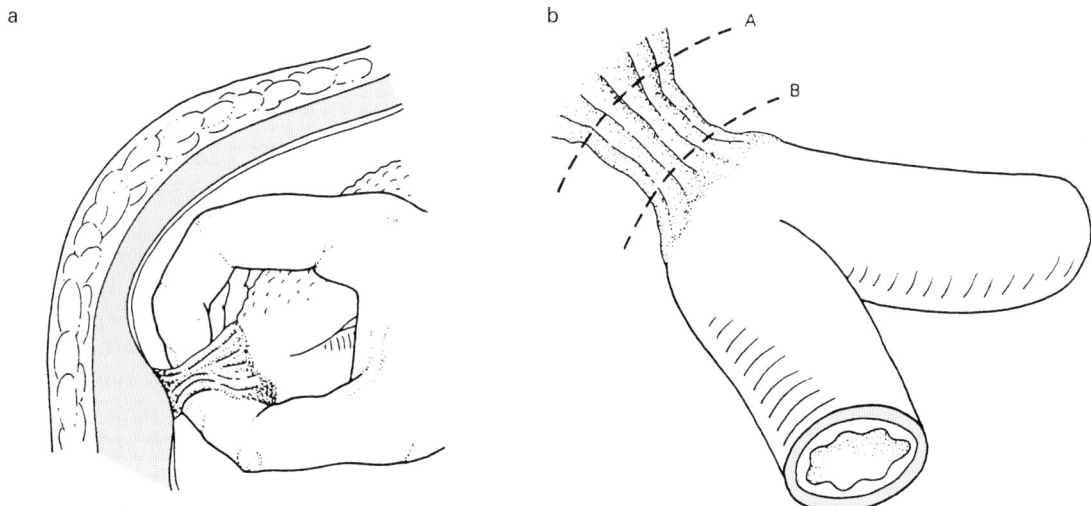

Fig. 80.1 a Adherent gut is gradually encircled until it is finally attached at its most adherent point: this is then pinched off between finger tip and thumb. b If it has to be divided because it is so firm or fibrous, it should be divided close to the parietes (A) not close to the gut (B). Reproduced with permission from Kumar D, Alexander-Williams J (eds) 1993 Crohn's disease and ulcerative colitis: surgical treatment. Springer-Verlag, London.

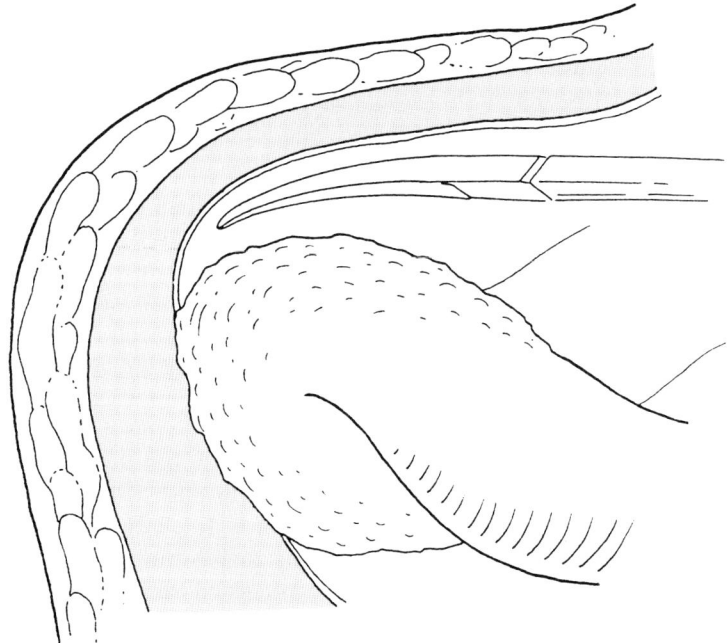

Fig. 80.2 'Tyre lever' maneuve, using closed scissors to create a plane of cleavage between edematous gut and abdominal wall. Reproduced with permission from Kumar D, Alexander-Williams J (eds) 1993 Crohn's disease and ulcerative colitis: surgical treatment. Springer-Verlag, London.

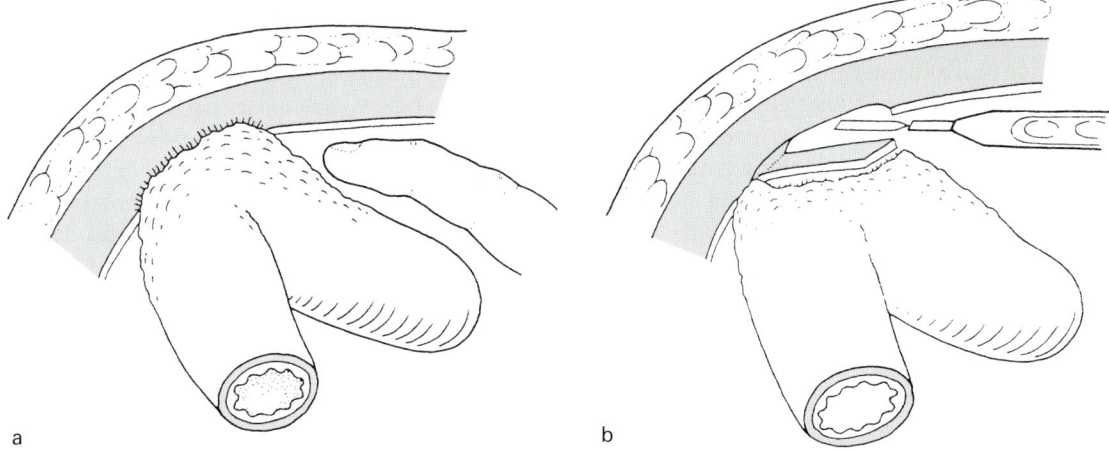

Fig. 80.3 a When the gut is so densely adherent that it may be damaged if it is levered off the parietes. b A portion of the attached parietes is cut off with diathermy: the 'postage-stamp' manoeuvre. Reproduced with permission from Kumar D, Alexander Williams J (eds) 1993 Crohn's disease and ulcerative colitis: surgical treatment. Springer-Verlag, London.

dioxide under low pressure, delivered from the pneumoperitoneum apparatus used in laparoscopy, is connected via a tube to a 21 gauge needle. The needle can be inserted between the tissue planes and the gas allowed to force itself along the plane of least resistance. This plane can then be followed easily and safely by diathermy dissection.

I also use carbon dioxide insufflation to inflate the lumen of loops of bowel. The needle can be passed obliquely through the muscle wall of the bowel and the lumen distended with carbon dioxide. Distension of two adjacent loops of gut with gas makes it much easier to find a plane of cleavage between them. Gas inflation also has the advantage of demonstrating any holes or damage to the gut wall that have been made inadvertently. I use these technical aids whenever operating on recurrent Crohn's disease.

A decade or so ago, it was my custom to resect a block of gut en masse when several loops were stuck firmly together, perhaps with intervening enteroenteric fistulae. I now follow a policy of maximum conservation of functioning gut so that even the most matted and adherent loops are carefully separated one from another; en masse resections are never performed. It is often gratifying to be able to conserve 10 cm lengths of normal functioning gut between stenotic or even fistulating areas, which in earlier years might have been sacrificed along with the severely diseased areas.

HOW MUCH TO RESECT?

The general principle is to conserve as much as possible by resecting as little as possible. I only resect severely stenotic, thickened lengths of gut. If there is a short stricture then I perform strictureplasty (see below). If possible I try not to anastomose actively ulcerated mucosa, but sometimes there is no option. The best way of determining from the outside whether the gut has mucosal ulceration is to feel gently along the mesenteric border with the finger and thumb. If the mesenteric edge of the gut feels thickened, mucosal ulceration is usually present. If soft, mesenteric ulceration is uncommon.

I do not usually preserve the ileocecal junction because ileal disease extends up to the junction. In the past, when at the first operation I have retained a centimeter or two of the terminal ileum and the ileocecal junction, I have found that this has been followed by an early recurrence. For all primary terminal ileal Crohn's disease I now perform ileocecal resection and anastomose the ileum, end-on, to the ascending colon.

When operating on more proximal small bowel it is important to ensure that there is no residual stenosis distal to the anastomosis. A recipe for disaster is to perform an anastomosis or a strictureplasty on an obviously thickened stenotic loop of gut and fail to detect a tight distal stenosis. To ensure that no distal stenosis is missed, I now always thread a balloon catheter along the whole length of small gut distal to the anastomosis or strictureplasty. I then inflate the balloon with 8 mls of fluid so that it has a diameter of 25 mm, and then pull it back through the gut. By this means I often encounter unsuspected strictures, which I then treat by strictureplasty. When multiple dissections or multiple strictureplasties have been performed, I always check that all the anastomoses are gas-tight by finally reinflating the gut with carbon dioxide and milking it of the bolus of gas proximally. At one time I used to do this under saline, so that any bubbles indicating leaks would be detected, but now I can easily hear or see any minute leaks unaided.

STRICTUREPLASTY

There is nothing novel about the concept, or mysterious about the technique of strictureplasty. The idea was born from the observation that small-bowel strictures are often multifocal, with 'skip' areas of relatively normal bowel between, and that Crohn's disease is an incurable disease with frequent recrudescence. If the concept of wide excision, such as might be applied in the management of lymphoma of the gut, is followed then there is the risk of causing a shortage of functioning gut. Surgeons in Oxford and Birmingham, in the UK, and Cleveland in the USA, therefore tried to simply widen the strictures by incising the gut longitudinally across the stricture and sewing it transversely to widen the lumen (Alexander-Williams & Haynes 1985, Dehn et al 1989, Fazio et al 1989). This technique was called either strictureplasty or stricturoplasty; I prefer the 'e' to the 'o'.

Between 1978 and 1992 I performed over 350 intestinal strictureplasties. There were no perioperative deaths and more than 80% of patients were completely relieved of their symptoms of recurrent subacute obstruction. This experience has taught me that the option of strictureplasty is technically feasible and that small bowel containing even active Crohn's disease will hold sutures and heal without leaking. The techniques have been described elsewhere (Alexander-Williams 1986). The principles of suturing are exactly the same as for intestinal anastomosis.

THE ANASTOMOSIS

There is an almost infinite variety of anastomotic techniques that have been used in the surgical treatment of Crohn's disease. The anastomoses can be fashioned end-to-end, end-to-side or side-to-side. They can be stapled, or sutured with absorbable or unabsorbable sutures, which may be interrupted or continuous and in either one or two layers.

After trying various types of anastomoses, I now adopt a simple universal technique. I use an end-to-end anastomosis with a single layer of interrupted absorbable sutures, using a continuous suture where it is easy so to do. The reasons for the choice of this technique are the wish to make the anastomosis as quick, cheap and as safe as possible, to prevent inverting layers of gut that might possibly produce mechanical narrowing, and also to ensure that there will be the minimal interference with the blood supply of the ends that are being anastomosed. In the early years of my experience I encountered some bizarre anatomical consequences of side-to-side or end-to-side anastomoses in which a huge distension of the blind end of the limb had occurred. The theoretical disadvantage of an end-to-end anastomosis is the possibility that the

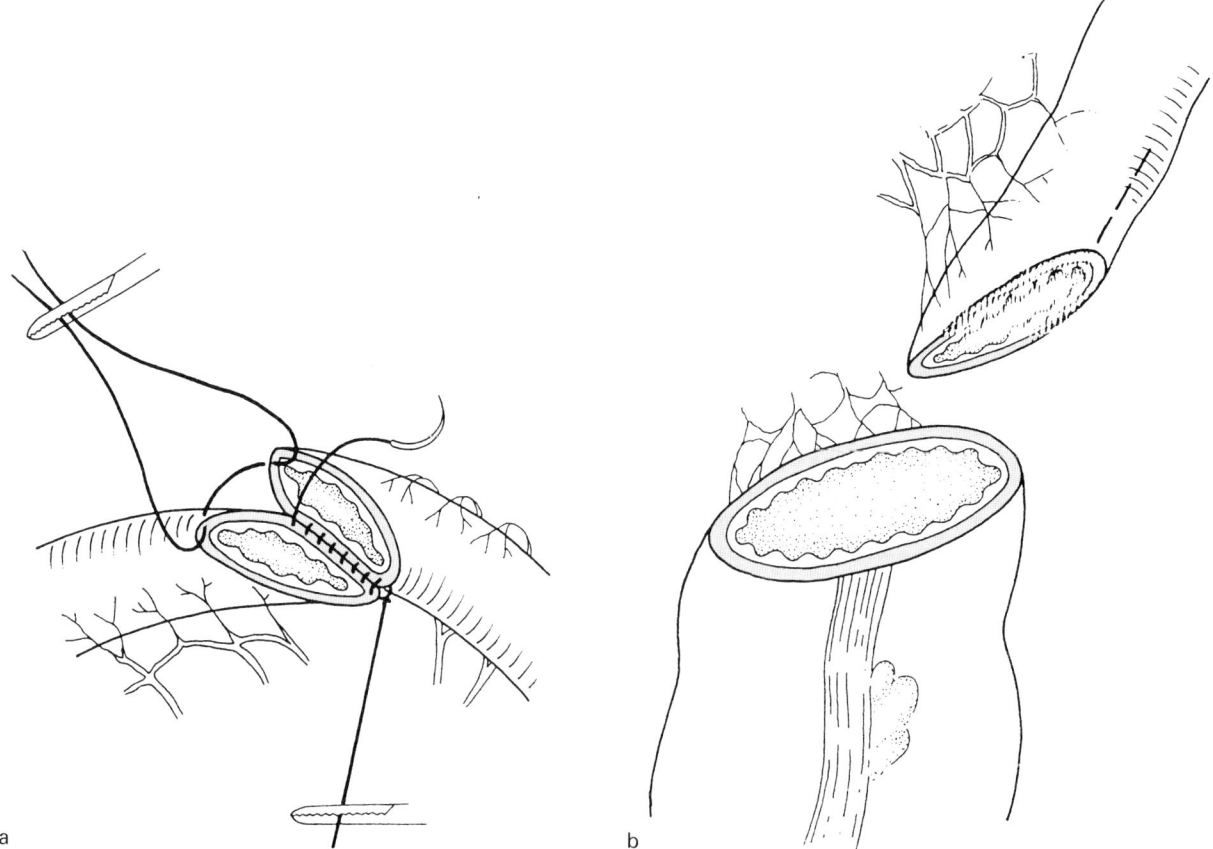

Fig. 80.4 **a** Small bowel to small bowel anastomoses are performed by rotating the obliquely cut gut end through 180°. **b** If there is still a size discrepancy between ileum and colon, a further animesenteric incision is made. Reproduced with permission from Kumar D, Alexander-Williams J (eds) 1993 Crohn's disease and ulcerative colitis: surgical treatment. Springer-Verlag, London.

diameters of the two ends of gut will be different. However, any discrepancy can be overcome by fashioning an oblique cut on the smaller-diameter bowel or making a relieving incision on its anterior mesenteric border (Fig. 80.4).

I have found staples to be unsuitable for anastomoses in Crohn's disease and no quicker than hand-sewn anastomoses. They are often unsuitable when edematous gut is being anastomosed, and can produce bizarre imaging artefacts in later investigations. Some surgeons advocate the use of non-absorbable sutures so that at subsequent operations they can see where the last anastomosis was performed. I do not find this knowledge to be particularly important since even when absorbable sutures have been used, it is usually easy to see where the last anastomosis was performed.

I am often asked about the appropriate distance between interrupted sutures. I believe that the fewer sutures that can be used to effect an anastomosis, the better: they are then likely to provide the least interference to blood supply. The distance apart will depend on the thickness of the tissue being sutured, but I generally aim to place interrupted sutures about 3 mm apart. I aim to put as few as possible and then, after completion, test the anastomosis by inflation with carbon dioxide. I add additional sutures wherever there is a leak. Using this technique, I find it surprising how few sutures are required to make an airtight suture of thickened bowel wall. I do not wrap an anastomosis with omentum. I close the hole in the mesentery and I never drain the peritoneal cavity. The abdominal wall is closed with a continuous mass suture of slowly absorbed suture material (PDS). The fat layer, which is frequently contaminated during the course of these operations, is gently washed with aqueous chlorhexidine or a similar antiseptic, and a loose monofilament absorbable suture is used as a subcuticular stitch. I do not drain even if there has been an abscess, provided the abscess cavity is draining freely into the peritoneal cavity.

If there has been a complex fistula, particularly with ramifications in the abdominal wall, I gently curette the track to make sure that no foreign material remains in it and that all ramifications are draining. No drain is placed in the fistula track, but the skin opening is made sufficiently large to ensure that it does not heal over before the drainage from the sinus has stopped.

COLONIC CROHN'S DISEASE

Most patients with colonic Crohn's disease who require surgical treatment prefer, if possible, to avoid a permanent stoma. I try, whenever possible, to preserve the rectum and make an ileorectal anastomosis. However, I have learned that if the rectal stump is less than 15 cm in length, or if it is indistensible and rigid from chronic disease, it rarely provides an adequate reservoir. I find that if the patient has frequent bowel movements after the operation they usually think that they would have been better off with a stoma.

If the ends of the bowel from which I wish to make an ileorectal anastomosis are so severely diseased that I am worried about the healing of the anastomosis, I prefer to bring out the ends as two end-stomas rather than make anastomosis and protect it by a proximal diversion ileostomy. If, after diversion for 3 months, the disease has settled, I then reanastomose. I have learned that an anastomosis in the presence of an abscess or in the presence of severe active disease at the suture line has a 30–40% chance of leakage, whereas the complications are minimal following a 12-week diversion and secondary reanastomosis.

TECHNICAL TIPS IN THE MANAGEMENT OF PERIANAL CROHN'S DISEASE

Perianal disease is common in patients with Crohn's disease but most are not severely troubled by symptoms. I maintain the principle that surgical intervention should only be used to treat symptoms, not to cure the disease. The symptoms in perianal Crohn's disease are caused either by pus under tension, a tight fibrous stenosis, or by perianal excoriation due to discharge.

The principal reason for surgical intervention is to relieve pain due to pus under tension. The difficulties are to precisely define the site of tension, and how effectively to drain the pus. In the operating room I find it helpful to ask the patient to point to the area of maximal pain and then, once the patient is anesthetized, to examine that area carefully. The site identified by the patient is usually the point of maximal induration, and squeezing the area will often cause pus to exude from one or more skin or anal canal openings. The skin between these openings can be divided to provide drainage, and there will be satisfactory healing. There will be no loss of continence provided no muscle fibers are divided. However, I have been referred many patients who have become incontinent after such tracks have been widely drained, and I presume that in them some muscle must have been divided. Furthermore, I often find it difficult to determine how much sphincter muscle is encircled by a fistula track, particularly when there is perianal scarring and deformity from recurrent sepsis. Once again therefore, I stress the importance of dividing tissues slowly in a bloodless field so that muscle can be identified and preserved. Whenever muscle tissue is encountered it is not divided but simply encircled with a soft silastic seton. This seton remains in position until the induration and discomfort have subsided. It is essentially a draining seton, not a cutting seton. I frequently leave setons in situ for many months, and so it is important that they are made of soft insert material such as sialastic tubing, and that the knot is reinforced with a soft non-absorbable suture. A stiff monofilament nylon seton knot will often cause some discomfort. I have been referred patients who have had such severe complex perianal sepsis that they have been advised to have a proctectomy. In some of them I have simply left draining setons through tracks around sphincters for years, with satisfactory control of symptoms.

Anal and low rectal strictures are often difficult to manage, particularly when associated with fistulae. However, it always surprises me to find how little trouble patients experience despite a stricture that will barely admit my little finger on examination. I have found that the most successful management of symptomatic strictures is a gentle, one index finger, dilatation under anesthesia, repeated if need be at 1- or 2-monthly intervals. Perseverance is needed, for in some patients it has taken five or six such dilatations before long-term successful control of symptoms has been achieved.

CONCLUSION

I pass on to you some of these practical tips in surgical management because they are not all orthodox surgical maneuvers: they have been acquired by repeated analysis of mistakes. I hope that surgeons of each generation should not have to repeat these mistakes. Most are peculiar to the management of Crohn's disease, a disease that most surgeons have to deal with only infrequently.

REFERENCES

Alexander-Williams J 1986 How I do it–the technique of intestinal strictureplasty. International Journal of Colorectal Disease 1: 54–57

Alexander-Williams J, Haynes I G 1985 Conservative operations for Crohn's disease of the small bowel. World Journal of Surgery 9: 945–951

Dehn T C B, Kettlewell M G W, Mortensen N J McC, Lee E C G, Jewell D P 1989 Ten-year experience of strictureplasty for obstructive Crohn's disease. British Journal of Surgery 76: 339–341

Fazio V W, Galandiuk S, Jagelman D G, Lavery I C 1989 Strictureplasty in Crohn's disease. Annals of Surgery 210: 621–625

81. Preserving anorectal function in surgery for inflammatory bowel disease

M. R. B. Keighley

It may not always be appropriate or even desirable to preserve the anorectum, particularly if it is severely diseased or if it is functionally incapable of preserving continence. Thus, in most patients with inflammatory bowel disease it is worthwhile carefully assessing anorectal function before any decision is taken as to whether or not to preserve the sphincters or the rectum, as opposed to performing radical ablative proctocolectomy.

CLINICAL ASSESSMENT

Clinical assessment is still extremely important in assessing the usefulness of the anorectum in maintaining continence for the future. A history of soiling suggests a gutter deformity or an incompetent sphincter; true incontinence of solid stool when the patient is unaware of a bowel evacuation suggests both sensory impairment and an incompetent sphincter and pelvic floor. On the other hand, a history of urgency indicates rectal disease and not necessarily an incompetent sphincter, since many will regain full continence when the inflammation is controlled or the diseased rectum is removed (Buchmann et al 1980, Ambrose et al 1984, Keighley et al 1993).

Inspection will reveal whether or not there is an intact anal sphincter ring as well as the presence of scars, a gutter defect, anal fistulae, skin tags, fissures or deficiency of the perineum. Asking the patient to contract the sphincter muscles and pelvic floor allows the observer to gauge the degree of contraction of the superficial fibers of the external sphincter when the perineum is observed. Similarly, careful digital examination will allow an assessment of resting tone, which is largely the function of the internal and external sphincters. The response to voluntary contraction can also be judged both within the sphincter ring itself and in the puborectalis sling. Digital examination will also identify areas of scarring, areas of deficiency in the sphincter, and induration as well as stenosis. These simple clinical measures are usually undertaken by most discerning clinicians. However, the sensory side of the reflex arch is often inadequately considered. Simply stroking the perianal skin with cotton wool allows a clinician to determine whether or not the sphincter contraction reflex is present. Careful assessment of perineal sensation is important, particularly in women who have previously had vaginal deliveries. After prolonged labor there may be impairment of pudendal nerve function, which may be associated with anesthesia around the vulva and anus. More extensive neurological deficiency involving the cauda equina will lead to blunting of perineal sensation and anesthesia of the buttocks. Crude assessment of sensation within the anal canal and rectum can be evaluated during digital examination and also by proctosigmoidoscopy.

Proctosigmoidoscopy is essential and is frequently not practised in an outpatient setting for fear of causing pain or discomfort. However, narrow proctoscopes and sigmoidoscopes are available and should be used in order to determine whether there is inflammatory change in the anal canal itself, and whether or not there is active proctitis.

Treat active proctitis

Both Crohn's disease patients and the occasional patient with ulcerative colitis who has perianal disease and active proctitis tend to do badly following attempted local anal surgery for conditions such as skin tags, fissures and fistulae. Under these circumstances therapy might be more appropriately directed against the inflammatory process in the rectum, leaving the anal disease alone, since in many cases these lesions resolve totally without any therapy. Furthermore, anal surgery particularly if wounds do not heal, may compromise continence and commit a patient to ablative proctocolectomy in the future (Alexander-Williams & Buchmann 1980).

SITUATIONS WHERE PRESERVATION OF ANAL FUNCTION REQUIRES CAREFUL CLINICAL AND PHYSIOLOGICAL EVALUATION

Colonic Crohn's disease

Crohn's disease of the large bowel is likely to require

rectal excision if the sphincter is destroyed from previous surgery or anal disease; if there is severe anorectal sepsis and multiple complex anorectal fistulae; in patients with large transeptal rectovaginal fistulae in severe rectal disease; or if there is a coexisting low rectal neoplasm. For patients with Crohn's colitis and relative rectal sparing, even in the presence of inactive perianal disease, rectal preservation may be an option, particularly if there is minimal small-bowel disease and provided that an extensive small-bowel resection has not been performed in the past (Lefton et al 1975, Weterman & Pena 1976). Under these circumstances rectal compliance and sphincter function will need to be assessed in order to determine whether anorectal preservation is likely to be associated with acceptable functional results. Our own experience clearly demonstrated that a large-capacity rectum was associated with the best long-term results following ileorectal anastomoses (Weaver & Keighley 1986).

Perianal Crohn's disease

If perianal Crohn's disease is associated with active rectal involvement, severe anorectal stenosis, multiple complex anorectal fistulae and sepsis, or if previous anal surgery has rendered the sphincters incompetent, rectal excision is likely to be the only available option. If there is active rectal inflammation in the presence of perianal disease every effort should be made to bring the proctitis under control by topical steroids or 5-ASA preparations.

If the problem is a rectovaginal fistula and the patient is totally incontinent as a result of a large septal defect, early defunctioning is mandatory; despite this, there are some whose rectal disease may improve and in whom a subsequent reconstruction may be possible. Many patients with low recto- or anovaginal fistulae have very few symptoms and only intermittently discharge; under these circumstances active surgical measures should probably be resisted for fear of rendering the patient worse. In symptomatic patients the exact location of the fistula should first be determined. The next step is to ensure that there is no sepsis requiring prior drainage. As many women have had previous vaginal deliveries it is wise to investigate whether there is any pudendal neuropathy or postobstetric pelvic floor or sphincter damage. Thus, advancement flaps or sphincter reconstructions would only be advised in the absence of a compromised pelvic floor, pudendal neuropathy, coexisting sepsis and rectal inflammation in symptomatic patients (Givel et al 1982, Bauer et al 1991).

If the problem is an anorectal fistula, the same considerations apply. Critical anatomical assessment is likely to require anorectal ultrasonography, MRI scans and gentle probing of the fistula under anesthetic (Keighley & Williams 1993). The first consideration is complete elimination of anorectal sepsis using soft mushroom catheters, taking great care to ensure that there are no residual collections in the intersphincteric space, the postanal spaces and the supralevator compartment (Pritchard et al 1990). Fistulotomy should only be contemplated in symptomatic patients without rectal disease; great care is needed to avoid dividing striated muscle and creating scars, and in this regard seton fistulotomy offers many advantages (White et al 1990).

Deep cavitating ulcers can be highly destructive and may require early defunctioning, particularly if topical steroid injection has not produced a remission (Hobbis & Schofield 1982). By contrast, anal fissures are often painless and may be left to heal spontaneously; certainly, open sphincterotomy and extensive anal stretching should be avoided. Anorectal stenosis may settle with topical therapy and repeated gentle dilatation, but the long-term results are generally poor and most patients require proctectomy or are defunctioned (Linares et al 1988).

Selection of patients for restorative proctocolectomy

All potential pouch patients should be carefully counselled: they should be well motivated as well as well informed. Results are poor if there is perianal disease or sepsis preoperatively, or if the sphincters are damaged from obstetric injury or previous anorectal surgery (Braun et al 1992). The very short rectal stump is often associated with a poor functional outcome. These patients should be investigated by anal manometry, anal mucosal electrosensitivity, pudendal nerve latency and anal ultrasonography to ensure that they do not have a postobstetric neuropathy, sphincter damage or an incompetent continence mechanism.

Incontinent patients with inflammatory disease being considered for rectal excision

Incontinence may be due to a localized sphincter defect or postobstetric damage in the absence of rectal disease; provided the patient is not suffering from severe diarrhea, and provided there is no evidence of gross neuropathy, sphincter repair or pelvic floor repair may preserve continence but a defunctioning stoma may be advisable, particularly in Crohn's disease (Scott et al 1989). If the rectum is very narrow and diseased but the sphincters are intact, rectal excision may restore continence in ulcerative colitis. In Crohn's disease severe anorectal stenosis, sepsis and fistulae usually necessitate rectal excision, but in ulcerative colitis anorectal function should be assessed since reconstructions may restore continence in appropriately selected patients.

ASSESSMENT OF ANORECTAL FUNCTION USING PHYSIOLOGICAL TESTS

It is not necessary to have a full physiological anorectal laboratory in order to treat patients with inflammatory bowel disease. On the other hand, it is an advantage and it does lead to better selection of particular procedures. Possibly the most important aspect of assessing anorectal function using physiological tests is an opportunity for the clinician to more thoroughly evaluate the pathophysiological process and to increase his or her level of communication with the patient. Consequently, where possible these anorectal physiological studies should be performed by the doctor and not by a technician. The following tests may prove useful in the selection of patients, justifying preservation of the anorectum in inflammatory bowel disease:

1. **Anal manometry.** Anal manometry will simply assess maximum resting and maximum squeeze pressures on command. Very low resting pressures and poor voluntary components are nearly always associated with disappointing function, and in such patients serious consideration should be given to removing the anorectum if it is not functioning satisfactorily or if it is diseased (Yoshioka et al 1988).
2. **Anal sensation.** Anal sensation allows the afferent side of the reflex arc of the pudendal nerve to be assessed. If there is gross anal anesthesia true incontinence is more common, as stool cannot be appreciated and in the presence of poor motor function anorectal preservation usually achieves little (Rogers et al 1988).
3. **Pudendal nerve latency.** Women who have had long traumatic vaginal deliveries have compromised pelvic floor and pudendal nerve function. If, in addition, they suffer from ulcerative colitis or anorectal Crohn's disease, sphincter preservation may prove of little worth. Thus, assessment of pudendal nerve latency provides an opportunity to predict outcome. Gross delay is associated with poor results (Laurberg & Swash 1989).
4. **Evacuation studies.** Impairment of rectal evacuation is also quite common after difficult and traumatic vaginal deliveries. Therefore, some assessment of rectal emptying may be beneficial. In the past we have used videoproctography, but this is associated with a high radiation dose and we no longer advise such a method for merely assessing rectal emptying (Womack et al 1985). The insertion of a semisolid contrast material into the rectal ampulla, followed by asking the patient to evacuate over a period of a minute, allows a reasonably reproducible assessment of rectal evacuation and is non-invasive. There are, however, a few occasions where videoproctography may be extremely helpful and entirely justified. If there are complex fistulae in the rectovaginal septum, or if there is incontinence from prolapse coexisting with inflammatory bowel disease, or if there has been obstetric trauma causing incontinence in association with inflammatory bowel disease, contrast radiology in the seated position during contraction and evacuation may prove useful. Under these circumstances we introduce a semisolid barium paste into the rectum; we also delineate the vagina with a viscous contrast material and we inject 'Omnipaque' into the peritoneal cavity so as to delineate the rectovaginal pouch. In this way, the anatomy and physiology of the anorectum can be usefully screened and played back on video.
5. **Rectal compliance.** Assessment of compliance can be very helpful in deciding whether it is worth preserving the rectal stump in patients with colitis. In our experience ileorectal anastomosis for Crohn's colitis has proved an extremely effective surgical procedure, provided the rectum is macroscopically normal and the rectal ampulla is compliant. Crude assessment of rectal compliance may be achieved by distending a balloon within the rectum and noting when a particular volume is no longer tolerated. For more formal and reproducible measurement, change in pressure with change in volume has to be assessed by incremental increases of volume with simultaneous intraballoon pressure measurements (Oresland et al 1990).
6. **Anal ultrasonography.** Anal ultrasonography can prove extremely useful in detecting undisclosed intersphincteric abscesses. It may delineate some anorectal and rectovaginal fistulae; it certainly provides evidence of an intact sphincter ring. Furthermore, functional evaluation of the sphincters and puborectalis during attempted contraction can also be visualized (Nielsen et al 1992).
7. **MRI.** Conventional MRI may prove the best method of assessing complex anorectal fistulae. However, the technique gives little information on function. In the future MRI coils within the rectal ampulla may provide more functional as well as anatomical information.
8. **Conventional electromyography.** Conventional electromyography has almost disappeared from the armamentarium of the anorectal physiologist. Needles are painful, they are poorly tolerated, they give less information than anal ultrasonography, and the most valuable information can now be obtained from conduction studies which cause far less patient discomfort.

CONCLUSIONS

The demonstration of severe unresolved inflammation or destroyed function is usually an indication either for proctocolectomy or for fecal diversion. There are, however, a few situations in which reconstructive surgery should be contemplated. The following rules are important:

1. Reconstruction should not be performed in the presence of active inflammation in the rectum or in the presence of coexisting anorectal sepsis.

2. Reconstructions always take longer to heal and there is a greater risk of sepsis in Crohn's disease than in the non-Crohn's population.

3. There should be a low threshhold for raising a proximal stoma to achieve fecal diversion for patients undergoing anorectal reconstructive procedures in Crohn's disease.

4. A measure of realism must be communicated to the patients, since the long-term results of many forms of reconstruction are poor.

REFERENCES

Alexander-Williams J, Buchmann P 1980 Perianal Crohn's disease. World Journal of Surgery 4: 203–208

Ambrose N S, Keighley M R B, Alexander-Williams J, Allan R N 1984 Clinical impact of colectomy and ileo-rectal anastomosis in the management of Crohn's disease. Gut 25: 223–227

Bauer J J, Sher M E, Jaffin H, Present D, Gelerent I 1991 Transvaginal approach for repair of rectovaginal fistulae complicating Crohn's disease. Annals of Surgery 213: 151–158

Braun J, Treutner K-H, Harder M, Lerch M M, Tons Chr, Schumpelick V 1992 Anal sphincter function after intersphincteric resection and stapled ileal pouch–anal anastomosis. Diseases of the Colon and Rectum 34: 8–16

Buchmann P, Mogg G A G, Alexander-Williams J, Allan R N, Keighley M R B 1980 Relationship of proctitis and rectal capacity in Crohn's disease. Gut 21: 137–140

Givel J C, Hawker P, Allan R N, Alexander-Williams J 1982 Enterovaginal fistulas associated with Crohn's disease. Surgery, Gynecology and Obstetrics 155: 494–496

Hobbis J H, Schofield P F 1982 Management of perianal Crohn's disease. Journal of the Royal Society of Medicine 75: 414–417

Keighley M R B, Grobler S P, Bain I M 1993 An audit of restorative proctocolectomy. Gut 34: 680–684

Keighley M R B, Williams N S 1993 Surgery of the anus, rectum and colon. WB Saunders, London

Laurberg S, Swash M 1989 Effects of aging on the anorectal sphincters and their innervation. Diseases of the Colon and Rectum 32: 737–742

Lefton H B, Farmer R G, Fazio V 1975 Ileorectal anastomosis for Crohn's disease of the colon. Gastroenterology 69: 612–617

Linares L, Moreira L F, Andrews H, Allan R N, Alexander-Williams J, Keighley M R B 1988 Natural history and treatment of anorectal strictures complicating Crohn's disease. British Journal of Surgery 75: 653–655

Nielsen M B, Hauge C, Rasmussen O O, Pedersen J F, Christiansen J 1992 Anal endosonographic findings in the follow-up of primarily sutured sphincteric ruptures. British Journal of Surgery 79: 104–106

Oresland T, Fasth S, Akervall S, Mordgren S, Hulten L 1990 Manovolumetric and sensory characteristics of the ileonal J pouch compared with healthy rectum. British Journal of Surgery 77: 803–806

Pritchard T J, Schoetz D J Jr, Roberts P L, Murray J J, Coller J A, Veidenheimer M C 1990 Perirectal abscess in Crohn's disease: drainage and outcome. Diseases of the Colon and Rectum 33: 933–937

Rogers J, Henry M M, Misiewicz J J 1988 Combined sensory and motor deficit in primary neuropathic faecal incontinence. Gut 29: 5–9

Scott A, Hawley P R, Phillips R K S 1989 Results of external sphincter repair in Crohn's disease. British Journal of Surgery 76: 959–960

Weaver R M, Keighley M R B 1986 Measurement of rectal capacity in the assessment of patients for colectomy and ileorectal anastomosis in Crohn's colitis. Diseases of the Colon and Rectum 29: 443–445

Weterman I T, Pena A S 1976 The long term prognosis of ileorectal anastomosis and proctocolectomy in Crohn's disease. Scandinavian Journal of Gastroenterology 11: 185–191

White R A, Eisenstat T E, Rubin R J, Salvati E P 1990 Seton management of complex anorectal fistulas in patients with Crohn's disease. Diseases of the Colon and Rectum 33: 587–589

Womack N R, Williams N S, Holmfield J H, Morrison J F B, Simpkins K D 1985 New method for dynamic assessment of anorectal function in constipation. British Journal of Surgery 72: 994–998

Yoshioka K, Hyland G, Keighley M R B 1988 Physiological changes after postanal repair and parameters predicting outcome. British Journal of Surgery 75: 1220–1224

82. The role of laparoscopy
M. J. Hershman   R. S. Kiff

INTRODUCTION

The first laparoscopic intestinal resection was reported in 1991 (Cooperman et al 1991, Jacobs et al 1991, Schlinkert 1991). As expertise in laparoscopic surgery has increased, it has become apparent that laparoscopic colonic mobilization and resection can be performed safely and adequately (Quattlebaum et al 1993, Scoggin et al 1993, Tate et al 1993, Beart 1994, Mathis & MacFadyen 1994, Musser et al 1994, Van Ye et al 1994, Fowler et al 1995, Scott & Spencer 1995). Currently all colorectal procedures which are performed at open surgery can and have been performed laparoscopically (Table 82.1). These rapid advances in laparoscopic techniques and equipment have been part patient, part professional and part industry driven.

Laparoscopic colorectal surgery is still in its infancy and remains a controversial subject. In cases of malignancy, concerns focus on the adequacy of 'oncological clearance' and the small number of port site recurrences that have occurred (Cuschieri 1995; Wexner & Cohen 1995). These concerns will only be answered with clinical studies, and such prospective studies are currently taking place.

There is little doubt that laparoscopic colorectal surgery for benign disease is appropriate, provided the well-established principles of conventional colorectal surgery, such as tension-free anastomoses, are adhered to. However, even for benign disease controversy remains as to when it is safe and appropriate. This chapter reviews the potential role of laparoscopic surgery in inflammatory bowel disease.

GENERAL PRINCIPLES

Laparoscopic surgery may be diagnostic, laparoscopic assisted or totally laparoscopic. Diagnostic laparoscopy may enable a differentiation to be made between Crohn's disease and ulcerative colitis, as transmural inflammation is usually easily visible. In addition, laparoscopic ultrasonography can diagnose lesions in the liver or other organs. In a laparoscopic-assisted procedure the bowel is mobilized laparoscopically and delivered through a 4–5 cm incision, then resected and anastomosed externally. The size of incision is determined by the size of the specimen. In a completely laparoscopic procedure the bowel is internally mobilized, resected and anastomosed. The resected specimen may be delivered via the rectum, the vagina, a large port, or through a stoma site. Mentges et al (1995) have reported the use of transanal endoscopic microsurgery in combination with laparoscopic surgery for specimen retrieval and anastomosis. Totally laparoscopic procedures are time-consuming and provide little advantage over laparoscopic-assisted procedures, and therefore the majority of resections performed are laparoscopic assisted.

The inflammatory process of inflammatory bowel disease makes dissection difficult, even for open surgery. As with all laparoscopic surgery, the success of the operation depends on a team approach and, in particular, the skill of the surgeon, the skill of the assistant and the quality of the equipment used. Surgical assistants present the bowel to the surgeon by providing an appropriate camera image and by using delicate instruments for traction and counter traction. There is no doubt that operating time will reduce with increased availability of skilled assistants in the next few years.

Table 82.1 Minimal-access colorectal procedures

Adhesiolysis
Ileostomy
Feeding jejunostomy
Right hemicolectomy
Transverse colectomy
Left hemicolectomy
Subtotal colectomy
Hartmann's operation
Reversal of Hartmann's operation
Colostomy
Rectopexy
Anterior resection
Abdominoperineal resection
Panproctocolectomy
Restorative proctocolectomy
Transanal endoscopic microsurgery

When performing laparoscopic surgery for inflammatory bowel disease, several important principles should be adhered to. The first is careful patient selection. Certainly, early in the surgeon's experience laparoscopic-assisted procedures should be reserved for the 'easiest' cases, such as thin patients. In patients with Crohn's disease the area to be resected should have been identified preoperatively, with complete upper and lower gastrointestinal imaging. Positioning the patient in the modified Lloyd Davis position permits maximal flexibility for repositioning the surgeon and assistants. In addition, it allows intraoperative access to the uterus and rectum to permit repositioning of these organs. It further allows intraoperative colonoscopy if required. Moving the patient to quite extreme positions allows gravity to aid exposure of the operative field.

In cases of Crohn's disease the entire small bowel should be inspected using atraumatic instruments and a two-handed technique. The use of a three-dimensional camera may aid depth perception. Good-quality instruments should be available, including an angled laparoscope. During dissection the direct grasping and handling of diseased bowel loops should be avoided, to prevent incidental enterotomies. In cases of ulcerative colitis the bowel may be very friable, and in this situation conversion to an open operation is preferable. The decision to convert to an open operation should be made rapidly to avoid a dangerous and time-consuming dissection. There is some evidence that patients with converted laparoscopic surgery do worse than those with standard open procedures (Slim et al 1995), perhaps because of the delay in converting. Conversion is good surgical judgement and should not be considered as a failure. In Crohn's disease the mesentery is often very thick and friable, and it is the authors' opinion that extracorporeal division of the mesentery is safer and more expeditious.

POTENTIAL BENEFITS AND INDICATIONS

The aims of laparoscopic surgery are a reduction in pain scores, early mobilization, a virtual eradication of wound sepsis, a rapid return of gastrointestinal function, early discharge and return to normal activity, and finally cosmesis (Table 82.2).

There is a large and increasing number of series of laparoscopic colonic procedures being reported, with minimal associated mortality and morbidity, and careful scrutiny of the published data suggests that overall, laparoscopic colorectal surgery is associated with a reduction in minor morbidity such as chest-related sepsis and wound infections (Quattlebaum et al 1993, Scoggin et al 1993, Tate et al 1993, Mathis & MacFadyen 1994, Musser et al 1994, Van Ye et al 1994, Beart 1994, Fowler et al 1995, Scott & Spencer 1995). In addition, pain scores are generally reduced, with a possible modest

Table 82.2 Advantages of minimal-access gastrointestinal surgery

Generic
Reduced postoperative pain
Reduced length of stay
More prompt return to work
Cosmesis
Biological
Lack of opening of abdominal cavity with decreased fluid replenishment
Accurate surgery
- Reduced blood loss
- Reduced tissue edema
- Reduced intestinal manipulation (preserving peristalsis)
Fewer wound complications
- Infections and hematomas
- Ventral hernias
Maintenance of immunological status

reduction in length of hospital stay. There is of course a clear cosmetic and psychological advantage for these patients.

One interesting effect of laparoscopic surgery is that it has had a major effect on the re-evaluation of open surgical practice, and earlier feeding, mobilization and discharge from hospital have all become much more common than previously. There is no doubt that previously the length of stay following colorectal surgery in the UK was far too long. Many traditional surgical habits are currently being called into question and subjected to critical review. It is likely to lead to an overall reduction in hospital stay, and perhaps a reduction in morbidity, thereby achieving advantages thought to be exclusively in the domain of laparoscopic surgery. Careful prospective comparative studies are required.

Finally, better pain relief with patient-controlled analgesia systems has improved patient care in the immediate postoperative period. Many patients are now told to return to work early, after both open and laparoscopic surgery. The ultimate determinant of medical discharge from hospital after major gastrointestinal surgery is the return of gut function. It may yet be proved that laparoscopic-assisted surgery leads to an earlier return of gut function, but any gain here is going to be at best marginal and difficult to assess. The ultimate advantages of laparoscopic surgery may well be an earlier return to full mobility and less postoperative pain.

POTENTIAL RISKS AND DISADVANTAGES

Most surgeons would agree that in inflammatory bowel disease minimal-access surgery is contraindicated in patients with intra-abdominal abscesses, multiple previous bowel operations, short bowel syndrome, acute intestinal obstruction, perforation and toxic colitis. Although it is possible that minor morbidity is reduced by laparoscopic surgery, this is unlikely to be the case for major morbidity. Performing the same operation using a small abdominal wound is unlikely to affect operative mortality or anastomotic leak rate; consequently, minimal-access surgical procedures must prove to be as safe as open operations if they are to become standard care.

There is current concern about complication rates. Surgeons need new technical skills, such as intracorporeal knot tying, and few at present have the skills for complex laparoscopic surgery. There may be difficulty in establishing pneumoperitoneum, and as the bowel cannot be palpated intracorporeally there is a risk that some disease could be missed. It is likely that a number of serious complications of minimal-access colorectal surgery may occur, and probably go unreported, rather like the early situation following the introduction of laparoscopic cholecystectomy. One series reports an increase in major complications, including bowel perforation and arterial laceration (Falk et al 1993). In addition, Slim et al (1995) emphasize that laparoscopic conversions do worse than open procedures.

A further area of concern is bleeding. Some proponents of laparoscopy claim a reduction in intraoperative bleeding when laparoscopy is employed (Senagore et al 1993). However, individual surgeons' estimate of blood loss has proved to be inaccurate during standard laparotomy (Ha & Weiler 1986). Peters & Bartels (1993) objectively compared patients undergoing laparoscopic-assisted colectomy with patients undergoing standard colectomy, and found that there was actually more blood loss in patients undergoing laparoscopy. Clearly, further studies are needed in this area.

Although the majority of reports in the laparoscopic literature show no evidence of an increase in postoperative thromboembolism, one series has reported a significant increase of thromboembolic complications (Monson et al 1995). It is difficult to avoid the concern that the combination of prolonged pneumoperitoneum with the possible reduction in venous blood flow, together with the almost unavoidable calf compression generated by the Lloyd Davis position, is significant. Therefore, in addition to the usual antithrombosis prophylaxis, routine use of Flowtron boots may be appropriate. It is the authors' own practice to deflate the abdomen approximately every 45 minutes in order to increase venous blood flow.

Another disadvantage relates to the cost of laparoscopic surgery. The length of hospital stay probably represents mainly different pressures on different surgeons and different communities. However, most series report a slight reduction in hospital stay in patients who have undergone laparoscopic surgery (Beart 1994), although not all (Wexner & Johansen 1992). However, it is not necessarily true that the reduced hospital stay results in reduced total hospital costs, because of increased operating time and expensive instrumentation (Falk et al 1993; Musser et al 1994). The longer operating time for minimal-access surgery will need to be justified in order to make minimal-access colorectal surgery economically viable. However, it is to be hoped that with increased experience and increasingly improved instrumentation, operating time will come down. Costs may further reduce with frequent use of basic video equipment and instruments.

SURGERY FOR CROHN'S DISEASE

Abdominal surgery for Crohn's disease is not curative and forms only part of a lifetime management of the patient. Most patients with ileocecal Crohn's disease will eventually come to surgery, and indeed delaying surgery can result in increased complications, for example fistulae. Therefore, most surgeons and gastroenterologists recommend early surgery, and for this reason and the fact that these resections are often relatively straightforward, they are ideally suited to minimal-access surgery. To date there has been only a small series of laparoscopic ileocecal resections for Crohn's disease, but all report good results (Milsom et al 1993, Kreissler-Haag et al 1994, Bauer et al 1995). The mean overall hospitalization was 5–7 days, and there was no morbidity and no conversion rate. However, one series of 31 cases of resections for colorectal surgery included 15 ileocecal resections and had a 16% conversion rate (Reissman et al 1995). It is not clear what the conversion rate for ileocecal resections was. When attempting either laparoscopic or open procedures for ileocecal Crohn's disease, unexpected findings such as fistulae, abscesses or strictures may be found. Therefore, particularly for minimal-access surgery, a full evaluation of the upper and lower gastrointestinal tract is essential. Laparoscopic procedures may be attempted according to the level and experience of the surgical team, but as with all laparoscopic surgery there must be low threshold for conversion to an open procedure. The entire small bowel can and should be inspected, so that the surgeon can decide whether there is other disease and whether resection or strictureplasty is appropriate. It is likely that strictureplasty may be repeated laparoscopically, if necessary (Stebbing et al 1995). In Crohn's disease the mesentery is thick and friable, and therefore in the authors' opinion extracorporeal resection is safer and more expeditious. Unlike open surgery, most laparoscopic anastomoses are performed side-to-side. Scott et al (1995) have shown that anastomotic configuration does not affect outcome. Occasionally Crohn's masses can be seen in the right iliac fossa, and as these are confined to a limited area they can usually be resected with ease (Fig. 82.1).

For recurrent and complex ileocecal disease, open surgery can be very exacting and difficult. In addition, other organs, such as the duodenum, bladder and ureter, can be adherent or have fistulae with or without abscesses. It is unlikely that these procedures will have a major place in minimal-access surgery.

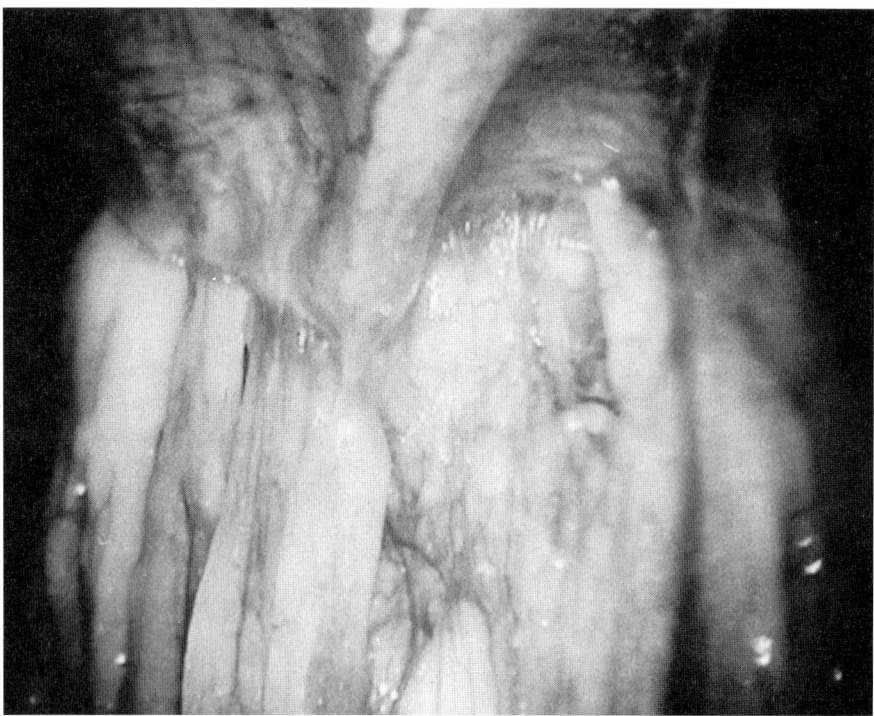

Fig. 82.1 Crohn's disease mass adherent to previous appendicectomy wound.

CURRENT STATE OF MINIMAL-ACCESS COLORECTAL SURGERY FOR INFLAMMATORY BOWEL DISEASE

To date approximately 500 colorectal resections have been published in the world literature (Quattlebaum et al 1993, Scoggin et al 1993, Tate et al 1993, Mathis & MacFadyen 1994, Musser et al 1994, Van Ye et al 1994, Beart 1994, Fowler et al 1995, Scott & Spencer 1995). A recent literature review of papers which included more than 10 cases (assumed to be the learning curve) reported 460 resections, approximately half of which were due to malignancy (Mathis & MacFadyen 1994). The overall mortality rate was 1%, which compares favorably with a 2–5% mortality reported by Goligher for open procedures (Goligher 1981). The rate of conversion to an open procedure was 15%, with an average operating time of 158 minutes (range 40–310). The reasons for conversion included uncertain anatomy, intra-abdominal abscess, bleeding, adhesions or extensive malignant disease. The overall morbidity was 17%, which compared favorably with a 21% morbidity for open procedures (Enker et al 1979). In addition, laparoscopic colectomy appears safe in elderly patients (Peters & Fleshman 1995). Figure 82.2 shows a laparoscopically assisted subtotal colectomy for ulcerative colitis.

There are very few data on resections for inflammatory bowel disease. Schmitt et al (1994) report a series of 16 laparoscopic-assisted ileal pouch–anal anastomoses for ulcerative colitis and compared them to 15 conventional operations for ulcerative colitis, and found that the length of time for ileus resolution and length of hospitalization was equal in the two groups. They concluded that laparoscopic ileal pouch–anal anastomosis conferred none of the advantages associated with other laparoscopic procedures. Similarly, there are reports of total laparoscopic proctocolectomy and laparoscopic-assisted proctocolectomy (Thibault & Poulin 1995) with small numbers of patients undergoing this procedure, and although the authors felt that the patients had a smoother and less painful postoperative course, no improved quantitative benefits were found. However, these techniques have a steep learning curve and so a definitive decision about these procedures should await further trials. One procedure that is very simple and straightforward to perform is laparoscopic colostomy and ileostomy, and there are reports of this procedure for perianal Crohn's disease (Romero et al 1992).

COMBINED ROLE OF ENDOSCOPIST AND SURGEON

Conversions to open procedures have been reported because of inability of the surgeon to visualize the area of disease. Similarly, there are instances in which the wrong area of the bowel has been removed (Hill et al 1993). Therefore, full preoperative assessment is essential in all cases. In some situations preoperative colonoscopic 'tattooing' can be achieved using indian ink, and the

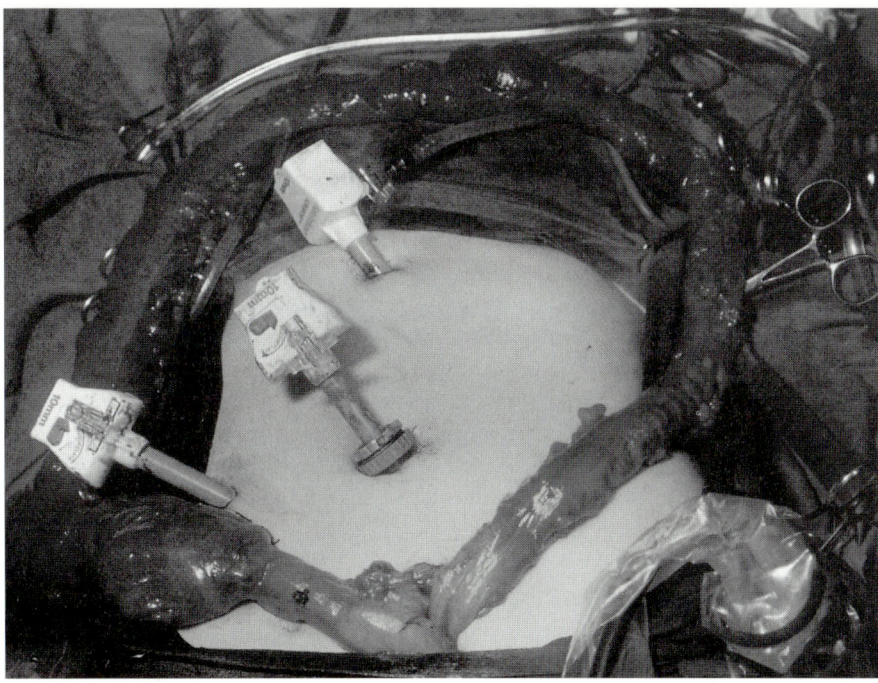

Fig. 82.2 Laparoscopic-assisted subtotal colectomy for ulcerative colitis.

endoscopist can mark the area of resection for the surgeon. In addition, there are instances during laparoscopic surgery when colonoscopy can intraoperatively aid the identification of lesions to be removed. Conversely, sometimes the endoscopist cannot pass a tortuous sigmoid colon, and laparoscopy has been used to help by manipulating the colon (Dwarakanath et al 1995).

Finally, endoscopic stricture dilatation is an extremely effective minimal-access endoscopic tool. Unfortunately, this always carries the risk of overstretching and hence perforation of the gut. It is likely that in the future, as an increasing number of these procedures are performed, many will be performed under laparoscopic guidance in order to help identify the appropriate limit of dilatation.

TRAINING AND ACCREDITATION

The learning curve for any new procedure is well known, and its ascent and length are variable (Monson et al 1992, Wexner & Reissman 1994, Van Ye et al 1994). Unfortunately, it is the patient that suffers. Adequate training and accreditation of surgeons in training, as well as of experienced general and colorectal surgeons, is essential to reduce complications. Unlike US surgeons, many British colorectal surgeons have a mixed practice and therefore have had the opportunity to develop laparoscopic skills before applying them to colorectal surgery. The same cannot be said of purely colorectal surgeons, who have not had an initial learning experience on simpler procedures. Animal courses provide a useful forum for learning colorectal surgery; unfortunately, these are not available in the UK and enthusiastic surgeons have had to travel abroad for such courses. Initial training could be performed on simulator boxes and then experienced colleagues could act as proctors. Training should be formalized, with privileging rights being granted. In the future this will be mandatory, with consequent restrictions of trade and implicit medicolegal aspects, as in the USA. In the UK, advances in simulator training are occurring, with sophisticated model systems even including pulsatile blood flow. Virtual reality training systems are also being developed.

THE FUTURE

Minimal-access surgery is here to stay, and its use for colorectal surgery, and in particular inflammatory bowel disease, is just beginning to evolve. However, at present it should not be considered as a standard care. It needs to be demonstrated through audit and randomized prospective clinical studies that minimal-access colorectal surgery gives at least equivalent – and hopefully better – care to the patient. This must be assessed with regard to both the disease process and patient mortality and morbidity. Certainly, length of hospital stay may not be the best indicator of morbidity. Long-term morbidity and time off work needs to be assessed. There must be constant evaluation at national level.

Advances will come with improvements in training, optical systems and instrumentation. The issue of training has been addressed and clearly must be formalized at both national and local level. The instrument technology industry is exploding with ideas, and developments such as articulating and steerable instruments are on the way. It is currently possible to perform laparoscopy in the absence of pneumoperitoneum, and this may eradicate tumor implantation (Paolucci et al 1995). Dissection techniques are improving, with advances such as pneumatic and ultrasonic dissection. Robotic technology exists, and already a robotic laparoscope manipulating arm is in clinical use. Instruments are even being developed to give the surgeon tactile sensation. The pace of change will be fast, and it must be met by the surgical community and not be industry driven. Inevitably these developments will lead to reduced operating times and, ultimately, cost reduction as cheaper, reusable instruments are developed.

In the field of optical systems the resolution of images is being improved with the use of three-chip cameras; in addition, there are available a number of systems using three-dimensional optics (Mitchell et al 1993). The author's own hospital has been using such a system for the last 18 months. Developments currently being worked on are face mask systems to enable the surgeon to perceive the internal organs while looking directly at the abdomen through a face mask. Audiovisual systems which enable live interactions between centers, at considerable distances, are valuable for teaching.

The further development of laparoscopic techniques and technology may result in obvious benefits to patients, but until then it behoves surgeons to concentrate on prospective randomized trials to assess objectively any possible advantages of laparoscopic colorectal surgery. Those of us who wish to perform minimal-access colorectal surgery must approach the future with enthusiasm, but also with caution and critical evaluation.

REFERENCES

Bauer J J, Harris M T, Grumbach N M, Gorfine S R 1995 Laparoscopic-assisted intestinal resection for Crohn's disease. Diseases of the Colon and Rectum 38: 712–715

Beart R W Jr 1994 Laparoscopic colectomy: status of the art. Diseases of the Colon and Rectum 37: S47–S49

Cooperman A M, Katz V, Zimmon D, Botero G 1991 Laparoscopic colon resection: a case report. Journal of Laparoendoscopic Surgery 1: 221–224

Cuschieri A 1995 Laparoscopic management of cancer patients. Journal of the Royal College of Surgeons of Edinburgh 40: 1–9

Dwarakanath A D, Chua E, Rhodes J M, Hershman M J 1995 Inspecting the colon from inside and out to solve pyrexia of unknown origin. Journal of the Royal Society of Medicine 88: 661–662

Enker W E, Laffa U T, Block G E 1979 Enhanced survival of patients with colon and rectal cancer is based upon wide anatomic resection. Annals of Surgery 190: 350–357

Falk P M, Beart R W Jr, Wexner S D et al 1993 Laparoscopic colectomy: a critical appraisal. Diseases of the Colon and Rectum 36: 28–34

Fowler D L, White S A, Anderson C A 1995 Laparoscopic colon resection: 60 Cases. Surgical Laparoscopy and Endoscopy 5: 468–471

Goligher J 1981 Results of operations for large bowel cancer. In: DeCosse J J (ed) Large Bowel Cancer. Churchill Livingstone, New York, pp 154–165

Ha H C, Weiler R L 1986 Estimation of blood loss in the operating room. Canadian Anaesthetics Society Journal 3: 685

Hill A D K, Banwell P B, Darzi A 1993 Laparoscopic colonic surgery: the unseen lesion. Minimally Invasive Therapy 2: 171–172

Jacobs M, Verdeja J C, Goldstein H S 1991 Minimally invasive colon resection (laparoscopic colectomy). Surgical Laparoscopy and Endoscopy 1: 144–150

Kreissler-Haag D, Hildebrandt U, Pistorius G, Schuder G, Lindermann W, Feifel G 1994 Laparoscopic surgery in Crohn's disease. Surgical Endoscopy 8: 1002 (Abstract)

Mathis C R, MacFadyen B Jr 1994 Laparoscopic colorectal resection: a review of the current experience. International Surgery 79: 221–225

Mentges B, Buess G, Schafer D, Becker H D 1995 Combined laparoscopic transanal rectosigmoid resection. Minimally Invasive Therapy 4: 75–80

Milsom J W, Lavery I C, Bohm B, Fazio V W 1993 Laparoscopically assisted ileal colectomy in Crohn's disease. Surgical Laparoscopy and Endoscopy 3: 77–80

Mitchell T N, Robertson J, Nagy A G, Lomax A 1993 Three-dimensional endoscopic imaging for minimal access surgery. Journal of the Royal College of Surgeons of Edinburgh 38: 285–292

Monson J R T, Darzi A, Carey P D, Guillou P J 1992 Prospective evaluation of laparoscopic-assisted colectomy in an unselected group of patients. Lancet 340: 831–833

Monson J R T, Hill A D K, Darzi A 1995 Laparoscopic colonic surgery. British Journal of Surgery 82: 150–157

Musser D J, Boorse R C, Madera F, Reed J F III 1994 Laparoscopic colectomy: at what cost? Surgical Laparoscopy and Endoscopy 4: 1–5

Paolucci V, Schaeff B, Gutt C M 1995 Gasless laparoscopy – why and how? Minimally Invasive Therapy 4: 165–172

Peters W R, Bartels T L 1993 Minimally invasive colectomy: are the potential benefits realized? Diseases of the Colon and Rectum 36: 751–756

Peters W R, Fleshman J W 1995 Minimally invasive colectomy in elderly patients. Surgical Laparoscopy and Endoscopy 5: 477–479

Quattlebaum J K Jr, Flanders H D, Usher C H III 1993 Laparoscopically assisted colectomy. Surgical Laparoscopy and Endoscopy 3: 81–87

Reissman P, Pfeifer J, Wexner S D 1995 Role of laparoscopic surgery in the management of Crohn's disease. Techniques in Coloproctology 3: 121–123

Romero C A, James K M, Cooperstone L M, Mishrick A S, Ger R 1992 Laparoscopic sigmoid colostomy for perianal Crohn's disease. Surgical Laparoscopy and Endoscopy 2: 148–151

Schlinkert R T 1991 Laparoscopic-assisted right hemicolectomy. Diseases of the Colon and Rectum 34: 1030–1031

Schmitt S L, Cohen S M, Wexner S D, Nogueras J J, Jagelman D G 1994 Does laparoscopic-assisted ileal pouch–anal anastomosis reduce the length of hospitalisation? International Journal of Colorectal Disease 9: 134–137

Scoggin S D, Frazee R C, Snyder S K et al 1993 Laparoscopic-assisted bowel surgery. Diseases of the Colon and Rectum 36: 747–749

Scott H J, Spencer J 1995 Colectomy: the role of laparoscopy. Surgical Laparoscopy and Endoscopy 5: 382–386

Scott N A, Sue-Long H M, Hughes L E 1995 Anastomotic configuration does not affect recurrence of Crohn's disease after ileocolonic resection. International Journal of Colorectal Disease 10: 67–69

Senagore A J, Luchtefeld M A, Mackeigan J M, Mazier W P 1993 Open colectomy versus laparoscopic colectomy: are there differences? American Surgery 59: 549–553

Slim K, Pezet D, Riff Y, Clark E, Chipponi J 1995 High morbidity rate after converted laparoscopic colorectal surgery. British Journal of Surgery 82: 1406–1408

Stebbing J F, Jewell D P, Kettlewell M G W, Mortensen N J McC 1995 Long-term results of recurrence and reoperation after strictureplasty for obstructive Crohn's disease. British Journal of Surgery 82: 1471–1474

Tate J J T, Kwok S, Dawson W, Lau W Y, Li A K C 1993 Prospective comparison of laparoscopic and conventional anterior resection. British Journal of Surgery 80: 1396–1398

Thibault C, Poulin E C 1995 Total laparoscopic proctocolectomy and laparoscopy-assisted proctocolectomy for inflammatory bowel disease:

operative technique and preliminary report. Surgical Laparoscopy and Endoscopy 5: 472–476

Van Ye T M, Cattey R P, Henry L G 1994 Laparoscopically assisted colon resections compare favorably with open technique. Surgical Laparoscopy and Endoscopy 4: 25–31

Wexner S D, Cohen S M 1995 Port site metastases after laparoscopic colorectal surgery for cure of malignancy. British Journal of Surgery 82: 295–298

Wexner S D, Johansen O B 1992 Laparoscopic bowel resection: advantages and limitations. Annals of Medicine 24: 105–110

Wexner S D, Reissman P 1994 Laparoscopic colorectal surgery. A provocative critique. International Surgery 79: 235–239

SECTION 10

Surgical treatment of ulcerative colitis

83. Emergency colectomy for fulminant colitis

J. J. Tjandra

The terms 'acute', 'severe', 'toxic' and 'fulminant' have been used to describe seriously ill patients with ulcerative or Crohn's colitis. In practice they are almost synonymous. Acute colitis is characterized by abrupt onset of bloody diarrhea, urgency, anorexia and abdominal colic. Patients often are ill, with severe anemia and dehydration.

FULMINANT COLITIS: DEFINITION

In general we consider a patient to be toxic when, in addition to severe colitis, there is evidence of at least two of the following:

1. Tachycardia > 100/min
2. Temperature > 38.6°C
3. Leukocytosis > $10.5 \times 10^9/l$
4. Hypoalbuminemia < 3.0 g/100 ml.

Other features commonly present include stool frequency greater than nine per day, abdominal distension, tenderness, mental changes, dehydration, anemia, electrolyte imbalance (hyponatremia, hypokalemia) and alkalosis (Buckell & Lennard-Jones 1979).

TOXIC DILATATION AND IMPENDING PERFORATION

Abdominal distension often indicates colonic dilatation, and abdominal tenderness suggests impending perforation. However, it is important to recognize that colonic perforation can occur without any colonic dilatation or abdominal distension. Toxic dilatation or megacolon is usually defined as a diameter exceeding 5.5 cm in the transverse colon. However, dilatation may also affect the cecum, descending and sigmoid colon. Toxic dilatation and perforation is more common in ulcerative colitis than in Crohn's disease (Edwards & Truelove 1963, Farmer et al 1975). Signs of septicemia are often delayed and masked by the use of steroids.

Development of toxic colonic dilatation is perhaps the most serious and life-threatening complication that can occur in patients with severe acute colitis. This is part of the spectrum of disease in severe attacks of colitis, rather than a separate entity. Although toxic megacolon is more common in patients with pancolitis, it does occur in left-sided disease. It is important that the definition of fulminant colitis is not too rigid. Patients may develop toxicity without megacolon or megacolon without severe toxic signs. Many patients may not comply with all the necessary criteria, but are no less ill and require the same aggressive management. When toxic megacolon occurs in a patient with previously undiagnosed colitis, less common causes such as infection, ischemia and pseudomembranous colitis need to be excluded.

NATURAL HISTORY

Acute fulminating colitis may occur as an acute exacerbation of inflammatory bowel disease, but in more than 60% of patients it develops as an initial manifestation (Campiesi et al 1987). In ulcerative colitis the acute attacks tend to occur after a longer duration of disease, and at an older age than with Crohn's colitis (Fazio & Verschueren 1992).

The outcome following an acute fulminating colitis depends upon the severity of the attack and the extent of the disease (Edwards & Truelove 1963). Historically, acute fulminating colitis has carried a high mortality. With the adoption of more aggressive resuscitation a coordinated plan of management and an early operative approach, the operative mortality has fallen to less than 3% (Albrechtsen et al 1981, Hawley 1988). Colonic dilatation correlates closely with the depth of ulceration (Buckell et al 1980) and carries a risk of perforation. Colonic dilatation complicated by perforation still carries a mortality of 33% (Greenstein & Aufses 1985, Heppell et al 1986).

Properly managed, about half of patients with acute fulminating colitis respond to medical treatment, thereby avoiding emergency surgery. However, the ultimate prospect of retaining the colon is low (Grant & Dozois 1984). The majority of patients develop repeated episodes of toxic dilatation or incapacitating chronic symptoms (Albrechtsen et al 1981).

MEDICAL MANAGEMENT

Initial diagnosis and investigations

Patients with clinical manifestations of severe colitis are admitted to hospital. Initial investigations include a complete blood count, a serum biochemical profile, blood cultures and coagulation studies. Plain abdominal and erect chest radiographs are obtained to check whether there is any colonic dilatation and/or free intraperitoneal gas from colonic perforation.

In patients in whom an infective etiology is suspected an urgent stool culture must be collected to exclude Salmonella, Campylobacter, Shigella, pathogenic *Escherichia coli*, ameba, *Clostridium difficile* and cytomegalovirus, especially in immunocompromised patients. This group of colitides will not be considered further in this chapter. A limited sigmoidoscopic (preferably flexible) examination with minimal insufflation of air is helpful in previously undiagnosed patients, to exclude pseudomembranous colitis and ischemic colitis. Unless the diagnosis of inflammatory bowel disease is in doubt, it is unwise to delay therapy awaiting the results of stool culture and, if taken, biopsies. Barium enema and colonoscopy are absolutely contraindicated in the presence of acute fulminating colitis.

Resuscitation

Intravenous fluids are initiated to correct dehydration, hyponatremia and hypokalemia. Blood transfusion is sometimes necessary for extreme anemia. A central venous catheter is often inserted for hyperalimentation. Nasogastric suction is not used routinely unless there is severe vomiting or colonic dilatation.

Antibiotics

These may reduce the consequences from infection associated with microperforations from the friable bowel. Antibiotics effective against aerobic and anerobic organisms are used. The ones we prefer are cefotaxime and metronidazole, given intravenously.

Steroids

Intravenous steroids have clearly been shown to be effective in treating acute fulminating colitis. Hydrocortisone 100 mg intravenously is given every 6 hours. A total of 400 mg per day is rarely exceeded. In patients in whom a satisfactory response is obtained the intravenous steroid dose is reduced after 5 days and changed to oral prednisolone. Immunosuppressive agents have little place in the treatment of toxic colitis, and particularly, if surgery may be indicated.

Other measures

Narcotics are used with caution because of their potential to exacerbate toxic megacolon and obscure the signs of peritonitis. Antidiarrheal agents may exacerbate toxic dilatation and are contraindicated.

MONITORING

Careful and regular clinical evaluation, together with monitoring of heart rate, temperature, stool frequency, abdominal girth, leukocyte count and albumin level, indicates clinical response to treatment (Lennard-Jones et al 1975). Serial plain abdominal radiographs daily or twice daily will detect progressive colonic dilatation (Greenstein et al 1986).

INDICATIONS FOR SURGERY

Evidence of free perforation, generalized peritonitis, septic shock and massive colonic hemorrhage indicates the need for emergency surgery.

Surgery is indicated with clear signs of deterioration, as for instance worsening signs of toxicity, increasing colonic dilatation and peritonitis at any time after initiation of adequate medical management, or if there has not been a clear improvement within 24–72 hours of admission. A rapid worsening of colonic dilatation is a sinister event and should be regarded as an absolute indication for surgery. A reduction in stool frequency resulting from progressive ileus often heralds the development of megacolon rather than an overall improvement. Development of toxic megacolon is usually, but not always, an indication for early surgery.

If after 5 days the patient has shown only minor improvement and still has signs of toxicity, such as tachycardia, fever, raised leukocyte count or frequent bloody diarrhea, the likelihood of sustaining a remission is slight. In most of these cases surgery is also indicated.

Some patients respond reasonably well to medical treatment but continue to have manifestations of low-grade smoldering disease. Conversion to oral medications and a normal diet frequently exacerbates the symptoms. Some of these patients ultimately require elective surgery.

SURGICAL MANAGEMENT

Preoperative preparation

The patient and family are counselled jointly by the gastroenterologist and colorectal surgeon. The need for a stoma is discussed. Unless there is clear evidence of Crohn's disease, with severe anorectal problems, a permanent stoma may not be necessary. The stoma site is marked preoperatively. Steroids are continued and intravenous antibiotics are given preoperatively and continued postoperatively for 1–5 days, depending on the operative findings. Mechanical bowel preparation is contraindicated.

Antiembolic stockings are used but subcutaneous heparin is generally avoided as postoperative bleeding can be troublesome in these malnourished patients. Total parenteral nutrition is often started preoperatively and continued postoperatively until resolution of abdominal ileus occurs.

Choice of operations

The optimal operation is subtotal colectomy with end ileostomy because of its simplicity. The diagnosis of ulcerative colitis and Crohn's disease is often not clear, even following histopathologic examination of the colectomy specimen (Price 1978). With the development of ileoanal reservoir surgery, this option becomes even more attractive.

The principal alternative is total proctocolectomy and a permanent ileostomy. Rarely, a loop ileostomy with a decompressive 'blowhole' colostomy may have a role in patients with toxic megacolon complicated by walled-off perforations. In the editor's experience decompression alone has never been necessary.

Subtotal colectomy and ileostomy

Principle

Subtotal colectomy and ileostomy with either oversewing of the rectal stump or mucus fistula is the most widely used and the safest procedure in these ill patients. It preserves the anorectum and has the major advantage of allowing a second-stage operation to be undertaken in a healthy patient who is no longer on steroid therapy. The risk of damaging the pelvic nerves is also eliminated during the emergency operation. Occasionally, persistent bleeding from the retained rectal stump may occur in some patients in whom the principal indication for surgery is massive colonic hemorrhage. In most cases the rectal bleeding can be controlled by topical steroids. If bleeding persists, an ultralow Hartmann's closure of the rectum at the level of the levator floor, preserving the anal sphincters, is preferable to a complete proctectomy, unless the tissue of the rectum is so friable that a safe stapled or sutured closure cannot be obtained. If a low rectal closure cannot be performed the anal stump may simply be left open, hemostasis being secured by leaving a 30 F Foley catheter with the balloon inflated in the pelvis through the anal stump. A delayed ileoanal reservoir will be a future consideration in ulcerative colitis if the patient wishes to avoid a permanent stoma. Other future options are rectal excision or a secondary ileorectal anastomosis if there is rectal sparing, as in Crohn's disease (Longo et al 1992). Definitive diagnosis of either ulcerative colitis or Crohn's disease can be difficult in the toxic colectomy specimen or the retained rectal stump. Histopathologic changes in the defunctionalized rectum may mimic Crohn's disease (Warren et al 1993).

If secondary restorative surgery is unlikely, either because the patient is elderly or if the rectum has severe Crohn's disease, the ultralow Hartmann's closure of the rectum at the level of the levator floor can be performed as the primary surgery, provided that operative factors for a pelvic dissection are favorable. Subsequent completion proctectomy and rectal mucosectomy may simply be performed as a perineal procedure (Dean & Celestin 1983).

Practice

The operation is performed with the patient in the Lloyd-Davies position to provide access to the rectum. A midline incision is used, so as not to compromise potential future stoma sites. Extreme care must be taken when handling the colon. At laparotomy any serosal attachment of the colon to the parietes, omentum or other viscera is noted. Careless mobilization of the colon in this situation constitutes a risk of colonic disruption and fecal spillage. Often, occult sealed perforations can exist on the posterior aspect of the colon, only becoming obvious when the colon is mobilized.

The colectomy is started by mobilizing the right colon, then the transverse colon. The sigmoid and descending colon is next mobilized, prior to taking down the splenic flexure. Several large mops are placed in the left paracolic gutter and over the small bowel to quarantine the splenic flexure region prior to its mobilization. This is a common site for iatrogenic perforation, particularly if the splenic flexure is high and there is massive colon dilatation. In this situation preliminary gentle decompression of the colon with a long rectal tube or through a colotomy in the transverse colon may be helpful. Careful quarantine of the surrounding structures is essential prior to decompressive colotomy, as the pursestring suture may not hold in the friable colon.

If the omentum is adherent to the colon, or if the peritoneum adjacent to the colon is adherent to the bowel, the omentum and a segment of the pericolic peritoneum are resected together with the colon to minimize iatrogenic perforation.

During mobilization of the bowel care is taken to preserve the main ileocolic and superior mesenteric vessels for future pouch construction, with the branches divided close to the cecum (Fazio et al 1993). The terminal ileum is mobilized only enough to allow the bowel to reach the anterior abdominal wall as an end ileostomy. None of the terminal ileum is removed, particularly if construction of a pouch in the future is contemplated. The individual sigmoid branches, rather than the main trunk or the inferior mesenteric vessels, are divided. This avoids bunching of the tissues and facilitates easy reach of the distal sigmoid colon to the anterior abdominal wall. It is important not to open the planes of dissection in the pelvis, with the attendant risk of sepsis and impotence.

Our preferred technique is to staple-transect the distal sigmoid colon using a linear stapler, at a level that will lie without tension in the subcutaneous plane at the lower end of the midline incision. The seromuscular layer of the bowel wall is then sutured circumferentially to the peritoneum, with further sutures to the surrounding abdominal wall fascia. The skin over the bowel end is left partly open. This technique of 'subcutaneous implantation' effectively quarantines the end of the distal sigmoid colon from the peritoneal cavity, so that if the rectosigmoid stump dehisces intraperitoneal abscess is avoided and drainage can easily occur through the skin wound. This procedure avoids a troublesome discharging mucous fistula and allows the rectum to be easily identified at a future laparotomy.

Less commonly, the sigmoid colon is so severely diseased that a formal mucous fistula at the lower end of the abdominal incision is preferred. Rarely, the bowel wall is so friable that it will not hold sutures. In this situation, the sigmoid stump is left protruding 2–3 inches beyond the skin level and wrapped snugly with a gauze roll to anchor it to the abdominal wall. In 7–10 days' time the sigmoid stump becomes sufficiently adherent to the abdominal wall to allow amputation at the skin level and maturation of the mucous fistula.

Emergency proctocolectomy

This was once advocated as the operation of choice for acute colitis (Binder et al 1975), but there is now little place for this procedure in the acute setting. There is increased morbidity and mortality as the surgery is more prolonged and demanding, especially in the presence of toxic megacolon (Hosking et al 1985). The pelvic dissection is more vascular, and the risk of pelvic sepsis, small-bowel obstruction and damage to the pelvic autonomic nerves is increased. It is also desirable to preserve the sphincter mechanism for possible later ileoanal reservoir surgery. Emergency proctocolectomy may occasionally have a role in patients with profuse colorectal bleeding, or in the less severely ill patient who is not a candidate for later sphincter-saving restorative procedures. Techniques of close rectal dissection to avoid damage to the autonomic nerves, and perineal excision in the plane between the internal and external anal sphincters, are discussed in Chapter 86.

Diverting loop ileostomy and decompressive 'blowhole' colostomy

This technique was described by Turnbull and colleagues from the Cleveland Clinic for long-standing toxic megacolon complicated by walled-off perforations (Fazio & Verschueren 1992). Definitive colectomy is carried out 4–6 months later. It was argued that colonic decompression might be safer than a colectomy, with the attendant risk of major fecal spillage when the walled-off perforation was disturbed. Nowadays, with more effective coordinated medical management and earlier surgical intervention, emergency colectomy can and should be performed safely in most patients.

Rarely, when multiple sealed-off perforations are found at laparotomy, or when the patient is critically ill, especially in the presence of comorbid factors such as massive distension of the colon, high splenic flexure and relative lack of experience of the surgeon, the lesser procedure with ileostomy–colostomy should be considered.

The abdomen is explored through a small lower midline incision and a loop ileostomy is constructed through a transrectus incision in the intended stoma site. The lower midline incision is then closed. The surface of the transverse colon is marked preoperatively using a supine radiograph of the abdomen with a radio-opaque marker in the umbilicus. A separate vertical left paramedian incision 4–6 cm long is then made over the dilated transverse colon. Quarantining sutures are placed between the parietal peritoneum of the abdominal wall and both the omentum and the seromuscular layer of the transverse colon. The colon is deflated by placing a 14-gauge needle through the taenia in the line of the planned colostomy. A vertical incision is made in the transverse colon, within the quarantined area. A skin-level colostomy is then constructed. If the patient is obese, or if there is excessive tension, the colonic edges are sutured to the subcutaneous fat only. Ileostomy and colostomy appliances are placed over the stomas.

Emergency colectomy with ileorectal anastomosis

In rare circumstances subtotal colectomy with an ileorectal anastomosis is performed, but only if the patient is not severely ill and if the rectal disease is minor, as in Crohn's disease.

Emergency restorative proctocolectomy and diverting ileostomy

This is associated with a higher operative morbidity and a higher incidence of anastomotic leakage, especially in patients on high-dose steroids (Heyvaert et al 1994). As a general rule such extensive surgery is unwise and should be avoided (Tjandra & Fazio 1993).

Follow-up

Emergency colectomy should be regarded as the first phase of a two-stage procedure. Later surgical options include restorative proctocolectomy, completion proctectomy and end ileostomy or continent ileostomy and ileorectal anastomosis. An accurate diagnosis (ulcerative colitis versus Crohn's disease) and careful counselling will decide on the most appropriate future surgical procedure. At the Cleveland Clinic (Oakley et al 1985) many patients had no further surgery because of lack of symptoms, poor general health, short rectal stump or refusal to have any further operation. Nine of these patients (3%) developed malignancy in the retained rectal stump, highlighting the importance of careful surveillance.

REFERENCES

Albrechtsen D, Bergan A, Mygaard K et al 1981 Urgent surgery for ulcerative colitis: early colectomy in 132 patients. World Journal of Surgery 5: 607–615

Binder S C, Miller H H, Deterling R A Jr 1975 Emergency and urgent operations for ulcerative colitis. Archives of Surgery 110: 284–289

Buckell N A, Lennard-Jones J E 1979 How district hospitals see ulcerative colitis. Lancet ii: 1226–1229

Buckell N A, Williams G T, Bartram C P et al 1980 Depth of ulceration in colitis. Correlation with outcome and clinical and radiological features. Gastroenterology 79: 19–25

Campiesi M, Gionchetti P, Belluzzi A et al 1987 Efficiency of 5-aminosalicylic acid enemas versus hydrocortisone enemas in ulcerative colitis. Digestive Diseases and Sciences 32 (Suppl): 67S–70S

Dean A M, Celestin R L 1983 Rectocolectomy with anal conservation in inflammatory colitis. Annals of the Royal College of Surgeons of England 65: 32–34

Edwards F C, Truelove S C 1963 The course and prognosis of ulcerative colitis. Gut 4: 299–308

Farmer A R G, Hawk W A, Turnbull R B 1975 Clinical patterns in Crohn's disease: a statistical study of 615 cases. Gastroenterology 68: 627–635

Fazio V W, Tjandra J J, Lavery I C 1993 Techniques of pouch construction. In: Nicholls J, Bartolo D, Mortensen N (eds) Restorative proctocolectomy. Blackwell, Oxford, pp 18–33

Fazio V W, Verschueren R C J 1992 Ileostomy–colostomy for toxic megacolon. In: Nyhus L M, Baker R J, Fischer J E (eds) Mastery of surgery. Little Brown, Boston, pp 1227–1234

Grant C S, Dozois R R 1984 Toxic megacolon: ultimate fate of patients after successful medical treatment. American Journal of Surgery 147: 106–110

Greenstein A J, Aufses A H 1985 Differences in pathogenesis, incidence and outcome of perforation in inflammatory bowel disease. Surgery, Gynecology and Obstetrics 160: 63–69

Greenstein A J, Bawrth J A, Sachar D B et al 1986 Free colonic perforation without dilatation in ulcerative colitis. American Journal of Surgery 152: 272–275

Hawley P R 1988 Emergency surgery for ulcerative colitis. World Journal of Surgery 12: 169–173

Heppell J, Farkouh C, Dube S et al 1986 Toxic megacolon: an analysis of 70 cases. Diseases of the Colon and Rectum 28: 789–792

Heyvaert G, Penninckx F, Filez L et al 1994 Restorative proctocolectomy in elective and emergency cases of ulcerative colitis. International Journal of Colorectal Disease 9: 73–76

Hosking S W, Kane S P, Cour-Palais I J 1985 Reducing the surgical mortality of acute colitis. A district hospital experience. Journal of the Royal College of Surgeons of Edinburgh 30: 255–257

Lennard-Jones J E, Ritchie J K, Hilder W et al 1975 Assessment of severity in colitis: a preliminary study. Gut 16: 579–584

Longo W E, Oakley J R, Lavery I C et al 1992 Outcome of ileorectal anastomosis for Crohn's colitis. Diseases of the Colon and Rectum 35: 1066–1071

Oakley J R, Lavery I C, Fazio V W et al 1985 The fate of the rectal stump after subtotal colectomy for ulcerative colitis. Diseases of the Colon and Rectum 28: 394–396

Price A B 1978 Overlap in the spectrum of non-specific inflammatory bowel disease: colitis indeterminate. Journal of Clinical Pathology 31: 567

Tjandra J J, Fazio V W 1993 Indication for and results of ileal pouch. Current Practice in Surgery 4: 22–28

Warren B F, Shepherd N A, Bartolo D C C et al 1993 Pathology of the defunctioned rectum in ulcerative colitis. Gut 34: 514–516

84. Ulcerative colitis – indications for elective colectomy

J. J. Murray

INTRODUCTION

Proctocolectomy remains the sole curative option for patients with ulcerative colitis. The surgical approach to the treatment of ulcerative colitis continues to evolve: the technique for restorative proctocolectomy with ileal pouch–anal anastomosis has overcome some of the functional and psychosocial disadvantages associated with a permanent ileostomy, and is currently the procedure of choice for the majority of patients with ulcerative colitis who require surgery. Additional surgical options include proctocolectomy with Brooke ileostomy, proctocolectomy with continent ileostomy, subtotal colectomy with ileostomy and Hartmann pouch, and subtotal colectomy with ileorectal anastomosis. These options provide a spectrum of treatment alternatives that differ in the extent to which the disease is eradicated and the degree to which normal physiology is altered.

The price for cure can be substantial. Although improvement in perioperative care has reduced operative mortality, 25–50% of patients experience one or more postoperative complications (Leijonmarck et al 1989, Marcello et al 1993). Moreover, problems with ileostomy dysfunction, small-bowel obstruction, incomplete healing of perineal wounds, or a variety of pelvic pouch complications may require additional surgery (Phillips et al 1989, Marcello et al 1993). Owing to the imperfect results achieved with surgery, pharmacologic palliation of the symptoms of the disease remains the mainstay of treatment for the majority of patients with total ulcerative colitis. However, population-based studies indicate that 25–45% of patients with ulcerative colitis ultimately require surgery (Leijonmarck et al 1989, 1990a, Sedgwick et al 1991). Most of these undergo operation within 5 years of diagnosis (Leijonmarck et al 1990a). The extent of disease at the time of diagnosis is the factor that correlates most closely with subsequent need for operation.

Population-based studies and reports from specialized referral centers confirm a 5-year cumulative colectomy rate of 35–40% for patients whose disease extends proximal to the splenic flexure at the time of diagnosis (Ritchie et al 1978, Sinclair et al 1983). The 25-year cumulative colectomy rate in this cohort of patients is reported to range as high as 65% (Leijonmarck et al 1990a). In 35–40% of patients who require operation, colectomy is performed on an urgent or emergency basis as a life-saving measure to treat active or fulminant colitis (Leijonmarck et al 1989). Elective colectomy is undertaken in the remainder of patients for therapeutic or prophylactic purposes.

The indications for elective colectomy have not changed substantially, despite the availability of less toxic aminosalicylate preparations, more effective immunosuppressive agents, or alternative surgical procedures that reduce the functional disadvantages associated with traditional proctocolectomy. Elective operation is recommended to alleviate the debilitating consequences of chronic illness, to avoid the distressing side effects that may accompany long-term medical treatment, and to prevent the development of colorectal carcinoma. Choosing the appropriate surgical option for a patient with ulcerative colitis requires close collaboration between patient and physician. The decision is influenced by the patient's age and general health, the severity of the disease, the indication for operation, and the quality of anal sphincter function.

INTRACTABLE DISEASE

Elective colectomy is undertaken most frequently to relieve symptoms of chronic disease that cannot be adequately controlled with medical therapy. Intractable ulcerative colitis may have a variety of manifestations (Table 84.1). It is important to distinguish intractable disease from intractable patients who are unable or unwilling to comply with

Table 84.1 Manifestations of intractable ulcerative colitis

Persistent active disease
Recurring acute colitis
Corticosteroid dependence
Chronic fecal urgency
Growth retardation

the treatment prescribed for their colitis. Included in the intractable disease category are individuals who suffer persistent symptoms of active colitis despite months of aggressive treatment with anti-inflammatory or immunosuppressive medications. The inability to achieve remission of symptoms in these patients results in an insidious, progressive deterioration in health and performance status. Patients whose symptomatic remission is punctuated by frequently recurring attacks of acute colitis, despite maintenance therapy with aminosalicylate preparations, also qualify for a designation of intractable disease. An additional category of refractory disease includes individuals who require continuous treatment with corticosteroids to keep the symptoms of colitis in remission. Typically, these patients experience a flare in the symptoms of colitis as the dose of corticosteroids is decreased or withdrawn. Treatment with topical steroid preparations and immunosuppressive agents such as 6-mercaptopurine may permit gradual withdrawal of systemic steroids in some of these patients, but prolonged treatment with corticosteroids to sustain clinical remission may be complicated by cataract formation, osteoporosis and osteonecrosis (Adler & Korelitz 1990, Blodgett et al 1956). Fecal urgency is a characteristic symptom of active colitis, but may occasionally become a disabling symptom in patients with chronic, mildly active disease. These patients have a foreshortened tubular colon on radiographic examination. Fecal urgency reflects the consequences of chronic mucosal inflammation and scarring. At this stage it is unlikely that fecal urgency will respond to treatment with anti-inflammatory agents, but antiperistaltic medications may provide some degree of symptomatic relief by reducing the frequency of bowel movements.

Unfortunately, these descriptions of symptoms of intractable disease do not define the frequency of acute attacks, the duration of steroid dependence, or the severity of chronic fecal urgency that warrants surgical intervention. Criteria for defining the limits of medical therapy in the long-term management of chronic ulcerative colitis have not been established. Active disease that fails to subside following 3 months of medical therapy, or corticosteroid dependence for more than 12 months, are reasonable criteria upon which to base a decision to proceed with elective colectomy. In many instances, however, the patient decides when the disease has reached an intractable stage. The physician must advise the patient of the potential therapeutic options, as well as the possible complications and functional consequences that accompany various alternatives. With this information the patient can determine when the limitations imposed by continued medical palliation are more burdensome than the consequences of elective colectomy.

GROWTH RETARDATION

Growth retardation and delayed sexual maturation are additional manifestations of intractable disease in children with inflammatory bowel disease. Growth failure is more commonly a complication of Crohn's disease, but has been reported to occur in 7–21% of children with ulcerative colitis (Berger et al 1975, Kirschner et al 1978, Telander et al 1981, Trudel et al 1987, Orkin et al 1990). Distinguishing growth retardation from genetically determined short stature or constitutionally delayed growth may be difficult, especially during the early stages of growth arrest. Linear growth curves and growth velocity curves constructed from serial height measurements can be compared to standards for normal children. Under normal circumstances growth progresses along a standard height percentile line, and rarely shifts from one major percentile curve to another. The growth curves of children with genetic short stature parallel those of normal children. Children with growth retardation will experience a decrease or cessation of growth velocity that is often accompanied by a shift to a lower height percentile curve. Although growth velocity curves provide the most sensitive method for identifying growth retardation, the diagnosis can also be confirmed by radiographs of the hands and wrists in children for whom there are insufficient data to construct growth curves. In growth-retarded children the skeletal age is at least 1 year behind chronological age (Kirschner et al 1978). If growth arrest persists through puberty the growth spurt that accompanies sexual maturation will be blunted. Subsequent closure of the epiphyseal growth plates will prevent a child from achieving the full potential for skeletal growth. Although a variety of factors may contribute to growth retardation, the problem appears to be caused primarily by malnutrition, specifically, inadequate caloric intake (Kirschner et al 1978, 1981, Kirschner & Sutton 1986). This is the most consistent nutritional abnormality identified in children with growth retardation (Adler & Korelitz 1990). Patients with ulcerative colitis have increased caloric requirements to compensate for energy losses engendered by the chronic inflammatory process. Nutritional therapy designed to correct this deficiency will accelerate linear growth, especially when combined with appropriate treatment for the colitis. Whether catch-up growth will restore patients to their premorbid linear growth potential depends on the time available before the epiphyseal growth plates close. Long-term treatment with corticosteroids is an additional factor that may adversely influence linear growth in children. Corticosteroids exert an inhibitory effect on DNA synthesis, which may impair epiphyseal growth (Blodgett et al 1956, Kusonoki et al 1992). Growth suppression can be detected within weeks of initiating treatment with prednisone at a dose of 5 mg/m^2/day (Berger et al 1975). Alternatively, some patients with arrested development may experience a growth spurt if corticosteroid treatment results in disease remission. Therefore, the net effect of steroid treatment on growth potential is unpredictable. A compensatory growth spurt will occur as the dose of corticosteroids is reduced, and there should be no adverse impact on a child's ultimate height as long as steroids are discontinued prior to the pubertal growth spurt.

The potential for correcting growth retardation is greatest when colectomy is performed prior to the onset of puberty. Berger and colleagues, from Mount Sinai Hospital in New York, reported dramatic growth spurts within 1 year of surgery in ten of 12 patients undergoing elective colectomy for ulcerative colitis. The accelerated growth rate shifted six of the ten patients to a higher height percentile curve (Berger et al 1975). Telander and colleagues (1981), from the Mayo Clinic, reported an increase in height percentile in 84% of patients undergoing colectomy for colitis. When growth retardation was the primary indication for operation, a significant growth spurt was identified in 18 of 22 patients. In many cases the improvement in height percentile was not evident for more than 2 years following surgery, however, and may have reflected the impact of the pubertal growth spurt rather than a direct consequence of elective colectomy.

Growth retardation is rarely the sole indication for operation in children with ulcerative colitis. More commonly, growth arrest is one of several manifestations of intractable disease that in the aggregate prompt the decision to proceed with elective colectomy. Children with chronic ulcerative colitis should be monitored closely for any sign of growth failure, and those who fail to demonstrate a rapid response to aggressive medical therapy with nutritional supplementation should be referred for elective colectomy. Similarly, patients whose growth retardation accompanies treatment with corticosteroids should undergo curative resection if the medication cannot be withdrawn.

Surgical intervention for growth retardation is most effective when delay is minimized, so that the interval between surgery and epiphyseal closure is maximized. When ulcerative colitis is complicated by growth retardation, prolonged medical therapy is unwarranted. Although long-term parenteral hyperalimentation may represent a reasonable option for palliative treatment of children with Crohn's disease who suffer growth retardation, the potential morbidity as well as the psychological, social and financial consequences of such therapy are difficult to justify for patients with ulcerative colitis who might otherwise be cured by proctocolectomy (Kirschner et al 1981).

EXTRAINTESTINAL MANIFESTATIONS

Although extraintestinal manifestations of ulcerative colitis may cause significant morbidity, they rarely serve as an indication for elective colectomy. Extraintestinal manifestations are best categorized by the extent to which their expression is influenced by the activity of the underlying colitis (Table 84.2). Unfortunately, the more serious and disabling extraintestinal manifestations of ulcerative colitis

Table 84.2 Extraintestinal manifestations of chronic ulcerative colitis

Colitis independent
Sclerosing cholangitis
Ankylosing spondylitis
Sacroiliitis
Pyoderma gangrenosum

Colitis dependent
Peripheral arthritis
Erythema nodosum
Thromboembolic complications
Uveitis, iritis, episcleritis

have a course and prognosis unrelated to the severity of the patient's disease. Proctocolectomy will not alter or alleviate the symptomatic expression of these associated disorders. The remaining extraintestinal manifestations have a natural history that correlates more directly with the activity of ulcerative colitis. The disability caused by extraintestinal manifestations is rarely sufficient to warrant elective colectomy. Primary sclerosing cholangitis is estimated to occur in 5–7.5% of patients with chronic ulcerative colitis, and a subclinical form of biliary tract disease may be responsible for the chronic hepatic abnormalities that afflict an additional 8–10% of patients (Olsson et al 1991, Jewell 1993). Primary sclerosing cholangitis is a slowly progressive disorder, leading ultimately to cirrhosis, portal hypertension and chronic liver failure. Proctocolectomy will not alter the course or prognosis of the disease.

Sacroiliitis and ankylosing spondylitis are destructive arthropathies involving the axial skeleton in approximately 5% of patients with ulcerative colitis. Although the clinical course is variable, the severity of these arthropathies appears to be unrelated to the activity of the colitis. The symptoms of sacroiliitis and ankylosing spondylitis are not improved with elective colectomy (Jewell 1993, Mayer & Janowitz 1988). An additional 10–15% of patients with active colitis experience a seronegative non-destructive large joint arthropathy that characteristically has an asymmetric distribution (Jewell 1993, Mayer & Janowitz 1988). The arthritis is frequently confined to the hips and lower extremities. The severity of the arthropathy correlates with the activity of the colitis and typically responds to medical treatment for inflammatory bowel disease. Given the non-destructive nature of the joint involvement, symptomatic relief of colitic arthritis is generally not an indication for elective colectomy.

Among the variety of dermatoses that may accompany ulcerative colitis, pyoderma gangrenosum is the most debilitating (Levitt et al 1991). The disorder is characterized by painful pustules that ulcerate and coalesce. This process may result in extensive soft tissue necrosis. Although the anterior tibial surface of the lower extremities is the most common site of involvement, pyoderma gangrenosum can also involve the trunk, where it has a predilection for developing at sites of traumatic injury. In many cases the severity of the skin disease parallels the activity of the underlying colitis, but the response to elective colectomy is often unpredictable (Levitt et al 1991). Indeed, pyoderma gangrenosum may develop along the midline abdominal scar or adjacent to the ileostomy many years following proctocolectomy.

Thromboembolic complications involving both arterial and venous systems have been reported to develop in 1–2% of patients with inflammatory bowel disease. These complications have been attributed to a hypercoagulable state (Johns 1991). Although the mechanism for spontaneous thrombosis has not been defined, active inflammatory bowel disease has been associated with thrombocytosis and elevated levels of several components of the coagulation cascade, including fibrinogen, clotting factor VIII and thromboplastin (Johns 1991, Talbot et al 1986). A deficiency of antithrombin III has also been identified as a contributing factor (Johns 1991, Talbot et al 1986). Deep vein thrombophlebitis and pulmonary emboli are the most common thrombotic complications afflicting patients with ulcerative colitis. Thrombosis of cerebral vessels, retinal arteries, peripheral arteries and portions of the portal–venous system have been recorded. The potential for hemorrhagic complications makes therapeutic anticoagulation particularly hazardous in patients with active or smoldering colitis. The risk of recurring pulmonary emboli can be minimized by placing a filter in the inferior vena cava. Elective colectomy is preferable to long-term anticoagulation for patients with active or intractable ulcerative colitis who experience recurring thromboembolic complications.

COMPLICATIONS OF MEDICAL THERAPY

The medical treatment of ulcerative colitis carries a risk of serious morbidity resulting from adverse reactions to medications. Occasionally these adverse reactions may necessitate withdrawal of therapy. Elective colectomy may be required if disease remission cannot be achieved with alternative medications. This situation arises most frequently in patients who are intolerant of corticosteroids (Table 84.3). Patients with active colitis who cannot be treated with steroids have a limited range of therapeutic options. The complications of corticosteroid therapy include a variety of side effects, such as skin lesions, edema and dysmenorrhea, which are distressing but do not require active intervention (Kusonoki et al 1992). Supportive care for the duration of corticosteroid therapy is usually sufficient. Potentially more serious side effects, such as hypertension, hyperglycemia, peptic ulcer disease, growth retardation, or mild agitation, may respond to a reduction in the dose of steroids as well as treatment with adjunctive medications (Kusonoki et al 1992, Talbot et al 1986). A small proportion of patients treated with corticosteroids may experience severe or disabling complications that require immediate withdrawal of the medication. There is no reliable correlation between the mean daily dose of corticosteroids or duration of treatment and the subsequent risk of developing osteoporosis, osteonecrosis, steroid myopathy or steroid psychosis (Kusonoki et al 1992, Skalka & Prchal 1980, Zizil et al 1985, Ellis 1985). When corticosteroids are withdrawn, recovery from these complications may be incomplete. Even if the underlying colitis can be controlled with alternative medications, elective colectomy should be considered to avoid the possibility that an acute flair in the symptoms of colitis will require further treatment with steroids.

Table 84.3 Complications of corticosteroid therapy

Complications requiring supportive care
Skin lesions
Edema
Dysmenorrhea
Hypertrichosis

Complications requiring dose adjustment or adjunctive therapy
Diabetes
Peptic ulcer disease
Hypertension
Growth retardation
Glaucoma
Osteoporosis
Agitation/psychosis

Complications requiring discontinuation
Osteonecrosis
Myopathy
Cataracts
Psychosis
Growth retardation

CANCER PROPHYLAXIS

Colorectal carcinoma is the most serious long-term complication of chronic ulcerative colitis. The risk of developing carcinoma is influenced by the extent and duration of disease (Katzka et al 1983, Lennard-Jones et al 1990, Gyde et al 1988, Ekbom et al 1990, Langholz et al 1992, Lashner et al 1989). Although patients with pancolitis are at greatest risk, patients with a long duration of disease confined to the left colon have also been reported to be at considerable risk for developing carcinoma (Nugent et al 1991, Greenstein et al 1979). Whether age at onset of colitis is an independent risk factor for carcinoma is controversial. A number of studies have identified onset of colitis in childhood as an additional risk factor (Gyde et al 1988, Ekbom et al 1990, Devroede et al 1971). The extent to which this correlation reflects simply a longer duration of disease is uncertain, however (Sufita et al 1991). When cancer incidence is standardized for duration of disease, the risk of malignancy may be greater in patients who develop symptoms of colitis at an older age (Lashner et al 1989).

Treatment of carcinoma or cancer prophylaxis is the indication for operation in 15–30% of patients who undergo elective colectomy (Leijonmarck et al 1989). Although there is agreement that patients with ulcerative colitis have a greater risk of developing colorectal carcinoma than the normal population, estimates of this risk have varied widely. Devroede and colleagues reported that patients having ulcerative colitis for more than 30 years had a 43% cumulative risk of developing carcinoma (Devroede et al 1971). More recent reports have estimated the risk of cancer complicating ulcerative colitis to range from 3 to 30% for a similar duration of disease (Table 84.4). Hospital-based studies from specialized referral centers have tended to exaggerate the risk of colon cancer (Greenstein et al 1979, Devroede et al 1971). Population-based studies suggest that the cumulative risk of developing colorectal carcinoma increases by no more than 0.5–1.0% per year after 10 years of disease for patients with extensive colitis (Lennard-Jones et al 1990, Ekbom et al 1990, Langholz et al 1992). Patients who are minimally symptomatic from colitis are usually unwilling to submit to prophylactic proctocolectomy for a risk of this magnitude. Based on the observations of Morson and Pang that multifocal mucosal dysplasia accompanies colitis-associated carcinoma in 70–90% of cases, routine colonoscopic surveillance for mucosal dysplasia in patients with colitis for more than 8 years has become a commonly employed strategy for identifying patients at risk of developing carcinoma (Morson & Pang 1967). Elective colectomy has been recommended if surveillance reveals high-grade dysplasia, dysplasia associated with a mass lesion, or persistent low-grade dysplasia on multiple examinations. Colonoscopic surveillance is costly, however, and its success in controlling the risk of carcinoma in ulcerative colitis has probably been exaggerated (Gyde 1990).

Although the practice is widely endorsed, its merits have never been confirmed in a randomized prospective trial. There are several factors that make colonoscopic surveillance for dysplasia an imperfect strategy for managing the risk of carcinoma in patients with ulcerative colitis. Criteria for defining and grading dysplasia have been standardized, but interobserver variation in the assessment of dysplasia by experienced pathologists ranges from 4 to 8% (Collins et al 1987). Dysplasia cannot be diagnosed reliably in the presence of active inflammation because the histologic features of dysplasia and regenerative atypia may be indistinguishable. Moreover, colorectal carcinoma need not be preceded by multifocal mucosal dysplasia. Analysis of surgical specimens from patients undergoing proctocolectomy for ulcerative colitis complicated by carcinoma has failed to identify dysplasia in 26% of cases (Ransohoff et al 1985, Taylor et al 1992). In addition, the technique of obtaining four-quadrant biopsies at 10 cm intervals during withdrawal of the colonoscope samples less than 1% of the surface area of the large intestine, and introduces the possibility of substantial sampling error (Collins et al 1987, Taylor et al 1992). The lead time between the development of high-grade dysplasia and subsequent progression to invasive cancer may be too short to reliably permit intervention before a life-threatening carcinoma has developed. An undiagnosed synchronous carcinoma of the colon is identified in 15–46% of patients who undergo elective colectomy for a finding of high-grade mucosal dysplasia (Nugent et al 1991, Collins et al 1987). Although there is evidence to support the notion that colonoscopic surveillance for dysplasia identifies carcinomas at an earlier pathologic stage, a significant proportion of carcinomas identified through surveillance ultimately prove fatal (Lennard-Jones et al 1990, Sugita et al 1991, Collins et al 1987, Choi et al 1993). The natural history of low-grade mucosal dysplasia is uncertain. Repeat examination in 6–12 months has been recommended as an alternative to elective proctocolectomy in patients found to have low-grade dysplasia. Repeat biopsies often reveal no evidence of dysplasia. Although regression of low-grade mucosal dysplasia is a potential explanation for the absence of dysplasia on follow-up biopsies, sampling error is an equally plausible explanation. Reports from St Mark's Hospital in London and Lenox Hill Hospital in New York reveal that 15–18% of patients found to have low-grade dysplasia on initial screening will develop colorectal carcinoma within 2–10 years regardless of the results of subsequent surveillance examinations (Lennard-Jones et al 1990, Woolrick et al 1993). If mucosal dysplasia is a premalignant lesion, then any degree of dysplastic change should be considered an indication for elective

Table 84.4 Cumulative risk of carcinoma in ulcerative colitis

Reference (no. of patients)	Disease duration (years)				
	20	25	30	35	40
Katzka et al 1983 (258)		6.6%	11.4%		
Lennard-Jones et al 1990 (401)	5%	9%			
Gyde et al 1988 (823)	7.2%		16.5%		
Ekbom et al 1990 (3117)				30%	
Langholz et al 1992 (1161)		3.1%			
Lashner et al 1989 (99)		4%*		13%*	20%*

* High-grade dysplasia or carcinoma

colectomy. Low-grade dysplasia is the most appropriate criterion for a positive screening examination because of the significant risk of synchronous carcinomas in patients with high-grade mucosal dysplasia.

Screening for carcinoma or dysplasia is more complicated when ulcerative colitis is accompanied by stricture or extensive pseudopolyp formation. Colonic strictures are found in 3–11% of patients with ulcerative colitis (Gunaste et al 1992). A minority of these strictures are caused by an underlying carcinoma. (Gunaste et al 1992, Lashner et al 1990). Distinguishing benign from malignant strictures can be difficult. Endoscopic biopsy of malignant strictures is frequently unreliable because the carcinoma is often an infiltrating intramural lesion covered by intact mucosa. The false negative rate for endoscopic biopsy of malignant strictures has been reported to range from 40 to 65% (Gunaste et al 1992, Lashner et al 1990, Reiser et al 1993). Clinical features associated with an increased risk of carcinoma in patients with a stricture of the colon include duration of disease greater than 20 years, location of the stricture proximal to the splenic flexure, and the presence of symptoms of colonic obstruction (Gunaste et al 1992). Remembering that the goal of treatment is to save lives, not colons, elective colectomy should be carefully considered when any patient develops a stricture of the colon while under observation for ulcerative colitis, regardless of the results of endoscopic biopsy. Extensive pseudopolyp formation in patients with longstanding disease precludes adequate inspection of the mucosal surface and increases the risk of sampling error with endoscopic biopsies. Despite its limitations, colonoscopic surveillance for dysplasia is currently the only alternative to prophylactic colectomy for controlling the risk of cancer in patients with ulcerative colitis. Elective colectomy is advisable for those individuals who cannot be adequately screened because of extensive pseudopolyp formation, colonic stricture or patient refusal.

A search for more objective and more sensitive markers for the risk of cancer in patients with ulcerative colitis has met with limited success to date. Investigators have studied the relationship between mucosal dysplasia or carcinoma and the presence of mucin-associated antigens, alterations in mucosal DNA content, alleic deletion of the *p53* tumor suppressor gene, and a variety of oncogenic byproducts. As yet, these efforts have not influenced the indications for elective colectomy in patients with ulcerative colitis (Melville et al 1988, Lofberg et al 1992, Rubin et al 1992, Burmer et al 1992, Yin et al 1993, Dean & Vernava 1992).

FATE OF THE RETAINED RECTUM

Patients undergo colectomy with ileostomy and mucous fistula or Hartmann closure of the rectum as the initial operative procedure for fulminating colitis, or if their disease has features suggestive of Crohn's colitis. This approach restores patients to good health, minimizes postoperative morbidity, and preserves the option for ileal pouch–anal anastomosis if a diagnosis of ulcerative colitis or indeterminant colitis is confirmed. Although the majority of patients proceed with pouch–anal anastomosis when their postoperative recovery is complete, some choose to delay operation indefinitely. Typically, these patients are unwilling to jeopardize their new-found good health for the sole benefit of avoiding the often minor inconvenience that accompanies life with an ileostomy. Younger individuals who have not completed their family may wish to postpone proctectomy to avoid potential problems with infertility or sexual dysfunction. The symptoms of residual proctitis are generally inconsequential, and patients typically respond to treatment with topical steroids or topical aminosalicylates if therapy is required.

Individuals with an ileorectal anastomosis represent an additional category of patients with a retained rectum following surgery for ulcerative colitis. Colectomy with ileorectal anastomosis has never been a widely performed operation for the treatment of ulcerative colitis, because of concerns regarding the quality of the functional result and the potential risk of developing carcinoma of the rectum. The risk of malignancy requires that all patients with an ileorectal anastomosis or a defunctionalized rectum be monitored closely. Based on results of long-term follow-up in patients with an ileorectal anastomosis it is estimated that 3–6% of individuals with ulcerative colitis will develop carcinoma if the rectum is preserved (Table 84.5). Surveillance examination with random biopsy to screen for dysplasia should be performed at 6–12-month intervals if the duration of colitis exceeds 8–10 years. Elective proctectomy is indicated if dysplasia or a mass lesion is identified. Occasionally, chronically inflamed mucosa in a defunctionalized rectum will fuse or a focal stricture of the rectum will develop, thereby precluding endoscopic surveillance. These developments require prophylactic proctectomy to minimize the risk of developing an undetectable carcinoma of the rectum.

FUTURE DIRECTIONS

New approaches to the treatment of patients with chronic ulcerative colitis include a search for more effective immunosuppressive agents as well as an investigation of alternative methods for modulating the immune response in patients with refractory disease. Owing to its more rapid onset of action, cyclosporin has been shown to be potentially useful in the management of patients with active severe colitis. Clinical remission can be achieved in more than 80% of patients receiving intravenous infusions of cyclosporin to treat disease that is unresponsive to parenteral corticosteroids (Sandborn & Tremaine 1992, Linn & Peppercorn 1992). Although a significant proportion of patients develop side effects related to cyclo-

Table 84.5 Risk of cancer in the retained rectum

Reference	No. of patients	Mean follow-up	Cancer (%)
Baker et al 1978	374	20	6*
Farrell et al 1980	63	8.4	0
Oakley et al 1985	288	8.2	3.1
Johnson et al 1986	183	27	14*
Mann et al 1988	85		3.5
Khubchandani et al 1989	26	8.4	0
Leijonmarck et al 1990	51	13	0†

* Cumulative probability of developing rectal carcinoma at duration of follow-up indicated
† 6% of patients required proctectomy for dysplasia

sporin infusion, serious irreversible toxicity is uncommon. Cyclosporin, may therefore reduce the need for urgent operation in patients with active or fulminant colitis. Whether long-term treatment with cyclosporin is safe or effective in maintaining remission remains to be proven. Preliminary reports suggest that sustained remission is maintained in fewer than 50% of patients following cessation of treatment with cyclosporin (Sandborn & Tremaine 1992). At present, the availability of cyclosporin and the potential availability of more effective, less toxic immunosuppressive agents have not altered the indications for elective colectomy in patients with intractable disease.

Until a cure for the disease is found, surgery will continue to play a central role in the treatment of patients with ulcerative colitis. Initial speculation that restorative proctocolectomy with ileal pouch–anal anastomosis would substantially alter the treatment protocol for ulcerative colitis has proved to be unfounded. Although the operation provides an option for cure that avoids the functional disadvantages associated with standard proctocolectomy, refinements in the procedure have failed to diminish the significant operative morbidity or to eliminate the long-term problems with diarrhea, soiling and pouchitis that may complicate the operation. The option of ileal pouch–anal anastomosis may make patients more willing to consider surgery, but it has not changed the indications for operation. Elective colectomy should be recommended to alleviate the symptoms of chronic intractable disease, to avoid the potentially harmful side effects that accompany long-term medical palliation of the disease, and to minimize the risk of developing fatal carcinoma of the colon or rectum.

REFERENCES

Adler D J, Korelitz B I 1990 The therapeutic efficacy of 6-mercaptopurine in refractory ulcerative colitis. American Journal of Gastroenterology 85: 712–722

Baker W N, Glass R E, Ritchie J K, Aylett S O 1978 Cancer of the rectum following colectomy and ileorectal anastomosis for ulcerative colitis. British Journal of Surgery 65: 862–868

Berger M, Gribetz D, Korelitz B I 1975 Growth retardation in children with ulcerative colitis: the effect of medical and surgical therapy. Pediatrics 55: 459–467

Blodgett F M, Burgin L, Iezzoni D, Gribetz D, Talbot N B 1956 Effects of prolonged cortisone therapy on the statural growth, skeletal maturation, and metabolic status of children. New England Journal of Medicine 254: 636–641

Burmer G C, Rabinovitz P S, Haggitt R C et al 1992 Neoplastic progression in ulcerative colitis: histology, DNA content, and loss of p53 allele. Gastroenterology 103: 1602–1610

Choi P M, Nugen F W, Schoetz D J, Silverman M S, Haggitt R C 1993 Colonoscopic surveillance reduces mortality from colorectal cancer in ulcerative colitis. Gastroenterology 105: 418–424

Collins R H, Feldman M, Fordtran J S 1987 Colon cancer, dysplasia and surveillance in patients with ulcerative colitis. New England Journal of Medicine 316: 1654–1658

Dean P A, Vernava A M 1992 Flow cytometric analyses of DNA content in colorectal carcinoma. Diseases of the Colon and Rectum 35: 95–102

Devroede G J, Taylor W E, Sauer W G, Jackman R J, Stickler G B 1971 Cancer risk and life expectancy of children with ulcerative colitis. New England Journal of Medicine 285: 17–21

Ekbom A, Helmick C, Zuck M, Adari H Q 1990 Ulcerative colitis and colorectal cancer. New England Journal of Medicine 323: 1228–1233

Ellis E F 1985 Steroid myopathy. Journal of Allergy and Clinical Immunology 37: 431–432

Farrell M B, VanHeerden J A, Beart R A, Weiland L H 1980 Rectal preservation in non-specific inflammatory disease of the colon. Annals of Surgery 192: 249–253

Greenstein A J, Sachar D B, Smith H et al 1979 Cancer in universal and left-sided ulcerative colitis: factors determining risk. Gastroenterology 77: 290–294

Gunaste V, Sachar D B, Greenstein A J 1992 Benign and malignant colorectal strictures in ulcerative colitis. Gut 33: 938–941

Gyde S 1990 Screening for colorectal cancer in ulcerative colitis: dubious benefits and high costs. Gut 31: 1089–1092

Gyde S N, Prior P, Allan R N et al 1988 Colorectal cancer in ulcerative colitis: a cohort study of primary referrals from three centers. Gut 29: 206–217

Jewell D P 1993 Ulcerative colitis. In: Sleisenger M H, Fordtran J S (eds) Gastrointestinal disease. WB Saunders, Philadelphia, p 1318–1320

Johns D R 1991 Cerebrovascular complications of inflammatory bowel disease. American Journal of Gastroenterology 86: 367–370

Johnson W R, Hughes E S R, McDermott F T, Katrivessis H 1986 The outcome of patients with ulcerative colitis managed by subtotal colectomy. Surgery, Gynecology and Obstetrics 162: 421–425

Katzka I, Brody R S, Morris E, Katz S 1983 Assessment of colorectal cancer risk in patients with ulcerative colitis: experience from a private practice. Gastroenterology 85: 22–29

Khubchandani I T, Sandfort M R, Rosen L, Sheets J A, Stasik J J, Riether R D 1989 Current status of ileoanal anastomosis for inflammatory bowel disease. Diseases of the Colon and Rectum 32: 400–403

Kirschner B S, Voinchet O, Rosenberg I H 1978 Growth retardation in inflammatory bowel disease. Gastroenterology 75: 504–511

Kirschner B S, Klick J R, Kalman S S, DeFavaro M V, Rosenberg I H 1981 Reversal of growth retardation in Crohn's disease with therapy emphasizing oral nutritional restitution. Gastroenterology 80: 10–15

Kirschner B S, Sutton M M 1986 Somatomedin-C levels in growth-impaired children and adolescents with chronic inflammatory bowel disease. Gastroenterology 91: 830–836

Kusonoki M, Moeslein G, Shoji Y et al 1992 Steroid complications in patients with ulcerative colitis. Diseases of the Colon and Rectum 35: 1003–1009

Langholz E, Munkholm P, Davidsen M, Binder V 1992 Colorectal cancer risk and mortality in patients with ulcerative colitis. Gastroenterology 103: 1444–1451

Lashner B A, Silverstein M D, Hanauer S B 1989 Hazard rates for dysplasia and cancer in ulcerative colitis. Digestive Diseases and Sciences 34: 1536–1541

Lashner B A, Turner B C, Bostwick D G, Frank P H, Hanauer S B 1990 Dysplasia and cancer complicating strictures in ulcerative colitis. Digestive Diseases and Sciences 35: 349–352

Leijonmarck C E, Brostrom O, Monson U, Hellers G 1984 Surgical treatment of ulcerative colitis in Stockholm County, 1955 to 1984. Diseases of the Colon and Rectum 32: 918–926

Leijonmarck C E, Persson P G, Hawley P R 1990a Factors affecting colectomy rate in ulcerative colitis: an epidemiologic study. Gut 31: 329–333

Leijonmarck C E, Lofberg R, Ost A, Heilers G 1990b Long-term results of ileorectal anastomosis in ulcerative colitis in Stockholm County. Diseases of the Colon and Rectum 33: 195–200

Lennard-Jones J E, Melville D M, Morson B C, Ritchie J K, Williams C B 1990 Pre-cancer and cancer in extensive ulcerative colitis: findings average 401 patients over 22 years. Gut 31: 800–806

Levitt M D, Ritchie J K, Lennard-Jones J E, Phillips R K S 1991 Pyoderma gangrenosum in inflammatory bowel disease. British Journal of Surgery 78: 676–678

Linn F V, Peppercorn M A 1992 Drug therapy for inflammatory bowel disease: Part II. American Journal of Surgery 164: 178–185

Lofberg R, Brostrom O, Karlen P, Ost A, Tribukait B 1992 DNA aneuploidy in ulcerative colitis: reproducibility, topographic distribution and relation to dysplasia. Gastroenterology 102: 1149–1154

Mann C V 1988 Total colectomy and ileorectal anastomosis for ulcerative colitis. World Journal of Surgery 12: 155–159

Marcello P W, Roberts P L, Schoetz D J, Coller J A, Murray J J, Veidenheimer M C 1993 Long-term results of the ileoanal pouch procedure. Archives of Surgery 128: 500–504

Mayer L, Janowitz H 1988 Extraintestinal manifestations of inflammatory bowel disease. In: Kirsner J B, Shorter R G (eds) Inflammatory bowel disease. Lea & Febiger, Philadelphia, p 299–318

Melville D M, Jass J R, Shepherd N A et al 1988 Dysplasia and deoxyribonucleic acid aneuploidy in the assessment of precancerous changes in chronic ulcerative colitis. Gastroenterology 95: 668–675

Messer J, Reitman D, Sacks H S, Smith H, Chalmers T C 1983 Association of adenocorticosteroid therapy and peptic-ulcer disease. New England Journal of Medicine 309: 21–24

Morson B C, Pang L S 1967 Rectal biopsy as an aid to cancer control in ulcerative colitis. Gut 8: 423–434

Nugent F W, Haggitt R C, Gilpin P A 1991 Cancer surveillance in ulcerative colitis. Gastroenterology 100: 1241–1248

Oakley J R, Lavery I C, Fazio V W, Jagelman D G, Weakley F L, Easley K 1985 The fate of the rectal stump after total colectomy for ulcerative colitis. Diseases of the Colon and Rectum 28: 394–396

Olsson R, Danielsson A, Jarnerot G et al 1991 Prevalence of primary sclerosing cholangitis in patients with ulcerative colitis. Gastroenterology 100: 1319–1323

Orkin B A, Telander R L, Wolff B G, Perrault J, Ilstrup D M 1990 The surgical management of children with ulcerative colitis. Diseases of the Colon and Rectum 33: 947–955

Phillips R K, Ritchie J K, Hawley P R 1989 Proctocolectomy and ileostomy for ulcerative colitis: the longer term story. Journal of the Royal Society of Medicine 82: 386–387

Ransohoff D F, Riddell R H, Levin B 1985 Ulcerative colitis and colonic cancer. Diseases of the Colon and Rectum 28: 383–388

Reiser J R, Waye J D, Janowitz H D, Harpaz N 1993 Adenocarcinoma in strictures of ulcerative colitis without antecedent dysplasia by colonoscopy. American Journal of Gastroenterology 89: 119–122

Ritchie J K, Powell-Tuck J, Lennard-Jones J E 1978 Clinical outcome of the first few years of ulcerative colitis and proctitis. Lancet 1: 1140–1143

Rubin C E, Haggitt R C, Burmer G C et al 1992 DNA aneuploidy in colonic biopsies predicts future development of dysplasia in ulcerative colitis. Gastroenterology 103: 1611–1620

Sandborn W J, Tremaine W J 1992 Cyclosporine treatment of inflammatory bowel disease. Mayo Clinic Proceedings 67: 981–990

Sedgewick D M, Barton J R, Hamer-Hodges D W, Nixon S J, Ferguson A 1991 Population-based study of surgery in juvenile onset ulcerative colitis. British Journal of Surgery 78: 176–178

Sinclair T S, Brunt P W, Mowat N G 1983 Nonspecific proctocolitis in northeastern Scotland; a community study. Gastroenterology 85: 1–11

Skalka H W, Prchal J T 1980 Effect of corticosteroids on cataract formation. Archives of Ophthalmic Medicine 98: 1773–1777

Sugita A, Sachar D B, Bodian C, Ribeiro M B, Aufses A H, Greenstein A J 1991 Colorectal cancer in ulcerative colitis: influence of anatomical extent and age at onset on colitis–cancer interval. Gut 32: 167–169

Talbot R W, Heppell J, Dozois R R, Beart R W 1986 Vascular complications of inflammatory bowel disease. Mayo Clinic Proceedings 61: 140–145

Taylor B A, Pemberton J H, Carpenter H A et al 1992 Dysplasia in chronic ulcerative colitis: implications for colonoscopic surveillance. Diseases of the Colon and Rectum 35: 950–956

Telander R L, Smith S L, Marciaek H M, O'Fallon W M, van Heerden J A, Perrault J 1981 Surgical treatment of ulcerative colitis in children. Surgery 90: 787–794

Trudel J L, Lavery I C, Fazio V W, Jagelman D G, Weakley F L, Oakley J R 1987 Surgery for ulcerative colitis in the pediatric population. Diseases of the Colon and Rectum 30: 747–750

Woolrick A J, DaSilva M D, Korelitz B I 1993 Surveillance in the routine management of ulcerative colitis: the predictive value of low-grade dysplasia. Gastroenterology 103: 431–438

Yin J, Harpaz N, Tong Y et al 1993 p53 point mutations in dysplastic and cancerous ulcerative colitis lesions. Gastroenterology 104: 1633–1639

Zizil T M, Marcoux C, Hungerford D S, Dansereau J V, Stevens M B 1985 Corticosteroid therapy associated with ischemic necrosis of bone in systemic lupus erythematosus. American Journal of Medicine 79: 596–604

85. Surgical treatment of ulcerative colitis – subtotal colectomy and ileorectal anastomosis

P. R. Hawley

INTRODUCTION

Colectomy and ileorectal anastomosis is the simplest sphincter-saving operation in ulcerative colitis and, until the ileoanal pouch became increasingly popular in the 1980s, was the only procedure which would allow a patient to avoid a permanent Brooke or continent Kock reservoir ileostomy. Although Devine (1943) and Corbett (1952) reported the procedure, Aylett, after performing the operation in 1952, became the leading proponent and carried out this procedure in 384 patients (Baker et al 1978). The first colectomy and ileorectal anastomosis was carried out at St Mark's Hospital in 1953, but after initial enthusiasm the number performed in the 1960s decreased. However, in the early 1970s a decision was made to promote this procedure in suitable patients. The question in the mid-1990s is, does this procedure still have a place in the surgical treatment of ulcerative colitis or has it been superseded by the ileoanal pouch (restorative proctocolectomy)?

MAIN INDICATIONS FOR ILEORECTAL ANASTOMOSIS

The main indication for ileorectal anastomosis is the wish of the patient to avoid a permanent stoma and to avoid an ileoanal pouch procedure, either temporarily or permanently. The advantage over the pouch is its ease and simplicity, and the fact that it is always a one-stage operation with a minimum hospital stay and complication rate. It also has the advantage of avoiding pelvic dissection and completely eliminates the risk of nerve damage, with sexual and urinary complications and bleeding from pelvic veins. Although the functional results of ileorectal anastomosis and ileoanal pouch procedures are similar as far as bowel frequency is concerned, and the latter may have less urgency, soiling is reduced, particularly at night and in females. The patient with marginal sphincter control may be better with an ileorectal anastomosis than a pouch procedure. After an ileorectal anastomosis, if the rectum requires excision at a later date all the other operative procedures are still available. It may be particularly useful in indeterminate colitis when an ileostomy can be avoided, and if the disease subsequently discloses itself as Crohn's, the optimum procedure for avoiding an ileostomy has been performed.

However, there are many contraindications. For the operation to be successful the rectum must retain its reservoir function and be distensible, without severe active colitis or a stricture. The anal sphincter must be adequate to control liquid stool and there must be no dysplasia or invasive carcinoma in the colon or rectum, unless the operation is purely palliative. It is not a suitable procedure for patients whose main symptom is frequency and uncontrolled bowel action, and for the few patients with severe distal colitis who require surgery.

TECHNICAL ASPECTS

Elective colectomy and ileorectal anastomosis is undertaken in one stage without a protective ileostomy. The anastomosis should be constructed at the level of the sacral promontory, which leaves the rectum 13–15 cm in length, and only 1 or 2 cm of terminal ileum are resected with the colon. The ileum is rotated 90° to the right with respect to the rectum and is matched to size with a Cheatle slit if necessary. My preference is to make a hand-sewn anastomosis with one layer of vertical mattress sutures using 4/0 woven polypropylene without drainage. Aylett believed that the inflammation in the retained rectum settled more quickly if the inferior mesenteric artery and vein were ligated rather than being retained with the rectum. This, however, has not been substantiated.

A two-stage operation is only undertaken when an ileorectal anastomosis is carried out after colectomy, ileostomy and a mucus fistula has been performed as an urgent or emergency procedure. A defunctioned ileostomy may be performed at the same time as the ileorectal anastomosis when a distal complication such as a rectovaginal fistula is repaired at the same time.

THE ST MARK'S SERIES

Between 1953 and 1984 125 patients had a colectomy and ileorectal anastomosis for ulcerative colitis (Hawley 1985). There were 11 deaths, four related to the disease or operation (one postoperative death early in the series, one due to small-bowel obstruction, one from carcinoma of the colon and one from carcinoma of the rectum).

The rectum was later excised in 33 patients (28%) and one patient has an ileostomy with the rectum still in place. The main reason for rectal excision has been an unsatisfactory functional result with frequent bowel actions in 18 patients. Technical failure occurred in five patients in the early part of the series, and bleeding in one. The rectum was removed for severe dysplasia in six patients and in two of these invasive carcinoma was found, and in three further patients with a clinically detected carcinoma.

The choice of surgical treatment for ulcerative colitis in the era of the ileoanal pouch shows that there has been a reduction in the percentage of ileorectal anastomoses that have been carried out. In 1976 the first ileoanal pouch was carried out by Parks, and from 1980 onwards increasing numbers of restorative proctocolectomies have been performed (Melville et al 1994). Between 1976 and 1990 there were 422 patients in whom all the surgery for ulcerative colitis was carried out at St Mark's Hospital.

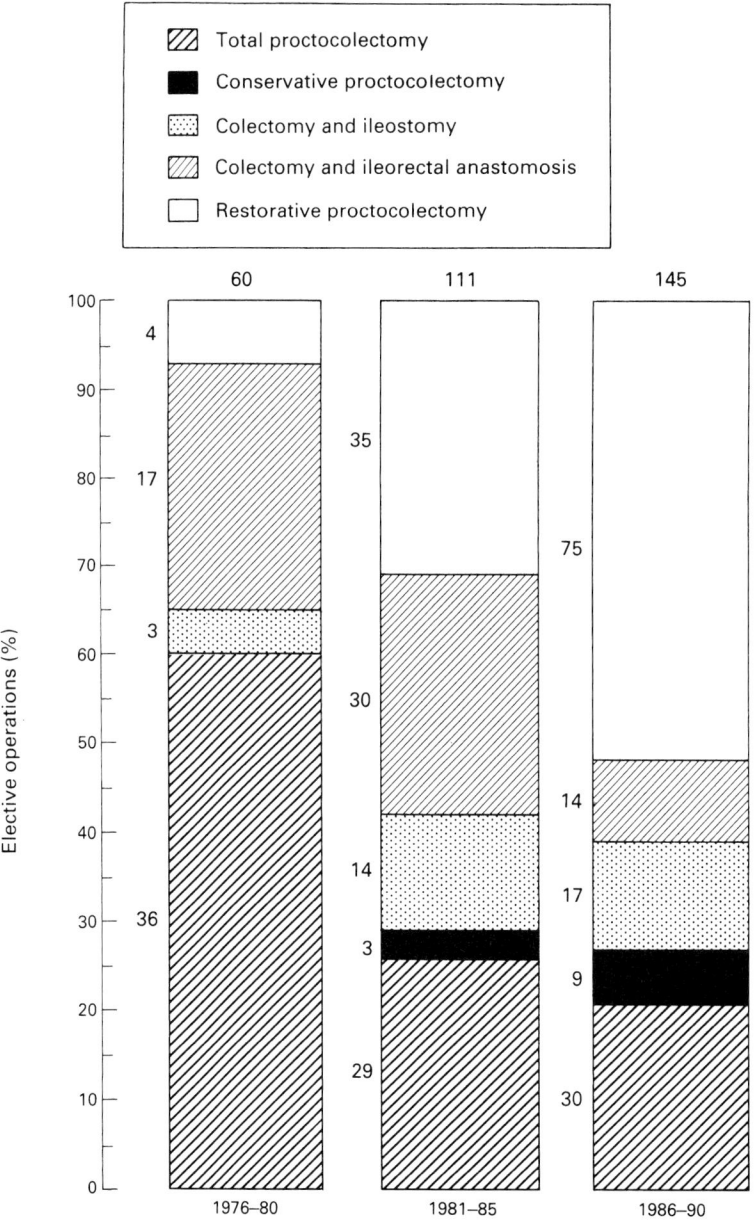

Fig. 85.1 Proportion of operations performed at St Mark's Hospital.

Elective surgery was carried out in 316 patients, with one postoperative death. The proportions of conventional proctocolectomy colectomy and ileorectal anastomosis and restorative proctocolectomy for the three quinquennia 1976–1980, 1981–1985 and 1986–1990 are shown in Fig. 85.1.

Sixty-one ileorectal anastomoses were performed, with no postoperative deaths. The percentage of patients treated by colectomy and ileorectal anastomosis remained constant over the first two periods, but fell considerably in the last. Colectomy and ileorectal anastomosis is not normally an operation performed for acute or fulminant colitis, but of the 106 patients treated urgently four had ileorectal anastomosis with no mortality. Of the urgent patients treated more conventionally by colectomy and ileostomy, ten subsequently had an ileorectal anastomosis performed, compared with 27 who had restorative proctocolectomy and 35 who had a rectal excision and ileostomy (Fig. 85.2). By the end of 1990, of the 61 patients who had this operation the ileorectal anastomosis was not functioning in 11 patients (18%). One patient with cirrhosis and gross ascites postoperatively was treated by a loop ileostomy, as the ascitic fluid drained out through the anastomosis and rectum and this has not since been closed.

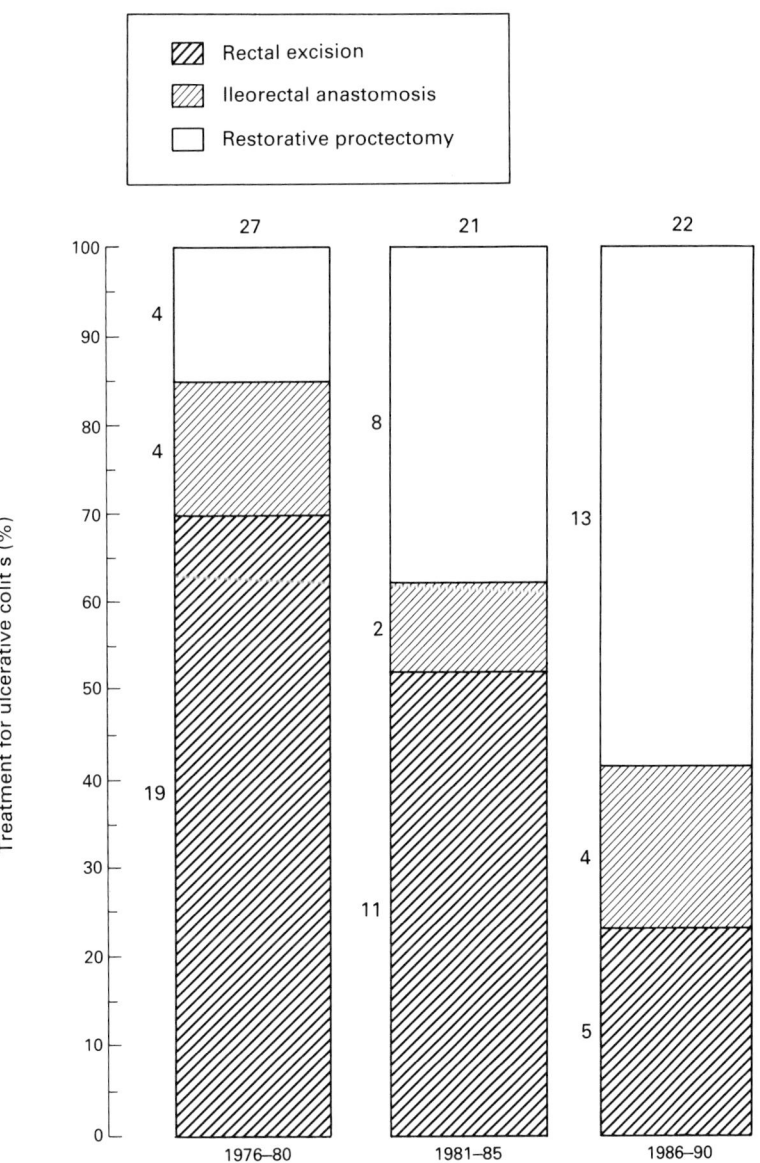

Fig. 85.2 Proportion of operations at St Mark's Hospital: urgent operations

POSTOPERATIVE COMPLICATIONS

The postoperative mortality was 0.8% at St Mark's and 0 in the era of the ileoanal pouch, and varies in most series between 0 and 6.9% (Williams & Johnson 1985). The complication rate is low compared with total proctocolectomy and the ileoanal pouch procedure. The mean hospital stay after operation was 17 days. Fifty-five percent of patients had no complication and stayed in a mean of 14 days after the operation, and 12 patients had complications: small-bowel obstruction in seven, four of whom required laparotomy, and sepsis in five. Minor complications occurred in 39% of the patients with an average stay of 28 days, and major complications in 6% of patients with a mean stay of 63 days. During the period of study proctectomy was carried out in six patients, of whom four had restorative proctocolectomies. Anastomotic leakage has occurred in a published series and varies from 0 to 15%, with a mean of 7% (Williams & Johnson 1985). The pelvic complications, mainly associated with pelvic sepsis after ileoanal pouch procedures, are considerably greater, resulting in prolonged hospital stay in a proportion of patients (Hawley 1985). However, the main problems arising after ileorectal anastomosis concern the functional results and the risk of carcinoma.

FUNCTIONAL RESULTS

The functional result will depend upon the degree of inflammation in the retained rectum, and this to some extent upon the indication for this particular surgical procedure. The results are generally good. In the St Mark's series 64 of 74 patients (84%) had a functioning ileorectal anastomosis, compared with 142 of 153 (93%) with a restorative proctocolectomy. There is a mean bowel frequency of 4.5 in 24 hours, 83% of patients having six or fewer actions in 24 hours and only 4% having a regular action at night. Urgency and soiling was not a problem, although 17% of patients had at least one episode of fecal soiling in the previous 12 months. Fifty-one percent of patients had regular medication, such as codeine phosphate, loperamide, co-phenotrope (Lomotil or methylcellulose). Nine percent used occasional medication for rectal inflammation (Newton & Baker 1975). These functional results accord well with other large series. Jagelman et al (1969) showed that 90% of patients had fewer bowel movements per day postoperatively than preoperatively, and 40% had three or fewer. Parc et al (1985), in a series of 193 patients, found that mean stool frequency was also 4.5 a day. Of 31 patients who had more than six bowel actions a day, nine eventually had a completion proctectomy for poor functional results. Normal continence was reported in 99% of patients but three had social limitations because of urgency. Nocturnal evacuation occurred in 35% of their patients. Fifty percent took antidiarrheal medication.

Leijonmark and colleagues (1990) in Stockholm, reported the long-term results of ileorectal anastomosis in 60 patients: 51 remained for evaluation at a mean follow-up of 13 years and 22 (43%) were successes. The cumulative probability of having a functional ileorectal anastomosis at 10 years was 51%, and at 20 years 32%. The most common cause for failure was severe diarrhea of inflammation of the rectum. Although a significant number of ileorectal anastomoses have to be taken down for poor function, they state that in the remainder the bowel frequency, nocturnal evacuation, continence and continence rates are somewhat better than the results published from ileoanal pouch procedures.

Failure is usually defined as the necessity to take down the ileorectal anastomosis and excise the rectum. Aylett (1978) reported that 11% of 374 patients underwent rectal excision; Hughes, in Melbourne, 25% of 155 patients; at St Mark's 28% of 125; and at the Cleveland Clinic 31% of 109. At St Goren Hospital in Stockholm 57% of 51 patients had the rectum excised, but the authors make the point that their follow-up is longer than some other series. Although there is some disagreement as to the reasons for the increased risk of eventual proctectomy, this occurs more commonly when the ileorectal anastomosis is carried out in a younger age group and there is significant inflammation in the rectum.

DYSPLASIA AND CARCINOMA IN THE RETAINED RECTUM

The main fear of the surgeon carrying out an ileorectal anastomosis is that cancer may develop in the retained rectum and lead to the death of the patient. Patients who have this procedure need careful follow-up, with regular sigmoidoscopy and biopsies from the rectal mucosa and any raised areas, and these are evaluated for dysplasia. The incidence of carcinoma increases with time and, although significant, is not sufficient to invalidate the procedure. The cancer risk is in the order of 5% at 15–20 years. In the largest series of Aylett, reported by Baker et al in 1978 22 (6%) cancers arose in 374 patients. The cumulative risk was 6% at 20 years, 15% at 30 years and 18% at 35 years. Many tumors were advanced: 18% were poorly differentiated, 12 were Duke's C cases, and four were inoperable at operation. Grundfest et al (1981), from the Cleveland Clinic, reported on 89 patients, with rectal cancer in 4.8%, with a cumulative risk of 2.1% at 15 years, 5% at 20 years and 12.9% at 25 years. Five of seven patients with cancer or severe dysplasia in the resected colon ultimately developed cancer or severe dysplasia in the rectum. In the St Mark's series, with careful follow-up and regular pathological monitoring by rectal biopsy, five (4%) patients out of 124 developed carcinoma, but unlike many of the published series where the carcinoma proved fatal, only one patient died, an incidence of less than 1%.

Tonelli et al (1991) have shown that proliferative activity and polyamine levels in rectal epithelium increase in ulcerative colitis compared with control patients, but that after an ileorectal anastomosis patients showed that the labeling index and distribution of labeled cells in the crypts approached normal. The level of polyamines was also decreased compared to unoperated patients. Increased cell proliferation and higher polyamine levels are related to an increased risk of colorectal carcinoma in ulcerative colitis: these parameters indicate that ileorectal anastomosis may reduce the risk compared to the patient with unoperated colitis. Lofberg et al (1991) looked at mucosal dysplasia and DNA aneuploidy, and have suggested that this may be an adjunct to dysplastic changes in early malignancy after ileorectal anastomosis.

However, with increasing length of follow-up of patients with ileorectal anastomosis the surgeon needs to be aware of the cumulative risk of cancer. In the last year I have operated upon three patients with early carcinoma in the rectum after ileorectal anastomosis, carried out in two patients 15 and 20 years previously, and in the other patient only 6 years after an ileorectal anastomosis. However, he had had total colitis for 10 years preoperatively and was on large doses of cyclosporin A, after having had a liver transplant 18 months ago for sclerosing cholangitis. All these patients had excision of the rectum and a one-stage restorative proctocolectomy.

CONCLUSION

Provided that the indications for colectomy and ileorectal anastomosis are adhered to, this operation remains a very satisfactory procedure. The operation is simple, with a mortality, complication and morbidity rate at least comparable to any other procedure. The patient avoids an ileostomy and every other option is available later if necessary. If a young person has a satisfactory ileorectal anastomosis for 10 or more years, this must be regarded as a success even if rectal excision is eventually required. The operation would seem to be appropriate in children, as stressed by Jones and Orr (1983) but this is at variance with the Mayo Clinic view.

The functional results are comparable with those obtained by restorative proctocolectomy, bowel frequency is similar, and nocturnal evacuation and soiling is less. For the patient with marginal sphincter function, provided the rectum is compliant, continence will be superior. There are two long-term problems with ileoanal pouches: pouchitis, which occurs in 15–20% of patients but is only severe and intractable in 5%, is a more difficult condition to treat than the residual colitis in the retained rectum after ileorectal anastomosis. The second complication is enteropathic arthropathy, which is often transitory but can be protracted and severe. The etiology is uncertain but patients may require steroid therapy for long periods. If the pouch is excised, the arthropathy rapidly improves.

It used to be said that the gold standard for surgical treatment of ulcerative colitis was total proctocolectomy and ileostomy, but this has been superseded by the one-stage restorative proctocolectomy without a defunctioning ileostomy. Ileorectal anastomosis still has a place in the treatment of ulcerative colitis, and can provide excellent results in the right patient. It has rather gone out of fashion and is probably waiting to be rediscovered.

REFERENCES

Baker W N W, Glass R E, Ritchie J K, Aylett S O 1978 Cancer of the rectum following colectomy and ileorectal anastomosis for ulcerative colitis. British Journal of Surgery 65: 862–867

Corbett R S 1952 Recent advances in the surgical treatment of chronic ulcerative colitis. Annals of the Royal College of Surgeons of England 10: 21–32

Devine H 1943 A method of colectomy for desperate cases of ulcerative colitis. Surgery, Gynecology and Obstetrics 76: 136–138

Grundfest S F, Fazio V W, Weiss R A, et al 1981 The risk of cancer following colectomy and ileorectal anastomosis for extensive mucosal ulcerative colitis. Annals of Surgery 193: 9–14

Hawley P R 1985 Ileorectal anastomosis. British Journal of Surgery (Suppl) S75–82

Jagelman D G, Lewis C G, Rowe-Jones D C 1969 Ileorectal anastomosis: appreciation by patients. British Medical Journal 1: 756–757

Jones P F, Orr G 1983 Colectomy and ileo-rectal anastomosis. In: Allan R N et al (ed) Inflammatory Bowel Diseases. Churchill Livingstone, pp 268–273

Leijonmarck C E, Lofberg R, Ost A, Hellers G 1990 Long-term results of ileorectal anastomosis in ulcerative colitis in Stockholm County. Diseases of the Colon and Rectum 33.3 195

Lofberg R, Leijonmarck C E, Brostrom O et al 1991 Mucosal dysplasia and DNA content in ulcerative colitis patients with ileorectal anastomosis. Diseases of the Colon and Rectum 34.7.566–571

Melville D M, Ritchie J K, Nicholls R J, Hawley P R 1994 Surgery for ulcerative colitis in the era of the pouch: The St Mark's Hospital experience. Gut 35: 1076–1080

Newton C R, Baker W N H 1975 Comparison of bowel function after ileo-rectal anastomosis for ulcerative colitis and colonic polyposis. Gut 16: 785–791

Orkin B A, Trelander R L, Wolff B G 1990 The surgical management of children with ulcerative colitis. Diseases of the Colon and Rectum 33.11.947

Parc R, Levy E, Frileux P et al 1985 Current results: ileorectal anastomosis after total abdominal colectomy for ulcerative colitis. In: Dozois R R (ed) Alternatives to conventional ileostomy. Chicago: Year Book Medical Publishers, pp 81–99

Tonelli F, Bianchini F, Lodovici M et al 1991 Mucosal cell proliferation of the rectal stump in ulcerative colitis patients after ileorectal anastomosis. Diseases of the Colon and Rectum 34.5.385–90

Williams N S, Johnston D 1985 The current status of mucosal proctectomy and ileoanal anastomosis in the surgical treatment of ulcerative colitis and adenomatous polyposis. British Journal of Surgery 72: 159–168

86. Surgical treatment of ulcerative colitis – proctocolectomy and permanent ileostomy

A. P. Meagher   B. G. Wolff

INTRODUCTION

Proctocolectomy and permanent end ileostomy was advocated for the treatment of ulcerative colitis as early as 1931 (Rankin 1931). Improvements in operative morbidity and the introduction of the everted (Brooke) ileostomy (Brooke 1952), ensured that this procedure became the standard surgical therapy for ulcerative colitis for several decades. Since then there has been considerable evolution in the surgical options available for the treatment of ulcerative colitis. The more recently introduced alternative surgical procedures, including ileorectal anastomosis, continent ileostomy and ileal pouch–anal anastomosis, each have their advantages and disadvantages when compared to proctocolectomy with ileostomy. Although in many major centers the ileal pouch–anal procedure now is performed in the majority of patients undergoing elective surgery for ulcerative colitis, even in such centers proctocolectomy with ileostomy remains the treatment of choice in a substantial proportion of patients (Fig. 86.1).

Proctocolectomy with permanent ileostomy results in the removal of all large-bowel mucosa, so that there can be no further symptoms due to inflammation of this mucosa, and no risk of subsequent carcinoma. It can be performed safely as a one-stage procedure by the majority of well trained surgeons, without major complications. Following surgery there is generally a rapid restoration of the patient's health. The overriding disadvantage of this procedure is the creation of a permanent ileostomy. Patients, particularly the young patients often faced with operative management of ulcerative colitis, frequently are willing to accept the increased risks of alternative procedures so as to avoid the disadvantages, both real and perceived, of a permanent stoma.

INDICATIONS

Elective

In patients with ulcerative colitis in whom operative intervention is considered appropriate, most commonly for failure of medical therapy or the risk of carcinoma, all the various surgical options available should be outlined. The final decision will depend on the individual patient's medical

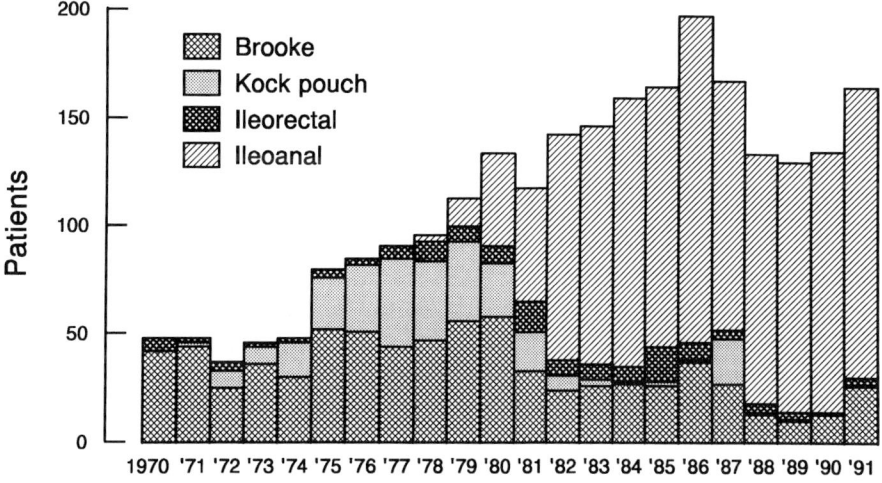

Fig. 86.1 Evolution of the surgical treatment of ulcerative colitis at the Mayo Clinic between 1970 and January 1992.

condition and wishes, and the expertise of the surgeon. There are a number of factors which may influence the decision-making towards proctocolectomy with end ileostomy.

Few patients over the age of 60 years have been treated with ileal pouch–anal anastomosis. Although functional results in older patients can be only marginally worse than in younger patients (Pemberton et al 1987, Lewis et al 1993), it should be recognized that the older patients in these series represent a very select, medically fit, motivated group. In the majority of patients over 60 proctocolectomy with permanent ileostomy remains the treatment of choice.

Both ileal pouch–anal and ileorectal anastomoses result in fluid or semiformed stool, placing substantial stress on the anal sphincters. Patients with anal sphincter damage, most commonly resulting from obstetric trauma or previous surgery, are unlikely to achieve a satisfactory functional outcome. It is not possible, at present, to state the anorectal physiological parameters required for good functional outcome following ileal pouch–anal anastomosis (Morgado et al 1994). None the less, examination of the anal sphincters, using anorectal physiological tests when indicated, should be part of the evaluation of patients in whom surgical management of ulcerative colitis is considered.

Patient choice remains one of the most common reasons for the performance of proctocolectomy and ileostomy. Some patients are not over concerned by the thought of a permanent ileostomy, and are keen to avoid the possible short-term and long-term complications of an ileal pouch–anal procedure, such as the risk of pelvic sepsis, the need for a second surgical procedure of loop ileostomy closure in most cases, the risk of pouchitis, the risk of poor function, and the long-term risk of pouch failure. Likewise, they are anxious to avoid the complications of ileorectal anastomosis, such as the risk of worsening proctitis and the fear of carcinoma. The patient's occupation may also be an important determinant when deciding the most favorable operative procedure. Although bowel function following ileal pouch–anal or ileorectal anastomosis is usually considered adequate by people eager to avoid an ileostomy, in some occupations the frequency and urgency often accompanying these operative procedures are unacceptable.

Patients who have advanced colorectal carcinoma complicating ulcerative colitis may also be best treated by initial proctocolectomy with permanent ileostomy. In particular, patients with advanced rectal carcinoma, who often undergo postoperative radiation therapy, may benefit from this procedure, as outcome following ileal pouch–anal anastomosis is poor when postoperative radiotherapy is employed (Fozard et al 1992).

Concomitant medical conditions may be relative contraindications to the performance of procedures other than proctocolectomy and ileostomy, as these other procedures are associated with increased operative time and increased risk of postoperative complications.

The patient's habitus can also play an important role in decision making. In very obese patients it can be difficult to anastomose an ileal pouch to the anus. Obesity is also considered a relative contraindication to the formation of a continent (Kock) ileostomy (Dozois 1990).

Occasionally there remains real doubt about whether the primary pathology is Crohn's disease or ulcerative colitis, even following laparotomy and frozen section. Some patients with 'indeterminate colitis' have a long-term outcome following ileal pouch–anal anastomosis almost as favorable as that in patients with confirmed chronic ulcerative colitis (McIntyre et al 1993), whereas others behave much more as if they had Crohn's disease. However, in certain circumstances, especially in centers where frozen section is not routinely performed, significant doubt about the primary pathology found at operation may influence the surgeon towards performing ileorectal anastomosis or, if the rectum is significantly diseased, proctocolectomy and ileostomy, rather than an ileal pouch–anal procedure.

Finally, patients who have had small-bowel resections in the past may have unacceptable frequency following ileorectal or ileal pouch–anal anastomosis, and may be treated best with an end ileostomy.

Emergency

The majority of patients requiring urgent operative treatment for ulcerative colitis should undergo subtotal colectomy with preservation of the rectum, generally with formation of a mucous fistula (Keighley 1993). This allows for restoration of continuity at a later date. Only very occasionally, in patients in whom later restoration of continuity would not be considered appropriate, such as elderly patients, total proctocolectomy may be performed at the initial procedure. However, the increased risks of performing this procedure on a medically compromised patient should be borne in mind. The advantages are the prevention of occasionally troublesome inflammation or bleeding in the rectal remnant, which may require eventual proctectomy, and avoidance of the risk of subsequent carcinoma. If emergency surgical treatment is required in a patient in whom later restoration of continuity is not contemplated, then a reasonable alternative is to divide the rectum low in the pelvis, at the level of the levator muscles. This avoids the complications of a perineal wound and, if the short stump of remaining rectum does continue to cause symptoms, then mucosectomy or proctectomy via a perineal approach can be performed at a later date (Dean & Celestin 1983).

PREOPERATIVE PREPARATION

Preoperative assessment by a stoma therapist is especially important. Full discussion of the management of an ileostomy is often reassuring to the patient, and careful preoperative siting of the stoma is essential. Furthermore, preoperative discussion with someone of the same age, sex and background who has an ileostomy is often helpful, and can usually be arranged by the stoma therapist.

As the colon is excised and no anastomosis performed, the unpleasant traditional full mechanical bowel preparation may be omitted. However, a modified preparation (for example just 1 l of polyethylene glycol solution the evening before the procedure) does prevent any substantial fecal loading, thereby facilitating the operation. Prophylaxis against venous thrombosis and perioperative antibiotics are both integral to modern colectomy. Patients often are, or recently have been, taking corticosteroids, so that perioperative intravenous steroids should be given. Patients presenting for elective resection may be markedly malnourished. It is not currently possible to state clear criteria for the use of nutritional supplementation, but consideration should be given to the use of preoperative and/or perioperative parenteral nutrition in malnourished patients, especially those who have lost 15% of their body weight in the month prior to operation, or who have a markedly low serum albumin (Hill et al 1977).

OPERATIVE PROCEDURE

Under general anesthesia the patient is positioned in the modified lithotomy Trendelenburg position and a urinary catheter is inserted. A nasogastric tube may be placed, although it can safely be removed at the end of the procedure in most cases (Wolff et al 1989). An anal pursestring suture to prevent contamination of the perineal wound should be placed at this stage. Colectomy is performed in the usual way with preservation of the omentum, and the ileum is transected just proximal to the ileocecal junction, to preserve ileal length.

The rectal dissection should be performed so that there is preservation of the pelvic autonomic nerves supplying the bladder and genitalia. In inflammatory bowel disease this may be accomplished in two ways. Starting above the sacral promontory the dissection may be performed close to the posterior wall of the rectum, leaving the mesorectum and inferior mesenteric vessels intact. This ensures preservation of the presacral autonomic plexus, which lies posterior and posterolateral to the mesorectum, but dissection in this plane can be sanguinary, due to division of multiple small branches of the inferior mesenteric artery supplying the rectum. This may make identification of the anterior plane of dissection more difficult, and thus preservation of the autonomic nerves lying anterolateral to the rectum. In the alternative method posterior dissection is performed in the relatively bloodless plane immediately behind the mesorectum. However, this is immediately anterior to the presacral autonomic plexus, so that the plane must be identified precisely because any posterior deviation may injure the plexus and compromise the function of the bladder and genitalia.

The anterior and anterolateral planes of dissection should lie on the front wall of the rectum, ensuring preservation of the autonomic nerves anterior to Denonvilier's fascia, which are important for sexual function. The majority of the rectal dissection is performed by the abdominal operator.

In original descriptions the rectal dissection, in particular the perineal dissection, was similar to that described for rectal carcinoma and hence poor perineal wound healing and problems with bladder and sexual function were common. With the introduction of perimuscular dissection of the rectum (Lee & Dowling 1972) and, later, excision of the anus through the intersphincteric plane (Lyttle & Parks 1977), these complications have decreased substantially. The perineal dissection should now be performed through a small perianal incision. The plane between the internal and external anal sphincters is identified, and upward dissection is carried out in this plane until the pelvis is entered, connecting with the abdominal dissection. The colon and rectum are removed, and the resulting small perineal wound is usually closed primarily. One or two closed suction drains are placed in the pelvis.

At the predetermined ileostomy site a disc of skin and subcutaneous fat is excised, a cruciate incision made in the anterior fascial sheath of the rectus muscle, the rectus muscle is split longitudinally, and the posterior sheath and peritoneum are divided. The previously divided terminal ileum is brought out through this wound. After closure of the midline wound the terminal ileum is everted so that there is a spout 2–3 cm in lenght, and the ileal mucosa is sutured to the skin.

POSTOPERATIVE MANAGEMENT

Careful fluid management is essential in the postoperative period. If excessive ileostomy loss continues for more than a few days, and the patient is tolerating a diet, then a stool bulking agent, or oral loperamide or codeine, can be helpful in decreasing the output.

Early attention should be paid to teaching the patient to manage the ileostomy. In the elderly population who often undergo this procedure it may take over a week to learn to care for the stoma, and unless teaching is begun early this may prolong the period of postoperative hospitalization.

SPECIFIC COMPLICATIONS

Perineal wound

Poor healing of the perineal wound, often related to pelvic sepsis, is a common complication. Delayed healing was reported in over half of all cases in earlier series, although this appears to have decreased with the introduction of intersphincteric dissection (Lyttle & Parks 1977, Berry et al 1986). Poor initial healing of the perineal wound can result in long-term morbidity, with one survey of 273 patients who underwent proctocolectomy finding that 8% had chronic unhealed perineal wounds (McLeod et al 1986).

Sexual dysfunction

The effect of proctocolectomy and ileostomy on sexual function is difficult to define precisely. On the one hand sexual function is often impaired in patients with chronic ulcerative colitis, and is enhanced postoperatively because of improved overall wellbeing related to removal of the diseased colon (Metcalf et al 1986, Pemberton et al 1987). Nevertheless, sexual function may be adversely affected because of damage to the pelvic autonomic nerves at operation, the occurrence of dyspareunia following pelvic surgery, and the psychological and physical effects of the stoma. It is often not possible to separate the individual importance of these various factors on sexual function, especially when comparing past and recent publications examining sexual function following the different operations for ulcerative colitis. Increased surgical attention to preserving the pelvic autonomic nerves is likely to have been responsible for improved results. Whereas impotence occurred in about one in ten men who underwent proctocolectomy (Watts et al 1966, Burnham et al 1977), it now occurs in only 1–2% of patients following perimuscular excision of the rectum with ileostomy (Berry et al 1986, Lee & Truelove 1980), or ileal pouch–anal anastomosis (Meagher et al, in preparation). A similar decrease in the prevalence of retrograde ejaculation has been noted (Watts et al 1966, Burnham et al 1977, Meagher et al, in preparation). Following proctectomy females also may suffer owing to damage to the pelvic autonomic nerves, for example complaining of loss of genital sensation (Gruner et al 1977). Although difficult to quantify, and likely to lessen with length of follow-up, the presence of an ileostomy can be a serious impediment to sexual relations. One survey found that one-third of ileostomates reported that intercourse was more difficult physically or psychologically because of the ileostomy, and half felt less desirable sexually (Rolstad et al 1983). Finally some degree of dyspareunia can be a chronic problem following proctectomy and ileostomy, and has been reported in 12–30% of women (Burnham et al 1977, Gruner et al 1977).

Stomal complications

The esthetic unpleasantness of a permanent ileostomy may be foremost in the mind of a patient contemplating the surgical alternatives. Although the surgical morbidity of the more complex operative procedures may be more immediately striking, it should be recognized that the Brooke ileostomy is associated with considerable long-term morbidity. In an actuarial analysis of 150 patients with permanent end ileostomies, the cumulative incidence of stomal complications at 20 years in patients undergoing surgery for ulcerative colitis was 76% (Leong et al 1994). The authors included adhesive small-bowel obstruction (cumulative probability at 20 years of 23%) as a stomal complication, although the obstruction was related to the stoma in only a minority of patients. Overall, the most common stomal complications were skin problems (cumulative probability of 34%), retraction (17%), parastomal herniation (16%) and prolapse (11%). The cumulative probability of undergoing revisional surgery at least once for a stomal complication (excluding operations for intestinal complications) was 23% at 20 years. Similarly high reoperation rates have been noted previously (Ritchie 1971, Phillips et al 1989).

Urologic complications

Patients who have undergone proctectomy for inflammatory bowel disease have often been found to suffer long-term bladder dysfunction. One-quarter of 37 patients studied for a mean period of 4 years postoperatively complained of urinary symptoms, predominantly incomplete emptying, straining and poor stream (Neal et al 1982). Furthermore, evidence of denervation of the bladder, including capacious bladders with poor detrusor function and large residual volumes, was significantly more common than in a control group. Again, it is likely that a meticulous operative technique with precise attention to preservation of the pelvic autonomic nerves will decrease the incidence of bladder and sexual dysfunction.

A number of studies have shown that patients treated for ulcerative colitis with proctocolectomy and permanent ileostomy have an increased incidence of urolithiasis (Kennedy et al 1982, Bennett & Hughes 1972, Maratka & Nedbal 1964). It has been suggested that this is more common in males with hyperuricemia, a low urinary volume and low urinary pH (Kennedy et al 1982). The consumption of ample quantities of fluid and salt may be helpful and allopurinol has been suggested for hyperuricemic patients (Kennedy et al 1982).

Adhesive small-bowel obstruction

Although adhesive small-bowel obstruction may complicate any intraperitoneal procedure, it is perhaps most common following proctocolectomy. The cumulative probability of developing bowel obstruction following proctocolectomy and ileostomy in one series was 23% at 20 years (Leong et al 1994); in another series the cumulative probability of developing bowel obstruction following proctocolectomy and ileal pouch–anal procedure was 22% at 10 years

(Meagher et al, in preparation). It is likely that the greater incidence after the pouch procedure is related to the high incidence of obstruction in the interval between the pouch procedure and ileostomy closure.

COMPARISONS WITH ALTERNATIVE SURGICAL PROCEDURES

Each of the operations available for ulcerative colitis have both advantages and disadvantages compared to the alternative procedures. Colectomy and ileorectal anastomosis should only be performed when the rectum is relatively spared. The surgical dissection does not extend into the pelvis, so that the risk of sexual or urinary dysfunction is minimal. Postoperative morbidity is low and functional outcome is generally acceptable. However, about one-third of patients eventually require proctectomy because of progressive disease or carcinogenesis in the rectal stump (Goligher 1980, Johnson et al 1986). The creation of a continent Kock ileostomy requires considerable surgical expertise, and even in experienced hands commonly requires revision (Dozois et al 1980, Fazio & Church 1988). Pouchitis can be troublesome. Although patients with a continent ileostomy usually prefer it to a standard ileostomy, anal defecation is not achieved. The ileal pouch–anal procedure does allow anal defecation, along with complete removal of the large-bowel mucosa. Although some early reports noted high operative morbidity, with increasing experience the incidence of pelvic sepsis has fallen, to 4% in one series, and the mortality was 0.2% (Meagher et al, in preparation). In this series of 1091 patients who underwent ileal pouch–anal procedure with a J shaped pouch and who had at least 1 year of follow-up, the mean stool frequency was seven per 24 hours, and 90% of patients had no incontinence or only occasional minor incontinence. Ninety percent of patients had a functioning pouch after 9 years. During this prolonged follow-up bowel function was stable. Among the males 1.6% reported impotence at the last follow-up, and 2.3% reported retrograde or lack of ejaculation. Among the females 3.3% reported dyspareunia and 2.3% reported fear of leakage during intercourse. The cumulative probability of suffering at least one episode of clinical pouchitis at 9 years was 44%.

The different merits and problems of these alternative procedures are difficult to compare. The alternative procedures are performed in markedly disparate patient populations, so that direct comparison of surgical morbidity rates is not meaningful. Likewise, comparison of the results of more modern procedures with large series of patients undergoing proctocolectomy and ileostomy several decades ago is flawed. Furthermore, the complications of the different procedures are different, so that value judgments are necessary, for example the morbidity of a permanent stoma versus the morbidity of pouchitis and minor incontinence.

Some investigators have examined the outcome of these procedures in terms of quality of life. First, overall satisfaction with proctocolectomy and ileostomy is high (McLeod et al 1986). In particular, in the patients over 60 who often undergo this treatment, the overall incidence of satisfaction has been found to be 97% (Stryker et al 1985). None the less, it has been found that after ileal pouch–anal anastomosis patients experienced significant advantages in performing daily activities compared to patients with Brooke ileostomy, and thus may experience a better quality of life (Pemberton et al 1989). Likewise, it has been found that patients with an ileal pouch–anal anastomosis have fewer restrictions in sports and sexual activities than those with Koch pouches or Brooke ileostomies (Köhler et al 1991).

CONCLUSION

Proctocolectomy and ileostomy has proved to be a safe, reliable surgical treatment for chronic ulcerative colitis. Moreover, this relatively straightforward procedure generally results in a rapid restoration of health. Nevertheless, like all alternative operations available for ulcerative colitis, it is associated with substantial, specific, surgical morbidity. Delayed perineal wound healing and long-term complications of the ileostomy are foremost. However, proctocolectomy with ileostomy is now only utilized in a minority of patients in most major centers, primarily because patients prefer the opportunity to live without a permanent ileostomy.

REFERENCES

Bennett R C, Hughes E S R 1972 Urinary calculi and ulcerative colitis. British Medical Journal 2: 494–496

Berry A R, DeCampos R, Lee A C G 1986 Perineal and pelvic morbidity following perimuscular incision of the rectum for inflammatory bowel disease. British Journal of Surgery 73: 675–677

Brooke B N 1952 Management of ileostomy including its complications. Lancet ii: 102

Burnham W R, Lennard-Jones J E, Brooke B N 1977 Sexual problems among married ileostomists. Survey conducted by the Ileostomy Association of Great Britain and Ireland. Gut 18: 673–677

Dean A M, Celestin R L 1983 Rectocolectomy with anal conservation in inflammatory colitis. Annals of the Royal College of Surgeons of England 65: 32–34

Dozois R R 1990 Ulcerative colitis: surgical alternatives. In: Fazio V W (ed) Current therapy in colon and rectal surgery. B. C. Decker Inc, Toronto, pp 166–173

Dozois R R, Kelly K A, Beart R W, Beahrs O H 1980 Improved results with continent ileostomy. Annals of Surgery 192: 319–323

Fazio V W, Church J M 1988 Complications and function of the continent ileostomy at the Cleveland Clinic. World Journal of Surgery 12: 148–154

Fozard J B J, Nelson H, Pemberton J H, Dozois R R 1992 Primary ileal pouch–anal anastomosis and colorectal cancer – results and contraindications. Diseases of the Colon and Rectum 35: P22

Goligher J C 1980 Surgery of the anus, rectum and colon. Baillière-Tindall, London

Gruner O N, Naas R, Fretheim B, Gjone E 1977 Marital status and sexual adjustment after colectomy. Results in 178 patients operated on for ulcerative colitis. Scandinavian Journal of Gastroenterology 12: 193–197

Hill G L, Blackett T C, Pickford L et al 1977 Malnutrition in surgical patients. Lancet i: 689–692

Johnson W R, Hughes E S R, McDermott F T, Pihl E A, Katrivessis H 1986 The outcome of patients with ulcerative colitis managed by subtotal colectomy. Surgery, Gynecology and Obstetrics 162: 421–425

Keighley M R B 1993 Acute fulminating colitis and emergency colectomy. In: Keighley M R B, Williams N S (eds) Surgery of the anus, rectum and colon. WB Saunders, London, pp 1379–1397

Kennedy H J, Fletcher E W L, Truelove S C 1982 Urinary stones in subjects with a permanent ileostomy. British Journal of Surgery 69: 661–664

Köhler L W, Pemberton J H, Zinsmeister A R, Kelly K A 1991 Quality of life after proctocolectomy. A comparison of Brooke ileostomy, Kock pouch, and ileal pouch–anal anastomosis. Gastroenterology 101: 679–684

Lee E C G, Dowling B L 1972 Perimuscular dissection of the rectum for Crohn's disease and ulcerative colitis. British Journal of Surgery 59: 29–32

Lee E C G, Truelove S C 1980 Proctocolectomy for ulcerative colitis. World Journal of Surgery 4: 195–201

Leong A P K, Londono-Schimmer E E, Phillips R K S 1994 Life-table analysis of stomal complications following ileostomy. British Journal of Surgery 81: 727–729

Lewis W G, Sagar P M, Holdsworth P J, Axon A T R, Johnston D 1993 Restorative proctocolectomy with end-to-end pouch–anal anastomosis in patients over the age of fifty. Gut 34: 948–952

Lyttle J A, Parks A G 1977 Intersphincteric excision of the rectum. British Journal of Surgery 64: 413–416

McIntyre P B, Pemberton J H, Wolff B G, Dozois R R, Beart R W, Kelly K A 1993 Indeterminate colitis: long-term outcome in patients after ileal pouch–anal anastomosis. Diseases of the Colon and Rectum 36: P37

McLeod R S, Lavery I C, Leatherman J R et al 1986 Factors affecting quality of life with a conventional ileostomy. World Journal of Surgery 10: 474–478

Maratka Z, Nedbal J 1964 Urolithiasis as a complication of the surgical treatment of ulcerative colitis. Gut 5: 214–217

Meagher A P, Dozois R R, Kelly K A et al Ileal pouch–anal canal anastomosis: complication rate and long-term functional results. (In preparation)

Metcalf A M, Dozois R R, Kelly K A 1986 Sexual function in women after proctocolectomy. Annals of Surgery 204: 624–627

Morgado P J, Wexner S D, James K, Nogueras J J, Jagelman D G 1994 Ileal pouch–anal anastomosis: is preoperative anal manometry predictive of postoperative functional outcome? Diseases of the Colon and Rectum 37: 224–228

Neal D E, Parker A J, Williams N S, Johnston D 1982 The long term effects of proctectomy on bladder function in patients with inflammatory bowel disease. British Journal of Surgery 69: 349–352

Pemberton J H, Kelly K A, Beart R W, Dozois R R, Wolff B G, Ilstrup D M 1987 Ileal pouch–anal anastomosis for chronic ulcerative colitis. Long-term results. Annals of Surgery 206: 504–511

Pemberton J H, Phillips S F, Ready R R, Zinsmeister A R, Beahrs O H 1989 Quality of life after Brooke ileostomy and ileal pouch–anal anastomosis. Comparison of performance status. Annals of Surgery 209: 620–626

Phillips R K S, Ritchie J K, Hawley P R 1989 Proctocolectomy and ileostomy for ulcerative colitis: the longer term story. Journal of the Royal Society of Medicine 82: 386–387

Rankin F W 1931 Total extirpation of colon and rectum: six consecutive successful cases. Proceedings of Staff Meeting Mayo Clinic 6: 436–440

Ritchie J K 1971 Ileostomy and excisional surgery for chronic inflammatory disease of the colon: a survey of one hospital region. Gut 12: 528–540

Rolstad B S, Wilson G, Rothenberger D A 1983 Sexual concerns in patients with an ileostomy. Diseases of the Colon and Rectum 26: 170–175

Stryker S J, Pemberton J H, Zinsmeister A R 1985 Long-term results of ileostomy in older patients. Diseases of the Colon and Rectum 28: 844–846

Watts J M, de Dombal F T, Goligher J C 1966 Long-term complications and prognosis following major surgery for ulcerative colitis. British Journal of Surgery 53: 1014–1023

Wolff B G, Pemberton J H, Van Heerden J A et al 1989 Elective colon and rectal surgery without nasogastric decompression. A prospective, randomized trial. Annals of Surgery 209: 670–673

87. Surgical treatment of ulcerative colitis – continent ileostomy

J. G. Peiser   Z. Cohen   R. S. McLeod

There are four surgical procedures from which a patient with ulcerative colitis may choose. These are total proctocolectomy and conventional Brooke ileostomy, total proctocolectomy and the continent ileostomy, colectomy and ileoproctostomy, and restorative proctocolectomy (pelvic pouch procedure). This chapter will focus on the continent ileostomy.

HISTORICAL EVOLUTION OF KOCK'S CONTINENT ILEOSTOMY

Early skin-level ileostomies were unsatisfactory owing to complications such as stomal stenosis, prolapse, fistula, parastomal hernia and, in particular, skin excoriation. Almost all of these complications were encountered by at least 90% of the patients during their early postoperative years (Bargen 1956). With the advance of the Brooke ileostomy and the resultant improvement in appliance technology, quality of life with a stoma was much improved (Brooke 1952). However, despite these improvements, patients with a conventional Brooke ileostomy still encounter both mechanical and psychosocial difficulties. Some of the complications include leakage of ileal effluent beneath the appliance, resulting in skin excoriation or ulceration, psychosocial and sexual problems, noise, odor, and stomal prolapse or retraction. Body image and sexual attractiveness, particularly in women, as well as sexual function, are further factors resulting in psychosocial impairment in these patients (Thompson & Lennard-Jones 1977).

In order to improve the quality of life of ileostomates and potential ileostomates, Professor Nils Kock devised a method of creating a reservoir from the terminal ileum, which would enable the patient to have voluntary control over their own bowel function. The first reservoir ileostomy was constructed by Kock in 1967. A 40 cm segment of terminal ileum was used to create the reservoir and an isoperistaltic outlet was brought out obliquely through the abdominal wall (Kock et al 1977). The stoma was matured at the skin level. Subsequently an antiperistaltic outlet was used, the hypothesis being that the unidirectional peristaltic waves of the small bowel would be negated and continence would be maximized. Thus intestinal content would remain in the pouch until voluntary catheterization was performed, and full continence could be achieved (Kock 1971).

However, these initial modifications resulted in only partial continence. The creation of an intussuscepted segment of the outlet known as the 'nipple valve' achieved full continence. In the creation of a nipple valve a 10 cm segment of terminal ileum is intussuscepted on itself, thereby creating a 5 cm valve (Fig. 87.1). With this continent system patients emptied the reservoir themselves three to four times a day and remained completely continent at night. Skin irritation did not occur and patients were not restricted in their activity or diet. However, despite the early encouraging results with the 'nipple valve', extrusion of the valve or desusception was encountered, usually within the first 3 months after the operation, in approximately 30% of cases. When extrusion or slippage occurred there was difficulty in catheterization, and often incontinence. Other complications, such as fistulization, valve necrosis and prolapse of the valve, were also encountered. A series of modifications was introduced in an attempt to stabilize the valve and prevent slippage. These included stripping of the mesentery along the segment of ileum to be used for valve construction; the use of fascia or mesh (Marlex, Mersilene, Dexon) around the outlet (Kock et al 1980a); scarification of the valve segment by creating numerous transverse incisions with cautery in the seromuscular layer of the intestinal segment to encourage fibrous adhesions between the intussuscepted layers (Gelernt et al 1977, Cranley 1983); and finally, stapling of the valve itself and stapling of the valve to the pouch (Kock 1971, Steichen 1977). Despite all of these modifications, slippage of the nipple valve remains a common problem and difficult corrective surgery is often required. Nevertheless, patients who do have a well functioning continent ileostomy are extremely pleased with the outcome.

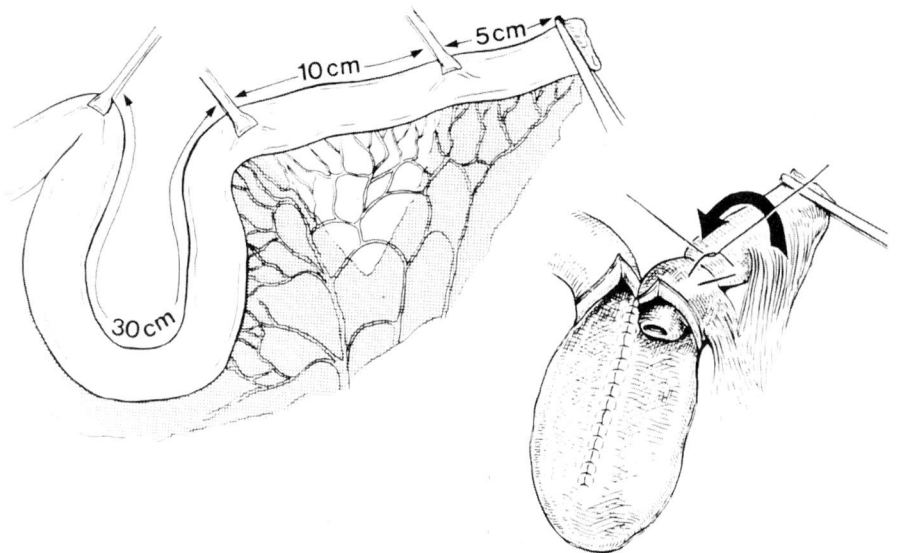

Fig. 87.1 Construction of the Kock pouch using a 45 cm segment of terminal ileum, 5 cm for the outlet, 10 cm for the nipple valve and 30 cm for pouch construction. The nipple valve is intussuscepted over a 5 cm segment.

INDICATIONS AND CONTRAINDICATIONS FOR KOCK POUCH IN ULCERATIVE COLITIS

Indications

Indications for the continent ileostomy are similar to those for patients undergoing a pelvic pouch procedure. A firm, histologically proven diagnosis of ulcerative colitis is mandatory. In 1994 the most frequent indications are patients who are seeking an alternative to a conventional ileostomy owing to skin problems or psychosocial and sexual difficulties, or failed ileoanal pouch procedures. Anal sphincter dysfunction or the presence of a low rectal cancer in conjunction with ulcerative colitis are contraindications to the pelvic pouch, and may make the patient a candidate for continent ileostomy (McLeod 1993).

Contraindications

Crohn's disease is considered a specific contraindication to pouch surgery, as such patients tend to experience a very high complication rate (Kock et al 1980b, Myrvold 1987). Handelsman et al reviewed 100 consecutive patients with a continent ileostomy after a minimum follow-up time of 2.5 years. Seven of these patients were diagnosed as having Crohn's disease or indeterminate colitis at the time the pouch was constructed, and all developed severe complications within 12 months of surgery. Fistula formation, obstruction, leakage and symptomatic Crohn's disease were reasons for removal of the pouch. One patient developed obstruction of the small bowel proximal to the pouch 14 years after pouch construction, and examination of the ileal segment along with the pouch led to a pathologic diagnosis of ileitis of indeterminate type. Conversely, of 87 patients with ulcerative colitis in this study only 17 (20%) had complications, six of which were readily and simply corrected (Handelsman et al 1993). These results are in agreement with earlier reports by Kock, who stated that complications of all categories were markedly higher in patients with Crohn's disease. In his series the reservoir had to be removed in 17% of patients with Crohn's disease, compared to 2% of patients with ulcerative colitis (Kock et al 1980b).

Further relative contraindications for the construction of a continent ileostomy include previous resection of a significant amount of small bowel, age of the patient over 60 and patients who have coexisting serious medical illness (McLeod 1993). Schrock, in 1979, and Dozois in 1981, reported a higher complication rate among obese patients and suggested that obesity should be considered to be a relative contraindication.

OPERATIVE PROCEDURE

We have used many modifications since 1977. The authors' current preferred operative technique to construct a continent ileostomy is as follows. Following removal of the colon and rectum, approximately 45 cm of terminal ileum is measured, of which approximately 5 cm will be used for the outlet, 10 cm for the nipple valve, and three 10 cm segments for the reservoir. An S-shaped reservoir is constructed by suturing the three limbs together using 3/0 vicryl. The limbs of the 'S' are opened along the antimesenteric border. A second suture layer is inserted to complete the posterior wall of the pouch. The mesentery and fat overlying the vascular supply to the nipple valve segment is stripped away. The distal ileum is then intussuscepted over at least a 5 cm segment to create the nipple valve, which is secured in position by three rows of staples using the SGIA stapler without the blade. The intestinal plate is folded over on itself to create the reservoir, and the sides are completed using two layers of absorbable suture material. A strip of Mersilene mesh (2 cm wide) is then passed through a previously created window in the mesentery at a position approximately at the base of the outlet. The reservoir is sutured to the lower edge of the Mersilene mesh using absorbable sutures, and the corners of the mesh are secured to the anterior rectus sheath using interrupted 2/0 Prolene. The lateral aspect of the reservoir is then anchored to the lateral aspect of the undersurface of the ileostomy opening and the outlet is brought out through the stomal aperture. The medial aspect of the pouch is then anchored to the medial surface of the undersurface of the ileostomy opening. The excess outlet is trimmed away and a stoma is made flush with the skin. A 30 Fr ileostomy catheter (A. B. Medena, Kungsbacka, Sweden) is placed within the reservoir and attached to a straight drainage system.

SPECIFIC COMPLICATIONS

Stability of the nipple valve

Slippage or desusception of the nipple valve has been the most common complication of the continent ileostomy procedure. It usually occurs within the first 3 months following surgery, but may occur years later. Slippage of the valve usually presents with difficulty or even inability to intubate the pouch. In addition the pouch usually becomes at least partially incontinent. When patients state that they have difficulty with intubation, it almost always signifies partial or complete slippage of the nipple valve. The diagnosis can be confirmed by digital examination of the outlet, by ileoscopy, or by intubation by the surgeon. A hypaque study of the outlet and valve will usually confirm the 'hockey-stick' deformity which is characteristic of slippage (Fig. 87.2). Placement of a tube to achieve continuous drainage may relieve the problem temporarily, but a definitive solution usually requires surgical intervention. The pouch must be taken down from the abdominal wall and the nipple valve anchored into position once again. Occasionally the valve must be resected and a new one constructed from the afferent limb. The pouch must then be turned through 180° and a new afferent entrance made to complete the operation (McLeod 1993).

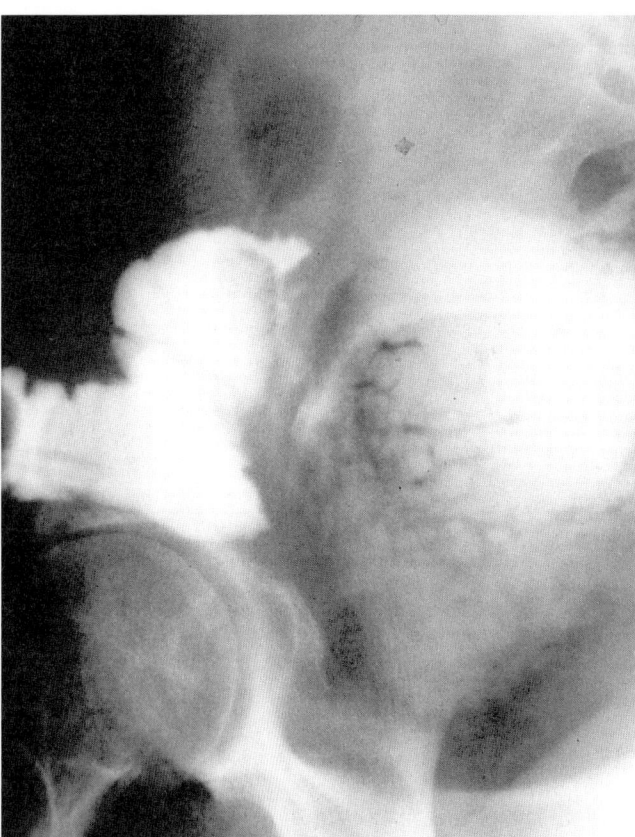

Fig. 87.2 This outlet injection demonstrates the 'L'-shaped hockey-stick deformity of an intact valve which has slipped out of the pouch. Manual digital replacement of the valve within the pouch is required prior to pouch intubation. Surgical correction and fixation is definitive treatment.

Fistulae

These can occur internally or externally and are encountered in 8–10% of patients. A fistula through the base of the valve or from the reservoir to the abdominal wound or ileostomy opening may be encountered, particularly if mesh is utilized. A fistula through the base of the valve usually causes incontinence but, unlike slippage of the valve, the patient has no difficulty with intubation. A fistula may be encountered at any time after operation. Fistulae from the reservoir to the abdominal wound or to the stoma site can be caused by a leak from full-thickness sutures used to secure the reservoir to the abdominal wall. Mesh, used to stabilize the valve, may erode at the base of the outlet and result in fistulization. Fazio and Church (1988) reported their experience in 168 patients. They encountered 17 fistulae, 12 of which required surgical revision of the continent ileostomy. In six of their 17 fistulae no associated predisposing factor could be established, whereas Crohn's disease and the mesh were considered the cause in four and three patients, respectively (Fazio & Church 1988). Treatment of valve fistulae usually consists of reoperation and excision of the valve and construction

Table 87.1 Comparison of the complications reported in various large series

Reference	No. of patients in series	Complication									
		Early				Late						
		Intest. obtruct.	Slough of valve	Anast. leakage	Mortal.	Abd. reop.	Sepsis	Valve slipp	Rec. Crohn's disease	Fistula	Rev. of stoma	Rev. of pouch
Schrock (1979)	39	2(5.1)	2(5.1)	2(5.1)	0	4(10)		13(33)	2(5.1)	2(5.1)		
Dozois et al (1980)	299 149 early	11			0	15(10)	5(3.3)	64(43)	5(3.3)	N/A	10(6.7)	5(3.3)
	150 late	9				5(3.3)	3(2)	33(22)	0		20(13)	4(2.7)
Gerber et al (1983)	100	1	2		1		2		5	5*		
Leijonmarck et al (1992)	88 (91 pouches)	13	2	2				50		2	25	21
Fazio & Church (1988)	168	13	4	3	1		12	32	15	23		61
Toronto	130 (176 pouches)	10	2(1.6)		2(1.6)		5(3.8)	36(20)		18(10)		37(28)

* All five patients with ileocolonic Crohn's disease developed a fistula
Numbers in parentheses designate percentages

of a new one using a technique similar to that described above. Fistulae are more often encountered in those patients with Crohn's disease. They tend to recur and may require pouch excision.

Intestinal obstruction

This commonly reported complication is usually secondary to adhesions and is not specific to the procedure. However, early in the postoperative period a food bolus may obstruct the indwelling catheter (Beart et al 1979). In addition there may be a volvulus of small bowel around the continent ileostomy, causing obstruction, perforation and peritonitis. The overall incidence of intestinal obstruction is 6–15%, which is comparable to the rate encountered after total proctocolectomy and conventional ileostomy.

Pouchitis

This disorder is a syndrome characterized by crampy abdominal pain, increased watery ileostomy output, bloody discharge, bloating and general malaise. In severe circumstances the condition may also be associated with weight loss, fever, arthralgias, anemia, increased sedimentation rate and low serum iron and albumin. The clinical presentation can vary from a minor flu-like illness to severe ileitis with general toxicity. The diagnosis should be considered on the basis of the history taken from the patient and confirmed by endoscopy and histology. The endoscopic appearance usually reveals various degrees of reddened edematous mucosa, with contact bleeding and sometimes numerous small ulcerations. The etiology of this condition is unknown, but its prompt response to broad-spectrum antibiotics such as metronidazole suggests it to be bacterial. Reports on the incidence of pouchitis vary considerably, from 8 to 42%. Variability in definition, small numbers of patients or short follow-up are among the possible explanations for this wide range of incidence reports. The risk of developing an episode of pouchitis seems to be highest during the first 2 years after surgery, and patients who have not experienced an episode during the first 4–5 years following surgery are likely to represent a low-risk group (Svaninger et al 1993).

Valve necrosis

This complication is attributed to ischemia resulting from excision of peritoneum and fat from the mesentery of the segment of ileum forming the valve, or to the placement of staples across the mesentery supplying the nipple valve (Palmu & Sivula 1978, Goligher 1980).

Volvulus of the reservoir

Volvulus of the pouch has been described owing to imperfect closure of the lateral gutter and the paraileostomy space, which may result in rotation and necrosis of the pouch. It is therefore of the utmost importance to fix the reservoir circumferentially to the anterior abdominal wall, and to close the paraileostomy space (Arges et al 1981).

Crohn's disease and the continent ileostomy

Crohn's disease may recur in the reservoir, necessitating its ultimate excision. Series from several institutions suggest that the complication rate among patients with Crohn's disease is significantly higher than in patients undergoing this procedure for chronic ulcerative colitis. In the Mayo Clinic series the rate of excision of the reservoir was markedly reduced following better selection of patients, and exclusion of those with Crohn's disease from having this procedure performed (Dozois et al 1980). In Myrvold and Kock's review of their 52 patients who had continent ileostomies with Crohn's disease, two mortalities due to complicated Crohn's disease were encountered. In eight patients the pouch had to be removed owing to postoperative complications, recurrence of Crohn's disease, enterocutaneous fistula and ileus (Myrvold & Kock 1981). In Fazio and Church's report, Crohn's disease in the pouch occurred in 15 patients (9%), 11 of whom were referred after proctocolectomy or continent ileostomy construction had been performed elsewhere; three of the remaining four had originally presented with toxic megacolon. Crohn's disease manifested itself as pouchitis in 11 patients (recurrent in six) and fistulae in four. Treatment consisted of removal of the pouch in eight and systemic and topical steroids in six (Fazio & Church 1988). In Gerber's (1983) series 16 patients with Crohn's disease were operated upon. Five of these had ileocolonic disease and the remaining 11 had pure colonic disease. All five patients with ileocolonic disease developed fistulae postoperatively, whereas all patients with pure colonic involvement with Crohn's disease did well (Gerber et al 1983). Bloom et al have carefully selected for the operation patients with quiescent Crohn's disease, who have been off medications for 5 years, and have produced good results (Bloom et al 1986). The mainstay of treatment of this complication is to avoid its occurrence by carefully selecting the patients for the continent ileostomy procedure and not to perform it in patients with histologically established Crohn's disease, or in those who are clinically suspected of having Crohn's disease despite a histological diagnosis of ulcerative colitis. In cases where Crohn's disease is diagnosed after construction of the pouch and complications are encountered, excision of the pouch may have to be considered.

Outflow tract problems

Stenosis and stricture of the outflow tract usually occur at the skin level. These complications can also occur at the junction of the afferent limb and the pouch. If symptomatic, the patient may require a skin-level revision or a resection (strictureplasty) of the bowel. Prolapse and eversion of the valve with incontinence and foreshortening, or loss of adequate length of the ileal outflow tract, are further complications encountered.

Prolapse of the valve results in incontinence. It occurs in the presence of a large discrepancy between the diameter of the outflow tract at the base of the valve, where the pouch meets the abdominal wall, and the diameter of the ileostomy itself. Fascia and mesh have been used to stabilize the circumference and to ensure a constant diameter. Stretching of the abdominal wall, as in excessive weight gain or pregnancy, may result in prolapse of the valve because of a larger than normal stomal aperture. To deal with this troublesome but infrequent problem, surgical intervention is often necessary. In these situations the pouch is opened and the valve secured in its normal position. In addition, if warranted, the stomal aperture should be made smaller (Fazio & Church 1988, Gottlieb & Handelsman 1991).

COMPARISON WITH OTHER PROCEDURES

Leijonmarck et al (1992) recently reviewed their results with 514 patients who underwent colectomy for ulcerative colitis. Twenty-two of their patients died following colectomy, and in nine patients Crohn's disease was diagnosed in a later review. Of the 483 patients remaining after excluding the above 31 patients, only 33% had not been admitted for further surgery during the study period.

Intestinal obstruction

Intestinal obstruction was a frequent complication requiring surgery, the cumulative, probabilities for intestinal obstruction being 11% after 2 years and 23% after 15 years, irrespective of the procedure performed. The annual risk of a first small-bowel obstruction was 1 in 25 for patients having had a pelvic pouch, 1 in 49 in patients with a continent pouch, 1 in 71 in patients with a colectomy and ileorectal anastomosis, and 1 in 66 for patients with a total proctocolectomy and conventional Brooke ileostomy. Watts et al reported an incidence of 2–3% per year for the first 3 years after proctocolectomy (Watts et al 1966). In a review of reports of small-intestinal obstructions after ileorectal anastomosis or total proctocolectomy and Brooke ileostomy by François et al, the rate of small-bowel obstruction requiring surgery varied from 5 to 17%, and the incidence of small-bowel obstruction requiring surgery after a pelvic pouch procedure ranged from 5 to 30% (François et al 1989). In the study by Leijonmarck et al the probability of a first small-bowel obstruction was as high as 23% after 15 years (Leijonmarck et al 1992).

Ileostomy dysfunction

Another late surgical complication following total proctocolectomy is ileostomy dysfunction in the form of retraction or stenosis of the stoma. Carlstedt et al reported their results with 104 patients treated by proctocolectomy: the probability of a first ileostomy revision was reported to be 40% after 8 years (Carlstedt et al 1987). Jacob et al reported an ileostomy revision rate of 44% after 9 years (Jacob et al 1969). Leijonmarck et al reported 99 ileostomy revisions in 70 (16%) of 437 patients who had 450 Brooke ileostomies constructed, and calculated a cumulative probability of a first ileostomy revision of 19% at 15 years (Leijonmarck et al 1992).

Revision rates

A study from the Mayo Clinic showed that the probability of a first revision of a Kock pouch was 35% after 2 years (Dozois et al 1980). The findings of Leijonmarck et al show an even higher rate of revision after Kock pouch, with a 52% probability of a first revision after 2 years. Lack of surgical experience has been incriminated. Kock reported only a 10% revision rate with the technique of stapling of the nipple valve, and it seems that after 5 years with a well-functioning Kock pouch the need for revision is very low (Kock et al 1985). The revision and excision rate for the pelvic pouch are much lower according to Leijonmarck's data from Sweden, and our data from Toronto. Fazio and Tjandra described a technique for nipple valve fixation. In addition to the two to three longitudinal stapled rows applied to the nipple valve, a 2 cm transverse enterotomy is made in the anterior pouch wall, just beyond the point where the intussuscepted nipple would comfortably lie. The nipple valve is then aligned to the anterior pouch wall away from the main anterior suture line. A single application of a linear stapler without a knife blade was used to anchor the nipple valve to the anterior pouch wall. The anvil of the stapler was brought through the transverse enterotomy from outside the pouch to pass along the inside of the nipple valve to effect a stapled anchorage. This stapled three layers of the bowel: the anterior wall of the pouch and two layers of the intussuscepted nipple. This procedure was carried out on 31 patients, with a mean follow-up of 20 months, and there has been no subsequent slippage or necrosis of the nipple valve (Fazio & Tjandra 1992).

Pouchitis

Svaninger et al (1993) prospectively studied the incidence and characteristics of pouchitis in 84 patients with a continent ileostomy and 96 patients with a pelvic pouch. Median follow-up for the Kock pouch patients was 8.5 years and for pelvic pouch patients 5 years. Pouchitis, with symptoms severe enough to require treatment, was encountered in 33% of continent ileostomy patients and in 47% of pelvic pouch patients. The cumulative risk of developing one or more episodes of pouchitis over a 5-year follow-up was 34% in continent ileostomy patients and 51% in pelvic pouch patients. The median time of the first appearance of pouchitis was 5 and 12 months, respectively. Eighty-six percent of continent ileostomy patients with pouchitis and 71% of pelvic pouch patients experienced their initial episode of pouchitis within the first 2 years after surgery. Most of the patients responded promptly to metronidazole treatment. Eighteen percent of the continent ileostomy group and 6% of the pelvic pouch group had long-lasting episodes, with poor response to treatment. However, in that study only three patients had their pouch removed because of treatment failure (Svaninger et al 1993).

Evacuation frequency and continence

In almost 90% of the patients in whom a continent ileostomy is constructed complete continence is achieved. McLeod and Fazio reported the Cleveland Clinic experience with 71 patients having a Kock pouch, and found that patients emptied their pouch on average 3.2 times daily (McLeod & Fazio 1984). Köhler et al from the Mayo Clinic, reported that in their group of 313 Kock pouch patients the pouch was emptied a median of five times per day. Patients who had a conventional Brooke ileostomy had to empty their appliances six times a day, and patients with ileal pouch–anal anastomosis had a median stool frequency of six per 24 hours, including one at night. Among patients with ileal pouch–anal anastomosis, 77% reported no incontinence during the day, whereas 22% reported one to two episodes per week and 1% reported more than twice a week (Köhler et al 1991).

Dietary restriction

In both the Cleveland Clinic and the Mayo Clinic studies, Kock pouch patients experienced dietary restriction. According to the Mayo Clinic series, 46% of patients with the continent ileostomy experienced restriction in food intake, compared to the Brooke ileostomy group (28%) and to the ileal pouch–anal anastomosis group (22%). The Cleveland Clinic study, however, suggests that in their patients the restrictions in diet were similar in frequency and severity to those experienced by patients with conventional ileostomies.

Regarding the type of operation, no differences were found concerning attitude and overall satisfaction. However, in the Mayo Clinic study, of the patients who had knowledge of alternative procedures, more with conventional ileostomies (39%) and Kock pouches (14%) desired changes than did those with ileal pouch–anal anastomosis.

Quality of life

In a recent study comparing quality of life between Brooke ileostomy, Kock pouch and ileal pouch–anal anastomosis, Kock pouch patients performed better than their Brooke ileostomy counterparts in terms of sports and sexual activity (Köhler et al 1991). This might be supported by the study of Nilsson et al, who reported that 98% of their patients had felt embarrassed or inhibited by the conventional ileostomy, but only 24% had these feeling after conversion to continent ileostomy. Eighty percent thought that their sexual lives were disturbed by the conventional ileostomy, whereas none of them felt inhibited by the

Kock pouch (Nilsson et al 1981). Ojerskog et al reported that 64% of their patients felt that their overall sexual satisfaction was improved after construction of a continent ileostomy (Ojerskog et al 1988). In the Cleveland Clinic series, 80% of the patients felt that their body image was improved after conversion of their conventional ileostomies to continent ileostomies. However, in Köhler's study patients with ileal pouch–anal anastomosis scored higher than both Brooke ileostomy and Kock pouch patients, in terms of sports and sexual activity. The main reason for this difference is likely to be the stoma itself, although the appliance, leakage, odor and noise of the Brooke ileostomy were eliminated by the Kock pouch.

Most surveys have estimated quality of life using mailed or interviewer-administered questionnaires, in which measurements were not quantitative, but McLeod et al recently assessed quality of life of patients with ulcerative colitis preoperatively and postoperatively using the time trade-off technique and the direct questioning of objectives. These tests provide a global quantitative assessment of quality of life. Patients with conventional ileostomies were compared to these with Kock continent ileostomies or ileal pouch–anal anastomoses, taking into consideration their physical, social and emotional wellbeing. In this study the quality of life was high in all three groups of patients, with mean utilities ranging from 0.87 to 0.97, irrespective of the surgical procedure performed (McLeod et al 1991).

CONCLUSIONS

Overall satisfaction with the Kock pouch is high, despite the multitude of complications which can occur. It is a useful procedure in selected patients, and in particular in those who seek an alternative to a conventional ileostomy. Presentation of all options to ulcerative colitis patients is essential. Specific knowledge of reconstructive surgery for Kock pouch patients is also mandatory. Patients with a well-functioning Kock pouch can expect an excellent quality of life with an appliance-free existence. The only major disadvantage apart from the risk of complications is of mucus discharge from the exit conduit, which can be troublesome.

REFERENCES

Arges M V, Dozois R R, Beahrs O H 1981 Volvulus of the Kock pouch with obstruction and perforation: a case report. Australia and New Zealand Journal of Surgery; 51: 311–313

Bargen J A 1956 Complications and problems associated with the management of ulcerative colitis. Gastroenterologica 86: 674–683

Beart R W, Beahrs O H, Kelly K A, Dozois R R, Wolf S A 1979 The continent ileostomy. A viable alternative. Mayo Clinic Proceedings 54: 643–645

Bloom R J, Larsen C P, Watt R, Oberhelman H A 1986 A reappraisal of the Kock continent ileostomy in patients with Crohn's disease. Surgery, Gynecology and Obstetrics 162: 105–108

Brooke B N 1952 The management of an ileostomy, including its complications. Lancet ii: 102–104

Carlstedt A, Fasth S, Hultén L, Nordgren S, Palselius I 1987 Long term ileostomy complications in patients with ulcerative colitis and Crohn's disease. International Journal of Colorectal Disease 2: 22–25

Cranley B 1983 The Kock reservoir ileostomy: a review of its development, problems and role in modern surgical practice. British Journal of Surgery 70: 94–99

Dozois R R, Kelly K A, Beart R W, Beahrs O H 1980 Improved results with continent ileostomy. Annals of Surgery 192: 319–324

Dozois R R, Kelly K A, Ilstrup D, Beart R W, Beahrs O H 1981 Factors affecting revision rate after continent ileostomy. Archives of Surgery 116: 610–613

Fazio V W, Church J M 1988 Complications and function of the continent ileostomy at the Cleveland Clinic. World Journal of Surgery 12: 148–154

Fazio V W, Tjandra J J 1992 Technique for nipple valve fixation to prevent valve slippage in continent ileostomy. Diseases of the Colon and Rectum 35: 1177–1179

François Y, Dozois R R, Kelly K A et al 1989 Small intestinal obstruction complicating ileal pouch–anal anastomosis. Annals of Surgery 209: 46–50

Gelernt I M, Baner J J, Kreel I 1977 The reservoir ileostomy. Early experience with 54 patients. Annals of Surgery 185: 179–184

Gerber A, Apt M K, Craig P H 1983 The Kock continent ileostomy. Surgery, Gynecology and Obstetrics 156: 345–350

Goligher J C 1980 Surgery of the anus, rectum and colon, 4th edn. Baillière Tindall, London, p 782

Gottlieb L M, Handelsman J C 1991 Treatment of outflow tract problems associated with continent ileostomy (Kock pouch). Report of six cases. Diseases of the Colon and Rectum 34: 936–940

Handelsman J C, Gottlieb L M, Hamilton S R 1993 Crohn's disease as a contraindication to Kock pouch (continent ileostomy). Diseases of the Colon and Rectum 36: 840–843

Jacob R A, Pace W G, Thomford N R 1969 The hazards of permanent ileostomy. Archives of Surgery 99: 549–552

Kock N G 1971 Ileostomy without external appliances: a survey of 25 patients provided with intra-abdominal intestinal reservoir. Annals of Surgery 173: 545–550

Kock N G, Darle N, Hultén L, Kewenter J, Myrvold H E, Philipson B 1977 Ileostomy. Current Problems in Surgery 24. 1–52

Kock N G, Myrvold H E, Nilsson L O, Ahrén C 1980a Construction of a stable valve for the continent ileostomy. Annales Chirurgiae Gynecologica 69: 132–143

Kock N G, Myrvold H E, Nilsson L O 1980b Progress report on the continent ileostomy. World Journal of Surgery 4: 143–148

Kock N G, Myrvold H E, Nilsson L O, Philipson B M 1985 Achtzehn Jahre mit der Kontinenten Ileostomie. Chirurgie 56: 299–304

Köhler L W, Pemberton J H, Zinsmeister A R, Kelly K A 1991 Quality of life after proctocolectomy. A comparison of Brooke ileostomy, Kock pouch and ileal pouch–anal anastomosis. Gastroenterology 101: 679–684

Leijonmarck C E, Liljeqvist L, Poppen B, Hellers G 1992 Surgery after colectomy for ulcerative colitis. Diseases of the Colon and Rectum 35: 495–502

McLeod R S 1993 Chronic ulcerative colitis. Traditional surgical techniques. Surgical Clinics of North America 73: 891–908

McLeod R S, Fazio V W 1984 Quality of life with continent ileostomy. World Journal of Surgery 8: 90–95

McLeod R S, Churchill D N, Lock A M, Vanderburgh S, Cohen Z 1991 Quality of life of patients with ulcerative colitis preoperatively and postoperatively. Gastroenterology 101: 1307–1313

Myrvold H E 1987 The continent ileostomy. World Journal of Surgery 11: 720–726

Myrvold H E, Kock N G 1981 Continent ileostomy in patients with Crohn's disease. Gastroenterology 80: 1237

Nilsson L O, Kock N G, Kylberg F, Myrvold H E, Palselius I 1981 Sexual adjustment in ileostomy patients before and after conversion to continent ileostomy. Diseases of the Colon and Rectum 24: 287–290

Ojerskog B, Hallstrom T, Kock N G, Myrvold H E 1988 Quality of life in ileostomy patients with ulcerative colitis before and after conversion to the continent ileostomy. International Journal of Colorectal Disease 3: 166–170

Palmu A, Sivula A 1978 Kock's continent ileostomy: results of 51 operations and experiences with correction of nipple valve insufficiency. British Journal of Surgery 65: 645–648

Schrock T R 1979 Complications of continent ileostomy. American Journal of Surgery 138: 162–169

Steichen F M 1977 The creation of autologous substitute organs with stapling instruments. American Journal of Surgery 134: 659–673

Svaninger G, Nordgren S, Öresland T, Hultén L 1993 Incidence and characteristics of pouchitis in Kock continent ileostomy and the pelvic pouch. Scandinavian Journal of Gastroenterology 28: 695–700

Thompson J P S, Lennard-Jones J E 1977 Life with an ileostomy. Part III. Clinical Gastroenterology 6: 699–708

Watts J M, deDombal F T, Goligher J C 1966 Early results of surgery for ulcerative colitis. British Journal of Surgery 53: 1005–1014

88. Surgical options – ileoanal pouch

P. A. Dean   R. R. Dozois

INTRODUCTION

Chronic ulcerative colitis is an inflammatory disease of the mucosa limited to the colon and rectum, which varies in severity from an intermittent mild process requiring little or no treatment, to an acute fulminant life-threatening process demanding intensive emergency therapy. The disease may involve the rectum only (ulcerative proctitis), or extend more proximally to involve part or all of the colon. Management of patients with ulcerative colitis is determined by several factors, including the extent, severity and duration of disease; response and tolerance to medication; patient age and comorbid conditions; and preference regarding surgical therapy. Although there is no specific medical treatment for ulcerative colitis, a wide variety of non-specific immunosuppressive and anti-inflammatory agents are available to control the disease activity. Medical treatment adequately controls the disease in many patients, although eventual failure of medical therapy and the long-term risk of cancer may lead to the consideration of surgical alternatives for some patients (Farmer et al 1993).

The underlying rationale for surgical treatment of ulcerative colitis is that since the disease is confined to the large bowel, proctocolectomy is uniquely curative. Reluctance to consider curative surgery for ulcerative colitis by patients and referring physicians in the past has been based on the unacceptability of a conventional incontinent ileostomy (Brooke ileostomy). Fear of the ileostomy and its social, physical and psychological consequences has often caused significant delay in surgical treatment, in spite of strong indications. These fears have been addressed with advances in the understanding of the role of surgery, newer surgical sphincter-saving and continence techniques, and improvement in the care of stomas, which improves the quality of life for patients after proctocolectomy. There are now several established surgical options for patients with ulcerative colitis, including the traditional proctocolectomy with Brooke ileostomy, the continent ileostomy (Kock pouch), subtotal colectomy with ileorectal anastomosis, and ileal pouch–anal anastomosis (ileoanal pouch).

Of the many surgical options available the ileoanal pouch procedure comes closest to the ideal: safe removal of the disease, preservation of physiologic anorectal function, and restoration of normal lifestyle (Kelly et al 1992). Complete removal of the colon, rectum and proximal anal mucosa effectively eliminates the disease in patients with ulcerative colitis. The creation of an ileal pouch anastomosed to the anal canal provides an adequate fecal reservoir capacity and voluntary transanal defecation with fecal continence not offered by the other surgical options following proctocolectomy for ulcerative colitis. In addition, since the distal rectum is removed transanally, the chance of damage to the innervation of the bladder and genitalia is minimized and a perineal wound with its associated healing difficulties is avoided. For a complex and varied disease such as ulcerative colitis no single surgical procedure will be suitable for every patient, and all viable options should be considered for a given patient and the choice based on the patient's lifestyle, expectations, needs and preference. Because it cures the disease and avoids a permanent ileostomy, however, the ileoanal pouch is currently the operation of choice for most patients with ulcerative colitis.

This chapter discusses the factors affecting selection of the ileoanal pouch procedure, in the context of other surgical options, for patients with ulcerative colitis considering a surgical cure of their disease. Appropriate indications, as well as relative and absolute contraindications for this procedure, are presented. The functional outcome, potential problems with the ileoanal pouch, and quality of life issues (discussed in detail in subsequent chapters) are presented here for comparison with alternative surgical and medical treatments, in an attempt to facilitate the therapeutic decisions for each individual patient.

PATIENT SELECTION

Surgical treatment of ulcerative colitis is considered for

complications of the disease or failure of medical treatment, and the ileoanal pouch procedure is generally considered the operation of choice because it removes the disease and preserves anal defecation and continence. This procedure is more complex than other options, and careful consideration must be given to selecting the appropriate patients to provide an acceptable outcome. The ileoanal pouch procedure is usually performed in two stages (Ballantyne et al 1985). First, proctocolectomy is performed and an ileal pouch is created and anastomosed to the anal canal, with a temporary diverting loop ileostomy. At a second stage, typically 2–3 months later, the ileostomy is closed, restoring intestinal continuity. In carefully selected patients the procedure can be safely completed in one stage (Galandiuk et al 1991, Cohen et al 1992, Grobler et al 1992); conversely, acutely ill or debilitated patients may require a three-stage procedure. Consideration should be given to the overall health of the patient before selection of this complex procedure over other, simpler alternatives.

Indications

The ileoanal pouch may be considered whenever surgery is indicated for ulcerative colitis. The most common indication is intractable ulcerative colitis that has failed to respond adequately to medical therapy (Farmer et al 1993). Although the initial response rate for intensive medical treatment is good for mild to moderate disease (Jarnerot et al 1985), surgery is needed in one-quarter of patients by 5 years and in one-third after 10 years of medical therapy (Farmer et al 1993). Some patients will be unresponsive, or have an inadequate response, to medical treatment. In others the response to treatment may be adequate, but excessive doses of steroids may be required to maintain the response. Still other patients will experience complications or intolerable side effects related to medication, or be non-compliant with medical regimens (Kusunoki et al 1992). Lifestyle choices and medical costs may lead some patients to request surgical therapy in long-standing disease (Hay & Hay 1992).

Complications of ulcerative colitis are the next most common indication for surgical therapy, and include both acute life-threatening complications and chronic sequelae of the disease process. Fulminant colitis, toxic megacolon, colonic perforation and massive hemorrhage are severe, but fortunately uncommon, complications of ulcerative colitis that require urgent or emergency surgical therapy to minimize mortality (Greenstein et al 1985, Hawley 1988, Robert et al 1990). Because of the severity of disease, colectomy and ileostomy is the procedure of choice in most of these patients, and few if any should be offered a primary ileoanal pouch procedure (Hawley 1988). If proctectomy is not required in the emergency situation, however, the rectum should be preserved to allow the possibility of subsequent proctectomy with endorectal mucosectomy and ileoanal pouch as a two- or three-stage procedure in an appropriate candidate (Greenstein et al 1985, Hawley 1988, Penna et al 1993).

One of the most dreaded intestinal complications of ulcerative colitis is the development of colon cancer. With the increasing risk of cancer in patients who have extensive and long-standing disease (Kewenter et al 1978, Ekbom et al 1990), there is general agreement that after patients have had the disease for 8–10 years they are candidates for either prophylactic proctocolectomy or a close surveillance program (Nugent et al 1991). Surveillance programs are not without problems, since they require frequent (biannual) colonoscopy, abnormal areas of mucosa may be missed, and dysplasia may not always precede carcinoma (Ransohoff et al 1985, Taylor et al 1992). Total colectomy with ileorectal anastomosis is a poor surgical approach for this indication, since cancer may still develop in the rectum (Baker et al 1978). Given the expense and difficulties associated with surveillance, the ileoanal pouch is an acceptable alternative to surveillance in long-standing ulcerative colitis.

Other, less frequent complications of chronic ulcerative colitis may be indications for an ileoanal pouch procedure. Chronic recurrent hemorrhage necessitating repeated blood transfusion can be alleviated with a proctocolectomy and ileoanal pouch. Many patients with ulcerative colitis have extraintestinal manifestations of their disease, and some of these, such as migratory arthritis, skin changes and uveitis, will improve following proctocolectomy, and are an indication for proctocolectomy with ileoanal pouch reconstruction. Other extraintestinal manifestations, such as ankylosing spondylitis, rheumatoid arthritis (Gravallese & Kantrowitz 1988) and primary sclerosing cholangitis (Cangemi et al 1989), are not usually affected by proctocolectomy, although ileoanal pouch is not contraindicated when these manifestations are present. Because of portal hypertension and parastomal varices, ileoanal pouch is in fact the procedure of choice in patients with primary sclerosing cholangitis and ulcerative colitis requiring surgical treatment (Fucini et al 1991, Kartheuser et al 1993).

Contraindications

Although the ileoanal pouch provides excellent functional results the procedure is not for every patient with ulcerative colitis. Since the ileoanal pouch is designed to restore continent anal defecation, the most important contraindication is ineffective anal sphincter function. Patients should be carefully assessed preoperatively to ensure competency of anal sphincter function and adequate continence. Since most patients with ulcerative colitis have frequent liquid stools, similar to those following the ileoanal pouch procedure, this is usually easy to determine with a careful history, although in selected cases anorectal manometry may be useful. This is particularly true in older patients (> 50 years), women with a history of multiple pregnancies and/or difficult deliveries, and patients with diminished sphincter tone on digital rectal examination.

Patients with Crohn's colitis do poorly after ileoanal pouch construction, and known or active Crohn's disease at the time of proctocolectomy is an absolute contraindication (Deutsch et al 1991). The ability to distinguish Crohn's disease from ulcerative colitis is often difficult, however, and approximately 5% of patients operated on for colitis will be classified as 'indeterminate colitis' (Pezim et al 1989). These patients do not appear to differ from patients with ulcerative colitis after ileoanal pouch, therefore 'indeterminate colitis' should not necessarily constitute a contraindication to the procedure.

Cancer of the rectum or anus at the time of proctocolectomy poses a special problem. If the cancer is in the distal rectum or anus, mucosectomy with anal preservation will not provide adequate oncologic margins, and ileoanal pouch is contraindicated. Patients with cancer in the mid rectum, for whom postoperative radiation therapy is a consideration, may also have a poor outcome if the ileoanal pouch is placed and subjected to radiation, making these patients poor candidates for the procedure. These two groups of patients are better suited for proctocolectomy with Brooke or continent ileostomy (Kock pouch) to provide optimum cancer treatment. In contrast, for those patients with early cancers of the mid rectum or cancer of the more proximal large bowel, ileoanal pouch appears to be an acceptable option at the time of proctocolectomy (Taylor et al 1988), although the proctectomy should be more radical than in normal patients with ulcerative colitis to provide an optimal oncologic resection.

Ileoanal pouch is technically more difficult to perform and physiologically more demanding to the patient than some of the other surgical alternatives, and for these reasons several patient-related factors offer a relative contraindication to this particular procedure. Older patients should be carefully selected based on general overall health and anal sphincter function. Older patients generally experience deterioration of the anal continence mechanism, and the larger volume of softer stool resulting from an ileoanal pouch may lead to troublesome fecal incontinence. Children and young adults have excellent results following ileoanal pouch construction (Telander et al 1990), and with careful selection patients over 50 years of age may have nearly as good a result (Lewis et al 1993). Patients over the age of 65, however, are less likely to be good candidates and may be better suited to one of the other surgical procedures available for ulcerative colitis.

Other patient-related factors in addition to age may be relative contraindications to an ileoanal pouch procedure. Short obese patients and very tall patients represent a technical challenge in that the small-bowel mesentery may not allow the pouch to reach the anal canal. Long periods of heavy steroid use or malnutrition may also result in suboptimal outcomes (Scott et al 1988). Patients who are psychologically impaired, emotionally unstable, unmotivated or non-compliant may have difficulty adjusting to the physiologic changes associated with an ileoanal pouch, and should be carefully evaluated before deciding on the best surgical therapy. More frequent bowel movements and occasional minor leakage may create difficult problems for patients with limited access to toilet facilities and so occupational concerns should be taken into account in choosing surgical therapy. However, these factors should not necessarily preclude attempted ileoanal pouch in an otherwise acceptable candidate.

CLINICAL OUTCOME

Although the ileoanal pouch is the newest surgical option for the treatment of ulcerative colitis, it has been extensively analyzed since its widespread use began in 1980, with the results from several thousand patients reported in more than 20 published series. Because the ileoanal pouch is safe, restores intestinal continuity with the normal route of defecation, and cures the disease, it has become the preferred procedure for most patients requiring surgery for ulcerative colitis. The safety, potential complications, functional outcomes and patient satisfaction are outlined below for comparison with other surgical and medical therapeutic options. These results are discussed in greater detail in subsequent chapters.

Operative results

Mortality

The ileoanal pouch procedure is very safe, with only rare deaths being reported. Overall mortality in large series ranges from 0 to 1% (Table 88.1), in spite of the fact that the ileoanal pouch is a complex, often multistage procedure typically performed on malnourished, debilitated, immunosuppressed patients with complications of ulcerative colitis. In our own series of over 1500 ileoanal pouch

Table 88.1 Operative morbidity and mortality following ileoanal pouch procedures

Reference	No. of patients	Morbidity (%)	Mortality (%)
Becker & Raymond (1986)	100	13	0
Oresland et al (1989)	100	24	0
Wexner et al (1990)	180	50	0
Cohen et al (1992)	483	19	0
Grotz & Pemberton (1993)	1400	39	0.1
Marcello et al (1993)	460	58	0.4

procedures at the Mayo Clinic in the last 12 years we have had only two postoperative deaths. Mortality is similar for proctocolectomy with either Brooke or Kock pouch ileostomy (Schrock 1979, McLeod 1993), and for colectomy and ileorectal anastomosis (Oakley et al 1985), as would be expected since a major common denominator in each surgery is the extirpative proctocolectomy.

Morbidity

In contrast to mortality, the considerable morbidity following ileoanal pouch procedures has been a continued source of concern (Table 88.1). The overall complication rates ranging from 13 to 58% are reported in the literature. Although this may reflect in part the debilitated and immunosuppressed condition of many patients undergoing the operation (Scott et al 1988), many complications, such as bowel obstruction, are related primarily to operative manipulation, and suggest that the rate of complications should be taken into account when opting for surgical therapy for ulcerative colitis. High complication rates are not unique to this particular procedure, with similar complication rates for proctocolectomy and Brooke ileostomy or Kock pouch (Fazio & Church 1988, Schrock 1979, McLeod 1993). Oakley et al (1985) reported a lower major complication rate of 8% for colectomy and ileorectal anastomosis, but an additional 9% were unable to have their temporary ileostomy closed owing to persistent disease.

Postoperative complications typically occurring in patients following ileoanal pouch procedures are shown in Table 88.2.

Obstruction

The most frequent complication encountered is small-bowel obstruction, which occurs in 10–22% of patients (François et al 1989, Fischer et al 1993, Marcello et al 1993) and requires reoperation in slightly less than half of these. Obstruction in this setting is most often due to problems at the ileostomy site or adhesions, and the risk of obstruction is greater in patients who have had a previous operation (François et al 1989). Serious pelvic infections develop in 5–6% of patients (Pemberton et al 1987, Marcello et al 1993). Approximately half of these require surgical treatment for the infection, and pouch failure and excision is high in this group (Scott et al 1988). Wound infections and urinary retention are uncommon, and rarely cause serious long-term problems (Pemberton et al 1987).

Most patients undergoing proctocolectomy with ileoanal pouch reconstruction have a temporary diverting ileostomy, and such patients are subject to a second set of complications following ileostomy closure. Again, small-bowel obstruction is the most common complication after closure of the ileostomy (Pemberton et al 1987, Salemans et al 1992). Most of these bowel obstructions are caused by adhesions (François et al 1989), and approximately half of these will require operative treatment.

Anastomotic leakage

Another complication occurring after ileostomy closure is anastomotic leakage, with an incidence of 2–3% (Pemberton et al 1987, Fischer et al 1993), which may require a repeat temporary ileostomy but with eventual restoration of intestinal continuity. These problems are also associated with proctocolectomy and Kock pouch (Schrock 1979) or ileorectostomy (Oakley et al 1985), but are much less common after proctocolectomy and Brooke ileostomy alone (Phillips et al 1989).

Although these complications pose a significant problem for patients undergoing an ileoanal pouch procedure, they are spared the risk of some of the serious postoperative complications following other forms of surgical therapy for ulcerative colitis. Patients having a total proctocolectomy with either Brooke ileostomy or Kock pouch have a significant risk of perineal wound complications (McLeod 1993), and these wounds may take months to years to heal completely (Morowitz & Kirsner 1981). Anastomotic leakage is not uncommon following colectomy with ileorectal anastomosis, often resulting in the need for further surgical intervention (Oakley et al 1985, Backer et al 1988). It should be kept in mind that although each

Table 88.2 Complications following ileoanal pouch procedure and ileostomy closure

Reference	No. of patients	Small-bowel obstruction (%)	Sepsis/leak (%)	Wound infection (%)
Becker & Raymond (1986)	100	15	8	0
Pemberton et al (1987)	390	22	7	3
Oresland et al (1989)	100	6	13	–
Wexner et al (1990)	180	11	7	4
de Silva et al (1991)	61	11	7	4
McMullen et al (1991)	73	16	5	–
Cohen et al (1992)	483	–	18	–
Fischer et al (1993)	205	12	2	–
Marcello et al (1993)	460	20	8	10

therapeutic surgical alternative for ulcerative colitis is associated with a small risk of complication, the underlying disease itself is subject to significant morbidity with medical therapy alone, particularly in the type of patient often selected for surgical management (McLeod et al 1991, Farmer et al 1993).

Long-term results

The ileoanal pouch procedure has been performed extensively in many centers for more than 12 years, and the functional results of patients undergoing proctocolectomy and ileoanal pouch have been studied in depth. Both the early and late overall functional results are good, with few patients requiring a permanent ileostomy and thus failing the procedure, even 10 years later (McIntyre et al 1994). The majority of failures occur within 1 year of the procedure (Pemberton et al 1987), and most late failures are associated with evidence of Crohn's disease (McIntyre et al 1994).

Physiologic changes

Extensive physiologic measurements of the ileoanal pouch have been made to assess the alterations in physiologic function that occur in the pouch and the anal canal which may alter the pattern of defecation. The ileal pouch is designed to function as a neorectum, that is to say, a reservoir for stool. Testing has shown the pouch to be as distensible and capacious as a normal rectum (O'Connell et al 1987a, Oresland et al 1990). This does not appear to be determined by pouch design alone, with similar capacity being shown for the various designs of ileoanal reservoirs (de Silva et al 1991). The ileoanal pouch is able to adapt to its function as a reservoir with an increase in capacity over 1–2 years following construction (Becker et al 1991).

Reservoir emptying

Contraction and evacuation of the ileoanal pouch is an important factor in stool frequency and continence following an ileoanal anastomosis (Stryker et al 1986). The pattern of contraction in the ileoanal pouch differs from that in the normal rectum (Stryker et al 1985), with strong contractions in the pouch as it distends, rather than the relative lack of such contractions in the normal rectum. These contraction waves are associated with the urge to evacuate. In spite of these differences in the response to distension, evacuation of the ileoanal pouch is nearly as complete as that of the normal rectum (Ambroze et al 1991). An exception to this finding is that evacuation after construction of an S-pouch is significantly less effective than after other types of pouches (de Silva et al 1991), and this type of pouch is more likely to require intubation to facilitate emptying.

Sensation sphincter function

Sensation and function of the anal canal and sphincter are critical to normal anal defecation. Anal canal sensation following ileoanal pouch construction is intact enough to allow most patients to discriminate between gas, liquid or solid stool, thus facilitating continence (Pemberton et al 1987, Wexner et al 1989). Mean resting pressure of the anal canal is lower following the ileoanal pouch procedure, but returns toward normal over 1–2 years (Becker et al 1991). The anal squeeze mechanism is not usually impaired following mucosectomy, and ileoanal pouch with anal squeeze pressure is normal in most patients (Becker et al 1991). Those patients who do have a decrease in maximum squeeze pressure, however, are more likely to experience incontinence (O'Connell et al 1988). The precise role of the rectal inhibitory reflex in continence and evacuation is unclear, since O'Connell et al (1988) found that it was abolished in their patients after ileoanal pouch, whereas Becker et al (1991) found that the normal rectal inhibitory reflex may be lost early after ileoanal pouch, but returns in most patients within 1–2 years.

Pouch function

The ileoanal pouch serves to replace the rectum following proctocolectomy, and pouch function can be assessed based on the normal functions of the rectum. Extensive effort has gone into the design and construction of the pouch, as discussed in subsequent chapters. Although there are functional differences between pouch designs, these are relatively minor (de Silva et at 1991, Liljeqvist et al 1988, Nicholls & Pezim 1985). Since modification of the initial technique of Parks et al (1980), which frequently required intubation to empty, nearly all ileoanal pouches can be evacuated spontaneously (Pemberton et al 1987, Liljeqvist et al 1988). With today's techniques ileoanal pouch function is best determined by stool frequency, patterns of continence, the ability to discriminate gas from stool, and the requirement for bowel-regulating medication.

Frequency

Stool frequency is typically five to seven times per day following ileoanal pouch reconstruction (Table 88.3), including one bowel movement per night or less. The frequency of stools is higher in older patients, but there is no difference between men and women (Pemberton et al 1987, Lewis et al 1993). Daytime and night-time stool frequency may improve slightly over the first year after the procedure (Becker & Raymond 1986, Liljeqvist et al 1988, Oresland et al 1989), but remain stable thereafter for at least 10 years (McIntyre et al 1994). This early decrease in stool frequency over time is probably the

Table 88.3 Long-term stool function following ileoanal pouch procedures

Reference	No. of patients	No. stools (mean)		Gas/stool discrimination (%)	Leakage (%)		Antidiarrheal medication (%)
		Day	Night		Day	Night	
Becker & Raymond (1986)	100	5.4*	0.6	–	–	25	59
Pemberton et al (1987)	389	6.2	1.1	77	9	13	30
Liljeqvist et al (1988)	82	4.9*	–	58	–	–	58
Oresland et al (1989)	100	4.9	0.5	–	20	22	79
Wexner et al (1989)	114	5.4	1.5	–	9	24	30
Marcello et al (1993)	460	5	1	75	–	6	39
Sagar et al (1993)	103	5*	1	68	–	–	52

*Denotes stools per 24 hours in these series

result of adaptation of the pouch, with an increase in capacity during the first 2 years (Becker et al 1991).

The increased frequency of stools observed with an ileoanal pouch is probably related to an increase in stool volume after removal of the colon and rectum (O'Connell et al 1987a), and attempts to alter the fecal volume may have a significant effect on stool frequency. Dietary changes, such as the number, timing and composition of meals, can significantly affect the frequency of stools (Tyus et al 1992, Michelassi et al 1993). Some patients reduce stool output by the use of antidiarrheal medication to improve stool frequency (Emblem et al 1989), but the need for this appears to decrease with time (Pemberton et al 1987, Oresland et al 1989). Bulking agents may thicken the stool, and are also used by some patients to decrease stool frequency (Pemberton et al 1987, Mowschenson et al 1993).

Continence

Perhaps the most significant measurement of success for ileoanal pouch patients is continence. The majority of patients experience perfect or near perfect daytime continence for solid stool in all series (Table 88.3), but many will experience occasional minor leakage at night. Only rarely do patients experience gross fecal incontinence either during the day or at night. Most are able to discriminate gas from stool, and pass gas independently (Pemberton et al 1987, Wexner et al 1989, Marcello et al 1993). Nocturnal continence (Pemberton et al 1987, Becker et al 1991), the ability to distinguish gas from stool (Pemberton et al 1987) and the ability to delay defecation (Marcello et al 1993) all appear to improve with time early on, though over the long term there appears to be a slight, but not clinically significant, deterioration in continence (McIntyre et al 1994). Pemberton et al (1987) found continence problems were more common in women than men, and also that the frequency of incontinence was higher with increasing frequency of stools. Although patients over 50 years of age have a higher frequency of stools (Pemberton et al 1987), the age of the patient (at least below age 60) does not appear to affect the ability to achieve continence after ileoanal pouch (Lewis et al 1993).

Pouch function following ileoanal anastomosis compares favorably with anorectal function in medically treated ulcerative colitis patients, as shown by Sagar et al (1993). Although frequency of bowel actions was higher in ileoanal pouch patients and those using antidiarrheal medication more frequently, there was no difference in continence between the two groups. Urgency was much more common in medically treated patients with ulcerative colitis, and many required steroid use to control the disease. Similarly, Parc et al (1989) found that in spite of leaving the rectum behind, with the potential for disease, ileorectal anastomosis offered no functional advantage over the ileoanal pouch. For patients with ulcerative colitis, the ileoanal pouch procedure appears to offer long-term functional results comparable to the other options that preserve anal defecation, including medical treatment.

Late complications

Ileoanal pouch construction following total proctocolectomy involves replacing the complex physiologic functions of the normal rectum with a small-intestinal pouch not designed for this capacity, and while the vast majority of patients do well with this neorectum, complications can arise months to years after the operation. These include anastomotic stricture, fistulae, pouchitis, malignancy, and poor pouch function. Athough many of these can be treated conservatively, reoperation is required in some cases and the overall risk of pouch failure (excision or permanent ileostomy) is a consideration (Galandiuk et al 1990).

Stricture

Stricture of the pouch–anal anastomosis occurs in 4–16% of patients, and is usually the result of tension (with or without ischemia), or sepsis with anastomotic dehiscence (Fleshman et al 1988, Wexner et al 1990, de Silva et al 1991, Marcello et al 1993). These may appear either before or after closure of the ileostomy, and may be associated with outlet obstruction symptoms, diarrhea, anal pain or obstructive-type abdominal pain (Galandiuk et al 1990).

Most strictures can be treated with outpatient dilatation, often requiring anesthesia (Marcello et al 1993), although 60% need repeated dilatations and a small number may eventually require a diverting ileostomy or pouch excision (Galandiuk et al 1990).

Fistulae

Pouch fistulae occur in approximately 5% of patients (Wexner et al 1990, Marcello et al 1993), with an external opening most commonly to the perineum or vagina. Evidence of Crohn's disease should be sought, particularly in the absence of anastomotic dehiscence or stricture, which suggests a poor prognosis (Hyman et al 1991). Many fistulae can be treated with simple fistulotomy, although for deep fistulae diverting ileostomy may be required. Galandiuk et al (1990) found that pouch excision was ultimately required in 17% of patients because of persistent complications.

Pouchitis

Another difficult problem with the ileoanal pouch is pouchitis, which is essentially inflammatory disease of the ileoanal pouch. The true incidence of pouchitis is unclear owing to variations in the definition of the process, but what is clear is that the incidence rises steadily with the length of follow-up, with the most recent incidence of 31% in our series of patients (Lohmuller et al 1990). The etiology of pouchitis remains an enigma, but it appears to be disease related, with a much higher incidence in ulcerative colitis patients than familial adenomatous polyposis after ileoanal pouch. Ulcerative colitis patients with evidence of more extensive immunologic dysfunction, such as primary sclerosing cholangitis, are at an even greater risk of pouchitis (Karthcuser et al 1993). Symptoms include abdominal cramps, frequent stools, watery or bloody diarrhea, urgency, incontinence, malaise, and fever. Symptoms are usually not severe, and most patients can be treated rapidly and successfully with metronidazole (Lohmuller et al 1990). Recurrent episodes can usually be treated successfully with metronidazole or, more recently, ciprofloxacin, and pouch loss for this condition is quite uncommon. Pouchitis is also seen in patients following proctocolectomy and Kock pouch reconstruction, and this similarly responds well to conservative management with antibiotics and pouch drainage (Vernava & Goldberg 1988).

Malignancy

One of the reasons for proctocolectomy and ileoanal pouch construction in patients with ulcerative colitis is to remove the risk of malignancy by removing all of the involved bowel. Following mucosectomy and ileoanal anastomosis, however, there do appear to be small microscopic remnants of rectal mucosa retained in a minority of patients (O'Connell et al 1987b), and although rare, cancer has been observed in this rectal cuff (Stern et al 1990, Puthu et al 1992). This risk of cancer may even be slightly higher in patients in whom preservation of the entire anal transition zone with a double-stapled technique is employed, although further long-term follow-up is necessary to substantiate this supposition. This extremely low risk of cancer, however, is orders of magnitude lower than in those patients in whom the entire diseased colon is left in place, or those with an ileorectal anastomosis. The risk of cancer in medically treated patients with ulcerative colitis is 30% after 35 years with pancolitis, and even higher if ulcerative colitis began at an early age (Ekbom et al 1990). Colectomy and ileorectostomy reduce this risk by removing the majority of the susceptible bowel, but even after ileorectal anastomosis the cumulative risk of cancer is approximately 5% after 20 years, and 15% after 30 years (Baker et al 1978, Grundfest et al 1981).

Crohn's disease

Although extensive efforts are made to confirm the diagnosis of ulcerative colitis in patients undergoing proctocolectomy and ileoanal pouch reconstruction, a small number of patients will subsequently be proved to have Crohn's disease in the pouch or small bowel (Deutsch et al 1991, Hyman et al 1991). Complications are much more common in this group of patients, usually related to reactivation of the underlying disease, and excision of the pouch may be required for extensive disease or intractable symptoms (Galandiuk et al 1990). McIntyre et al (1994) found that subsequently confirmed or suspected Crohn's disease was the indication for late (< 1 year) pouch excision in 75% of cases.

Pouch failure

Eventual pouch failure (excision of the ileoanal pouch or permanent ileostomy) is infrequent in spite of these complications, occurring in only 2–12% of patients (Table 88.4). The most common reasons for pouch failure are pelvic sepsis, gross fecal incontinence and Crohn's colitis (Galandiuk et al 1990). Failure of ileoanal pouch reconstruction leads primarily to the creation of a permanent Brooke ileostomy, although a Kock pouch should be considered an option in motivated patients without Crohn's disease (Handelsman et al 1993, Hulten et al 1992).

Sexual function

As with any operative procedure in the pelvis, the impact of total proctocolectomy with or without ileoanal pouch

Table 88.4 Cumulative risk of pouch excision or permanent diverting ileostomy following ileoanal pouch procedure

Reference	No. of patients	Pouch failure (%)
Liljeqvist et al (1988)	82	5
Oresland et al (1989)	100	3
Wexner et al (1989)	114	13
de Silva et al (1991)	88	11
McMullen et al (1991)	73	3
Kelly (1992)	1193	5
Marcello et al (1993)	460	5

on sexual function is an important consideration for patients. This is particularly true in ulcerative colitis, since many of the patients who require surgery are in their reproductive years. In spite of the extent of the operation, however, sexual problems are uncommon. The incidence of postoperative sexual dysfunction is difficult to analyze, since many patients with ulcerative colitis have significant sexual dysfunction with medical management alone (Sagar et al 1993). A small percentage of patients report a deterioration in sexual function after operation (Pemberton et al 1987), but most actually report an improvement in sexual function following ileoanal pouch construction (Oresland et al 1989, Kohler et al 1991).

Men. Although sexual dysfunction occurs in over 40% of men treated medically for ulcerative colitis, serious or permanent sexual dysfunction is rare following ileoanal pouch reconstruction (Sagar et al 1993). The incidence of impotence is 0–1% in most series (Pemberton et al 1987, Wexner et al 1990, Becker et al 1991), with a slightly higher rate of retrograde ejaculation which usually resolves. Improvement is much more common than deterioration in men following ileoanal pouch reconstruction (Oresland et al 1989).

Women. Sexual dysfunction is also frequent in women treated medically for ulcerative colitis. The incidence of dyspareunia decreases following ileoanal pouch reconstruction, although it remains a problem in 7–19% of patients, rarely prohibiting intercourse (Metcalf et al 1986). Another problem occurring in women following ileoanal pouch reconstruction is leakage of stool with intercourse occurring in 3–4% of patients, which is largely improved by emptying the pouch beforehand (Pemberton et al 1987, Oresland et al 1989, Sagar et al 1993). Sexual function in both men and women appears to be better following ileoanal pouch reconstruction after proctocolectomy than either Kock pouch or Brooke ileostomy (Metcalf et al 1986, Pemberton et al 1989, Kohler et al 1991), although this may primarily represent an enhanced body image owing to the absence of an abdominal wall stoma with the ileoanal pouch.

Pregnancy and delivery. Many women undergoing surgical treatment for ulcerative colitis are in their childbearing years, and subsequent conception and safe delivery is a concern. A number of women in several large series of patients undergoing ileoanal pouch reconstruction after proctocolectomy have become pregnant and delivered a healthy child, either by cesarean section or by vaginal delivery (Nelson et al 1989, Wexner et al 1990, Becker et al 1991). Although the frequency of nocturnal stooling increased during pregnancy, neither daytime stool frequency nor continence appear to be adversely affected, and neither route of delivery appears to significantly alter postpartum pouch function (Nelson et al 1989). Based on this information, it appears that pregnancy and delivery are both possible and safe for the mother and child following proctocolectomy and ileoanal pouch reconstruction.

Quality of life

These clinical and functional data support the observation that proctocolectomy and ileoanal pouch reconstruction is a safe, effective operation that achieves its goal of removing the disease and restoring the normal route of defecation. Even though serious complication rates are low, pouch function is excellent and long-term success is high after ileoanal pouch reconstruction, these data would be meaningless if patients were not able to have a normal lifestyle after this or any other procedure for the treatment of ulcerative colitis.

Surgical versus medical therapy

Ulcerative colitis is a disease marked by a continual progression of symptoms and risks, necessitating surgical treatment in as many as 50% of patients within 10 years (Farmer et al 1993). Although the treatment of those with mild disease and minimal symptoms may remain conservative for many years, a significant number of patients are faced with the choice of surgery as their disease progresses. McLeod et al (1991) found that for patients who required surgery, the overall quality of life was improved postoperatively over the immediate preoperative status. Physical, social and emotional wellbeing was better following total proctocolectomy with either Brooke ileostomy, Kock pouch or ileoanal pouch reconstruction. Sagar et al (1993), in comparing medically treated patients with ulcerative colitis to those with proctocolectomy and ileoanal pouch, found a similar functional outcome for both groups, but significant fewer social restrictions and less depression in the group treated surgically. These results suggest that in patients with significant symptoms of ulcerative colitis, surgical therapy offers an improvement in quality of life, along with removing the disease and its associated risks.

Comparison of surgical procedures

The standard Brooke ileostomy following proctocolectomy for ulcerative colitis is well accepted, with 93% of patients happy and living a normal lifestyle (Awad et al 1993). Ileoanal pouch reconstruction is a newer, more complex alternative, and should offer an improved quality of life over that of an ileostomy to be an acceptable operation. In a direct comparison between ileostomy and ileoanal pouch reconstruction, Pemberton et al (1989) found that patient satisfaction with both procedures was excellent (93% for ileostomy, 95% for ileoanal pouch). Over 95% of ileoanal pouch patients would not prefer to change to an ileostomy, but 36% of ileostomy patients would prefer to have an ileoanal pouch, given the option. Patients with the ileoanal pouch had significant advantages over those with an ileostomy in performing daily activities such as sports, work, recreation, travel and social life.

Similar advantages can be demonstrated for ileoanal pouch reconstruction over Kock pouch reconstruction (Kohler et al 1991). Although slightly more patients were satisfied with the Kock pouch than an ileoanal pouch (98% vs. 96%), Kock pouch patients were three times more likely to have dietary restrictions, and more Kock pouch patients desired a change, given an alternative. Patients with an ileoanal pouch had better performance scores for sports and sexual activity, but were no different for other lifestyle activities. These results indicate that the presence of an abdominal stoma results in some degree of deterioration in the quality of life after proctocolectomy, and suggest that the ileoanal pouch reconstruction may provide a better alternative in the appropriately selected patient with ulcerative colitis.

The other surgical option for ulcerative colitis which does not necessitate a permanent abdominal stoma is the ileorectostomy. This procedure has functional results comparable to the ileoanal pouch reconstruction as discussed previously, and Oakley et al (1985) found that over 95% of patients experienced improved quality of life following the procedure. Direct lifestyle comparison with ileoanal pouch reconstruction is not available, although patients appear to do well after both procedures. One limitation with the ileorectostomy is the persistence of disease in the rectum, which often requires subsequent excision, either for symptoms or for cancer (Grundfest et al 1981), limiting its attractiveness to young and middle age patients with a long life expectancy.

SUMMARY

The ultimate goal of surgical therapy for ulcerative colitis is to remove the disease with as little alteration of normal physiologic functions and lifestyle as possible. A number of acceptable surgical options are available for the treatment of ulcerative colitis, and each has its unique advantages and disadvantages (Table 88.5). Abdominal colectomy and ileorectostomy, by leaving the rectal reservoir in place, maintains the normal anorectal defecation route with as little alteration as possible, and thereby avoids the need for a permanent ileostomy. This procedure does not, however, remove all the diseased bowel, and so the risks of disease recurrence and rectal cancer remain a significant problem. Continued follow-up evaluation and possibly treatment may be required. In spite of this, the procedure may be particularly useful as a temporizing measure in a young patient unwilling to accept the surgical risk of bladder or sexual dysfunction associated with removal of the rectum, or in patients unwilling to live with a permanent ileostomy who are not candidates for an ileoanal pouch.

Total proctocolectomy, on the other hand, has the advantage of removing the involved bowel entirely and thus eliminating the risk of cancer or colitis, but because of the extensive pelvic dissection and removal of the rectum is associated with a higher risk of sexual and urinary dys-

Table 88.5 Summary of surgical options for ulcerative colitis

Procedure	Benefits	Risks
Colectomy–ileorectostomy	No pelvic dissection Maintains rectal reservoir No perineal wound No stoma	Persistent proctitis Rectal cancer
Proctocolectomy–Brooke ileostomy	Removes disease Prevents cancer	Permanent stoma Perineal wound Sexual/bladder dysfunction
Proctocolectomy–Kock pouch	Removes disease Prevents cancer Controlled fecal continence	Permanent stoma Perineal wound Continent stoma complications Pouchitis Sexual/bladder dysfunction
Proctocolectomy–ileoanal pouch	Removes disease Prevents cancer No permanent stoma Continent transanal defecation	Pouchitis Sexual/bladder dysfunction

function, and requires the reconstruction of a new mechanism of fecal elimination. Of the options for reconstruction following proctocolectomy, the simplest and most reliable is Brooke ileostomy, which is tolerated well by most patients but leaves them completely and permanently incontinent and subject to the complications of an ileostomy as well as a perineal wound. This is the ideal option in an older patient with severe rectal disease, and for patients with inadequate anal sphincter function.

Total proctocolectomy with Kock pouch reconstruction is associated with all the benefits of a proctocolectomy and ileostomy but with the added advantage of maintaining fecal continence. Although an abdominal stoma is required, fecal content can be controlled. Complications involving the nipple valve are not uncommon, however, often requiring reoperation, and pouchitis occurs not infrequently, though it is usually easy to control. The perineal wound can also be a difficult healing problem, as with a Brooke ileostomy. This procedure has an important role as an option for patients who have already had a proctocolectomy but desire to have control of the fecal content, and in those patients for whom an ileoanal pouch reconstruction has been unsuccessful or is not technically possible.

Proctocolectomy with ileoanal pouch reconstruction comes closest to the ideal goal of surgical therapy for ulcerative colitis by not only removing the entire diseased bowel, but restoring the normal route of controlled, continent anal defecation as well. As discussed in this chapter, the procedure can be performed safely in most patients under the age of 65, and eliminates the need for a permanent abdominal stoma. Functional results compare favorably with those of medically treated ulcerative colitis but without the need for toxic immunosuppressive agents, and results in a near normal lifestyle for most patients. The risks of sexual and bladder dysfunction along with other complications associated with proctocolectomy are low but present, but long-term failure is less than 10%. As with the Kock pouch, pouchitis is a common, though usually easily controlled, complication. Ileoanal pouch reconstruction is the procedure of choice for most patients requiring surgery for ulcerative colitis with an intact anal sphincter mechanism, and should be considered as an alternative to long-term medical management of the disease.

REFERENCES

Ambroze W L, Pemberton J H, Bell A M et al 1991 The effect of stool consistency on rectal and neorectal emptying. Diseases of the Colon and Rectum 34: 1–7

Awad R W, El-Gohary T M, Skilton J S, Elder J B 1993 Life quality and psychological morbidity with an ileostomy. British Journal of Surgery 80: 252–253

Backer O, Hjortrup A, Kjaergaard J 1988 Evaluation of ileorectal anastomosis for the treatment of ulcerative proctocolitis. Journal of the Royal Society of Medicine 81: 210–211

Baker W N W, Glass R E, Ritchie J K, Aylett S O 1978 Cancer of the rectum following colectomy and ileorectal anastomosis for ulcerative colitis. British Journal of Surgery 65: 862–868

Ballantyne G H, Pemberton J H, Beart R W, Wolff B G, Dozois R R 1985 Ileal J pouch–anal anastomosis. Current technique. Diseases of the Colon and Rectum 28: 197–202

Becker J M, Raymond J L 1986 Ileal pouch–anal anastomosis: a single surgeon's experience with 100 consecutive cases. Annals of Surgery 204: 375–381

Becker J M, McGrath K M, Meagher M P, Parodi J E, Cunnegan D A, Soper N J 1991 Late functional adaptation after colectomy, mucosal proctectomy, and ileal pouch–anal anastomosis. Surgery 110: 718–725

Cangemi J R, Weisner R H, Beaver S J et al 1989 Effect of proctocolectomy for chronic ulcerative colitis on the natural history of primary sclerosing cholangitis. Gastroenterology 96: 790–794

Cohen Z, McLeod R S, Stephen W, Stern H S, O'Connor B, Reznick R 1992 Continuing evolution of the pelvic pouch procedure. Annals of Surgery 216: 506–511

de Silva H J, de Angelis C P, Soper N, Kettlewell M G M W, Mortensen M J, Jewell D P 1991 Clinical and functional outcome after restorative proctocolectomy. British Journal of Surgery 78: 1039–1044

Deutsch A A, McLeod R S, Cullen J, Cohen Z 1991 Results of the pelvic-pouch procedure in patients with Crohn's disease. Diseases of the Colon and Rectum 34: 475–477

Ekbom A, Helmick C, Zack M, Adami H 1990 Ulcerative colitis and colorectal cancer: a population based study. New England Journal of Medicine 323: 1228–1233

Emblem R, Stein R, Morkrid L 1989 The effect of loperamide on bowel habits and anal sphincter function in patients with ileoanal anastomosis. Scandinavian Journal of Gastroenterology 24: 1019–1024

Farmer R G, Easley K A, Rankin G B 1993 Clinical patterns, natural history, and progression of ulcerative colitis: a long-term follow-up of 1116 patients. Digestive Diseases and Sciences 38: 1137–1146

Fazio V W, Church J M 1988 Complications and function of the continent ileostomy at the Cleveland Clinic. World Journal of Surgery 12: 148–152

Fischer J E, Nussbaum M S, Martin L W et al 1993 The pull-through procedure: technical factors in influencing outcome, with emphasis on pouchitis. Surgery 114: 828–835

Fleshman J W, Cohen Z, McLeod R S, Stern H, Blair J 1988 The ileal reservoir and ileoanal anastomosis procedure: factors affecting technical and functional outcome. Diseases of the Colon and Rectum 31: 10–16

François Y, Dozois R R, Kelly K A et al 1989 Small intestinal obstruction complicating ileal pouch–anal anastomosis. Annals of Surgery 209: 46–50

Fucini C, Wolff B G, Dozois R R 1991 Bleeding from peristomal varices: perspectives on prevention and treatment. Diseases of the Colon and Rectum 34: 1073–1078

Galandiuk S, Scott N A, Dozois R R et al 1990 Ileal pouch–anal anastomosis: reoperation for pouch-related complications. Annals of Surgery 212: 446–452

Galandiuk S, Wolff B G, Dozois R R, Beart R W 1991 Ileal pouch–anal anastomosis without ileostomy. Diseases of the Colon and Rectum 34: 870–873

Gravallese E M, Kantrowitz F G 1988 Arthritic manifestations of inflammatory bowel disease. American Journal of Gastroenterology 83: 703–709

Greenstein A J, Sachar D B, Gibas A, Heimann T, Hanowitz H D, Aufses A H 1985 Outcome of toxic dilatation in ulcerative and Crohn's colitis. Journal of Clinical Gastroenterology 7: 137–144

Grobler S P, Hosie K B, Keighley M R B 1992 Randomized trial of loop ileostomy in restorative proctocolectomy. British Journal of Surgery 79: 903–906

Grotz R L, Pemberton J H 1993 The ileal pouch operation for ulcerative colitis. Surgical Clinics of North America 73: 909–932

Grundfest S F, Fazio V, Weiss R A et al 1981 The risk of cancer following colectomy and ileorectal anastomosis for extensive mucosal ulcerative colitis. Annals of Surgery 193: 9–14

Handelsman J C, Gottlieb L M, Hamilton S R 1993 Crohn's disease as a contraindication to Kock pouch (continent ileostomy). Diseases of the Colon and Rectum 36: 840–843

Hawley P R 1988 Emergency surgery for ulcerative colitis. World Journal of Surgery 12: 173–196

Hay A R, Hay J W 1992 Inflammatory bowel disease: Medical cost algorithms. Journal of Clinical Gastroenterology 14: 318–327

Hulten L, Fasth S, Hallgren T, Oresland T 1992 The failing pelvic pouch conversion to continent ileostomy. International Journal of Colorectal Disease 7: 119–121

Hyman N H, Fazio V W, Tuckson W B, Lavery I C 1991 Consequences of ileal pouch–anal anastomosis for Crohn's colitis. Diseases of the Colon and Rectum 34: 653–657

Jarnerot G, Rolny P, Sandberg-Gertzen H 1985 Intensive intravenous treatment of ulcerative colitis. Gastroenterology 89: 1005–1013

Kartheuser A H, Dozois R R, Wiesner R H, LaRusso N F, Ilstrup D M, Schleck C D 1993 Complications and risk factors after ileal pouch–anal anastomosis for ulcerative colitis associated with primary sclerosing cholangitis. Annals of Surgery 217: 314–320

Kelly K A 1992 Anal sphincter-saving operations for chronic ulcerative colitis. American Journal of Surgery 163: 5–11

Kelly K A, Pemberton J H, Wolff B G, Dozois R R 1992 Ileal pouch–anal anastomosis. Current Problems in Surgery 29: 59–131

Kewenter J, Ahlman H, Hulten L 1978 Cancer risk in extensive ulcerative colitis. Annals of Surgery 188: 824–828

Kohler L W, Pemberton J H, Zinsmeister A R, Kelly K A 1991 Quality of life after proctocolectomy: a comparison of Brooke ileostomy, Kock pouch, and ileal pouch–anal anastomosis. Gastroenterology 101: 679–684

Kusunoki M, Moeslein G, Shoji Y et al 1992 Steroid complications in patients with ulcerative colitis. Diseases of the Colon and Rectum 35: 1003–1009

Lewis W G, Sagar P M, Holdsworth P J, Axon A T R, Johnston D 1993 Restorative proctocolectomy with end-to-end pouch–anal anastomosis in patients over the age of fifty. Gut 34: 948–952

Liljeqvist L, Lindquist K, Ljungdahl I 1988 Alterations in ileoanal pouch technique, 1980 to 1987: complications and functional outcome. Diseases of the Colon and Rectum 31: 929–939

Lohmuller J L, Pemberton J H, Dozois R R et al 1990 Pouchitis and extraintestinal manifestations of inflammatory bowel disease after ileal pouch–anal anastomosis. Annals of Surgery 211: 622–629

McIntyre P B, Pemberton J H, Wolff B G, Beart R W, Dozois R R 1994 Comparing functional results one year and ten years after ileal pouch–anal anastomosis for chronic ulcerative colitis. Diseases of the Colon and Rectum 37: 303–307

McLeod R S 1993 Chronic ulcerative colitis. Traditional surgical techniques. Surgical Clinics of North America 73: 891–908

McLeod R S, Churchill D N, Lock A M, Vanderburgh S, Cohen Z 1991 Quality of life of patients with ulcerative colitis preoperatively and postoperatively. Gastroenterology 101: 1307–1313

McMullen K, Hicks T C, Ray J E, Gathright J B, Timmicke A E 1991 Complications associated with ileal pouch–anal anastomosis. World Journal of Surgery 15: 763–767

Marcello P W, Roberts P L, Schoetz D J, Coller J A, Murray J J, Veidenheimer M C 1993 Long-term results of the ileoanal pouch procedure. Archives of Surgery 128: 500–504

Metcalf A M, Dozois R R, Kelly K A 1986 Sexual function in women after proctocolectomy. Annals of Surgery 204: 624–627

Michelassi F, Stella M, Block G E 1993 Prospective assessment of functional results after ileal J pouch–anal restorative proctocolectomy. Archives of Surgery 128: 889–895

Morowitz D A, Kirsner J B 1981 Ileostomy in ulcerative colitis: a questionnaire study of 1803 patients. American Journal of Surgery 141: 370–373

Mowschenson P M, Critchlow J F, Rosenberg S J, Peppercorn M A 1993 Factors favoring continence, the avoidance of a diverting ileostomy and small intestinal conservation in the ileoanal pouch operation. Surgery, Gynecology and Obstetrics 177: 17–26

Nelson H, Dozois R R, Kelly K A, Malkasian G D, Wolff B G, Ilstrup D M 1989 The effect of pregnancy and delivery on the ileal pouch–anal anastomosis functions. Diseases of the Colon and Rectum 32: 394–388

Nicholls R J, Pezim M E 1985 Restorative proctocolectomy with ileal reservoir for ulcerative colitis and familial adenomatous polyposis: a comparison of three reservoir designs. British Journal of Surgery 72: 470–474

Nugent F W, Haggitt R C, Gilpin P A 1991 Cancer surveillance in ulcerative colitis. Gastroenterology 100: 1241–1248

Oakley J R, Jagelman D G, Fazio V W et al 1985 Complications and quality of life after ileorectal anastomosis for ulcerative colitis. American Journal of Surgery 149: 23–29

O'Connell P R, Pemberton J H, Brown M L et al 1987a Determinants of stool frequency after ileal pouch–anal anastomosis. American Journal of Surgery 153: 157–163

O'Connell P R, Pemberton J H, Weiland L H et al 1987b Does rectal mucosa regenerate after ileoanal anastomosis? Diseases of the Colon and Rectum 30: 1–5

O'Connell P R, Stryker S J, Metcalf A M et al 1988 Anal canal pressure and motility after ileoanal anastomosis. Surgery, Gynecology and Obstetrics 166: 47–54

Oresland T, Fasth S, Nordgren S, Hulten L 1989 The clinical and functional outcome after restorative proctocolectomy. International Journal of Colorectal Disease 4: 50–56

Oresland T, Fasth S, Nordgren S et al 1990 Pouch size: the important functional determinant after restorative proctocolectomy. British Journal of Surgery 77: 265–269

Parc R, Legrand M, Frileux P, Tiret E, Ratelle R 1989 Comparative clinical results of ileal pouch–anal anastomosis and ileorectal anastomosis in ulcerative colitis. Hepatogastroenterology 36: 235–239

Parks A G, Nicholls R J, Belliveau R 1980 Proctocolectomy with ileal reservoir and anal anastomosis. British Journal of Surgery 67: 533–538

Pemberton J H, Kelly K A, Beart R W, Dozois R R, Wolff B G, Ilstrup D M 1987 Ileal pouch–anal anastomosis for chronic ulcerative colitis. Annals of Surgery 206: 504–511

Pemberton J H, Phillips S F, Ready R R, Zinmeister A R, Beahrs O H 1989 Quality of life after Brooke ileostomy and ileal pouch–anal anastomosis: comparison of performance status. Annals of Surgery 209: 620–626

Penna C, Caude F, Parc R et al 1993 Previous subtotal colectomy with ileostomy and sigmoidostomy improves the morbidity and early functional results after ileal pouch–anal anastomosis in ulcerative colitis. Diseases of the Colon and Rectum 36: 343–348

Pezim M E, Pemberton J H, Beart R W et al 1989 Outcome of 'indeterminant' colitis following ileal pouch–anal anastomosis. Diseases of the Colon and Rectum 32: 653–658

Phillips R K S, Ritchie J K, Hawley P R 1989 Proctocolectomy and ileostomy for ulcerative colitis: the longer term story. Journal of the Royal Society of Medicine 82: 386–387

Puthu D, Rajan N, Rao R, Rao L, Venugopal P 1992 Carcinoma of the rectal pouch following restorative proctocolectomy: Report of a case. Diseases of the Colon and Rectum 35: 257–260

Ransohoff D F, Riddel R H, Levin B 1985 Ulcerative colitis and colonic cancer: problems in assessing the diagnostic usefulness of mucosal dysplasia. Diseases of the Colon and Rectum 28: 383–388

Robert J H, Sachar D B, Aufses A H, Greenstein A J 1990 Management of severe hemorrhage in ulcerative colitis. American Journal of Surgery 159: 550–555

Sagar P M, Lewis W, Holdsworth P J, Johnston D, Mitchell C, MacFie J 1993 Quality of life after restorative proctocolectomy with a pelvic ileal reservoir compares favorably with that of patients with medically treated colitis. Diseases of the Colon and Rectum 36: 584–592

Salemans J M J I, Nagengast F M, Lubbers E J C, Kuijpers J H 1992 Postoperative and long-term results of ileal pouch–anal anastomosis for ulcerative colitis and familial polyposis coli. Digestive Diseases and Sciences 37: 1882–1889

Schrock T R 1979 Complications of continent ileostomy. American Journal of Surgery 138: 162–167

Scott N A, Dozois R R, Beart R W, Pemberton J H, Wolff B G, Ilstrup D M 1988 Postoperative intra-abdominal and pelvic sepsis complicating ileal pouch–anal anastomosis. International Journal of Colorectal Disease 3: 149–152

Stern H, Walfisch S, Mullen B et al 1990 Cancer in an ileoanal reservoir: a new late complication. Gut 31: 473–475

Stryker S J, Borody T J, Phillips S F et al 1985 Motility of the small intestine after proctocolectomy and ileal pouch–anal anastomosis. Annals of Surgery 201: 351–356

Stryker S J, Kelly K A, Phillips S F et al 1986 Anal and neorectal function after ileal pouch–anal anastomosis. Annals of Surgery 203: 55–61

Taylor B A, Pemberton J H, Carpenter H A et al 1992 Dysplasia in chronic ulcerative colitis: implications for colonoscopic surveillance. Diseases of the Colon and Rectum 35: 950–956

Taylor B A, Wolff B G, Dozois R R et al 1988 Ileal pouch–anal anastomosis for chronic ulcerative colitis and familial polyposis coli complicated by adenocarcinoma. Diseases of the Colon and Rectum 31: 358–362

Telander R L, Spencer M, Perrault J, Telander D, Zinsmeister A R 1990 Long-term follow-up of the ileoanal anastomosis in children and young adults. Surgery 108: 717–723

Tyus F J, Austhof S I, Chima C S, Keating C 1992 Diet tolerance and stool frequency in patients with ileoanal reservoirs. Journal of the American Dietetic Association 92: 861–863

Vernava A M, Goldberg S M 1988 Is the Kock pouch still a viable option? International Journal of Colorectal Disease 3: 135–138

Wexner A D, Jensen L, Rothenberger D A, Wong W D, Goldberg S M 1989 Long-term functional analysis of the ileoanal reservoir. Diseases of the Colon and Rectum 32: 275–281

Wexner S D, Wong W D, Rothenberger D A, Goldberg S M 1990 The ileoanal reservoir. American Journal of Surgery 159: 178–183

89. The role of ileoanal anastomosis – patient assessment and counseling

L. Hultén L. W. Köhler T. Öresland

Restorative proctocolectomy, i.e. the construction of a reservoir of distal ileum and an ileoanal anastomosis, is currently the most popular option for surgical treatment of ulcerative proctocolitis. There is no stoma or need for an external bag, and the normal route of defecation is preserved, leaving the patient with a normal body image. It has become the first-choice operation to be recommended in most specialized centers in the world. In the conventional technique colectomy is combined with endoanal mucous proctectomy and the ileal pouch is hand-sewn to the pectinate line (Hultén 1994a). In analogy with the traditional total proctocolectomy procedure it is curative, since all diseased mucosa is completely removed. At first sight restorative proctocolectomy therefore seems to be an unmistakable opportunity, but when looking at the results in more detail and objectively it is quite clear that the pelvic pouch is a demanding operation with a high potential for complications, sometimes with a protracted postoperative course. The complication rate amounts to about 25–30% (Pemberton et al 1987, Öresland et al 1989), with a reoperation risk of about 15–20% (Hultén 1994b). Moreover, although the overall functional results are comparatively good, functional imperfections are common, with a high defecation frequency and continence problems, mucous soiling and sore perianal skin. The pelvic pouch is by no means a return to normal.

PATIENT ASSESSMENT – WHICH PATIENTS SHOULD BE OFFERED THE OPERATION

The pelvic pouch may be offered to most patients with ulcerative colitis today, provided that they are well motivated and prepared to take the risks and accept the functional imperfections. However, a range of issues, such as the indications for doing the operation at all, nutritional status, body configuration (habitus), uncertainty of diagnosis, patient age, and present or subsequent employment prospects, family and social situation etc. has to be seriously considered.

As part of the counseling the patient should be carefully informed about the complication risks and warned that even when performed selectively the operation should be staged, covered by a loop ileostomy to be closed when the construction has healed safely. A three-stage procedure, colectomy and ileostomy with preservation of the rectum in the first stage, is to be recommended in patients admitted for an acute attack or in those with a poor general condition. Apart from minimizing the trauma in severely ill patients, a staged procedure might have other advantages. The availability of the whole specimen allows the pathologist to establish a more reliable histological diagnosis before the final decision as to a restorative pouch procedure is decided upon. The inflammation in the excluded rectum might heal, to allow for a subsequent ileorectal anastomosis. This is a specially attractive option in the young, greatly diminishing the risk of sexual dysfunction (see below).

Preoperative factors

Age

The patient's age at the time of operation does correlate to overall functional outcome (Fig. 89.1). Elderly patients exhibit more pronounced defects in continence compared to the young (Öresland et al 1989, Metcalf et al 1985, Liljeqvist et al 1988). Although the functional outcome for women and men does not differ (Pemberton et al 1987, Öresland et al 1989), elderly women tend to have a slightly worse functional outcome – an observation that is in keeping with the general knowledge that fecal incontinence is especially prone to affect multiparous women in the upper middle ages. There is no established upper age limit for restorative proctocolectomy with a pelvic pouch, but there are many reasons why elderly patients should probably be discouraged from having the operation. One important aspect is whether he or she will be fit for another major operation should it be necessary to remove the pouch owing to poor function or complications.

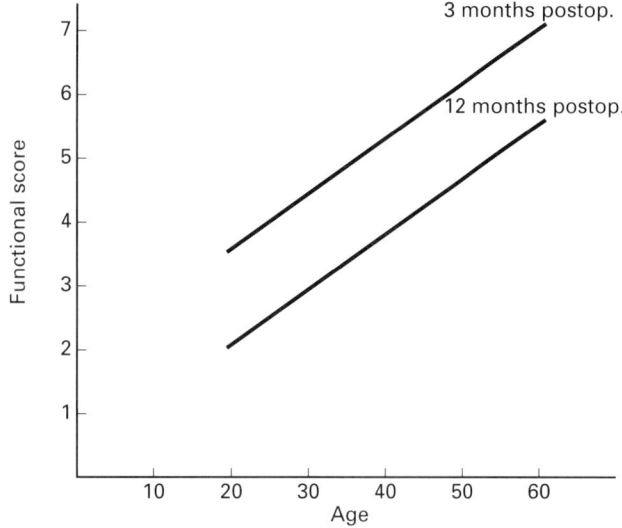

Fig. 89.1 Overall functional outcome vs. patient's age at the time of operation. A higher score denotes a worse function. (For details see Öresland et al 1989.)

Obesity

Obesity (both females and males) and tall patients (particularly males) have proved to be factors that can make construction of an ileal pouch–anal anastomosis technically difficult or even impossible as the small-bowel mesentery is either too bulky or too short to allow for construction of the anastomosis. It may be worthwhile to recommend that the obese patient loses weight, and a continent ileostomy may be an alternative for patients with a short mesentery. The continent ileostomy pouch will expand with the passage of time, and conversion to a pelvic pouch may subsequently be successful (Hultén et al 1992). With the introduction of the stapling technique for the ileoanal anastomosis these technical problems may well be slighter, but since pelvic dissection still can be difficult in obese patients, and to avoid undue tension in those with a short mesentery, the stapled anastomosis may not be as intended – a pouch–anal – but rather a pouch–rectal anastomosis.

Anal sphincter function

Good anal sphincter function is essential for a satisfactory functional result. It is well known that sphincter tone deteriorates after operation, with an approximate 25% reduction in anal resting tone. Preoperative manometry is therefore advisable to assess sphincter status. Special attention should be directed towards patients with a history of previous anal surgery or anal sphincter injury. Apart from manometry, anal endosonography might add valuable information in these patients. Patients in whom abnormalities can be demonstrated should probably be advised against restorative proctocolectomy. It should be emphasized, however, that sphincter pressures as measured preoperatively do not necessarily predict postoperative function. Opinions on this matter are widely different between authors (Scott et al 1989). In fact, the relative importance of anal sphincter function is less than one would expect, and neither preoperative nor postoperative anal pressures correlate significantly to functional outcome (Öresland et al 1990).

PATIENT COUNSELING

Psychological assessment and psychological preparation of the patient

Patients who are emotionally unstable and/or psychologically disturbed should probably be advised against a restorative proctocolectomy. In principle, only patients who are highly motivated, psychologically stable and determined to avoid a permanent stoma should be considered for an ileal pouch–anal operation.

A clear and concise description of the disease and the surgical options should be given and the advantages and disadvantages of the different operations should be explained and discussed, preferably with the patient and their family together. A booklet with printed information and schematic illustrations explaining the procedure may be helpful. The patient has to be informed without being confused or frightened. It is advisable for all patients to speak to others who have had the operation, and opportunities should be offered to speak to individuals of the same sex and background. Patients should see individuals who have had both a good and a poor result from restorative proctocolectomy. The first information will usually be given in the outpatient environment, and when patients are admitted to hospital for the operation they may have forgotten much of what they have been told. Patients have to be informed again, preferably by both the surgeons and a stoma therapist, who plays a particularly important role in counseling these patients.

When counseling patients coming to surgery we should always remember that the failure of medical therapy is mostly the primary indication of surgery (Jagelman 1986). This failure is accompanied by deterioration of the patient's wellbeing and restriction in their lifestyle. Therefore, the patients will ask the surgeon how life will be after surgery. They do not ask about manometric data after operation, but want to know if they can do sports, if they are allowed to travel, if they can live a normal lifestyle etc. Moreover, patients want to know which different operative procedures are available and what the results and the risks are.

While counseling surgeons should keep the ancient medical laws in mind:

1. Primum non nocere – first of all do no harm to the patient.
2. Primum utilis esse – first of all help the patient.
3. Salus aegroti suprema lex – the welfare of the patient is principal law.
4. Voluntas aegroti suprema lex – the wish of the patient is principal law.

Keeping these statements in mind, the results that can be obtained by the three major surgical procedures for ulcerative colitis: total proctocolectomy with ileal pouch anastomosis, Brooke ileostomy, or Kock pouch construction should be carefully explained. The ileal pouch–anal anastomosis maintains transanal defecation, avoids long-term ileostomy and offers reasonable fecal continence. In contrast, Brooke ileostomy and the Kock pouch procedure result in an ileostomy, even though the latter procedure offers stool continence to the patient. Therefore, the patient has to choose between the condition stoma yes/no and continence yes/no. It is obvious that the patient will immediately choose the option without a permanent ileostomy. But in the end is this the right choice, or does it conflict with the first and second laws: first of all do no harm to the patient and do help the patient?

Ileal pouch–anal anastomosis, as well as the continent ileostomy, are demanding operations with a substantial peri- and postoperative morbidity (Hultén & Svaninger 1984). Moreover, although the functional results of the ileal pouch are good they are far from perfect. Therefore, the patient and the doctor have to consider whether the risks of the procedure can be justified by the gain, i.e. a better quality of life. A risk–benefit analysis is necessary.

Preoperative quality of life

To assess the influence of different operative techniques on the patient's quality of life it is important first of all to consider their preoperative situation. For example, patients with familial adenomatous polyposis (in contrast to chronic ulcerative colitis) have few or no symptoms, and restorative proctocolectomy per se would not contribute to the quality of life. However, they will be relieved of the fear of cancer, so their quality of life must not, of necessity, deteriorate. Mitchell and co-workers (1988) investigated quality of life in 43 patients with ulcerative colitis. Stool frequency, abdominal cramps, general malaise and the lack of strength had the strongest influence on quality of life. Psychological factors such as frustration, depression and hopelessness were also important. About 25% of the patients had a diminished interest in sex. According to Morowitz and Kirsner (1981), 56% of 1803 patients with colitis felt ill all or most of the time.

Preoperatively most patients are afraid that a conventional ileostomy will interfere with their social life. They fear losing their attractiveness, that others may notice their ileostomy, or smell the odor. Many patients fear that they may become impotent or sterile. Others are afraid to lose their job or are afraid to handle the stoma appliances (Pemberton et al 1987).

Quality of life with an ileostomy

Studies have shown that patients with a good functioning ileostomy do not differ from 'healthy' people physically. The improvement of operative techniques and stoma appliances has improved the psychic and physic wellbeing of these patients, so that most are rehabilitated and lead a nearly normal life (Ray et al 1970, Bone & Sorensen 1974, Kennedy et al 1982, McLeod et al 1986, Pemberton et al 1989).

As most patients are tormented by persistent symptoms preoperatively, most of them feel improved postoperatively. Morowitz and Kirsner (1981) showed that 74% of the patients with a Brooke ileostomy felt much better, 14% better, 1% unchanged, 9% improved in some parts and deteriorated in others; 89% stated that their health was excellent or good, 10% were satisfied, and 96% were able to return to work (Roy et al 1970).

Although social activities were seldom restricted because of the stoma, physical activities, especially sports, seemed to have deteriorated in 43% of the patients (Pemberton et al 1983). Thirty percent of the patients with an ileostomy stated that their sexual life had deteriorated with the stoma; 55% did not notice any changes, and 15% stated that sex life was improved (Pemberton et al 1985, 1989, Grüner et al 1977). Although functional results after Brooke ileostomy are good, patients' subjective assessment is often divergent (Bone & Sorensen 1974, Kennedy et al 1982). Psychological problems are present, such as the fear of odor, problems with the stoma appliances, loss of attraction and deterioration of sex life. Patients also worry about the loss of the bowel and their ability to control defecation (Prudden 1971).

Quality of life after ileal pouch–anal construction

According to an extensive questionnaire, although patients with a conventional ileostomy were satisfied, nearly 40% wanted a change, even though some had had up to 9 years to become familiar with the stoma (Köhler et al 1991). Sagar and co-workers (1993) compared quality of life in patients who had undergone restorative procto-colectomy with that of patients with ulcerative colitis on long-term medical treatment. The principal finding in this study was that the quality of life after successful restorative proctocolectomy with a pelvic ileal reservoir was good, and appeared to be no worse than that of patients with long-standing ulcerative colitis on medical treatment in remission. Pouch patients reported fewer symptoms of anxiety or depression, and were less restricted socially than their medically treated counterparts.

Comparing patients after ileal pouch procedure with a 'healthy' control group (patients after cholecystectomy), no difference was found in regard to patients' assessment of qualify of life, health status and satisfaction with personal life (Köhler et al 1992). The scores for the quality of life dimensions, namely family life, social life, recreational activities, sex life, occupational work, housework, sports and travel, showed no difference (Table 89.1). It was concluded that, despite functional results being not ideal, pouch patients have a good quality of life and do not differ from the 'normal' population. These results remained stable over an 8-year period. However, one should realize that only patients with a functioning pouch participated in the study: 6% of the patients were excluded because the protecting ileostomy was never closed, or had to be re-established during follow-up. These patients took the gamble but lost.

Quality of life in comparison

When quality of life after the ileal pouch procedure was compared with that after a Brooke ileostomy or Kock pouch procedure, it was demonstrated that patients with an ileal pouch–anal anastomosis had fewer restrictions in sports and sexual activities than those with a Kock pouch. Patients with Kock pouches in turn had fewer restrictions in these activities, but more restrictions in travel than those with Brooke ileostomies. No difference was seen in the categories of social life, housework, recreational activities and family life (Köhler et al 1991). No differences were found concerning attitudes towards the type of operation and overall satisfaction. None the less, of the patients who had knowledge of alternative procedures, more patients with Brooke ileostomies and Kock pouches desired a change than did those with an ileal pouch (Table 89.2). Several studies have investigated the effect of converting a Brooke ileostomy to a Kock pouch, and demonstrated that more than 50% of the patients stated that their ability to work, their sex life and their social life were all improved (Gerber et al 1984, McLeod & Fazio 1984, Öjerskog et al 1988). However, Köhler et al (1991) could not demonstrate such an effect in 137 patients who had been converted. Pemberton et al (1989) compared quality of life after Brooke ileostomy and ileal pouch procedure, and showed that the ileal pouch was superior in seven performance areas.

Sexual function and fertility

Whether, and if so to what extent, restorative proctocolectomy may have influence on the patient's sexual life and fertility is of major concern for young men and

Table 89.1 Results of the different dimensions of quality of life. No difference was seen between the pouch procedure and the cholecystectomy. Results remained stable over the 8-year period (Köhler et al 1992)

	Ileal pouch	Cholecystectomy	Ileal pouch vs. cholecystectomy over an 8-year period
Stool frequency	5 stools/day	1,5 stools/day	Stable
Bowel medication	40%	12%	Stable
Episodes of fecal soiling	68%	13%	Stable
Wearing of protective pads	46%	6%	Stable
Ability to postpone defecation longer than 30 min	15%	18%	Stable
Restriction of daily living due to incontinence	32%	13%	Stable
Worry about stool habits	65%	26%	Stable

Table 89.2 Patient satisfaction after creation of Brooke ileostomy, Kock pouch or ileal pouch–anal anastomosis (Köhler et al 1991)

Categories	Ileostomy $n = 406$ (%)	Kock pouch $n = 313$ (%)	Ileal pouch anal anastomosis $n = 298$ (%)
Attitude since operation			
Improved	60	60	62
No change	35	36	34
Deteriorated	5	4	4
Overall satisfaction	93	98	96
Desired change but satisfied	33	11	3
Definitely desired change	6	3	1

women. It is often stated that conventional proctocolectomy interferes greatly with these functions in both men and women, whereas such disturbances can be avoided or are less pronounced after restorative proctocolectomy. These opinions are controversial, however. Patients should, therefore, irrespective of sex, be carefully informed that sexual disturbances may still occur. A 1–2% risk of partial or complete impotence is equal to that after conventional proctocolectomy in men. Women may suffer from dyspareunia and fecal leak during intercourse (Öresland et al 1989). Moreover, a 5–10% risk of retrograde ejaculation and reports on abnormalities of hysterosalphingography and difficulties in becoming pregnant are other factors that should be considered (Öresland et al 1994). In a young population such sequelae have to be seriously considered and individual advice should be given to the patient. Whenever possible a colectomy and ileorectal anastomosis should probably be recommended to the young, to buy time and postpone the curative operation until a later occasion.

Functional considerations

There is a wide variation in functional outcome after pelvic pouch surgery. The average patient will ultimately have about five bowel movements per day; less than half will have night evacuations. One-third will now and then suffer from seepage and need to use a protective pad. Most patients will prefer to use retarding drugs (Fig. 89.2).

Patients should be informed that the initial period after loop ileostomy closure may be distressing, with a high frequency of bowel movements and leaks. We have no way in which we can predict the severity and durability of such problems. Our policy is to inform patients that it may take as long as a year before the bowel function become stable, and even after the first year further improvement can often be expected, although it may not be very dramatic. In the initial period it is very important that great care is taken to protect the perianal skin, as the pouch output is very irritant and often watery. Even if the patient does not experience leaks minimal amounts of ileal contents will inevitably come into contact with the skin, so they are advised to use a barrier cream for skin protection. Retarding drugs such as loperamide are prescribed to all patients and a majority will find this very useful. Protective pads are also prescribed, as many patients will experience some soiling, usually at night, at least in the early period. Some patients prefer the use of psyllium seeds to increase the consistency of stools, others find that the stool volume increases too much. In some

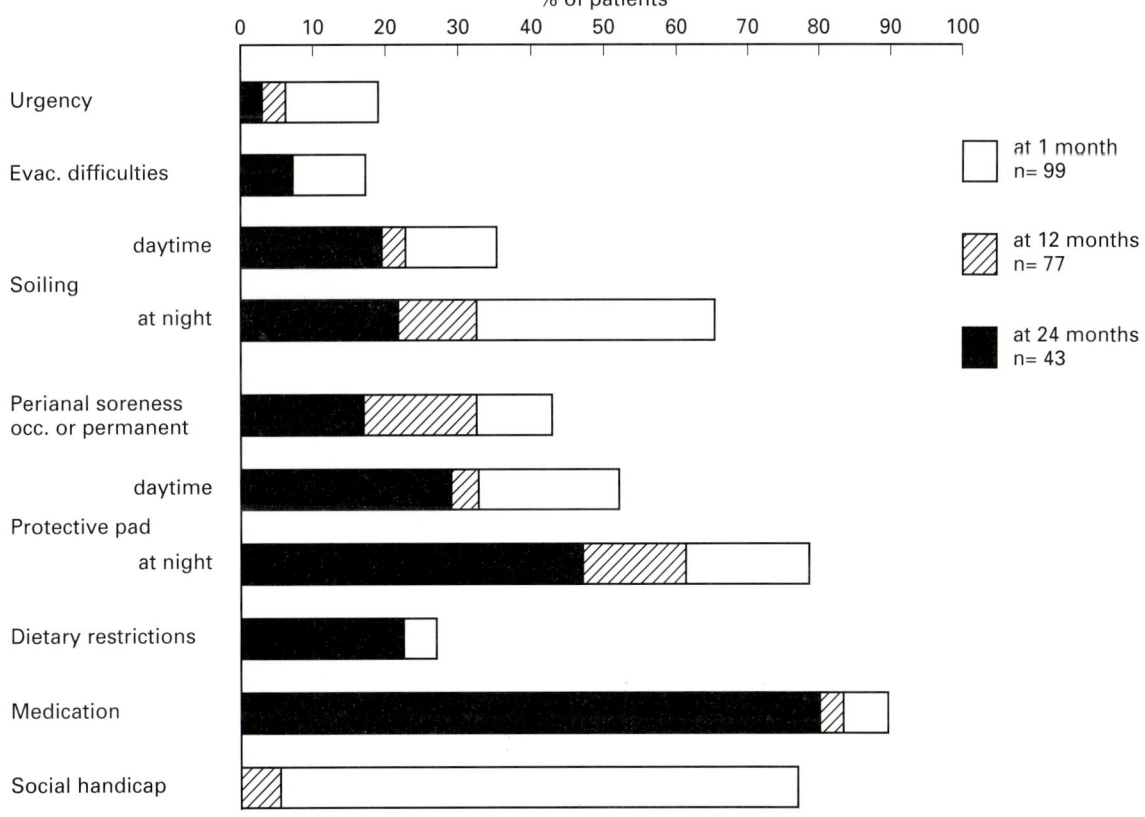

Fig. 89.2 Details of functional outcome at different time intervals after the operation. (For details see Öresland et al 1989.)

patients with frequent night evacuations an evening dose of an anticholinergic drug may be useful, but during the daytime the side effects are usually too prominent to be acceptable. It is our experience that those patients who have to empty their loop ileostomy appliance during the night are the same ones that with a pelvic pouch will have bowel movements during the night.

It seems that there is no consistent pattern in the foods that should be omitted, so each patient is advised to test this on an individual basis. Most patients state that they have no or very minor dietary restrictions. Normally, however, late meals will result in night evacuations or leakage during the night – this is more evident if wine or alcohol has been consumed in quantities. From a homeostatic point of view a patient with a pelvic pouch will be in the same situation as a patient with an ileostomy. In case of gastroenteritis they are likely to suffer excessive losses of fluid and salt. It is important to make patients aware of this, especially when travelling. Should it happen, extra intake of fluids and salt is recommended. Our patients carry Oralyte WHO, as this composition of salt and glucose will give the best possible absorption of fluids. Patients may sometimes ask if there is anything else they can do themselves to improve continence. Some years ago Telander et al (1981) showed that in young patients with straight ileoanal anastomosis dilatation of the ileum above the anastomosis improved the early postoperative functional outcome. Others have suggested that patients should do sphincter exercises in the early period after the operation. While this action seems logical and reasonable, we have not been able to show any effect either of pouch dilatation or of sphincter exercises (Öresland et al 1988).

Pouchitis

Pouchitis, an unspecific inflammation of the ileal mucosa, is the most frequent complication of pouch surgery (Svaninger et al 1993). The syndrome is not exactly defined but is characterized by an increase in defecation frequency, with concomitant defects in continence, watery blood-stained stools and urgency being most distressing. Although most patients respond promptly to treatment with metronidazole, with restoration of function, recurrent episodes or chronic therapy-resistant pouchitis has a considerable impact on quality of life in those afflicted. Giving preoperative information about this syndrome might be wise as it may contribute considerably to long term morbidity.

SUMMARY

Many investigators have tried to measure physiological variables and correlate these to the ultimate functional result after operation, but it seems that only a fraction of the variability in function can be explained by these methods. It is reasonable to assume that the unexplained variability in functional outcome is dependent on the personality of each patient, in terms of previous experiences, degree of anxiety, prospects for the future etc. Both the surgeon and the nursing staff should be very much aware of these factors, and inform and support patients on an individual basis. It is crucial to start this procedure early, before the operation, allowing the patient to obtain as much information as possible. Preferably you should give the patient a feeling that the final decision has been made by him- or herself, and then make it clear that you strongly support this decision. It is also worthwhile recommending that the patient seeks further information and counseling from one who has already been operated upon. The essence of this would be that a well motivated and well informed patient might cope better with the problems arising both during the postoperative hospital stay and later in the rehabilitation phase.

REFERENCES

Bone J, Sorensen F H 1974 Life with a conventional ileostomy. Diseases of the Colon and Rectum 17: 194–199

Gerber A, Apt M K, Craig P H 1984 The improved quality of life with the Kock continent ileostomy. Journal of Clinical Gastroenterology 6: 513–517

Grüner O P N, Naas R, Fretheim B, Gjone E 1977 Marital status and sexual adjustment after colectomy: results in 178 patients operated on for ulcerative colitis. Scandinavian Journal of Gastroenterology 12: 193–197

Hultén L, Svaninger G 1984 Facts about Kocks continent ileostomy. Diseases of the Colon and Rectum 27: 553–557

Hultén L, Fasth S, Hallgren T, Öresland T 1992 The failing pelvic pouch conversion to continent ileostomy. International Journal of Colorectal Disease 7: 119–121

Hultén L 1994a Koch pouch ileoanal anastomosis. In: Surgery of the colon, rectum and anus. Rob & Smith's operative surgery, 5th edn. Chapman & Hall, London, pp 604–614

Hultén L 1994b Problems after ileopouch anal anastomosis for ulcerative colitis. How can we prevent it? Netherlands Journal of Medicine 45: 80–85

Jagelman D G 1986 Mucosal ulcerative colitis. Futura Publishing Company, Mount Kisco, New York

Kennedy H J, Lee E D G, Claridge G, Truelove S C 1982 The health of subjects living with a permanent ileostomy. Quarterly Journal of Medicine 203: 341–357

Köhler L W, Pemberton J H, Zinsmeister A R, Kelly K A 1991 Quality of life after proctocolectomy. A comparison of Brooke ileostomy, Kock pouch, and ileal pouch–anal anastomosis. Gastroenterology 101: 679–684

Köhler L W, Pemberton J H, Hodge D O, Zinsmeister A R, Kelly K A 1992 Long-term functional results and quality of life after ileal pouch–anal anastomosis and cholecystectomy. World Journal of Surgery 16: 1126–1132

Liljeqvist L, Lindqvist K, Ljungdahl I 1988 Alterations in ileoanal pouch technique, 1980 to 1987 Complications and functional outcome. Diseases of the Colon and Rectum 31: 929–938

McLeod R S, Fazio V W 1984 Quality of life with the Kock continent ileostomy. World Journal of Surgery 8: 90–95

McLeod R S, Lavery I C, Leatherman J R 1986 Factors affecting quality of life with a conventional ileostomy. World Journal of Surgery 10: 474–480

Metcalf A M, Dozois R R, Kelly K A, Beart R W Jr, Wolff B G 1985

Ileal 'J' pouch–anal anastomosis: clinical outcome. Annals of Surgery 202: 735–739

Mitchell A, Guygatt G, Singer J 1988 Quality of life in patients with inflammatory bowel disease. Journal of Clinical Gastroenterology 10: 306–310

Morowitz D A, Kirsner J B 1981 Ileostomy in ulcerative colitis: a questionnaire study in 1803 patients. American Journal of Surgery 141: 370–375

Öjerskog B, Hellström T, Kock N G, Myrvold H E 1988 Quality of life in ileostomy patients before and after conversion to the continent ileostomy. International Journal of Colorectal Disease 3: 166–170

Öresland T, Fasth S, Hultén L, Nordgren S, Swensson L, Åkervall S 1988 Does balloon dilatation and sphincter training improve ileoanal pouch function? International Journal of Colorectal Disease 3: 153–157

Öresland T, Fasth S, Nordgren S, Hultén L 1989 The clinical and functional outcome after restorative proctocolectomy. A prospective study in 100 patients. International Journal of Colorectal Disease 4: 50–56

Öresland T, Fasth S, Nordgren S, Åkervall S, Hultén L 1990 Pouch size: the important functional determinant after restorative proctocolectomy. British Journal of Surgery 77: 265–269

Öresland T, Palmblad S, Ellström M, Berndtsson I, Crona N, Hultén L 1994 Gynaecological and sexual function related to anatomical changes after restorative proctocolectomy. International Journal of Colorectal Disease 9: 77–81

Pemberton J H, Beahrs O H 1987 Brooke ileostomy. In: Nelson RCNLJ (ed) Surgery of the small intestine. Appelton-Century-Crofts, Norwalk, pp 449–458

Pemberton J H, van Heerden J A, Beart R W 1983 A continent ileostomy device. Annals of Surgery 197: 618–626

Pemberton J H, Phillips S F, Dozois R R 1985 Current clinical results of conventional ileostomy. In: Dozois R R (ed) Alternatives to conventional ileostomy. Year Book Medical Publishers, Chicago: pp 40–50

Pemberton J H, Kelly K A, Beart R W, Dozois R R, Wolff B G, Ilstrup D M 1987 Ileal pouch–anal anastomosis for chronic ulcerative colitis. Long-term results. Annals of Surgery 206: 504–511

Pemberton J H, Phillips S F, Ready R R, Zinsmeister A R, Bears O H 1989 Quality of life after Brooke ileostomy and ileal pouch–anal anastomosis. Annals of Surgery 209: 620–628

Prudden J F 1971 Psychological problems following ileostomy and colostomy. Cancer 28: 236–238

Roy P H, Sauer W G, Beahrs O H, Farrow G M 1970 Experience with ileostomies. Evaluation of long-term rehabilitation in 497 patients. American Journal of Surgery 119: 77–86

Sagar P M, Lewis W, Holdsworth P J, Johnston D, Mitchell C, MacFie J 1993 Quality of life after restorative proctocolectomy with a pelvic ileal reservoir compares favourably with that of patients with medically treated colitis. Diseases of the Colon and Rectum 36: 584–592

Scott N A, Pemberton J H, Barkel D C, Wolff B G 1989 Anal and ileal pouch manometric measurements before ileostomy closure are related to functional outcome after ileal pouch–anal anastomosis. British Journal of Surgery 76: 613–616

Svaninger G, Nordgren S, Öresland T, Hultén L 1993 Incidence and characteristics of pouchitis in the Kock continent ileostomy and the pelvic pouch. Scandinavian Journal of Gastroenterology 28: 695–700

Telander R L, Perrault J, Hoffman A D 1981 Early development of the neorectum by balloon dilations after ileoanal anastomosis. Journal of Pediatric Surgery 16: 911–916

90. Role of the ileal pouch procedure – pouch construction, and the ileoanal anastomosis

P. M. Sagar   J. H. Pemberton

Ileal pouch-anal anastomosis is now the optimal surgical procedure for most patients with chronic ulcerative colitis (Williams 1989). These patients need no longer live with the fear that their ultimate surgical fate is to be a permanent ileostomy, with its associated psychological, social, physical and sexual problems; indeed, the procedure confers a good quality of life. The purpose of this chapter is to review the technical details, the types of ileal pouch and ileoanal anastomosis available, and, finally, its complications and their sequelae.

OVERVIEW OF THE OPERATION

The operation is usually performed in two stages (Utsunomiya et al 1980). First, the cecum, colon and rectum are mobilized and removed. The ileum is preserved in its entirety. A reservoir is constructed from 30–40 cm of distal ileum and anastomosed to the anal canal at or just above the dentate line. This anastomosis can be performed with sutures or staples and can be fashioned with or without mucosectomy to the mucosa immediately above the dentate line. A temporary ileostomy is used to protect this anastomosis and is closed 8–12 weeks later. All diseased tissue is removed and yet normal defecation and fecal continence are maintained. Experience with the procedure and simplifications in technique have led to an improved outcome. Quality of life in patients with a pelvic ileal reservoir is better than that of patients with Brooke ileostomies, continent Kock ileostomies and medically treated colitis (Pemberton et al 1989, Sagar et al 1993).

WHICH POUCH?

The pelvic ileal reservoir may be constructed from two, three or four limbs of distal ileum which are anastomosed in a side-to-side fashion (Fig. 90.1) (Sagar & Taylor 1994). There is no ideal configuration because there is no difference in functional outcome among the several available designs of pouch. However, some pouches are easier to construct than others.

Three-limbed pelvic ileal reservoirs

This was the first pelvic ileal reservoir to be described (Fig. 90.1a) (Parks & Nicholls 1978) and was a modification of the reservoir originally described by Kock for use as a continent ileostomy (Kock 1969). It was constructed from 30 cm of distal ileum. A 25 cm segment was opened along the antimesenteric border, folded three times and the adjacent edges sutured together. The most distal 5 cm were not incorporated into the reservoir but rather acted as an efferent conduit or spout. Unlike the Kock reservoir, there was no inverted nipple valve. Self-catheterization was needed to empty the pouch in four of the original five patients (Parks et al 1980), but this problem was largely overcome by reducing the length of the efferent spout and by avoiding a long rectal muscular cuff. A long efferent limb (4–6 cm) will tend to impede evacuation because of acute angulation between the pouch and the efferent spout. The longer the limb, the more likely it is to angulate and hence obstruct (Pescatori et al 1983).

Although it is not widely used, the S pouch is of value in the patient in whom it is difficult to mobilize the ileum sufficiently to allow the apex of a conventional two-limbed pelvic ileal reservoir to reach the anal canal without tension. In this situation, the most distal part of the ileum can usually be made to reach low enough in the pelvis to allow a tension-free anastomosis to be constructed.

There is no firm rule with regard to the length of ileum used to construct the S pouch, or indeed any pouch. After the initial descriptions, most S pouches have been constructed from three limbs of 15 cm of ileum. If too large a pouch is made, however, there is a tendency for it to become distended and atonic. Although such pouches may be both capacious and compliant, the tone of the muscular wall may be low. This leads to stasis and incomplete evacuation. Furthermore, the efferent spout possesses peristaltic activity which is independent of that of the body of the ileal reservoir, and this may further impede emptying (Schraut et al 1983). The S pouch can

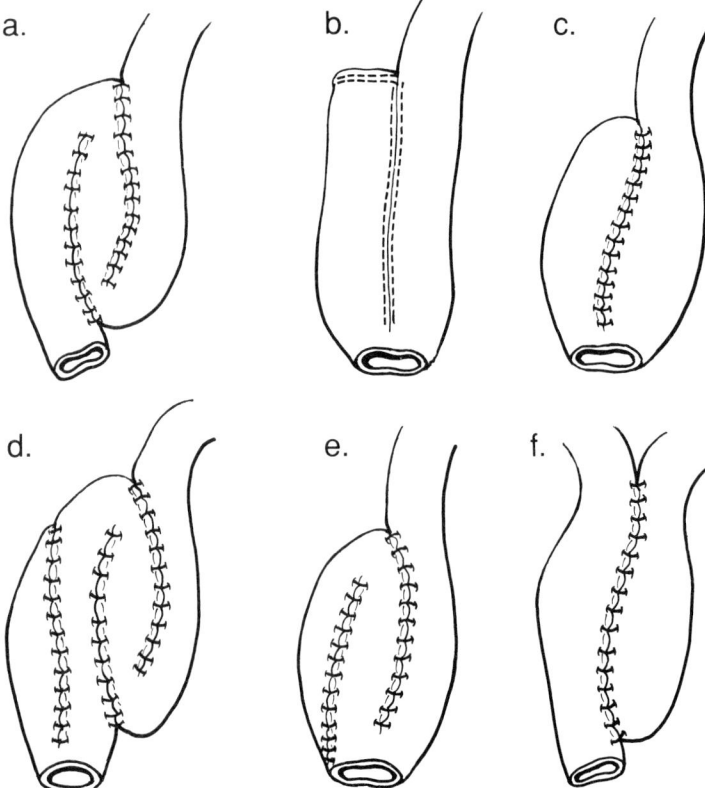

Fig. 90.1 Types of ileal reservoir: a = sutured S; b = stapled J; c = sutured J; d = sutured W; e = sutured S, no efferent limb. Maneuver to bring a pouch under tension to the dentate line.

be constructed with no efferent spout (Fig. 90.1e). The distal end of the ileum is oversewn and an enterotomy made at the apex of the first and second loops at the most dependent part. The ileal pouch–anal anastomosis is constructed side-to-end between the most dependent part of the reservoir and the anal canal. This permits spontaneous evacuation. Although the S pouch is usually hand sutured, linear stapling instruments can be used with no increase in morbidity (Stern et al 1987).

The efficiency of evacuation of S pouches is less than that of J and W pouches, and a small minority of patients still need to self-catheterize (Sagar et al 1992a). Self-catheterization is not popular with patients as it is messy, time-consuming and unpleasant (Vasilevsky et al 1987). Such pouches can be revised, particularly if the efferent limb is too long, either because of the original construction or because the spout has lengthened with time after the operation. A small group of patients, who have an efferent spout of only 1 cm at the time of operation, return with a spout of 4 or 5 cm. Revision of the segment, without changing the configuration of the pouch, can restore satisfactory function (Galandiuk et al 1990). Long efferent limbs may be shortened, excised, or the S pouch may be converted to a J pouch (Galandiuk et al 1990). Resection of a long efferent limb and reanastomosis may be performed endoanally but the success rate is low (Nicholls & Gilbert 1990). Revision usually requires complete mobilization of the reservoir and its efferent conduit by a transabdominal approach, a procedure that is not easily accomplished. The ileoanal anastomosis is taken down and the entire efferent spout excised. The ileal pouch–anal anastomosis is then re-established. Most of the small number of patients who have undergone such revisional surgery have been able to evacuate their reservoir spontaneously (Liljeqvist et al 1988). Alternatively, the septum between pouch and efferent limb may be divided transanally by the linear stapler (Schoetz et al 1988), or the efferent spout may be shortened by inserting a circular staple gun into the pouch and positioning it such that when the gun is closed part of the efferent spout is trapped. When the gun is subsequently fired the spout is shortened and the ileal pouch–anal anastomosis simultaneously recreated. Nonetheless, the difficulties of revisional surgery to the ileal pouch–anal anastomosis must not be underestimated and only about 50% of these patients will eventually have good function (Galandiuk et al 1990).

Two-limbed pelvic ileal reservoirs

J-shaped pouch

The two-limbed J-shaped reservoir was introduced by Utsunomiya in 1980 (Fig. 90.1c) and is currently the most popular pouch. It is fashioned from a long side-to-side anastomosis along the antimesenteric border of the ileum, with the limbs arranged in an isoantiperistaltic fashion. The apex of the ileal loop which reaches to the level of the anal canal without tension is chosen to form the most dependent part of the reservoir. The ileocecal artery often must be divided to increase the mobility of the ileal mesentery. The length of the two limbs is variable and depends partly on the amount of fat in the ileal mesentery and the distribution of the ileal arcades. There is no difference in functional outcome between J pouches constructed from two 10 cm limbs or two 20 cm limbs (Williamson et al 1993). The J-shaped reservoir is simple and quick to construct, particularly if linear stapling devices are used (Fig. 90.1b).

Difficulty may be experienced in mobilizing the ileum to permit the apex of the ileal loop to reach down to the anal canal without tension. In this event, two maneuvers are useful. First, an efferent limb may be constructed by division of the apex of the ileal loop. The two ileal limbs are then anastomosed in the usual isoantiperistaltic fashion with a 2 cm efferent spout emerging from the isoperistaltic limb (Fig. 90.1f). This facilitates the creation of a longer reservoir and reduces the possibility of tension on the anastomosis. Alternatively, the ileal loop may be divided at a point proximal to the apex. An efferent spout is fashioned with the ileal spout positioned in an antiperistaltic manner, which results, at least theoretically, in improved continence and reduced fecal leakage, although this might be outweighed by a tendency for the antiperistaltic efferent limb to impede evacuation. In practice, careful division of the ileocolic vessels will usually permit a tension-free anastomosis. Division of the visceral peritoneum on either side of the ileal mesentery allows the mesentery to stretch, but this can be risky since tension on the pouch as it is brought down to the anal canal may tear the terminal branches of the superior mesenteric arcades at the apex of the J, which are now unsupported by their protective mesentery. Generally, if the most dependent part of the pouch will reach to a level of 5 cm below the upper border of the symphysis pubis, then there is sufficient length to allow a tension-free anastomosis.

H-shaped pouch

The idea of the lateral isoperistaltic pelvic ileal reservoir was introduced by Peck in 1980. The procedure was performed in two stages. The first stage involved total colectomy, excision of the rectal mucosa, preparation of a rectal mucosal graft and placement of the graft within a rectal muscular cuff. This grafted rectal tube was closed at the proximal end and the divided ileum was brought out as an end ileostomy. The second stage was performed 3 months later, and involved a longitudinal incision along the antimesenteric border of the grafted rectum and a similar incision along the antimesenteric border of the distal ileum after disconnection of the ileostomy. A two-layered anastomosis was used to create a two-limbed, iso-isoperistaltic reservoir. The rectal mucosal graft sloughed, however. Fonkalsrud adapted this concept and constructed a reservoir from two limbs of ileum with a side-to-side anastomosis of 25-30 cm. A 5-7 cm efferent spout of single-lumen ileum projected from the lower end and was anastomosed to the anal sphincter. There was no ileal graft. The hypothetical advantage of this lateral isoperistaltic reservoir was that the orientation of the limbs of the reservoir was in an aboral direction, which should promote emptying while providing adequate storage capacity. Unfortunately, the efferent spout again caused problems (Stone et al 1986) and led to gross distension and elongation of the reservoir. Shortening the efferent limb to 2 cm has led to improved evacuation and functional outcome (Fonkalsrud 1987).

It is possible to construct an H reservoir in patients who have had an unsuccessful functional result with a straight ileoanal anastomosis (Fonkalsrud et al 1988). This is a procedure which has been met with success in children, in whom considerable adaptation has been observed (Martin et al 1985), but the results in adults have been poor (Taylor et al 1983). Conversion from straight ileoanal anastomosis to H pouch is associated with significant improvement in the functional result, with a reduction in the frequency of daytime and night-time bowel actions of 50 and 60% respectively.

Inverted U pouch

A variant on this theme is the conversion from straight ileoanal anastomosis to an inverted U pouch. This is achieved by dividing the ileum 30 cm above the anal canal and folding the distal ileum over itself to allow the level of division to reach to the pelvic floor. The two limbs of folded ileum are anastomosed side-to-side with a linear stapler to fashion a reservoir and the proximal ileum is then anastomosed to the top of this new pouch (an inverted U) (Nelson et al 1991).

B pouch

The pelvic ileal reservoir may become inflamed by pouchitis. (Madden et al 1990). The B pouch, which is essentially a J pouch with two or three interrupted anastomoses within the lumen, has been described as an attempt to overcome the effects of fecal stasis on the mucosa (Slors et al 1989). Although circulation of the contents of a B pouch may be greater than that observed within a J pouch, the clinical relevance of this finding and any potential influence on the incidence of pouchitis is unclear.

Quadruplicated pelvic ileal reservoirs

The W pouch was introduced in 1985 in an attempt to answer the problems of incomplete evacuation of the S pouch and to improve the functional results obtained with the J pouch (Nicholls & Lubowski 1987, Harms et al 1987). It was constructed from four 12 cm lengths of ileum which were sutured in a W arrangement (Nicholls & Pezim 1983). The ileal pouch–anal anastomosis was side-to-end between the most dependent part of the reservoir and the top of the anal canal.

Esthetically this is a pleasing alternative, as the spheroidal design gives the greatest volume for a given length of ileum (Thompson et al 1987), the pouch sits well within the confines of the pelvis, and the horizontal diameter of the W pouch is similar to that of the normal rectal ampulla (Hatakayama et al 1989). The bulky nature of this pouch may, however, cause difficulty, particularly in an obese male with a narrow pelvis. The design of the reservoir may be modified such that the distal two limbs are each 11-12 cm in length, with the more proximal two limbs being 9-10 cm long (Fig. 90.1d). The reservoir is then effectively two J-shaped reservoirs anastomosed together and slightly offset. This allows the reservoir to sit more comfortably within the bony confines of the pelvis while maintaining its large capacity.

Comparative studies have suggested that W pouches have some benefits over other designs in terms of capacity, compliance and evacuation characteristics (Nicholls & Pezim 1985, Sagar et al 1992a) but, importantly, prospective randomized studies have not shown a significant benefit in functional outcome (Keighley et al 1988). In addition, W pouches are sutured and therefore take much longer to construct than the J pouch, which is stapled quickly.

Single-lumen ileum

Anastomosing the end of the ileum to the anal sphincter was performed early in the development of the ileoanal procedure. A single-lumen ileum, functioning as a neorectum, has the advantage of simplicity. The clinical outcome has been disappointing, however, because high-pressure waves generated within the ileal wall often exceeded both resting and squeeze pressures of the anal sphincter, with consequent leakage of feces, particularly at night. In addition, the frequency of bowel actions is high as the distal ileum is principally designed to be a conduit rather than a reservoir. Comparative studies between single-lumen ileum and J pouches have shown a significantly higher rate of failure and patient dissatisfaction with single-lumen ileum (Taylor et al 1983). Interestingly, the results of straight ileoanal anastomosis in children are much better. The functional outcome steadily improves in the 3 years after operation (Martin et al 1985, Morgan et al 1987). There appears to be considerably more adaptation of the ileum in children compared to adults (Telander & Perrault 1981), and this procedure continues to have a role in the pediatric setting.

Alternative approaches

Preservation of the colon

Ulcerative colitis is limited to the rectum and sigmoid in about 30% of patients. The cecum and ascending colon may be macroscopically and microscopically normal, and attempts have been made to preserve this 'normal' colon as an alternative form of neorectum. This has the possible advantage of maintaining the storage capacity and distensibility of the cecum, which are similar to those of the rectum. However, resection of the rectosigmoid with construction of an end colostomy is associated with a high rate of recurrent disease in the residual colon, and 25% of patients require further resection (Clarke & Ward 1980). Similarly, the results of coloanal anastomosis in patients with ulcerative colitis have been variable at best (Roediger et al 1982). Again, recurrence of disease is common and completion colectomy is required in 75% of patients (Varma et al 1987). Cecoanal anastomosis was found to fail in over 80% of cases (Johnston et al 1981), and preservation of the colon in these situations cannot be recommended.

Two-sphincter operation

The ileocecal valve combines with the terminal ileum to form a highly specialized region which provides an effective brake to the flow of gastrointestinal content. If this functional unit could be kept intact, then its absorptive, motor and valvular effects could be utilized, with a reduction in gastrointestinal transit and frequency of bowel actions. This idea was tested by isolating a 50 cm ileal segment on its vascular pedicle, which was then interposed between the ileocecal valve upstream and the anal sphincter downstream (Fig. 90.2a) (Johnston et al 1989). The muscular component of the ileocecal valve was preserved but the mucosa was excised. The ileocecal sphincter protruded into the single-lumen ileal segment as a nipple valve. Although the early functional outcome in eight of 12 patients in a pilot study was not dissimilar to that of patients with conventional pouches, the authors abandoned the procedure because of the high long-term failure rate.

Ileal myectomy

Myectomy of single-lumen ileum (Fig. 90.2b), excising strips of the muscular wall and serosa, is an attractive concept because it changes the compliance and capacity characteristics of the terminal ileum completely: the ileum becomes highly compliant and capacious, characteristics similar to an ileal pouch. Both the frequency and amplitude of peristaltic waves are diminished (Sagar et al 1990). Studies in animals have demonstrated that the functional outcome of single-lumen ileum with myectomy is similar to that of the J pouch. Double myectomy gives superior results compared to single myectomy (Sagar et al 1990). To date, there are only anecdotal reports of its use in humans (Accarpio et al 1983), and it is unlikely to become popular. Myotomy alone – simple incision of the seromuscle – is unsuccessful (Aly & Fonkalsrud 1988) because the incision heals promptly and no benefit is obtained.

Miscellaneous

Telander and Perrault described the insertion of a 10–15 cm balloon attached to a catheter into the ileal

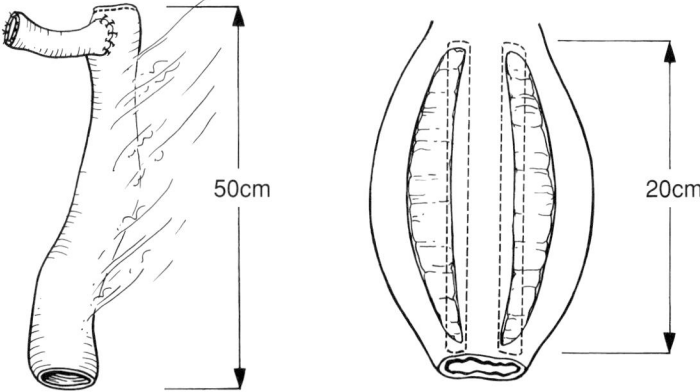

Fig. 90.2 Two-sphincter operation (left) and ileal myectomy (right).

lumen of young patients after ileoanal anastomosis. Patients could then inflate the balloon and so stretch the ileum. Graduated balloon dilatation over a period of weeks was associated with a steady decrease in the frequency of bowel actions (Telander & Perrault 1981). Most patients failed to dilate the balloon sufficiently, however, and as a result noticed little change in their frequency of bowel action.

Reversal of ileal segments (Barros D'Sa 1979) to slow intestinal transit and the construction of ileal 'valves' (Williams & King 1985) have also been unsuccessful.

Comment

The perfect pouch has not been described. The choice of design of the pouch depends on the characteristics of the patient and the surgeon's preference. The functional outcome varies little between the basic options, and most patients will find that they will have a frequency of bowel action of between four and seven times per 24 hours, with perhaps one nocturnal evacuation (Table 90.1). They will experience a normal urge to defecate, will be able to defer defecation, and to discriminate between flatus and feces.

THE ILEOANAL ANASTOMOSIS

The method used to construct the ileal pouch–anal anastomosis is debatable. There are two options:

1. An endoanal mucosal resection with hand-sutured anastomosis between the pouch and the internal anal sphincter, fashioned at the level of the dentate line
2. A double-stapled technique, with construction of the ileoanal anastomosis at a slightly higher level (Kmiot & Keighley 1989).

The advantages of transanal mucosectomy are that all diseased mucosa is removed, so that there can be no symptoms from residual diseased mucosa and the risk of cancer occurring in retained rectal mucosa is eliminated. Postoperative surveillance is therefore unnecessary. Resting anal pressure falls after restorative proctocolectomy irrespective of the surgical technique used to construct the ileal pouch–anal anastomosis (Johnston et al 1987). However, a significant recovery of the anal sphincter, with a rise in the resting anal pressure, return of the rectoanal inhibitory reflex and improvement in clinical outcome is seen to occur for at least 12 months after stapled restorative proctocolectomy (Sagar et al 1991). A similar recovery

Table 90.1 Complications after restorative proctocolectomy

Reference (No. of Patients)	Center	Mortality	Pelvic sepsis	Anastomotic dehiscence	Small-bowel obstruction		Anastomotic stricture
					Op.	No op.	
Schoetz et al 1988 (91)	Burlington USA	0	2	1	7	3	1
Fleshman et al 1988 (179)	Toronto	0	25	18	16	18	14
Keighley et al 1988 (65)	Birmingham	0	16	–	5	4	12
Becker & Raymond 1986 (100)	Salt Lake	0	0	–	2	5	–
Fonkalsrud et al 1987 (184)	Los Angeles	1	4	–	16	–	38
Nicholls & Lubowski 1987 (152)	London	1	25	–	18	–	11
Wexner et al 1990 (178)	Minneapolis	0	20	–	5	15	–
Pemberton et al 1987 (390)	Rochester	1	23	–	20	31	20
Oresland et al 1989 (100)	Gothenberg	0	5	10	6	0	4
Skarsgard et al 1989 (75)	Vancouver	1	–	6	–	14	17

	Fistula	Wound infection	Bleeding	Failure
Schoetz et al 1988	–	2	2	5
Fleshman et al 1988	5	28	1	23
Keighley et al 1988	3	11	2	9
Becker & Raymond 1986	–	0	–	2
Fonkalsrud et al 1987	2	–	–	6
Nicholls & Lubowski 1987	–	16	3	10
Wexner et al 1990	9	7	9	7
Pemberton et al 1987	–	12	–	24
Oresland et al 1989	2	–	–	3
Skarsgard et al 1989	1	6	1	10

has not been reported in patients after mucosectomy by some (Becker & Raymond 1986) but not all authors (Kelly et al 1992). Surgeons in favor of the double-stapled technique suggest that it is a technically simpler operation, with improved functional outcome. This latter point is debatable, however, as most reports of studies in which comparisons have been made between the two techniques have not been randomized, and have included historical controls which have invariably been taken from the 'learning curve' of the surgeon's experience. The few randomized trials (Seow-Choen et al 1991) and case control studies (McIntyre et al 1994) published to date, although small in numbers, show no functional differences.

Mucosal resection

In order to preserve normal rectal sensation it was long thought necessary to preserve a long muscular cuff of rectum. Preservation of a 10–12 cm rectal cuff denuded of its mucosa was very tedious and difficult, especially in the presence of severe disease, and often required a combination of both abdominal and transanal dissection. Transanal mucosal resection required a long period of anal retraction, which was associated with significant functional impairment of the anal sphincter (Johnston et al 1987), although this was minimized if the amount of anal retraction was reduced (Heppell et al 1982). Extensive rectal mucosectomy was also associated with a high incidence of postoperative pelvic sepsis in the form of cuff abscesses, despite meticulous hemostasis and drainage of the cuff space (Liljeqvist et al 1988). The realization that sensation of 'rectal' fullness and need to evacuate were preserved in the absence of a rectum allowed the length of mucosal resection to be shortened significantly. Transanal mucosal resection is now carried out for a distance of only 3–4 cm, and can be completed with minimal retraction on the anal sphincter, especially if a specifically designed ring retractor is used.

With the patient in the lithotomy position, retraction hooks are placed circumferentially into the dentate line to splay the mucosa of the anal canal (Lone Star retractor, Lone Star Company, Texas, USA) (Fig. 90.3). The submucosal plane is infiltrated with a solution of 1 in 100 000 adrenaline and the mucosa dissected off the underlying rectal wall with either scissors or diathermy. This is continued to the level of the pelvic floor, at which point the muscularis is incised and a finger pushed through into the presacral space. The rectum is fully divided at this level and the mucosectomy specimen retrieved through the anus. The pouch is then delivered into the pelvis and its apex brought down to the pelvic floor. The perineal operator inserts four quadrant sutures to approximate the seromuscular layer of the pouch to the puborectalis, and the apex of the pouch is then opened transanally. Full-thickness absorbable sutures are inserted through the pouch wall, the internal anal sphincter and into the anoderm to complete the ileal pouch–anal anastomosis (Fig. 90.4).

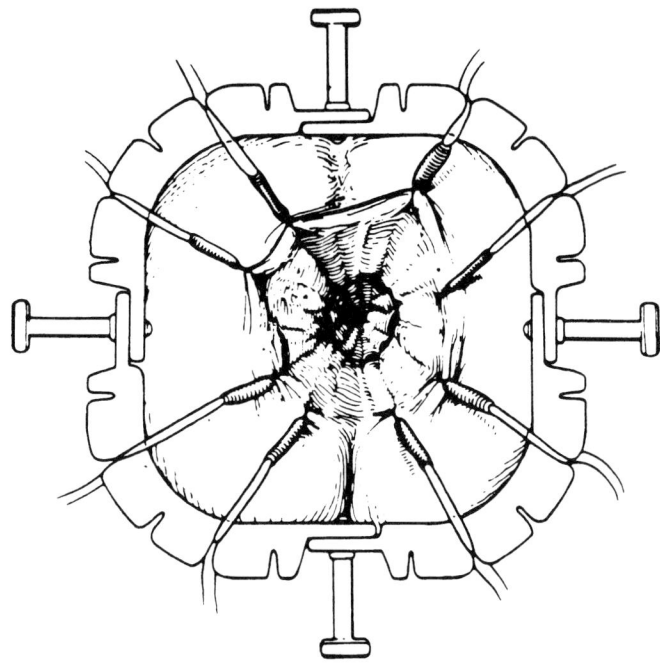

Fig. 90.3 Lone Star retractor for mucosal resection.

Double-stapled technique

This technique, in which the anal canal is cross-stapled about 2 cm above the dentate line and a circular stapling device inserted into the anal stump to perform the

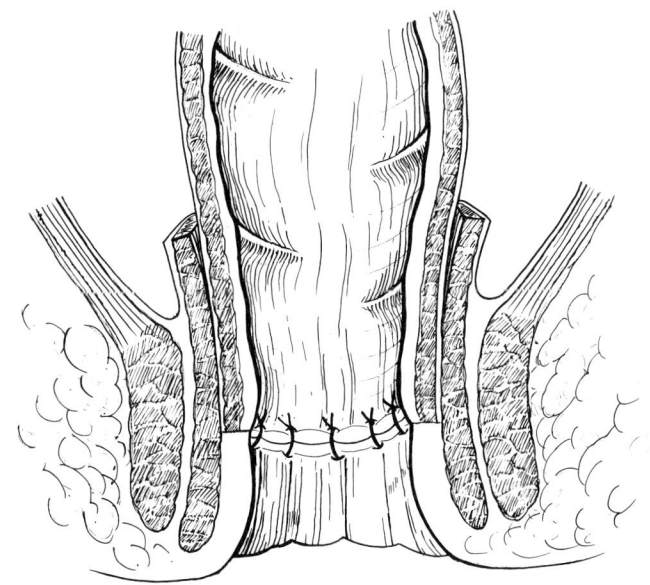

Fig. 90.4 Ileopouch and anastomosis, lower rectal cuff preserved.

anastomosis, has acquired wide popularity, as the technical difficulties of transanal mucosal resection and hand-sutured pouch–anal anastomosis are eliminated

An early stimulus to the development of this procedure was the high incidence of nocturnal incontinence after mucosectomy and hand-sutured anastomosis. The anal transitional zone is richly innervated and seems to be important in the discrimination between flatus and feces (Duthie & Gairns 1960, Duthie & Bennet 1963). Preservation of the zone improves anal sensation (Holdsworth & Johnston 1988), and several authors have demonstrated recovery of the motor function of the anal sphincter

The cecum, colon and rectum are mobilized in the usual manner, with care being taken to preserve the pelvic nerves. The rectum is mobilized fully to the pelvic floor and a small (35 mm) linear cross-stapler maneuvered into the lower pelvis. When the surgeon is confident that the stapler is in the correct position, confirmed by measuring the distance above the dentate line by insertion of a digit, it is closed, fired and the high anal canal divided. A circular stapling device is then inserted into the anal stump and the central trocar advanced through the cross-staple line. The detached head of the gun, positioned within the ileal pouch, is manipulated into line with the shaft of the circular gun. The gun is closed, fired and the double-stapled ileal pouch–anal anastomosis is complete (Fig. 90.5).

The exact distance between the level of the ileoanal anastomosis and the dentate line may be critical in terms of functional outcome. A comparison of ileoanal anastomoses made at the dentate line, at the top of the anal columns of Morgagni and at a level 1 cm above the columns, showed the importance of this region in terms of fecal continence and fine control of defecation (Martin et al 1985). Construction of the ileoanal anastomosis at the dentate line was associated with a higher incidence of seepage and soilage than when the anastomosis was made at the top of the anal columns. If the anastomosis was made too far proximal, however, recurrence of disease occurred. It can be very difficult to accurately place the linear stapler, particularly if the patient is a thick-set male with a narrow pelvis. However, it is surprising just how low the stapler can be placed even in such large patients. Conversely, in a thin female with an accessible pelvis, the linear stapler may be positioned too low on the rectum, such that the 'doughnuts' of the stapling device may include part of the internal sphincter. In order to permit direct inspection of the upper border of the anal transitional zone, the anorectum can be everted by fully mobilizing the rectum to the level of the upper anal canal. The rectum is then transected at mid-body. Stay sutures are inserted into the lateral walls of the rectal stump and passed transanally to the perineal operator. Strong distal traction on the anorectum everts it through the anal canal and allows direct visualization of the zone and accurate

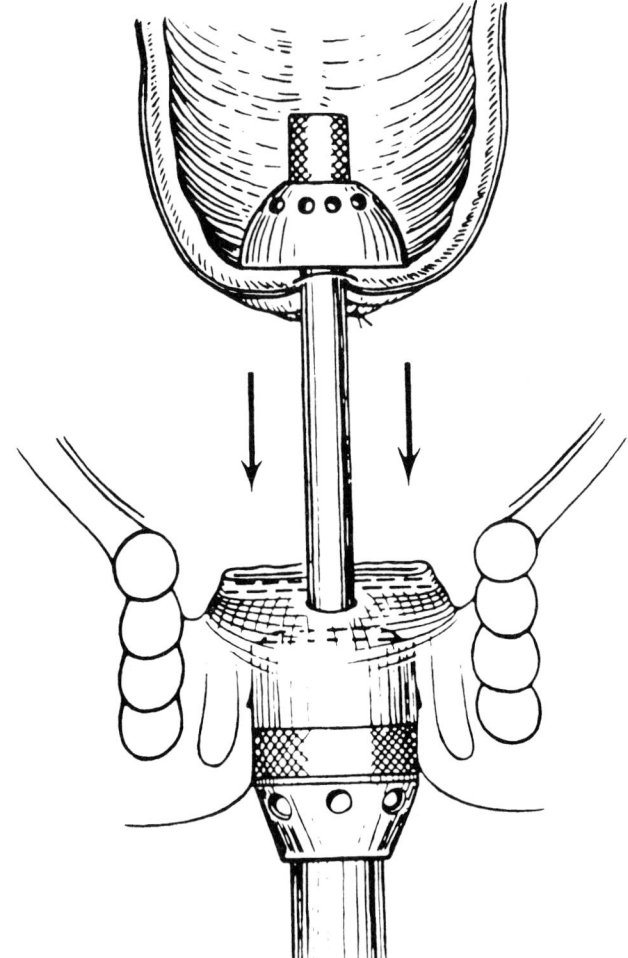

Fig. 90.5 Double-stapled technique for ileal pouch–anal anastomosis.

placement of the cross-stapler. The residual rectal sleeve is then removed and the 'blind' anal stump allowed to return to the pelvis. The ileal pouch–anal anastomosis is then stapled into position in the usual manner (Lewis et al 1993). This technique is more likely to result in a true ileal pouch–anal anastomosis than an ileal pouch–rectostomy.

Despite full rectal mobilization, quite firm traction is required by the perineal operator to achieve complete eversion. Early reports of this technique suggested that the functional results between everted and non-everted ileoanal anastomoses were similar (Brough & Schofield 1989). However, objective measurements of anal sphincter function have shown increased pudendal nerve latency times and blunted electrosensation after double-stapled anastomosis with anorectal eversion (Lewis et al 1992). This appears to result in some impairment of anal sensation, and a greater tendency of patients to experience seepage than in those who have undergone conventional ileal pouch–anal anastomosis.

Fate of residual anorectal mucosa

Preservation of the anal transitional zone may be associated with a potential for proctitis, dysplasia and cancer to develop. The upper border of the zone is irregular. Fingers of transitional zone and true rectal columnar mucosa interdigitate. The rectal tongues may extend all the way down to the dentate line. Ulcerative colitis has been shown to be present within the transitional area in 90% of specimens resected by conventional proctocolectomy (Ambroze et al 1993). Mucosal columnar epithelial cells may remain within the zone in up to 20% of patients after mucosectomy (O'Connell et al 1987). However, mucosectomy does not guarantee elimination of the disease (Heppell et al 1983). Indeed, the only reports to date of rectal cancer after restorative proctocolectomy have been in patients who had undergone mucosectomy with hand-sutured anastomoses and preservation of a rectal cuff (Stern et al 1990). Most patients with a stapled ileal pouch–anal anastomosis will have inflammation at the margin of the staple line (Sugarman et al 1991). The incidence of dysplasia in mucosal strippings from the anal stump studied in a series of 118 patients with ulcerative colitis was 2.5% (Tsunoda et al 1990). A retrospective study of 254 patients who underwent restorative proctocolectomy for ulcerative colitis with a stapled ileal pouch–anal anastomosis revealed low-grade dysplasia in eight (3.1%) (Ziv et al 1994). Neither high-grade dysplasia nor cancer were identified in the anal transitional zone. However, biopsies of the zone taken 6 months later revealed dysplasia in only two patients, in one of whom the initial diagnosis was chronic ulcerative colitis with concurrent colon cancer (T3, N0, M0), whereas the other patient had chronic ulcerative colitis with concurrent high-grade dysplasia. Both subsequently underwent completion mucosal resection. Although the incidence of low-grade dysplasia in the anal transitional zone is low after restorative proctocolectomy with stapled ileal pouch–anal anastomosis (Ziv et al 1994), and it remains to be determined whether or not low-grade dysplasia always progresses to high-grade dysplasia and cancer, it is probably wiser to perform total mucosectomy with hand-sutured anastomosis in patients with a preoperative diagnosis of concurrent colon carcinoma or dysplasia.

Any potential benefit in terms of functional outcome achieved by preservation of the anal transitional zone must be balanced against the potential need for intervention if symptomatic inflammation or malignancy develops. The majority of patients who undergo restorative proctocolectomy are young adults. They are likely to require good anal sphincter function for many years but, conversely, any residual rectal mucosa will potentially have that long to undergo malignant degeneration. This may be dealt with by reoperation, with transanal dissection of the residual mucosa, disconnection of the ileal pouch–anal anastomosis and resection of any rectal cuff and reanastomosis (Fazio & Tjandra 1994).

USE OF A DIVERTING ILEOSTOMY

Pelvic sepsis is the bête noire of ileal pouch–anal anastomosis. Leakage from either the pouch or the anastomosis is associated with a high rate of eventual failure and excision of the pouch (Scott et al 1988, Galandiuk et al 1990). This understandable fear of sepsis has meant that most centers routinely use a temporary diverting ileostomy to divert the fecal stream away from the pouch and anastomosis until they have healed.

The temporary ileostomy is itself, however, a potential source of morbidity (Feinberg et al 1987). Intestinal obstruction, before and after closure of the stoma, is more common in patients with a temporary ileostomy than in patients in whom restorative proctocolectomy is completed as a one-stage procedure. Inevitably, the stoma is sited more proximally than a conventional ileostomy, and is therefore more commonly associated with dehydration secondary to high stomal losses. The stoma may also be associated with peristomal skin breakdown, retraction, stenosis and prolapse.

Several reports have presented the results of restorative proctocolectomy without a temporary stoma (Thow 1985, Metcalf et al 1986, Everett & Pollard 1990, Sugarman et al 1991, Sagar et al 1992b). These studies suggest that a one-stage procedure is safe. Selection of patients is important. The acutely unwell colitic patient who is malnourished and receiving high-dose steroids should not be considered for a one-stage procedure. If a surgeon opts for a one-stage operation, even when all factors are favorable, a heavy burden is assumed. The surgeon must have a low threshold to reoperate if signs suggestive of pelvic peritonitis develop. Patients who undergo this one-stage procedure should not be taking high dose steroids, should undergo an uneventful operation, and should be in good general health. The postoperative course is more difficult for the patient as they must adapt to the ileal reservoir at the same time as recovering from their operation.

Several measures can be used to reduce the chances of complications after one-stage ileal pouch–anal anastomosis. The distal ileum should be irrigated with a solution of antibiotics prior to construction of the pouch. Likewise, the anorectum should be irrigated before division of the rectum and construction of the ileoanal anastomosis. Finally, at the end of the operation, a size 24 Fr urinary catheter should be placed into the pouch and brought out through the anal canal to allow drainage of accumulated blood, mucus and other secretions.

There have been no randomized trials of sufficient power to adequately address the question of the advantages and disadvantages of one-stage versus two-stage restorative proctocolectomy. Although several studies have shown that the one-stage procedure may be carried out safely, the routine use of temporary ileostomy remains the preferred option of most experienced surgeons in this field. Most patients and surgeons would rather deal with the complications of the temporary ileostomy than with the sequelae of feces in the pelvis.

SUMMARY

The vast majority of patients, if carefully selected, can expect a good outcome after ileal pouch–anal anastomosis. Two factors are critical: an anal sphincter capable of providing an adequate high-pressure zone to act as a barrier to pouch content, and the construction of a pouch with adequate capacity to act as a reservoir. All factors considered, it is likely that the J pouch with a stapled ileal pouch–anal anastomosis is set to become the most widely practised variant of the procedure. The operation is undoubtedly complex and this is illustrated by the relatively high rates of associated morbidity (Table 90.2) and the reoperation needed for pouch complications (Table 90.3). Nevertheless, ileal pouch–anal anastomosis is now an established procedure which offers cure of disease and good quality of life.

Table 90.2 Influence of design of the ileal reservoir on frequency of bowel action

Reference	Design of ileal reservoir	No. of patients	Length of follow up (mo)	Bowel actions per 24 h	Bowel actions at night
Morgan et al (1987)	Straight ileoanal	72	12	9.6	–
Pemberton et al (1987)	Dup J	389	6–60	7.0	1.0
Fonkalsrud et al (1987)	Dup lateral ileal	172	46	5.2	–
Becker & Raymond (1986)	Dup J	100	12	5.4	0.6
Wexner et al (1990)	Trip S	114	16–88	6.9	1.5
Schoetz et al (1986)	Dup J	69	>3	5.1	0.2
	Trip S	23			
Fleshman et al (1988)	Dup J	72	>12	6.2	–
	Trip S	107			
Oresland et al (1989)	Dup J	90	12	5.0	40%
	Trips S	10			
Skarsgard et al (1989)	Dup J	9	15	6.0	1.0
	Trip S	66			
Nasmyth et al (1986)	Dup	22	12	7.0	50%
	Trip S	17		5.0	
Hatakayama et al (1989)	Quad W	16	24	3.3	–
Nicholls et al (1987)	Trip S	58	48	3.6	21%
	Dup J	17	29.7	5.5	57%
	Quad W	51	14.8	3.3	14%
Keighley et al (1988)	Dup J	18	12	5.0	1.0
	Quad W	15		4.0	1.0
Harms et al (1990)	Trip S	12	14	5.6	0.6
	Quad W	38		4.4	0.6
Sagar et al (1992a)	Trip S	20	12	6.0	0
	Quad W	20	12	3.5	0

Table 90.3 Reoperation for pouch-related complications. (From Galandiuk et al 1990, with permission)

	Complication (%)			
	Anastomotic stricture (n=42)	Perianal fistula or abscess (n=30)	Intra-abdominal fistula or abscess (n=29)	Poor function (n=13)
Dilatation of stricture	42 (100)		9 (30)	
Fistulotomy		17 (57)	4 (14)	
Closure of fistula		3 (10)	3 (10)	
Drainage of abscess		5 (17)	18 (62)	
Diverting ileostomy		3 (10)	6 (21)	
Redo IPAA			5 (17)	4 (31)
Division of pouch septum				4 (31)
Shorten or excise efferent limb				2 (16)
Convert to different pouch type				4 (31)
More than 1 op. for pouch complications	25 (60)	22 (73)	17 (59)	5 (38)

REFERENCES

Accarpio G, Scodamaglia R, Mignone D, Pozzatti A, Accarpio V 1983 Total colectomy with ileoanal anastomosis and myotomy in the treatment of patients with colonic diseases. Coloproctology 5: 263–265

Aly A, Fonkalsrud E W 1988 Construction of ileal reservoir with longitudinal ileal myotomy. American Surgeon 54: 475–478

Ambroze W L, Pemberton J H, Dozois R R, Carpenter H A, O'Rourke J S, Ilstrup D M 1993 The histologic pattern and pathologic involvement of the anal transition zone in patients with ulcerative colitis. Gastroenterology 104: 514–518

Barros D'Sa A A B 1979 An experimental evaluation of segmental reversal after massive small bowel resection. British Journal of Surgery 66: 493–500

Becker J M, Raymond J L 1986 Ileal pouch–anal anastomosis: a single surgeon's experience with 100 cases. Annals of Surgery 204: 375–381

Brough W A, Schofield P F 1989 An improved technique of J pouch construction and ileoanal anastomosis. British Journal of Surgery 76: 350–351

Clarke C G, Ward M W M 1980 The place of isolated rectal excision in the treatment of ulcerative colitis. British Journal of Surgery 67: 653–654

Duthie H L, Bennett R C 1963 The relation of sensation in the anal canal to the functional anal sphincter: a possible factor in anal continence. Gut 4: 179–182

Duthie H L, Gairns F W 1960 Sensory nerve-endings and sensation in the anal region of man. British Journal of Surgery 47: 585–595

Everett W G, Pollard S G 1990 Restorative proctocolectomy without temporary ileostomy. British Journal of Surgery: 77: 621–622

Fazio V W, Tjandra J J 1994 Transanal mucosectomy: ileal pouch advancement for anorectal dysplasia or inflammation after restorative proctocolectomy. Diseases of the Colon and Rectum 37: 1008–1011

Feinberg S M, McLeod R S, Cohen Z 1987 Complications of loop ileostomy. American Journal of Surgery 153: 102–107

Fleshman J W, Cohen Z, McLeod R S, Stern H, Blair J 1988 The ileal reservoir and ileoanal anastomosis procedure: factors affecting technical and functional outcome. Diseases of the Colon and Rectum 31: 10–16

Fonkalsrud E W 1987 Update on clinical experience with different surgical techniques of the endorectal pull-through operation for colitis and polyposis. Surgery, Gynecology and Obstetrics 165: 309–316

Fonkalsrud E W, Stelzner M, McDonald N 1988 Construction of an ileal reservoir in patients with a straight anorectal ileal pullthrough. Annals of Surgery 208: 50–55

Galandiuk S, Scott N A, Dozois R R et al 1990 Ileal pouch–anal anastomosis: reoperation for pouch-related complications. Annals of Surgery 212: 446–454

Harms B A, Pellett J R, Starling J R 1987 Modified quadruple-loop (W) ileal reservoir for restorative proctocolectomy. Surgery 101: 234–237

Harms B A, Pahl A C, Starling J R 1990 Comparison of clinical and compliance characteristics between S and W ileal reservoirs. American Journal of Surgery 159: 34

Hatakayama K, Yamai K, Muto T 1989 Evaluation of ileal W pouch–anal anastomosis for restorative proctocolectomy. International Journal of Colorectal Disease 4: 150–155

Heppell J, Kelly K A, Phillips S F, Beart R W, Telander R L, Perrault J 1982 Physiologic aspects of continence after colectomy, mucosal proctectomy and endorectal ileo-anal anastomosis. Annals of Surgery 195: 435–443

Heppell J, Weiland H, Perrault J, Pemberton J H, Telander R I, Beart R W 1983 Fate of rectal mucosa after rectal mucosectomy and ileoanal anastomosis. Diseases of the Colon and Rectum 26: 768–771

Holdsworth PJ, Johnston D 1988 Anal sensation after restorative proctocolectomy for ulcerative colitis. British Journal of Surgery 75: 993–996

Johnston D, Holdsworth P J, Smith A H 1989 Preservation of the ileocecal junction and entire anal canal in surgery for ulcerative colitis – a 'two-sphincter' operation. Diseases of the Colon and Rectum 32: 555–561

Johnston D, Williams N S, Neal D E, Axon A T R 1981 The value of preserving the anal sphincter in operations for ulcerative colitis and polyposis: a review of 22 mucosal proctectomies. British Journal of Surgery 68: 874–878

Johnston D, Holdsworth P J, Nasmyth D G et al 1987 Preservation of the entire anal canal in conservative proctocolectomy for ulcerative colitis: a pilot study comparing end-to-end ileo-anal anastomosis without mucosal resection with mucosal protectomy and endo-anal anastomosis. British Journal of Surgery 74: 940–944

Keighley M R B, Yoshioka K, Kmiot W 1988 A prospective randomized trial to compare the stapled double lumen pouch and the sutured quadruple pouch for restorative proctocolectomy. British Journal of Surgery 75: 1008–1012

Kelly K A, Wolff B G, Pemberton J H, Dozois R R 1992 Ileal pouch–anal anastomosis. Current Surgical Problems 29: 59–132

Kmiot W A, Keighley M R 1989 Totally stapled abdominal restorative proctocolectomy. British Journal of Surgery 79: 961–964

Kock N G 1969 Intra-abdominal 'reservoir' in patients with permanent ileostomy. Preliminary observations on a procedure resulting in faecal 'continence' in five ileostomy patients. Archives of Surgery 99: 223–230

Lewis W, Holdsworth P J, Sagar, P M, Johnston D 1992 Is the anal sphincter damaged by anorectal eversion and double stapling of the pouch–anal anastomosis? Diseases of the Colon and Rectum 35: P40

Lewis W G, Holdsworth P J, Sagar P M, Holmfield J H, Johnston D 1993 Effect of anorectal eversion during restorative proctocolectomy on anal sphincter function. British Journal of Surgeons 80: 121–123

Liljeqvist L, Lindqvist K, Ljungdahl I 1988 Alterations in ileoanal pouch technique, 1980–1987: complications and functional outcome. Diseases of the Colon and Rectum 31: 929–938

McIntyre P B, Pemberton J H, Beart R W Jr, Devine R M, Nivatvongs S 1994 Double-stapled vs. handsewn ileal pouch–anal anastomosis in patients with chronic ulcerative colitis. Diseases of the Colon and Rectum 37: 430–433

Madden M V, Farthing M J G, Nicholls R J 1990 Inflammation in ileal reservoirs: 'pouchitis'. Gut 31: 247–249

Martin L W, Torres A M, Fischer J E, Alexander F 1985 The critical level for preservation of continence in the ileoanal anastomosis. Journal of Pediatric Surgery 20: 664–667

Metcalf A M, Dozois R R, Beart R W, Kelly K A, Wolff B G 1986 Ileal pouch–anal anastomosis without temporary diverting ileostomy. Diseases of the Colon and Rectum 29: 33–35

Morgan R A, Manning P B, Coran A G 1987 Experience with the straight endorectal pullthrough for the management of ulcerative colitis and familial polyposis in children and adults. Annals of Surgery 206: 595–599

Nasmyth D G, Williams N S, Johnston D 1986 Comparison of function of triplicated and duplicated pelvic ileal reservoirs after mucosal proctectomy and ileoanal anastomosis for ulcerative colitis and adenomatous polyposis. British Journal of Surgery 73: 361–366

Nelson R L, Prasad M L, Pearl R K, Abcarian H 1991 Inverted U-pouch construction for restoration of function in patients with failed straight ileoanal pullthroughs. Diseases of the Colon and Rectum 34: 1040–1042

Nicholls R J, Gilbert J M 1990 Surgical correction of the efferent ileal limb for disordered defaecation following restorative proctocolectomy with the S ileal reservoir. British Journal of Surgery 77: 152–154

Nicholls R J, Lubowski D Z 1987 Restorative proctocolectomy: the four loop (W) reservoir. British Journal of Surgery 74: 564–566

Nicholls R J, Pezim M E 1985 Restorative proctocolectomy with ileal reservoir for ulcerative colitis and familial adenomatous polyposis: a comparison of three reservoir designs. British Journal of Surgery 72: 470–474

O'Connell P R, Pemberton J H, Weiland L H 1987 Does rectal mucosa regenerate after ileoanal anastomosis? Diseases of the Colon and Rectum 30: 1–5

Oresland T, Fasth S, Nordgren S, Hulten L 1989 the clinical and functional outcome after restorative proctocolectomy. A prospective study in 100 patients. International Journal of Colorectal Disease 4: 50–56

Parks A G, Nicholls R J 1978 Proctocolectomy without ileostomy for ulcerative colitis. British Medical Journal 2: 85–88

Parks A G, Nicholls R J, Belliveau P 1980 Proctocolectomy with ileal reservoir and anal anastomosis. British Journal of Surgery 67: 533–538

Peck D A 1980 Rectal mucosal replacement. Annals of Surgery 91: 294–303

Pemberton J H, Kelly K A, Beart R W Jr, Dozois R R, Wolff B G, Ilstrup D M 1987 Ileal pouch–anal anastomosis for chronic ulcerative colitis. Long term results. Annals of Surgery 206: 504–513

Pemberton J H, Phillips S F, Ready R R, Zinsmeister A R, Beahrs O H 1989 Quality of life after Brooke ileostomy and ileal pouch–anal anastomosis. Comparison of status. Annals of Surgery 209: 620–628

Pescatori M, Manhire A, Bartram C I 1983 Evacuation pouchography in the evaluation of ileoanal reservoir function. Diseases of the Colon and Rectum 26: 365–368

Roediger W E W, Pihl E, Hughes E 1982 Preserving the ascending colon as an alternative surgical option in ulcerative colitis. Surgery, Gynecology and Obstetrics 54: 348–350

Sagar P M, Taylor B A 1994 Pelvic ileal reservoirs: the options. British Journal of Surgery 81: 325–332

Sagar P M, Holdsworth P J, Salter G V, King R F G J, Johnston D 1990 Single lumen ileum with myectomy: an alternative to the pelvic reservoir in restorative proctocolectomy? British Journal of Surgery 77: 1030–1035

Sagar P M, Holdsworth D, Johnston D 1991 Correlation between laboratory findings and clinical outcome after restorative proctocolectomy: serial studies in 20 patients after end to end pouch–anal anastomosis. British Journal of Surgery 78: 67–70

Sagar P M, Holdsworth P J, Godwin P G R, Quirke P, Smith A N, Johnston D 1992a Comparison of triplicated (S) and quadruplicated (W) pelvic ileal reservoirs. Studies on manovolumetry, fecal bacteriology, fecal volatile fatty acids, mucosal morphology and functional results. Gastroenterology 102: 520–528

Sagar P M, Lewis W G, Holdsworth P J, Johnston D 1992b One stage restorative proctocolectomy without temporary defunctioning ileostomy. Diseases of the Colon and Rectum 35: 582–588

Sagar P M, Lewis W, Holdsworth P J, Johnston D, Mitchell C, MacFie J 1993 Quality of life after restorative proctocolectomy with a pelvic ileal reservoir compares favorably with that of patients with medically treated colitis. Diseases of the Colon and Rectum 36: 584–592

Schoetz D J, Coller J A, Veidenheimer M C 1988 Can the pouch be saved? Diseases of the Colon and Rectum 31: 671–675

Schraut W H, Rosemurgy A S, Wang C H, Block G E 1983 Determinants of optimal results after ileoanal anastomosis: anal proximity and motility patterns of the ileal reservoir. World Journal of Surgery 7: 400–408

Scott N A, Dozois R R, Beart R W, Pemberton J H, Wolff B G, Ilstrup D M 1988 Postoperative intra-abdominal and pelvic sepsis complicating ileal pouch–anal anastomosis. International Journal of Colorectal Disease 3: 149–152

Seow-Choen A, Tsunoda A, Nicholls R J 1991 Prospective randomized trial comparing anal function after handsewn anastomosis with mucosectomy versus stapled ileoanal anastomosis without mucosectomy in restorative proctocolectomy. British Journal of Surgery 78: 430–434

Skarsgard E D, Atkinson K G, Bell G A, Pezim M E, Seal A M 1989 Function and quality of life results after ileal pouch surgery for chronic ulcerative colitis and familial polyposis. American Journal of Surgery 157: 467–471

Slors J F M, Taat C W, Brummelkamp W H 1989 Ileal pouch–anal anastomosis without rectal muscular cuff. International Journal of Colorectal Disease 4: 178–181

Stern H, Bernstein M, Killam S, Cohen Z, McLeod R 1987 A stapled S-shaped ileoanal reservoir. Diseases of the Colon and Rectum 30: 214–219

Stern H, Walfish S, Mullen B, McLeod R, Cohen Z 1990 Cancer in an ileo-anal reservoir: a new late complication? Gut 31: 473–475

Stone M M, Lewin K, Fonkalsrud E W 1986 Late obstruction of the lateral ileal reservoir after colectomy and endorectal ileal pullthrough procedures. Surgery, Gynecology and Obstetrics 162: 411–417

Sugarman H J, Newsome H H, Decosta G, Zfass A M 1991 Stapled ileoanal anastomosis for ulcerative colitis and familial polyposis without temporary diverting ileostomy. Annals of Surgery 213: 606–619

Taylor B M, Beart R W, Dozois R R, Kelly K A, Phillips S F 1983 Straight ileoanal anastomosis vs. ileal pouch–anal anastomosis after colectomy and mucosal proctectomy. Archives of Surgery 118: 696–701

Telander R L, Perrault J 1981 Colectomy with rectal mucosectomy and ileoanal anastomosis in young patients: its use for ulcerative colitis and familial polyposis. Archives of Surgery 116: 623–629

Thompson W H F, Simpson A H R W, Wheeler J L 1987 Mathematical prediction of ileal pouch capacity. British Journal of Surgery 74: 567–568

Thow G B 1985 Single-stage colectomy and mucosal proctectomy with stapled antiperistaltic ileoanal reservoir. In: Dozois R R (ed) Alternatives to conventional ileostomy. Year Book Medical Publishers, Chicago, pp 420–432

Tsunoda A, Talbot I C, Nicholls R J 1990 Incidence of dysplasia in the anorectal mucosa in patients having restorative proctocolectomy. British Journal of Surgery 77: 506–508

Utsunomiya J, Iwama T, Imajo M et al 1980 Total colectomy, mucosal proctectomy and ileo-anal anastomosis. Diseases of the Colon and Rectum 23: 459–466

Varma J S, Browning G G P, Smith A N, Small W P, Sircus W 1987 Mucosal proctectomy and colo-anal anastomosis for distal ulcerative proctocolitis. British Journal of Surgery 74: 381–383

Vasilevsky C, Rothenberger D A, Goldberg S M 1987 The S ileal pouch–anal anastomosis. World Journal of Surgery 11: 742–750

Wexner S D, Wong W D, Rothenberger D A, Goldberg S M 1990 The ileoanal reservoir. American Journal of Surgery 159: 178–183

Williams N S 1989 Restorative proctocolectomy is the first choice elective surgical procedure for ulcerative colitis. British Journal of Surgery 76: 1109–1110

Williamson M E R, Lewis W, Sagar P M, Holdsworth P J, Johnston D 1993 Prospective randomised trial of pouch design in restorative proctocolectomy: early results of J vs W: big vs little. Diseases of the Colon and Rectum 36: P38

Williams N S, King R F G J 1985 The effect of a reversed ileal segment and artificial valve on intestinal transit and absorption following colectomy and low ileorectal anastomosis in the dog. British Journal of Surgery 72: 169–174

Ziv Y, Fazio V W, Sirimarco M T, Lavry I C, Goldblum J R, Petras R E 1994 Incidence, risk factors, and treatment of dysplasia in the anal transitional zone after ileal pouch–anal anastomosis. Diseases of the Colon and Rectum 37: 1281–1285

91. Complications after ileal pouch–anal anastomosis

D. A. Rothenberger   B. T. Gemlo   K. I. Deen

The reintroduction of the ileal pouch–anal anastomosis (IPAA) procedure in the early 1980s provided patients with an alternative to life with an abdominal stoma. For many patients the negative body image of a stoma and the physical and psychosocial aspects of adjusting to an ileostomy seem overwhelming. To overcome those problems, surgeons and patients give high priority to the preservation of anal sphincter function and normal defecation. Unfortunately, this perceived improvement in quality of life is achieved at the expense of higher morbidity than that associated with traditional operative alternatives. None the less, restorative proctocolectomy with IPAA is now one of the standard operative options for patients with ulcerative colitis or familial adenomatous polyposis (Rothenberger et al 1992).

It is appropriate to review the complications associated with IPAA, since both physician and patient must weigh the potential risks before undertaking a major operation predicated on lifestyle rather than medical necessity. Complications common to all major operations performed in the pelvis under a general anesthetic will not be discussed. These include cardiopulmonary complications, such as atelectasis, pneumonia and arrhythmias, deep vein thrombosis and pulmonary embolism; infective complications specific to indwelling intravascular or urinary catheters; and metabolic problems such as confusion, depression, steroid or alcohol withdrawal or mild azotemia (Pemberton 1993). First we review the literature on complications specifically related to the IPAA procedure, and then we present a detailed analysis of our own experience.

LITERATURE REVIEW

Mortality

Operative mortality is low for such a major operation as the IPAA. The Mayo Clinic, which has the largest institutional series, has reported only two deaths in over 1200 cases (Pemberton 1993): neither was related to the anastomosis. Other authors have reported similarly low mortality (Leijonmarck et al 1992, Keighley et al 1993, Wettergren et al 1993). This favorable experience probably reflects the fact that most patients undergoing IPAA are young and free of comorbid diseases. Additionally, the reported literature is from specialized centers that have a high volume of colorectal operative cases and considerable expertise to perform such surgery efficiently and safely.

Small-bowel obstruction

The reported incidence of small-bowel obstruction after IPAA varies from 10 to 20%. Partial or complete small-bowel obstruction may result from postoperative adhesions, volvulus, internal herniation of the bowel, or torsion of an ileostomy. In addition, obstruction may occur shortly after closure of a temporary ileostomy owing to luminal stenosis or adhesions at the takedown site.

Senapati et al (1993), from St Mark's Hospital in London, England, reported obstruction complicating IPAA in 30 (9.7%) of 310 patients. Twenty-two (7.2%) patients were treated successfully by conservative measures. Furthermore, it was noted that 17 patients required operative decompression of obstructed bowel due to the ileostomy. Small-bowel obstruction was also significant after ileostomy closure: 4.2% of patients required reoperation. Marcello et al (1993) reported on 460 patients undergoing IPAA at the Lahey Clinic. Ninety-two (20%) patients presented with 109 episodes of small-bowel obstruction. Just under half required operative intervention. The ileostomy was found to be the site of obstruction in just over half of these patients. Rotation of the stoma during its construction so that the functional limb was inferiorly located was the only statistically significant risk factor for obstruction ($P=0.0005$). Mathey et al (1993), reporting on a cumulative Swiss experience, had a 13% incidence of small-bowel obstruction in 213 patients. In a randomized controlled trial of loop ileostomy for pouch–anal anastomosis, Grobler et al (1993) found a high incidence of ileostomy-related complications (52%), which prompted these authors to terminate the trial prematurely. However, the incidence

Table 91.1 Comparison of leak rates after ileal pouch–anal anastomosis

Reference	Center	No. of patients	Pouch design	Overall leak rate (%)
Mathey et al 1993	Cumulative Swiss Experience	213	J/S/W	11
Sugarman & Newsome 1994	Virginia Medical School	75	J	5
Tjandra et al 1993	Cleveland Clinic	100	J	18
Cohen et al 1992	University of Toronto	483	J/S	12
Wettergren et al 1993	University of Copenhagen	144	J	13
Marcello et al 1993	Lahey Clinic	460	J	9
Pemberton 1993	Mayo Clinic	390	J	5

of bowel obstruction was not dissimilar to those without an ileostomy.

Leaks

The reported overall leak rate after IPAA varies between 5 and 18%, as noted in Table 91.1. Leaks may develop shortly after operation from the pouch–anal anastomosis and, less commonly, from the pouch itself. Leakage has also been reported as a complication after closure of a loop ileostomy (Feinberg et al 1987). Well known factors contributing to leakage are anastomotic tension and bowel ischemia. Tjandra et al (1993), from the Cleveland Clinic, reported that pouch–anal anastomotic leakage was greater in patients undergoing IPAA without a diverting ileostomy. In addition, Cohen et al (1992) found that elderly patients, males and those on corticosteroids were at a greater risk for developing leaks, especially if restorative proctocolectomy was performed in a single stage. They subdivided 483 patients undergoing restorative proctocolectomy with IPAA into three groups. Group I consisted of patients having hand-sewn IPAA with loop diversion; group II consisted of patients having stapled IPAA and loop diversion; and group III consisted of those with stapled IPAA without diversion. Leak rates were 12%, 7% and 18%, respectively. Those without diversion therefore had a greater leak rate, but only two (15%) patients who had a leak required reoperation. The remaining 85% were successfully treated by simple tube drainage of their pouches. Furthermore, in all patients with a leak who subsequently healed, pouch–anal function was comparable to those with no leak.

Some studies (Sagar et al 1992, Senapati et al 1993) have shown no difference in leak rates between selected pouch patients with and without diverting stomas. In a small series of eight patients, Launer and Sackier (1991) demonstrated the benefit of an intraluminal bypass device (Coloshield: Deknetel, Fall River, MA) in complementing single-stage restorative proctocolectomy and IPAA. In this study no anastomotic leaks were encountered. Furthermore, the intraluminal device was reported to have been passed between 18 and 26 days after operation without incident. Although this technique may be useful in protecting the pouch–anal anastomosis, it does not militate against leakage from the pouch itself.

Sepsis

Pelvic sepsis may complicate restorative proctocolectomy and IPAA in both the short and the long term. When sepsis occurs early after IPAA it usually does so between the third and sixth postoperative days, and is manifested by pelvic pain or discomfort, fever with tachycardia and a leukocytosis. Alternatively, pelvic sepsis may result from infection of a hematoma adjacent to the anastomosis. Symptoms may resolve with antibiotic therapy or progress to pelvic abscess formation, which may either drain spontaneously through the anastomosis or require formal CT-guided or operative drainage.

There is a wide variation in the reported incidence of pelvic sepsis after this operation. Sugarman and Newsome (1994) reported a 5% incidence of pelvic sepsis in 75 patients undergoing a one-stage procedure. By contrast, Jarvinen and Luukkonen (1993) reported a 33% incidence of pelvic septic complications in 201 patients. Sepsis was due to either hemorrhage or anastomotic leakage; 21% of patients required reoperation. In both of these studies ulcerative colitis was the indication for operation in over 95% of the patients. Mathey et al (1993) reported septic complications in 17 of 157 patients (11%). One hundred and twenty-seven (81%) patients had ulcerative colitis. Although it seems logical that septic complications would be greater in patients with ulcerative colitis compared to those with familial adenomatous polyposis, no trials have been reported that confirm this hypothesis.

Delayed sepsis and fistula

Although a fistula may occur in the first few days after IPAA, chiefly due to anastomotic dehiscence, it is more frequently identified as a late complication some months after pouch construction (Wexner et al 1989). The etiology of a delayed fistula following IPAA may be an occult leak or dehiscence from the pouch or pouch–anal anastomosis, anastomotic stenosis, or underlying Crohn's disease. A pouch–cutaneous fistula may result from adhesions of the pouch to the anterior abdominal wall with a leak or as a consequence of true cryptoglandular infection in the anal canal. Keighley et al (1993) have reported fistula complications in 27 (16%) of 168 patients undergoing IPAA. Rarely, a fistula may be due to previously undiagnosed Crohn's disease. The common sites of fistula are as follows:

from ileoanal anastomosis to vagina, abdominal wall or perineum; from the pouch to the abdominal wall; from the pouch appendage to the abdominal wall with or without bladder involvement; and from the loop ileostomy closure site to the abdominal wall.

Bleeding

Bleeding from the anus after restorative proctocolectomy and IPAA may occur from the suture line or from pouch ischemia (Nicholls 1993). In the former, bleeding is often bright red and anoscopy may reveal an arterial pumping vessel. In the case of pouch ischemia, bleeding is often heavier and consists of dark red blood with clots. Bleeding may also occur from inflamed retained columnar epithelium, although this does not appear to be a significant problem. Nicholls (1993) reported one case of pouch ischemia occurring in 406 patients, whereas Keighley et al (1993) have reported a 6% incidence of pouch ischemia. Most of these pouches were excised.

Peristomal varices have been a significant cause of morbidity in patients with primary sclerosing cholangitis complicating ulcerative colitis who undergo proctocolectomy with a permanent ileostomy (Wiesner et al 1986). Such patients now have the option of hepatic transplantation, providing longevity and an improved quality of life, thus making them suitable candidates for restorative proctocolectomy. To assess bleeding complications from varices in patients having IPAA, Kartheuser et al (1993) studied 40 patients with ulcerative colitis and primary sclerosing cholangitis. Although postoperative complications were high and directly proportional to the state of the liver disease in these patients, there were no cases of bleeding from the anastomosis, indicating the safety of the IPAA in this group of patients. However, such patients require preoperative clotting studies to assess the risks of bleeding.

Pouchitis

Pouchitis is the most frequently reported late complication of restorative proctocolectomy with IPAA (deSilva et al 1991, McIntyre et al 1994, McMullen et al 1991, Rothenberger & Wiltz 1993). It is characterized by bloody diarrhea with macroscopic inflammation and/or ulceration of the pouch. Histology reveals an acute granulocyte infiltration. Extraintestinal manifestations may be present, for example arthritis, iritis and pyoderma gangrenosum. Some studies indicate that pouchitis may not be a significant complication in patients with familial adenomatous polyposis. Penna et al (1994) reported no episodes of pouchitis in 41 patients with familial adenomatous polyposis. Salemans et al (1992) compared the incidence of pouchitis in 72 patients with either ulcerative colitis or familial polyposis undergoing restorative proctocolectomy with IPAA. Pouchitis occurred in 44% of patients with colitis and no patients with familial polyposis ($P<0.005$). Tjandra et al (1992) reported a 33% incidence of pouchitis in patients with ulcerative colitis compared to 10% in familial polyposis patients ($P<0.05$) at a median follow-up of 32 months. Most episodes of pouchitis are mild and resolve with a single course of antibiotic therapy (Keighley et al 1993, Rothenberger & Wiltz 1993). However, some may be protracted, which may lead to poor pouch function, patient dissatisfaction and ultimately pouch excision. Subramani et al (1993), at the Mount Sinai Hospital, studied 15 cases of refractory pouchitis where the original diagnosis was ulcerative colitis. Patients were compared with 18 matched controls without pouchitis. They found that extraintestinal symptoms were more common in pouchitis patients than in the control group (38% versus 5%). Furthermore, there was a male preponderance in pouchitis patients. They concluded that refractory pouchitis did not tend to reflect underlying Crohn's disease, but may indeed reflect an underlying immunological disorder in these patients. Furthermore, Lofberg et al (1991) have postulated an association between DNA aneuploidy, dysplasia in the pouch, and refractory pouchitis.

Anastomotic stricture

Stenosis at the ileoanal anastomosis has been reported, with a frequency of 9% by Marcello et al (1993), 15% by Keighley et al (1993), and up to 30% by Dozois et al (1986), depending on the definition of stenosis. It may result from fibrosis following partial dehiscence of the IPAA or ischemia at the margins of the pouch to anal canal anastomosis. It is not uncommon to encounter a stenotic web at the site of IPAA in a defunctioned pouch. The latter has no serious consequences and may be easily dealt with by digital dilatation.

The consequences of anastomotic stenosis are proximal pouch dilatation and bacterial overgrowth as a result of stasis. This may lead to pouchitis-like symptoms. A grossly dilated pouch has been known to perforate. Data from the Mayo Clinic (Tsao et al 1992) seem to indicate that stenotic complications may have been underreported in the literature: they reported a 33% incidence of IPAA stricture in patients undergoing routine pouchography.

Dysplasia and malignancy

Dysplasia and malignancy are longer-term complications of restorative proctocolectomy and IPAA. Dysplasia in the retained columnar epithelium has been reported in up to 14% of patients (Schmitt et al 1991). It has been postulated that the subsequent risk of cancer developing in these patients is negligible. However, three cases of adenocarcinoma have now been reported with a maximum of 20 years' follow-up after pouch constructions (King et al 1989, Puthu et al 1992, Stern et al 1990). All these

Table 91.2 Reporting of function after ileal pouch–anal anastomosis

Reference	No. of patients	Median follow-up	Frequency of defecation (median)		Incontinence (%)		Urgency (%)	Pads (%)
			Daytime	Nocturnal	Daytime	Nocturnal		
McIntyre et al 1994	61	10 years	7		78	52		
Keighley et al 1993	168	5 years	6		7			
Mathey et al 1993	157	Variable	5.5		6	27	3	
Jarvinen & Luukkonen 1993	150	1 year	6					11
Tjandra	78	3 years	5	1	13	51		
Marcello et al 1993	460	5 years	6			13		

patients had undergone mucosectomy. It is not certain whether malignancy arose from the retained islands of columnar epithelium hidden from mucosal surveillance, the pouch epithelium, or anal canal glandular epithelium. Thus it is recommended that patients undergo surveillance examinations regularly with mucosal biopsy to identify underlying areas of dysplasia and/or carcinoma. More recently, Ziv et al (1994) have recommended circumferential completion mucosectomy in patients with dysplasia in whom some columnar mucosa may have been retained.

The incidence of desmoid tumors is low after the ileoanal pouch procedure (Ambroze et al 1992). There is concern, however, that operation in patients with familial polyposis, particularly before the age of 20, may predispose these patients to develop desmoid tumors in the mesentery.

Poor pouch function

Function of the ileal pouch is the ultimate subjective measure of the success of restorative proctocolectomy and IPAA. In the Mayo Clinic series over 90% of patients had satisfactory pouch function (Pemberton 1993, McIntyre et al 1994). The degree of patient satisfaction following IPAA from other centers is similar (Cohen et al 1992, Keighley et al 1993, McIntyre et al 1994).

Poor pouch–anal function may result from a number of factors. Underlying irritable bowel may result in incoordinate pouch contractions, despite satisfactory anal canal pressures (Keighley et al 1993). Pouch capacity may be diminished, leading to frequency and urgency. The pouch–anal pressure gradient is all-important in the preservation of continence (Farouk et al 1994). Abnormalities of this gradient, because of either high intrapouch pressure or low anal canal pressures, may result in incontinence (Grotz et al 1994). There is evidence that proctectomy alone may result in reduced resting anal pressure, chiefly due to internal sphincter denervation (Hallgren et al 1993). Endoanal mucosectomy and endoanal IPAA were thought to result in significant damage to the internal anal sphincter, hence the development of the double-stapled procedure (Wexner et al 1991). There is evidence, however, that the double-stapled technique does not confer added protection to the internal sphincter. Anorectal division, particularly at the dentate line, will remove proximal internal sphincter muscle, thus reducing the length of the high-pressure zone (Deen et al 1994). Intersphincteric dissection to achieve a low anastomosis may denervate the internal sphincter. Recent data (Deen et al 1995) indicate that even the striated muscle components of the anal sphincter complex may be incorporated in the stapled anastomosis, although the implications of the latter remain unclear. Excision of sensory mucosa from the upper anal canal has been thought to be associated with impaired discrimination (Johnston et al 1987).

The consequences of such alteration in anorectal physiology in terms of function are increased frequency of defecation, nocturnal evacuation, soiling (particularly at night), urgency, and frank incontinence, for which some require a protective pad. In some patients the sensation of impending evacuation may be diminished or absent. Table 91.2 is a comparison of pouch–anal function from centers around the world. Unfortunately, most of these studies have failed to report in a uniform manner that would make comparison meaningful.

Pouch failure

Pouch failure, judged by the number of patients relegated to a permanent ileostomy which may or may not be accompanied by pouch excision, is the final objective measure of the outcome of the IPAA procedure. A multitude of factors, discussed earlier, may lead to poor pouch function and ultimately to a permanent stoma. Reports of pouch failure have been 2.5% (Jarvinen & Luukkonen 1993), 3.5% (Marcello et al 1993), 6% (Mathey et al 1993), 11% (deSilva et al 1991), 11% (Pemberton 1993) and 13% (Keighley et al 1993). Some studies have indicated that pouch failure is more likely when the original diagnosis was ulcerative colitis rather than familial polyposis. More recently, several authors have undertaken either pouch salvage operations or redo pouches in an attempt to improve the results of this operation even further (Poggioli et al 1993).

Sexual dysfunction

Most patients undergoing restorative proctocolectomy and IPAA are sexually active. Sexual function after IPAA is thus an important consideration for both men and women. Both complain of loss of libido and sexual drive in the early postoperative period. Retrograde ejaculation has been reported in up to 10% of men undergoing IPAA, but erectile difficulties have been less common, at 2%. Dyspareunia has been reported in up to 8% of women (Keighley et al 1993, Mathey et al 1993). Subfertility has been ascribed to pelvic adhesions in women. Oresland et al (1994) undertook a detailed radiological study of the reproductive system in women after IPAA to identify a possible underlying anatomical abnormality causing either dyspareunia or subfertility. Abnormalities identified were occlusion of the fallopian tubes, hydrosalpinx, and adhesions between fallopian tubes and pelvic floor. However, vaginal displacement after IPAA was not a problem. Comparison between patients having a conventional ileostomy after proctocolectomy and an ileal pouch in this study revealed vaginal displacement in 100% of ileostomy patients compared to none in the IPAA group.

Metabolic abnormalities

The terminal ileum is the site of absorption of bile salts and vitamin B_{12}. A number of studies have indicated that absorption from the terminal ileum may be impaired in the pouch in its adaptive role as a neorectum (Max et al 1987, Lerch et al 1989, Harvey et al 1991). Furthermore, studies have also indicated that carbohydrate, amino acid and short-chain fatty acid absorption may be impaired (Stelzner et al 1990). The degree of impairment is directly related to length of ileum used to construct the pouch, thus W pouches are associated with the greatest impairment of absorption. Liljeqvist et al (1988) and Nicholls et al (1981) have reported low levels of B_{12} in pouch patients who subsequently needed replacement therapy. Microcytic anemia caused by iron deficiency, and impaired lactose and xylose absorption, have also been reported in some patients.

Cholesterol concentration and cholesterol saturation index are impaired in some patients, who may thus be prone to gallstone formation. Nasmyth et al (1989) have reported gallstones in three of 20 patients undergoing total colectomy. Keighley et al (1993) found gallstones in eight of 168 patients having an ileal–anal pouch. However, the incidence of gallstones in these patients is not greater than in the general population.

Nephrolithiasis may occur in up to 10% of patients having proctocolectomy and conventional ileostomy (Stelzner et al 1990). Ileal reservoir patients are known to have increased urinary volumes that make them less susceptible to nephrolithiasis.

Other complications

A number of other rare complications have been reported after IPAA: superior mesenteric artery syndrome, solitary pouch ulcer and adrenal insufficiency (Bubrick et al 1985, Wexner et al 1990, Tjandra et al 1992).

UNIVERSITY OF MINNESOTA RESULTS

Overview

Complications associated with our first 301 ileoanal procedures, performed between 1981 and 1992, were recently reviewed. Functional results have been reported elsewhere and adverse functional results such as high stool frequency and incontinence will not be included in this review unless they resulted in pouch excision or permanent diversion. The complications of IPAA have been defined as major or minor, the distinction being that a major complication necessitated hospitalization or reoperation, whereas a minor complication did not prolong hospitalization or require admission.

There was one death and 339 complications in 197 (65%) of 301 patients undergoing IPAA (Table 91.3.) One hundred and forty-eight major complications occurred in 108 patients (36%), and 191 minor complications occurred in 132 patients (44%). Forty patients had more than one

Table 91.3 Major and minor morbidity after ileal pouch–anal anastomosis procedure

	No. of patients	Patients with Complications		Number of Complications	
		Major	Minor	Major	Minor
Total patients	301	108 (36%)	132 (44%)		
Complications	339	43 (14%) with both		148 (44%)	191 (56%)
S pouches	231	87 (38%)	100 (43%)		
Complications	263			123 (47%)	140 (53%)
J pouches	68	18 (26%)	30 (44%)		
Complications	68			21 (31%)	47 (69%)
H pouches	2	3 (100%)	4 (100%)		
Complications	7			3 (43%)	4 (57%)
Elective cases	209	80 (38%)	91 (44%)		
Complications	242			113 (47%)	129 (53%)
Urgent cases	76	22 (29%)	33 (43%)		
Complications	81			26 (32%)	55 (68%)
Emergency cases	4	3 (75%)	2 (50%)		
Complications	7			5 (71%)	2 (29%)

Table 91.4 Annual morbidity after ileal pouch–anal anastomosis procedure

Year	No. of patients	Number of patients with complications	
		Major	Minor
1980	1	0	0
1981	25	11 (44%)	6 (24%)
1982	18	10 (56%)	7 (39%)
1983	21	9 (43%)	10 (48%)
1984	25	17 (68%)	12 (48%)
1985	25	7 (28%)	11 (48%)
1986	18	6 (33%)	10 (56%)
1987	32	7 (22%)	10 (31%)
1988	20	8 (40%)	11 (55%)
1989	45	9 (20%)	18 (40%)
1990	32	9 (28%)	16 (50%)
1991	40	9 (23%)	14 (35%)
1992	16	6 (38%)	7 (44%)

major complication, and 43 had both major and minor complications. Patients in whom an S pouch was constructed did not have a significantly different overall complication rate (38% major, 43% minor) than those patients who had J pouches (26% major, 44% minor, $P=0.09$). However, J-pouch patients did have a significantly lower proportion of major complications ($P=0.018$). Procedures performed electively had complication rates similar to those done urgently (defined as requiring surgery during a hospitalization for a flare-up of colitis when medical management was unsuccessful). There were only four emergency cases, and the numbers were too small for comparison.

Only 21% of major and 14% of minor complications occurred during the 30-day postoperative period, so most of the observed morbidity was late. Direct comparison between groups is difficult, since we have much longer follow-up on our S-pouch patients than the J-pouch patients (85 versus 37 months mean follow-up).

Evaluation of the learning curve, if it exists, is also difficult (Wexner et al 1990). Table 91.4 demonstrates a

Table 91.5 Details of complications after ileal pouch–anal anastomosis procedure in 301 patients

	No.	Treatment	No.	Total
Major complications				
Abscess		Drainage		11
Cuff	1			
Intra-abdominal	2			
Pelvic	5			
Perianal	2			
RV septum	1			
Anal stricture				7
		EUA dilation	1	
		Stricturotomy	2	
		Stricturoplasty	4	
Anastomotic leak		Local therapy		4
Desmoids				3
Enterocutaneous fistula				2
Small-bowel obstruction		Enterolysis		34
Fistula in ano				6
		Fistulotomy	3	
		Seton	3	
Pouch failure				30
		Pouch excision		22
		Crohn's	2	
		Fistula	4	
		Pouchitis	5	
		Pelvic sepsis	3	
		Stricture	1	
		Frequency	3	
		Incontinence	1	
		Infarction	1	
		Perforation	1	
		Obstruction	1	
		Permanent diversion		8
		Crohn's	3	
		Frequency	1	
		Obstruction	1	
		Pouch leak	1	
		Pouch perf.	1	
		Pouchitis	1	
Transient pouch failure		Temporary diversion		7
		Pouch leak	3	
		Intra-abdom	1	
		Abscess	1	
		Pouchitis	1	
		Frequency	1	
		Bowel perf.	1	
Incisional hernia		Repair		4
Takedown site		Exploration		11
Obstruction	7			
Perforation	2			
Leak	2			
Postoperative hemorrhage		Re-exploration		6
Pouch perforation		Oversew		2
In X-ray	1			
During flexible endoscopy	1			
Pouch fistula				7
Buttock	1			
Perneal	1			
Vaginal	5			
Psychotic episode				2
Pulmonary embolus				2
Minor complications				
Abscess		Drainage		9
Intersphincteric	3			
Perianal	2			
Perineal	1			
Perirectal	2			
Recurrent	1			
Anal stricture				15
		Noted	3	
		Dilated	12	
Dehydration				11
		Noted	2	
		Admitted	9	
Deep vein thrombosis				3
Imperfect anastomosis (revised intraop.)				2
Partial small-bowel obstruction		Conservative therapy		64
Adhesive	62			
At ileostomy	1			
At takedown site	1			
Pneumothorax				2
Pouchitis				55
		Antibiotics	54	
		Admitted, antibiotics	1	
Steroid insufficiency		Replacement therapy		2
Wound infection		Open wound		4
Midline	2			
Takedown site	2			

fall in the major complication rate with time, but this has to be qualified by the fact that follow-up is shorter. None the less, our initial experience was almost exclusively with hand-sewn S pouches before the evolution of several technical modifications which have simplified the operation and presumably decreased morbidity (Heald & Allen 1986). A breakdown of complications encountered is presented in Table 91.5.

Bowel obstruction

Admission to hospital for partial or complete small-bowel obstruction was our most common major complication, occurring in 29% of patients. The obstruction was partial in 73% of patients and only a minority (11% of patients overall) required exploration and enterolysis. Patients typically presented with crampy abdominal pain, nausea, vomiting and decreased stool or ileostomy output. Time of presentation ranged from the immediate postoperative period to years after ileostomy takedown, with 31% of episodes occurring during the interval between creation of the pouch and ileostomy takedown.

Pouch failure

Pouch failure was our second most common major complication (Gemlo et al 1992). Thirty (10%) of 301 patients eventually underwent pouch excision or permanent ileostomy for reasons listed in Table 91.5. This 9.9% failure rate is similar to other reported series (Lukkonen & Jarvinen 1988, Keighley et al 1989, Marcello et al 1993). Although Crohn's disease contributed to a large number of failures, nine patients had their diagnosis changed from ulcerative colitis to Crohn's disease after surgery but still have functional ileal pouches. The subsequent diagnosis of Crohn's does not necessitate pouch excision, but ileal pouches are not recommended for patients with known Crohn's disease.

Ileostomy complications

After early success with temporary diversion with IPAA, an ileostomy was not constructed in five patients. Four of the five patients developed pelvic septic complications necessitating pouch excision. Since then we have advocated the use of a temporary ileostomy after IPAA. This policy, however, has resulted in significant morbidity. One patient developed volvulus at the ileostomy site and 13 have had complications associated with the takedown procedure, including a leak or obstruction at the takedown site and wound infection. One patient experienced a perforation during a preileostomy takedown radiographic contrast study of the ileal reservoir and proximal stapled split ileostomy, necessitating urgent takedown. Many surgeons now advocate avoiding a temporary ileostomy, a policy change we are cautiously assessing.

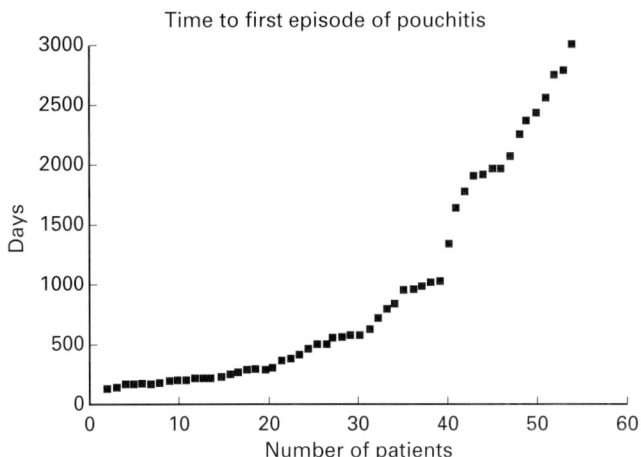

Fig. 91.1

Pouchitis

The most common minor complication in our series is pouchitis, characterized by fever, malaise, anorexia, abdominal cramps and bloody diarrhea. As discussed, the etiology is uncertain. Pouchitis has developed between 2 months and 8 years after IPAA surgery. As Figure 91.1 shows, the majority of pouchitis cases occur within the first few years, and there is a diminishing risk with the passage of time.

CONCLUSION

Morbidity following IPAA remains significant, but the increase in experience, successful negotiation of the learning curve, better understanding of anorectal physiology, and several technical modifications have contributed to an overall improvement in results (Keighley et al 1993). Cuff sepsis appears to have been reduced following recognition that a long cuff of anorectum is not essential for preservation of continence. Functional results improved with the adoption of pouch designs without long efferent limbs to promote spontaneous pouch evacuation (Rothenberger et al 1992). Stapling technology seems to have decreased operative time, and the double-stapling technique may have decreased the incidence of internal sphincter damage, anastomotic stenosis and minor seepage and incontinence. When appropriate, elimination of a temporary ileostomy may further minimize morbidity.

All surgeons would probably agree that attention to detail and significant operative experience are crucial to a successful outcome. The pelvic surgeon with only occasional cases is encouraged to refer patients in need of an IPAA to appropriate centers of expertise. Preoperative knowledge of underlying pathology, sphincter morphology and function, gender and physical stature of the patient can help the surgeon anticipate difficulties and alter the specifics of the operation. A patient with prior pelvic sepsis, a muscular male patient with a narrow pelvis, or an obese patient with a fat-laden short mesentery may present technical challenges for even the most experienced colorectal surgeon. Intraoperative damage to other organs, such as the ureters, pelvic autonomic nerves and pelvic venous plexus, must be avoided. A tension-free anastomosis is the goal, but at times the surgeon may be forced to compromise on the ideal. Restorative proctocolectomy with IPAA calls for dynamic decision making during the operation. The appropriate configuration of the pouch, type and site of the pouch–anal canal anastomosis, the necessity to perform a mucosectomy and the need for a staged procedure are decisions that must be made during the operation.

REFERENCES

Ambroze W L, Dozois R R, Pemberton J H, Beart R W, Ilstrup D M 1992 Familial adenomatous polyposis: results following ileal pouch–anal anastomosis and ileorectostomy. Diseases of the Colon and Rectum 35: 12–15

Bubrick M P, Jacobs D M, Levy M 1985 Experience with endorectal pull through and J pouch for ulcerative colitis and familial polyposis in adults. Surgery 89: 689–699

Cohen Z, McLeod R S, Stephen W, Stern H S, O'Connor B, Reznick R 1992 Continuing evolution of the pelvic pouch procedure. Annals of Surgery 216: 506–512

Deen K I, Hubscher S, Bain I, Patel R, Keighley M R B 1994 Histological assessment of the distal doughnut in patients undergoing stapled restorative proctocolectomy with high or low anastomosis. British Journal of Surgery 81: 900–903

Deen K I, Kumar D, Williams J G, Grant E A, Keighley M R B 1995 Randomized trial of internal anal sphincter plication with pelvic floor repair for neuropathic fecal incontinence. Diseases of the Colon and Rectum 38: 14–18

deSilva H J, de Angelis C P, Soper N, Kettlewell M G, Mortensen N J, Jewell D P 1991 Clinical and functional outcome after restorative proctocolectomy. British Journal of Surgery 78: 1039–1044

Dozois R R, Goldberg S M, Rothenberger D A et al 1986 Restorative proctocolectomy with ileal reservoir. International Journal of Colorectal Disease 1: 2–19

Farouk R, Duthie G S, Bartolo D C C 1994 Recovery of the internal anal sphincter and continence after restorative proctocolectomy. British Journal of Surgery 81: 1065–1068

Feinberg S M, McLeod R S, Cohen Z 1987 Complications of loop ileostomy. American Journal of Surgery 153: 102–107

Gemlo B T, Wong W D, Rothenberger D A 1992 Ileal pouch anal anastomosis: patterns of failure. Archives of Surgery 127: 784–786

Grobler S, Hosie K B, Keighley M R 1992 Randomised trial of loop ileostomy in restorative proctocolectomy. British Journal of Surgery 79: 903–906

Grotz R, Pemberton J H, Ferrara A, Hanson R 1994 Ileal pouch pressures after defecation in continent and incontinent patients. Diseases of the Colon and Rectum 11: 1073–1075

Hallgren T, Fasth S, Delbro D, Nordgren S, Oresland T, Hulten L 1993 Possible role of the autonomic nervous system in sphincter impairment after restorative proctocolectomy. British Journal of Surgery 80: 631–635

Harvey P R C, McLeod R S, Cohen Z, Strasberg S M 1991 Effect of colectomy on bile composition, cholesterol crystal formation and gallstones in patients with ulcerative colitis. Annals of Surgery 214: 396–402

Heald R J, Allen D R 1986 Stapled ileo-anal anastomosis: a technique to avoid mucosal proctectomy in the ileal pouch operation. British Journal of Surgery 73: 571–572

Jarvinen H J, Luukkonen P 1993 Experience with restorative proctocolectomy in 201 patients. Annales Chirurgiae et Gynaecologiae 82: 159–164

Johnston D, Holdsworth P J, Nasmyth D G et al 1987 Preservation of the entire anal canal in conservative proctocolectomy for ulcerative colititis: a pilot study comparing end to end ileoanal anastomosis without mucosal resection with mucosal proctectomy and endoanal anastomosis. British Journal of Surgery 74: 940–944

Kartheuser A H, Dozois R R, Wiesner R H, LaRusso N F, Ilstrup D M, Schleck C D 1993 Complications and risk factors after ileal pouch–anal anastomosis for ulcerative colitis associated with primary sclerosing cholangitis. Annals of Surgery 217: 311–320

Keighley M R, Winslet M, Flinn R, Kmiot W 1989 Multivariate analysis of factors influencing the results of restorative proctocolectomy. British Journal of Surgery 76: 740–744

Keighley M R B, Grobler S, Bain I 1993 An audit of restorative proctocolectomy. Gut 34: 680–684

King D W, Lubowski D Z, Cook T A 1989 Anal canal mucosa in restorative proctocolectomy for ulcerative colitis. British Journal of Surgery 76: 970–972

Launer D P, Sackier J M 1991 Pouch anal anastomosis without diverting ileostomy. Diseases of the Colon and Rectum 34: 993–998

Leiljonmarck C E, Liljeqvist L, Poppen B, Hellers G 1992 Surgery after colectomy for ulcerative colitis. Diseases of the Colon and Rectum 80: 628–630

Lerch M M, Braun J, Harder M, Hofstadter F, Schumpelick V, Matern S 1989 Postoperative adaptation of the small intestine after total colectomy and J pouch anal anastomosis. Diseases of the Colon and Rectum 32: 600–608

Liljeqvist L, Linquist K, Ljungdahl J 1988 Alterations in ileoanal pouch technique, 1980–1987: complications and outcome. Diseases of the Colon and Rectum 31: 929–938

Lofberg R, Liljequist L, Lindquist K, Veress B, Reinholt F P, Tribukait B 1991 Dysplasia and DNA aneuploidy in a pelvic pouch. Diseases of the Colon and Rectum 34: 280–284

Luukkonen P, Jarvinen H 1988 Restorative proctocolectomy for ulcerative colitis. Annales Chirurgiae et Gynaecologiae 77: 1988

McIntyre P B, Pemberton J H, Wolff B G, Beart R W, Dozois R R 1994 Comparing functional results one year and ten years after ileal pouch–anal anastomosis for chronic ulcerative colitis. Diseases of the Colon and Rectum 37: 303–307

McMullen K, Hicks T C, Ray J E, Gathright J B, Timmcke A E 1991 Complications associated with ileal pouch–anal anastomosis. World Journal of Surgery 78: 1039–1044

Marcello P W, Roberts P L, Schoetz D J, Coller J A, Murray J J, Veidenheimer M C 1993 Long-term results of the ileoanal pouch procedure. Archives of Surgery 128: 500–503

Mathey P, Ambrosetti P, Morel P et al 1993 The Swiss experience of the ileoanal anastomosis with reservoir: complications and functional results. Annales de Chirurgie 47: 1020–1025

Max E, Trabanino G, Reznick R K, Bailey H R, Smith K W 1987 Metabolic changes during the defunctioned stage after ileal pouch–anal anastomosis. Diseases of the Colon and Rectum 30: 508–512

Nasmyth D G, Johnston D, Williams N S, King R F, Burkinshaw L, Brooks K 1989 Changes in absorption of bile acids after total colectomy in patients with ileostomy or pouch–anal anastomosis. Diseases of the Colon and Rectum 32: 230–234

Nicholls R J 1993 Controversies and practical problem solving. In: Restorative proctocolectomy. Blackwell Scientific Publications, Oxford, pp 53–82

Nicholls R J, Belliveau P, Neill M, Wilks M, Tabaqchali S 1981 Restorative proctocolectomy with ileal reservoir: a patholophysiological assessment. Gut 22: 462–468

Oresland T, Palmblad S, Ellstrom M, Berndtsson I, Crona N, Hulten L 1994 Gynaecological and sexual function related to anatomical changes in the female pelvis after restorative proctocolectomy. International Journal of Colorectal Disease 2: 77–81

Pemberton J H 1993 Complications, management, failure and revisions. In: Restorative proctocolectomy. Blackwell Scientific Publications, Oxford, pp 34–52

Penna C, Tiret E, Daude R, Parc R 1994 Results of Ileoanal J pouch anal anastomosis in familial adenomatous polyposis complicated by rectal carcinoma. Diseases of the Colon and Rectum 37: 157–160

Poggioli G, Marchetti F, Selleri S, Laureti S, Stocchi L, Gozzetti G 1993 Redo pouches: salvaging of failed ileal pouch–anal anastomoses. Diseases of the Colon and Rectum 36: 492–496

Puthu D, Rajan N, Rao R et al 1992 Carcinoma of the rectal pouch following restorative proctocolectomy: report of a case. Diseases of the Colon and Rectum 35: 257–260

Rothenberger D A, Wiltz O 1993 Etiology of pouchitis. Annales de Chirurgie 47: 1043–1046

Rothenberger D A, Wong W D, Buls J G, Goldberg S M 1992 The 'S' ileal pouch–anal anastomosis. In: Alternatives to conventional ileostomy. Year Book Medical Publishers, Chicago, pp 345–362

Sagar P M, Lewis M, Holdsworth P J, Johnston D 1992 One-stage restorative proctocolectomy without temporary defunctioning ileostomy. Diseases of the Colon and Rectum 35: 582–588

Salemans J M, Nagengast F M, Lubbers E J, Kuijpers J H 1992 Postoperative and long-term results of ileal pouch–anal anastomosis for ulcerative colitis and familial polyposis coli. Digestive Diseases and Sciences 37: 1882–1889

Schmitt S K, Wexner S D, Lucas F V, James K, Nogueras J J, Jagelman D G 1991 Retained mucosa after double stapled ileal reservoir and ileoanal anastomosis. Diseases of the Colon and Rectum 35: 1051–1056

Senapati A, Nicholls R J, Ritchie J K, Tibbs C J, Hawley P R 1993 Temporary loop ileostomy for restorative proctocolectomy. British Journal of Surgery 80: 628–630

Stelzner M, Fonkalsrud E W, Buddington R K, Phillips J D, Diamond J M 1990a Adaptive changes in ileal mucosal nutrient transport following colectomy and endorectal ileal pull through with ileal reservoir. Archives of Surgery 125: 586–590

Stelzner M, Phillips J D, Saleh S, Fonkalsrud E W 1990b Experience with endorectal pull through and J pouch for ulcerative colitis and familial polyposis in adults. Surgery 48: 552–556

Stern H, Walfisch S, Mullen B, McLeod R, Cohen Z 1992 Cancer in the ileoanal reservoir: a new late complication? Gut 31: 473–475

Sugarman H J, Newsome H H 1994 Stapled ileoanal anastomosis without a temporary ileostomy. American Journal of Surgery 167: 159–164

Subramani K, Harpaz N, Bilotta J et al 1993 Refractory pouchitis: does it reflect underlying Crohn's disease? Gut 34: 1539–1542

Tjandra J J, Fazio V W, Church J M, Lavery J C, Oakley J R, Milsom J W 1992 Clinical conundrum of solitary rectal ulcer. Diseases of the Colon and Rectum 35: 227–234

Tjandra J J, Fazio V W, Milsom J W, Lavery I C, Oakley J R, Fabre J M 1993 Omission of temporary diversion in restorative proctocolectomy – is it safe? Diseases of the Colon and Rectum 36: 1007–1014

Tsao J I, Galandiuk S, Pemberton J H 1992 Pouchogram: predictor of clinical outcome following ileal pouch–anal anastomosis. Diseases of the Colon and Rectum 35: 547–551

Wettergren A, Gyrtrup H J, Grosmann E et al 1993 Complications after J-pouch ileoanal anastomosis: stapled compared with handsewn anastomosis. European Journal of Surgery 159: 121–124

Wexner S D, Rothenberger D A, Jensen L et al 1989 Ileal pouch vaginal fistulas: incidence, etiology and management. Diseases of the Colon and Rectum 32: 460–465

Wexner S D, Wong W D, Rothenberger D A, Goldberg S M 1990 The ileoanal reservoir. American Journal of Surgery 159: 178–183

Wiesner R H, LaRusso N F, Dozois R R, Beaver S J 1986 Peristomal varices after proctocolectomy in patients with primary sclerosing cholangitis. Gastroenterology 90: 316–322

Ziv Y, Fazio V W, Goldblum J R, Sinmarco M T, Lavery I C, Petras R E 1994 ATZ dysplasia post IPAA: incidence, risk factors and treatment. Diseases of the Colon and Rectum 37: 4 Abstract

92. Pouchitis

D. P. Jewell   N. J. McC. Mortensen

The term 'pouchitis' was first used by Kock (1977) to describe an acute inflammation in the ileal reservoir of patients who had had a continent ileostomy fashioned following proctocolectomy. Subsequently it has been described in pelvic pouches in patients who have had a proctocolectomy with ileal pouch–anal anastomosis. Since continent ileostomies are now rarely performed this chapter will review data pertaining to pelvic pouches, although the clinical features, diagnosis and treatment are similar for both.

INCIDENCE

The incidence of pouchitis reported in the literature is highly variable, ranging from 7 to 45% (Dozois et al 1986). This variability is largely dependent on diagnostic criteria, which has led to a much stricter definition of pouchitis. As a result most major centers are now reporting a 15–25% frequency (Zuccaro et al 1989, Mortensen & Madden 1993, Luukkonen et al 1994, de Silva et al 1991a, Oresland et al 1989). It occurs almost exclusively in patients who have had the surgery for ulcerative colitis and very rarely in those who have had a pouch formed following proctocolectomy for familial adenomatous polyposis. The first attack of pouchitis usually occurs within the first 2 years following the establishment of a functioning pouch, and may even occur as early as 3 months (Oresland et al 1989, Setti-Carraro et al 1994). The cumulative risk of developing pouchitis over a 7–10-year period is about 35%. Recurrent episodes occur in around half of the patients (Lohmuller et al 1990), but many investigators, although not all, suggest that the frequency of episodes falls with time.

CLINICAL FEATURES AND DIAGNOSIS

Patients with pouchitis present with diarrhea, with an increase in frequency of pouch emptying. They may pass blood and can experience urgency and incontinence. Pelvic as well as abdominal pain can occur, and the patient may also complain of bloating and excess wind. More severe attacks of pouchitis may be associated with fever, malaise, anorexia and occasionally extraintestinal manifestations such as an acute arthropathy, iritis, conjunctivitis and skin lesions such as erythema nodosum or pyoderma gangrenosum (Oresland et al 1989, Meuwissen et al 1989). In other words, patients may feel that they are yet again suffering from an attack of ulcerative colitis.

To make the diagnosis of pouchitis, there must be both endoscopic and histological evidence of inflammation. The endoscopic appearances are similar to those of ulcerative colitis and, in mild attacks, can be patchy, with the most marked changes occurring on the posterior wall of the pouch. Initially the mucosa becomes more erythematous and edematous, but with increasing inflammation there is friability and then frank ulceration and spontaneous hemorrhage. The importance of endoscopic examination is emphasized by the fact that only about half of the patients presenting with clinical features of pouchitis actually have endoscopic inflammation (Shepherd et al 1987, Meuwissen et al 1989).

Even in healthy non-inflamed pouches the ileal mucosa is rarely normal. There is some loss of villus height, with an increase in crypt depth and a chronic inflammatory cell infiltrate (Shepherd et al 1987, Warren & Shepherd 1993) (Fig. 92.1). The severity of these changes is variable over time, and also between biopsies taken from different sites within the pouch. The inflammatory infiltrate consists predominantly of lymphocytes and plasma cells, but eosinophils can be prominent. The architectural changes can be sufficiently severe for the mucosa to appear colonic rather than ileal. Furthermore, there are changes in mucus composition (colonic-type sulfamucin predominates over the sialomucin typically seen in ileal mucosa) as well as the expression of colonic antigens, supporting the concept of colonic metaplasia. When the pouch mucosa becomes inflamed, there is a marked increase in both acute and chronic inflammatory cells (Farrands et al 1988) (Fig. 92.2). Polymorphonuclear leukocytes are particularly prominent and migrate across the epithelium, causing epithelial cell destruction and crypt abscesses. There are varying degrees

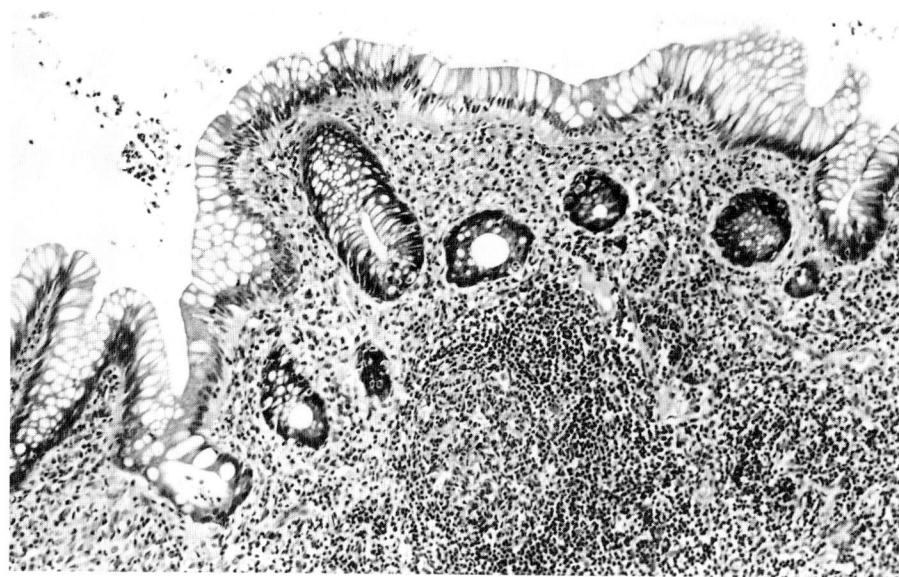

Fig. 92.1 Section of a healthy pouch showing loss of villus height indicating colonic phenotypic change. There is some increase in chronic inflammatory cells and a lymphoid follicle but no acute inflammation. (Courtesy of Dr Bryan Warren)

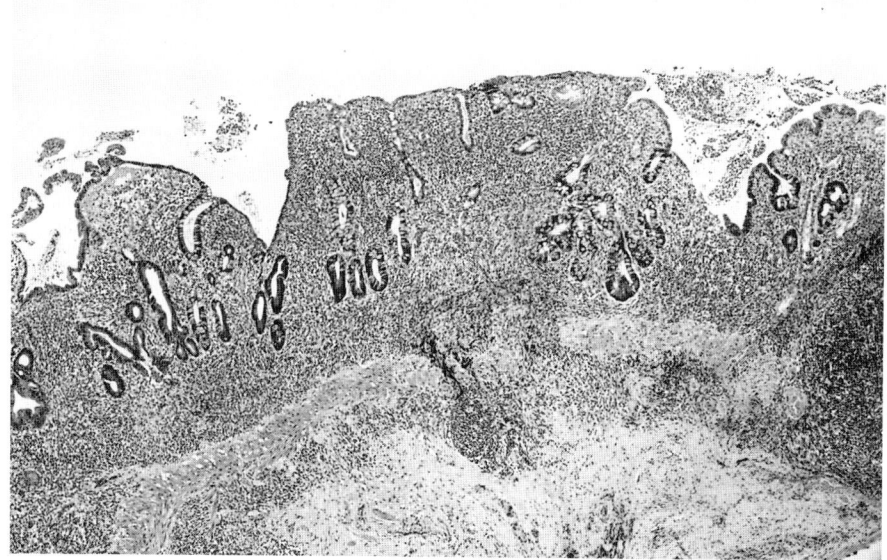

Fig. 92.2 Acute pouchitis showing loss of villus height, increase in crypt depth and dense inflammatory infiltrate. The surface epithelium has become attenuated and irregular. (Courtesy of Dr Bryan Warren)

of mucosal ulceration. In common with ulcerative colitis, the intraepithelial lymphocytes are not increased and may even be low, when expressed as a density count with respect to the number of epithelial cells.

For clinical purposes it is useful to grade the degree of architectural change and the increase in both acute and chronic inflammatory cells, as shown in Table 92.1. A combined score of nine or more defines histological evidence of pouchitis (Warren & Shepherd 1993).

Stool cultures are necessary for all patients presenting with symptoms of pouchitis, as pathogens are occasionally isolated and treatment will clearly differ. Campylobacter, salmonellae and *Clostridium difficile* are the most common pathogens to be isolated.

Digital examination of the anal canal is also an essential part of the assessment in order to exclude significant stenosis at the level of the ileoanal anastomosis.

FACTORS PREDISPOSING TO POUCHITIS

Infection with an enteric pathogen, ischemia as a result of surgical manipulation, and chronic stasis resulting from

Table 92.1 Scoring system for pathological changes in the ileal reservoir mucosa (From Shepherd et al 1987)

	Score
Acute changes	
Acute inflammatory cell infiltrate	
None	0
Mild and patchy infiltrate in the surface epithelium	1
Moderate with crypt abscesses	2
Severe with crypt abscesses	3
Ulceration	
None	0
Mild superficial	1
Moderate	2
Extensive	3
Maximum total	6
Chronic changes	
Chronic inflammatory cell infiltrate	
None	0
Mild and patchy	1
Moderate	2
Severe	3
Villus atrophy	
None	0
Minor abnormality of villus architecture	1
Partial villus atrophy	2
Subtotal villus atrophy	3
Maximum total	6

anal stenosis are well defined and clearly recognized causes of acute inflammation in an ileoanal pouch. However, these probably only account for 10% of pouchitis episodes at the most, but factors predisposing to the rest are much more speculative.

The most obvious factor predetermining susceptibility to pouchitis is the nature of the original disease. Very few cases of pouchitis, as defined on clinical, endoscopic and histological criteria, have been documented in patients with familial polyposis. Thus, ulcerative colitis is the major risk factor and it is an interesting speculation that whatever rendered the patient originally susceptible to ulcerative colitis also makes him or her susceptible to pouchitis when the ileal mucosa undergoes colonic metaplasia.

Nevertheless, pouchitis only affects 15–25% of patients, implying that other factors must be operative. It occurs with equal frequency irrespective of pouch design (S, J or W). Several series have reported a higher incidence of pouchitis in patients who had previously had extensive colitis than in those who had had left-sided disease (de Silva et al 1991a, de Silva et al 1991d), but there is no association with the so-called 'backwash ileitis' (Luukkonen et al 1994, de Silva et al 1991a, de Silva et al 1991d, Gustavsson et al 1987). Patients who had extraintestinal manifestations prior to proctocolectomy are also more prone to developing pouchitis (Oresland et al 1989). However, since the extraintestinal manifestations tend to occur more frequently in patients with extensive colitis, there may be confounding variables. Of particular interest is the recent observation that smoking appears to protect a patient from pouchitis (Merrett et al 1995). Duration of the colitis prior to surgery is not a risk factor, but whether disease severity might predict pouchitis risk is not so clear. Some studies show data suggesting that there is a tendency for pouchitis to be more common in patients undergoing colectomy for severe disease unresponsive to medical therapy, than in those who were having surgery for other reasons. Whether this tendency is statistically significant will only be proved when larger numbers of patients are studied.

TREATMENT (Fig. 92.3)

In the absence of a specific pathogen, treatment of acute pouchitis is entirely empirical in the virtual absence of controlled clinical trials. For the majority of patients a 10–14-day course of an antibiotic will rapidly control symptoms. Metronidazole, ciprofloxacin or augmentin (amoxycillin with clavulanic acid) can be used, with metronidazole usually being first-line treatment. The value of metronidazole compared with placebo has just been confirmed in the first randomized controlled trial to report in pouchitis (Madden et al 1994). For patients who are having frequent episodes a more prolonged course may be helpful, and a few patients will benefit from continuous antibiotics given on a rotational basis.

The major challenge is those few patients (5–10%) who have a chronic persistent pouchitis which is either not affected by antibiotics or who rapidly cease to derive benefit from them. These form a particularly difficult group, and some of them ultimately come to pouch excision with the formation of an end ileostomy. Two questions need to be answered when assessing these patients, namely, is there histological inflammation, and is pouch emptying adequate?

For patients who have histological evidence of persistent pouchitis the original colectomy specimen should be reviewed for evidence of Crohn's disease, although this is an uncommon cause of refractory pouchitis (Subramani et al 1993). Secondly, pouch emptying should be measured using isotope scans (Oresland et al 1989), although these are not widely available. If pouch evacuation is incomplete (>10% of counts remaining), then patients are encouraged to intubate the pouch with a Kock pouch catheter or similar (Medena) every 2 hours to obtain complete drainage. This maneuver can, of course, be tried in the absence of an isotope scan. If evacuation is good, or the patient fails to respond to drainage, then further medical therapy is required. This comes back to the treatment of ulcerative colitis. Thus, topical 5-aminosalicylic acid or corticosteroids can be used, and if there is still no response oral therapy with these drugs should be commenced. In a few patients it may be necessary to defunction the pouch with an ileostomy in order to obtain every chance of healing before excising the pouch.

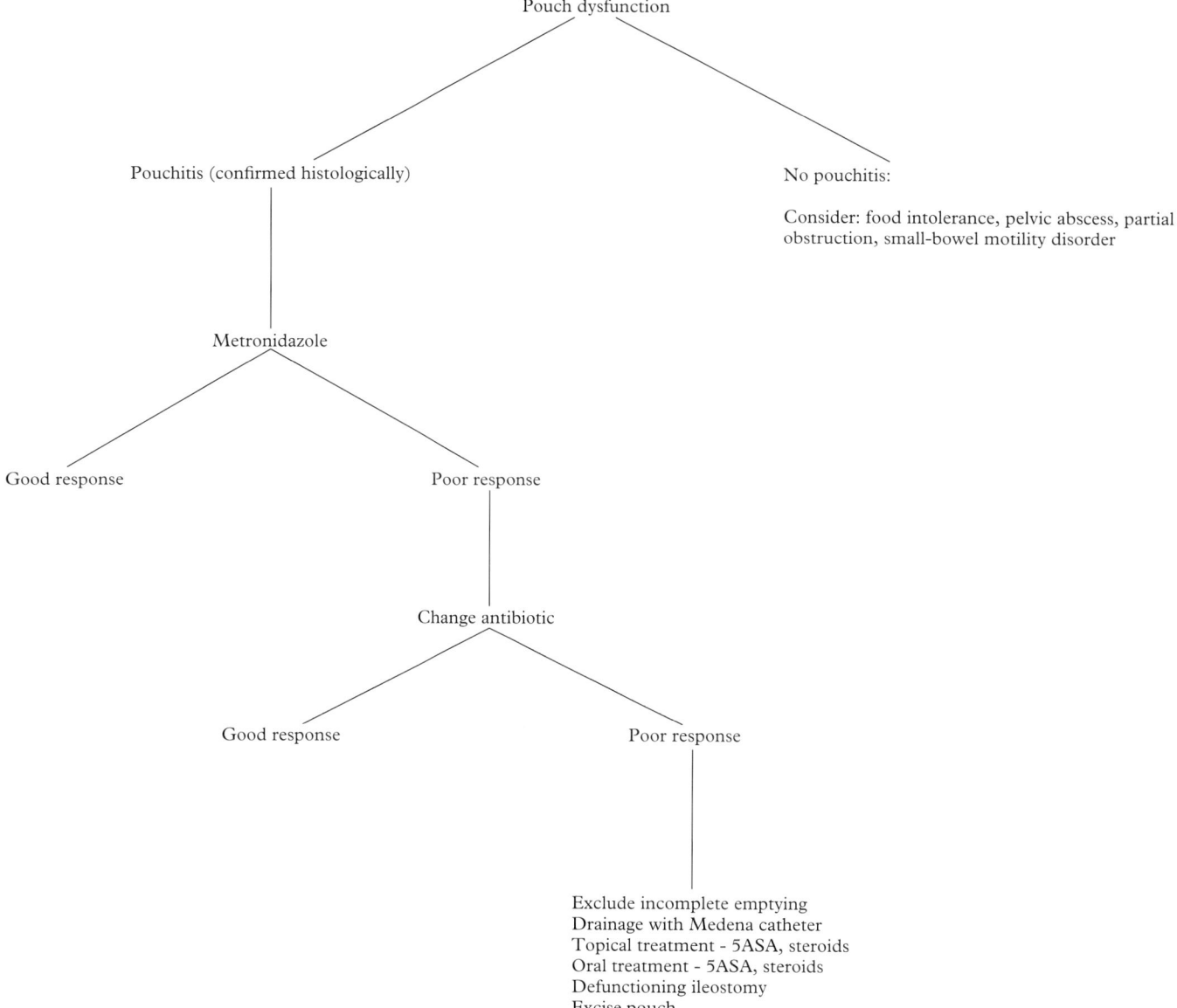

Fig. 92.3 An algorithm for the management of pouch dysfunction.

Some patients with 'refractory pouchitis' do not have any significant histological inflammation and yet have severe diarrhea, frequent incontinence and discomfort. They do not have pouch stasis. The following questions need to be addressed:

1. Is there a pelvic abscess?
2. Is there partial obstruction of the ileum?
3. Is there a small-bowel motility disturbance?
4. Is there dietary intolerance?

Sepsis and obstruction are usually easy enough to exclude by barium radiology, CT scans or ^{99m}Tc-HMPAO labeled white cell counts. However, the others are difficult. It is useful to determine whether the diarrhea is secretory, i.e. whether the 24-hour volume exceeds 500 ml when the patient is strictly nil by mouth. Hypolactasia should be considered, as it can be revealed once the colon is removed. Other dietary influences can best be determined by the use of exclusion diets and subsequent challenge or, at the most extreme, by starting with an elemental diet. If there is stool frequency but without a secretory component, then treatment as for an irritable bowel syndrome can be helpful. Antidiarrheals such as loperamide or codeine phosphate alone usually have minimal effect, but combinations of tricyclic antidepressants, antispasmodics such as mebeverine or alverine citrate, and bulking agents are worth trying. Cholestyramine can also be tried.

PATHOGENESIS

Pouchitis is undoubtedly a heterogeneous disorder. As

implied above, it may be caused by intercurrent enteric infection, ischemia or stasis secondary to anal stenosis. Ischemia probably accounts for the uncommon occurrence of pouchitis in patients who have recently had their pouch created and may even still have a defunctioning ileostomy. There is no convincing evidence, from a histological point of view, that ischemia causes recurrent acute pouchitis or even the chronic refractory form. Nevertheless, mucosal blood flow is reduced in the presence of pouchitis compared to a healthy pouch, as measured by a laser Doppler probe, and so ischemia may be a contributory factor (Hosie et al 1989).

The cause of most cases of pouchitis is completely unknown. The majority of patients will have had ulcerative colitis as their original diagnosis, which is likely to have affected the whole colon. Patients who have occasional episodes of acute pouchitis responding well to antibiotics are clearly different from the 10% or so who have much more refractory disease. However, there are no obvious differences between these two groups in terms of their original disease or pouch design, although the numbers of patients with refractory pouchitis in any one series is small.

Whether a pouch has been formed for ulcerative colitis or familial polyposis, the ileal mucosa undergoes a variable degree of colonic metaplasia (Warren & Shepherd 1993, Nasmyth et al 1989a, de Silva et al 1991b). This involves loss of villus height, with a corresponding increase in crypt depth, a change in mucin composition from sialomucin to sulfomucin, and the expression of colonic antigens on epithelial as well as goblet cells (Campbell et al 1994). These changes are accompanied by an increase in crypt cell proliferation rate, but the stimuli to this increase in epithelial cell turnover are unknown (de Silva et al 1990). It frequently occurs in the absence of histological evidence of inflammation, which makes it unlikely that it is merely a response to growth-regulating cytokines released during immunological activation. Serial observations in patients undergoing staged pouch formation have shown that the fecal stream is an important stimulus, since colonic metaplasia only occurred following ileostomy closure (de Silva et al 1991c). Furthermore, similar metaplastic change can occur proximal to small-intestinal strictures, suggesting that stasis may play a role (Merrett et al 1991). Nevertheless, the colonic metaplasia is incomplete since a healthy pouch epithelium continues to express sucrose-isomaltase (de Silva et al 1991b), a small-intestinal brush border enzyme, and is able to absorb xylose, vitamin B_{12} and bile acids (Jagenburg et al 1975, Gadacz et al 1977, Nasmyth et al 1989b). Furthermore, metaplastic change in epithelial cells, as opposed to goblet cells, may occur prior to ileostomy closure and may therefore not be dependent on the fecal stream (Campbell et al 1994).

The main hypotheses that have been suggested are as follows.

Crohn's disease

A few patients with refractory pouchitis will have had a misdiagnosis of ulcerative colitis on review of the colectomy specimen. This is reported in most of the large series that have been published, but is uncommon. Furthermore, in a controlled study from Mount Sinai Hospital, a missed diagnosis of Crohn's disease was no more common in the pouchitis group than the non-pouchitis group (Subramani et al 1993). Histological assessment of pouch mucosa alone may be misleading, since granuloma and fissures may be seen in pouchitis occurring in patients who have no other evidence of Crohn's disease (Farrands et al 1988, Shepherd 1989).

Stasis and bacterial overgrowth

A major functional factor distinguishing a pouch from an ileostomy is that of stasis. Its role in causing pouchitis, however, is unclear. Both isotope and non-isotopic methods have documented stasis in some patients, but there has been no correlation between incomplete emptying and the occurrence of pouchitis (Oresland et al 1989). Furthermore, there is no reason to presume that there is more stasis in pouches formed for ulcerative colitis than in those formed for familial polyposis, and yet pouchitis rarely, if ever, occurs in the latter situation. Nevertheless, histological changes of pouchitis are more severe on the posterior wall (Shepherd et al 1992), which is the most dependent part of the pouch, and rarely occur in a defunctional pouch. Therefore, there is strong prima facie evidence that the fecal stream has a role.

Even in a perfectly functioning pouch, emptying studies show a small residual volume following evacuation. Since stasis allows bacterial overgrowth, the possible role of bacteria has been investigated (Luukkonen et al 1988, Go et al 1988, Santavirta et al 1991). In general, bacterial cell counts are higher than those in ileostomy fluid but lower than in normal feces. There is a predominance of anerobes in pouches, but microbiological studies have failed to demonstrate significant quantitative or qualitative changes in the pouch contents of patients with or without pouchitis. Metronidazole predictably lowers the *Bacteroides* counts in patients treated for pouchitis, without altering the counts of other organisms, but whether that is the mechanism by which its therapeutic effect on pouchitis is mediated is unknown.

Changes in bacterial flora within the pouch may affect bile acid metabolism (Go et al 1988). Increased concentrations of secondary bile acids have been measured in pouch effluent, suggesting bacterial degradation of primary bile acids. Since bile acids may be toxic to epithelial cells leading, for example, to changes in permeability, they may have an important role to play. However, cholestyramine has not been notably successful in treating pouchitis.

Short-chain fatty acids

Short-chain fatty acids (acetic, butyric and propionic acids) are formed from dietary fiber and other carbohydrates by bacterial action, principally by anerobes. The epithelium of the left colon uses short-chain fatty acids as a fuel substrate, rather than glucose, and it is a low luminal concentration of these acids which is thought to be the cause of diversion colitis. Short-chain fatty acid concentrations have been measured in pouch effluent but the results are conflicting (Nasmyth et al 1989a, Onderdonk et al 1992). Some authors have reported concentrations similar to ileostomy fluid or normal feces, but others have reported reduced concentrations. More recently, a marked reduction has been found in patients with pouchitis compared to healthy pouches (Clausen et al 1992). However, attempts to treat pouchitis with butyrate enemas have not been successful (de Silva et al 1989). Since epithelial cells of the distal colon are reported to metabolize butyrate poorly, it is possible that the epithelial cells of the pouch, having undergone colonic metaplasia, may also have reduced butyrate metabolism, but this has yet to be demonstrated.

Colonic metaplasia – implications for inflammation

As described above, the epithelium of the pouch develops many characteristics of colonic mucosa once there is contact with the fecal stream (de Silva et al 1991c). Furthermore, the metaplastic change is usually maximal on the posterior wall (Shepherd et al 1992), where fecal contact is greatest, and similar changes can be seen in small-intestinal strictures proximal to a stricture (Merrett et al 1991). However, the mechanisms involved in colonic metaplasia are unknown and many factors may be involved, including intestinal hormones, polyamines, cytokines and growth factors. Very few studies have been made on any of these potential mechanisms. Recent studies on TGFα and TGFβ$_1$ have shown altered expression of mRNA and protein in metaplastic mucosa (Campbell et al 1995). In healthy ileal mucosa, mRNA for TGFα or TGFβ is maximal in the crypts, whereas maximal protein expression occurs in the villi. In metaplastic mucosa less mRNA was seen in the crypt cells, but there was increased expression in villus cells. For protein, there was much greater expression on the crypt cells than in healthy mucosa. Crypt cell proliferation tended to correlate with TGFβ$_1$ expression. Whether those changes in growth factor expression are merely secondary to the metaplasia, or whether they might reflect a negative feedback mechanism inducing the change, is unknown.

Whatever the precise mechanisms involved in the metaplastic change, they appear to operate in all pouches regardless of the initial diagnosis of colonic disease. However, pouchitis only occurs in patients who have previously had ulcerative colitis. Thus, the possibility that pouchitis represents ulcerative colitis occurring in metaplastic mucosa has frequently been suggested. If this is true, then it follows that the pathogenesis of pouchitis is similar to that of the original disease. Many features of pouchitis are similar to ulcerative colitis. For example, smokers have less pouchitis than non-smokers (Merrett et al 1995) and immunological features (Merrett & Jewell, unpublished observations) such as an increase in IgG1 and 3 and an infiltration of RFD9$^+$ macrophages are seen in both situations. Whether there is a genetic susceptibility to pouchitis, or whether the 'colonic' epithelial cells of a pouch have an abnormal cell biology similar to that of the resected colonic epithelial cells, is not known.

REFERENCES

Campbell A P, Merrett M N, Kettlewell M G W, Mortensen N J, Jewell D P 1994 Expression of colonic antigens by goblet and columnar epithelial cells in ileal pouch mucosa: their association with inflammatory change and faecal stasis. Journal of Clinical Pathology 47: 834–838

Campbell A P, Smithson J E, Lewis C et al 1995 Altered expression of TFα and TGFβ$_1$ in the mucosa of a functioning pelvic ileo-anal pouch. Journal of Pathology (in press)

Clausen M R, Tuede M, Mortensen P B 1992 Short-chain fatty acids in pouch contents with and without pouchitis after ileal pouch–anal anastomosis. Gastroenterology 103: 1144–1153

de Silva H J, Ireland A, Kettlewell M, Mortensen N, Jewell D P 1989 Short-chain fatty acid irrigation in severe pouchitis. New England Journal of Medicine 321: 1416–1417

de Silva H J, Gatter K C, Millard P R, Kettlewell M, Mortensen N J, Jewell D P 1990 Crypt cell proliferation and HLA-DR expression in pelvic ileal pouches. Journal of Clinical Pathology 43: 824–828

de Silva H J, de Angelic D P, Soper N, Kettlewell M G W, Mortensen N J, Jewell D P 1991a Clinical and functional outcome after restorative proctocolectomy. British Journal of Surgery 78: 1039–1044

de Silva H J, Millard P R, Kettlewell M, Mortensen N J, Prince C, Jewell D P 1991b Mucosal characteristics of pelvic ileal pouches. Gut 32: 61–65

de Silva H J, Millard P R, Soper N, Kettlewell M G W, Mortensen N J, Jewell D P 1991c Effects of faecal stream and stasis on the ileal pouch mucosa. Gut 32: 1166–1169

de Silva H J, Mortensen N J, Jewell D P 1991d Review: Acute inflammation in ileal pouches (pouchitis). European Journal of Gastroenterology and Hepatology 3: 343–349

Dozois R, Goldberg S M, Rothenberger D A 1986 Restorative proctocolectomy with ileal reservoir. International Journal of Colorectal Disease 1: 14–15

Farrands P A, Shepherd N A, Nicholls R J 1988 Ileal reservoir inflammation (pouchitis) after restorative proctocolectomy. Gut 29: A1486

Gadacz T R, Kelly K A, Philips S F 1977 The continent ileal pouch: absorptive and motor features. Gastroenterology 72: 1287–1291

Go P M N Y H, Dieijon-Visser M P, Davies B I, Lens J, Brombacher P J 1988 Microbial flora and bile acid metabolism in patients with an ileal reservoir. Scandinavian Journal of Gastroenterology 23: 229–236

Gustavsson S, Weiland L H, Kelly F A 1987 Relationship of back-wash ileitis to pouchitis after ileal pouch–anal anastomosis. Diseases of the Colon and Rectum 30: 25–28

Hosie K, Sachaguchi M, Tudor R, Gourevitch D, Kmiot W, Keighley M R B 1989 Pouchitis following proctocolectomy is associated with mucosal ischaemia. Gut 30: A1471–1472

Jagenburg R, Kock N G, Philipson B 1975 Vitamin B$_{12}$ absorption in patients with continent ileostomy. Scandinavian Journal of Gastroenterology 10: 141–144

Kock N G, Darle N, Hulten L, Kewenter J, Myrvolol H, Philipson B 1977 Ileostomy. Current Problems in Surgery 14: 36–38

Lohmuller J L, Pemberton J H, Dozois R R, Illstrup D, van Heerden J 1990 Pouchitis and extra-intestinal manifestations of inflammatory bowel disease after ileal pouch–anal anastamosis. Annals of Surgery 211: 622–627

Luukkonen P, Valkonen V, Sivonen A, Sipponen P, Jarvinen H 1988 Faecal bacteriology and reservoir ileitis in patients operated on for ulcerative colitis. Diseases of the Colon and Rectum 31: 864–867

Luukkonen P, Järvinen H, Tanskanen M, Kahri A 1994 Pouchitis – recurrence of the inflammatory bowel disease? Gut 35: 243–246

Madden M V, McIntyre A S, Nicholls R J 1994 Double-blind crossover trial of metronidazole versus placebo in chronic unremitting pouchitis. Digestive Diseases and Sciences 39: 1193–1196

Merrett M N, de Silva H J, Rhodes J M et al 1991 Colonic type mucin occurs in the ileal pouch and small intestinal Crohn's strictures, but not in coeliac disease. Gut 32: A1254–1255

Merrett M, Mortensen N, Kettlewell M, Jewell D P 1995 Smoking may prevent pouchitis in patients with restorative proctocolectomy for ulcerative colitis. Gut (in press)

Meuwissen S G M, Hoitsma H, Boot H, Seldonrijk C A 1989 Pouchitis (pouch ileitis). Netherlands Journal of Medicine 35: 554–566

Mortensen N J M, Madden M V 1993 Pouchitis – acute inflammation in ileal pouches. In: Nicholls J, Bartolo D, Mortensen N (eds) Restorative proctocolectomy. Blackwell Scientific Publications, Oxford, pp 119–131

Nasmyth D G, Godwin P G R, Dixon M F, Williams N S, Jokuston D 1989a Pouch ecology after pouch–anal anastomosis or ileostomy. A study of mucosal morphology, fecal bacteriology, fecal volatile fatty acids and their interrelationship. Gastroenterology 96: 817–824

Nasmyth D G, Johnston D, Williams N S, King R F G J, Burkinshaw I, Brooks K 1989b Changes in the absorption of bile acids after total colectomy in patients with an ileostomy or pouch–anal anastomosis. Diseases of the Colon and Rectum 32: 230–234

Onderdonk A B, Dvorak A M, Cismeros R L et al 1992 Microbiologic assessment of tissue biopsy samples from ileal pouch patients. Journal of Clinical Microbiology 30: 312–317

Oresland T, Fasth S, Nordgren S, Hulten L 1989 The clinical and functional outcome after restorative proctocolectomy. International Journal of Colorectal Disease 4: 50–56

Santavirta J, Matille J, Kokki M, Matikainen M 1991 Mucosal morphology and fecal bacteriology after ileo-anal anastomosis. International Journal of Colorectal Disease 6: 38–41

Setti-Carraro P, Ritchie J K, Wilkinson K H, Nicholls R J, Hawley P R 1994 The first ten years of restorative proctocolectomy for ulcerative colitis. Gut 35: 1070–1075

Shepherd N A, Jass J R, Duval J, Moskowitz R L, Nichols R J, Morson B C 1987 Restorative proctocolectomy with ileal reservoir: pathological and histochemical study of mucosal biopsy specimens. Journal of Clinical Pathology 40: 601–607

Shepherd N A 1989 The pathology of the ileal reservoir. Pouchitis. International Journal of Colorectal Disease 5: 206–208

Shepherd N A, Healey C J, Warren B F, Thompson W H F, Wilkinson S P 1992 The distribution of pathological changes and an assessment of colonic phenotypic change in the pelvic ileal reservoir. Gut 34: 101–105

Subramani K, Harpaz N, Bilotta J et al 1993 Refractory pouchitis: does it reflect underlying Crohn's disease? Gut 34: 1539–1542

Warren B F, Shepherd N A 1993 Pouch pathology. In: Nicholls R J, Bartolo D, Mortensen N (eds) Restorative proctocolectomy. Blackwell Scientific Publications, Oxford, pp 147–162

Zuccaro G, Fazio V W, Church J M, Lavery I C, Ruderman W B, Farmer R G 1989 Pouch ileitis. Digestive Diseases and Sciences 34: 1505–1510

93. Quality of life after restorative proctocolectomy

S. D. Wexner   S. L. Glorsky

Unlike Crohn's disease, mucosal ulcerative colitis is surgically curable. Three of the four operations for elective resection entail disease eradication: total proctocolectomy with Brooke ileostomy, total proctocolectomy with Kock's continent ileostomy, and restorative proctocolectomy. Only the latter preserves the normal route of evacuation, and has therefore become the preferred surgical alternative. The fourth operation, total abdominal colectomy with ileoproctostomy, also preserves anal bowel emptying, but does so at the expense of preservation of the diseased rectum.

Patients who are surgical candidates include those with intractable disease, side effects from medication, dysplasia, carcinoma or lifestyle compromise. In general, however, most patients with colitis have a relatively non-compliant rectum which functions as a conduit rather than a reservoir, and challenges rather than assists the sphincters. Patients with mucosal ulcerative colitis may have tenesmus, urgency and frequent bloody or mucoid stools, often while receiving high-dose steroids and suffering the ill-effects of these steroids. Restorative proctocolectomy offers them an opportunity to preserve sphincter function with improved neorectal capacity and compliance.

Improvement of the quality of life for patients with ulcerative colitis constitutes a goal which significantly motivates the election and continued technical enhancement of the ileoanal reservoir procedures. Manifesting in such diverse areas as anorectal, sexual, reproductive, psychosocial and vocational function, restorative proctocolectomy offers clear advantages over those procedures which involve permanent ileostomy construction. Thus, the ileoanal reservoir has emerged as the most frequent choice in the elective surgical management of ulcerative colitis.

However, as will be subsequently detailed, the current state of the art does not yet offer a panacea for these patients. Although significantly improved postoperatively, gastrointestinal function does not attain parity with that of the normal population. Moreover, there are subgroups to whom restorative proctocolectomy cannot be offered, such as elderly and debilitated patients, individuals with severe anorectal sphincter dysfunction, and those with distal rectal adenocarcinoma. Crohn's disease must be specifically and convincingly excluded. Additionally, this procedure is not appropriate in the emergency setting for complications such as fulminant colitis, toxic megacolon and massive hemorrhage (Wexner 1991). Restorative proctocolectomy is preferably performed on an elective basis, following complete physiologic stabilization, the histopathologic confirmation of disease identity, and the completion of patient counselling with regard to therapeutic options. Patients should be afforded the opportunity to discuss outcome, not only with the surgeon but also with patients who have had each of the four above-cited operations.

Subsequent to the earlier history of restorative proctocolectomy (Martin et al 1977), the incidence of operative complications and procedural failures has steadily declined owing to technical modifications and extensive surgical experience. Postoperative continence and bowel frequency reflect prominently upon the overall success of this operation. Consideration of this parameter is inherently biased by variance in definitions, functional assessment measures, surgical experience and technique, as well as by patient psychologic factors.

Patient accuracy in reporting postoperative bowel function is questionable unless they log this activity daily (Michelassi et al 1993); such detailed data are not available from most clinical series. Surgical experience varies and there is a significant learning curve associated with this technically challenging procedure (Fischer et al 1993). Length of follow-up at the time of reporting affects functional outcome; this variable has also differed significantly among studies. Lastly, definitions of continence vary. Some surgeons discuss subjective parameters such as 'perfect', 'near-perfect', or 'acceptable'. Others rate the type of accident, such as 'seepage', 'staining' or 'soiling'. The most reproducible parameters are based upon an incontinence scale (Jorge & Wexner 1993).

Age further affects outcome. Martin ascribes the superior results in younger patients to fewer associated medical problems and a shorter disease duration, as well as better adaptability and muscular function (Martin et al 1993). Conversely, older patients may suffer impairment of anal sphincter function (Kelly et al 1992). Other investigators have not found a difference in function between older and younger patients (Jorge et al 1994). In fact, recent data have shown that the double-stapled ileoanal reservoir is associated with good functional results even in patients over age 60 years (Reissman et al 1996). Finally, qualitative and quantitative aspects of continence are strongly influenced by reservoir anatomy and physiology. This in turn reflects upon constructional technique, another variable which often differs markedly among surgical investigators (Martin 1993). All of these factors challenge the comparative interpretation of outcome studies of restorative proctocolectomy.

The alterations in lower gastrointestinal anatomy and physiology which occur subsequent to subtotal proctocolectomy and ileoanal pouch anastomosis have been extensively described. Colectomy poses a limitation upon the ability of the gastrointestinal tract to reduce fecal fluid volume and consistency. This change causes a four-fold increase in the quantity of stool presented for evacuation, resulting in a commensurate rise in stool frequency (Kelly et al 1992). This semisolid stool is caustic and may promote perianal skin irritation. Stool consistency may be altered postoperatively through dietary manipulation and the use of bulk forming agents such as psyllium seed preparations. Additionally, loperamide hydrochloride is often employed to slow enteric transit, improve fluid absorption and increase anal sphincter tone, thus decreasing fecal frequency and urgency (Emblem et al 1989, Kelly et al 1992, Grotz & Pemberton 1993).

Pouch volume is intimately associated with stool frequency and continence (Pemberton et al 1987). Physiologic testing can determine the maximum tolerable volume or threshold of reservoir fecal volume at which patients develop the urge to evacuate. This variable, in turn, relates directly to pouch compliance (Kelly 1992, Kelly et al 1992). Greater pouch capacity and compliance theoretically correlate inversely with stool frequency (Tuckson & Fazio 1991, Michelassi et al 1993).

Several reservoir configurations, including S, W, H and K types, have been conceived with the goal of accomplishing compliance characteristics which are superior to the popular J-pouch design. Although some retrospective studies have attested to lower 24-hour stool frequencies, better compliance and improved continence with these configurations (Tuckson & Fazio 1991), this claim has not been borne out (Keighley et al 1988). Furthermore, all pelvic reservoir designs, including the J pouch, exhibit significant increases in capacity and compliance within the first 2 postoperative years, with associated improvements in function (Harms et al 1990, 1992, Becker 1993). Ease of evacuation is an additional, design-related aspect of reservoir function with implication for continence and fecal frequency (Kelly et al 1992).

There are aspects of postoperative pelvic outlet function which directly affect surgical outcome. Mean and maximal internal anal sphincter resting pressures may be moderately diminished for the first 12 months (Grotz & Pemberton 1993, Reissman et al 1995). Anorectal dilatation in the course of mucosectomy may exacerbate this effect (Keighley et al 1993, Binderow & Wexner 1994). Although external anal sphincter squeeze pressure is insignificantly altered by surgery, allowing the patient to consciously defer defecation during sleep, especially in the early postoperative period, the effective total sphincteric barrier to stool passage can become critically low, predisposing to nocturnal soilage. The anorectal sphincter may also be challenged by the frequent large-amplitude propulsive pouch contractions which are characteristic of reservoir response to filling (Kelly et al 1992). Finally, mucosectomy techniques which resect the anal transitional zone may disturb anal discrimination between solid, liquid and gas, as well as local continence reflex mechanisms (Kelly et al 1992, Fischer et al 1993, Mowschenson et al 1993).

A collective review of the outcomes of more than 3000 patients from 20 clinical series who underwent ileoanal pouch anastomosis revealed 90% daytime and 60% nocturnal continence, with an incidence of gross continence of 4% (Stryker 1992). Procedural failure, requiring conversion to a permanent ileostomy, occurred in 6%. However, significant variability is observed among series that have analyzed functional outcome in the treatment of ulcerative colitis (Pemberton et al 1987, Wexner et al 1990, Miller et al 1990). Less often discussed is relative success in alleviation of urgency, which may be more significant than stool frequency (Kelly et al 1992).

The largest single clinical series, representing the Mayo Clinic experience, comprises 1400 patients operated upon over an 11-year period (Kelly et al 1992, Grotz & Pemberton 1993). In this group of largely J-pouch recipients, the average daytime stool frequency was six, and the nighttime one. This figure remained stable over a 5-year follow-up period; however, the need for loperamide therapy decreased from 26 to 4% and psyllium use declined 16%. Becker and Raymond (1986) showed a decrease in daily bowel movements from 7.5 1 month after ileostomy closure to 5.4 11 months later. Schoetz et al (1986) observed similar improvement in their series. Thus, most authors have shown that the daily number of evacuations after restorative proctocolectomy does decrease for at least 12 months after bowel continuity is re-established, regardless of pouch configuration. This has largely been ascribed to a significant increase in pouch capacity during this period of adaptation (Becker 1993).

Significant fecal incontinence was observed in the Mayo series in 5% of patients during the daytime and in

Table 93.1 Functional results of the ileoanal reservoir

Reference	No. of patients	Follow-up (months)	Frequency of evacuation no. of times		Leakage (%)		Incontinence (%)	
			Day	Night	Day	Night	Day	Night
Becker & Raymond 1986	100	24	5.4		–	25	–	
Wexner et al 1989a	114	60	5.4	1.5	12	29	2	1
Harms et al 1992	109	33	4.9	0.3		10	4	
Marcello et al 1993	460	60	5.8	1		10		
Grotz & Pemberton 1993	1400	60	6	1		20–30	5	12
Reissman et al 1995	140	24	5.4	1.2			5	8

Table 93.2 Objective physiologic results of the ileoanal reservoir

Reference	No. of patients	Follow-up (months)	Mucosectomy (+/–)	Mean internal anal sphincter (resting) pressure (mmHg)	Maximal external anal sphincter (squeeze) pressure (mmHg)	Rectoanal inhibitory reflex (+/–)	High-pressure zone (cm)
Lindquist 1990	42	12	+	46	130	+13%	2.9
Oresland et al 1990	67	24	+	52	150	+26%	
Tuckson & Fazio 1991	35	14	+	51	225		
Harms et al 1992	57	12	+	57	142		
Mowschenson et al 1993	22	9.5	–	40	109	+22%	
Reissman et al 1995	124	24	–	55	138		2.9

12% during sleep. Episodes of minor incontinence occurred in 20–30%, with 28% of patients wearing protective pads (Grotz & Pemberton 1993), although many continent patients wear a pad at night to ensure confidence. Higher stool frequencies were noted for patients with greater preoperative frequency and in patients over the age of 50. Conversely, pediatric series reveal a comparably lower stool frequency, for reasons noted above (Martin et al 1993). In the Mayo series, women suffered more episodes of nocturnal fecal soilage than did men (Grotz & Pemberton 1993). The latter has also been observed by others (Michelassi et al 1993). Physiologic adaptation accounted for improvements in all aspects of incontinence over the first 4 years (Pemberton et al 1987). In addition, at 5 years 86% of patients could distinguish flatus from stool (Kelly et al 1992). However, the incidence of pouchitis increases with the duration of postoperative follow-up and may confound progress towards total continence (Fischer et al 1993). The University of Minnesota series, including 129 patients with S pouches, at a mean follow-up of 5 years, revealed a mean number of evacuations of 5.4 during the day and 1.5 at night, with improvement noted over the ensuing 2 years (Wexner et al 1990). Daytime continence was good at 91%, but decreased to 76% at night. Continence for gas was complete or near complete in 81%. Other clinical series, employing a variety of pouch configurations, have produced comparable results (Harms et al 1992, Grotz & Pemberton 1993, Fischer et al 1993, Keighley et al 1993, Marcello et al 1993, Reissman et al 1995) (Tables 93.1 and 93.2).

More recent efforts to improve subsequent bowel function, through retention of the anal transitional zone (ATZ) and the avoidance of interoperative anorectal dilatation, have resulted in the double-stapled ileoanal reservoir technique. In a recent review of 140 patients in whom this technique was employed exclusively, mean daytime bowel movements were 5.4 per 24 hours. The nocturnal frequency was 1.2. Most significantly, 95% and 92% of the patients reported perfect or almost perfect continence during day and night, respectively (Reissman et al 1995). The procedure offers superior function and has not been associated with the development of either intractable 'anusitis' or carcinoma, as feared by its opponents (Schmitt et al 1992). Conversely, three patients with rectal muscular cuff carcinoma have been reported after mucosectomy (Stern et al 1990, Puthu et al 1992, Rodriguez-San Juan et al 1995). Thus both procedures are associated with the potential for subsequent carcinoma. The difference is that after the double-stapled reservoir technique the residual anal transitional zone can be seen, palpated and readily biopsied, whereas after mucosectomy the potentially neoplastic tissue, present in 21% of patients (Horgan et al 1989), is inaccessible. The effects of the various ileoanal reservoir procedures on anal sphincter function are shown in Table 93.2.

Regardless of the technique of reservoir construction, imperfect continence can contribute to the troublesome symptoms and signs of perianal skin irritation. As mentioned above, these inflammatory changes occur secondary to exposure to caustic enteric contents. This has been reported to occur in 22–63% of patients (Grotz & Pemberton 1993, Marcello et al 1993). Beyond pharmacologic treatment to increase stool consistency, local therapy with emollients such as Desitin, A and D ointment and aloe assists in skin protection.

Although the implications for gastrointestinal function following restorative proctocolectomy are less than perfect, they offer substantial improvements over the preoperative disease state as well as the functional outcome following Brooke ileostomy construction. Even when compared to a population of ulcerative colitis patients in medical remission, ileoanal reservoir recipients enjoy less fecal urgency. There is no significant reduction in their ability to discriminate flatus from feces, nor an increased incidence of perianal fecal soilage, perianal pad usage or perianal skin irritation (Sagar et al 1992). They are further spared from the complications of steroid therapy. Alternatively, ileostomy patients are completely incontinent of stool and suffer an incidence of peristomal skin complications which may range as high as 74% (Awad et al 1993).

Dietary intake exerts a significant effect upon postoperative bowel function after restorative proctocolectomy. Certain indiscretions predispose to increase stool frequency and soilage. Specific examples include excessive intake of fluids such as coffee, beer, fruit juice or milk, and the consumption of fatty foods or certain green vegetables (Fujita et al 1992). Conversely, high-fiber diets promote more solid stools (Fischer et al 1993). Patients who eat immediately prior to bedtime are more likely to have their sleep interrupted by a nocturnal bowel movement (Martin 1993). Despite these constraints, requirements for dietary restriction after restorative proctocolectomy are still less than after Brooke ileostomy (Kohler et al 1991), and remain an issue in medically treated ulcerative colitis.

One might feel that sphincter-strengthening exercises would further improve function. However, a recent prospective randomized series failed to show any benefit from such exercises (Jorge et al 1994). Nonetheless, the patients in that trial had undergone a non-mucosectomy double-stapled reservoir procedure, and thus had relatively little operative sphincter trauma. Had they instead undergone mucosectomy with markedly lower postoperative resting pressures, the impact might have been more dramatic.

Few studies address vocational function after restorative proctocolectomy in an isolated fashion. Kohler et al (1991) stated that 94% of patients had returned either to their previous employment or to school after ileal pouch–anal anastomosis. Wexner et al (1990) found that 98% of their ileoanal patients attributed no limitation in their daily activities to their operation. Moreover, return to work can be achieved within 2 or 3 months after hospital discharge (Fujita et al 1992). Conversely, in a recent review, 16% of Brooke ileostomy recipients were required to change employment after surgery (Awad et al 1993).

Social reintegration is more complete after restorative proctocolectomy than after Brooke ileostomy (Kohler et al 1991), with more than 86% of patients noting this aspect of their lifestyle to be improved or unchanged (Kohler et al 1991, Reissman et al 1995). Patients in remission under medical treatment for ulcerative colitis still suffered a 46.3% limitation in their social activities, compared to 21.4% of patients after restorative proctocolectomy. Moreover, the medically treated patients exhibited higher anxiety and depression scores on psychological testing (Sagar et al 1992).

As Kohler et al (1991) have observed, the achievement of continence results in improvements in functional areas where close but uncontrollable contact with other individuals occurs. Specific examples are sexual activity and sports. The appearance of an ileostomy, as well as the risks of leakage, odor and noise, is an operative factor. Because patients afflicted with ulcerative colitis are relatively young, such issues figure prominently in the determination of their quality of life.

Nilsson et al (1981) reported that 83% of women and 72% of men found the Brooke ileostomy to be a hindrance to their sexual life. All of the women and 92% of the men took precautions prior to intercourse, such as emptying, changing or covering the ileostomy bag. Moreover, 52% of the women and 31% of men reported their sexual activity to be reduced or absent. These findings have been corroborated by others (Awad et al 1993). Patients with medically treated colitis also suffer a significant degree of sexual dysfunction, with men reporting a 26% incidence of impotence and a 16% incidence of ejaculatory failure. Dyspareunia is a complaint in approximately 9% of women (Sagar et al 1992). Similarly, the Mayo Clinic experience reports sexual dysfunction in 49% prior to surgery (Kelly et al 1992), which is probably due to poor general health as well as proctitis.

Theoretically, the avoidance of pelvic dissection and successful extirpation of chronic disease in the course of restorative proctocolectomy should contribute to preservation if not the improvement of sexual function for male and female patients alike. This feature has been widely borne out (Binderow & Wexner 1994, Reissman et al 1995). In the Mayo Clinic experience, 11% of men and

12% of women reported postoperative sexual dysfunction, with a 1.5% incidence of impotence and a 4% incidence of retrograde ejaculation. Dyspareunia affected 7% of women. Soiling during intercourse occurred in 3% (Pemberton et al 1987). Similar findings are noted elsewhere (Becker 1992, Fischer et al 1993, Mowschenson et al 1993, Marcello et al 1993).

Impotence and dyspareunia may eventually resolve in a modest percentage of patients (Marcello et al 1993). Moreover, dyspareunia and fecal soilage may be partially mitigated by emptying the reservoir prior to sexual intercourse (Sagar et al 1992).

Frequent concerns of female patients were their future fertility and other issues related to pregnancy and parturition after restorative proctocolectomy. These concerns are often shared by obstetricians. However, rates of conception are unaffected by this procedure (Metcalf et al 1986). During and after pregnancy, pouch function is minimally altered, with a notable increase in the frequency of nocturnal evacuation which normally resolves within the first 3 months postpartum. Daytime frequency and the incidence of incontinence, perineal leakage and skin irritation remains unchanged (Kelly et al 1992). Although the pelvic location of the ileoanal reservoir creates obstetrical concerns for its anatomic or functional disruption during vaginal delivery, these have not been realized (Wexner et al 1990, Kelly et al 1992, Keighley et al 1993). In the Mayo Clinic experience, 88 childbirths have been successfully completed after ileoanal reservoir procedures, all without pouch disruption; 75% of these deliveries were vaginal (Grotz & Pemberton 1993). It is felt that the usual obstetric decisions in the choice between vaginal delivery and cesarian section should be maintained after restorative proctocolectomy. A mediolateral episiotomy is recommended during vaginal delivery in order to avoid damage to the pelvic pouch or anal sphincters (Kelly et al 1992). If pouch–vaginal fistulae do occur, they can be difficult to treat (Wexner et al 1989).

Participation in sports is significantly enhanced after the ileoanal reservoir procedure. Some patients feel that frequent sports activity actually effects further improvements in their bowel function (Fujita et al 1992). After restorative proctocolectomy 17% of patients report restriction in their ability to participate in sports, compared to 42% after Brooke ileostomy. The presence of a stoma is considered to be a significant factor in the ability to tolerate physically strenuous activities (Kohler et al 1991).

Judgment regarding overall patient satisfaction after restorative proctocolectomy constitutes a summation of the component issues described above, including general state of health, anal and neorectal function, medication requirements, degree of dietary restriction, social and vocational rehabilitation, sexual and reproductive function, as well as the ability to participate in recreational activities.

Individual conclusions regarding overall satisfaction significantly correlate with patient personality factors and lifestyle (Fujita et al 1992). In addition, patients are biased towards reporting satisfaction because of the time they and their surgeon have invested in the procedure (Sagar et al 1992), as well as a strong desire to please their physicians (Michelassi et al 1993). Most significant, however, is the marked improvement in health and general sense of wellbeing that occurs following the surgical cure of ulcerative colitis (Kelly et al 1992, Awad et al 1993). Patients are no longer shackled to the toilet, suffering deterioration in their social and professional lives, nor dependent upon pharmacologic agents which extract a high cost in untoward side effects. Thus, patients who have undergone Brooke ileostomy, Kock pouch construction and ileoproctostomy as well as the ileoanal reservoir procedures following colectomy for ulcerative colitis, indicate a high degree of overall satisfaction (Kohler et al 1991, Michelassi et al 1993, Fischer et al 1993, Marcello et al 1993, Awad et al 1993). Kohler et al (1991) reported overall satisfaction in 93% of Brooke ileostomy, 98% of Kock pouch and 96% of restorative proctocolectomy recipients. However, further analysis reveals that after ileal pouch–anal anastomosis patients suffer fewer restrictions in sports and sexual activities than within the two other surgical groups (Kohler et al 1991). Thus, although restorative proctocolectomy does not offer perfect bowel function to the sufferers of ulcerative colitis, it offers a significant improvement over the preoperative state and superior results towards the goal of improved life quality by achieving reliable continence without the requirement for a stoma.

REFERENCES

Awad R W, El-Gohary T M, Skilton J S, Elder J B 1993 Life quality and psychological morbidity with an ileostomy. British Journal of Surgery 80: 252–253

Becker J M 1992 Surgical treatment of ulcerative colitis: the role of the ileoanal pull-through operation. Surgical Rounds January: 25–40

Becker J M 1993 Ileal pouch–anal anastomosis: current status and controversies. Surgery 113: 599–602

Becker J M, Raymond J L 1986 Ileal pouch–anal anastomosis. Annals of Surgery 204: 375–383

Binderow S R, Wexner S D 1994 Current surgical therapy for mucosal ulcerative colitis. Diseases of the Colon and Rectum 37: 610–624

Emblem R, Stien R, Morkrid L 1989 The effect of loperamide on bowel habits and sphincter function in patients with ileoanal anastomosis. Scandinavian Journal of Gastroenterology 24: 1019–1024

Fischer J E, Nussbaum M S, Martin L W et al 1993 The pull-through procedure: technical factors in influencing outcome with emphasis on pouchitis. Surgery 114: 828–835

Fujita S, Kusunoki M, Shoji Y et al 1992 Quality of life after total proctocolectomy and ileal J-pouch–anal anastomosis. Diseases of the Colon and Rectum 35: 1030–1039

Grotz R L, Pemberton J H 1993 The ileal pouch operation for ulcerative colitis. Surgical Clinics of North America 73: 909–932

Harms B A, Anderson A B, Starling J R 1992 The W ileal reservoir: long term assessment after proctocolectomy for ulcerative colitis and familial polyposis. Surgery 112: 638–647

Harms B A, Pahl C, Starling J R 1990 Comparison of clinical and compliance characteristics between S and W ileal reservoirs. American Journal of Surgery 159: 34–40

Horgan P G, O'Connell P R, Shinkain L A, Kirwan W O 1989 Effect of anterior resection on anal sphincter function. British Journal of Surgery 76: 783–786

Jorge J M N, Wexner S D 1993 Etiology and management of fecal incontinence. Diseases of the Colon and Rectum 36: 77–97

Jorge J M N, Wexner S D, Morgado P J Jr 1994 Optimization of the sphincter function after the ileoanal reservoir procedure: a prospective randomized trial. Diseases of the Colon and Rectum 37: 419–423

Jorge J M N, Wexner S D, James K, Nogueras J J, Jagelman D G 1994 Recovery of anal sphincter function after the ileoanal reservoir procedure in patients over the age of 50. Diseases of the Colon and Rectum 37: 1002–1005

Keighley M R B, Grobler S, Bain I 1993 An audit of restorative proctocolectomy. Gut 4: 680–684

Keighley M R B, Yoshioka K, Kmiot W 1988 Prospective randomized trial to compare the stapled double lumen pouch and the sutured quadruple pouch for restorative proctocolectomy. British Journal of Surgery 75: 1009–1011

Kelly K A 1992 Anal sphincter-saving operations for chronic ulcerative colitis. American Journal of Surgery 163: 5–21

Kelly K A, Pemberton J H, Wolff B G, Dozois R R 1992 Ileal pouch–anal anastomosis. Current Problems in Surgery 29: 59–131

Kohler L W, Pemberton J H, Zinsmeisler A R, Kelly K A 1991 Quality of life after proctocolectomy: a comparison of Brooke ileostomy, Kock pouch and ileal pouch–anal anastomosis. Gastroenterology 101: 679–684

Lindquist K 1990 Anal manometry with microtransducer technique before and after restorative proctocolectomy: sphincter function and clinical correlations. Diseases of the Colon and Rectum 33: 91–98

Marcello P W, Roberts P L, Schoetz D J, Coller J A, Murray J J, Veidenheimer M C 1993 Long-term results of the ileoanal pouch procedure. Archives of Surgery 128: 500–504

Martin L W 1993 Current surgical management of patients with chronic ulcerative colitis. Journal of Pediatric Gastroenterology and Nutrition 17: 121–131

Martin L W, Lecoultre C, Shubert W K 1977 Total colectomy and mucosal proctectomy with preservation of continence. Annals of Surgery 186: 477–486

Martin L W, Warner B W, Brockmeier M 1993 Long-term evaluation of the endorectal Soave operation performed for ulcerative colitis or polyposis in the pediatric patient. Surgery 114: 893–896

Metcalf A M, Dozois R R, Kelly K A 1986 Sexual function in women after proctocolectomy. Annals of Surgery 204: 624–627

Michelassi F, Stella M, Block G 1993 Prospective assessment of functional results after ileal J-pouch anal restorative proctocolectomy. Archives of Surgery 128: 889–895

Miller R, Bartolo D C C, Orrom W J, Mortensen N J, Roe A M, Cervero F 1990 Improvement of anal sensation with preservation of the anal transition zone after ileoanal anastomosis for ulcerative colitis. Diseases of the Colon and Rectum 33: 414–418

Mowschenson P M 1993 Inflammatory bowel disease. Part I: pathophysiology and management: new surgical approaches. Seminars in Colon and Rectal Surgery 4: 25–36

Mowschenson P M, Critchlow J F, Rosenberg S J, Peppercorn M A 1993 Factors favoring continence, the avoidance of a diverting ileostomy and small intestinal conservation in the ileoanal pouch operation. Surgery, Gynecology and Obstetrics 177: 17–26

Nilsson L O, Kock N G, Kylberg F, Myrvold H E, Palselius I 1981 Sexual adjustment in ileostomy patients before and after conversion to continent ileostomy. Diseases of the Colon and Rectum 24: 287–290

Oresland T, Fasth S, Nordgren S, Akervald S, Hulten L 1990 Pouch size: the important functional determinant after restorative proctocolectomy. British Journal of Surgery 77: 265–269

Pemberton J H, Kelly K A, Beart R W Jr, Dozois R R, Wolff B G, Ilstrup D M 1987 Ileal pouch–anal anastomosis for chronic ulcerative colitis: long term results. Annals of Surgery 206: 504–513

Puthu D, Rajon N, Rao R et al 1992 Cancer of the rectal pouch following restorative proctocolectomy: report of a case. Diseases of the Colon and Rectum 35: 257–260

Reissman P, Piccirillo M, Ulrich A, Daniel N, Nogueras J J, Wexner S D 1995 Functional results of the double-stapled ileoanal reservoir. Journal of the American College of Surgeons 181: 444–450

Reissman P, Teoh T-A, Weiss E G, Nogueras J J, Wexner S D 1996 Functional outcome of the double-stapled ileoanal reservoir in patients over 60 years of age. American Surgeon 12(3): 178–183

Rodriguez-San Juan J C, Polavieja M G, Naranjo A, Castillo J 1995 Adenocarcinoma in an ileal pouch for ulcerative colitis. Diseases of the Colon and Rectum (editorial) 38(7): 779–780

Sagar P M, Lewis W, Holdsworth P J, Johnston D, Mitchell C, MacFie J 1992 Quality of life after restorative proctocolectomy with a pelvic ileal reservoir compares favorably with that of patients with medically treated colitis. Diseases of the Colon and Rectum 36: 584–592

Schmitt S L, Wexner S D, James K et al 1992 The retained mucosa after double-stapled ileal reservoir and ileoanal anastomosis. Diseases of the Colon and Rectum 35: 1051–1056

Schoetz D J, Coller J A, Veidenheimer M C 1986 Ileoanal reservoir for ulcerative colitis and familial polyposis. Archives of Surgery 121: 404–409

Stern H, Walfish S, Mullen B et al 1990 Cancer in the ileoanal reservoir: a new late complication. Gut 31: 473–475

Stryker S 1992 Crohn's and Colitis Foundation Third Annual RMAC/CMAC Meeting. October 1992 (unpublished data)

Tuckson W B, Fazio V W 1991 Functional comparison between double and triple ileal loop pouches. Diseases of the Colon and Rectum 34: 17–21

Wexner S D 1991 General principles of surgery in ulcerative colitis and Crohn's disease. Seminars in Gastrointestinal Disease 2: 90–106

Wexner S D, Jensen L, Rothenberger D A, Wong W D, Goldberg S M 1989a Long-term functional analysis of the ileoanal reservoir. Diseases of the Colon and Rectum 32: 275–281

Wexner S D, Rothenberger D A, Jensen L 1989b Ileal pouch–vaginal fistulae: incidence, etiology and management. Diseases of the Colon and Rectum 32: 460–465

Wexner S D, Wong W D, Rothenberger D A, Goldberg S M 1990 The ileoanal reservoir. American Journal of Surgery 159: 178–185

SECTION 11

Surgical treatment of Crohn's disease

94. Gastroduodenal Crohn's disease

P. L. Roberts

DUODENAL CROHN'S DISEASE

Although Crohn's disease most commonly affects the small bowel and colon, it has been recognized with increasing frequency in the stomach and duodenum. In a comprehensive review of 600 patients with Crohn's disease, van Patter et al (1954) cited a frequency of duodenal involvement of 0.5%. Since then, a number of authors (Jones et al 1966, Legge et al 1970, Fielding et al 1970, Frandsen et al 1980, Sandler & Golden 1986) have added new cases, demonstrating a frequency of primary gastroduodenal Crohn's disease of 0.5–4.0% of patients with Crohn's disease. In the largest single institutional experience, Nugent and Roy (1989) reported 89 cases of primary gastroduodenal Crohn's disease.

Clinical features

Gastroduodenal Crohn's disease characteristically occurs in association with established disease elsewhere in the gastrointestinal tract. In one series, distal gastrointestinal involvement was previously diagnosed in 51.7% of patients at the time that gastroduodenal disease was diagnosed (Nugent & Roy 1989). The median interval between the diagnosis of intestinal disease and gastroduodenal involvement was 4 years. An additional 30.3% of patients were found to have unsuspected intestinal disease during gastrointestinal tract evaluation for duodenal disease. Only 7.9% of patients had isolated gastroduodenal Crohn's disease with a median follow-up of 11.7 (range 6–14) years. The median age of patients with gastroduodenal Crohn's disease was 26 (range 5–70) years.

Upper abdominal pain is the most common presenting complaint of patients with gastroduodenal Crohn's disease. This symptom is non-specific and may be attributed to acid-peptic disease or more distal Crohn's disease. Nausea, vomiting and weight loss are also reported in almost two-thirds of patients (Nugent & Roy 1989). Although many patients with gastroduodenal Crohn's disease will have evidence of occult blood in the stool, upper gastrointestinal hemorrhage is less common, occurring in 17% (Nugent & Roy 1989). Bleeding of sufficient magnitude to require surgical intervention is rare (<2%) (Nugent & Roy 1989). Free perforation (Katz et al 1983) and acute pancreatitis (Legge et al 1971) complicating gastroduodenal Crohn's disease are uncommon.

The differential diagnosis of patients with suspected gastroduodenal Crohn's disease includes peptic ulcer disease, primary pancreatic and duodenal tumors, and lymphoma. In particular Crohn's disease should be considered in the differential diagnosis of patients with atypical symptoms for peptic ulcer disease, especially those who fail to respond to H_2 blockers and those who are biopsy negative for *Helicobacter pylori*.

The most common distribution of disease is contiguous antral and duodenal involvement, which occurs in 60%. The duodenum is involved and the stomach unaffected in 40% (Nugent & Roy 1989). Proximal extension of the disease to the esophagus is rare. The distribution of other sites of extraduodenal disease is similar to the distribution typically seen in Crohn's disease.

Radiographic findings

Contrast studies of the upper gastrointestinal tract are abnormal in over 90% of patients with gastroduodenal Crohn's disease. The early findings include edema, aphthous ulceration and irregular mucosal thickening (Miller et al 1979). With progression of the disease other radiographic abnormalities, such as stricture or a string sign (Fig. 94.1), deformed duodenal bulb, evidence of ulceration and cobblestoning, and pseudodiverticula may be present. Fistula formation is uncommon, but fistulae involving the duodenum may occur from segments of distal disease adherent to the duodenum. Many of these findings, such as deformation of the duodenal bulb, are not specific to Crohn's disease but may also be seen in patients with peptic ulcer disease.

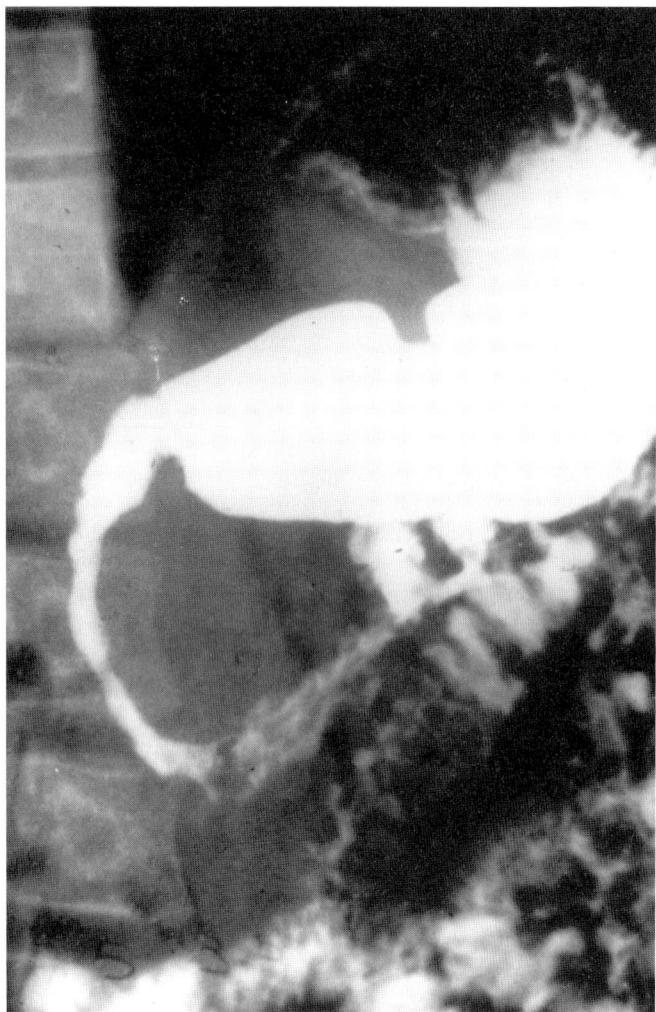

Fig. 94.1 Upper gastrointestinal series showing long duodenal stricture.

Endoscopic findings

The endoscopic findings of gastroduodenal Crohn's disease include granularity, friability and nodularity of the antrum and duodenum. Serpiginous ulcerations are occasionally seen. Severe stricture or stenosis may make intubation of the duodenum impossible. Granulomas appear to be more common at the mucosal level in gastroduodenal Crohn's disease than other sites of Crohn's disease (Haggitt & Meissner 1973), and have been seen in 15–68% of biopsy specimens (Rutgeerts et al 1980, Nugent & Roy 1989). Acute and chronic inflammation, however, is the most common finding on endoscopic biopsy (Nugent & Roy 1989).

Medical therapy

As with Crohn's disease elsewhere in the gastrointestinal tract, the first form of treatment is medical therapy and surgery is reserved for complications. Many patients will undergo successful initial treatment with a combination of antacids and H_2 blockers. Systemic corticosteroids provide symptomatic relief in over 90% of patients with non-obstructing gastroduodenal Crohn's disease (Nugent & Roy 1989). Recently, 5-ASA medications, such as Pentasa (Marion Merrill Dow, Kansas City, MO), which is released in the proximal gastroduodenal tract, have also been used.

Surgical treatment

Approximately one-third of patients with gastroduodenal Crohn's disease require surgical intervention, the most common indication for which is unrelenting obstruction followed by pain and upper gastrointestinal bleeding (Table 94.1). Preoperatively it is important to distinguish between peptic ulcer disease and gastroduodenal Crohn's disease, since bypass without resection is generally the preferred procedure for Crohn's disease. Indeed, gastroduodenal Crohn's disease is the one location where bypass, either by gastrojejunostomy or Roux-en-Y duodenojejunostomy, instead of resection, is recommended. The morbidity of resection is four times higher than bypass for gastroduodenal Crohn's disease (Murray et al 1984).

The issue of whether or not to perform a vagotomy at the time of gastrojejunostomy is controversial. Gastroenterostomy is an ulcerogenic operation, and therefore, if it is carried out for peptic ulcer disease, vagotomy is usually performed. However, truncal vagotomy may be associated with diarrhea, which is already a potential problem in patients with distal Crohn's disease. In one series marginal ulceration was noted in three patients, all of whom had undergone a truncal vagotomy as part of their initial operation (Murray et al 1984), whereas in another series four of ten patients surgically treated developed marginal ulcerations and/or gastric erosions. All of these patients underwent a gastrojejunostomy without vagotomy as the primary procedure (Ross et al 1983). Highly selective vagotomy may be considered, although the edema and thickening in the lesser omentum in patients with gastroduodenal Crohn's disease may make performance of the procedure difficult (Murray et al 1984). Vagotomy should probably be considered on a patient by patient basis.

Isolated pyloric or duodenal strictures may also be treated by strictureplasty. This procedure has the advantage of avoiding a blind loop syndrome or stomal ulceration (Shepherd et al 1985). However, complications such as duodenal fistulae may cause appreciable potential morbidity.

Table 94.1 Indications for surgery for gastroduodenal Crohn's disease ($n=37$) – Lahey Clinic data (From Nugent & Roy 1989)

Indication	Number	Percent
Obstruction	23	70
Pain	9	27
Hemorrhage	1	3

Isolated strictures may also be treated by endoscopic balloon dilatation, but the long-term results are not known and repeated dilatations are often necessary (Williams & Palmer 1991).

Recently, a laparoscopic approach has been used to perform the gastrojejunostomy and highly selective vagotomy. With this approach, examination of the distal bowel for unsuspected Crohn's disease may be difficult as tactile sensation and examination are limited with laparoscopy. The long-term results of laparoscopic procedures for Crohn's are unknown.

GASTRODUODENAL FISTULAE

Clinical features

Fistulae involving the stomach and duodenum in patients with Crohn's disease are relatively rare, with a reported incidence of 0.6% and 0.5% respectively (Klein et al 1987). Fistulae involving the stomach or duodenum appear to arise almost exclusively from distal bowel (small bowel or colon) involved with Crohn's disease that secondarily involves the stomach or duodenum. Symptoms of duodenal or gastric fistulae include diarrhea, weight loss, abdominal pain and feculent vomiting. Diarrhea may result in profound nutritional and electrolyte disturbances, and is the result of a combination of factors, including the presence of Crohn's disease, the irritant effect of hydrochloric acid on the colonic mucosa, the regurgitation of fecal contents into the small bowel leading to bacterial contamination, and the presence of unconjugated bile salts in the colon (Abcarian & Udezue 1978). Associated signs include anemia, fever and abdominal mass. Duodenal fistulae generally involve the second or third portion of the duodenum because of its proximity to the colon or small bowel (Lee & Schraut 1989). Gastric fistulae complicating Crohn's disease arise from the transverse colon in the majority of patients, and extend by means of the gastrocolic ligament to secondarily involve the greater curvature of the stomach (Greenstein et al 1989).

Radiographic findings

Gastric and duodenal fistulae are more likely to be demonstrated on barium enema examination than on upper gastrointestinal series, because of the greater intraluminal pressure of the colon (Fig. 94.2). Fistulae may have a nodular or spiculated appearance, with thickened folds in the area.

Medical treatment

The presence of a gastrocolic or gastroduodenal fistula does not mandate operation (Broe et al 1982). Symptoms are treated with corticosteroids or sulfa compounds, depending

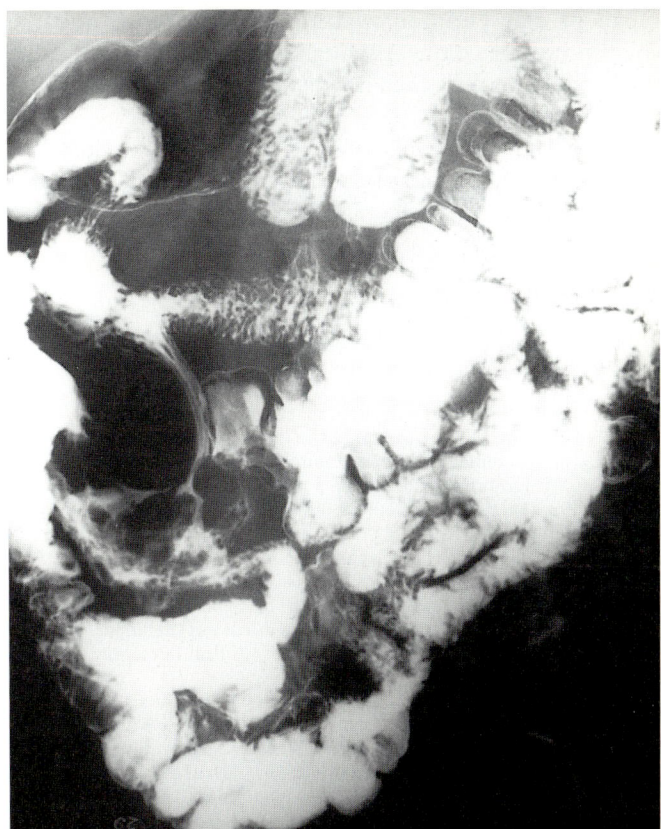

Fig. 94.2 Duodenocolic fistula is shown on barium enema examination in a patient who underwent a prior ileocolic resection for Crohn's disease. (Reprinted with permission from Roberts & Schoetz 1994)

on the site of disease. Inability to control symptoms, progressive weight loss, malnutrition, obstruction and sepsis are indications for operative intervention. In patients who are profoundly malnourished, a short course of preoperative total parenteral nutrition may be helpful.

Surgical treatment

The surgical treatment of the patient with a gastrocolic or duodenocolic fistula is aimed at the primary intestinal source of disease. When a fistula is known to be present preoperatively, the presence of gastric or duodenal Crohn's disease should be excluded. In most patients the stomach and duodenum are normal, and the treatment is disconnection of the fistula, resection of the diseased segment, and suture closure of the duodenal or gastric defect. The defect is generally small and the edges of the bowel may be excised, freshened and sutured. A secure closure is effected by adherence to careful dissection and meticulous hemostasis.

When the duodenal defect is close to the pancreatic border, care must be taken to avoid injury to the pancreas. If present, the omentum may be used to buttress the repair or may be interposed between the repair and the small bowel or colon. Although not proven scientifically, this may prevent the development of a subsequent duodenocolic fistula.

When the duodenal defect is large, the options for closure include simple suture closure, duodenojejunostomy or a serosal onlay patch. Simple suture closure of the defect must be performed with good hemostasis and without tension on the anastomosis. If the defect cannot be safely primarily closed, serosal onlay patch is our preference, as duodenojejunostomy may bypass an appreciable amount of the small bowel in a patient with Crohn's disease who has already undergone small-bowel resection.

REFERENCES

Abcarian H, Udezue N 1978 Coloenteric fistulas. Diseases of the Colon and Rectum 21: 281–286

Broe P J, Bayless T M, Cameron J L 1982 Crohn's disease: are enteroenteral fistulas an indication for surgery? Surgery 91: 249–253

Fielding J F, Toye D K M, Beton D C, Cooke W T 1970 Crohn's disease of the stomach and duodenum. Gut 11: 1001–1006

Frandsen P J, Jarnum S, Malmstrøm J 1980 Crohn's disease of the duodenum. Scandinavian Journal of Gastroenterology 15: 683–688

Greenstein A J, Present D H, Sachar D B et al 1989 Gastric fistulas in Crohn's disease: report of cases. Diseases of the Colon and Rectum 32: 888–892

Haggitt R C, Meissner W A 1973 Crohn's disease of the upper gastrointestinal tract. American Journal of Clinical Pathology 59: 613–622

Jones G W Jr, Dooley M R, Schoenfield L J 1966 Regional enteritis with involvement of the duodenum. Gastroenterology 51: 1018–1022

Katz S, Talansky A, Kahn E 1983 Recurrent free perforation in gastroduodenal Crohn's disease. American Journal of Gastroenterology 78: 722–725

Klein S, Greenstein A J, Sachar D B 1987 Duodenal fistulas in Crohn's disease. Gastroenterology 89: 1347–1352

Lee K K, Schraut W H 1989 Diagnosis and treatment of duodenoenteric fistulas complicating Crohn's disease. Surgery, Gynecology and Obstetrics 124: 712–715

Legge D A, Carlson H C, Judd E S 1970 Roentgenologic features of regional enteritis of the upper gastrointestinal tract. American Journal of Radiology 110: 355–360

Legge D A, Hoffman H N II, Carlson H C 1971 Pancreatitis as a complication of regional enteritis of the duodenum. Gastroenterology 61: 834–837

Miller E M, Moss A A, Kressel H Y 1979 Duodenal involvement with Crohn's disease: a spectrum of radiographic abnormality. American Journal of Gastroenterology 71: 107–116

Murray J J, Schoetz D J Jr, Nugent F W, Coller J A, Veidenheimer M C 1984 Surgical management of Crohn's disease involving the duodenum. American Journal of Surgery 147: 58–65

Nugent F W, Roy M A 1989 Duodenal Crohn's disease: an analysis of 89 cases. American Journal of Gastroenterology 8: 160–165

Roberts P L, Schoetz D J Jr 1994 Gastroduodenal Crohn's disease. Seminars in Colon and Rectal Surgery 5: 199–203

Ross T M, Fazio V W, Farmer R G 1983 Long-term results of surgical treatment for Crohn's disease of the duodenum. Annals of Surgery 197: 399–406

Rutgeerts P, Onette E, Vantrappen G, Geboes K, Broeckhert L, Talloen L 1980 Crohn's disease of the stomach and duodenum. A clinical study with emphasis on the value of endoscopy and endoscopic biopsies. Endoscopy 12: 288–294

Sandler R S, Golden A L 1986 Epidemiology of Crohn's disease. Journal of Clinical Gastroenterology 8: 160–165

Shepherd A F I, Allan R N, Dykes P W, Keighley M R B, Alexander-Williams J 1985 The surgical treatment of gastroduodenal Crohn's disease. Annals of the Royal College of Surgeons of England 67: 382–384

Van Patter W N, Bargen J A, Dockerty M B, Feldman W H, Mayo C W, Waugh J M 1954 Regional enteritis. Gastroenterology 26: 347–350

Williams A J K, Palmer K R 1991 Endoscopic balloon dilatation as a therapeutic option in the management of intestinal strictures resulting from Crohn's disease. British Journal of Surgery 78: 453–454

95. Small-bowel Crohn's disease – localized/diffuse disease

V. W. Fazio

RESECTIONAL SURGERY FOR CROHN'S DISEASE OF THE SMALL BOWEL

Introduction

There is general acceptance – albeit not total – that surgery for Crohn's disease of the small bowel is for specific complications of the disease. The clinical/anatomical pattern of disease is the main determinant of the type of surgery used, although the extent of disease and the presence or absence of comorbidity as well as factors adverse to intestinal wound healing, will figure prominently in the decision process. Perforative, septic or fistulous disease will usually mandate resective surgery. Obstructive patterns of disease, which may or may not be accompanied by local penetration will also require resective surgery. In certain cases, however, for example where foreshortening of the small bowel has occurred due to previous small-bowel resection, or diffuse disease where the short bowel syndrome is a consideration, non-resective surgery such as stricture-plasty is appropriate. This is discussed in Chapter 80. Since Crohn's disease is inherently panenteric and not curable by current modalities of therapy, and since the specter of recurrence after surgery looms large in the natural history of the disease, it behoves the clinician to hold a strategic view of the patient's illness – the natural history of both the disease and its complications for this particular patient.

This view is applied with the knowledge that surgery has a capacity to harm as well as help; that conservative, i.e. limited, surgery is increasingly the trend in most centers. Yet, when the patient has acquired a chronic disability owing to a complication of Crohn's disease, and where this is not responding to or is inappropriately treated by medical therapy, the informed clinician will rapidly refer the patient for surgical consideration. Generally, patients with Crohn's disease are managed non-surgically until complications of the disease or failure to thrive or significant side effects of medication occur. Surgery is usually offered at this point. The short-term gains include improvement in the patient's presenting symptoms and overall state of health, usually with a reduction or cessation of steroid medication. The price paid by the patient commonly includes a variable amount of diarrhea, occasional metabolic disturbance and, as mentioned earlier, the risk of disease recurrence.

Early descriptions of regional enteritis and resective surgery implied the possible goal of curative surgery (Ward et al 1954). Yet, since cumulative surgical recurrence rates approach 50–60% with the passage of time, surgeons rapidly became disillusioned. At long-term follow-up

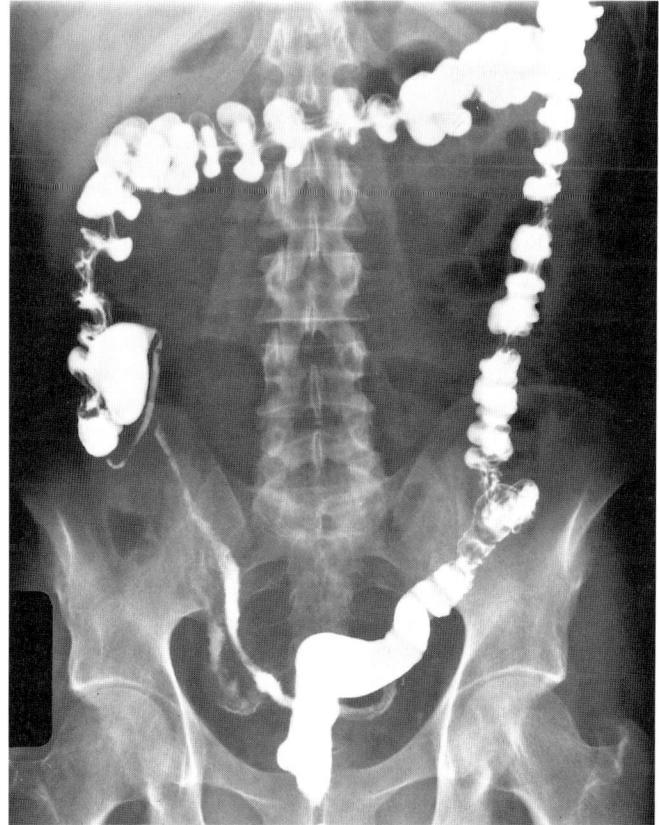

Fig. 95.1 Long stricture of terminal ileum affected by Crohn's disease.

(15 years), recurrence rates of 60% after primary surgery and 80% after multiple resections were reported (Chardavanayne et al 1986). Garlock and Crohn (1954) reported a 16.4% mortality rate and a 19.5% recurrence rate in 55 patients treated by resection. Thus, there was a trend towards bypass surgery because of the high morbidity and mortality rates of bowel resection in the 1950s. These same authors reported a very successful experience with bypass surgery in 65 patients undergoing this procedure. There was no mortality and only a 13.8% recurrence rate.

As other reports occurred (Schofield 1965, Atwell et al 1965) resection became the preferred method of surgical treatment for Crohn's disease, as the inherent problems of bypass surgery were realized.

The recognition of Crohn's colitis as an entity (Lockhart-Mummery & Morson) was followed by the observation that subpatterns of small-bowel Crohn's disease occurred. These included Crohn's disease of the terminal ileum (Fig. 95.1); jejunal or midileal Crohn's disease with or without colonic involvement and with (Fig. 95.2) or without sparing of the terminal ileum; diffuse jejunoileitis (Fig. 95.3); skip lesions; duodenal Crohn's disease; ileal recurrence (Fig. 95.4) after colonic resections, as well as the patterns of ileal disease occurring when an ileal pelvic (Fig. 95.5) or Koch pouch was done inadvertently in a patient with Crohn's disease.

Indications for surgery

The majority of patients with Crohn's disease will require surgery in the course of their illness. The probability that this is so after 20 and 30 years of Crohn's disease was 78% and 90%, respectively, in the National Cooperation Crohn's Disease Study (NCCDS) (Mekhijan et al 1979). Rates of surgery with disease of 5 years' duration were 75% for ileocolitis, 50% for ileal disease and 50% for colitis, at the Cleveland Clinic (Whelan et al 1985). By 10 years' duration of disease, over 90% of patients with ileocolitis had undergone surgery and almost 70% of those with ileal or colonic Crohn's disease underwent resection.

Farmer, at the Cleveland Clinic, reported on a cohort of 615 patients seen from 1966 to 1969 (Farmer et al 1975). It was clear from the study that the anatomical/clinical pattern of disease had an impact on the indications for surgery, clinical course and recurrence rates. Crohn's disease of the small intestine was reported in 176 patients; Crohn's disease of the small and large bowel (ileocolitis) occurred in 252 patients. When the small intestine was involved, either alone or in association with the colon, bowel obstruction and internal fistula with or without abscess occurred as the two major indications for surgery. Poor response to medical therapy (Fig. 95.6) was an infrequent indicator for surgery in ileal disease, which is in contrast to patients with Crohn's colitis.

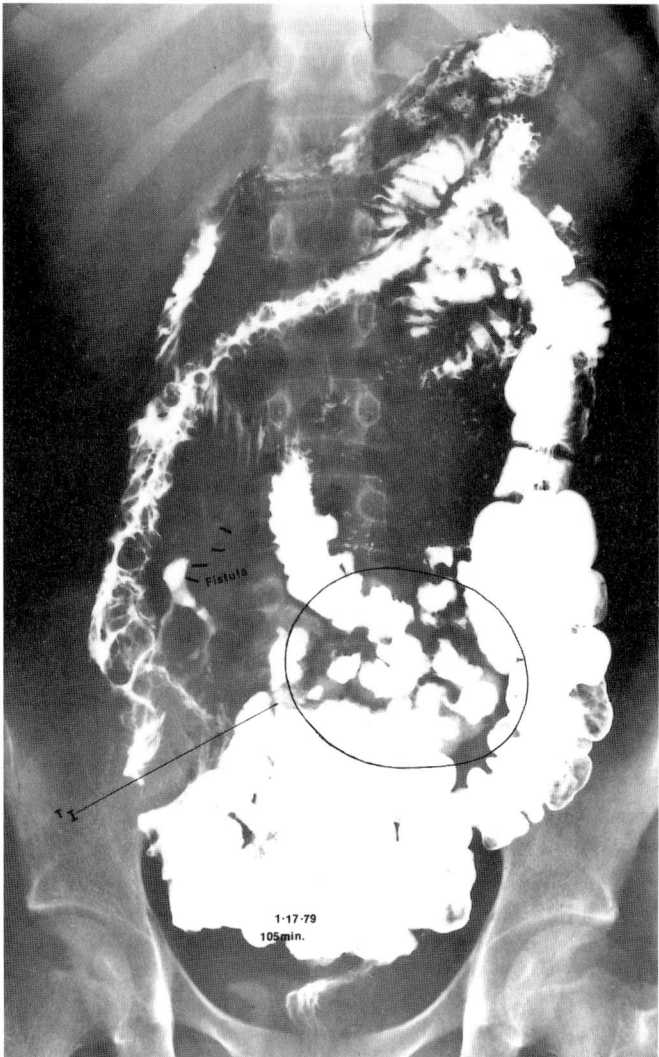

Fig. 95.2 Extensive jejunal and ileal Crohn's disease with multiple mid-small bowel strictures, ileoileal fistulae and Crohn's disease affecting the right and transverse colon.

Surgery for Crohn's disease is mostly an elective undertaking, one in which close cooperation between the gastroenterologist and the surgeon is required in deciding whether a particular situation constitutes an indication for surgery, and secondly, in agreeing on the timing of such surgery. It is therefore critical to identify the patient in whom surgical delay is potentially disastrous. This has been stated well by Alexander-Williams, who noted that whereas surgery of Crohn's disease is generally reserved for the complications, one should not delay excessively. Once a complication has developed, 'don't wait for this to become further complicated'. The experience of the clinician will determine when a particular complication merits early or urgent intervention. Bowel obstruction, for example, commonly can be managed conservatively with expectation of obstruction relief. The decision for later surgery is based upon a number of factors, including

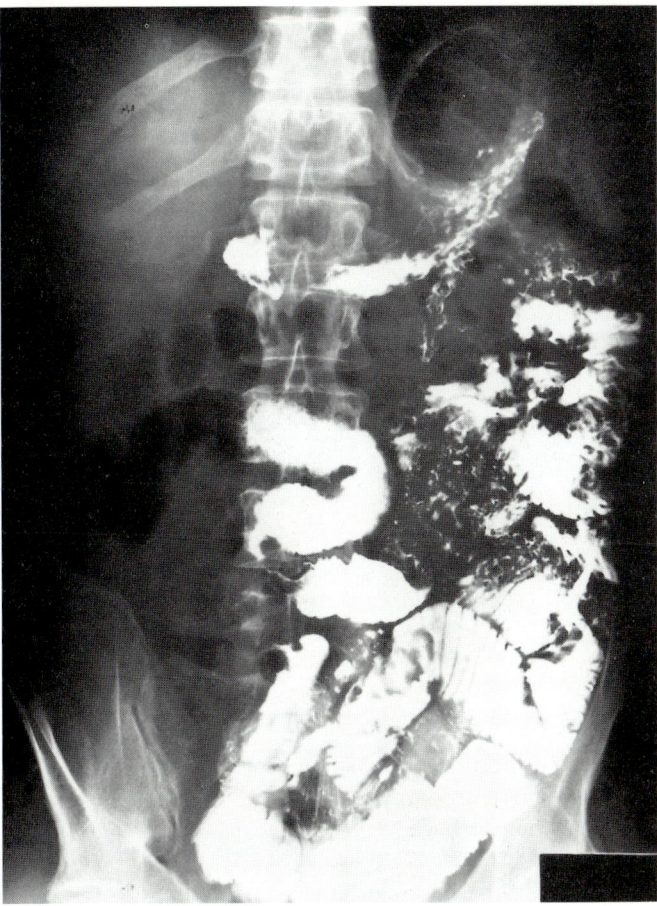

Fig. 95.3 Diffuse jejunoileitis.

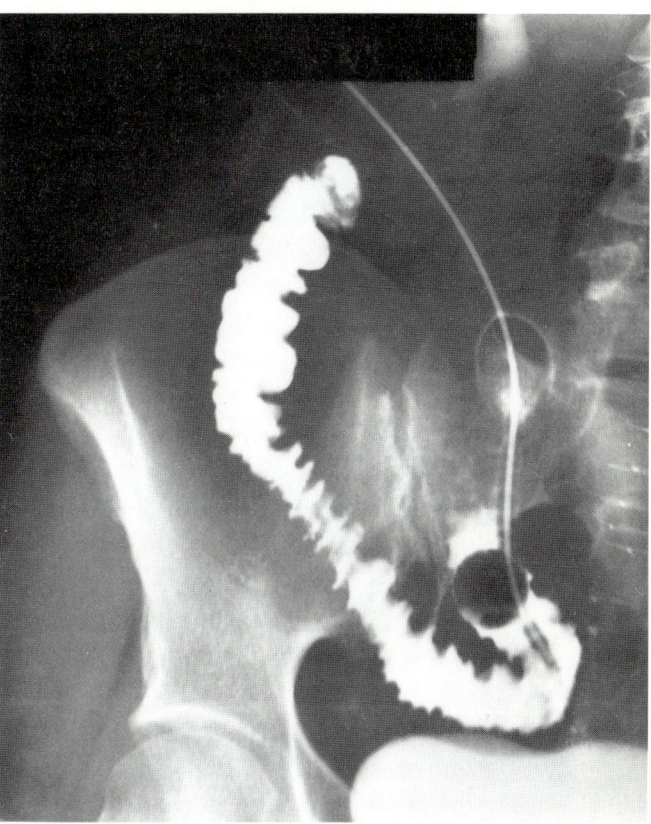

Fig. 95.4 Recurrent Crohn's disease in the ileostomy and terminal ileum following colectomy.

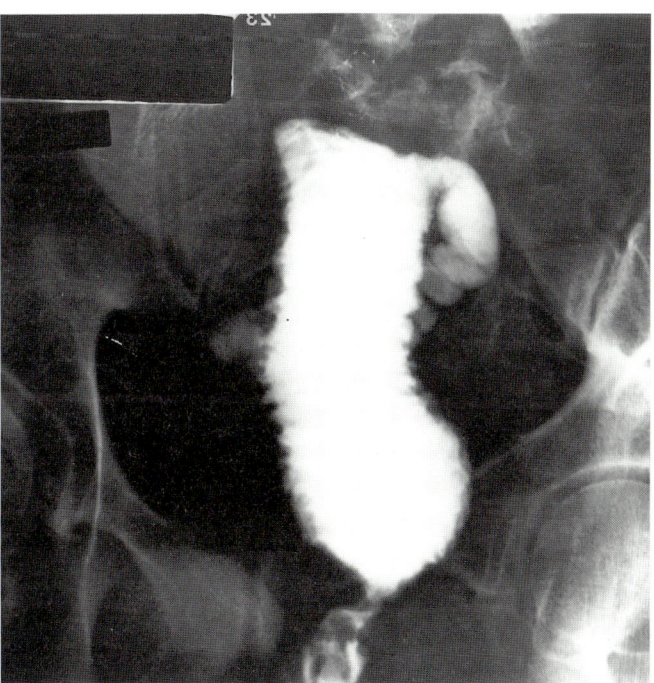

Fig. 95.5 Ileal pelvic pouch with diffuse ulceration due to emergence of Crohn's disease.

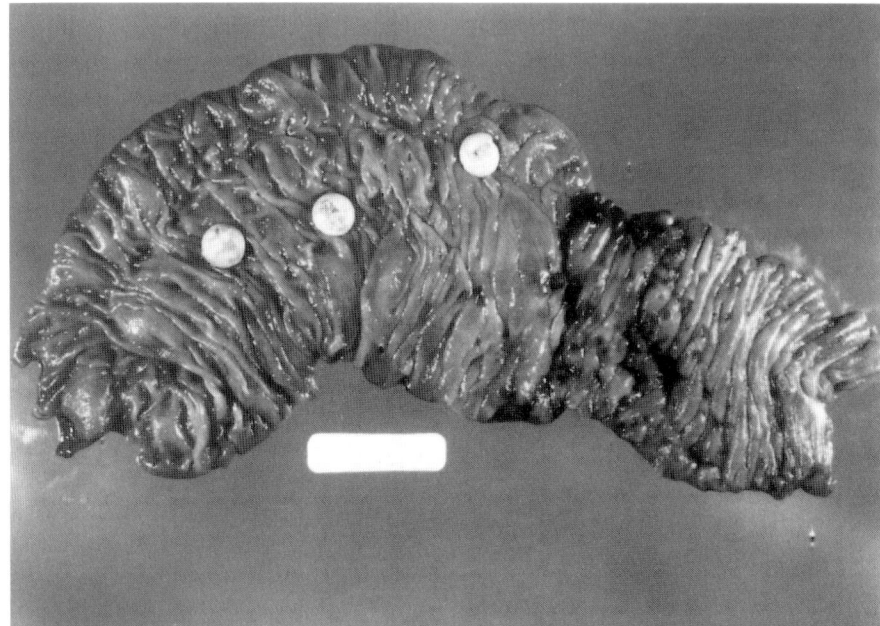

Fig. 95.6 Recurrent Crohn's disease at ileocolic anastomosis manifested by deep serpiginous ulcers; anti-inflammatory medications failed to sustain a remission.

responsiveness to therapy, comorbid conditions, and whether or not the patient had been on adequate medical therapy preoperatively.

It should be noted that a contrary view exists with respect to the general tenet of avoiding surgery until complications have occurred. This philosophy, espoused by some Swedish surgeons, favors the use of operative intervention early in the course of the disease, before serious, or especially septic, complications develop (Hulten 1988). Hulten found that when operating on advanced Crohn's disease (usually associated with abscess or fistula) there is a 49% complication rate. In contrast, operating on non-complicated Crohn's disease was associated with a 12% complication rate. At present, the early-intervention practice is not usually used in North America.

Complications commonly requiring operation

The complications can be listed as follows:

1. Small-bowel obstruction
2. Abdominal abscess
   (a) enteroparietal
   (b) interloop
   (c) intramesenteric
   (d) psoas or retroperitoneal
3. Fistula
   (a) enterocutaneous
   (b) enteroenteric
   (c) enterovesical
   (d) enterogenital
   (e) other
4. Free perforation of the small bowel
5. Obstructive uropathy
6. Major hemorrhage
7. Carcinoma
8. Failure to thrive, including extraintestinal manifestations
9. Recurrent Crohn's disease.

Operative techniques

Counseling

Prior to operation a complete and full discussion with the patient is required, particularly concerning the alternatives to surgery and the attendant risks associated with a variety of surgical procedures. The risks and sequelae are discussed with the patient, preferably with a family member in attendance, as recall by an anxious patient is often incomplete. Included in this interview is discussion of the specific risks attendant with surgical resection of the intestine and anastomosis, such as sepsis, peritonitis, anastomotic leak, postoperative fistula and risks of blood transfusion. In particular, the risks of disease recurrence is explained.

Stoma site marking

One must be cautious about discussions relating to stoma site marking, as this may cause some anxiety in the patient. None the less, in certain patients who will be undergoing intestinal resection there may be the possibility that a temporary stoma will be required. Such patients may include those that are malnourished or who have major intra-abdominal septic problems. The most important aspect of rehabilitation of a stoma patient, whether temporary or permanent, is the accurate preoperative siting and intraoperative construction of the stoma. The principles of siting include visibility of the stoma site to the patient; leaving a zone of 5.0 cm of undisturbed skin around the stoma site; use of the summit of the infraumbilical fat mound; the site should be located within the surface marking of the rectus abdominus muscle; the stoma incision should be made remote from bony prominences or skin creases or scars.

Restoration of deficits

Those deficits that can be made good in the short term are attended to. These include correction of anemia, electrolyte imbalance and correctable comorbid conditions such as heart failure or arrhythmia. Nutritional deficit, on the other hand, is common in patients with Crohn's disease. Except in patients needing reoperation for enterocutaneous fistulae, opinion is divided as to whether or not malnutrition increases morbidity (Higgens et al 1981). In the immediate preoperative phase nutritional supplementation adds little to reverse protein malnutrition, unless sepsis is present (Irving 1990). We have used hyperalimentation when treating acute Crohn's disease, in an attempt to reverse the catabolic state and facilitate remission sufficiently to allow for elective surgery (Fazio et al 1976). Decisions are often difficult when it comes to selecting particular patients for adjuvant hyperalimentation. In practice, intravenous nutritional supplementation is not used if there is an urgent or emergency indication for surgery, if grip strength is reasonable; or if the patient has an absence of anergy. In the elective situation, and where malnutrition is severe, hyperalimentation may be used for 5–7 days, with a possible boost of intravenous albumin for a day or two prior to surgery if hypoalbuminemia remains severe and resistant to treatment.

Steroids

The patient who has been taking steroids in the 6-months prior to surgery is generally given stress dose therapy in the pre- and postoperative periods. This consists of intravenous hydrocortisone 100 mg every 8 hours for three doses. On day two, 100 mg every 12 hours is given, and this is reduced further to 50 mg every 12 hours on day three. Further reductions are determined by institution of oral intake. A tapering program is then given when resective surgery has been completed.

Mechanical bowel preparation

Some patients with Crohn's disease of the small bowel will have or exhibit obstructive features which may preclude the usual mechanical bowel preparation chosen for elective non-obstructive cases. In many circumstances a modified preparation can be used, with dietary restriction of fluids and modified elemental diets for several days prior to surgery. Over and above this, however, the patient may be able to tolerate what might be called moderate catharsis, using 5–12 ounces of magnesium citrate solution. In the patient who has evidence of obstruction, our preference has been to use polyethylene glycol.

Antibiotic preparation

A variety of agents may be used. Our preference has been to use cefotaxime 1.0 g and metronidazole 500 mg intravenously on call to the operating room. This is continued 8-hourly for three doses postoperatively. Antibiotics may be continued for 3 days if any intraoperative contamination occurs.

Other factors

Patients will be given pneumatic compression stockings throughout the intraoperative and postoperative course until they are fully ambulant. Patients who have a history of thrombophlebitis will be managed with minidose heparin. A Foley catheter is placed in the bladder and a nasogastric tube in the stomach.

Incision

A midline abdominal incision has been used. In most cases it has been our preference to use the old incision rather than create a new one. An important consideration is the preservation of the infraumbilical right and left lower quadrants for potential stoma siting in the future.

Intraoperative recognition of Crohn's disease

In the classic state, regional ileitis will exhibit certain overt features that characterize the disease. These include thickening of the bowel wall, narrowing of the lumen and rigidity of the segment. The serosal surface is commonly inflamed, with a tortuous corkscrewing appearance of serosal vessels. Fat wrapping is commonly present, with a variable degree of obliteration of the mesentery/bowel angle. The mesentery is quite thick as a rule, owing to increased fat deposition as well as lymph node enlargement. In certain cases a phlegmon or peri-intestinal abscess may be present. Adherent loops of small intestine may present a matted appearance. This may further disguise the presence of an occult enteroenteric fistula. In this state the disease process is easy to identify. The open specimen will exhibit classic features of longitudinal ulcers, deep penetrating fissures, and focal 'cobblestoning' of the mucosal lining owing to a combination of deep longitudinal and slit transverse fissures. In the milder cases aphthoid ulcers may be found. The bowel mucosa immediately adjacent to the proximal line of resection is commonly edematous and may exhibit such fissures.

In patients with chronic bowel obstruction the classic features of Crohn's disease may be absent. It is then difficult to distinguish the thickening of the bowel wall due to chronic bowel obstruction from that underlying Crohn's disease. It is not always advantageous for the patient to undergo surgical opening of the small intestine at this point with resultant contamination, just to be sure where the lines of demarcation should be. In practice, it is useful to use the palpation of the mesenteric bowel angle as a fairly accurate indicator of proximal extent of the disease. An inbuilt comparison is possible because of the ability to palpate the upper small intestine, which is clearly free of Crohn's disease. Thus, when the mesenteric margin of the overtly affected segment is palpated, as one extends in a cephalad direction so the decreasing thickness of the mesenteric angle associated with return of the scalloped appearance between the vasa recti, signals the merging into normal intestine.

Margins and extent of resection

There is controversy regarding the optimal margin of resection, i.e. how much apparently normal intestine proximal and distal to the diseased segment should be removed. There is an increasing trend among surgeons to use conservative resection margins based upon reports, some of which are discussed below. We have favored conservative resection margins, with proximal clearances of 5–10 cm beyond the apparent disease, and distal clearances of 5 cm. In a report from Berman and Krause (1977), those cases in which extensive resections were done fared best of all. In this non-controlled and multi-institutional trial there was a recurrence rate of 29% after radical resection. This contrasted with an 84% recurrence rate with conservative procedures, a result unsupported by most studies. Karesan and colleagues (1981) studied 54 patients in whom a crude recurrence rate of 66% occurred in 12 with microscopic evidence of disease at the resection margin. This contrasted with 42 patients where normal margins were found, and in whom a recurrence rate of 14% was found (Karesan et al 1981). A study of 110 patients compared outcomes in those with normal, minor or major inflammatory changes at the resection margins. The cumulative recurrence rates at 10 years were 37%, 44% and 73%, respectively (Lindhager et al 1989).

This notwithstanding, the fact remains that there has been no consistent reporting of a relationship between inflammation at resection margins and recurrence rates (Papaioannou et al 1979, Speranza et al 1986). Additionally, Heuman and colleagues found no value in the use of frozen sections to assess the status of margins (Heuman et al 1983). In this case, recurrence rates were not affected by disease margins as determined by frozen section. In a study by Hamilton and colleagues (1985), frozen section was used in 38 patients for defining resection margin and compared with resection where the margin chosen was based upon clinical inspection of the resection site. Clinical recurrence rates were 37% and 50%, respectively, in the frozen section and non-frozen section groups 5 years postresection. At 10 years they were 60% and 66%. At 5 years, reoperation rate was identical (18% and 18%), and was similar at 10 years (36% and 32%). Thus, the practice of frozen section is not proved to be of value and is not recommended. In a study by Pennington et al (1980), some 108 specimens were reviewed in 97 patients, and the presence or absence of inflammation at the resection margins was recorded. Recurrence rates were similar in both those with involved and those with non-involved margins. In a similar study at the Cleveland Clinic we reviewed 100 patients who underwent resection and anastomosis for small-bowel Crohn's disease (Kotanagi et al 1991). There was no significant difference in recurrence rates between the various subcategories that were rated according to the degree of inflammatory change at the resection margins. Thus, the evidence to date would indicate that wide resection lines are unnecessary. At operation, one may see aphthous ulceration at sites remote from the major ulcerative component of the disease. The practical implication of this is that wide resections to include such aphthous ulcerations are not only unnecessary, but may lead to substantial shortening of the gut. It is, however, desirable to perform anastomoses in 'normal' bowel. However, in patients who have substantial previous intestinal loss, anastomoses may in fact have to be made with overt Crohn's disease in the bowel ends. One tenet is that anastomosis should not be made in bowel ends that have undergone stricturing.

Operative procedures

There is currently no serious challenge to the belief that intestinal resection is the preferred method of surgical management of Crohn's disease of the small bowel in most circumstances. Although in the past attitudes may have questioned this because of perceived increased rates of morbidity and indeed mortality, this is not the case today. Homan and Dineen (1978) compared outcomes in three groups of patients who had undergone intestinal resection, intestinal bypass in continuity, and exclusion bypass procedures for Crohn's disease. This series was characterized by having similar indications for surgery in the subgroups, and the series selection, although not randomized, was done in sequence with few exceptions. With a 15-year follow-up in 115 patients, recurrence rates for resection, bypass with exclusion and simple bypass

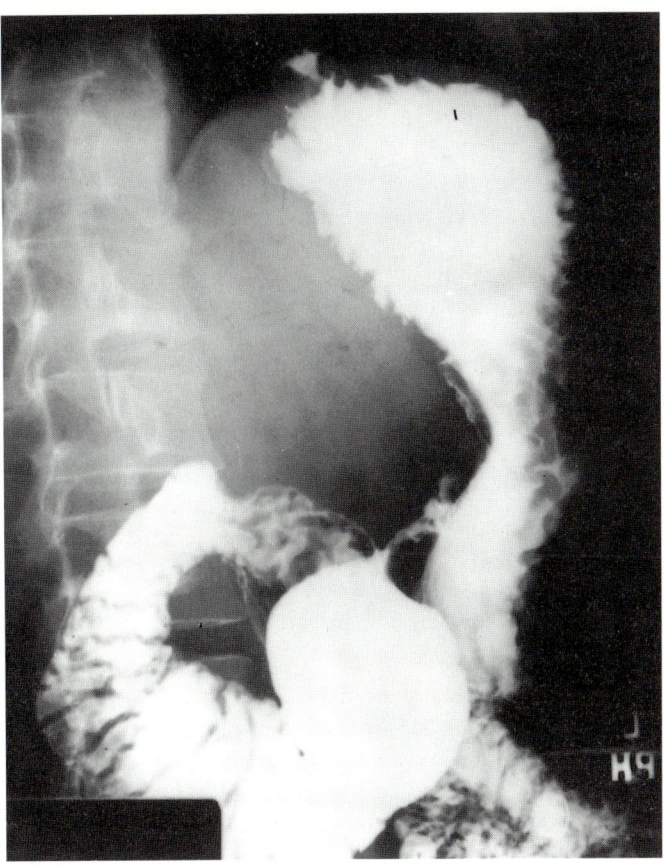

Fig. 95.7 Gastroduodenal Crohn's disease with prepyloric stricture.

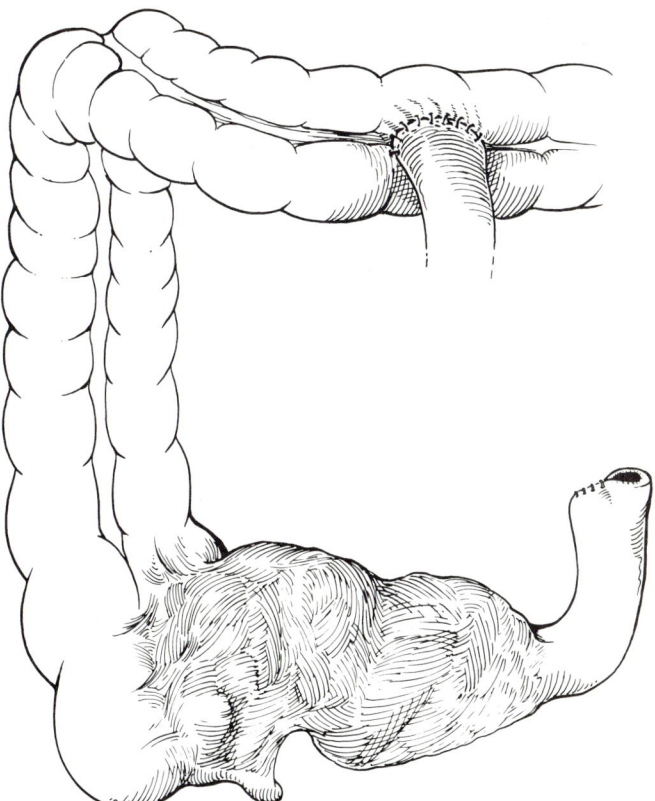

Fig. 95.8 Unilateral exclusion bypass with end of ileum to midtransverse colon anastomosis. The proximal matured segment is sutured to the skin of the abdomen as a mucus fistula to minimize the risk of blowout of this segment from an infected mucocele.

were 65%, 82% and 94%, respectively (Homan & Dineen 1978).

In certain cases small bowel resection may be passed over in favor of a bypass procedure. Such situations include gastroduodenal Crohn's disease (Fig. 95.7) and patients with perforative ileocecal Crohn's disease where dense adherence to the pelvic vasculature may be present (in such cases unilateral exclusion bypass is a reasonable alternative). Here, the excluded small-bowel segment is decompressed by placing the proximal end of the bypassed segment into the wound as a mucus fistula (Fig. 95.8). Subsequent elective resection of the bypassed segment can and should be carried out, as this area, no longer under good surveillance, may have malignant potential.

Technique of resection

The principles utilized here include mobilization of the diseased segment as well as the adjacent normal intestine. This will allow for resection and the fashioning of a subsequent tension-free anastomosis or stoma. Whichever technique of anastomosis will be subsequently used, it is critical to minimize contamination in the patient who has partial or total small-bowel obstruction where the proximal bowel is still filled with fecal material. It is critical to apply certain principles to minimize the effects of such contamination and spill during the anastomotic construction. The contents of the small intestine may be milked in a cephalad or caudad direction beyond the margins of the planned anastomosis and, using a linen tape, the bowel segment can be occluded and quarantined from the rest of the fecal stream (Fig. 95.9). In addition, the operative area is packed off to minimize the effect of any inadvertent spill. Should ileostomies be planned, the bowel can be occluded at the proximal resection line by linear stapler. Thus, the bowel can be exteriorized through the ileostomy aperture without wound contamination.

For patients with ileal or ileocecal disease, adjacent matted loops of small intestine or omentum may be encountered. Separation of ileal loops is often difficult in the abdominal cavity; thus, there is value in attempting to mobilize the right colon or ileocolic anastomosis sufficiently that the loops matted together may be delivered through the abdominal incision. When the entire mass of loops is brought outside the abdominal cavity, one can proceed to separate them by a combination of sharp dissection or teasing apart. This also allows for a closer examination of which segments of bowel have to be resected and which may be preserved. For example, an enteroenteric or ileo-

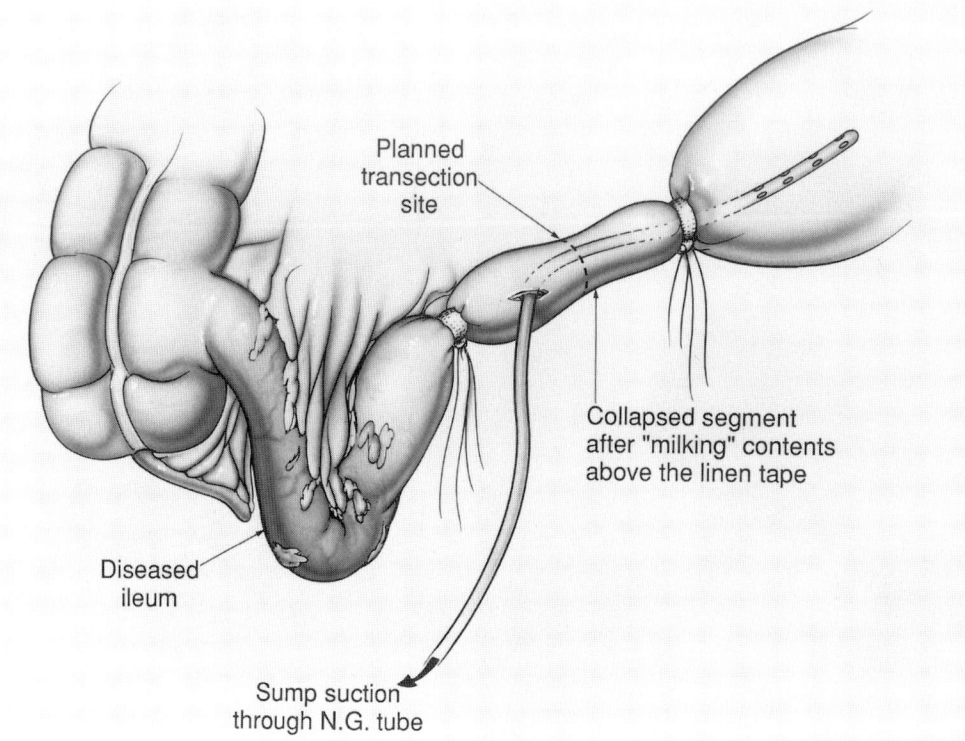

Fig. 95.9 Decompression of proximal dilated small bowel secondary to an obstructing diseased ileum to minimize intraoperative contamination. Make-and-break suction is established through a sterile nasogastric tube passed into the dilated segment through an occluding tape.

transverse or sigmoid fistula may be identified. In such cases, the offending originating diseased segment is usually the terminal ileum. The other component of the fistula is commonly free of Crohn's disease. In such cases a simple wedge resection of the secondarily affected target organ may be achieved without recourse to a formal secondary complete bowel resection. Margins of resection are chosen along the previously mentioned lines.

When transecting the bowel and the mesentery, attention is directed to the mesenteric margin (Fig. 95.10). A curved forceps is placed at the mesenteric margin and separated to allow for initial electrocautery dissection of the mesenteric fat in a fan-shaped fashion. The ileal mesentery (Fig. 95.11), however, is commonly thickened due to excessive fat deposition and enlarged, sometimes massively enlarged, mesenteric lymph nodes. These tend to follow the course of the ileocolic and sometimes superior mesenteric vessels in a cephalad direction towards the third part of the duodenum and head of the pancreas. Traditional techniques to divide the mesentery in patients with carcinoma of the right colon include the placement of ligatures around isolated vascular pedicles. However, in patients with Crohn's disease, especially in the terminal ileum, there is excessive thickening of the fat, which commonly precludes the safe fashioning of convenient pedicles for such ligatures. This carries a serious risk of injuring the vessels, leading to an alarming rapidly developing hematoma that extends towards the pancreas. Thus, one can start up a chain of events that could culminate in serious vascular injury and further bowel ischemia, as a result of excessive attempts to control hematomas.

Our preferred technique has been to use an overlapping Kocher clamp technique (Fig. 95.12). Using this straddling technique (Fazio & Strong 1995), the vascular pedicles are suture-ligated using 1/0 chromic catgut so that the pedicles are serially underrun, thereby eliminating the risk of a spreading hematoma.

One might comment at this point on enlarged lymph nodes. It is not a stated goal of resectional surgery in Crohn's disease to perform a 'lymphadenectomy'. There is no evidence that removal of lymph nodes will reduce the risk of recurrent disease, but these lymph glands are commonly infected and it is often undesirable to leave a large mass of such nodes in close proximity to a planned anastomotic line. In the event that such nodes can be removed without extending the margins of resection, one should do so (Fig. 95.13).

Laparoscopic-assisted resection of the small bowel in Crohn's disease has been increasingly reported. In our experience with 35 patients, there have been no significant complications. Intracorporeal anastomosis has not been attempted. In essence, the mobilization of the base of the small-bowel mesentery and the right colon is carried out using conventional laparoscopic techniques. The terminal

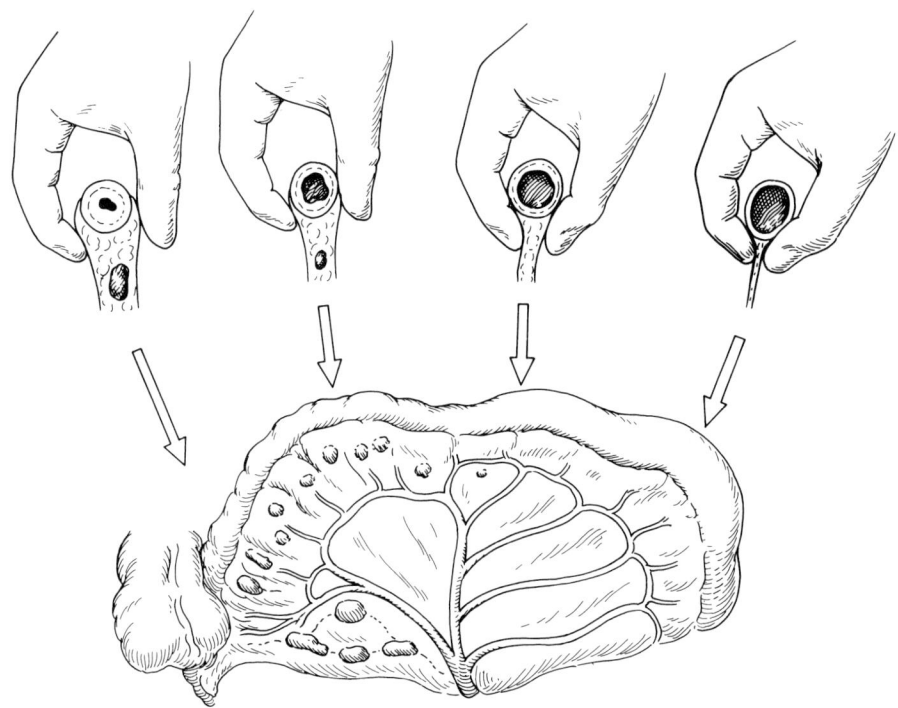

Fig. 95.10 Assessment of proximal margin of resection. Palpation of the mesenteric margin is a useful technique to aid in the clinical recognition of appropriate margins of resection. Serosal surface of the bowel may appear normal although an occult mucosal ulcer is present on the mesenteric aspect.

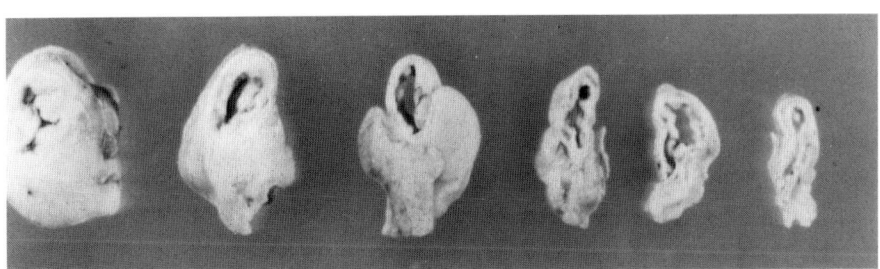

Fig. 95.11 Serial cross-sections of ileum affected by Crohn's disease. Bowel-wall thickening and encasement of the mesenteric margin by fat deposition is seen in these serial sections, ranging from grossly diseased to normal bowel.

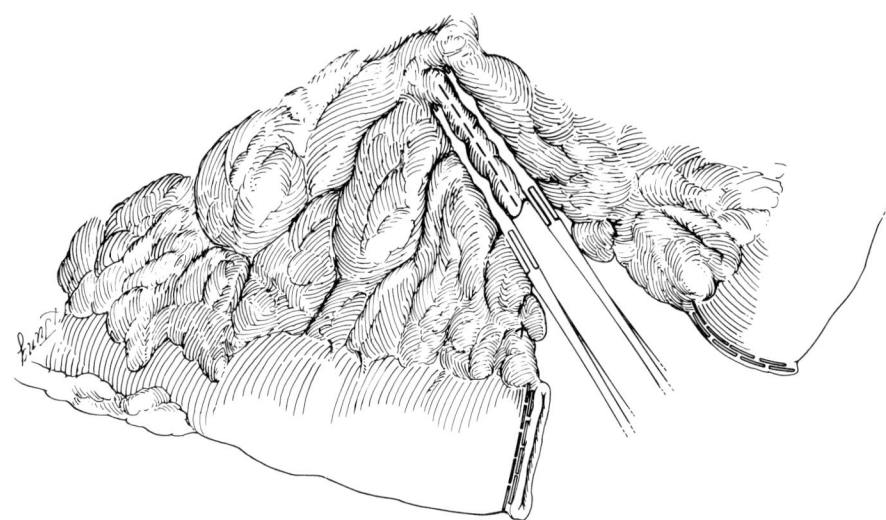

Fig. 95.12 Dividing the mesentery in patients with very thick mesentery due to enlarged lymph nodes. Serial clamping is done using Kocher clamps and after division of the tissue, 1/0 chromic catgut is used to provide suture ligation of the newly fashioned pedicle.

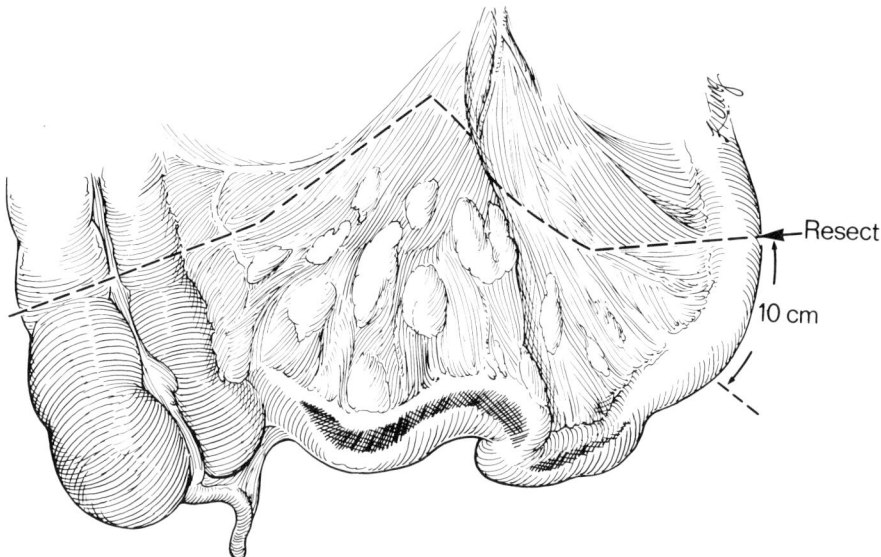

Fig. 95.13 Margins of resection for Crohn's disease of the small bowel: 5–10 cm margins are taken both proximally and distally to the overt disease. If most of the enlarged nodes can be resected without enforcing further bowel resection, then this is done.

ileum and cecum are then delivered through a 2–3 in right lower quadrant transverse incision, and ligation of the vascular pedicles and transection of the cecum/ascending colon junction and proximal small bowel is carried out extracorporeally; a stapled anastomosis is effected.

Technique of anastomosis

A variety of techniques exist, individual preference favoring either hand-sewing or stapling. With either technique it is important to inspect the lumen on both sides of the anastomosis. As mentioned earlier, the presence of aphthoid ulcers in supple, otherwise healthy, bowel does not constitute a reason for further resection. With patients who have deep longitudinal ulcers, and provided there is adequate length of remaining small bowel, it would be important to eliminate such ulceration by extending the margin of resection further. In certain cases there are compelling reasons not to do so, such as those patients who have a substantial shortening of the small bowel, e.g. less than 150 cm. As mentioned earlier, there is no circumstance under which suturing of a stricture to another portion of bowel in an end-to-end fashion is justified. Assessment of the distal line of resection may also be difficult, especially if this is in the midtransverse or distal colon. There may then be value in performing intraoperative colonoscopy to avoid leaving a substantial segment of ulcerated colon that has occurred in a skip fashion. This is especially the case if preoperative study of the colon has been incomplete.

In the patient who has substantial dilated proximal small bowel, where the dilatation may be due to both gas and enteric content, it is important to decompress the distended intestine as return of the dilated segment to the abdomen may preclude safe closure of the abdominal wall. Such decompression, however, runs the risk of intraoperative contamination of stool. This can be minimized by the use of occluding tapes around the proximal bowel. A sterile nasogastric tube may be passed through the opening of the bowel and the proximal bowel can then be decompressed, by make and break suction of the tube.

The principles of bowel anastomosis are similar in that one will obtain a good blood supply to the bowel ends, that the anastomosis will be conducted in a tension-free manner, that there will be equilibration of the lumen caliber for both proximal and distal sides, that no twists in the bowel will be allowed, and that the mesenteric defect will be obliterated. In patients who undergo stapled operations our preference has been to use side-to-side GIA-60 (Fig. 95.14) anastomosis (US Surgical, Norwalk, Connecticut). In such cases the defect into which the limbs of the stapler have been introduced is closed with two layers of 3/0 polyglycolic acid suture.

Operative tactics for certain clinical entities

Bowel obstruction

This is the major indication for surgery in patients with Crohn's disease of the small intestine in the Cleveland Clinic series (Farmer et al 1975). Bowel obstruction was the primary indication for surgery in 54% of our patients with small-bowel pattern of disease among 500 patients undergoing surgery. In those with ileocolitis pattern, bowel obstruction was the prime indicator for surgery in 37% of cases. Rarely will a patient present with acute total

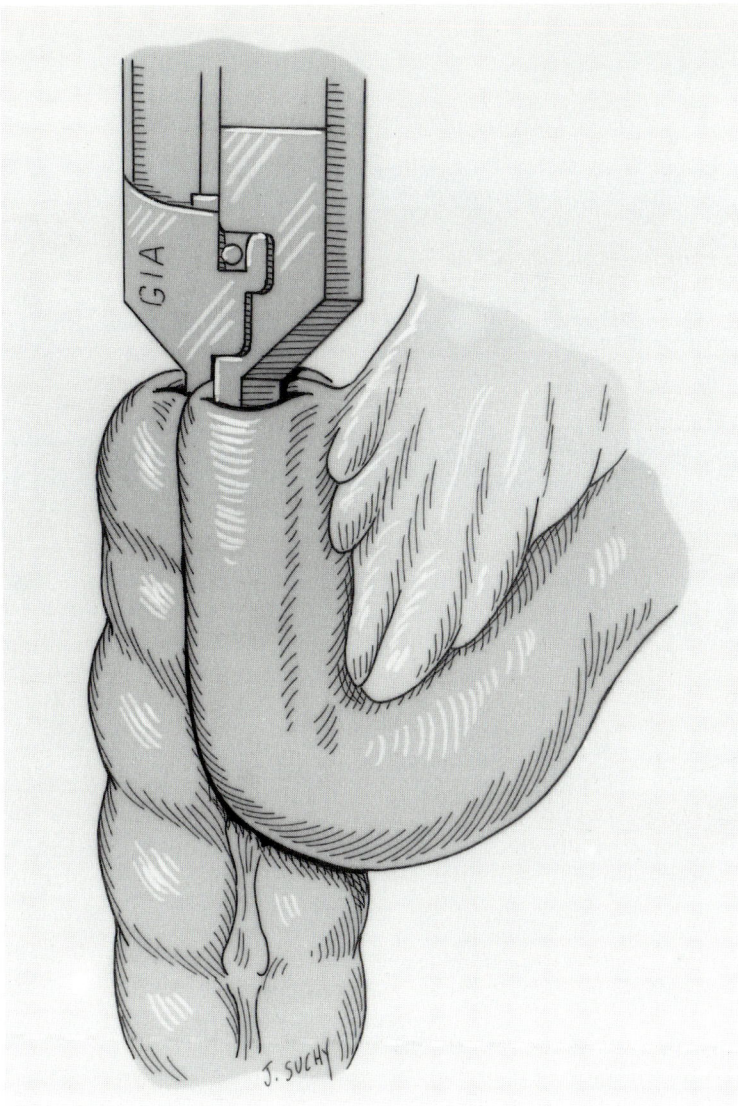

Fig. 95.14a One common method of anastomosis is the side-to-side linear cutter/stapler technique.

obstruction. Usually, they will have had several episodes of partial obstruction manifested as cramping abdominal pain, abdominal distension and nausea. Vomiting is uncommon, as is absolute constipation. Patients learn to minimize their symptoms by lessening their oral intake. When obstructive episodes have failed to respond adequately to medical therapy, or the frequency of the episodes indicates a fibrotic type of tight obstruction, then surgery is performed. Surgery is advised if, in addition to the obstructive features, there are one or more of the following features:

1. Abdominal mass
2. Obstructing bouts occurring with increased frequency
3. Recovery from successive bouts is taking longer
4. Associated fever – leukocytosis
5. Malnutrition, especially with hypoalbuminemia
6. Internal/external fistula (Fig. 95.15)
7. Side effects of medication
8. Chronic fatigue, chronic malaise and disturbance of socioeconomic state.

In the patient who presents with acute small-bowel obstruction, medical therapy will usually be successful in relieving the acute obstruction to allow for elective surgery, should this be indicated. If obstruction of this nature has occurred without the patient being on medical therapy in the past, then a trial of medical therapy is usually offered, especially if subsequent small-bowel radiology demonstrates a lack of evidence of obstruction. The subject of strictureplasty in diffuse small-bowel disease is discussed later.

Resective surgery is almost always the preferred method of management. In rare circumstances bypass procedures, either in the form of ileostomy alone or internal bypass

834 INFLAMMATORY BOWEL DISEASES

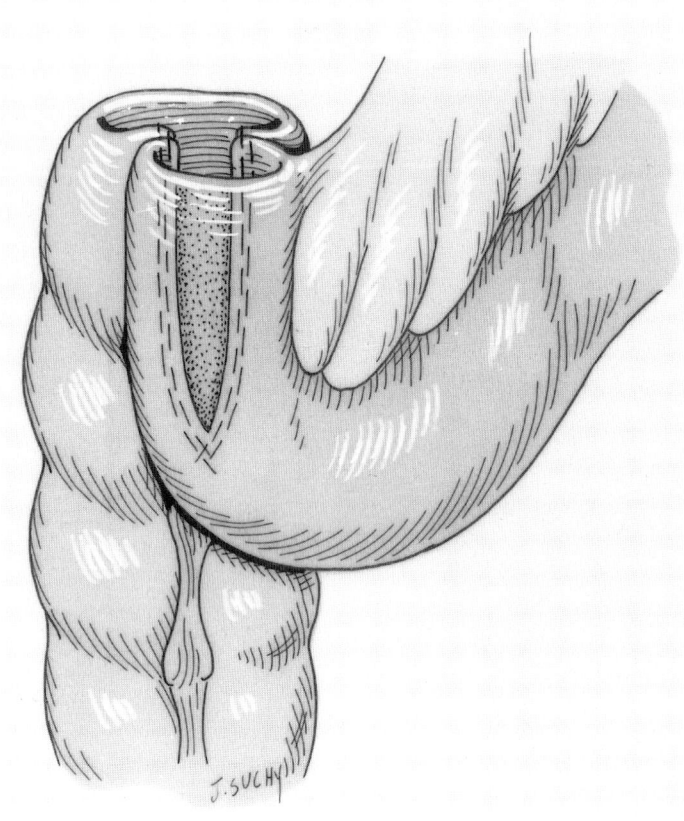

Fig. 95.14b

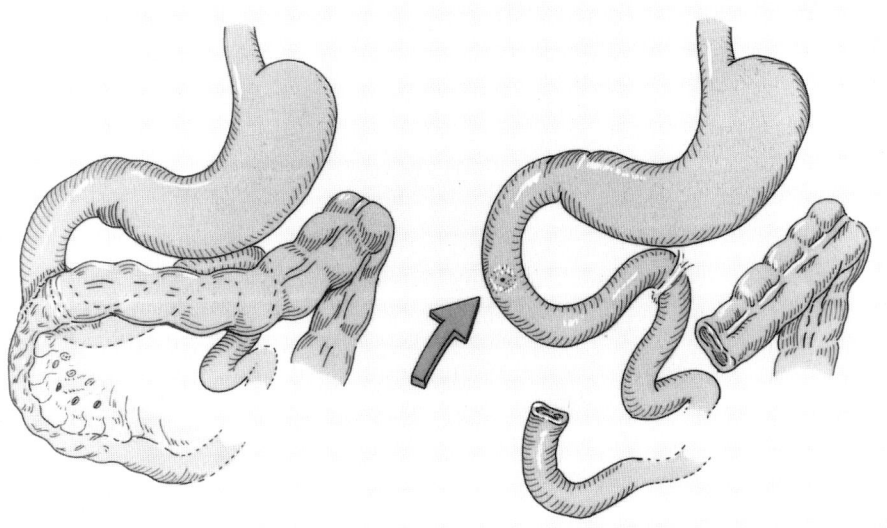

Fig. 95.15a Internal fistula between the ileocolic anastomosis and the anterior duodenum due to recurrent Crohn's disease. After resecting the recurrence, including margins of small bowel and colon, the anterior duodenal defect is inspected. Active septic process or inflammatory induration of the duodenal defect may preclude safe closure of the duodenum except by side-to-side duodenojejunostomy

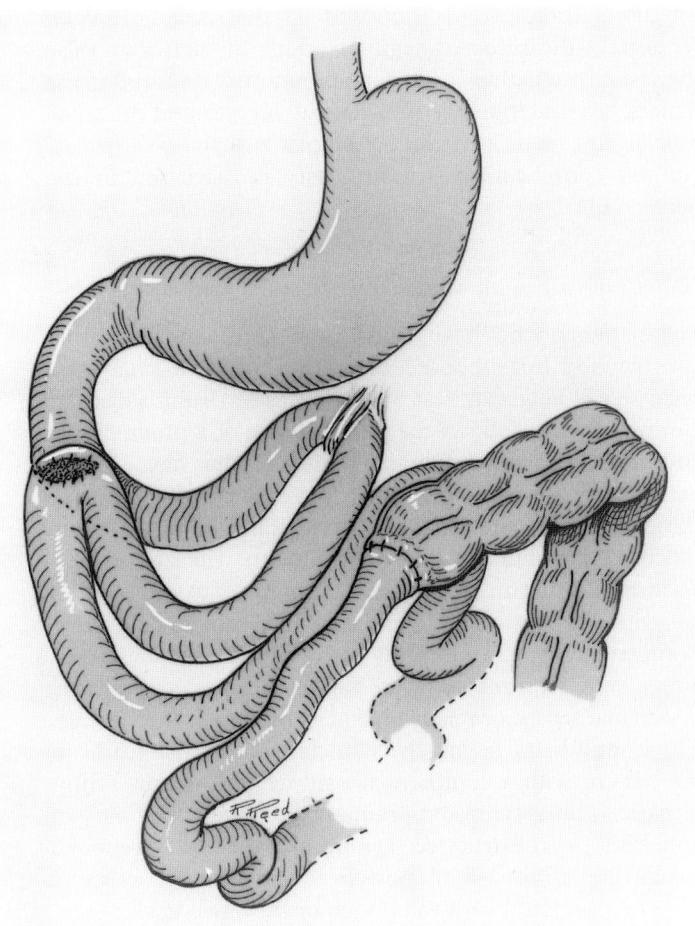

Fig. 95.15b Internal fistula between the ileocolic anastomosis and the anterior duodenum due to recurrent Crohn's disease. After resecting the recurrence, including margins of small bowel and colon, the anterior duodenal defect is inspected. Active septic process or inflammatory induration of the duodenal defect may preclude safe closure of the duodenum except by side-to-side duodenojejunostomy.

such as enteroenteric or enterocolic anastomosis, is appropriate. These latter circumstances may include patients who are so ill, malnourished, have substantial comorbid conditions and be such anesthesia risks that resectional surgery is considered excessively risky. In such cases ileostomy may be used as a staging mechanism. In other patients, where there is a fixed ileocecal phlegmon and dense attachments to the right retroperitoneum and common iliac vessels, unilateral exclusion bypass is a reasonable procedure, with a plan to resect the outer circuit segment 6 months later. This is done to reduce the risk of cancer developing in the excluded segment.

Greenstein and colleagues (1988) proposed two major types of clinical or pathological entity in Crohn's disease, namely, a perforative type associated with sepsis or fistula, and a non-perforating type (obstruction). They found singular concordance between the initial type of presentation and the same presentation when disease recurred. We failed to find such concordance in a similar study at the Cleveland Clinic (McDonald et al 1989).

Abscess fistula

These complications are discussed in subsequent chapters. For patients with an intra-abdominal or retroperitoneal abscess that lends itself to percutaneous drainage, such a procedure should be used, in order to lessen the toxicity of the patient preoperatively, as well as to minimize the risk of spreading sepsis at the time of laparotomy. In certain cases intra-abdominal abscesses may 'self-drain' as, for example, in a patient with an ileocecal phlegmon in whom the mass becomes impalpable with the use of antibiotics due to the paraileal septic process draining back through the perforation into the intestinal lumen itself. More often than not, however, such a process is incomplete, necessitating surgery, especially when the septic process has abutted against another organ structure, producing an enteroenteric fistula or a communication between the small bowel and a hollow viscus, such as the urinary bladder. In such circumstances resectional surgery is the procedure of choice. Should there be local and systemic factors conducive to intestinal healing, then the anastomosis is made in such a way that it remains quarantined or at a distance from the septic or fistulous area. This can be achieved by placing omentum between the anastomosis and the site of the sepsic fistulous process.

Obstructive uropathy

This subject is also discussed in another chapter. Obstructive uropathy was described by Hyams et al in 1943. The incidence has been reported to be as high as 25% (Block et al 1973). In our department's report on this same subject we found a 4.7% incidence among 958 patients with Crohn's disease who had undergone intravenous pyelography (Siminovitch & Fazio 1980). With obstructive uropathy complicating Crohn's disease, there is usually a predominance of gastrointestinal symptoms and relatively few genitourinary symptoms. In the Cleveland Clinic series, 44% had an abdominal mass or fistula. Present et al (1989) drew attention to the psoas spasm associated with retroperitoneal inflammation. Usually, an ileocecal phlegmon or abscess causes direct obstruction to the ureter, with ensuing hydronephrosis. Block (1973) felt that periureteric fibrosis may also occur, necessitating formal ureterolysis at the time of surgery to relieve the obstruction. This, however, is not uniformly or indeed commonly present in our experience. Because ureterolysis may be associated with devascularization injury and ultimate nephrectomy, we have not used it to any extent in the management of this condition. In our study of 49 patients with obstructive uropathy due to Crohn's disease, intestinal resection proved to be the procedure of choice without necessitating ureterolysis.

Hemorrhage

Major small-bowel hemorrhage is an uncommon indication for surgery in Crohn's disease of the small bowel. Crohn and Yarnis (1958) reported a 0.9% instance of bleeding in 540 patients. In 1976, Homan et al found a 1.4% incidence in 503 patients. In 1980, Rubin and others performed a small-bowel resection in seven of eight patients with massive hemorrhage complicating small-bowel Crohn's disease (Rubin et al 1980). We have reported the Cleveland Clinic experience of 14 patients with massive hemorrhage from the small bowel (Fazio). Rebleeding has been reported as a cause of significant morbidity following resection of small-bowel Crohn's disease. However, this remains the treatment of choice and is used for patients who have failed to respond to medical therapy, following restoration of any coagulopathy defect and exclusion of other causes of bleeding, such as peptic ulcer. To minimize the risk of resecting a segment of bowel that is not the cause of the bleeding, intraoperative superior mesenteric angiography may be helpful (Fazio et al 1980). Thus, resection is advised when the patient's hemodynamic state is not sustainable by transfusion; if severe bleeding exists in addition to another indication for resection; if the patient is stable but continues to bleed after receiving four to six units of blood; or if the patient has recurrent major hemorrhage.

Carcinoma

Carcinoma of the small intestine is an uncommon complication of Crohn's disease. This is discussed elsewhere in the book. Factors that seem to be associated with a high risk include diffuse segmental disease of the small intestine; longevity of disease; and bypassed ileocecal segments of Crohn's disease. Thus, from a preventive standpoint patients who have bypassed segments, especially those that are impossible to keep under surveillance, are best treated by resectional surgery. It may not be an easy matter to persuade the patient to undergo such surgery as they may very well be asymptomatic. None the less, the patient must be strongly encouraged to do so. Another clinical problem is the patient with long-standing Crohn's disease, for example a 20-year history, and who has an identifiable stricture of the small bowel on contrast studies. In the absence of significant symptoms it is difficult to persuade the patient to undergo surgery because of a dearth of literature reports on the precise level of risk. This may be rendered all the more difficult if there are several strictured segments. None the less, it would seem prudent to raise the issue of malignant disease with the patient and to give strong consideration to resectional surgery for individual strictured segments of long duration, provided there is minimal risk of producing short bowel syndrome. When carcinoma is found at surgery in a segment of strictured small intestine, this is usually recognized by the pathologist (as opposed to the surgeon) when sectioning the resected segment. This in turn may raise the issue of whether a further operation is required if the patient has undergone a 'non-radical' resection of the small bowel. The issue of stricture biopsy and the risk of carcinoma complicating strictureplasty is discussed in the next section.

Crohn's disease in the continent ileostomy

For patients who have undergone continent ileostomy construction for supposed ulcerative colitis, a small percentage will later manifest with features of Crohn's disease. Commonly this follows the performance of a proctectomy and continent ileostomy in patients who have had a preliminary subtotal colectomy for toxic colitis. Notwithstanding the diagnosis of ulcerative colitis in the resected specimen, a small percentage of patients will later exhibit features of Crohn's disease. The same can be said of patients who have had a delayed ileal pouch–anal anastomosis or a proctocolectomy with primary pelvic reservoir, where such features as severe ulceration, previous history of perianal sepsis, or relative rectal sparing were in evidence. The conundrum facing the clinician is of what to do in the patient with a continent ileostomy who is now symptomatic. These symptoms range from recurring bouts of pouchitis to obstructive symptoms due to prepouch stricturing of the small bowel, to perforative or septic disease associated with the pouch or the valve itself.

Patients with recurring pouchitis, having diffuse ulceration of the reservoir with bleeding diarrhea and peristomal pain, have usually been treated with antibiotics such as metronidazole, as well as with intraluminal steroids and even systemic anti-inflammatory agents. By the time these drugs have failed to improve the patient's condition, resectional surgery with construction of an end ileostomy (pouch removal) is the treatment of choice. For patients with Crohn's disease in the proximal bowel, either in the jejunum or distally near the afferent loop of the pouch, then resectional surgery and anastomosis or strictureplasty is often feasible, thus retaining the pouch. The rationale behind this is that such patients usually have a well-functioning continent ileostomy and are most reluctant to lose their pouch. In such cases resection and anastomosis can be regarded in much the same light as in patients who do not have a continent ileostomy. In patients who have perforating disease in the pouch, either in the form of a valve–cutaneous fistula or a pouch–cutaneous fistula, then reconstructive surgery is essentially ineffective and pouch excision is the preferred method of management.

Crohn's disease in the pelvic ileal pouch (Fig. 95.5)

Such patients have a number of different clinical presentations. For the patient who has undergone proctocolectomy and ileal pouch–anal anastomosis, but who subsequently has had a diagnosis of Crohn's disease made from the colorectal resection, it is our practice to close the temporary ileostomy. This decision is taken on the basis that pouch function may be successful and the pouch preserved in 70% of patients for at least 3 years (Fazio et al 1994). The rationale of this is that the patient has already borne most of the complication risks at the time of the restorative proctocolectomy. The relative risk of reversal of the ileostomy is small by comparison. In some ways this is analogous to an ileorectal anastomosis, which is commonly done for Crohn's disease of the colon.

A second clinical entity is the patient in whom the diagnosis of Crohn's disease is made many months or years after the time of pouch construction. The patient may present with episodic recurrent resistant pouchitis, with varying degrees of responsiveness to medical therapy. The medical treatment is as for recurrent Crohn's disease. When the patient has failed to thrive or has developed side effects of medication, or the complications of the disease prove to be disabling, then pouch resection with neo-end ileostomy is usually advised. Another presentation is of a stricture of ileum just proximal to the pouch or in the pouch itself. Under these circumstances, strictureplasty may be feasible, particularly in patients who wish to avoid an ileostomy or pouch excision. A further manifestation of Crohn's disease in the pelvic pouch is that of fistulous disease from the pouch to the perineum or the vagina. This may be associated with an apparently normal pouch but with active inflammation of the anal canal and extensive perianal fistulous disease. In such circumstances, conservative measures usually consist of seton drainage, antibiotics, steroids, and sometimes immunosuppression. In selected cases, e.g. pouch–vaginal fistula associated with an apparently normal pouch, a neo-ileal pouch–anal anastomosis can be performed after resecting the anal canal and repairing the fistula. Although this is a successful procedure in patients with ulcerative colitis who develop pouch–cutaneous or pouch–vaginal fistulae, only 25% of patients in our series with Crohn's disease had a successful outcome.

Recurrent Crohn's disease (Fig. 95.16)

Common definitions for recurrent disease include recurrent symptoms; recurrent symptoms with radiological and/or surgical evidence of recurrent disease; and further resection with histological proof of Crohn's disease recurrence. As one might expect, the more stringent the criteria the lower the rates of recurrence reported. Furthermore, the reporting of crude rather than cumulative recurrence rates will make for differences depending on the methodology used. Other factors reported to influence recurrence rates include the age of the patient (the younger the age, the more likely is recurrence), previous operations for Crohn's

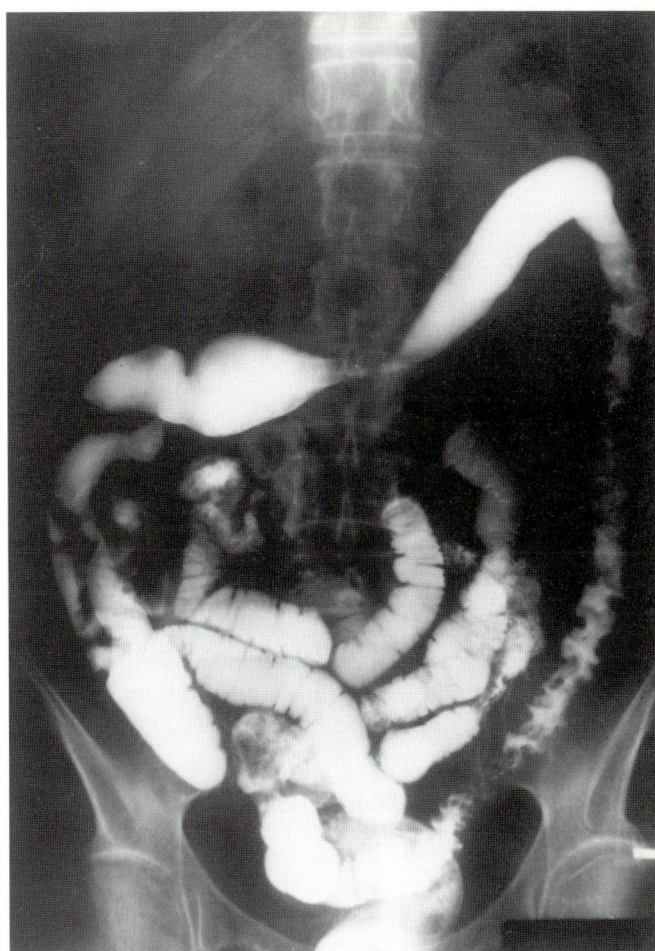

Fig. 95.16 Recurrent Crohn's disease at an ileocolic anastomosis. The transverse colon has developed a stricture due to Crohn's disease.

disease, the site of the disease (clinical anatomical pattern), the use of bypass surgery, the extent of disease in the small intestine, the leaving behind of enlarged lymph nodes, and finally the preservation of residually diseased bowel.

The higher recurrence rate in younger patients was reported by deDombal et al in 1971. Goligher (1971) also reported that a short presection history of Crohn's disease favored a higher recurrence. Higgens and Allan (1980) refuted the earlier reports that surgical procedures themselves favored recurrence.

Farmer and others (1975) had noted a better outcome for patients with ileitis or colitis as opposed to those with ileocolic disease. Gump and others, in 1972, found that there was a higher risk of recurrence if patients had perianal disease.

There is general agreement that recurrence rates are related to the length of follow-up. Lock and others (1981) reviewed the Cleveland Clinic experience of patients undergoing their initial definitive surgery at this institution. Recurrence, defined as the need for further resection, occurred in 35% of patients after a mean follow-up of

11.4 years (Lock et al 1981). Recurrence rates varied at different sites. At 14 years after the first procedure the cumulative recurrence risk for patients with ileocolitis was 50% (±9.6%), whereas for terminal ileal disease alone it was only 38% (±6%), and for large bowel disease alone it was 32% (±7%).

Greenstein and others showed that reoperation rates diminished with each succeeding operation, from 58% after the first operation to 47% after the fourth. However, actuarial analysis showed that with 3 years of follow-up, the cumulative chance of reoperation increased from 37% after the first resection to 60% after the fourth. This pessimistic view of an inexorable tendency for recurrence was challenged by Higgens and Allan, who reported similar reoperation rates after the first, second and third resections.

In general, surgery for recurrent disease follows the same guidelines as those for the first procedure. Concern, especially in those who have had multiple reoperations, for patients developing short bowel syndrome has resulted in a more cautious approach to repeated-resection, and in such patients strictureplasty is often favored. None the less, for obstruction or for intra-abdominal sepsis, further operation is almost always required using resectional surgery.

DIFFUSE SMALL-BOWEL DISEASE

Diffuse jejunoileitis is an uncommon entity, most frequently seen in adolescents and young adults. There is a general trend towards avoiding resectional surgery in such patients for as long as possible, because of natural concerns about inducing a short bowel syndrome. In 1974, Cook and Swan reported 18 cases of diffuse jejunoileitis among 330 in their series with Crohn's disease. Thirteen underwent a surgical procedure, usually for obstruction. Abscesses and fistulae were rarely seen. Common accompanying deficiencies included iron, folic acid and other vitamins. Patients were usually malnourished. Although radiological features are initially relatively minimal, with the passage of time extensive involvement with multiple and diffuse stenotic areas was demonstrated in the series report by Cook and Swan. Six patients, all men, died at intervals ranging from between 2 and 18 years from the onset of disease. Surgical resection, usually for obstruction, was associated with a better outcome when short rather than long segments were removed.

In a study of 27 patients with diffuse jejunoileitis Allan and Andrews (1990) found that one-third of the patients died: three patients died of small-bowel cancer, three from sepsis, one from thromboembolism, and one from metabolic causes.

Historically, patients with extensive jejunoileitis would normally be managed medically for many years with combinations of steroids, antimicrobials to minimize bacterial overgrowth, and periodic hospitalization. In addition, nutritional support by oral alimentation as well as intravenous nutrition would be required. Resectional surgery was commonly required when bowel obstruction, unresponsive to conservative measures, occurred. Such surgery was usually selective, involving limited resections of small segments, possibly in combination with selective bypass of obstructed segments. Since the colon is usually spared of Crohn's disease, patients could tolerate even major resections (> 50%) of the small bowel. However, recurrence was common and served notice on the limitations of major resective surgery in patients with diffuse disease.

With the advent of hyperalimentation it was felt that this might be particularly appropriate for patients with short bowel syndrome secondary to Crohn's disease or resectional surgery for the condition. In a review of the Cleveland Clinic experience, Galandiuk and colleagues (1990) found that although this is of value, home hyperalimentation was by no means a panacea for this condition. They found that eight of 40 patients died while on hyperalimentation, mostly due to the progressive nature of the disease or to line sepsis.

The decision to operate in diffuse jejunoileitis is generally reached only after careful consideration, and when obstruction persists despite intensive medical management.

Although diffuse jejunoileitis may be manifested as a non-obstructive ulcerative process, more usually segments of narrowing are seen, especially with progression of the disease. This may manifest itself as skip lesions, which can occur in both the small and the large bowel. Binder and Katz (1977) reviewed the literature and found skip lesions occurring in 12–35% of patients with small-bowel Crohn's disease. The operative strategy usually depended upon the proximity of the skip lesion or lesions to the terminal ileal disease. In general, if these were concentrated within 100 cm of the ileocecal valve, then a single or double resection was usually the recommended procedure. For patients with multiple skip lesions (Fig. 95.17) diffusely located throughout the small bowel, traditional management called for resection of the most distal obstructing ileal lesion and individual assessment of the others. With proximal skip lesions, particular attention was paid to dilatation of the segment above them and to the assessment of whether or not these might be capable of producing obstruction. In such cases, throughout the 1960s and 1970s, limited individual resections would be done or, if multiple, then side-to-side enteroenteric bypass would be used above and below the skip lesion. The disadvantage of this, was that of leaving behind partial closed loops, along with the possible detrimental effects of leaving residual strictures in situ. None the less, this was the standard practice as an alternative to inducing the short bowel syndrome.

DEVELOPMENT OF STRICTUREPLASTY

The stimulus for the application of strictureplasty in patients with Crohn's disease of the small bowel came about as a

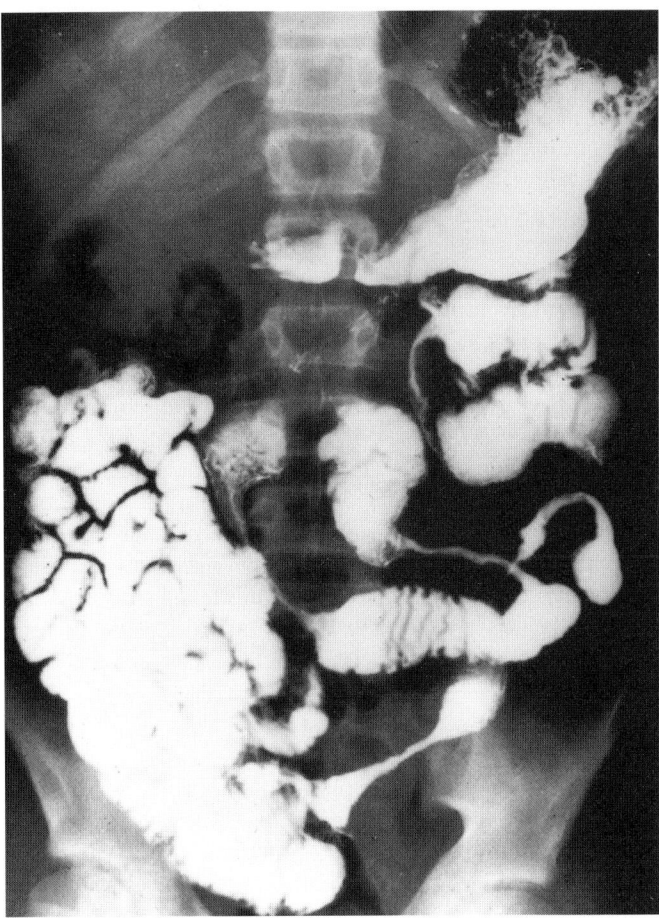

Fig. 95.17 Multiple small-bowel strictures of jejunum and ileum due to Crohn's disease.

result of the pioneering work of Katariya and colleagues (1977), who applied this technique to patients with tuberculous strictures of the small intestine. Recognizing the high risks of inducing the short bowel syndrome with massive resection of the small intestine for tuberculous strictures, these Indian surgeons successfully performed strictureplasty on strictured segments with preservation of the intestinal tract. The late Emanuel Lee, from Oxford, was the first to apply the procedure to patients with Crohn's disease strictures of the small bowel (Lee & Papaioannou 1982). Subsequently, strictureplasty has been used more or less routinely in patients with short fibrotic strictures in Crohn's disease, especially where there was the risk of developing short bowel syndrome as a result of multiple resections. The Birmingham group, under the leadership of Alexander-Williams, provided much of the guidelines for the application of this modality.

Techniques of strictureplasty

At operation, the laparotomy includes examination of the stomach, duodenum, small and large bowel. The small intestine is traced from the duodenojejunal junction down to the ileocecal valve and suture tags are placed on segments affected by the disease. The small intestine is measured out, as are the number, location and length of the strictures. Diseased sections may be manifested by gross fat wrapping or by only subtle changes, in which there is some increased vascularity or fatty deposition along a somewhat tortuous vessel on the serosal surface. The mesenteric margin is palpated carefully for thickening. This may be the only sign indicating the presence of

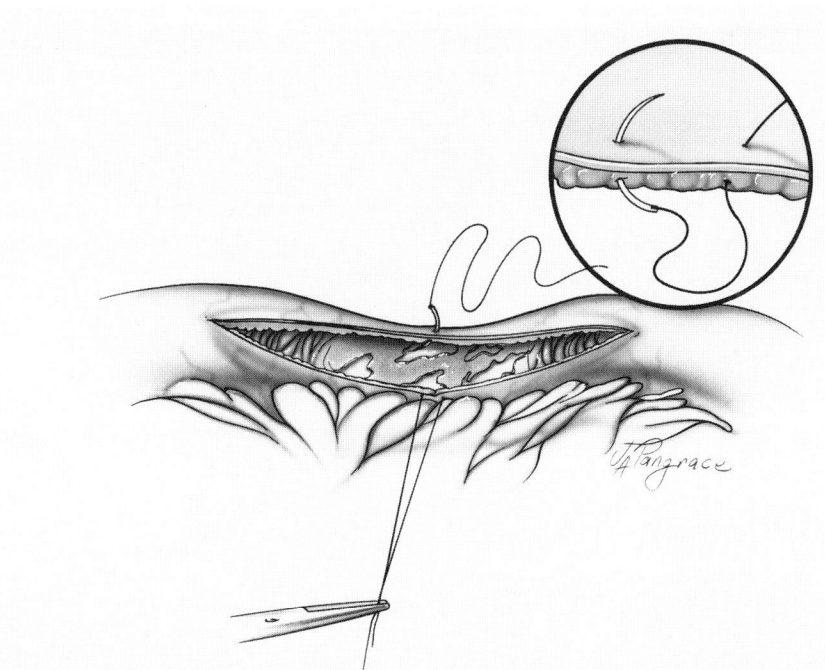

Fig. 95.18 Technique of strictureplasty for short strictures. An antimesenteric incision is made extending 3 cm on either side of the diseased segment into 'normal' bowel. Transverse lateral stay sutures are placed.

Crohn's disease. In the early experience of the surgeon, strictures may be difficult to identify and quantify in terms of caliber. In such cases, techniques including tracing a marble throughout the intestinal tract have been used to identify the strictures. Other techniques, including Foley catheter placement, have been used to identify the location of problematic strictures. As experience is gained, so there is probably less need for such quantification. Contamination is a hazard when using the Foley catheter technique.

For short strictures (<10 cm) a linear antimesenteric incision is used which extends for 3 cm on either side of the stricture (Tjandra & Fazio 1992). Stay sutures are placed at both edges of the enterotomy site in the midportion (Fig. 95.18) and lateral traction is applied (Fig. 95.19). This converts the defect into a rhomboid shape. Biopsy of the stricture is carried out, which may identify an occult carcinoma, although there have been no reports in the literature to confirm this. Hemostasis of the wound edges is necessary, as perioperative transfusion rates may be quite high owing to continued oozing. The wound is closed transversely using a single layer of interrupted 3/0 polyglycolic acid sutures. At the end of the strictureplasty a radio-opaque clip is placed on the mesenteric margin (Fig. 95.20) to facilitate monitoring of the strictureplasty site in the future during contrast radiological examination for evidence of site-specific recurrence.

Longer strictures are treated by a similar enterotomy (Fig. 95.21). The most common method of management is the Finney-type strictureplasty. The bowel is arranged in a U-shape and the antimesenteric incision is made, as mentioned before. The side-to-side 'anastomosis' is then constructed using similar suture material (Figs 95.22). This configuration is only feasible when the bowel wall is supple enough to allow for a tension-free side-to-side closure to be effected. Other authors have used the linear staple cutter to construct this type of anastomosis. The concern here is that of a diverticulum or blind loop syndrome developing in which bacterial overgrowth may occur. At present this seems to be more theoretical than real. Notwithstanding, attempts to construct an 'in-line' strictureplasty have been made using the combination strictureplasty (Heineke Mikulicz combined with Finney) technique (Figs 95.23) (Fazio & Tjandra 1993), as well as the isoperistaltic side-to-side anastomosis technique. Strictureplasty may be applied to strictures of the small bowel or for recurrence at an ileocolic or ileorectal anastomosis and for short duodenal strictures. At present, strictureplasty is not recommended for colonic strictures.

Indications for strictureplasty

The indications for strictureplasty include clinical situations where the patient is symptomatic from bowel obstruction that has failed to respond to medical therapy, and is vulnerable to development of the short bowel syndrome (Fig. 95.24). Thus, patients who have evidence of extensive

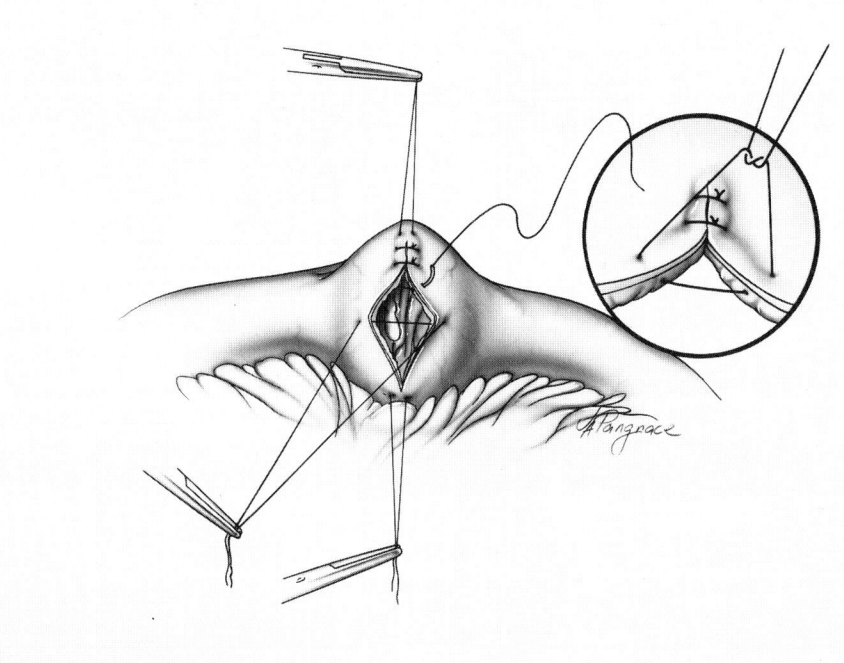

Fig. 95.19 With lateral traction, seromuscular sutures of 3/0 polyglycolic acid are used to close the defect transversely.

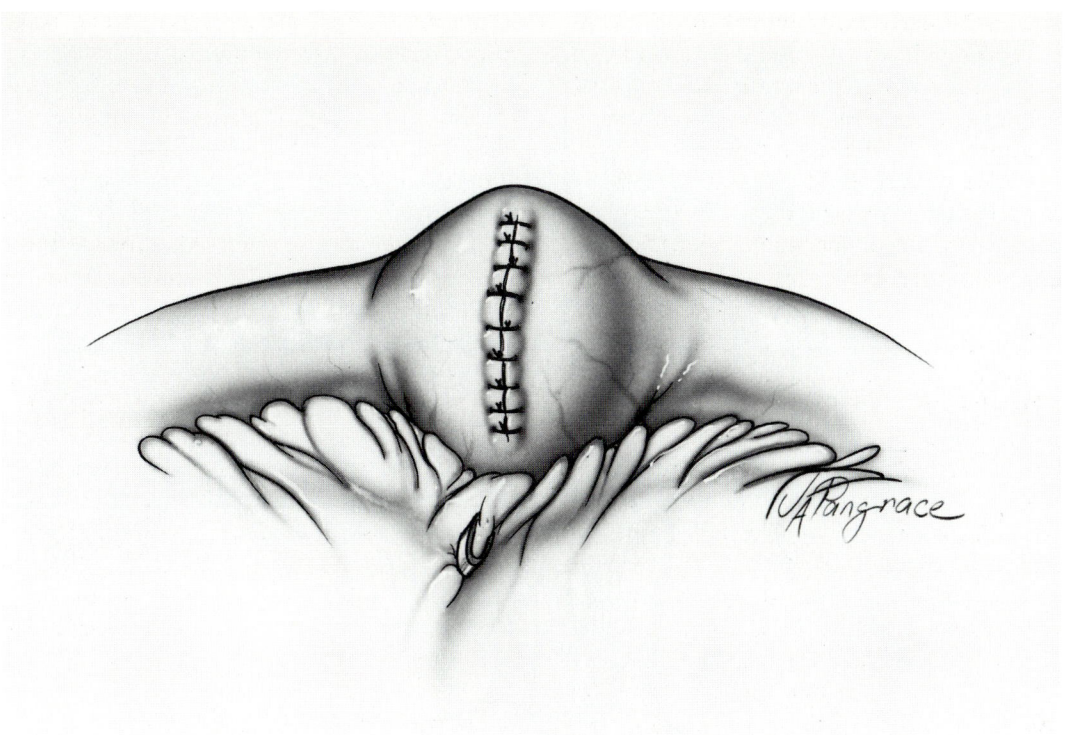

Fig. 95.20 On completion of the strictureplasty, a radio-opaque clip is placed on the mesenteric edge.

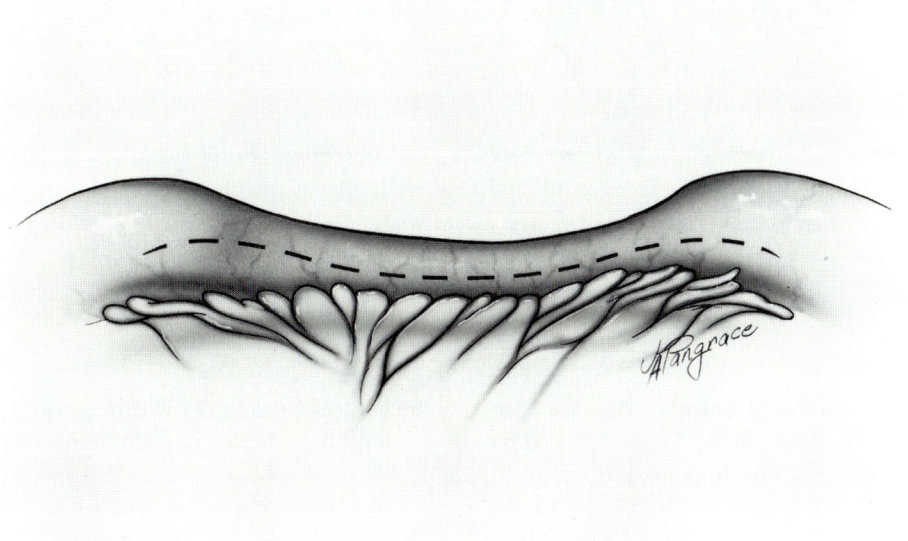

Fig. 95.21 Longer strictures are treated by using a similar antimesenteric incision.

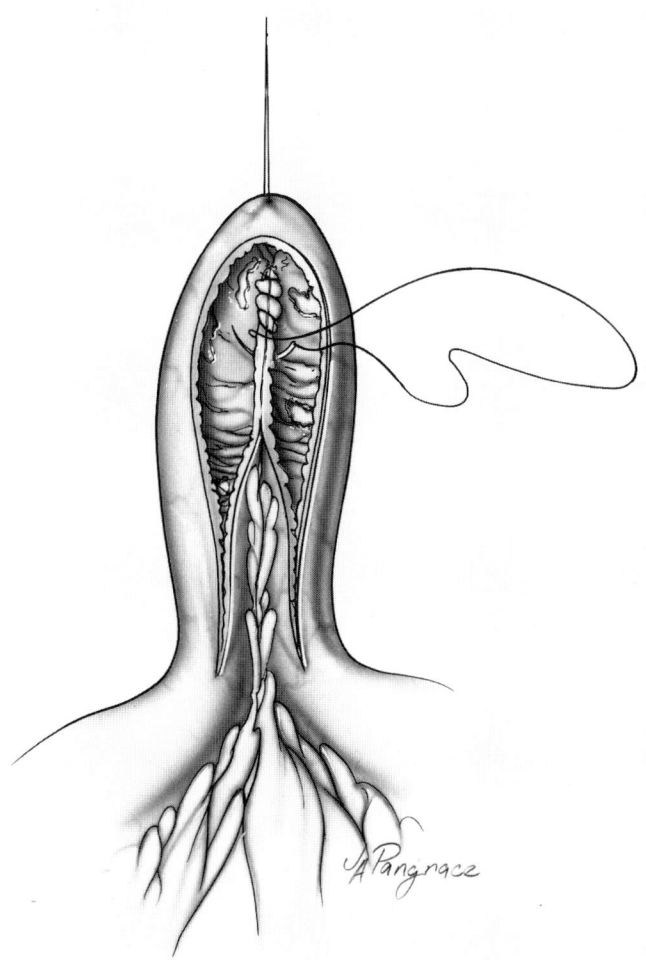

Fig. 95.22a The strictured segment is converted into a U-shape. The posterior edges are brought together by a continuous 3/0 polyglycolic acid suture. Selected areas are chosen for reinforcement with interrupted suture as extra security. The anterior layer is closed in an interrupted fashion similar to the Heineke–Mikulicz technique.

short fibrotic strictures on small-bowel series are particularly suitable for this procedure. Those who have already had a major resection or multiple resections of the small intestine, who have concurrent stricturing of the small bowel, are also suitable for such a procedure. There are patients with longer strictures of the small intestine where it may be appropriate to use strictureplasty.

Contraindications for strictureplasty include the following:

1. Paraintestinal sepsis
2. Perforation
3. Phlegmon
4. Fistula (enteroenteric or enterocutaneous)
5. Long strictured segments (> 20 cm)
6. Multiple strictures within a short segment that might lend itself better to a single resection
7. Patients who have a short stricture in close proximity to a distal ileal phlegmon which will require resection
8. Patients who have a hemorrhagic, fragile mucosa with gross ulceration at the planned strictureplasty site
9. Severe malnutrition, hypoalbuminemia
10. Colonic stricture
11. Carcinoma.

The natural concern of the surgeon when embarking on strictureplasty is that it apparently flies in the face of the traditional principles of surgery, in calling for incisions into diseased intestine and then suturing of diseased bowel to diseased bowel. The rationale behind the procedure

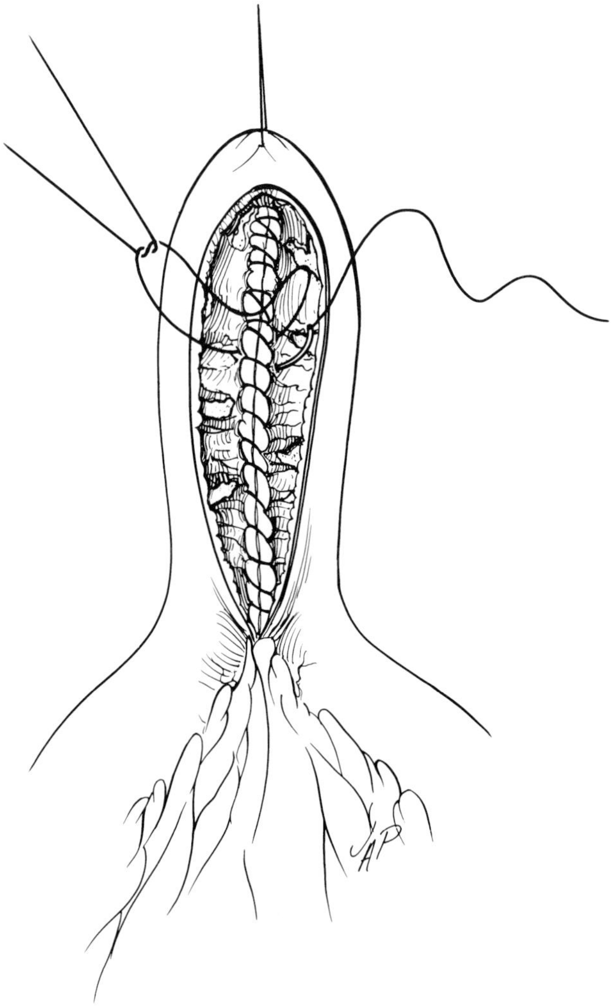

SMALL-BOWEL CROHN'S DISEASE   843

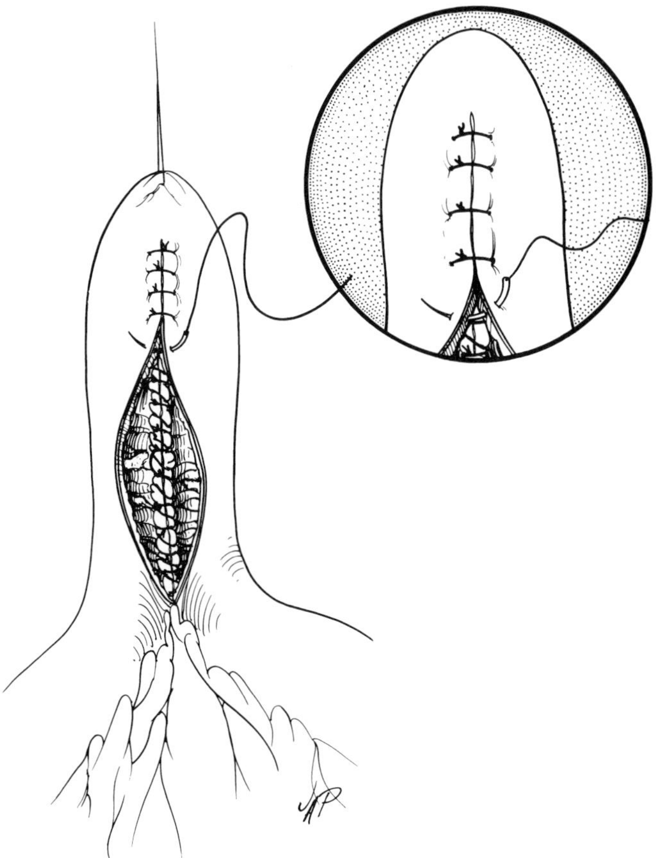

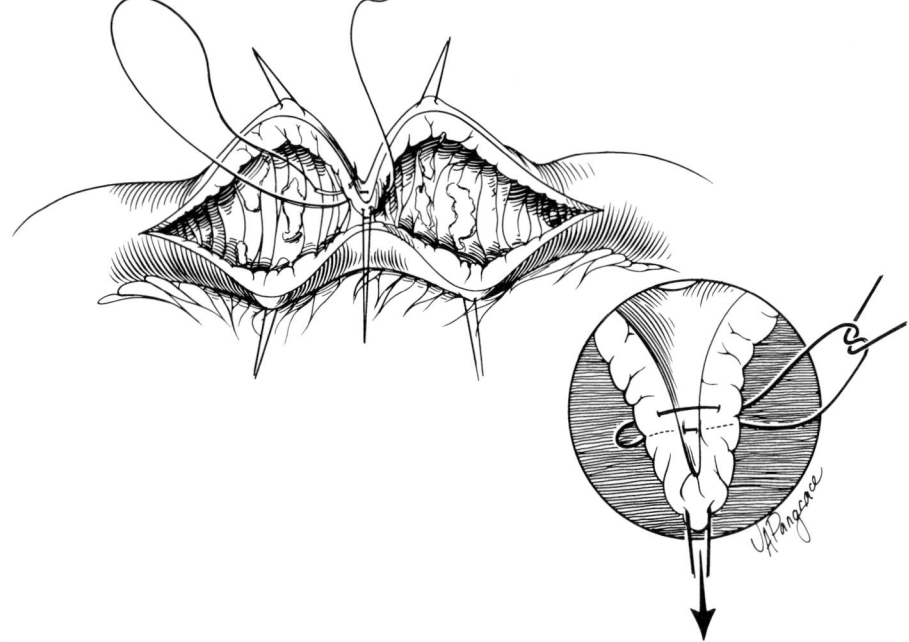

Fig. 95.22b,c

Fig. 95.23a Technique of combination strictureplasty for multiple medium-length strictures in close proximity to one another. An antimesenteric incision is made. The posterior wound edges are approximated as for a Finney strictureplasty in a 'north' and 'south' fashion as these sutures are placed, so that the midportions of the antimesenteric margins are able to come closer together. The anterior layer is then closed as for the other strictureplasties. This technique eliminates the need for creation of a large laterally placed diverticulum, which concerns some critics of strictureplasty on a score of possible bacterial overgrowth.

844   INFLAMMATORY BOWEL DISEASES

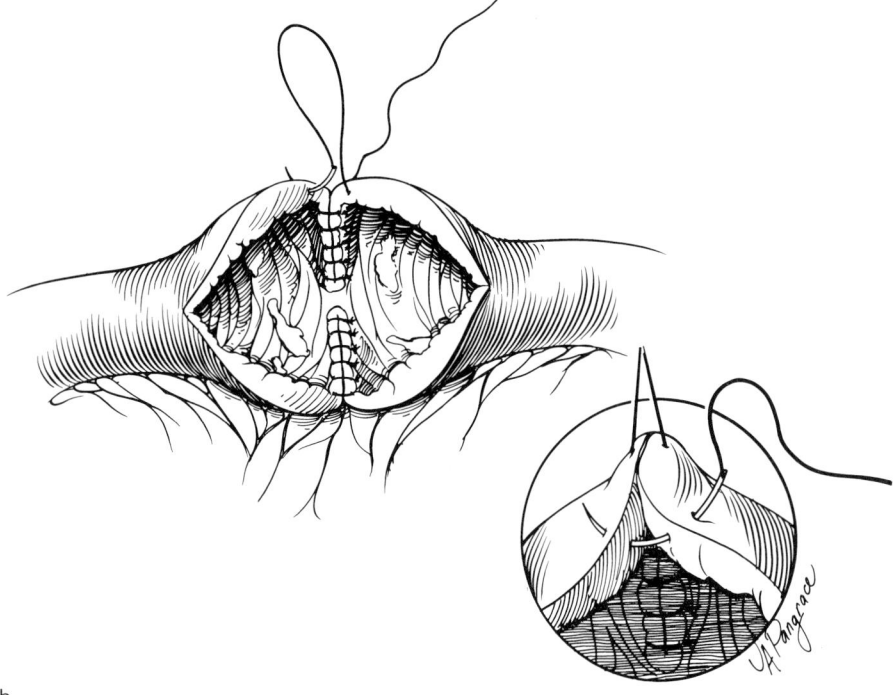

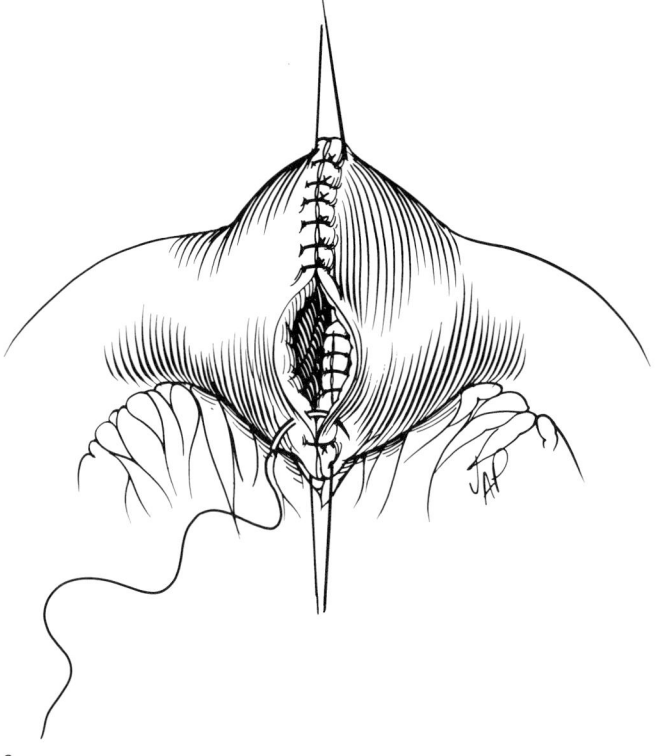

Fig. 95.23b, c

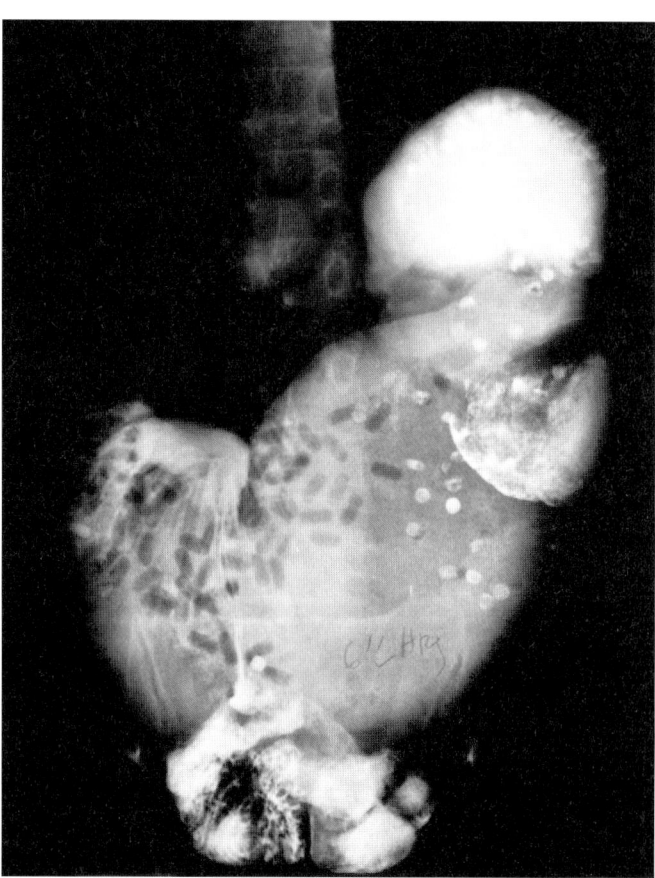

Fig. 95.24 Patient with a long-standing bowel obstruction due to multiple strictures that have failed to respond to 5-aminosalicylic acid capsules.

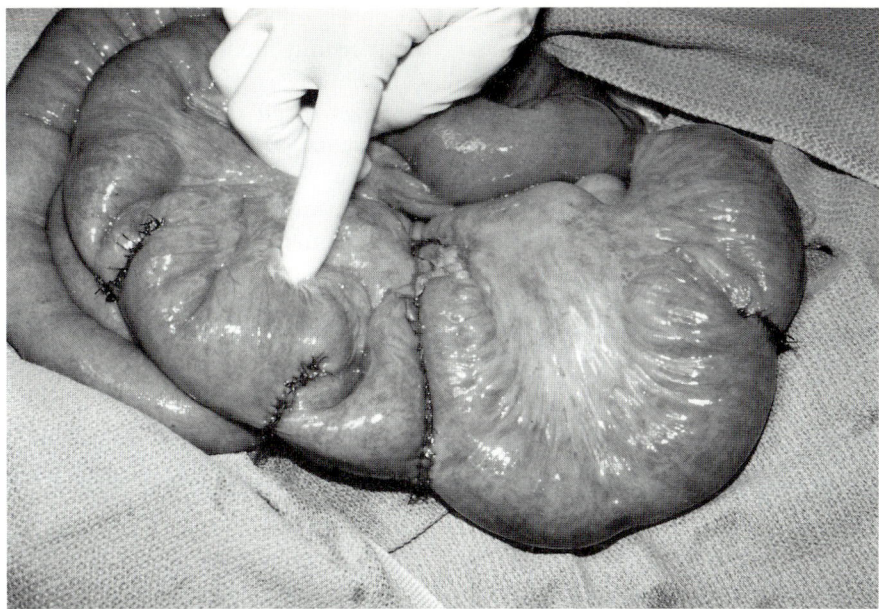

Fig. 95.25 Operative photograph of multiple strictureplasty segments. The surgeon points to a Heineke–Mikulicz strictureplasty located in close proximity to a long Finney strictureplasty.

stems from the fact that the bulk of the disease process in the small intestine is located at the mesenteric margin, as opposed to the antimesenteric margin. Clearly, however, should the surgeon deem the approximation of the bowel edges to be under excessive tension, after beginning the strictureplasty, then the procedure must be abandoned. With strictures that have been the site of perforating disease in the form of enterocutaneous or enteroenteric fistulae, there would be added concern about strictureplasty, in that the patient may develop a leak or fistula from the strictureplasty site. Accordingly, this is regarded as a major contraindication to such a procedure.

For patients with long strictures there is difficulty in obtaining a tension-free anastomosis. None the less, in certain supple strictures in which a chain of lakes appears, it is often possible to align these respective segments of bowel together to create a long strictureplasty (Fig. 95.25). Common sense would indicate that if multiple strictures are present in a short segment of bowel, then the patient would not be well served by several strictureplasties. In addition, there is no good information about the function of such long segments that have been subject to strictureplasty. There also remains the remote risk of cancer. Vigorous attempts to preserve these long strictures are reserved for patients whose intestinal foreshortening is of such a degree that the risk is justified by the potential benefit of preserving intestinal length.

There are now numerous reports in the literature of substantial groups of patients that have been subjected to strictureplasty (Table 95.1). These reports show a remarkable concordance with results. Specifically, the procedure has been proved safe, with a zero reported mortality. In

Table 95.1 Major series reporting strictureplasty for Crohn's disease

Center	Year	No. of patients	No. of strictureplasties
Birmingham	1987	52	148
Oxford	1989	24	86
Toronto	1989	14	37
Boston	1990	13	55
Cleveland	1993	116	452

Table 95.2 Complications related to strictureplasty ($n=452$) in 116 patients at the Cleveland Clinic

Complication	No. of patients	(%)
Mortality	0	0
Fistula, abscess, or leak	7	6
Prolonged ileus without sepsis	4	3
Hemorrhage (transfusion ≥ 3U)	5	4
Reoperation for sepsis	2	2

addition there has been a septic complication rate, particularly enterocutaneous fistula rate, that ranges from 0 to 10% averaging at about 6%.

The operation has also proved to be effective in overcoming obstruction and obstructive symptoms. Weight gain and restoration of nutritional parameters such as albumin levels is the rule rather than the exception. Accompanying this is improved appetite and food tolerance. Steroid medications can usually be withdrawn or substantially reduced.

We reported our experience with 116 patients undergoing 452 strictureplasties (Fazio et al 1993) (Table 95.2), with complications in 15%.

Septic complications were associated with hypoalbuminemia. However, no such association of sepsis with other factors such as number of strictures, stricture length, steroid dosage or synchronous resection could be found. Hemorrhage was a challenging complication following surgery. In all patients operation was avoided by either transfusion alone or the combination of transfusion and intra-arterial pitressin (two cases). This situation could prove a major challenge if operative intervention were required for major hemorrhage, in that it would be difficult to identify which of the strictureplasty sites was bleeding. It could prove necessary to resect all such strictureplasty sites to be certain of removing the bleeding point.

In the group of patients studied, approximately two-thirds required synchronous resection of the distalmost phlegmonous segment of Crohn's disease in the small intestine. In the study of 116 patients at a mean follow-up of 36 months 99% were relieved of their obstructive symptoms, and two-thirds discontinued taking steroids. Medium weight gain was 4 kg. Reoperation was required in 15% of patients. In the majority this was for new stricture formation or perforative disease at a location remote from the original strictureplasty site. Asymptomatic restricturing occurred in only 2.8% of the 452 stricture-plasties. Nine percent of patients with recurrent obstructive symptoms were managed medically.

One of the curious phenomena associated with the operation of strictureplasty is the frequent observation that sites treated by strictureplasty appear to undergo resolution of overt inflammatory change. Thus, when patients undergo repeat surgery for such conditions as 'recurrent' Crohn's disease or obstruction, gallstones or ventral hernia repair, an opportunity exists for the surgeon to check on the previously treated strictures. These are fairly readily identified when radio-opaque clips are placed on the mesenteric margin. It is remarkable that the findings of all those who report on their strictureplasty experience, that many, if not most, of the treated segments appear to lack any features of Crohn's disease. The mechanism by which this regression of inflammation might occur remains conjectural. One hypothesis states that by relieving the obstructed site, where mucosal and transmural fissuring is often present, the enteric content is not under such high pressure to drive the material into the interstices of the bowel wall. Thus, an infective component to the enteritis might be eliminated by relief of the obstruction.

With respect to the cancer risk in patients undergoing strictureplasty, there are two major forms of clinical concern. The first is that a strictured segment may already have undergone malignant change; this concern has been partly answered by the advice of the Birmingham group in performing biopsies of strictured sites. To date, there has not been a single case report of cancer occurring in such a biopsy specimen. Indeed, the only previous report of cancer occurring in association with a strictureplasty was that of Alexander-Williams. Recently, we identified a case of adenocarcinoma occurring at a strictureplasty site some 8 years following the construction of the stricture-plasty (Fig. 95.26). Biopsy of the original stricture was negative for carcinoma. The patient may have had a contributing added risk for small-bowel carcinoma in that she had adult-onset celiac disease. The patient is now 2 years from undergoing resection of the malignant segment. The risks of malignancy remain in patients with strictures that have been present for many years. The

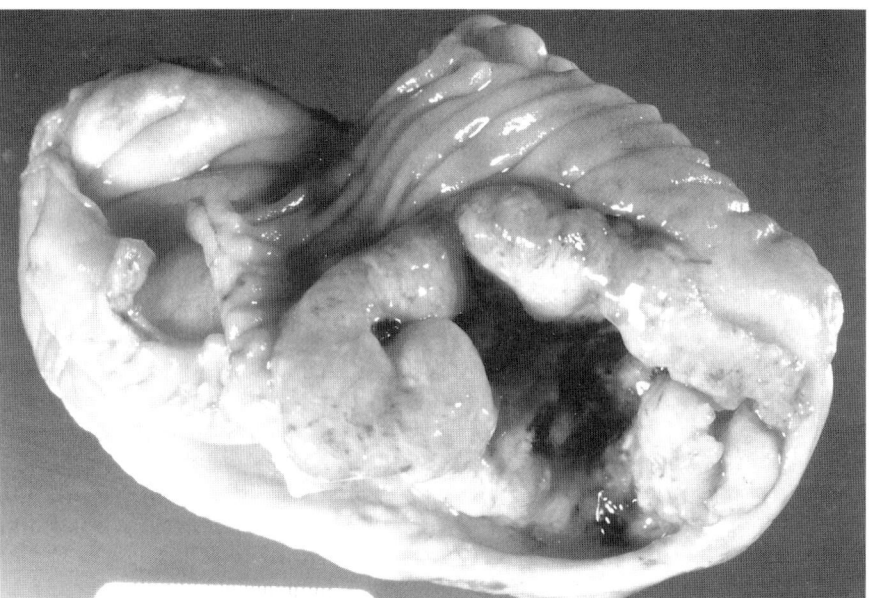

Fig. 95.26 A resected specimen of carcinoma complicating small-bowel Crohn's disease. A strictureplasty had been performed 8 years earlier.

level of this risk remains unknown, but it is likely to be very low and at present one can still advocate strictureplasty on the basis of the rarity of the complication.

Future directions for research in this area will include assessment of the strictureplasty segment in terms of the morphological, histological and physiological changes that occur in the diseased bowel following strictureplasty. In addition, the microbiology and function of the side-to-side strictureplasty segments deserves investigation, as well as those procedures to eliminate the diverticulum-inducing operations in favor of the 'in-line' strictureplasty.

REFERENCES

Andrews H A, Allan R N 1990 Crohn's disease of the small intestine. In: Allan R N, Keighley M R, Alexander-Williams J, Hawkins C (eds) Inflammatory bowel disease 2nd edn. Churchill Livingstone, Edinburgh

Atwell J D, Duthie H L, Goligher J C 1965 The outcome of Crohn's disease. British Journal of Surgery 52: 966–972

Berman I, Krause U 1977 Crohn's disease: a long-term study of a clinical course. Scandinavian Journal of Gastroenterology 12: 937

Binder S C, Katz B 1977 Regional enteritis, a review of the intestine. Ohio State Medical Journal 73: 661–666

Block G E, Inker W E, Kersner J B 1973 Significance in treatment of occult obstructive uropathy complicating Crohn's disease. Annals of Surgery 178: 322–330

Chardavanayne R, Flint G W, Pollack S, Wise L 1986 Factors affecting recurrence following resection for Crohn's disease. Diseases of the Colon and Rectum 29: 495

Cook W T, Swan C H 1974 Diffuse jejunoileitis of Crohn's disease. Quarterly Journal of Medicine 43: 583–601

Crohn B B, Yarnis H 1958 Regional ileitis, 2nd edn. Grune & Stratton, New York, pp 71–72

deDombal F T, Burton I, Goligher J C 1971 Recurrence of Crohn's disease after primary excisional surgery. Gut 12: 519–527

Farmer R G, Hawk W A, Turnbull R B Jr 1975 Clinical patterns in Crohn's disease: a statistical study of 615 cases. Gastroenterology 68: 627–635

Fazio V W The surgery of Crohn's disease of the small bowel. In: Keighley M R, Alexander-Williams J, Hawkins C (eds) Inflammatory bowel disease. Churchill Livingstone, London, pp 452–461

Fazio V W, Strong S A 1995 The surgical management of Crohn's disease. In: Kirsner J B, Shorter R G (eds) Inflammatory bowel disease, 4th edn. Williams & Wilkins, Baltimore, pp 830–887

Fazio V W, Tjandra J J 1993 Strictureplasty for Crohn's disease with multiple long strictures. Diseases of the Colon and Rectum 36: 71–72

Fazio V W, Kodner I, Jagelman D G et al 1976 Parenteral nutrition as primary or adjunctive treatment. Diseases of the Colon and Rectum 19: 574

Fazio V W, Tjandra J J, Lavery I C, Church J M 1993 Long-term follow-up for strictureplasty in Crohn's disease. Diseases of the Colon and Rectum 36: 353

Fazio V W, Zelas P, Weakley F L 1980 Intraoperative angiography in the localization of bleeding from the small intestine. Surgery, Gynecology and Obstetrics 151: 637–640

Fazio V W, Ziv Y, Church J M et al 1994 The ileal pouch–anal anastomosis: complications and function in 1005 patients. Annals of Surgery (in press)

Galandiuk S, O'Neill M, McDonald P, Fazio V W 1990 A century of home parenteral nutrition for Crohn's disease. American Journal of Surgery 159: 540–544

Garlock J H, Crohn B B 1954 An appraisal of the results of surgery in the treatment of regional ileitis. Journal of the American Medical Association 127: 205–208

Goligher J C, deDombal F T, Burton I 1971 Surgical treatment and its results. In: Engel A, Larssont (eds) Regional enteritis (Crohn's disease). Scandia International Symposium, Stockholm, Nord, Bokhandelns Forlag, pp 166–176

Greenstein A J, Lachman P, Sachar D B et al 1988 Perforating and nonperforating indications for repeated operations in Crohn's disease. Gut 29: 588–592

Gump F E, Sakellariadis P, Wolff M, Broell J R 1972 Clinical pathological investigation of regional enteritis as a guide to prognosis. Annals of Surgery 176: 233–242

Hamilton S R et al 1985 The role of resection margin and frozen section in the surgical management of Crohn's disease. Surgery, Gynecology and Obstetrics 160: 57

Heuman R, Boeryd B, Bolin T, Sjodahl R 1983 The influence of disease at the margin of resection on the outcome of Crohn's disease. British Journal of Surgery 70: 519

Higgens C S, Keighley M, Allan R N 1981 Impact of preoperative weight loss on postoperative morbidity. Journal of the Royal Society of Medicine 74: 571

Higgens C S, Allan R N 1980 Crohn's disease of the distal ileum. Gut 21: 933–940

Homan W P, Dineen P 1978 Comparison of the results of resection, bypass and bypass with exclusion for ileocecal Crohn's disease. Annals of Surgery 187: 530–535

Homan W P, Tang C S, Thorbjarnarson B 1976 Acute massive hemorrhage from intestinal Crohn's disease: report of seven cases and review of the literature. Archives of Surgery 111: 901–905

Hulten L 1988 Surgical treatment of Crohn's disease of the small bowel or ileocecum. World Journal of Surgery 12: 180–185

Hyams J A, Weinberg S R, Alley J L 1943 Chronic ileitis with concomitant ureteritis, case report. American Journal of Surgery 61: 117–120

Irving M H 1990 The management of surgical complications in Crohn's disease – abscess and fistula. In: Allan R N, Keighley M R, Alexander-Williams J, Hawkins C (eds) Inflammatory bowel disease, 2nd edn. Churchill Livingstone, Edinburgh

Karesan R, Serch-Hansen A, Thorensen B O, Hertzberg J 1981 Crohn's disease: long-term results of surgical treatment. Scandinavian Journal of Gastroenterology 16: 57

Katariya R N, Sood S, Rao P G et al 1977 British Journal of Surgery 64: 496–498

Kotanagi H, Kramer K, Fazio V W, Petras R E 1991 Do microscopic abnormalities at resection margins correlate with increased anastomotic recurrence in Crohn's disease? Retrospective analysis of 100 cases. Diseases of the Colon and Rectum 34: 909

Lee E C, Papaioannou N 1982 Minimal surgery for chronic obstruction in patients with extensive or universal Crohn's disease. Annals of the Royal College of Surgeons of England 64: 229–233

Lindhager T et al 1989 Crohn's disease in a defined population: course and results of surgical treatment. Acta Chirurgica Scandinavica 149: 407

Lock M R, Farmer R G, Fazio V W, Jagelman D G, Lavery I C, Weakley F L 1981 Recurrence and reoperation for Crohn's disease (the role of disease location in prognosis). New England Journal of Medicine 304: 1586–1588

Lockhart-Mummery H E, Morson B C Crohn's disease (regional enteritis) of the large intestine and its distinction from ulcerative colitis. Gut 1: 87–105

McDonald P J, Fazio V W, Farmer R G, Jagelman D J et al 1989 Perforating and nonperforating Crohn's disease; an unpredictable guide to recurrence after surgery. Diseases of the Colon and Rectum 32: 117–129

Mekhijan H S, Sweitz D M, Watts H D et al 1979 National Cooperative Crohn's Disease Study: Factors determining recurrence of Crohn's disease after surgery. Gastroenterology 77: 907–913

Papainoannou N, Piris J, Lee E C, Kettlewell M G 1979 The relationship between histological inflammation and the cut-ins after resection of Crohn's disease and recurrence. Gut 20: A916

Pennington J et al 1980 Surgical management of Crohn's disease: influence of disease at margin of resection. Annals of Surgery 192: 311

Present D H, Raninowitz J G, Banks P A, Janowitz H D 1989 Obstructive hydronephrosis. New England Journal of Medicine 280: 523–528

Rubin M, Crecelius D A, Hudson J B 1980 Regional enteritis with major gastrointestinal hemorrhage at the initial manifestation. Archives of Internal Medicine 140: 217–219

Schofield P F 1965 The natural history and treatment of Crohn's disease. Annals of the Royal College of Surgeons of England (London) 36: 258–279

Siminovitch J M, Fazio V W 1980 Ureteral obstruction secondary to Crohn's disease: a need for ureterolysis? American Journal of Surgery 139: 95–98

Speranza V, Zimi M, Leardi S, DelPap M 1986 Recurrence of Crohn's disease: are there any risk factors? Journal of Clinical Gastroenterology 8: 640

Tjandra J J, Fazio V W 1992 Techniques of strictureplasty. In: Schrock T R (ed) Perspectives – focus on technique. W B Saunders, Philadelphia, pp 189–198

Ward N, Van Patter W V, Bargen J A et al 1954 Regional enteritis. Gastroenterology 26: 347–450

Whelan G, Farmer R G, Fazio V W, Goormastic M 1985 Recurrence after surgery in Crohn's disease: relationship to location of disease (clinical pattern) and surgical indication. Gastroenterology 88: 1826–1833

96. Crohn's disease of the colon – segmental resection

S. A. Strong

Lockhart-Mummery and Morson (1960) are credited with establishing Crohn's disease of the colon and rectum as a distinct disease pattern. This particular distribution of Crohn's disease was subsequently divided into two subgroups: total colonic involvement (70%) and segmental disease distribution (30%). Based on disease distribution, Farmer et al (1975) analyzed 615 consecutive patients presenting to the Cleveland Clinic with Crohn's disease. They determined that more than a quarter of patients initially present with involvement of the large intestine without small bowel disease.

INDICATIONS AND OPTIONS FOR OPERATION

Despite multiple options in the medical treatment of patients with large-bowel Crohn's disease, most will require operative treatment during their lifetime. Moreover, 50% and 75% of patients will require an operation within 5 and 10 years of disease onset, respectively.

The specific operative indications for Crohn's colitis can be categorized as elective or non-elective (Tables 96.1, 96.2). Although few clinicians will debate the place for operative intervention in those patients with Crohn's colitis

Table 96.1 Elective indications for surgery

Internal fistula
External (colocutaneous) fistula
Chronic abscess
Stricture
Malignancy
Growth retardation
Extraintestinal manifestations
Failed medical therapy
Cancer prophylaxis and dysplasia

Table 96.2 Non-elective indications for surgery

Abscess
Toxic colitis and toxic megacolon
Perforation (contained)
Peritonitis
Hemorrhage

experiencing internal or colocutaneous fistula, intra-abdominal abscess, colonic obstruction, concomitant malignancy, growth retardation, toxic colitis, free perforation or massive colonic hemorrhage, two of the indications – failed medical therapy and carcinoma prophylaxis – generate some controversy.

The choice of operation for large-intestinal Crohn's disease depends on many variables, including patient age; previous resections; disease distribution; rectal compliance; fecal continence; urgency of operation; and conduct of operation (Tables 96.3, 96.4). Some would argue, however, that proctosigmoidectomy and colostomy for anorectal disease carries a high risk of recurrence in the proximal colon. Many purists would never advocate pouch construction knowingly for Crohn's disease, even if it appears confined to the colon.

Fistula

Crohn's disease of the large intestine frequently (16%) results in internal fistulae requiring laparotomy (Farmer et al 1975). The transmural nature of the disease causes inflammatory adhesions that may progress by fistulous extension into adjacent viscera (e.g. bladder, skin, small bowel, stomach, ureter, uterus, vagina). Because these fistulae rarely heal with bowel rest, hyperalimentation or immunosuppression, operative intervention is often warranted. Surgery is directed at resection of the diseased segment of colon and closure of the secondarily involved organ. Occasionally, the inflammatory process is severe enough to warrant en bloc resection of the adjacent viscera.

Abscess

An intra-abdominal abscess complicating Crohn's colitis typically originates from a sealed perforation. Computerized tomography-assisted percutaneous drainage, coupled with intravenous antibiotics, has obviated the need for emergency laparotomy in many of these cases. In those instances where radiographic drainage is not possible, or

Table 96.3 Elective surgery for Crohn's disease of the large bowel

Site	Indication or comment	Procedure
Right colon	Anastomosis overlying duodenum risks complex fistula with recurrence	Right colectomy, ileodistal transverse colostomy, wrap anastomosis with omentum
Right and transverse colon	Ileodescending colostomy has a large mesenteric defect	Extended colectomy with ileosigmoid colostomy
Segmental colon (transverse, descending, or sigmoid)	Older (>50) patients; previous enterectomy (>30 cm). High recurrence rate	Segmental resection, colocolic or cecocolic anastomosis
	Younger (<50) patients; minimal or no previous enterectomy	Resect diseased segment *plus* proximal colon with ileocolostomy
Rectum with colon sparing	Older (>50) patients; previous enterectomy (>30 cm)	Proctosigmoidectomy and colostomy
	Younger (<50) patients; minimal or no previous enterectomy	Proctocolectomy and ileostomy
Total colon disease	Rectum essentially normal; good rectal compliance; good continence; no perianal sepsis	Total colectomy and ileorectal anastomosis
	Above *plus* proximal rectal disease. High recurrence rate	Total colectomy, partial proctectomy, ileal (10 cm) pouch–rectal anastomosis

Table 96.4 Non-elective surgery for Crohn's disease of the large bowel

Site	Indication or comment	Procedure
Right or segmental colitis	Toxic or severely malnourished patient with perforation and peritonitis	Resect disease, exclude distal bowel, proximal diversion
Rectal disease	Perforation or abscess with signs of sepsis	Drain abscess, colostomy; staged resection 6 months later
Total colon disease	Toxic megacolon with perforation; toxic colitis	Subtotal colectomy with ileostomy and extraperitoneal rectosigmoid stump or mucus fistula
	Toxic megacolon with contained perforation; dangerous colectomy due to high splenic flexure, pregnancy or comorbid disease	Ileostomy and blowhole colostomy; staged resection 6 months later
	Colonic hemorrhage	Subtotal colectomy with ileostomy and extraperitoneal rectosigmoid stump or mucus fistula
	Rectal hemorrhage	Proctocolectomy and ileostomy
	Colonoscopic perforation with quiescent colitis	Oversew or resect perforation with ileostomy

the patient's clinical picture worsens despite drainage, operative intervention is warranted, with extensive drainage of the infected cavity, resection of the involved colon, and proximal diversion. If the abscess cavity and sepsis can be controlled, eventual resection is usually necessary for significant intestinal symptoms or a colocutaneous fistula.

Stricture

The incidence of Crohn's colonic stricture ranges from 5 to 17% (Yamazaki et al 1991). Although luminal narrowing in Crohn's colitis is usually benign, carcinoma can arise in long-standing benign strictures, presumably secondary to chronic inflammation. In 132 patients with colonic stricture complicating their Crohn's disease, nine (6.8%) harbored a malignancy in the strictured segment (Yamazaki et al 1991). Although malignant strictures tend to be shorter than benign strictures, the clinical symptoms are typically identical.

Most strictures secondary to Crohn's colitis can be managed non-operatively if they are not causing obstructive symptoms. However, even the asymptomatic stricture must be thoroughly assessed by colonoscopy and exclusion of malignant degeneration attempted. If a standard colonoscope cannot pass through the stricture, a 9 mm pediatric endoscope should be used. The mucosa of the strictured segment must be inspected, with multiple biopsies taken from the margins and from within the stricture. Furthermore, cytological brushings should be obtained from a stricture, especially if the segment cannot be easily passed. Fibrotic strictures tend to be short and web like; inflammatory strictures are concentric, with erythematous, edematous and ulcerated mucosa; malignant strictures have a rigid, abrupt edge with an eccentric lumen. Resection is indicated for biopsy- or cytologically proven malignancy, a malignant appearance despite biopsy results, and high-grade obstruction, particularly with worsening symptoms.

Malignancy

The risk of colonic malignancy complicating Crohn's disease ranges from four to 20 times that of the general population, although the site distribution is similar to that of ordinary colorectal cancers (Weedon et al 1973, Gyde et al 1980, Ekbom et al 1990, Greenstein et al 1990). Savoca et al (1990) reviewed the literature and reported that Crohn's tumors tend to have worse histologic differentiation, but do not usually show an increased propensity for regional or distant metastasis.

Weedon et al (1973), at the Mayo Clinic, were among the first to examine the association between Crohn's disease and colorectal carcinoma. Of patients with extensive Crohn's colitis who were less than 22 years of age when first evaluated, the incidence of colorectal cancer, particularly of the proximal colon, was found to be approximately 20 times greater than seen in a demographically matched control population.

Gyde et al (1980), of the Cancer Epidemiology Research Unit in Birmingham, England, similarly evaluated individuals with long-standing Crohn's disease extensively involving the large intestine. They reported that this select patient population was nearly four times more likely to develop cancer of the alimentary tract than a non-diseased cohort. Although a long duration of Crohn's disease was a significant antecedent factor, juvenile onset was not a necessary requisite.

Greenstein et al (1980), at Mount Sinai Hospital, studied 579 people with Crohn's disease who presented over a 16-year period; their findings substantiated those mentioned. Moreover, they found that colon cancers associated with pre-existing Crohn's disease occasionally occur in sites that are only microscopically involved with inflammation, and surgically excluded portions of the intestine were at particular risk for malignant degeneration. Subsequently, other series have supported the notion that patients with bypassed segments of colon are at an increased risk for the development of a malignancy within that segment (Victor et al 1982, Shorter 1983, Hamilton 1985). Lavery and Jagelman (1982) found the same to be true of excluded rectal stumps.

Most recently, Ekbom et al (1990) closely studied the increased relative risk of colorectal cancer in 1655 Swedish patients with Crohn's disease. Over a 30-year follow-up period they found the excess risk to be not significantly different between cancer of the colon and cancer of the rectum, nor did gender influence the likelihood of malignancy. However, the distribution of disease at the time of diagnosis was an important determinant of this risk. The relative risk was 1.0 for those people with Crohn's disease limited to the terminal ileum at diagnosis, 3.2 for patients with ileocolitis, and 5.6 for persons who had isolated colonic involvement. Patients under 30 years of age when initially diagnosed with Crohn's disease carried a significantly higher risk for colorectal malignancy than their older counterparts. In fact, individuals younger than 30 years when diagnosed with any type of colonic involvement had the greatest relative risk, at 20.9.

Unfortunately, colorectal carcinoma complicating Crohn's disease is difficult to diagnose preoperatively or intra-operatively, even though 80% of tumors occur in diseased segments (Hamilton 1985). Because the X-ray features of Crohn's colitis include patchy disease distribution, asymmetry of the bowel lumen and markedly narrowed strictures, a superimposed malignancy is often difficult to appreciate. Endoscopically the tumor may not appear as an ulcerated exophytic lesion, but instead as a flat plaque or polypoid growth. These subtleties explain why intestinal carcinoma was not recognized by pathologists in more than half of their Crohn's specimens until the mucosa was microscopically evaluated (Flemming & Pollock 1975).

The operative treatment of a colorectal malignancy arising in a diseased Crohn's colon obviously requires resection, with high ligation of the associated lympho-vascular pedicle. However, as synchronous lesions have been described in up to 35% of patients, consideration is given to resection beyond the directly involved segment of colon (Savoca et al 1990). In young patients with long-standing large-bowel disease of an extensive nature, or in those in whom future surveillance would be difficult, the discovery of a colonic carcinoma requires either an abdominal colectomy with ileorectal anastomosis or panproctocolectomy with ileostomy.

Growth retardation

Severe growth retardation is a well known complication of chronic Crohn's disease. Cessation of linear growth, lack of weight gain, retarded bone development and delayed onset of sexual maturation occurs in approximately 30% of children with Crohn's disease. Of 28 children and adolescents with colonic disease, catch-up growth following disease resection occurred only in those operated on before the onset of puberty, and those in whom there was no recurrence during the 2 years following their initial resection (Homer et al 1977). Therefore, growth failure is considered an important operative indication in the prepubertal child with Crohn's colitis, but is probably not an indication after the onset of puberty.

Extraintestinal manifestations

Extraintestinal manifestations are twice as common in patients with Crohn's disease of the large bowel compared to small-bowel involvement. Moreover, the activity of the colitis is closely associated with the severity of the extra-intestinal manifestations. Accordingly, with the exception of primary sclerosing cholangitis, cirrhosis and ankylosing spondylitis, the extraintestinal manifestations of Crohn's colitis typically improve after disease resection. Operative resection may be warranted if medical therapy fails to provide symptomatic control of incapacitating manifestations.

Failed medical therapy

Intractability to appropriate medical therapy is among the most common indications for the operative treatment of

Crohn's colitis. The controversy surrounding this indication, however, lies in what criteria are accepted to define medical intractability. Failure to respond to conventional non-operative therapy is dependent upon the dosing and the duration of treatment with established agents, either individually or in combination. Typically, sulfasalazine (2–4 g/day) should demonstrate clinical improvement within 2–4 weeks or be considered ineffective. Within a similar time period, oral metronidazole (10–20 mg/kg/day) will either improve or have no impact on the patient's clinical course. A response to either of these drugs warrants a 4–6-month treatment course unless troublesome side effects develop, intestinal complications mandate operative treatment, or the disease flares again. If a response to sulfasalazine or metronidazole is not achieved or maintained, prednisone (30–60 mg/day) is initiated, preferably in combination with one of the other conventional agents as a synergistic effect can occur. After 10–14 days of high-dose prednisone the disease flare should have abated and tapering can begin at 5 mg/week, with ultimate discontinuation. If the colitis is refractory to oral prednisone, the patient is hospitalized for high dosages of intravenous corticosteroids and a diagnosis of toxic colitis is considered. Those patients who cannot be tapered below moderate dosages of prednisone may experience a steroid-sparing effect with the initiation of 6-mercaptopurine or azathioprine (1–2 mg/kg/day). If no positive response is achieved by 6 months, the immunosuppressive is stopped; if a response is noted, therapy should not exceed 12 months. Failure of the patient with Crohn's colitis to respond to the initiation of the medications detailed by this regimen, or demonstrated inability to be weaned from the agents as described, is considered a failure of medical management and the patient deserves resection of his disease. The principal symptoms prompting surgery in this group are lethargy and tiredness from anemia and hypoproteinemia, urgency, diarrhea, weight loss, anorexia and coexisting sepsis.

Cancer prophylaxis and dysplasia

As discussed earlier, the incidence of colorectal cancer complicating pre-existing Crohn's colitis is markedly elevated above that of the general population. In an attempt to counteract the effects of this increased risk, the question of prophylactic resection has been raised by some clinicians. Although the predisposition to malignancy does not warrant such an aggressive approach, the need for a routine colonoscopic surveillance program may be justified in select patients. However, the rationale for surveillance in ulcerative colitis (i.e. dysplasia–carcinoma sequence) cannot be extrapolated to Crohn's disease (Lofberg et al 1990). In Crohn's disease involving the large intestine, the dysplasia–carcinoma sequence is not well documented, with large series reporting a relatively low incidence of dysplastic findings. Warren and Barwick (1983) found dysplasia in only 2% of 47 consecutive specimens from patients with non-malignant ileocolic or colonic Crohn's disease. Petras et al (1987) evaluated 3500 patients with Crohn's disease over a 10-year period and discovered dysplasia in five of six patients with colonic carcinoma. Although the dysplastic mucosa was typically located in proximity to the cancer, four patients (67%) demonstrated additional dysplasia remote from the tumor site. Similarly, Hamilton (1985) reported a series of nine patients with resectable colorectal cancer complicating their Crohn's colitis; all harbored high-grade dysplasia near the tumor and six (67%) had dysplasia distant from the index lesion. Richards et al (1989) also found high-grade dysplasia in all five specimens from their Crohn's patients with colon cancer. Simpson et al (1981) studied four patients with colonic Crohn's disease and colorectal carcinoma: two (50%) had dysplasia remote from the tumor.

Lofberg et al (1991) used colonoscopic biopsy to follow 24 patients with long-standing Crohn's colitis. Although none showed evidence of dysplasia, three displayed DNA aneuploidy with the subsequent discovery of an ascending colon cancer in one. Korelitz et al (1990) prospectively evaluated 356 patients with intestinal Crohn's disease for evidence of rectal dysplasia and synchronous or metachronous colorectal cancer. Over a 10-year period, rectal dysplasia was found in 18 patients. Of these two (11%) subsequently developed large-bowel cancer. Another four of the study patients, who had not demonstrated dysplasia, also developed a malignancy. Therefore, dysplasia, as noted on routine rectal biopsy, correctly identified one-third of the patients who would develop a carcinoma.

In summary, mucosal dysplasia is often observed when a malignancy is present, in both remote and adjacent mucosa. Given the difficult task of diagnosing colorectal cancer associated with long-standing Crohn's colitis, and the relationship between dysplasia and carcinoma in this setting, the finding of dysplasia on colonoscopic biopsy or brushing, particularly in a worrisome area, warrants colonic resection. Moreover, albeit controversial, a colonoscopic surveillance program should be considered in Crohn's disease patients at particularly high risk for the development of a colorectal malignancy.

Toxic colitis and toxic megacolon

Toxic colitis, with or without megacolon, is a relatively uncommon, but potentially fatal, complication of Crohn's colitis that can occur any time during the course of the disease. Initial therapy consists of intravenous hydration, correction of electrolyte imbalances, high doses of intravenous corticosteroids and, occasionally, bowel rest with nasogastric decompression. Although the use of parenteral antibiotics is somewhat controversial, it would seem justified to use broad-spectrum coverage to minimize the morbidity associated with the infection that may result from transmural inflammation or microperforation. Narcotics, anticholinergics and antidiarrheals are avoided, as they may mask a worsening clinical course or aggravate colonic dysmotility (Fazio 1980). Hyperalimentation is often started once the initial resuscitation is completed. Unless the patient requires immediate operation because of free perforation, peritonitis, septic shock or drastic deterioration, he is closely observed with serial examinations and abdominal X-rays over the ensuing 24–72 hours. Worsening clinical signs or lack of improvement are indications for an urgent operation. Operation is also recommended after 5–7 days if the patient has demonstrated only minimal improvement.

Perforation

Free perforation of the colon is a rare complication of Crohn's colitis. Bundred et al (1985) reported an incidence of 3% over a 10-year study period of 198 patients with Crohn's colitis. Although colonic perforation may occur spontaneously, toxic megacolon and distal obstruction secondary to fibrotic or malignant stricture must be considered.

Hemorrhage

The incidence of patients with Crohn's disease who bleed massively is low, ranging from 1.4 to 13% (Renison et al 1983). Hemorrhage in Crohn's colitis probably arises from deep ulcerations that extend into the mucosal or submucosal layers and erode moderate-sized vessels. Operative treatment of such hemorrhage is considered only after thorough evaluation of the stable patient with radiography and endoscopy to identify and initiate therapeutic control of the bleeding site. If the patient remains unstable despite aggressive resuscitative efforts, requires continued transfusions, or experiences a rebleed following initial control of the site, laparotomy is required. If the source of colonic hemorrhage is located, segmental resection is advocated. If the source is unidentified panendoscopy is performed intraoperatively, with subtotal colectomy reserved for those situations where the bleeding site remains undetected.

PREOPERATIVE ASSESSMENT

Barium enema radiography was traditionally used to diagnose Crohn's colitis. The most characteristic radiographic features of severe Crohn's colitis include skip lesions, longitudinal and transverse ulceration, cobblestoning of the mucosa, narrowing or stricture, haustral thickening, and terminal ileal involvement. However, the subtle changes associated with mild and early disease are often difficult to appreciate with contrast enema studies. Therefore, endoscopy is considered a more sensitive tool for diagnostic evaluation. Proctoscopic examination provides valuable information (e.g. degree of mucosal inflammation, bowel compliance) necessary to assess the rectum's suitability for preservation with concomitant bowel anastomosis. Obviously, proximal large-bowel involvement can only be diagnosed by complete colonoscopy. The earliest endoscopic abnormalities of Crohn's colitis are erythematous punctate spots, which then progress to aphthoid erosions and ulcerations. As the disease worsens further, deep excavating ulcers appear with raised nodular borders sometimes accompanied by fibrotic strictures. Unfortunately, in some individuals with pan-proctocolitis the endoscopist can have difficulty distinguishing the gross findings of Crohn's disease from those of ulcerative colitis. In these instances biopsy may assist in discriminating between the two disease entities. However, focal granulomas or microgranulomas with giant cells of the Langhans type, typical of Crohn's disease, are recognized in only 30% of patients, thereby making the certainty of most microscopic differentiations impossible (Poulsen et al 1984). To further assist in differentiating Crohn's disease from ulcerative colitis, upper gastrointestinal endoscopy may reveal asymptomatic lesions typical of Crohn's disease in 30% of cases.

In addition to appropriately diagnosing the patient afflicted with Crohn's colitis, the extent of the intestinal involvement is assessed to exclude extracolonic disease. The oral cavity should be examined for aphthoid ulceration of the buccal mucosa, soft palate, gingiva, tongue and lips. The anal canal and perianum may be involved, as evidenced by edematous skin tags, cyanotic discoloration, fissures or canal ulceration, abscesses, fistulae and anorectal stricture. An upper gastrointestinal series with small-bowel follow-through using barium contrast is necessary to exclude concomitant esophageal, gastric and/or small-intestinal disease. An eye examination and a radiographic skeletal survey are obtained if symptoms implicate areas of extraintestinal involvement.

OPERATIVE PREPARATION

Counseling

Although most patients with Crohn's disease are under medical supervision, many have only a limited knowledge of their condition. Still fewer know much about the common operative procedures. Therefore, a discussion about hospitalization and the rationale for nasogastric tubes, intravenous lines, urinary catheters and drains may help allay anxiety. The risk of recurrence also needs to be discussed from the outset.

Stoma site marking

Any discussion about stomas will naturally evoke anxiety for the patient unless he has been living with this possibility for some time. Patients with proctocolitis who require surgery will usually need a permanent ileostomy. In others, complicating conditions (e.g. fulminant colitis or megacolon, severe hypoalbuminemia, free perforation, intra-abdominal abscesses) may mandate a temporary stoma. Whether the stoma is intended to be permanent or temporary, preoperative marking of the site is essential. The major factor influencing satisfactory rehabilitation of a stoma patient is the correct siting and construction of the stoma. The principles of stoma siting include:

1. The site should be clearly visible to the patient
2. The surrounding zone of skin is undisturbed for a distance of 5 cm
3. The site is located at the summit of the infraumbilical fat mound
4. The surface marking is within the rectus abdominis muscle
5. The site is away from bony prominences, skin creases or scars.

Restoration of physiologic deficits

It is common for patients with Crohn's disease to present with varying degrees of malnutrition. Although nearly all reports on the preoperative use of total parenteral nutrition in Crohn's disease show some positive changes in nutritional parameters, a comprehensive review of the literature will conclude that there is no significant reduction in the rate of postoperative complications. Therefore, hyperalimentation is omitted if an non-elective indication for surgery exists, or in the absence of an anergic state. Despite the above findings, TPN is used preoperatively for 5–7 days in cases where surgery is elective or semielective and malnutrition is considered severe. If significant hypoalbuminemia (i.e. <2.5 g/dl) persists, a bowel anastomosis is avoided in favor of a temporary ileostomy after resectional surgery.

Other deficits, such as anemia, electrolyte deficiencies, dehydration or coagulation defects can be readily restored, even in emergencies. Comorbid conditions (e.g. diabetes, respiratory disorders, cardiovascular disease) may require assistance from medical colleagues.

Steroids

Unless the patient has taken steroids or adrenocorticotropic hormone (ACTH) during the previous 6 months, no stress dosing of steroids is necessary. Many patients are taking these drugs at the time of presentation for surgery, and so the dosages are increased during the perioperative period. The author's preference is to place patients on intravenous hydrocortisone immediately prior to operation and continue this dose at 100 mg every 8 hours for six doses. On day three, 100 mg of intravenous hydrocortisone in the morning is prescribed. Further reductions depend on whether oral intake is possible, as well as the preoperative dosage and duration of such therapy. For example, if steroids were used in low dosages or only a few weeks prior to surgery, the tapering regimen can be completed within 2–3 weeks. Otherwise, the tapering period may be longer, up to 12 weeks in some cases.

Mechanical preparation

Under ideal circumstances, mechanical cleansing of the intestine is used. However, many patients with Crohn's disease involving the large bowel will present with obstructive symptoms that vary in degrees of chronicity and severity. In these patients mechanical bowel preparation is modified or omitted and the patient's diet is restricted to modified elemental diets for 3–5 days, with supplemental oral or intravenous fluids. Understandably, some patients with chronic obstruction may require days of hospitalized treatment prior to elective surgery. Magnesium citrate solutions may be used over several days to help clean the bowel in partially obstructed patients, as this is usually better tolerated than polyethylene glycol.

For elective cases when there are few or no symptoms suggestive of obstruction, a conventional polyethylene glycol preparation is used in the afternoon preceding the day of surgery. Such patients usually take this preparation at home and are admitted on the day of surgery. Despite apparently excellent patient compliance with the mechanical bowel preparation, a warm saline washout of the rectum through a large rectal (34 Fr) catheter is performed after the patient has been anesthetized.

Antibiotic preparation

Opinions vary as to the optimal antibiotic prophylactic regimen. The author's practice is to use a third-generation cephalosporin or ciprofloxacin in combination with metronidazole systemically. A common regimen is that of cefotaxime 1000 mg and metronidazole 500 mg given intravenously to the patient on call to the operating room and continued every 8 hours postoperatively for two doses. If intraoperative contamination occurs, antibiotics are prescribed for 5 days and then their continued use is reassessed. At operation, septic foci are cultured and antibiotics are continued postoperatively, to be changed after sensitivities have been reported. Free perforation or gross fecal soiling may indicate a need for added coverage with ampicillin or imipenem.

For patients who are septic preoperatively, computerized tomography with or without needle aspiration may help locate, treat and identify the nature of an abscess. Antibiotic selection is based on likely flora pending the outcome of cultures and sensitivities.

Other

After the patient has been anesthetized a nasogastric tube is passed and a Foley catheter placed in the bladder. Central venous lines and peripheral arterial lines may be placed after conferring with the anesthesiologist. Ureteric stents are not routinely used, but can be helpful with reoperative pelvic surgery.

SEGMENTAL RESECTION

Indications

Although the use of limited resection for Crohn's disease of the small intestine is widely accepted, the place of segmental resection in colonic Crohn's disease is more ambiguous. Among the large intestine's physiologic roles, the absorption of water and salt, particularly in the right colon, acts to protect against systemic dehydration and electrolyte imbalance; therefore, attempts at colon preservation are justified. Although a panproctocolectomy with ileostomy may eventually be performed, a patient may be adequately palliated for a number of years with a segmental resection, thereby lessening the portion of his life that he is burdened with an ileostomy. In the younger patient especially, a sphincter-preserving operation may prevent the psychological and social embarrassment that occasionally accompanies a stoma during the formative years.

Crohn's disease of the transverse, descending or sigmoid colon presents a situation where segmental resection and colocolic or colorectal anastomosis are most commonly employed. Segmental resection is particularly ideal for older individuals (>50 years) and colitics who have previously undergone significant small-bowel resection (>30 cm). In both instances, maximal preservation of the colonic absorptive surface may dramatically improve the functional results. In addition, maintenance of the ileocecal valve may afford some protective effect against diarrheal stools. Resection with colorectal anastomosis is used for selected patients with left-sided disease. Care must be taken in disease confined to the sigmoid colon simulating diverticular disease. In some of these patients local resection and anastomosis may be associated with a very high leakage rate. A cecorectal anastomosis is created if the transverse colon is also involved. In the younger patient and those without prior small-bowel resection, the diseased segment and uninvolved proximal colon are typically resected with the construction of an ileosigmoid or ileorectal anastomosis.

Operative technique

Almost without exception, the abdomen is opened through a midline incision to provide adequate exposure without compromising potential stoma sites. The abdominal cavity is explored and the entire gastrointestinal tract examined for evidence of disease involvement (e.g. adenopathy, fat wrapping, prominent vascular serositis, mesenteric thickening). Additionally, intraoperative colonoscopy may help delineate the extent of disease involvement. The adjacent viscera and retroperitoneum are inspected for possible fistulae and abscesses. If the preoperative and intraoperative evaluations are conducive, segmental resection with primary anastomosis is performed.

The optimal length of 'normal' intestine to be resected proximal and distal to the diseased segment remains controversial. Historically a wide resection was advocated, taking 30 cm of non-involved bowel and all of the enlarged lymph nodes (Crohn et al 1932). Wolff et al (1983) recommend frozen sections on the resection margins to search for evidence of microscopic disease. They cite concerns of an associated high risk for anastomotic recurrence if margins are not clear. Contrarily, other authors contend that if the transected bowel and its mucosa are grossly uninvolved, an anastomosis can be safely performed without threat of undue recurrence (Pennington et al 1980, Heuman et al 1983). Taking the issue further, Alexander-Williams and Haynes (1985) have safely performed anastomoses in bowel that was mildly ulcerated.

The author's general approach is to recommend conservative resection margins of 5–10 cm. Lymphadenectomy is not routinely performed; however, any suppurative nodes that can be safely included without vascular compromise of the remaining bowel are excised. Often the mesentery is markedly thickened with enlarged nodes, making the resection difficult as uncontrolled hemorrhage can result from transected vessels retracting into the fatty tissue. If the mesentery has this inflammatory appearance the resection is best carried out between paired clamps using a heavy absorbable suture ligature to secure the vessels. High ligation of the mesenteric vessels is unnecessary unless a malignancy is suspected. Instead, in order to prevent injury to the retroperitoneal organs and remaining bowel, the named vessels are divided distal to their branching. Following resection of the diseased intestine, the open limbs of bowel are inspected without microscopic sections for edema, ulceration or stricture. An anastomosis is subsequently constructed, avoiding any overtly diseased intestine.

In patients with disease limited to the ascending colon, with or without ileal disease, resection of the involved bowel can leave the anastomosis overlying the second portion of the duodenum. Given the nature of Crohn's disease, an anastomotic recurrence may result in a complex fistula that secondarily involves the duodenum or retroperitoneum. To obviate this disastrous complication, the transverse colon is divided at the level of the middle colic vessels so that the root of the mesentery can be interposed between the retroperitoneal structures and the ileocolic anastomosis. Alternatively, a more proximal anastomosis may be wrapped by a pedicle of omentum, thereby preventing the anastomosis from lying in direct contact with the duodenum.

Disease contiguously involving the ascending and transverse colon is treated in a manner similar to isolated ascending colon disease. In this instance, however, resection limited to the diseased segment will result in an anastomosis between the ileum and descending colon, with a mesenteric defect that can be difficult to manage. Therefore, an extended right colectomy is recommended, as the mesenteric leaves of the ileum and sigmoid colon are more easily approximated. Resection of the additional colonic segment prevents the development of an internal hernia and usually does not adversely affect the functional outcome.

Outcome and recurrence

Over the past three decades a number of institutions have published their results with segmental colon resection for Crohn's disease of the large bowel (Table 96.5). Although the majority of patients will experience symptomatic recurrence, over 75% will maintain intestinal continuity for more than a decade after their initial resection with anastomosis.

The recurrent Crohn's disease often occurs in the ileal or colonic segments just proximal to an anastomosis. Typically, these stricture sites require operative resection and neoanastomosis, although strictureplasty has been reported for ileocolic strictures. More recently an endoscopically placed balloon catheter has been used to dilate the narrowed lumen in selected patients. Blomberg et al (1991) reported on 27 Crohn's patients with anastomotic strictures that measured 0.5–3 cm in length and had predilatation diameters of 5–8 mm. All lumina were successfully expanded by balloon dilatation to a size of at least 12 mm, with complications encountered in three patients: one bowel perforation and two cases of hemorrhage requiring transfusion. With a median follow-up of 15 months, 67% of the patients were free of symptoms. Although more than one dilatation session was typically required, all of the patients preferred this to repeat laparotomy. Breysem et al (1992) successfully dilated strictures in 16 patients, of 17 attempted, without complication. Half of the group remained asymptomatic an average of 25 months later. Hydrostatic dilatation was noted to be most successful in those patients with a short (<8 cm) fibrotic stricture, but without active disease involvement. Long-term experience will help define the usefulness of this new non-operative therapy.

In the rare patient whose large-bowel disease is confined to the rectum, proctectomy with end colostomy may be considered if operative treatment is needed. Ritchie and Lockhart-Mummery (1973) reported on a series of 26 patients with such a presentation who were treated by proctectomy and sigmoid colostomy. Overall the results were favorable, with recurrence noted in a single patient (3.8%). Stern et al (1984) reported a subgroup of 11 patients who had Crohn's disease limited to the rectum and sigmoid colon; seven underwent proctosigmoidectomy with colostomy and four had a panproctocolectomy with ileostomy. Of these patients with proctosigmoiditis, none experienced a recurrence and ten had a good quality of life.

COLECTOMY AND ILEORECTAL ANASTOMOSIS

Indications

A population of patients with symptomatic Crohn's colitis exists where segmental resection is not feasible because of extensive colonic involvement. However, a subgroup of this population (25%) demonstrates relative rectal sparing, adequate fecal continence, and absence of active perianal sepsis; these individuals are considered candidates for colectomy with ileoproctostomy.

Many surgeons rely on subjective evidence of rectal compliance as witnessed by distension with proctoscopic air insufflation, to select patients suitable for ileorectal anastomosis. In an effort to add objective criteria, Keighley et al (1982) analyzed the physiologic function of these patients with Crohn's colitis. Although quantitation of anal canal pressures was of no value in predicting functional outcome, patients whose maximum tolerated rectal volume measured less than 150 ml did poorly.

Rarely a patient will present with pancolonic Crohn's disease and significant upper rectal involvement, with a normal mid- and distal rectum. An ileoproctostomy is technically feasible but, as the anastomosis lies only 8–10 cm above the anal verge, function may be excessively impaired secondary to compromised compliance. In this instance, an ileal J pouch is configured with 10 cm limbs and

Table 96.5 Recurrence and enteric continuity following segmental colonic resection

Reference		Colon segment resected (No. of patients)			Recurr (%)	Continuity (%)	F/U (years)
		Right	Transverse	Left			
deDombal et al	1971	35	–	7	32	–	15
Sanfey	1984	5	1	6	29	88	7
Longo et al	1988	9	–	8	62	81	5
Allan et al	1989	1	7	28	66	74	15

Table 96.6 Recurrence and enteric continuity following ileorectal anastomosis

Reference		No of patients	Morbidity (%)	Recurr (%)	Continuity (%)	F/U (years)
Baker	1971	26	8	84	–	6
Flint et al	1977	37	–	41	80	6
Ambrose et al	1984	63	16	52	66	10
Longo et al	1992	118	15	65	61	10

anastomosed to the disease-spared mid-rectum after total colectomy and proximal proctectomy. Although the recurrence rate is undoubtedly greater than that associated with total panproctocolectomy and ileostomy, the patient may enjoy several years without an ileostomy.

Operative technique

The procedure itself is carried out with the patient placed in a modified lithotomy position. After exploring the abdominal cavity, the ascending and descending segments of the large intestine are mobilized by incising along the lateral peritoneal reflections, with careful sweeping of the mesentery off the retroperitoneal structures. Because the transmural nature of Crohn's colitis can cause retroperitoneal inflammation and mesenteric shortening, it is particularly important to identify the right ureter and duodenum while mobilizing the ascending colon, with the left ureter similarly protected during sigmoid colon mobilization. As with segmental resection, the entire lymphovascular drainage basin need not be resected unless a carcinoma is complicating the colitis. With division of the right colonic blood vessels, the integrity of the ileocolic artery is maintained to ensure adequate perfusion of the terminal ileum. Similarly, the terminal branches of the inferior mesenteric artery (superior rectal arteries) are left intact. The ileorectal anastomosis is created between the terminal ileum and the large bowel just beyond the most distal extent of Crohn's disease, as determined by endoscopy. An end-to-end anastomosis is fashioned using a circular stapling device or absorbable suture; the hand-sewn anastomosis is created by approximating the posterior walls with vertical mattress sutures and, anteriorly, an interrupted, single-layer closure of the seromuscular layers. The completed anastomosis is then leak-tested using betadine instilled through the anus and proctoscopic air insufflation with the anastomosis submerged in saline.

Outcome and recurrence

The principal difficulties of this operation concern anastomotic leakage, severe diarrhea, disease recurrence, and surveillance of the retained rectum. Longo et al (1992) reviewed the Cleveland Clinic's experience utilizing this technique. Of 131 patients operated on over a 26-year period, only four (3.6%) anastomotic leaks occurred. After an average 10 years of follow-up, 118 patients (61%) maintained intestinal continuity with a functioning ileorectal anastomosis. The patients who maintained their ileorectal anastomosis averaged 4.2 stools/day, with only 28 of these (23%) being on steroids or antidiarrheals. The success of this operation was independent of patient age and duration of symptoms, but inversely linked, in part, to the presence of concomitant small-bowel disease at the time of anastomosis. Many other authors have reported similar favorable findings (Table 96.6).

COLECTOMY AND ILEOSTOMY

Indications

Non-emergency colectomy and ileostomy are indicated for patients with large-bowel Crohn's disease that would be ideally treated by panproctocolectomy and ileostomy or colectomy and ileorectal anastomosis, but where coexisting factors mandate otherwise. In such cases the patient is well enough to undergo a colectomy but the more stressful proctectomy may be associated with prohibitive morbidity. In addition, these patients typically have significant rectal disease or fecal incontinence that prevents restoration of bowel continuity.

Emergency colectomy and ileostomy are indicated for patients with toxic colitis or toxic megacolon that is not associated with a contained perforation or clinical characteristics that would complicate colectomy (i.e. pregnancy, high-lying splenic flexure, significant comorbid conditions). Moreover, the procedure should be used when perforation or colonic hemorrhage complicates these toxic disease states.

Operative technique

The elective operation is conducted in a manner similar to colectomy and ileorectal anastomosis. In order to reduce operative morbidity, the individual sigmoid vessels, instead of the major vascular trunk, are divided to facilitate delivery of the distal limb to the anterior abdominal wall. The sigmoid colon is then divided and closed with sutures or staples, so that it can lie without tension in the subcutaneous fat of the lower midline wound. Prior to closure of the incision the seromuscular layers of the now-closed bowel are circumferentially sutured to the surrounding fascia, so as to quarantine the rectosigmoid stump from the peritoneal cavity. If the closure dehisces during the postoperative period, a mucus fistula develops; if the divided bowel is instead left intraperitoneal, as in a Hartmann's procedure, a pelvic abscess would probably result.

The ileostomy is usually fashioned as an end stoma. Alternatively, an end-loop stoma can be created if an end ileostomy would risk ischemia (e.g. in obese patients). In either case a 3.5 cm aperture is created in the skin with the subcutaneous fat and rectus abdominus fascia incised longitudinally. If the stoma is to be permanent, the defect between the mesentery and abdominal wall is closed to prevent internal herniation. After closure of the abdominal wound, the ileostomy is primarily matured.

For an end ileostomy the everting sutures pass through the full thickness of the ileal wall and then the dermis of the skin; an additional 'bite' of the seromuscular layer proximal to the bowel end is avoided to lessen the likelihood of a postoperative enterocutaneous fistula. Additional sutures are placed to ensure circumferential approximation of the mucosa and dermis: exposed serosa causes stoma fibrosis and stricturing. For an end-loop ileostomy, a linen tape is passed through the mesentery to assist in tension-free delivery of the ileal loop above the skin level. If possible, the bowel is oriented so the non-functional lumen is rostral to the everted functional limb. The loop is matured by incising the bowel from mesenteric margin to mesenteric margin eccentrically and everting the functional limb with interrupted sutures.

For emergency operations in patients with toxic megacolon, the dilated colon is decompressed upon entering the abdomen to minimize the risk of iatrogenic perforation. A large-bore needle is inserted through a tinea into the bowel lumen, and intermittent suctioning of the luminal gases performed. Following decompression the colon is mobilized and its mesentery divided, as previously described. The most difficult aspect of the procedure is managing the distal bowel stump: the friable nature of the severely inflamed colon wall risks dehiscence of any stump closure. In those instances when the bowel wall is too friable to hold sutures or staples, a mucus fistula is created primarily. Rarely, instead of creating the fistula, the rectosigmoid stump must be exteriorized and wrapped in gauze to prevent retraction, with a mucus fistula safely fashioned 7–10 days later.

Outcome and recurrence

Following subtotal colectomy and end ileostomy, the patient is normally able to recover to good health without short-term problems from the retained rectum. In fact, of 32 patients with toxic colitis undergoing subtotal colectomy and subcutaneous sigmoid stump closure, only two required operative intervention for postoperative complications (Ng et al 1992). Generally, less than 10% of patients require completion proctectomy for continued mucosal inflammation or hemorrhage during the immediate postoperative period.

Six months postoperatively, the patient has the option of ileorectal anastomosis if the disease involvement is minimal, sphincter function appears adequate, and rectal compliance is acceptable. If an ileorectal anastomosis is contraindicated, the patient is counseled as to the risk of malignancy and annual surveillance recommended. However, in those individuals where the rectum remains unused, ongoing inflammation with stricturing can make adequate inspection impossible. In this instance, the patient is allowed a 3–4-year period of observation from the time of last successful surveillance. If recurrent small-bowel disease necessitates laparotomy during the observation interval, proctectomy is performed concomitantly. Conversely, completion proctectomy is suggested for cancer prophylaxis at the end of the allotted observation period.

Unfortunately, it appears that many patients never undergo restoration of their intestinal tract. Mortensen et al (1984) found that rectal excision was necessary in ten of 16 patients (63%) who underwent an emergency rectum-preserving colectomy for acute Crohn's colitis; the average time interval between colectomy and proctectomy was 22 months. Harling et al (1991) reported that, of 79 patients undergoing emergency colectomy and ileostomy for Crohn's colitis, 25 underwent subsequent ileorectal anastomosis, with another 24 being considered for the same operation. Of the 25 patients that underwent ileorectal anastomosis, nine required takedown and 16 patients retain a functioning ileorectal anastomosis after an average follow-up of 19 months. Lock et al (1981) reported similar findings in 101 patients with Crohn's colitis treated by colectomy and rectal exclusion.

PANPROCTOCOLECTOMY

Indications

Elective panproctocolectomy and ileostomy are reserved for those Crohn's disease patients whose large-bowel disease is complicated by proctitis, severe perianal diseases or fecal incontinence too severe for rectal preservation and ileorectal anastomosis.

In patients with a diagnosis of Crohn's disease, panproctocolectomy and the creation of an ileal pouch with ileal pouch–anal anastomosis is contraindicated. In a patient with ulcerative or indeterminant colitis treated by ileal pouch–anal anastomosis, where the postoperative pathology review indicates the disease process to actually be Crohn's disease, the ileal pouch is not to be excised. Rather, the patient is informed of the histologic finding and counseled as to its meaning. If no symptoms or signs of extracolonic Crohn's disease develop during the ensuing 3 months, loop ileostomy closure is performed.

Hyman et al (1992) published the Cleveland Clinic's experience with 24 patients treated by ileal pouch–anal anastomosis in whom the postoperative diagnosis was reported as Crohn's colitis rather than mucosal ulcerative colitis. Of the nine with preoperative symptoms suggestive of Crohn's disease, eight ultimately underwent pouch excision or diversion. Of the 16 remaining patients, in whom suspicious symptoms were absent, only one had lost his pouch with a mean follow-up of 3 years.

Emergency panproctocolectomy with ileostomy is rarely indicated in the severely ill toxic colitic because of the high associated mortality (9–30%) and morbidity rates (Scott et al 1974, Binder et al 1975, Koudahl & Kristensen 1975). The pelvic dissection increases the complexity of the procedure and inherently risks the occurrence of pelvic abscess, enteric fistula and autonomic nerve damage. However, the operation may have a place in the individual with rectal perforation, profuse colorectal hemorrhage, or in the less severely ill patient who would not be a candidate for future ileorectal anastomosis. The surgeon must be cautioned, however, that the differentiation of ulcerative colitis from Crohn's proctocolitis is especially difficult in the fulminant case. Primary panproctocolectomy would nullify the future option of a pelvic pouch procedure in the ulcerative colitic.

Operative technique

The colon and its mesentery are excised as described earlier. In the absence of malignancy or dysplasia, the rectum is mobilized so as to avoid damage to the autonomic innervation of the bladder and reproductive organs. After the distal sigmoid colon has been mobilized, the presacral sympathetic nerves are swept posteriorly at the level of the sacral promontory before division of the superior rectal vessels. With mobilization of the rectum, electrocautery and a little blunt dissection is used to minimize blood loss and reduce the potential subsequent pelvic abscess. The lateral parietal peritoneum is incised to the apex of the genitorectal cul de sac, remaining close to the rectal wall, and the anterior peritoneal reflection is incised outside Denonvilliers' fascia, thereby avoiding the seminal vesicles and prostate or vagina. Posteriorly, the mesorectum and its overlying fascia propria are sharply dissected from the presacral fascia. Waldeyer's fascia is then incised and mobilization continued posteriorly to the level of the levator ani muscles. Laterally, the dissection cones down on to the muscularis propria of the rectum as the superior aspect of the lateral stalks is encountered. From this point on, the lateral and anterior dissection is continued close to the wall of the rectum until the levator hiatus is reached. Many times during the course of the lateral dissection a large clamp is passed perpendicularly through the stalks, creating 'pseudopedicles' of tissue. By spreading the jaws of the clamp, the vessels within the tissue are compressed by traction. Electrocautery, coupled with this technique, ensures better hemostatic division of the lateral stalks. Any bleeding that cannot be controlled with cautery is stopped with suture ligation. If the lateral dissection accidentally wanders out to the pelvic side walls, the nervi erigentes risk needless injury. Once the levator ani muscles are reached circumferentially, the abdominal portion of the procedure is complete.

Following mobilization of the rectum, the author prefers to use an intersphincteric (endoanal) approach to the anorectal excision. Perianal sutures are used to efface the anal canal, revealing the palpable intersphincteric groove. Using electrocautery once again, a circumferential incision is made just outside the anoderm and the intersphincteric plane is developed. The dissection is carried proximally to the level of the levators, meeting the previous plane of transabdominal rectal mobilization. The specimen, including the internal sphincter, is then delivered from the operative field. Primary closure of the perineal wound, as opposed to healing by secondary intention, is performed because of its association with improved healing. In all cases the levators and puborectalis are approximated; if perineal sepsis is absent the external sphincter and perianal skin are also closed. Otherwise, the remaining wound is packed after mushroom catheter drainage of any abscesses and unroofing, with curettage of fistulae. Utilizing this technique, Leicester et al (1984) reported only a 4% incidence of permanent ejaculation difficulty, with no instances of parasympathetic dysfunction.

Prior to abdominal wound closure every effort is made to fill the pelvic dead space. The pelvic parietal peritoneum is left open and the small bowel adequately mobilized so that it can migrate into the pelvis. A pedicle of omentum can often be created, with an arterial supply based on the left gastroepiploic vessel, and secured at the level of the levator hiatus. A transabdominally placed suction drain is positioned in the depths of the pelvis to prevent the collection of serosanguinous fluid, an ideal culture medium for infection and pelvic abscess. The purpose of these maneuvers is to avoid the unfortunate complication of an unhealed perineal wound with recalcitrant sinus. However, despite careful operative technique and attention to the above details, some wounds will not readily heal, but early reoperative therapy is not warranted in the majority of cases as many of these wounds will gradually heal over the ensuing 6–12 months. Instead, local wound care is recommended. Gauze packing and use of a Water Pik provides gentle tissue debridement on a daily basis, which can often complement more formal curettage in the office setting.

Instead of primary panproctocolectomy, Sher et al (1993) advocate a low Hartmann's closure of the rectum, thereby allowing subsequent perineal proctectomy to be performed in less inflamed tissues. Of 25 patients treated by a low Hartmann's pouch, ten continued to demonstrate disease that required intersphincteric perineal proctectomy. Despite this staged approach, three of the ten proctectomy patients continued to suffer from an unhealed perineal wound.

Outcome and recurrence

As mentioned, one of the most common frustrating complications of panproctocolectomy and ileostomy for Crohn's disease is the occurrence of an unhealed perineal wound. Perineal wounds in which the healing process has completely stopped after 6–12 months require aggressive management. Conventional sinogram and small-bowel follow-through radiographs are necessary to exclude the possibility of an enteroperineal fistula. If a pelvic abscess is suspected, a CT scan is indicated. Often an examination of the perineum under anesthesia is warranted to adequately evaluate the region. Biopsies of the sinus tract are reviewed for the presence of granulomas indicative of local Crohn's disease involvement. Concomitantly, the wound can be debrided of necrotic tissue and epithelium. Much like the initial operative intent, treatment of a persistent perineal sinus is aimed at obliteration of the thick-walled cavity that is incapable of collapse. The fibrotic walls are completely excised to expose the softer peripheral tissue. Unfortunately, simple debridement alone, or with simultaneous skin grafting, is often unsuccessful. In the past, coccygectomy and distal sacrectomy permitted adequate mobilization of the perineal soft tissue into the pelvic space by eliminating the posterior bony boundary. However, this extensive procedure fell into disfavor as muscle and musculocutaneous flaps were described (Mann & Springall 1986). These vascular-based grafts have afforded the benefits of a single-stage procedure with a relatively high success rate and low morbidity. Only those muscles whose use will not produce functional impairment are utilized. The gracilis, gluteus maximus (inferior or superior half), gluteal thigh and rectus abdominis muscle flaps are recommended for perineal reconstruction after thorough wound debridement. The particular flap of choice depends on muscle availability, wound size and necessary skin coverage. Muscle flap availability is determined by the patient's position during the procedure, the status of the individual muscle's vascular pedicle, and the operative wound approach.

Recurrent Crohn's disease after panproctocolectomy manifests itself as disease in the ileostomy or remaining small bowel. Scammell et al (1987) reported a 24% and 35% cumulative reoperative rate for recurrence at 5 and 10 years, respectively. The majority (89%) of recurrences occurred within 25 cm of the stoma. Although the rates vary, these values largely agree with the experience of others (Lock et al 1981, Ritchie and Lockhart-Mummery 1973, Goligher 1985).

FECAL DIVERSION

Indications

The role of fecal diversion alone in the management of Crohn's colitis is limited to the initial management of the sick or debilitated patient who has failed to improve with aggressive medical therapy. Subsequently, definitive therapy may be performed 6 months later when the patient is more fit, with less morbidity and mortality.

Historically, Turnbull et al (1970) had championed the creation of a loop ileostomy combined with decompression 'blowhole' colostomy for select patients with toxic colitis complicated by megacolon, pregnancy, contained perforation or significant comorbid conditions. Contraindications to the procedure are associated colonic hemorrhage, free perforation, or the colon that is 'easy' to excise. With improved medical recognition and more sophisticated management of toxic colitis, the use of this procedure has declined. In the past decade, of the 50 Crohn's disease patients undergoing operation at the Cleveland Clinic for toxic colitis, only eight (16%) were sick enough to require loop ileostomy and blowhole colostomy; seven of the eight individuals treated by this procedure had concomitant megacolon. Overall, only four operative mortalities (8%) occurred in these toxic patients with Crohn's disease of the large bowel, all of whom had toxic megacolon.

Technique

The decision to create an ileostomy and blowhole colostomy is typically made preoperatively based upon the criteria mentioned above. Consequently, a relatively small infraumbilical midline incision is made for abdominal exploration. If no reason for a major laparotomy is detected, a segment of terminal ileum is selected and delivered through a transrectus incision in the right lower quadrant for the creation of a loop ileostomy. The location of the dilated transverse colon is marked on the epigastric midline and the lower abdominal wound closed. A separate vertical incision measuring 4–6 cm in length is then made over the colon. The incision is carried down into the peritoneal cavity, with the seromuscular layer of the dilated colon sutured to the linea alba so as to quarantine the wound and a segment of colonic serosa from the remaining peritoneal cavity. The colon is then deflated with a large-bore needle as described earlier, and opened transversely. The mucosa is gently pulled to the skin margins or subcutaneous fat, and the blowhole colostomy created. The loop ileostomy is then matured in an everting fashion. In elective cases, particularly in patients with severe rectal and perianal disease, loop ileostomy or split ileostomy alone may be used for fecal diversion.

Outcome and recurrence

The complications specific to this procedure include those associated with an ileostomy, as mentioned earlier. Moreover, the diverted segment is associated with an increased incidence of malignant degeneration that mandates periodic endoscopic surveillance or resection in the event that premalignant or malignant changes develop, surveillance is impossible due to stricturing or poor patient compliance, or laparotomy is necessary for preileostomy disease.

Winslet et al (1993) reported their experience with 32 patients who underwent fecal diversion alone solely for Crohn's proctocolitis. After a median diversionary period of 22 months, sustained disease remission was attained in 71%, but 16% had no response to proximal diversion. Unfortunately, the overall outcome after a median 99 months of follow-up, is less optimistic, with intestinal continuity restored in only four of the initial 32 patients; 11 patients remained defunctioned because of associated clinical conditions or personal preference. Burman et al (1971) demonstrated that, despite an overall improvement in 28 of 29 patients who underwent diversion for Crohn's colitis, 15 patients (52%) required excision of the defunctionalized bowel after approximately 3 years. Many of the other reports dealing with this issue are skewed by short follow-up and the inclusion of patients who underwent synchronous resection.

REFERENCES

Alexander-Williams J A, Haynes I G 1985 Conservative operations for Crohn's disease of the small bowel. World Journal of Surgery 9: 945–951

Allan A, Andrews M B, Hilton C J, Keighley M R B, Allan R N, Alexander-Williams J 1989 Segmental colonic resection is an appropriate operation for short skip lesions due to Crohn's disease in the colon. World Journal of Surgery 13: 611–616

Ambrose N S, Keighley M R B, Alexander-Williams, J, Allan R N 1984 Clinical impact of colectomy and ileo-rectal anastomosis in the management of Crohn's disease. Gut 25: 223–227

Baker W N 1971 Ileorectal anastomosis for Crohn's disease of the colon. Gut 12: 427–431

Binder S C, Miller H H, Deterling R A Jr 1975 Emergency and urgent operations for ulcerative colitis; the procedure of choice. Archives of Surgery 110: 284–289

Blomberg B, Rolny P, Jarnerot G 1991 Endoscopic treatment of anastomotic strictures in Crohn's disease. Endoscopy 23: 195–198

Breysem Y, Janssens J F, Coremans G, Vantrappen G, Hendrickx G, Rutgeerts P 1992 Endoscopic balloon dilation of colonic and ileocolonic Crohn's strictures: Long-term results. Gastrointestinal Endoscopy 38: 142–147

Bundred N J, Dixon J M, Lumsden A B, Gilmour H M, Davies G C 1985 Free perforation in Crohn's colitis. A ten-year review. Diseases of the Colon and Rectum 28: 35–37

Burman J H, Thompson H, Cooke W T, Alexander-Williams J 1971 The effects of diversion of intestinal contents on the progress of Crohn's disease of the large bowel. Gut 12: 11–15

Crohn B B, Ginzburg L, Oppenheimer G D 1932 Regional ileitis. Journal of the American Medical Association 99: 214–220

deDombal F T, Burton I, Goligher J C 1971 Recurrence of Crohn's disease after primary excisional surgery. Gut 12: 519–527

Ekbom A, Helmick C, Zack M, Admami H O 1990 Increased risk of large bowel cancer in Crohn's disease with colonic involvement. Lancet 336: 357–359

Farmer R G, Hawk W A, Turnbull R G 1975 Clinical patterns in Crohn's disease: a statistical study of 615 cases. Gastroenterology 68: 627–635

Fazio V W 1980 Toxic megacolon in ulcerative colitis and Crohn's colitis. Clinical Gastroenterology 9: 389–407

Flemming K A, Pollock A C 1975 A case of 'Crohn's carcinoma'. Gut 16: 533–537

Flint G, Strauss R, Platt N, Wise L 1977 Ileorectal anastomosis in patients with Crohn's disease of the colon. Gut 18: 236–239

Goligher J C 1985 The long-term results of excisional surgery for primary and recurrent Crohn's disease of the large bowel. Diseases of the Colon and Rectum 28: 51–55

Greenstein A J, Sachar D B, Smith H, Janowitz H D, Aufses A H Jr 1980 Patterns of neoplasia in Crohn's disease and ulcerative colitis. Cancer 46: 403–407

Gyde S N, Prior P, McCartney J C, Thompson H, Waterhouse J A, Allan R N 1980 Malignancy in Crohn's disease. Gut 21: 1024–1029

Hamilton S R 1985 Colorectal carcinoma in patients with Crohn's disease. Gastroenterology 89: 398–407

Harling H, Hegnhoj J, Rasmussen T N, Jarnum S 1991 Fate of the rectum after colectomy and ileostomy for Crohn's colitis. Diseases of the Colon and Rectum 34: 931–935

Heuman R, Boeryd B, Bolin T, Sjodahl R 1983 The influence of disease at the margin of resection on the outcome of Crohn's disease. British Journal of Surgery 70: 519–521

Homer D R, Grand R J, Colodny A H 1977 Growth, course and prognosis after surgery for Crohn's disease in children and adolescents. Pediatrics 59: 717–725

Hyman N H, Fazio V W, Tuckson W B, Lavery I C 1991 Consequences of ileal pouch–anal anastomosis for Crohn's colitis. Diseases of the Colon and Rectum 34: 653–657

Keighley M R B, Buchmann P, Lee J R 1982 Assessment of anorectal function in selection of patients for ileo-rectal anastomosis in Crohn's colitis. Gut 23: 102–107

Korelitz B I, Lauwers G Y, Sommers S C 1990 Rectal mucosal dysplasia in Crohn's disease. Gut 31: 1382–1386

Koudahl G, Kristensen M 1975 Toxic megacolon in ulcerative colitis. Scandinavian Journal of Gastroenterology 10: 417–421

Lavery I C, Jagelman D G 1982 Cancer in the excluded rectum following surgery for inflammatory bowel disease. Diseases of the Colon and Rectum 25: 522–524

Leicester R J, Ritchie J K, Wadsworth J, Thompson J P S, Hawley P R 1984 Sexual function and perineal wound healing after intersphincteric excision of the rectum for inflammatory bowel disease. Diseases of the Colon and Rectum 27: 244–248

Lock M R, Farmer R G, Fazio V W, Jagelman D G, Lavery I C, Weakley F L 1981 Recurrence and reoperation for Crohn's disease: the role of disease location in prognosis. New England Journal of Medicine 304: 1586–1588

Lock M R, Fazio V W, Farmer R G, Jagelman D G, Lavery I C, Weakley F L 1981 Proximal recurrence and the fate of the rectum following excisional surgery for Crohn's disease of the large bowel. Annals of Surgery 194: 754–760

Lockhart-Mummery H E, Morson B C 1960 Crohn's disease (regional enteritis) of the large intestine and its distinction from ulcerative colitis. Gut 1: 87–105

Lofberg R, Brostrom O, Karlen P, Tribukait B, Ost A 1990 Colonoscopic surveillance in longstanding total ulcerative colitis – a fifteen year follow-up study. Gastroenterology 99: 1021–1031

Lofberg R, Brostrom O, Karlen P, Ost A, Tribukait B 1991 Carcinoma and DNA aneuploidy in Crohn's colitis – a histological and flow cytometric study. Gut 32: 900–904

Longo W E, Ballantyne G H, Cahow E 1988 Treatment of Crohn's colitis. Segmental or total colectomy? Archives of Surgery 123: 588–590

Longo W E, Oakley J R, Lavery I C, Church J M, Fazio V W 1992 Outcome of ileorectal anastomosis for Crohn's colitis. Diseases of the Colon and Rectum 35: 1066–1071

Mann C V, Springall R 1986 Use of a muscle graft for unhealed perineal sinus. British Journal of Surgery 73: 1000–1007

Mortensen N J, Ritchie J K, Hawley P R, Todd I P, Lennard-Jones J E 1984 Surgery for acute Crohn's colitis: results and long term follow-up. British Journal of Surgery 71: 783–784

Ng R L H, Davies A H, Grace R H, Mortensen N J 1992 Subcutaneous rectal stump closure after emergency subtotal colectomy. British Journal of Surgery 79: 701–703

Pennington L, Hamilton S R, Bayless T M, Cameron J L 1980 Surgical management of Crohn's disease. Influence of disease at margin of resection. Annals of Surgery 192: 311–318

Petras R E, Mir-Madjilessi S H, Farmer R G 1987 Crohn's disease and intestinal carcinoma. Gastroenterology 93: 1307–1314

Poulsen S S, Pedersen N J, Jarnum S 1984 'Microerosions' in rectal biopsies in Crohn's disease. Scandinavian Journal of Gastroenterology 19: 607–612

Renison D M, Forhouhar F A, Levine J B, Breiter J R 1983 Filiform polyposis of the colon presenting as massive hemorrhage. An uncommon complication of Crohn's disease. American Journal of Gastroenterology 78: 413–416

Richards M E, Rickert R R, Nance F C 1989 Crohn's disease-associated carcinoma: a poorly recognized complication of inflammatory bowel disease. Annals of Surgery 209: 764–773

Ritchie J K, Lockhart-Mummery H E 1973 Non-restorative surgery in the treatment of Crohn's disease of the large bowel. Gut 14: 263–269

Sanfey H, Bayless T M, Corman J L 1984 Crohn's disease of the colon. Is there a role for limited resection? American Journal of Surgery 147: 38–42

Savoca P E, Ballantyne G H, Cahow C E 1990 Gastrointestinal malignancies in Crohn's disease: a 20-year experience. Diseases of the Colon and Rectum 33: 7–11

Scammell B E, Andrews H, Allan R N, Alexander-Williams J, Keighley M R B 1987 Results of proctocolectomy for Crohn's disease. British Journal of Surgery 74: 671–674

Scott H W, Sawyers J L, Gobbel W G Jr, Graves H A, Shull H W 1974 Surgical management of toxic dilatation of the colon in ulcerative colitis. Annals of Surgery 179: 647–656

Sher M E, Bauer J J, Gorfine S, Gelernt I 1992 Low Hartmann's procedure for severe anorectal Crohn's disease. Diseases of the Colon and Rectum 35: 975–980

Shorter R G 1983 Risk of intestinal cancer in Crohn's disease. Diseases of the Colon and Rectum 26: 686–689

Simpson S, Traube J, Ridell R H 1981 The histologic appearance of dysplasia (precancerous change) in Crohn's disease of the small and large intestine. Gastroenterology 81: 492–501

Stern H S, Goldberg S M, Rothenberger D A 1984 Segmental versus total colectomy for large bowel Crohn's disease. World Journal of Surgery 8: 118–122

Turnbull R B, Weakley F L, Hawk W A, Schofield P 1970 Choice of operation for the toxic megacolon phase of nonspecific ulcerative colitis. Surgical Clinics of North America 50: 1151–1169

Victor D W Jr, Thompson H, Allan R N, Alexander-Williams J 1982 Cancer complicating defunctioned Crohn's disease. Clinical Oncology 8: 163–165

Warren R, Barwick K W 1983 Crohn's colitis with carcinoma and dysplasia. American Journal of Surgical Pathology 7: 151–159

Weedon D D, Shorter R G, Ilstrup D M, Huizenga K A, Taylor W F 1973 Crohn's disease and cancer. New England Journal of Medicine 289: 1099–1103

Winslet M C, Andrews H, Allan R N, Keighley M R B 1993 Fecal diversion in the management of Crohn's disease of the colon. Diseases of the Colon and Rectum 36: 757–762

Wolff B G, Beart R E Jr, Frydenberg H B, Weiland L H, Agrz M V, Ilstrup D M 1983 The importance of disease-free margins in resections for Crohn's disease. Diseases of the Colon and Rectum 26: 239–243

Yamazaki Y, Ribeiro M B, Sachar D B, Aufses A H, Greenstein A J 1991 Malignant strictures in Crohn's disease. American Journal of Gastroenterology 86: 882–885

97. Perianal Crohn's disease

I. J. Kodner

GENERAL CONSIDERATIONS

Incidence of anal and perianal involvement

In patients with Crohn's disease both the anus and perianal tissue are frequently involved, although rarely is this the only manifestation of disease. It is not clear, based on the pathophysiology of Crohn's, why the anus should be involved so frequently but it may be related to an immunologic abnormality. When dealing with Crohn's disease it is important to differentiate the anus and the anal canal from the rectum. The surgical anal canal consists of the mucocutaneous junction and the adjacent 2 cm proximal and distal, an area of intense activity in Crohn's disease and of critical importance for the physician who will be managing these patients. Loss of the anal sphincter mechanism due to Crohn's disease necessitates surgery and sometimes stoma construction. It is therefore a very important functional area, which can be evaluated by digital examination and by anoscopic visualization. Approximately 5% of patients with Crohn's disease present with anal lesions only. The vast majority of these go on to develop other intestinal manifestations. One-third of all Crohn's patients will have anal lesions at some time during the course of their disease. Because of the need to preserve sphincter function, sometimes to its maximum, the surgical management of anal disease due to Crohn's must be safe and conservative, making every effort to preserve the sphincter mechanism.

Spectrum of anal and perianal involvement

In a review from the Lahey Clinic of the incidence of anal complications in Crohn's disease (Table 97.1), Williams showed that there was a much higher incidence of anal involvement with colonic rather than small-intestinal Crohn's disease. In a review of our own patient series, we found that, although Crohn's disease is described as an entity involving Caucasians, especially those with a Jewish ethnic background, the African-American population showed a very high percentage of destructive Crohn's disease of the anus and perineum (Table 97.2). Comparing the time of onset of the anal disease with the diagnosis of other intestinal Crohn's disease, a review of our patient population showed that the anal manifestations often preceded the intestinal diagnosis by several years (Fig. 97.1).

Table 97.1 Incidence of anal complications in Crohn's disease. (From Williams et al, Lahey Clinic, 1981)

Primary site	No. of patients	Anal complications
Small bowel	878 (80%)	127 (14%)
Colon	220 (20%)	115 (52%)
Total	1098 (100%)	242 (22%)

Table 97.2 Comparison of major complications with Crohn's disease

	Perineal disease (%)	Intestinal fistulae (%)
Whites	48	35
Blacks	67	20

In order to understand the management of anal and perineal Crohn's disease, it is important to consider the spectrum of disease which can present in this limited anatomic area (Table 97.3). Crohn's can present with complications also seen in non-Crohn's patients, such as ulcer/fissure and abscess/fistula, which must be handled in a safer, more conservative fashion. The unusual manifestations seen in Crohn's disease involve diffuse destruction of the anus and perineum, and the unhealed perineal wound, which can result after ultimate removal of the rectum.

MANAGEMENT OF SPECIFIC MANIFESTATIONS

Crohn's ulcer/fissure

The patient who presents with a painful anal fissure and is suspected of having Crohn's disease should be treated

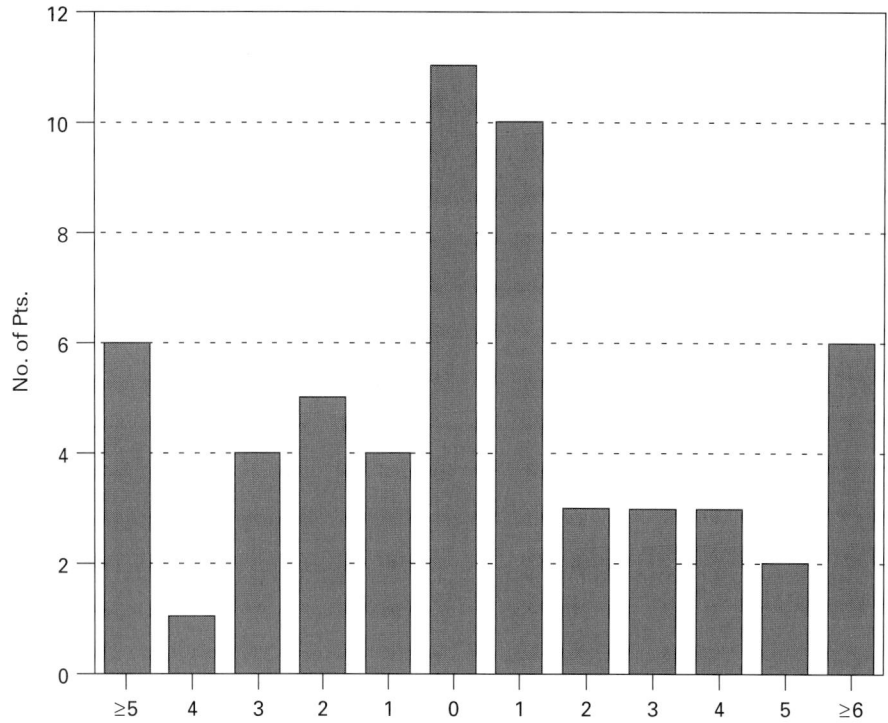

Fig. 97.1 Time of onset of anal disease compared with time, in years, of diagnosis of intestinal Crohn's disease.

Table 97.3 Spectrum of anal and perianal Crohn's disease

Ulcer/fissure
Abscess/fistula
　simple
　complex
　rectovaginal fistula
　anal incontinence
Diffuse destruction
Unhealed perineal wound

with intensive medical management as long as there is evidence of activity of Crohn's disease within the anal canal. Even a painful burrowing ulcer can be treated with the medications which have now been shown to be effective for this type of disease. Medications such as metronidazole, 5-ASA compounds in enema or suppository form, and some of the immunosuppressive drugs are very effective at putting the anal disease into remission. Only in the rare situation, where the Crohn's disease is in remission and specific hypertrophy of the lower third of the internal sphincter muscle can be demonstrated, should consideration ever be given for sphincterotomy. Even this limited incision in the sphincter mechanism can place the patient with Crohn's disease in jeopardy, perhaps much later in life. The appearance of the boggy edematous anal tags sometimes related to an anal ulcer from Crohn's disease represents an excellent source of biopsy to look for the presence of granulomata and thus help confirm the diagnosis of Crohn's disease.

Crohn's abscess/fistula

In managing an abscess or fistula in the patient with active Crohn's disease in the anal canal, surgical treatment should be limited to a non-destructive and conservative approach. The presence of pain in such patients often indicates the accumulation of pus and an abscess. It is disturbing to see the magnitude and severity of abscesses which can occur in patients with Crohn's disease. This can often lead to destruction of the surrounding tissue and the formation of horseshoe abscess/fistulae as the septic process dissects in the tissue of the perianum and perineum. Our preference is to drain these abscesses using indwelling mushroom-tipped catheters, because the internal opening is frequently caused by the Crohn's disease, the condition is chronic in nature, and may not close until much later in treatment, when advancement closure of the internal defect can be undertaken. A classic fistulotomy should be performed only if the disease is in remission and the fistula tract is very superficial. In most cases it is necessary to examine the patient under anesthesia, so that the complex nature of the dissecting Crohn's disease can be identified, abscesses can be drained with indwelling catheters, and fistula tracts can be kept open with setons. Only then can aggressive medical treatment be undertaken, so that definitive surgery can be carried out later without risk of injury to the sphincter mechanism (Fig. 97.2). It is especially important to note that, in Crohn's disease, the appropriate management of

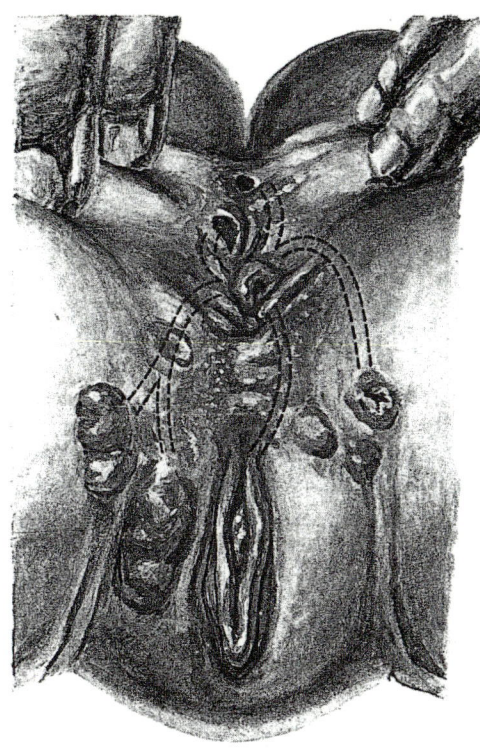
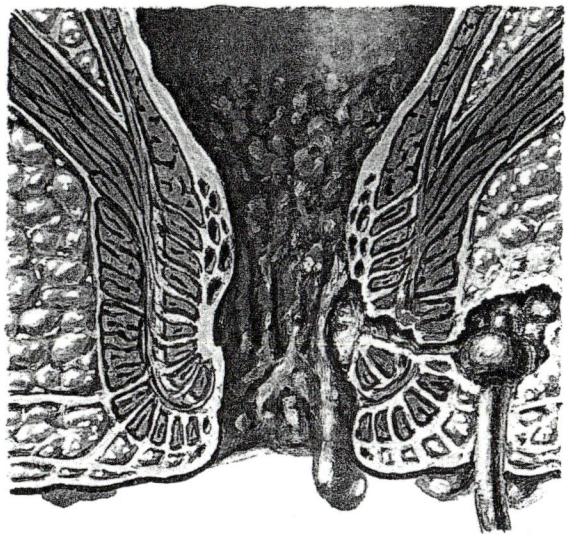
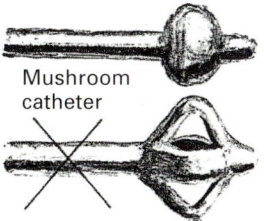
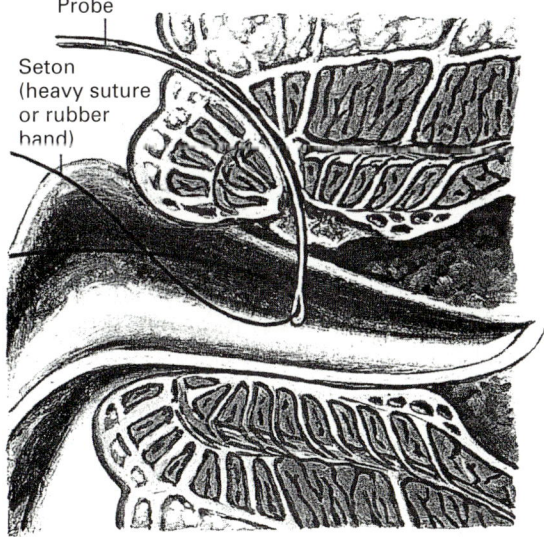
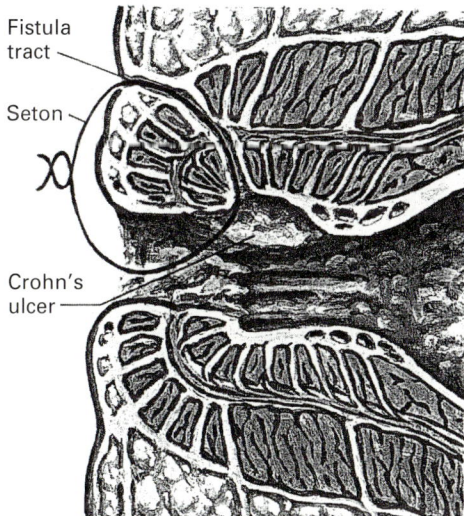
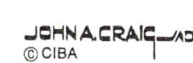

Fig. 97.2 Appearance and management of anorectal Crohn's disease. (From Kodner & Fry 1982, with permission)

an abscess/fistula is incision, and not excision, of the tissue. There is no place for anal fistulectomy in the patient with Crohn's disease who has the potential to maintain sphincter function. On the other hand, in the person with known Crohn's disease not all abscesses/fistulae of the perineum are attributable to the disease. Occasionally, a patient with a remote history of Crohn's disease will present with a cryptoglandular abscess/fistula which can be managed by a simple anal fistulotomy. It is still inappropriate to perform any procedure which could jeopardize the sphincter function.

Crohn's stricture

Patients with Crohn's disease involving the anus and lower rectum occasionally present with circumferential inflammation and scarring, resulting in stricture formation. These strictures are rarely symptomatic unless there is a perforation or an abscess associated with them. In these cases the stricture can be dilated. However, the primary management must involve treatment of the septic process, including drainage and perhaps subsequent reconstruction. Reconstruction becomes especially difficult in the patient with a stricture because the fibrotic nature of the stricture precludes mobilization of an endorectal flap. In our practice we occasionally dilate the anal stricture in patients with Crohn's disease. This is done initially in the operating room under anesthesia, and can subsequently be done at approximately 6-week intervals in the office. These patients often respond well to local applications of corticosteroids or 5-ASA compounds in suppository form. The stricture must be treated symptomatically until the Crohn's disease goes into remission, usually with advancing age. As long as the rectum is not totally destroyed, protectomy can usually be avoided.

Successful sphincter and rectal preservation

We evaluated 73 patients treated at Washington University Medical Center over a 10-year period for the type of surgical management of anal and perineal Crohn's disease and for success in preserving anorectal function. The site of intestinal disease in those patients who presented with anorectal complications is described in Table 97.4. There were 156 operations performed in these 73 patients, as indicated in Table 97.5. It can be seen that by using the conservative and often frequently repeated techniques with intensive medical treatment, the need for fecal diversion and the need for removal of the rectum was very low (Table 97.6). This study again showed that the need for fecal diversion and the need for removal of the rectum were based on the geographic location of the disease, with colonic and rectal involvement being the most powerful determinant of disease severity. In general, the more distal the intestinal disease the lower the chance of successful

Table 97.4 Site of intestinal Crohn's disease in patients treated by anorectal operations

Site of disease	No. of patients	(%)
Small intestine	7	6
Ileocolic	27	40
Colon	31	42
Small intestine and colon	7	6
Anus	1	1

Table 97.5 Anorectal operations in 73 patients with Crohn's disease

Operation	Procedures
Incision and drainage of perianal abscess	130
Anal fistulotomy	13
Placement of seton	6
Endorectal advancement flap	6
Primary closure of rectovaginal fistula	1
Total	156

Table 97.6 Results of treatment of anal and perianal Crohn's disease

	Number (%)
Healed after initial treatment	8 (11)
Healed after two or more procedures	30 (41)
Incomplete healing, condition acceptable	17 (23)
Healed after fecal diversion	9 (12)
Required protectomy	9 (12)

preservation of the rectum. Our figures were confirmed by those of Wolff at the Mayo Clinic, who in 1985 reported the probability of avoiding proctectomy for anal Crohn's disease to be 92% at 10 years and 83% at 20 years. It was concluded, from our series and others, that most patients with anal or perineal Crohn's disease respond to local treatment. In the few who required diversion, the disease improved after operation. Situations where local treatment or diversion failed were generally confined to patients with severe rectal and anal involvement. Under these circumstances proctectomy was performed, with radical excision of septic tracts and primary closure of the perineum.

MANAGEMENT OF RECTOVAGINAL AND COMPLICATED ANOPERINEAL FISTULAE IN CROHN'S DISEASE

Principles

Patients who develop rectovaginal, anovaginal, or complex anoperineal fistulae with Crohn's disease must be managed using special surgical considerations. The rectovaginal fistula in Crohn's disease is frequently anoperineal and extends into the low vagina or labia, and is related to severe activity of the disease within the anal canal. The other form of rectovaginal fistula involves ileal or colonic disease which extends into the upper vagina, usually the vaginal cuff, after hysterectomy has been performed in

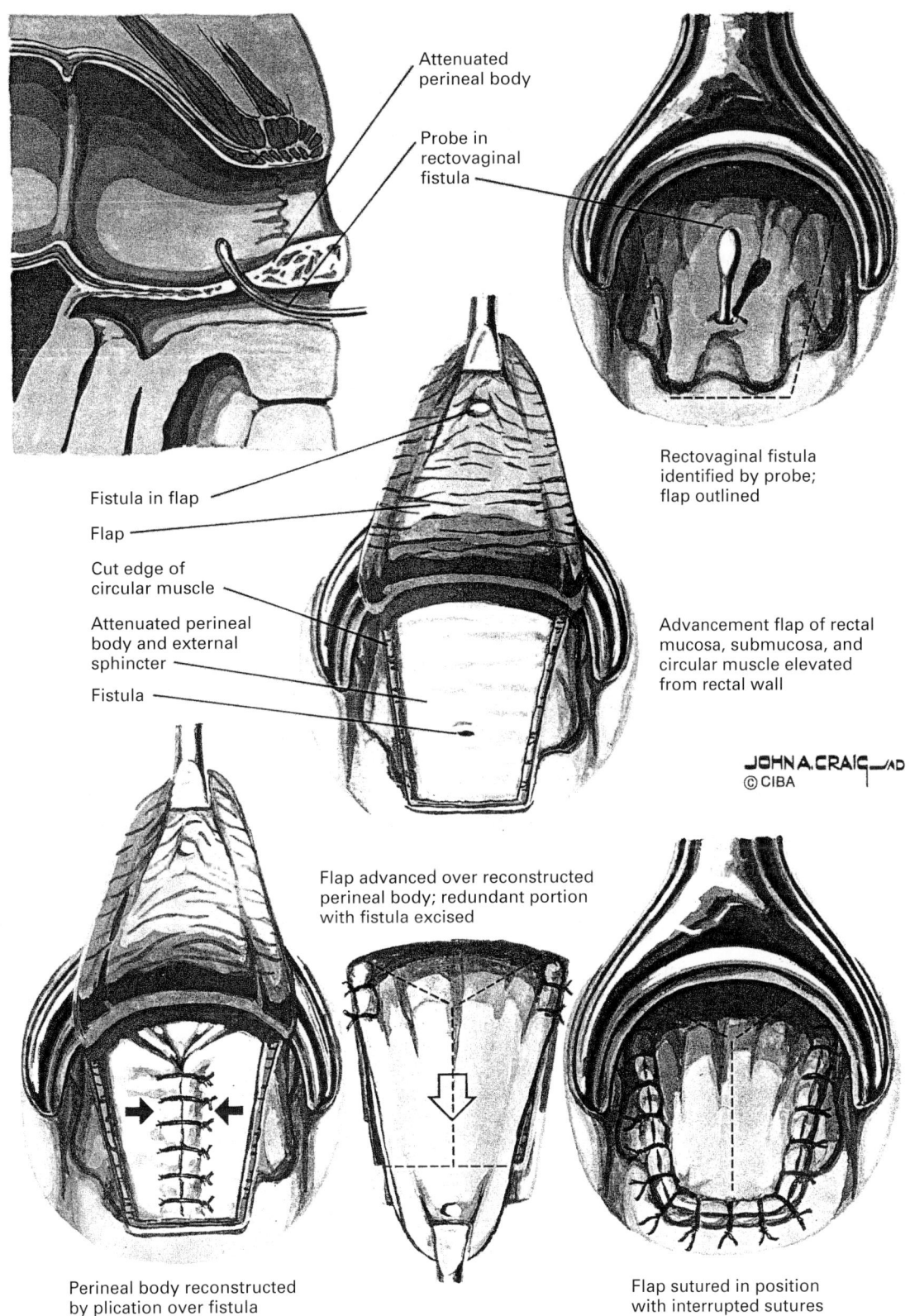

Fig. 97.3 Rectovaginal fistula repair. (From Fry & Kodner 1985, with permission)

Table 97.7 Techniques of advancement flap repair

Bowel preparation	Mechanical cleansing
	Antibiotics
Anesthesia	Spinal or epidural
Urinary catheter	
Position	Prone flexed
Local infiltration	0.5% Bupivacaine
	+
	1: 200 000 epinephrine

earlier years. These high vaginal fistulae from ileal or colonic Crohn's disease require resection of the diseased segment, usually with restoration of continuity and no special management of the vagina. The vagina will heal by itself once the active segment of Crohn's disease is removed. A low rectovaginal, anovaginal or anoperineal fistula due to Crohn's disease can be repaired once the abscess is drained and the Crohn's disease is in remission. The first step in management involves examining the patient under anesthesia and providing long-term chronic drainage of the septic process, as previously described, so that intensive medical management can be undertaken, the tissue returned to its normal state and, eventually, consideration given to dealing with the internal opening that resulted from the Crohn's ulcer. The management of these fistulae in previous years was frustrating because of the repair technique of perineorrhaphy. This surgical technique had a low success rate because of excessive tension on the repair and the apposition of multiple suture lines. Also, consideration was not given to protecting the rectal side of the repair which, because of going to high pressure, was most at risk for infiltration of fecal content into the repair. The results from our institution of advancement flap repair for complicated anal, rectovaginal and perineal fistulae were reported on 107 patients over a 10-year period (Fig. 97.3, Table 97.7). The advantages of the endorectal advancement flap are attributed to the prone-flexed position and preparation of the patient; to the approach from the rectal side; to better visualization, to there being no overlapping suture lines; and to avoidance of a diverting colostomy. We extended this technique of repair for rectovaginal fistulae to the complicated anal or low rectoperineal fistulae as well. These usually present as either a fistula in an anterior anatomic location or as a transsphincteric fistula high enough to place the sphincter muscle in jeopardy. We stressed the importance of the anatomic consideration for an anterior fistula, especially in a woman, because the sphincter mechanism contains only one loop of muscle, it is shorter and weaker than posterior sphincter and, if transected, will cause incontinence (Fig. 97.4). The anatomic location of the repaired fistulae is summarized in Table 97.8, and the results of management for these complicated fistulae by advancement flap repair are summarized in Table 97.9 ultimately with a 93% success rate. Specifically, the results of managing the patient with complicated fistulae secondary to

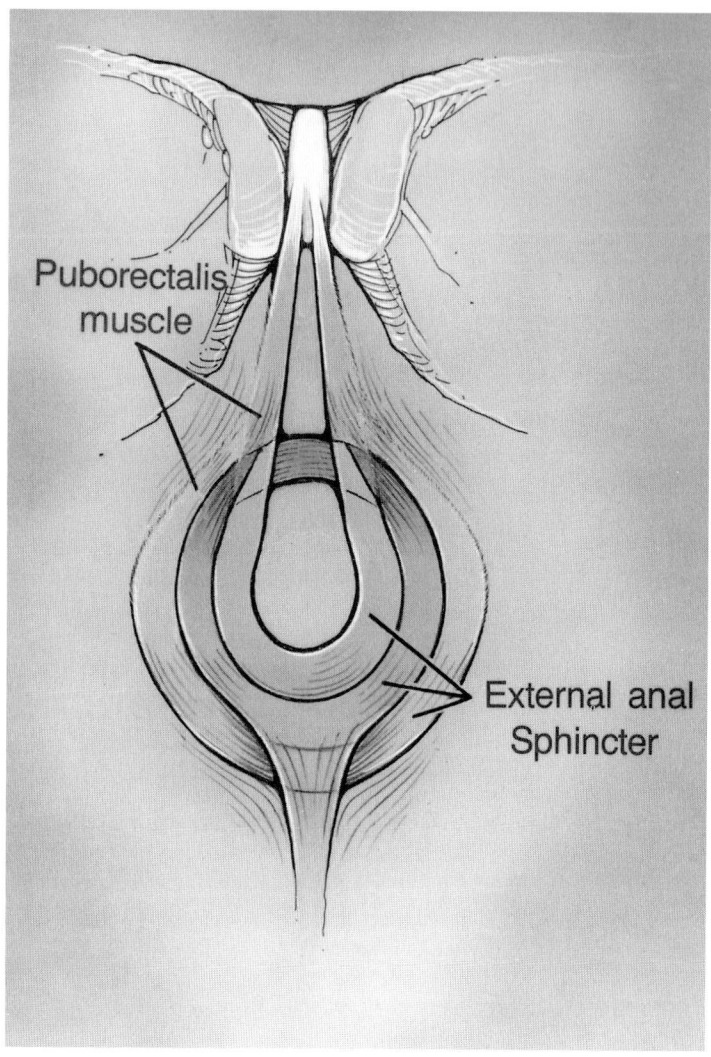

Fig. 97.4 The puborectalis muscle and external sphincter.

Table 97.8 Advancement flap repair of fistulae

Location of fistula	No. of patients
Low rectovaginal	71
Anterior anoperineal	28
Posterior anoperineal	8
Total	107

Table 97.9 Advancement flap repair of fistulae: results by etiology ($n=107$)

Etiology	Healed primarily	Healed after further treatment
Obstetrical injury	88% (42/48)	94% (45/48)
Cryptoglandular	87% (27/31)	92% (30/31)
Crohn's	71% (17/24)	92% (22/24)
Trauma (two post-sphincterotomy)	100% (4/4)	
Totals	84% (90/107)	93% (99/107)

Table 97.10 Crohn's disease: results of advancement flap repair of fistulas (*n*=24)

71% (17/24)	Healed after initial repair
92% (22/24)	Healed after more than one procedure
8% (2/24)	Had unhealed fistulae
Long-term results	
13% (3/24)	Lost anorectal function
	1 fecal diversion
	2 required proctectomy

Crohn's disease are summarized in Table 97.10; and with an advancement flap, satisfactory management is provided for the internal opening resulting from the Crohn's ulcer. This certainly does not indicate a cure of the Crohn's disease, but merely a technique which, coupled with intensive medical management, can preserve sphincter function and avoid proctectomy in many cases. We have been amazed occasionally to see that the patient who presents with severe anoperineal disease can be brought into remission and have the sepsis controlled, sometimes for months or years until a single internal opening remains, which can eventually be closed by the endorectal advancement technique.

When undertaking repair of these complicated fistulae, the surgeon must consider the following key points: Is the tissue normal? Does the sphincter function? Is systemic evaluation necessary? One must also always consider the presence of active inflammatory bowel disease or cancer. If there has been radiation to the pelvis, one must always completely rule out the possibility of cancer before embarking on any of these repairs.

MANAGEMENT OF FECAL INCONTINENCE IN THE PATIENT WITH CROHN'S DISEASE

Etiology of incontinence

The patient with Crohn's disease who presents with anal incontinence represents a very challenging management problem. The incontinence can be multifactorial, and all aspects must be considered in the evaluation of the patient before specific management is undertaken. The etiology of incontinence in Crohn's disease is summarized in Table 97.11. It is especially important to understand the biphasic nature of Crohn's disease and the fact that, in the chronic stage, when severe fibrosis of the rectum occurs and there is loss of reservoir function, the patient may have incapacitating diarrhea and incontinence based on the scarring deformity of the anus and rectum (Fig. 97.5). In this situation intensive medical management is

Table 97.11 Anal incontinence in Crohn's disease

Diffuse muscle destruction by anoperineal Crohn's
Distinct muscle injury from fistulotomy or childbirth
Fibrosis of muscle from chronic Crohn's
Loss of rectal capacity from fibrotic Crohn's
Diarrhea from colonic disease or short bowel syndrome

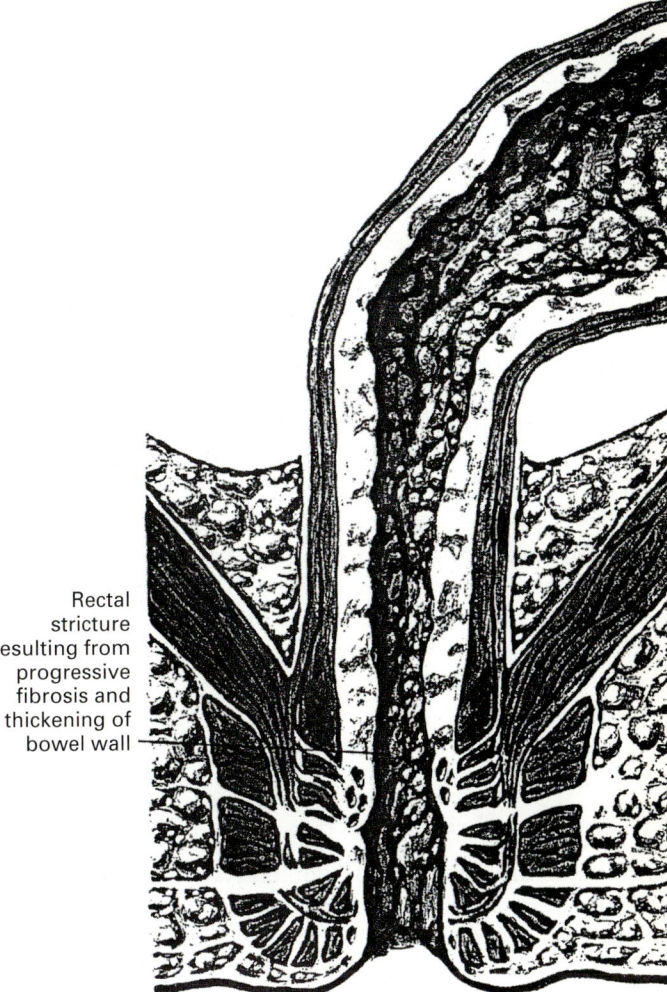

Rectal stricture resulting from progressive fibrosis and thickening of bowel wall

Fig. 97.5 Crohn's disease. (From Kodner & Fry 1982, with permission)

not effective. In fact, the patient may actually be placed in jeopardy by being treated with corticosteroids or immunosuppressive agents. These patients need at least fecal diversion and probably proctectomy, as the situation is incapacitating and irreversible. The same situation exists in the patient who presents with severe muscle destruction due to Crohn's disease. If the disease is limited to the low rectum and anus, with severe destruction and incontinence, this may represent one of the few cases where colostomy alone is used in treatment. These patients are usually significantly helped and returned to a normal lifestyle by the construction of a colostomy in the sigmoid or descending colon, which should be constructed using an ileostomy technique, in that the location should be chosen with extreme care and the stoma constructed with an everted nipple, in the anticipation of a higher output from the colon, which is potentially involved with the Crohn's disease. With the availability of sophisticated anal physiology laboratories in referral centers, the patient who presents with incontinence and Crohn's disease should be accurately evaluated with manometry, electromyography and transrectal ultrasound to define the nature of the incontinence. We have found that ultrasound helps to accurately define the nature of these defects or destruction. We caution the surgeon against embarking on sphincter reconstruction in a patient who has had injury to the pudendal nerves supplying the anus.

In our series of patients with Crohn's disease treated surgically for anal incontinence, we have found a subset where there has been a distinct muscle injury from fistulotomy or episiotomy which can be repaired once the Crohn's disease is in remission. These are difficult clinical situations because the diarrhea of the Crohn's disease stresses the capacity of the injured sphincter mechanism. It should be noted that in patients with Crohn's disease and severe muscle destruction, our tendency has been to construct a diverting stoma before undertaking the sphincter repair. We have not hesitated to create endorectal advancement flaps for fistulous disease, but have been hesitant in the Crohn's patients to undertake extensive reconstruction without diversion.

MANAGEMENT OF SEVERE ANOPERINEAL DESTRUCTION DUE TO CROHN'S DISEASE

Diversion and reconstruction

As previously described, the patient who has severe destruction of the anus and perineum requires fecal diversion, usually by colostomy, or by colectomy and ileostomy. Construction of an ileostomy, allowing the colon to remain in place, does not provide adequate relief for the patient with a severely destroyed anus or perineum: the presence of the colon and its secretions does not give enough protection for disease resolution to proceed sufficiently to allow eventual anal sphincter reconstruction. It is only the rare patient who has severe anal perineal destruction from Crohn's disease who can eventually be returned to normal function, even with diversion and subsequent reconstruction. However, in a population involving young adults who wish to be spared the change in body image caused by a permanent stoma, it is sometimes a useful undertaking. We should stress that the surgical, and often the medical, management of patients with Crohn's disease of the anus and perineum should be directed to centers where these problems are seen frequently. These patients require long-term, detailed, conservative, and often tedious and frustrating management, which should not be undertaken by someone unfamiliar with the physical, emotional, medical and surgical implications of dealing with such patients.

Resection: radical

Although everything previously described has been aimed at the preservation of anorectal function, if this battle is lost and the rectum must be removed, the treatment of the disease in the perineum should be radical. Although the dissection of the rectum itself should be limited to the rectal wall, in order to preserve normal neurologic and sexual function, the treatment of the perineal disease should include debridement and opening of all of the infected tracts. Our practice has been to close the levator muscle, preserving as much of the external sphincter and puborectalis as possible, and then to carry out the radical debridement of the perineum. Sometimes this is so extensive that it requires the use of vascularized muscle flaps to fill the defect. The surgeon should never hesitate to perform a staged resection of the rectum if there is severe destructive disease.

Prevention and treatment of unhealed perineal wound

Although the postoperative complication of unhealed perineal wound and perineal sinus from Crohn's disease remains unsolved, the author's suspicion is that this results from retained rectal mucosa from the time of proctectomy, especially in the patient who has active fistula tracts or severe inflammation of the rectum. Therefore, the author's preference, in most cases, is to carry out a Hartmann resection of the rectosigmoid (or total colec-

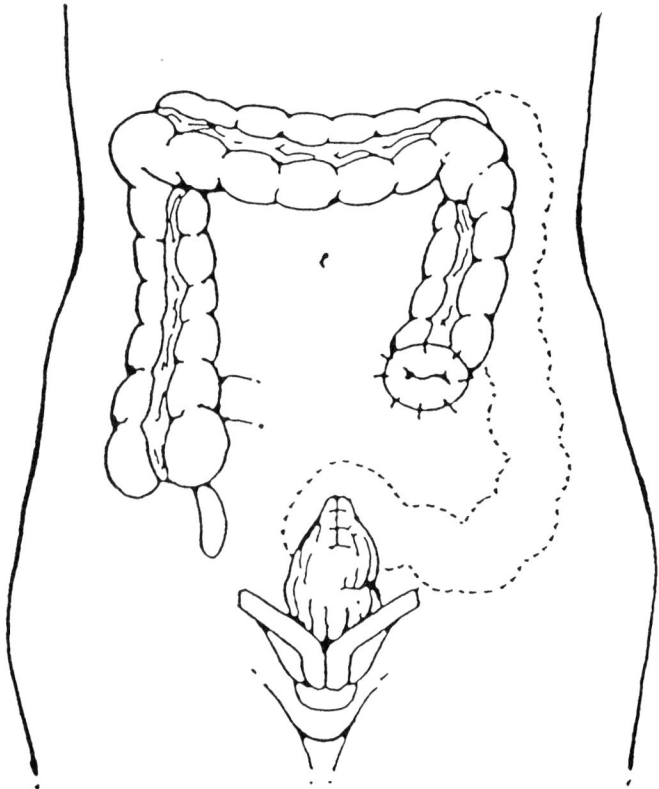

Fig. 97.6 Hartmann resection. (From Kodner & Fry 1993, with permission)

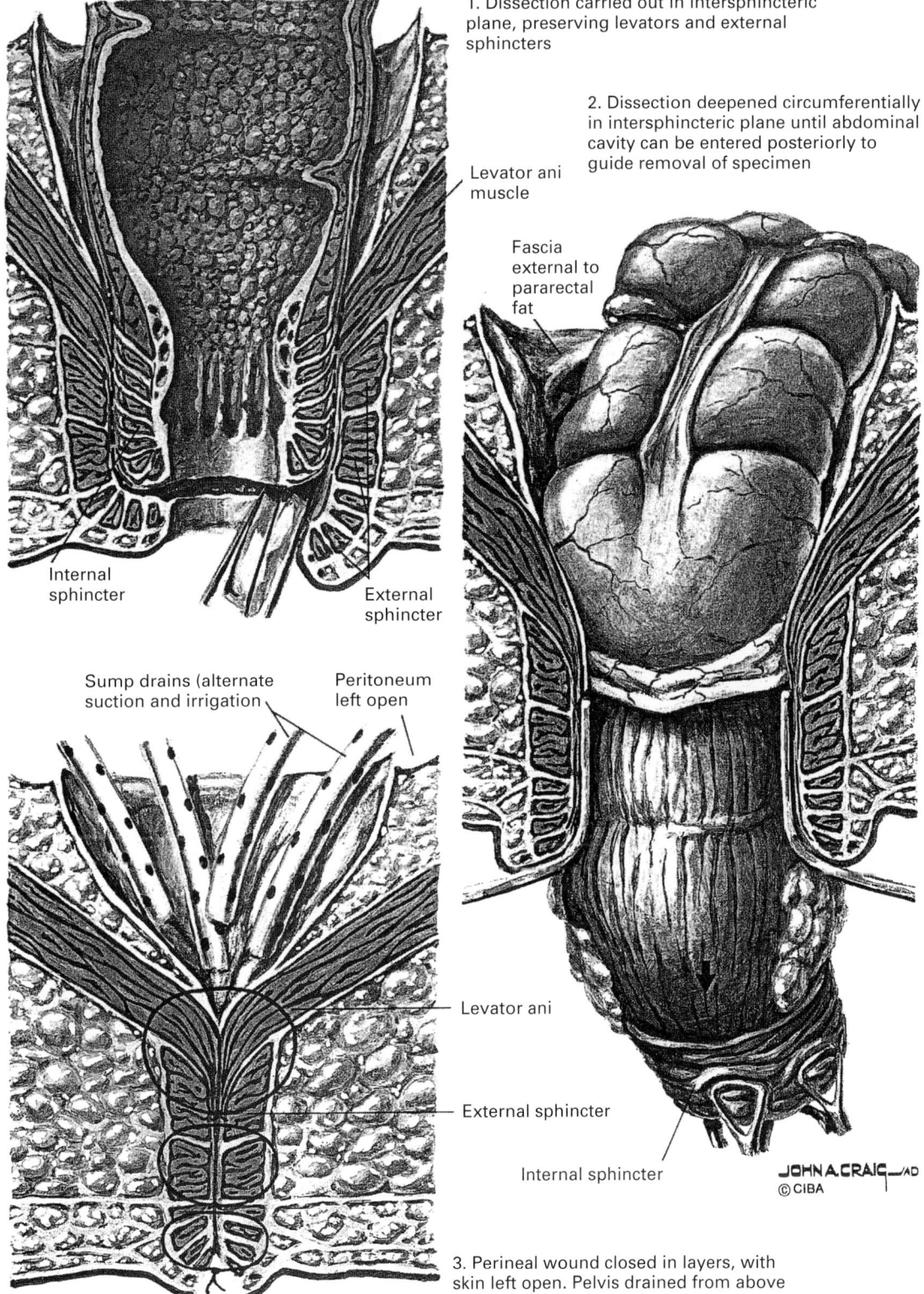

Fig. 97.7 Surgical removal of the rectum: perineal phase. (From Kodner & Fry 1982, with permission)

Table 97.12 Treatment of persistent perineal sinus

Total excision of wound
Repair of fistulae (example: perineal–vesical)
Primary reconstruction
   Skin graft
   Z-plasty

tomy with ileostomy) as illustrated in Fig. 97.6, and then return at a later date for delayed proctectomy. At that time the resection should be limited to the rectum, preserving the levators and external sphincters. The peritoneum and skin should be left open, drainage should be from above, and the remaining Crohn's disease should be totally excised (Fig. 97.7).

The treatment of the persistent perineal sinus is summarized in Table 97.12. Because of the possibility of retained secreting rectal mucosa, we stress again that all of the perineal wound must be completely excised and the reconstruction be undertaken with either split-thickness or Z-plasty reconstruction. Our own preference is to do this in collaboration with the plastic surgery service, to be sure of the best chance for the reconstruction of the perineum.

In summary, this specific aspect of Crohn's disease is very tedious and difficult to manage, but results in enormous gratification when normal anoperineal function can be preserved in a group of young adults with a long and productive life expectancy.

REFERENCES AND FURTHER READING

Allan A, Keighley M R B 1988 Management of perianal Crohn's disease. World Journal of Surgery 12: 198–202

Fleshman J W, Kodner I J, Fry R D, Birnbaum E H. Anal incontinence. In: Zuidema G (ed) Shackleford's surgery of the alimentary tract, 4th edn. W B Saunders, Philadelphia 1995

Fry R D, Kodner I J 1985 Anorectal disorders. Ciba Clinical Symposia 37: 1–32

Fry R D, Kodner I J 1989 Management of anal and perineal Crohn's disease. Infections in Surgery 8: 209–220

Fry R D, Shemesh E I, Kodner I J, Timmcke A 1989 Techniques and results in the management of anal and perianal Crohn's disease. Surgery, Gynecology and Obstetrics 168: 42–48

Goldman C D, Kodner I J, Fry R D, MacDermott R P 1986 Clinical and operative experience with non-caucasian patients with Crohn's disease. Diseases of the Colon and Rectum 29: 317–321

Gray B K, Lockhart-Mummery H E, Morson B C 1965 Crohn's disease of the anal region. Gut 6: 515–524

Kodner I J, Fry R D 1982 Inflammatory bowel disease. Ciba Clinical Symposia 34: 1–32

Kodner I J, Fry R D, Fleshman J W 1992 Surgical management of Crohn's. In: Inflammatory bowel disease: current topics in gastroenterology. Elsevier Science, New York, pp 615–642

Kodner I J, Fry R D, Fleshman J W, Birnbaum E H 1993 Colon, rectum and anus. In: Schwartz S I (ed) Principles of surgery, 6th edn. McGraw-Hill, New York, p 1282

Kodner I J, Mazor A, Shemesh E I, Fry R D, Fleshman J W, Birnbaum E H 1993 Endorectal advancement flap repair of rectovaginal and other complicated anorectal fistulas. Surgery 114: 682–690

Williams J G, Rothenberger D A, Nemer F D, Goldberg S M 1991 Fistula-in-ano in Crohn's disease: results of aggressive surgical treatment. Diseases of the Colon and Rectum 34: 378–384

Williams D R, Collier J A, Corman M L, Nugent F W, Veidenheimer M C 1981 Anal complications in Crohn's diseases. Diseases of the Colon and Rectum 24: 22–24

Wolff B G, Culp C E, Beart R W Jr, Ilstrup D M, Ready R L 1985 Anorectal Crohn's disease: a long-term perspective. Diseases of the Colon and Rectum 28: 709–711

98. Perianal Crohn's disease: rectovaginal fistula

T. L. Hull

Discharge of stool or gas from the vagina signals an abnormal internal opening between the rectum or anus and the vagina. This tract is termed a rectovaginal or anovaginal fistula. Symptoms may be tolerable for some women, but incapacitating for others. Crohn's disease, presumably owing to its transmural inflammation, can lead to anovaginal or rectovaginal fistula.

CLASSIFICATION

Most fistulae are really anovaginal because the internal opening is located in the anal canal. The anal opening may be associated with a deep anterior ulcer. Anovaginal fistulae from a cryptoglandular source are rare, but do occur.

Rectovaginal fistulae have their internal opening above the anorectal ring. They are usually associated with deep ulceration in the rectum and severe proctitis.

One additional type of fistula occurs in some women, particularly after a hysterectomy. Diseased ileum or sigmoid colon, can form a fistula into the vagina, resulting in an enterovaginal fistula. The vaginal opening is located in the upper third of the vagina.

CLINICAL PRESENTATION

Symptoms from these fistulae vary. Up to two-thirds of afflicted women may not be aware of their symptoms because of more severe intestinal symptoms or anorectal suppuration (Richie & Lennard-Jones 1976). There may be passage of frank stool or flatus from the vagina, or drainage of purulent foul-smelling liquid. Some women experience dyspareunia, perineal pain, difficulty with hygiene, or yeast infections. Diarrhea may exacerbate the symptoms.

ASSESSMENT

Treatment depends on multiple factors that must be evaluated by history and physical examination to plan the best treatment for the patient. The degree of distress due to the symptoms must initially be assessed. For example, fistulae with minimal symptoms need no treatment. The extent of other disease in the gastrointestinal tract should be determined, particularly the degree of proctitis and associated anal disease, such as strictures. Sphincter tone should be noted as this may influence the treatment. Women should be aware that any treatment does not 'cure' the Crohn's disease but rather that the aim is to control the symptoms.

TREATMENT: PRINCIPLES

All treatments start with adequate drainage of sepsis. Insertion of a seton and/or mushroom drain is usually adequate and provides pain relief. Some women with minimal symptoms may find an increase in stool and/or flatus through the vagina after drain insertion, and should be forewarned. If symptoms are minimal, drainage of the sepsis may be the only treatment needed and the drains can remain in situ indefinitely.

Medical therapy consists of steroids, sulfasalazine (and other 5-ASA) compounds, metronidazole and immunosuppressives. This treatment option is covered elsewhere.

Resection

When the fistula is the result of proximal disease penetrating into the upper vagina, the extent of the disease must first be assessed. If there is ileal disease only and the colon and rectum are normal, resection of the diseased ileum with closure (if possible from the abdominal side) of the vaginal defect is carried out. A pedicle of omentum is placed between the vaginal repair and the resected bowel. When diseased colon (usually sigmoid) is the culprit, with impaired sphincter muscles, segmental resection is sometimes entertained if the remainder of the colon and rectum are normal. If the remainder of the colon is diseased, a subtotal colectomy with an ileorectal anastomosis is an attractive option, provided the sphincter muscles are adequate. If there is associated rectal and colonic disease proctocolectomy should be considered.

Diversion

The fecal stream may be diverted with an ileostomy or colostomy in patients with symptomatic fistulae, especially if there is proximal disease that must be addressed in the small bowel. Usually an ileostomy is preferable, because there may be colonic involvement. With diversion alone the chance that the fistula will resolve is almost zero, so women must be aware that other surgical treatment will be needed to obtain healing (Grant et al 1986) For some women, when a stoma is inevitable this provides an adjustment period before any bridges have been burned.

Proctocolectomy

Proctocolectomy was advocated by Goligher (1975) as the gold standard of treatment for Crohn's-related rectovaginal fistula with significant proctitis or colitis. If there is perineal sepsis or severe proctitis, a colectomy with preservation of the rectum and an ileostomy may be performed initially because perineal wound healing may be affected by the sepsis and inflammation (Ward et al 1982). A completion proctectomy can be done at a later date. At the Cleveland Clinic we perform an intersphincteric proctectomy (Turnbull & Fazio 1975). The internal sphincter is excised and the external sphincter, levator muscles and puborectalis are retained. The levators are closed from the abdominal side and from the perineal aspect. The vaginal defect is cored out and closed with absorbable sutures. If a proctectomy is performed when there is active sepsis in the perineal area, all fistula tracts must be excised and the skin edges left open. When the levators are sutured closed a shallow wound may form, but this usually heals within 6–9 months. If the wound does not close, re-excision and closure or application of a split-thickness skin graft is considered.

Closure of the fistula can be accomplished in several ways. An episioproctotomy entails opening all the tissue superior to the fistula tract, then closing the layers (similar to obstetrical repair of a fourth-degree perineal laceration). This approach is attractive if not much muscle need be divided during the procedure, or if repair of a previous obstetric injury needs to be addressed.

Advancement flap

Perhaps the most popular repair is a sliding advancement flap (Jones et al 1987), but this should only be considered if there is no rectal disease and only minimal anal canal disease. Although this repair can be approached either transvaginally or transanally, we at the Cleveland Clinic agree with Greenwald and Hoexter (1978) and prefer the transanal approach, because it addresses the problem from the area of high pressure, the anal canal. A flap of mucosa, submucosa and a few circular muscle fibers is elevated in curvilinear fashion for several centimeters. The fistula tract is cored out and closed in layers, leaving the vaginal mucosa open for drainage. The distal end of the flap, where the fistula tract penetrated into the anal canal, is trimmed and the flap is advanced over the repaired defect and closed. For patients with failed repairs or a mild anal stricture, a sleeve advancement flap should be considered. The layers of the flap and the handling of the fistula tract are the same as for the curvilinear flap, but the circumference of the flap is greater (90–100%). With a previously failed flap, or if the surgeon is not satisfied with the technical conduct of the operation (with either type of repair), a temporary stoma should be considered. Our results at the Cleveland Clinic with all types of advancement flaps for Crohn's-related anovaginal and rectovaginal fistulae showed that 24 out of 35 had healing of their fistula (Hull & Fazio, unpublished data).

In conclusion, surgical treatment for anovaginal and rectovaginal fistula in Crohn's disease must be planned according to the degree of symptoms and the presence of associated Crohn's disease elsewhere in the gastrointestinal tract.

REFERENCES

Goligher J C 1975 Rectovaginal fistula and irradiation proctitis and enteritis: In: Surgery of the anus, colon, and rectum, 3rd edn. Charles C. Thomas, Springfield, Illinois, pp 205–255

Grant D R, Cohen Z, McLeod R S 1986 Loop ileostomy for anorectal Crohn's disease. Canadian Journal of Surgery 29: 32–35

Greenwald J C, Hoexter B 1978 Repair of rectovaginal fistulas. Surgery, Gynecology and Obstetrics 146: 443–445

Jones I T, Fazio V W, Jagelman D G 1987 The use of transanal rectal advancement flap in the management of fistulas involving the anorectum. Diseases of the Colon and Rectum 30: 919–923

Ritchie J K, Lennard-Jones J E 1976 Crohn's disease of the distal large bowel. Scandinavian Journal of Gastroenterology 11: 433–436

Turnbull R B, Fazio V 1975 Advances in the surgical technique of ulcerative colitis surgery: endoanal proctectomy and two-directional myotomy ileostomy. Surgery Annual 7: 315–329

Ward M W N, Morgan B G, Clark C G 1982 Treatment of persistent perineal sinus with vaginal fistula following proctocolectomy for Crohn's disease: a long-term perspective. Diseases of the Colon and Rectum 28: 709–711

> SECTION 12

Management of surgical complications in inflammatory bowel disease

99. Percutaneous drainage of Crohn's abscesses

E. Lee   R. Bleday

Percutaneous drainage under computed tomography (CT) or ultrasound guidance is an established method of treatment for intra-abdominal abscesses (Haaga 1990, Hemming et al 1991, Lambiase et al 1992, McLean et al 1993). As interventional radiologists and surgeons become more experienced with this technology, limitations to the percutaneous drainage of complicated abscesses have gradually decreased. Now even multiloculated abscesses, abscesses with fistulae, or multiple abscesses can be approached with percutaneous catheter drainage. Depending on the location and etiology of intra-abdominal or retroperitoneal abscesses, percutaneous drainage can be a curative procedure or, more often, a temporizing measure of controlling infection.

Patients with inflammatory bowel disease, especially Crohn's disease, have an increased risk for abscess formation: up to one-quarter of patients with Crohn's disease present with abdominal abscesses at some point in their life (Biller et al 1987, Cybulsky & Tam 1990, Ribeiro et al 1991). Furthermore, abscesses can develop after bowel surgery owing to anastomotic leakage or inability to clear intra-abdominal contaminations (Casola et al 1987, Lambiase et al 1992, Lango et al 1993). Surgery for intra-abdominal abscesses in patients with inflammatory bowel disease has many potential problems, since these patients are steroid dependent, nutritionally depleted and immunocompromised. Because of the complexity of abscesses associated with inflammatory bowel disease, there has been some reluctance to drain them percutaneously. However, with improvements in imaging and interventional skills, percutaneous drainage has become the procedure of choice in selected patients. When patients are clinically stable, percutaneous catheter drainage can be useful as a temporizing procedure before definitive resection of inflamed bowel, and can often change a two-stage procedure with an initial resection and stoma to a one-stage procedure with definitive resection or anastomosis. Percutaneous drainage can also be used as a therapeutic maneuver in patients who develop abscesses postoperatively.

This chapter will discuss two different clinical settings in which intra-abdominal abscesses are frequently encountered in patients with inflammatory bowel disease: patients with Crohn's disease who present with intra-abdominal abscess de novo and patients with inflammatory bowel disease whose postoperative course is complicated by an intra-abdominal abscess.

CROHN'S DISEASE

More than half of all patients affected by Crohn's disease will need to have at least one surgical intervention in their lifetime (Summers et al 1979). The three most common indications for surgery are intestinal obstruction, septic complications and the failure of medical management. The presence of an inflammatory phlegmon or abscess is often a marker of severe disease. These complications are unlikely to respond to medical therapy and are therefore an indication for surgical treatment.

On presentation the signs and symptoms of intra-abdominal abscess are difficult to distinguish from an exacerbation of the disease. Steroid therapy may mask the signs of sepsis and inflammation. An abdominal mass may be either a phlegmon or an abscess. A phlegmon, without an abscess, is due to inflammatory edema of the acutely affected intestinal segment and surrounding tissues. An abscess is the result of a walled-off perforation. The mechanism of abscess formation can be considered as an extension of transmural fissuring through the serosa. Generalized peritonitis is prevented by adhesions that form between loops of bowel as a result of serosal inflammation. The CT scan has become a valuable test to validate clinical suspicion and distinguish between a phlegmon and an abscess (Jabra et al 1991, Shokouh-Amiri et al 1989).

After an abscess has been documented, the physician needs to decide on the best treatment option. Antibiotics need to be started but successful treatment of an intra-abdominal abscess depends on providing adequate drainage. The two treatment options are percutaneous drainage or operative drainage. Even though there have not been controlled prospective randomized trials, the percutaneous approach seems to offer a number of advantages. Many of these poor surgical risk patients are immunocompromised and malnourished, and delaying the stress of general anesthesia and exploratory laparotomy gives time for restoration of a positive nitrogen balance with total parenteral nutrition (TPN). Percutaneous drainage, intravenous antibiotics and TPN allow for control of the infection, which may also permit a one-stage procedure with resection and anastomosis of the diseased bowel in a non-infected field, instead of a two-stage procedure with resection and stoma followed in a delayed fashion by a takedown of the stoma.

The published results of percutaneous drainage of intra-abdominal abscesses have recorded the results of the different causes of intra-abdominal abscess and have reported varying degrees of success. Good results are recorded in patients who present with diverticulitis, in whom the disease has progressed to a pericolic or pelvic abscess. The current standard of care is CT or ultrasound-guided percutaneous drainage of the abscess, followed in 5–10 days by operation (Ambrosetti et al 1992, Hemming et al 1991, Stabile et al 1990). With percutaneous drainage, a catheter is connected to passive drainage until drainage ceases and the pain and fever resolve. With this method of treatment the patient can undergo elective resection of the diseased bowel, thus obviating the need for colostomy and multiple-stage surgery. This treatment plan of preoperative drainage followed by resection and primary anastomosis can be completed in about 75% of patients presenting with large diverticular abscesses (Stabile et al 1990).

Because the pathophysiology of Crohn's disease is different from that of diverticular abscess, there has been some scepticism about the prospects of success of percutaneous drainage of intra-abdominal abscesses as the primary treatment in patients with Crohn's disease (Greenstein et al 1987, Ribeiro et al 1991). Transmural inflammation with bowel perforation is commonly associated with downstream bowel stricture or stenosis which makes percutaneous drainage more difficult (Fig. 99.1). Patients often have multiple and interloop abscesses that are not easily accessible to percutaneous drainage. However, if patients are selected carefully, percutaneous drainage can be used to advantage in seriously ill patients as a temporary measure that may delay and facilitate subsequent surgical intervention (Fig. 99.2).

Although there are many reports of percutaneous abscess drainage the total number of patients in any particular category of abscess is small (Casola et al 1987, Doemeny et al 1988, Flancbaum et al 1990, Lambiase et al 1988, Moss 1989, Safuit et al 1987).

In most of these series clinical assessment and inclusion criteria are not clearly defined and there is little or no

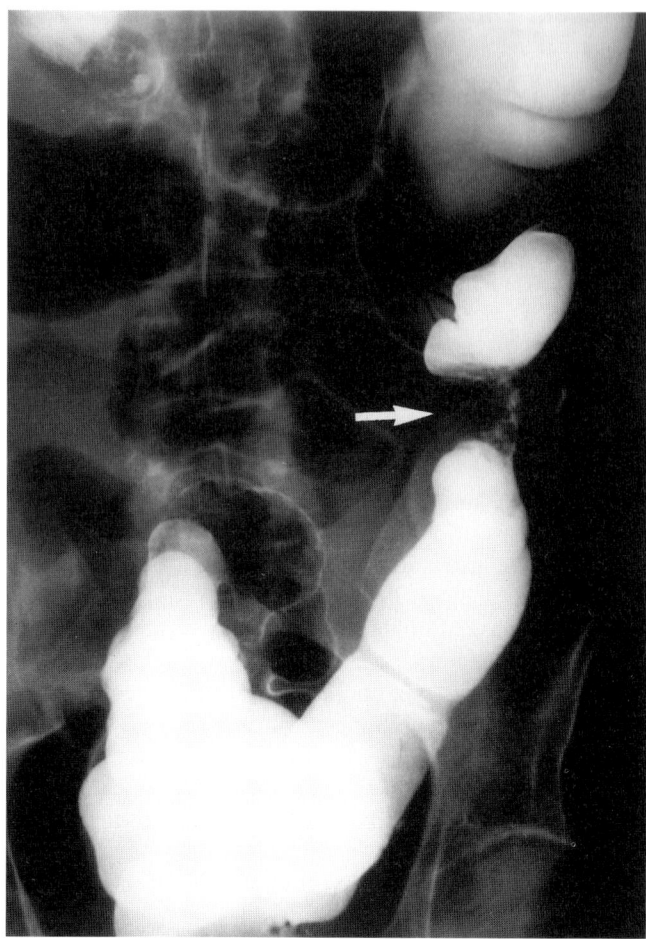

Fig. 99.1 Air contrast barium enema showing a Crohn's stricture with extraluminal barium lateral to the colon. The patient had a walled-off perforation from the proximal sigmoid along with an associated abscess.

clinical follow-up. Therefore, it is difficult to form firm conclusions from anecdotal, retrospective case reports on the treatment of abscesses in patients with Crohn's disease. However, from the retrospective evidence several common guidelines can be formulated.

When a patient with Crohn's disease is admitted with possible spontaneous intra-abdominal abscess, a CT scan of the abdomen and pelvis with double contrast (intravenous and gastrointestinal) should be performed without delay (Fig. 99.2). If the patient is hemodynamically stable, and the abscess appears to be amenable to percutaneous drainage, it should be drained under CT guidance with the placement of a large (12–14 Fr) percutaneous catheter. However, if the patient is septic or shows signs of generalized peritonitis then, after rapid resuscitation, they should be taken to the operating room from open drainage of the abscess (Fig. 99.3).

Once the percutaneous catheter is in place it should be irrigated with 10–20 ml of normal saline two to three times per day to keep it patent. The drainage output is recorded every 8 hours. Should the patient become

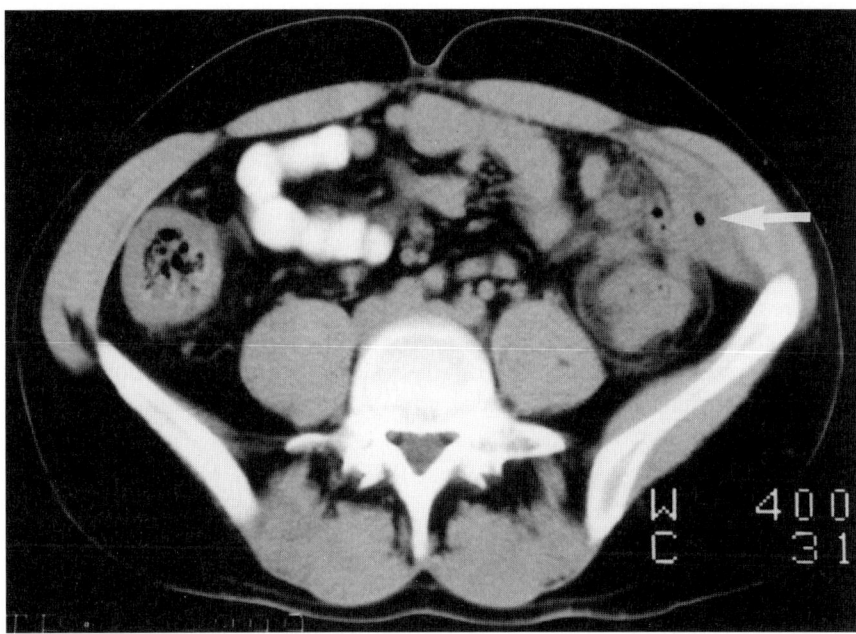

Fig. 99.2 Extraluminal fluid and air is seen between the abdominal wall and the colon. The abscess correlated with the barium enema findings, which showed a walled-off perforation from the proximal sigmoid that tracked both superiorly and inferiorly along the left gutter. The patient was treated with percutaneous drainage, which then led to a colocutaneous fistula. After a period of percutaneous drainage, intravenous antibiotics and bowel rest with total parenteral nutrition, the patient underwent a one-stage segmental resection of this diseased area of bowel. Both the rectum and proximal bowel had little or no inflammatory changes.

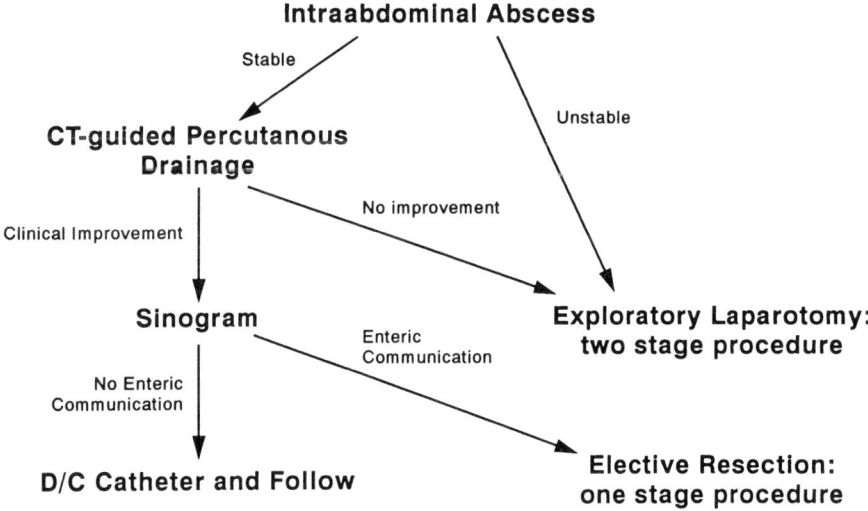

Fig. 99.3 Algorithm for the treatment of intra-abdominal abscesses in patients with Crohn's disease. Exploratory laparotomy should be performed in unstable patients or patients who remain septic even with percutaneous drainage. Stable patients and those who improve with drainage should then have a follow-up sinogram to determine enteric communication. Treatment is then dependent upon the sinogram results (surgery vs. conservative treatment).

clinically worse at any point during this conservative treatment period, they should be taken to the operating room for open drainage. If the patient continues to improve, a sinogram via the catheter can be obtained within a week to investigate the size, extension and possible enteric communication of the abscess cavity. Subsequent sinograms are obtained as needed, especially if the output increases.

If an abscess has an enteric communication, complete resolution without bowel resection is unlikely (Fig. 99.3).

Lambiase et al reported nine patients with intra-abdominal abscesses in Crohn's disease who were treated initially with percutaneous drainage, six of whom developed a fistula to the skin and all six had to undergo bowel resection (Lambiase et al 1988). However, because of the preoperative percutaneous drainage, all six could have resection of involved bowel with primary anastomosis. In the remaining three patients, there was no intestinal communication and they had percutaneous drainage only. Complete resolution of enteric fistulae with percutaneous drainage alone is unlikely. Therefore, if a sinogram reveals an enteric communication elective surgical resection of the involved bowel should be planned, after resolution of the sepsis and conversion from a catabolic to an anabolic state. However, if a sinogram does not reveal enteric communication and the drainage is minimal, the catheter can be removed and the patient followed closely for possible recurrence. (Fig. 99.3).

POSTOPERATIVE COMPLICATIONS

The development of a postoperative intra-abdominal abscess is a potentially life-threatening complication. Inadequate drainage of an abscess has been said to lead to a mortality of 40–50% (Longo et al 1993, McLean et al 1993). Postoperative abscess is most often a result of an anastomotic leak, but a significant minority are due to contamination during surgery, inadequate hemostasis or ischemia. Since patients with inflammatory bowel disease are often immunocompromised they have an increased risk for this complication. CT-guided drainage of postoperative intra-abdominal abscess has been offered as an alternative to open surgical drainage, with lower morbidity and mortality rates (Haaga 1990). The success of percutaneous drainage depends on the cause and location of the abscess. Many postoperative abscesses are amenable to percutaneous drainage and the rate of cure is higher than that with spontaneous transmural abscess. If anastomotic dehiscence is the cause of the abscess then the patient should be ultimately managed surgically. However, initial localization of the abscess should be achieved by either CT or ultrasound. If the abscess is amenable to percutaneous drainage, it should be attempted since sometimes this will treat the abscess successfully and occasionally even obviate the need for surgical drainage.

Unlike spontaneous abscesses, in Crohn's disease, most postoperative abscesses do not communicate with the intestine. Doemeny et al reviewed nine patients with intra-abdominal abscesses drained percutaneously, of whom seven had had postoperative complications (Doemeny et al 1988). Six of these seven resolved completely with percutaneous drainage only, whereas both patients with spontaneously formed abscesses had to undergo a single-stage bowel resection. All the abscesses with enteric communication needed subsequent bowel resection, but the simple abscesses were cured with percutaneous drainage. Many of the reported postoperative abscesses were located away from bowel, i.e. perihepatic. Therefore, depending on the etiology of postoperative abscesses, results are similar to the ones found in non-inflammatory bowel disease patients.

As can be seen from Figure 99.3, the likelihood of cure from the drainage is very high in this subgroup, since the majority of abscesses do not communicate with the bowel.

CONCLUSION

Percutaneous abscess drainage has now become the procedure of choice in inflammatory bowel disease patients with intra-abdominal abscess. Percutaneous drainage procedures are usually temporary, as most abscesses have enteric communication. However, even in these cases temporary palliation by percutaneous drainage can delay an operation on high-risk, underresuscitated patients.

In abscesses without bowel communication, percutaneous drainage can be used as a therapeutic procedure. Many abscesses that form postoperatively do not have enteric communications, as many occur as a result of intraoperative contamination. Therefore, if a patient with an intra-abdominal abscess is hemodynamically stable and the abscess is amenable to percutaneous drainage, then CT-guided drainage should be attempted with the expectation of avoiding exploratory laparotomy.

REFERENCES

Ambrosetti P, Robert J, Witzig J A et al 1992 Incidence, outcome, and proposed management of isolated abscesses complicating acute left-sided colonic diverticulitis. Diseases of the Colon and Rectum 35: 1072–1076

Biller J A, Grand R J, Harris B H 1987 Abdominal abscesses in adolescents with Crohn's disease. Journal of Pediatric Surgery 22: 873–876

Casola G, van Sonnenberg E, Neff C C, Saba R M, Withers C, Emarine C W 1987 Abscesses in Crohn's disease: percutaneous drainage. Radiology 163: 19–22

Cybulsky I J, Tam P 1990 Intra-abdominal abscesses in Crohn's disease. American Surgeon 56: 678–682

Doemeny J M, Burke Dr, Meranze S G 1988 Percutaneous drainage of abscesses in patients with Crohn's disease. Gastrointestinal Radiology 13: 237–241

Flancbaum L, Nosher J L, Brolin R E 1990 Percutaneous catheter drainage of abdominal abscesses associated with perforated viscus. American Surgeon 56: 52–56

Greenstein A J, Sachar D B, Mann D, Lachman P, Heimann T, Aufses A H 1987 Spontaneous free perforation and perforated abscess in 30 patients with Crohn's disease. Annals of Surgery 205: 72–76

Haaga J R 1990 Imaging intra-abdominal abscesses and nonoperative drainage procedures. World Journal of Surgery 14: 204–209

Hemming A, Davis N L, Robins R E 1991 Surgical versus percutaneous drainage of intra-abdominal abscesses. American Journal of Surgery 161: 593–595

Jabra A A, Fishman E K, Taylor G A 1991 Crohn's disease in the pediatric patient: CT evaluation. Radiology 179: 495–498

Lambiase R E, Cronan J J, Dorfman G S, Paolella L P, Haas R A 1988 Percutaneous drainage of abscesses in patients with Crohn's disease. American Journal of Radiology 150: 1043–1045

Lambiase R E, Deyoe L, Cronan J J, Dorfman G S 1992 Percutaneous drainage of 335 consecutive abscesses: results of primary drainage with 1-year follow-up. Radiology 184: 167–179

Longo W E, Milsom J W, Lavery I C, Church J C, Oakley J R, Fazio V W 1993. Pelvic abscess after colon and rectal surgery – what is optimal management? Diseases of the Colon and Rectum 36: 936–941

McLean T R, Simmons K, Svensson L G 1993 Management of postoperative intra-abdominal abscesses by routine percutaneous drainage. Surgery, Gynecology and Obstetrics 176: 167–177

Moss A A 1989 Critical review: percutaneous drainage of abscesses in patients with Crohn's disease. Investigative Radiology 24: 334–336

Ribeiro M B, Greenstein A J, Yamazaki Y, Aufses A H 1991 Intra-abdominal abscess in regional enteritis. Annals of Surgery 21: 32–36

Safrit H D, Mauro M A, Jaques P F 1987 Percutaneous abscess drainage in Crohn's disease. American Journal of Radiology 148: 859–862

Shokouh-Amiri M H, Hansen C P, Moesgaard F, Bulow S 1989 Psoas abscess complicating Crohn's disease. Acta Chirurgica Scandinavica 155: 409–412

Stabile B E, Puccio E, van Sonnenberg E, Neff C C 1990 Preoperative percutaneous drainage of diverticular abscesses. American Journal of Surgery 159: 99–105

Summers R W, Switz D M, Sessions J T et al 1979 National Cooperative Crohn's disease study: results of drug treatment. Gastroenterology 77: 847–869

100. Enterocutaneous fistula: conservative and surgical management

S. T. O'Dwyer

Safe and timely surgical intervention is the key to minimizing complications in patients with refractory colitis and Crohn's disease. Despite this, enterocutaneous fistulae can still occur and, because they are associated with intra-abdominal sepsis they remain one of the most serious complications of Crohn's disease. Even today the prospect of treating a patient with an enterocutaneous fistula can seem daunting, but a concentration of knowledge and experience within specialist groups has allowed the principles of management to be defined, and their application undoubtedly leads to an improved outcome for these patients.

CLASSIFICATION AND INCIDENCE OF FISTULA

An external fistula is an abnormal communication between the gastrointestinal tract and the body surface and is seen in 15–20% of patients with Crohn's disease. Enterocutaneous fistulae occur spontaneously when they are associated with a chronic intra-abdominal inflammatory process, or develop acutely after operations, usually due to a leak from an anastomosis or strictureplasty. Traditional surgical teaching supported the belief that postoperative fistulae were common following resection in Crohn's disease, but we now know that anastomotic leaks can be avoided with better understanding of the physiological response to injury and infection, advances in perioperative nutrition, and improved surgical technique. Recent publications suggest that in expert hands postoperative fistulae occur in approximately 6% of Crohn's patients (Fazio et al 1989, Alexander-Williams 1993, Michelassi et al 1993, Tjandra et al 1993), but this figure may not reflect the true incidence as the rate in non-specialized units is not known.

Postoperative enterocutaneous fistula

The vast majority of postoperative fistulae arise from a small defect at the anastomosis: most are preventable by careful technique and sound judgment. As with any intestinal closure a leak will occur if there is ischemia or tension at the suture line, if there is inadequate approximation of the seromuscular layers of the bowel, and if an anastomosis has been attempted when there is contamination of the abdominal cavity, established sepsis or severe malnutrition. In reoperative surgery for recurrent Crohn's disease it is imperative to mobilize and examine the remaining small bowel along its entire length: failure to do so may lead to missed strictures or adhesions causing distal obstruction, which will increase intraluminal pressure and compromise a proximal suture line.

Surgical technique is usually at fault if a leak occurs following primary terminal ileal resection, where an anastomosis is fashioned in macroscopically normal bowel. More commonly a leak occurs from a strictureplasty which has been fashioned in the presence of active inflammatory disease, or from the site of closure of an internal fistula.

In some instances a postoperative fistula arises from a loop of bowel that has been traumatized during mobilization when there are dense adhesions due to previous leaks and intra-abdominal sepsis. Again, careful dissection, inspection of the bowel and repair of any defect is mandatory. Perhaps the only non-preventable postoperative fistula is that associated with an exacerbation of residual Crohn's disease, but this is rare (Steinberg et al 1973).

Clinical presentation

An acute postoperative fistula usually presents with a discharge through the abdominal wound between the seventh and tenth postoperative days. Until that time the leak has been contained with adhesion of small bowel loops and the formation of a perianastomotic abscess. The patient may seem generally well, having opened the bowel satisfactorily in the preceding days, but will complain of abdominal pain (rather than wound pain), and there may be asymmetrical fullness in the abdomen with a persistent low-grade fever. In the 24 hours before discharge there is often a localized ileus in the small bowel loops that are adherent to the developing fistula track: the patient will be anorexic, nauseous and lethargic until the fistula discharges.

Spontaneous fistulae

The development of a spontaneous enterocutaneous fistula is often an early indicator of recurrent Crohn's disease, and the majority open on to the anterior abdominal wall through a previous abdominal incision (Fig. 100.1). Spontaneous fistulae through a virgin abdominal wall and the umbilicus have been recorded but are rare (Greenstein 1987, Veloso et al 1989). Occasionally a penetrating fistula develops when a loop of inflamed bowel becomes adherent to the bladder, vagina, or even the salpinx. Intestinal contents then discharge through the urethra or vagina. When there is a fistula associated with a chronic pelvic or retroperitoneal abscess the fistula can progress along an anatomical plane, tracking through the obturator foramen into the buttocks or perineum (Fig. 100.2), or along the ileopsoas muscle into the hip and thigh. These latter examples are uncommon, but often go unrecognized until the patient is severely malnourished, with evidence of chronic sepsis.

Spontaneous fistulae in close proximity to an established ileostomy occur in approximately 1% of patients, and are indicative of a short stricture or recurrent disease immediately proximal to where the ileum exits through the rectus abdominis. Peri-ileostomy fistulae interfere with the fitting of the stoma appliance and usually require early surgical intervention to prevent skin excoriation.

Pathogenesis of fistulae in Crohn's disease

The presence of transmural inflammation distinguishes Crohn's disease from ulcerative colitis, and it is attractive to propose that the deep fissuring ulceration in Crohn's disease penetrates through to the serosa, where the inflammatory reaction promotes adherence of the bowel to adjacent viscera or the abdominal wall. Once a full-thickness fissure has developed, small abscesses lead to

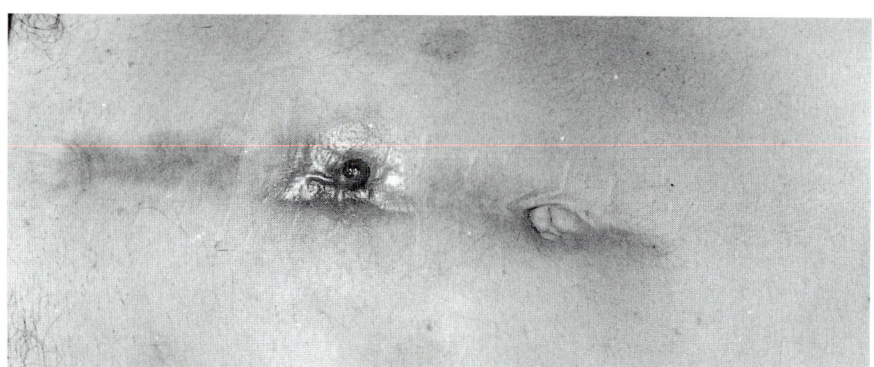

Fig. 100.1 Classic presentation of a spontaneous fistula through an old midline abdominal scar in a patient with recurrent Crohn's disease.

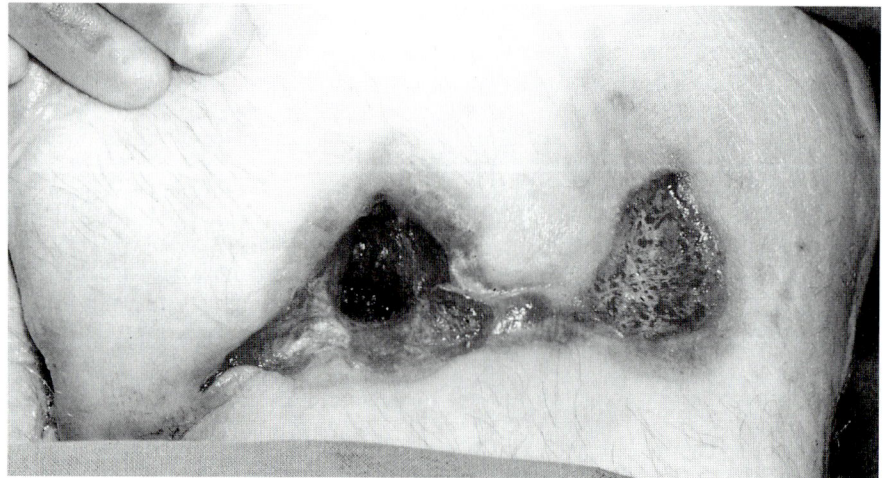

Fig. 100.2 Fistula presenting on to the buttock in a patient with small- and large-bowel Crohn's disease. The fistula originated from recurrence at a previous ileosigmoid anastomosis and tracked through the obturator foramen, presenting as a deep gluteal abscess.

localized tissue necrosis, further penetration and fistula formation. This is supported in part by the observation that fistulae usually arise from an area of florid active disease, and although the disease process leads to stricture formation (which will undoubtably prevent an established fistula from healing), it is extremely rare to observe perforation of macroscopically normal bowel proximal to the stricture. On the other hand, it is puzzling to find evidence of aggressive disease with long inflammatory strictures of the mid small bowel without adherence or fistula formation. Some authors have noted a group of patients who, at initial surgery, had fistulating disease and tended to develop recurrent fistulae requiring reoperation more frequently than patients initially undergoing surgery for obstructing, non-fistulating disease. This observation led Greenstein and colleagues (1988) to propose a distinction between perforating and non-perforating Crohn's disease, although there is some support for this clinically (Irving, personal communication), it remains debatable whether fistulating disease simply reflects aggressive ulceration and inflammation in the bowel wall or whether there are other distinguishing factors.

Measurable differences in zinc and ascorbate metabolism have been reported between patients with fistulating and those with non-fistulating disease. Collagen deposition is also abnormal in these patients with fistulae (Alexander & Irving 1990). Zinc levels are notably lower than normal in patients with fistulae (Kruis et al 1985). Although total body ascorbate does not differ in fistulating and non-fistulating Crohn's patients, tissue levels in fistulating intestine are 50% less than in non-fistulating disease (Pettit & Irving 1987). Substrates such as zinc influence fibroblastic activity, protein synthesis and collagen deposition, which is integral to satisfactory regeneration and repair of the inflammatory injury in the bowel wall. Micronutrient abnormalities may contribute to fistula formation in patients with aggressive disease.

Clinical presentation

Because of the insidious nature of the chronic inflammatory process in Crohn's disease spontaneous fistulae vary in their complexity. Classically the patient presents with a swelling beneath an old abdominal scar which is red, hot and tender, and there is often a small area of skin necrosis at the dome of the swelling which, when probed, releases pus and occasionally gas. The patient may have been constitutionally unwell for 48 hours, with a fever, but rarely is there evidence of intestinal obstruction. To the experienced physician or surgeon the discharging fistula is a manifestation of recurrent disease and, if recognized as such, allows for timely assessment and intervention. Once the initial abscess has been drained the volume discharged from the fistula is usually low, granulation tissue develops around the exit site, and the patient is then probably eating, with apparently normal gastrointestinal function. Further investigations can be organized on an outpatient basis.

In some cases both patient and doctor fail to acknowledge the significance of a spontaneous fistula and recurrent disease goes untreated. Progression of the inflammatory process enhances stricture formation, which in turn prevents healing of the fistula. The exit site may seal superficially, only to break down again weeks later. Further loops of bowel become involved in the reactive inflammatory process and a complex mass of bowel loops adheres to the abdominal wall. At this stage the patient will often have had intermittent episodes of subacute obstruction and will limit their dietary intake to avoid provoking abdominal pain. The patient gradually loses weight, becomes anemic and feverish, and abdominal examination reveals a palpable mass. Without intervention the patient usually deteriorates; a localized ileus of the intestinal loops develops and secondary intra-abdominal abscesses form. In neglected cases chronic intra-abdominal sepsis leads to severe malnutrition and metabolic disturbance, which can only be reversed once all the abscesses have been drained.

ASSESSMENT AND INVESTIGATION

The evaluation of a patient with an enterocutaneous fistula is similar whether the fistula is postoperative or spontaneous, and should be directed along three paths simultaneously: the general and nutritional state of the patient; the anatomical assessment of the fistula; and a search for occult sepsis.

General and nutritional evaluation

The majority of patients who develop a postoperative fistula should have reasonable nutritional reserve: if there was significant malnutrition or infection before operation an anastomosis should have been avoided and a stoma fashioned (Irving & O'Dwyer 1993).

When a patient develops a postoperative fistula there is always intra-abdominal infection, transient ileus, poor intake and an increased nutritional requirement to support the acute-phase response. Persistent catabolism rapidly reduces lean body mass, decreases the patient's ability to combat infection, and promotes steady nutritional deterioration. The overall condition of the patient will also depend upon the level of the fistula: high-output fistulae arising from the stomach, duodenum or proximal jejunum will lead to rapid dehydration, severe electrolyte disturbance and circulatory collapse.

The majority of spontaneous external fistulae in Crohn's disease arise from the lower small bowel and are not usually a source of large fluid loss. However, postoperative fistulae can arise from any site that has been manipulated surgically, and will include those with a high output. If there are large-volume losses careful determination of fluid balance, measurements of serum sodium, potassium, urea and creatinine, and assessment of acid–base status will be necessary.

All patients should have baseline hematological and serological measurements. Patients are usually anemic, with Hb < 10 g/dl, and have low serum iron and folate values. Blood transfusion alone may be inadequate to replace these deficits, as iron stores are constantly depleted and remain low until the sepsis has cleared. Chronic vitamin B_{12} deficiency may also exist as a result of previous terminal ileal resection. The white cell count will usually be elevated, but may be below normal if there is endotoxemia or if the patient is receiving immunosuppressants such as azathioprine. Liver function tests usually reveal a low albumin, and chronic sepsis is reflected by a high alkaline phosphatase, raised bilirubin and abnormal triglyceride levels. Malabsorption of trace minerals is common in Crohn's disease patients, resulting in low levels of zinc and magnesium (Rosenberg et al 1985), and in the chronically ill selenium levels are often as low as one-third of normal values (personal observation).

Examination of the patient often reveals clinical evidence of weight loss, with wasting of the deltoid in the upper arms and quadriceps muscles in the thighs. Baseline and twice-weekly measurements of body weight are essential, and measurements of skin-fold thickness and determination of muscle circumference are useful in the patient needing prolonged nutritional support.

Anatomy of the fistula

When evaluating a postoperative fistula it is important to determine whether it is simple or complicated. A simple fistula, where there is a single track connecting the skin with the bowel lumen, will almost always heal without surgical intervention unless there is distal obstruction. Complicated fistulae are those where the communication involves more than one loop of bowel, where there are numerous tracks connecting interloop abscesses (Fig. 100.3), or when there are intra-abdominal, pelvic or retroperitoneal collections. More aggressive intervention is necessary in complex fistulae and imaging must be planned so as to achieve the maximal useful information with the lowest radiation exposure to the patient. This is of particular importance in the young, who are likely to be subjected to repeated radiation exposure in future. Using a team approach with physicians, surgeons and radiologists experienced in the management of inflammatory bowel disease, radiation exposure can be minimized and the optimal imaging sequence for an individual patient can be achieved.

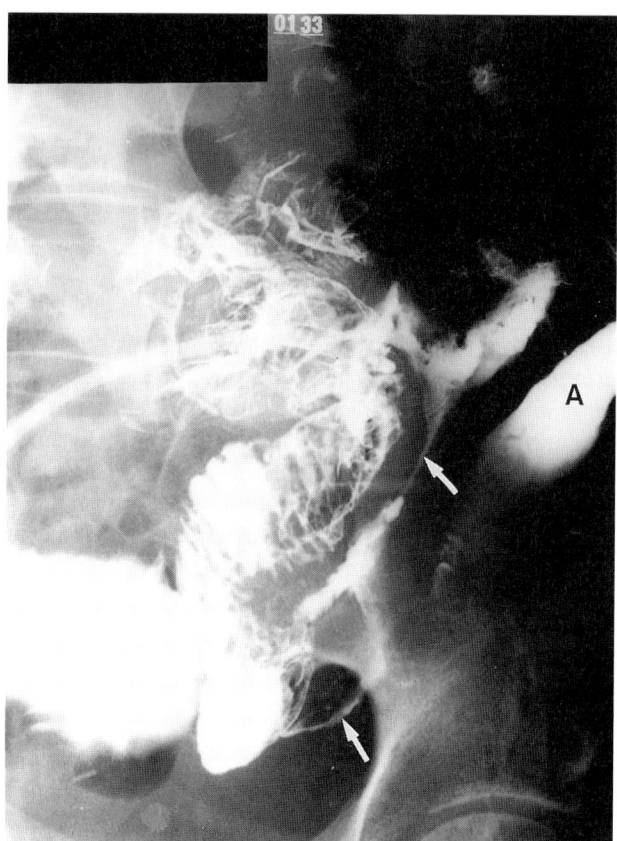

Fig. 100.3 Contrast X-rays of a patient with complex postoperative fistula following iatrogenic injury to the small bowel during mobilization and adhesiolysis. Multiple tracks (arrows) connect with the small bowel and an interloop abscess (A).

'Home-grown' postoperative fistulae should be relatively easy to investigate because the surgeon knows the anatomy as a result of his or her recent laparotomy, or from reference to previous operation records. In such patients, once the fistula has discharged through the wound, attention is directed towards localization and drainage of abscesses.

It is always more difficult to manage a patient who has been transferred from another unit and these patients usually need more extensive investigation. Contrast studies will provide much of the required information; direct fistulography will outline the tracks, but it may be necessary to perform synchronous imaging of the bowel both proximal and distal to the fistula by means of a small-bowel enema, in addition to a conventional enema (Glick 1987). Distal imaging is important in outlining sites of recurrent disease or other causes of obstruction which would prevent closure of the fistula.

CT scanning with oral contrast may prove to be the most effective means of imaging a complex fistula when one is suspicious of collections or concerned that the fistula involves organs other than the gastrointestinal tract (Orel et al 1987, Jabra et al 1991). When communication with the urinary tract is suspected intravenous urography may be helpful, but usually this is only necessary in rare cases of ureteric involvement. Colovesical fistulae can usually be diagnosed using a combination of luminal contrast, CT and endoscopic techniques.

Both contrast radiology and CT scanning should be used wisely to provide the team with information to aid in planning radiological and surgical intervention, and allow the surgeon to give the patient and relatives an outline of the treatment plan and an indication of the expected length of hospitalization and time to recovery. There is no doubt that finding a sympathetic and interested radiologist will make this task much easier.

Endoscopy has a limited place in the assessment of fistulae, but occasionally colonoscopy is helpful in determining disease activity in the colon if barium studies have outlined an ileocolic or jejunocolic fistula, and flexible cystourethroscopy can demonstrate an obscure colovesical or urethral fistula. In the author's opinion direct fistuloscopy of enterocutaneous fistulae is of little value, but it has been used by some who support the application of fibrin glue to enhance occlusion of the fistula (Eleftheriadis et al 1990, Lange et al 1990).

Searching for occult sepsis

Failure to identify abscesses in patients with fistulae leads to a relentless decline in the nutritional state of the patient and undoubtedly contributes to an increased risk of mortality. In the initial stages all fistulae are associated with some degree of infection and abscess formation, but once there is discharge through the abdominal wall many collections will drain satisfactorily. More complex fistulae fail to discharge completely externally and become the source of intra-abdominal abscesses, which can be pelvic, subphrenic, subhepatic and intrahepatic, paracolic and retroperitoneal. More difficult to detect are interloop abscesses, particularly in postoperative cases; also collections in the pelvis that track into the perineum or gluteal regions and retroperitoneal collections which have tracked into the ileopsoas or lumbar muscles.

CT and ultrasound are complementary when investigating the fistula patient with occult sepsis (Cybulsky & Tam 1990). Many interventional radiologists define the anatomy of the abscess using CT but prefer to drain the cavity using realtime ultrasound (McGahan et al 1986, Safrit et al 1987). Portable ultrasound can be particularly helpful in the highly dependent patient requiring ventilatory and circulatory support (Casola et al 1987). Endoanal and endovaginal ultrasound is also useful in the detection of small pelvic collections and enables aspiration or secondary external drainage through the abdominal wall or to the perineum (Tio et al 1990). Magnetic resonance imaging has not been used widely in fistula patients, but it may have a role in the investigation of complex pelvic fistulae where the perineum and gluteal regions are involved (Koelbel et al 1989).

When dealing with immunosuppressed patients it can be difficult to decide whether there is an abscess or whether the main source of inflammation is recurrent Crohn's disease within the bowel wall. In such cases scintographic scanning using technetium-labeled granulocytes can be helpful in determining the sites of active inflammation in the bowel itself, and has a high sensitivity in detecting abscesses and fistulae (Sciarretta et al 1993). This technique can also be useful in the postoperative patient, when it is difficult to be sure whether an intra-abdominal or pelvic fluid collection is an organizing hematoma, seroma or pus.

The majority of abscesses can be drained using radiological techniques and surgical drainage is reserved for the few cases where the cavity is inaccessible or the abscess is multiloculated and where, despite percutaneous drainage, the patient shows persistent signs of sepsis. If radiological support is weak it is far better to operate on a sick patient early and drain the infection surgically, rather than observe their steady decline.

DEFINITIVE TREATMENT OF FISTULAE

The practical management of all patients with fistulae should include care of the wound, nutritional support and control of infection. All three aspects of care must be addressed early or the patient will deteriorate and what was a straightforward problem will become difficult to manage, with increased hospitalization and exaggerated cost. Although almost 70% of postoperative fistulae will close using the conservative approach outlined in Table 100.1, spontaneous fistulae rarely close without additional intervention.

Drug therapies are directed toward reducing gastroenteric and pancreatic secretions and modifying the inflammatory

Table 100.1 Management plan for patients with external fistulae. (Adapted from Alexander-Williams & Irving 1982)

Phase 1:
0–24 hours
Skin protection
Fluid & electrolyte replacement

Phase 2:
24–48 hours
Nutritional assessment
Abscess localization/drainage

Phase 3:
2–4 days
Define fistula anatomy
Enteral or parenteral nutrition

Phase 4:
5+ days
Eliminate infection
Improve nutritional status

response in acute Crohn's disease. Surgery is required for patients who do not respond to conservative measures or where there is stricture formation, distal mechanical obstruction and uncontrolled infection.

Care of the wound

An enterocutaneous fistula is an uncontrolled stoma: when a fistula develops postoperatively it is imperative that the skin around the exit site is protected as soon as it discharges: early involvement of the stoma therapist is mandatory. If the fistula communicates with the upper gastrointestinal tract the fluid contains bile and pancreatic secretions which cause severe contact dermatitis. It is usually possible to apply a standard stoma bag to the wound at the site where the fistula discharged and allow simple drainage, emptying the bag intermittently. When there are large-volume losses it may be necessary to apply intermittent suction or use continuous drainage devices to prevent pooling of small-bowel contents and erosion of the skin. Even when the fistula has a low output or connects with the colon it is better to apply a stoma bag, as this contains the secretions, allows accurate measurement of losses, and is more comfortable for the patient. Sometimes it is necessary to open the wound to allow satisfactory drainage of pus or bowel contents that have collected beneath the skin. On rare occasions, when there is gross contamination, drainage by laparostomy may be necessary (Irving & O'Dwyer 1993). If this measure is taken the application of stomadhesive around the wound edge will prevent ulceration and allow granulation tissue to be laid down, with secondary contraction of the wound.

Spontaneous fistulae associated with recrudescence of Crohn's disease usually discharge very little: many do not need a stoma appliance and can be managed with a simple non-adherent dressing. Peri-ileostomy fistulae can be troublesome, however, and usually require early surgical treatment for skin protection because of interference with the application of a satisfactory stoma appliance.

Nutritional support

Many clinicians who have limited experience of patients with fistulae instinctively and erroneously believe that administration of enteral nutrition is contraindicated, particularly soon after operation. Wherever possible the gut should be used for nutrient administration because failure to do so leads to loss of absorptive capacity, altered mucosal permeability and an increased tendency to absorption of luminal macromolecules and endotoxin (O'Dwyer et al 1990). There are a number of high-protein low-residue formulae which are absorbed in the proximal small bowel and can be safely administered to patients with mid or low small-bowel and colonic fistulae.

In some cases it is necessary to use the parenteral route, particularly in the early stages when there is a transient ileus. Traditional teaching has been to use the central route, but more recently peripheral parenteral nutrition has proved to be a safe and effective alternative to central feeding in patients who are likely to require parenteral supplementation for less than 3 weeks (Nordenstrom et al 1991). The majority of postoperative fistula patients fall into this group, the exception being those with high-output fistulae who need large volumes of fluid and electrolytes in addition to nitrogen and calories. These patients are best managed with total parenteral nutrition (TPN) administered by the central route, but as a psychological boost to their morale they should be allowed to drink clear fluids.

Gastric, duodenal or high jejunal fistulae are most difficult to manage, and it is often necessary to use proton pump inhibitors to decrease gastric acid production and somatostatin analogs to inhibit pancreatic secretion while maintaining nutrition and hydration with TPN and high-volume electrolyte replacement. It may be necessary to prolong TPN in these patients for 6 months, and this can be administered by the patient at home after a period of in-hospital training in a specialized unit (Stokes et al 1988).

Patients with complicated Crohn's disease are often malnourished (Rosenberg et al 1985, Stokes 1991) and many with spontaneous fistulae will have measurable nutritional deficiencies (Hill et al 1988). Urgent surgery is rarely necessary and, unless there is established sepsis, most deficiencies can be corrected rapidly. There is divided opinion about the benefit of preoperative nutrition in surgical patients in general, but the author's personal view, supported by the literature, is that perioperative nutritional support is advantageous in patients with complicated Crohn's disease (Hill 1992a, b).

Preoperative correction of fluid losses with replacement of vitamin and mineral deficiencies is certainly worthwhile, and iron treatment will often avoid the need for preoperative blood transfusion. The patient benefits from consultation with a dietitian, who should advise a low-residue high-protein enteral intake, which can lead to measurable physiological improvement within 2 weeks (Stokes 1991). Thus nutrition can be improved at home for a short time before surgery, but when there is recurrent Crohn's disease nutritional manipulation alone will not result in permanent closure of a fistula.

In a few neglected cases when there is severe protein calorie malnutrition, as in Fig. 100.4, preoperative parenteral nutrition is necessary. However, one often finds that these are the cases where there is occult sepsis, when early surgery and aggressive postoperative nutritional support is the key to recovery. Detailed practical advice for managing and administering enteral and parenteral nutrition can be obtained from the specialized texts of Rombeau and Caldwell (1990) and Hill (1992c).

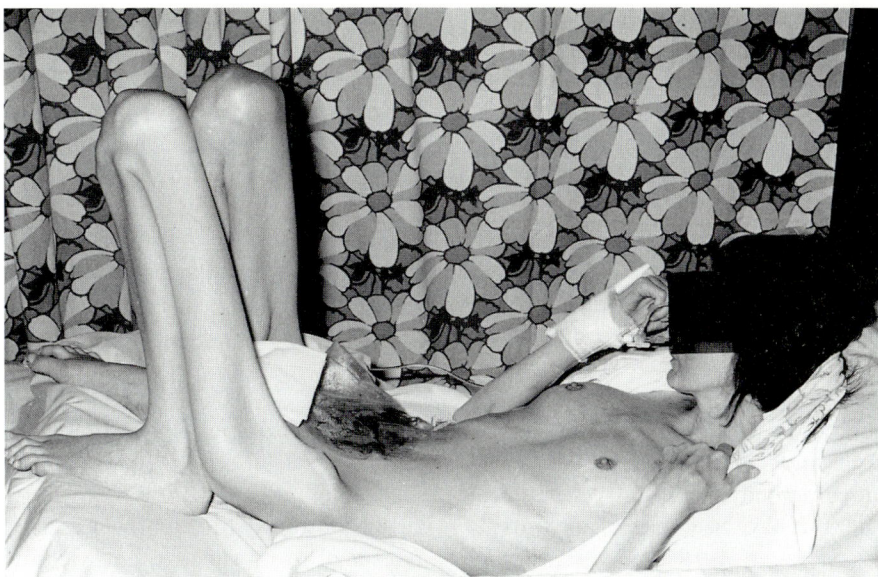

Fig. 100.4 Severe malnutrition and loss of lean body mass in a Crohn's patient with unrecognized chronic pelvic and intra-abdominal sepsis and small bowel fistulae.

Control of infection

Persistent infection, which prevents healing of postoperative fistulae, is associated with chronic hypercatabolism and a relentless deterioration in the patient's general condition. The malnourished patient is also immunocompromised and, if sepsis is not cleared, sequential organ failure leads to death. In the last decade much has been learnt of the immunological response to infection and the metabolic effects of immune mediators such as TNF (tumor necrosis factor), the interleukins, leukotrienes and prostaglandins (Fong & Lowry 1990). Endotoxin is a potent stimulus for the release of cytokines, which in turn have profound effects on the neuroendocrine response and on capillary permeability, leading to a decrease in systemic vascular resistance, hypotension and shock (Michie et al 1988). Circulating endotoxin also increases mucosal permeability of the gut (O'Dwyer et al 1988) and promotes translocation of bacteria from the gut lumen to mesenteric lymph nodes: a phenomenon known to occur in patients with Crohn's disease (Ambrose et al 1984). Thus even when abscesses have been drained the inflammatory response may persist until active disease has been controlled, either by resection or with the use of drugs aimed at modifying the immune response. Recent therapeutic additions include antibodies directed against individual mediators and against endotoxin. Although anti-IL2 and anti-TNF antibodies can prevent many cytokine effects in the controlled experimental setting, their application in the treatment of clinical infection has yet to be realized and initial hopes generated by the development of antiendotoxin antibody (Ziegler et al 1991) have so far failed to render a significant clinical impact.

Elimination of the inflammatory source, multisystem organ support and careful use of antibiotics are still the mainstay of infection control. Antibiotics are most useful when administered so as to achieve bacteriocidal activity at a time when organisms are likely to flood the circulation. This will inevitably occur when abscesses are drained, either surgically or percutaneously, and when the bowel is manipulated at operation. The author's preference is to use high-dose intraoperative antibiotics and only extend treatment postoperatively where there has been overwhelming abdominal sepsis. In this situation antibiotic treatment is adjuvant and cannot substitute for surgical drainage. The injudicious or long-term use of antibiotics is dangerous and promotes the development of resistant strains, pseudomembranous colitis and opportunistic pulmonary infections, which can be life-threatening.

DRUG THERAPIES IN THE TREATMENT OF FISTULAE

Manipulation of enteric secretions using H_2 antagonists, proton pump inhibitors and somatostatin analogs has particular application in the management of postoperative fistulae, whereas immunosuppressant drugs are used when there is active inflammation of the bowel in Crohn's fistulae. Success rates of fistula closure vary and, because of difficulties in recruiting satisfactory numbers of patients from an individual center and the wide variation in disease activity in fistula patients, there remains a lack of controlled trials comparing the different drug therapies.

Altering enteric secretion

Gastric acid secretion can be decreased by the administration of H_2 antagonists, or eliminated completely using oral preparations of the proton pump inhibitors. If the fistula arises from the stomach or duodenum intravenous preparations are available, and the dose can be titrated according to the acidity of the fluid emanating from the fistula. Somatostatin analogs are administered by subcutaneous injection up to three times a day. They act by inhibiting the secretion of pancreatic polypeptide, gastrin, secretin and motilin (Bharucha & Simon 1993). Dosage requirements vary widely between patients, which may be one reason for the variability in reported response rates from different groups. The most recently reported double-blind randomized controlled trial of octreotide in 19 postoperative enterocutaneous fistulae showed no differences in volume output and closure rates (Scott et al 1993); others have documented decreased output and earlier closure of fistulae, but have used historical controls for comparison (Sitges-Serra et al 1993, Spiliotis et al 1990). The greatest benefit of octreotide is seen in patients with pancreatitis and pancreatic fistulae, rather than in those with Crohn's fistulae (Rosenberg & Brown 1991).

Immunosuppresant therapy

In addition to corticosteroids, immunosuppressants such as azathioprine, 6-mercaptopurine and cyclosporin A have been used in the treatment of Crohn's fistulae. All of these agents have side effects which can be serious, and patients must be carefully monitored during treatment. Azathioprine has proved to be safe in the treatment of perineal disease but does not have a major role in enterocutaneous fistulae. Favorable effects have been documented using 6-mercaptopurine for external and internal fistulae (Korelitz & Present 1985, Margolin & Korelitz 1989). In these series almost 40% of fistulae closed, but treatment had to be continued for 6 months, the response rate was slow, and withdrawal of the treatment led to recurrence of the fistula. Recent studies using intravenous cyclosporin have shown rapid responses in fistula output provided high circulating levels are maintained (Hanauer & Smith 1993, Present & Lichtiger 1994). In approximately 40% of patients there is long-term improvement when the patient is continued on oral therapy, but side effects are common and there is a tendency for the fistulae to recur when the drug is withdrawn. In some cases these agents may allow temporary closure and rehabilitation of the patient if surgery is to be deferred.

PRINCIPLES OF SURGICAL TREATMENT

Fistulae that do not close using conservative measures are invariably associated with recurrent disease, distal obstruction, abscess formation, mucocutaneous continuity or discontinuity of the bowel ends. The timing of surgery is crucial to its success, and definitive surgery should be deferred for at least 3 months. Before this time the peritoneal reaction leads to the formation of dense inflammatory adhesions which encase the bowel, rendering dissection extremely difficult. Mobilization of the bowel in these circumstances often leads to iatrogenic injury, with shredding of the seromuscular layers or devascularization of the gut. In a few exceptional cases, where a fistula drains through a site which is difficult to contain, or when there is severe metabolic disturbances or uncontrolled sepsis, earlier surgery is necessary. In these circumstances definitive surgery should not be contemplated, and mobilization should be limited to allow drainage of infection and the formation of a proximal defunctioning stoma.

Detailed descriptions of surgical technique can be obtained from specialized texts (Alexander-Williams & Irving 1982, Hill 1992c, Kumar & Alexander-Williams 1993) but are best learnt by watching and assisting an operator experienced in reoperative surgery and inflammatory bowel disease. The general principles of fistula

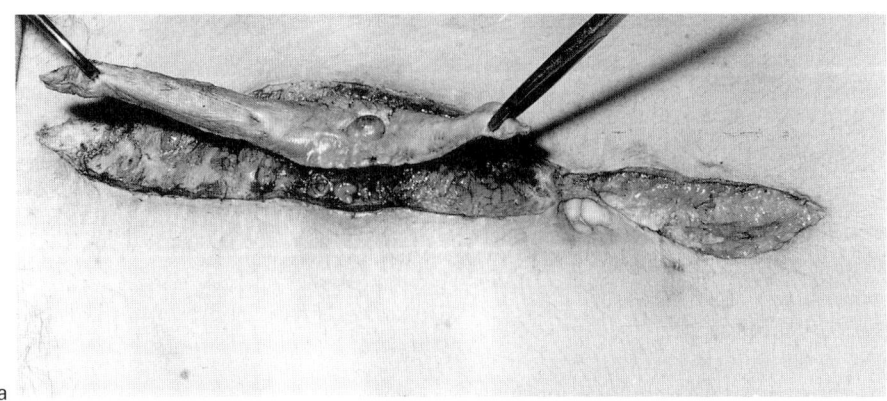

Fig. 100.5a Surgical approach extending the original wound above the umbilicus, entering the abdominal cavity away from dense adhesions which surround the fistula.

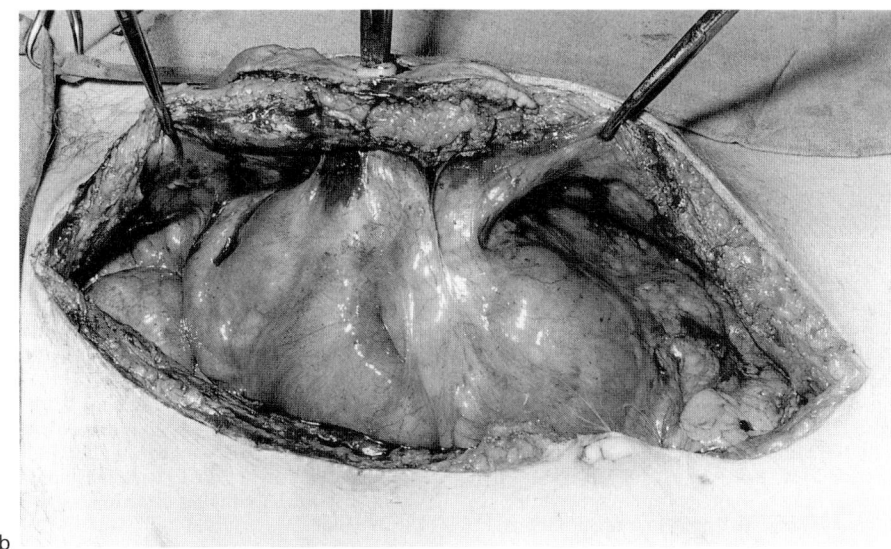

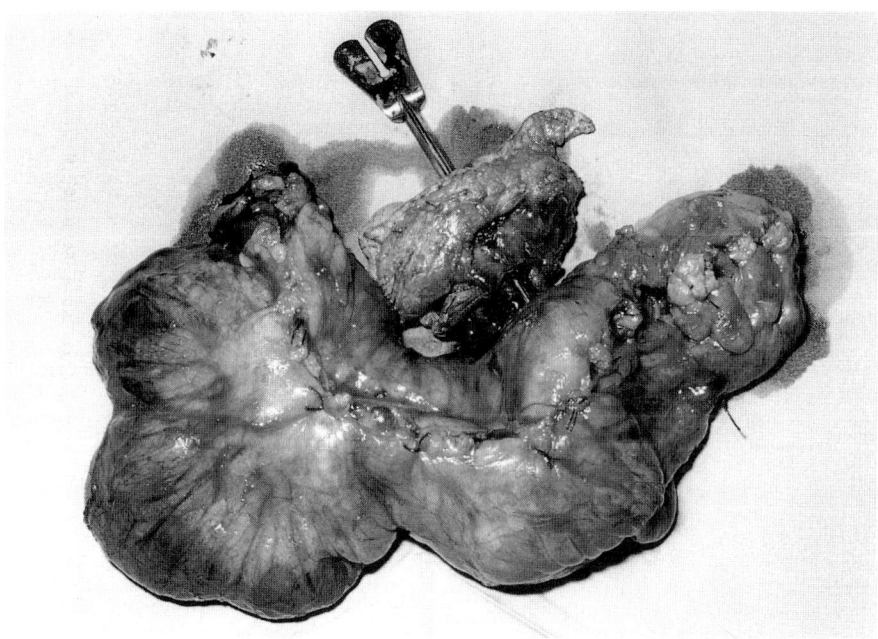

Fig. 100.5b The peritoneal adhesions are cleared above, below and behind the small-bowel fistula, the skin and scar tissue are circumcised from the abdominal wall, and adherent loops are carefully separated. **c** Careful surgical technique allows conservative resection of the small-bowel fistula and an associated distal stricture (probe demonstrates enterocutaneous track).

surgery include complete mobilization of the gut, resection of the fistulous bowel, and elimination of distal obstruction by conservative resection or strictureplasty. Provided the patient is well nourished, primary anastomoses can be performed and gastrointestinal continuity achieved even if multiple resections and strictureplasties are necessary. In the majority of cases the mid small bowel is adherent to the abdominal wall, but often in addition to the primary external fistula there is secondary involvement of further bowel loops, which may be the site of internal fistulae. The author's approach is usually by extension of the original abdominal wound, with lateral dissection of peritoneal adhesions (Fig. 100.5a,b). Patience and persistence are essential, so that adherent bowel loops are freed without injury and conservative resection of the fistula and small bowel loop is achieved (Fig. 100.5c). Gastric and duodenal fistulae can be particularly difficult to manage, and it is often necessary to perform a distal gastrectomy with a Roux-en-Y bypass and jejunal patch repair. Secondary internal fistulae can be closed by simple suture, but when the colon is involved extra care is necessary and should there be a chronic abscess cavity it is always safer to defunction proximal to the site of repair (Pettit & Irving 1988).

CONCLUSION

Treating patients with enterocutaneous fistulae is extremely demanding of healthcare resources, as multiple procedures are often necessary to achieve gastrointestinal continuity and restore the patient to health. There is no doubt that prevention is better than cure, but when a fistula develops it should be remembered that an experienced team can achieve excellent results with the majority of these relatively young patients, who can ultimately achieve their professional goals and return to full social activity.

REFERENCES

Alexander A C, Irving M H 1990 Accumulation of pepsin solubility of collagens in the bowel of patients with Crohn's disease. Diseases of the Colon and Rectum 33: 956–962

Alexander-Williams J 1993 Strictureplasty. In: Alexander-Williams J, Kumar D (eds) Crohn's disease and ulcerative colitis: surgical management. Springer-Verlag, London, pp 89–102

Alexander-Williams J, Irving M 1982 Intestinal Fistulas. Wright, Bristol

Ambrose N S, Johnson M, Burdon D W, Keighley M R B 1984 Incidence of pathogenic bacteria from mesenteric lymph nodes and ileal serosa during Crohn's disease surgery. British Journal of Surgery 71: 623–625

Bharucha S B, Simon D 1993 Somatostatin for enterocutaneous fistula: a silver bullet? American Journal of Gastroenterology 88: 963–964

Casola G, van Sonnenberg E, Neff C C, Saba R M, Withers C, Emarine C W 1987 Abscesses in Crohn's disease: percutaneous drainage. Radiology 163: 19–22

Cybulski I J, Tam P 1990 Intra-abdominal abscesses in Crohn's disease. American Surgery 56: 678–682

Eleftheriadis E, Tzartinoglou E, Kotzampassi K, Aletras H 1990 Early endoscopic fibrin sealing of high output postoperative enterocutaneous fistulas. Acta Chirurgica Scandinavica 156: 652–658

Fazio V W, Galandiuk S, Jagelman D G, Lavery I C 1989 Strictureplasty in Crohn's disease. Annals of Surgery 210: 621–625

Fong Y, Lowry S F 1990 Cytokines and the cellular response to injury and infection. In: Care of the surgical patient. American College of Surgeons vol 1, 7: 1–17

Glick S N 1987 Crohn's disease of the small intestine. Radiological Clinics of North America 25: 25–45

Greenstein A J 1987 The surgery of Crohn's disease. Surgical Clinics of North America 67(3): 573–596

Greenstein A J, Lachman P, Sachar D B et al 1988 Perforating and non perforating indications for repeated operations in Crohn's disease: evidence for two clinical forms. Gut 29: 588–592

Hanauer S B, Smith M B 1993 Rapid closure of Crohn's fistulas with continuous intravenous cyclosporin A. American Journal of Gastroenterology 88: 646–649

Hill G L 1992a Metabolic physiological and pharmacological effects of nutritional therapy. In: Hill G L (ed) Nutrition and metabolism in clinical surgery. Churchill Livingstone, Edinburgh, pp 85–103

Hill G L 1992b Perioperative nutrition. In: Hill G L (ed) Nutrition and metabolism in clinical surgery. Churchill Livingstone, Edinburgh, pp 233–245

Hill G L 1992c Nutrition and metabolism in clinical surgery. Churchill Livingstone, Edinburgh

Hill G L, Bourchier R G, Witney G B 1988 Surgical and metabolic management of patients with external fistulas of the small intestine associated with Crohn's disease. World Journal of Surgery 12: 191–197

Irving M, O'Dwyer S T 1993 Surgical management of anastamotic leakage and intrabdominal sepsis. In: Fielding P, Dudley H (eds) Rob and Smith's Operative Surgery, 5th edn. Butterworth-Heinemann New York, pp 93–104

Jabra A A, Fishman E K, Taylor G W 1991 Crohn's disease in the pediatric patient: CT evaluation. Radiology 179: 495–498

Koelbel G, Schmiedl U, Majer M C et al 1989 Diagnosis of fistulae and sinus tracts in patients with Crohn's disease. American Journal of Roentgenology 152: 999–1003

Korelitz B I, Present D H 1985 Favorable effect of 6-mercaptopurine on fistulas of Crohn's disease. Digestive Diseases and Sciences 30: 58–64

Kruis W, Rindfleisch G E, Weinzierl M 1985 Zinc deficiency as a problem in patients with Crohn's disease and fistula formation. Hepatogastroenterology 32: 133–134

Kumar D, Alexander-Williams J 1993 Crohn's disease and ulcerative colitis: Surgical management. Springer-Verlag, London

Lange V, Meyer G, Wenk H, Schindberg F W 1990 Fistuloscopy – an adjuvant technique for sealing gastrointestinal fistulae. Surgical Endoscopy 4: 212–216

McGahan J P, Anderson M W, Walter J P 1986 Portable real time sonographic and needle guidance systems for aspiration and drainage. American Journal of Roentgenology 147: 124–126

Margolin M L, Korelitz B I 1989 Management of bladder fistulas in Crohn's disease. Journal of Clinical Gastroenterology 11: 399–402

Michelassi F, Stella M, Balestracci T, Giuliante F, Marogna P, Block G E 1993 Incidence, diagnosis and treatment of enteric and colorectal fistulae in patients with Crohn's disease. Annals of Surgery 218: 660–666

Michie H, Spriggs D R, Manogue K et al 1988 Tumour necrosis factor and endotoxin induce similar metabolic effects in humans. Surgery 104: 280–286

Nordenstrom J, Jeevanandam M, Elwyn D H et al 1991 Peripheral parenteral nutrition: effect of standardised compounded mixture on infusion phlebitis. British Journal of Surgery 78: 1391–1394

O'Dwyer S T, Michie H, Zeigler T R, Revhaug A, Smith R J, Wilmore D W 1988 A single dose of endotoxin increases intestinal permeability in healthy humans. Archives of Surgery 123: 1459–1464

O'Dwyer S T, Smith R J, Rombeau J L 1990 New fuels for the gut. In: Rombeau J, Caldwell L (eds) Clinical nutrition, enteral and tube feeding, 2nd edn, Saunders, New York, pp 540–555

Orel S G, Rubesin S E, Jones B, Fishman E K, Bayless T M, Siegelman S S 1987 Computer tomography vs barium studies in the acutely symptomatic patient with Crohn's disease. Journal of Computer Assisted Tomography 11: 1009–1016

Pettit S H, Irving M H 1987 Does local intestinal ascorbate deficiency predispose to fistula formation in Crohn's disease? Diseases of the Colon and Rectum 30: 552–557

Pettit S, Irving M H 1988 The operative management of fistulating Crohn's disease – experience with 100 consecutive cases. Surgery, Gynecology and Obstetrics 167: 223–228

Present D H, Lichtiger S 1994 Efficacy of cyclosporine in treatment of fistula of Crohn's disease. Digestive Diseases and Sciences 39: 374–380

Rombeau J L, Caldwell M D 1990 Enteral and tube feeding, 2nd edn. WB Saunders, Philadelphia

Rosenberg I H, Bengoa J M, Sitrin M D 1985 Nutritional aspects of inflammatory bowel disease. In: Annual Review of Nutrition, Annual Reviews inc., Palo Alto, pp 463–484

Rosenberg L, Brown R A 1991 Sandostatin in the management of neuroendocrine gastrointestinal and pancreatic disorders: a preliminary study. Canadian Journal of Surgery 34: 223–229

Safrit H D, Mauro M A, Jaques P F 1987 Percutaneous abscess drainage in Crohn's disease. American Journal of Roentgenology 148: 859–862

Sciarretta G, Furno A, Mazzoni M, Basile C, Malaguti P 1993 Technetium-99m hexamethyl propylene amine oxime granulocyte scintigraphy in Crohn's disease. Gut 34: 1364–1369

Scott N A, Finnegan S, Irving M H 1993 Octreotide and postoperative enterocutaneous fistulas: a controlled prospective study. Acta Gastroenterologica Belgica 56: 266–270

Sitges-Serra A, Guirao X, Pereira J A, Nubiola P 1993 Treatment of gastrointestinal fistulas with Sandostatin. Digestion 54 (Suppl 1): 38–40

Spiliotis J, Vaganas K, Panagopoulos K, Kalfarentzos F 1990 Treatment of enterocutaneous fistulas with TPN and somatostatin compared with patients who received TPN only. British Journal of Clinical Practice 44: 616–618

Steinberg D M, Cooke W T, Alexander-Williams J 1973 Abscess and fistulae in Crohn's disease. Gut 14: 865–869

Stokes M A 1991 The malnutrition of Crohn's disease. ChM Thesis, University of Dublin

Stokes M A, Almond D J, Pettit S H et al 1988 Home parenteral nutrition: a review of 100 patient years of treatment in 76 consecutive cases. British Journal of Surgery 75: 481–483

Tio T L, Mulder C J, Wijers O B, Sars P R, Tytgat G N 1990 Endosonography of peri-anal and peri-colorectal fistula and/or abscess in Crohn's disease. Gastrointestinal Endoscopy 36: 331–336

Tjandra J J, Fazio V W, Lavery I C 1993 Results of multiple strictureplasties in diffuse Crohn's disease of the small bowel. Australia and New Zealand Journal of Surgery 63: 95–99

Veloso F T, Cardoso V, Fraga J, Carvalho J, Diaas L M 1989 Spontaneous umbilical fistula in Crohn's disease. Journal of Clinical Gastroenterology 11: 197–200

Ziegler E J, Fisher C J, Sprung C L et al 1991 Treatment of Gram-negative bacteremia and septic shock with HA-1A human monoclonal antibody against endotoxin. New England Journal of Medicine 324: 429–436

101. Management of the persistent perineal sinus

N. A. Scott

INTRODUCTION

Proctectomy and the resulting perineal wound is still necessary for some patients with Crohn's disease (Van Dongen & Lubbers 1986, Fry et al 1989, Levien et al 1989), ulcerative colitis and low rectal cancer. The initial management of the perineal wound can be either primary suture or healing by granulation. Satisfactory perineal wound healing can be achieved by either approach in the majority of patients.

A significant minority of patients encounter problems with delayed healing of the perineal wound after proctectomy, especially those requiring proctectomy for perianal Crohn's disease (Keighley & Allan 1986, Nordgren et al 1992). In a series of 68 patients having rectal excision for Crohn's disease, 29 (43%) still had unhealed perineal wounds 6 months later (de Dombal et al 1971). No fewer than 23 of these were noted to have perineal sepsis before operation (de Dombal et al 1971). So notorious are the problems of healing of the perineum after Crohn's proctectomy that some have even advocated a low Hartmann's procedure to avoid the perineal wound (Sher & Bauer 1992).

Management options for the postproctectomy persistent perineal sinus (non-healing after 6 months) range from conservative measures alone through local surgical revision to muscle flap perineal reconstruction.

CONSERVATIVE MEASURES

The mere presence of a persistent perineal sinus does not mandate surgical intervention. In many patients with incomplete perineal healing after rectal excision, the symptoms encountered are trivial or non-existent. The sinus may be a small pit or opening only evident to the surgeon on examination, and of no consequence to the patient. Some patients with a small amount of discharge may need to wear a pad to avoid soiling of the underwear. In others, the unhealed wound may persist for years, making sitting painful and producing a distressing, irritating discharge. These are the patients in whom surgical revision of the non-healing sinus should be considered.

LOCAL SURGICAL PROCEDURES

Curettage

In patients with small symptomatic perineal wounds the simplest local surgical procedure is curettage to remove granulation tissue. Those who advocate this method stress that frequent supervision of the wound packing is required to maximize the chances of success, and they state that curettage of the wound can be repeated on several occasions until healing is achieved (Kasper 1984).

For more extensive perineal wounds some used to recommend a combination of curettage and skin grafting (Anderson & Turnbull 1976). The unhealed perineal sinus was widely saucerized and 2–3 days later the granulating surface was covered with a split-skin graft. Of 48 patients with a non-healing perineal wound after proctectomy, 35 required a single grafting procedure and 13 required two procedures. Although 44 of these patients were judged to have had a good result and four a poor result, only a few patients achieved complete healing of the perineum (Anderson & Turnbull 1976). The technique was described in the 1970s and has not been popular in the United Kingdom.

Excision of the perineal sinus

This approach is well suited to the small sinus that can be adequately excised locally. If the wound produced can be closed without tension, then primary healing may be obtained (Ferrari & den Besten 1980). Alternatively, the cone-shaped cavity left by excision can be allowed to heal by granulation (Silen & Glotzer 1974). However, the deeper the sinus the less likely is limited local excision of the track to succeed. Under these circumstances the presence of the immovable sacrum and coccyx keeps the perineal wound cavity from collapsing and closing. Also in the 1970s this 'space problem' of the perineal wound was recommended to be tackled by resection of part of the coccyx and sacrum, allowing free drainage of the apex of the cavity. Healing of the cavity then occurs by wound contraction and ingrowth of epithelium from the buttocks (Silen & Glotzer 1974).

Although satisfactory healing of the persistent perineal sinus can be achieved in some patients by local surgical procedures alone, a significant number of patients do not heal using these techniques. In one series of 21 patients with persistent perineal sinus, satisfactory wound healing had not been achieved despite an average of 6.8 local surgical procedures (range 1–25) (Pezim et al 1987). In such patients reconstruction of the perineum with a muscle flap should be considered (Anthony & Mathes 1990).

MUSCLE FLAP PERINEAL RECONSTRUCTION

The well vascularized muscle flap provides a good blood supply to the perineal wound, and tissue bulk to fill the cavity of the persistent sinus (Chang & Mathes 1982). Before this type of reconstruction is performed active perineal sepsis must be adequately treated. The muscle flaps that are available to close the persistent perineal sinus are based on the gluteal muscles, the hamstrings (semimembranosus and gracilis) or the rectus abdominis muscles.

Gluteal muscle flaps

Flaps based on the gluteus maximus muscle have to be raised with the patient in the prone position. The presence of both superior and inferior gluteal arteries means that it is possible to split the muscle and use either its superior or inferior half as a flap, with an associated skin island (Anthony & Mathes 1990, Shaw & Futrell 1978).

The gluteal thigh flap (Anthony & Mathes 1990, Hurwitz 1980), can be raised with the patient in either the prone or the lithotomy position. This flap is supplied by the descending branch of the inferior gluteal artery. Its primary use is in perineal wounds with extensive skin defects (Achauer et al 1983).

Hamstring muscle flaps

Semimembranosus muscle (Mann & Springall 1986)

An incision is made along the semimembranosus muscle, which is divided at its distal end. The muscle is then swung into the wound, preserving vessels which enter the muscle close to its origin on the ischial tuberosity. The perineal skin is then sutured primarily. Mann and Springall (1986) reported on five patients (one Crohn's, four ulcerative colitis) with a persistent perineal sinus (average duration 4.2 years) who achieved complete healing with a semimembranosus muscle flap.

Gracilis muscle flap

The gracilis muscle (supplied by the medial femoral circumflex vessels) is usually mobilized with the patient in the lithotomy position (Bartholdson & Hulten 1975). In this technique the gracilis muscle is mobilized through a long incision in the medial portion of the thigh. The distal end of the muscle is divided and then transposed as high as possible into the perineal wound. Of four patients (three Crohn's, one ulcerative colitis) with persistent perineal sinus, two healed and two failed (Bartholdson & Hulten 1975). The failures resulted from necrosis of the gracilis muscle flap.

Greater success with perineal gracilis muscle reconstruction was seen in a Mayo Clinic series of 21 patients with persistent perineal sinus (Crohn's disease ten, ulcerative colitis seven, trauma two, cancer two), (Pezim et al 1987). A single gracilis flap was used in 16 patients, six of which had a skin island attached to the muscle. A further four patients had bilateral gracilis flaps, one with a skin island. At a mean follow-up of 47 months the sinus had healed completely in 14 patients (66%). The average time to wound healing in this successful group was 2.3 months. Among the one-third of patients with an unhealed perineal sinus after gracilis muscle repair, no association was found between healing and the primary disease, previous radiotherapy, postoperative sepsis or type of flap (Pezim et al 1987).

Rectus abdominis muscle flap

Transposition of the rectus abdominis muscle to the perineum, based on the inferior epigastric vessels, is best done through the abdomen. This muscle flap is usually employed with a combined abdominoperineal approach to the postproctectomy perineal wound (Young et al 1988, Cox et al 1991).

The perineal sinus is excised by abdominal and perineal dissection and the rectus abdominis muscle is isolated on the inferior epigastric artery and detached from the costal margin. The upper end of the rectus is then led through the dissected tract and delivered into the perineum, with suture of the perineal skin over it (Young et al 1988). The rectus sheath is repaired with a non-absorbable suture. Later abdominal wall weakness does not appear to be a problem.

SUMMARY

Non-healing of the perineum after proctectomy occurs in up to 40% of patients with Crohn's disease. It is less common with ulcerative colitis. In most patients conservative measures alone or simple curettage or wound excision will achieve a satisfactory outcome. For more recalcitrant perineal wounds extensive curettage with skin grafting or sacrococcygeal excision was advocated but is now rarely used, as muscle flap reconstruction offers a better alternative. Gluteus maximus or the gracilis muscle is used in a purely perineal approach and the rectus abdominis muscle for a combined abdominoperineal approach.

REFERENCES

Achauer B M, Turpin I M, Furnas D W 1983 Gluteal thigh flap in reconstruction of complex pelvic wounds. Archives of Surgery 118: 18–22

Anderson R, Turnbull R B 1976 Grafting the unhealed perineal wound after coloproctectomy for Crohn's disease. Archives of Surgery 111: 335–338

Anthony J P, Mathes S J 1990 The recalcitrant perineal wound after rectal extirpation. Applications of muscle flap closure. Archives of Surgery 125 1371–1377

Bartholdson L, Hulten L 1975 Repair of persistent perineal sinuses by means of a pedicle flap of musculus gracilis. Scandinavian Journal of Reconstructive Surgery 9: 74–76

Chang N, Mathes S J 1982 Comparison of the effect of bacterial inoculation in musculocutaneous and random pattern flaps. Plastic and Reconstructive Surgery 70: 1–9

Cox M R, Parks T G, Hanna W A, Leonard A G 1991 Closure of persistent post-proctectomy perineal sinus using a rectus muscle flap. Australia and New Zealand Journal of Surgery 61: 67–71

de Dombal F T, Burton I, Goligher J C 1971 The early and late results of surgical treatment for Crohn's Disease. British Journal of Surgery 58: 805–816

Ferrari B T, den Besten L 1980 The prevention and treatment of the persistent perineal sinus. World Journal of Surgery 4: 167–171

Fry R D, Shemesh E I, Kodner I J, Timmcke A 1989 Techniques and results in the management of anal and perianal Crohn's disease. Surgery, Gynecology and Obstetrics 168: 42–48

Hurwitz D J 1980 Closure of a large defect in the pelvic cavity by an extended compound myocutaneous flap based on the inferior gluteal artery. British Journal of Plastic Surgery 33: 256

Kasper R 1984 Persistent perineal sinus. Surgical Clinics of North America 64: 761–768

Keighley M R, Allan R N 1986 Current status and influence of operation on perianal Crohn's disease. International Journal of Colorectal Disease 1: 104–107

Levien D H, Surrell J, Mazier W P 1989 Surgical treatment of anorectal fistula in patients with Crohn's disease. Surgery, Gynecology and Obstetrics 169: 133–136

Mann C V, Springall R 1986 Use of muscle graft for unhealed perineal sinus. British Journal of Surgery 73: 1000–1001

Nordgren S, Fasth S, Hulten L 1992 Anal fistulas in Crohn's disease: incidence and outcome of surgical treatment. International Journal of Colorectal Disease 7: 214–218

Pezim M E, Wolf B G, Woods J E, Beart R W, Ilstrup D M 1987 Closure of postproctectomy perineal sinus with gracilis muscle flaps. Canadian Journal of Surgery 30: 212–214

Shaw A, Futrell J W 1978 Cure of chronic perineal sinus with gluteus maximus flap. Surgery, Gynecology and Obstetrics 147: 417–420

Sher M E, Bauer J J 1992 Low Hartmann's procedure for severe anorectal Crohn's disease. Diseases of the Colon and Rectum 35: 975–980

Silen W, Glotzer D J 1974 The prevention and treatment of the persistent perineal sinus. Surgery 75: 535–542

van Dongen L M, Lubbers E J 1986 Perianal fistulas in patients with Crohn's disease. Archives of Surgery 121: 1187–1190

Young M R A, Small J O, Leonard A G, McKelvey S T D 1988 Rectus abdominis muscle flap for persistent perineal sinus. British Journal of Surgery 75: 1228

102. Management of fecal incontinence complicating inflammatory bowel disease

R. D. Madoff

Diarrhea and urgency are among the cardinal symptoms of inflammatory bowel disease. Troublesome as these complaints are, the distress they cause increases exponentially when they are combined with the inability to maintain continence.

NORMAL FUNCTION

Normal continence depends upon an intact neuroanatomic arc that extends from the cerebral cortex to the anal sphincter. Defects in this pathway, alone or in combination, lead to incontinence (Madoff et al 1992). Fecal incontinence is frequently due to a combination of factors.

The normal sphincter mechanism comprises the puborectalis, the external anal sphincter and the internal anal sphincter. The puborectalis is a sling-shaped muscle which, as its name implies, originates on the pubis and loops posteriorly behind the rectum. This muscle, innervated by pelvic branches of S3 and S4 (Percy et al 1981), is easily appreciated posteriorly on digital rectal examination as the anorectal ring. Puborectalis contraction pulls the anorectal junction anteriorly and superiorly and sharpens the anorectal angle. The physiologic importance of an acute anorectal angle is a contentious issue. Although this has been postulated to be the anatomic basis of a 'flap valve' mechanism (Parks 1975) combined radiologic and manometric studies have failed to demonstrate a physiologic 'valve' (Bartolo et al 1986, Bannister et al 1987).

The internal anal sphincter is the thickened distal portion of the circular smooth muscle layer of the rectum; it provides approximately 80% of resting anal pressure (Frenckner & Guler 1975, Schweiger 1979). The internal anal sphincter is surrounded by the external sphincter, a skeletal muscle which accounts for the remaining 20% of resting pressure and all additional 'squeeze' anal pressure generated by voluntary contraction. The external anal sphincter is innervated by branches of the pudendal nerve (S2,3,4) (Percy et al 1981). Despite the fact that the external anal sphincter is composed of predominantly slow twitch, fatigue-resistant muscle fibers, maximum voluntary contraction pressures can generally be maintained only for 1 minute or less before fatigue sets in and pressures diminish (Pemberton & Kelly 1986).

Intact rectal and anal sensation are important components of normal continence. There is a well documented physiologic 'sampling' reflex whereby rectal distension leads to internal sphincter relaxation and subsequent external anal sphincter contraction. The absence of this 'sampling' reflex correlates with poor control (Miller et al 1988). None the less, the exact function of the reflex remains unproven, despite the suggestive presence of many sensory receptors in the transitional anal mucosa.

Colonic transit and stool volume and consistency can also be important factors in the maintenance of continence. An entirely normal sphincter can be overcome by severe diarrhea of any cause. Normal rectal reservoir function is also important. Although many laboratories attempt to quantify this function by determining rectal 'compliance', the significance of this measurement (as opposed to the significance of reservoir function) is questionable (Madoff et al 1990).

ABNORMALITIES WITH INFLAMMATORY BOWEL DISEASE

Inflammatory bowel disease is associated with a number of problems that can lead to fecal incontinence. These frequently may be compounded by additional unrelated abnormalities (Table 102.1) (Madoff et al 1992). Common factors include anal sphincter disruption (due to trauma, childbirth or anorectal surgery), peripheral neuropathy (due to diabetes mellitus) and pudendal neuropathy (due to childbirth, chronic straining at stool and rectal prolapse).

As already noted, diarrhea predisposes to incontinence because of the large stool volume, liquid consistency and high pressure at which they enter the rectum. Frequent causes of diarrhea in inflammatory bowel disease include active disease, extensive surgical bowel resection and,

Table 102.1 Causes of fecal incontinence. (From Madoff et al 1992, with permission)

Congenital anorectal abnormalities
Spina bifida/myelomeningocele
Anorectal malformations

Overflow
Impaction
Encopresis
Rectal neoplasms
Constipating drugs

Incontinence with a normal pelvic floor
  Diarrheal states
    Infectious diarrhea
    Inflammatory bowel disease
    Short gut syndrome
    Laxative abuse
    Radiation enteritis
  Neurologic conditions
    Multiple sclerosis
    Dementia/strokes/tabes dorsalis
    Neuropathies (e.g., diabetes)
    Neoplasms of brain/spinal cord/cauda equina
    Injuries to brain/spinal cord/cauda equina

Incontinence with an abnormal pelvic floor
  Trauma
    Accidental injuries (impalement, pelvic fractures)
    Anorectal surgery
    Obstetrical injury
  Aging
  Pelvic floor denervation (idiopathic neurogenic incontinence)
    Prolonged vaginal delivery
    Chronic straining at stool
    Rectal prolapse
    Descending perineum syndrome

occasionally, an internal fistula (e.g. ileosigmoid). Active proctitis leads to increased rectal irritability, with an associated decreased ability to tolerate distension.

Anal operations, with or without inflammatory bowel disease, can lead to disordered continence. Lateral internal sphincterotomy for anal fissure causes minor incontinence in up to 30% of otherwise normal patients (Garcia-Aguilar et al 1996). Anal fistulotomy, which may require division of larger quantities of sphincter muscle than does sphincterotomy, alters control in 45% of patients (Garcia-Aguilar et al 1994). The adverse effects on continence of sphincter division can be expected to be magnified in the presence of diarrhea or proctitis. Furthermore, because patients with Crohn's disease are predisposed to perianal suppuration, they often develop multiple fistulae that may need surgical attention. Because of this, surgical conservatism with muscle preservation and liberal use of setons is mandatory for fistula management when Crohn's disease is known or suspected. The adage that the surgeon and not the disease leads to incontinence in Crohn's disease is, unfortunately, for the most part correct. However, it is equally true that patients with anorectal Crohn's disease may develop fecal incontinence as the result of chronic sepsis and fibrosis, even in the absence of surgical intervention.

Impaired continence is common after proctocolectomy with ileal pouch–anal anastomosis (see Chapter 90) (Wexner et al 1990). This is due in part to the physiology of pouch motility, which generates high-pressure contractile waves after a threshold volume of distension is reached. Compared to patients who are continent following ileoanal pouch surgery, incontinent pouch patients have higher large pressure wave contractions and increased basal and phasic pouch pressures at night and following evacuation (Grotz et al 1994). The sampling reflex is lost after operation but returns over the course of 1 year; this is associated with renewed ability to discriminate flatus from stool (Sagar et al 1991). In addition, sphincter pressures decrease following anal mucosectomy, presumably owing to excessive traction on the sphincter mechanism. Because of this, many surgeons have abandoned anal mucosectomy in favor of an extended low double-stapled anastomosis performed at or just above the dentate line. Although the double-stapled technique avoids anal dilatation and preserves sphincter pressure, it is also associated with a shortened high-pressure zone due to low transsection of the internal anal sphincter (Wexner et al 1991). Studies using retrospective controls have suggested that there are better functional results using the two-stage technique; prospective trial data are unfortunately still lacking.

CLINICAL EVALUATION

A detailed clinical history and careful physical examination are the mainstays of evaluation for patients with inflammatory bowel disease who develop incontinence. Because these patients often have complicated histories and have had many operations, every effort should be made to obtain old charts and operative notes.

True fecal incontinence must be differentiated from simple fecal urgency and from perianal soiling, which can be caused by poor hygiene, mucus leakage or fistula drainage. Pseudoincontinence may be caused by vaginal drainage due to colo-, recto- or anovaginal fistulae.

Once the diagnosis of true fecal incontinence is established, it is important to assess the severity of the disorder and its impact on the patient. Patients should be questioned as to the nature, frequency and timing of their accidents. Because solid stool is the easiest to control, loss of solid stool denotes the most severe level of incontinence. Conversely, gas is the most difficult substance to control and the loss of flatus alone indicates mild incontinence. Liquid stool incontinence occupies an intermediate position. Frequency of incontinent events is a simple and important measure of incontinence severity. In addition, because control is generally best by day, when volitional reflexes are intact, diurnal incontinence is considered to be more severe than nocturnal. Another good indication of incontinence severity is the need to wear protective pads and the number of pads used per day.

Much can be learned from a simple physical examination. Perineal inspection may reveal staining of the underwear, perianal excoriation and anal deformity. A careful search should be made for perianal disease, including anal ulcers and fistulae. Digital examination gives a good qualitative evaluation of resting and squeeze anal pressures, and bidigital examination should be performed when a rectovaginal fistula is suspected.

DIAGNOSTIC EVALUATION

Diagnostic evaluation should have two goals: to assess the activity of the inflammatory bowel disease and to evaluate the function of the pelvic floor. Gastrointestinal evaluation is performed by endoscopy and contrast radiography. Endoscopic evaluation of the large-bowel mucosa is essential. Directed studies such as CT and vaginogram for fistula may be needed.

Specialized tests are necessary to evaluate the pelvic floor and anal sphincters. Although these tests are not always essential, they are often helpful in confirming a suspected diagnosis, demonstrating associated abnormalities and providing quantification of the dysfunction.

Anal manometry uses a pressure transducer to create a four-quadrant pressure profile of the anal canal (Smith et al 1990, Felt-Bersma et al 1990). These studies are usually performed with the patient at rest and during maximum voluntary squeeze effort. Resting and maximum voluntary contraction anal pressures indicate the functional status of the internal and external anal sphincters respectively. Vector manometry, which assesses cross-sectional pressures in the anal canal, is occasionally useful to identify the site of a sphincter defect (Perry et al 1990).

Anal ultrasonography is increasingly used in the assessment of sphincter anatomy. The technique utilizes a rotating 7.5 or 10 mHz probe that is inserted into the anal canal and provides a 360° scan. The technique precisely delineates the normal anatomy of the internal and external anal sphincters and identifies anatomic disruptions, as well as concomitant pathology such as abscess and fistula (Law et al 1990, Cuesta et al 1992, Burnett et al 1991). Anal ultrasonography is particularly useful to define the sphincter anatomy of patients who have had many anorectal operations.

Sphincter innervation is evaluated using electromyography to assess the conduction time along the pudendal nerve from the level of the ischial spine to the anal sphincter (pudendal nerve terminal motor latency, PNTML) (Snooks & Swash 1985). This technique is painless and uses a glove-mounted electrode. Use of the needle EMG, to assess innervation (Neill & Swash 1980) and to map the location of sphincter defects (Bartolo et al 1983), has now been supplanted by a combination of PNTML studies and anal ultrasonography. Assessment of pudendal nerve conduction is important to rule out nerve injury from previous surgery or from the traction neuropathy that is commonly associated with prolonged vaginal childbirth.

Dynamic radiologic studies of rectal evacuation (cinedefecography) are frequently used in the evaluation of incontinent patients, particularly to assess impaired evacuation and when associated pathology (e.g. internal intussusception, rectocele) is suspected (Mahieu et al 1984). They are not always necessary when evaluating patients with inflammatory bowel disease.

TREATMENT

Treatment of incontinence associated with inflammatory bowel disease depends upon the severity of the problem, the specific cause of the incontinence and the status of the proximal gastrointestinal tract. In general, the first step in managing the incontinence is to treat the inflammatory bowel disease. This may require additional medical therapy, surgery or a combination. The importance of abdominal (rather than anorectal) surgery to improve bowel function in inflammatory bowel disease patients deserves emphasis. Resection of intra-abdominal (e.g. segmental Crohn's disease or ileosigmoid fistula) often cures incontinence by managing the underlying diarrhea. Similarly, patients with severe colitis may have unacceptable fecal urgency or incontinence which improves when the inflamed rectum is replaced with a healthy ileoanal reservoir.

Minor incontinence of any cause often responds to simple conservative therapy. Antimotility drugs (given in moderation) and stool bulking agents are often beneficial to alleviate the effects of diarrhea. Minor leakage is often controlled by placing a small cotton wad between the buttocks adjacent to the anal orifice. A barrier cream may prevent skin excoriation.

For patients with more severe degrees of incontinence, choice of therapy is dictated by the presence or absence of pelvic floor or sphincter abnormalities. The most straightforward of these to correct is an anterior sphincter defect, such as that caused by childbirth injury. Repair follows mobilization of the entire anterior sphincter to the level of the levators by way of an anterior U-shaped incision. Dissection is not performed posterior to the midline as the nerve supply enters the muscle posterolaterally. The scar tissue is divided but not excised. A snug overlapping plication is performed. Although in the absence of inflammatory bowel disease patients do not normally need a proximal stoma, fecal diversion may be reasonable in patients with Crohn's disease.

Unfortunately, sphincter division secondary to sphincterotomy is frequently off the midline and sphincter repair under these circumstances is more difficult. Overlapping repair may be impossible, in which case simple apposition with absorbable sutures is performed (Pezim et al 1987, Arnaud et al 1991). Particular care must be taken when mobilizing the sphincter edges laterally to avoid injury to the pudendal nerve branches. Results of sphincter repair following fistula treatment are not as good as those following obstetrical injury.

There are few collected series of sphincter repairs in the presence of Crohn's disease. The largest series is of six patients treated over 15 years at St Mark's Hospital in London. Five of the six were women. Incontinence was due to abscess or fistula surgery in five patients and one patient became incontinent following obstetrical injury. All patients had perianal disease (quiescent in five), and all but one had had intestinal disease resected. All had an overlapping sphincteroplasty and all but one had a proximal diverting stoma, either before or at the time of the repair. Five of the six patients were rendered fully continent with a mean follow-up of almost 8 years. One patient remained incontinent and required permanent colostomy.

Biofeedback is an increasingly popular treatment for fecal incontinence, whatever the cause. An instrument (manometer or EMG) quantifies and displays the magnitude of external anal sphincter contraction. Patients are trained to recognize decreasing volumes of rectal distension, to increase sphincter contraction in response to this distension, and then to maintain this response as the instrumental feedback is gradually withdrawn. A typical patient requires three or four weekly sessions of 10–45 minutes, and performs exercises at home, sometimes with a home training unit.

Candidates for biofeedback must be well motivated, able to follow instructions, have some degree of rectal sensation and some ability to contract their sphincter muscle. The technique works poorly in patients with dementia, marked neurologic disease or absent rectal sensation. The technique also works poorly in patients with 'keyhole' anal deformities. In patients with inflammatory bowel disease active proctitis is associated with poor results (Wald 1994).

Biofeedback has the advantage of being painless and causes no morbidity. Reported success rates, depending upon patient selection and definition of success, range from 65 to 90%. At the University of Minnesota, 154 of 188 incontinent patients (82%) treated with biofeedback had a successful outcome, defined as at least a 90% decrease in incontinent events (Jensen & Lowry 1994). The technique is useful both as primary therapy and as an adjunct to unsuccessful or partially successful sphincter repair.

Anal encirclement has been used as a salvage procedure for incontinent patients in whom direct sphincter repair was impossible or has failed. Prosthetic materials are associated with a high incidence of local complications and are rarely recommended (Vongsangnak et al 1985). However, a limited but largely successful experience with inflatable artificial anal sphincters has been reported (Wong & Rothenberger 1990).

Transposed gracilis and gluteus muscles have also been used in patients without inflammatory bowel disease. Reasonable results have been reported for control of solid stool, but control of liquid stool and flatus are often poor (Corman 1985, Devesa et al 1992). This technique has been improved by the addition of an implantable electrical pulse generator. This is used first to convert the muscle from type 2 (fast twitch, fatiguable) to type 1 (slow twitch, fatigue resistant) fibers by means of a graded stimulation protocol (Konsten et al 1993, Williams et al 1991). The converted muscle is then maintained in a tonically contracted state until the patient wishes to defecate, at which time the pulse generator is deactivated by a handheld magnet and the muscle relaxes. This technique has been successful in roughly two-thirds of patients treated (Konsten et al 1993, Williams et al 1991, Baeten et al 1991). Results in patients with inflammatory bowel disease are unknown.

Creation of a stoma is often the best option for patients whose inflammatory bowel disease is complicated by incontinence. When severe or rectal or perianal disease is present, proctectomy should be performed. Although many patients are reluctant to accept a stoma despite severe ongoing incontinence, it should be emphasized that quality of life improves markedly when a manageable incontinent anus is converted to an abdominal stoma. Once the patient agrees to have a stoma, it is critical that the surgeon creates a well vascularized, nicely everted and properly sited ostomy. A stoma therapist should be consulted before operation to educate the patient in stoma care and to mark a suitable site that is visible to the patient and away from abdominal scars, deformities and bony protuberances. Unfortunately, 'optimal' stoma sites can be hard to find in Crohn's disease patients who have already had many abdominal operations, and a compromise location must sometimes be accepted.

REFERENCES

Arnaud A, Sarles J C, Sieleznef I et al 1991 Sphincter repair without overlapping for fecal incontinence. Diseases of the Colon and Rectum 34: 744–747

Baeten C G M I, Konsten J, Spaans F et al 1991 Dynamic graciloplasty for treatment of faecal incontinence. Lancet 338: 1163–1165

Bannister J J, Gibbons C, Read N W 1987 Preservation of faecal continence during rises in intraabdominal pressure: is there a role for the flap valve? Gut 28: 1241–1245

Bartolo D C, Jarrat J A, Read N W 1983 The use of conventional electromyography to assess external sphincter neuropathy in man. Journal of Neurology Neurosurgery and Psychiatry 46: 1115–1118

Bartolo D C C, Roe A M, Locke-Edmunds J C, Virjee J, Mortensen N J M 1986 Flap-valve theory of anorectal continence. British Journal of Surgery 73: 1012–1014

Burnett S J, Speakman C T, Kamm M A, Bartram C I 1991 Confirmation of endosonographic detection of external anal sphincter defects by simultaneous electromyographic mapping. British Journal of Surgery 78: 448–450

Corman M L 1985 Gracilis muscle transposition for anal incontinence: late results. British Journal of Surgery 72 (Suppl): S21–S22

Cuesta M A, Meijer S, Derksen E J, Boutkan H, Meuwissen S G 1992 Anal sphincter imaging in fecal incontinence using endosonography. Diseases of the Colon and Rectum 35: 59–63

Devesa J M, Vicente E, Enriquez J M 1992 Total fecal incontinence – a new method of gluteus maximus transposition: preliminary results in reported previous experience with similar procedures. Diseases of the Colon and Rectum 35: 339–349

Felt-Bersma R J, Klinkenberg-Knol E C, Meuwissen S G 1990 Anorectal function investigations in incontinent and continent patients: differences and discriminatory value. Diseases of the Colon and Rectum 33: 479–486

Frenckner B, Euler C H R V 1975 Influence of pudendal block on the function of the anal sphincters. Gut 16: 482–489

Garcia-Aguilar J, Belmonte C, Wong W D, Lowry A C, Madoff R D 1996 Open vs. closed sphincterotomy for chronic anal fissure: long-term results. Diseases of the Colon and Rectum 39: 440–443

Garcia-Aguilar J, Belmonte C, Wong W D, Goldberg S M, Madoff R D 1994 Surgical treatment of fistula-in-ano: factors associated with recurrence and incontinence. Diseases of the Colon and Rectum 37: P8

Grotz R L, Pemberton J H, Ferrara A, Hanson R B 1994 Ileopouch pressures after defecation in continent and incontinent patients. Diseases of the Colon and Rectum 37: 1073–1077

Jensen L L, Lowry A C 1994 Biofeedback for incontinence and constipation. Principles of Colon and Rectal Surgery (syllabus) University of Minnesota

Konsten J, Baeten C G, Spaans F, Havenith M G, Soeters P B 1993 Follow-up of anal dynamic graciloplasty for fecal continence. World Journal of Surgery 17: 404–409

Law P J, Kamm M A, Bartram C I 1990 A comparison between electromyography and anal endosonography in mapping external anal sphincter defects. Diseases of the Colon and Rectum 33: 370–373

Madoff R D, Orrom W I, Rothenberger D A, Goldberg S M 1990 Rectal compliance: a critical reappraisal. International Journal of Colorectal Disease 5: 37–40

Madoff R D, Williams J G, Caushaj P F 1992 Fecal incontinence. New England Journal of Medicine 326: 1002–1007

Mahieu P, Pringot J, Bodart O 1984 Defecography. II. Contribution to the diagnosis of defecation disorders. Gastrointestinal Radiology 9: 253–261

Miller R, Bartolo D C, Cervero F, Mortensen N J 1988 Anorectal sampling: a comparison of normal and incontinent patients. British Journal of Surgery 75: 44–47

Neill M E, Swash M 1980 Increased motor unit fibre density in the external anal sphincter muscle in anorectal incontinence: a single fibre EMG study. Journal of Neurology Neurosurgery and Psychiatry 43: 343–347

Parks A G 1975 Anorectal incontinence. Proceedings of the Royal Society of Medicine 68: 681–690

Pemberton J H, Kelly K A 1986 Achieving enteric continence: principles and applications. Mayo Clinic Proceedings 61: 586–599

Percy J P, Neill M E, Swash M, Parks A G 1981 Electrophysiological study of motor nerve supply of the pelvic floor. Lancet 1: 16–17

Perry R E, Blatchford G J, Christensen M A, Thorson A G, Attwood S E 1990 Manometric diagnosis of anal sphincter injuries. American Journal of Surgery 159: 112–117

Pezim M E, Spencer R J, Stanhope C R et al 1987 Sphincter repair for fecal incontinence after obstetrical or iatrogenic injury. Diseases of the Colon and Rectum 30: 521–525

Sagar P M, Holdsworth P J, Johnson D 1991 Correlation between laboratory findings and clinical outcome after restorative proctocolectomy: studies in 20 patients with end to end pouch–anal anastomosis. British Journal of Surgery 78: 67–69

Schweiger M 1979 Method for determining individual contributions of voluntary and involuntary anal sphincters to resting tone. Diseases of the Colon and Rectum 22: 415–416

Smith L E (ed) 1990 Practical guide to anorectal testing. Igaku-Shoin, New York

Snooks S J, Swash M 1985 Nerve stimulation techniques. In: Henry M M, Swash M (eds) Coloproctology and the pelvic floor. Butterworths, London, pp 112–128

Vongsangnak V, Varma J S, Smith A N 1985 Reappraisal of Thiersch's operation for complete rectal prolapse. Journal of the Royal College of Surgeons of Edinburgh 30: 185–187

Wald A 1994 Biofeedback treatment for fecal incontinence In: Kuijpers H C (ed) Colorectal physiology: fecal incontinence. CRC Press, Boca Raton, pp 173–177

Wexner S D, James K, Jagelman D G 1991 The double-stapled ileal reservoir and ileoanal anastomosis. A prospective review of sphincter function and clinical outcome. Diseases of the Colon and Rectum 34: 487–494

Wexner S D, Wong W D, Rothenberger D A, Goldberg S M 1990 The ileoanal reservoir. American Journal of Surgery 159: 178–185

Williams N S, Patel J, George B D, Hallan R I, Watkins E S 1991 Development of an electrically stimulated neoanal sphincter. Lancet 338: 1166–1169

Wong W D, Rothenberger D A 1990 Surgical approaches to anal incontinence. In: Bock G (ed) The neurobiology of incontinence. John Wiley and Sons, London, pp 246–266

103. Sexual dysfunction in inflammatory bowel disease

A. C. Lowry   K. I. Deen

Sexual dysfunction secondary to chronic illness is always troublesome. It is particularly so in patients with inflammatory bowel disease, as the peak incidence is in young adults. To successfully help patients cope with their illness clinicians must be aware of the potential impact of the disease and its treatment on sexual function.

SEXUAL DYSFUNCTION COMPLICATING INFLAMMATORY BOWEL DISEASE

Sexual function has both physical and psychological components, both of which may be affected by inflammatory bowel disease. Reduced sexual interest, dyspareunia and impotence all occur in patients with inflammatory bowel disease. The exact incidence of sexual dysfunction is unknown as the patient may not tell the doctor about sexual difficulties because of embarrassment or because they fail to associate it with the disease. Moody et al (1992) conducted a prospective case control study in 50 women with Crohn's disease using a structured questionnaire to assess sexual dysfunction. They found that women with Crohn's disease described sexual difficulties more often than age-matched controls (27% of Crohn's patients compared with 4% of controls). A number of contributory factors were found in this study: abdominal pain during intercourse, diarrhea and the fear of fecal incontinence.

Sexual desire may be reduced by generalized debility and nutritional depletion. Patients with perianal disease or fecal incontinence may avoid sexual encounters for fear of embarrassment. Emotional support, appropriate medical or surgical treatment, and nutritional support are necessary.

Dyspareunia affects both males and females with inflammatory bowel disease. Dyspareunia in patients with Crohn's disease is commonly related to perianal disease or the juxtaposition of the diseased segment of ileum to the uterus and posterior fornix. In ulcerative colitis patients proctitis or apposition of inflamed colon to the uterus may result in dyspareunia. Metastatic Crohn's disease in the form of skin lesions distant from the intestinal tract may occur on male and female genitalia, leading to dyspareunia (Hamilton et al 1997). Studies show that dyspareunia is more common in women with Crohn's disease than in controls. In the study by Moody et al (1992) dyspareunia was significantly more common in patients than controls (60% vs. 34% respectively), independent of the site of intestinal disease. Furthermore, they found a greater incidence of vaginal candidiasis in patients with Crohn's disease, which may contribute to dyspareunia. Sagar and colleagues (1993) used questionnaires to assess the quality of life in patients with medically treated colitis compared to patients with restorative proctocolectomies. Four of the 45 medically treated women (8.9%) reported dyspareunia. In a study of 71 women undergoing proctocolectomy for either ulcerative colitis or Crohn's disease, Wikland and colleagues (1990) found that 8 of 66 women (12%) reported dyspareunia preoperatively. The data were not sorted by type of disease.

Impotence is an important cause of sexual dysfunction in males with inflammatory bowel disease treated medically (Ireland & Jewell 1989). One cause is treatment with sulfasalazine. In such cases withdrawal of the drug has usually resulted in improvement of symptoms. In the study by Sagar and colleagues (1993) already cited, 13 of 50 males (26%) were impotent on medical therapy. Eight others (16%) reported frequent failure of ejaculation. The authors speculate that increased age, higher anxiety scores and the use of steroids might be contributory.

The few studies available for analysis indicate that sexual dysfunction is more common among patients with medically treated inflammatory bowel disease than previously thought. It may be that increased awareness by clinicians has helped patients identify the problem.

Treatment of sexual dysfunction varies according to the cause. Some forms may respond to a change in medication. Aggressive treatment of perianal disease may be necessary to alleviate dyspareunia. If dyspareunia is secondary to the apposition of a diseased intestinal segment to the uterus or vagina, it may be an indication for surgical resection.

SEXUAL DYSFUNCTION COMPLICATING SURGICAL MANAGEMENT OF INFLAMMATORY BOWEL DISEASE

As resection of diseased bowel generally results in improved general health, sexual function typically improves after operation (Damgaard et al 1995). In a study of 180 patients who underwent colectomy and ileoanal reservoir construction, 44 (23%) reported an increase in sexual activity. Metcalf et al (1986), in their study of 100 women, found that 78% described increased frequency of intercourse postoperatively, which most attributed to improved overall health. Most sexually active women were able to achieve orgasm both before (78%) and after (89%) surgery.

However, sexual dysfunction is a known complication of surgery for inflammatory bowel disease. Normal sexual function is dependent on intact parasympathetic and sympathetic nerves, both of which are vulnerable to injury during dissection of the rectum. The parasympathetic supply from the nervi erigentes originates from the second, third and fourth sacral nerves. The sympathetic supply derives from the first three lumbar segments of the spinal cord, giving rise to the preaortic plexus from which the presacral nerve arises. The presacral nerve divides into two branches which pass laterally where they join the parasympathetic nerves to form the pelvic plexus. The branches of the presacral nerve lie between the ureters, behind the inferior mesenteric vessels. They descend adjacent to the posterolateral aspect of the rectum and can be injured during mobilization of the rectum. The pelvic plexus lies on the pelvic side walls and is vulnerable if the lateral stalks are divided too far laterally. The periprostatic plexus arises from the pelvic plexus and travels anteriorly to supply the prostate, seminal vesicles, corpora cavernosa, urethra and ejaculatory ducts.

Erection involves both parasympathetic and sympathetic nervous systems. In addition, sympathetic nerves control ejaculation of semen from the ducts, seminal vesicles and prostate. Depending on the nerves injured, incomplete erection, lack of or retrograde ejaculation, or impotence may result (Nivatvongs & Gordon 1992). In addition to nerve damage, psychological factors, the patient's age and relationship, and the presence of a stoma may all contribute to sexual dysfunction.

Sexual dysfunction in males

Historically, when proctocolectomy was warranted in young males, a staged procedure was performed, removing the colon and leaving the rectum. The strategy was to defer proctectomy until the patient had achieved his procreative ambitions. The disadvantages were that it left potentially symptomatic residual disease and committed the individual to a second major procedure. Corman et al (1978) reviewed 151 patients at the Lahey Clinic to identify the incidence of male sexual dysfunction following proctectomy. They reported no instances of impotence in their study; however, their review of the literature revealed a 2% incidence of impotence. At approximately the same time as this review the techniques were described of perimuscular dissection of the rectum and intersphincteric dissection of the rectum (Lee & Dowling 1972, Lyttle & Parks 1977). Both techniques aim to avoid injury to the pelvic nerves. Leicester et al (1984), in a review of 23 male patients at St Mark's Hospital who underwent proctectomy employing a close perimuscular dissection, found that seven of the 23 reported transient sexual difficulties, including pain during intercourse, loss of desire, difficulty with penetration, premature ejaculation, failed ejaculation, and diminution in the intensity of orgasm. All of these symptoms resolved at least partially with time. Review at 6 years after operation revealed that four of 23 men had permanent erectile difficulty, and one had failure of ejaculation. Two of these patients felt that their stomas were a contributing factor to their difficulties.

In a study of proctectomy with perimuscular and intersphincteric dissection, Bauer et al (1986) reported permanent impotence in one of 187 men, whereas transient impotence was reported in two. These authors reported full recovery in one man who had been impotent for 3 years after operation. Yeager and Van Heerden (1980) compared sexual dysfunction in 25 men undergoing proctocolectomy for inflammatory bowel disease with 20 age-matched men who underwent abdominoperineal excision for cancer, where there is a much wider pelvic resection. The incidence of erectile impotence at a similar length of follow-up was 4% following proctocolectomy and 15% after abdominoperineal excision. This study supports the use of perimuscular and intersphincteric dissection whenever possible in inflammatory bowel disease. Compared to proctocolectomy alone, restorative proctocolectomy with ileal pouch–anal anastomosis for ulcerative colitis does not appear to be associated with a different incidence in these complications (Pemberton et al 1989).

These data indicate that the incidence and severity of sexual dysfunction in men is reduced but not completely abolished by conservative proctectomy. Although some of the dysfunction may be temporary, it is essential during preoperative counseling to inform patients undergoing proctectomy of the possibility of sexual dysfunction.

Evaluation of sexual dysfunction

Although postoperative impotence is most often neurogenic other possible causes need to be excluded, such as vascular or hormonal factors. Psychological causes may be distinguished from organic causes through a detailed medical and sexual history. Postoperative depression, which can be secondary to the creation of a stoma, contributes to sexual dysfunction. Vascular disease, generalized neurologic illness and hormonal imbalance may be identified with a careful history and physical examination.

In addition to the combined history and physical, Aboseif and colleagues (1990) outlined a protocol for further testing. Prostaglandin E_1 is injected intracavernously in the penis and the onset, extent and duration of erection are noted. A full erection obtained within 15 minutes and lasting at least 20 minutes makes arterial or venous insufficiency unlikely. A nocturnal penile tumescence test is undertaken to distinguish neurogenic from psychologic impotence. If ejaculatory disorders are identified in the patient's history, the presence of sperm in the urine separates retrograde ejaculation from failure of ejaculation.

Management of impotence and ejaculatory failure

If the patient does develop permanent erectile dysfunction, a penile prosthesis is the obvious therapeutic option. A less invasive alternative is intracavernous injection of vasoactive agents which bypass the neurologic mechanism. Papaverine, with or without phentolamine, is the most widely used agent. Prostaglandin E_1 has also been shown to be effective and safe. Sidi (1986) reported a 100% response in patients with neurologic impotence. Complications include dizziness, pain, penile fibrosis and priapism.

It is possible to treat retrograde ejaculation, but this may be less rewarding. The use of sympathomimetic agents such as ephedrine sulfate (25–50 mg) four times a day, phenylpropanolamine hydrochloride (75 mg) twice daily, or imipramine hydrochloride (25 mg) twice daily has been shown to improve ejaculation by maintaining an increase in the smooth muscle tone of the vas deferens and internal sphincter urethra (Sigman & Howards 1992). When treatment of retrograde ejaculation is undertaken to improve fertility there should be an improvement in ejaculatory volume and sperm count within 2 weeks. Lack of improvement within this period indicates a poor chance of success. Infertility due to retrograde ejaculation not responding to medical treatment may be treated by recovery of sperm from the bladder and intrauterine insemination (Shargold et al 1990). Transrectal electrostimulation of the perioprostatic plexus has also been described (Brindley 1981), but its efficacy is uncertain.

Sexual dysfunction in females

Dyspareunia is the most common complaint in women after operation for ulcerative colitis or Crohn's disease. Often this symptom may not be recognized as having an association with the operation itself. The etiology of dyspareunia after surgical intervention is an important consideration. Historically, when abdominoperineal excision was necessary for inflammatory bowel disease of the anorectum, the posterior wall of the vagina was incorporated in the excision. This led to vaginal stenosis, which may have resulted in painful penetration. Since the development of the intersphincteric dissection technique for inflammatory bowel disease there has probably been a reduction in the incidence of vaginal stenosis, although no comparative data are available. However, even intersphincteric proctectomy does not completely prevent dyspareunia. Bauer et al (1986) reported temporary dyspareunia in two women who underwent proctectomy with an intersphincteric dissection. In both patients laceration of the vagina had occurred during proctectomy. This study raises the questions of the association of intraoperative vaginal injury with postoperative dyspareunia. In another study (Wikland et al 1990) 18 of 66 women (27%) complained of dyspareunia after proctocolectomy. No operative injury to the vagina was reported.

Translocation of the vagina after proctectomy is another possible cause of dyspareunia. Studies have shown that the vagina may be displaced horizontally after proctectomy, which may result in dyspareunia in both partners (Sjodahl et al 1990). Horizontal angulation of the vagina results in poor drainage of vaginal secretions and menstrual blood. Stasis causes vaginitis, further increasing dyspareunia in these women. Often, women need to wear pads to protect themselves from unexpected discharge of vaginal secretions.

Wikland and coworkers (1990) confirmed the problem of unexpected episodic discharge of vaginal secretions and found that 35 of 71 women (49%) had trouble with abnormal vaginal secretions after proctocolectomy, compared to 8 of 71 women (9%) preoperatively. Heavy vaginal secretions without vaginal infection were confirmed by gynecological examination in 32 of 35 women. The finding was associated in most patients (68%) with what they described as a caudally fixed vagina.

Restorative proctocolectomy, in which the pouch of ileum is interpositioned between vagina anteriorly and sacrum posteriorly, should prevent vaginal angulation. In a recent report of 21 women after restorative proctocolectomy, Oresland et al (1994) reported a normal position of the uterus and vagina in all patients, demonstrated by contrast vaginography. Metcalf et al (1986) compared sexual function in 50 women who had an ileal pouch for ulcerative colitis with age-matched women who had a proctectomy and a Kock pouch. The authors found less postoperative dyspareunia (18% vs. 38%) in women with an ileoanal reservoir. Patients with a Kock pouch had more episodic vaginal discharge (18% vs. 0%). This study supports the concept that the presence of an ileal reservoir reduces horizontal vaginal translocation.

Septic complications following proctectomy or ileoanal anastomosis may also cause dyspareunia, particularly when the focus of sepsis is adjacent to the vagina or cervix.

Management of dyspareunia

Most dyspareunia complicating proctectomy for inflammatory bowel disease can be prevented. Dissection in the rectovaginal septum should leave the posterior vaginal wall intact. The vaginal introitus should be preserved during operation and vaginal laceration should be avoided. In women opting for an end ileostomy rather than an ileal reservoir horizontal angulation of the vagina may be prevented by interposition of omentum in the space between the vagina and sacrum.

To improve dyspareunia in patients with horizontal translocation of the vagina, Kylberg and Johnson (1982) described an operation in which the posterior wall of the vagina was dissected free of its adhesions to the coccyx, which was then excised. Bilateral flaps of gluteus maximus muscle were interposed between the posterior part of the vagina and the sacrum, and sutured to the sacrum in an attempt to restore the vagina to its original anatomic position. In a follow-up study of nine women who underwent this procedure for dyspareunia (Sjodahl et al 1990) normal drainage of vaginal secretions and menstrual blood occurred in all women. Eight were relieved of dyspareunia on follow-up 2 years later.

Sexual concerns in patients with a stoma

Patients with inflammatory bowel disease who have a stoma may have problems related to their sexuality (Lyons 1975), caused by the physical alteration in their body image; other concerns are psychological in origin. Rolstad et al (1983), in a study of 50 patients with an ileostomy, revealed that approximately half considered the presence of a stoma a psychological deterrent to sexual intercourse. One-third of the patients stated that the stoma made intercourse more difficult physically; 36 of 50 (72%) blamed the appliance for their sexual difficulty, and eight of them attributed it to the stoma. Burnham et al (1977) revealed that 12% of 376 married ileostomists described marital tension related to the stoma. Patients also indicated that concealing the stoma was helpful in improving sexual desirability. Subsequently, Nilsson et al (1981) surveyed 48 patients who underwent conversion of a Brooke ileostomy to a continent stoma with a Kock pouch. They found that 85% of patients reported an improved quality of sexual life after the conversion.

The development of stoma care facilities has enabled the provision of ongoing support for these patients. Sexual rehabilitation should not only be provided for the patient but also for the partner, in order to improve the outlook for these patients. Rehabilitation should begin preoperatively with education and proper stoma site location. The appliance must be unobtrusive, free of odor and leakproof to minimize its impact on body image. Long-term interaction with a stoma therapist and confidence gained from managing one's own stoma resolves most patients' anxiety.

CONCLUSION

Although the incidence of sexual dysfunction is low in patients with inflammatory bowel disease, the problems are quite troublesome. Aggressive medical and surgical treatment of disease corrects many problems. Counseling is essential, as sexual dysfunction has a psychological component. Patients should be encouraged because in general sexual function improves as their overall health improves.

REFERENCES

Aboseif S, Matzel K E, Lue T F 1990 Sexual dysfunction after rectal surgery. Perspectives in Colon and Rectal Surgery 3: 157–172

Bauer J J, Gelernt I M, Salk B A, Kreel I 1986 Proctectomy for inflammatory bowel disease. American Journal of Surgery 151: 157–162

Brindley G S 1981 Electro-ejaculation: its technique, neurological implications and uses. Journal of Neurology Neurosurgery and Psychiatry 44: 9

Brooke B N 1979 Dyspareunia: a significant symptom in Crohn's disease. Lancet 1: 1199

Burnham W R, Lennard-Jones J E, Brooke B N 1977 Sexual problems among married ileostomists. Gut 18: 673–677

Corman M L, Vedenheimer M C, Coller J A 1978 Impotence after proctectomy for inflammatory disease of the bowel. Diseases of the Colon and Rectum 21: 418–419

Damgaard B, Wettergren A, Kirkegaard P 1995 Social and sexual function following ileal pouch–anal anastomosis. Diseases of the Colon and Rectum 38: 286–289

Ireland A, Jewell D P 1989 Sulfasalazine-induced impotence: a beneficial resolution with olsalazine? Journal of Clinical Gastroenterology 11: 711

Kylberg F, Johnson P 1982 Extirpation of coccyx and perineal plasty with a muscle flap in vaginal dislocation after proctocolectomy. Svensk Kirurgi 41: 61

Lee E C G, Dowling B L 1972 Perimuscular excision of the rectum for Crohn's disease. British Journal of Surgery 59: 29

Leicester R J, Ritchie J K, Wadsworth J, Thomson J P, Hawley P R 1984 Sexual function and perineal wound healing after intersphincteric excision of the rectum for inflammatory bowel disease. Diseases of the Colon and Rectum 27: 244–248

Lyons A S 1975 Sex after ileostomy and colostomy. Medical Aspects of Human Sexuality 9: 107–108

Lyttle J A, Parks A G 1977 Intersphincteric excision of the rectum. British Journal of Surgery 64: 413–416

Metcalf A M, Dozois R R, Kelly K A 1986 Sexual function in women after proctocolectomy. Annals of Surgery 204: 624–627

Moody G, Probert C S J, Srivastava E M, Rhodes J, Mayberry J F 1992 Sexual dysfunction amongst women with Crohn's disease: a hidden problem. Digestion 52: 179–183

Nilsson L O, Kock N G, Kylberg F, Myrvold H E, Paselius I 1981 Sexual adjustment in ileostomy patients before and after conversion to continent ileostomy. Diseases of the Colon and Rectum 24: 287–290

Nivatvongs S, Gordon P H 1992 Surgical anatomy. In: Gordon P H, Nivatvongs S (eds) Colon, rectum and anus. Quality Medical Publishing, St Louis, pp 31–37

Oresland T, Palmblad S, Ellstrom M, Berndtsson I, Crona N, Hulten L 1994 Gynaecological and sexual function related to anatomical changes in the female pelvis after restorative proctocolectomy. International Journal of Colorectal Disease 9: 77–81

Pemberton J H, Phillips S F, Ready R R, Zinsmeister A R, Beahrs O H 1989 Quality of life after Brooke ileostomy and ileal pouch–anal anastomosis: comparison of performance status. Annals of Surgery 206: 620–626

Rolstad B S, Wilson G, Rothenberger D A 1983 Sexual concerns in the patient with an ileostomy. Diseases of the Colon and Rectum 26: 170–171

Sagar P M, Lewis W, Holdsworth P J, Johnson D, Mitchell D, Macfie J 1993 Quality of life after restorative proctocolectomy with a pelvic ileal reservoir compares favorably with that of patients with medically treated colitis. Diseases of the Colon and Rectum 36: 584–592

Shargold G A, Cantor B, Schreiber J R 1980 Treatment of infertility due to retrograde ejaculates: a simple, cost-effective method. Fertility and Sterility 34: 175

Sidi A A, Cameron J S, Duffy L M, Lange P H 1986 Intracavernous drug-induced erections in the management of male erectile dysfunction: experience with 100 patients. Journal of Urology 135: 704

Sigman M, Howards S S 1992 Male infertility. In: Walsh P C, Retik A B, Stamey T A, Vaughan E D (eds) Campbell's urology, 6th edn, vol 1. WB Saunders, Philadelphia, pp 661–705

Sjodahl R, Nystrom P O, Olaison G 1990 Surgical treatment of dorsocaudal dislocation of the vagina after excision of the rectum. Diseases of the Colon and Rectum 33: 762–764

Wexner S D, Jensen L, Rothenberger D A, Wong W D, Goldberg S M 1989 Long-term functional analysis of the ileoanal reservoir. Diseases of the Colon and Rectum 32: 275–281

Wikland M, Jansson I, Asztely M et al 1990 Gynaecological problems related to anatomical changes after conventional proctocolectomy and ileostomy. International Journal of Colorectal Disease 5: 49–52

Yeager E S, Van Heerden J A 1980 Sexual dysfunction following proctocolectomy and abdominoperineal resection. Annals of Surgery 191: 169–170

SECTION 13

Stoma management

104. Running a stomaltherapy service

P. J. d'E. Stevens

INTRODUCTION AND HISTORY

The specialty of stomaltherapy nursing was pioneered in the early 1960s to provide practical and emotional support for people with intestinal stomas. It has become an integral part of a colorectal and gastroenterological service. In the past three decades the scope of practice has broadened to include the management of fistulae, draining wounds, incontinence and potential or actual loss of tissue integrity. The key function is to be a support resource for patients and their families, and for medical and paramedical staff.

Skilled and informed trained nursing staff, having graduated from a formal postgraduate stomaltherapy education program, work as part of a multidisciplinary team. For the stomaltherapy nurse to play a major part in the orientating and counseling team they have to understand the precipitating diseases and the options for medical and surgical management. They have to have experience in the practical management of stomas, fistulae, draining and chronic wounds and incontinence, and they require a knowledge of available products, skills in application, and the ability to assist the patient to become independent and to take control of their own care.

Fifty-two countries have now established stomaltherapy nursing services, 21 of which have one or more accredited stomaltherapy nursing programs.

Credit for the original concept of a stomaltherapy service goes to Dr Rupert Turnbull of the Cleveland Clinic Foundation, who in 1958 invited Mrs Norma Gill, a rehabilitating ostomate, to join with him in advising and supporting patients undergoing stoma surgery. Together they established the first educational program for nurses at the Cleveland Clinic. Since then the clinic programs have educated graduates from all over the world. Two other pioneering services of note were begun in 1966: in England by Sir Ian Todd and Sister Barbara Saunders at St Bartholomew's Hospital, and in Melbourne, Australia, by Sir Edward Hughes and Sister Eleanor Kyte of the Royal Alfred Hospital. In 1978 16 countries joined together to form the World Council of Enterostomal Therapists which, apart from promoting international communications, has formulated standards of stomaltherapy nursing and quality assurance to ensure optimal care for stoma patients.

CODE OF PRACTICE FOR STOMALTHERAPY NURSES

The stomaltherapy nurse has a professional obligation to adhere to the code of practice established by the World Council:

1. The stomaltherapy nurse will provide needed services to persons irrespective of race, color, creed, sex, sexual preference, age, political or social status.
2. The stomaltherapy nurse respects the beliefs, values and customs of individuals and maintains their rights to privacy by maintaining confidentiality, sharing with others only that information relevant to care.
3. Stomaltherapy nurses will practice according to the standards of their national code of nursing ethics.
4. The stomaltherapy nurse must maintain competency by keeping abreast of new developments, theory, practices of stoma care and related fields.
5. The stomaltherapy nurse must at all times maintain the highest professional standards of nursing care and professional conduct.
6. The stomaltherapy nurse participates actively in professional, interprofessional and community endeavors to meet the highest professional standards.

FUNCTION OF A STOMALTHERAPY SERVICE

The key to a first-class service is a highly motivated and professional staff with good communication skills and interpersonal relationships, able to integrate their activities within multidisciplinary teams. Staffed by trained stomaltherapy nurses and ancillary staff, including a receptionist and an enrolled or assistant nurse, the service provides care for both in- and outpatients in the normal working week, with an emergency service for difficult practical or counseling problems after hours and at weekends.

The key functions of a stomaltherapy service are: orientation and counseling; preoperative stoma siting; practical stoma, fistula, wound and continence care; provision of and advice on products; education, research and administration.

Orientation and counseling

This is one of the most important roles of the stomaltherapy nurse. It is vital that a potential stoma patient, before giving informed consent, is made fully conversant with their underlying condition and the planned surgical intervention.

Assessing new patients is a skill requiring the therapist to interpret many signals given by both patient and family as they respond to the diagnosis, current symptoms and proposed intervention. Many factors influence the response, including age, marital status, personality, intelligence and comprehension, ethnicity, religion and sexuality. Social issues may be economic or related to family or work. Other agencies may need to be involved, such as social workers, personnel managers, ministers of religion, GPs and community nurses. These needs can all be assessed before operation, thereby removing some of the hidden obstacles that could influence recovery.

The diagnosis tends to influence the emotional response, as does whether the stoma, fistula or incontinence will be permanent or temporary. Chronic incurable conditions such as advanced malignancy require an empathic approach. The family and general nursing staff may also need support as the fluctuating mood swings and associated complications can be very stressful.

The advent of new surgical techniques add to the dimension of stomaltherapy practice; these include sphincter-saving procedures, low transanal anastomosis, ileoanal pouches and laparoscopic colonic procedures. They also include management of complications and assistance during learning curves associated with evacuation and control once temporary stomas are closed.

Preparing the patient for operations requiring a stoma

This requires time and privacy. It is also ideal to counsel both the patient and a chosen family member or friend. Clarity is essential. We use the spoken word, in language and terminology understood by the patient; simple drawings, visual aids and explanatory booklets. We need to give relevant information on normal anatomy and physiology, the underlying condition and the proposed surgery and stoma. We must provide the opportunity to ask and answer questions regarding lifestyle, diet, sexual function and practical issues associated with pouches, skin care and waste disposal. Meeting a rehabilitated stoma patient can be a wonderful adjunct to preparation, but care must be taken to select a patient with the same condition, same type of stoma and, if possible, from the same social and ethnic background.

Stoma siting

A stoma site is chosen before operation following discussion between the therapist and the surgeon regarding the surgical plan and any other relevant issues. The site is then clearly marked with an indelible pen.

Practical nursing care

There are many products available for managing all types of stoma, fistula and wounds. The task of a stomaltherapy service is to ensure that a wide range of equipment is available to cope with all potential situations. For stoma patients we usually have a standard postoperative system until such time as a change is required. The newly formed stoma will be measured and future recommendations will be dictated by the diameter, site, type of stoma and the amount of efflux, skin integrity and possible complications. The patient will be gradually involved in the practicalities of self-care and, once they are mobile, will be given the opportunity of assisted education away from the ward in the privacy of the stomaltherapy unit. Once they are competent and the therapist feels they can cope alone at home, discharge is planned. A supply of equipment is provided to last until the first follow-up appointment. A basic starter pack includes bags, skin-care products, disposal bags, a cleaning agent and deodorant. All colostomates are taught how to apply both a closed and a drainable pouch so they can cope with an attack of diarrhoea. They are also given details of where to call for help in the event of problems.

Using the same follow-up date for both surgeon and stoma therapist will save extra trips to hospital. The patient is given a card with details of their diagnosis, operative procedure, type of stoma, medications, special considerations, complications and ostomy equipment. This is useful for patients returning home or traveling a long distance from the hospital, and can be shown to other health professionals in the event of illness or need for assistance.

Fistulae or draining wounds

In the management of fistulae the primary function of the stomaltherapy service is to provide adequate skin protection and efficient pouches to contain the efflux. There must be good communication with other disciplines. For example when radiological investigation necessitates removal of the pouch to gain access for sinography. Immediate reapplication of skin protection and the pouch after X-ray means that the stomaltherapist must be available at any time in order to avoid lengthy exposure of the surrounding skin to corrosive effluent.

Wound care

To ensure the most efficient and economical use of resources the stomaltherapist must know the wide variety of products available for debridement, cleaning and protection of wound granulation.

Continence care

Urinary and fecal continence management requires the stomaltherapist to be familiar with the principles of urodynamics, anal manometry and biofeedback techniques. They need to give practical instruction on low-volume rectal washouts and intermittent self-catheterization. They are also needed for counseling and assistance in decision making should a stoma be recommended as an alternative to conservative measures. They are responsible for ordering and supplying continence aids and consumable products for continence control.

Ordering, storing and dispensing of continence products

Consumable products for stoma, fistula and wound care are manufactured and distributed worldwide by many companies. The stomaltherapy nurse must be familiar with the types of equipment available and with the ordering and storage methods required. The nurse should meet regularly with manufacturers to keep abreast of developments and be able to make recommendations.

Education

In 1980 the World Council of Enterostomal Therapists decreed that only trained nurses who had undertaken and passed a recognized program of stomaltherapy nursing could practice as stomaltherapists. Many excellent services are associated with such programs, providing education in conjunction with departments of nursing and medical and surgical faculties. The basic courses for registered nurses are a minimum of 320 hours. Some centers also offer BScN programs and an opportunity to complete a master's degree in stomaltherapy nursing.

In-service education is continuous for all grades of nurses, medical students, medical staff and paramedical staff. Regular attendance at workshops, conferences and seminars is important.

Patient education begins before operation and continues afterwards for both the patient and the family. Educational materials can be obtained from many sources, including commercial companies, ostomy associations and other stomaltherapy services.

Administration

Immaculate and accurate records are essential; these include patient records, statistics and data relating to diagnosis, surgical procedures, types of stoma, complications etc. Most units have a budget: good records and tight budget control are needed to prevent deficits.

Senior personnel must keep open communication with the nursing administration and their peers as they assess staff members. They should support their staff and pay attention to the role of the stomaltherapist within the hospital and community.

Research

Accurate records and statistics are vital for giving staff the opportunity to produce original work and mutual projects with other disciplines. Computer programs for specific projects and training give an added dimension.

FACILITIES NEEDED BY A STOMALTHERAPY UNIT

Much of the success of a unit depends on its location within the hospital complex as well as the facilities available. Ideally the unit should be sited within the departments of colorectal surgery and gastroenterology; it should be close to the wards, X-ray department, operating theatres, pharmacy and intensive care units. There should be car parking close by for outpatients and a good porter service.

The reception area should be welcoming, providing access to information and the opportunity to meet other patients as well as a comfortable waiting area. Patients' records can be kept on the unit and the receptionist can make appointments and communicate with other areas of the hospital to save patients time and trouble.

Two clinic rooms are needed to enable smooth running. These should be adequately ventilated and furnished, and preferably have air extraction facilities for freshness.

The clinical nurse specialist's office is the nerve center of the clinic. Here there is privacy for daily reports, consultations with staff, and telephone communication with patients at home, GPs and other community services. It can also be a safe place to store educational and reference materials.

An assisted toilet is useful so that patients can receive training in the care of their stomas, and for ostomy washouts and rectal irrigation. The service assists with mechanical cleansing of the bowel before radiological or endoscopic examinations and provides appropriate pouches to accommodate large volumes from the proximal bowel associated with oral preparation.

A cool, well lit storage room is required for supplies of equipment: staff should ensure that stock is rotated so they do not expire or deteriorate. A wide range of stock is necessary and administrators should be aware of budgetary constraints; recording and monitoring of stock is essential.

A seminar room is invaluable for conducting regular tutorials and meetings for ongoing education of staff.

THE SURVIVAL OF PROFESSIONAL STOMALTHERAPY SERVICES

In the belief that fewer stomas are being created, there is a tendency in some hospitals to curtail stoma services. A clinical nurse specialist has been perceived as a luxury, but the traumas experienced by patients denied such a service cannot be quantified in monetary terms. Although excellent support groups exist in many countries these cannot replace the expertise provided by professionals working in a multidisciplinary team. We believe that there is a firm future for gastroenterological specialist nursing services incorporating the skills of stomaltherapy for the management of stomas, fistulae, draining wounds and incontinence, and in the preparation of the bowel for X-ray and endoscopy.

FURTHER READING

Broadwell D, Jackson B 1982 Role of the enterostomal therapy practitioner. Principles of ostomy care. Mosby, New York, pp 8–13

Keighley M R B 1993 Running a stoma therapy service. In: Keighley M R B, Williams N S (eds) Surgery of the anus, rectum and colon. W B Saunders, London, pp 288–292

WCET Standards of nursing practice (1992) Members' handbook

105. Counseling of patients with inflammatory bowel disease

J. Alexander-Williams

THE IMPORTANCE OF COUNSELING

If I were asked to define the prerequisite for a specialist in inflammatory bowel diseases, I would say that one of the most important skills needed is that of a sensitive counselor. Counseling is needed whenever a patient is concerned about the risks and the future.

Counseling means the proffering of advice after careful consideration of the patient's needs and expectations. To know what those are we have to listen carefully to their account of their problems and fears. Counseling is a highly professional activity, requiring skills no less than those of technical endoscopy or surgery. Counseling may be needed on many occasions in the lifetime of a patient with inflammatory bowel disease, particularly because these are diseases of unknown cause, unpredictable course and punctuated by complications and the need for surgery. The surgery is sometimes dangerous and sometimes disfiguring, leading to a radical alteration of body image.

My own views on the subject of counseling derive much from my mentor, Professor Bryan Brooke, who spent a lot of time teaching counseling skills to medical students and surgical trainees and putting them into practice with patients.

I have spent 30 years in befriending patients with inflammatory bowel disease, talking to them and operating on their complications. I have worked closely with many devoted stoma therapists and have been involved, every week, in what we used to call a stoma clinic. This has increasingly become a counseling clinic in inflammatory bowel disease. About 10 years ago we submitted a questionnaire to 100 of our patients, asking questions relating to counseling. The details of this questionnaire have been published elsewhere, and the results will be referred to often.

WHO BREAKS THE NEWS?

The imparting of such important information cannot easily be delegated. It is no mean task, and can be delegated only to those we know to be specifically trained. The episodes that require particularly sensitive counseling include telling the patient the definitive diagnosis, the need for surgery, or the need for a change of body image.

It is important for doctors to realize that whoever imparts important information to patients must assume a counseling role and be prepared to spend time and to exhibit sensitivity to the patient's needs. You cannot simply say, 'We have found out what is the matter with you – it is Crohn's disease'. Or, 'You are going to need to have an operation and we will do it tomorrow'. Such shattering information must only be imparted when there is ample time for explanation and discussion.

THE EFFECT OF BEING TOLD THE DIAGNOSIS: HOW MUCH DO THEY KNOW AND HOW MUCH CAN THEY UNDERSTAND?

Patients often know very little about the diagnosis, particularly of Crohn's disease. In our own survey 93% of our patients said that they did not know anything about Crohn's disease before they were told the diagnosis and 85% did not know anyone else suffering from it. When asked whether they were given a satisfactory explanation about the disease at the time they were given the diagnosis, I am sorry to report that 45% said No. This survey was performed 10 years ago and was answered by many patients who had been diagnosed 20 or even 30 years ago. I hope that the answers today would be more favorable to the medical profession than those I have quoted.

When patients were asked about their predominant emotion on learning the diagnosis, most cited relief (47%), then bewilderment (37%), interest (27%), depression (26%), and horror in only 10%. A skilled counselor should be able to ensure that interest and relief are the prominent emotions.

I find that it is difficult to make an instant or rapid assessment of the effect on the family of the patient of the diagnosis of Crohn's disease or ulcerative colitis. Much depends on their level of education and their ability to understand what these diseases are and what their effects. Their reaction is likely to be affected by a knowledge of someone else who has the disease. As Crohn's disease and ulcerative colitis have a familial tendency, I expect that nowadays about 20% know of someone else with one of these diseases. This is, of course, often detrimental to their morale because, as we know it is bad news that is more likely to make the headlines than good news, and they are likely to know little or nothing about friends or relatives with mild inflammatory bowel disease. I am fond of quoting a headline from the *Sunday Express* in 1978 which read, 'A doctor's error made him steal'. It was a story from New York advanced in mitigation of a larceny case and it continued: 'He had never heard of Crohn's disease. But that, he was told, was what was killing him'. The first part of this sentence might have been true and, sadly, the second half may be something that he had been led to believe. Further reading of the article indicated that the sufferer was using this diagnosis as an excuse to claim leniency in a criminal charge; so perhaps there was selective reporting all round! This parable emphasizes that, even if our patients claim to know something about inflammatory bowel disease, we must find out what their concepts are and counter their misconceptions. We must find out what they know already and where they have learned it. This underlines the importance of listening to the patient. It seems to me wisest to assume that most patients will be in total ignorance of their disease, and even if they know people who have the same diagnosis, it is unlikely that they have been adequately informed, particularly of the good news about longevity and overall high quality of life.

THE AIMS OF COUNSELING

In this context counseling has three aims: to give information, to give hope and to give strength. I believe that the purpose of counseling patients with inflammatory bowel disease is to give them enough information for them to have hope for the future and strength to live with the disease. I believe, also, that the keynote of counseling should be optimism: it is important not to overwhelm them with information, particularly information that can be misconstrued. I think that for patients with inflammatory bowel disease health education is as important as is sex education for children. It deserves as much careful thought in planning and care in execution as does sex education, yet it is something that is rarely considered deeply and seldom taught.

Although most of our patients claimed to have felt initial relief on hearing the diagnosis, this was probably because they had been afraid of something more serious and life-endangering, such as malignant disease. However, the relief that they feel is likely to be short-lived, whereas the emotions of interest, bewilderment or depression are likely to be long-lasting.

HOW MUCH ARE PATIENTS ABLE TO COMPREHEND?

Because I have been keen to impart as much information as possible, I think that in the past I may have been guilty of trying to give too much information initially, so that the patients possibly became more confused than enlightened.

I have come to realize that most sufferers are eventually capable of assimilating a lot of information and achieving much understanding about their disease. However, they rarely achieve this in their first counseling session, and it is a mistake to try to tell them too much. Unfortunately, such is the patient's thirst for knowledge that they can rarely be satisfied by the initial consultation, which often lasts less than half an hour. At the end of such an interview most patients still want further information and, if not satisfied, will seek it from medical or surgical textbooks that are written for a sophisticated medical readership and often seem to emphasize the complications and the death rates, or the development of cancer.

HOW MUCH TO TELL, PARTICULARLY ABOUT CANCER RISKS

The doctor informing patients about their disease has a difficult task. The patient has to be informed without being confused or frightened, and this is sometimes difficult for the doctor to understand. If doctors speak to the patient as they would speak to other members of the medical profession, they are likely to refer to such concepts as the risk of the development of cancer. Although medical colleagues will understand it in statistical terms, to a patient the emotive words 'cancer' and 'the risk' will be heard entirely out of context. I rarely make any reference to malignancy unless specifically asked. If asked, I can only answer with the truth.

I believe that in our present state of knowledge, we are wise if we dismiss or play down the risk of cancer developing in Crohn's disease and, provided we have an efficient method of surveillance for patients with long-standing ulcerative colitis, I think it wise to defer this risk for discussion in future years.

Those of us interested in Crohn's disease tend to quote the evidence from Mount Sinai Hospital in New York, of the greatly increased risk of cancer developing in bypassed small bowel (Greenstein et al 1978). Fascinating though this information may be to researchers in the field, I believe that it should not be discussed with patients simply to cover ourselves against the risk of litigation. I believe that we should emphasize that ulcerative colitis and Crohn's disease are *not* a form of cancer. We know that any form of chronic epithelial inflammation in the body may be associated with a small risk of the development of malignant disease many years or decades later. I think that this risk is a very small one, and is much less than the risk of developing lung cancer if you smoke, or of women developing cervical cancer if they have many partners. I think it creates more problems than it solves if we try to explain a complex disease process to someone who has less scientific knowledge. The saying 'A little knowledge is a dangerous thing' could well have been coined to describe patients' awareness of chronic inflammatory diseases of the bowel.

DO WE GIVE THEM BOOKS OR PAMPHLETS?

Our market research showed that a small majority (53%) of our patients thought that the initial explanation they were given about their disease was too superficial or too limited; 43% thought that the explanation they were given was adequate and only 4% considered that it was too detailed or too complex for them to understand. A large majority (95%) stated that they would like to have had more information than they received; 62% felt that they would like to have read a book or pamphlet giving further details about the disease from which they were suffering.

Some of the printed information that is available to patients about inflammatory bowel diseases is listed and reviewed in a later section of this chapter. All I would like to say here is to advise all those engaged in counseling to read and critically review the level of information provided in the booklets and books, then consider carefully whether any of that information could possibly do more harm than good.

WHEN SHOULD PATIENTS BE COUNSELED AND WHO SHOULD DO IT?

The diagnosis of inflammatory bowel disease almost always results from hospital investigations, usually including X-rays and histological examination of biopsies. Therefore, it is usually the hospital doctor who is the first to confront the patient with the definitive diagnosis. In a review of our practice, it appears that in only about 10% of our patients was the definitive diagnosis given to them by their GP or community doctor: almost all were by the hospital consultant.

I think that it is sensible for the patients to be told the diagnosis immediately it is confirmed. Therefore, it would usually be the physician in charge in the office or outpatient clinic who will impart the news. In public hospital practice this could be a junior member of the medical team. If the doctor is inexperienced in the art of counseling patients with inflammatory bowel disease, it is important to consider carefully what is expected. There must be a plan before starting, and not just a plunge into an explanation that may confuse rather than inform and lead to questions that cannot be answered satisfactorily. I think that it is important that anyone who has to impart the information to the patient must be well aware of what the news may mean, and to be in a position to give a satisfactory and comprehensive explanation. The doctor who does so, however junior, has to be trained and prepared to assume the role of counselor and should remember the three precepts of giving information, hope and strength. They should be aware that the impact of the diagnosis could have a serious and disturbing emotional effect on the patient. They should take care where and when the news is given. It is generally inappropriate that the diagnosis should be imparted to the patient over the telephone, or even in writing. It is undoubtedly better given when there can be eye contact. I find that such important news is best imparted after some form of physical contact, in the form of either a handshake or a physical examination.

I believe that it is important that the specialist or the deputy in charge of the case should have the first opportunity of imparting information, before any misconceptions have been planted in the patient's mind by unsolicited lay advice or studies of medical texts, even those specifically designed for the lay patient.

I am sure that the patients must be given as much explanation and reassurance as possible at the time the diagnosis is imparted, but we must remember that they will not be able to take in much detail at this first interview. Nevertheless, it is important to have time available for the patient, preferably in the presence of a close or supportive relative or friend.

WHERE TO COUNSEL AND WITH WHOM?

Our survey showed that 57% of our patients had no other member of the family present at the time of the first explanation of the disease; 69% felt that a relative or friend should have been there. As 14% felt that they did not wish anyone else to know about the diagnosis, it is clearly important to be sensitive to the patient's wishes.

I believe it is best, if possible, to have the spouse or partner present, and when the patient is a child the parents will naturally be present. If this is impractical a special discussion consultation should be arranged as soon as possible. As the information is often first imparted in the outpatient or clinic environment, some privacy is desirable.

I recommend a team approach at the first counseling session. When there was a possibility of a stoma being required, the counselling on our unit was always shared with the enterostomal therapist; with the changing role of the enterostomal nurses it is now usually the specialist gastrointestinal nurse.

The role of the specialist nurse is rapidly evolving into one of equal partnership with the consultant. It is often easier for the nurse to establish rapport with the patient than it is for the consultant, of whom the patient may be in awe. Nevertheless, I feel that the consultant has the ultimate responsibility for counseling and for teaching the skills to the junior staff. I think that the consultant and specialist nurse act best as a team, with the doctor giving the news about diagnosis and management and imparting confidence. The nurse adds reassurance and answers questions and allays fears.

Experienced doctors have to train others in counseling and I often had a resident or a medical or nursing student present also. I believe that any more than three professional personnel will seem to the patient to be a crowd.

SHOULD WE TELL ALL?

In deciding how much to tell the patient initially, we must judge their background, character and powers of comprehension – often a difficult task. We have to make a decision about what would be appropriate for the particular patient: how much science, how much analogy and how much poetic licence. Perhaps the most important attribute of the counselor is empathy. Attitudes concerning the breaking of bad news to patients have changed: to tell or not to tell is no longer the issue, but rather what information is appropriate for a particular patient.

The full details of diagnosis, prognosis and possible complications, as is required by many American trial protocols, are as inappropriate for the average patient as is bland reassurance. Although a degree of paternalism may be an ingredient of compassionate care, if it is associated with lack of empathy then it becomes destructive arrogance. I think that the tone of the first interview should be light on science, heavy on analogy and rich in sympathy.

OPTIMISTIC ANALOGIES

I explain to patients that they have a chronic inflammatory disease that is usually not particularly severe and one with which most patients can live a normal span of life without great inconvenience. I commonly use the analogies of chronic nasal sinusitis and chronic eczema, because the patient usually knows of someone suffering from one or other of these common disorders. I explain that chronic sinusitis is a combination of infection and nasal blockage which may give many patients a persistent purulent runny nose. However, for most of the time it is a relatively easy disease to live with, although most would rather be without it. It is only occasionally that sinusitis flares up with an acute symptomatic exacerbation that requires drugs, time off work and occasionally surgical intervention. When I use the analogy of eczema, I explain that much of the time the disease is quiescent. Occasionally, for some reason which we understand rather better with dermatitis than we do with ulcerative colitis or Crohn's disease, the disease flares up and the skin becomes inflamed. It may then require antibiotics to combat secondary infection, or cortisone to suppress the inflammatory response. I tell them that most patients with chronic eczema can live a long and useful life with few limitations. I point out that in many patients the eczema can become totally quiescent, even if it was once so severe as to have been almost incapacitating. The same is true for Crohn's disease or ulcerative colitis. I find that one or both of these analogies is easily understood by most patients, and tends to put their own disease into perspective.

CROHN'S DISEASE AND ULCERATIVE COLITIS IN PERSPECTIVE

I often explain to them that, in our inflammatory bowel disease clinic, we have in our care some 500 patients with Crohn's disease, and that for most of the time some 425 have few symptoms, requiring only a little dietary management and vitamin supplementation. At any one time some 60 are undergoing exacerbations of the disease sufficiently severe to warrant powerful therapy with such things as steroids, other inflammatory drugs or antibiotics. There are only about 15 of the 500 patients whose disease is causing any concern, enough to require weekly supervision or even inpatient treatment. Most of these 15 have some complication of the disease that warrants consideration of surgical treatment or temporary complete bowel rest. I explain that when this complication has been dealt with, we expect all 15 to go back and join the 425 with minimal inconvenience. Of course, statistics have an element of 'poetic licence' but the key features is to tinge the initial consultation with optimism.

REFERENCES

Alexander-Williams J 1993 Psychosis, psychology, stress and counselling. In: Kumar D, Alexander-Williams J (eds) Crohn's disease and ulcerative colitis: surgical management. Springer-Verlag, London, pp 27–34

Greenstein A J, Sachar D, Pucillo A 1978 Cancer in Crohn's disease after diversionary surgery. A report of seven carcinomas occurring in excluded bowel. American Journal of Surgery 135: 86–90

PATIENT INFORMATION

W. K. Pringle, M. C. White

The *Patient's Charter* (1995) states that every patient has the right, prior to making a decision, to 'have any proposed treatment, including any risks involved in that treatment and any alternatives, clearly explained'. Ill health can cause feelings of anxiety, fear and depression, leading to denial and refusal to seek help. Information is therefore necessary for the patient and their family to make an informed choice about treatment (Lowry 1995). Janis (1958) says that information and explanations of what to expect may enable patients to prepare both physically and emotionally for treatment, facilitating a reduction in anxiety. Anderson (1987) reiterates this point by saying: 'understanding of conditions and treatments enhances recovery and/or ability to cope with a situation'. Information has a beneficial effect on postoperative recovery, reducing pain (Hayward 1975) and stress (Boore 1978).

Disseminating information has traditionally been the doctor's responsibility (Faulkner 1984). However, all members of the multidisciplinary team have a role to play in informing patients. It is important that members of the team are aware of each other's contributions in order to 'minimize conflicting and contradictory statements which might confuse patients' (Lowry 1995).

Wilson Barnett (1988) defines information giving as a 'process of provision' and expresses concern that there is so little emphasis on how the information is provided. Heron (1990) reinforces this message by saying: 'Informative interventions seek to impart to the client new knowledge, information and meaning that is relevant to their needs and interests, in terms that the person can understand, and in a manner that enhances the person's need to participate in the learning process with self directed activity.' He states that two important issues are the quantity and quality of the information given, and whether to give the information or to place the onus on the patient to seek it for himself or herself.

The quality of information given can affect recall at a later date, particularly when the information is given only once (Castledine 1988). Retention of information can be enhanced by using simple, short sentences. However, a balance is required between using language that is too simple and conveying a patronizing attitude (Dobree 1989). Information should be tailored to the patient's individual lifestyle and incorporate social, spiritual and cultural elements (Breckman 1986).

Written material must be readable, clear and pertinent. Lowry (1995) suggests that the information should provoke further enquiry by the patient and provide a resource for the patient and their family. There is a proliferation of patient information booklets freely available, which include information regarding treatment and management of inflammatory bowel disease. These booklets should complement existing knowledge, rather than introduce new and unfamiliar facts. Dobree (1989) analyzed pre-admission booklets for patients awaiting surgery. Her study revealed that the quality of information was inadequate and some topics were only dealt with superficially. A more recent study (Coey 1995) has evaluated stoma care information booklets. The author found that only 36% of the population would understand the contents. Written information must therefore match reading ability and other strategies should be implemented for ensuring the dissemination of information.

Several stages have been identified in the process of giving information (Kagan & Evans 1995). An assessment of prior knowledge determines what information is required and how it should be delivered. First, information giving can be verbal, non-verbal or recorded. Secondly, the salient points need to be highlighted and presented in the correct order. Thirdly, these points should be reinforced by examples and illustrations. Fourthly, any restrictions limiting 'what can and cannot be said' should be identified (Kagan & Evans 1995). The final stage involves summarizing the information given, and checking whether it has been understood and is appropriate.

For some inflammatory bowel disease patients surgery is inevitable, possibly resulting in the formation of a stoma, which may greatly affect their emotional, psychological and social wellbeing (Whates & Irving 1984, Rubin & Devlin 1987). Information for this group of patients is crucial, yet needs to be specific in order to meet their needs. Kelly (1987) advocates that clinical nurse specialists in stoma care, who are regularly available for consultation at a very stressful time, help to alleviate some of the anxieties surrounding this taboo subject. Following diagnosis patients will require certain information and counseling about their proposed surgery. Early referral of the patient to the stoma care nurse can ensure that information can be given and clarification sought. 'This time lag appears to be critical in determining, among other things, how people subsequently felt about their surgery, and the way they had been treated postoperatively' (Kelly 1992).

Wade (1989) confirms that the stoma care nurse is the main provider of written information in districts where they are employed. In districts where there is no stoma care nurse, ward nurses are more involved in the information-giving process.

Kelly's (1992) study indicates that patients' concerns are practical at this stage. Information regarding lifestyle issues was required, rather than deep psychological interventions. He also raises an interesting point regarding 'credible' information, stating that information supplied by ostomists was viewed very positively. It should be remembered that voluntary associations can provide valuable first-hand information on a personal level or in the form of booklets.

Several experimental studies evaluating information strategies, based on stress-provoking situations, have indicated that lack of information causes anxiety. Wilson Barnett (1988) suggests that it is more beneficial for the patient to be told of the sensations or feelings they will experience, rather than learning practical coping strategies. Johnson's (1983) study has shown this to be the case with some surgical patients.

As the patient's advocates, all members of the team involved in the delivery of care must ensure that the patient has adequate opportunity, not only to be given information but for it to be clearly explained and tailored to suit. The essence of informed consent is to offer the patient as much or as little information as he requires. It would be denying them their autonomy to do less (Faulder 1985). However, forcing information on patients who indicate that they do not want it, is equally to deny them their autonomy.

REFERENCES

Anderson E A 1987 quoted in Lowry M 1995 Knowledge that reduces anxiety: creating patient information leaflets. Professional Nurse 10: 318–320
Boore J 1978 Information: a prescription for recovery. Royal College of Nursing, London
Breckman B 1986 Success by stages. Senior Nurse 5: 14–19
Castledine G 1988 Preoperative information. Surgical Nurse 1: 11–13
Coey L R 1995 Readability formulas and printed educational materials used to inform ostomates. Queen Elizabeth College of Nursing, Birmingham (Unpublished Project ENB 216)
Department of Health 1995 NHS: The Patient's Charter. DOH, London
Dobree L 1989 Pre admission booklets for patients awaiting surgery. Nursing Times 85: 42–44
Faulder L 1985 Whose body is it? The troubling issue of informed consent. Virago Press, London
Faulkner A 1984 (ed) Communication. Recent Advances in Nursing Series, 7. Churchill Livingstone, Edinburgh
Hayward J 1975 Information: a prescription against pain. RCN Study of Nursing Care Series: Royal College of Nursing, London
Heron J 1990 Helping the client: a creative practical guide. Sage Publications, London
Janis I 1958 quoted in Dobree L 1990 Pre-operative advice for patients. Nursing Standard 4: 28–30
Johnson J E 1983 Preparing patients to cope with stress while hospitalized. In: Wilson Barnett J (ed) Patient teaching. Recent Advances in Nursing Series 6. Churchill Livingstone, Edinburgh
Kagan C, Evans J 1995 Professional interpersonal skills for nurses. Chapman & Hall, London
Kelly M 1987 Adjusting to ileostomy. Nursing Times 83: 29–31
Kelly M 1992 Colitis. Tavistock/Routledge, London
Lowry M 1995 Knowledge that reduces anxiety (creating patient information leaflets). Professional Nurse 10: 318–320
Rubin G, Devlin H 1987 The quality of life with a stoma. British Journal of Hospital Medicine 38: 300–306
Wade B 1989 A stoma is for life. Scutari Press, Middlesex
Whates P, Irving M 1984 Return to work following ileostomy. British Journal of Surgery 71: 619–622
Wilson Barnett J 1988 Patient teaching or patient counselling? Journal of Advanced Nursing 13: 215–222

APPENDIX

Sources of information

Voluntary associations (registered charities)

British Colostomy Association (BCA)

15 Station Road, Reading, Berkshire RG1 1LG, UK
Tel: 01734 391537

The association provides support, reassurance, practical information and home and hospital visiting. Formal group meetings are not organized but open days in cooperation with stoma care nurses and manufacturing companies are arranged locally. A telephone and letter helpline is available.

Written information is provided in the form of:

Living with a Colostomy (publication date and author unknown)

A 16-page A5 illustrated booklet describing the role of the BCA and including basic lifestyle issues. Also offered in Spanish, Turkish, Chinese, French, Gujarati, German, Polish and Tamil.

A5 leaflets covering particular topics (publication dates and authors unknown):

1. Travel advice
2. Wind, constipation and diarrhea
3. The personal carer
4. If you are about to have a colostomy
5. Directory of area organizers

The Ileostomy and Internal Pouch Support Group (Formerly IA)

IA National Office, Amblehurst House, PO Box 23, Mansfield, Nottinghamshire NG18 4TT, UK
Tel/Fax: 01623 28099

The association publishes a quarterly journal containing news and views, articles of interest and correspondence. Members will visit new ostomists at home or in hospital to offer support and build confidence. Local meetings are held for members at which a guest speaker, medical adviser or stoma care nurse may be present. These meetings may also include representations by manufacturing companies. An advisory service is available for topics such as employment, housing, insurance, pensions, financial difficulties, marriage, pregnancy, sexual problems and personal relationships. IA contribute greatly to the field of medical research, raising funds to study various aspects of bowel disease.

Written information is presented in the form of 12 A4 information sheets (published 1994):

1. This is IA (author unknown)
2. Introducing you to your ileostomy: Eades, D

3. Publications available from IA (author unknown)
4. Travel tips (author unknown)
5. Medical aspects of an ileostomy: Kellock, D
6. Ulcerative colitis – a surgeon's view: Irving, M
7. Skin problems associated with ileostomies: Beck, M H
8. Self image: Snow, B
9. Ileostomies and eating habits (author unknown)
10. Please read the label: Eyles, A
11. Pregnancy, contraception, infertility and the ileostomy: Setchell, M
12. The ileoanal pouch operation: Maxwell, R

Publications available from IA

Bosanko S (ed) 1988 The ileostomy book. IA, Mansfield
A 98-page A5 booklet containing articles which have previously been published in the IA journal, giving information on all aspects of living with an ileostomy. Available from IA price £2.50.

Mullen B D, McGinn K A 1992 The ostomy book. Bull Publishing Co, California. A 330-page book written by an ostomist and her daughter, it offers a practical guide and a personal insight into life with a stoma. Price £9.50 from IA.

Jeter K F 1982 These special children. Bull Publishing Co, California. A 192-page book written by the mother of a child with a stoma, it offers support and advice to parents about equipment, information regarding anatomy and physiology, schooling and family relationships. Price £8.95 from IA.

IA 1993 Video: Our present your future? A 30-minute video produced by the Leicestershire division of the IA including a series of personal interviews discussing various aspects of everyday living, as well as showing members involved in recreational activities. The video is aimed at potential stoma or pouch patients.

National Association for Colitis and Crohn's Disease (NACC)
4 Beaumont House, Sutton Road, St Albans, Hertfordshire
AL1 5HH, UK
Tel/Fax: 01727 844296

The association provides information through newsletters, booklets and local meetings. It offers support to both patients and their families and raises money for research. Written information is provided in the form of nine A5 booklets; contributors include members of NACC's National Council of Medical Advisers:

1. The role of diet (1991)
2. Pregnancy in inflammatory bowel disease (1991)
3. Crohn's disease (1991)
4. Ulcerative colitis (1990)
5. Glossary of terms used or the language of inflammatory bowel disease (1991)
6. Inflammatory bowel disease in childhood: a parent's guide (1991)
7. Drugs used in ulcerative colitis and Crohn's disease: the pros and cons (1991)
8. Living with inflammatory bowel disease (1993)
9. Is there a risk of cancer in inflammatory bowel disease? (1994)

National Advisory Service for Parents of Children with a Stoma (NASPCS)
51 Anderson Drive, Valley View Park, Darvel, Ayrshire
KA17 0DE, UK
Tel: 01560 22024

The association provides practical advice, reassurance, information and contacts about the day-to-day care of a child or baby with a stoma. Written information is supplied in the format of a 24-page A5 illustrated booklet entitled *Our special children*. It describes the anatomy and physiology of the digestive and genitourinary tracts, types of stoma and appropriate appliances and lifestyle issues.

Crohn's in Childhood Research Association (CICRA)
Parkgate House, 356 West Barnes Lane, Motspur Park, Surrey KT3 6NB, UK
Tel: 0181 949 6209

CICRA is dedicated to providing funds for research into Crohn's disease, and it also publishes a newsletter. Written information is provided:

1. Judy can only concentrate on the pain: How can the school help? (Publication date and author unknown)
   An A5 leaflet giving basic information about inflammatory bowel disease and its effects on lifestyle. (Sponsored by SmithKline Beecham.)
2. Chronic inflammatory bowel disease in childhood: Crohn's disease and ulcerative colitis. (Rossiter M, Walker-Smith J A, publication date unknown)
   A 16-page A5 booklet containing information regarding symptoms and treatment for inflammatory bowel disease.

An important source of information is available in the form of booklets, videos and audio tapes supplied free by manufacturing and pharmaceutical companies.

Pharmaceutical companies

Pharmacia

1. Living with ulcerative colitis (Reprinted 1994) (Mani, V)
   A 19-page A5 booklet outlining the anatomy, nature of the disease, investigations, treatment and complications with relevant, clear diagrams to clarify the information given.
2. Living with Crohn's disease. (Reprinted 1994) (Mayberry J, Rhodes J)

An 11-page A5 booklet outlining anatomy, disease, investigations, treatment and complications, with clear diagrams.

SmithKline and French Laboratories

A series of five booklets covering various aspects of inflammatory bowel disease:

1. 20 Questions about ulcerative colitis (1992) (Mayberry J, Rhodes J)
2. 20 Questions about proctitis and distal colitis (1991) (Mayberry J, Mayberry M)
3. 20 Questions about Crohn's disease (1990) (Mayberry J, Mayberry M)
4. Diet, Crohn's disease and colitis (1992) (Mayberry J, Leonard C)
5. My operation: surgery in ulcerative colitis and Crohn's disease (1992) (Muir I, Mayberry J)

Stafford Miller

Five leaflets outlining various aspects of ulcerative colitis:

1. Screening in ulcerative colitis (1994) (Mayberry J, Mayberry M)
2. Ulcerative colitis – surgical options (1994) (author unknown)
3. How is ulcerative colitis treated? (1993) (author unknown)
4. What is ulcerative colitis? (1993) (author unknown)
5. Can I lead a normal life with ulcerative colitis? (1993) (author unknown)

Manufacturing companies

Clinimed Ltd, Cavell House, Knaves Beech Way, Loudwater, High Wycombe, Buckinghamshire HP10 9QY, UK
Tel: 0800 585125

1. Colostomy: a practical guide to stoma care
2. Ileostomy: a practical guide to stoma care
   Two 25-page A5 booklets containing practical advice about stoma care and lifestyle issues. No known author or publication date.
3. Temporary loop ileostomy: A guide for patients.
   An A5 leaflet with basic information regarding a loop ileostomy and preparation for closure. No known author or publication date.
4. The ileoanal pouch: an alternative to a permanent ileostomy (1992) (Jameson H) A 12-page A5 booklet containing information about the stages of pouch surgery, adaptation, diet and complications.

Coloplast Ltd., Peterborough Business Park, Peterborough PE2 6BR, UK
Tel: 0800 220622

1. Your colostomy operation and afterwards
2. Your ileostomy operation and afterwards
   Two 16-page A5 booklets containing practical advice about stoma care and lifestyle issues. No known author or publication date.
3. The ileoanal pouch: an alternative to a permanent ileostomy. Contributions made by several stoma care nurses and Mr R J Nicholls, Consultant, St Mark's Hospital, London. No publication date.
   A 14-page A5 booklet including details about the stages of pouch surgery, pre- and postoperative care and returning to normal activity. Clear diagrams enhance the written information.
4. The transverse colostomy: an explanatory guide. Contributions made by several stoma care nurses. No publication date.
   A 14-page A5 booklet containing information on all aspects of care.
5. Your guide to healthy eating and drinking.
6. Your guide to keeping fit and staying healthy.
7. Your guide to carefree travel and holidays.
   Three A5 booklets regarding the above issues. No known authors or publication date.

Convatec Ltd., Harrington House, Milton Road, Ickenham, Uxbridge UB10 8PU, UK
Tel: 0800 282254

1. Understanding colostomy: a guide for new patients (Foulkes, B)
2. Understanding ileostomy: a guide for new patients (Foulkes, B)
   Two 30-page A5 booklets (publication date unknown). *Understanding ileostomy* is also published in Urdu and available via the freephone number. Other translations are obtainable upon request. Audio tapes of these booklets, lasting approximately 50 minutes, are particularly useful for the blind and visually impaired. These are entitled *Understanding and caring for your colostomy/ileostomy*.
3. Ulcerative colitis: a guide for patients (Nicholls R J, Harocopos C J) (Publication date unknown).

Information is also available in the form of video tapes:

1. What you really need to know about . . . colostomies, ileostomies and urostomies (1993)
   A 30-minute video including interviews with patients giving accounts of life with a stoma and advice from a stoma care nurse, including aspects such as diet, travel and sexual function. Presented by Dr Robert Buckman and John Cleese.
2. In the picture series (1995)
   Three 30-minute videos covering colostomy, ileostomy and urostomy, containing patient interviews, practical stoma care advice and contributions from a stoma care nurse.

Hollister Ltd, Rectory Court, 42 Broad Street, Wokingham, Berkshire RG11 1AB, UK
Tel: 0800 521377

1. Lifestyle for colostomists (1994)
2. Lifestyle for ileostomists (1994)
   Two 19-page booklets with contributions from several stoma care nurses. The Lifestyle series continues with five 11-page booklets dealing with specific lifestyle issues:
   a) Sport and fitness (1993)
   b) Travel and holidays (1993)
   c) Relationships (1993)
   d) Love and sex (1993)
   e) Pregnancy and childbirth (1991)
   Contributions made by stoma care nurses, patient associations and other healthcare professionals.

Salt and Son Ltd Saltair House, Lord Street, Heartlands, Birmingham B7 4DS, UK
Tel: 0800 626388

1. Your colostomy and you: a guide to living your life to the full
2. Your ileostomy and you: a guide to living your life to the full
   Two 15-page A5 booklets, author and publication date unknown.

Book

Kelly M 1992 Colitis. Tavistock/Routledge, London
A 127-page book written by Professor Michael Kelly, a sociologist and himself an ostomist, describing his experience of ulcerative colitis and examining the social and psychological issues surrounding the disease.

106. Stoma construction

Kong-Weng Eu   J. R. Oakley

INTRODUCTION

Almost all patients who require a stoma for inflammatory bowel disease (IBD) will have an ileostomy. A colostomy is rarely indicated or advisable because many patients have unsatisfactory stoma function, usually because of the stoma size or appliance problems because of the high output of liquid stool. A colostomy should therefore be avoided wherever possible. Loop ileostomy is the preferred option should diversion of the distal bowel be required.

TYPES OF ILEOSTOMY AND THEIR INDICATIONS

The types of ileostomy most commonly constructed are end ileostomy, loop ileostomy and loop–end ileostomy. Continent ileostomy is a further option for ulcerative colitis, which is discussed in Chapter 87. Each type of ileostomy has different characteristics and different applications.

End ileostomy

An end ileostomy is constructed from the divided terminal ileum, which is then brought through an anterior abdominal wall aperture, everted and sutured to the surrounding skin to form a short spout with a single aperture. An end ileostomy may be indicated after completion of total abdominal colectomy or proctocolectomy for mucosal ulcerative colitis or Crohn's disease; as a temporary stoma after ileal or ileocecal resection for Crohn's disease, complicated by perforation or abscess formation; or to provide total diversion to allow resolution of severely inflamed Crohn's disease with associated sepsis in preparation for a later definitive resection.

Loop ileostomy

A loop ileostomy is constructed from a loop of ileum on which the antimesenteric wall is opened in an eccentric fashion and everted to form a short spout stoma, with the afferent (functioning) limb opening at its apex and a second opening to the efferent (non-functioning) limb close to the mucocutaneous junction.

The loop ileostomy is usually a temporary stoma. In inflammatory bowel disease a loop ileostomy may be indicated as a temporary diversion following ileal pouch–anal anastomosis or ileorectal anastomosis; as a temporary diversion after the construction of a continent ileal reservoir (continent ileostomy); proximal to an enterocutaneous fistula, before or after surgical resection; proximal to an intestinal anastomosis where the anastomosis is felt to be at increased risk of leakage because of poor nutrition, in the proximity of local sepsis, or from the long-term effects of steroids or immunosuppressive drugs; in certain cases of severe perianal Crohn's disease, or following some rectal advancement flap repairs for perianal fistulae or stenosis; or in association with decompressing blowhole colostomy in very severe cases of toxic megacolon or fulminant colitis.

Loop–end ileostomy

A loop–end ileostomy is similar to a loop ileostomy except that the efferent limb is divided and closed several centimeters distal to the stoma aperture.

The loop–end ileostomy may be preferred to end ileostomy in the obese patient, where a thick abdominal wall may make it difficult to prepare a sufficient length of well vascularized bowel, once the bowel and its mesenteric blood supply has been divided. By using a loop of bowel approximately 10 cm proximal to the divided end, there is less disturbance to the blood supply of the segment of bowel used to construct the stoma. The same technique may also be used in Crohn's disease, where edema and fibrosis produce a thickened, shorter and less mobile small-bowel mesentery, which restricts the bowel from reaching skin level.

A previously constructed (temporary) loop ileostomy may be converted to a (permanent) loop–end ileostomy by dividing and closing the efferent limb just inside the peritoneal cavity. This is usually done at the time of a subsequent abdominal colectomy or proctocolectomy.

PREOPERATIVE PREPARATION

Patient education and instruction

The preoperative psychological preparation is one of the most important aspects of stoma construction. The stoma nurse, surgeon, and sometimes a trained lay ostomy visitor, should discuss the implications of the operation. They must describe life with a stoma, not just for the patient but also for the family. They must provide reassurance and encouragement. Although many patients are not emotionally able to absorb or remember detailed preoperative teaching, they have a right to be given a broad overview of their postoperative stoma function and care.

Siting of the stoma

Accurate preoperative selection of a stoma site is essential. In some patients alternative sites may also need to be marked. In most patients the preferred site will be over the infraumbilical fat mound, but in some cases, such as the obese, a stoma in an upper quadrant may be preferred.

The stoma should be at least 3 cm from the planned incision, and preferably pass through the middle of the rectus abdominis muscle, where the abdominal skin is usually more convex and where the bulk and support of the rectus and the strength of the rectus sheaths may reduce the risk of parastomal herniation. The stoma should also be sited away from all previous scars, skin creases and bony prominences, and should be easily visible to the patient (Fig. 106.1). It is important to site the stoma with the patient in both the lying and the sitting positions to ensure that all these principles are observed.

Once the stoma site has been chosen, it is indelibly marked by placing a small drop of indian ink or methylene blue over the site. Several needle pricks through the ink produce a small tattoo which cannot be washed away.

Bowel preparation

A full mechanical bowel preparation is usually performed if colectomy or proctocolectomy is planned. This may be avoided if large-bowel resection is not being performed: then, clear liquids orally for 12–24 hours will usually suffice. Peroperative intravenous antibiotics are given to cover both aerobic and anerobic organisms.

Anesthesia

Although these procedures can be performed under local or regional anesthesia, general anesthesia with muscle relaxation and endotracheal intubation is preferred because traction on the mesentery may cause pain and nausea.

THE OPERATION

The techniques of stoma construction for end ileostomy, loop ileostomy and loop–end ileostomy are similar, with many steps being common to all three. However, there are clear differences in the way in which the bowel segment is initially prepared and subsequently sutured to the skin.

Incision

The surgeon's choice of incision will be influenced by the operation for which the stoma is required. In most cases a midline incision is preferred because it preserves all potential stoma sites through the rectus muscles bilaterally. This is particularly so in Crohn's disease, where there is a high incidence of recurrent disease in the ileostomy, and of parastomal abscesses and fistulae, which may necessitate stoma relocation.

Making the stoma aperture

The abdominal wall aperture is the same for all types of stoma. The linea alba and dermis in the midline incision at the level of the stoma site are grasped with strong clamps and retracted medially. A circular incision, 2–2.5 cm in diameter, is made around the tattooed stoma site. Only

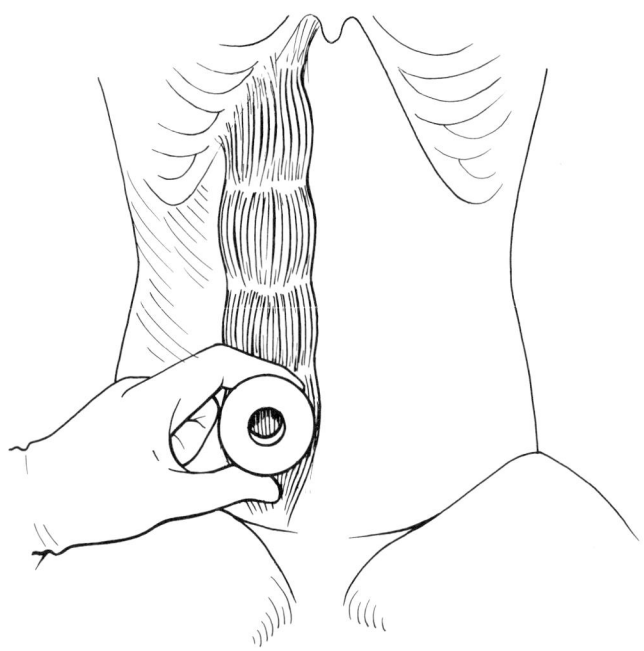

Fig. 106.1 The stoma is sited, with the patient both sitting and lying, so that the gut will pass through the belly of the rectus muscle.

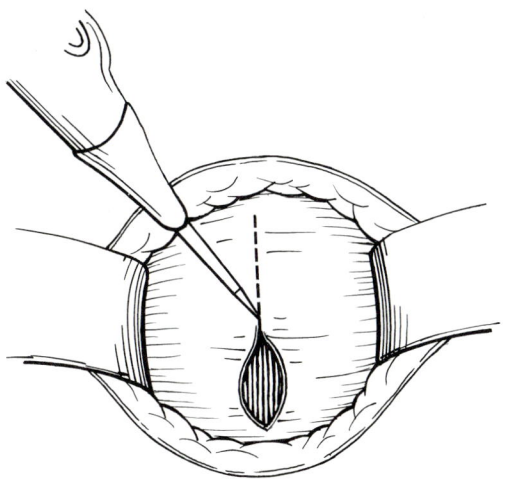

Fig. 106.2 The stoma aperture is created using right-angled retractors to progressively retract the subcutaneous fat and the anterior rectus sheath is incised.

the disc of skin is removed: the subcutaneous fat is preserved to lessen the chance of a dead space, resulting in a parastomal seroma or abscess. The fat also gives external support to the bowel wall. The fat is pushed aside with retractors and a vertical incision, approximately 3–3.5 cm long, is made in the anterior rectus sheath, exposing the fibers of the rectus muscle (Fig. 106.2). A vertical muscle split, rather than a transverse cutting procedure, separates the muscle and exposes the posterior rectus sheath, which is also divided vertically (Fig. 106.3). We do not use cruciate incisions in the rectus sheaths. The aperture in the abdominal wall should fit two fingers snugly. These technical details reduce the chance of stoma herniation and prolapse (if too large an aperture) or obstruction (if too small an aperture).

End ileostomy

The loop of bowel to be used for the stoma is prepared by dividing the terminal ileum approximately 6–10 cm from the ileocecal valve (Fig. 106.4). A linear stapling and cutting instrument facilitates this process and minimizes contamination during later delivery of the bowel through the abdominal wall.

The mesentery of the terminal ileum is divided and the vessels suture-ligated to prevent subsequent slipping of the ligatures. The mesentery to the terminal 5–8 cm of the bowel is divided about 1 cm from the bowel wall, preserving a vascular arcade close to the bowel. This reduces the bulk of the mesentery and straightens the terminal ileum (Fig. 106.5).

A soft, non-crushing forceps is then passed through the stoma aperture and the prepared ileum is drawn gently through the abdominal wall (Fig. 106.6). The optimal length of bowel to be exteriorized is 5–6 cm, in order to construct a satisfactory everted stoma. Ideally the final spout should be about 2 cm in length, with a slight downward angulation.

The bowel wall is then sutured to the peritoneum surrounding the internal stoma aperture. The previously divided free edge of the small-bowel mesentery is sutured to the back of the abdominal wound, approximately 3–4 cm from, and parallel to, the midline incision (Fig. 106.6). This suture line, which may be continued

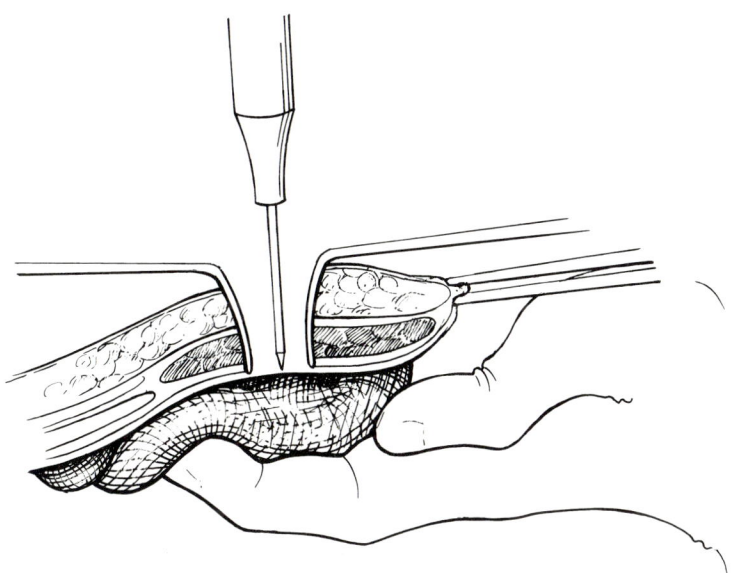

Fig. 106.3 Rectus muscle fibers, posterior rectus sheath and peritoneum as each is divided or separated in a longitudinal direction.

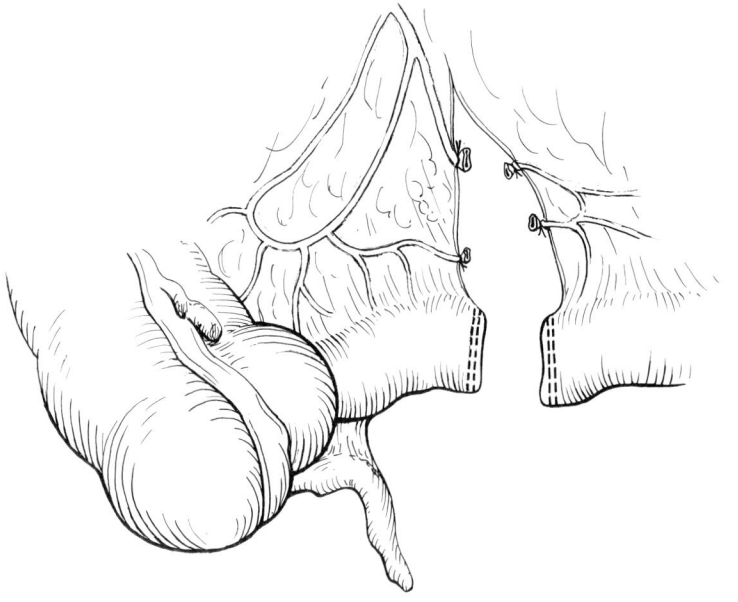

Fig. 106.4 For end ileostomy the terminal ileum and its mesentery are divided close to the ileocecal valve.

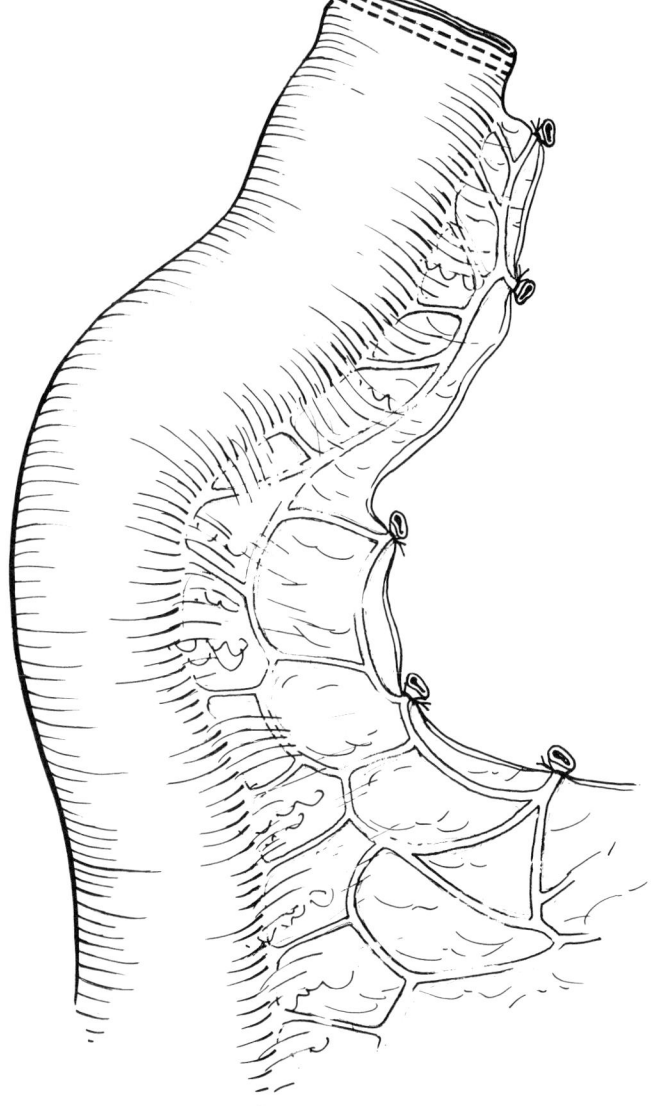

on to the free edge of the falciform ligament, serves to fix the small-bowel mesentery and helps to prevent stoma prolapse, internal small-bowel herniation, and volvulus of the small bowel around the point where it passes through the abdominal wall aperture.

After closure of the abdominal incision, the end of the bowel is trimmed to the required length. Good arterial bleeding from the cut end is an important sign of bowel viability. Radial sutures of fine absorbable material such as catgut are placed at the four 'compass points' of the stoma, passing through the full thickness of the bowel wall, but only through the subcuticular part of the skin edge of the stoma aperture (Fig. 106.7a). The needle should not pass through the external surface of the skin so as to minimize any risk of ileal mucosal implantation, which could cause premature separation of the stoma appliance. Four additional sutures are placed before all are tied, everting the bowel wall to produce a spouting stoma (Fig. 106.7b).

Loop-ileostomy

The loop of bowel chosen for a loop ileostomy will usually be 15–20 cm proximal to the ileocecal valve, new anastomosis or newly constructed pouch. In pelvic pouch surgery this distance may need to be considerably longer, because the more distal small-bowel loops close to the pouch may not be able to reach the skin level without tension.

At the apex of the selected loop a cotton tape is brought through a small 'window' made in the mesentery adjacent to the bowel wall. The afferent and efferent

Fig. 106.5 The mesentery of the terminal ileum is trimmed, preserving a vascular arcade to supply the distal bowel which will become the end ileostomy.

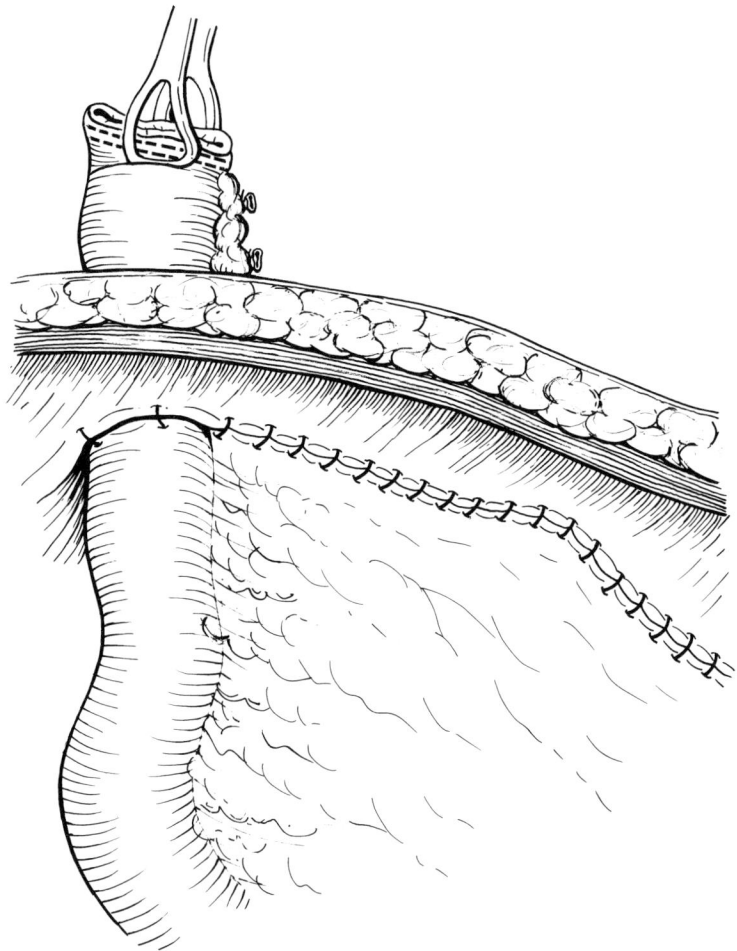

Fig. 106.6 The bowel is brought through the stoma aperture and the mesentery is sutured to the back of the abdominal wall and falciform ligament.

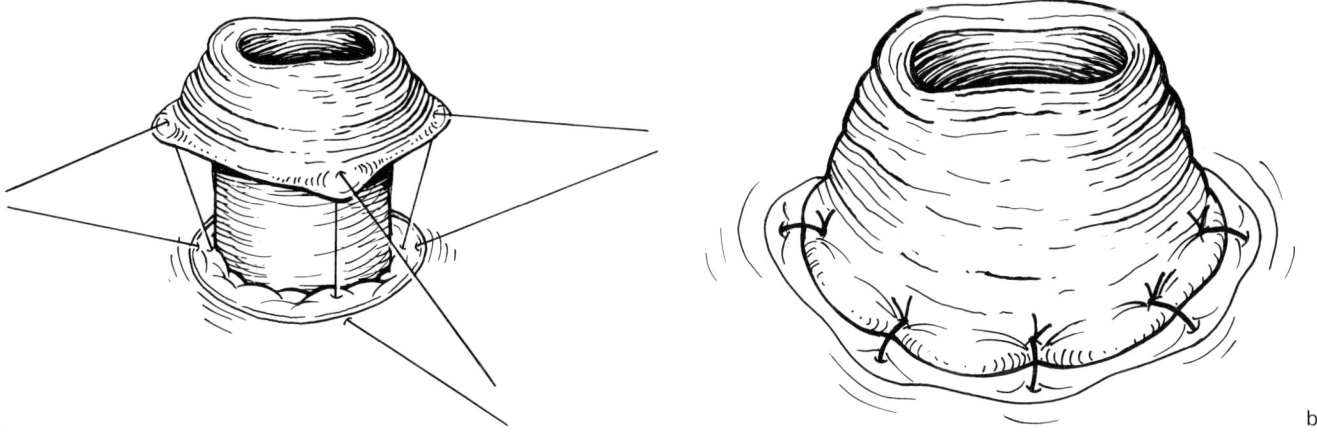

Fig. 106.7a Eight absorbable sutures are placed. **b** The bowel is everted and the sutures tied down to produce a spouting end ileostomy.

limbs of the loop are tagged with sutures of different materials or colors to avoid confusion when the loop is brought through the abdominal wall aperture.

A pair of forceps is placed through the stoma aperture, grasping the ends of the tape, which is used to draw the bowel through the abdominal wall (Fig. 106.8). The preferred orientation of the loop is with the proximal (afferent) loop lying caudad and the distal (efferent) limb cephalad.

A short ileostomy rod is placed under the bowel, replacing the tape, and holding the bowel in place while the abdominal incision and skin are closed.

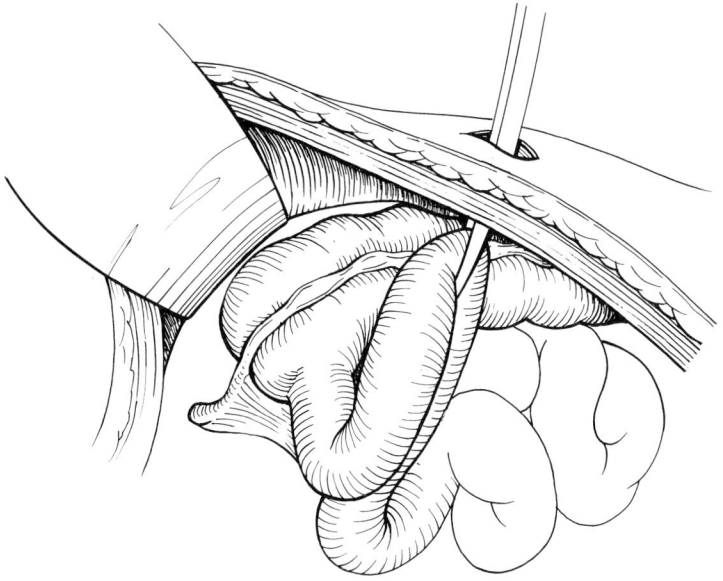

Fig. 106.8 A loop of bowel is drawn through the stoma aperture using a cotton tape passed through the mesentery at the chosen site for a loop ileostomy.

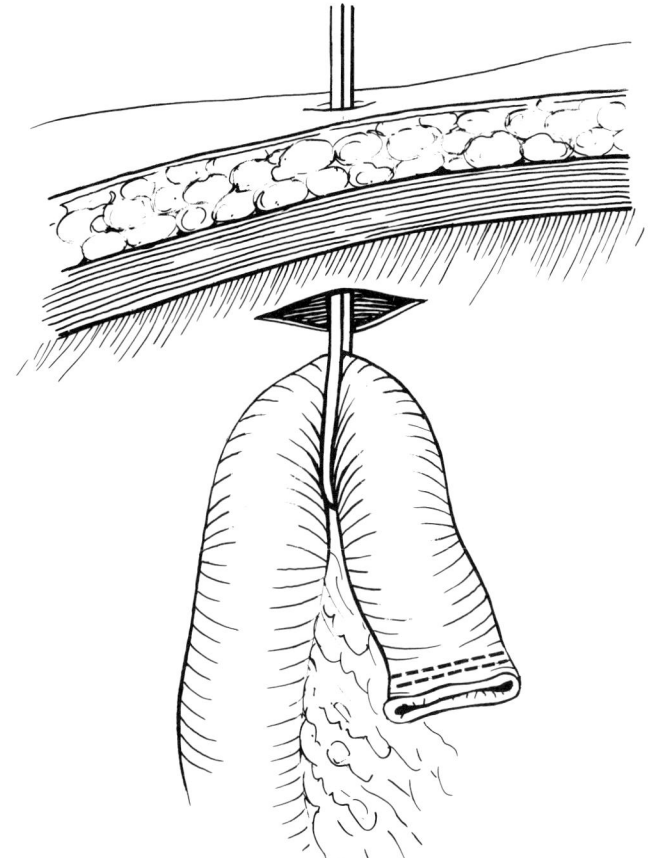

Fig. 106.9 For loop-end ileostomy, the divided and stapled bowel is drawn through the stoma aperture so that the divided end will lie just inside the peritoneal cavity.

The identifying suture tags are now removed and a transverse antimesenteric incision made in the distal (efferent) small-bowel limb, approximately 0.5 cm above and parallel to the skin surface (Fig. 106.10). The incision will involve 70–80% of the circumference of the bowel wall and start and end near the mesentery on each side, adjacent to the rod.

Fine absorbable sutures are then placed through the full thickness of the bowel edges and the subcuticular skin. Three sutures are usually placed on the distal (efferent) side and five on the proximal (afferent) side (Fig. 106.11). They are not tied down until all have been inserted, with the distal (efferent) limb sutures being tied first. The blunt end or handle of a pair of forceps is used to evert the proximal (afferent) bowel wall (Fig. 106.12a,b) while the remaining sutures are tied, thereby producing a stoma spout.

Loop–end ileostomy

The terminal ileum and its mesentery are divided as for an end ileostomy, but the mesentery and blood supply to the distal few centimeters of the bowel are left undisturbed. A small mesenteric window is made 7–10 cm proximal to the transected margin after estimating the length of the small bowel that is needed to traverse the (often thickened) abdominal wall, such that the divided distal end lies just inside the peritoneal cavity (Fig. 106.9). A cotton tape is passed through the mesenteric window and used to draw the bowel through the abdominal wall aperture. Differently colored suture tags are used to maintain the correct orientation. The functional (afferent) end should lie caudad, with the non-functional (efferent) end cephalad, as this will allow the divided mesenteric edges to be easily aligned with the anterior abdominal wall. The tape is then replaced with a short ileostomy rod.

The free, divided, edge of the small-bowel mesentery may then be sutured to the anterior abdominal wall, parallel to the main incision, which is then closed. The stoma is matured to the skin in the same way as with a loop ileostomy (Figs 106.10–106.12).

EARLY POSTOPERATIVE CARE OF THE STOMA

The skin surrounding the stoma is covered by a skin barrier in the operating room. The most used barrier is a karaya ring or disc which can be applied over the stoma and its rod (if present). A transparent pouch with adhesive backing is then attached to the skin barrier and surrounding skin. The transparent bag allows for easy inspection of the stoma in the early days after operation.

With a loop or loop–end stoma the rod may be removed after 3–5 days, at which time the permanent pouch is selected and the patient given detailed instruc-

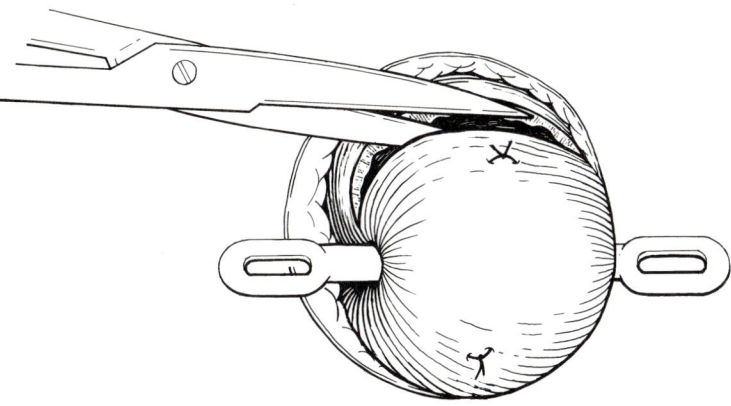

Fig. 106.10 For loop ileostomy and loop–end ileostomy, the tape is replaced by an ileostomy rod before the distal (efferent) limb is opened.

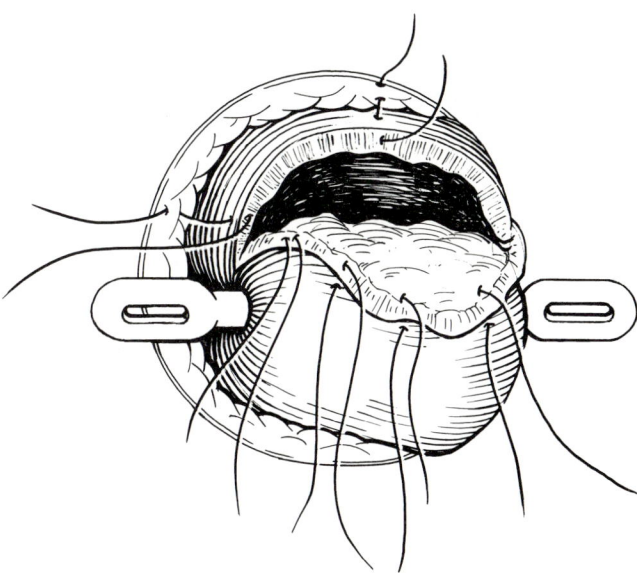

Fig. 106.11 Three sutures are placed on the efferent side and five on the afferent side.

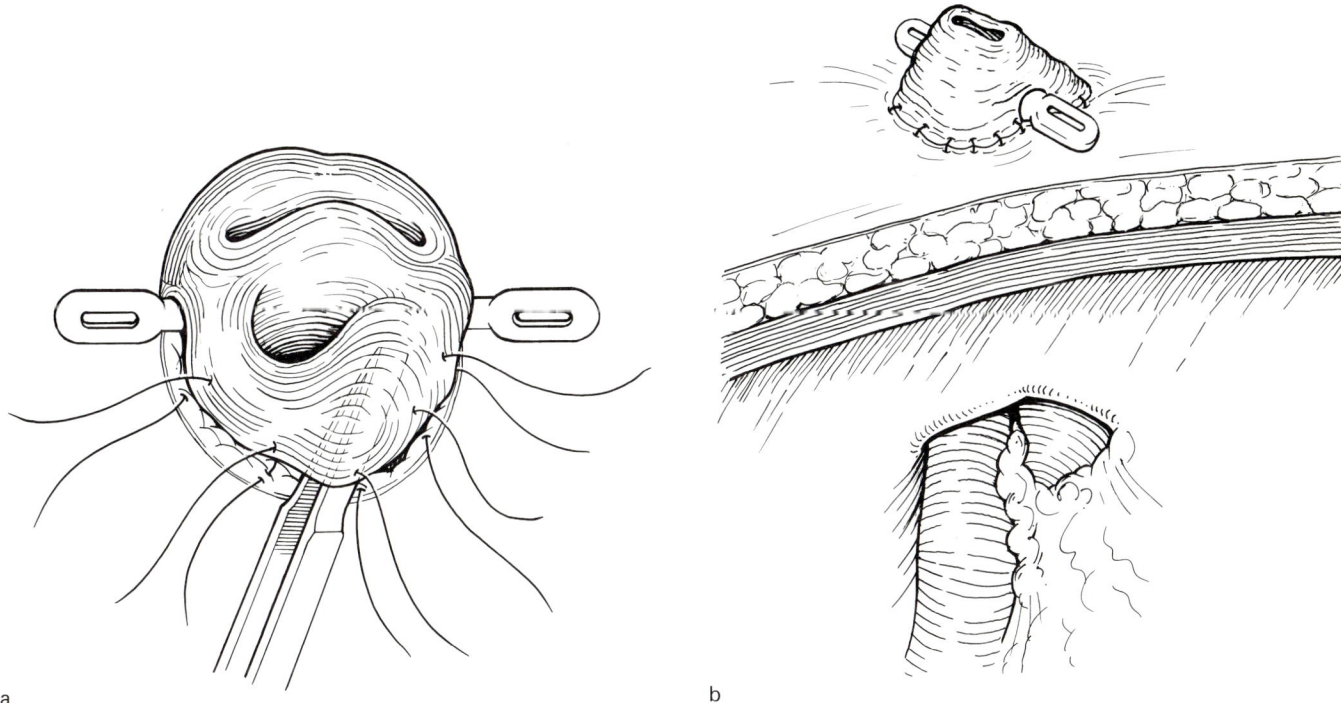

Fig. 106.12a The afferent bowel wall is everted and the sutures tied, producing a stoma spout (**b**).

tions on emptying and changing the appliance, and on skin care and diet.

A loop ileostomy, which is intended to be temporary, may be closed after about 3 months. Earlier closure is associated with a higher incidence of complications because of residual edema friability of the tissues.

107. Complications of stomas and their management

J. G. Williams   S. M. Goldberg

Many patients with inflammatory bowel disease will require a stoma at some time during the course of their life, either temporarily or permanently. Complications related to the stoma can mar the improvement in quality of life expected of surgical intervention. For this reason great attention should be given to stoma construction, which should not be regarded as an afterthought at the end of a long operation.

Many different stomal complications have been described (Table 107.1), with over two-thirds of ileostomy patients experiencing at least one of these (Leong et al 1994). Stomal complications often are interrelated, with one arising as a result of another. An example of this is appliance leakage, which may be caused by poor appliance technique, but in many patients is caused by another stoma complication, such as inappropriate siting, parastomal hernia, ileostomy retraction or fistula formation. Careful assessment is important if correct identification of the primary problem is to be made and appropriate treatment instituted.

ISCHEMIA

Satisfactory healing of the mucocutaneous junction of a stoma depends on an adequate blood supply to the end of the gut. Ischemia is more common in an end stoma than a loop stoma, because it has a more tenuous blood supply. It is important not to denude the terminal part of the bowel of its blood supply during mobilization. Similarly, the hole through the abdominal wall should not be too small or the blood supply will be compromised. It is useful to prepare the bowel for stoma formation early in the operation, as inadequate perfusion will be evident by the time the stoma is constructed. A stoma which is obviously ischemic during or immediately after construction should be revised before the patient wakes from the anesthetic. A more proximal segment of bowel, with a better blood supply, may need to be used.

A minor degree of ischemia is usual in the early postoperative phase, with edema and darkening of the exposed mucosa, but this usually resolves in a few days. More profound ischemia may result in necrosis of part or all of the circumference of the bowel used to form the stoma. Complete necrosis of an ileostomy requires relaparotomy and the creation of a new stoma. Necrosis of a colostomy does not necessarily require stomal revision. Healing by secondary intention may occur if the necrotic segment is short. However, this usually results in stenosis.

Table 107.1 Incidence of common complications of intestinal stomas

Complication	Ileostomy* 150 patients		Colostomy† 126 patients	
	n	%	n	%
Necrosis	1	1	–	–
Stenosis	6	5	11	9
Prolapse	12	11	4	3
Retraction	19	17	–	–
Obstruction	27	23	9	7
Fistula	11	12	3	2
Hernia	16	16	14	11
Skin problems	44	34	17	14

* Data from St Mark's Hospital (Leong et al 1994). All complications recorded at clinic review. Complication rate expressed as a cumulative probability from life-table analysis
† Data from Porter et al 1989. Retrospective review of all patients having end colostomy formed

STENOSIS

Stomal stenosis is a consequence of ischemia in the bowel used to form the stoma (see above). A tight stenosis will cause subacute intestinal obstruction. Local revision of the stoma is sometimes possible without laparotomy by excising the stenosed mucocutaneous junction, mobilizing the distal intestine and resuturing the fresh, mobilized bowel to the widened skin edge. A laparotomy will be required if insufficient bowel can be mobilized to create the new anastomosis without tension.

STOMAL PROLAPSE

Transverse loop colostomies are most frequently affected by stomal prolapse, especially if constructed for acute large-bowel obstruction, where the hole in the abdominal fascia needs to be large to accommodate the obstructed bowel (Burns 1970, Saha et al 1973). Prolapse may affect both limbs of the colostomy, but more often it is the distal limb that prolapses. The appearances are often alarming, but symptoms may be few and usually are related to difficulties in fitting an appliance. Treatment options include closing the stoma (if feasible), dividing the loop and closing the distal end and returning it to the abdomen, and revision of the stoma, carefully fixing the emerging bowel to the abdominal fascia.

Ileostomy prolapse may be fixed or sliding. A sliding prolapse will retract flush with the abdominal wall when the patient lies down, predisposing to leakage. Symptomatic ileostomy prolapse will require revision of the stoma. The mucocutaneous junction is taken down and the everted ileum is unfolded. The emerging ileum is fixed to the abdominal fascia with interrupted non-absorbable seromuscular sutures. The redundant prolapsed ileum is excised and the stoma refashioned. Ileostomy prolapse does not appear to be prevented by ensuring that the stoma is brought out through the rectus abdominis, or by fixing the mesentery to the abdominal wall (Leong et al 1994).

RETRACTION

Colostomy retraction usually results from insufficient mobilization of the colon used to form the stoma. Fitting an appliance to a sunken colostomy can be difficult, and leakage and skin problems may develop. Retraction of an ileostomy usually results from poor adhesion between the emerging ileum and the abdominal fat and fascia. Fixing the mesentery to the abdominal wall does not appear to prevent ileostomy retraction (Leong et al 1994). Another cause of stomal retraction is a parastomal hernia. A flush ileostomy is difficult to manage and skin problems often arise. Fixed ileostomy retraction will require laparotomy and stomal revision by mobilizing a proximal length of ileum. This usually necessitates a laparotomy. Mobile ileostomy retraction can be dealt with in a number of ways. Inserting a series of interrupted sutures through the full thickness of the everted stoma will fix the two walls of the stoma together. An alternative method is to evert the bowel with tissue forceps and apply a number of rows of staples along the stoma to keep it everted (Fig. 107.1) (Winslet et al 1990). Care must be taken not to occlude the blood supply. Recurrences are common after any sort of retraction fixation.

PARASTOMAL HERNIA

An abdominal stoma requires an abnormal opening in the abdominal wall, which is a weak point through which a hernia may form alongside the emerging bowel. Great emphasis is placed on the technique of stomal construc-

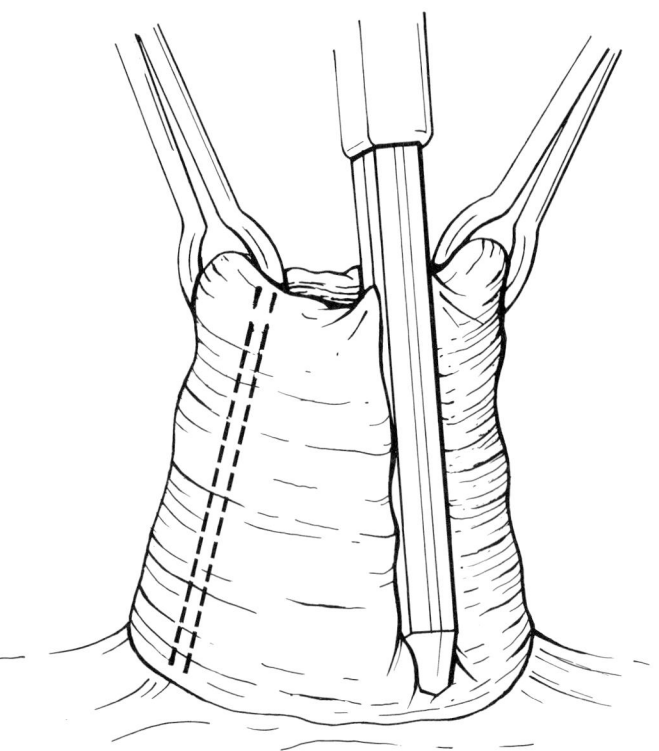

Fig. 107.1 Stabilization of a retracted ileostomy using a linear stapler. The ileostomy is prolapsed with Babcock forceps. A linear stapler, without a blade, is inserted into the ileostomy and fired. This is repeated with a fresh cartridge at a further two sites round the circumference of the stoma, avoiding the area of the mesentery. The procedure can be performed under intravenous sedation.

tion in preventing parastomal hernia formation. Care must be taken not to make the fascial incision too large. An incision which admits the tips of two fingers is usually sufficient. The risk of hernia formation is stated to be less if the stoma is brought out through the rectus abdominis muscle (Rosin & Bonardi 1977, Goligher 1984, Sjödahl et al 1988). However, a radiological study using CT scanning showed a similar incidence of parastomal hernia formation in stomas brought out through the rectus muscle and those which were lateral to the muscle (Williams et al 1990). A similar conclusion has been reached by other authors (Leong et al 1994). However, there have been no randomized controlled trials.

The most common type of parastomal hernia is subcutaneous, which may contain small bowel, large bowel or omentum. An interstitial hernia has a sac which lies between the layers of the abdominal wall. An intrastomal hernia lies between the emerging bowel wall and the everted bowel of an end ileostomy (Devlin 1988). The reported incidence of parastomal hernia is shown in Table 107.2. It is generally accepted that paracolostomy hernia is more common than paraileostomy hernia. The true incidence of parastomal hernia formation is probably higher than that quoted, as a parastomal hernia may be asymptomatic and may develop many years after surgery.

Table 107.2 Incidence of parastomal hernia formation

Reference	Date	Stoma type	Follow-up (years)	Total patients	No. with hernia	%
Burns (1970)[1]	1970	Colostomy	1–21	307	16	5.2
Saha et al (1973)[1]	1973	Colostomy	1–6	200	2	1.0
Kronborg et al (1974)[3]	1974	Colostomy	1–10	362	42	11.6
Harshaw et al (1974)[2]	1974	Colostomy	1–7	99	9	9.1
Marks and Richie (1975)[2]	1975	Colostomy	1–6	227	23	32.6[6]
Burgess et al (1984)[3]	1984	Colostomy	1–10	124	6	4.8
Carlstedt et al (1987)[5]	1987	Ileostomy	1–26	203	3	1.5
Sjödahl et al (1988)[4]	1988	All stomas	1–36	130	9	6.9
Porter et al (1989)[2]	1989	Colostomy	<8	130	14	10.7
Williams et al (1990)[7]	1990	Ileostomy	1–16	46	13	28.2
Hoffman et al (1992)[2]	1992	Colostomy	<10	111	5	4.5
Leong et al (1994)[3]	1994	Ileostomy	<20	150	16	16.0[6]
Martin et al (1994)[4]	1994	All stomas	N/A	242	15	6.2

[1] Details of follow-up method not provided
[2] Retrospective study of patients undergoing stoma construction
[3] Prospective follow-up of patients undergoing stoma construction
[4] Patients presenting to a specialist stoma clinic
[5] Incidence based on reoperation rate
[6] Cumulative rate, based on life-table analysis
[7] Patients specifically reviewed for hernia formation

A recent clinical and radiological study of 46 patients with an ileostomy, revealed a hernia incidence of 28%. Limited CT scanning of the stoma in 28 patients demonstrated 10 paraileostomy hernias; two of these were not evident on clinical examination (Williams et al 1990).

A parastomal hernia may present as a bulge at the stoma site, which makes appliance fitting difficult. Alternative presentations include leakage, skin excoriation and difficulty irrigating a colostomy. Rarely the patient will present with complications of the parastomal hernia, such as intestinal obstruction or strangulation of a loop of bowel within the hernia. Diagnosis of a parastomal hernia is usually straightforward, but difficulty may be encountered if the hernia is small or the patient obese; CT scanning is useful in such situations (Williams et al 1990).

For most patients a parastomal hernia is an inconvenience, making appliance fitting difficult, with occasional leakage. However, many patients can manage by wearing a special appliance with a belt. Surgical intervention should be considered if symptoms are incapacitating. The suggestion of bowel strangulation within a parastomal hernia is an absolute indication for surgery.

Three surgical approaches are possible.

1. **Local repair.** This is the simplest approach, but probably the least effective. The stoma is mobilized and the hernial sac dissected free. The defect in the abdominal wall is narrowed round the emerging stoma with a series of non-absorbable sutures (Fig. 107.2) and the stoma is recreated. Failure of local repair is likely (Horgan & Hughes 1986, Allen-Mersh & Thomson 1988, Devlin 1988). For this reason, other surgical options have evolved.

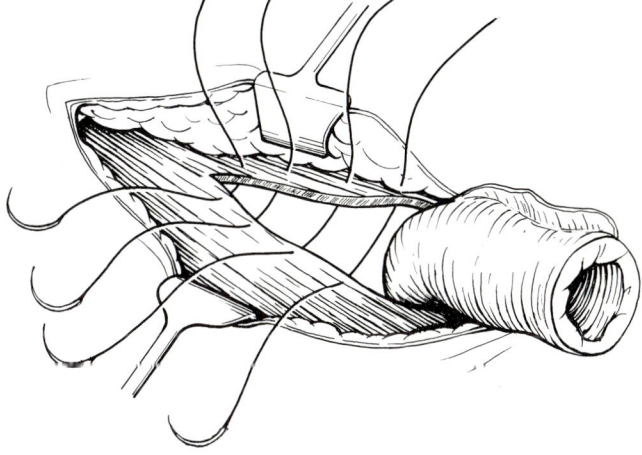

Fig. 107.2 Local repair of a parastomal hernia. An incision is made adjacent to the stoma and the enlarged defect in the fascia is defined and cleaned. The defect is narrowed round the stoma with a series of non-absorbable sutures.

2. **Repair with prosthetic material.** Prosthetic mesh can be used to support the abdominal wall surrounding the stoma, with a hole just sufficient to accommodate the emerging bowel cut in the mesh. Three methods have been employed. The most invasive is intraperitoneal mesh repair (Sugarbaker 1985, Byers et al 1992). A preperitoneal placement requires laparotomy (Fig. 107.3), with the mesh inserted behind the abdominal wall and in front of the peritoneum (Devlin 1988). An alternative technique is to suture the mesh to the abdominal wall in the subcutaneous plane (Leslie 1984). An L-shaped incision away from the stoma site is used to prevent scarring and deformity of the skin underneath the

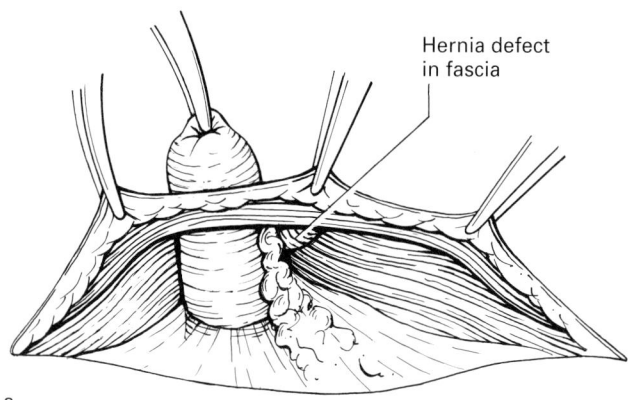 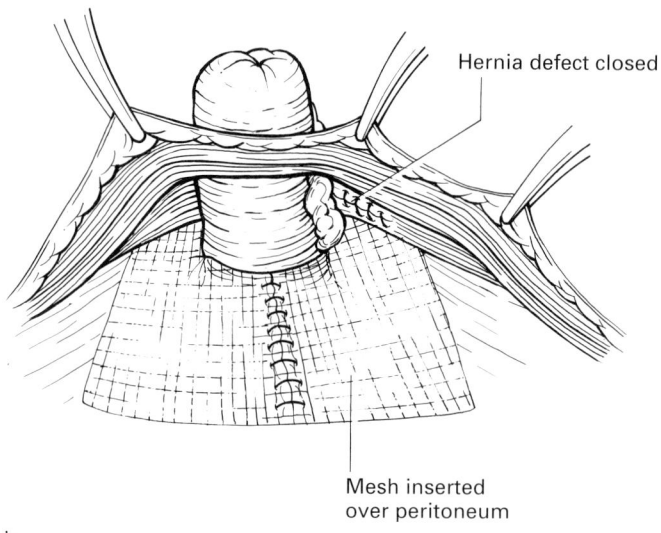

Fig. 107.3a Preperitoneal mesh repair of a parastomal hernia. The main abdominal incision is opened and the preperitoneal plane is developed around the stoma. The enlarged fascial defect is defined.
b A precut sheet of mesh is placed round the emerging stoma and sutured to the peritoneum. The defect in the fascia is narrowed from within by a series of interrupted sutures.

appliance. The advantage of the former technique is that the risk of infection in the mesh is less. The advantage of the extraparietal technique is that laparotomy is avoided.

3. **Stoma relocation.** Relocating the stoma to another site is often the best way of dealing with a parastomal hernia. This can be achieved without laparotomy, by mobilizing the stoma fully, making a new hole in the abdominal wall, developing a plane below the anterior abdominal wall and passing the mobilized stoma out through the new stoma site (Kaufman 1983). If difficulties are encountered a laparotomy will be required. The original stoma site is closed with non-absorbable sutures. Incisional hernia is common, especially if the original defect is large.

Unfortunately, a recurrent hernia may follow repair of a parastomal hernia, however performed. A large series of 105 parastomal hernia repairs reported from the Cleveland Clinic had a cumulative recurrence rate of 48%. Recurrence was slightly more frequent after local repair (57%) than after stomal transposition (46%) (Mellbring et al 1988).

OBSTRUCTION

Intestinal obstruction may occur for a number of reasons in a patient with an intestinal stoma.

1. Stenosis of the stoma, if profound, will cause subacute obstruction and require stomal revision.
2. A parastomal hernia, especially an incarcerated hernia, may obstruct the emerging stoma.
3. Intestinal obstruction may be caused by postoperative adhesions. The incidence of adhesive obstruction following proctocolectomy is between 10 and 20% (Phillips et al 1989, Leong et al 1994).
4. In a patient with Crohn's disease obstruction may represent recurrent disease, which usually develops just proximal to the stoma. A retrograde contrast study, or examination with a flexible sigmoidoscope, will establish the diagnosis.

FISTULA

A fistula between the emerging bowel and the peristomal skin is a rare complication. Persistent seepage from the fistula can cause skin problems and make appliance fitting difficult, thereby compounding the problem. There are three possible causes of fistula formation:

1. Inadvertent full-thickness penetration of the emerging bowel wall by a suture placed between the fascia and the bowel
2. Pressure necrosis from a tight-fitting ileostomy appliance may erode through the ileostomy to form a skin-level fistula
3. In Crohn's disease a peristomal fistula may arise from recurrent disease in the emerging bowel. One series reported an incidence of 7% in 214 patients who had an ileostomy formed for Crohn's disease (Greenstein et al 1983).

Surgical treatment usually requires laparotomy and formation of a new stoma.

MISCELLANEOUS COMPLICATIONS

Bleeding from a stoma is usually due to trauma, either from a poorly fitting appliance or from inflammatory polyps, which sometimes develop on the exposed mucosa. However, other causes which should be considered are recurrent Crohn's disease and portal hypertension, where a caput medusae may form in the skin surrounding a stoma (Conte et al 1990).

With colostomies perforation proximal to the stoma may be traumatic in origin, related to stoma irrigation. Cases of stercoral perforation have been described, secondary to scybala in a loaded proximal colon (Serpell et al 1991).

Pyoderma gangrenosum may develop in the peristomal skin, but few cases have been described in patients with ulcerative colitis and Crohn's disease (Keltz et al 1992). Skin ulceration develops within a few months of stoma construction. Differential diagnosis includes suture reaction, contact dermatitis, peristomal abscess and enzymatic digestion secondary to a poorly fitting appliance. Treatment with steroids is recommended, but topical ointments can be messy and make appliance fitting difficult. Alternatives include systemic steroids and intralesional steroid injections.

Adenocarcinoma is an unusual stoma complication. A carcinomatous deposit in a stoma formed during resection of large-bowel cancer represents tumor implantation, tumor recurrence following inadequate resection, or a second primary, either synchronous or metachronous, depending on the time interval. Over the last few years there have been an increasing number of reports of adenocarcinoma developing in an ileostomy formed after colonic resection for inflammatory bowel disease (Gadacz et al 1990, Carey et al 1993, Starke et al 1993). The interval between stoma construction and the development of cancer is usually many years. One possible explanation is that ileal mucosa undergoes metaplastic change to 'colonic' mucosa, in which dysplasia eventually develops into invasive cancer. Certainly these cases of late-onset cancer are worrying, especially as many patients have an ileostomy constructed during early adult life and would be expected to survive for many decades.

REFERENCES

Allen-Mersh T, Thomson J P S 1988 Surgical treatment of colostomy complications. British Journal of Surgery 75: 416–418

Burgess P, Matthew V V, Devlin H B 1984 A review of terminal colostomy complications following abdominoperineal resection for carcinoma. British Journal of Surgery 71: 1004

Burns F J 1970 Complications of colostomy. Diseases of the Colon and Rectum 13: 448–450

Byers J M, Steinberg J B, Postier R G 1992 Repair of parastomal hernias using polypropylene mesh. Archives of Surgery 127: 1246–1247

Carey P D, Suvarna S K, Baloch K G et al 1993 Primary adenocarcinoma in an ileostomy: a late complication of surgery for ulcerative colitis. Surgery 113: 712–715

Carlstedt A, Fasth S, Hultén L et al 1987 Long-term ileostomy complications in patients with ulcerative colitis and Crohn's disease. International Journal of Colorectal Disease 2: 22–25

Conte J V, Arcomano T A, Naficy M A et al 1990 Treatment of bleeding stomal varices. Report of a case and review of the literature. Diseases of the Colon and Rectum 33: 308–314

Devlin H B 1988 Parastomal hernia. In: Management of abdominal hernias. Butterworths, London, pp 177–186

Gadacz T R, McFadden D W, Gabrielson E W et al 1990 Adenocarcinoma of the ileostomy: the latent risk of cancer after colectomy for ulcerative colitis and familial polyposis. Surgery 107: 698–703

Goligher J C 1984 Complications relating to the colostomy. In: Surgery of the anus rectum and colon. Baillière Tindall, London, pp 702–705

Greenstein A J, Dicker A, Meyers S et al 1983 Periileostomy fistulae in Crohn's disease. Annals of Surgery 197: 179–182

Harshaw D H, Gardner B, Vives A et al 1974 The effect of technical factors upon complications from abdominal perineal resections. Surgery, Gynecology and Obstetrics 139: 756–758

Hoffman M S, Barton D P J, Gates J et al 1992 Complications of colostomy performed on gynecology cancer patients. Gynecologic Oncology 44: 231–234

Horgan K, Hughes L E 1986 Para-ileostomy hernia: failure of a local repair technique. British Journal of Surgery 73: 439–440

Kaufman J J 1983 Repair of parastomal hernia by translocation of the stoma without laparotomy. Journal of Urology 129: 278–279

Keltz M, Lebwohl M, Bishop S 1992 Peristomal pyoderma gangrenosum. Journal of the American Academy of Dermatology 27: 360–364

Kronberg O, Kramhöft J, Backer O et al 1974 Late complications following operations for cancer of the rectum and anus. Diseases of the Colon and Rectum 17: 750–753

Leong A P K, Londono-Schimmer E E, Phillips R K S 1994 Life-table analysis of stomal complications following ileostomy. British Journal of Surgery 81: 727–729

Leslie D 1984 The parastomal hernia. Surgical Clinics of North America 64: 407–415

Marks C G, Ritchie J K 1975 The complications of synchronous combined excision for adenocarcinoma of the rectum at St Mark's Hospital. British Journal of Surgery 62: 901–905

Martin L, Lightfoot C, Foster G 1994 Parastomal hernia: adding insult to injury. Proceedings of the Association of Coloproctology of Great Britain and Ireland, Poster 18.

Mellbring G, Fazio V W, Lavery I C et al 1988 The results of surgery for parastomal hernia. Abstract, American Society of Colon and Rectal Surgeons, Scientific Meeting, Anaheim

Phillips R K S, Ritchie J K, Hawley P R 1989 Proctocolectomy and ileostomy for ulcerative colitis: the longer term story. Journal of the Royal Society of Medicine 82: 386–387

Porter J A, Salvati E P, Rubin R J et al 1989 Complications of colostomies. Diseases of the Colon and Rectum 32: 299–303

Rosin J D, Bonardi R A 1977 Paracolostomy hernia repair with marlex mesh: a new technique. Diseases of the Colon and Rectum 20: 229

Saha S P, Rao N, Stephenson S E 1973 Complications of colostomy. Diseases of the Colon and Rectum 16: 515–516

Serpell J W, Sen M, Giddings G et al 1991 Stercoral perforation of the colon proximal to an end colostomy. Postgraduate Medical Journal 67: 299–300

Sjödahl R, Anderberg B, Bolin T 1988 Parastomal hernia in relation to site of the abdominal stoma. British Journal of Surgery 75: 339–341

Starke J, Rodriguez-Bigas M, Marshall W et al 1993 Primary adenocarcinoma arising in an ileostomy. Surgery 114: 125–128

Sugarbaker P H 1985 Peritoneal approach to prosthetic mesh repair of paraostomy hernias. Annals of Surgery 201: 344–346

Williams J G, Etherington R, Hayward M W J et al 1990 Paraileostomy hernia: a clinical and radiological study. British Journal of Surgery 77: 1355–1357

Winslet M C, Alexander-Williams J, Keighley M R B 1990 Ileostomy revision with a GIA stapler under intravenous sedation. British Journal of Surgery 77: 647

SECTION 14

Social and psychological aspects of disease

108. Psychological factors including sexual function

F. A. Frizelle   H. Nelson

RELATIONSHIP BETWEEN PSYCHOSOCIAL AND PHYSICAL ASPECTS OF IBD

Although it is well recognized that physical symptoms can cause stress, it is perhaps less well recognized that stress can aggravate physical symptoms, as in pre-existing IBD. Certainly behavioral problems that result in non-compliance with medical or surgical therapies can directly aggravate IBD. Despite there being a recognized dynamic interaction between physical manifestation and psychosocial problems in IBD, a true cause and effect relationship has not been established. Since the interactions between the psychosocial and physical aspects can make the management of IBD patients more difficult, it is probably most rewarding to consider them together, regardless of cause and effect.

A model to aid conceptualization of the dynamic between the physical and psychosocial aspects of disease was described by Lask in 1986 (Fig. 108.1).

Although this model was developed for children and adolescents, who are in the process of development, it can be applied to adults as well. Since the physical manifestations of IBD are well covered in other chapters, this chapter will focus on what is known about the psychological and social profiles of patients with IBD, including an examination of psychosocial aspects of surgical therapy, stomas and sexual function.

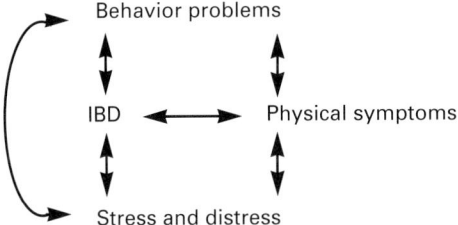

Fig. 108.1 Model of interaction of psychosocial and physical factors in IBD. (Lask 1986)

PSYCHOLOGICAL PROFILE OF PATIENTS WITH IBD

The impression that psychiatric illness is common in patients with IBD is only partly accurate. Although extreme psychiatric disorders, as measured by frequency of suicide, divorce, psychosis or use of psychotropic medications, have been reported to be the same in ulcerative colitis as in the general population (Gruner et al 1978), less severe disorders appear more common (Engstrom & Lindquist 1991).

Engstrom and Lindquist (1991) studied the prevalence of psychiatric disorders in adolescent patients aged 9–18 years. Using classifications according to the revised third edition of the *Diagnostic and statistical manual*, they found that 60% of IBD patients had psychiatric disturbances compared to 15% in a matched control group ($P=0.009$), mainly depression or anxiety disorders. This study also revealed a tendency towards more frequent psychiatric disturbances in patients with ulcerative colitis than those with Crohn's disease, despite the fact that Crohn's patients were more seriously disturbed physically and had been ill for longer periods of time (Engstrom & Lindquist 1991). At least one author reports that the symptoms of malaise and fatigue, which are generally attributed to the underlying inflammatory process, can be relieved when depression is treated medically (Andrews et al 1987). As the complications of anxiety and depression can be identified using a self-administered questionnaire and can respond to drug therapy, these should be considered useful adjuncts in the care of IBD patients.

The chronic and unpredictable nature of inflammatory bowel disease dramatically affects the social and psychological wellbeing of patients and their families. There are many interactions that occur between the disease, therapies and the patient's mental state. Understanding the interactions of physical disease, social and psychological components is critical for developing comprehensive plans for the care of patients with IBD. Providing such comprehensive care can, in theory, avoid problems with compliance, denial and displaced aggression. In addition to improving the professional relationship and alleviating patient anxieties, comprehensive patient care may improve health-related outcomes, since stress is thought to affect disease activity. To develop such an all-encompassing approach to the IBD patient, it is probably most useful to consider the behavioral and psychological problems of patients with IBD as manifestations of chronic disease in an otherwise normal population. Successful management of a patient with a chronic disease requires the early development of a solid, trusting relationship. A surgeon can gain the patient's confidence early in the relationship by providing reassurance and education about the surgical therapies, as well as information about available support services.

SOCIAL PROFILE

Another measure of the psychological wellbeing of a population is its integration into contemporary cultural and social activities. When patients with Crohn's disease and age- and gender-matched controls were compared in a study from Copenhagen, the two populations exhibited similar levels of social interaction, including cultural, sporting, educational and private social arrangements (Sorensen et al 1987). In a separate study examining the effects of Crohn's disease on academic success, Mayberry and colleagues demonstrated that, despite the fact that these patients experienced significantly more school day absences than the controls ($P<0.001$), they achieved similar academic success (Mayberry et al 1992). In this Welsh study, academic success was measured as passing scores on examinations and attendance at tertiary institutes of education (Mayberry et al 1992).

Work, which is less a social and more an essential activity, is generally normal in IBD patients, despite the fact that they may be hampered by diarrhea, urgency (requiring access to appropriate facilities), fatigue and the occasional need for hospitalization (Wyke 1988). A study from Copenhagen showed that 65% of patients with Crohn's disease were employed compared to 64% of age- and gender-matched controls. The same study showed that Crohn's patients had retained their jobs for more than 5 years (77% versus 64%) (Sorensen et al 1987). Similar results were reported from the United Kingdom, where 72% of patents with IBD were reported as employed, 1% as unemployed, with 75% retaining the same job over 6 years (Wyke et al 1988). It is unfortunate that, despite these favorable employment records, at least a few patients considered that they were not promoted or were demoted as a result of their disease (Whates & Irving 1984). It might be assumed that work-related problems would arise due to illness-related absences, but in fact overall these patients generally have good work attendance records.

The number of sick days was reported as being similar in patients with Crohn's disease and controls, with 72% and 69% respectively having fewer than 11 sick days (Sorensen et al 1987). Even though overall attendances are similar, differences in time off work may be demonstrated based on the need for therapy. For example, in IBD patients that require surgery, proctocolectomy with ileostomy resulted in more patients requiring lengthy absences compared to colectomy and ileorectal anastomosis, with 35% and 17% respectively absent from work for 12 months following surgery (Wyke 1988). Despite higher initial postoperative absences, patients with an ileostomy ultimately experienced fewer problems and less sick leave (Wyke 1988). Additional work-related impairments may be job specific, since it has been reported that impairment of the ability to work is more common in white collar workers than in blue collar workers (Sonnenberg 1989). Since at least one report claims that employment status can be improved by 72% with rehabilitation, this should be considered an option for patients who are experiencing employment difficulties as a result of their illness and/or therapy (Sonnenberg 1992).

Finally, it should be recognized that some patients may face less than optimal attitudes at work. Even though the attitude of employers to patients with IBD is often better than other chronic diseases, up to 25% would not continue to employ people if they developed IBD, and 30% said they would not provide time off work to attend hospital clinics (Moody et al 1992). The attitudes of colleagues is more encouraging, with 80% considered 'helpful', 18% 'neutral', and only 2% 'unhelpful'. The presence or absence of a stoma did not influence the attitude of colleagues (Wyke 1988).

PSYCHOSOCIAL AND SEXUAL FUNCTION CONSIDERATIONS IN THE MANAGEMENT OF IBD

Patients with IBD are generally concerned about the need for surgery, and are specifically concerned about the need for a stoma, yet are unlikely to volunteer their fears (Mitchell et al 1988). Since true psychiatric morbidity from a stoma is rare (<5%: Lask et al 1987), and improving the patient's ability to cope with their illness is best achieved by effectively treating the underlying disease, the need to create a stoma as part of optimal surgical management should not be deferred for fear of adverse psychological consequences (Lask et al 1987). Instead, patients' anxieties should be anticipated and their concerns addressed. Patient concerns will range from the impact of surgery and a stoma on sexual and social activities to its impact on employment and family matters. Providing preoperative educational materials and stoma therapy counseling will aid the patient through this difficult time, and assist in their ultimate adjustment.

Surgical consultation should be sought early in the course of a patient's care. Results of surgery on quality of life should be reviewed with the patient and family. The literature suggests that patients who require surgery and a stoma have an improvement in their quality of life, with overall satisfaction rates as high as 93% for Brooke ileostomy and 96% for ileal pouch–anal anastomosis (Kohler et al 1991). In the same series 98% of patients with a Brooke ileostomy and 94% of those with an ileal pouch–anal anastomosis returned to work or school following surgery (Kohler et al 1991).

Although the vast majority of patients return to work or school, a change of employment may be necessary for some (16%), according to a report by Awad and colleagues (Awad et al 1993). Further, in adult patients requiring stomas it is reported that sport and leisure activities are only minimally impaired (Awad et al 1993) – 12 and 21%, respectively, yet housework and holidays were restricted in 34% and 37%, respectively (Awad et al 1993).

In addition to their concerns regarding work, schooling and quality of life, patients will have fears regarding the impact of surgery and a stoma on sexual function. Such fears may range from concerns about the appliance, including malfunction, with spillage and odor, or about physical impairment, such as sexual inadequacy or undesirability. Patients may grieve for real or presumptive loss of body image (Levin & Pemberton 1989). The most important first step is to provide factual information regarding sexual function following surgery.

Although sexual function is rarely altered after abdominal procedures, it can be adversely affected after procedures involving pelvic dissections. In males the rate of erectile dysfunction following pelvic surgery is 5%, with retrograde ejaculation reported as 6% (Walsh & Schlegel 1988). Dyspareunia in females, which may result from anatomic alterations due to surgery or from the disease process, has not been as well characterized. Overall, 14% of patients experience a severe degree of morbidity with respect to sexual activity, and a total of 49% experience at least a mild degree of morbidity. Long-term sexual limitations are less common following the ileal pouch–anal anastomosis (14%) than following the Brooke ileostomy (29%) (Kohler et al 1991). When overall sexual function in patients undergoing surgery for IBD was compared to the general population, no differences in frequency of marriage, divorce or coital practices were identified (Gruner et al 1977). Patients and their partners should be assured that sexual function and sexual interest generally return following recovery from surgery.

Counseling about the physical influence of surgery on sexual function should be complemented with further advice on practical approaches to living with a stoma. Many psychological barriers to intimacy with a stoma may be overcome by proper preparation. The pouch should be emptied, cleansed, and perhaps deodorized as necessary. The application of extra adhesive tape may secure the bag and prevent slippage. Men may find that wearing a cummerbund or boxer shorts provides intimacy without complete exposure. Women may find that a short nightdress accomplishes the same end. Dietary adjustments may help reduce gas and stool production. Despite all these measures, leaks will occur from time to time and it is essential that the patient feels confident and self-assured enough to cope. At these times a sense of humor and a shower may be all that is needed.

Another patient concern that requires thoughtful approach is that of the reproductive aspect of sexual function. Fertility, pregnancy and childbirth are important to the often youthful IBD patient. Although female fertility was originally thought to be reduced in patients with ulcerative colitis (deDombal et al 1965), recent studies suggest that this is not the case (Willoughby & Truelove 1980). In contrast, several reports indicate that fertility is reduced in women with Crohn's disease (Fielding & Cooke 1970, deDombal et al 1972). There are, however, difficulties associated with defining and studying fertility (Khosla et al 1984). Although female infertility is only rarely a result of pelvic inflammation and scarring (Burakoff 1993), it is more commonly due to active disease and/or poor nutritional status. Reasons other than decreased female fertility may explain reduced birth rates in Crohn's patients. Interest in childbearing may be low during times of acute or prolonged illness, and sexual intercourse may be infrequently practised at times when dyspareunia is experienced (Gazzard et al 1978). Women with IBD who are trying unsuccessfully to bear children should be referred for fertility investigations, including testing of their male partners.

Male fertility, although not reduced by the IBD process itself, may be reduced by medical and surgical therapies. Sulfasalazine produces several reversible forms of spermatozoa abnormalities, including oligospermia, reduced motility, and an increase in abnormal forms. Fortunately, these problems resolve when the medication is discontinued (Levi et al 1979, Toovey et al 1981). The use of 5-aminosalicylic acid (5-ASA) compounds avoids the need for sulfasalazine hence the spermatozoa dysfunction (Burakoff 1993).

For those IBD patients who become pregnant most (>80%) will experience a normal full-term delivery. In patients with ulcerative colitis the incidence of congenital abnormalities, low birthweight and spontaneous abortion is the same as in the general population (Willoughby & Truelove 1980, Levy et al 1981, Porter & Stirrat 1986). Although the outcome of pregnancy is particularly good in patients in whom IBD is in remission at the time of conception, those with active Crohn's disease do not often experience normal childbirth (Willoughby & Truelove 1980, Nielson et al 1983). Women with severely active Crohn's disease are twice as likely to have a stillbirth, spontaneous abortion or premature delivery (Neilson et al 1983, Khosla et al 1984).

Although the effect of IBD on pregnancy appears to be minimal in most cases, the effects of pregnancy on the course of IBD is not so straightforward. For patients with ulcerative colitis in remission at the time of conception, 10–54% will relapse (mean 34%). This is a comparable figure with a non-pregnant group of patients with ulcerative colitis (deDombal et al 1965, Nielson et al 1983). Recurrent symptoms usually occur in the first trimester (Crohn et al 1956, deDombal et al 1965, McEwan 1972, Willoughby & Truelove 1980). In patients with active colitis at the time of conception one-third will improve, two-thirds will not (Abramson et al 1951, MacDougall 1956, Banks et al 1957, McEwan 1972, Willoughby & Truelove 1980, Neilson et al 1983). Therapeutic abortion does not alter the course of the disease (deDombal et al 1965, Willoughby & Truelove 1980).

The effects of surgery on childbirth have been incompletely studied. There is now an increasing number of women who have had a normal vaginal delivery after an ileoanal pouch procedure without significant complications (Juhasz et al 1994). The rate of complications during pregnancy appears to be lower for this (0%) than for either ileostomy (9%) or Kock pouch (19%) (Juhasz et al 1994). Overall, IBD patients wishing to bear children should not be discouraged but should be counseled on the optimum timing, according to other health-related issues.

REFERENCES

Abramson D, Jankelson I R, Milner L R 1951 Pregnancy in idiopathic ulcerative colitis. American Journal of Obstetrics and Gynecology 61: 121–129

Andrews H, Barczak P, Allan R N 1987 Psychiatric illness in patients with inflammatory bowel disease. Gut 28: 1600–1604

Awad R W, El-Gohary T M, Skilton J S et al 1993 Life quality and psychological morbidity with an ileostomy. British Journal of Surgery 80: 252–253

Banks B M, Korelitz B I, Zetzel L 1957 The course of nonspecific ulcerative colitis: review of twenty years' experience and late results. Gastroenterology 32: 983–1012

Burakoff R 1992 Inflammatory bowel disease: fertility and pregnancy. In: Inflammatory bowel disease. Elsevier Science, Amsterdam pp 431–438

Crohn B B, Yarnis H, Crohn E B et al 1956 Ulcerative colitis and pregnancy. Gastroenterology 30: 391–403

deDombal F T, Burton I L, Goligher J C 1972 Crohn's disease and pregnancy. British Medical Journal 2: 550–553

deDombal F T, Watts J M, Watkinson G et al 1965 Ulcerative colitis and pregnancy. Lancet 25: 599–601

Engstrom I, Lindquist B L 1991 Inflammatory bowel disease in children and adolescents: a somatic and psychiatric investigation. Acta Paediatrica Scandinavica 80: 640–647

Fielding J F, Cooke W T 1970 Pregnancy and Crohn's disease. British Medical Journal 2: 76–77

Gazzard B G, Price H L, Libby G W et al 1978 The social toll of Crohn's disease. British Medical Journal 2: 1117–1119

Gruner O P N, Naas R, Fretheim B et al 1977 Marital status and sexual adjustment after colectomy: results in 178 patients operated on for ulcerative colitis. Scandinavian Journal of Gastroenterology 12: 193–197

Gruner O P N, Naas R, Gjone E et al 1978 Mental disorders in ulcerative colitis: suicide, divorce, psychosis, hospitalization for mental abuse, alcoholism, and consumption of psychotropic drugs in 178 patients subjected to colectomy. Diseases of the Colon and Rectum 21: 29–37

Juhasz E S, Fozard B, Dozois R R et al Ileal pouch–anal anastomosis function following childbirth: an extended evaluation. Diseases of the Colon and Rectum (in press)

Khosla R, Willoughby C P, Jewell D P 1984 Crohn's disease and pregnancy. Gut 25: 52–56

Kohler L W, Pemberton J H, Zinsmeister A R et al 1991 Quality of life after proctocolectomy: a comparison of Brooke ileostomy, Kock pouch, and ileal pouch–anal anastomosis. Gastroenterology 101: 679–684

Lask B 1986 Psychological aspects of inflammatory bowel disease. Wiener Klinische Wochenschrift 98: 544–547

Lask B, Jenkins J, Nabarro L et al 1987 Psychosocial sequelae of stoma surgery for inflammatory bowel disease in childhood. Gut 23: 1257–1260

Levi A J, Fisher A M, Hughes L et al 1979 Male infertility due to sulphasalazine. Lancet 11: 276–278

Levin K E, Pemberton J H 1990 Quality of life after ileostomy surgery. Practical Gastroenterology 14: 16–35

Levy N, Roisman I, Teodor I 1981 Ulcerative colitis in pregnancy in Israel. Diseases of the Colon and Rectum 24: 351–354

MacDougall I 1956 Ulcerative colitis and pregnancy. Lancet 29: 641–643

McEwan H P 1972 Anorectal conditions in obstetrical practice. Section of Proctology With Section of Obstetrics and Gynaecology 65: 279–283

Mayberry M K, Probert C, Srivastava E 1992 Perceived discrimination in education and employment by people with Crohn's disease: a case control study of educational achievement and employment. Gut 33: 312–314

Mitchell A, Guyatt G, Singer J et al 1988 Quality of life in patients with inflammatory bowel disease. Journal of Clinical Gastroenterology 10: 306–310

Moody G A, Probert C S J, Jayanthi V et al 1992 The attitude of employers to people with inflammatory bowel disease. Social Science and Medicine 34: 459–460

Nielsen O H, Andreasson B, Bondesen S et al 1983 Pregnancy in ulcerative colitis. Scandinavian Journal of Gastroenterology 18: 735–742

Porter R J, Stirrat G M 1986 The effects of inflammatory bowel disease on pregnancy: a case-controlled retrospective analysis. British Journal of Obstetrics and Gynaecology 93: 1124–1131

Sonnenberg A 1989 Disability from inflammatory bowel disease among employees in West Germany. Gut 30: 367–370

Sonnenberg A 1992 Disability and the need for rehabilitation among patients with inflammatory bowel disease. Digestion 51: 168–178

Sorensen V Z, Olsen B G, Binder V 1987 Life prospects and quality of life in patients with Crohn's disease. Gut 28: 382–385

Toovey S, Hudson E, Hendry W F 1981 Sulphasalazine and male infertility: reversibility and possible mechanism. Gut 22: 445–451

Walsh P C, Schlegel P N 1988 Radical pelvic surgery with preservation of sexual function. Annals of Surgery 208: 391–400

Whates P D, Irving M 1984 Return to work following ileostomy. British Journal of Surgery 71: 619–622

Willoughby C P, Truelove S C 1980 Ulcerative colitis and pregnancy. Gut 21: 469–474

Wyke R J 1988 Capacity for work and employment record of patients with inflammatory bowel disease. International Disability Studies 10: 176–179

Wyke R J, Edwards F C, Allan R N 1988 Employment problems and prospects for patients with inflammatory bowel disease. Gut 29: 1229–1235

109. Social consequences of inflammatory bowel disease

G. Moody   J. F. Mayberry

The social consequences of chronic illnesses can have a major impact on patients' lives. Personal relationships may be destroyed, employment difficulties arise and sufferers face discrimination from insurance companies, adoption agencies and immigration authorities (Shivananda et al 1984, Smith et al 1993). Many of these problems are common to people with various chronic illnesses, but sometimes specific difficulties can relate to conditions such as inflammatory bowel disease (IBD). Recent studies have shown that patients are largely concerned with issues of prognosis, risk to family members and learning to cope with the consequences of their disease (Rees et al 1988, Martin et al 1993). Medical and surgical gastroenterologists often fail to give a high priority to these aspects, and concentrate rather on etiology and treatment. One consequence of this divergence of views is that doctors can fail to understand those patients' difficulties which impinge directly on quality of life (Moody et al 1993). Medical and surgical treatments may alter the clinical course of a disease, but usually have little impact on employment, life insurance and personal relationships. These differences of opinion may explain the antagonism felt by some patients towards junior doctors who care for them (Moody et al 1993).

FAMILY LIFE

Inflammatory bowel disease can impair interpersonal relationships, reduce fertility and cause concern about the health of children.

Interpersonal relationships

Sexual activity is directly affected by inflammatory bowel disease owing to the fear of fecal incontinence and pain (Moody & Mayberry 1993, Moody et al 1992). A substantial number of women with Crohn's disease in a stable relationship completely abstain from sexual intercourse. Those who have sexual intercourse do so with similar frequency to their healthy peers. Where fear and pain dominate sexual activities the treatment of rectal disease or unsuspected vaginal involvement may help. However, there are no clinical trials to assess the benefits of sympathetic treatment. Such programs will require considerable psychological input, as it is fear of fecal incontinence rather than incontinence itself that leads to abstention.

The social effects of stoma surgery can present an additional problem for people with IBD. There is some anecdotal evidence to suggest that young people are keen to avoid a stoma and prefer the more esthetically desirable pouch. The effect of a stoma on body image can be disastrous, particularly for women from ethnic minorities, for whom it can end marriage prospects. The messages from various studies on the effect of stomas on sexual activity are conflicting. The generally accepted view is that couples adjust well to this form of surgery, but few reviews have used in-depth interviewing techniques or studied partners as well as patients.

Effects on fertility

Crohn's disease leads to reduced fertility in both men (Burnell et al 1986) and women (Mayberry & Weterman 1986). After diagnosis women have half the expected number of children. It seems likely that reduced sexual activity (Lichtarowicz & Mayberry 1987, Moody & Mayberry 1993) and an early menopause (Lichtarowicz et al 1989, 1991) contribute substantially to this effect. In the case of women this infertility is clearly not voluntary, whereas in men there is some evidence that concerns about ability to support a family play some part. Detailed case control studies of fertility among patients with ulcerative colitis have yet to be published.

Concerns about the safety of medications in pregnancy and the puerperium have no basis, and sulfasalazine and the newer 5-ASA compounds can be safely prescribed. However, the effects of sulfasalazine on sperm are now well known. Clearly, male patients must be advised of these effects and, if they fail to achieve a pregnancy within 6 months, the drug should be withdrawn.

Concerns about children

Inflammatory bowel disease clearly has an increased frequency within families (Mayberry et al 1980a). However, lay people usually consider inheritance to have a dominant or recessive pattern and patients often believe many of their children will develop the disease. Reassurance that the vast majority of relatives will *not* develop Crohn's disease or ulcerative colitis can be a relief. The effects of such beliefs and the consequences of chronic inflammatory bowel disease on interfamily dynamics have yet to be investigated.

The relative infertility seen in IBD has prompted some patients to consider adoption. Although there are no formal studies of adoption societies and their specialist social workers, anecdotal evidence from patients would suggest that these diseases generally lead to rejection of applications.

EMPLOYMENT DIFFICULTIES

Some years ago work in South Wales (Mayberry et al 1988) showed people with Crohn's disease to have as good a work record as the local healthy population. Despite such observations, a later study from Cardiff showed that patients believed themselves to be actively discriminated against (Mayberry et al 1992). This took the form of failure to offer jobs to patients, delaying promotions and an unwillingness to provide time off to attend specialist clinics. Such attitudes existed against a background of academic qualifications equivalent to their peers. Similar discrimination was seen in other studies, but there may be some truth to the suggestion that it is perceived rather than real. Despite this, patients do often feel discriminated against.

Employers' awareness of these difficulties is blunted (Moody et al 1992, Probert et al 1993). Many believe they give people with chronic illness equal employment opportunities. However, in practice this is not the case and the IBD sufferer is significantly underrepresented in the workforce (Mayberry et al 1992). Any 'discrimination' is usually due to failure at the pre-employment medical examination. Clearly, a more optimistic but equally disturbing interpretation is that patients hide their illness from employers. There is some evidence that this approach is adopted in the belief that discrimination is practised. The need to educate employers about the academic achievements and work record of people with IBD is paramount. Factual errors about infectiousness in IBD are often quoted as reasons for excluding patients from a number of posts. The easy suggestion that patients with IBD could be registered disabled and so fitted into 'protected' posts is unacceptable.

INSURANCE PROBLEMS

About 70% of insurance companies in the UK either refuse patients cover or offer it with significant weighting. This attitude is seen across the board, and includes life insurance, mortgage protection and health insurance. The underlying philosophies are based on either old data (Mayberry et al 1980b) or studies irrelevant to the United Kingdom. The belief that mortality is increased in IBD has not been substantiated in the most recent and largest studies from Copenhagen, Uppsala and Leicester. Indeed, some older studies (Mayberry et al 1988) also failed to find evidence for a raised mortality in Crohn's disease. Additional weighting on life insurance premiums is no longer appropriate. In addition, the good work record of patients with IBD should be reflected in a more sympathetic assessment for mortgage protection schemes. However, insurance is a commercial activity motivated by profit, and any change in weightings will depend more on demonstrating a potential for increased profit, rather than just low morbidity and mortality from IBD. Such arguments can be made and the contrasting views of insurance company doctors and underwriters gives hope for such review, as does the fact that such attitudes are not universal in the insurance world.

SOCIAL CONSEQUENCE OF A STOMA

At its beginning, the era of the ileostomy was characterized by concerns about leakage, skin irritation and smell (Mayberry & Rhodes 1978), whereas at its end the need was to distinguish Crohn's colitis from ulcerative colitis. The successful surgical management of stomas has not been paralleled by equally successful social management (Bhakta et al 1992, Foulis & Mayberry 1990). Although all doctors pay lip service to the need for preoperative counseling, in practice it is often inadequate or inappropriate. A national review of stoma care found major discrepancies between what stoma therapists thought they offered and what patients themselves believed they received (Bhakta et al 1992). Again, patients' perceptions and doctors' understanding of their needs are at variance. Within this study there was some evidence of discrimination against ethnic minorities, who also were seen one-third as frequently as other patients. Counseling and postoperative support must deal with problems of body image, personal relationships and cultural difficulties. Clearly, elderly people (Foulis & Mayberry 1990) experience difficulty in coming to terms with a stoma and physically handling it. For women who wear saris the siting is critical: indeed, with the more ready availability of 'pouching' this should always be available for young people and those from ethnic minorities. It goes almost without saying that the procedure should not be done unsupervised by an inexperienced surgeon.

REFERENCES

Bhakta P, Probert C S J, Jayanthi V, Mayberry J F 1992 Stoma anxiety: a comparison of the attitudes of Asian migrants and the indigenous population in the United Kingdom to abdominal surgery and the role of intestinal stomas. International Journal of Colorectal Disease 7: 1–3

Burnell D, Mayberry J, Calcraft B J, Morris J S, Rhodes J 1986 Male fertility in Crohn's disease. Postgraduate Medical Journal 62: 269–272

Foulis W, Mayberry J F 1990 Elderly ileostomies and their social problems. Journal of Clinical Gastroenterology 11: 276–278

Lichtarowicz A M, Mayberry J F 1987 Sexual dysfunction in women with Crohn's disease. British Medical Journal 295: 1065–1066

Lichtarowicz A, Norman C, Calcraft B, Mooris J S, Rhodes J, Mayberry J F 1989 A study of the menopause, smoking and contraception in women with Crohn's disease. Quarterly Journal of Medicine 72: 623–632

Lichtarowicz A, Srivastava E, Norman C et al 1991 A study of the menopause in women with ulcerative colitis. Journal of Obstetrics and Gynaecology 11: 361–364

Martin A, Leone L, Naccarato R 1993 Quality of life in functional and organic intestinal diseases. Gut 34 (Suppl 4): S14

Mayberry J F, Rhodes J 1978 Aspects of the ileostomy appliance. A survey of the patient's difficulty. Practitioner 220: 958–961

Mayberry J F, Rhodes J, Newcombe R C 1980a Familial prevalence of inflammatory bowel disease in relatives of patients with Crohn's disease. British Medical Journal 1: 84

Mayberry J F, Newcombe R C, Rhodes J 1980b Mortality in Crohn's disease. Quarterly Journal of Medicine 49: 63–68

Mayberry J F, Weterman I T 1986 European survey of fertility and pregnancy in women with Crohn's disease: a case control study by European collaborative group. Gut 27: 821–825

Mayberry J F, Dew M J, Morris J S, Powell D B 1988 An audit of Crohn's disease in a defined population. Journal of the Royal College of Physicians of London 17: 196–198

Mayberry M K, Probert C, Srivastava E, Rhodes J, Mayberry J F 1992 Perceived discrimination in education and employment by people with Crohn's disease; a case controlled study of educational achievement and employment. Gut 33: 312–314

Moody G A, Gillespie C, Mayberry J F 1993 What doctors need to know about their patients with IBD. Gut 34 (Suppl 4): S56

Moody G A, Mayberry J F 1993 Perceived sexual dysfunction amongst patients with inflammatory bowel disease. Digestion 54: 256–260

Moody G A, Probert C S J, Jayanthi V, Mayberry J F 1992 The attitude of employers to people with inflammatory bowel disease. Social Science and Medicine 34: 459–460

Moody G, Probert C S J, Srivastava E M, Rhodes J, Mayberry J F 1992 Sexual dysfunction amongst women with Crohn's disease: a hidden problem. Digestion (Suppl 2): 179–181

Probert C S J, Mayberry M, Mayberry J F 1992 Education and young people with inflammatory bowel disease. Journal of the Royal Society of Health 113: 112–113

Rees J E P, Mayberry J F, Calcraft B 1988 What the patient wants to know about Crohn's disease. Journal of Clinical Gastroenterology 5: 221–222

Shivananda S, van Blankenstein M, Hordijk J L, Mayberry J F, Themans V, van Does E 1984 Factors influencing quality of life in patients with Crohn's disease – interim results of a case-controlled study. Scandinavian Journal of Gastroenterology 24 (Suppl 158): 29–32

Smith G D, Eastwood M A, Palmer K R 1993 Quality of life in inflammatory bowel disease: morbidity may be greatly underestimated. Gut 34 (Suppl 4): S221

110. Inflammatory bowel disease and insurance

R. Driscoll

Patients who have been diagnosed with inflammatory bowel disease frequently report that they have had difficulty in obtaining insurance cover or have had to pay increased premiums. In 1992 a survey of 5000 randomly selected members of the National Association for Colitis and Crohn's Disease was undertaken in the United Kingdom: 3103 members responded, or whom 2250 (73%) had applied for some form of insurance. Of these, 42% reported having had difficulties owing to their illness. Patients with Crohn's disease were significantly more likely to have experienced difficulty than those with ulcerative colitis (49% vs 38%; $P<0.01$).

Obtaining insurance cover becomes an important issue when patients are diagnosed with a chronic and incurable illness. A sense of the unpredictability of colitis and Crohn's perhaps encourages patients and their families to seek protection against the future financial consequences of increasing ill health and possible loss of employment prospects.

Some forms of insurance have become almost mandatory to participate fully in normal daily activities (e.g. motor insurance, and travel insurance for package holidays), and others are increasingly being required by financial institutions (e.g. mortgage protection assurance, income protection plans). There is also an evident trend in many countries towards encouraging greater reliance on private insurance provision for health, sickness, housing and pension needs, so that Governments may defray the economic burden of high levels of public provision. It is therefore to be expected that problems of access to insurance at a fair and reasonable cost will become an even more important issue for patients in the coming years.

THE REALITIES OF INSURANCE COVER

Different considerations apply to the various forms of insurance that patients seek. Life assurance can be obtained on competitive terms by seeking insurance companies that are sympathetic in their attitudes towards inflammatory bowel disease and the considered life expectancy of patients. Insurance against the consequences of ill health is understandably more difficult to obtain. This includes private medical insurance, holiday and travel insurances, permanent health insurance, income protection plans (for redundancy, sickness and accident) and mortgage premium protection policies. Since there is an obvious risk of the person falling ill, being absent from work and requiring medical treatment, it is understandable that underwriters will normally include in the conditions of the policy an exclusion clause for inflammatory bowel disease, and for any conditions arising as a direct result.

Although such an exclusion might nullify the primary purpose of a patient seeking these types of policies, it is sensible before rejecting a policy altogether to consider the disadvantages of the exclusion clause against the advantage of all other forms of illness, accident or injury being covered. Patients who have been trouble-free for 2 years should be able to obtain cover without exclusions for short-term insurances such as holiday cover.

In respect of motor insurance, the decision as to whether a proposal is declined or a higher than normal premium is demanded depends on the guidance given to underwriters by their medical advisers, and whether the insurance company is seeking to increase or reduce the proportion of its business that carries 'increased risk'. Patients will get very different responses from different companies and should search for the best offer.

CONSTRAINTS IN CHANGING INSURANCE COMPANIES' RATINGS

The decisions of insurance companies about all types of insurance are governed by their commercial duty to provide a profit for their shareholders or, in the case of mutual societies, to look after the interests of their policy holders.

Taking life assurance as an example, the primary objectives of a life assurance underwriter are to offer life assurance to as many people as possible while ensuring that any medical rating for 'impaired lives' is commensurate with the additional risk. The underwriter must also ensure that the overall mortality of the 'normal risk' lives insured is no worse than the mortality assumed in calculating premium rates. An insurance company accepting a disproportionate amount of 'substandard' business would unbalance the calculation for its normal premium rates. These would then have to be increased, making the company less competitive and deterring 'healthy lives' from applying to the company.

Since the willingness to consider 'impaired lives' is essentially a commercial decision, it follows that the terms offered by companies do not remain constant. This means that professional advisers need to be vigilant in seeking the most competitive terms, and that people who have a chronic illness should not accept high medical ratings without checking whether they can obtain less expensive life assurance elsewhere.

Insurance companies differ in their assessment of risks, and where one company might decline a proposal another, better informed, one may offer competitive or even standard terms. It has been suggested that a consumer guide giving information about the different companies' ratings for different medical conditions would enable people with impaired health to approach the best insurer. In practice, companies are very reluctant to openly express their view of different illnesses, and will seek to avoid 'antiselection', where, for example, everyone suffering from inflammatory bowel disease would go to a particular company because it offered better terms than all the others.

The approach must therefore be to try to ensure that each company is basing its underwriting on the best possible information. This is an area in which patients' associations can exert influence by writing to all companies, and one in which individual doctors who act as advisers to insurance companies can also help. The results of recent population-based epidemiological studies show that, with modern patterns of diagnosis and management, mortality for most patients with inflammatory bowel disease is not increased. However, it has to be borne in mind that when underwriters talk of a comparison to 'normal risk' they are not referring to the risk of a background-matched population, such as that used in the Copenhagen studies. Their normal tables are those for 'insured lives', not the population as a whole. Socio-economic factors and the effects of selection by insurance companies mean that the underlying mortality assumed on lives to be insured is significantly lower than that for the general population as a whole. It is this lower mortality figure that is used to calculate the basic premiums, and therefore patients with inflammatory bowel disease may have a mortality risk that is worse than the risk for 'insured lives', even though it is very similar to that for the population as a whole.

WHAT CAN BE DONE TO REDUCE DISADVANTAGE FOR IBD PATIENTS?

Primary factors used by companies for risk assessment are:

1. Severity of disease and age at the time of onset
2. Current oral corticosteroid treatment
3. Frequency of attacks and the date of the last attack
4. The extent of the disease, particularly the extent of colonic involvement
5. Whether surgery has been performed recently or is contemplated
6. Associated complications
7. Duration of disease, which can indicate an increasing risk of malignancy.

It is to be hoped that advice from those who are medical advisers to insurance companies will gradually improve the factors on which companies assess the risks. For example, ongoing treatment with steroids is usually regarded as warranting an increased rating, whereas many specialists would regard the frequency of blood in the stools as a better indicator of severity for ulcerative colitis.

Doctors who are asked to produce reports for individual patients can also help. If they feel that the factors listed above might result in an assessment of risk which was inappropriately high, they should clearly state their own assessment of the severity of the patient's condition.

HELPFUL ADVICE FOR PATIENTS

1. Patients should 'shop around' for quotations from different companies, and should seriously consider using a broker who specializes in insurance for 'impaired lives' (patients' associations should be able to help with this).
2. It can save time and frustration to enquire from insurance companies at the outset whether they are likely to decline or to impose special terms on a proposer who has inflammatory bowel disease. (It is helpful to try and avoid a situation where a proposal is submitted and then rejected by a company, since future proposal forms are likely to ask if insurance has ever been declined.)
3. Applying for life assurance in the first year after diagnosis may result in a higher premium than would apply in later years, as it is more difficult for the degree of risk to be assessed at that early stage.

Patients should carefully consider which type of life assurance they choose, because the medical loading is converted into increased premiums in different ways. For temporary or fixed-term policies any increased risk is applied as a multiple of the basic premium, perhaps at double or triple the rate. With permanent assurance such as whole-life or endowment policies, the medical loading is converted into additional years, which are added to the proposer's age (e.g. a loading of 100%, normally double the premium, could equate to an additional 7 years on the proposer's age). This would be negligible for younger proposers, and far less penal for those who are older.

Since whole-life policies also have a cash surrender value, it therefore makes sense for the patient to assess carefully which type of life insurance offers the best value for money. Another factor to be considered here is whether the policy has an option to be increased or extended without further evidence of health status. This is particularly important where future deterioration in health is likely.

I wish to acknowledge the help received in preparing this article from Paul Robinson of Baskeyfields, and Dr S.P.L. Travis of Plymouth Hospitals NHS Trust.

SECTION 15

Follow-up

111. Follow-up in inflammatory bowel disease

R. N. Allan

This chapter examines the most appropriate facilities for the long-term care of patients with ulcerative colitis and Crohn's disease, particularly in an era when the cost-effectiveness of routine 'follow-up care' is being evaluated. No outcome audit of different approaches has been published. Traditional and alternative approaches are explored which require further evaluation.

ROUTINE FOLLOW-UP

Much routine follow-up has acquired a bad name, and deservedly so. Repeated 6-monthly appointments where the individual patient is seen by a different newly qualified houseman each time, are only gradually becoming a thing of the past. Any active follow-up policy is an active process requiring clear plans and guidelines to ensure that the visit is worthwhile.

Nature of disease process

Ulcerative colitis and Crohn's disease are characterized by chronic relapsing symptoms where appropriate medical or surgical treatment can only be determined by careful evaluation.

Potential advantages of regular follow-up clinic

Ulcerative colitis and Crohn's disease are uncommon conditions, so that most hospital doctors and family practitioners see few such patients. A follow-up clinic provides a focus for them and the accumulated experience provides the background for rational and consistent advice and care. The resources of medical and surgical follow-up can be linked to stoma care, first-class radiology, histopathology and laboratory services. The provision of outpatient and inpatient services in adjacent areas familiarizes the patient with the available inpatient facilities should they need them in the future.

Some patients are fortunate and run an uncomplicated course. Most have intermittent exacerbations of their disease, often with unusual but associated complications where the appropriate selection of dietary, medical or surgical treatment may require careful evaluation.

CHARACTERIZATION OF PATIENT GROUP

Patients with ulcerative colitis or Crohn's disease pose a wide variety of problems masquerading under these two specific labels. All patients subject to review should be characterized in more precise terms.

Patients with ulcerative colitis should be grouped according to the extent of disease (proctitis, left-sided disease, extensive disease or total colitis). Each of these groups can then be further subdivided according to the pattern of their symptoms: asymptomatic, chronic intermittent, chronic persistent, and the small but important group with severe acute colitis.

Patients with Crohn's disease can be grouped according to the site and extent of macroscopic disease and the presence or absence of local complications, such as fibrous stricture, abscess or fistula formation. The possibility of other complications, including anemia, malnutrition, fluid and electrolyte imbalance, or associated disorders such as peptic ulcer, gallstones or renal stones must also be considered.

PATIENTS' RECORDS

The records of each patient are headed by a problem sheet summarizing these features, including previous surgical treatment, the present site and extent of disease, associated complications and current therapy. Biochemical, hematological, endoscopic, radiological and pathology data are filed separately to ensure ready access to this important information. The file should also include sequential outpatient follow-up records and a separate area for filing correspondence in date order.

OUTPATIENT VISITS

Each outpatient follow-up visit opens with a brief review of the problem sheet, previous visit notes, correspondence and recent laboratory data, so that the nature of the patient's previous problems can be categorized to provide the background to evaluate current symptoms.

The patient's symptoms can then be summarized, characterized and the likely cause determined. Thus, patients with proctitis are likely to have diarrhea, urgency and rectal bleeding; the patient with distal ileal disease recurrent obstructive symptoms; and the patient with extensive colitis diarrhea, malaise and lethargy. The frequency, duration and severity can all be assessed and symptoms may be quantified for clinical trials with one of the indices of disease activity.

Abnormal physical signs are uncommon, but include evidence of weight loss, an abdominal mass or perianal disease.

Laboratory evaluation of disease activity

There are a number or readily available laboratory indices for assessing disease activity. Anemia occurs from a variety of causes, including bone marrow depression in the severely ill patient, overt bleeding, or malabsorption of iron, B_{12} or folate. Measurement of serum albumin is helpful, since a low level indicates a source of protein loss in the gut, usually associated with extensive colitis, or depression of albumin synthesis in the liver in the severely ill patient.

Measurement of acute-phase proteins is helpful. The erythrocyte sedimentation rate reflecting increased fibrinogen release from the liver, is variably elevated in active inflammatory bowel disease so that C-reactive protein or serum orosomucoids are more useful for evaluating disease activity.

The symptomatic patient with normal indices usually has mechanical problems such as a fibrous stricture in distal ileal Crohn's disease. The symptomatic patient with abnormal laboratory indices has severe or extensive disease, which will probably need further evaluation and a change in medical treatment.

Radiological assessment

Once the initial diagnosis has been established, the frequency and nature of radiological evaluation is determined by the nature and severity of new symptoms.

Thus the asymptomatic patient is unlikely to need further assessment, except perhaps for the individual with extensive colitis entering a surveillance program for colorectal cancer, when a further barium enema examination or colonoscopy would be appropriate.

The frequency of investigation is determined by the severity of symptoms and the rate of change. Radiological investigation may be required quite frequently in the early years following the diagnosis of Crohn's disease, when the macroscopic site and extent of disease can change rapidly. The need for re-evaluation becomes less frequent with time for both ulcerative colitis and Crohn's disease.

Endoscopic evaluation

Endoscopy is used primarily to assess the severity of mucosal inflammation, to explain the nature of new symptoms such as diarrhea and bleeding, and to confirm during an exacerbation whether the symptoms are due to the underlying disease. Endoscopic assessment complements the symptoms, signs and laboratory indices in determining the appropriate therapy, or complications such as carcinoma, particularly in patients with long-standing colitis. Upper gastrointestinal endoscopy may be appropriate in patients suspected of having peptic ulcer.

EVALUATION OF MEDICAL THERAPY

Most patients are fit and well either without medication or with maintenance therapy alone. Except for maintenance therapy in ulcerative colitis, medical treatment is needed only for the symptomatic patient. At each visit the physician must decide whether the present regimen and dose is appropriate, or whether alternative therapy is required, either alone or in combination with other drugs.

Medical/surgical collaboration

Some patients, particularly those with perianal or distal ileal Crohn's disease and those with extensive Crohn's colitis, have persistent or recurrent symptoms despite medical treatment, and need to be considered for surgery. It is particularly appropriate for these patients to have both a medical and surgical opinion at the same visit, so that appropriate management can be planned.

Stoma care

The stoma clinic should be held concurrently, so that patients in whom surgical treatment, including a stoma, is being considered can be counseled. The problems of any stoma patients can be discussed with the stoma therapist and resolved. The role of the stoma clinic has been extended recently to include the counseling of patients who are being considered for pouch operations for the surgical treatment of ulcerative colitis.

Newly diagnosed patients

For the newly diagnosed patient, the follow-up clinic provides an excellent opportunity to explain the nature of their disorder, for both them and their families, the possible medical and surgical treatment involved, the prognosis and the likely impact on their work and family life. These newly diagnosed patients are also encouraged to contact the clinic between regular review appointments should any unexpected problems arise, which overcomes the problems of a disorder characterized by unpredictable exacerbations and remissions.

Symptomatic patients

For the symptomatic patient each follow-up visit is an opportunity to assess the nature of their symptoms and signs, to initiate or amend treatment, and to arrange appropriate laboratory, radiological and endoscopic investigations as outlined above. A clear distinction has to be drawn between organic and functional symptoms.

Asymptomatic patients

For asymptomatic individuals the follow-up clinic is a useful occasional point of contact, with the reassurance of direct access between appointments, should the need arise.

Special problems

The follow-up clinic enables patients with special problems to be identified, particularly pregnancy, patients with long-standing ulcerative colitis for screening, and complications such as hepatobiliary disorders and other extraintestinal manifestations.

The follow-up clinic should provide consistent informed advice to counter often misleading, although well-intentioned, advice from family, friends, newspapers and journals, who offer a myriad of alternative solutions and generate many unnecessary anxieties.

NUMBER OF PATIENTS FOR FOLLOW UP

If one is providing a first-class service with informed, consistent advice, then regular outpatient follow-up is a counsel of perfection. In the context of the individual patient, regular review seems sensible. In the context of cost-effective care this blanket approach may need re-evaluation.

The prevalence of ulcerative colitis in Europe is of the order of 100:100 000 population and Crohn's disease 50:100 000. A district hospital serving a population of 400 000 would see 400 patients with ulcerative colitis and some 200 patients with Crohn's disease annually, or 12 000 patients for a biannual visit. In the UK alone, with a population of 60 million, this is equivalent to 90 000 annual visits or 180 000 biannual visits per year. In 1994 the South Birmingham Health Authority outpatient visits were costed at £35 per visit, which on an annual national basis would be an expenditure of £6,300,000.

Selective follow-up

A few centers will need to follow-up all patients for the purposes of determining natural history, cancer risk and to select patients for drug trials and other research studies. In recent years we have been developing alternative strategies to maintain a first-class service but with a more cost-effective follow-up program. The principle is that patients should be reviewed according to the severity of their disease and the follow-up pattern modified appropriately.

ULCERATIVE COLITIS

Two-thirds of patients with ulcerative colitis (Hendriksen et al 1985) have distal disease, of whom the majority run a benign course. This group of patients have been placed on an annual mailing list with clear instructions to the patient and their doctor as to whom to contact in the event of relapse.

In order to ascertain the severity of a relapse, we have developed a 'really useful simple colitis activity index', which can be calculated based on symptoms alone but which compares with other, more complex, indices which have included physical examination, blood tests and sigmoidoscopic appearances. In relapse the patient can thus evaluate their own score and assess the severity of their disease and know whether it is appropriate to contact their own doctor or the hospital, and whether electively or urgently (Walmsley & Allan 1995).

The annual mailing list is currently carried out by mail, with self-addressed stamped envelopes included in the enquiry, but we plan to introduce a 'colitis call' with regular contact annually by telephone.

Using the annual mailing list we contact patients with ulcerative colitis treated by panproctocolectomy and ileostomy and encourage them to attend should their symptoms recur or new symptoms develop.

Finally, we have reduced the frequency of follow-up for those who are symptomatic, leaving time for regular review of those patients who have severe persistent symptoms. With this approach we have reduced the outpatient attendance by more than 50%, but maintained the quality of service.

CROHN'S DISEASE

Crohn's disease is uncommon and more unpredictable, but even in this group certain patients can be selected for contact by annual mailing list. This applies particularly to those with distal ileal disease treated by resection, who might be expected to remain well for many years before developing recurrent disease. This group are informed of the likely symptoms should their disease recur, and are encouraged to seek further medical advice at that time.

PUBLISHED LITERATURE

The follow-up clinic is a useful source of the excellent publications from the NACC and Ileostomy Association, which further contributes to the receipt of consistent advice.

GRADUATE TRAINING

A regular follow-up clinic for inflammatory bowel disease provides an important focus for training of graduates, in both general medicine and gastroenterology. The natural history and prognosis of a wide range of problems in inflammatory bowel disease can be appreciated within the course of a few months, and appropriate management discussed. This clinical training can be combined with regular meetings of the medical and surgical teams to discuss specific problems.

CLINICAL RESEARCH

Regular review of all patients with inflammatory bowel disease enables the center to collate data and to determine optimal medical and surgical treatments and long-term prognosis. Appropriate management of different groups of patients can be analyzed and published, and individual patients can be identified for inclusion in controlled drug trials and other studies into the underlying mechanisms of pathogenesis.

THE WAY AHEAD

Extending the annual mailing list to include patients with relatively few symptoms should enable the clinic to focus on those individuals with persistent symptoms and yet maintain contact with the whole group.

Much of the clinical information is already entered into a computer database, and it should be possible within the next few years to record most of the clinical data in this way and develop online communication with the patient's family practitioner.

There are a number of other possible developments, including guidelines for patients and their family practitioners, based on the nature of their disease and severity of symptoms. It may well be that the development of outreach clinics will also have a place in the follow-up of some patients with inflammatory bowel disease.

CONCLUSION

An appropriately organized follow-up clinic should minimize the number of patients requiring hospital care and yet identify those few where inpatient care is essential.

A well organized follow-up clinic should minimize morbidity by appropriate medical and surgical treatment and the provision of consistent advice.

One outpatient session each week for medical and surgical patients with inflammatory bowel disease and the annual mailing list provides care for a total of 3500 outpatient attendances per year, enabling us to look after 1000 patients with ulcerative colitis and a similar number with Crohn's disease. It seems the minimum to offer to patients, usually young adults, who are unlucky enough to develop either ulcerative colitis or Crohn's disease in the prime of life.

REFERENCES

Hendriksen C, Kreiner S, Binder V 1985 Long term prognosis in ulcerative colitis. Gut 26: 158–163

Walmsley R S, Ayres R S C, Allan R N 1995 A really useful simple colitis activity index. (Submitted for publication)

112. Assuring the quality of care

B. T. Collopy

Whilst it is human to err, it is inhuman not to try, if possible, to protect those who entrust their lives into our hands from avoidable failures and danger. Max Thorek 1937

HISTORICAL REVIEW

The value of statistics in medical science has been appreciated for many years (Simpson 1847). However, there was little demand for the systematic review and scientific evaluation of medical care until early in the 20th century, and although a plea for a national register of operative results was made in England (Hey-Groves 1908), a formal system was first developed in America. A report to the Carnegie Foundation (Flexner 1910) brought to light the poor training of many of the 5000 physicians graduating annually from 154 medical schools in the previous decade. This stimulated the American College of Surgeons in 1916 to survey hospitals, and found that less than 15% of hospitals met acceptable standards. The College continued its surveys until 1952, when the then Joint Commission on Accreditation of Hospitals started a program requiring hospitals to have a formal system of review which was termed medical audit.

It was regarded as a peer review exercise and an early method which the Joint Commission encouraged was criteria auditing (Lembcke 1956). It remains an appropriate form of clinical review and is time saving for busy clinicians provided that the criteria for evaluation are precise enough for non-medical personnel such as medical records clerks to produce data for clinical analysis (Collopy 1980).

In the 1970s the terms peer review and medical/surgical audit gave way to quality assurance (QA) to highlight the importance of being able to demonstrate the quality of care. Further changes in terminology in the United States occurred in the late 1980s, quality improvement (QI) replacing QA to highlight the need to strive for further improvement in patient care through audit activities. In parallel with programs in other industries, hospitals now speak of continuous quality improvement (CQI) and total quality management (TQM), emphasizing a role for senior management as well as clinicians, and combining the concepts of a review of the quality of care and the utilization of resources (utilization review). Not all clinicians, however, will agree that the principles applied so successfully in the manufacturing industry by Deming and others apply in clinical practice (Collopy 1993). Programs under development in the 1990s in Australia and in the United States, which involve the development of clinical performance measures (clinical indicators), are more acceptable to clinicians (Collopy & Balding 1993).

In the United Kingdom, apart from some long-standing formal review programs, such as the West Lothian/Edinburgh surgical audit (Gruer et al 1986), which most importantly included a committee structure, widespread interest in the formal assessment of the quality of medical care has developed around 80 years after the plea by Hey-Groves. There is no doubt that a major influence has come from government (Working Paper No 6 1989), but also from individuals and particular disciplines, especially the proceduralists (Hoile 1993).

QUALITY ASSURANCE PRINCIPLES

Quality activities is the author's preferred terminology for the formal process of reviewing clinical performance, as it encompasses all of the terms discussed and recognizes that many methods exist for assessing the effectiveness and efficiency of the delivery of health care, such as retrospective medical record review, computerized audit of short- and long-term outcomes, and even direct observation of clinical performance. Furthermore, quality is not always assured by a review process, and indeed the objective of a review should be to detect problems that can be resolved.

The quality of care can be assessed as the degree of excellence of the process (or management) and outcome of care. There are three essentials for a successful quality activity in any healthcare facility. These are documentation, discussion and action.

Documentation

Data may be collected on a regular basis (monitoring of major diseases/procedures) or on a 'one off' basis. The former is more suited to procedural units and is facilitated by the ready availability of software programs. Non-procedural care, which more often addresses the process rather than the outcome, is more suited to an occasional review because of the time-consuming and detailed inquiry required. The system of documentation should have the capacity to review the care given by all providers for all patients, but be selective in its application, focusing on the ability to detect problem areas for discussion.

Discussion

The documented information obtained should be presented to an appropriate peer group, either department or discipline specific or hospital wide, depending on the size and complexity of the facility. Where problems in management or patient outcome are perceived discussion should address the case mix and illness severity of the patient group and the likelihood of chance occurrence. The larger the audience for discussion the more important is the preservation of confidentiality for both providers and patients, particularly where legal protection for QA documentation does not exist.

Action

This is the most important aspect but is commonly overlooked. The data may reveal that no action is necessary, or the message is clear, prompting clinicians to react appropriately to improve performance without being directed to do so (Collopy 1990). Action in general, however, is enhanced if there is a QA committee to make recommendations concerning alterations in the management of a condition or performance of a procedure, the conduct of an educational program, a restriction of privileges (this should rarely be invoked, apart from during the introduction of new invasive procedures) or a further clinical study. Where recommendations have been made following discussion of the documentation a further review is required to ensure that they were implemented – audit is never ending.

Relationship between audit/QA and research

The difference between audit and research has been described thus: 'research extends scientific knowledge, audit determines whether practitioners are utilizing that knowledge' (Bull 1993). They are complementary. Where the QA process has identified a problem and the cause of that problem is clear, recommendations can be made to correct it. Where the cause of the problem is not identifiable, but is possibly correctable, a clinical research study should be developed.

AUDITING IN INFLAMMATORY BOWEL DISEASE

Although publications on inflammatory bowel disease in the context of formal QA programs (as outlined above), are rare there have been many publications auditing the results of treatment, leading to an increase in knowledge of these uncommon but fascinating disorders and thus improving outcomes, i.e. QI. There have been many outstanding contributions, from individuals and from institutions such as St Mark's, the Birmingham General Hospital and the Mayo and Cleveland Clinics, establishing standards in care. Some of the difficulties facing those establishing standards of care are that the etiology of ulcerative colitis and Crohn's disease remains unknown, patients are subject to exacerbation and remission, acute and chronic forms of the diseases exist, there are no curative agents, medical treatment frequently fails, and surgical treatment is complex.

Further difficulties for those institutions and providers of care wishing to reach the standards of the major centers are the relatively small number of patients they encounter, the lack of a single diagnostic entity (apart from granulomata in Crohn's), the complexity of illness, the compromised state of some patients, and once again the high failure rate of medical treatment and the complexity of surgery.

A case could be made for all complex or critically ill patients to be referred to centers dealing with a high volume of IBD (Flood et al 1984), but all facilities would benefit from a more formal program of management and outcome review, if only to replace clinical impression with fact. For example, with regard to conservatism or aggression in the management of anal lesions in Crohn's disease, of 129 patients presenting with anal disease to one facility only 3.8% of the fistulae were complex and of all fistulae treated 90% achieved primary healing after fistulotomy (Platell et al 1996). As in other series experience of the high complex fistula was limited and no firm conclusions could be drawn from it, but for the majority of patients presenting to that facility a surgical policy was appropriate. Where clinicians have no ideal guide to the best treatment and therefore the best outcome, as with a complex fistula, a QA study will be of limited value. A more global approach by clinicians is required, through such techniques as consensus meetings or meta-analysis.

SPECIFIC AREAS TO ADDRESS FOR INFLAMMATORY BOWEL DISEASE

For each discipline involved in the management of patients with inflammatory bowel disease there are a number of areas in which performance may be less than optimal, and the following provides some guide as to what could be addressed when reviewing the quality of patient management to determine whether events might have been avoidable.

Diagnosis

Although the separation of Crohn's disease from ulcerative colitis may require consideration of clinical as well as macroscopic and microscopic determinants, pathologists should endeavor to maintain the 'indeterminate group' at about 10% or lower (Lee et al 1979), to reduce the risks of performing an inappropriate restorative proctocolectomy in patients with Crohn's disease. Histological misinterpretation of dysplasia should also be kept to a minimum (Riddell et al 1983).

The cost of surveillance programs in ulcerative colitis should also be borne in mind. In view of uncertainties concerning the effectiveness and efficiency of surveillance programs, again a global approach to surveillance would be an appropriate quality activity. The colonoscopist should remain conscious of the invasive nature of the procedure, and the patient should be warned of the risk of perforation, which is of the order of 0.1–0.2% (Arblaster et al 1992).

Medical management

Before initiating treatment for acute colitis with corticosteroids it is important to exclude the infective and pseudomembranous forms of colitis. Clinicians should therefore have a protocol for investigation which includes stool culture, sigmoidoscopy, biopsy and toxin assay (where appropriate), and compliance with a protocol should form part of a review program.

Timeframes for medical management should be considered at the start of treatment, particularly with acute colitis as delays, either in admission to hospital, diagnosis of toxic megacolon, or referral for surgery, can adversely affect outcome. Compliance with the timeframes established should be included in a review of the management. With chronic disease also timeframes for treatment should be established, so that delays in referral for surgery are kept to a minimum. It should be possible to anticipate deterioration and not wait until patients are nutritionally deficient or toxic.

Drug side effects

Clearly, monitoring should occur for side effects of the more toxic drugs such as azathioprine. Monitoring should also take place for the complications of long-term steroid administration, such as osteoporosis (Kusunoki et al 1992).

Surgical management

Quality activities would obviously take the form of a surgical audit, with particular reference in inflammatory bowel disease to postoperative infection, as the risk is high in patients who are nutritionally compromised at the time of surgery. Similarly, the risk of fistula formation is high, either through damage to the small intestine after repeated laparotomies or breakdown of the anastomosis in a compromised patient. A review discussion should take into account the experience of the operator and whether nutritional support was adequate.

Following resection for Crohn's disease it is appropriate to monitor recurrence rates, which may be as high as 30% at 5 years. Knowledge of the recurrence rate enables a patient to be better informed about the options for treatment and prognosis.

Newer procedures, such as strictureplasty in Crohn's disease, should be audited for morbidity and their effectiveness in both the short and the long term (Tjandra et al 1993). Restorative proctocolectomy in ulcerative colitis is now accepted as the ideal operation, particularly for patients under 50, but even in experienced hands postoperative morbidity may be as high as 30–40% (Phillips 1991).

Patient satisfaction

A health facility QA program is not complete unless it has a mechanism for reviewing patient satisfaction. This is usually through a patient questionnaire, which is distributed either routinely, randomly or intermittently.

In the management of inflammatory bowel disease such questionnaires should include questions relating to the following:

1. Adequacy of information about the nature of the disease, its long-term effects and the options for treatment
2. Adequacy of instruction before and after the establishment of a stoma. The move to 'day of admission' surgery and a short postoperative stay is a threat in this regard (Jeter 1992)
3. The quality of life for patients with stomas. Reliable information on this aspect of outcome is probably not obtainable from routine questionnaires, but it is appropriate for a major gastroenterological service to intermittently perform such a review. Several examples are now available in the literature (McLeod et al 1991).

REFERENCES

Arblaster M J, Collopy B T, Elliott P R, Mackay J R, Ryan P J Woods R J 1992 Colonoscopy in a private hospital: continuous quality improvement in practice. Australian Clinical Review 12: 71–76

Bull A R 1993 Audit and research: complementary but distinct. Annals of the Royal College of Surgeons 75: 308–311

Collopy B T 1980 A pilot study in surgical audit: evaluation of criteria auditing and a comparison with other systems. St Vincent's Hospital, Melbourne

Collopy B T 1990 Quality assurance: Much ado, much to do. Australian Clinical Review 10: 141–144

Collopy B T 1993 Do doctors need Deming? Quality Assurance in Health Care 5: 3–5

Collopy B T, Balding C M 1993 The Australian development of national quality indicators in health care. Joint Commission Journal on Quality Improvement 19: 510–516

Flexner A 1910 Medical education in the United States and Canada. Report to Carnegie Foundation for Advancement of Teaching. Updike, New York

Flood A B, Scott W R, Ewy W 1984 Does practice make perfect? Part II: The relation between volume and outcomes and other hospital characteristics. Medical Care 22: 115–124

Gruer R, Gordon D S, Gunn A A, Ruckley C V 1986 Audit of surgical audit. Lancet 1: 23–26

Hey-Groves E 1908 A plea for uniform registration of operation results. British Medical Journal 2: 1008

Hoile R W 1993 The national confidential inquiry into peri-operative deaths (NCEPOD). Australian Clinical Review 13: 11–16

Jeter K R 1992 Perioperative teaching and counselling. Cancer 70 (Suppl): 1346–1349

Kusunoki M, Moeslein G, Shoji Y 1992 Steroid complications in patients with ulcerative colitis. Diseases of the Colon and Rectum 35: 1003–1009

Lee K S, Medline A, Shoskey S 1979 Indeterminate colitis in the spectrum of inflammatory bowel disease. Archives of Pathology and Laboratory Medicine 193: 173–176

Lembcke P 1956 Medical auditing by scientific methods. Journal of the American Medical Association 162: 646

McLeod R S, Churchill D N, Lock A M, Vanderburg S, Cohen Z 1991 Quality of life of patients with ulcerative colitis pre operatively and post operatively. Gastroenterology 101: 1307–1313

Phillips R K S 1991 Pelvic pouches. British Journal of Surgery 78: 1025–1026

Platell C, Mackay J, Collopy B T, Fink R, Woods R 1996 Anal pathology in patients with Crohn's disease. Australia and New Zealand Journal of Surgery 66: 10–13

Riddell R, Goldman H, Ransohoff D F et al 1983 Dysplasia in inflammatory bowel disease. Standardised classification with provisional clinical applications. Human Pathology 14: 931–968

Simpson J Y 1847 Value and necessity of the numerical method of investigation as applied to surgery. Monthly Journal of Medical Science XVII: 313–333

Thorek M 1937 Surgical errors and safeguards. J P Lippincott, Philadelphia: p ix

Tjandra J J, Fazio V W, Lavery I C 1993 Results of multiple strictureplasties in diffuse Crohn's disease of the small bowel. Australia and New Zealand Journal of Surgery 63: 95–99

Index

Abdominal pain, *see* Pain; Pseudoappendicitis
Abdominal wall, closure, 711
Abdominoperineal resection
    dyspareunia, 905
    impotence, 904
Abortion, therapeutic, 944
Abscesses
    communicating, isotope scanning, 263
    computed tomography, 249, 250–251, 252
    Crohn's disease, 477
        colitis, 847–848
        perianal, 617, 711, 862–864
        surgery, 833
    diffuse jejunoileitis, 598
    endoluminal ultrasound, 288, 289–290
    fistulae, 885
    liver, 637 (Table), 644
    percutaneous drainage, 251, 875–879
    radiolabeled leukocyte scans, 590
Academic success, IBD on, 942
Accreditation, minimal-access surgery, 721
Acetarsol, 556
Acetic acid, experimental colitis, 168
Acetyl CoA, xenobiotic metabolism, 205
Acid phosphatase, macrophages, 82, 83
Acidosis, intraluminal, ischemic colitis, 422
Acquired immunodeficiency syndrome, 399–403
    acute infectious-type colitis, 366
    cytomegalovirus, 550
    granuloma-producing organisms, 380
    HIV enteropathy, 402
    tuberculosis, 391
Activated partial thromboplastin time, therapy monitoring, 699
Active ulcerative colitis, histology, 292–298
Activity index, colitis, 957
Acute colitis, 274–275
Acute-phase proteins
    Crohn's disease, children, 653
    follow-up, 956
    ulcerative colitis, children, 662
Acute-phase response, 329–331
    Crohn's disease *vs* ulcerative colitis, 345
Acute severe colitis, *see* Fulminant colitis
Acyclovir, herpes simplex virus, 401
Adenomatous dysplasia, 317
Adenomatous polyps
    antigens, 146
    colonoscopy, 282
    management, 681
    ulcerative colitis, 320

Adenosine deaminase, tuberculous ascites, 392–393
Adenosine monophosphate, 77–78
Adenosine triphosphate, mucus secretion, 150
Adherence proteins, *Entamoeba histolytica*, 410
Adhesion, neutrophils, 73, 75–76
Adhesion molecules, 81, 135–136, 146, 522
Adhesions
    enterocutaneous fistula surgery, 888, 889
    fulminant colitis, 727
    management, 707–708
    proctocolectomy, 748–749
Adolescents, diffuse jejunoileitis, 598
Adoption of children, 946
Adrenal failure, ileal pouch–anal anastomosis, 795
Adrenocorticotrophic hormone, 506
    adrenal hemorrhage, 568
    children, 655 (Table)
    fulminant colitis, 567
Advancement flaps, perineal fistulae, 866–867, 872
Aeromonas spp., IBD, 366–367
African-Americans, Crohn's disease, perianal disease, 861
Agammaglobulinemia, 65
Age, 13–14, 37
    cancer risk, 470, 676
    colorectal carcinoma in cotton-top tamarins, 162
    Crohn's disease recurrence, 478
    ileal pouch–anal anastomosis outcome, 809–810
Agglutinating antibodies, *vs* bacteria, 118–119
Aggressive Crohn's disease, 479
Agranulocytosis
    azathioprine, 607
    sulfasalazine, 558
AIDS, *see* Acquired immunodeficiency syndrome
Air contrast studies, 215, 243
Albinism, Hermansky–Pudlak syndrome, 16
Albumin (levels), 332, 956
    acute-phase response, 329, 331
    Crohn's disease
        children, 653
        colitis, 603
        surgery, 852
    NSAID enteropathy, 437
    sepsis and stricturoplasty, 843
    tuberculosis, 392
Alcohol

    intestinal permeability, 178
    metronidazole reaction, 618
    and smoking, 42, 49
Aldosterone, colonic electrolyte transport, 183–184
Alkaline phosphatase, primary sclerosing cholangitis, 640
Alkalosis, 186
    fulminant colitis, 565
Allchin, W., on ulcerative colitis, 4
Allergic proctocolitis, babies, 277
Allopurinol
    with DMSO, 531
    and immunosuppressants, 559, 574
    postoperative, 748
    pouchitis, 113
$\alpha\beta$ T cells, 54
α_1-acid glycoprotein, 329, 330–331
α_1-antitrypsin, 143, 329, 331
Amebapore, 410
Amebiasis (colitis), 356–357, 409–412
    colonoscopy, 275
    vs Crohn's disease, 242–243
    diagnosis, 549
    IBD, 366
Amebomas, 410
Amiloride-sensitive sodium absorption, 183
Amino acid radicals, tissue damage, 78
Amino acids, elemental diets, 537
Aminoglycosides, 694
Aminosalicylates, 487–501, *see also named drugs*
    adverse effects, 557, 558
    Crohn's disease, trials, 607
    on inflammatory mechanisms, 523
    maintenance therapy, 571–574
    ulcerative colitis, 553
    worsening disease, 557
Aminosalicylic acid (4-ASA), 489, 497–498, 572–573
Ampicillin, fulminant colitis, 568
Amyloidosis, 628–629, *see also* Serum amyloid A
    Behçet's disease, 388
    vs collagenous colitis, 371
    Crohn's disease, 606
        children, 651
        vs ulcerative colitis, 344
    liver, 637 (Table), 644
Anal canal, 861
Anal encirclement, prosthetic, 900
Anal fistulotomy, 898
Anal irritation, from enemas, 574

Anal lesions
    Crohn's disease, 615
    ulcerative colitis, 304
Anal physiology measurements, 867
Anal sphincter, see also Sphincterotomy
    denervation, 794
    endoluminal ultrasound, 289
    exercises, 776, 812
    function, ileal pouch–anal anastomosis,
        760–761, 763, 772, 775–776, 810
    mechanism, 897
    repair, 899–900
    transanal mucosectomy, 783–784
Anal squeeze pressure, ileal pouch–anal
        anastomosis, 763
Anal stenosis, 343
Anaphylactic shock
    ischemic colitis from, 421
    mucus secretion, 150
Anastomoses, 692, see also Ileorectal
        anastomoses
    Crohn's disease, 710–711, 830
        recurrence at, 138–139, 313
    fistulae from, 853–854, 881
    ileal pouch–anal anastomosis
        leakage, 762–763, 792
        technique, 779, 784–785
    laparoscopic, 719
    radiation bowel disease surgery, 428
    strictureplasty, 838
    strictures, 593–594
    testing, 711, 855
Anatomy, echoendoscopy, 285–287
Anemia, 44
    Crohn's disease, 176–177, 594, 627,
        652–653
        colitis, 605
    diffuse jejunoileitis, 598
    enterocutaneous fistulae, 884
    ileal pouch–anal anastomosis, 795
    NSAID enteropathy, 437
    sulfasalazine, 490, 558
    ulcerative colitis, children, 662
Anergy
    cutaneous, 57
    T cells
        cyclosporin A, 64
        induction, 30
Anerobic bacteria, surgical infection, 693–694
Anesthesia, 926
Aneuploidy, see DNA aneuploidy
Angiography, 139
Angiotensin-converting enzyme, 114
Angular cheilitis, 634
    triamcinolone, 656
Animal models
    B lymphocytes, 65, 66–67, 70
    butyrate on colonic epithelium, 203
    experimental, 167–171
    infective agents, 121, 167–168
    molecular genetics, 27
    natural, 157–165
    vascular factors, 138–139, 169–170
    yersiniosis, 414
Ankylosing spondylitis, 16–17, 452, 453–455,
        624
    HLA associations, 276
    theories, 457
    ulcerative colitis, 733
Anorectal angle, 897
Anorectal excision, intersphincteric, 857, 905
Anorectal region, see also Perianal region
        cancer

Crohn's disease, 325–326, 679–680
    surgery, 685–686
Crohn's disease, 198–199
    function, 195–197
        assessment, 714–715
        preserving, 713–716
    mucosa after ileal pouch–anal anastomosis,
        786
    radiation, 427
    reconstruction, 715–716, 868
    strictures, 712, 714, 864
    surgical access, 691
    tuberculosis, 395
Anorexia nervosa, Crohn's disease, 481, 649
Antabuse effect, metronidazole, 618
Antacids, gastroduodenal Crohn's disease,
        586
Anterior uveitis, see Uveitis
Antibiotic-associated colitis, 355–356, see also
        Pseudomembranous colitis
    colonoscopy, 275
Antibiotics, 8, 121–122, 557
    Campylobacter spp., 350
    chronic granulomatous disease, 382
    enterocutaneous fistulae, 887
    fulminant colitis, 567–568, 726
    irrigation, ileal pouch–anal anastomosis,
        786
    malakoplakia, 383
    perianal fistulae, 618
    pouchitis, 803
    primary sclerosing cholangitis, 642
    salmonellosis, 352
    spondylarthropathies, 457
    surgery, 693–696
        Crohn's disease, 825, 852
    toxic megacolon, 850–851
    ulcerative colitis, 560–561
Antibodies, see also Autoantibodies;
        Monoclonal antibodies and named
        antibodies
    vs bacteria, 118–119
    therapeutic, enterocutaneous fistula, 887
Antibody-dependent cytotoxicity (ADCC),
        55, 67–68
Anticardiolipin antibody, Crohn's disease,
        627
Anti-CD4 therapy, 519
Anticholinergic drugs, for night evacuation
        frequency, 776
Anticoagulants, 698–700
Anticolon antibodies, 67–68
    IL-2 gene knockout mice, 66
Anticytokines, therapy, 98
Antidiarrheal agents, 552–553, 726
    and colonic dilatation, 194
    ileal Crohn's disease 591
    ulcerative colitis, maintenance therapy,
        577
Antiendothelial antibodies, 138
Antierythrocyte antibodies, 68, 69 (Table)
Antigen presentation, 63
    by macrophages, 83
    to T cells, 28
Antihistamines, 90
Antimycobacterial therapy
    Crohn's disease, 129
    drugs, 396
Antineutrophil cytoplasmic antibodies, 27, 28,
        68–69, 332–333, see also Perinuclear
        antineutrophil cytoplasmic antibodies
    Behçet's disease, 388
    Crohn's disease vs ulcerative colitis, 345

primary sclerosing cholangitis, 640
Antioxidants, 112–113, 531
Antiplatelet therapy, 699
Antireticulin antibodies, celiac disease, 375
Antithrombin III
    Crohn's disease, 627
    deficiency, 103, 697, 734
Antituberculous drugs, see Antimycobacterial
        therapy
Anxiety, 481, 941
Aortic surgery, ischemic colitis, 422
Aphthous ulcers, 226, 229–230 (Fig.), 311,
        312
    colon, 237, 239
        histology, 305
    endoscopists' definitions, 307
    esophagus, 270
    infections, 363
    mouth, 625, 634, 662
        triamcinolone, 656
    stomach and duodenum, 234
Apomucin core sequences, 143
Apoptosis, epithelium, 205, 206
Appendix, see also Pseudoappendicitis
    tuberculosis, 394
Arabs, Bedouin, 15
Arachidonic acid (metabolism), 109, 489,
        522–523, 527
    dietary n-3 fatty acids, 42
    eosinophils, 90
    mast cells, 88
    steroids on metabolism, 504
    therapeutic target, 528, 560
Argentaffin cells, quiescent ulcerative colitis,
        298
Arginine
    dietary, 537
    small intestinal nutrition, 202
Arsenic absorption, acetarsol, 556
Arterial thrombosis, 697
    Crohn's disease, 627–628
Arthralgia, azathioprine and 6-MP, 516
Arthritis, 624–625, see also
        Spondylarthropathies and named
        arthritides
    bacterial infections, 119
    with collagenous colitis, 369, 370
    colon changes, 276
    Crohn's disease
        children, 650
        colitis, 602–603
        vs ulcerative colitis, 344
    ileal pouch–anal anastomosis, 743
    incidence, 623 (Table)
    and pseudopolyps, 304
    spondylarthropathies, 451
    ulcerative colitis, children, 661
Arthritogenic peptide model,
        spondylarthropathies, 457
Asacol, 488, 571 (Table)
    maintenance therapy
        Crohn's disease trials, 495–496
        ulcerative colitis, dosage, 572
    vs placebo, 492
    renal toxicity, 558
    vs sulfasalazine, 491, 492
    trials, 493
Ascites, tuberculosis, 391, 392
Ascorbic acid
    deficiency, fistulae, 883
    for malakoplakia, 383
Ashkenazi Jews, 13, 14, 15, 16
    HLA antigens, 27, 30

Asian migrants
  tuberculosis, 392
  to United Kingdom, 15, 37, 38
Aspergillosis, colon, 275
Aspiration, *see also* Drainage
  endoluminal ultrasound, 289–290
Aspirin
  on cancer risk, 471
  on thromboxanes, 529
Asthma, mortality in ulcerative colitis, 472
Atherosclerosis, ischemic colitis, 421
Athletes, ischemic colitis, 423
Atopy, 17
  oral Crohn's disease, 635
Audit, 694, 959, 960
'Auer' procedure, 170
Augmentin, pouchitis, 803
Autoagglutination, *Yersinia* spp., 414
Autoantibodies, 65, 67–69
  Behçet's disease, 387–388
Autoimmune disorders, 16–17
  collagenous colitis, 372
  cotton-top tamarin colitis, 163
  Crohn's disease, 627
Axial arthropathy, 624–625, *see also*
  Ankylosing spondylitis; Reiter's
  syndrome; Sacroiliitis
Azathioprine (Imuran), 513–517
  adverse effects, 559
  children, 655
  Crohn's disease, 592, 607–608
  diffuse jejunoileitis, 598
  enterocutaneous fistula management, 888
  fulminant colitis, 568
  on inflammatory mechanisms, 523
  lymphocyte function, 57
  on mast cells, 90
  perianal fistulae, 618
  pregnancy, 516–517, 578, 673
  response failure, Crohn's colitis, 850
  ulcerative colitis, 554–555
    children, 664
    maintenance therapy, 574–576, 577
  ulcerative jejunoileitis, 434
Azo-bond prodrugs, 488

Bacillary dysentery, *see* Shigellosis
Bacille Calmette-Guerin, 128, 523
Bacillus pyliformis, mouse colitis, 158
Backwash ileitis, 223, 226 (Fig.), 239, 297
Bacteremia
  Campylobacter spp., 350
  salmonellosis, 351–352
  yersiniosis, 416
Bacteria, 117–120
  experimental colitis, 169
  mucus breakdown, 150
  overgrowth
    Crohn's disease, 176, 198
    on fat absorption, 175
    pouchitis, 805
  translocation, 202, 887
Bacterial antigens, 56, 629
  reactive arthritis, 453
  spondylarthropathies, 456
Bacterial lipopolysaccharide, macrophage activation, 82
Bacterium necrophorum, 117
Bacteroides vulgaris overgrowth, experimental colitis, 169
Bad news, 915–916
Balloon catheters, finding strictures, 709

Balloon dilatation of strictures, 281
  Crohn's disease, 854
    gastroduodenal, 819
  ileoanal anastomoses, 782–783
Balsalazide, 488, 571 (Table)
  maintenance therapy, 577
    dosage, 572
Banks, Isabella, Crohn's disease *vs* homicide, 3
Barium enemas, 219–223
  collagenous colitis, 370
  and colonic dilatation, 194
  vs colonoscopy, 277
  Crohn's disease
    children, 652, 653
    colitis, 604, 851
    vs ulcerative colitis, 344–345
  distal ileum imaging, 219
  diverticular disease, 443
  fistulae, 819
  ischemic colitis, 423
  preoperative, 273–274
  radiation doses, 266
  ulcerative colitis
    children, 662
    extent, 467
Barium meals
  and follow-through, 216, *see also*
    Enteroclysis; Small-bowel barium meals
  gastroduodenal Crohn's disease, 817
  radiation doses, 266
Barium sulfate, 215
Basal plasmacytosis, 304, 360–361
Basophils, *vs* mast cells, 87–88
B cells, 63–65
  function, 55
  granulomata, 380
  vs T lymphocytes in mucosa, 54
B-cell/T-cell ligand pairs, 63–64
BCG, 128, 523
Beclomethasone dipropionate, 508, 554
Bedouin Arabs, 15
Beer Sheva district, ethnic studies, 15
Behçet's disease, 387–390
  children, 665–666
  vs Crohn's disease, 242, 243, 315
  extraintestinal manifestations, 623
Benign lymphoid hyperplasia, 273, 277
Benzalazine, 488
  vs sulfasalazine, 491
Beryllium, granulomata, 379
β_1-3Gal-GalNAc transferase, 147
β_2 integrins, neutrophil adhesion, 75
β_2 microglobulin, genes, *vs* HLA B27, 456–457
β-glucuronidase, 82
Betamethasone, 505
β-thromboglobulin, plasma levels, 104
Bethanecol, malakoplakia, 383
Bf-F complement allotype, 20
Bicarbonate, colon, 182
Bile acids, salts
  absorption
    Crohn's disease, 177, 594
    ileal resection, 187
  catharsis, 177, 594, 605
  metabolism, pouchitis, 805
  toxic, theory, 639
Biliary diversion, cyclosporin absorption, 517
Biliary tract
  disease, 637–646
  lavage, prednisolone, 642

obstruction
  AIDS, 400, 403
  Mycobacterium avium intracellulare, 402
sludge
  Crohn's disease, 594
  primary sclerosing cholangitis, 642
  total parenteral nutrition, 544
Bilirubin
  displacement, sulfasalazine, 578
  primary sclerosing cholangitis, 640
Biofeedback, for incontinence, 900
Biopsies
  acute infectious-type colitis, 360
  cancer surveillance, 680
  colonoscopy, 274
    Crohn's disease, 601
    current practice, 291–292
    malignant strictures, 281
  culture, 365–366
  drug levels, 488
  gastroduodenal Crohn's disease, 586
  ischemic/radiation colitis, 276
  macroscopically-normal areas, 295–297, 306–307
  mouth, 635
  number required for dysplasia, 677
  pouchitis, 801
  primary sclerosing cholangitis, 641
  ulcerative colitis, 278
    children, 662
  ulcerative jejunoileitis, 431–432
Birds
  Campylobacter spp., 350
  Crohn's disease models, 158
Bisacodyl, electrolyte secretion, 183
Bismuth salts, ulcerative colitis, 151
  enemas, 556
Bladder
  computed tomography, 254
  fistulae, Crohn's disease, 606, 628
  and surgery, 692, 748
Blood flow, intestinal, 139
Blood group antigens, *see also* Pk antigen
  cancer-associated, 146
  sequences similar to mucins, 144, 148
Blood transfusion, infection, 693
Bloody diarrhea
  Crohn's disease, 649
  diagnosis, 291, 549
  fulminant colitis, 565
Bloody flux of Sydenham, 3
'Blowhole' colostomy
  Crohn's colitis, 858–859
  fulminant colitis, 728
Body image, stomas, 943, 945
Bone age, 653, 732
Bone marrow
  azathioprine and 6-MP, 516, 559, 574, 576
  magnetic resonance imaging, 249
  transplantation, *see* Hemopoietic stem cell transplantation
Books, 917, 919, 920–923
Bouginage, esophagus, 585
Bowel flora, 118–119
  elemental diets on, 536
  ulcerative colitis, 560
Bowel preparation
  Crohn's colitis surgery, 852
  endoscopy, 273, 680
  surgery, 694, 926
    Crohn's disease, 825
Bowel rest, 541–542, *see also* Medical bypass
Boxer dogs, 158–159

Brain stem lesions, 399
Bran, diverticular disease, 446
Bread, 42
Breakfast cereals, 42
Breastfeeding
  drug therapy, 578
  sulfasalazine, 673
British Colostomy Association, 920
Broad-spectrum antibiotics, 121
Brokers, insurance, 950
Bronchial disease
  Crohn's disease, 626–627
  mortality in ulcerative colitis, 472
Bronchial mucin genes, 144
Bronchiolitis obliterans, 627
Brooke, Professor Bryan, 915
Bruel and Kjaer rectal probe, 285
Budesonide, 505
  CIR, 509–510, 591–592
  enemas, 508, 554
  gastroduodenal Crohn's disease, 586
Buffalo hump, 503
Bulking agents, on stool frequency, 764, 810
Butyrate
  on colonic epithelium, 202–204, 205, 449, 521
  enemas, 450, 609
    diversion colitis, 277
    refractory proctitis, 556
  mucin synthesis, 149
Bypass operations, 8, 822, 826–827, see also Medical bypass
  Crohn's disease
    gastroduodenal, 818
    obstructive, 831–833

Caco-2 model, butyrate on colonic epithelium, 203
Caecum, see Cecum
Calcium
  absorption
    colon, 182
    Crohn's disease, 176
  colonic secretory mechanisms, 184
  metabolism, steroids, 503
  mucus secretion, 149, 150
  NSAID enteropathy, 441
  serum levels, 44
Calcium-calmodulin pathway, colonic secretory mechanisms, 184
Calcium dependence, *Yersinia* spp., 414
Calcium ionophores, 150
Calcospherites (Michaelis-Gutmann bodies), 383
Calculi, see Gallstones; Kidneys, stones
Callitrichidae family, 160
cAMP pathway, mucus secretion, 150
Campylobacter (spp.), 349–352
Campylobacter fetus, ferrets, 157
Campylobacter jejuni, 119, 364
  arthritis, 453
  colonoscopy, 274–275
  cotton-top tamarins, 160–161
  course of infection, 359
  enterocolitis
    antierythrocyte antibodies, 68
    incidence, 349
  histology, 305
  ulcerative colitis, 304
Campylobacter sputa, pigs, 158
Cancer risk, 675–682, see also Surveillance for cancer risk
  azathioprine and 6-MP, 516, 559, 576
  counseling, 916–917
  Crohn's disease, 480, 654, 679–680, 681, 683
    colitis, 679, 848–849, 850
    dysplasia, 320, 322, 676–677
    fecal diversion, 859
    ileal pouch–anal anastomosis, 760, 786, 811
    oxidants, 113
    prostaglandins, 109–110
    reduction, 463
    strictureplasty, 844–845
  ulcerative colitis, 683
    children, 665
    colectomy for, 734–736
    effect of treatment, 470–471
    prophylaxis, 675–679, 680–681
    St Mark's experience, 472
Candidiasis
  colon, 275
  esophagus, 399
Capetown Index, 339
Capillary thromboses, 697
Carbachol, mucus secretion, 150
Carbenoxolone, colonic mucin synthesis, 149
Carbohydrates
  absorption, 44
    Crohn's disease, 174–175
  metabolism, steroids, 503
  refined, 38, 41–42, 609
Carbon dioxide
  gas contrast studies, 215
  testing anastomoses, 711
  use in dissection, 708–709
Carbonic anhydrase, chloride absorption, 182
Carcinoembryonic antigen, 320
Carcinoid tumor
  with collagenous colitis, 369
  vs Crohn's disease, 237
Carcinoma, see also Cancer risk; Colorectal carcinoma; Rectum, retained after surgery
  of cervix, radiation bowel disease on survival, 428
  computed tomography, 250
  cotton-top tamarins, 162
  Crohn's disease, 324–326
  vs Crohn's disease, 235, 241
  from DALM, 320
  vs diverticular disease, 443–444
  glycosylation, 146–147, 151
  ileal pouch–anal anastomosis, 761, 765, 793–794
  and ischemic colitis, 423
  radiology, 223, 226 (Fig.)
  recurrence *vs* radiation bowel disease, 427
  stomas, 937
  strictureplasty, 844–845
  in strictures, 281
  surgery, 683–688
  terminal ileum, bypass operations, 8
  ulcerative colitis, 323–324
    sporadic *vs*. 324
Cards, stoma patients, 912
Carrageenan, 42–43, 169
Caseation, 392
Catalase, 113
Cathepsin G autoantibodies, 69
Catheters, see Balloon catheters; Self-catheterization
Cats, colitis, 159
Cattle, *Salmonella* spp., 351

Caustic agents, experimental colitis, 168–169
CD4 antigens, monoclonal antibodies, 526, 560
CD4/CD8 ratios, lymphocytes, 53, 54
CD4 T cells, granulomata, 380
CD8+ T cells, activation, 57
CD11/CD18 integrins, neutrophil adhesion, 75–76
CD18 monoclonal antibodies, for TBNS-induced colitis, 169
CD40/CD40 ligand pair, 63–64
Cecoanal anastomoses, 782
Cecum
  Crohn's disease, 477
    radiology, 235
  tuberculosis, 392, 393–394
Cefotaxime, 694
  Crohn's colitis surgery, 852
  Crohn's disease surgery, 825
Cefuroxime, 694
Celiac disease, 17–18
  HLA haplotypes, 30
  lymphocytic/collagenous colitis, 375
  ulcerative jejunoileitis, 431, 433, 434
Cell death, epithelium, 205, 206
Cell differentiation, epithelium, 206
Cell proliferation, dysplasia, 321
Cell shedding, epithelium, 205
Cell surface glycoproteins, T cells, 31
Cell surface markers, peripheral blood lymphocytes, 53
Cell surface proteases, epithelium, 206
Cell-wall defective bacteria, 119, see also Spheroplast-like agents
  mycobacteria, 125
Cement, colostomy bag (Koernig), 5
Centrifugation, see Density-gradient centrifugation
Cephalosporins, 694, see also named drugs
Cereals (breakfast cereals), 42
Cerebral lymphoma, azathioprine and 6-MP, 516
Cerebrovascular thrombosis, Crohn's disease, 628
Cervical lymph nodes, orofacial granulomatosis, 633
Cervix, carcinoma, radiation bowel disease on survival, 428
Chancre, 404
Charcot-Leyden crystals, 90
Cheilitis granulomatosa, triamcinolone, 635
Chemical-induced colitis, 168–169
Chemokines, 96
Chemotactic factors, mast cells, 88 (Table)
Chemotaxis inhibitors, Crohn's disease, 77
Chickens
  Crohn's disease models, 158
  Salmonella spp., 351
Childbirth
  Crohn's disease, 943
  ileal pouch–anal anastomosis, 766, 813
Children, 647–670
  clinical indices, 339
  computed tomography, 255
  Crohn's disease
    diets, 538
    psychiatric symptoms, 481
    surgery, 477, 657–658
    upper gastrointestinal tract, 583
  differential diagnosis, 277
  diffuse jejunoileitis, 597–598
  extraintestinal manifestations, 624
  fluoroquinolones, 353

Children (contd)
  growth retardation, 732–733
  ileoanal anastomoses, 781, 811
  therapeutic trials, Crohn's disease, 493–494
  ulcerative colitis, cancer risk, 676
China, diverticular disease, 445
Chlamydia spp., 119–120
  arthritis, antibiotics, 457
  granulomata, 363
Chloride
  absorption in colon, 182
  loss
    Crohn's disease, 174 (Table)
    IBD, 186
  secretion
    colon, 183
    eosinophils, 91
    neutrophil-generated oxidants, 77
    prostaglandins, 109
Chloroquine, arachidonic acid release inhibition, 528
Cholangiocarcinoma, 637 (Table), 639, 643–644
  cross-sectional imaging, 259
Cholangiography, primary sclerosing cholangitis, 641
Cholecystitis, AIDS, 400
Choleglycine, Crohn's disease, 177
Cholestasis
  Crohn's disease, 478
  cyclosporin, 519 (Table)
  management, 642
  primary sclerosing cholangitis, 640
  total parenteral nutrition, 544
Cholesterol
  ileal pouch–anal anastomosis, 795
  serum levels, steroids, 503
Cholesterol emboli, 421
Cholestyramine, 594
  for collagenous colitis, 371
  microscopic colitis, 276
  primary sclerosing cholangitis, 642
Cholinergic agonists, on mucus secretion, 150
Cholinomimetic drugs, on mucus secretion, 150
Cholorrhetic diarrhea, *see* Bile acids, salts, catharsis
Chromium-51 EDTA, intestinal permeability, 178
Chromosomal abnormalities, 16, 23 (Fig.)
Chromosomal markers, cancer surveillance, 679
Chromosomal properties, *Yersinia* spp., 415
Chronic active hepatitis, 637 (Table), 643
  ulcerative colitis, children, 662
Chronic active ulcerative colitis, histology, 298–299
Chronic amebiasis, 409
Chronic dry peritonitis, 391
Chronic granulomatous disease, 77, 381–382, 652
Chronic inflammatory infiltrate, ulcerative colitis, 294–295
Chronic obstructive airways disease, mortality in ulcerative colitis, 472
Chronic phlegmonous ileitis, 6
Chymase staining, mast cells, 88
Cinedefecography (videoproctography), 715, 899
CIN medium, *Yersinia* spp., 414
Ciprofloxacin, 121, 694
  gonorrhea, 404
  perianal fistulae, 618

Circulating granulocyte pool, 262
Cirrhosis, 637 (Table), 640, 643
Citrobacter freundii, mouse colitis, 158
Classification
  cytokines, 95–96
  dysplasia, 319
  radiation bowel disease, 426
Claversal (Salofalk), 488, 571 (Table)
  Crohn's disease
    after resection, 593
    trials, 494, 495
  maintenance therapy, 495
  dosage, 572
  vs sulfasalazine, 491, 492
Cleveland Clinic, stomaltherapy training, 911
Clinical indices, 335–341, 550, 957, *see also* Grading
Clinical nurse specialists, *see* Nurse specialists
Clinimed Ltd, publications, 922
Clonal expansion, dysplasia, 322
Clonidine, 531
Clostridium difficile, 119, 355–356, 364
  colonoscopy, 275
  course of infection, 359
  horses, 159
  ulcerative colitis, 304
  yersiniosis, 416
Clostridium perfringens type A, enterotoxemia in horses, 159
Closure, Crohn's disease surgery, 711
Clubbing, 625
  Crohn's disease
    children, 650
  vs ulcerative colitis, 344
Clustering, Crohn's disease, 117
Coagulation factors, 697
  XIII, 102–103
Coagulation system, 101–105
  Crohn's disease, 627
Cobblestone mucosa, 228 (Fig.), 239, 311, 601
  mouth, 634
Coccyx, resection, 894
Codeine phosphate, ileal Crohn's disease, 591
Code of practice for stomaltherapy nurses, 911
Cod liver oil enemas, 300
Coeliac disease, *see* Celiac disease
Coffee, 42
Cogan's syndrome, 18, 140
Colazide, *see* Balsalazide
Colchicine, amyloid, 629
Cold enrichment, *Yersinia* spp., 414
Colectomy
  on cancer risk, 470–471
  Crohn's disease, 478, 854–855
  laparoscopic, 720
  risk in ulcerative colitis, 471–472, 665
  stools, output, 810
  ulcerative colitis, elective, 731–738
Coliforms, 118
Colitic arthritis, 624
Colitis (Kelly), 923
Colitis cystica profunda, 276
Colitis polyposa, 304
Colitis X (horses), 159
Collagen
  collagenous colitis, 371–372
  fistulous Crohn's disease, 883
Collagen layer, collagenous colitis, 370–371
Collagenous colitis, 186, 275–276, 307, 369–373

  vs lymphocytic/microscopic colitis, 373–375
  treatment, 372–373
Collar-stud ulcers, radiology, 220
Colleagues at work, attitudes to IBD, 942
Colon
  absorptive capacity, 185
  Crohn's disease, 7
    motility, 198–199
  dilatation, *see also* Toxic megacolon
    ischemic colitis, 422
  fluid and electrolyte absorption, 181–190
  mucin synthesis, drug effects, 149
  mucosa, endoscopic appearance, 273
  as neorectum, 782
  nutrition of epithelium, 202–203
  remnant, cancer risk, 676, 680
  resection with ileal resection, 187
  transit, ulcerative colitis, 192–194
  tuberculosis, 394–395
Colonic metaplasia, pouches, 805, 806
Colonic protein (40 kDa), 68
Colonic reserve, 185
Colonoscopists, variation, 307
Colonoscopy, 273–284, *see also* Biopsies, colonoscopy
  bias, 305
  Crohn's disease
    children, 653
    colitis, 279–281, 604, 851
  echoendoscope (Olympus CF-UM20), 285
  excluding collagenous colitis, 370
  fistulae, 885
  fulminant colitis, 566
  intraoperative, 830
  quality of care, 961
  'tattooing', 720–721
  ulcerative colitis, 278, 550
    children, 662
    vs Crohn's disease, 277, 279
    upper limit in bowel, 467
Colony-stimulating factors, 527
Coloplast Ltd, publications, 922
Color Doppler ultrasound, deep vein thrombosis, 699
Colorectal carcinoma
  azathioprine, 576
  Crohn's disease, 325, 480
    colitis, 848–849
  after liver transplantation, 643
  surgery, 684–685, 746
  survival rates, 688
  ulcerative colitis, 663
Colostomies, *see also* 'Blowhole' colostomy
  endoscopy of, 280
  historical aspects, 4
  for incontinence, 867
  perforation, 937
  prolapse, 933–934
  retraction, 934
Common variable immunodeficiency, 65
Complement
  activation alterations, 67
  Crohn's disease, 629
  mast cell activation, 88
  therapeutic target, 530
  vascular damage, 138
Complement C_3, 329
Complement haplotypes, 20
Compliance (with treatment), 557, 731–732
Compliance, rectum, 715, 897
Complicated fistulae, *vs* simple fistulae, 884
Compression stockings, graduated, 698, 727

Computed tomography, 249, 250–257
　Crohn's disease
　　abscesses, 876
　　colitis, 604
　　vs ulcerative colitis, 345
　　vs endoluminal ultrasound, perianal lesions, 289
　　enterocutaneous fistulae, 884
Condylomata lata, 404
Congenital chloridorrhea, 182
Congo Red absorption, *Yersinia* spp., 415
Conjunctivitis, ulcerative colitis, children, 662
Connective-tissue type mast cells, 87
Constipation
　collagenous colitis, 369
　Crohn's disease, children, 649–650
　proximal, ulcerative colitis, 556–557
　ulcerative colitis, 194
Contagion, 38
Contamination, Crohn's disease surgery, 827
Continence, *see also* Incontinence
　after reservoir surgery, 756, 809, 810–811
　role of stomaltherapists, 913
　saline infusion studies, 194–195
Continent ileostomies, 5, 751–758, *see also* Kock's continent ileostomy
　Crohn's disease in, 834
Continuous quality improvement, 959
Contraceptives, *see* Oral contraceptives
Contrast studies, 215–247
Controlled ileal release budesonide, 509–510, 591–592
Convatec Ltd, publications, 922
Cooke, W.T., steroid therapy, 8
Copper, primary sclerosing cholangitis, 639, 642
Coronaviruses, cotton-top tamarins, 163
Corticosteroids, 8, 503–511
　adverse effects, 558–559
　arachidonic acid release inhibition, 528
　arthropathy from, 624
　for Behçet's disease, 388–389
　on butyrate oxidation, 204
　cheilitis granulomatosa, 635
　colonic electrolyte transport, 183–184
　colonic mucin synthesis, 149
　cotton-top tamarin colitis, 161–162
　Crohn's disease
　　children, 655
　　colitis, response failure, 850
　　esophagus, 584
　　vs 5-ASA, 494
　　gastroduodenal, 586, 818
　　ileal, 591–592
　　surgery, 825, 852
　　topical, 496
　　trials, 606–607
　diffuse jejunoileitis, 598
　enemas, children, 663
　eye lesions from, 626
　fulminant colitis, 567, 569, 726
　growth retardation, 655, 732–733
　on inflammatory mechanisms, 523
　insurance ratings, 950
　on leukocyte counts, 331
　lymphocyte function, 57
　on mast cells, 89–90
　microscopic colitis, 276
　pouchitis, 803
　primary sclerosing cholangitis, 642
　and sepsis, 693
　tuberculosis, 396
　ulcerative colitis, 506–508, 553–554, 560

　children, 663
　　maintenance therapy, 577
　　steroid-dependent, 554
Cortisone, 504
Costs
　follow-up, 957
　laparoscopic surgery, 719
　stoma care, 914
Cotton-top tamarins, 160–163
　E-selectin, 74
Counseling, 551, 915–918
　Crohn's disease surgery, 824
　colitis, 851
　ileal pouch–anal anastomosis, 772–776
　stoma care, 912
Cow's milk sensitivity, 41
Cramps, prostaglandins, 109
C-reactive protein, 329, 330
　Crohn's disease
　　children, 653
　　recurrence, 478
　　vs ulcerative colitis, 345
　follow-up, 956
　ulcerative colitis, children, 662
Crescentic fold disease of sigmoid colon, 276
Crest syndrome, *see* CRST syndrome
Crohn's colitis, 477–478, 601–613
　anal function, 713–714
　cancer risk, 679, 848–849, 850
　children, management, 657–658, 659
　colectomy specimens, 311
　colonoscopy, 279–281, 604, 851
　elemental diets, 609
　histology, 314–316
　radiology, 237–243
　surgery, 847–860
　　children, 657–658
　　techniques, 711
　ultrasound, 287, 604
Crohn's disease, 581–620, *see also* Abscesses, Crohn's disease; Crohn's colitis
　vs acute infectious-type colitis, 363
　AIDS, 403
　anastomotic recurrence, 138–139, 313
　animal models, 157–158
　autoantibodies, 69
　azathioprine and 6-MP, 513–515, 517
　cancer, 324–326
　　differentiation between, 235, 241
　　indications for surgery, 683
　　risk, 480, 654, 679–680, 681, 683
　childbirth, 943
　children, 647–660
　clinical indices, 336–339
　clustering, 117
　computed tomography, 250–256
　continent ileostomy
　　contraindication, 752
　　recurrent, 754–755
　corticosteroids, 508–510
　cytokine production, 66
　diets for, 535–539
　vs diversion colitis, 450 (Table)
　and diverticular disease, 446
　vs diverticular disease, 242, 243, 315
　enterocutaneous fistulae, 882–883
　eosinophils, 91
　epithelial nutrition, 203
　erythrocyte sedimentation rate, 330
　extraintestinal manifestations, incidence, 623 (Table)
　fertility, 480–481, 671
　follow-up, 957

4-ASA, 498
granulomata, *see* Granulomata, Crohn's disease
histology, 311–316
historical aspects, 6–8
HLA associations, 29, 276
ileal pouch–anal anastomosis, 765, 856–857
　contraindication, 761
intestinal dysfunction, 173–180
intraoperative recognition, 825–826
laparoscopic surgery, 719
magnetic resonance imaging, 257–259
mast cells, 89
motility disturbances, 197–199
mucus breakdown, 151
mycobacteria, 125–131
natural history, 475–483
non-steroidal anti-inflammatory drugs, 439
　vs NSAID enteropathy, 441
obstetric parity, 673
peripheral arthritis, 452
pouchitis, 805
primary sclerosing cholangitis, 639
proctocolectomy, 685
radiology, 226–245
recurrence, 243, 478, 835–836
resolution at strictureplasty, 844
sexual dysfunction, 903
smoking, 48–49, 347, 479, 602, 648
surgery, *see* Surgery, Crohn's disease
terminology, 7–8
therapeutic trials, 493–496
transmission experiments, 121
vs tuberculosis, 235, 236, 241, 313–314, 395
vs ulcerative colitis, 343–347
　colon, 601
　colonoscopy, 277, 279
　cytokines, 97, 345
　histology, 305–306, 315
　insurance, 949
　MHC genes, 27
　psychiatric illnesses, 941
　radiology, 224–226, 344–345
　same disease?, 346–347
　ulcerative colitis, in same patient, 306
vs ulcerative jejunoileitis, 433–434
vascular etiology proposed, 697
yersiniosis
　differentiation between, 417
　negative correlation, 416
Crohn's Disease Activity Index, 337–338
Crohn's in Childhood Research Association, 921
Cromoglycate, *see* Disodium cromoglycate
Crosby capsule, 7
CRST syndrome, with collagenous colitis, 369
Cryoproteins, Crohn's disease, 629
Cryptosporidiosis, AIDS, 401
Crypt rupture granulomata, 312
Crypts
　abscesses, 73, 76
　　active ulcerative colitis, 293–294
　　ulcerative colitis
　　　and Crohn's disease, 346
　　　vs infectious colitis, 304–305
　active ulcerative colitis, 292–294
　atrophy, *vs* acute infectious-type colitis, 363
　Crohn's disease, 312
　density, IBD, 206
　distortion, *vs* acute infectious-type colitis, 361–362

Crypts (contd)
  quiescent ulcerative colitis, 298
  restitution, 207
Culture-negative acute infectious-type colitis, 364–366, 367
Cultures, see also Stools, culture
  biopsies, 274, 365–366
Culture studies, mycobacteria, 126–127
Curettage, perineal sinuses, 893
Cutaneous anergy, 57
Cutting diathermy, 707
Cyclo 3 fort (phlebotonic drug), collagenous colitis, 372
Cyclo-oxygenase inhibitors, 110
Cyclo-oxygenase pathway, 489
Cyclosporin, 8, 517–519
  Behçet's disease, 666
  CD40 ligand expression, 64
  Crohn's disease, 608
    children, 656
    esophagus, 585
    vs ulcerative colitis, 523
  enterocutaneous fistula management, 888
  fulminant colitis, 567, 568, 569
  on inflammatory mechanisms, 523, 526
  lymphocyte function, 57
  mast cells, 90
  perianal fistulae, 618–619
  refractory ulcerative proctitis, 555–556
  ulcerative colitis, 559–560, 736–737
    children, 664
    maintenance therapy, 576
Cystic fibrosis, 18, 22
Cysts, Entamoeba histolytica, 409
Cytokines, 95–100, 522
  acute-phase response, 329
  aminosalicylates on, 489
  on B cells, 63
  in blood, 332
  corticosteroids on production, 504
  on C-reactive protein, 330
  Crohn's disease
    children, 654
    vs ulcerative colitis, 97, 345
  and cytotoxicity, 55
  effects on mucosa, 97–98
  on eosinophils, 90
  genes, 21–22, 27
  immunoglobulin production, 65, 66
  localization, 97
  from macrophages, 82
  mast cell activation, 88
  and receptors, 31
  Shigella spp., 352
  therapy, 98
Cytological atypia, 317
Cytology, cancer detection, 681
Cytomegalovirus, 120, 141
  AIDS, 400–401, 550
  IBD, 366
Cytoplasmic antineutrophil cytoplasmic antibody, Wegener's granulomatosis, 68
Cytoskeletal proteins, autoantibodies vs, 69
Cytotoxicity, cell-mediated, 55–56
Cytotoxic T lymphocytes, 28
  response, spondylarthropathies, 457
Cytotoxin, Clostridium difficile, 356

Decompression, see also 'Blowhole' colostomy
  Crohn's disease surgery, 830
  toxic megacolon, 568, 856

Deep vein thrombosis, 698–700
  Crohn's disease, 628
Defecation, see Evacuation
Degree of illness, 335
Delayed-release 5-ASA, renal toxicity, 558
Dendritic cells on T lymphocytes, 83
Denmark, incidence of IBD, 36
Density-gradient centrifugation, granulocyte isolation, 261
Dental treatment, Behçet's disease, 387
Dentate line, relation of ileoanal anastomosis, 785
Deoxycholic acid, Crohn's disease, 177
Depressive illness, 904–905, 941
  Crohn's disease, 481
Desferrioxamine, 113
Desmoid tumors, ileal pouch–anal anastomosis, 794
Developing countries, infectious colitis, 349
Dexamethasone, 505
  on mast cells, 89–90
Dextran preparations, 699
Dextran sulfate sodium, experimental colitis, 169
Diabetes mellitus
  HLA class II molecules, 28
  infection, 693
Diacylglycerol esters, 150, 184
Diapedesis, 76
'Diaphragm' disease, 438, 440–441
Diarrhea, see also Bile acids, salts, catharsis
  acute infectious colitis, 359
  AIDS, 400
  aminosalicylates, 557, 558
  azathioprine and 6-MP, 516, 576
  vs bloody diarrhea, 291
  collagen layers, 371
  collagenous colitis, 369, 372
  Crohn's disease, 649
  developing countries, 349
  fatty acid diarrhea, 187
  5-ASA, 572
  fulminant colitis, 565
  IBD, 183–186
  ileal Crohn's disease, 591
  ileal resection, 187
  incontinence, 897–898
  inflammatory vs non-inflammatory, 349
  interleukin-1, 98
  olsalazine, 490, 558, 572
  pouchitis, 804
  prostaglandins, 109
    therapeutic, 110
  right hemicolectomy, Crohn's disease, 174
  ulcerative colitis, children, 661
Diathermy, cutting, 707
Diclofenac, enteropathy, 438, 440
Dietary factors, 41–43
  diverticular disease, 445
  food bolus obstruction, 589, 594
  on stool frequency, 764
  sucrose, 38, 41–42, 609
Dietary restriction, reservoir surgery, 756, 776, 812
Dieticians, 706
Diets (management), see also Nutritional therapy
  Crohn's disease, 535–539
  enterocutaneous fistula patients, 886
  ulcerative colitis, 553
Diffuse jejunoileitis, 597–599, 836
Digital examination, 713
  vs endoluminal ultrasound, 289

pouchitis, 802
Dihydroxy bile acids, electrolyte secretion, 183
Di-iodohydroxyquinoline, amebiasis, 411
Dilatation (procedures), see also Balloon dilatation of strictures
  anal strictures, 864
  endoscopic, 271–272, 721
  ileum, ileal pouch–anal anastomosis, 776
Diloxanide furoate, amebiasis, 411
Dimethyl PGE_2, 530
Dimethylsulfoxide, with allopurinol, 531
Dinitrochlorobenzene, experimental colitis, 169
Dinitrogen trioxide, 79
Dioctyl sodium sulfosuccinate, electrolyte secretion, 183
Dipentum, see Olsalazine
Diphenoxylate, ileal Crohn's disease, 591
Disaccharide absorption, Crohn's disease, 175
Discoid lupus, with collagenous colitis, 369
Discrimination, employment, 946
Disease activity indices, see Clinical indices
Disodium cromoglycate, 8, 90, 577
  ulcerative proctitis, 556
Dissection, Crohn's disease, 707, 708–709, 827–828
Diversion, fecal see Diverting loop ileostomy
Diversion colitis, 276–277, 449–450
Diverticular disease, 443–447
  and Crohn's disease, 446
    colitis, 603
    vs Crohn's disease, 242, 243, 315
  extraintestinal manifestations, 623
  percutaneous abscess drainage, 876
  segmental colitis, 276
  vs ulcerative colitis, 307
Diverting loop ileostomy
  construction, 925
  Crohn's colitis, 858–859
  fulminant colitis, 728
DMSO, with allopurinol, 531
DNA, steroid binding, 503
DNA aneuploidy, 321
  cancer surveillance, 679
  pouchitis, 793
  primary sclerosing cholangitis, 639
Dogs, ulcerative colitis models, 158–159
Doppler ultrasound, deep vein thrombosis, 699
Dosage
  aminosalicylates, maintenance therapy, 572
  cyclosporin, 517–518
  5-ASA, 492
  steroids, ulcerative colitis, 554
Double-contrast barium studies, vs single-contrast studies, 215
Double halo, Crohn's disease, 250
Double-stapled anastomosis, ileal pouch–anal anastomosis, 784–785, 794, 797, 811, 898
Downregulating mechanisms, inflammation, 522
Drainage
  abscesses, 251, 875–879
    perianal, 289–290, 862
  infection, 693
  rectovaginal fistulae, 871
  stomaltherapy, 912–913
Drug resistance, tuberculosis, 396
Drugs
  adverse effects, 558–559, 734
    aminosalicylates, 489–490, 557, 558

Drugs (contd)
  azathioprine and 6-MP, 516–517, 575–576
  on cancer risk, 471
  on cyclosporin levels, 518
  on histology, 307
  masking fulminant colitis, 565
  toxic megacolon, 301, 566
  ulcers, colon, 315
Duodenum
  Crohn's disease, 7, 476–477, 583, 585–587, 817
    children, 650
    radiology, 232–235
  endoscopy, 271
  fistulae, 271, 819, 886
  tuberculosis, 393
Duration of disease, ulcerative colitis, cancer risk, 676
Dye-spraying, endoscopy, 282
Dysenteric arthritis, 453
Dysentery, see Amebiasis; Shigellosis
Dyspareunia, 903
  Crohn's disease, 481
  surgery, 749, 905–906, 943
    ileal pouch–anal anastomosis, 766, 795, 812–813
    proctocolectomy, 748
Dysphagia, 399
  Crohn's disease, 584
Dysplasia
  and cancer risk, 320, 322, 676–677
  colonoscopy, 735–736
  Crohn's disease, 325, 480, 679
    colitis, 850
  histology, 317–326
  polyps associated, 282
  primary sclerosing cholangitis, 639
  vs resolving ulcerative colitis, 297, 298
  retained rectum, 742
  surgery, 681
    ileal pouch–anal anastomosis, 786, 793–794
Dysplasia-associated lesion or mass (DALM), 320, 322

Echoendoscopes, 285
Echoendoscopy, see Endoluminal ultrasound
Eczema, 17
Edema
  Crohn's disease, 226
  ulcerative colitis, computed tomography, 256
Education, see also Training
  of patients, 551, see also Counseling
    'hour-long explanation', 705
    stoma care, 912, 913, 926
  school performance, 942
Effective dose equivalents, radiation, 266
Eggs
  albumin, immune complex-induced colitis, 170
  Salmonella spp., 351
Ehrlichia risticii, horses, 159
Eicosanoids, 109–111
  colonic electrolyte secretion, 184
  cotton-top tamarin colitis, 161
  metabolism, 489
  smoking, 50 (Table)
  therapeutic target, 527
Eicosapentanoic acid, 528
Ejaculation, see also Retrograde ejaculation
  impairment after panproctocolectomy, 857
ELAM-1, see E-selectin
Elastase (neutrophil elastase), 331
Elasticity coefficient, rectum, 196
Elderly patients
  Crohn's colitis, 602
  and ileal pouch–anal anastomosis, 761, 771
  ischemic colitis, 421
  laparoscopic surgery, 720
  proctocolectomy, 746
Electrically stimulated transposed muscle, implantable, 900
Electrocautery, panproctocolectomy, 857
Electrogenic sodium absorption, colon, 182
Electrolytes
  absorption, 173–174
    colon, 181–190
  loss, 44
  secretion, colon, 183
Electromyography, 715, 899
Electroneutral sodium absorption, colon, 182
Electrostimulation, transrectal, periprostatic plexus, 905
Elemental diets, Crohn's disease, 535–539, 592, 608–609
  children, 656–657
  perianal, 617
Elevated lesions, dysplasia, 677
Elimination diets, 43
Emergency hospital admission, 703
Emergency surgery
  fulminant colitis, 726–729, 746
  toxic megacolon, 856
Emphysema, mortality in ulcerative colitis, 472
Employers, attitudes to IBD, 942
Employment, 942, 946, see also Occupation; Working capacity
  Crohn's disease, 481
  ileal pouch–anal anastomosis, 812
  surgery, 943
Encephalopathy, hemorrhagic colitis, 354
End ileostomies, 5, 856
  construction, 925, 927–928
End-loop ileostomies, 856, see also Loop–end ileostomies
Endoanal endoscopic microsurgery, 717
Endoanal ultrasound, 259, 282, 616, 715, 885, 899
  fecal incontinence, 867–868
Endoluminal ultrasound, 285–289
  Crohn's disease
    colitis, 604
    esophagus, 584
Endoscopic retrograde cholangiography, primary sclerosing cholangitis, 641
Endoscopy, 269–284, see also named investigations
  Crohn's disease
    vs ulcerative colitis, 344
    upper gastrointestinal tract, 818
    colitis, 851
    vs radiology, 585–586
  follow-up, 956
  indices of disease, 339
  lower intestinal tract, 273–284
  pouchitis, 280, 801
  therapy via, 271–272
Endothelin-1, 136
Endothelium, see also Adhesion molecules
  inflammatory process, 135
  isotope scanning, 267
  and neutrophils, 73–76
Endothelium-derived relaxing factor, see Nitric oxide
Endotoxemia, glutamine uptake, 203
Endotoxins, effects, 887
Endovaginal ultrasound, 289, 885
End-to-end anastomoses, Crohn's disease, 710–711
Enemas, 557, see also named substances
  anal irritation from, 574
  Crohn's disease, 496–497
  cyclosporin, 518
  fulminant colitis, 567
  pH, 488, 573
Energy-deficiency disease, 556
Energy expenditure, 44
Entamoeba dispar, 356, 409
Entamoeba histolytica, 356–357, 409
  vs Crohn's disease, 242, 243
  mucus secretion, 150
Enteral nutrition
  Crohn's disease, 535–539, 592
    children, 656–657
    diffuse jejunoileitis, 598
    enterocutaneous fistulae, 886
Enteric-coated steroids, 554
Enteric hyperoxaluria, 188
Enteric nervous system, 184
Enteroaggregative E. coli, 355
Enteroclysis, 216–217
  vs CT, radiation doses, 255
  NSAID enteropathy, 438
Enterocolic fistulae, 232, 236
Enterocutaneous fistulae, 881–891
  management, 885–889
  results of neglect, 883
Enteroenteric fistulae, 232, 236, 590
  Crohn's colitis, 605
Enterohemorrhagic E. coli, 353–355
Enterohepatic recirculation, Crohn's disease, 177
Enteroinvasive E. coli, 355
Enteroscopy, 269–270, 271, see also Ileoscopy
  intraoperative, 281
Enterotoxins
  Clostridium difficile, 356
  mucus secretion, 150
  Yersinia spp., 415
Enterovaginal fistulae, 871
Enthesopathy, 451
Eosinophil cationic protein, 90
Eosinophilia, 90–91, 331
Eosinophil peroxidase, 90
Eosinophils, 87, 90–91
  colitis, 295
  peripheral blood, 90–91
Ephedrine, for retrograde ejaculation, 905
Epidemiology, 35–52
  and genetics, 13–23
  infective agents, 117–118
Epidermal growth factor, 531
  on crypt restitution, 208
  on glutamine uptake, 203
  in mucus, 143
  protective effect, 207
Episcleritis, 626
Episioproctotomy, 872
Episiotomy, ileal pouch–anal anastomosis, 813
Epithelial cell antigen, antibody cross-reaction, 629
Epithelial cell-associated components (ECAC), on mast cells, 89
Epithelial mucin, membrane-bound (MUC1), 144

Epithelioid cells, 275
Epithelioid granulomata, 380
    infections, 363
Epithelium
    antigen presentation, 57
    barrier function, 77
    cells
        and neutrophils, 76–78
        proliferation, pouchitis, 805
    colon, 181
    cytotoxicity against, 56
    hierarchical organization, 205–207
    nutrition of, 201–204
    ulcerative colitis
        active, 292–293
        resolving, 297–298
Epstein-Barr virus, 120
    HLA molecules on response, 29
Erection testing, 905
Erythema nodosum, 344, 625–626
    bacterial infections, 119
    ulcerative colitis, children, 661
    Yersinia enterocolitica, 355
Erythrocyte antigen, *see* Antierythrocyte antibodies
Erythrocytes
    neutrophil displacement, 74
    radiolabeled, deep vein thrombosis, 699
Erythrocyte sedimentation rate, 329–330, 332
    Crohn's disease
        children, 653
        colitis, 604
    ulcerative colitis, children, 662
Erythropoietin therapy, 605
Escherichia coli, 118, 521
    colonoscopy, 274
    vs Crohn's disease, 363
    enterotoxins, mucus secretion, 150
    infective colitis, 535–355
E-selectin, 74–75, 136
Esophagus
    candidiasis, 399
    Crohn's disease, 583–585
        radiology, 232
    endoscopy, 270–271
    tuberculosis, 393
Ethambutol, 396
Ethics, stomaltherapy, 911
Ethnic groups, *see also* named ethnic groups
    Crohn's disease, 648
        perianal disease, 861
    stomas, 945, 946
    studies, 15, 37
Eudragit-S, -L, -L100, 488
Euglobulin lysis time, 104
European Cooperative Crohn's Disease Study, 493, 606
    steroids, 508–509
    sulfasalazine maintenance therapy trial, 494–495
Evacuation
    frequency after reservoir surgery, 756, 763–764
    ileoanal pouch performance, 763
    studies, 715
Exclusion diets
    Crohn's disease, 537–538
    oral Crohn's disease, 635
    pouchitis, 804
    ulcerative colitis, 553, 557
Exercise, diverticular disease, 445
Experimental animal models, 167–171
Explanation, *see also* Counseling

'hour-long', 705
Extent of disease, ulcerative colitis, 466–469, 550
    cancer risk, 676, 680
External anal sphincter, 897
Extraintestinal manifestations, 139–140, 623–632
    Crohn's disease, 7, 478
        colitis, 602–603, 849
        vs ulcerative colitis, 344
    cross-sectional imaging, 259
    experimental animals, 168
    ileal pouch–anal anastomosis, 760
    isotope scanning, 266–267
    pouchitis, 793, 803
    ulcerative colitis, 733–734
        children, 661–662
        management, 557
    yersiniosis, 416, 417
Extrinsic allergic encephalomyelitis, 31
Eye lesions, *see also* Uveitis
    Crohn's disease, 626
    vs ulcerative colitis, 344
    incidence, 623 (Table)

Face-mask optics, minimal-access surgery, 722
Familial Behçet's disease, 665
Familial polyposis, ileal pouch–anal anastomosis, 346, 794
Family history, 946
    Crohn's disease, 648
Family practitioners, 705
Family studies, 13–14, 15, 117, *see also* Heredity patterns
    autoantibodies, 68
Faroe Isles, incidence of IBD, 36
Fast foods, 42
Fats
    absorption, 44
        Crohn's disease, 175–176
        ileal resection, 187
    enteral diets, 537
    metabolism, steroids, 503
Fatty acid diarrhea, 187
Fatty acids, *see also* Free fatty acids
    aminosalicylates on oxidation, 489
    dietary, 42
Fatty liver, 259, 637 (Table), 644
    nutrition risk, 544
Fat wrapping, Crohn's disease, 157, 311
Fears, delaying surgery, 759
Fecal collections, indium-111, 265–266
Fecal diversion, *see also* Diverting loop ileostomy
    rectovaginal fistulae, 872
Fecal extracts, mucus breakdown, 150–151
Fecal stream, on mucosa, 805
Fecal vomiting, colic fistulae, 605
Feces, *see* Stools
Feeding tubes, endoscopic placement, 272
Ferrets, Crohn's disease models, 157
Fertility, 671–672, 943, 945
    Crohn's disease, 480–481
    ileal pouch–anal anastomosis, 774–775, 795, 813
    sulfasalazine, 490, 558, 572
Fetal intestinal explants, modeling HIV enteropathy, 402
Fetus, 672
    bone marrow suppression, azathioprine and 6-MP, 516–517
Fiber, 42, 43

diverticular disease, 445, 446
    on mucosal barrier function, 203
Fibrin deposition, 103, 133
Fibrinogen, 697
    iodine-125-labeled, imaging, 699
    as laboratory marker, 329
Fibrinolysis, impaired, 103–104
    Crohn's disease, 627
Fibrinolytic drugs, 700
Fibrinopeptide A, 101–102
    Crohn's disease, 627
Fibrosing alveolitis, 626–627
Fibrosis, radiology
    Crohn's disease, 230–232, 239
    ulcerative colitis, 220–223
Filiform inflammatory polyps, 282
Finney-type strictureplasty, 838
First attacks, ulcerative colitis, 463–464
Fish oils, 528, 576, *see also* Cod liver oil enemas
Fissuring
    Crohn's disease, 311, 312
        anal, 615, 617, 714, 861–862
    fulminant colitis, 300–301
Fistulae, *see also* Rectovaginal fistulae
    anal
        Crohn's disease, 615–616, 617–619, 711, 862–864, 864–867
        tuberculosis, 395
    from anastomoses, 853–854, 881
    anorectal region, incontinence, 714
    bacterial overgrowth from, 176
    bladder, Crohn's disease, 606, 628
    cancer, 686
    Crohn's disease
        abscesses, 833
        barium studies, 232, 236
        colitis, 605, 847
        gastroduodenal, 476, 477, 586
        ileum, 590, 592, 594
        vs ulcerative colitis, 343–344
        water-soluble contrast studies, 244–245
    cyclosporin for, 608
    diffuse jejunoileitis, 598
    diverticular disease, 443, 444
    duodenum, 271, 819, 886
    endoluminal ultrasound, 288
    esophagus, 270
    gastroduodenal, 819–820
    ileal pouch–anal anastomosis, 765, 792–793
    isotope scanning, 263
    Kock's pouch, 753–754
    perianal
        Crohn's disease, 478
        magnetic resonance imaging, 257
    and quality activities, 961
    radiation, 427
        surgery for, 428
    stomach, 271
    stomas, 936
    stomaltherapy, 912–913
    surgical technique, 711
    total parenteral nutrition, 543
    ulcerative colitis, 223
Fistulography, team approach, 704
Fistuloscopy, 885
Fistulotomy, audit results, 960
5-ASA, 8, 487–497
    adverse effects, 490, 557
    CIR, renal toxicity, 558
    cotton-top tamarin colitis, 161, 162
    crescentic fold disease of sigmoid colon, 276

5-ASA (contd)
　Crohn's disease
　　ileal, 591, 592
　　　maintenance therapy trials, 495
　　　after resection, 593
　　　topical, 496–497
　fulminant colitis, 568
　maintenance therapy, 571–572
　on mast cells, 89
　microscopic colitis, 276
　pouchitis, 803
　pregnancy, 672
　renal toxicity, 572
　ulcerative colitis, 491, 492, 553
　　endoscopic improvement, 277
5-lipoxygenase inhibitors, 528–529
Fixed-neutrophil ELISA, pANCA detection, 69
FK506 (immunosuppressant), on mast cells, 90
FLAP inhibitor, 529, 560
Flask-shaped ulcers
　amebic colitis, 410
　Behçet's disease, 665
Flexical, 656–657
Flora, see Bowel flora
Flow cytometry, cancer surveillance, 679
Fluorescent treponemal antibody test, 404
Fluoroquinolones
　salmonellosis, 352
　shigellosis, 353
Fluticasone propionate, 505, 560
Foam preparations
　children, 663
　Crohn's disease, 496
　ulcerative colitis, 508, 553, 554
Folate deficiency, 44, 331–332, 627, 652
　Crohn's disease, 176–177
　sulfasalazine, 558, 577–578
Follicular lymphoid hyperplasia, diversion colitis, 449
Follicular proctitis or colitis, 295
Follow-up, 953–962, see also Surveillance for cancer risk
　Crohn's disease, children, 659
　radiology, 243–244, 956
　ulcerative colitis, cancer risk, 680
Food, see also Dietary factors; Diets; Nutritional therapy
　on colonic motility, 196–197
Food additives, 42–43
Food bolus obstruction, 589, 594
Food intolerance, 43
　oral Crohn's disease, 635
　pouchitis, 804
Food poisoning, *Salmonella* spp., 351
Foreign-body granulomata, 379
　fulminant colitis, 300
Formaldehyde-sensitive mast cells, 87
Formalin
　immune complex-induced colitis, 170
　mast cell investigation, 89
Forskolin, 150
Foscarnet, cytomegalovirus, 401
4-ASA, 489, 497–498, 572–573
France, incidence of IBD, 36
Free fatty acids, serum levels, steroids, 503
Free protein S, 103
Free radicals, 112, see also Oxidants
　mucus scavenging, 143
Free radical scavengers, 489, 531
Frequency of examination, cancer surveillance, 680–681
Frequency of stools, 764

anticholinergic drugs, 776
　reservoir surgery, 756, 763–764, 809, 810
Frozen sections, 313
Fruit, 42
Frusemide (furosemide), chloride secretion, 183
Fucosylated carbohydrates, 74
Fucosyltransferases, 148
Fulminant colitis, 565–570, 725–729
　children, 663–664
　histology, 299–301, 305, 314–316
Functional post-dysenteric colitis, 366
Functional zone, epithelium, 205
Furosemide, chloride secretion, 183

Galβ1-3GalNAc expression, 147, 320
Gallstones, 259, 637 (Table)
　Crohn's disease, 177, 594, 644
　　vs ulcerative colitis, 344
　　ileal pouch–anal anastomosis, 795
　primary sclerosing cholangitis, 642
　total parenteral nutrition, 544
γ δ T cells, 54
Gamma globulins, serum levels, 66
γ-interferon, see Interferon-γ
Ganciclovir, cytomegalovirus, 401
Gangrenous ischemic colitis, 421–422
Gastric acid secretion, fistulae to skin, 887–888
Gastric outlet obstruction, Crohn's disease, 477
Gastroduodenal Crohn's disease, 476–477, 583, see also Duodenum, Crohn's disease; Stomach, Crohn's disease
　surgery, 817–820
Gastroenteritis
　colon changes, 276
　ileal pouch–anal anastomosis, 776
　salmonellosis, 351
Gastroenterologists, view of pathologists, 307
Gastrointestinal echoendoscope (Olympus GF-UM20), 285
Gastrointestinal hemorrhage
　colonoscopy, 281
　Crohn's disease, 585, 834
　　colitis, 851
　　gastroduodenal, 817
Gastrojejunostomy, 818
Gastro-esophageal reflux, 270
Gastroscopes, pediatric, pouch endoscopy, 280
Gay bowel syndrome, 403
Genetic markers, cancer surveillance, 679
Genetics, 13–33, see also Family studies; Molecular genetics
　IBD, 346–347
　marker studies, 18–22
Genomic transcription, steroids on, 503–504
Geographical distribution
　Crohn's disease, 648
　ulcerative colitis, 660
Giardia lamblia, arthritis, 453
Gibbons, stress-induced dysentery, 159
Gingival hyperplasia
　Crohn's disease, 634
　cyclosporin, 519 (Table)
Ginsberg, L., Crohn's disease, 6–7
GlcNAc-GalNAc transferase, 147
Globotriasylceramide (Pk antigen), 354
Glomerular filtration rate, cyclosporin, 518
Glomerulonephritis, yersiniosis, 416
Glucocorticoids, 503–506
　colonic electrolyte absorption, 184
Glucose-6 phosphate dehydrogenase, dysplasia, 321

Glutamine
　dietary, 537
　enemas, pouchitis, 204
　epithelial nutrition, 201–202, 203
Glutathione peroxidase, 112
Gluteal muscle flaps, 894
　for fecal incontinence, 900
　vaginal restoration, 906
Glycogen storage disease type Ib, 16
Glycosaminoglycans, sulfated, 137
Glycosidases, mucus breakdown, 150
Glycosylation, mucins, 143, 146–147, 148, 151
Glycosyl transferases, 146–147
Gm 1,2,10 immunoglobulin marker genes, 20
Goblet cells, 149, 151
Golgi apparatus, mucin synthesis, 148
Gonococcal proctitis, 403–404, 550
Gorillas, colitis, 159
Gp91-*phox*, 382
Gracilis muscle flap, 894
　for fecal incontinence, 900
Grading, see also Clinical indices
　Crohn's colitis, 279, 603
　dysplasia, 319
　endoscopy for, 339
　pouchitis, 802
　ulcerative colitis, 277
Graduated compression stockings, 698, 727
Grafting, see also Muscle flaps
　perineal wounds, 893
Granulocytes, radiolabeled, 261
Granulomata, 83, 379–381, see also Foreign-body granulomata
　chronic granulomatous disease, 382
　Crohn's disease, 312, 314, 380–381
　　diagnosis, 652
　　gastroduodenal, 818
　　vs ulcerative colitis, 345, 346, 601
　endoscopy, 270
　liver, 637 (Table), 644
　skin, 626
　tuberculosis, 314, 391–392
　vascular studies, 133
Granulomatous synovitis, 453
Greece, incidence of IBD, 36
GRO (chemokine), 96
Grouping of patients, 955
Growth factors, see also named growth factors
　on epithelial repair, 207
　in mucus, 143
　pouchitis, 806
　for ulcerative jejunoileitis, 434
Growth hormone
　levels, 653–654
　mucus secretion, 149
Growth retardation, 543
　corticosteroids, 655, 732–733
　Crohn's disease, 43–44, 477, 650, 653–654
　　colitis, 849
　diets and, 538
　diffuse jejunoileitis, 597–598
　steroids, 503
　surgery effects, 658 (Fig.)
　ulcerative colitis, 661, 732–733
Guanidinium thiocyanate pretreatment, PCR, 128–129
Guillain-Barré syndrome, *Campylobacter* spp., 350

H_2-receptor antagonists, gastroduodenal Crohn's disease, 586

Habershon, on pseudopolyps, 4
Haemo-, *see headings starting* Hemo-
Hamsters, Crohn's disease models, 158
Hamstring muscle flaps, 894
Hapten-induced colitis, 168–169
Hartmann resection of rectosigmoid, 870
Harvey and Bradshaw Crohn's disease index, 338
Haustra
  colonoscopy, 273
  radiology, 223
HBsAG carrier state, AIDS, 400
Headache, cyclosporin, 519 (Table)
Heaf testing, 392
Healing, mucosa, 207
Health status measurement, 335, 339–400
Heat shock proteins, 207–208
  Behçet's disease, 387
  in mucus, 143
Heinz body hemolytic anemia, sulfasalazine, 558
Helicobacter pylori, treatment, 587
Helminths
  experimental infection, 168
  intestinal permeability, 178
Helper T lymphocytes, 28, 63–64, 65, 66, 98
Hematoma, Crohn's disease surgery, 828
Heme, activated, 78
Hemicolectomy, right, electrolyte absorption, 174
Hemochromatosis
  HLA associations, 29
  yersiniosis, 415
Hemoglobin, 331, 332
Hemolysis
  autoimmune, 18
  Crohn's disease, 627
  sulfasalazine, 44, 490
    Heinz body anemia, 558
Hemolytic uremic syndrome, 352, 353–354
Hemophilia, protective effect *vs*, 140
Hemopoietic stem cell transplantation, chronic granulomatous disease, 382
Hemorrhage, *see also* Bloody diarrhea; Rectal bleeding
  Crohn's disease, 649
    colitis, 605
  diverticular disease, 444
  fulminant colitis, 567
  ileal pouch–anal anastomosis, 793
  laparoscopic surgery, 719
  stomas, 936
  strictureplasty, 844
  ulcerative colitis, 471
Hemorrhagic colitis, *E. coli*, 353–354
Hemorrhoids, 617
Henderson County chronic diarrhea outbreak, 359, 363–364
Heparins (therapy), 139, 698–699
  and fulminant colitis, 727
Hepatic acute-phase response, 98
Hepatitis B, AIDS, 400
Hepatitis C, 643
Hepatocellular carcinoma, 637 (Table)
Hepatocyte growth factors, on crypt restitution, 207
Heredity patterns, 15–16, 648, 660, 946, *see also* Family studies
Hermansky–Pudlak syndrome, 16
Hernias, parastomal, 934–936
Herpes simplex virus
  AIDS, 401
  Behçet's disease, 387
  proctitis, 404–405
Herpesviruses, 120
  colon histology, 305
Hexamethyleneamine oxime (HMPAO), 261
High-fiber diets
  diverticular disease, 446
  ulcerative colitis, 553
High-risk group, cancer in ulcerative colitis, 680
Hirschsprung's disease, diversion colitis complicating treatment, 277
Histamine, 88 (Table)
  collagenous colitis, 372
Histiolytic colitis, boxer dogs, 158–159
Histocompatibility antigens, 18–20, 22, 27–30
  cotton-top tamarins, 163
Histopathology, 291–328
  children, 652 (Table)
  Crohn's disease *vs* ulcerative colitis, 345, 601
Histoplasmosis, 314
Historical aspects, 3–10
Hit-and-run mechanisms, 125
HIV enteropathy, 402
HLA-B27 antigen, 17
  vs β2 microglobulin genes, 456–457
  similar molecule in cotton-top tamarins, 163
  spondylarthropathies, 451–452, 453, 454–455, 456, 457, 625
HLA-B27 transgenic rats, infective agent experiments, 121
HLA Bw62, spondylarthropathies, 453, 456
HLA haplotypes, 18–20
  ANCA positivity, 69
  Behçet's disease, 387
  disease risk, 276
  lymphocytic colitis, 373
  primary sclerosing cholangitis, 18, 346, 639–640
  ulcerative colitis *vs* Crohn's disease, 346
Hockey-stick deformity, Kock's pouch slippage, 753
Hodgkin's lymphoma, with collagenous colitis, 369–370
Holland, incidence of IBD, 36
Hollister Ltd, publications, 923
Hope Hospital, 703
  intestinal failure unit, 704–705
Hormone replacement therapy, 558–559
Horses, IBD models, 158, 159
Hosepipe thickening, 226, 228 (Fig.)
Hospital admission, 703–704
  rates, 35–36
'Hour-long explanation', 705
Housing, 37
H pouches, 781
Human immunoglobulin, radiolabeled, 266–267
Humoral immunity, 63–72
Hydrocortisone, 504
  Crohn's colitis surgery, 852
  fulminant colitis, 567, 726
  oral Crohn's disease, 656
  topical therapy, children, 655 (Table)
  toxic megacolon, children, 664
Hydrogen peroxide, 78, 112
Hydronephrosis, Crohn's disease, 628
Hydroxychloroquine, 528
Hydroxyl ions, 112
Hypercoagulability, 697–698, 734
Hyperoxaluria, Crohn's disease *vs* ulcerative colitis, 344
Hyperparathyroidism, 44
  steroids, 503
Hypersensitivity, azathioprine and 6-MP, 516, 575
Hypertension, cyclosporin, 519 (Table)
Hypertrichosis, cyclosporin, 519 (Table)
Hypertrophic pulmonary osteoarthropathy, 625
Hypochlorous acid, 78, 79, 112
Hypokalemia
  and colonic dilatation, 194
  toxic megacolon, 301
Hypopituitarism, 653

IA (Ileostomy and Internal Pouch Support Group), 920
IBMX (mucus secretagogue), 150
ICAM-1, 69, 136
  and ICAM-2, neutrophil adhesion, 75, 76
ICE inhibitors, 524
Idiopathic proctitis, 295, 549
IgA, 64, 65–66, 331
  secretory, 143
IgE receptors, mast cells, 88
IgG, 65, 66, 331
IgG-producing cells, ulcerative colitis, 295
IgG receptors, macrophages, 83
IgM, 331
  primary sclerosing cholangitis, 640–641
IL-1 receptor antagonist, 98
  gene, ulcerative colitis, 346
IL-2 gene knockout mice
  anticolon antibodies, 66
  infective agent experiments, 121
Ileal pouch–anal anastomosis, 759–770, *see also* Pelvic pouches
  benefits and risks, 767 (Table)
  children, 664–665
  complications, 791–799
  counseling, 772–776
  Crohn's disease, 761, 765, 856–857
  drug therapy, 577
  failure rate, 765
  familial polyposis, 346, 794
  fulminant colitis, 569
  incontinence, 764, 775–776, 785, 898
  indeterminate colitis, 345, 478, 761
  laparoscopic-assisted, 720
  outcome, 961
  patient selection, 771–772
  pouch function, 749
  pregnancy, 672, 766, 813
  publications on, 922
  quality of life, 809–813, 943
  repeat operation, 835
  sexual dysfunction, 765–766, 774–775, 794–795, 943
    impotence, 775, 812, 904
  St Mark's series, 740
  technical aspects, 779–789
  ulcerative colitis, 737
Ileal pouches, *see* Continent ileostomies; Pouches; Pouchitis
Ileitis
  spondylarthropathies, 451–460
  Yersinia enterocolitica, 119
Ileoanal anastomoses, 5–6, 781, 782, *see also* Ileal pouch–anal anastomosis
Ileocecal masses, *see also* Toxic masses
  Crohn's disease, 477, 590, 592
    children, 592, 649
Ileocecal valve, two-sphincter operation, 782

Ileocecoplasty, tuberculosis, 397 (Fig.)
Ileopsoas muscle, fistula tracking, 882
Ileorectal anastomoses, 5
  benefits and risks, 767 (Table)
  Crohn's disease, 711
    colitis, 854–855, 856
    leakage, 855
    technique, 739
  ulcerative colitis, 739–743
    cancer risk, 736
Ileoscopy, 280 see also Enteroscopy
Ileostomies, 3, 5–6, 745–750, see also Continent ileostomies
  benefits and risks 767 (Table)
  cancer at sites, 686
  clinical indices, 339
  complications, 748
  construction, 747, 925–932
  Crohn's disease, 609
  diverting, 786–787, 797
  dysfunction, 755
  endoscopy of, 280
  enterocutaneous fistulae, 882
  fear of, 759
  fulminant colitis, 727–728
  historical aspects, 4–6
  intestinal obstruction, 791
    after closure, 762
  pregnancy, 672
  prolapse, 934
  quality of life, 766–767, 773, 943
  retraction, 934
  sexual dysfunction, 943
  St Mark's series, 741
  subtotal colectomy, Crohn's colitis, 854–856
Ileostomy and Internal Pouch Support Group, 920
Ileostomy book (Bosanko), 921
Ileum
  biopsies, culture, 274
  Crohn's disease, 589–595
    cancer, 325
    radiology, 235–236
  flow, 185
  radiation bowel disease surgery, 428
  resection, diarrhea, 187
Imipenems, 694
Imipramine, for retrograde ejaculation, 905
Immune complexes, Crohn's disease, 629
Immune complex-induced colitis, experimental, 170
Immune responses, 122, 346
  aminosalicylates on, 489
  defects in primary sclerosing cholangitis, 640
  enterocutaneous fistulae, 887
  macrophages, 81–82
  pouchitis, 806
  smoking, 50 (Table)
Immunocompromized patients
  colonoscopy, 275
  fistulae, 885
  infection, 693
Immunoglobulin gene libraries, 68
Immunoglobulin marker genes, 20
Immunoglobulins, 63, see also Human immunoglobulin, radiolabeled
  production patterns, 55, 65–66
  V_H segments, 67
Immunohistochemistry, vascular studies, 133–136
Immunology, 53–72

Immunoprotection, yersiniosis, 415
Immunoregulation, 57
Immunoregulatory cytokines, 96–97
Immunosuppressants, 8, 513–520
  anorectal cancer, 326
  Crohn's disease, 607–608
    colitis, response failure, 850
    ileal, 592
  enterocutaneous fistula management, 888
  fulminant colitis, 568
  on leukocyte counts, 331
  on mast cells, 90
  ulcerative colitis, 554–555, 559–560, 736–737
    children, 664
    maintenance therapy, 574–576
Immunosuppression, steroids, 503
Immunotherapy, 31, 146
Implantable electrically stimulated transposed muscle, 900
Impotenance, 903
  ileal pouch–anal anastomosis, 775, 812, 904
  nerve damage, 904
  after surgery, 748, 749, 766, 795, 904, 943
Imuran, *see* Azathioprine
Incidence, 36–37
Incisions, 691
  Crohn's disease surgery, 707, 825
  stoma construction, 926–927
Inclusion bodies, 120
Incontinence, 713, 714, 897–901
  Crohn's disease, 199
    management, 867–868
  ileal pouch–anal anastomosis, 764, 775–776, 785, 898
  of Kock's pouch, endoscopy, 280
  ulcerative colitis, 191
Indeterminate colitis, 343, 345–346
  change to Crohn's colitis, 478
  children, 666
  endoluminal ultrasound, 288
  fissuring, 301
  fulminant colitis, 316
  histology, 306
  ileal pouch–anal anastomosis, 345, 478, 761
  pathology performance, 961
  surgery, 746
Indian subcontinent, ulcerative colitis, 660
Indigo carmine, endoscopy, 282
Indirect immunofluorescence, pANCA detection, 69
Indium-111-labeled leukocytes, 261
  excretion, 332
  NSAID enteropathy, 441
  migration to lungs, 627
  quantification studies, 265–266
Indolent Crohn's disease, 479
Indomethacin, 110
Infantilization, 651
Infarction, Behçet's disease, 388
Infection, immunosuppressants, 516
Infectious colitis, 274–275, 349–358
  acute, 359–368
    change to IBD, 366–367
  vs Crohn's disease, 315
  extraintestinal manifestations, 623
  vs ulcerative colitis, 304–305, 549–550
  histology, 292–297
Infectious-type colitis, 359
Infective agents, 117–155
  animal models, 121, 167–168

vascular factors, 133–142
Infective ulcerative typhlocolitis (pigs), 159
Inferior mesenteric artery
  ligation, ileorectal anastomoses, 739
  territory, Crohn's colitis, 602
Inferior vena cava interruption, 698
Inflammation, 73
  active ulcerative colitis, 293
  acute, infectious colitis, 363
  collagenous colitis, 371
  resolution at strictureplasty, 844
Inflammatory cells, intravascular, 133
Inflammatory diarrhea, 349
Inflammatory mediators, 107–116, 521–534
  electrolyte secretion, 173–174
  intestinal permeability, 178
Inflammatory mucosal Crohn's disease, 479, 589–590
  ileum, 591
  management, 598
  recurrence, 594
Inflammatory polyps, *see* Pseudopolyps
Influenza-like illness, azathioprine, 655
Information, for patients, 917–923
Informed consent, 920
Inheritance, *see* Heredity patterns
Insertion sequences, mycobacterial DNA, 127
Instant barium enema, 219
Insulin-dependent diabetes mellitus, HLA class II molecules, 28
Insulin-like growth factors
  Crohn's disease, children, 654
  IGF-1 on epithelial repair, 207
Insurance, 946, 949–951
Integrins, 81
  neutrophil adhesion, 75
  transepithelial lymphocytes migration, 77
Interferon-γ, 96–97
  chronic granulomatous disease, 382
  Crohn's disease, 66
  macrophage priming, 82
  steroids on production, 504
Interferons
  effects, 98
  mucosal lymphocyte response, 55
  redundancy, 95
  therapy, 523
    potential for, 526–527
Interleukin-1, 96, 522
  aminosalicylates on, 489
  effects on mucosa, 98
  localization, 97
  mucus secretion, 150
  and prostaglandin secretion, 184
  therapy target, 524
Interleukin-1 receptor antagonist (HL-1ra), 524
  gene, 21, 22, 522
Interleukin-2, 70, 96–97, 522
  Crohn's disease, 66
  therapy, 523
  therapy target, 525–526
Interleukin-2 receptor, peripheral blood lymphocytes, 53
Interleukin-4, 97
Interleukin-5, on immunoglobulin synthesis, 65
Interleukin-6, 96
  production, 66
  therapy target, 524
Interleukin-8, 96, 527
  localization, 97
  salmonellosis, 351

Interleukin-10, 97
  therapy, 98
Interleukin-13, 97
Interleukins
  acute-phase response, 329
  in blood, 332
  on C-reactive protein, 330
  redundancy, 95
  steroids on production, 504
Intermediate colitis, 237
Internal anal sphincter, 897
International Study Group for Behçet's Disease, 387
Intersphincteric anorectal excision, 857, 905
Interstitial hernias, 934
Interstitial matrix, and neutrophils, 76
Intestinal adenomatosis complex, pigs, 158
Intestinal failure unit, Hope Hospital, 704–705
Intestinal intraepithelial lymphocytes, 54
  cytolytic potential, 56
  IgA suppression factor, 66
  suppressor function, 57
Intestinal obstruction
  after colectomy, 755
  colonic gangrene, 422
  Crohn's disease, 313, 589, 590
    ileal, 591
    operative appearance, 826
  diffuse jejunoileitis, 598–599
  ileal pouch–anal anastomosis, 762, 791–792, 797
  at ileostomies, 748, 936
  Kock's pouch, 754
  on motility, 198
  NSAID enteropathy, 438
  proctocolectomy, 748–749
  radiotherapy, 426, 427
  surgery for, 830–833
  tuberculosis, 396–397
Intestinal permeability, 22, 186, 441
  AIDS, 403
  Crohn's disease, 177–178, 629
  elemental diets on, 536–537
  laboratory tests, 332
  psoriasis, 17
  smoking, 50 (Table)
  spondylarthropathies, 457
Intestinal tubes, toxic megacolon, 568
Intractable Crohn's colitis, 849–850
Intractable enterocolitis of infancy, 666
Intractable ulcerative colitis, 731–732
Intraluminal pressures, ulcerative colitis, 194
Intraoperative enteroscopy, 281
Intrastomal hernias, 934
Intrathoracic sepsis, isotope scanning, 265
Intravenous antibiotic prophylaxis, 694–695
Intravenous urography, fistulae, 885
Invasion plasmid antigens, *Shigella* spp., 352
Inverted U pouches, 781
Iodine-125-labeled fibrinogen, imaging, 699
Iodine-based contrast studies, 215
IOIBD index (Oxford index), 338
I pouch, 197
Ipsalazide, 488
Iritis, *see* Uveitis
Iron
  chelation, 531
  deficiency (anemia)
    Crohn's colitis, 605
    Crohn's disease, 176, 594, 627
    laboratory markers, 331–332
    outpatient treatment, 552
  overload, yersiniosis, 415
  serum levels, 44
  total parenteral nutrition, 544
Irrigation, *see also* Lavage
  antibiotics, ileal pouch–anal anastomosis, 786
  whole bowel, 694
Irritable bowel syndrome
  biopsy results, 276
  excluding collagenous colitis, 370
  vs IBD, 332–333
  ileal pouch–anal anastomosis, 794
Irritants, mucus secretion, 150
IS*900* gene
  Crohn's disease, 129
  and IS*901* gene, mycobacteria, 127–128
Ischemia
  acute insults, 138–139
  Behçet's disease, 388
  vs Crohn's disease, 237, 241–242
  motility inducing, 195
  pelvic pouches, 793, 805
  stomas, 933
Ischemic bowel disease, *vs* Crohn's disease, 313, 602
Ischemic colitis, 421–424
  vs collagenous colitis, 371
  colonoscopy, 276
  vs ulcerative colitis, 305, 306
Ischiorectal fossa, computed tomography, 251
Isoniazid, 396
Isoperistaltic pelvic ileal reservoirs (H pouches), 781
Isospora belli, AIDS, 401
Isotope scanning, *see* Radionuclide scanning
Israel
  ethnic studies, 15
  family studies, 14
  incidence of IBD, 36, 37
Itraconazole, 382

Jackdaws, *Campylobacter* spp., 350
Japan
  Behçet's disease, 387
  Crohn's disease, upper gastrointestinal tract, 583
  diverticular disease, 445
Japanese, HLA antigens, 27
Japanese waltzing mice, ulcerative colitis models, 158
Jarisch-Herxheimer reaction, 404
Jaundice, AIDS, 400
Jejunoileitis
  cancer, 686
  diffuse, 597–599, 836
Jejunum
  aspiration for bacterial overgrowth, 176
  Crohn's disease, 477
    radiology, 235–236
Jews, 37, 118, *see also* Ashkenazi Jews
  Crohn's disease, 648
Johne's disease, 125–130, 157
J pouches, 780–781, 787, 796
  ileorectal anastomoses, 854–855
Junior doctors, 917, 945
Juvenile chronic arthritis, 456

Kallikreins, 114
Kaposi's sarcoma, 399, 400, 402–403
Kelly, M., *Colitis*, 923
Keratopathy, 626
Kernicterus, 578, 673
Ketone bodies, nutrition of colonic epithelium, 202
Ketotifen, 90
Kidneys
  amyloid, Crohn's disease, 606
  damage avoidance, 692
  disease and infection risk, 693
  drug toxicity
    cyclosporin, 518–519
    5-ASA, 490, 558
    mesalazine, 572
  stones, 595
    Crohn's disease, 606, 628
      children, 650–651
    ileal pouch–anal anastomosis, 795
    postoperative, 748
Killer cells, 55
Kinins, 109 (Table), 110 (Table), 114
Ki-*ras* mutations, 322
Klebsiella pneumoniae
  ankylosing spondylitis, 456
  cotton-top tamarins, 161
Klemperer, P., Crohn's disease, 7
Knockout mice, *see* Mice, knockout
Kocher clamp technique, Crohn's disease, 828
Kock's continent ileostomy, 5, 751–758
  benefits and risks 767 (Table)
  endoscopy of, 280
  function, 187–188
  revision rates, 756
  sex life improvement, 906
Koernig, colostomy bag, 4–5

Laboratory markers, 329–334, 550
  sepsis, enterocutaneous fistulae, 884
Lactic acid dehydrogenase isoenzymes, dysplasia, 320–321
Lactoferrin, 143, 331
Lactose absorption/malabsorption, 44
  Crohn's disease, 175
  ulcerative colitis, 553, 557
Lactulose, 557
  absorption, 22, 178
Lactulose/mannitol test, intestinal permeability, 178
Lamina propria, 53–54
  neutrophils, ulcerative colitis, 294
Langhans giant cells, 275
Laparoscopy, 717–723
  Crohn's disease surgery, 828–830
  gastrojejunostomy and vagotomy, 819
  tuberculous peritonitis, 393
Laparostomy, 695
  for enterocutaneous fistulae, 886
Laparotomy
  Crohn's disease, 707
  tuberculosis, 396
  ulcerative jejunoileitis, 432
Larynx, tuberculosis, 393
Lateral internal sphincterotomy, 898
Lateral isoperistaltic pelvic ileal reservoirs (H pouches), 781
Lavage, *see also* Irrigation
  tetracyclines, 694
Laxatives, electrolyte secretion, 183
Leaflets, 917, 919, 920–923
Lean body mass, 44
Learning curve, ileal pouch–anal anastomosis, 796–797
Lectin antigens, 146
Lectins
  dietary, mucin interactions, 147, 149, 151

Lectins (contd)
  Entamoeba histolytica, 356
  mucosal lymphocyte response, 55
Left-sided ulcerative colitis, cancer incidence, 323
Leishmaniasis, cytokines, 95
Leprosy, cytokines, 95
Leptospirosis, arthritis, 453
Leucine metabolism, whole-body, 44
Leukemia, colonic surgery, 685
Leukemia wards, *Clostridium difficile*, 355–356
Leukocytes, *see also* Indium-111-labeled leukocytes; Radolabeled leukocytes *and named types*
  counts, 331
  polymorphonuclear, pouchitis, 801
Leukopenia, azathioprine and 6-MP, 576
Leukotriene B4
  synthesis, 522
    dietary *n*-3 fatty acids, 42
  therapeutic target, 527–529
Leukotrienes, 109, 110 (Table), 111, 489
  colonic electrolyte secretion, 184
  cotton-top tamarin colitis, 161
  fish oils on, 576
  steroids on production, 504
Leukotriene synthesis genes, immunosuppressants on, 90
Levamisole, 523
L-forms, *see* Cell-wall defective bacteria
Life assurance, 949–951
Lignocaine (lidocaine)
  arachidonic acid release inhibition, 528
  ulcerative proctitis, 556
Linear array systems, rectal probes, 285
Linked genes, 29
Linoleic acid, 537
Lipid peroxidation, 112, 113
Lipocortin, 528
  steroids on production, 504
Lipopolysaccharides
  spondylarthropathies, 456
  Yersinia spp., 415
Lipoxygenase pathway inhibitors, 90, 111
Lipoxygenases, 109, 111
  inhibition, 489, *see also* 5-lipoxygenase inhibitors
Liver, *see also* Fatty liver; Liver disease
  abscesses, computed tomography, 251
  function tests
    AIDS, 400
    total parenteral nutrition, 543–544
    ulcerative colitis, children, 662
  metastases, lack in cotton-top tamarins, 162
  sulfasalazine on, 490
  toxicity
    cyclosporin, 519 (Table)
    methotrexate, 519, 576
  transplantation, 642–643, 793
Liver disease, 637–646
  cotton-top tamarins, 163
  Crohn's disease, children, 650
  ulcerative colitis, children, 662
Living with a colostomy (BCA), 920
Lloyd Davies position, 691, 718, 719
Local anesthetics, *see* Lignocaine
Lockhart-Mummery, J.P., 4
Lone Star retractor, 784
Long-chain fatty acids
  diarrhea, 185
  on oxalate absorption, 176
Long-term follow-up, Crohn's disease

  recurrence, 821–822
Loop–end ileostomies, construction, 925–926, 930–932, *see also* End-loop ileostomies
Loop ileostomies, construction, 925, 928–930
Loperamide
  ileal Crohn's disease, 591
  ileal pouch–anal anastomosis, 810
Loss of heterozygosity, 321–322
Low-affinity IgG receptors, macrophages, 83
Low-dose subcutaneous heparin, 698–699
Low-dose warfarin, 699
Lowland gorilla colitis, 159
Low-molecular-weight heparins, 699
L-selectin, 74–75
LTB$_4$, on eosinophils, 90
Lungs
  collagenous colitis, 369
  Crohn's disease, 626–628
  isotope scanning, 266–267, 627
  vasculitis, 139
Lymphangiectasia, 331
Lymphangiography, tuberculosis, 393
Lymph nodes
  cervical, orofacial granulomatosis, 633
  Crohn's disease surgery, 828
  Kaposi's sarcoma, 403
  ulcerative jejunoileitis, 432
Lymphocytes, 53–61, *see also* B cells; T cells
  azathioprine, 574
  epithelioid granulomata, 380
  non-specific function, 56–57
Lymphocytic colitis, 275–276, 307, 369, 373–375
Lymphocytic gastritis, 375
Lymphocytic plasmacytic colitis, dogs, 159
Lymphoid aggregates
  Crohn's disease, 312, 314
  fulminant colitis, 315
Lymphoid follicles, ulcerative colitis, 295
Lymphoid hyperplasia, 243, *see also* Benign lymphoid hyperplasia follicular, diversion colitis, 449
Lymphoid nodular hyperplasia, 652
Lymphomas
  AIDS, 399
  azathioprine and 6-MP, 516
  colorectal, 324
  computed tomography, 250
  vs Crohn's disease, 236
  cyclosporin, 519 (Table)
  Hodgkin's, with collagenous colitis, 369–370
  non-Hodgkin's, from azathioprine, 559
  surgery, 685
  T-cell, oral lesions, 633
  and ulcerative jejunoileitis, 432, 434
Lymphopenia, 53
Lyophosphatase, Charcot-Leyden crystals, 90
Lysosomal acid hydrolases, 82, 83
Lysozyme, 143

Macrophage inflammatory protein-1β, 96
Macrophage membrane transporter protein gene, salmonella protection, 352
Macrophages, 81–85
  activation, 82, 521–522
  downregulation in intestine, 83
  in granulomata, 379–380
  mast cell activation, 88
  Mycobacterium avium intracellulare, 402
  vascular damage by, 136

Magnesium
  absorption
    colon, 182
    Crohn's disease, 176
  deficiency, Crohn's disease, 594, 605–606
  serum levels, 44
Magnesium citrate, 825, 852
Magnesium oxalate agar, *Yersinia* spp., 414
Magnesium sulfate catharsis, 694
Magnetic resonance imaging, 249
  anorectal region, 715
  Crohn's disease, 257–259
    perianal, 616
    vs ulcerative colitis, 345
  sepsis and fistulae, 885
Magpies, *Campylobacter* spp., 350
Mailing list, ulcerative colitis follow-up, 957
Maintenance therapy
  Crohn's disease, 606–607
    ileal, 592
    topical, 496–497
    trials, 494–496
  cyclosporin, 518
  ulcerative colitis, 571–580
    trials, 492–493
Major histocompatibility antigens, *see* Histocompatibility antigens
Malabsorption, 44, *see also* Lactose absorption/malabsorption
  Crohn's disease, 173–177, 594
  HIV enteropathy, 402
  ileal pouch–anal anastomosis, 795
  radiotherapy, 426
  ulcerative jejunoileitis, 432
Malakoplakia, 383
Malaria, reverse genetics, 28
Malnutrition, 43–45, 537, 541
  Crohn's disease, 608, 825
    colitis surgery, 852
  enterocutaneous fistulae, 883, 884, 886
  growth retardation, 732
  infection, 693
  ulcerative colitis, 551–552
  ulcerative jejunoileitis, 434
Mannitol absorption, 22, *see also* Lactulose/mannitol test
Manometry, anal, 715, 899
Manufacturers, publications, 922–923
Marginated granulocyte pool, 262
Marker studies, genetic, 18–22
Marmosets, 160
Married couples, spouse studies, 15, 117–118
Masses, *see also* Dysplasia-associated lesion or mass (DALM); Ileocecal masses
  toxic, resection, 657
Mast cell mediators, 88
Mast cells, 87–90
  collagenous colitis, 372
  and prostaglandin secretion, 184
Mayo-Robson, A.W., Crohn's disease, 7
MCC/APC gene, 321–322
MCP-1 (chemokine), 96
  localization, 97
Measles virus, 120, 141, 521
Mechanical bowel preparation, *see* Bowel preparation
Medical bypass, 536
Medical ethics, 772–773
Medical management
  fulminant colitis protocol, 569 (Table)
  ulcerative colitis, 549–564
Medical practitioners, team role, 705

Medical records, 955
Meetings, weekly, 704
Megacolon, see Toxic megacolon
Membrane-associated NADPH-oxidase system, 380
Membrane-bound epithelial mucin (MUC1), 144
Membrane-bound polymorphic epithelial mucin (PEM), 144
Membrane b-type cytochrome, Crohn's disease, 16
Membrane pumps, colonic epithelium, 182
Menopause, 945
Mersilene mesh, Kock's pouch, 753
Mesalazine, 558, 571 (Table)
　absorption, 205
　on butyrate oxidation, 204
　Crohn's disease
　　children, 654
　　trials, 607
　pregnancy, 578
　renal toxicity, 572
　ulcerative colitis, children, 663
Mesasal, see Claversal
Mesenteric lymph nodes
　Crohn's disease, 311
　yersiniosis, 314
Mesentery
　computed tomography, 250
　Crohn's disease surgery, 828, 853
Mesh, see Prosthetic mesh
Metallothionein, 112
Metaplasia, mucin sulfation, 147
Metastases, liver, lack in cotton-top tamarins, 162
Metastatic Crohn's disease, 7, 626
Metasulfobenzoate, prednisolone enemas, 508, 560
Methotrexate, 519
　Crohn's disease, 608
　vs ulcerative colitis, 523
　fulminant colitis, 568
　on IL-1, 523
　on mast cells, 90
　ulcerative colitis, 560
　　maintenance therapy, 576
Methylene blue, endoscopy, 282
Methylprednisolone, 505
　Crohn's disease, 508–509
　European Cooperative Crohn's Disease Study, 606
　fulminant colitis, 567
　pulse therapy, 506
Metronidazole, 8, 121, 694
　amebiasis, 357, 411
　children, 655 (Table), 656
　Crohn's colitis
　　response failure, 850
　　surgery, 852
　Crohn's disease, 607
　　vs sulfasalazine 494
　　surgery, 825
　　fulminant colitis, 568
　　perianal fistulae, 618
　　pouchitis, 803, 805
　　pregnancy, 672
　　pseudomembranous colitis, 356
Mice
　knockout, 66–67, 158
　　cytokine studies, 96
　　IL-2 gene disruption, 66, 526
　　infective agent experiments, 121
　ulcerative colitis models, 158

Michaelis-Gutmann bodies, 383
Microagglutination assay, Yersinia spp., 414
Microbiologists, 706
Microcytic anemia, Crohn's colitis, 605
Microgranulomata, 83, 312
Microinfarction, 697
Micronutrients, total parenteral nutrition, 544
Microperforations, fulminant colitis, 566
Microscopic colitis, 186–187, 275–276, 307, 369, 373–375
　children, 666
Microspheres
　Pentasa, 488
　vascular experiments, 138–139, 170
Microsporidiosis, AIDS, 401, 402
Microsurgery, transanal endoscopic, 717
Microvascular thromboses, 101, 133
Midline incisions, 691
Migrating motor complexes, ileoanal reservoirs, 197
Miliary nodules, 393
Milk
　Campylobacter spp., 350
　Crohn's disease
　　etiology, 41
　　worsening, 175
Milk-free diets, ulcerative colitis, 553
Mineralocorticoids
　colonic electrolyte absorption, 184
　effects, 503
Minimal-access surgery, see Laparoscopy
Minimal change colitis, 373
Minimal excision, 8
Miniresections, 692
Minnesota University, ileal pouch–anal anastomosis results, 795–797
Misoprostol, 530
Mitogen-induced cytotoxicity (MICC), 55
Mitogen-induced proliferation, lymphocytes, 56
Mitogens, on epithelium, 205
Mixed lymphocyte reaction, 57
Molecular genetics, 27–33
Molecular mimicry hypothesis, spondylarthropathies, 457
Monobactams, 694
Monoclonal antibodies
　CD4 antigens, 526, 560
　mast cell investigation, 89
　studies of CD11/CD18 integrins, 75
　therapy, 519
　tumor necrosis factor, 525, 560
Monocyte chemotactic and activating factor (MCAF), 81
Monocyte procoagulant activity, 103
Monocytes, granulomata, 380
Monokines, 96
Mononuclear cells, 54, 55–56, 65, 66, 81–85
　CD11/CD18 integrins, 75
　ICAM-1 expression, 76
Monosaccharide absorption, Crohn's disease, 174–175
Moon face, 503
　CIR budesonide, 509
Morale, 705
Mortality, 35
　carcinoma, 677
　Crohn's disease, 475, 610
　　children, 660
　diarrhea, developing countries, 349
　diffuse jejunoileitis, 599
　ileal pouch–anal anastomosis, 761–762, 791
　laparoscopic surgery, 720

and life assurance, 950
　proctocolectomy, Crohn's disease, 603
　total parenteral nutrition, 543
　ulcerative colitis, 463, 464, 472, 507, 665
Motility
　and absorption, colon, 185
　disturbances, 191–200
　　ulcerative colitis, 191–197, 556–557
Motor insurance, 949
Mount Sinai Hospital, Crohn's disease, 6
Mouth, see Oral lesions
Mouth-to-cecum transit
　Crohn's disease, 198
　ulcerative colitis, 192
Moxon, W., on ulcerative colitis, 3
Moynihan, B.J.A., Crohn's disease, 7
Mucin-associated protease inhibitor, 143
Mucin core-protein genes, 144–145
Mucinous carcinoma, cotton-top tamarins, 162
Mucins, 143–145, 521
　colitis in cotton-top tamarins, 161
　depletion, ulcerative colitis, 295–297
　dysplasia, 320
　genetics, 22
　pouchitis, 801
　synthesis, 148–149
　twin studies, 207
Mucin secretagogue, from macrophages, 83
Mucin sulfatases, fecal, 151
Mucosa, see also Epithelium
　colon, endoscopic appearance, 273
　defenses, 143–155
　echoendoscopy, 287
　lymphocytes, 53–55
　metabolism, 201–211
　pH, ischemic colitis, 422
　pouches, colonic metaplasia, 805
Mucosal atrophy, diffuse, 305
Mucosal B lymphocytes, 64–65
Mucosal islands, see Pseudopolyps
Mucosal proctectomy with ileoanal anastomosis, 197
Mucosal resection, rectal cuff, 784
Mucosal T-cell receptors, 31
Mucosectomy, transanal, 783–784
　cancer risk, 811
　on sphincter function, 810, 898
Mucus
　enzymatic breakdown, 150–151
　secretion, 149–150
　smoking, 50 (Table)
Mucus fistulae, subtotal colectomy, 856
Mucus secretagogues, 150
Multiparous women, and ileal pouch–anal anastomosis, 771
Multiple adhesion molecules, 81
Multiple biopsies, 306
Multiple regression analysis, activity index, 336
Multiple sclerosis, 18
Murder trial of T. Smethurst, 3
Muscarinic receptors, on mucus secretion, 150
Muscle flaps
　for fecal incontinence, 900
　perineal reconstruction, 858, 894
　vaginal restoration, 906
Muscle injury, incontinence, 868
Muscle mass, 44
Muscularis mucosae, quiescent ulcerative colitis, 298
Muscularis propria, echoendoscopy, 287

Myasthenia gravis, 18
Mycobacteria, 125–131, see also Tuberculosis
  antibodies vs, 69
  antigens, 56
  atypical, 521
  vasculitis, 141
Mycobacterial stress protein, oral Crohn's disease, 635
Mycobacterium avium, 126
  AIDS, 391
Mycobacterium avium intracellulare, AIDS, 401–402
Mycobacterium bovis strain BCG, 128, 523
Mycobacterium 'linda', 157
Mycobacterium paratuberculosis, 125–130, 157
  experimental animals, 167
Mycoplasma spp., 119
Myectomy, ileoanal anastomoses, 782
Myeoperoxidase-derived oxidants, 78
Myelotoxicity, azathioprine and 6-MP, 516, 559, 574, 576
Myocytolysis, toxic megacolon, 301
Myoelectrical studies
  colonic contractility, 196–197
  electromyography, 715, 899
  rectosigmoid contractility, 194

N-acetyl-5-aminosalicylic acid, 488, 497
N-acetyl-β-glucosaminidase, 82
  dysplasia, 321
NADPH oxidase, 380, 382
Nailbed capilloscopy, 140
National Advisory Service for Parents of Children with a Stoma, 921
National Association for Colitis and Crohn's Disease, 921
  insurance survey, 949
National Cooperative Crohn's Disease Study, 493, 606–607
  perianal Crohn's disease, 615
  steroids, 508
  sulfasalazine maintenance therapy trial, 494–495
  surgery requirement, 822
Natural killer cells, 55
  azathioprine, 574
Nausea
  AIDS, 400
  azathioprine and 6-MP, 516
  cyclosporin, 519 (Table)
N-chloramines, 78
Necrosis, stomas, 933
Nematodes, intestinal permeability, 178
Neonates
  Behçet's disease, 665
  virus infections, 120
Neoplasia, see also Carcinoma; Leukemia; Lymphomas
  vs dysplasia, 317
Neopterin, 331
Neorectum, see also Ileal pouch–anal anastomosis
  colon as, 782
Nephrotoxicity, see Kidneys, drug toxicity
Nervi erigentes, preserving, 692
Neuroanatomic arc, 897
Neuropeptides, 184
  on mast cells, 88
Neurotensin, mucus secretion, 150
Neurotoxic products, eosinophils, 91
Neutrophil elastase, 331

Neutrophils
  Crohn's disease, 16, 305, 315
  infectious colitis, 304
  lamina propria, ulcerative colitis, 294
  pathogenesis, 73–80, 522
N-formyl-methionyl-leucyl-phenylalanine (FMLP), on interstitium, 76
Nicotinamide-adenine-dinucleotide phosphate oxidase, 78
Nicotine, 47, 48
  colonic mucin synthesis, 149
  therapy, 531, 560
Night, see headings beginning Nocturnal . . .
Night sweats, fulminant colitis, 565
Nipple valve, 751, 753
  fixation technique, 756
Nippostrongylus brasiliensis, experimental infection, 168
Nitric oxide, 109 (Table), 110 (Table), 113–114, 136–137
  granulomata, 380
  and oxidants, 78
  therapeutic target, 530–531
Nitric oxide synthase, 113–114
  induction, Rhesus macaques, 159–160
Nitrites, on butyrate oxidation, 204
Nitroblue tetrazolium microscope test, 382
Nitroblue tetrazolium test, 652
Nitrogen absorption, Crohn's disease, 175
Nitrogen balance, 44
Nitrogen dioxide, 79
Nitrogen oxides, 78–79
Nitroimidazoles, amebiasis, 411
Nitro-L-arginine-methyl ester, 114
Nitrosamines, from nitric oxide, 113
Nocadazole, on mucus secretion, 149
Nocturnal defecation, ulcerative colitis, 191
Nocturnal evacuation frequency, anticholinergic drugs for, 776
Nocturnal feeding, 44
Nocturnal incontinence, ileal pouch–anal anastomosis, 785
Nocturnal penile tumescence test, 905
Nodular lesions, colon carcinoma, 324
Non-dysenteric intestinal amebiasis, 409
Non-Hodgkin's lymphoma, from azathioprine, 559
Non-ionic diffusion, short-chain fatty acids in colon, 183
Non-relapsing colitis, see Infectious-type colitis
Non-specific esterase, macrophages, 82
Non-specific ulcerative colitis, 360
Non-steroidal anti-inflammatory drugs, 110, 557
  vs ankylosing spondylitis, 454
  for Behçet's disease, 388–389
  on butyrate oxidation, 204
  colitis, 226, 276, 315
    experimental, 169
  collagenous colitis, 372
  endoscopy, 270
  enteritis, 437–442
  provoking ulcerative colitis, 489
  terminal ileum, 236
  for ulcerative colitis, 530
Normal flora, see Bowel flora
Nosocomial infection, *Clostridium difficile*, 355–356
Nucleotides, small intestinal nutrition, 202
Nurse specialists, 703
  counseling, 917–918, 919
  nutritional support, 705
  stoma care, 705, 913

Nursing care, stomas, 705, 912
Nursing staff, 705
Nutrition, mucosal, 201–204
Nutritional deficiencies, see Malnutrition
Nutritional support nurses, 705
Nutritional therapy, see also Diets
  Crohn's disease, 608–609
    children, 654
  enterocutaneous fistulae, 886
  ulcerative colitis, children, 664

O-acetylation loss, sialomucin, 147
O-acetyl sialic acid dysplasia, 320
O-acyl esterases, 151
Obesity
  ileal pouch–anal anastomosis, 761, 772
  infection, 693
  surgery, 746
Obliterative cholangitis, 642
Obstetrics, see Childbirth; Parity
Obstructive uropathy, see Ureteric obstruction
Obturator foramen, enterocutaneous fistulae, 882
Occupation, see also Employment; Working capacity
  choice of surgery, 746
  ileal pouch–anal anastomosis, 812
Octreotide, for enterocutaneous fistula management, 888
Ocular lesions, see Eye lesions
Odynophagia, 399
Oedema, see Edema
Oesophagus, see Esophagus
Ofloxacin, gonorrhea, 404
O-glycosylation, mucins, 148
Oleic acid, vs 10-OH stearic acid, 187
Oligopeptide-based diets, 536
Oligosaccharides, mucins, 143, 145, 148
Olsalazine, 488, 571 (Table)
  diarrhea, 490, 558, 572
  maintenance therapy, 577
    dosage, 572
  pregnancy, 578
  topical, 496
  trials, 491, 492, 493, 553
Olympus echoendoscope, 285
ω-3 fatty acids, 576
Omental buttress, fistula surgery, 819–820
Omeprazole, 434
  Crohn's disease
    esophagus, 585
    gastroduodenal, 476, 586–587
Oncosuppressor genes, 321–322
Ophthalmic lesions, see Eye lesions
Opiates, on colon, 194
Oppenheimer, G.D., Crohn's disease, 6–7
Optical systems, minimal-access surgery, 722
Optimistic analogies, 918
Oral contraceptives, 38, 50–51, 671
  colitis, 315
    ischemic, 423
  Crohn's disease and smoking, 480
Oral lesions, 633–636
  Behçet's disease, 388, 389
  Crohn's disease, 7, 584, 602, 625, 633
    children, 650, 656
    vs ulcerative colitis, 344
  Kaposi's sarcoma, 400
  ulcerative colitis, 557
Oral pneumocolon, 219
Oralyte WHO, 776
Ornithine, small intestinal nutrition, 202

Orocecal transit time, *see* Mouth-to-cecum transit
Orofacial granulomatosis, 633
Orosomucoid-α_1-acid glycoprotein, 330–331
Orosomucoids
 Crohn's disease recurrence, 478
 follow-up, 956
O-serogroups, *E. coli*, 353
Osmotic agents, bowel preparation, 694
Osmotic gap, Crohn's colitis, 174
Osteomalacia, 44, 625
 Crohn's disease, 606
Osteoporosis, 558–559, 625
 Crohn's disease, 606
 primary sclerosing cholangitis, 642
 steroids, 503
Ostomy book (Mullen and McGinn), 921
Ouabain, chloride secretion, 183
Our present your future? (video), 921
Our special children (NASPCS), 921
Outer membrane proteins, *Yersinia* spp., 415
Outflow tract problems, Kock's pouch, 755
Outlet view, pelvis, 262
Outpatient management
 consultations, 703
 follow-up 955–956
 ulcerative colitis, 551–561
Oxalate absorption
 Crohn's disease, 175–176
 enteric hyperoxaluria, 188
Oxalate stones, 188
 Crohn's disease, 606, 628
 children, 650–651
Oxford index, *see* IOIBD index
Oxidants, 109 (Table), 110 (Table), 112–113
 on endothelium, 74
 macrophages, 82
 from neutrophils, 77, 78
Oxidases, granulomata, 380
Oxine (labeling complex), 261
Oxygen burst, granulomata, 380, 382
Oxygen free radicals, 489
 ischemic colitis, 421
 therapeutic target, 531

p53 gene, 321–322
Pain, *see also* Pseudoappendicitis
 AIDS, 399
 Crohn's disease, 649
  gastroduodenal, 817
  vs ulcerative colitis, 343
 enterocutaneous fistulae, 881
 ischemic colitis, 423
 ulcerative colitis, children, 661
Palliative surgery, colorectal carcinoma, 685
p-aminobenzoic acid, benzalazine, 488
Pamphlets, 917, 919, 920–923
Pancolectomy, *see also* Proctocolectomy
 Crohn's disease, 609
  colitis, 856–858
  staged procedure, 904
Pancolitis
 cancer risk 470, 680
 colectomy, 471
 Crohn's disease, 602
 mortality, 472
 ulcerative colitis, 468
Pancreatic secretion
 autoantibodies *vs*, 69
 Crohn's disease, 175
Pancreatitis
 azathioprine and 6-MP, 516, 575

Crohn's disease, 478, 595, 629
 5-ASA, 572
Paneth cells
 metaplasia, 361
 quiescent ulcerative colitis, 298
Para-aminosalicylic acid (4-ASA), 489, 497–498, 572–573
Paracetamol
 mucosal injury, 205
 ulcerative colitis relapse, 530
Paramedian incisions, 691
Paramyxoviruses, 120
Pararectal incisions, 691
Parasites, experimental infection, 168
Parastomal hernias, 934–936
Parasympathetic supply, sexual function, 904
Paresthesia, cyclosporin, 519 (Table)
Parity (obstetric)
 Crohn's disease, 673
 ileal pouch–anal anastomosis, 771
Paramomycin, amebiasis, 411
PAS (4-ASA), 489, 497–498, 572–573
Passive smoking, 49
 Crohn's disease, 648
 recurrence, 479
Patchy distribution, collagenous colitis, 371
Pathology, performance, 961
Patient position, surgery, 691–692
Patients
 grouping, 955
 satisfaction, 961
Patient's Charter, 919
Peanut agglutinin reactivity, dysplasia, 320
Peanut lectin
 cotton-top tamarin colitis, 161
 TF antigens, 146
Pediatric gastroscopes, pouch endoscopy, 280
Pelvic plexus, 904
Pelvic pouches
 Crohn's disease in, 834–835
 endoscopy of, 280
Pelvis
 computed tomography, 251–252
 dead space filling, 857
 magnetic resonance imaging, 257
 outlet view, 262
Penicillin
 resistance of *Yersinia enterocolitica*, 417
 sexually transmitted diseases, 404
Pentasa, 488, 571 (Table)
 Crohn's disease
  ileal, 591
  trials, 493, 494
   maintenance therapy, 495
  enemas, absorption from, 573
  maintenance therapy, 577
  dosage, 572
  steroid sparing, 494
 ulcerative colitis, trials, 492
Pentax FG-32UA echoendoscope, 285
Peptic ulcer
 vs Crohn's disease, 235, 587
 and resections, 595
Peptide-based diets, 536
Peptide factors, *see* Cytokines
Peptidergic nerves, and mast cells, 89
Peptides, HLA antigen binding, 30
Peptidoglycan-polysaccharide complex,
 animal experiments, 167–168
Percutaneous drainage, abscesses, 251, 875–879
Percutaneous feeding tube placement, 272
Perforating Crohn's disease, 479, 833, 883

Perforation
 colonoscopy, 273, 961
 colostomies, 937
 Crohn's colitis, 851
 diverticular disease, 444
 fulminant colitis, 566, 568
  steroids, 565
 radiotherapy, 426, 427
 toxic megacolon, 662–663
 tuberculosis, 397
 ulcerative colitis, 301, 725
Perfusion-fixation, vascular studies, 133
Perianal region
 Crohn's disease, 615–620, 861–872
  anal function, 714
  cancer, 679–680
  children, 649, 650
  endoluminal ultrasound, 288–290
  rectovaginal fistulae, 871–872
  surgery, techniques, 711–712
  vs ulcerative colitis, 343, 346
 dyspareunia management, 903
 fistulae
  Crohn's colitis, 605
  Crohn's disease, 478
  magnetic resonance imaging, 257
 skin irritation, ileal pouch–anal anastomosis, 812
 ulcerative colitis, children, 661
Pericarditis, 627
 5-ASA, 572
Pericholangitis (small-duct PSC), 637 (Table), 643
Perinatal virus infection, 120
Perineal Crohn's disease, endoluminal ultrasound, 289
Perineorrhaphy, 866
Perineum
 destruction by Crohn's disease, 868
 sensation, 713
 wound complications, 747–748, 762, 857–858, 868–870, 872
 management, 893–895
Perinuclear antineutrophil cytoplasmic antibodies (pANCA), 22, 68–69, 70
 primary sclerosing cholangitis, 640
Periodontal infection, *Wolinella* spp., Crohn's disease, 77–78
Periostosis, 625
Peripheral arthritis, 452–453
Peripheral blood lymphocytes, 53
Peripheral parenteral nutrition, enterocutaneous fistulae, 886
Periprostatic plexus, 904
 transrectal electrostimulation, 905
Perirectal abscesses, computed tomography, 251
Peristomal cancer, 686
Peristomal fistulae, 882, 886, 936
Peristomal varices, 642, 793, 936
Peritoneum
 amebic colitis, 410
 antibiotic lavage, 695
 surgical access, 707
 toxic megacolon, 662–663
 tuberculosis, 391
Peroxynitrite, 78
 on rats, 113
Peyer's patches, macrophages, 82
pH
 enemas, 488, 573
 mucosa, ischemic colitis, 422
 profiles, gastrointestinal tract, 488

Phagocytic labeling, 267
Pharmaceutical companies, publications, 921–922
Pharmacia, publications, 921
Pharmacists, 705
Pharmacokinetics
 cyclosporin, 517
 prednisolone, 504
Pharynx, Crohn's disease, 7
pH-dependent aminosalicylates, 487–488, 572
Phenol extraction, PCR, 128
Phenols, mucosal injury, 205
Phenylpropanolamine, for retrograde ejaculation, 905
Phlegmons, 875
Phorbol esters, 150
 colonic secretory mechanisms, 184–185
Physical signs, fulminant colitis, 567
Picket fence appearance, 237
Picolax, 694
Picotamide, 111
 on thromboxanes, 529
Pigs
 Crohn's disease models, 157–158
 ulcerative colitis models, 159
Pinch biopsies, cytokine studies, 96
Pinching technique, 692, 708
Pk antigen, 354
Placebo effect, Crohn's disease, 476
Plain films
 fulminant colitis, 565–566
 ulcerative colitis, 223–224, 550
Plaque-like lesions, colon carcinoma, 324
Plasma cells, azathioprine, 574
Plasmacytosis, basal, 304, 360–361
Plasmids
 Shigella spp., 352
 Yersinia spp., 415
Plasmin, on epithelia, 206
Plasminogen activator inhibitor, 103
Platelet-activating factor, 90, 109 (Table), 110 (Table), 111, 522, 527
 antagonists, 90, 529–530
 intestinal permeability, 178
 mast cells, 88
 steroids on production, 504
Platelet counts, 331
 Crohn's disease, 627
 colitis, 603
 radiation bowel disease, 427
Platelets, 104, 697, 698
Pneumatic compression boots, 698
Pneumonitis, methotrexate, 576
Polyacrylates, ulcerative colitis, 151
Polyamine levels, cancer risk, 743
Polyarteritis nodosa, 140
Polyethylene glycols, intestinal permeability, 178, 181
Polyethylene glycol solution, 747, 825
Polylactosamine structures, blood group antigens, 146
Polymerase chain reaction
 mycobacteria studies, 126–128
 tuberculosis, 392
Polymeric diets, 536, 657
 Crohn's disease, 609
 fats, 537
Polymorphic epithelial mucin, membrane-bound (PEM), 144
Polymorphonuclear leukocytes, pouchitis, 801
Polypectomy, endoscopy, 271
Polyps, *see also* Adenomatous polyps; Postinflammatory polyps;

Pseudopolyps
 colonoscopy, 282
 ulcerative colitis, radiology, 223
Population studies, cancer incidence, 323, 325
Pore size, colonic epithelium, 181, 186
Portal hypertension
 colitic changes, 276
 cross-sectional imaging, 259
 stomal bleeding, 936
Portal vein, infection theory, 639
Position of patient, surgery, 691–692
'Postage stamp' maneuver, 708
Postenteric arthritis, 453
Postinfectious colitis, 366–367
Postinflammatory polyps, radiology
 Crohn's disease, 235, 239
 ulcerative colitis, 223, 225 (Fig.)
Postoperative abscess, 878
Postoperative care, stomas, 932
Postoperative enterocutaneous fistulae, 881–882
Postoperative infection, 693
Postoperative recurrence, Crohn's disease, 480
Potassium
 deficiency, Crohn's disease, 594, 605
 loss
  Crohn's disease, 174 (Table)
  IBD, 186
 serum levels, 44
 transport, aldosterone, 184
Potential difference, colonic transepithelial, 181, 186
Potomac horse fever, 159
Pouches, 5, 197, *see also* Continent ileostomies; Pelvic pouches
 computed tomography, 257
 epithelium, 204
  mucin sulfation, 147
 evacuation, 803
 failure, ileal pouch–anal anastomosis, 797
 function, 187–188, 763
 volume, 810
Pouchitis, 197, 743, 749, 801–806
 allopurinol, 113
 ANCA, 69
 endoscopy, 280, 801
 glutamine enemas, 204
 ileal pouch–anal anastomosis, 765, 776, 793, 797, 835
 incidence, 569
 Kock's pouch, 754
 vs pelvic pouch, 756
 mast cells, 89
 RFD9-positive macrophages, 83
 smoking, 48, 803, 806
 surgery, 834
Poultry, *Salmonella* spp., 351
Powell-Truck activity index, 336, 550
Prednisolone, 504
 vs Asacol, ulcerative colitis, 493
 biliary lavage, 642
 children, 663
 Crohn's disease
  absorption, 607
  children, 655
  ileocecal masses, 592
  diffuse jejunoileitis, 598
  with immunosuppressants, Crohn's disease, 513–514
  metasulfobenzoate enemas, 508, 560
  toxic megacolon, children, 664
  ulcerative colitis, 506, 507

Prednisone, 504
 Crohn's disease, 508
  esophagus, 584
  response failure in colitis, 850
  trials, 606
Predsol, children, 655 (Table)
Pregnancy, 672–673, 943–844, *see also* Parity
 azathioprine, 559, 578
 and 6-MP, 516–517
 Crohn's disease, 481
 ileal pouch–anal anastomosis, 672, 766, 813
 ulcerative colitis, maintenance therapy, 577–578
Premature birth, Crohn's disease, 481
Preoperative period
 colonoscopy, 273, 280
 stoma construction, 926
 total parenteral nutrition, 542–543
Prepro-von Willebrand factor, sequence similar to mucins, 144
Presacral nerve, 904
Presacral space, ulcerative colitis, computed tomography, 256–257
Pressure gradient, ileal pouch–anal anastomosis, 794
Primary biliary cirrhosis, 18, 637 (Table), 644
Primary sclerosing cholangitis, 18, 637, 638–643
 cancer risk, 676
 Crohn's disease *vs* ulcerative colitis, 344
 cross-sectional imaging, 259
 HLA class II molecules, 28
 HLA haplotypes, 18, 346, 639–640
 ileal pouch–anal anastomosis, 760, 793
 model in cotton-top tamarins, 163
 peristomal varices, 642, 793, 936
 ulcerative colitis, 638, 733
Primates, ulcerative colitis models, 159–163
Primer sequences, mycobacterial DNA, 127
Priming, macrophages, 82
Proctectomy
 Crohn's disease, 609
  after colitis surgery, 856
  pancolectomy for colitis, 857
  after ileorectal anastomoses, 740, 742, 749
 ulcerative colitis, 736
 wound problems, 893
Proctitis
 gonococcal, 403–404, 550
 herpes simplex virus, 404–405
 idiopathic, 295, 549
 incontinence, 898
 and perianal disease, 713
 syphilitic, 404
 ulcerative colitis
  cancer risk, 680
  management, 555–557
  progression, 467
Proctocolectomy, 683–685, 745–750, *see also* Pancolectomy
 benefits and risks, 767 (Table)
 fulminant colitis, 728
 laparoscopic, 720
 mortality, Crohn's disease, 603
 for rectovaginal fistulae, 872
Proctoscopy, 344, 467, 851
Progression, ulcerative colitis, 467–469
Progressive systemic sclerosis, *vs* collagenous colitis, 371
Prolapse
 Kock's pouch valve, 755
 stomas, 933–934

Proliferative hemorrhagic enteropathy, pigs, 158
Proliferative zone, epithelium, 205
Proline, mucins, 148
Promotion prospects, effect of IBD, 942
Prone position, toxic megacolon, 569
Prophylaxis
　cancer, Crohn's colitis, 850
　surgical infections, 694–695
　thromboembolism, 698–699
Propranolol, on colonic secretion, 187
Prostacyclin, detection, 109
Prostaglandin analogues, 110
Prostaglandin E_1, penis injection, 905
Prostaglandins, 109–110, 114
　aminosalicylates on production, 489
　colonic electrolyte secretion, 184
　cotton-top tamarin colitis, 161
　electrolyte secretion, 183
　steroids on production, 504
　therapeutic target, 530
Prosthesis, primary sclerosing cholangitis, 642
Prosthetic anal encirclement, 900
Prosthetic mesh
　Kock's pouch, 753
　parastomal hernia repair, 935–936
Protease inhibitor, mucin-associated, 143
Proteases, see also Cell surface proteases
　mucus breakdown, 150
Proteinase/antiproteinase balance, oxidants on, 79
Proteinases, mast cells, 88 (Table)
Protein C activity, 103
Protein kinase C cascade, colonic secretory mechanisms, 184
Protein-losing enteropathy
　α_1-antitrypsin, 331
　laboratory tests, 332
Proteins
　deficiency, 44
　loss, 175
　　and calcium balance, 176
　　elemental diets on, 537
Protein S deficiency, 697
　Crohn's disease, 627
Proteoglycans, mast cells, 88
Prothrombin fragments, 102
Protocols
　local, 704
　medical investigation, 961
Proton pump inhibitors, for enterocutaneous fistula management, 888
Proximal constipation, ulcerative colitis, 556–557
Pruritus, 642
P-selectin, 74–75, 136
Pseudoappendicitis
　Crohn's disease, 590, 649
　salmonellosis, 351
　yersiniosis, 355, 416
Pseudoincontinence, 898
Pseudomembranes, 356, 363
　Crohn's disease, 313
　ischemic/radiation colitis, 276
Pseudomembranous colitis, see also Antibiotic-associated colitis
　cotton-top tamarins, 161
　vs Crohn's disease, 243
　histology, 304, 305
Pseudo-obstruction, small intestine, ulcerative colitis, 192
Pseudopolyps, 299–300
　colonoscopy, 282, 736

Crohn's disease vs ulcerative colitis, 344, 601
　Habershon on, 4
　radiology, 223
　toxic megacolon, 303–304
　ulcerative colitis, radiology, 223
Pseudosacculation, 239
Psoas muscle, fistula tracking, 882
Psoriasis, 17
　Crohn's disease, 478
Psoriatic arthritis, 455–456
Psychiatric illness, 941
　Crohn's disease, children, 651
　diffuse jejunoileitis, 599
Psychological effects, 941–944
　Crohn's disease, 481, 610
　sexual dysfunction, 904–905
Psychosis, steroids, 567
Psychotherapy, 4
Psyllium seeds, 775, 810
Publications, 920–923
Puborectalis muscle, 897
Pudendal nerve
　function, 713
　　latency, 715
　injury, 868
　terminal motor latency, 899
Puerto Rico, Hermansky–Pudlak syndrome, 16
Pull through examination, 244
Pulmonary disease, Crohn's disease, 626–627
Pulmonary embolism, Crohn's disease, 628
Pulmonary fibrosis, with collagenous colitis, 369
Pulmonary vasculitis, 139
Pulse therapy, methylprednisolone, 506
Push-type enteroscopes, 270
Pyoderma gangrenosum, 139, 344, 626, 733–734
　children
　　Crohn's disease, 650
　　ulcerative colitis, 662
　peristomal, 937
Pyostomatitis vegetans, 634–635
Pyrazinamide, 396
Pyrexia
　Crohn's disease, children, 650
　fulminant colitis, 565
Pyridoxine, with isoniazid, 396

Quadruplicated pelvic ileal reservoirs, 781–782
Quails, Crohn's disease models, 158
Quality activities, 959–962
Quality assurance, 959–960
Quality of life
　Crohn's disease, 481, 610
　　children, 660
　measurement, 339–340
　stomas, 943, 961
　surgery, 749, 943
　　operations compared, 773–774
　　reservoir surgery, 756–757, 766–767
Quiescent ulcerative colitis, histology, 298
Quinolones, 694
　traveler's diarrhea, 352
Qulcc index, 340

Rabbit-pellet stool, 443
Rachmilewitz, D., endoscopic index, 339, 550
Radiation bowel disease, 425–429

　colonoscopy, 276
Radiation doses
　CT vs enteroclysis, 255
　radionuclide scanning, 266
Radiolabeled leukocytes, 261–267, 550, see also Indium-111-labeled leukocytes
　Crohn's disease
　　colitis, 604
　　gastroduodenal, 586
　　vs ulcerative colitis, 345
　ileocecal masses, 590
　lungs, 627
　sepsis, 885
Radiologists, 704
Radiology, 215–268, see also Plain films
　Crohn's disease vs ulcerative colitis, 224–226, 344–345
　vs endoscopy, gastroduodenal Crohn's disease, 585–586
　enterocutaneous fistulae, 884–885
　follow-up, 243–244, 956
　fulminant colitis, 565–566
　spondylarthropathies, 451
Radionuclide scanning, 261–268, see also Radiolabeled leukocytes
　abscesses, 263, 590
　deep vein thrombosis, 699
　extraintestinal manifestations of IBD, 266–267
　leukocyte migration to lungs, 627
　pouchitis, 803
Radionuclide studies
　leukocyte excretion, 332, 441, 604
　mucus breakdown, 151
Radiotherapy, 425, see also Radiation bowel disease
　and ileal pouch–anal anastomosis, 761
'Ramshorn' deformity, 234–235
Ranitidine, Crohn's disease, esophagus, 585
RANTES peptide, 81, 96
Rapid mucus secretion, 149
Rats
　HLA B27 transgenic, infective agent experiments, 121
　peroxynitrite on, 113
Rb gene, 321–322
Reactive arthritis, 453, 457–458
　with collagenous colitis, 369
　Crohn's disease, 478
　yersiniosis, 416
Reactive oxygen metabolites, see Oxidants
Recall bias, 47
Recessive gene, Crohn's disease, 16
Recombinant erythropoietin therapy, 605
Recombination-activating gene (RAG-1), deficient mice, 67
Records, medical, 955
Recovery, labeled granulocytes, 262
Rectal bleeding
　Crohn's disease vs ulcerative colitis, 343
　radiation bowel disease, 426
　ulcerative colitis, children, 661
Rectal cuff, mucosal resection, 784
Rectal inhibitory reflex, 763
Rectal mucosal grafts, H pouches, 781
Rectosigmoid contractility, ulcerative colitis, 194
Rectovaginal fistulae, 304, 871–872
　Crohn's disease, 478, 616, 864–865
　fecal incontinence, 714
　ulcerative colitis, 344
Rectum
　blood flow, smoking, 50 (Table)

Rectum (contd)
  compliance, 715, 897
  computed tomography, 251
  dialysis, 332
  excision, 747, 868–870
    indications, Crohn's disease, 714
  gonorrhea, 403–404
  Hartmann's closure
    Crohn's colitis surgery, 857–858
    fulminant colitis, 727–728
  reservoir function, 185
  retained after surgery, 736
    cancer risk, 676, 680, 729, 742–743
  sensitivity, 195–196
  sparing, 344, 601
    fulminant colitis, 300
    ulcerative colitis, children, 660
  ulcerative colitis
    histology, 295
    radiology, 223
  ultrasound probes, 285
  washout, 852
Rectus abdominis
  hernia prevention, 934
  muscle flap, 894
Recurrence, see also Relapses
  Crohn's disease, 243, 478, 835–836
    anastomotic, 138–139, 313
    associations, 479
    colon, 610
      segmental resection, 854
    definitions, 476 (Table)
    extent of resection, 826
    ileal, 593–594
    panproctocolectomy, 609
    postoperative, 480
    surgical experience, 821–822
  drugs on risk, 464
  from pregnancy, 944
  ulcerative colitis, 550
Red blood cells, see Erythrocytes
Redundancy, cytokines, 95
Refeeding syndrome, 544
Refined sugar, 38, 41–42, 609
Refractory pouchitis, 804
Refractory sprue, 431
Refractory ulcerative proctitis, 555–556
Regenerative mucosa, 317
  O-acetyl sialic acid, 320
  resolving ulcerative colitis, 297–298
Regional ileitis (term), 6, 7
Reiter's syndrome, 453
Relapses, see also Recurrence
  assessing severity, 957
  endoscopic prediction
    Crohn's colitis, 279–280
    ulcerative colitis, 278
  laboratory markers of risk, 332
  from pregnancy, 944
  ulcerative colitis, children, 661
Relatives, presence at counseling, 917
Remission, see also Maintenance therapy
  Crohn's disease, spontaneous, 479
  ulcerative colitis, rates, 465–466
Renin, mucus secretion, 149
Reovirus type III, primary sclerosing cholangitis, 639
Research, see also Trials
  and audit, 960
  follow-up clinics, 958
Resections, 8
  Crohn's disease, 313, 709, 826
  ileal Crohn's disease, 593, 821–836

peptic ulcer and, 595
segmental, Crohn's colitis, 853–854
with strictureplasty, 844
Reservoir functions, colon and rectum, 185
Reservoirs, see Pouches
Resin-casting vascular studies, 139
Restitution, 207
Restorative proctocolectomy, see Ileal pouch–anal anastomosis
Restriction fragment length polymorphism, linkage studies, 22
Retinal vasculitis, 139
Retraction, stomas, 934
Retraction technique
  ileoanal anastomoses, 785
  rectal mucosectomy, 784
Retrograde ejaculation
  ileal pouch–anal anastomosis, 766, 795, 812
  postoperative, 748, 749, 943
  treatment, 905
Retrograde ileography, 280
Retrograde imaging of small intestine, 217–219
Retroperitoneal disease, see Ureteric obstruction
Retrospective cohort studies, cancer incidence, 323
Reverse genetics, malaria, 28
Review processes, care quality, 959
Revision, pelvic ileal reservoirs, 780
RFD9-positive macrophages, 83
Rhamnose absorption, 22
Rhesus macaques, nitric oxide synthase induction, 159–160
Rheumatoid arthritis
  with collagenous colitis, 369
  HLA class II molecules, 28
Ricinoleic acid, 187
  electrolyte secretion, 183
Ridogrel, 111
  on thromboxanes, 529
Rifampicin, 396
Right iliac fossa masses, see Ileocecal masses
Rioprostil, 530
RNHC1 (N-chloramines), 78
Robotics, minimal-access surgery, 722
Rodents, see also Mice; Rats
  ulcerative colitis models, 158
Rolling, neutrophils, 73–75
Rolling technique, toxic megacolon, 569
Rope-way enteroscopy, 269–270
Rosethorn ulcers, 230, 243
Routine follow-up, 955
Rowasa, 488
Rural populations, 37

Sacral syndrome, 405
Sacroiliitis, 452, 625
  colon changes, 276
  ulcerative colitis, 733
Sacrum, partial resection, 894
Saguinus spp. (tamarins), 160
Salazopyrine, see Sulfasalazine
Salicylates, see Aminosalicylates
Salicylazosulfadimidine, 491
Saline, use in dissection, 708
Saline infusion studies, ulcerative colitis, 194–195
Salmonella enteritidis, 351
Salmonella typhi, crypt distortion (case), 362
Salmonella typhimurium, 351

Salmonellosis, 351–352
  arthritis, 456
  colonoscopy, 274–275
  course, 359
  histology, 304
  horses, 159
  IBD, 366, 367
  incidence, 349
  with ulcerative colitis, 549
Salofalk, see Claversal
Salt and Son Ltd, publications, 923
Sampling reflex, 197, 897, 898
Sarcoid granulomata, monocytes, 380
Sarcoidosis, vs Crohn's disease, 235
Saris, 946
Schistosomiasis
  colon, 275
  ischemic colitis, 421
School performance, Crohn's disease, 481
Scintigraphy, see Radionuclide scanning
Scleroderma, with collagenous colitis, 369
Sclerosing cholangitis, see Primary sclerosing cholangitis
Scoring
  Crohn's colitis, 279
  ulcerative colitis, 277
Screening, for cancer risk, 675, 678
Seasonal incidence, yersiniosis, 416
Secretory component, dysplasia, 320
Segmental colonic transit, ulcerative colitis, 193
Segmental resection, Crohn's disease, 685
  colitis, 853–854
Segregation analysis, genetic, 15–16
Selectins, 74–75, 136
  radiolabeling, 267
Selective follow-up, 957
Selenium
  enterocutaneous fistulae, 884
  total parenteral nutrition, 544
Self-catheterization
  pelvic ileal reservoirs, 780
  pouchitis, 803
Self-help groups, 920–921
Semimembranosus muscle flap, 894
Sepsis, 692, 693
  Crohn's colitis, 605
  enterocutaneous fistula, management, 887
  glutamine uptake, 203
  ileal pouch–anal anastomosis, 786, 792–793
  intrathoracic, isotope scanning, 265
  laboratory markers, enterocutaneous fistulae, 884
  occult, 885
  before proctectomy, 893
  strictureplasty, 843–844
  total parenteral nutrition, 543
Sequential isotope imaging, 265
Seronegative polyarthritis (spondylarthropathies), 451–460, 733
Serosa
  Crohn's colitis, 311
  echoendoscopy, 287
  fulminant colitis, 299
  toxic megacolon, 301
Serotonin, 88 (Table), 174, 184, 194
Serum amyloid A, 329, 330
  Crohn's disease vs ulcerative colitis, 345
Serum resistance, Yersinia spp., 415
Setons, perianal surgery, 711–712
Severe acute colitis, see Fulminant colitis
Sex incidence, 37
Sexual abuse, vs perianal Crohn's disease, 650

Sexual dysfunction, 903–907, 945
   ileal pouch–anal anastomosis, 765–766, 774–775, 794–795, 812, 943
   ileostomies, 773
   postoperative, 748, 749, 756–757, 904–906, 943–944
     minimizing, 692, 747
Shear stress, neutrophil rolling, 75
Sheep, Crohn's disease models, 158
Shiga-like toxins, *see* Verocytotoxins
Shigella dysenteriae, 117
Shigellosis, 117, 352–353
   arthritis, 453, 456
   colonoscopy, 274–275
   histology, 304, 305
   IBD, 366
   incidence, 349
Short bowel syndrome, 509, 659
   total parenteral nutrition, 543
Short-chain fatty acids, 609
   colon absorption, 182–183
   Crohn's disease, 176
   intestinal nutrition, 202–203, 449
   pouchitis, 806
Shortening of colon, ulcerative colitis, 298
Sialic acid/sulfate ratio, dysplasia, 320
Sialomucin
   cotton-top tamarins, 161
   O-acetylation loss, 147
Sialyl-dimeric-Le^x antigen, 146
Sialyl-Lewis x, 74
Sialyl-Tn antigens, tumours, 146–147, 148
Siamang gibbons, stress-induced dysentery, 159
Sick leave, 942
Sickle cell disease, ischemic colitis, 421
Sickness Impact Profile, 339
Side-to-side anastomoses
   Crohn's disease surgery, 830
   strictureplasty, 838
Sigmoid colon
   crescentic fold disease, 276
   surgery for fulminant colitis, 728
Sigmoid motility, ulcerative colitis, 194, 197
Sigmoidoscopy
   diverticular disease, 445
   fulminant colitis, 726
   normal biopsies, 307
   ulcerative colitis, follow-up, 680
   without preparation, 550
Sigmoid tanometer, 422
Simple fistulae, *vs* complicated fistulae, 884
Single contrast barium studies, 215
Single-dose antibiotic prophylaxis, 694–695
Single-lumen ileum (ileoanal anastomosis), 5–6, 781, 782
Sinograms, abscesses, 877, 878
Sinuses
   on barium studies, 232
   computed tomography, 252, 254
   diverticular disease, 444
6-mercaptopurine, 513–514
   adverse effects, 559
   Crohn's disease, 607–608
   enterocutaneous fistula management, 888
   fulminant colitis, 568
   on mast cells, 90
   perianal fistulae, 618
   pregnancy, 578
   response failure, Crohn's colitis, 850
   ulcerative colitis, 554–555
     maintenance therapy, 574–576, 577
Skin, anergy, 57

Skin grafting, perineal wounds, 893
Skin lesions, *see also* Enterocutaneous fistulae
   Crohn's disease, 7, 625–626
     children, 650
     perianal, 615
     squamous cell carcinoma, 480
   ileostomies, 812
   incidence, 623 (Table)
   ulcerative colitis, 733
Skin tags, perianal, 343, 615, 617
   vs condylomata lata, 404
'Skip' areas, Crohn's disease, 226, 836
Slim disease, 400
Slow acetylators, 558
Slow baseline mucus secretion, 149
Small-bowel barium meals, 216–217, *see also* Enteroclysis
   Crohn's disease, children, 652, 653
   vs ileoscopy, 280
   radiation doses, 266
Small-duct primary sclerosing cholangitis, 637 (Table), 643
Small intestine
   barium studies, 216–219, 235–236
   cancer
     Crohn's disease, 325, 480, 834
     surgery, 685
     survival rates, 688
   distension, fulminant colitis, 566
   enteroscopy, 269–270, 271
   nutrition of, 201–202
   pseudo-obstruction, ulcerative colitis, 192
   resections, subsequent surgery, 746
   surgery, 821–846
   transit time, ulcerative colitis, 192
Smethurst, T., murder trial, 3
Smith Kline and French Laboratories, publications, 922
Smoking, 38, 42, 47–50, 531
   Crohn's disease, 48–49, 347, 602, 648
     recurrence, 479
   fulminant colitis, 566
   and pouchitis, 803, 806
   twin studies, 11
Social effects, 942, 945–947
   Crohn's disease. 610
   ileal pouch–anal anastomosis, 812
SOD (antioxidant), 112, 113
Sodium
   colonic absorption, 182
   loss
     Crohn's disease, 174
     colitis, 605
     IBD, 186
     ileal pouch–anal anastomosis, advice, 776
   serum levels, 44
Sodium cromoglycate, *see* Disodium cromoglycate
Sodium-potassium ATPase, colon, 182
Soiling, 713, 775, 899
   sexual intercourse, 812–813
Solitary rectal ulcer syndrome, 276
Soluble antigen fluorescent antibody, 393
Soluble IL-2 receptor (neopterin), 331
Somatomedin-C
   deficiency, Crohn's disease, 477
   levels, 44
Somatostatin analogues, for enterocutaneous fistula, 888
Sonde endoscopes, 270
Soybean trypsin inhibitor, on fecal proteases, 151
Sperm, sulfasalazine, 558, 671–672, 943, 945

Spheroplast-like agents, 126–127, *see also* Cell-wall defective bacteria
Sphincter contraction reflex, 713
Sphincterotomy
   Crohn's disease, 862
   lateral internal, 898
Spike ulcers (rosethorn ulcers), 230, 243
Spine, spondylarthropathies, 451
Spirochetes, 404
Splenic flexure, ischemic colitis, 423
Spondylarthropathies, 451–460, 733
Spontaneous cytotoxity (SCMC), 55
Spontaneous enterocutaneous fistulae, 882–883
Sports, ileal pouch–anal anastomosis, 813
S pouches, 779–780, 796
Spouse studies, 15, 117–118
Sprue, refractory, 431
Squamous cell carcinoma
   anus, 685–686
   skin, 480
SR2640 (leukotriene antagonist), 111
Stafford Miller, publications, 922
Staged procedures
   ileal pouch–anal anastomosis, 771, 779, 786
   pancolectomy, 904
Staging
   carcinoma, 677
   esophageal Crohn's disease, 584
   primary sclerosing cholangitis, 641–642
Stapling, 692, 711, *see also* Double-stapled anastomosis
   ileal pouch–anal anastomosis, 772, 797
   Kock's pouch, 753
Starter pack, stoma care, 912
Stasis, pouchitis, 805
Steatorrhea, 44
Stem cells
   epithelium, 205
   transplantation, chronic granulomatous disease, 382
Stenosis
   anal, 343
   stomas, 933
Stenting, primary sclerosing cholangitis, 642
Steroid-dependent ulcerative colitis, 554
Steroids, *see* Corticosteroids
St Mark's Crohn's Disease Index, 337
St Mark's series, ileorectal anastomoses, 740–743
Stockings, graduated compression, 698, 727
Stomach
   Crohn's disease, 7, 476–477, 583, 585–587, 817–819
     motility, 198
     radiology, 232–234
   endoscopy, 270, 271
   fistulae to skin, 886, 887
   mucus, 143
   tuberculosis, 393
   ulcerative colitis, stasis, 192
Stomas, 5, 900, *see also* Colostomies; Ileostomies
   on body image, 943, 945
   complications, 933–937
   management, 909–937, *see also* Stomaltherapy
   quality of life, 943, 961
   relocation, 936
   sexual dysfunction, 906, 943
   social effects, 942–943
   stoma care nurses, 705
     early referral, 919

Stoma sites
  marking, 824–825, 851–852, 912, 926
  preserving, 692
Stomaltherapy
  at follow-up, 956
  services, 911–914
  specialists, 746
    enterocutaneous fistulae, 886
    perceptions, 946
  units, 913–914
Stools
  amebiasis, 410–411, 549
  culture, 274
    children, 662
    failure, 364–366
    pouchitis, 802
  diverticular disease, 443
  fulminant colitis, 567
  infectious colitis *vs* ulcerative colitis, 304
  laboratory markers, 332
  osmolality, Crohn's colitis, 174
  output
    colectomy, 810
    ulcerative colitis, 191–192
  radionuclide leukocyte excretion, 332, 441, 604
  water and electrolytes, *vs* ileal flow, 185
Storage rooms, stomaltherapy units, 913–914
Streptococcus spp.
  Behçet's disease, 387
  cell wall fragments, animal experiments, 167–168
  group D, 118
Streptomycin, 396
Stress, 941
  colonic motility, 195
  Crohn's disease, 481, 610
Stress-induced dysentery, gibbons, 159
Stress protein, mycobacterial, *see also* Heat shock proteins
  oral Crohn's disease, 635
Strictureplasty, 8, 709–710, 836–845
  gastroduodenal Crohn's disease, 818
  ileal Crohn's disease, 593
  laparoscopic, 719
  and quality activities, 961
  tuberculosis, 397, 837
Strictures
  anastomoses, 593–594
  anorectal region, 712, 714, 864
  cancer, 686, 834
  colonoscopy, 281
  Crohn's disease
    colitis, 679, 848
    gastroduodenal, 587
  esophagus, 584
  finding at surgery, 709
  ileal pouch–anal anastomosis, 764–765
  ischemic colitis, 423
  NSAID, 437–438, 440
  transforming growth factor, 98
  ulcerative colitis, 303
    cancer risk, 676
    radiology, 223
  ulcerative jejunoileitis, 432
String sign, 235, 653
Stroke, Crohn's disease, 628
Stump-tailed macaques, *Mycobacterium 'linda'*, 157
Subclinical genetic markers, 22
Subcutaneous fat, stoma construction, 927
Subcutaneous heparin, low-dose, 698–699

Subcutaneous lesions, Crohn's disease, 7
Submucosa, echoendoscopy, 287
Submucosal vasculitis, tissue factor, 103
Subtotal colectomy
  children, 658, 664
  colon cancer, 685
  Crohn's colitis, 854–856
  fulminant colitis, 727–728
  laparoscopic, 720
  ulcerative colitis, 684
Sucralfate
  Crohn's disease, esophagus, 585
  ulcerative colitis, 556
Sugar (sucrose), refined, 38, 41–42, 609
Sulfapyridine, 487
Sulfasalazine, 8, 487
  adverse effects, 489–490, 557, 558
  ankylosing spondylitis, 457
  Behçet's disease, 389
  breastfeeding, 673
  on cancer risk, 471
  cotton-top tamarin colitis, 161–162
  crescentic fold disease of sigmoid colon, 276
  Crohn's disease
    children, 654–655
    esophagus, 584–585
    ileal, 592
    maintenance therapy, 494–495
    after resection, 593
    topical, 496
    trials, 493, 607
  fibrosing alveolitis, 627
  vs 5-ASA, 574
  on folate absorption, 177
  fulminant colitis, 568
  on *Helicobacter pylori*, 587
  hemolysis, 44, 490, 558
  impotence, 903
  lymphocyte function, 57
  on mast cells, 89
  vs metronidazole, 121
    Crohn's disease, 494
  pregnancy, 672
  response failure, Crohn's colitis, 850
  sperm, 558, 671–672, 943, 945
  spondylarthropathies, 457
  ulcerative colitis, 491, 492, 553
    children, 663
    maintenance therapy, 571–572, 577
Sulfated polysaccharides, experimental colitis, 169
Sulfation, mucins, 147, 151, 152
Sulfides, on butyrate oxidation, 204
Superantigens, 30–31, 56–57
Superinfection, 693
Superior mesenteric angiography, 834
Superior mesenteric artery syndrome, ileal pouch–anal anastomosis, 795
Superoxide, 112
  granulomata, 380
  and nitric oxide, 113
Superoxide dismutase, 531
Supervision, clinical, 675, 677–678
Suppositories
  Crohn's disease, 496
  ulcerative proctitis, 497, 553, 554
Suppressor function, lymphocytes, 57
Surgery, 689–723
  aorta, ischemic colitis, 422
  Behçet's disease, 389
  for cancer risk, 675
  carcinoma, 683–688

  Crohn's disease, 609, 692, 815–872
    children, 477, 657–658
    colitis, risks, 603
    gastroduodenal, 817–820
    ileal, 592–593
    indications, 479
    maneuvers, 707–712
    rates, 610
  diffuse jejunoileitis, 599
  diverticular disease, 446
  for enterocutaneous fistulae, 888–889
  historical aspects, 8
  NSAID enteropathy, 441
  for perineal sinuses, 893–894
  quality activities, 961
  for radiation bowel disease, 427–428
  rectovaginal fistulae, 871–872
  social effects, 942–943
  stoma construction techniques, 926–932
  tuberculosis, 396–397
  ulcerative colitis, 471–472, 725–814
    for cancer risk, 681
    children, 664–665
Surveillance for cancer risk, 675, 678–679, 680–681, 760
  cancer patients not included, 679
  colonoscopy, 273, 735
  trials of, 681
Survival rates, cancer, 687–688
Sutures, 711
Svartz, N., salicylates and sulfas, 487
Sweden
  Crohn's disease in children, 647
  incidence of IBD, 36
  twin studies, 14
Swine dysentery, 159
Swiss-Webster mice, ulcerative colitis models, 158
Switzerland, incidence of IBD, 36
Sydenham, T., bloody flux of, 3
Sympathetic supply, sexual function, 904
Synovial fluid
  peripheral arthritis, 452
  reactive arthritis, 453
Syphilis
  colon histology, 305
  proctitis, 404
Syrian hamsters, Crohn's disease models, 158

Taenia coli, diverticular disease, 445
Takayasu's disease, 140
Tall patients, ileal pouch–anal anastomosis, 761, 772
Talsted and Gjone Crohn's disease index, 337
Tamarins, ulcerative colitis models, 160–163
Tandem balloon system, rectosigmoid contractility, 194
TAP genes, 29
'Tattooing', colonoscopy, 720–721
T-cell antigen receptors
  deficient mice, 67
  genetics, 20–21
  mucosa, 54
  repertoire selection, 28–29, 30–31
T-cell lymphoma, oral lesions, 633
T cells, *see also named types*
  anergy induction, 30
  vs B lymphocytes, mucosa, 54
  CD4, granulomata, 380
  CD8+, activation, 57
  collagenous colitis, 371
  dendritic cells on, 83

T cells (contd)
　IL-2 from, 331
　on immunoglobulin isotype secretion, 64–65
　presentation of antigens, 28
　primary sclerosing cholangitis, 640
　Vβ 8+, Crohn's disease, 57
Team approach, 703–706
　following-up, 956
　patient information, 919
Technetium-99m, 261
　quantification of disease, 266
Tenesmus
　antidiarrheal agents, 577
　Crohn's disease vs ulcerative colitis, 343
Teratogenicity, azathioprine, 559
Terminal ileitis (term), 7
Terminal ileum, radiology, 219, 223, 233 (Fig.), 234 (Fig.), 235
Terminology, Crohn's disease, 7–8
Tertiary referral centers
　intestinal failure unit, 704–705
　surveillance and cancer risk, 679
Tetracyclines, 694
Th 1 cytokines, 95, 96–97
Th 2 cytokines, 95, 97, 98
Thalidomide, Behçet's disease, 389
Theatre discipline, 694
Theophylline, chloride secretion, 183
These special children (Jeter), 921
Thiopurine-methyltransferase deficiency, 559, 574
Thomsen–Friedenreich antigens, 146–147
　tumours, 146–147
Three-dimensional optics, minimal-access surgery, 722
Three-limbed pelvic ileal reservoirs, 779–780
Thromboembolism, 101, 140, 697–701, 734
　laparoscopic surgery, 719
Thrombosis, Crohn's disease, 627–628
Thromboxanes, 110–111
　A_2, detection, 109
　B_2, 104, 109 (Table), 110 (Table)
　therapeutic target, 529
Thumbprinting, 243
Thyroid disease
　autoimmune, 18
　with collagenous colitis, 370
Tight junctions
　colon, 181
　intestinal permeability, 177
Timeframes for management, 961
Time trends, 37
Tine testing, 392
Tissue factor (procoagulant), 103, 136
Tissue injury neutrophil-mediated, 78
Tissue plasminogen activator, 103, 104, 136
Tixocortol, 505–506, 508, 554
Tn antigens, tumours, 146–147
Tobramycin, 561
Toilets, stomaltherapy units, 913
Toluidine blue, mast cell investigation, 87, 89
Tongue, tonsils, tuberculosis, 393
Toothpaste, 43
Topical therapy, see also Enemas; Foam preparations; Suppositories
　children, 655 (Table)
　Crohn's disease, trials, 496–497
　cyclosporin, 518
　5-ASA, 553, 573–574
　steroids, 554
　　Crohn's disease, 505, 509–510
　　ulcerative colitis, 508

ulcerative colitis, 558
Total colitis, see Pancolitis
Total parenteral nutrition, 535, 541–548
　Crohn's disease, 567, 608
　　children, 659
　　perianal, 617
　　surgery, 825
　　colitis, 852
　diffuse jejunoileitis, 598, 836
　enterocutaneous fistulae, 886
　ulcerative colitis, children, 664
　ulcerative jejunoileitis, 434
Total proctocolectomy, see Proctocolectomy
Total quality management, 959
'Toxic appearance', Crohn's disease, children, 650
Toxic colitis, ulcerative colitis, 471
Toxic masses, see also Ileocecal masses
　resection, 657
Toxic megacolon, 568, 725, 850–851
　amebic colitis, 410
　children, 662–663, 663–664
　Crohn's disease, 239, 478
　emergency surgery, 856
　endoscopic decompression, 281
　proximal colonic stasis, 194
　radiology, 224, 227 (Fig.), 566
　ulcerative colitis, 301
Tracheobronchial mucin genes, 144
Training
　follow-up clinics, 958
　minimal-access surgery, 721
　stomaltherapy, 913
Transanal endoscopic microsurgery, 717
Transanal mucosectomy, 783–784
Transanal ultrasound, see Endoanal ultrasound
Transcription, genomic, steroids on, 503–504
Transdermal nicotine patches, 48
Transendothelial migration, neutrophils, 76
Transferrin, 331
　acute-phase response, 329
Transforming growth factor-β
　on C-reactive protein, 330
　on crypt restitution, 207
　effects, 98
　on immunoglobulin synthesis, 65
Transforming growth factors, 96
Transgenic technology, 31
Transit times, ulcerative colitis, 192–194
Translations, publications, 922
Translocation
　bacteria, 202, 887
　vagina, 905, 906
Transmission experiments, infective agents, 120–121
Transmural inflammation, Crohn's disease, 312
Transrectal electrostimulation, periprostatic plexus, 905
Transrectal ultrasound, see Endoanal ultrasound
Transverse incisions, 691
Traveler's diarrhea, antibiotics, 352
Treatment-resistant, IBD, 69
Trefoil peptides, 96
　on crypt restitution, 207
　in mucus, 143
Treponema pallidum, 404
Trials (clinical)
　aminosalicylates, 490–497, 553
　corticosteroids, 606–607
　surveillance for cancer risk, 681

Trials (criminal), 3
Triamcinolone, 505
　with balloon dilatation, 281
　oral Crohn's disease, 635, 656
Trichinella spiralis, experimental infection, 168
Trinitrobenzene sulfonic acid, experimental colitis, 168–169
Trophozoites, *Entamoeba histolytica*, 409
Tropical countries, travelers from, 549
Tropical sprue, with collagenous colitis, 369
Tropolonate (labeling complex), 261
Truelove and Witts index, 335–336
Tryptase, mast cells, 89
　staining, 88
Tuberculosis, 391–398
　colonoscopy, 275
　vs Crohn's disease, 235, 236, 241, 313–314, 395
　strictureplasty, 397, 837
　vasculitis, 141
Tubular colon, 243, 566
Tumor necrosis factor-α, 96
　on C-reactive protein, 330
　Crohn's disease
　　children, 654
　　vs ulcerative colitis, 346
　humanized antibodies, 98
　therapy target, 525
　vascular damage by, 136
Tumor necrosis factor-β, Behçet's disease, 387
Tumor necrosis factors
　effects on mucosa, 98
　genes, 21–22, 27, 29
　localization, 97
　monoclonal antibodies, 525, 560
　steroids on production, 504
Turnbull, R.
　ileostomies, 5
　stomaltherapy services, 911
Turner's syndrome, 16
24-hour cover, antibiotic prophylaxis, 694–695
Twin studies, 14–15
　mucins, 207
Two-limbed pelvic ileal reservoirs, 780–781
Two-sphincter operation, ileoanal anastomoses, 782
'Tyre lever' maneuver, 708
Ulcerative colitis, 547–580, see also
　　Colonoscopy, ulcerative colitis;
　　Crohn's disease, vs ulcerative colitis
　vs acute infectious-type colitis, 359
　AIDS, 403
　aminosalicylates, trials, 491–493
　animal models, natural, 158–163
　autoantibodies, 68–69
　azathioprine, 515–516
　　and 6-MP, 517
　barium studies, 219–226
　cancer, 323–324, see also Cancer risk, ulcerative colitis
　　indications for surgery, 683
　change to Crohn's disease, 278, 306, 345
　children, 660–665
　coexisting with Crohn's disease, 306
　computed tomography, 256–257
　corticosteroids, 506–508, 553–554, 560
　vs diversion colitis, 450 (Table)
　dysplasia, 317–326
　epithelial nutrition, 203–204
　extraintestinal manifestations, incidence, 623 (Table)

Ulcerative colitis (contd)
  fertility, 671
  on fetus, 672
  follow-up, 957
  4-ASA, 497–498
  histopathology, 291–309
  historical aspects, 3–9
  HLA associations, 29
  intractable, 731–732
  mast cells, 89
  motility disturbances, 191–197, 556–557
  mucin abnormalities, 145–146
  mucus breakdown, 151
  natural history, 463–473
  peripheral arthritis, 452
  pouchitis, 803
  primary sclerosing cholangitis, 638, 733
  smoking, 47–48
  surgery, see Surgery, ulcerative colitis
  ultrasound, 287
  vascular studies, 133
Ulcerative jejunoileitis, 431–435
Ulcerative post-dysenteric colitis, 366
Ulcers
  active ulcerative colitis, 292
  amebic colitis, 410
  anal, 714, 861–862
  colon
    drugs, 315
    radiology, 220
  Crohn's disease, radiology, 226–227
  detection by palpation, 709
  after gastrojejunostomy, 818
  ileal pouch–anal anastomosis, 795
  NSAID, 437, 438, 439
  segmental or isolated, colonoscopy, 276
  severity, 335
  toxic megacolon, 301
  yersiniosis, 416
Ulex europaeus agglutinin reactivity, 320
Ultrasound, 249–250, 287, see also Endoanal ultrasound; Endoluminal ultrasound
  Crohn's disease
    colitis, 287, 604
    vs ulcerative colitis, 345
  deep vein thrombosis, 699
Undifferentiated spondylarthropathies, 455
  sulfasalazine, 457
Unilateral exclusion bypass, 827, 833
United Kingdom
  Asian migrants, 15, 37, 38
  Crohn's disease in children, 647
  incidence of IBD, 36
United States
  vs Europe, Crohn's disease studies, 476
  incidence of IBD, 36
Urate stones
  Crohn's disease, 606, 628
  postoperative, 748
Urban populations, 37
Urdu, publication, 922
Ureteric obstruction, Crohn's disease, 628, 833
  vs ulcerative colitis, 344
Ureterolysis, 833
Ureters, and surgery, 692, 855
Urgency of defecation, 713, 732
Urinary tract malakoplakia, 383
Urokinase, on epithelia, 206
Urokinase plasminogen activator, 103, 104
Ursodeoxycholic acid, 544
  Crohn's disease, 177
  primary sclerosing cholangitis, 642

Uveitis, 626
  Behçet's disease, 389
  Crohn's disease, children, 650
  ulcerative colitis, 557
    children, 662

Vagina
  endoluminal ultrasound, 289, 885
  fistulae, 871, see also Rectovaginal fistulae
  postoperative deformations, 905
  secretions, episodic discharge, 905
Vagotomy, and gastrojejunostomy, 818
Valve necrosis, Kock's pouch, 754
Vancomycin, 119, 356, 568
Van Hees Crohn's disease index, 338
Vanishing bile duct syndrome, 642
Varices, peristomal, 642, 793, 936
Vasa recta, 139
Vascular effects
  granulomata, 83
  oral contraceptives, 50, 51
  smoking, 50 (Table)
Vascular endothelium, see Endothelium
Vascular factors, infective agents, 133–142
Vascular occlusion, experimental colitis, 169–170
Vascular pattern, colonoscopy, 273
Vascular volume, 139
Vasculitis, 139
  Behçet's disease, 388
  Crohn's disease, 312
  fulminant colitis, 300
  submucosal, tissue factor, 103
Vasoactive intestinal peptide
  cholera diarrhea, 183
  inactivation, mast cells, 89
  on mucus secretion, 150
Vβ 8+ T cells, Crohn's disease, 57
VCAM-1, 136
Vector manometry, 899
Vegetables, 42
Venereal Diseases Research Laboratory test, 404
Venography, 699
Venous thrombosis
  Crohn's disease, 627–628
  recurrent, 140
Verocytotoxins
  E. coli, 354
  Shigella spp., 352
Very-low-dose warfarin, 699
V_H immunoglobulin marker genes, 20
V_H segments, immunoglobulins, 67
Vibrio cholerae toxins
  electrolyte secretion, 183
  mucus secretion, 150
Video cameras, minimal-access surgery, 722
Videoproctography, 715, 899
Video tapes, patient information, 921, 922, 923
Villous atrophy
  HIV enteropathy, 402
  intestinal permeability, 178
Villous configuration
  vs acute infectious-type colitis, 362–363
  dysplasia, 317
Virulence, *Yersinia enterocolitica*, 414–415
Viruses, 117, 120
  T-cell response, 31
Virus theory, primary sclerosing cholangitis, 639
Vitamin A deficiency, eye lesions from, 626
Vitamin B_{12} malabsorption, 44, 331, 594

Crohn's disease, 177, 627
  children, 652–653
  ileal pouch–anal anastomosis, 795
Vitamins
  antioxidant, 531
  deficiencies, 44
  total parenteral nutrition, 544
Vocational function, see Occupation
Volcano lesions, 275
Vomiting
  AIDS, 400
  azathioprine and 6-MP, 516
Von Hansemann cells, 383
Von Willebrand's disease, protective effect vs, 140
Von Willebrand's factor, 138

Wangensteen, O., ileoanal anastomosis, 5
Ward rounds, 704
Wards, 703
  for leukemia, *Clostridium difficile*, 355–356
Warfarin, 699–700
Water absorption
  colon, 181–190
  Crohn's disease, 173–174
Water loss
  Crohn's disease, 594
    colitis, 605
  enterocutaneous fistulae, 883–884
  IBD, 186
  ileal pouch–anal anastomosis, advice, 776
Water secretion, colon, 183
Watery diarrhea–colitis syndrome, 374
Weekly meetings, 704
Wegener's granulomatosis, antineutrophil cytoplasmic antibody, 68
Weight loss, enterocutaneous fistulae, 884
Weight retardation, 43–44, see also Growth retardation
Whipple's disease, 117
White cells, see Leukocytes *and named types*
Whole-body counting, indium-111, 265–266
Whole-body leucine metabolism, 44
Whole-bowel irrigation, 694
Wilks, S., 3–4
Wolinella spp., 119
  periodontal infection, Crohn's disease, 77–78
Working capacity, 469–470
World Council of Enterostomal Therapists, 911
Wound healing, steroids on, 503
W pouches, 197, 781–782

X chromosome abnormalities, 16
Xenobiotic metabolism, 204–205
Xylose malabsorption, 44, 175

Yersinia (spp.), 413
  arthritis, 453, 456
  course of infection, 359
Yersinia enterocolitica, 119, 355, 413–419
  colonoscopy, 275
  vs Crohn's disease, 314
  radiology, 236
Yersinia pseudotuberculosis, pigs, 159

Zileuton, 111, 489, 504
  trials, 529, 560

Zinc
- absorption
  - colon, 182
  - Crohn's disease, 176
- deficiency, 45, 606
- fistulae, 883
- total parenteral nutrition, 544

Zirconium, granulomata, 379